Textbook of
PEDIATRIC DENTISTRY

5 Edition

Textbook of
PEDIATRIC DENTISTRY

Editor

Nikhil Marwah BDS MDS PhD
Associate Dean (Research)
Mahatma Gandhi University of Medical Sciences and Technology
Jaipur, Rajasthan, India
Professor and Head
Department of Pediatric and Preventive Dentistry
Mahatma Gandhi Dental College and Hospital (MGUMST)
Jaipur, Rajasthan, India

Co-editors

Satish Vishwanathaiah
Associate Professor
Department of Pediatric Dentistry
Jazan University
Jazan, Saudi Arabia

Ravi GR
Assistant Professor
Department of Pediatric Dentistry
King Faisal University
Al-Ahsa, Saudi Arabia

Forewords

Figen Seymen U
Radhika Muppa
Varinder Goyal

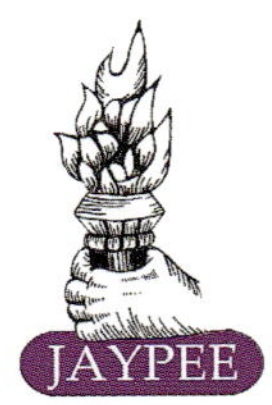

JAYPEE BROTHERS MEDICAL PUBLISHERS
The Health Sciences Publisher
New Delhi | London

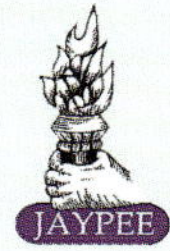

Jaypee Brothers Medical Publishers (P) Ltd

Headquarters

Jaypee Brothers Medical Publishers (P) Ltd
EMCA House, 23/23-B
Ansari Road, Daryaganj
New Delhi 110 002, India
Landline: +91-11-23272143, +91-11-23272703
+91-11-23282021, +91-11-23245672
Email: jaypee@jaypeebrothers.com

Corporate Office

Jaypee Brothers Medical Publishers (P) Ltd
4838/24, Ansari Road, Daryaganj
New Delhi 110 002, India
Phone: +91-11-43574357
Fax: +91-11-43574314
Email: jaypee@jaypeebrothers.com

Overseas Office

J.P. Medical Ltd
83 Victoria Street, London
SW1H 0HW (UK)
Phone: +44 20 3170 8910
Fax: +44 (0)20 3008 6180
Email: info@jpmedpub.com

Website: www.jaypeebrothers.com
Website: www.jaypeedigital.com

Textbook of Pediatric Dentistry

First Edition: 2006

Second Edition: 2009

Third Edition: 2014

Fourth Edition: 2019

Fifth Edition: 2023, Reprint: **2024**

ISBN: 978-93-5696-101-2

Printed at: Samrat Offset Pvt. Ltd.

Contributors

Aayushi Bansal
Pediatric Dentist
Jaipur, Rajasthan, India

Abhilasha Agarwal
Postgraduate
Department of Pediatric and Preventive Dentistry
King George Medical College
Lucknow, Uttar Pradesh, India

Abhinav Talekar
Associate Professor
MA Rangoonwala Dental College
Pune, Maharashtra, India

Abhishek Khairwa
Professor
Department of Pediatric and Preventive Dentistry
Jaipur Dental College
Jaipur, Rajasthan, India

Abhishek Soni
Pediatric Dentist
Vanilla Smiles
Pune, Maharashtra, India

Ahmad Faisal Ismail
Associate Professor
Kulliyyah of Dentistry
International Islamic University
Malaysia

Ajay Parihar
Professor and Head
Department of Oral Medicine and Radiology
Government College of Dentistry
Indore, Madhya Pradesh, India

Ajay Yadav
Professor and Head
Department of Periodontology
Mahatma Gandhi Dental College
Mahatma Gandhi University of Medical Sciences and Technology (MGUMST)
Jaipur, Rajasthan, India

Akash Patodia
Pediatric Dentist
Ahmedabad, Gujarat, India

Amanpreet Singh
Director
Baba Jaswant Singh Dental College
Ludhiana, Punjab, India

Amit Bhamboo
Reader
Department of Oral and Maxillofacial Surgery
Mahatma Gandhi Dental College
Mahatma Gandhi University of Medical Sciences and Technology (MGUMST)
Jaipur, Rajasthan, India

Amit Khatri
Professor
Department of Pediatric and Preventive Dentistry
University College of Medical Sciences, Dental College
New Delhi, India

Amita Hegde
Professor and Head
Department of Pediatric and Preventive Dentistry
AB Shetty Dental College
Mangaluru, Karnataka, India

Ambika Joshi
Postgraduate
Department of Pediatric and Preventive Dentistry
Mahatma Gandhi Dental College
Mahatma Gandhi University of Medical Sciences and Technology (MGUMST)
Jaipur, Rajasthan, India

Amita Rai
Assistant Professor
Department of Pediatric Dentistry
Peoples Dental College
Kathmandu, Nepal

Amol Suresh Patil
Reader
Department of Pediatric and Preventive Dentistry
MA Rangoonwala College of Dental Science and Research Centre
Pune, Maharashtra, India

Amrish Bhagol
Associate Professor
Department of Oral and Maxillofacial Surgery
Government Dental College
Rohtak, Haryana, India

Anant Nigam
Professor
Department of Pediatric and Preventive Dentistry
Mahatma Gandhi Dental College
Mahatma Gandhi University of Medical Sciences and Technology (MGUMST)
Jaipur, Rajasthan, India

Anita Hooda
Associate Professor
Department of Oral Anatomy
Government Dental College
Rohtak, Haryana, India

Anshula Deshpande
Professor
Department of Pediatric and Preventive Dentistry
KM Shah Dental College
Vadodara, Gujarat, India

Anshuman Jamdade
Professor and Head
Department of Oral Medicine and Radiology
Mahatma Gandhi Dental College
Mahatma Gandhi University of Medical Sciences and Technology (MGUMST)
Jaipur, Rajasthan, India

Anup Panda
Professor and Head
Department of Pediatric and Preventive Dentistry
Ahmedabad Dental College
Ahmedabad, Gujarat, India

Anupma Sharma
Professor
Department of Community Dentistry
Government Dental College and Hospital
Jaipur, Rajasthan, India

Anuradha Pathak
Ex-Professor and Head
Department of Pediatric and Preventive Dentistry
Government Dental College
Patiala, Punjab, India

AR Prabhakar
Ex-Professor and Head
Department of Pediatric and Preventive Dentistry
Bapuji Dental College and Hospital
Davangere, Karnataka, India

Archana Agnihotri
Professor
Department of Pediatric and Preventive Dentistry
Harvansh Singh Judge Institute of Dental Sciences and Hospital
Chandigarh, India

Arun Bhupathi
Assistant Professor
Vishnu Dental College
Bhimavaram, Andhra Pradesh, India

Arvind Sridhara
Reader
Department of Pediatric and Preventive Dentistry
Subbhaiah Dental College
Shimoga, Karnataka, India

Ashish Saxena
Professor and Head
Department of Pediatric and Preventive Dentistry
Government College of Dentistry
Indore, Madhya Pradesh, India

Ashwin M Jawdekar
Vice Principal
Bharati Vidyapeeth Deemed to be University Dental College
Navi Mumbai, Maharashtra, India

Ashwin Rao
Professor
Department of Pediatric and Preventive Dentistry
Manipal College of Dental Sciences
Mangaluru, Karnataka, India

Asmita Sharma
Pediatric Dentist
Jaipur, Rajasthan, India

Avantika Tuli
Professor and Head
Department of Pediatric and Preventive Dentistry
Seema Dental College
Rishikesh, Uttarakhand, India

Bhagyashree M Thakur
Pediatric Dentist
Miniso Centre for Dental Excellence
Mumbai, Maharashtra, India

Bharat Suneja
Professor and Head
Department of Pediatric and Preventive Dentistry
Baba Jaswant Singh Dental College
Ludhiana, Punjab, India

Bhavna Dave
Professor and Head
Department of Pediatric and Preventive Dentistry
KM Shah Dental College
Vadodara, Gujarat, India

Bhavna Gupta Saraf
Professor and Head
Department of Pediatric and Preventive Dentistry
Sudha Rastogi Dental College
Faridabad, Haryana, India

Bhawna Kaul
Professor
Department of Pediatric and Preventive Dentistry
Indira Gandhi Government Dental College
Jammu, Jammu and Kashmir, India

Chaitanya P
Reader
Department of Pediatric and Preventive Dentistry
Drs Sudha and Nageswara Rao Siddhartha Institute of Dental Sciences
Gannavaram, Andhra Pradesh, India

Chaitanya Ram
Reader
Department of Pediatric and Preventive Dentistry
Drs Sudha and Nageswara Rao Siddhartha Institute of Dental Sciences
Gannavaram, Andhra Pradesh, India

Chandrashekar Yavagal
Professor and Head
Department of Pediatric and Preventive Dentistry
Maratha Mandal's Nathajirao G Halgekar Institute of Dental Sciences
Belagavi, Karnataka, India

Chitrita Gupta Mukherjee
Professor and Head
Department of Pediatric and Preventive Dentistry
Buddha Institute of Dental Sciences and Hospital
Patna, Bihar, India

Debarchhana Jena
Pediatric Dentist
Childhood Smiles Dental Clinic
Bengaluru, Karnataka, India

Deeksha Khurana
Reader
Department of Conservative Dentistry and Endodontics
Mahatma Gandhi Dental College
Mahatma Gandhi University of Medical Sciences and Technology (MGUMST)
Jaipur, Rajasthan, India

Deepak Raisinghani
Professor and Head
Department of Conservative Dentistry and Endodontics
Mahatma Gandhi Dental College
Mahatma Gandhi University of Medical Sciences and Technology (MGUMST)
Jaipur, Rajasthan, India

Deepesh Prajapati
Pediatric Dentist
Sudeep Dental Clinic
Jaipur, Rajasthan, India

Deval Kumar Arora
Department of Dentistry
Pt Ram Prasad Bismil Autonomous State Medical College
Shahjahanpur, Uttar Pradesh, India

Dhanraj Kalaivanan
Associate Professor
Department of Pediatric and Preventive Dentistry
Sathyabama Dental College
Chennai, Tamil Nadu, India

Dimpal Parmar
Assistant Professor
Department of Pediatric and Preventive Dentistry
Narsinhbhai Patel Dental College
Sankalchand Patel University (SPU)
Visnagar, Gujarat, India

Disha Kumar
Pediatric Dentist
Pune, Maharashtra, India

Divya Gera
Postgraduate
Department of Pediatric and Preventive Dentistry
Mahatma Gandhi Dental College
Mahatma Gandhi University of Medical Sciences and Technology (MGUMST)
Jaipur, Rajasthan, India

Divya Prahlad
Pediatric Dentist
Aster CMI Hospital
Bengaluru, Karnataka, India

Divya Reddy
Professor
Department of Pediatric and Preventive Dentistry
Sri Rajeev Gandhi College of Dental Sciences
Bengaluru, Karnataka, India

Divya Singh
Assistant Professor
Department of Pediatric and Preventive Dentistry
Santosh Dental College
Ghaziabad, Uttar Pradesh, India

G Deepa
Professor
Department of Pediatric and Preventive Dentistry
Saveetha Dental College
Chennai, Tamil Nadu, India

Ganesh Jeevanandan
Reader
Department of Pediatric and Preventive Dentistry
Saveetha Dental College
Chennai, Tamil Nadu, India

Gargi S Murthy
Reader
Department of Pediatric and Preventive Dentistry
Dayanand Sagar College of Dental Sciences
Bengaluru, Karnataka, India

Gaurav Gupta
Professor
Department of Pediatric and Preventive Dentistry
Jaipur Dental College
Jaipur, Rajasthan, India

Girish AB
Pediatric Dentist
Queensland, Australia

Gopakumar R
Professor and Head
Department of Oral Medicine and Radiology
KD Dental College
Mathura, Uttar Pradesh, India

Gurvanit Kaur Lehl
Professor and Head
Department of Dentistry
Government Medical College
Chandigarh, India

Gyanender Saroj
Professor
Department of Pediatric and Preventive Dentistry
Maulana Azad Institute of Dental Sciences
New Delhi, India

Hind Pal Bhatia
Pediatric Dentist
New Delhi, India

IK Pandit
Principal, Professor and Head
Department of Pediatric and Preventive Dentistry
DAV (Centenary) Dental College
Yamuna Nagar, Haryana, India

Iqbal Musani
Professor
Department of Pediatric and Preventive Dentistry
Dr DY Patil Dental College and Hospital
Pune, Maharashtra, India

Isha Angne
Oral Pathologist
Children Dental and Myofunctional Centre
Mumbai, Maharashtra, India

Joby Peter
Professor and Head
Department of Pediatric and Preventive Dentistry
Annoor Dental College and Hospital
Muvattupuzha, Kerala, India

Jyothsna V Setty
Professor
Department of Pediatric and Preventive Dentistry
MR Ambedkar Dental College and Hospital
Bengaluru, Karnataka, India

Jyoti Sumi Issac
Professor and Head
Department of Pediatric and Preventive Dentistry
Azeezia College of Dental Science
Kollam, Kerala, India

Kanika Singh
Professor
Department of Pediatric and Preventive Dentistry
Kalinga Institute of Dental Sciences
Bhubaneswar, Odisha, India

Kanwalpreet Kaur
Postgraduate
Department of Pediatric and Preventive Dentistry
Baba Jaswant Singh Dental College
Ludhiana, Punjab, India

Karthik Krishna M
Principal, Professor and Head
Department of Periodontics
Rungta College of Dental Sciences
Bhilai, Chhattisgarh, India

Karuna YM
Assistant Professor
Department of Pediatric and Preventive Dentistry
Manipal College of Dental Sciences
Mangaluru, Karnataka, India

Kayalvizhi G
Professor
Department of Pediatric and Preventive Dentistry
Indira Gandhi Dental College
Puducherry, India

Keyur Chauhan
Postgraduate
Department of Pediatric and Preventive Dentistry
Ahmedabad Dental College
Ahmedabad, Gujarat, India

Kiran Hegde
Department of Pediatric Dentistry
School of Dental Medicine University of Colorado Denver
Colorado, USA

Kirthiga M
Assistant Professor
Department of Pediatric and Preventive Dentistry
Faculty of Dental Science
Shri Ramchandra Institute of Higher Education and Research
Chennai, Tamil Nadu, India

Kirti Asopa
Assistant Professor
Department of Pediatric and Preventive Dentistry
Rajasthan Dental College
Jaipur, Rajasthan, India

Koya Srikanth
Reader
Department of Pediatric and Preventive Dentistry
Drs Sudha and Nageswara Rao Siddhartha Institute of Dental Sciences
Gannavaram, Andhra Pradesh, India

Kshitij Rohilla
Oral Pathologist
New Delhi, India

Kunal Gupta
Pediatric Dentist
Children Dental Centre
Gurugram, Haryana, India

Lalitha Jairam
Assistant Professor
Department of Pediatric and Preventive Dentistry
Faculty of Dental Sciences
Ramaiah University of Applied Sciences
Bengaluru, Karnataka, India

Lumbini Pathivada
Associate Professor
Department of Pediatric and Preventive Dentistry
Rungta College of Dental Sciences and Research
Bhilai, Chhattisgarh, India

MH Raghunath Reddy
Professor and Head
Department of Pediatric and Preventive Dentistry
SJM Dental College
Chitradurga, Karnataka, India

Mahesh Ramakrishnan
Associate Dean
Saveetha Dental College
Chennai, Tamil Nadu, India

Mandeep Virdi
Principal
Professor and Head
Department of Pediatric and Preventive Dentistry
Prabhu Dayal Memorial (PDM) Dental College
Bahadurgarh, Haryana, India

Manish Madan
Professor
Department of Pediatric and Preventive Dentistry
Ponta Sahib Dental College
Himachal Pradesh, India

Manju Gopakumar
Professor and Head
Department of Pediatric and Preventive Dentistry
AB Shetty Memorial Institute of Dental Sciences
Mangaluru, Karnataka, India

Manohar Bhatt
Principal, Professor and Head
Department of Pediatric and Preventive Dentistry
Jaipur Dental College
Jaipur, Rajasthan, India

Manojit Mahato
Postgraduate
Department of Pediatric and Preventive Dentistry
Mahatma Gandhi Dental College
Mahatma Gandhi University of Medical Sciences and Technology (MGUMST)
Jaipur, Rajasthan, India

Manu Bansal
Professor
Department of Conservative Dentistry
Jaipur Dental College
Jaipur, Rajasthan, India

Maya Ramesh
Professor and Head
Department of Oral and Maxillofacial Pathology
Vinayaka Mission Sankarachariyar Dental College
Salem, Tamil Nadu, India

Megha Gupta
Associate Professor
Department of Pediatric and Preventive Dentistry
Vyas Dental College
Jodhpur, Rajasthan, India

Mihir Jha
Assistant Professor
Department of Pediatric and Preventive Dentistry
MGM Dental College
Navi Mumbai, Maharashtra, India

Mihir Shah
Pediatric Dentist
Department of Pediatric and Preventive Dentistry
Nair Hospital and Dental College
Mumbai, Maharashtra, India

Mili Meghpara
Postgraduate
Department of Pediatric and Preventive Dentistry
Mahatma Gandhi Dental College
Mahatma Gandhi University of Medical Sciences and Technology (MGUMST)
Jaipur, Rajasthan, India

Milind L Shah
Pediatric Dentist
Mumbai, Maharashtra, India

Mitakshra Nirwan
Assistant Professor
Department of Pediatric and Preventive Dentistry
Mahatma Gandhi Dental College
Mahatma Gandhi University of Medical Sciences and Technology (MGUMST)
Jaipur, Rajasthan, India

Mitesh Sanghvi
Pediatric Dentist
St. Clair Dental Practice Adelaide
Australia

MK Jindal
Professor
Department of Pediatric and Preventive Dentistry
Aligarh Muslim University Dental College
Aligarh, Uttar Pradesh, India

Mousumi Goswami
Professor and Head
Department of Pediatric and Preventive Dentistry
ITS Dental College
Greater Noida, Uttar Pradesh, India

Mridula Goswami
Professor and Head
Department of Pediatric and Preventive Dentistry
Maulana Azad Institute of Dental Science
New Delhi, India

Mridula Trehan
Principal, Professor and Head
Department of Orthodontics
MS Dental College
Jaipur, Rajasthan, India

Mrunal Bandiwar
Postgraduate
Department of Pediatric and Preventive Dentistry
Mahatma Gandhi Dental College
Mahatma Gandhi University of Medical Sciences and Technology (MGUMST)
Jaipur, Rajasthan, India

MS Muthu
Professor and Head
Department of Pediatric and Preventive Dentistry
Faculty of Dental Science, Shri Ramchandra Institute of Higher Education and Research
Chennai, Tamil Nadu, India

Mukul Jain
Pediatric Dentist
Brightsmiles Dental Care
Founder Kids-e-Dental
Mumbai, Maharashtra, India

Naveen Manuja
Professor
Department of Pediatric and Preventive Dentistry
Kothiwal Dental College
Muradabad, Uttar Pradesh, India

Navneet Grewal
Pediatric Dentist
Amritsar, Punjab, India

Neeraj Gugnani
Professor
Department of Pediatric and Preventive Dentistry
DAV (Centenary) Dental College
Yamuna Nagar, Haryana, India

Neha Aggarwal
Pediatric Dentist
Jaipur, Rajasthan, India

Neha Bhargava
Reader
Department of Pediatric and Preventive Dentistry
Rajasthan Dental College
Jaipur, Rajasthan, India

Nikhil Ghawate Patil
Postgraduate
Department of Pediatric and Preventive Dentistry
Mahatma Gandhi Dental College
Mahatma Gandhi University of Medical Sciences and Technology (MGUMST)
Jaipur, Rajasthan, India

Nikhil Srivastav
Principal, Professor and Head
Department of Pediatric and Preventive Dentistry
Subharti Dental College
Meerut, Uttar Pradesh, India

Nikita Gupta
Postgraduate
Department of Pediatric and Preventive Dentistry
Mahatma Gandhi Dental College
Mahatma Gandhi University of Medical Sciences and Technology (MGUMST)
Jaipur, Rajasthan, India

Nikita Sobti
Assistant Professor
Department of Pediatric and Preventive Dentistry
Mahatma Gandhi Dental College
Mahatma Gandhi University of Medical Sciences and Technology (MGUMST)
Jaipur, Rajasthan, India

Nilesh Rathi
Professor and Head
Department of Pediatric and Preventive Dentistry
Dr DY Patil Dental College
Pune, Maharashtra, India

Nirapjeet Kaur
Professor and Head
Department of Pediatric and Preventive Dentistry
Government Dental College
Amritsar, Punjab, India

Nirmala SVSG
Professor
Department of Pediatric and Preventive Dentistry
Narayana Dental College
Nellore, Andhra Pradesh, India

Nivedita Saxena
Assistant Professor
Department of Pediatric and Preventive Dentistry
Mahatma Gandhi Dental College
Mahatma Gandhi University of Medical Sciences and Technology (MGUMST)
Jaipur, Rajasthan, India

Noopur Kaushik
Professor
Department of Pediatric and Preventive Dentistry
Subharthi Dental College
Meerut, Uttar Pradesh, India

PR Geethapriya
Professor and Head
Department of Pediatric and Preventive Dentistry
KSR Institute of Dental Sciences
Tiruchengode, Tamil Nadu, India

Pallavi Pawar
Assistant Professor
Department of Pediatric and Preventive Dentistry
Rungta, College of Dental Sciences
Bhilai, Chhattisgarh, India

Parvind Gumber
Oral Pathologist
Jaipur, Rajasthan, India

Peeyush Shivhare
Senior Resident
Department of Dentistry
All India Institute of Medical Sciences
Patna, Bihar, India

Pooja Mishra
Pediatric Dentist
Switzerland

Pooja Yadav
Postgraduate
Department of Pediatric and Preventive Dentistry
Mahatma Gandhi Dental College
Mahatma Gandhi University of Medical Sciences and Technology (MGUMST)
Jaipur, Rajasthan, India

Prabhadevi C Maganur
Assistant Professor
Department of Pedodontics
Jazan University
Jazan, Saudi Arabia

Prachi Mital
Reader
Department of Conservative Dentistry and Endodontics
Mahatma Gandhi Dental College
Mahatma Gandhi University of Medical Sciences and Technology (MGUMST)
Jaipur, Rajasthan, India

Pradnya Kathe
Pediatric Dentist
Pune, Maharashtra, India

Pragati Kaurani
Professor
Department of Prosthodontics
Mahatma Gandhi Dental College
Mahatma Gandhi University of Medical Sciences and Technology (MGUMST)
Jaipur, Rajasthan, India

Prateek Agarwal
Reader
Department of Oral and Maxillofacial Surgery
Mahatma Gandhi Dental College
Mahatma Gandhi University of Medical Sciences and Technology (MGUMST)
Jaipur, Rajasthan, India

Pratik B Kariya
Associate Professor
Department of Pediatric and Preventive Dentistry
KM Shah Dental College
Vadodara, Gujarat, India

Pratima Swarnkar
Pediatric Dentist
New Delhi, India

Priya Nagar
Professor and Head
Department of Pediatric and Preventive Dentistry
Krishnadevaraya College of Dental Sciences
Bengaluru, Karnataka, India

Priya Verma
Pediatric Dentist
Dr. Joy Dental Clinic
Dubai, UAE

Priyanka Lekhwani
Postgraduate
Department of Pediatric and Preventive Dentistry
Mahatma Gandhi Dental College
Mahatma Gandhi University of Medical Sciences and Technology (MGUMST)
Jaipur, Rajasthan, India

Puneet Goenka
Professor
Department of Pediatric and Preventive Dentistry
Jaipur Dental College
Jaipur, Rajasthan, India

Rajesh Kumar
Professor
Department of Prosthodontics
Jaipur Dental College
Jaipur, Rajasthan, India

Rajesh Sharma
Professor
Department of Pediatric and Preventive Dentistry
Jaipur Dental College
Jaipur, Rajasthan, India

Raju OS
Professor and Head
Department of Pediatric and Preventive Dentistry
Bapuji Dental College and Hospital
Davangere, Karnataka, India

Ramanandvignesh P
Senior Resident
Department of Dentistry
Government Medical College
Chandigarh, Punjab, India

Ramesh K
Registrar Pedodontics
Armed Forces Hospital Southern Region
Khamis Mushayit
Kingdom of Saudi Arabia

Ravi GR
Assistant Professor
Department of Pediatric Dentistry
King Faisal University
Al-Ahsa, Saudi Arabia

Ravi Kumar Mahto
Assistant Professor
Department of Orthodontics
Kathmandu University School of Medical Sciences
Kathmandu, Nepal

Ravichandra KS
Professor and Head
Department of Pediatric and Preventive Dentistry
Drs Sudha and Nageswara Rao Siddhartha Institute of Dental Sciences
Gannavaram, Andhra Pradesh, India

Renuka C
Pediatric Dentist
Mumbai, Maharashtra, India

Rinku Mathur
Professor
Department of Pediatric and Preventive Dentistry
RUHS Government Dental College
Jaipur, Rajasthan, India

Rishi Tyagi
Professor
Department of Pediatric and Preventive Dentistry
University College of Medical Sciences Dental College
New Delhi, India

Ruchi Singhal
Associate Professor
Department of Pediatric and Preventive Dentistry
Government Dental College
Post Graduate Institute of Medical Sciences (PGIMS)
Rohtak, Haryana, India

Rupinder Bhatia
Ex-Professor and Head
Department of Pediatric and Preventive Dentistry
Dr DY Patil Dental College
Navi Mumbai, Maharashtra, India

Saima Yunus Khan
Professor
Department of Pediatric and Preventive Dentistry
Aligarh Muslim University Dental College
Aligarh, Uttar Pradesh, India

***Late* Sameer Dutta**
Ex-Professor and Head
Department of Pediatric and Preventive Dentistry
Government Dental College
Rohtak, Haryana, India

Sanchit Paul
Pediatric Dentist
Tooth Talez
Noida, Uttar Pradesh, India

Sangeetha Venkatesh
Pediatric Dental Surgeon
Department of Dentistry
Royal Oman Police Hospital
Sultanate of Oman

Sanjay Tewari
Principal, Professor and Head
Department of Conservative Dentistry and Endodontics
Government Dental College
Post Graduate Institute of Medical Sciences (PGIMS)
Rohtak, Haryana, India

Sapna Hegde
Pediatric Dentist
Dubai, UAE

Saranya Mony
Assistant Professor
Department of Dental Surgery
District Early Intervention Centre
Government Medical College
Coimbatore, Tamil Nadu, India

Saraswathi V Naik
Professor
Department of Pediatric and Preventive Dentistry
Bapuji Dental College and Hospital
Davangere, Karnataka, India

Satish Vishwanathaiah
Associate Professor
Department of Pediatric Dentistry
Jazan University
Jazan, Saudi Arabia

Satyapal Yadav
Reader
Department of Oral Medicine and Radiology
Mahatma Gandhi Dental College
Mahatma Gandhi University of Medical Sciences and Technology (MGUMST)
Jaipur, Rajasthan, India

Seema Bargale
Professor
Department of Pediatric and Preventive Dentistry
KM Shah Dental College
Vadodara, Gujarat, India

Seema Thakur
Professor and Head
Department of Pediatric and Preventive Dentistry
Government Dental College
Shimla, Himachal Pradesh, India

Senchhema Limbu
Head
Department of Pediatric Dentistry
Kantipur Dental College
Nepal

Shabnam Zahir
Professor and Head
Department of Pediatric and Preventive Dentistry
Guru Nanak Institute of Dental Sciences and Research
Kolkata, West Bengal, India

Sham S Bhat
Professor and Head
Department of Pediatric and Preventive Dentistry
Yenepoya Dental College
Mangaluru, Karnataka, India

Shantanu Jain
Professor
Department of Pediatric and Preventive Dentistry
Mahatma Gandhi Dental College
Mahatma Gandhi University of Medical Sciences and Technology (MGUMST)
Jaipur, Rajasthan, India

Sharath Asokan
Principal and Professor
Department of Pedodontics
KSR Institute of Dental Sciences
Tiruchengode, Tamil Nadu, India

Sharath Chandra
Reader
Department of Pediatric and Preventive Dentistry
SJM Dental College
Chitradurga, Karnataka, India

Shashibala Singh
Professor
Department of Periodontics
Government Dental College
Post Graduate Institute of Medical Sciences (PGIMS)
Rohtak, Haryana, India

Shavan Yadav
Pediatric Dentist
Mumbai, Maharashtra, India

Shefali Chaturvedy
Pediatric Dentist
Jaipur, Rajasthan, India

Shilpa Ahuja
Pediatric Dentist
New Delhi, India

Shilpy Singla
Pediatric Dentist
Ambala, Punjab, India

Shital Kiran DP
Professor and Head
Department of Pediatric and Preventive Dentistry
College of Dental Sciences
Bhavnagar, Gujarat, India

Shivani Mathur
Professor and Head
Department of Pediatric and Preventive Dentistry
ITS Centre for Dental Studies and Research (ITS-CDSR)
Muradnagar, Uttar Pradesh, India

Shobha Fernandes
Professor and Head
Department of Pediatric and Preventive Dentistry
Narsinhbhai Patel Dental College
Sankalchand Patel University (SPU)
Visnagar, Gujarat, India

Shradha Jain
Postgraduate
Department of Pediatric and Preventive Dentistry
Mahatma Gandhi Dental College
Mahatma Gandhi University of Medical Sciences and Technology (MGUMST)
Jaipur, Rajasthan, India

Siddharth Mehta
Professor
Department of Orthodontics
Mahatma Gandhi Dental College
Mahatma Gandhi University of Medical Sciences and Technology (MGUMST)
Jaipur, Rajasthan, India

Simran Vangani
Postgraduate
Department of Pediatric and Preventive Dentistry
Mahatma Gandhi Dental College
Mahatma Gandhi University of Medical Sciences and Technology (MGUMST)
Jaipur, Rajasthan, India

Sivakumar Nuvvula
Professor and Head
Department of Pediatric and Preventive Dentistry
Narayana Dental College and Hospital
Nellore, Andhra Pradesh, India

Sonali Saha
Professor and Head
Department of Pediatric and Preventive Dentistry
Sardar Patel Post Graduate Institute of Dental and Medical Sciences
Lucknow, Uttar Pradesh, India

Sonu Acharya
Professor
Department of Pediatric and Preventive Dentistry
Institute of Dental Sciences
Bhubaneswar, Odisha, India

Srinivas LS
Reader
Department of Pediatric and Preventive Dentistry
KLE Society Institute of Dental Sciences
Bengaluru, Karnataka, India

Srinivas Namineni
Pediatric Dentist
Rainbow Hospital
Hyderabad, Telangana, India

Srirang Sevekar
Professor and Head
Department of Pediatric and Preventive Dentistry
MGM Dental College and Hospital
Navi Mumbai, Maharashtra, India

Srishty Chalana
Postgraduate
Department of Pediatric and Preventive Dentistry
Mahatma Gandhi Dental College
Mahatma Gandhi University of Medical Sciences and Technology (MGUMST)
Jaipur, Rajasthan, India

Suhani Khanna
Assistant Professor
Department of Pediatric and Preventive Dentistry
Yerala Medical Trust Dental College
Navi Mumbai, Maharashtra, India

Sundeep Hegde K
Professor
Department of Pediatric and Preventive Dentistry
Yenopoya Dental College
Mangaluru, Karnataka, India

Suneet Sable
CEO and Founder
Brainiac IP Solutions
Mumbai, Maharashtra, India

Sunil Sharma
Pro-Vice-Chancellor
Professor and Head
Department of Oral Surgery
NIMS Dental College
Jaipur, Rajasthan, India

Sunny Priyatham Tirupathi
Assistant Professor
Department of Pediatric and Preventive Dentistry
Dr DY Patil Dental College
Pune, Maharashtra, India

Suresh K Sachdeva
Professor
Department of Oral Medicine
Surendra Dental College
Sriganganagar, Rajasthan, India

Suresh S
Professor and Head
Department of Preventive and Community Dentistry
Vishnu Dental College
Bhimavaram, Andhra Pradesh, India

Suruchi Juneja Sukhija
Professor and Head
Department of Pediatric and Preventive Dentistry
Surendra Dental College
Sriganganagar, Rajasthan, India

Sushil Beniwal
Assistant Professor
Department of Pediatric and Preventive Dentistry
Mahatma Gandhi Dental College
Mahatma Gandhi University of Medical Sciences and Technology (MGUMST)
Jaipur, Rajasthan, India

Suzan Sahana
Professor
Department of Pediatric and Preventive Dentistry
St Joseph Dental College
Eluru, Andhra Pradesh, India

Swathi Karkare
Pediatric Dentist
Nasik, Maharashtra, India

Swati Aggarwal
Pediatric Dentist
Jaipur, Rajasthan, India

Swati Sharma
Professor
Department of Periodontology
Mahatma Gandhi Dental College
Mahatma Gandhi University of Medical Sciences and Technology (MGUMST)
Jaipur, Rajasthan, India

T Pavani
CEO Medispaces

Tabassum Tayab
Specialist Pediatric Dentist
Al Hilal Hospital
Kingdom of Bahrain

Thejo Krishna Pammi
Pediatric Dentist
Mumbai, Maharashtra, India

Umme Azher
Professor
Department of Pediatric and Preventive Dentistry
Sri Rajiv Gandhi College of Dental Sciences
Bengaluru, Karnataka, India

Unnat Dhanwani
Assistant Professor
Department of Pediatric and Preventive Dentistry
Mahatma Gandhi Dental College
Mahatma Gandhi University of Medical Sciences and Technology (MGUMST)
Jaipur, Rajasthan, India

Vaibhav Kumar
Faculty
GD Pols Foundation YMT Dental College
Navi Mumbai, Maharashtra, India

Vaibhav Ravindra Wani
Professor and Head
Department of Pediatric and Preventive Dentistry
RR Kambe Dental College
Akola, Maharashtra, India

Vemina Paul
Pediatric Dentist
New Delhi, India

Vijay Lakshmi
Pediatric Dentist
Jaipur, Rajasthan, India

Vineet Dhar
Professor
Department of Pediatric Dentistry
University of Maryland Dental School
Baltimore, USA

Vineeta Nikhil
Professor and Head
Department of Conservative Dentistry and Endodontics
Subharti Dental College
Meerut, Uttar Pradesh, India

Vinita Goyal
Senior Lecturer
Department of Pediatric and Preventive Dentistry
ITS Centre for Dental Studies and Research (ITS-CDSR)
Muradnagar, Uttar Pradesh, India

Vinola Duraisamy
Professor and Head
Department of Pediatric and Preventive Dentistry
Vinayaka Mission Sankarachariyar Dental College
Salem, Tamil Nadu, India

Vipul Sharma
Postgraduate
Department of Pediatric and Preventive Dentistry
Mahatma Gandhi Dental College
Mahatma Gandhi University of Medical Sciences and Technology (MGUMST)
Jaipur, Rajasthan, India

Viral Maru
Associate Professor
Department of Pediatric and Preventive Dentistry
Government Dental College
Mumbai, Maharashtra, India

Virat Galhotra
Professor and Head
Department of Pediatric and Preventive Dentistry
All India Institute of Medical Sciences
Raipur, Chhattisgarh, India

Virinder Goyal
Professor and Head
Department of Pediatric and Preventive Dentistry
Guru Nanak Dev Dental College and Research Institute
Sunam, Punjab, India

Vivek Lath
Professor
Department of Prosthodontics
Maitri College of Dentistry
Durg, Chhattisgarh, India

Vritika Singh
Postgraduate
Department of Pediatric and Preventive Dentistry
Mahatma Gandhi Dental College
Mahatma Gandhi University of Medical Sciences and Technology (MGUMST)
Jaipur, Rajasthan, India

Yash Bafna
Professor
Department of Pediatric and Preventive Dentistry
Narsinhbhai Patel Dental College
Sankalchand Patel University (SPU)
Visnagar, Gujarat, India

Yash Shah
Assistant Professor
Department of Pediatric and Preventive Dentistry
KM Shah Dental College
Vadodara, Gujarat, India

Yogita Chaturvedi
Pediatric Dentist
Jaipur, Rajasthan, India

Foreword

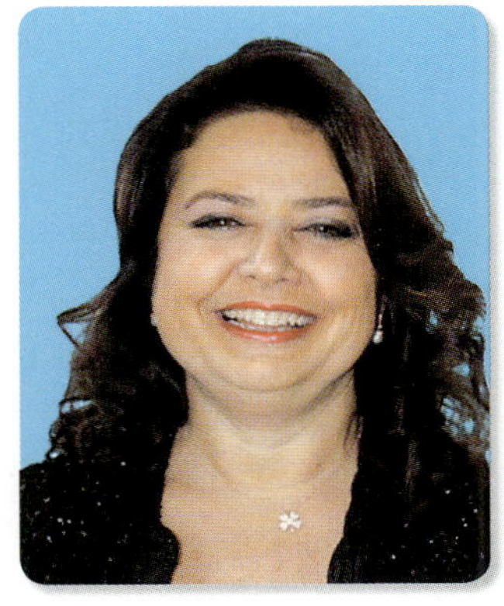

The fifth more comprehensive edition is the outcome of an enthusiastic response to the previous editions of *Textbook of Pediatric Dentistry*, edited by Nikhil Marwah who is Professor and Head of Department of Pediatric and Preventive Dentistry at Mahatma Gandhi Dental College and Hospital and Associate Dean (Research) at Mahatma Gandhi University of Medical Sciences and Technology, Jaipur, Rajasthan, India.

This new edition of the *Textbook of Pediatric Dentist*ry fulfills the need for a practical, clinical guide not only to the pediatric dental profession but also to all dental practitioners and students with the user-friendly adaptation with its quick revision format and questionnaire.

The textbook highlights the approach to diagnosis, developmental aspects, actual preventive treatment techniques, pediatric orthodontics, cariology, endodontics, periodontal and surgical procedures, oral pathology, lasers in pediatric dentistry, forensic pediatric dentistry, and dental care for patients with special healthcare needs, and all these existing chapters have been extensively revised and updated with new concepts like pediatric dental clinic, new techniques in digital radiographic diagnosis, new assessment scales in dental fear and anxiety, updated new methodologies in behavior management, nitrous oxide—oxygen anxiolysis, new types of space maintainers, concepts of minimal intervention, bioflex crowns, concepts of revascularization and pulp regeneration, rotary endodontics along with many others.

The inclusion of new actual interesting chapters which are parenting styles, molar incisor hypomineralization (MIH), remineralization, sleep-disordered breathing in children, teledentistry, patents and innovation, stem cells in pediatric dentistry, digital pediatric dentistry, infant cleft care, hypnosis enriched the content of the textbook.

The textbook is also including more than 1,000 illustrations and clinical photographs. The addition of these good-quality color illustrations and photographs is an important adjunct to the written descriptions and facilitates diagnosis and management.

The enlightenment about research studies, scientific references, and text provided in this edition has been updated and amended in accordance with the curriculum of Dental Council of India (DCI) with contributions from more than 200 stalwarts of Pediatric Dentistry.

Dental practitioners and students need information on all of these areas of dental care for children, on a daily basis. *Textbook of Pediatric Dentistry*, authored by Professor Dr Nikhil Marwah undoubtedly provides the excellent information necessary in a clear and readily retrievable form, at the same time providing guidance on the most appropriate texts or journals, where more detailed information may be found.

It is my great honor and pleasure to know Nikhil Marwah not only as a colleague but also as a friend. This edition of the *Textbook of Pediatric Dentistry*, which was prepared with great effort, will be very successful like the previous editions, and I offer my sincere congratulations and eagerly looking forward to the next edition.

Prof. Dr. Figen Seymen U
President-Elect, International Association of Pediatric Dentistry
President, Turkish Society of Pediatric Dentistry
Head, Department of Pediatric Dentistry
Director of Master of Dentistry, Pediatric Dentistry Graduate Program
Faculty of Dentistry Altınbaş University, Turkey

Foreword

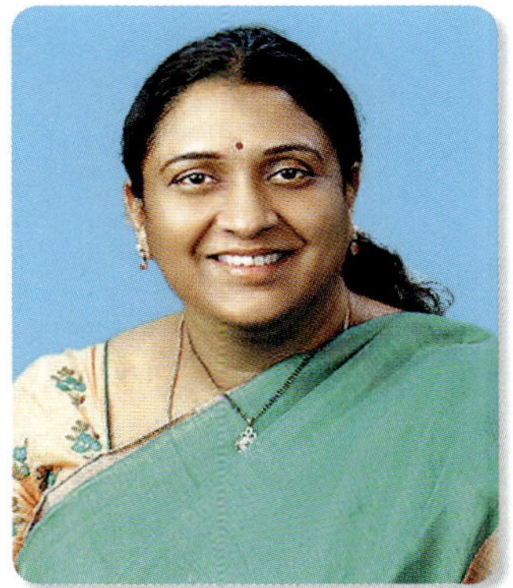

Touching other peoples life, being authentic and always open to receiving as well as giving, expanding the purview of our field of Pediatric Dentistry is the description of one of the most amazing and dynamic authors I have encountered—Dr Nikhil Marwah

- The present edition captures various aspects and essential steps required for grooming a graduate student in the subject of Pediatric Dentistry to a postgraduate level.
- All the existing chapters have been thoroughly revised and updated with new concepts.
- Contributions from more than 200 authors with recent literature till 2022.
- New techniques in digital diagnosis, latest assessment scales, and methodologies in behavior management along with recent concepts of minimal intervention, space maintainers, and bioflex crowns, pulp revascularization and regeneration are among the few.
- Student-friendly adaptation with 1,000 illustrations and clinical pictures along with quick revision format and questionnaire are the highlights of this book.

Textbook of Pediatric Dentistry is for all the students who are struggling to find excellence in Pediatric Dentistry and I'm sure it will live up to the reader's expectations. My heartfelt congratulations and best wishes to Dr Nikhil Marwah for his new 5th edition of the book and all his future endeavors.

Prof. Dr. Radhika Muppa
President, Indian Society of Pedodontics and Preventive Dentistry 2022-23
Professor
Drs Sudha and Nageswara Rao Siddhartha Institute of Dental Sciences
Gannavaram, Andhra Pradesh, India

Foreword

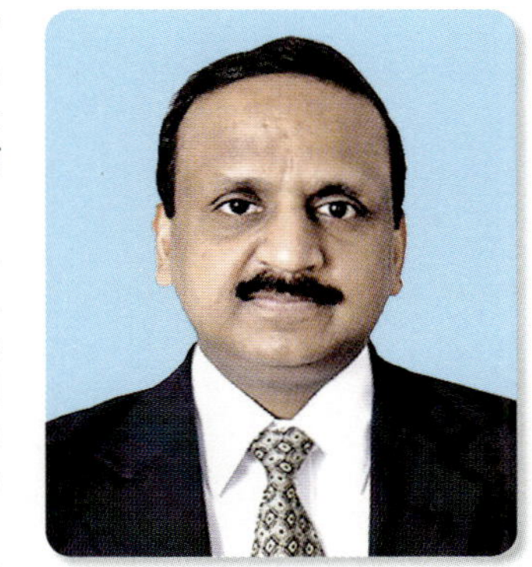

It is a delightful opportunity to introduce the fifth edition the *Textbook of Pediatric Dentistry* authored by Professor Dr Nikhil Marwah. I feel honored as it is my second foreword for this outstandingly composed book with thoroughly revised and updated chapters with recent advances and literature. Additionally, the author has augmented the existing content of the textbook with recent burning topics such as molar incisor hypomineralization (MIH), remineralization, sleep-disordered breathing in pediatric patients, teledentistry, digital pediatric dentistry and stem cells in Pediatric Dentistry. These topics are indeed the need of the hour as we all had faced the pandemic together and thus; this book may prove to be one of the best medium of knowledge and expertise to handle pediatric patients in clinical practice. This new edition appears to have more than 1,000 illustrations and clinical images which would be an added advantage for the undergraduate as well as postgraduate students aiding in better understanding of concepts.

The students could also revise and self-assess themselves with the summary and the questions available at the back of each chapter. The Editors have worked tirelessly towards the compilation of newer techniques under various chapters such as bioflex crowns, recent concepts of minimal intervention, revascularization and pulp regeneration, recent advances in radiographic diagnosis and many more. I am certain that the entire volume of this book would be able to guide and give deep insight to its readers into the vast field of Pediatric and Preventive Dentistry. I extend my appreciation and best wishes to the editor and all the contributors of this well-written textbook for their arduous task.

Prof. Dr. Varinder Goyal
Founder President, South Asian Association of Pediatric Dentistry
Member, Board of Directors, International Association of Pediatric Dentistry
Chair Education Committee, International Association of Pediatric Dentistry
Board Member, Pediatric Dentistry Association of Asia
Past President, Indian Society of Pedodontics and Preventive Dentistry
Member Faculty of Dental Surgery, Royal College of Physicians and Surgeons, Glasgow
Professor and Head, Department of Pediatric and Preventive Dentistry
Guru Nanak Dev Dental College and Research Institute, Sunam, Punjab, India

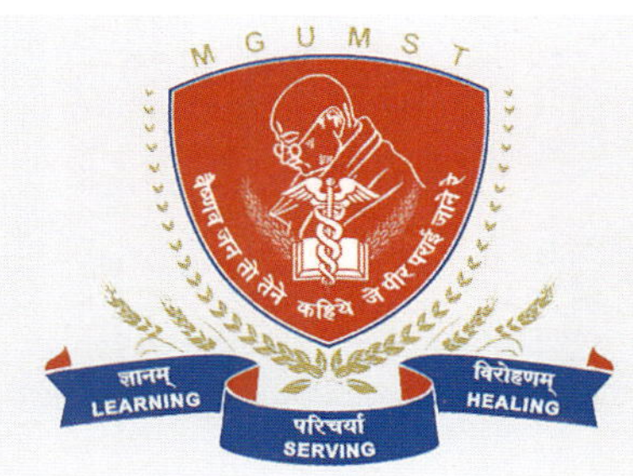

MAHATMA GANDHI UNIVERSITY
of
MEDICAL SCIENCES & TECHNOLOGY
JAIPUR

Message

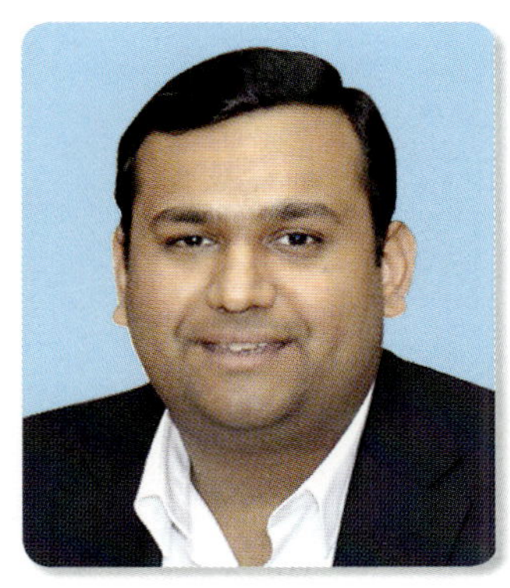

Dr Nikhil Marwah has been associated with Mahatma Gandhi University of Medical Sciences and Technology, Jaipur, Rajasthan, India for more than 15 years and has excelled in his academic contributions in all fields.

Pediatric and Preventive Dentistry is a continuously evolving field. It deals with the overall health of our younger generation who are the future of India. The fifth edition of '*Textbook of Pediatric Dentistry*' is a compilation of updated facts, recent studies and newer advancements in treatment modalities. It will surely help the graduates and post-graduates not only to study but to better understand and implement the theoretical and clinical aspects of Pediatric Dentistry. A stand out point for this book is the contributions from various renowned faculties from all over India.

My best wishes are with Dr Nikhil Marwah, for this book and also for the future endeavors.

With personal regards!

Vikas Chandra Swarankar MS (OBGYN) MS (Gen. Surgery)
Chairperson-Cum-Chancellor
Specialist in Reproductive Medicine and IVF
Mahatma Gandhi University of Medical Sciences and Technology
Jaipur, Rajasthan, India

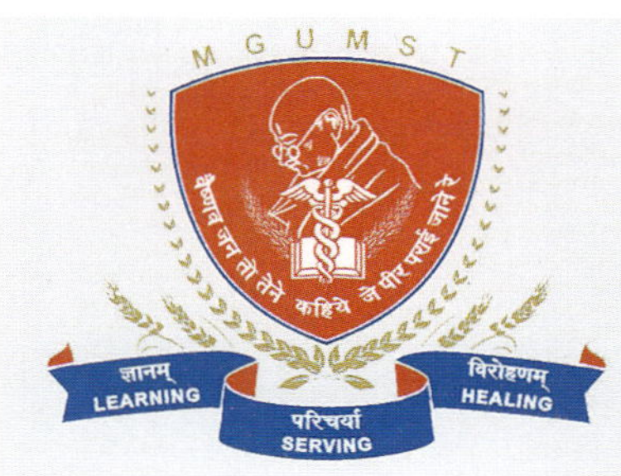

MAHATMA GANDHI UNIVERSITY
of
MEDICAL SCIENCES & TECHNOLOGY
JAIPUR

Message

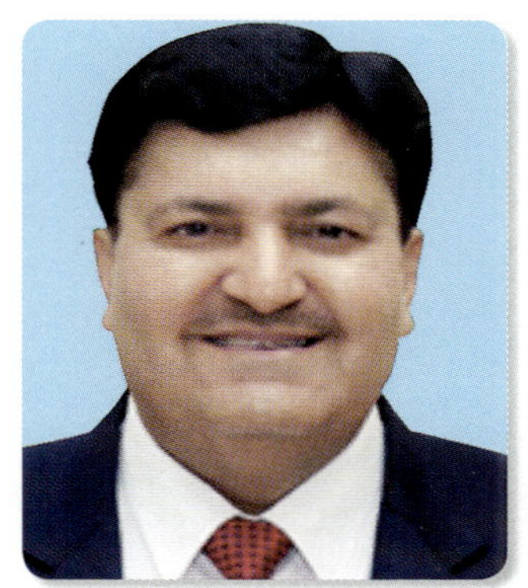

Pediatric Dentistry is a distinct branch of dentistry which deals with treating children from infancy through adolescence. Children seek special attention in diagnosis, prognosis and management of dental problems.

After the success of his first four editions, Dr Nikhil Marwah, has come out with the fifth edition of '*Textbook of Pediatric Dentistry*.' This edition is a well written book which provides much needed knowledge and recent updates. I am sure it would be the book of choice for graduate and postgraduate students in India and abroad.

I convey my best wishes and congratulations to Dr Nikhil Marwah, Associate Dean (Research) MGUMST; Professor and Head, Department of Pediatric and Preventive Dentistry, Mahatma Gandhi Dental College and Hospital, a unit of Mahatma Gandhi University of Medical Sciences and Technology, Jaipur, Rajasthan, India for the fifth edition of '*Textbook of Pediatric Dentistry*.'

Sudhir Sachdev MD FRCP (Edin.)
President/Vice Chancellor
Professor, Department of Anesthesiology
Mahatma Gandhi University of Medical Sciences and Technology
Jaipur, Rajasthan, India

Preface to the Fifth Edition

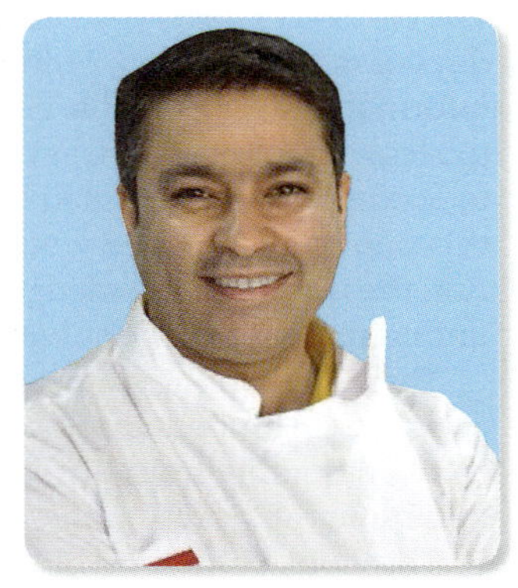

Revisions are often tedious and complicated tasks but the essence is to present a simplified picture not much different from the original one yet complete and updated on its own. We hope the new edition of *Textbook of Pediatric Dentistry* is appreciated by all students and faculty likewise just like the previous ones.

In this edition we have included newer chapters like parenting styles, molar incisor hypomineralization (MIH), Remineralization, sleep disordered breathing in children, teledentistry, patents and innovation, stem cells in pediatric dentistry, digital pediatric dentistry, infant cleft care, hypnosis, etc. Apart from this some major modifications are done and newer concepts are added in various chapters like pediatric dental clinic, new techniques in digital radiographic diagnosis, new assessment scales in dental fear and anxiety, updated new methodologies in behavior management, nitrous oxide—oxygen anxiolysis, new types of space maintainers, concepts of minimal intervention, bioflex crowns, concepts of revascularization and pulp regeneration, rotary endodontics along with many others. All the chapters have been updated with recent literature till 2022.

This textbook has numerous contributors not only from the stalwarts of academic fields but also from the private practitioners thereby lending solidarity to both theoretical and practical approach to Pediatric Dentistry. This edition will help all undergraduates, postgraduates and clinicians to understand the subject in a more comprehensive manner with elaborate flowcharts, descriptive photos and simplified text.

I hope we will continue to enjoy the same patronage and blessings from all faculty members and students across the globe and an even larger response to the fifth edition of *Textbook of Pediatric Dentistry*.

Nikhil Marwah

Preface to the First Edition

The curiosity I developed about the subject came out of my interest in search of precise text for pediatric dentistry. During the days of my graduation, I often found that it was difficult to understand and comprehend this text as no book with adequate information was available and I had to go through many books to satisfy my queries as the information in one book was either too less or too much. It was this time that a budding idea of writing this book struck my mind. But, I had to wait for many years to accomplish this, so as to have a complete knowledge and understanding of this vast subject. Many a times during writing this book, my patience would snap and thoughts that I will not be able to complete this task would often cross my mind. But, the quest for knowledge and the desire to share it with others propelled me to complete one of the exclusive books for undergraduates in the subject of pedodontics.

There is a well-known concept that it is always difficult to hit a moving target than a stationary one, this analogy seems appropriate for pedodontists who are dealing with growing children. Such practice involves comprehensive treatment of the child emanating from birth to adulthood and encompasses a wide-range of treatment modalities, ranging from preventive treatment replacement therapy.

This book comprises of 31 Chapters that have been uniformly divided into various sections. The first section explains the basics as applied to pedodontics such as the concepts of growth and nutrition. The second section helps in understanding and management of child in a dental clinic. The third section comprises of clinical pediatric dentistry that includes preventive and restorative protocol. The fourth section includes the conglomeration of orthodontics and pedodontics whereas the fifth section explains the effects of external or internal environment on oral tissues. The treatment and management of physically, mentally or medically compromised patients is covered in the sixth section. The last section includes some small but very informative topics like lasers, forensic pedodontics.

"I hear, I forget, I see, I learn." The human mind is brilliantly capable of remembering things that it visualizes and keeping this in mind we have tried to illustrate concepts with some of the best dental photographs that range from those commonly seen in clinical practice to may exceedingly rare conditions.

Textbook of Pediatric Dentistry especially takes note of the recently added concepts and maximum care has been taken to update this information for the readers. Some of the newly and exclusively added chapters include Lasers, Early Childhood Caries, Diet and Nutrition, Stainless Steel Crowns, Temporomandibular Joint (TMJ) Disorders, Pit and Fissure Sealant, Atraumatic Restorative Treatment (ART), Vaccination Schedule and Recently Prescribed American Academy of Pediatric Dentistry (AAPD) Guidelines.

The purpose of the book is many fold but in general it provides an organizational structure from which every student can learn about the concepts and complexity of this truly vast but astonishing subject.

Nikhil Marwah

Gratitude

To my parents and family for their blessings

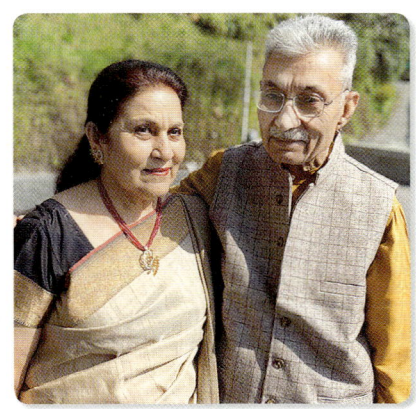

To my wife Kanupriya, who has always stood behind be as my pillar of strength

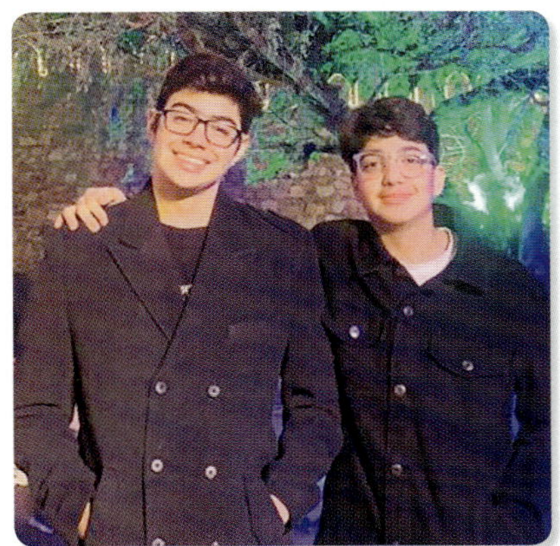

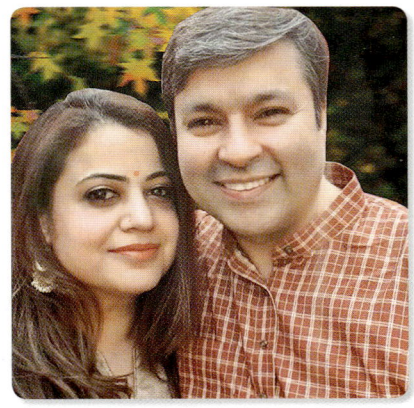

To my sons Aayushman & Ayaan, the essence of my life

Acknowledgments

I would like to express my gratitude to all my teachers, seniors, colleagues and friends who have helped me in compilation of the fifth edition of *Textbook of Pediatric Dentistry*.

Firstly, I would like to thank the Almighty God and my family, who have been my constant source of support, encouragement and motivation during the revision of the textbook.

I would like to express my sincere thanks to all the contributors of this book for sharing their immense knowledge, texts and photographs with me, which were truly helpful in revising the textbook.

I thank Dr ML Swarankar (Emeritus Chairperson, Mahatma Gandhi University of Medical Sciences and Technology, Jaipur, Rajasthan, India), Dr Vikas Swarankar (Chairperson, Mahatma Gandhi University of Medical Sciences and Technology, Jaipur, Rajasthan, India), Dr Sudhir Sachdev (Vice-Chancellor, Mahatma Gandhi University of Medical Sciences and Technology, Jaipur, Rajasthan, India), Dr GN Saxena (Pro-Vice-Chancellor, Mahatma Gandhi University of Medical Sciences and Technology, Jaipur), Shri RR Soni (CFO, Mahatma Gandhi University of Medical Sciences and Technology, Jaipur) for providing me with a congenial environment and adequate academic support to revise the textbook.

The revision of textbook is always a more tedious task as enormous time is spent trying to add the best possible literature into the textbook. I have to thank my academic team of Dr Satish V, Dr Ravi GR and my team of postgraduates in Department of Pediatric and Preventive Dentistry, Mahatma Gandhi Dental College, MGUMST, Jaipur, for their unending efforts.

I would like to whole heartedly thank my teachers and senior faculty members, who have taken time from their busy schedule not only to contribute academically to the book but also preview the book in such a short span of time.

My sincere thanks to Shri Jitendar P Vij (Group Chairman), Mr Ankit Vij (Managing Director), Mr MS Mani (Group President), Dr Madhu Choudhary (Director–Educational Publishing), Ms Pooja Bhandari (Production Head), Ms Sunita Katla (Executive Assistant to Group Chairman and Publishing Manager), Dr Sangeeta Yadav (Development Editor), Mr Rajesh Sharma (Production Coordinator), Ms Seema Dogra (Cover Visualizer), Mr Kulwant Singh (Typesetter), Ms Geeta Barik (Proofreader), Mr Manoj Pahuja (Senior Graphic Designer) and their team members, for all their support to work in this project and make it a success.

Contents

Section 14: Dentistry for the Differently-abled Child

Section 15: Pediatric Oral Pathology

Section 16: Forensic Pedodontics

Section 17: Lasers in Pediatric Dentistry

Section 18: Recent Concepts Associated with Pediatric Dentistry

Section 19: Research Methodology in Pediatric Dentistry

CHAPTER

Introduction and History of Pediatric Dentistry

Nikhil Marwah, Bhavna Gupta Saraf

Chapter Outline

- Importance of Primary Teeth
- Aims and Objectives of Pediatric Dentistry
- Pedodontic Triangle
- Indian Society of Pedodontics and Preventive Dentistry
- South Asian Association of Pediatric Dentistry
- Other International Pediatric Dentistry Association
- Scope of Pediatric Dentistry

Pediatric Dentistry is the art and science and that branch of dental science, which deals with comprehensive, preventive and interceptive oral health in children from childhood to adolescent age particularly and complete health in general. In other words, it is a branch of dentistry that includes training of a child to accept dentistry, restoring and maintaining primary, mixed, permanent dentitions and applying preventive methods for dental care. The value of a Pediatric Dentist always depends upon how carefully the child has been managed at a young age and so they should have a better understanding of the subject. The word Pedodontics is a part of American English whereas Paedodontics belongs to Commonwealth English.

The word pedodontics is made of two words, i.e., pedo + dontics. Pedo is derived from Greek word "*pais*" meaning child and "*dontics*" is the study of teeth.

Pediatric Dentistry has come a long way from its early days of extraction oriented beginning to the current comprehensive era with the emphasis on diagnosis and treatment planning. There was a time when dental clinics were biased against this specialty and considered it a waste of time and very often clinics displayed "No treatment for children under the age of 14 at this clinic." Most of the dentists also gave a negative knowledge influence to the parents and the most common excuse that was offered was, "These are milk teeth and fall on their own so treating them would be a waste of time and money."

As the years passed by, times changed and so did the schedule for the initial appointment for the child. The dentistry had now progressed significantly and it was thought that 3 years would be a good time for the child to visit the dentist. Recent knowledge in Pediatric Dentistry has enabled us to realize that age of 3 years is too old to initiate any type of preventive strategy as the disease will have already taken its toll on the teeth and it no longer remains preventive but becomes interceptive pedodontics. Therefore, it was realized that the first visit should be initiated as soon as the first tooth erupts in oral cavity and the preventive education should start much earlier, by parental counseling.

DEFINITIONS

Stewart 1982 defined *Pediatric Dentistry as the practice and teaching of comprehensive, preventive and therapeutic oral health care of child from birth to adolescence.* It is construed to include care for special patients who demonstrate physical, mental or emotional problems.

Pinkham: *Pediatric Dentistry is synonymous with dentistry for children. Pediatric Dentistry exists because children have dental and orofacial problems. The genesis of dentistry for children unquestionably is allied to dental decay, pulpitis, and the inflammation and pain associated with infected pulpal tissue and suppuration in alveolar bone.*

American Academy of Pediatric Dentistry (1999) defined "pediatric dentistry as an age defined specialty that provides both primary and comprehensive preventive and therapeutic oral health care for infants and children through adolescence, including those with special health care needs."

IMPORTANCE OF PRIMARY TEETH

It is very important that primary teeth are kept in place until they are lost naturally. These teeth serve a number of critical functions. Primary teeth:

- Maintain good nutrition by permitting your child to chew properly
- Involved in speech development
- Helps in the eruption of permanent teeth by saving space for them
- A healthy smile can help children feel good about the way they look to others.

AIMS AND OBJECTIVES OF PEDIATRIC DENTISTRY

- **Health of a child as a whole:** The pediatric dentist is a part of the health team concerned with the individuals,' that is, total physical, mental and emotional wellbeing of patient. We must be certain that our effort to improve dental health is always in accordance with the general health of patient.
- **More specifically we are concerned with oral health:** The other aim should be preventing disease. The earliest attempt at prevention is at expectant mother. She should be advised on dental health of her future child. After the child is born, we advise the mother to continue appointments. First dental appointment for a child is usually at 6 months.
- **Early diagnosis and prompt treatment:** Introduce and implement the principles of preventive dentistry from birth so that early diagnosis is initiated. Occlusal guidance and early treatment of developing malocclusion should be done to avoid complications.
- **Restoring the mouth to good health:** During restorative treatment first and foremost necessity is to convince the patient and parent that treatment is worthwhile. Only work of highest technical standards will succeed in primary teeth. However, this must be at the same time being enjoyable and at worst acceptable to patient. If dental treatment is unpleasant then the child will develop resistance and reluctance for further treatment. In order to overcome those problems, early diagnosis leading to proper treatment is required. Regular attendance, sound diagnosis, adequate local analgesia, modern-cutting equipment are important, but these only arrest the essential empathy that the dentist must have toward child.
- **To observe and control the necessary developing dentition of child patient:** A general dentist who sees the child every time is in an excellent position to study his oral development and to intervene himself or refer to a specialist for the necessary treatment.
- **Relief of pain:** As and when necessary bearing in mind the necessary treatment should be provided focusing on the patient's total well-being.
- **Increase the knowledge:** Following this, we will produce a service for the child as an individual population which is dentally educated which also leads to elevation of the profession.
- **Instill a positive attitude and behavior:** This not only will help in accomplishing the treatment in a desired manner but also make the child a good dental patient even in adulthood and will have a positive attitude.
- **Restore the lost tooth structure:** To maintain tissue harmony between the hard and soft tissue.
- **Management of special patients:** Managing physically and mentally disabled and medically compromised children in an efficient and orderly manner so as to avoid discomfort to the patient and at the same time avoiding any bias toward the special condition of the children.

PEDODONTIC TRIANGLE

*Pedodontic triangle was first explained and conceptualized by **Wright** in 1975 and was later modified by **McDonald** et al., in 2004.*

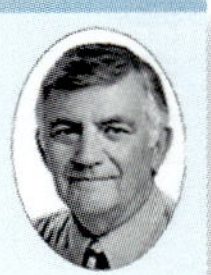

The differences between child and adults with respect to treatment have long been emphasized by **Hippocrates** in the 5th century BC and by **Celsius** in 4th century AD.

- An adult requires a service to be carried out in his mouth and if he is not satisfied he will seek satisfaction elsewhere, whereas the child attends the dental service because he is forced to do so and will have to return even if he does not like the treatment.
- We may expect the adult to put up with unavoidable discomfort; therefore, he has the freedom to choose his treatment and can also appreciate the outcome, whereas the child sees no good reason for dentist's attention.
- Child is in dynamic state of growth and development, whereas the adult is in static state.
- Consideration of behavior as an integral part of child oral health care and needs. The age appropriate behavior management and behavior shaping techniques are used to make the child comfortable.
- Attention to preventive care rather than rehabilitation.

Conventional Model

Patient-doctor relation in adults is linear, but in pedodontics, the relation is triangular. This is because in pedodontics, the parent and the child both are involved wherein the child is at the apex of triangle as he is the focus of attention. This was first elaborated best in the Pediatric Dentistry treatment triangle given by **Wright** in 1975.[1] Moreover, in **(Fig. 1.1)** the arrows

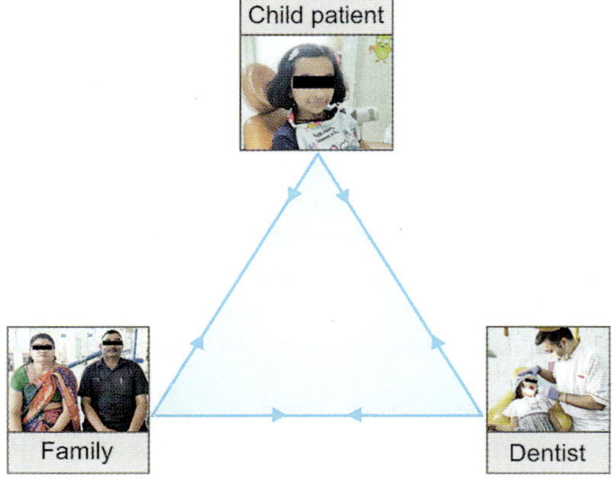

Fig. 1.1: Pedodontic triangle.

indicated that the communication is not only limited to the benefit of the child but is reciprocal in nature.

An authoritarian or over indulgent parent always tries to interfere in the conversation between the dentist and the child by answering on behalf of the child. As a consequence, there is more interaction between the parent and the dentist hence the equilateral triangle is replaced by isosceles triangle **(Fig. 1.2)**.

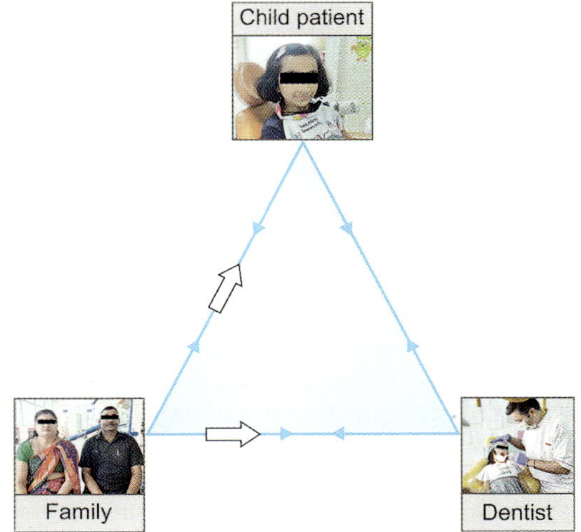

Fig. 1.2: Isosceles triangle—authoritarian parent.

On the contrary, if the parent is negligent or permissive, then the conversation between the parent and the dentist may not be reciprocal effectively; hence, right-angled triangle replaces the normal equilateral triangle **(Fig. 1.3)**.

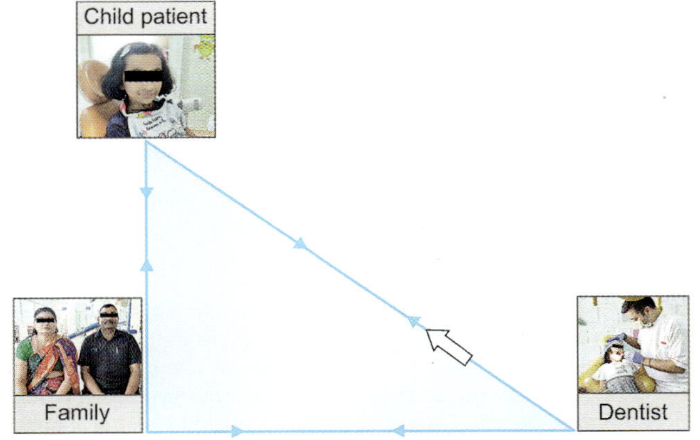

Fig. 1.3: Right angle triangle—neglectful or permissive parent.

Modified Model

As community has become a major part of all components of environment; therefore, recently, a new parameter has also been added, that is, society **(Fig. 1.4)**. This depiction looked complete with the fact that the communication is reciprocal and society came into the center of the triangle indicating that management methods acceptable to society and the litigiousness of society are important factors influencing treatment modalities.[2]

Since 2013, due to increased societal expectations the treatment in Pediatric Dentistry has seen an additional

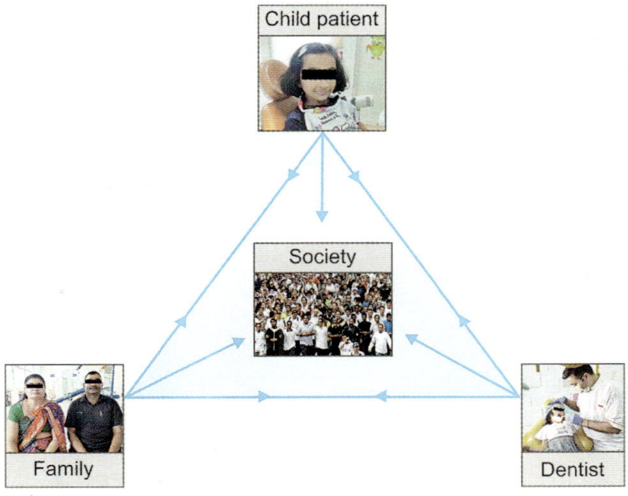

Fig. 1.4: Modified pediatric triangle.

impact of this component. Therefore, the pediatric triangle (earlier known as pedodontic triangle) no longer represents the isolated environment but society as a whole according to Wright 2014 **(Fig. 1.5)**.[3]

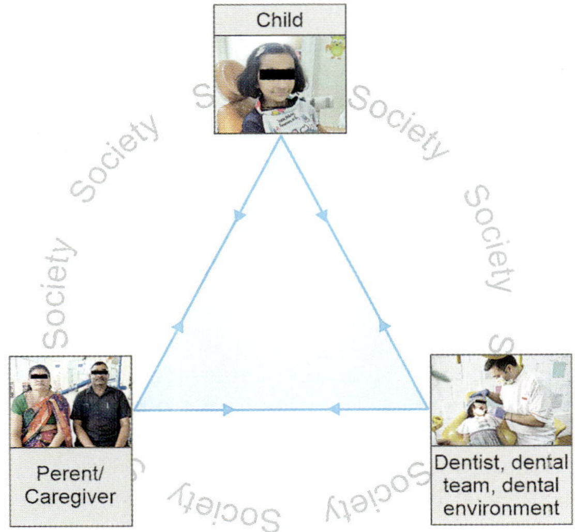

Fig. 1.5: Modified pediatric triangle according to Wright.

Pediatric Dentistry Treatment Model

Pediatric Dentistry is an amalgamation of all the branches of dentistry and most of its components have been either derived from or associated with other dentistry branches, but the four principles that stand out in this specialty are prevention, risk assessment and management, child psychology and behavior management. **Padmanabhan et al.**, have proposed a new model based on the pedodontic triangle and have termed it Pediatric Dentistry Treatment Model.[4] It presents the former triangle as a square which has the pediatric dentist, pediatrician, family and society playing important roles and definitely the child patient is the center of attention **(Fig. 1.6)**.

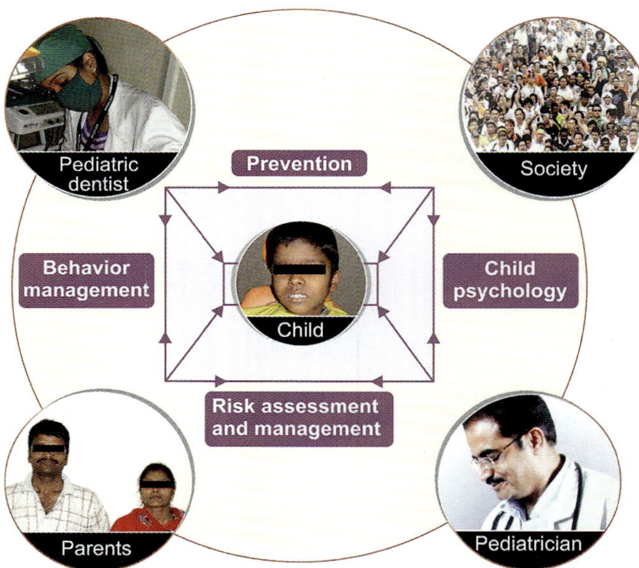

Fig. 1.6: Pediatric dentistry treatment model given by Padmanabhan et al.

INDIAN SOCIETY OF PEDODONTICS AND PREVENTIVE DENTISTRY

Indian Society of Pedodontics and Preventive Dentistry (ISPPD) is the national society specifically concerned with the oral health of children in India. It aims to improve oral health in children and encourage the highest standards of clinical care. The ISPPD has over 4,000 life members from university and hospital pediatric dental departments, pediatric dental practice and general dental practice. The emblem **(Fig. 1.7)** is based on the famous triad of **Keyes** (1960). One circle represents the tooth, the other the bacteria and the third diet. The shaded area of intersection of the circles represents dental caries. The stress given is that for caries to develop all the three factors are essential; caries cannot occur if one factor is missing. Incidentally, this area of intersection of circles takes the form of triangles. The triangle denotes two aspects—(1) it represents delta, which is the sign of dentistry, (2) it depicts the pedodontic triangle as given by Wright.[1]

The three corners of triangles are indicative of—(1) child, (2) mother (parent) and (3) dentist. This triangle represents 1:2 transactions for the management of children. The top circle of keys in the emblem carries symbols of the emblem of the Indian Dental Association (IDA)—Staff of Aesculpius with wings of serpents encircling around it. The Staff of Aesculapius stands of captor of authority and represents the professional authority of association. The serpents show the power of healing since serpents ages back have been used for healing. Hippocrates adopted this symbol and we have adopted it with two serpents entwined around the staff in opposite directions. The wings on the staff represent the spread of knowledge. The wings have six small and three large divisions as in the IDA emblem.

Attitudes of Pediatric Dentist

- Develop an attitude to adopt ethical principles in all aspects of pediatric dental practice.

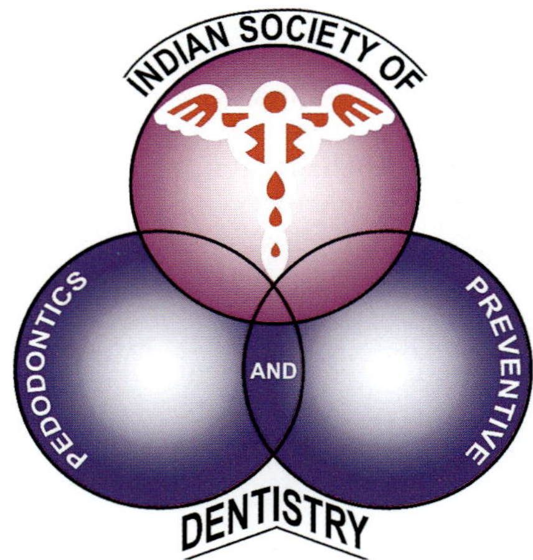

Fig. 1.7: Logo of Indian Society of Pedodontics and Preventive Dentistry (ISPPD).

- Professional honesty and integrity are to be fostered.
- Treatment care is to be delivered irrespective of the social status, cast, creed and religion of the patients.
- Willingness to share the knowledge and clinical experience with professional colleagues.
- Willingness to adopt, after a critical assessment, new methods and techniques of Pediatric Dentistry management developed from time to time, based on scientific researches, which are in the best interest of the child patient.
- Respect child patient's rights and privileges, including child patient's right to information and right to seek a second opinion.
- Develop an attitude to seek opinion from allied medical and dental specialties, as and when required.

Aims and Objectives of ISPPD

- The society is formed on the firm belief that "Every child in India has a fundamental right to total dental health." Every member of the dental profession in general and pediatric dentistry in particular have an obligation to uphold this right.
- The society shall have the solemn responsibility toward the maintenance of positive dental health of the children through prevention, involvement of the community and through other necessary measures to achieve this objective.
- The society shall make an endeavor to provide suitable medium for honoring the commitment it has so sacredly undertaken.
- The society shall be responsible for improvement of education, research and delivery of dental health care in the field pediatric and preventive dentistry and shall extend cooperation or collaborate with any person, persons or organizations; national or international with similar ideas, ideals and objectives.

To realize and attain above-mentioned goals the society may:

- Conduct dental health education programs in schools and in community for the promotion of better oral hygiene, better dental health awareness and prevention of dental diseases.
- Establish liaison with dental surgeons in general practice to carry the message of the society to term and also to keep them in contact with the new, relevant and advanced knowledge in the field through continuing education programs.
- To provide forum for the dental teachers to communicate and exchange knowledge on the current and recent advances in pediatric and preventive dentistry.
- Hold period meetings and conferences of the members of society.
- Organize courses on new techniques in the field of pediatric and preventive dentistry.

- To promote the publications of scientific literature including a journal of the society, which would be dynamic in character and shall have the possibility to adapt itself to the needs of the society from time to time. The publications shall not only be scientific in nature but shall also undertake publicity and propaganda as per the needs of the society and the community.
- Establish rapport with Dental Council of India, union and state governments and other national and international apex bodies to advise on the various aspects of pediatric and preventive dentistry including legislative and administrative areas.
- Accept endowments and grants from individuals or societies, official or nonofficial, governmental or nongovernmental, national or international.
- Make efforts to improve the basic curriculum of pediatric and preventive dentistry both at the undergraduate and postgraduate levels.
- Establish liaison with associations and societies of other allied sciences like pediatrics, psychiatry, psychology and basic sciences like biochemistry, microbiology and pathology.
- Encourage research in the specialty of pediatric and preventive dentistry and other related sciences by the establishment of scholarships, prizes and rewards, by publishing from time to time monographs embodying the results of the research conducted by members independently or under the auspicious of the society.
- Consider and express its views on all matters pertaining to public dental health, dental profession and dental education and take such steps from time to time as shall be deemed necessary.
- To collect, manage and disburse funds for all or any of the objects of the society.
- Do all such things and matters as are conducive to the attainment of the above objectives or any one of them which are subsidiary to the said objectives.

The Indian Society of Pedodontics and Preventive Dentistry has been formed on the firm belief that "Every child has a fundamental right to his total oral health."

SOUTH ASIAN ASSOCIATION OF PEDIATRIC DENTISTRY

The South Asian Association of Pediatric Dentistry is ardently devoted towards children's oral health care across the continent. An embodiment of constructive thinking specifically directed towards developing new methodologies while optimizing the use of traditional concepts aimed at building a future essentially free of oral ailments in children.

It is a platform for experts to congregate for effective exchange of ideas and skills relying on the belief that every child has a fundamental right to his total oral health. It is a consortium of dental professionals catering to a variety of populations with the goal of building healthy communities of children and with a vision that oral health is the key to general health and quality of life.

The South Asian Association of Pediatric Dentistry (SAAPD) **(Fig. 1.8)** is a nonprofit organization of individuals primarily concerned with area(s) of practice, education and research related to the field of Pediatric Dentistry. It provides a platform for the Pediatric Dentists of South Asia to work together in spirit of friendship, trust and understanding for benefit of the child's oral health.

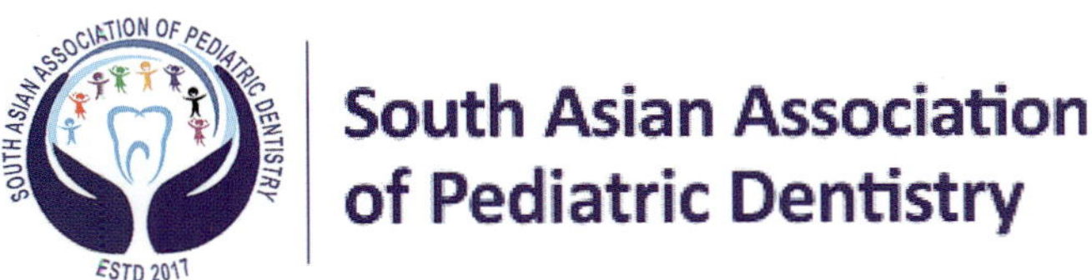

Fig. 1.8: Logo of South Asian Association of Pediatric Dentistry (SAAPD).

Objectives

- To constitute a forum for the exchange of relevant information concerning pediatric dentistry.
- To contribute to the progress and promotion of the oral health of children and to encourage research in this field.
- Provide patient/parent education, including anticipatory guidance in oral health promotion and disease.
- To arrange scientific meetings and summit.
- Strengthen cooperation with other developing countries.
- Strengthen cooperation among themselves in international forums on matters of common interest.

Goals

- To meet the oral health need of infants, children, adolescents and patients with special care needs.
- Able to collaborate in multidisciplinary teams concerned with the welfare of children.
- Promoting research in all aspects of pediatric dentistry and dissemination of knowledge in child's oral health.
- Continuing professional education for students pursuing pediatric dentistry among South Asian countries.

The mission of this body is working towards building a disease free and healthy community of children for holistic development of the South Asian countries. The society aims towards having the provision of optimal oral care to the pediatric population while maintaining the highest standards of ethics.

AMERICAN ACADEMY OF PEDIATRIC DENTISTRY

American Academy of Pediatric Dentistry (AAPD) was founded in 1947 **(Fig. 1.9)**. This nonprofit professional membership association endorses high ethical standards and safety of the patients. The head quarter is based in Chicago. The American Academy of Pediatric Dentistry focuses on the complete oral health care of the children. They have emphasized that the children should use fluoridated toothpaste as soon as the first tooth erupts so that adequate protection can be achieved from cavities from a very early age. AAPD emphasizes on providing optimal oral health for all children.

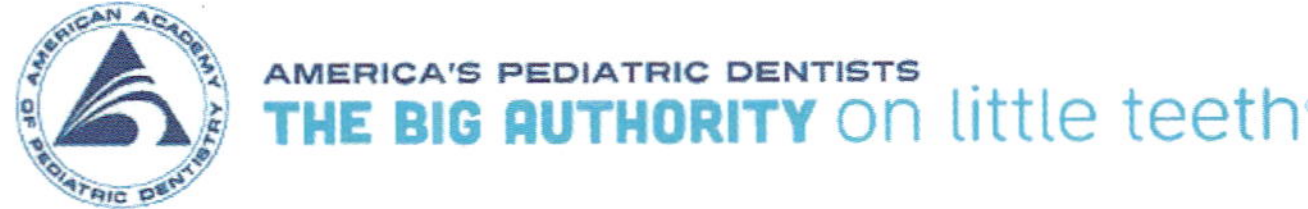

Fig. 1.9: Logo of American Academy of Pediatric Dentistry (AAPD).

INTERNATIONAL ASSOCIATION OF PAEDIATRIC DENTISTRY

The International Association of Paediatric Dentistry was founded in 1969 **(Fig. 1.10)**. It is nonprofit organization which promotes oral health to children across the world. Its major aim is to act as an International Forum for Pediatric Dentists and General Dentists who want to practice and treat children. They have 78 national member societies which represent over 20,000 dentists.

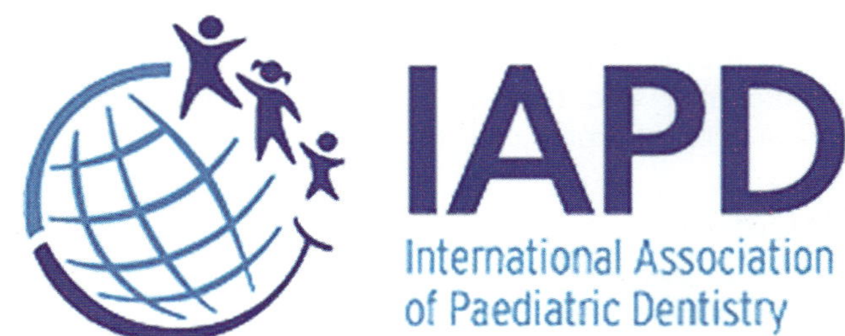

Fig. 1.10: Logo of International Association of Paediatric Dentistry (IAPD).

SCOPE OF PEDIATRIC DENTISTRY

Pediatric and preventive dentistry encompasses a variety of disciplines, techniques, procedures and skills that logically share a common basis with other specialties but are modified, transformed or adapted to the special needs of children and adolescence and those with special health care needs. Pediatric Dentistry concentrates on the integration of appropriate didactic and clinical knowledge from various specialties into a framework of quality oral health care for children. It deals with parents in their formative years, exhibiting rapid growth and development. Therefore, a pediatric dentist is in an excellent position to alter the growth pattern and resistance of oral tissues to diseases.

Pediatric dentists have extended services to fulfill the needs of the special child including the physically, mentally and medically handicapped. They also have the good fortune of being important team member in the children's hospital and in the management of cleft lip and palate patients and other such ailments.

Therefore, the scope of Pediatric Dentistry virtually includes the essence of all branches of dentistry like diagnosis, oral surgery, rehabilitation, endodontics, orthodontics, preventive dentistry and also includes the new era venues like lasers and nanodentistry.

WORLDWIDE HISTORY OF PEDODONTICS

1800 BC—Ancient Egypt: No caries in children's teeth

1563-64—Eustachius: Described and showed illustrations of both primary and permanent dentition

1737—Gerauldy: Writes about theories regarding tooth eruption and exfoliation

1763—Joseph Hurlock: Publishes book on children's dentistry

1764—Robert Bunon: "Father of Pedodontics" reiterates the importance of deciduous dentition

1865—First child dental clinic opened at Strasburg, Germany

1877—Ottofy: Became the first person in the history of dentistry to make a thorough dental examination of school children

1924—Book: First textbook of pedodontics was written

1926—Detroit Pedodontics Study Club: Dr Samuel D Harris Father of children's dentistry organizations worldwide, starts the Detroit Pedodontics Study Club

1927—AAPDC: Detroit Study club is now named the American Academy for Promotion of dentistry for Children

1935—Pedodontic Course: 6 undergraduates and 8 postgraduate courses in pedodontics were started

1940—ASDC: American Academy for Promotion of Dentistry for Children renamed as the American Society of Dentistry for Children

1947—AAP: American Academy of Pedodontics was founded

1967—CDH: First international symposium on child dental health conducted by British Pedodontic Society at the London Hospital Medical College

1969—IADC: International Association of Dentistry for Children was established and conducted its first congress in Sienna, Italy

1969—Journal: Concept of an IADC newsletter and Journal of the International Association of Dentistry for Children

1970—Journal of the IADC: The first issue was published in September with the Odore Levitas as editor and the first article published was "correlation between clinical and histological indications for pulpotomy of deciduous teeth" by Goran Koch and Hilding Nyborg (Sweden)

1984—AAPD: American Academy of Pedodontics was renamed as the American Academy of Pediatric Dentistry

1993—IAPD: First congress of International Association of Pediatric Dentistry, Chicago, USA

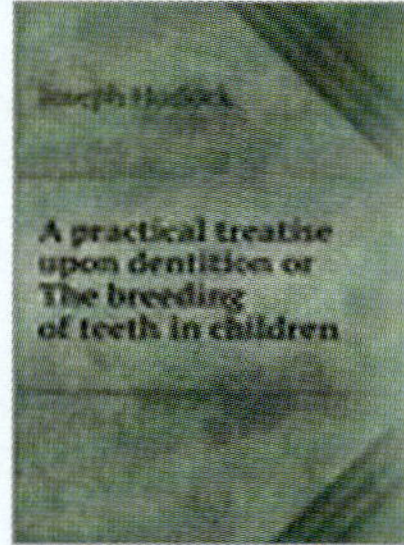

First book on children dentistry

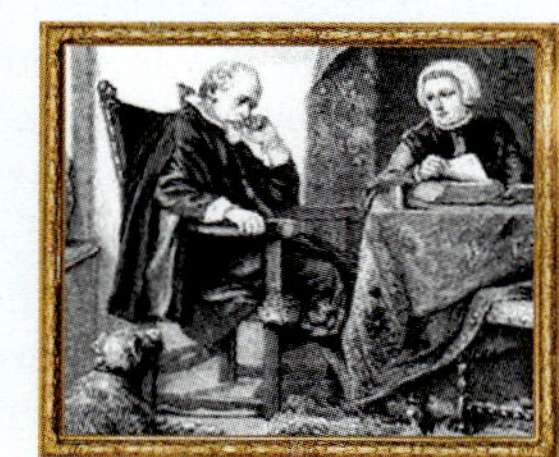

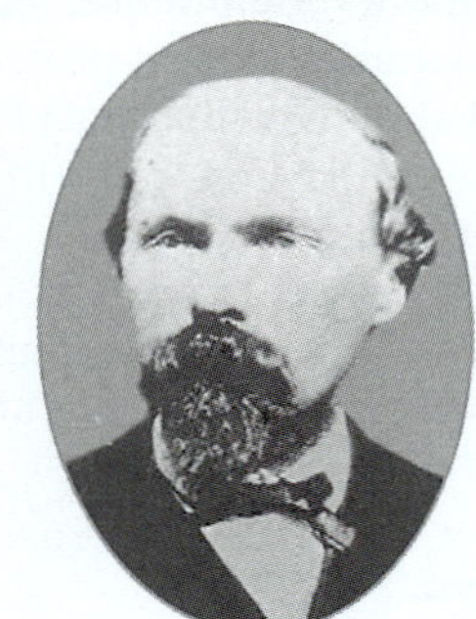

Samuel D Harris

EVOLUTION OF PEDODONTICS IN INDIA

1920—Calcutta Dental College and Hospital: 1st dental college started by Dr Rafiuddin Ahmed

1920—LDSC: Introduced as a 1-year course "Licentiate in Dental Science"

1926—Changed into 2-year course

1935—BBDS: Licentiate in Dental Science becomes Bachelor in Dental Surgery—4-year course

1950—Pedodontics is introduced: Government Dental College, Amritsar starts pedodontics as a specialty not as an independent specialty (one or two questions in operative dentistry) later—section "B" in orthodontics

1978—Pedodontics for undergraduates: Pedodontics was introduced as a specialty in the undergraduate curriculum

1979—Indian Society of Pedodontics and Preventive Dentistry: the Association of Indian Pedodontists holds the 1st conference. Dr BR Vacher is made the "Father of Pedodontics in India"

1982—Affiliated to IADC: Indian Society of Pedodontics and Preventive Dentistry becomes an affiliate member of International Academy for Dentistry for Children (IADC)

Dr R Ahmed

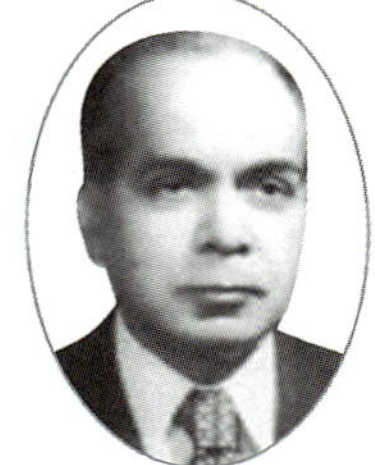

DR BR Vacher

HISTORY OF DENTISTRY

+100,000 BC: Homo Mousteriensis shows that prehistoric man had to contend with impacted teeth, the retention of deciduous teeth, caries, fractures and rickets

3000–525 BC: Confirmation of **Herodotus'** statements as to the specialization in medicine in Ancient Egypt that there were individuals who treated only the eye, or teeth, the earliest known dentist being **Hesi-Re**, great one (chief) of the others and the physicians

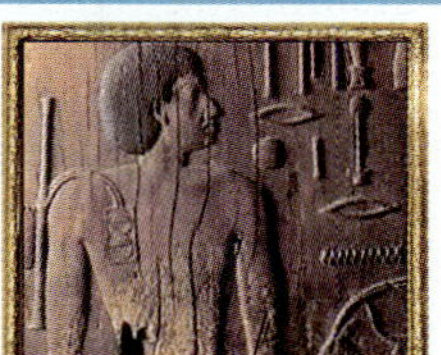

Hesi-Re

130–201 AD: Galen, the Prince of Physicians, born in Pergamos was the earliest to mention the nerves of teeth in removing the carious defect, and recommended the file

1498 AD: Invention of the modern toothbrush by the Chinese, June 24

1542 AD: Ambroise Paré, famous military surgeon, revived the old method of compression of nerve trunks to produce local anesthesia

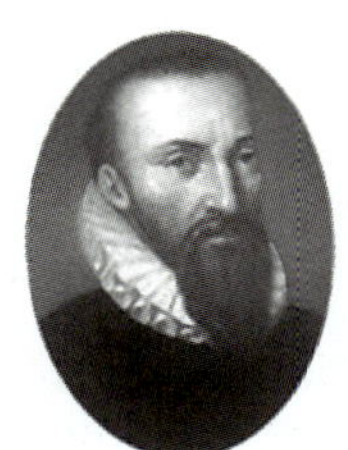

Ambroise Paré

1685: First dental textbook written in English was "operator for the teeth" by **Charles Allen**

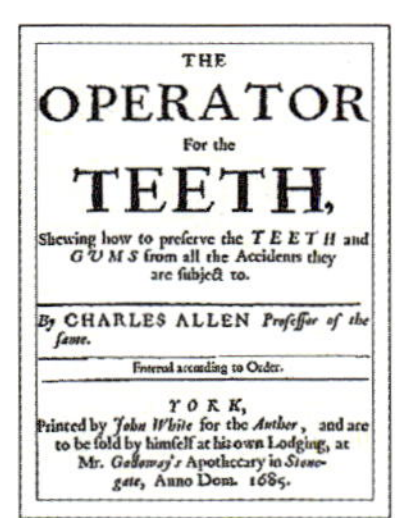

THE
OPERATOR
For the
TEETH,
Shewing how to preserve the *TEETH* and *GUMS* from all the Accidents they are subject to.

By CHARLES ALLEN *Professor of the same.*

Entered according to Order.

YORK,
Printed by *John White* for the *Author*, and are to be sold by himself at his own Lodging, at Mr. *Galloway's* Apothecary in *Stone-gate*, Anno Dom. 1685.

1723: Pierre Fauchard, a French surgeon publisher, "the Surgeon Dentist," a treatise on teeth

1790: Josiah Flagg, a prominent American dentist, constructed the first dental chair made specially for dental patients

1828: Dr John M Harris started the world's first dental school in Bainbridge, Ohio

1833: The **Crawcour brothers** introduced amalgam in the United States and advertised it as a substitute for gold restorations

1839: The American Journal of Dental Science, world's first dental journal, began its publications

1844: Horace Wells, a connection dentist, discovered that nitrous oxide can be used as an anesthesia and successfully used it to conduct several extractions in his clinic. In 1845, the public demonstration of the same failed

1864: Sanford C Barnum developed the rubber dam which solved the problem of isolating a tooth

1871: George F Green received the patent for the first electric dental engine, a self-contained motor and handpiece

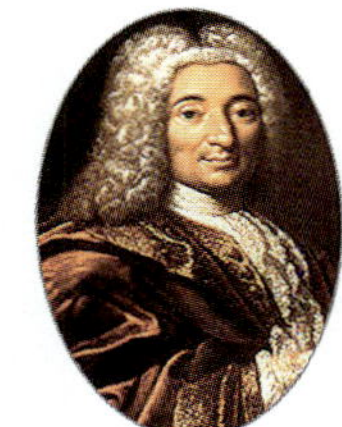

Pierre Fauchard

1895: Wilhelm Conrad Roentgen a German physicist discovered the X-ray

1899: Edward Hartley Angle classified the various forms of malocclusion

1900: FDI is formed

1913: Alfred C Fones opened the Fones Clinic for Dental Hygienists in Bridgeport, Connecticut, the world's first oral hygiene school. Dr Fones uses the term dental hygienist to become known as the Father of Dental Hygiene

1920: Dr R Ahmed founded the first dental college of India which was financed by starting the new York Soda Fountain in Calcutta

1931: Fluoride is identified by **HV Churchill** in new Kensington, Pennsylvania, **Smith Mc, Lantz EM, Smith HV** in Arizona and **Velu H and Balczet I** in France

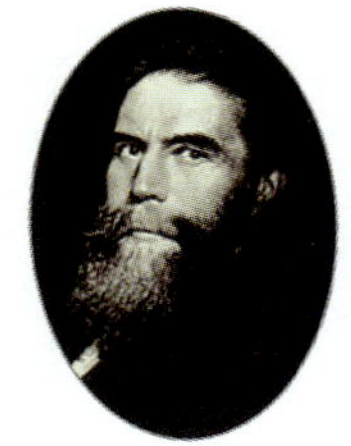

Wilhelm Roentgen

1933: The nylon toothbrush made with synthetic bristles was introduced by **DuPont**

1948: Dentist Act was passed by the Indian Parliament in close association with All India Dental Association on the 29th of March. This Act was introduced to regulate the profession of dentistry in India. The Act was amended on July 1, 1955 to make the law applicable to the state of Jammu and Kashmir

1957: John Borden introduced a high-speed air driven contra-angle handpiece. The airotor obtains speed up to 300,000 rotations per minute

1959: The first electric toothbrush, the Broxodent was introduced by Bristol-Myers company at the centennial of ADA

1960s: Lasers were developed and approved for soft tissue procedures

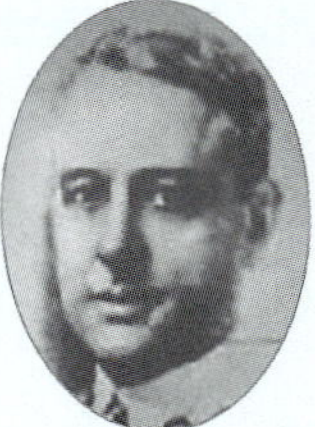

Alfred C Fones

POINTS TO REMEMBER

- Robert Bunon is Father of Pedodontics.
- BR Vacher is Father of Pedodontics in India.
- Samuel D Harris is Father of Children's Dentistry Organizations.
- First Dental College in India was established by Dr R Ahmed in Calcutta.
- Joseph Hurlock published first book on children's dentistry.
- Indian Society of Pedodontics and Preventive Dentistry is formed in 1979.
- American Academy of Pediatric Dentistry (1999) defined "Pediatric dentistry as an age-defined specialty that provides both primary and comprehensive preventive and therapeutic oral health care for infants and children through adolescence, including those with special health care needs".
- *Patient–doctor relation in pediatric dentistry:* The relation is triangular with the parent and the children; both are involved and child is at the apex of triangle as he is the focus of attention. This was first elaborated best in the pedodontic triangle given by Wright in 1975 which has been modified in 2014 as Pediatric Dentistry Treatment Triangle.

Clinical Significance

- As a clinician it is important to acknowledge the pediatric dentist and his clinical acumen.
- If we can assess the type of parent–patient relation based on pediatric dentistry triangle the management of child in the dental clinic becomes that much efficient.

Questionnaire

1. Define pediatric dentistry.
2. Give a brief history of pediatric dentistry.
3. What are the aims and objectives of pedodontics?
4. Importance of primary teeth in oral cavity.
5. Explain the concept of pedodontic triangle.
6. Name different Pediatric Dentistry societies and their main objectives

REFERENCES

1. Wright GZ. Behavior Management in Dentistry for Children, 1st ed. Philadelphia, PA: WB Saunders Co; 1975.
2. McDonald RE, Avery DR, Dean JA. Dentistry for the Child and Adolescent, 8th ed. Philadelphia, PA: CV Mosby Co; 2004.
3. Wright GZ, Kupietzky A, editors. Behavior management in dentistry for children. John Wiley & Sons; 2014
4. Padmanabhan V, Rai K, Hegde AM. Pediatric Dentistry treatment triangle—a review and a new model. J Health Sci Res. 2012;3(1):35-6.

FURTHER READING

1. De Civita M, Dobkin PL. Pediatric adherence as a multidimensional and dynamic construct, involving a triadic partnership. J Pediatr Psychol. 2004;29:157-69.
2. Gelbier S. 125 Years of developments in dentistry. Br Dent J. 2005;199:470-3.
3. Gelbier S. History of the International Association of Pediatric Dentistry Part 1: National associations and societies of dentistry for children. Int J Pediatr Dent. 1994;4: 281-7.
4. Gelbier S. History of the International Association of Pediatric Dentistry Part 2: Early events in the USA—the American Society of Dentistry for Children. Int J Pediatr Dent. 1995;5: 213-6.
5. Gelbier S. History of the International Association of Pediatric Dentistry Part 7: The International Forum of Dentistry for Children. Int J Pediatr Dent. 1996;6:289-93.
6. Gelbier S. History of the International Association of Pediatric Dentistry Part 9: Publications of the IADC. J Newsl Int J Pediatr Dent. 1997;7:49-55.
7. Pinkham JR, Casamassimo PS, McTigue DJ, editors. Pediatric Dentistry—Infancy through Adolescence, 4th edition. Saunders; 2008.
8. Suddick RP, Harris NO. Historical perspectives of oral biology: a series. Crit Rev Oral Biol Med. 1990;1:135-51.
9. Wilwerding T. History of dentistry, hosted on the Creighton University School of Dentistry.
10. www.isppd.org.in.
11. www.saapd.asia.
12. www.aapd.org.
13. www.iapdworld.org.

CHAPTER

First Dental Visit

Nikhil Marwah

Chapter Outline

Traditionally, the first visit of a child to dentist was scheduled around 3 years of age. This recommendation was based on the child's ability to cooperate in the dentist's office and the assumption that most children under 3 years of age did not have any cavities. According to **Nowak** (1997), a child's first visit to dentist should occur no later than 12 months of age so that the dentist can evaluate the infant's oral health, determine the child's risk for developing dental disease, intercept the potential problems, and educate parents in the prevention of dental disease in their child.

In 1986, the American Academy of Pediatric Dentistry (AAPD) adopted a position on infant oral health recommending that the first visit of the child to the dental clinic should occur within 6 months of the eruption of the first primary tooth. Recent knowledge in aspects of cariology and prevention has modified this further, and it is now stated that the first visit of the child to the dental office must be as soon as the tooth erupts in oral cavity, that is, 6 months of age.

The child's first dental visit should be organized in such a way that it becomes an enjoyable experience for him. The first visit is more or less a mutual assessment session during which the dentist assesses the child, and the child assesses the dentist and the dental environment. **Lenchner** (1975) postulated that the incorporation of attitudes and behavior patterns from parents, siblings, or peers is as common as contracting measles from a family member or friends. The main hypothesis for disruptive dental behavior were summarized by **Lenchner** as:

- Behavior contagion
- Threatening the child with the dentist as a punishment
- Well-intentioned but improper preparation of the child
- Discussing dentistry within hearing of the child
- Children's anxieties, generated both externally and internally, with respect to behavior contagion (a term used by **Wolking**, 1963).

PARENTS ROLE IN PREPARATION OF CHILD FOR FIRST DENTAL VISIT

The parents play an important role in the preparation of child for dental visit and also on the behavior which the child will exhibit at the time of appointment. Some of the common but necessary things which parents must perform before the child's appointment are:

- Before the visit, ask the dentist about the procedures of the first appointment so that there are no surprises.
- Plan a course of action for your child who may exhibit cooperative or non-cooperative behavior. Very young children may be fussy and may not sit still.
- Talk to your child about what to expect and build excitement as well as understanding about the upcoming visit.
- Bring with you to the appointment any records of your child's complete medical history.

PREAPPOINTMENT BEHAVIOR MODIFICATIONS

A child's first dental visit can be made successful by a few preappointment preparations which have been discussed in the following sections.

Preappointment Mailing

- Parents usually try in some way to prepare their child for the dental visit. Some parents, through their own fears or ignorance, do more harm than good in this attempt.

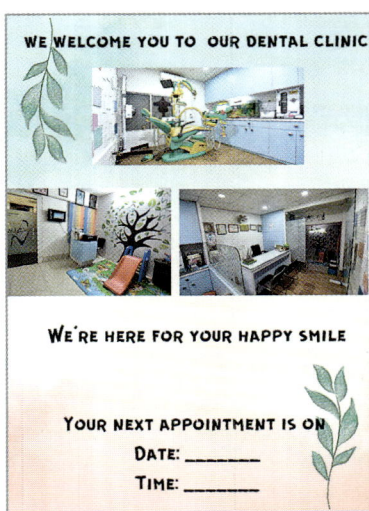

Fig. 2.1: Sample of preappointment mail.

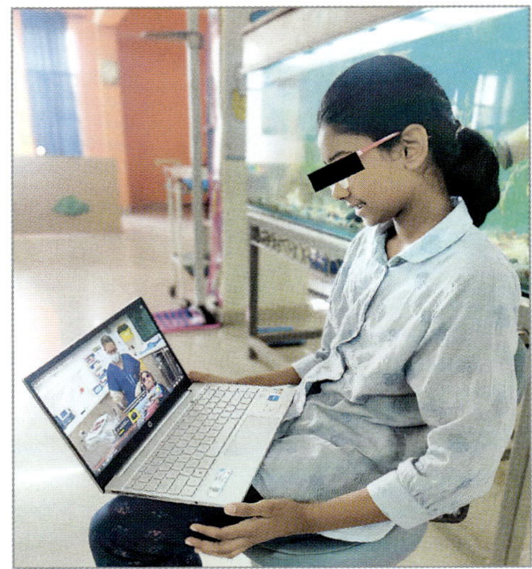

Fig. 2.2: Audiovisual modeling.

Contact with a child's parents before the first dental visit can alleviate some concerns.

- The precontact can provide directions for preparing the child patient for an initial dental visit and, therefore, increase the likelihood of a successful first appointment.
- Parents sometimes try to prepare their child for the visit by saying that "the dentist will not hurt," or by bribing them to be good with the promise of a toy (or even a sweet).
- It is suggested to the parents through mail **(Fig. 2.1)** to be as casual as possible. It is advised to simply inform the child, either on the morning of the appointment or on the day before, that he or she will be visiting the dentist. The child should be said that the dentist is going to count his/her teeth, and he will be helping the child to look after their teeth in a better way.
- Suggestion is also given to avoid conversation in the home that might include unfavorable references to dentistry.
- The parents are informed through the same mail about the procedures that will be carried out during the first visit. This will alleviate the anxiety and the concerns of the parents regarding the child's visit to the dental clinic to some extent.

Preappointment Modeling

Modeling is a type of behavior modification technique whereby a young patient can learn about the dental experience by viewing other children receiving treatment. Several authors have reported that this technique seems to improve the behavior of apprehensive patients who have no previous dental experience. The goal is for the patient to reproduce the behavior exhibited by a model (**Bandura**, 1967). Modeling is of two types, viz., audiovisual modeling and live modeling.

Audiovisual Modeling

- The child sees a video tape or film before proceeding to the dental clinic **(Fig. 2.2)**.
- This is done on the day of the appointment or perhaps at a previous visit.
- The presentation explains in terms the child can understand the dental equipment and the procedures to take place.
- The biggest advantage of an audiovisual modeling is that it is a prerecorded commercial presentation, thus nothing inadvertently creeps into the presentation that could influence the child negatively.
- The disadvantage of this technique is the need for special equipment and space for presentation which makes the technique expensive, and unless the procedure is developed by the dentist, it can be impersonal. In a few dental setups, some of the members of the dental team are employed to help the child understand the presentation and to draw their attention toward the important aspects of the presentation.

Live Modeling

- It can be achieved through siblings, other children, or parents.
- Since observing child will likely be initiated with a dental examination, a parent's recall visit offers an excellent modeling opportunity. On these occasions, many young children climb into dental chair following their parent's appointments.
- It has been found that sibling proves to be a better model as compared to their parents **(Fig. 2.3)**. At times, younger sibling can play the role of a model, but it is better to have the older sibling in this role. This is mainly because in the house an elder brother or sister plays the role of a role model for the younger ones. This is even better if the model is of the same sex.

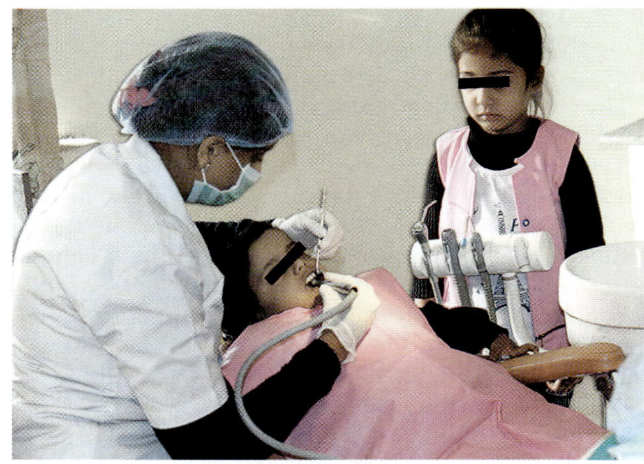

Fig. 2.3: Live modeling by sibling.

- When a cooperative sibling is not available, a non-related child may be used as a good model.
- The disadvantage of live modeling is that, sometimes the model himself/herself may show some disruptive behavior which may result into an improper impact over the behavior of the child. Thus, models should be selected carefully.

RECOMMENDED PROCEDURES TO BE CARRIED OUT ON FIRST VISIT

- Many first visits are nothing more than introductory ice-breakers to acquaint your child with the dentist and the practice.
- If the child is frightened, uncomfortable or non-cooperative, a rescheduling may be necessary.
- Patience and calmness on the part of the parent and reassuring communication with your child are very important in these instances.
- Short, successive visits are meant to build the child's trust in the dentist and the dental office and can prove invaluable if your child needs to be treated later for any dental problem.
- Appointments for children should always be scheduled earlier in the day, when the child is alert and fresh.
- For children under 2 years of age, the parent may have to sit in the dental chair and hold the child during the examination, whereas for older patients, parents may be asked to wait in the reception area so a relationship can be built between the child and the dentist.

Every effort should be made by the complete dental team to make the first dental visit of the child as comfortable and enjoyable as possible. For this reason, it is advisable not to carry out any invasive, stressful, painful or traumatic procedure on the first visit. Apart from taking history, the dentist can polish a few teeth on the first visit. If radiographs are required, it is logical to obtain them at the first visit, not only because they complement the clinical examination and contribute to the diagnosis but also because the procedures are not traumatic and therefore provide a suitable introduction to treatment **(Table 2.1)**.

Table 2.1: Common procedures carried out during the first visit.

1. History taking:
   - Social
   - Dental
   - Medical
2. Clinical examination:
   - Extraoral
   - Intraoral
3. Take radiographs if required
4. Explain aims of the treatment to the parents:
   - Emphasize the need for preventive as well as operative treatment
   - Request that the child's toothbrush be brought at the next visit
   - Inform about the financial aspects and the number of appointments required for the complete treatment of the child
5. Simple procedures:
   - Attend to any of the emergency present and treat for pain if present
   - *Prophylaxis:* Incisors only (in young child) or full mouth including removal of calculus if required
   - Topical fluoride application or other atraumatic procedure

EXAMINATION OF THE INFANT AND TODDLER

Objectives of the Infant Examination

- **Introduction to dentistry:**
  - Foundation for the development of a positive attitude towards dentistry should be built.
  - Pleasant, nonthreatening introduction to dentistry for the child and parents.
- **Risk assessment and oral examination:**
  - Medical history, current feeding and oral health practices, clinical findings, child's social and physical environment.
  - Evaluation of the head and neck and inspection of the oral cavity for early detection.
- **Prevention:** Parents' preventive counseling including diet, feeding and snatching practices, tooth cleaning, fluoride assessment is done.

Steps of the Infant Examination

- **Preappointment assessment:**
  - Obtain and preview information using a questionnaire.
  - Biographic data and family and social history to provide understanding of parent–child relationships.
  - Prenatal, natal, and neonatal history to explain dental abnormalities providing a means of documenting causative events such as high-risk pregnancies, medication ingested during pregnancy, preterm or low birth weight infants, and significant febrile episodes during early childhood.
  - Development history to discover significant growth alterations and basis for answering parent's queries.
  - Medical history regarding frequent episodes of otitis media, frequent ingestion of antibiotic suspensions containing high concentration of sucrose as it might influence recommendations for dietary management, tooth cleaning, and topical fluoride application.
  - Dental history regarding dental trauma, teething difficulties, non-nutritive sucking habits, current patterns of home oral health care for developing dentist.
  - Feeding history regarding breast and bottle feeding, frequency and duration, use of a night time bottle or pacifiers, contents of the bottle, weaning and transition to covered feeding cups.
- **Interview and counseling:**
  - Best accomplished prior to the examination
  - Specific concerns of the parents are identified
  - If the infant fusses during the examination (normal behavior), the parents predictability will direct their attention toward the child during the discussion that follows the examination and not toward the dentist.
  - The child can be occupied with toys in a nonthreatening environment prior to the examination.
- **The examination procedure (Figs. 2.4 and 2.5):**
  - Parent's assistance in a nonthreatening environment is taken
  - Use of dental chair is not necessary
  - A pleasant location away from operatory is recommended
  - Parent and dentist sit facing each other in a knee to knee position, supporting the child with the head cradled

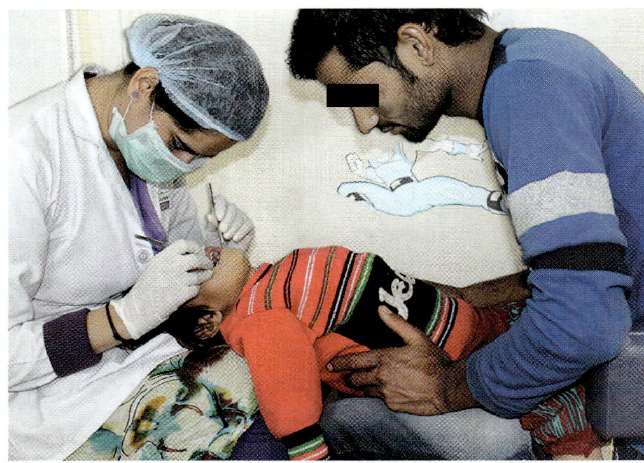

Fig. 2.4: Knee to knee examination.

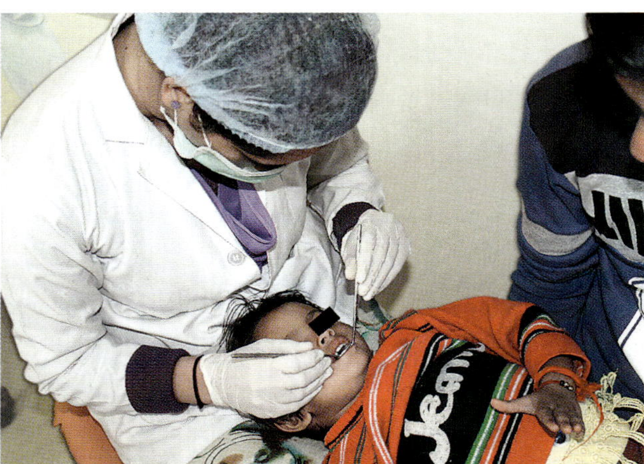

Fig. 2.5: Lap examination.

on the dentist's lap. The parent can restrain the child gently, and the dentist has a good visualization.

- This position is comfortable and parental contact has a calming reassurance to the child.
- Since the psychological development under 30–36 months is insufficient to facilitate cooperation, so crying and fussing should not interfere with examination.
- Dentist should begin with a general appraisal of the child, using a warm, gentle touch in a nonthreatening manner. The head-and-neck region should be evaluated for the presence of abnormalities in size, shape, and symmetry of the head, lymph nodes, facial symmetry, eyes, ears, nose, lips and mouth. Practitioner should be aware of possibility of child abuse and look for bruising. The examination of the mouth, with an artificial light source, if needed should begin with palpation of the lips, gingiva, and mucosa by placing a forefinger along the cheek and positioning it on the gum pad distal to the most posterior maxillary tooth. Evaluate soft tissues for presence of pathologic processes such as inclusion cysts, congenital epulis, submucous clefts, traumatic ulcers, frenum lacerations, gingivitis.
- Positioning and technique for tooth cleaning should be demonstrated. The child should then be positioned with the head on parents lap so that parent can practice tooth cleaning under supervision and appropriate suggestions can be offered. These findings are then collated with previous information, and risk is assessed based on which recommendations are made.

❖ **Determining a recall schedule:**

- Appointment should be individualized and not determined on a traditional 6-month interval.
- At the recall visit, in addition to the clinical examination, the practitioner assesses the parents tooth-cleaning efforts, evaluates feeding and snacking patterns, and investigates the degree to which the parents are following the recommended prevention program that was previously outlined.

TIPS TO PREPARE THE CHILD FOR FIRST DENTAL VISIT

Read a story and/or watch a movie with your child about going to the dentist: Children can relate to characters in a book or on the screen. If they see that their favorite character shows no fear and is having a good time at the dentist, it will help your child be less afraid when he/she visits the dentist for the first time.

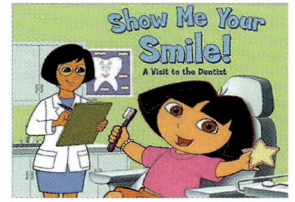

Make a dental appointment when the child is well rested and is generally a good time of day for them: Each child is different. Some children are much more receptive to new things and just generally in a better mood in the morning. Other children are not "morning people," and an appointment after an afternoon nap may be best. Schedule an appointment for a time of day that works best for your child.

Play "dentist" with your child: Sit down with your child and count his/her teeth, check the gum tissues, and just get your child comfortable with having fingers in his/her mouth. Let your child then be the dentist and allow the child to count your teeth and play with your mouth. Calling the dentist before your child's first dental visit will also prepare you for what takes place on the first visit and you can incorporate that into "playing dentist."

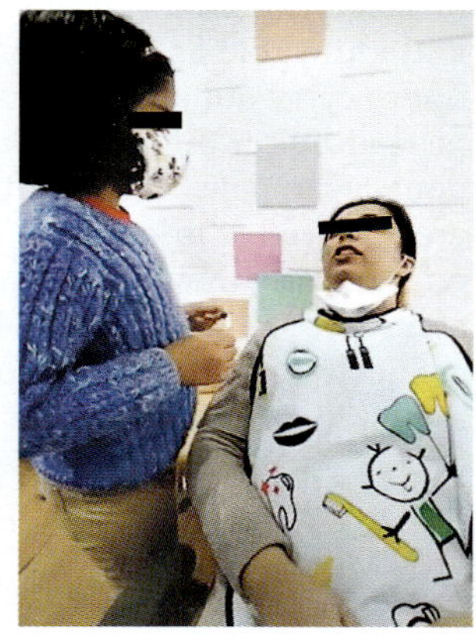

Let your dentist know of any psychological, mental, or physical disabilities your child may have: The more informed the dentist is about your child, the easier it will be for the dentist to work with your child to make the first dental visit a pleasant experience and not a traumatic one.

Do not be afraid to talk to your dentist: If you have any questions, do not be afraid to ask them. The more you know about your child's teeth, development, and how to best take care of your child's teeth and gums, and any treatment that may be needed, the better for your child. You will be able to help prevent cavities and/or other dental health issues, develop a good oral hygiene routine with your child that will most likely carry into adulthood, and also better prepare yourself and your child for any treatment that may be needed.

Do not convey anxiety to your child: Your child is very receptive to your moods, tones in your voice, facial movements, and just general body language. If your child senses any kind of fear that you may have, it will make your child more uncomfortable and fearful. Remain as calm and relaxed as you possibly can. Sometimes, it may be better if a spouse, older sibling, or someone close to the child attend your child's first dental visit, if you have a fear of the dentist and are concerned about whether or not your child will sense this.

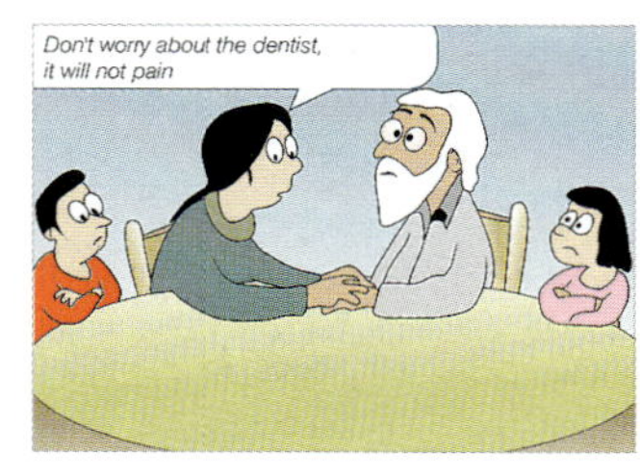

Watch what you say around your child: Never let your child hear of any past dental experiences that you may have had, or someone else experienced, that were traumatic or just generally bad experiences. Be careful not to use words like "shot," "needle," "hurt," "X-ray," or "drill." Instead, explain to your child that the "tooth doctor" will count his/her teeth and may be take pictures. Talk to your child about the first dental visit but keep it positive, short, and simple.

It's okay if your child cries during the first visit: Crying is perfectly normal during your child's first visit. Remain strong, supportive, and work with the dentist during this time. No parent enjoys seeing their child cry, but the parents should remain as positive and supportive as possible.

Allow some alone time for your child and dentist: When possible, let your child alone with the dentist and staff. Even if you just stand outside of the room so your child cannot see or hear you. By allowing your child some alone time with the dentist, this will help to create a bond between the dentist and your child. The dentist will create a comfortable environment for your child, one where the child can open up to asking questions or explore around the room on his/her own time. The dentist will talk to your child in terms that your child can relate to, as well as help create a positive experience for your child.

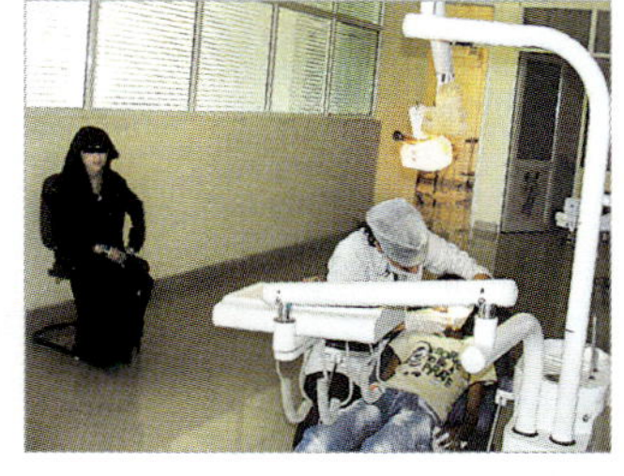

Toy support: If your child has a favorite toy, something small, allow them to bring it with them to their first dental visit.

The more positive and supportive you can remain before and after your child's first dental visit, the better. Each time your child visits the dentist, the easier it will be if they had a positive, enjoyable experience the first time. Your child will also be more likely to be willing to learn good oral hygiene skills and will want to take good care of their teeth. Children, who develop good oral hygiene routines, will most often carry these routines well into their adult life.

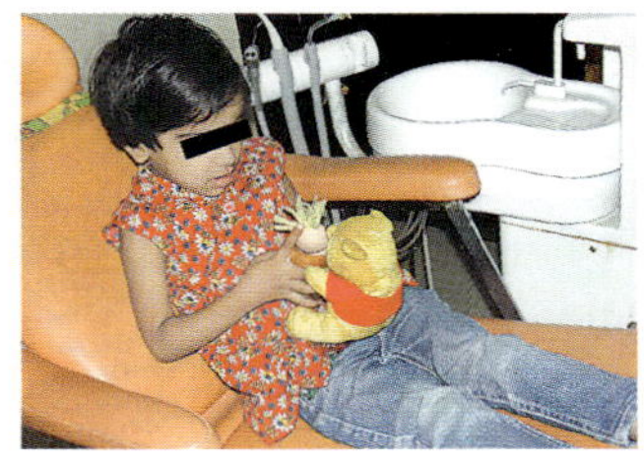

POINTS TO REMEMBER

- First visit of the child should occur within 6 months of the eruption of the first primary tooth.
- Preappointment behavior modifications include preappointment mailing and modeling.
- Live modeling by sibling is the best method to enhance positive behavior in a child.
- Simple procedures like examination, oral prophylaxis, and topical fluoride application should be carried out in the first dental visit.

Clinical Significance

First dental visit should occur:
- As soon as the first tooth erupt into the oral cavity (AAPD 2021 guidelines).
- At around 6 months of age.
- Never treat the child try to do the complex treatments at the first visit. It is advisable to first become friendly with the child and establish the rapport following which preliminary investigations like X-rays and oral prophylaxis can be initiated.
- Always make sure that you are providing the proper oral hygiene instructions and thoroughly explain the brushing technique to the patient/parent during the first visit.
- Include behavior shaping and modeling of the child.

Questionnaire

1. Explain the role of parent in behavior modification in children.
2. Define and explain modeling.
3. What should be the protocol for the first dental visit of child?
4. Explain some tips which may be useful for parents in alleviating the anxiety of their child.

FURTHER READING

1. Friedman LA, Mackler JG, Hoggard GJ, et al. A comparison of perceived and actual dental needs of a select group of children in Texas. Community Dent Oral Epidemiol. 1976;4:89-93.
2. Green M (Ed). Bright futures: guidelines for health supervision of infant, children and adolescents. Arlington, VA: National Center for Education in Maternal and Child Care; 1994. pp. 3-190.
3. Guidelines on Infant Oral Health Care. American Academy of Pediatric Dentistry Guidelines. American Academy of Pediatric Dentistry Reference Manual 2002–2003. Pediatr Dent. 2002;24:47.
4. Kleinknecht RA, Klepac RK, Aelxander LD. Origins and char- acteristics of fear in dentistry. J Am Dent Assoc. 1973;86:842.
5. Waldman HB. Oral health status of women and children in the United States. J Public Health Dent. 1990;50(6 Spec No):379-89.
6. Weinstein P, Nathan J. The challenge of fearful and phobic children. Dent Clin North Am. 1988;32:667-92.

CHAPTER

Dental Home: A Primary Care Oral Health Concept

Nikhil Marwah, Bhavna Gupta Saraf

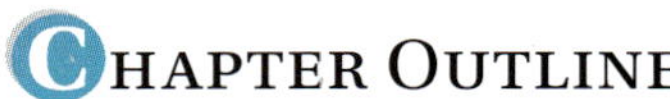

CHAPTER OUTLINE

- Medical Home Concept
- Dental Home Concept
- Specialized Care Referral

The concept of a dental home for children is new to most of the dental profession. For medical practitioners, however, the concept of identifying a child with a practitioner in a familiar and safe health supervision relationship is well established. The US general surgeon's recent concern about the low use of oral health services by children and the persistence of early childhood caries suggests that dentistry should consider taking a closer look at the potential benefits of an analogous concept of a "Dental Home." It could improve access to and provide children with a source of care and anticipatory guidance as early as 1 year of age.

MEDICAL HOME CONCEPT

The American Academy of Pediatrics (AAP) proposed a definition of a medical home in 1992 in the form of a policy statement. The essential concept is that medical care of children of all ages is best managed when there is an established relationship between a practitioner who is familiar with the child and the child's family. This relationship fosters care that is accessible, coordinated, and compassionate and that encourages mutual responsibility and trust. The medical home also presumes that the physician caring for the child is well-trained and capable of supervising health and managing illness. The medical home becomes the place where a child receives preventive instructions, immunizations, counseling, and anticipatory guidance.

DENTAL HOME CONCEPT

In an era in which access to oral health care has received such emphasis as a solution to oral health disparities, it would seem that the benefit of a dental home would not be questioned.

> Dental home according to American Academy of Pediatric Dentistry (AAPD) can be defined as "The dental home is the ongoing relationship between the dentist and the patient, inclusive of all aspects of oral health care delivered in a comprehensive, continuously accessible, coordinated, and family-centered way.
>
> Establishment of a dental home begins no later than 12 months of age and includes referral to dental specialists when appropriate."

The concept of a dental home, however, is too new to have been studied as a predictor of oral health.

- In 1999, **Nowak**[1] described the term in relation to the desired recurrence of preventive oral health supervisory services as propagated by the AAPD **(Fig. 3.1).**
- **Doykos**[2] **suggests** that early association with a dentist has the benefit of reduced cost of care, with the difference being attributed to an increased need for treatment services for those who delay the first dental visit.
- In a recent analysis of the Access to Baby and Child Dentistry, or ABCD, program in Washington State,

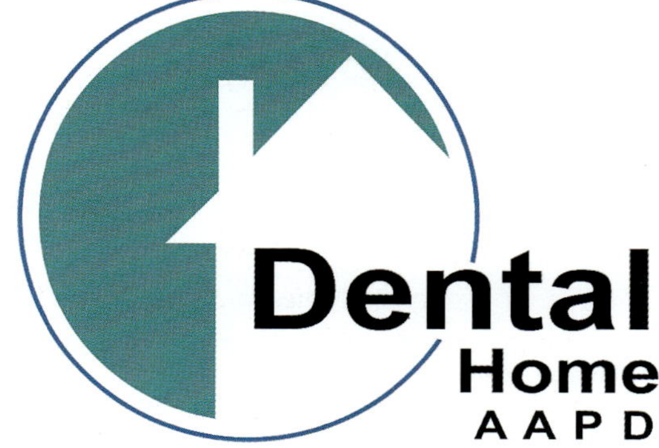

Fig. 3.1: Denotation of dental home.

Grembowski and **Milgrom**[3] found that children in the ABCD program had an increased use of services, particularly preventive services, compared with children not enrolled in the program. While the ABCD program is not a "dental home" program, it does train both families and dentists to manage young children and their oral health early and appears to have resulted in beneficial relationships between dentists and families sooner than traditional norms.

It is reasonable to ask whether establishment of a dental home by age 1 year—with the benefits of early detection, risk assessment, appropriate amounts of prescribed fluoride, sealants and early intervention of incipient disease—would reduce the prevalence of caries in preschoolers and ultimately reduce the 60% of 6–8 years old with dental caries. It could be argued that the concept of the dental home never has been studied. However, if access and utilization are used as indirect measures of the benefits of a dental home, then the concept has merit to improve oral health of children.

Characteristics of the Dental Home (Table 3.1)

Although a dental home most often connotes a building, place, or clinic, it also has to be a philosophy embraced by the dental practice. A practice that embraces children early and continues to follow them periodically throughout life would be ideal. The dental home may begin in the office of a pediatric dentist and then move to that of a family practitioner, once the child has matured and is more comfortable being treated by the parents dentist. As in medicine, the dental home should embrace prevention at the earliest time possible to prevent or at least reduce the effects of oral disease. It also should provide a place for children to be treated in case of emergency, where parents can feel comfortable and not have to worry that the management of their child's oral emergencies would be minimal.

Advantages of Dental Home

- Embraces the importance of early intervention with optimal preventive strategies chosen based on the risk of the patient.
- Encourage the first dental visit by approximately 1 year of age.
- Practitioners can provide personalized preventive approaches for children based on their family histories; the oral examination and the risk factors are identified. These risk factors include medical history, dietary habits, medication, fluoride availability, and parental attitudes.
- The AAPD's recommendations for periodic preventive care provide a framework for the practitioner to consider when developing office policies and recommendations.
- An important feature of a dental home is to provide anticipatory guidance to the parents so that they are aware of their children's growth and development, as well as possible risk factors that occur as children grow.
- Preventive intervention can be personalized to the needs of the child.

Table 3.1: Ideal characteristics and practical advantages of a dental home.

Characteristic	*Description*	*Practical advantages*
Accessible	• Care provided in the child's community • All insurance accepted and changes in coverage accommodated	• Source of care is close to home and accessible to family • Minimal Hassle encountered with payment • Office ready for treatment in emergency situations • Office is non-biased in dealing with children with special healthcare needs (CSHCN) • Dentist knows community needs and resources (fluoride in water)
Family centered	• Recognition of the centeredness of the family • Unbiased complete information is shared on an ongoing basis	• Low parent/child anxiety improves care • Care protocols are comfortable to family (behavior management) • Appropriate role of parents in home care is established
Continuous	• Same primary care providers from infancy through adolescence • Assistance provided with transitions (e.g., to school)	• Appropriate recall intervals are based on child's needs • Continuity of care is better owing to recall system versus episodic care • Coordination of complex dental treatment is possible (traumatic injury) • Liaison with medical providers for CSHCN is improved (congenital heart disease)
Comprehensive	• Health care available 24 hours/day, 7 days/week • Preventive, primary, tertiary care provided	• Emergency access is ensured • Care manager and primary care dentist are in same place
Coordinated	• Families linked to support, education, and community services • Information centralized	• Records centralized • School, workshop, therapy linkages established and known (cleft • palate care)
Compassionate	• Expressed and demonstrated concern for child and family	• Dentist–child relationship is established • Family relationship is established • Children less anxious owing to familiarity
Culturally competent	• Cultural background recognized, valued, respected	• Mechanism is established for communication for ongoing care • Specialized resources are known and proven if needed • Staff may speak other languages and know dental terminology

ALTERATION IN THE PEDODONTIC TRIANGLE IN RELEVANCE TO THE ESTABLISHMENT OF DENTAL HOME (FIGS. 3.2A AND B)

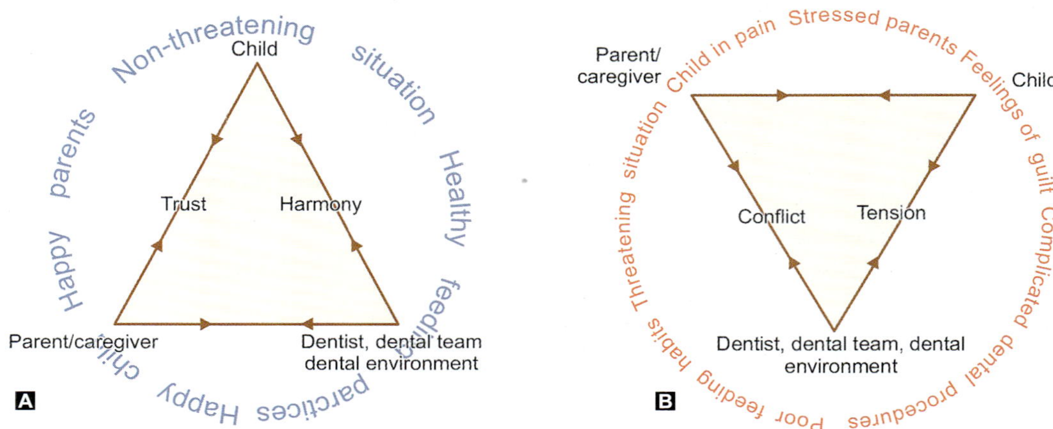

Figs. 3.2A and B: Alternation in Pediatric Dentistry triangle: (A) Diagrammatic representation of pediatric triangle during establishment of dental home under ideal circumstances till 1 year of age; (B) Diagrammatic representation of pediatric triangle during establishment of dental home during an emergency stage.

SPECIALIZED CARE REFERRAL

- Another feature of the dental home would be coordination of specialized care for the child. When a child has been observed over a period, appropriate recommendations can be made for other treatments such as orthodontic referral and observation. Using age-related guidelines and recommendations from the orthodontic community, appropriate scheduling of referrals can be made to optimize treatment and eliminate numerous referrals before treatment is initiated.
- It is known that after children are 2 or 3 years of age, dentists see them more frequently than do primary care medical providers. This provides a wonderful opportunity for the primary dental provider to recognize changes in growth and development that can be discussed with the parent, as well as make appropriate recommendations to seek further consultation from the child's physician.
- The continuous care provided by a dental team also would recognize other developmental milestones that may suggest needed attention.
- In a dental home, the office can track the sequencing of preventive interventions. For example, the timing of the placement of dental sealants on permanent first molars can be anticipated from previous appointments and scheduled appropriately, or primary tooth exfoliation and permanent tooth eruption can be monitored so that growth and development problems are reduced.
- Behavioral research supports a child's increased levels of comfort and reduced anxiety levels as familiarity increases with the dental environment. Being greeted cheerfully by the receptionist and staff in a non-threatening, child-friendly environment reduces anxiety and improves behavior. This becomes an important issue for many parents who do not want to see their children experience stress in a health provider's office.
- Lastly, the dental home can provide a personalized and individualized recall program for the child. Too frequently, recall programs are based on a schedule suggested by reports when caries was a normally distributed problem among all children, who thus needed close monitoring. Today, the majority of dental problems occur in high-risk populations, and all children may not require the same schedule of periodic supervision.
- Frequency of oral health supervisor visits also may need to be changed during the child's life, as there are times when more frequent observation and monitoring are necessary to ensure the child's health and to answer the parent's questions.
- Having a place to receive emergency treatment can be important. To be able to pick-up the telephone and immediately contact the office either during or after working hours and be sure that the dentist is available can be important to the family.
- Gaining access to dental care is a major health issue for children with special healthcare needs. Families with such children who have a dental home can know that an office is accessible and that the dentist and staff members are trained in and comfortable with treating special needs. All children with special healthcare needs should be welcomed in the dental office, and if the relationship is established early in the child's life, significant oral-systemic problems can be prevented or managed.

The dental home is an important concept for the dental profession to embrace. Evidence supports the advantages of receiving early professional dental care and intervention that are complemented by anticipatory guidance for parents, as well as periodic supervision visits based on the child's risk of dental disease. The dental home could increase opportunities for preventive oral health services for children that can reduce disease disparities. The dental home is a concept that deserves support, further investigation, and, in conjunction with the medical home, would provide the comprehensive health care to which all children are entitled.

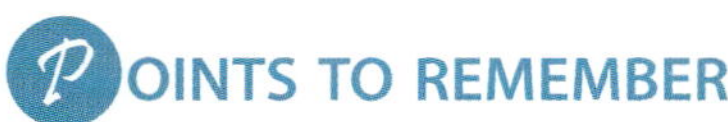

POINTS TO REMEMBER

- Dental home is an ongoing relationship between dentist and patient.
- AAP came out with the concept of medical home in 1992.
- Nowak advocated the concept of dental home.

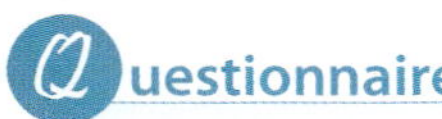

Questionnaire

1. Define dental home and give its advantages.
2. What are the characteristics of dental home?

REFERENCES

1. Nowak AJ. Dental home. In: Pinkham JR, Casamassimo PS, Fields HW, McTigue DJ, Nowak AJ (Eds). Pediatric Dentistry: infancy through adolescence, 3rd edition. Philadelphia: Saunders; 1999. pp. 187-8.
2. Doykos III JD. Comparative cost and time analysis over a two year period for children whose initial dental experience occurred between ages 4 and 8 years. Pediatr Dent. 1997;19:61-2.
3. Grembowski D, Milgrom PM. Increasing access to dental care for medical preschool children: The Access to Baby and Child Dentistry (ABCD) program. Public Health Rep. 2000;115:448-59.

FURTHER READING

1. American Academy of Pediatric Dentistry. Recommendations for preventive pediatric dental care. Pediatr Dent. 1999;21(special issue 5):80.
2. Saxena N, Hugar SM, Patil V, Gokhale NS, Joshi RS, Dialani PK. Assessment of Knowledge, Attitude, and Practices about Dental Home among Healthcare Professionals of Belagavi City: A Cross-sectional Study. International Journal of Clinical Pediatric Dentistry. 2022;15(2):164-7.
3. The American Academy of Pediatrics Ad Hoc Task Force on Definition of the Medical Home. The medical home. Pediatrics. 1992;90:774.

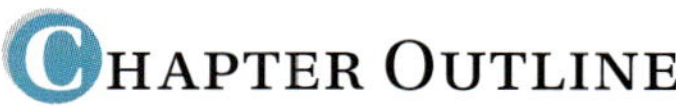

Pediatric Dental Clinic

Nikhil Marwah, Ashwin M Jawdekar, Sanchit Paul, Abhishek Soni

Chapter Outline

Dentistry for children is not difficult but is significantly different from what is practiced for adults routinely. This is due to the fact that children are not just miniature adults. They react differently to people and places around them. To treat them comfortably in a dental clinic environment, the approach of the dental clinic staff and the clinic atmosphere play an integral role in overall acceptance and positive experience. Children do have a "place memory." This can be both advantageous and disadvantageous. Also, they do like to be in places and interact with people that are fun and non-threatening for them. Often, medical set-ups are stereotype, designed to suit doctor's requirements and are not adapted to children's need.The environmental needs of children differ from those of adults, and it is preferable to plan a dental office that encourages feeling of care and familiarity for the child. In general, the area designed specifically for children should reflect the percentage of children in the entire practice. According to **Braham and Morris**, "The environment should encourage children to have the parents' side and well facilitate separation when child is transferred to the dental Operatory". It is important for dentists to know various aspects of dental experience that can have positive or negative impact on child behavior. Summarized in **Table 4.1** are a few such considerations.

PEDODONTIC CLINIC DESIGNING

As we already discussed, children perceive, express and adapt to the external environment way differently. Keeping this in mind, we have to design the set-up of the clinic as well as a system of a neat work flow and functioning. Pleasant visits to the dental office promote trust and confidence in a child that will last a life-time. The doctor's goal, along with the clinical staff, must be to help all children feel good about visiting the clinic. Since children constitute about 40% of the nation's population, the dental clinics must be made "child-friendly." Furthermore, we do live in a "child-centered" society today and, hence, in our clinics, children should be considered as important visitors. The design of pedodontic clinic should have four to five compartments as shown in **Figure 4.1**.

The dental operatory should be well isolated from other areas and the last place to be introduced to the child during the first visit. In this figure, the arrows indicate direction of movements toward operatory. The orange rectangular area is the front desk. The black area is a rest room. The white area is assistants' area, sterilization and storage place. To make our dental clinics child-friendly, the following aspects must be considered important:

- Space provision/play area with a spread of age specific games.
- Reception at the front desk
- Waiting area
- Attire and presentation of the clinic staff
- Child-friendly colors, smells and sounds
- Instructions for children/parents
- Readiness to accept children as they are
- Gifts and rewards
- Audiovisual aids for entertainment
- Child-friendly team with proper training and and approach including children with special healthcare needs

Table 4.1: Impact on child behavior.

Children like	***Children may not like***
Playful, colorful and vibrant environment	Clinic, hospital dull and non-friendly environment
Fresh, bright and bold colors like red, yellow, orange, blue	Dull, wooden, tiled walls; gray, black, brown colors
Open spaces to move around and explore	Restricted seating position
Being received with smile on faces who meet them, being called with their names, while also being displayed on a white board.	Being unnoticed, ignored or if not greeted well
To touch, feel and play with toys and games	Asked not to touch here and there
Humor, compliments, praise, positive comparisons from whole of team	Criticism, verbal ridicule, negative comparisons
Being termed as "grown-ups" (big boys/girls)	Being termed "small", immature, young
Shake-hands, patting on back, giving claps	Too little or too much of physical closeness
Eye-to-eye contact while talking	Indirect talks
Cartoon films, magic shows, favorite shows on TV	News, serials, films, other TV programs
Talking about games, friends, school, TV programs, movies, etc. Listening to stories, answering puzzles	Talking otherwise or related to dentistry
"I" message type communications such as "I like children who listen to me carefully and follow my instructions"; "I like children who do not move hands while I am working"	Communication styles such as "why do not you stop crying and listen to me" or "do not move your hands when I am working"
To be in a "comfort zone", e.g., a comfortable child engages himself in watching cartoon film while the dentist is treating him/her (and also follows all instructions like keeping mouth open, rinsing with water)	Too many instructions, orders, suggestions; too many distractions
To win prizes, rewards, stars	Being actually punished or verbally ridiculed (criticize the behavior and not the person)
Friendly gestures, child friendly attire of doctor/staff	Staff attire—apron, mask, gloves, caps, eye-shields
Dental chair moving up/down, ease of getting in and out of it, spittoon, tumbler operations, light buttons	Dental chair moving backward, too bright light, too many arms (of instrument tray, X-ray), too many noises (compressor, air-rotor drill, ultrasonic cleaner, suction)
Instrument tray with minimum things on it; only 1–2 mouth mirrors for initial examination	Tray loaded with sharp instruments—needles, root canal (RC) instruments, burs, scaler tips, being shown a needle while injecting
Simple words (see the list of euphemisms)	Words like pain, blood, injections, drill, pulling out teeth
Attention, quick and graceful approach to work	Too long appointments, too long waiting time, made to sit for long without interaction
Honest, clear and simple talks, e.g., being told that to clean the tooth, you need to put medicine near it to put it to sleep. It may pain only as much as an ant/mosquito bite	Cheating/lying; e.g., being told that he/she would not get pain at all before receiving injection (and actually experiencing it) or saying nothing will happen at all

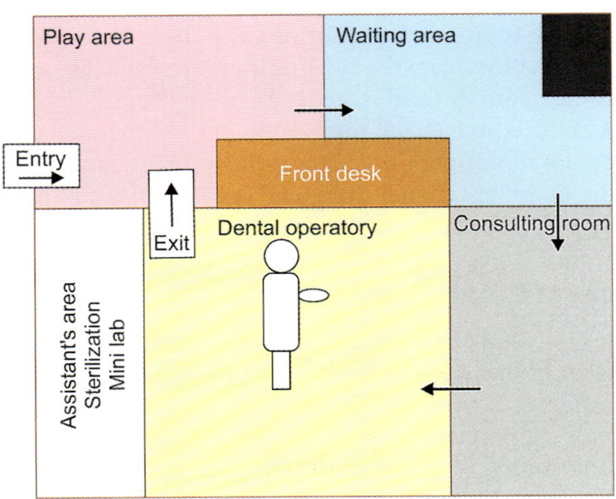

Fig. 4.1: Design of pedodontic clinic.

Space Provision/Play Area

- Children require free, empty spaces to move around. They usually do not sit in one place. They often stand near a window, move around reception or table or keep looking for interesting things around. Therefore, it is necessary to provide some empty space for them to move around.
- A fish aquarium or a slide may be kept (depending upon the space available) in such a vacant area. Keeping birds or parrots can also play a significant role in play therapy. Keeping therapy dogs is an internationally accepted concept worldwide especially with special needs children.
- Also, it is better to engage them in some interesting activity to relieve their anxiety before their turn comes for dental check-up or treatment **(Fig. 4.2)**. Story books, Montessorian toys, motor skills focused building blocks, Pictionary, drawing books or white wallpaper for scribbling can all be a great idea to implement. Using slider, music mat, keyboard player rather than just the screen also engages children much more effectively.
- It is prudent to keep sensory and fidgety toys which can be greatly utilized by children with special needs like ADHD, autism and intellectual delay.
- Behavior management and modification for us begins in the play area. Introduction to the mouth mirror on a dental hygiene demo puppet, pretend play, funny nose

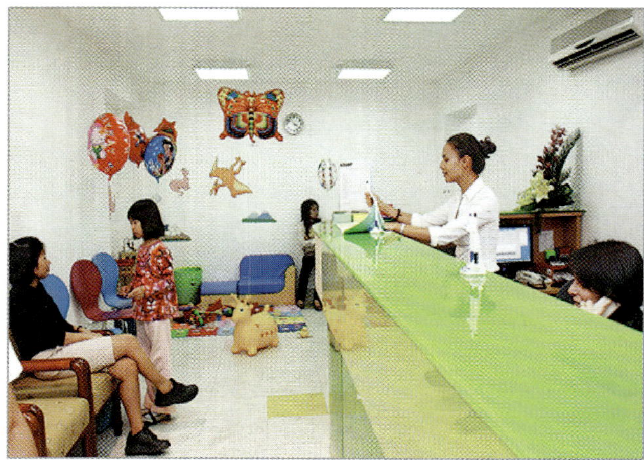

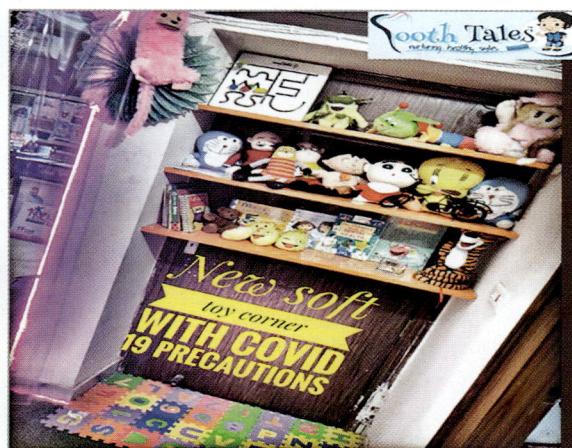

Fig. 4.2: Play room area for children.

introduction for inhalation sedation, presentation with happy children on dental chair playing its part in role modeling.

Front Desk

- The receptionist should possess good communication skills to deal with children and parents effectively.
- Understanding the mental make of not just children but also parents is equally essential. Front desk's role in alleviating the same is done by giving them a tab showcasing videos of children from different age groups being treated at your center.
- He/she must call each and every child by his/her name and converse about the topics of his/her interests. Often, lack of interest on the part of the clinic staff to deal with children fails to generate any excitement in the child.
- Also, many times children in our society are threatened by their parents of a doctor's visit or of injections, for not behaving properly (or a dentist's visit for eating too many chocolates, for example). Hence, before their initial dental visits they are unsure of what is going to happen. If a friendly welcome, cheerful conversation and playful atmosphere greet a child, the child feels that they are no longer brought for any punishment and that, in turn, makes the job of the clinician easy.
- The reception should be adjoining the play area so that not only can the receptionist keep a watch on behavior of child but also is able to engage them in conversation thereby alleviating their dental anxiety
- Identifying the frankel behavior rating for the child and communicating the same to the clinician helps preparing the dental operatory with requisite distractions. Depending on the age, past dental experiences, various sedation opinions are offered to parents to make it a playful visit for the children.
- After the procedure also, the front desk team shall be trained to receive the child and make them comfortable by ice-creams or juice in case they are tired, hungry or exhausted by the dental procedure. Giving them appropriate rewards and gifts is great way to appreciate their help and bring them back again for next appointment.

Waiting Area

- This is especially useful for children, who are big enough for the play area and would like to show their intellect and engage in smarter games
- This can comprise books and games for elder children and waiting parents.
- A tailor made approach can be made if adequate and explicit information about the child's favorites is deduced from the parents on call beforehand.
- Children like it when the dental office gives a personalized touch and shows eagerness, by mentioning their names on a white board alighted fastened in the waiting area.
- It is necessary that the waiting time of a child in the dental clinic is made pleasant. Often, children having to wait for long are bored by the time they are taken in for treatment. This can be avoided by giving prior appointments only with some additional time in between so that next kid does not have to wait in case previous appointment runs late.
- Also, 5–10 minutes of waiting time spent in playing can distract them from the fact that they have been brought for some treatment and is "refreshing" for them.
- A child, who is in a happy mood just before entering the dental clinic operatory, is more likely to be cooperative for the treatment than a child who is either bored of waiting in a dull room or is anxious about dentistry.

Attire and Presentation of the Clinic Staff

- A typical attire of dental staff comprising cap, apron, mask and gloves is certainly not child-friendly. In case of children, it is especially recommended to try and work with alternatives to apron as they have white coat anxiety **(Fig. 4.3).**
- Make an attempt to meet a child casually and preferably not around the dental chair. Informal conversations like around school, teacher, sibling or favorite shows builds around the rapport.
- The dentist first meets the child casually in the consulting room, takes a brief history, assesses the behavior and then directs the child to dental chair after showing around the clinic and meeting other staff.

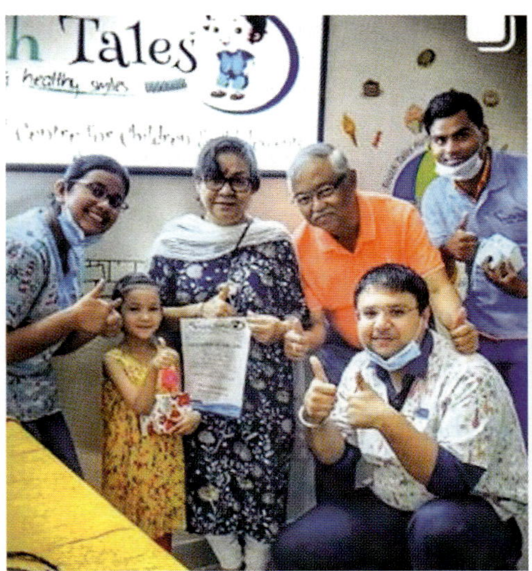

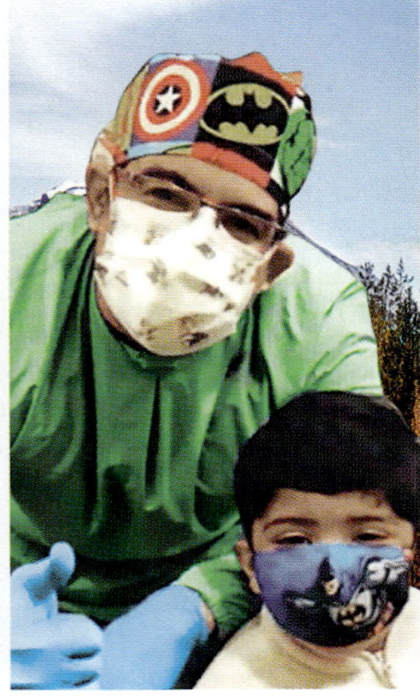
 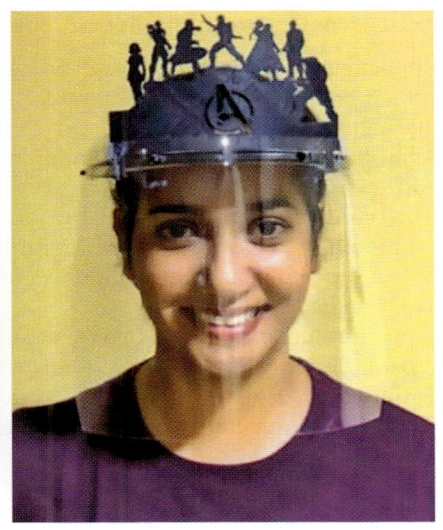

Fig. 4.3: Appearance of pediatric dentist. (*Pic courtesy:* Sanchit Paul, Nikhil Grober and Bhagyashree Thakur).

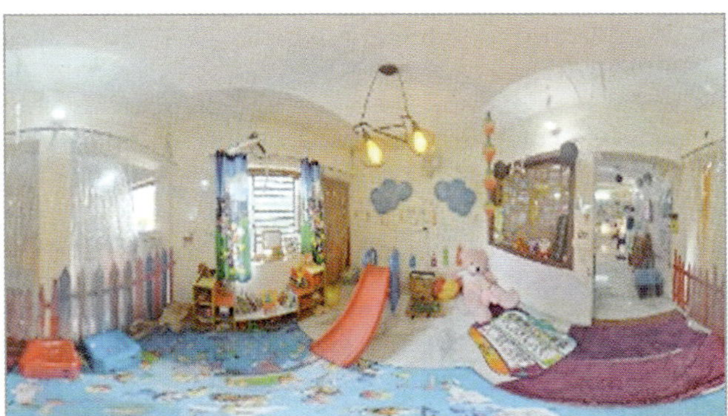
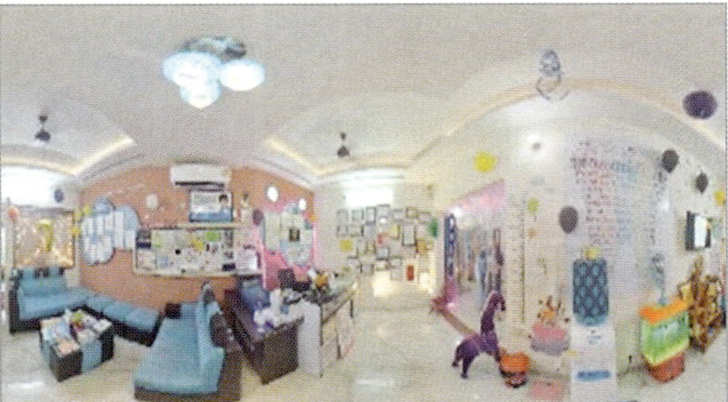

Fig. 4.4: Appearance of pediatric dental clinic.

Colors, Smells and Sounds

- Often clinics have roof-to-floor tiles for easy maintenance and cleanliness, and colors projecting office ambience.
- Children imagine and accept bold, bright fresh colors such as yellow, red, blue, green, orange, and pink and may dislike gray, black and white, wooden, and brown **(Fig. 4.4)**.
- Also, smell of spirit, eugenol, acrylic, waxes may not really go well with children. The noise of an air-rotor handpiece, suction apparatus, a compressor or an ultrasonic cleaner can be disturbing too. Hence, it is best to mask these sounds by use of light instrumental music; or running their favorite distraction shows on ceiling mount television streaming through the headsets.
- Recently, Snoezelen concept is getting hugely popular in Pediatric Dentistry. It is a unique model of multisensory adapted dental environment deemed to effectively and efficiently manage children with anxiety, apprehension or with special needs. This includes dimming or closing of other lights except head mounted lamp or mild dental light, using audiovisual aids or projector over ceiling, noise-free headphones, bubble maker, rhythmic music in background for parents and butterfly like wrap to give hugging effect etc. **(Fig. 4.5)**.

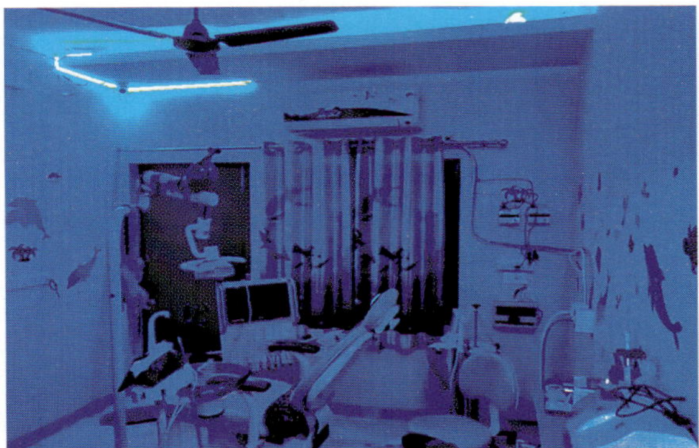
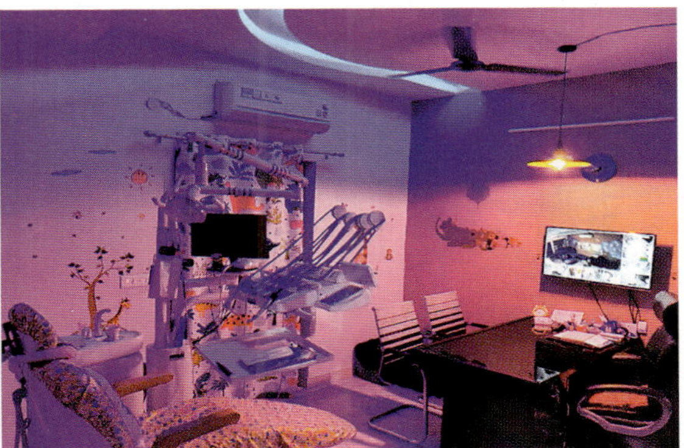

Fig. 4.5: Snoezelen or multisensory environment (MSE).

Instructions for Children and Parents

- A lot depends on how the children are prepared at home for their dental visits. It is important for us to inform and educate them well.
- The notice boards in the consultation room must carry instructions for parents before dental visits of children as well as certain post-treatment instructions. Also, a booklet or a brochure as a pretreatment communication can be mailed to parents beforehand or delivered to them soon as they enter.
- Certain instructions need to be given to parents for better preparation of them and their children for receiving dental treatments; such as:
  - Do not tell your child about pain, blood, and injections in the first place.
  - Do not tell him/her something like "... because you do not brush your teeth properly, doctor will give you an injection ..." or "because you eat chocolates, your spoiled teeth will be removed by doctor".
  - Do not voice your own fears about dentistry (pain, blood, etc.) in front of children. Your dentist can answer your queries separately.
  - Do not insist on starting the treatment in the first visit itself. Give your doctor enough time to talk to your child. The time spent initially on building rapport and gaining his/her confidence will in turn save the time required for treatment later.
  - Do not promise him/her in advance about the time the doctor would take to treat, the pain he/she might get, etc., which can mislead him/her. Simply say you do not know.
  - Report to the doctor any past negative experience.
- The discussion regarding the same may preferably take place in the absence of children; for example, in a consulting room while the child is busy in playing in the waiting area or watching cartoon films.

Readiness to Accept Children

- Children love fun, they enjoy being admired, interacting with others and making their "world" of people and non-living things such as places, toys, games and cartoon films. We have to accept them as they are and more importantly become a part of their world by communicating with them verbally as well as non-verbally (with an eye-to-eye contact, physical contact like shaking hands, patting on the back, giving a clap, etc.).
- According to **Pinkham**, no child is competent in language before the second birthday and all normal children are competent in language after fourth birthday. This is because between ages 3 and 6 years, fear of separation from parents, strangers, a new experience diminishes; control, conscience, aggression develop. Children learn interaction with peer, self-discipline; values (sexual as well as adult) develop. Thus, this age-group children are susceptible for distraction, friendship, feeling guilty, praise, emotions of other people, etc. Most of our behavior modification techniques in the linguistic domain (like Tell show do, modeling, voice control) are based on these basic observations. As discussed before, we can prepare the child before their first visit by set of previsit imageries and videos shot at our clinic so that they not only get familiar but also desensitize. These videos can be sent as social media links and parents are encouraged to prepare the child accordingly so that first visit can be as pleasant as possible. (https://youtu.be/aApyfbq-d0Y, https://youtu.be/VZ1r-m6reSQ).
- During initial visits, therefore, the dental team should focus on communicating with children properly to win their confidence and progress to carrying out treatments gradually.
- Also, children do cry at times we should not panic due to a child crying. A child may cry due to various reasons in a dental clinic. Noise of certain machines, taste of certain medicines, not wanting to get the treatment done, getting bored, are a few examples. As long as the child does not cry due to pain, there is nothing to worry at all and so we must be prepared to listen to it.
- Noise cancellation in your operatories, which are away from the waiting area is an important consideration in pediatric dental office.

Gifts and Rewards

- Give a child a token of appreciation for good work with a small gift at conclusion of a visit such as cars, dolls, pencil and medals **(Fig. 4.6)**.
- Even calling a child a "good boy" or a "good girl" or drawing a "star" on his/her hand can work like rewards and excite children and leave with them fond memories of dental visits.

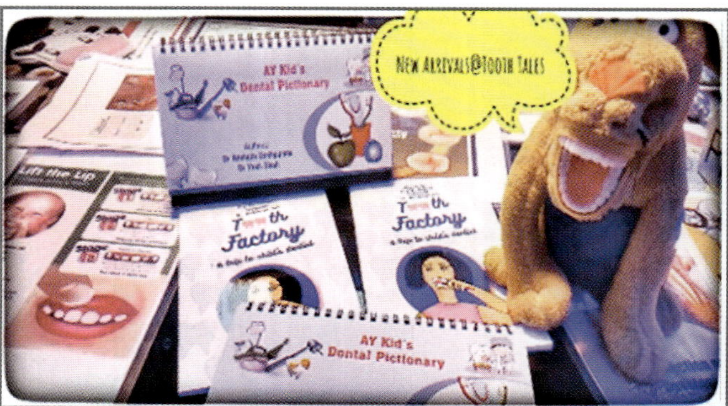

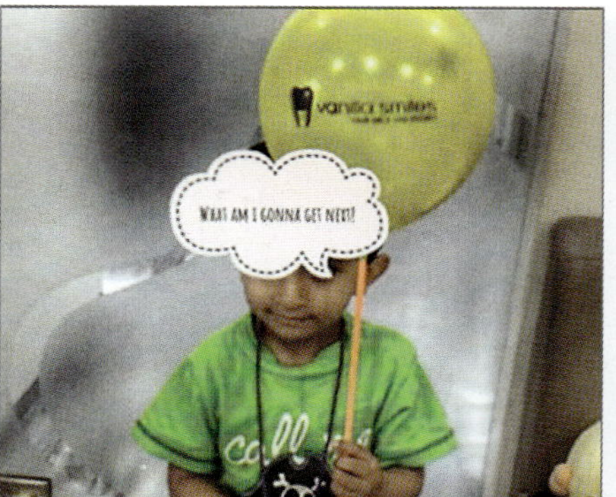

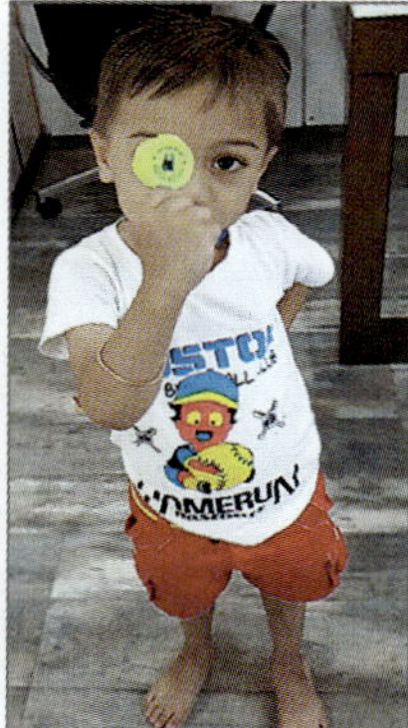

Fig. 4.6: Rewards and gifts. (*Pic courtesy:* Abhishek Soni).

- Bravery certificate; zero cavity certificates do their bit in leaving lasting impressions in the mind of the child. So much so that they look forward to their treatment visits.
- Never bribe the child before treatment.

Audiovisual Aids for Entertainment

- Children forget themselves while watching cartoon films. The TV set in front of dental chair can distract the child enough to forget the dental treatment while that being carried out **(Fig. 4.7)**.
- Also, once a child is cooperative, it reduces the need of talking on the part of the dental team. It is a good idea to have a camera attached to a TV set displaying the child on the chair as children do love watching themselves.

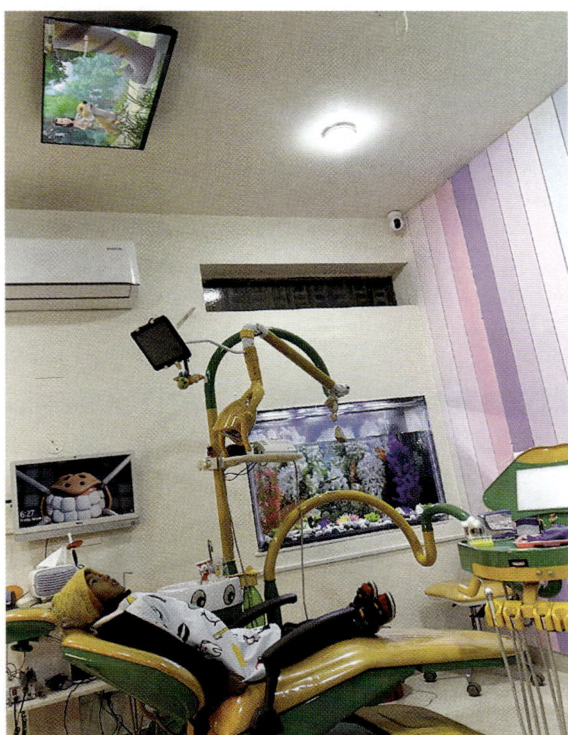

Fig. 4.7: Audiovisual set-up of children's dental operatory.

Team Approach

- The whole team should work with a plan for each visit of a child. The plans, however, should have certain flexibility.
- The initial visits are usually sufficient for ascertaining the child cooperation and diagnosis and treatment planning. Plan for the subsequent visit (if an uncooperative child is to be scheduled for his first restorative work), have his/her appointment after a cooperative child whom you can model for a certain procedure.
- Plan procedures requiring minimal cooperation initially and the complicated ones, later. It is a good idea to have a separate session of pediatric patients in a busy general practice.
- The team should work with a flexible approach, learn communication skills to deal with children effectively and be positive.

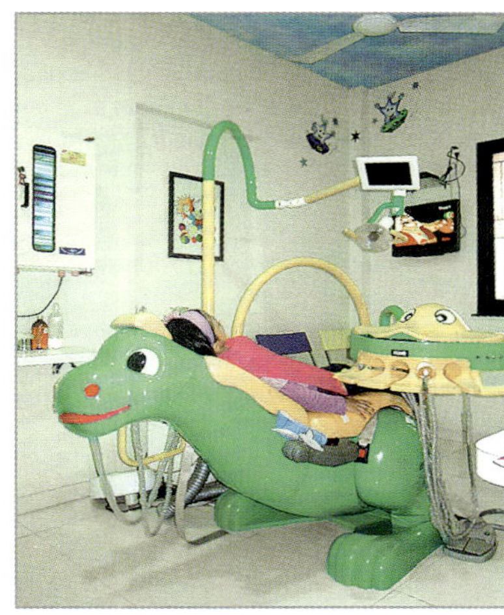

Fig. 4.8: A modern set-up of children's dental operatory.

Design of Equipment (Fig. 4.8)

- The sterilization equipment and area needs to be very accessible so as to cater to large volume of young children in dental office.
- Large size of multiple units for ultrasonic dug mat, steam or chemical mat sterilization.
- A sufficient number of instruments, mouth props and other restraints.
- Storage in every conceivable spot—under holding benches in the operatory, wall cabinets and under counter cabinets. Brush up sinks at graduated heights.
- Hard surface floor under operatory chairs.
- Foot controlled or automatic faucet for operatory sinks.
- Trash container in the operatory should be out of sight and out of reach from children's hands.
- A colorful towel to cover the restrained child.
- A camera to take first examination photograph.
- The equipment must be accommodated to the child not vice versa.
- Attractive mirror to demonstrate brushing.

ADDITIONAL CONSIDERATIONS IN A DENTAL CLINIC THAT TREATS YOUNG CHILDREN

- Ground or first floor location if possible; an elevator if above the first floor.
- Designated play area for young children in the reception rooms.
- Carpet on the wall makes the area more durable.
- Horse shoe traffic pattern in which children are called to the operation from one door and exit by a second.
- *Plenty of check out space:* Parents with multiple children need to be backed up at the check-out station, particularly in the peak hours.
- Marketing coordinator/dental health educator office/conference room to meet with parents for case presentation home care instruments and diet counseling.
- A small dental chair with a light in at least one conference rooms so that, if necessary, the patient can be shown something in the child's mouth.
- Door knobs on operatory doors approximately 5 ft from the floor, if building codes permit to prevent a child from wandering.
- At least one, preferable two quiet operatories for performing lengthy complicated procedures with sound proofing.
- Glass as a sound barrier, therefore constructed glass Patco doors make excellent enclosures for quiet room combining visibility and sound proofing. Patco doors are available with built in blinds between two planes.

- A large glass window in the dentist office looking on to the operation is very helpful. Blinds provide privacy when needed. Wallpaper to take the wear and tear of small hands better than painted walls.
- *Neat attention getter:* Small television with earphones in the ceiling over each choke showing tapes controlled from a central video cassette player.
- If individual TVs are impractical or too expensive, a TV/VCP in one location in operatory preferably mounted on a wall is a good alternative.
- Holding benches in the operatory that double as storage.
- Arcade style video games for the reception area or in the operatory index areas. Sound effects should be removed. The play must be such that it serves the interests of all ages.
- There are many varieties of stuffed animals, hand puppets and other toys which serve both as distraction and pleasure. Color is very significant for youngsters almost bright colors are preferredto pastels.
- Negative sound of any nature may arouse anxiety. Good sound insulation is essential. Carpeting very effectively reduces sound levels. Tones of voice of the dentist and staff may discourage confidence.
- The smell of medication such as eugenol or formaldehyde pervading the office can be particularly unpleasant.
- Cleanliness and neatness are important. They reflect the individuals, who administer therefore encourage or discourage confidence.
- Operatory should be designed to minimize potentials negative visual stimuli. Fear provoking instruments should be located in inconspicuous positions.
- Use of preparatory is especially helpful since the time required to prepare for each patient is reduced. This allows a quarter period of time for orientation.
- The location and size of the equipment must permit the dentist auxiliary and patient to remain comfortable for long period.
- Dental chairs which are narrow and thin backed enable the dentist and dental assistant to sit closer to the work.

"The foundation of practicing dentistry for children is the ability to guide them through their dental experiences." It is important to plant seeds for the future dental health early in life and to promote positive approach toward dentistry during childhood. A pediatric dentist or a dental surgeon has to play roles of a behavior therapist and a counselor in order to facilitate this, the clinical atmosphere must be child-friendly. A typical clinic set-up may not be liked by all children; however, there is no reason as to why adults should not like a child-friendly clinic. Also, the child-friendliness in a set-up can be a distinguishing feature of such a clinic and children may be brought to it by parents undergoing treatments a long with them. Such visits could help reduce fears related to dentistry in a child's mind and prepare him/her better for a treatment visit, if required, anytime later.

POINTS TO REMEMBER

- Pedodontic clinic should be distinctly designed with special provisions of play area for children.
- The receptionist should be pleasing and should converse with the child in their developmental age pattern.
- The attire of the pediatric dentist should be non-threatening as children have white coat fear.
- Sound of dental equipment should be well masked with music.
- The most important fear allaying mechanism is the role of parents and hence a prerequisite brochure should be mailed to them with detailed instructions.
- A reward is the best ensuring factor of a positive behavior in subsequent visit.
- Audiovisual distraction is the best method for distracting child.
- The dental clinic should have horse-shoe traffic pattern in which children are called to the operation from one door and exit by a second.
- Modifications of dental chair are also an important factor in removing the fear of child.

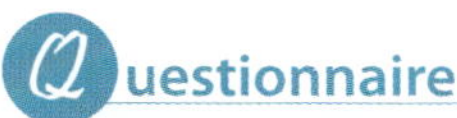

Questionnaire

1. Describe the design of a dental clinic.

FURTHER READING

1. Dent Clin North Am, 1995;39:4.
2. Jawdekar AM. Child management in clinical dentistry. New Delhi: Jaypee Brothers Medical Publishers, 2010.

CHAPTER

Parenting Styles Influencing Behavior in Pediatric Dentistry

Divya Gera

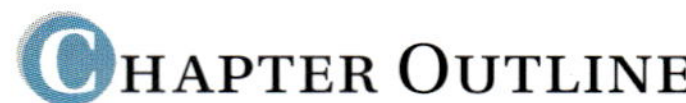

CHAPTER OUTLINE

- Authoritative Parenting
- Authoritarian Parenting
- Permissive Parenting
- Neglectful Parenting
- Other Parenting Styles
- Generation-wise Parenting
- Parents–Pedodontic Treatment Triangle Relation

Parenting or child rearing refers to the intricacies of raising a child and it is the process of supporting and promoting the emotional, social, intellectual and physical development of a child from infancy to adulthood.[1] The results of studies conducted by **Baumrind**, depict that preschoolers exhibited distinctly different types of behavior, highly correlates to a specific kind of parenting.[2] Based on these observation and analyses, **Baumrind** gave three parenting styles:

- Authoritative parenting
- Authoritarian parenting
- Permissive parenting

Among all the parenting theories most prevalent are **Diana Baumrind's** theory and **Maccoby & Martin** (1983) used two-dimensional framework to expand this three-dimensional parenting styles model.[3] Their research primarily focused on the configuration of the parenting styles their association with children's development.[4] They expanded Baumrind's permissive parenting style further into:

- *Authoritative*
- *Authoritarian (or disciplinarian)*
- *Permissive (or indulgent)*
- *Neglectful (or uninvolved)*

Statistically, 46% of parents use authoritative parenting style, 26% of parents use authoritarian parenting style, 18% of parents use permissive parenting style and 10% of parents use neglectful parenting style in the United States.[5] Although the distribution is relatively stable within the population, except that the European-American parents are about 2% more likely to have an authoritative style, while the Asian-American parents are 2% more likely to have an authoritarian style.[6]

AUTHORITATIVE PARENTING

- Parents have high expectations for achievement and maturity, but at the same time they are also warm and responsive.
- These parents set rules and boundaries by having an open discussion, providing guidance by using reasoning for their actions, which allow children to have a sense of awareness and teach children about values, morals, and goals.
- They have confrontive disciplinary methods, i.e., outcome-oriented, reasoned, negotiable and concerned with regulating behaviors.
- Authoritative parents encourage independence and provide their children with autonomy as they show their affectionate and supportive behavior to their children.
- They also allow bidirectional communication. This parenting style is also known as the democratic parenting style.
- According to Baumrind's research, this parenting styles helps the children in achieving higher academic success.

High Demandingness	High Responsiveness
Parents	**Children**
Sets clear rules and expectations for their kids while practicing flexibility and understanding	Good self-esteem
Communicates frequently	Interact using competent social skills
Allows natural consequences to occur	Have better mental health
Nurturing, supportive	Exhibit less violent tendencies
Open and honest discussions to teach values and reasoning	Securely attached
	Appear happy, content and more independent

AUTHORITARIAN PARENTING

- Authoritarian parenting are different from authoritative parenting styles as they have differences in parenting beliefs, demands, and approaches.
- Both parental styles demand high standards but authoritarian parents demand blind obedience using reasons such as "because I said so" and any attempts to reason with them are seen as backtalk.
- Parents use strict discipline and often employ harsh punishment to control children's behavior.
- Their disciplinary methods are coercive.
- Authoritarian parents are unresponsive to their children's needs and are generally not nurturing and usually justify their mean treatment as tough love.

High Demandingness

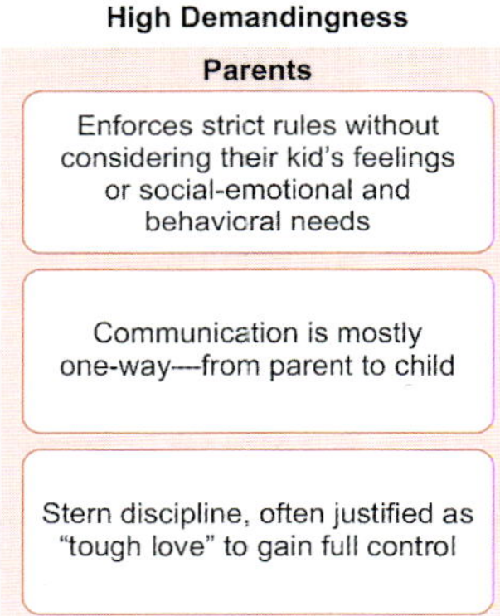

Parents
Enforces strict rules without considering their kid's feelings or social-emotional and behavicral needs
Communication is mostly one-way—from parent to child
Stern discipline, often justified as "tough love" to gain full control

Low Responsiveness
Offers little nurturance, guidance, and attention
Often struggles with their self-esteem issues

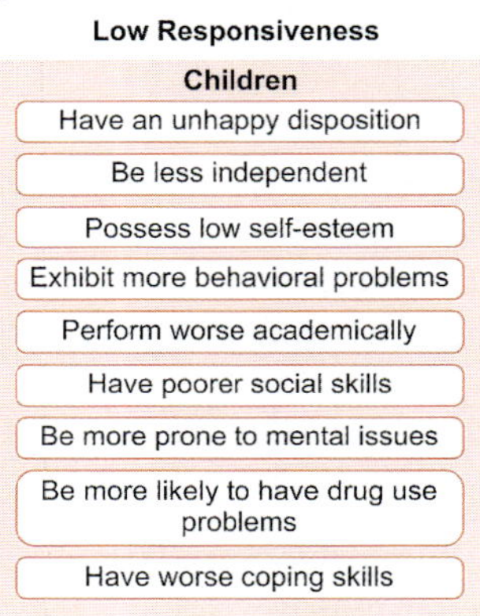

PERMISSIVE PARENTING (INDULGENT)

- Parents with permissive parenting style set very few rules and boundaries.
- They do not enforce rules.
- These parents are warm and indulgent.
- Child's freedom and autonomy are highly valued.
- Parents make children free from external constraints.
- More popular in middle-class than in working-class families.

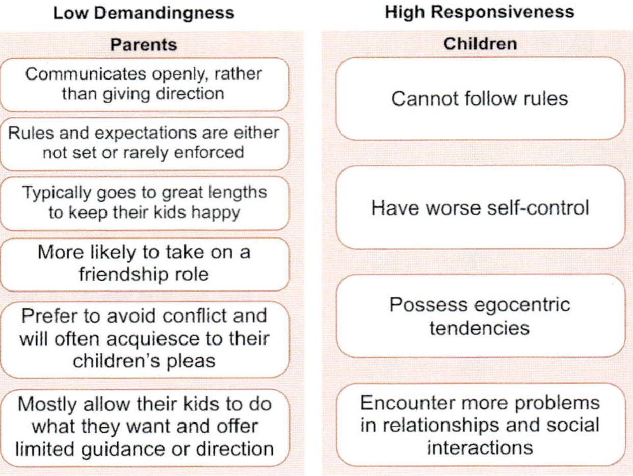

Low Demandingness
High Responsiveness
Parents
Communicates openly, rather than giving direction
Rules and expectations are either not set or rarely enforced
Typically goes to great lengths to keep their kids happy
More likely to take on a friendship role
Prefer to avoid conflict and will often acquiesce to their children's pleas
Mostly allow their kids to do what they want and offer limited guidance or direction
Can also be seen as cold and uncaring—but not always intentionally
Children
Have an unhappy disposition
Possess low self-esteem
More impulsive
Cannot self-regulate emotion
Encounter more delinquency and addiction problems
Cannot follow rules
Have worse self-control
Possess egocentric tendencies
Encounter more problems in relationships and social interactions

NEGLECTFUL PARENTING (UNINVOLVED)

- Neglectful parents do not set firm boundaries or high standards as they are uninvolved in their lives.
- These parents may have mental issues themselves such as child neglect, physical abuse, or depression when they were kids.
- Parents are often emotionally or physically absent.
- Often a large gap between parents and children with this parenting style.
- No regular communication between child and parent.

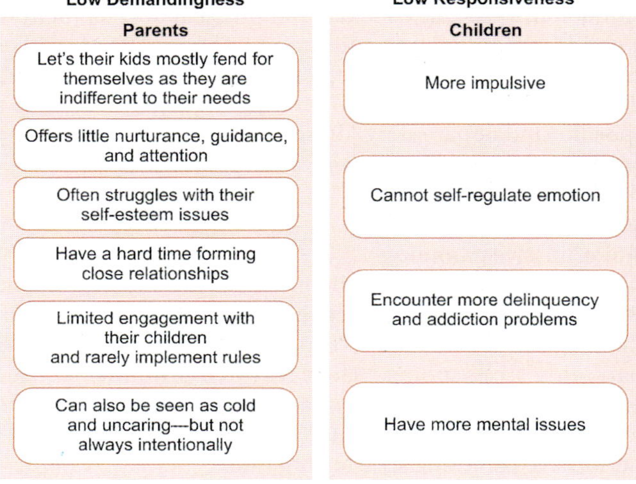

Classification system for categorization of parental behavior (CCPB): According to Simon Gamer	
Indifferent (0)	Obvious to the dentist interaction and who shows neither approval nor disapproval. They neither question the dentist nor they respond.
Dominant (1)	Respond to dentist interaction in a hostile manner. They challenge the authority of dentist. They question the treatment plan, overrule the authority of dentist and may advocate for child's denial to be fulfilled, overruling any proper reasoning.
Doubtful (2)	Respond to dentist action, question the treatment plan of child but they express doubt. They are wavy of dentist.
Reasonable (3)	Respond to dentist interaction in a respectable manner. They do not follow the treatment plan of the dentist blindly instead voice their questions though in a hostile manner (active partnership) and when convinced follow the direction cooperatively.
Submissive (4)	Respond to dentist interaction in a respectful manner. However they do not question the dentist treatment plan (blindly accept and follow). They idealize the dentist and show utter surrender to the dentist decision.
Apprehensive (5)	Respond to the dentist interaction but show signs of anxiety (shivering, crying, excessive speaking, constant reassurance to child). Not in a state of mind to question about the treatment plans of child in a healthy manner. They may either put up lots of questions or none at all.

OTHER PARENTING STYLES

Attachment Parenting

- This style of parenting aims at meeting the emotional needs of infants through close physical contact and emotional attachment.
- Parents create a positive, warm and safe environment where their children can develop trust, closeness and give their child enough time to feel comfortable and familiar with the world.
- In Baumrind's parenting style paradigm, attachment parenting emphasizes responsiveness. Since it focuses on a baby's early years, there are no references to parents' demands.[6]

Children tend to have:
- More cognitive competence
- Better communication
- Healthier social-emotional development

Helicopter Parenting

- These parents have over-protective attitude and tend to constantly involve with their children.
- A helicopter parent hovers over their child, monitors, and controls every aspect of their children's lives. They tend to control the environment and activities of their child, which mostly results in depriving them of the chance to learn things on their own.
- This parenting style often interferes with a child's development and leads to negative results.
- This parenting style does not fit under any of Baumrind's categories.
- Helicopter parents are insensitive to the child's emotional needs. This parenting style is close to authoritarian.

Children tend to have:
- Lower self-esteem
- Fear of failure
- More likely to develop mental and physical disorders
- Anxiety, depression, and drug abuse
- Poor stress coping skills
- Less independent

Tiger Parenting

- It is a strict parenting style which is a common parenting style among Chinese American families, but research has proven otherwise.
- It is characterized by a very strict and harsh set of rules and regulations.
- By creating a very rigid environment where the children have very little freedom or choices.
- Emotional abuse (shaming and insulting) is often used to force children to comply.
- A tiger parenting style is a typical example of the authoritarian parenting style.
- Tiger parenting focuses on raising driven, high-achieving kids.
- It often requires their kids to practice skills or study for lengthy periods.

Children tend to have:
- Lower academic performance
- Less sense of family obligation
- More depressive symptoms

Free-range Parenting

- Children are allowed to be more independent.
- It is directly opposite to helicopter parenting.
- Parents allow children to make decisions and develop a strong sense of responsibility and simply believe that children should be given more freedom and autonomy.
- In free-range parenting, there is less supervision, less control and more freedom as children can explore their environment and develop to make choices and learn from the consequences.

Children tend to be:
- Spoilt
- Would not take orders from anybody
- Right to make decisions

Concerted Cultivation Parenting

- This parenting style highlighted by a parent's attempts to foster their child's talents by incorporating organized activities in their children's lives.
- Children see adults as their equals and because of their early comfort they become more comfortable questioning adults, which in turn makes it easier for them to see themselves as equals.
- Parents start to encourage their children to learn how to speak with adults.

Children tend to:
- Express greater powers in social situations
- As increased experience with adults and power structure
- Overburdened sense of entitlement
- Disrespectful behavior toward authority figures
- The psychosomatic inability to play or relax

Little Emperor Parenting

- The little emperor syndrome (or little emperor effect) is an aspect/view where children of the modern upper class and wealthier Chinese families gain excessive amounts of attention from their parents and grandparents.
- Combined with increased spending power due to China's growing economic strength within the family unit and parents' general desire for their children to experience the benefits they themselves were denied, the phenomenon is generally considered to be controversial.
- Little emperors were primarily an urban phenomenon in which the one-child policy generally only applied to urban communities.

Children tend to be:
- Spoilt
- Submissive
- Easily irritated
- Anxious

Gentle Parenting

- It is an evidence-based approach to raising happy and confident children.
- It composed of four main elements: empathy, respect, understanding, and boundaries.
- Gentle parenting focuses on fostering the qualities you want in your child by being compassionate and enforcing consistent boundaries.
- It also encourages discipline. Discipline methods focus on teaching valuable life lessons rather than focusing on punishments.

Children tend to be:
- Well behaved
- Happy
- Cooperative

Child Centric Parenting

- Family's day-to-day activities and life revolve around the child's needs.
- These days, the average parent is much more attuned to the physical, emotional, spiritual, and psychosocial needs of each individual child.
- This type of parenting runs the risk of producing entitled, narcissistic children who cannot persevere and cope with difficulty, as there is a fine line between being 'loving' and being 'indulgent'.

Children tend to be:
- Spoilt child
- Over pampered
- Finds it hard to cope with dire situations
- Less cooperative in a dental setting

Soccer Parenting

The parents provide all type of facilities to the child (transportation, leisure, choice of food, other resource).

Children tend to be:
- Introvert
- Stoic behavior
- Tense cooperative

Snow Plough Parenting

- Parents remove any obstacles in their child's way.
- This type of parent does not want their child to experience any discomfort or problems, so the parent intervenes and fixes it for their child.

Children tend to:
- Trouble dealing with frustration
- Poor problem-solving skills
- Lack of self-efficacy
- Increased anxiety
- Prefers treatment under sedation

Guilty Parenting

- A guilty parent always lives in guilt for their past deeds where they could not fulfill their child's general and dental needs.
- They keep a track of the best dentists and hospitals around.

Children tend to:
- Throw temper tantrums
- Be over confident
- Search for outward validation

Lighthouse Parenting

- Focused on providing stability.
- They allow life to be experienced (like a boat experiences the ocean) but the parent is always visible and available to guide.
- This approach is a long-term practice for stability.
- A more positive approach than helicopter parenting.
- Parent trust their child and give them space to learn, grow and make mistakes themselves.
- Parent acknowledges children's growth and change.

Children tend to:
- More academically successful
- Take the fewest risks
- Have the closest relationships with their families

GENERATION-WISE PARENTING

Gen X	***Gen Y/Millenials***	***Gen Z***
1965–1979	1980–1995	1996–2010
Equilateral triangle relation	Isosceles triangle relation	Right angle triangle relation
The parent keeps a constant watch on the child but appears only when the child is in need	Parent places the child as first priority and giver over importance to looks	The parent becomes negligent towards the child as they are more involved in their own world
The child becomes: Bold, respectful, well mannered	The child becomes: Pampered, selfish, disrespectful, easily cries and not able to face hard situations	Child has less human values and respect

PARENTS–PEDODONTIC TREATMENT TRIANGLE RELATION

Equilateral triangle	***Isosceles triangle***	***Right angle triangle***
Authoritative	Authoritarian	Permissive
Gen X	Gen Y	Gen Z
Concerted cultivation	Helicopter	Negligent
Attachment parent	Tiger parent	Little emperor parent
Gentle parent	Child centric	Soccer parent
Self-motivated parent	Snow plough	Free range parent
	Google parent	
	Guilty parent	

REFERENCES

1. Darling N, Steinberg L. Parenting style as context: An integrative model. Psychological Bulletin. 1993;113(39):487-496.
2. Baumrind D. Effects of Authoritative Parental Control on Child Behavior, Child Development. 1966;37(4):887-907.
3. Maccoby EE, Martin JA. Socialization in the Context of the Family: Parent-Child Interaction. In: Handbook of Child Psychology. Socialization, Personality, and Social Development. ; 1983.
4. Baumrind D. Child care practices anteceding three patterns of preschool behavior. Genet Psychol Monogr. 1967;75(1):43-88.
5. ling PS, Johnston J, Chen V. Authoritarian Parenting and Asian Adolescent School Performance: Insights from the US and Taiwan. International Journal of Behavioral Development. Published online November 6, 2009:62-72.
6. Baumrind D. Differentiating between Confrontive and Coercive Kinds of Parental Power-Assertive Disciplinary Practices. Human Development. Published online 2012:35-51.

FURTHER READING

1. Baumrind D. The Influence of Parenting Style on Adolescent Competence and Substance Use. The Journal of Early Adolescence. Published online February 1991:56-95.
2. Chao RK. Beyond Parental Control and Authoritarian Parenting Style: Understanding Chinese Parenting Through the Cultural Notion of Training. Child Development. Published online August 1994:1111.
3. Chao RK. The Parenting of Immigrant Chinese and European American Mothers. Journal of Applied Developmental Psychology. Published online March 2000:233-48.
4. Chen X, Dong Q, Zhou H. Authoritative and Authoritarian Parenting Practices and Social and School Performance in Chinese Children. International Journal of Behavioral Development. Published online November 1997:855-73.
5. Gamer S, Tuch R, Garcia LT. (2003). MM House mental classification revisited: Intersection of particular patient types and particular dentist's needs. The Journal of Prosthetic Dentistry. 2003; 89(3):297-302.
6. Garcia F, Gracia E. Is always authoritative the optimum parenting style? Evidence from Spanish families. Adolescence. 2009;44(132):101.
7. Jackson C, Henriksen L, Foshee VA. The Authoritative Parenting Index: Predicting Health Risk Behaviors Among Children and Adolescents. Health Educ Behav. Published online June 1998:319-37.
8. Jain, Parul& Kaul, Rahul &Saha, Subrata. (2018). Reliability and validity of a newly proposed classification system for categorisation of parental behaviour (CCPB) in the dental setting. European Archives of Paediatric Dentistry. 19. 10.1007/s40368-018-0345-9
9. Jain P, Kaul R, Saha S. Reliability and validity of a newly proposed classification system for categorisation of parental behaviour (CCPB) in the dental setting. European Archives of Paediatric Dentistry. 2018;19(3).10.1007/s40368-018-0345-9
10. Landry SH, Smith KE, Swank PR. Responsive parenting: Establishing early foundations for social, communication, and independent problem-solving skills. Developmental Psychology. Published online July 2006:627-42.
11. LeMoyne T, Buchanan T. Does "hovering" matter? Helicopter parenting and its effect on wellbeing. Sociological Spectrum. Published online July 2011:399-418.
12. Locke JY, Campbell MA, Kavanagh D. Can a Parent Do Too Much for Their Child? An Examination By Parenting Professionals of the Concept of Overparenting. Aust j guidcouns. Published online December 2012:249-265.
13. Martin G, Waite S. Parental bonding and vulnerability to adolescent suicide. Acta Psychiatr Scand. Published online April 1994:246-254. doi:10.1111/j.1600-0447.1994.tb01509.x
14. McClun LA, Merrell KW. Relationship of perceived parenting styles, locus of control orientation, and self-concept among junior high age students. Psychol Schs. Published online October 1998:381-90. https://psycnet.apa.org/record/1998-12495-009
15. Miklikowska M, Hurme H. Democracy begins at home: Democratic parenting and adolescents' support for democratic values. European Journal of Developmental Psychology. Published online June 28, 2011:541-557.
16. Newman K, Harrison L, Dashiff C, Davies S. Relationships between parenting styles and risk behaviors in adolescent health: an integrative literature review. Rev Latino-Am Enfermagem. Published online February 2008:142-50.
17. Nyarko K. The influence of authoritative parenting style on adolescents' academic achievement. AJSMS. Published online September 2011:278-82.
18. Odenweller KG, Booth-Butterfield M, Weber K. Investigating Helicopter Parenting, Family Environments, and Relational Outcomes for Millennials. Communication Studies. Published online July 28, 2014:407-25.
19. Pimentel D. Criminal Child Neglect and the Free Range Kid: Is Overprotective Parenting the New Standard of Care. Utah Law Review. 2012;2012(947).
20. Polderman TJC, Benyamin B, de Leeuw CA, et al. Meta-analysis of the heritability of human traits based on fifty years of twin studies. Nat Genet. Published online May 18, 2015:702-9.
21. Rankin Williams L, Degnan KA, Perez-Edgar KE, et al. Impact of Behavioral Inhibition and Parenting Style on Internalizing and Externalizing Problems from Early Childhood through Adolescence. J Abnorm Child Psychol. Published online June 12, 2009:1063-75.
22. Rothrauff TC, Cooney TM, An JS. Remembered Parenting Styles and Adjustment in Middle and Late Adulthood. The Journals of Gerontology Series B: Psychological Sciences and Social Sciences. Published online January 1, 2009:137-46. doi:10.1093/geronb/gbn008
23. Smith JD, Dishion TJ, Shaw DS, Wilson MN, Winter CC, Patterson GR. Coercive family process and early-onset conduct problems from age 2 to school entry. Dev Psychopathol. Published online April 2, 2014:917-32.
24. Spera C. A Review of the Relationship Among Parenting Practices, Parenting Styles, and Adolescent School Achievement. Educ Psychol Rev. Published online June 2005:125-46.
25. Steinberg L, Dornbusch S. Ethnic differences in adolescent achievement: An ecological perspective. American Psychologist. 1992;47(6):723-9.
26. Steinberg L, Lamborn SD, Dornbusch SM, Darling N. Impact of Parenting Practices on Adolescent Achievement: Authoritative Parenting, School Involvement, and Encouragement to Succeed. Child Development. Published online October 1992:1266.
27. Strage A, Brandt TS. Authoritative parenting and college students' academic adjustment and success. Journal of Educational Psychology. Published online 1999:146-156.
28. Wolfradt U, Hempel S, Miles JNV. Perceived parenting styles, depersonalisation, anxiety and coping behaviour in adolescents. Personality and Individual Differences. Published online February 2003:521-32.
29. Zeinali A, Sharifi H, Enayati M, Asgari P, Pasha G. The mediational pathway among parenting styles, attachment styles and self-regulation with addiction susceptibility of adolescents. J Res Med Sci. 2011;16(9):1105-21.

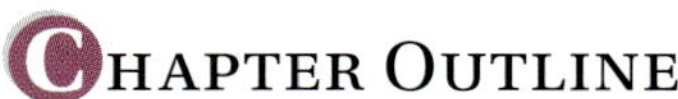

Oral Examination and Diagnosis

Ravi GR, Nikhil Marwah, Anshuman Jamdade, Suresh K Sachdeva

Chapter Outline

- Recording the History
- Clinical Examination
- Provisional Diagnosis
- Specialized Examination
- Final Diagnosis
- Comprehensive Treatment Plan

Successful dental treatment for children can be achieved by recording a detailed history, a complete clinical examination, appropriate investigations, a thoughtful diagnosis, and an appropriate treatment plan. It is very essential to obtain all relevant information about the patient and family along with an informed consent before embarking upon the comprehensive treatment plan for a child patient. In some circumstances, the diagnosis (i.e., an explanation for the patient's symptoms and identification of other significant disease process) may be self-evident.

When clinical data are more complex, the diagnosis may be established by:

- Reviewing the patient's history and physical, radiographic, and laboratory examination data.
- Listing those items that either clearly indicates an abnormality or that suggests the possibility of a significant health problem requiring further evaluation.
- Grouping these items into primary versus secondary symptoms, acute versus chronic problems, and high versus low priority for treatment.
- Categorizing and labeling these grouped items according to a standardized system for the classification of disease.

Components of oral examination and diagnosis

- Recording the history
- Examination of the patient
- Provisional diagnosis
- Special examination
- Final diagnosis
- Treatment plan (including medical referrals)

Emphasis on preventive dental care has taken the lead over the direct restorative intervention. Furthermore, recent information suggests that there is a more intimate relationship between oral and systemic health. Thus, the challenge dentists are facing in the 21st century is a rapidly growing population of patients who have chronic medical conditions, taking multiple medications (polypharmacy), yet still require routine, safe, and appropriate oral health care. This chapter addresses the rationale and method for gathering relevant medical and dental information (including the examination of the patient) and the use of this information for dental treatment.

RECORDING THE HISTORY

This can be further categorized for descriptive purposes into:

- Vital statistics
- Chief complaint
- History of present illness
- Family (social) history
- Medical history
- Drug history
- Dental history
- Natal, pre- and postnatal history
- Behavioral history
- Growth and development
- Diet history

Vital Statistics

It is a systematic approach to collect and compile all the information related to the vital events like birth, death, recognition, social structure, and legislation. Recording personal details of the child is required for both record purposes and for communication.

Table 6.1: Vital statistics of history.

Date	Name	Nick name	Age	Details of medical practitioner
It records the time the patient reported to the clinic and can be referred back during following appointments.	Knowing the name of the child will help in the following: • Establish good rapport with the child • Communication • Record purpose • Medicolegal issues	• To build rapport with the child • To alleviate apprehension	• As growth assessment parameter, e.g., dental age • To recognize the disparities between dental age, mental age, chronological age, and skeletal age, if any. • As an aid in treatment planning, e.g., growth spurts in girls are ahead of boys (based on chronological age) • Age-related diseases, e.g., tongue thrusting, cleft lip and palate. • For calculating a suitable dosage of the required drug, e.g., Young's rule.	Helps in diagnosing medical/ syndromic conditions
Gender	**Address**	**Source of information**	**Occupation of parents**	**Drugs**
• As an aid in treatment planning, e.g, growth spurts in girls are ahead of boys • Gender-related diseases, e.g., pubertal gingivitis is seen in adolescent females.	• Communication • Record purpose • Medicolegal issues • To rule out any endemic conditions, e.g., dental fluorosis.	To check whether the information provided is genuine or not.	Reflects the socioeconomic status of the family.	Helps to ascertain drug interactions and drug allergy.

All these details should be entered in the case sheet prior to the appointment. Details of the patient's medical practitioner should also be included **(Table 6.1)**.

Chief Complaint

- This is concerned about what made the patient to visit the dentist or what treatment they are seeking.
- It is better to ask the child about his/her chief complaint before involving the parent which helps to establish a good rapport with the child. But, it is mandatory to get an answer from the parent also regarding the child's complaint.
- It is recommended to record the chief complaint in patient's own words. When there are multiple complaints, they have to be recorded in chronological order (i.e., the problem which patient noticed first, should be recorded first followed by rest of the problems in sequence of their notice).

History of Present Illness

It is the elaboration/detailed description of the chief complaint.

- Several factors need to be evaluated regarding the chief complaint like duration, mode of onset (sudden/gradual), severity (mild/moderate/severe), nature (throbbing/burning/pricking), aggravating or relieving factors, associated symptoms (fever/difficulty in eating), diurnal variation (morning/evening), postural variation, any medications, investigations or treatment received for the same.
- Gives an insight toward the possible cause, progress and nature of the disease/condition.

Family (Social) History

- It provides relevant information about the social background of the child and his family.
- It should include factors like number of children in the family and their health condition, the child's attendance in the school, performance in the class, the housing conditions, and the parent's occupation.
- The family history should also include details of consanguineous marriage (if any), the occurrence of any genetic (e.g., Down syndrome) or hereditary (e.g., sickle cell disease) or endemic diseases (e.g., dental fluorosis).
- Furthermore, questions regarding family history must be neither offensive nor intrusive.

Medical History

- Various diseases or functional disturbances may directly or indirectly cause or predispose to oral problems and may affect the delivery of oral care.
- A comprehensive medical history should commence with information relating to pregnancy and birth, the neonatal period, and early childhood.
- Details about the previous hospitalization, surgery, illnesses, blood transfusion, and traumatic injuries should be recorded along with the information related to previous and current medical treatment.

Medical history should include information related to conditions affecting any of the below:

- Cardiovascular system (e.g., congenital heart disease, blood pressure, rheumatic fever)
- Central nervous system (e.g., seizures, cognitive delay)
- Endocrine system (e.g., diabetes)
- Gastrointestinal system (e.g., hepatitis)
- Respiratory system (e.g., asthma, respiratory tract infections)
- Hematological disorders (include family history of bleeding disorders)
- Urogenital system (e.g., nocturia, renal disease).

Prenatal, Natal, and Postnatal History

- Any infections, systemic conditions and history of drug intake (e.g., tetracyclines) during pregnancy.
- Immunization status during pregnancy.
- Whether received antiserum D vaccination or not—in case Rh +ve (father) and Rh –ve (mother).

Natal Events at Birth

- Time of birth—to rule out preterm birth.
- Type of delivery—normal/forceps/cesarean.
- Vaccinations given at birth.
- Forceps delivery—predisposed factor for temporomandibular joint (TMJ) disorder like TMJ ankylosis.

Postnatal Events after Birth

- Developmental milestones—crawling, sitting, walking, etc.
- Development of speech.
- Immunization schedule.

Drug History

- Details of the drugs being used for systemic ailments.
- Any adverse reaction/allergy to drugs.
- Any drugs already used for the condition.

Dental History

- The child's past experience with the dental treatment should be assessed.
- The kind of dental treatment received, including the pain control measures which has been offered, gives the dentist important information about the child's past behavior for dental treatment which might help us to modify the treatment appropriately.
- Dental history should also identify factors that have been responsible for the existing dental problems and those which might have an impact on future health.
- These include day-to-day oral hygiene measures like frequency of brushing and type of toothpaste used, the type, duration and frequency of sucking habits and dietary habits which should include duration of breastfeeding, bottle feeding at bed time, frequency of snacking between meals.
- Dental history should also give us explanation for the unusual conditions like rampant caries, erosion, and attrition.
- Finally by a thorough dental history, the dentist can evaluate the attitude of the parent to his/her child's dental treatment needs.

Dental history
- Helps in formulation of treatment plan.
- Knowledge about patient's habits.
- Helps to evaluate attitude of parents toward dentistry.
- Medicolegal purpose
- In addition, the survey of the previous dental records and radiographs may give important information for the treatment

Behavioral History

Any clues of negative or unpleasant behavior during the previous dental visit may call upon the need for behavior management or shaping.

Growth and Development

Developmental milestones, speech and language development, motor skills, and socialization should be evaluated.

Diet History

- Type of meal (vegetarian/mixed) influences the oral hygiene status.
- Habits of snacking between meals should be evaluated as they may be cariogenic.
- In case of high cariogenic patients, a diet diary with number of sugar exposures should be noted while taking diet history.

CLINICAL EXAMINATION

The clinical examination not only includes intra- and extraoral examination but also comprises of complete general examination.

General Examination

- **Height and weight**—both have a direct relation with developmental and nutritional status.
- **Gait**—look for any abnormality in gait, e.g., waddling gait, limping gait, hemiplegic gait.
- **Posture**—look for any abnormality, e.g., slumping posture.
- **Stature and built**—indicative of any malnutrition or other abnormality, e.g., poorly built, moderately or well built.
- **Vital signs**—pulse, heart rate, and respiratory rate differ in child at different ages till these reach the adult value. Hence, the clinician should have a thorough knowledge of these physiological variations.
- Any other data like illness, malaise.

Extraoral Examination

The extraoral examination should be one of the general appraisals of the child's well-being. The clinician should assess:

- Shapes of head **(Figs. 6.1A to C)** can be classified as:
  - Mesocephalic—average shape of head and arch **(Fig. 6.1A)**
  - Dolichocephalic—long and narrow head; narrow dental arches **(Fig. 6.1B)**
  - Brachycephalic—broad and short head; broad dental arches **(Fig. 6.1C)**
- Facial forms **(Figs. 6.2A to C)**—three common facial forms are:
  - Mesoprosopic—average facial form **(Fig. 6.2A)**
  - Euryprosopic—broad and short facial form **(Fig. 6.2B)**
  - Leptoprosopic—long and narrow face **(Fig. 6.2C)**
- Facial profile **(Figs. 6.3A to C)**—this is ascertained by examining the patient sideways. The three facial profiles are:
  - Straight **(Fig. 6.3A)**
  - Convex **(Fig. 6.3B)**
  - Concave **(Fig. 6.3C)**
- Facial swelling and asymmetry:
  - Bacterial or viral infections and trauma are the principal causes of facial swelling in a child.

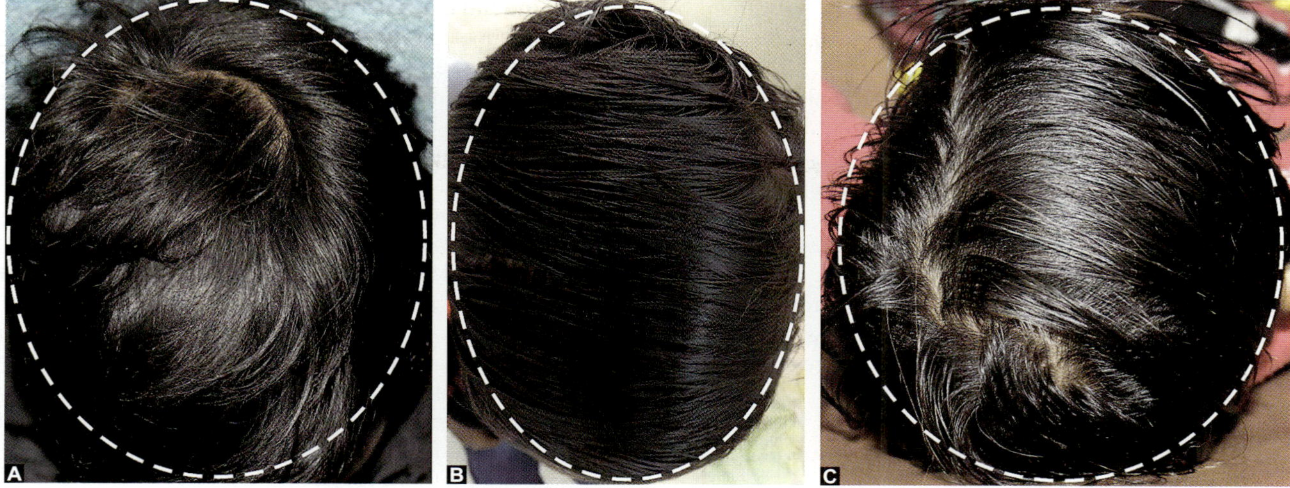

Figs. 6.1A to C: Head shapes: (A) Mesocephalic; (B) Dolichocephalic; (C) Brachycephalic.

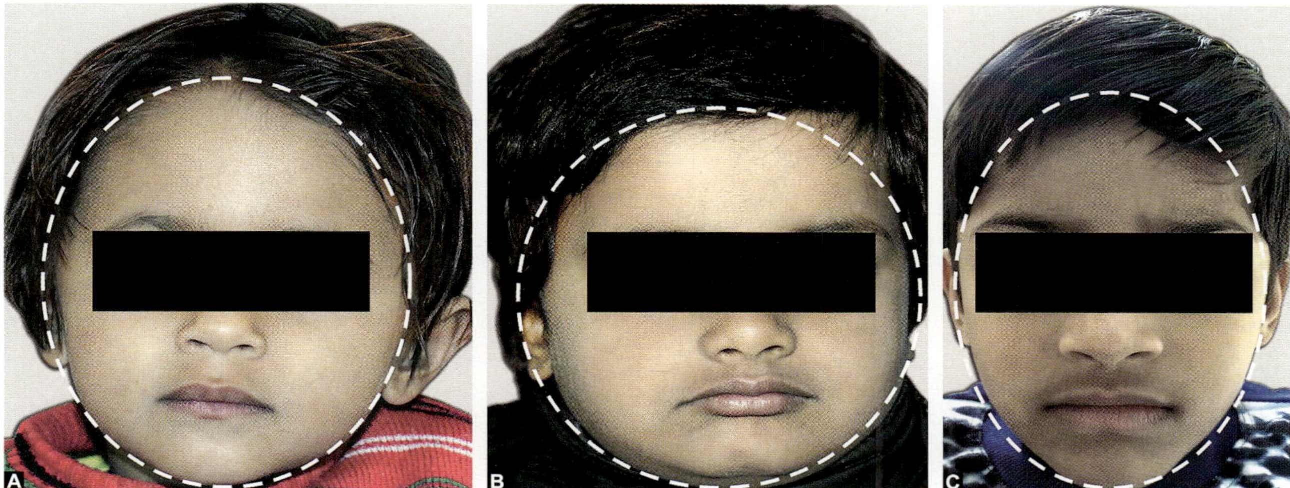

Figs. 6.2A to C: Facial forms: (A) Mesoprosopic; (B) Euryprosopic; (C) Leptoprosopic.

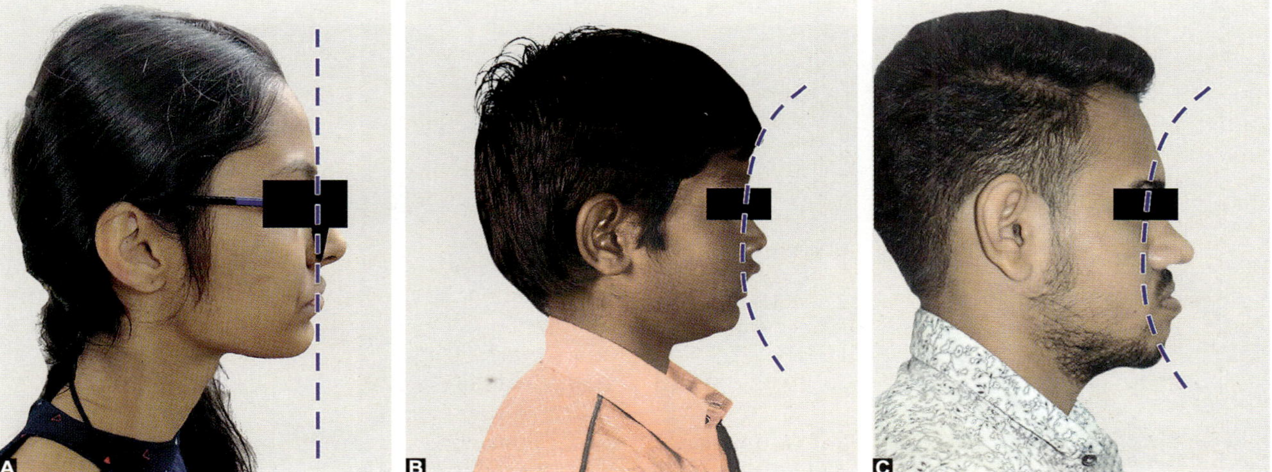

Figs. 6.3A to C: Facial profiles: (A) Straight; (B) Convex; (C) Concave.

- Pathological facial asymmetry may be produced by cranial nerve paralysis, fibrous dysplasia, and familial developmental disturbances.
- History and oral examination play a major role in the diagnosis of any swelling of the face.

❖ Examination of eyes:
- Eyes should be observed for any inflammation, swelling, or puffiness around the eye.
- Inflammation of maxillary teeth can cause swelling of the eyelids.
- Children with upper respiratory tract infection, sinusitis, and allergy have puffiness of eyelids.
- Congenital abnormalities can cause increased spacing between the two eyes (hypertelorism).

❖ Examination of nose:
- Nose should be examined for any abnormalities in size, shape, or color.
- Children who encounter nasal discharge indicate upper respiratory tract infection.
- Children with chronic upper respiratory tract infection will develop mouth breathing habit.
- Depression of nasal bridge (saddle nose) is seen in syphilis.

❖ Examination of skin:
- The skin of the face should be evaluated for the presence of primary and secondary skin lesions.
- Any scars, bruising, laceration, pallor, and birth marks should also be documented.

❖ Examination of chin:
- Prominence of chin and mentalis activity can indicate parafunctional habit and malocclusion.

❖ Examination of lips **(Figs. 6.4A and B)**:
- Lips should be examined for the presence of cold sores, swelling, or abnormal coloring.
- Competent—lips are in contact when musculature is relaxed.
- Incompetent—lip seal is not formed in normal circumstances, only hyperactivity of oral musculature can help in forming closure.

❖ Examination of TMJ **(Figs. 6.5A and B)**:
- Functional examination should include palpation and auscultation of TMJ and associated musculature.
- The patient should be examined for any clicking sound, crepitus, pain, gross deviation, and restricted condylar movements.

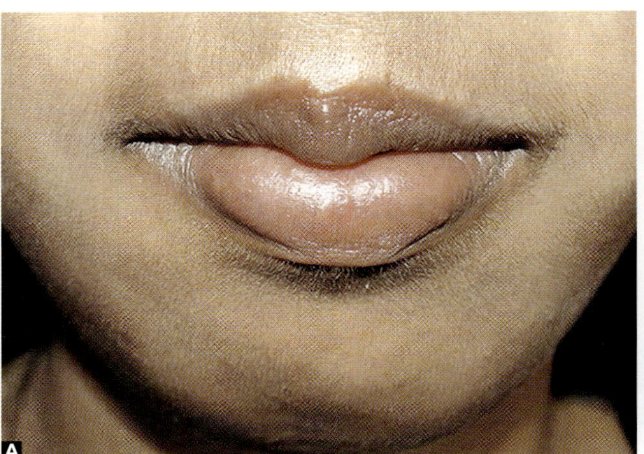

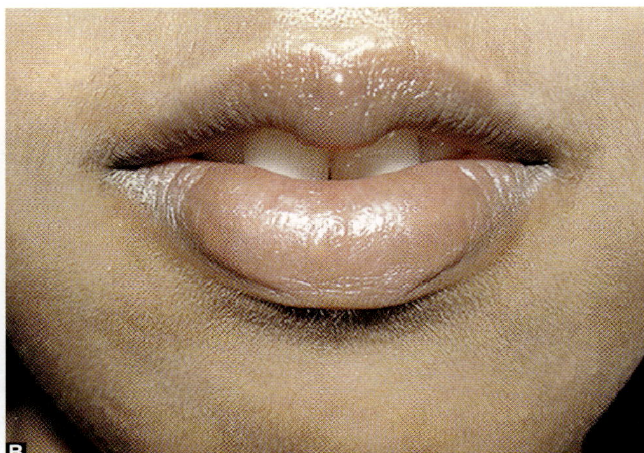

Figs. 6.4A and B: Competency of lip.

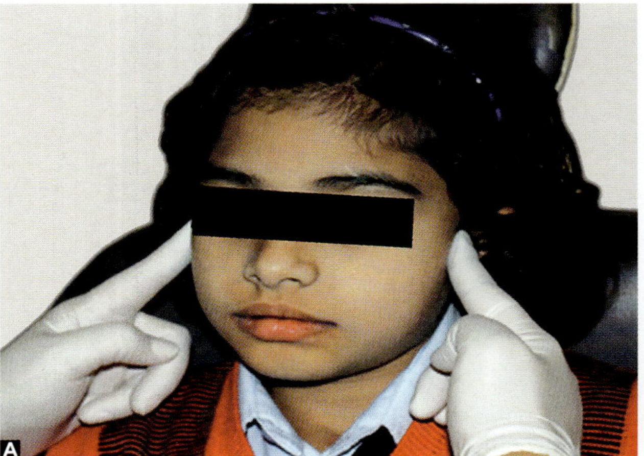

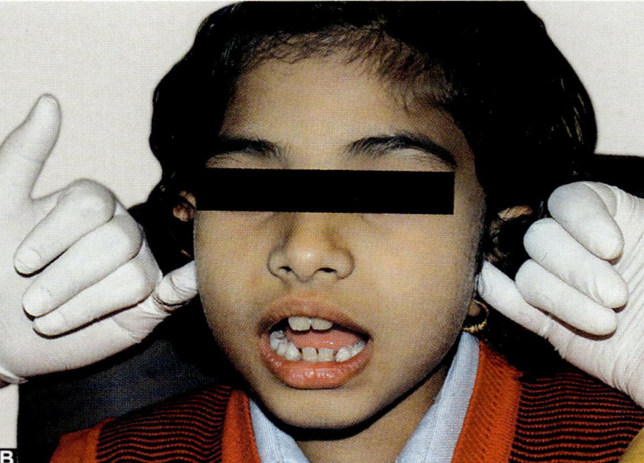

Figs. 6.5A and B: Method of examination of TMJ.

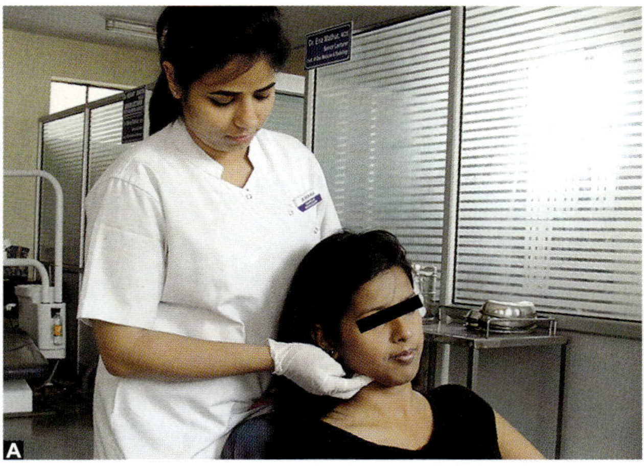

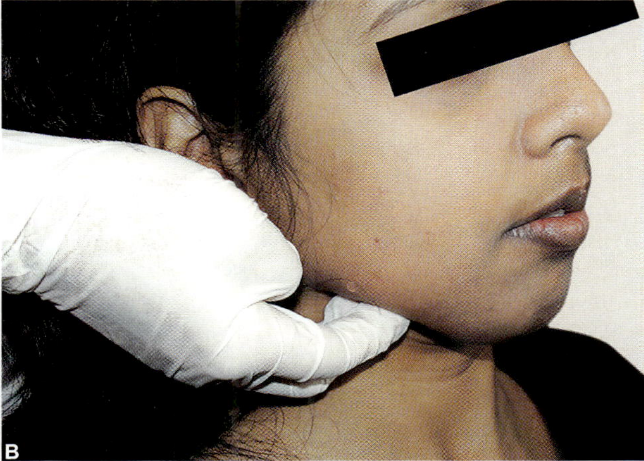

Figs. 6.6A and B: Examination of lymph nodes.

- Mouth opening is also related to TMJ function and should also be examined. Normal mouth opening is 40–45 mm.

TMJ examination
The function of TMJ is examined by palpating the head of mandibular condyle and observing the patient with mouth closed, open and during random (forward and lateral) movements.

- Lymph nodes examination **(Figs. 6.6A and B)**:
  - A complete examination of neck region including the lymph nodes is mandatory.
  - Lymphadenopathy is not uncommon in children due to frequent viral infections.
  - Ask the patient to bend his neck in forward and downward position to palpate the lymph nodes on the ipsilateral side and note the site, size, number, consistency, tenderness and fixity to the underlying structures.

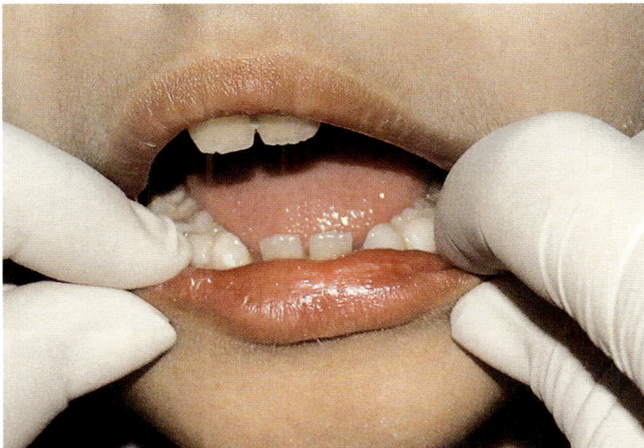

Fig. 6.7: Examination of lips.

Intraoral Examination

Intraoral examination for a young child should begin with the "tell-show-do" approach, i.e., by explaining the child what are you going to do; show him the examination instruments followed by intraoral examination. During and after the intraoral examination, explain the parents about the intraoral findings and discuss the treatment plan. This includes the examination of hard tissue as well as soft tissue.

- **Soft tissue:** It includes examination of the oral mucosa and examination of periodontal tissues. Complete inspection and palpation of all soft tissue oral structures is needed.
  - *Examination of oral mucosa:* An abnormal appearance of the oral mucosa may be indicative of an underlying systemic disease or nutritional deficiency. It is, therefore, very important to carefully examine the lips **(Fig. 6.7)**, palate and oropharynx, tongue **(Fig. 6.8)**, floor of the mouth **(Fig. 6.9)**, buccal mucosa **(Fig. 6.10)** and frenum attachments **(Figs. 6.11A to D)**.
  - During examination of intraoral soft tissues check the salivary flow rate and quality (thick, ropy).
  - Check for abnormal frenal attachment or tongue tie as it can have an effect on the development of speech.

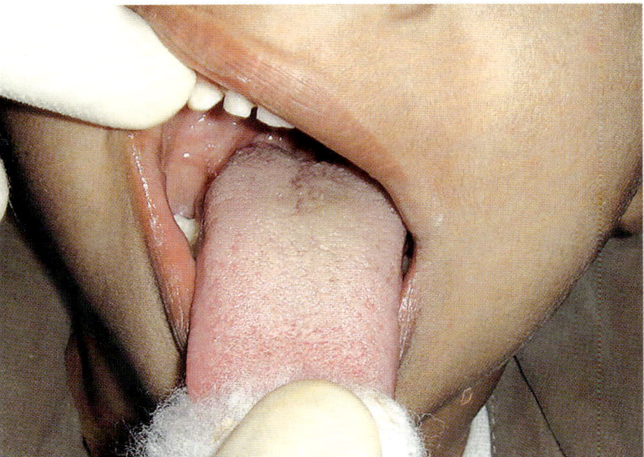

Fig. 6.8: Examination of tongue.

  - Since periodontal disease is very uncommon in children, examination of gingival tissues is indicated in young children.
  - Gingiva should be examined for redness, swelling, ulceration, and spontaneous bleeding.

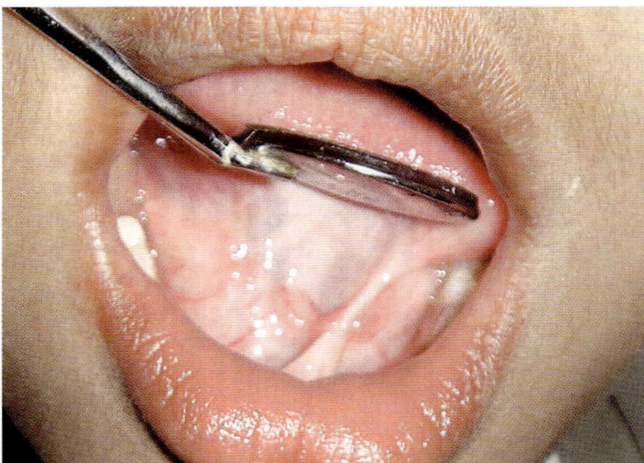

Fig. 6.9: Examination of floor of mouth.

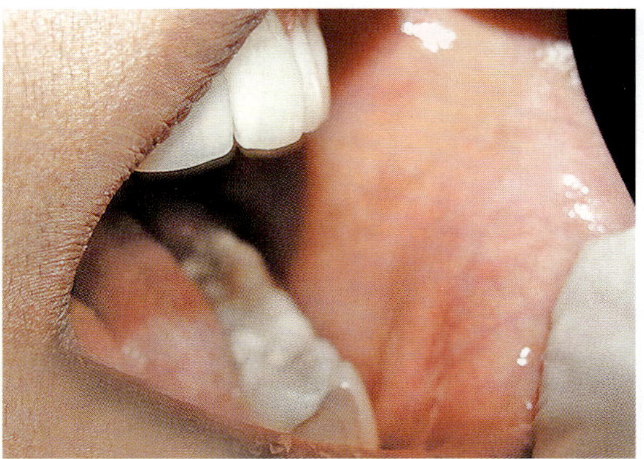

Fig. 6.10: Examination of buccal mucosa.

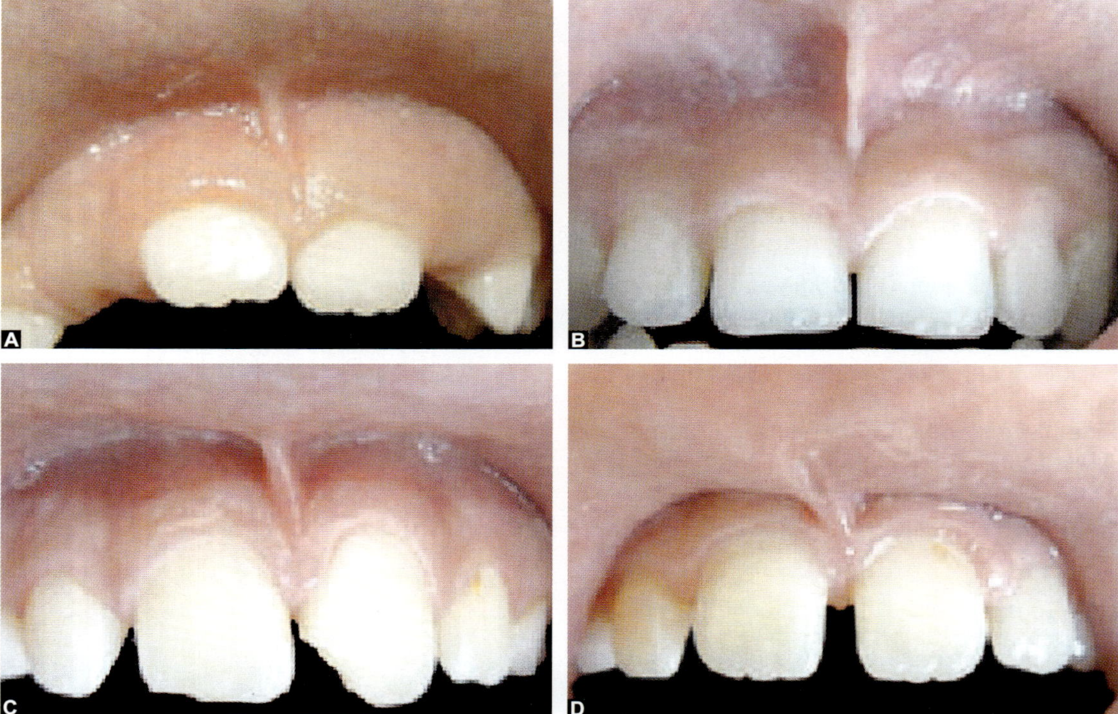

Figs. 6.11A to D: Examination of frenum attachments: (A) Mucosal—the frenal fibers are attached up to the mucogingival junction; (B) Gingival—the fibers are inserted within the attached gingiva; (C) Papillary–the fibers extend into the interdental papilla; (D) Papillary penetrating—the frenal fibers cross the alveolar process and extend up to palatine papilla.

- Assessment of the oral cleanliness and the presence of plaque and calculus should be done.
- The presence of profound gingival inflammation in the absence of gross plaque deposits, prematurely exfoliating teeth, or mobile permanent teeth may indicate a serious underlying disease.

❖ **Hard tissue:** Evaluation of the overall dentition can be made before the examination of individual teeth. These include variations in number, morphology, color, and surface structure. These should be observed under good light and after careful isolation and drying.

- Individual teeth should be evaluated for tooth number—any missing/extra teeth **(Fig. 6.12)**; caries—active/arrested **(Fig. 6.13)**; restorations—intact/deficient **(Fig. 6.14)**; trauma—note the extent, site, or signs of loss of vitality **(Fig. 6.15)**; tooth mobility **(Fig. 6.16)**—physiological/pathological; tooth structure—record any localized or generalized defect, for example, fluorosis **(Fig. 6.17)**.
- *Examination of occlusion* **(Fig. 6.18)***:* Occlusion of the child should be checked for molar and canine interdigitation. Early recognition of malocclusion will help to formulate a treatment plan in a very young age itself. The following should be analyzed: incisal relationship **(Fig. 6.19)**; canine relationship **(Figs. 6.20A to C)**; primary molar relationship **(Figs. 6.21 A to C)**; midline **(Figs. 6.22A and B)**; presence of crowding/spacing **(Fig. 6.23)**; and severe skeletal abnormalities.

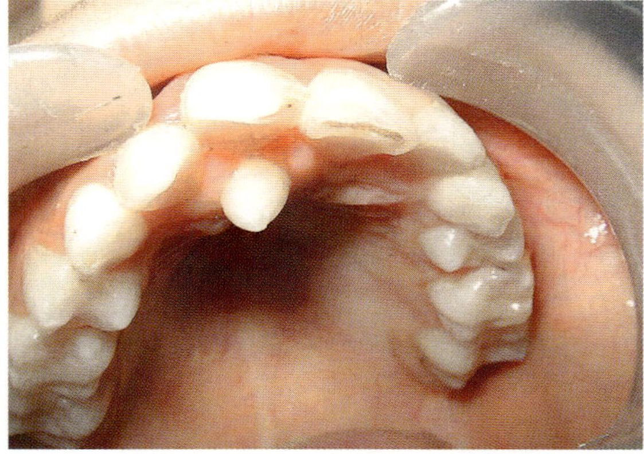

Fig. 6.12: Tooth number—any missing/extra teeth (mesiodens).

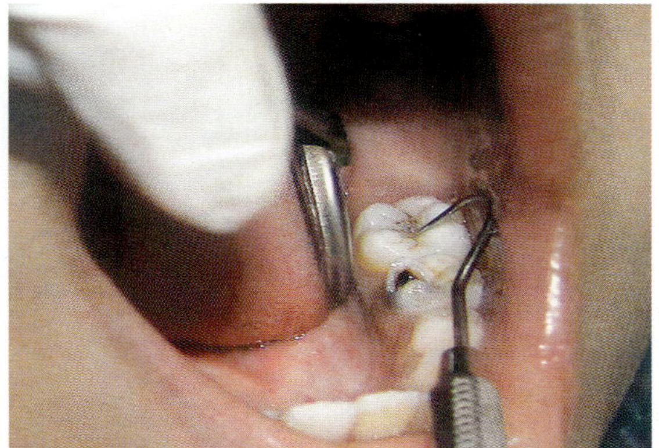

Fig. 6.13: Caries—active/arrested.

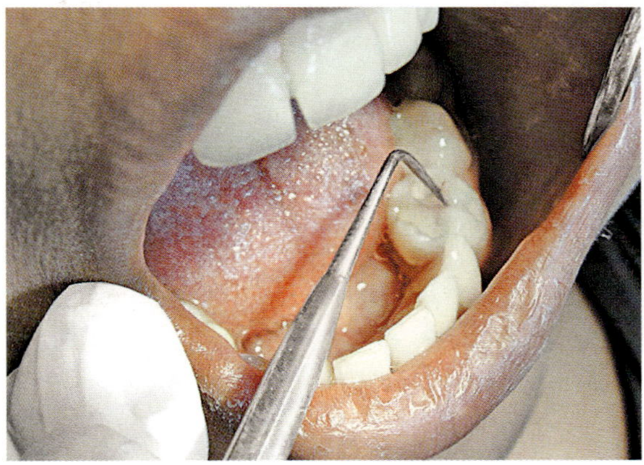

Fig. 6.14: Restorations—intact/deficient.

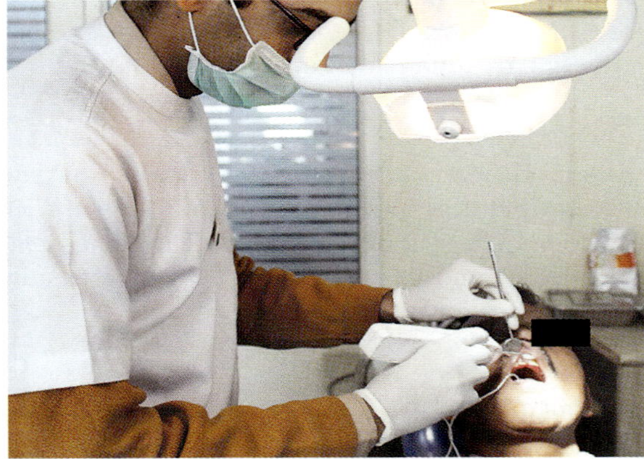

Fig. 6.15: Trauma—note the extent, site, or signs of loss of vitality.

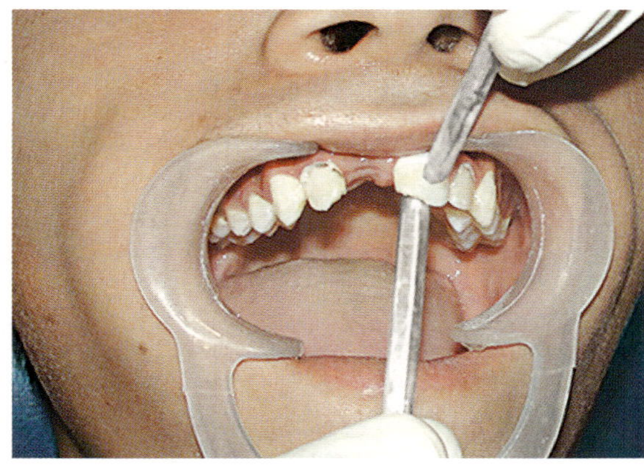

Fig. 6.16: Tooth mobility—physiological/pathological.

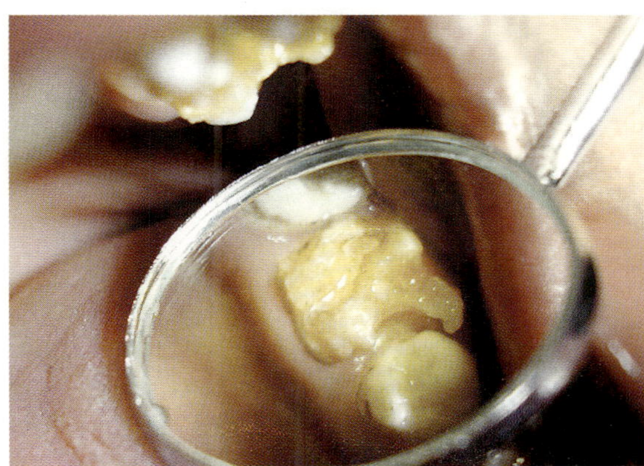

Fig. 6.17: Tooth structure—record any localized or generalized defect, e.g., fluorosis.

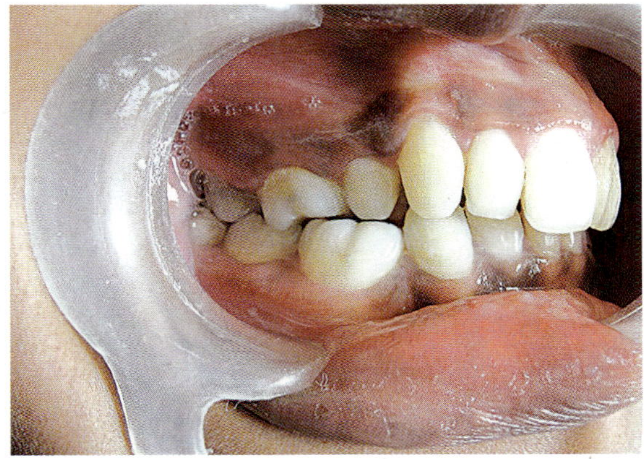

Fig. 6.18: Evaluation of occlusion.

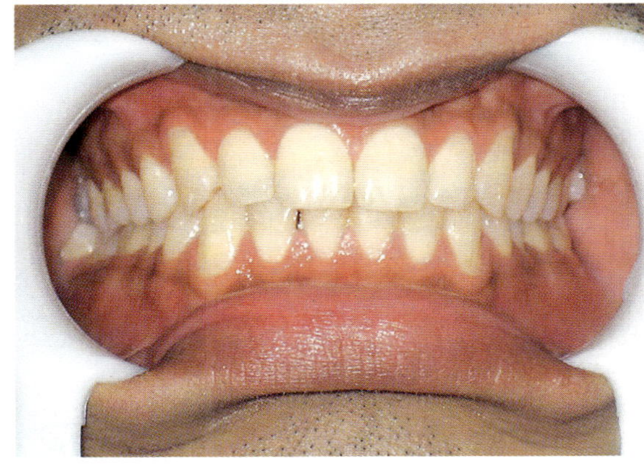

Fig. 6.19: Incisal relationship.

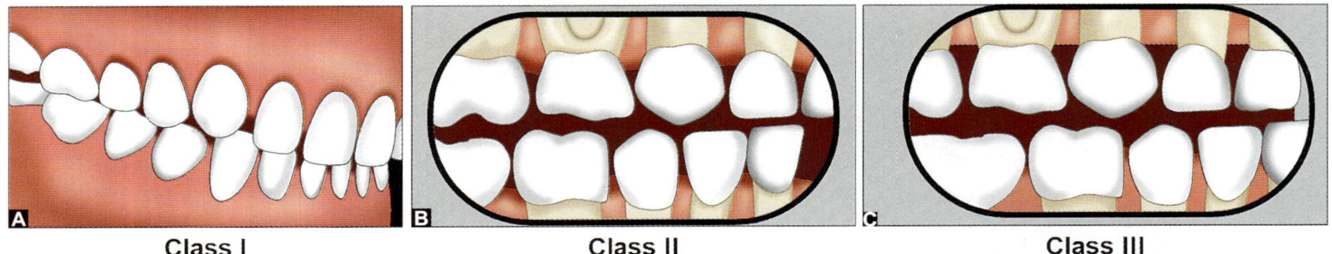

Figs. 6.20A to C: Canine relationship: (A) Class I: The cusp tip of primary maxillary canine is in the same vertical plane as the distal surface of the primary mandibular canine; (B) Class II: The cusp tip of primary maxillary canine is mesial to the distal surface of the primary mandibular canine; (C) Class III: The cusp tip of primary maxillary canine is distal to the distal surface of the primary mandibular canine.

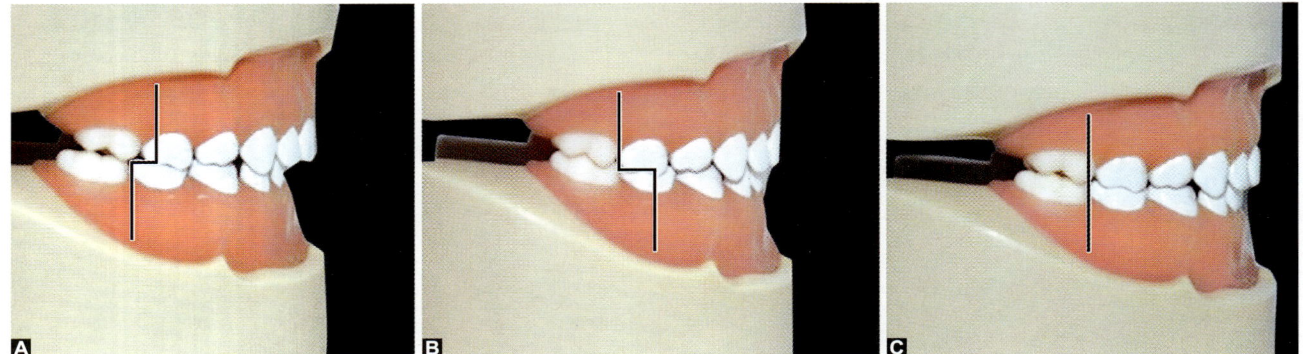

Figs. 6.21A to C: Primary molar relationship: (A) Distal step terminal plane; (B) Mesial step terminal plane; (c) Flush terminal plane.

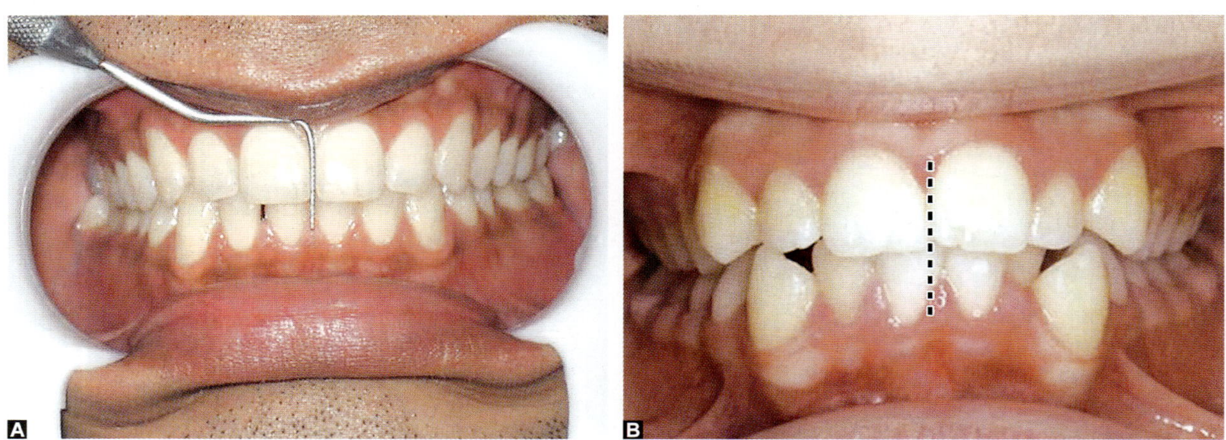

Figs. 6.22A and B: Midline: (A) Normal midline; (B) Teeth with midline shift.

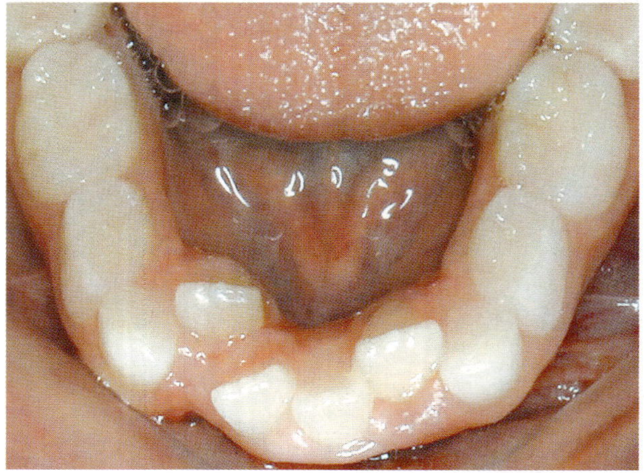

Fig. 6.23: Presence of crowding.

PROVISIONAL DIAGNOSIS

It is solely based on the history and clinical impression of the patient. This is followed by the special examinations, final diagnosis, and treatment planning.

SPECIALIZED EXAMINATION

This includes all necessary investigations that may be required to reach at final diagnosis like radiographs, pulp vitality testing, blood investigations, microbiological investigations, photography, diagnostic casts, caries activity tests, advance diagnosis, biopsy, etc.

FINAL DIAGNOSIS

This is the final conclusive answer that has been reached upon by applying investigative reports to our differential diagnosis options.

COMPREHENSIVE TREATMENT PLAN

This includes the following phases of treatment:

- **Emergency:** The first and foremost objective of the dentist is to relieve the patient of his acute pain and any other acute symptoms. For example, if a patient has reported with acute swelling and pain, the first task is to provide relief by performing emergency access opening.
- **Medical:** The patients should be referred to medical specialists through or by consultation with the family physician or paediatrician.
- **Preventive:** This phase includes risk assessment by caries diagnosis, dyes, diet charts and other preventive protocols like pit and fissure sealant, fluoride application, ART, etc.
- **Preparatory:** This includes behavior management and consultations with various other dental disciplines for interdisciplinary approach. Oral prophylaxis is also included in this phase.
- **Corrective:** Includes restorative, endodontic, surgical, orthodontic, periodontic, or prosthodontic treatments which are carried out as an active phase.
- **Maintenance:** Its variation depends on the patient's disease status and begins from one week up to 6 months or even 1 year.

To summarize, a clinician can be successful in rendering a comprehensive treatment by means of updating his knowledge timely. Nevertheless, the role of examination, diagnosis, and treatment planning still play the pivotal role in rendering the same even with the constant development of the science and technology. All the latest techniques do not yield the desired results if these three fundamentals are ignored.

POINTS TO REMEMBER

- Components of oral examination and diagnosis are recording the history, examination of the patient, provisional diagnosis, special examination, final diagnosis, and treatment plan (including medical referrals).
- History includes: History of present illness, family (social) history, medical history, drug history, dental history, pre- and postnatal history, behavioral history, and diet history.
- Use of name is to build rapport with child and to alleviate apprehension.
- Age is important to recognize the disparities between dental age, mental age, chronological age, and skeletal age, if any.
- Chief complaint should be in patient's own words.
- History of present illness is the elaboration of the chief complaint.
- Dental history mainly helps in formulation of treatment plan.
- Examination of oral mucosa is useful as any abnormal appearance of the oral mucosa may be indicative of an underlying systemic disease or nutritional deficiency.
- Examination of occlusion of the child will help in early recognition of malocclusion and will help to formulate a treatment plan in a very young age itself.
- Treatment plan includes emergency medical preventive preparatory corrective maintenance.

Clinical Significance

Taking proper history is the first and most important step towards correct diagnosis. Only with this can apt treatment plan can be set.

Questionnaire

1. Explain the role of vital statistics in case history.
2. Role of diet history in management of dental patient.
3. Explain the examination of TMJ and lymph nodes.
4. Describe the hard tissue examination.
5. Explain the phases of treatment plan.

FURTHER READING

1. Clerehugh V, Tugnait A. Diagnosis and management of periodontal diseases in children and adolescents. Periodontal. 2000;26:146-68.
2. Curcio RJ. The art of the dental examination. DCNA. 1978;22:209-28.
3. Curcio RJ. The first phone call. DCNA. 1978;22:197-208.
4. Jeffcoat MK. Diagnosing periodontal disease. New tools to solve old problems. J Am Dent Assoc. 1999:122-54.
5. Moskow BS, Barr CE. Examination of the patient. In: Goldman HM, et al. (Eds). Current Therapy in Dentistry (Vol. 4).St. Louis: Mosby; 1970.

CHAPTER

Teeth Identification and Numbering Systems

Chaitanya Ram, Nikhil Marwah, Srinivas LS

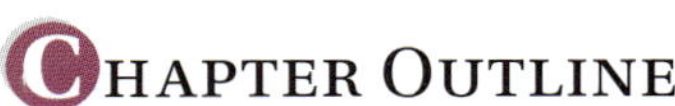

CHAPTER OUTLINE

Dental anthropologists and dentists who are building on a classic anatomic nomenclature will prefer a precise lexicon of terms for designating specific teeth. To say, there would be no confusion when describing a specific tooth as *primary human maxillary first molar*. However, in a dental clinic setting, when a dentist would have to extensively and expeditiously document voluminous details, this type of tag will prove to be lengthy and cumbersome.[1]

Thus, a practical need for conciseness, precision and succinctness has led dentists and clinicians to develop a variety of tooth-coding systems. The purpose of chapter is to delineate the common clinical systems of tooth nomenclature in order to familiarize dentists with a clinical nomenclature.[2] Before understanding the need for a tooth numbering, one has to understand different terms used in the context of this chapter. The etymology of teeth names are all from Latin. Incisor (Latin word *incidere* = to cut into) describes the function of incising and nipping. Canines (Latin word *canis* = dog, hound), derived from the prominent, well-developed teeth in the family *Canidae*. The name premolar is merely due to their position in relation to the molars. Since these teeth commonly possess two cusps, they are also known to be bicuspids.[3] Molars (Latin word *molaris* = millstone) refers to the triturating ability of these teeth with their substantial occlusal surfaces.

Tooth coding

When identifying a particular tooth, we should follow a specific pattern to name the tooth as mentioned below in the same order:

- Dentition—deciduous or permanent
- Arch—maxillary or mandibular
- Quadrant—right or left
- Tooth name—incisor, canine, molars

TRAIT CATEGORIES[4]

These are helpful in describing tooth similarities and differences. A trait can be defined as a distinguishing feature, characteristic, or an attribute. The trait can be classified as:

- **Set traits**—this distinguishes the teeth in primary dentition from permanent dentition. For example, primary central incisors are wider mesiodistally than cervicoincisally. This type of trait is also called dentition trait. Premolars do not have any set traits as they do not appear in the primary dentition.
- **Arch traits**—distinguish maxillary from mandibular arch, from maxillary incisors are larger than mandibular incisors, maxillary molars are wider buccolingually and mandibular molars wider mesiodistally
- **Class traits**—distinguish among individual teeth, that is, incisors, canines, premolars, and molars, for example, incisors have edges for cutting, canines have pointed cusps

for tearing, premolar cusps are modeled for grinding, and molars have flat cusps for chewing.

- **Type traits**—used for interclass differentiation like difference between central and lateral incisor or between first, second, and third molars. Canine although does not have a type trait as it is single in each arch.

DENTAL FORMULA

Denomination and number of teeth for all mammalian are expressed by a formula **(Table 7.1)**. Denomination of each tooth is noted as an initial letter like I for incisor and each letter is separated by a horizontal line, above which is written the maxillary teeth and below the mandibular teeth.

- Elephants have deciduous molars and no premolars
- Elephant tusks are central incisors and weigh about 440 lb
- Teeth of shrews wear out earliest as they have food every 1–2 hours
- Whales have no teeth

Dental formula expresses the number of teeth on one side, so total number of teeth is usually doubled.

Table 7.1: Dental formula for mammals.

S. No.	*Type of mammalian*	*Dental formula*
1.	Humans—primary teeth	I—2/2 C—1/1 M—2/2
2.	Humans—permanent teeth	I—2/2 C—1/1 P—2/2 M—3/3
3.	Apes	I—2/2 C—1/1 P—2/2 M—3/3
4.	Monkeys	I—2/2 C—1/1 P—3/3 M—3/3
5.	Dogs	I—3/3 C—1/1 P—4/4 M—2/3
6.	Cats	I—3/3 C—1/1 P—3/2 M—1/1
7.	Cows	I—0/3 C—0/1 P—3/3 M—3/3
8.	Horses	I—3/3 C—1/1 P—4/4 M—3/3
9.	Rabbits	I—2/1 C—0/0 P—3/2 M—3/3
10.	Elephants	I—1/0 C—0/0 DM—3/3 M—3/3
11.	Rats	I—1/1 C—0/0 P—0/0 M—3/3

TOOTH NUMBERING SYSTEMS

Tooth designation systems have been used for more than hundreds of years and were first reported in early literature of Latin America. The first comprehensive numbering system was developed by Viennese dentist **Adolf Zsigmondy** in 1861. He designated an eight tooth quadrant plan with the quadrant system symbolized by drawing one of four corners into which 1–8 tooth numbers were placed. In 1870, an Ohio dentist **Corydon Palmer** presented the same system at meeting of American Dental Association (ADA) and claimed it to be his original creation. Later in 1870 when **Zsigmondy** original article was published in British Journal of Dental Science and presented at 1889 International Dental Congress in Paris and also appeared in Ohio Journal of Dental Science and Dental Cosmos, it came as a great embarrassment to **Dr Palmer** who in America had taken credit for this system and claimed to discover it. In 1891, he wrote a complete article about his notation system in order to get complete recognition, but this was kept pending and never given official status. However, years after his death, ADA acknowledged his contributions in the field of numbering systems and began to associate his name with this system but never gave him official recognition as discoverer of quadrant numbering system.

Tooth numbering systems

- The first comprehensive numbering system was developed by Viennese dentist **Adolf Zsigmondy** in 1861, a Danish dentist
- Viktor Haderup added the symbols of "+" and "–" along teeth number to designate the jaws
- In 1882, a German dentist **Julius Parreidt** proposed a system of counting consecutive teeth called as Universal system
- In end of 1968, Federation Dentaire Internationale (FDI) came up with a unique two-digit system developed by Dr **Jochen Viohl** of Berlin, and this was introduced in 1970

Although accepted, this system underwent many modifications by various dentists all over the world. Out of them, the most distinguishing was by Danish dentist **Viktor Haderup** who added the symbols of "+" and "–" along teeth number to designate the jaws. However, none of these modifications ever sustained the test of time and none were implemented or accepted. Elsewhere in 1882, a German dentist **Julius Parreidt** proposed a system of counting consecutive teeth called as Universal system. He did this to simplify the quadrant system, but he later admitted that this universal system of counting 1–32 had many errors and was artificial when imposed upon permanent dentition. This system also did not include the primary teeth, and hence he was forced to abandon this system in 2 months. By the 1940s, there were many numbering systems that were being used. The committee on nomenclature was well versed with this problem and in 1947 recommended that 1–8 quadrant numbering system, that is, **Zsigmondy-Palmer** system will be universally used and accepted; the primary teeth were included as A–E. In the end of 1968, FDI came up with a unique two-digit system developed by **Dr Jochen Viohl** of Berlin, and this was introduced in 1970 and has since been widely accepted and used all over the world. However, **Zsigmondy-Palmer** system still continues to be the most dentist popular notational system of all time.

Tooth notation system

- **Alphabetical (letters) representation, e.g.,** primary teeth in universal system
- **Numerical (number) representation, e.g.,** FDI system
- **Alpha-numerical (letter number) representation system, e.g.,** Universal system
- **Symbolic, e.g.,** Zsigmondy-Palmer
- **Nonsymbolic, e.g.,** FDI

Zsigmondy-Palmer System

The most popular system of tooth designation for much of the 20th century was developed by the Viennese dentist ***Adolf Zsigmondy***.[5] *He broke with tradition, substituting numbers for the eight teeth in each quadrant in place of the lengthy Latin names used at that time.*[1,6]

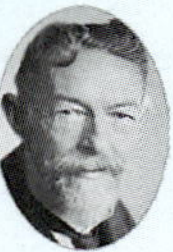

He combined his tooth numbering system with a graphical device to specify the quadrant of mouth also called angular and the grid system and also called eight numerical quadrant system.

- Primary teeth are represented by A–E and permanent by 1–8.
- The correspondence are **(Fig. 7.1):**
  - Central incisor
  - Lateral incisor
  - Canine (cuspid)
  - First premolar (bicuspid)
  - Second premolar (bicuspid)
  - First molar
  - Second molar
  - Third molar (dens sapientiae; wisdom tooth)
- Zsigmondy combined his tooth numbering system with a graphical device to specify the quadrant of the mouth. An L-shaped [L] mark was used, with the vertical line segment being the subject's midline and the horizontal segment his occlusal plane that separates the upper and lower arcades. The clinician could, then, easily code a specific tooth, such as the lower left canine as 3 or the upper right first molar.[6]
- Conflicts rose because an Ohio dentist **Corydon Palmer**[7] **(Palmer)** argued for his independent invention of the same coding system and said that the natural division of the dentition into quadrants was a well-known, obvious device. In fact, most American dentists in that era have been taught the notation as being **Palmer** (though also termed the "quadrant system" by some).[8]
- It also has been labeled the "angular system" and the "grid system" because of the horizontal and vertical line segments that denote the tooth's quadrant.
- However, the disadvantage for Zsigmondy-Palmer notation is that, even though it is easy to sketch, the tooth codes in a patient's record, it is tedious to type or verbalize them.

Indeed, it was the need to computerize the dental recording system that marshaled—in the FDI system—and incidentally promoted the use of the Universal system in the United States. Coding a tooth numerically, as no. 16 or no. 28, is easy and lends itself to word processing.

Palmer Analog for Primary Teeth

- Letters have commonly been used to denote the primary teeth; some systems use lower-case letters (perhaps mimicking the subadult nature of these teeth),[9] but capital letters are encountered more often. Again, the side and arcade are denoted by line segments: B is the maxillary right lateral incisor, and E is the mandibular left second molar.
- Primary teeth have also been designated by Roman numbers (I–V) **(Fig. 7.2)**, which can further confuse the novice[8,9] particularly since still other systems have used

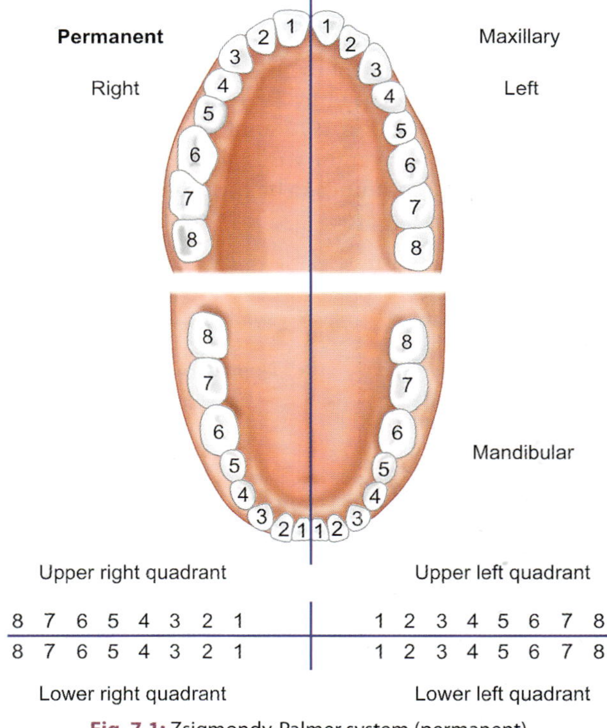

Fig. 7.1: Zsigmondy-Palmer system (permanent).

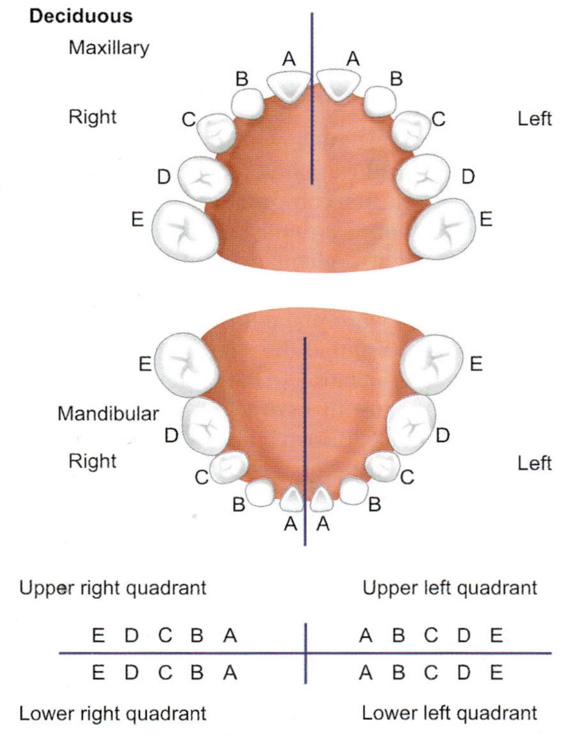

Fig. 7.2: Zsigmondy-Palmer designation (primary).

Roman numerals to designate quadrants in the permanent dentition.

Advantages of Zsigmondy-Palmer System

- Effective applicability
- Easy to use and understand
- Easy to record inpatient records and radiographic evidence

Disadvantages of Zsigmondy-Palmer System

- Takes more space in the patients' files
- Very difficult to type in electronic files
- Hard to convert it to HTML, the programming language of the Internet
- Like in Zsigmondy's method, the use of grid signs is significant obstacle to fast communication and data processing [10]
- Requires special software
- Needs private processing editor[11]

Fédération Dentaire Internationale System

- Excepting the United States dentists, all around the world now use the FDI two-digit system [Fédération Dentaire Internationale (FDI)].
- This was proposed by **Dr Jochen Viohl** of Berlin in 1970.
- This scheme was developed by a "Special Committee on Uniform Dental Recording" and passed as a resolution of the FDI General Assembly at its 1970 meeting in Bucharest, Romania.
- While the FDI labeled this the "Two-Digit System," it is more commonly referred to as the FDI system.
- According to this system, every tooth system is denoted with two digits, the first digit denoting the quadrant of the mouth, while the second digit defines the tooth's normal position in the mouth, front to back.
- Most dentists are right handed, so quadrant 1 (maxillary right) is closest to the dentist when examining a patient and is scored first, then the upper left quadrant, then one drops down to the lower left quadrant, finishing with teeth in the lower right quadrant. More formally, the quadrants are numbered "in a clockwise sequence... starting on the upper right side" when viewing the subject from the front[12]
- The FDIs description also suggests how to verbalize the system, namely, "The digits should be pronounced separately; thus, the permanent canines are teeth one-three, two-three, three-three, and four-three" **(Fig. 7.3).**

FDI System for Primary Teeth

- Even though developing first, the convention is that to use as numbers 5 through 8 to denote the primary teeth quadrants **(Fig. 7.4).**
- This numerical oddity was the subject of considerable discussion by the FDI committee, but it was reasoned, "mainly because deciduous teeth function for such a short time in comparison with permanent teeth that the bulk of dental data to be collected and computerized in the future would obviously concern permanent teeth".

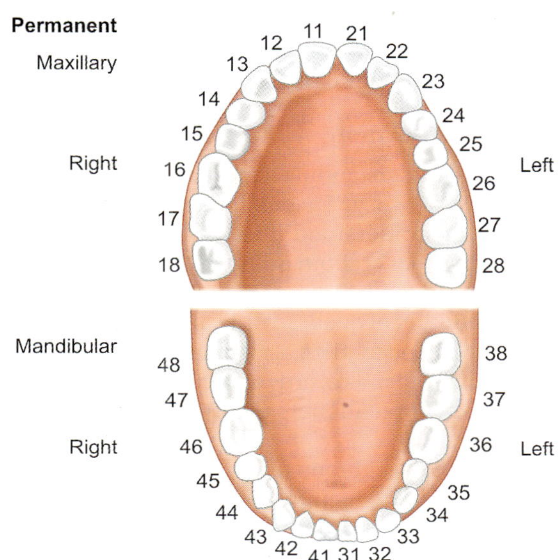

18	17	16	15	14	13	12	11	21	22	23	24	25	26	27	28
48	47	46	45	44	43	42	41	31	32	33	34	35	36	37	38

Fig. 7.3: FDI numbering system (permanent). (FDI: Federation Dentaire Internationale)

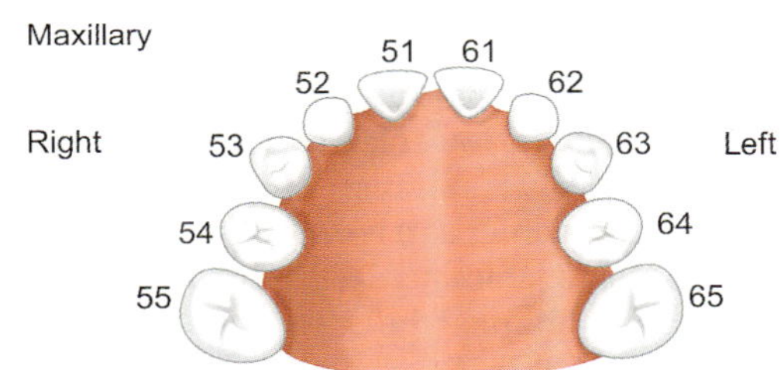

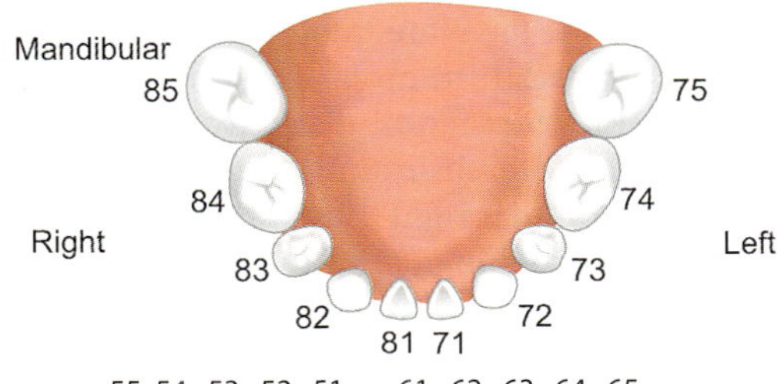

55	54	53	52	51	61	62	63	64	65
85	84	83	82	81	71	72	73	74	75

Fig. 7.4: FDI tooth numbering system for primary teeth. (FDI: Federation Dentaire Internationale)

- Given by **Dr Jochen Viohl**
- Also called as two-digit system
- Every tooth system is denoted with two digits, the first digit denotes quadrant of the mouth and second defines the tooth's position
- Quadrants are numbered clockwise starting from maxillary right. This system is simple, easy and more communicable

Advantages of FDI System

- Simple to understand and to teach
- Easy to pronounce in conversation and dictation

- ❖ Readily communicable in print
- ❖ Easy to translate into computer output
- ❖ Easily adapted to standard charts used in general practice

Disadvantages of FDI System

- ❖ Difficulty in understanding if the number written is FDI or Universal system, e.g., 12 sometimes between two doctors, it can be misunderstood if its tooth number twelve of Universal system or tooth number 2 of quadrant 1.
- ❖ Since the primary and permanent teeth are differentiated with the number of quadrants, it can be confusing for new learners to understand if it Is a primary tooth or permanent and can mislead the records.
- ❖ Some general practitioners reported they were confused by this system.
- ❖ In the case of deciduous teeth, there can be confusion, which is difficult to memorize.
- ❖ Common mistake in typing was transposition. As far as the FDI numbering system is concerned, there is a world of difference between tooth number 32 and tooth number.[13]

Universal Numbering System

The Universal system was proposed by **Julius Perreidt** in 1882 and endorsed by ADA in 1968.

- ❖ Perreidt disliked the redundancy repetition and potential confusion of Zsigmondy's use of tooth numbers 1–8 in all four quadrants. Instead, he numbered the permanent teeth 1–32, starting at the upper right and continuing to the upper left, then the lower left to the lower right.
- ❖ Today, the Universal system of tooth coding is an interesting misnomer as it is only used in the United States. The ADA by an unanimous decision of its Council on Dental Care Programs adopted the Universal System of numbering teeth on April 18, 1975.[1]
- ❖ Starting with the third molar in the upper right quadrant (tooth no. 1), the teeth are numbered around the arch, so the maxillary left third molar is tooth No. 16. One then drops down to the mandibular left third molar (No. 17) and numbers the teeth around the lower arcade, finishing with the mandibular right third molar (No. 32) **(Fig. 7.5).**
- ❖ The compelling value of the Universal system is the ease of computerizing the data, which is its singular selling point for automating office systems, thus accelerating communication.

> - Given by **Julius Perreidt** used only in USA
> - Numbered the permanent teeth 1–32, starting at the upper right and continuing to the upper left, then the lower left to the lower right
> - Ease of computerization

Universal System for Primary Teeth

- ❖ The 20 primary teeth are coded alphabetically from A to T.
- ❖ There is no anatomic parallel with this system.
- ❖ If using this system infrequently, it is of help that one remembers it by simply memorizing A, J, K and T are the second molars (at the distal ends of the quadrants) and that E, F, O and P are the central incisors **(Fig. 7.6).**

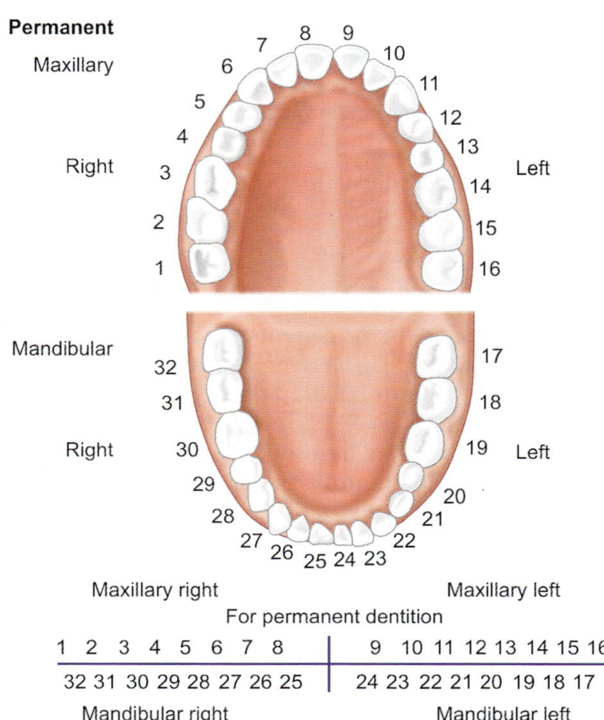

Fig. 7.5: Universal numbering system (permanent).

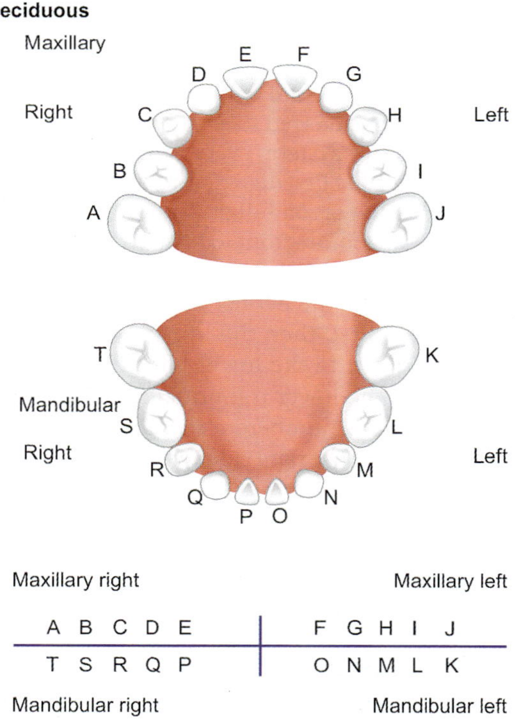

Fig. 7.6: Universal system for primary teeth.

Advantages of Universal System

- ❖ Convenient to write
- ❖ Convenient to record in the patients' records
- ❖ Every tooth has a separate number

Disadvantage of Universal System

- Its major drawback is the necessity for memorizing 32 digits and 20 characters and associating these 52 unrelated symbols with individual teeth.
- Difficult to count tooth without a picture present mainly in the absence of third molar.
- Need skill and training to build a habit of correct counting.
- In primary dentition, especially during mixed dentition, counting is difficult.
- In the universal tooth numbering system, it is difficult to memorize the tooth numbers, and there is no midline differentiation.[13]

Other tooth numbering systems
- Hillischer system
- Mons Dubois system
- MICAP system
- Woelfel system
- Victor Haderup system
- Frykolhm and Lysell system

There are two major motivations to develop a tooth-coding system. One is to conserve energy and communicate telegraphically. Writing or speaking (or typing) "the permanent mandibular right second premolar" is much more taxing than referring to this tooth as No. 29 or No. 45, especially if teeth consume one's professional life.

There is the need to be specific but also to be as concise as practical. The other recent driving force is to computerize ever-increasing masses of data and numeric codes (and their alphabetic equivalents) lend themselves to this end. A compilation of the tooth numbering system is explained in the schematic diagram **(Figs. 7.7 and 7.8)**.

One minor spin-off of the trend toward globalization is the need for standardization—so all of the participants understand the same set of "rules" and can communicate effectively. The FDI system seems to be the solution in terms of dental-coding systems. This leaves the US "Universal" system as an anachronism, but it doubtlessly will persist as a system paralleling the FDI system until the United States also converts to the metric system. In scientific circles, though, an increasing number of dental journals are requiring its authors to use of the FDI system for tooth designations.

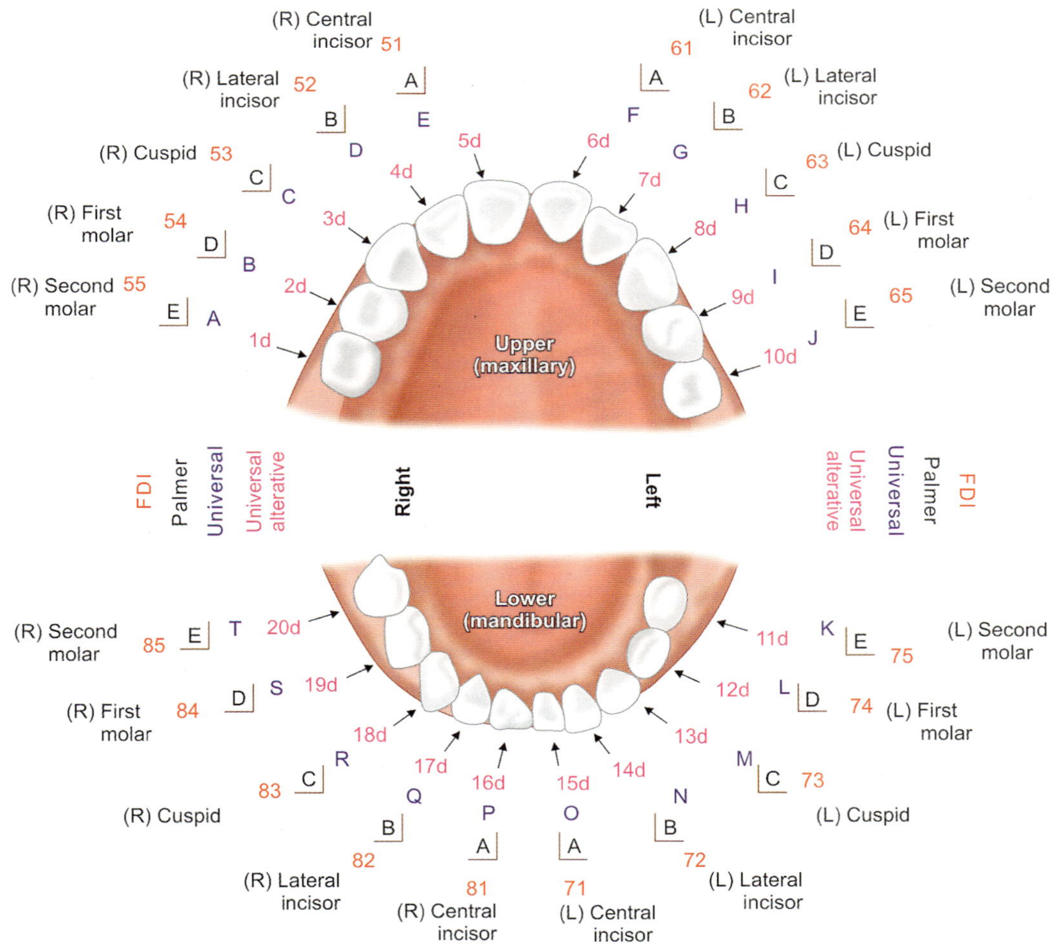

Fig. 7.7: Coding systems used while designating the primary teeth (Justi Educational Department Dental Numbering Systems Prim-Rev-9/03).

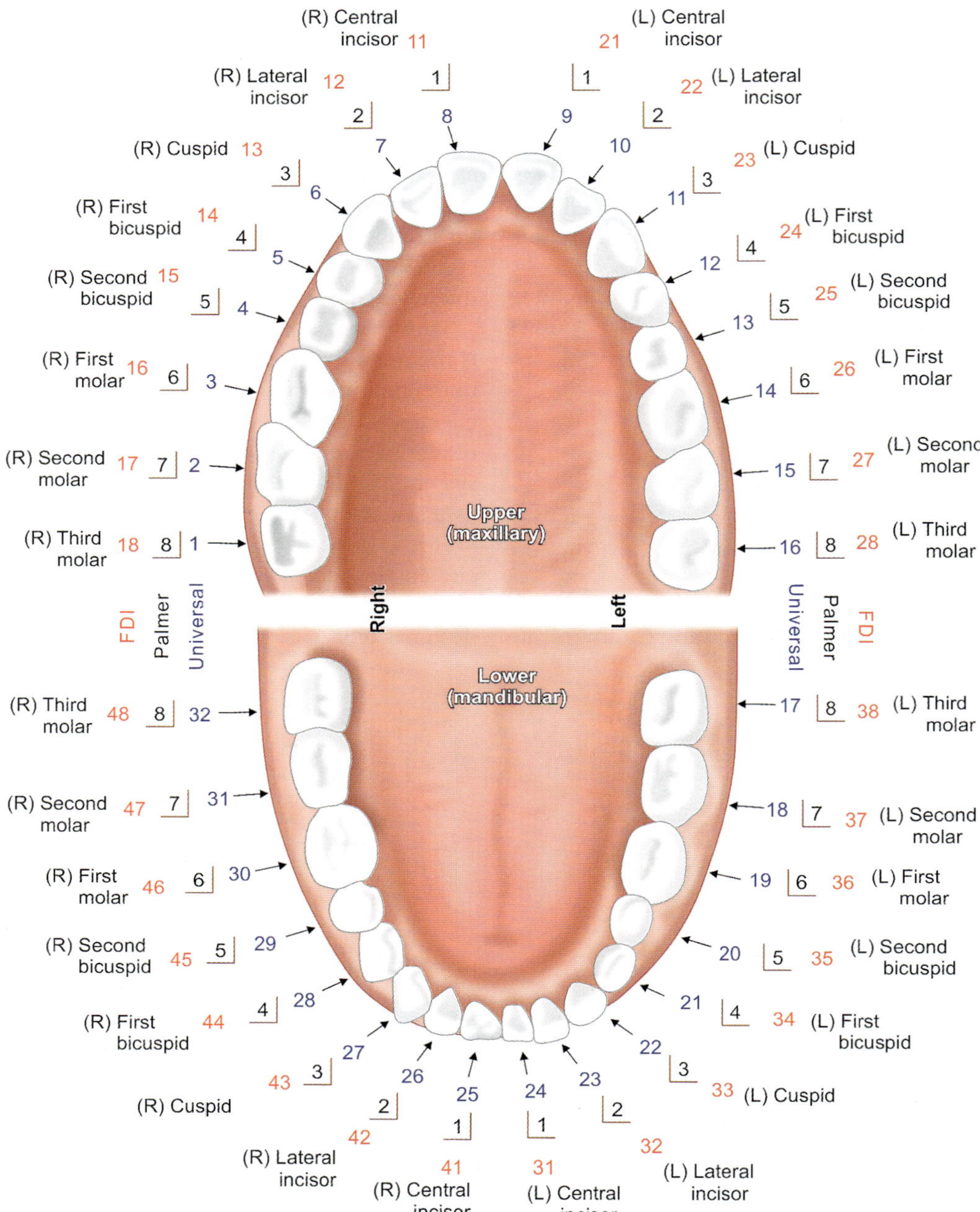

Fig. 7.8: A schematic diagram of the coding systems used while designating the permanent teeth (Justi Educational Department Dental Numbering Systems Perm-Rev-9/03).

POINTS TO REMEMBER

- When identifying a particular tooth, we should follow a specific pattern to name the tooth as mentioned below in the order dentition, arch, quadrant, tooth name.
- Dental formula for humans is primary teeth: I—2/2 C—1/1 M—2/2; permanent teeth I—2/2 C—1/1 P—2/2 M—3/3. The first comprehensive numbering system was developed by Viennese dentist Adolf Zsigmondy in 1861.
- Zsigmondy combined his tooth numbering system with a graphical device to specify the quadrant of mouth.
- In 1882, a German dentist Julius Parreidt proposed a system of counting consecutive teeth called as Universal system which numbered the permanent teeth 1–32, starting at the upper right and continuing to the upper left, then the lower left to the lower right.
- In end of 1968, FDI came up with a unique two digit system developed by Dr Jochen Viohl of Berlin, and this was introduced in 1970. Every tooth system is denoted with two digits, the first digit denotes quadrant of the mouth, and the second defines the tooth's position.

Clinical Significance

- It is important for the dentist to identify dentition and tooth as treatment protocol would exhibit a difference in case of primary and permanent teeth.
- Age related dentition assessment is of utmost importance to the dentist as it helps in identifying type of treatment indicated for the tooth.

Questionnaire

1. What are trait categories?
2. Explain mammalian dental formula.
3. Describe Zsigmondy-Palmer system.
4. Explain Universal system.
5. Describe FDI system.

REFERENCES

1. Schwartz S, Stege D. Tooth numbering systems: a final choice. Ann Dent. 1977;36:99-106.
2. Harris EF. Tooth-coding systems in the clinical dental setting. Dent Anthropol. 2005;18:43-9.
3. Kraus BS, Furr ML. Lower first premolars. I. A definition and classification of discrete morphologic traits. J Dent Res. 1953;32:554-64.
4. Scheid RC. Woelfel Dental Anatomy: Its Relevance to Dentistry, 7th ed. Wolters Kluwer, Lippincott Wiliams & Wilkins; 2007.
5. Zsigmondy A. A practical method for rapidly noting dental observations and operations. Br J Dent Sci. 1874;17:580-2.
6. Peck S, Peck L. A time for change of tooth numbering systems. J Dent Ed. 1993;57:643-7.
7. Palmer C. Palmer's dental notation. Dent Cosmos 1891; 33:194-8.
8. Sharma PS, Wadhwa P. Evaluation of the FDI two-digit system of designating teeth. Quintessence Int. 1977;8:99-101.
9. Churchill HR. Human odontography and histology. Philadelphia, PA: Lea & Febiger; 1932.
10. Erfan O, Qasemian E, Khan M, Niazi A. Introduction of New Tooth Notation Systems in Comparison with Currently In-Use Systems. European Journal of Dental and Oral Health. 2022;3(2):35-48.
11. Raghavendra H, Sheetal B, Patil R, Kumar R, Rajesh A, Inushekar K. Dental notation for primary teeth: A review and suggestion of a novel system. European Journal of Paediatric Dentistry. 2015;16:163-6.
12. Keiser-Nielsen S. Federation dentaire internationale. J Am Dent Assoc. 1971;82:1034-5.
13. Erfan O, Qasemian E, Khan M, Niazi A. Introduction of New Tooth Notation Systems in Comparison with Currently In-Use Systems. European Journal of Dental and Oral Health. 2022;3(2):35-48.

CHAPTER 8

Radiographic Techniques

Nikhil Marwah, Gopakumar R, Suresh K Sachdeva, Arvind Sridhara

CHAPTER OUTLINE

- Characteristics of an Ideal Radiograph
- X-ray Machine
- Intraoral Periapical Radiographic Techniques
- Supplementary Intraoral Radiographic Technique
- Radiographic Protocol
- Panoramic Radiography
- Specialized Radiography
- Radiation Protection
- Radiographic Infection Control
- Behavioral Considerations in Pedodontic Radiography

The radiographic examination is an essential part of the diagnosis of dental disease. Radiographs of children reveal many conditions that cannot be discovered by any other method. They help the practitioner to make an early diagnosis of carious lesions and development of eruption problems, and they enable him or her to confirm and evaluate a pathology diagnosed clinically. Moreover, the radiographic examination enables the clinician to establish a therapeutic decision. Radiography for children depends on three factors, that is, age of the child, size of oral cavity, and level of patient's cooperation.

HISTORY

The X-ray was discovered on November 8, 1895 by **Wilhelm Conrad Roentgen**, a professor of physics at the University of Würzburg in Germany. He was working with a vacuum tube called Crooke's tube. Since he was concerned with light, he was working in a darkened room with black cardboard covering the Crooke's tube, and there were many fluorescent plates in his laboratory **(Fig. 8.1)**. Thus, the stage was set for one of the most important discoveries that would aid medical and dental science.

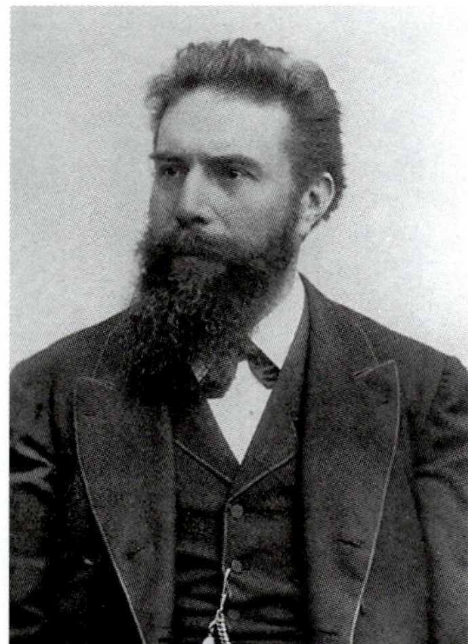

Fig. 8.1: Wilhelm Conrad Roentgen (1845-1925) with his X-ray apparatus.

One evening while working in his darkened laboratory, **Roentgen** noticed that one of the fluorescent plates at the far side of the room was glowing. He quickly realized that something coming from the Crooke's tube was striking the fluorescent plate and causing it to glow; since he did not know what it was, he called the phenomenon X-ray, X being the algebraic symbol for the unknown. He inadvertently placed his hand between the tube and the screen and saw the faint outline of the bones of his hand. He went on to expose and produce images on photographic plates of his wife **Bertha's** hand **(Fig. 8.2)** and his shotgun **(Fig. 8.3)**.

Terminologies

- **Radiation:** Emission and propagation of energy through space and matter in the form of waves or a stream of particles.
- **X-radiation:** A high energy radiation produced by the collision of a beam of electrons with a metal target in an X-ray tube.
- **X-ray:** A beam of energy that has the power to penetrate substances and record image shadows on photographic film.
- **Radiology:** The science or study of radiation as used in medicine, a branch of medical science that deals with the use of X-rays, radioactive substances, and other form of radiant energy in the diagnosis and treatment of disease.
- **Dental radiograph:** A photographic image produced on film by the passage of X-ray through teeth and related structure.
- **Dental radiography:** The making of radiographs of the teeth and the adjacent structures by the exposure of film to X-ray.
- **Dental radiographer:** A person, who positions, exposes, and processes dental X-ray film.
- **Density:** The overall degree of darkening of exposed film.
- **Latitude:** Measure of range of exposure that will produce distinguishable densities on film.
- **Film speed:** Amount of radiation needed to produce a standard density.
- **Contrast:** The difference in densities between various areas on radiograph.
- **Resolution:** Ability to distinguish between small objects that are close together.
- **Radiographic mottle:** Appearance of uneven densities of an exposed film.
- **Sharpness:** Ability of a radiograph to define an edge.

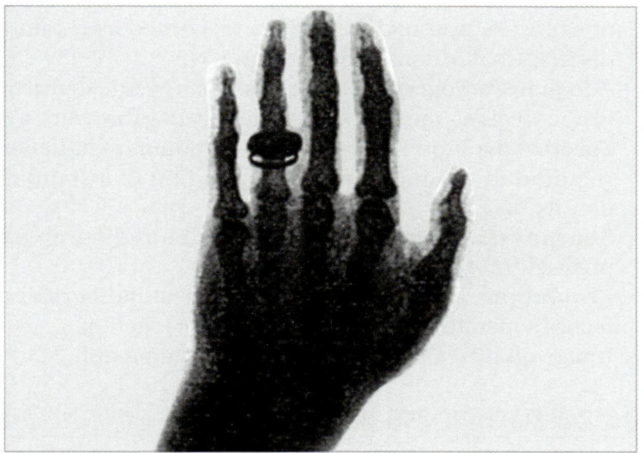

Fig. 8.2: Image of Wilhelm Conrad Roentgen wife's hand.

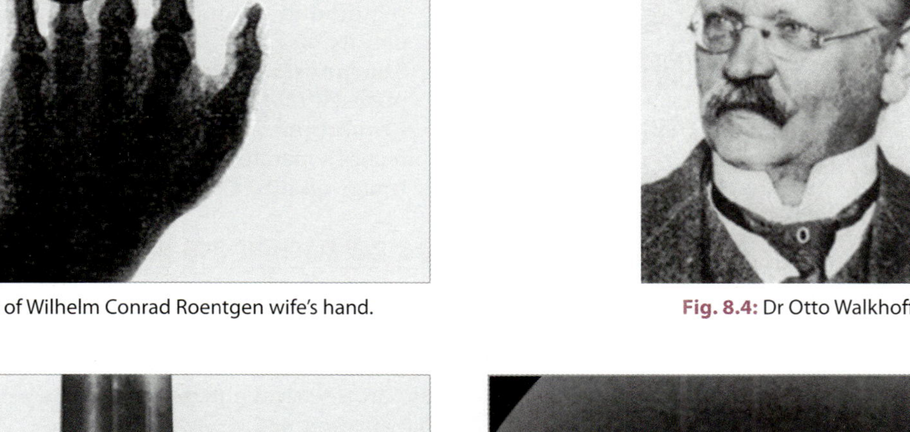

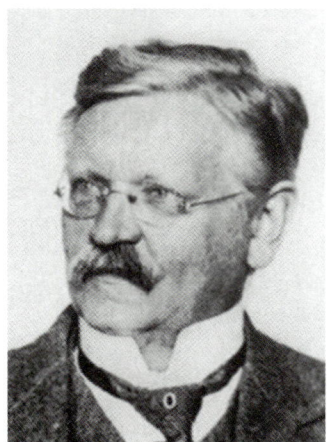

Fig. 8.4: Dr Otto Walkhoff.

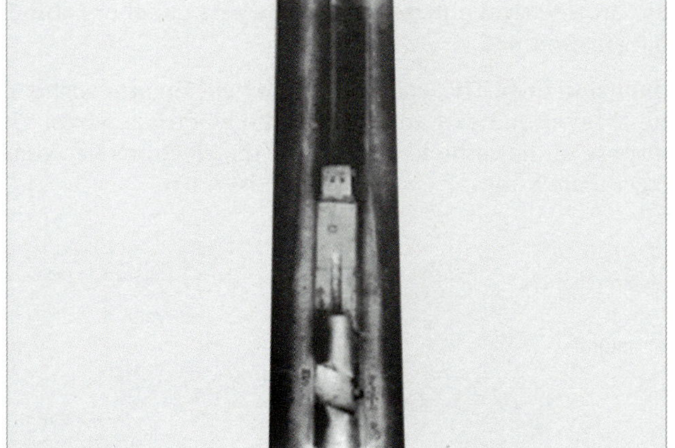

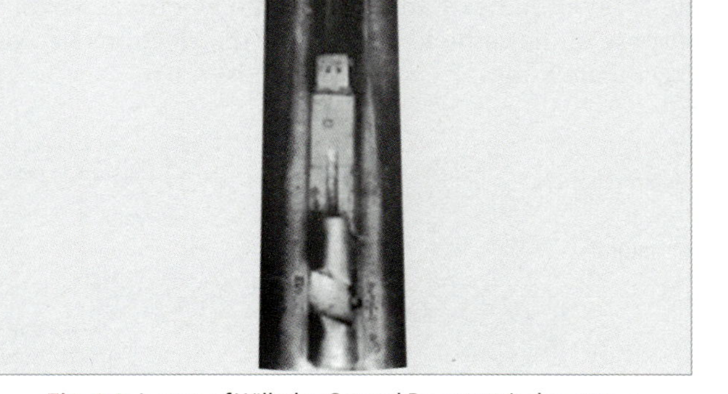

Fig. 8.3: Image of Wilhelm Conrad Roentgen's shotgun.

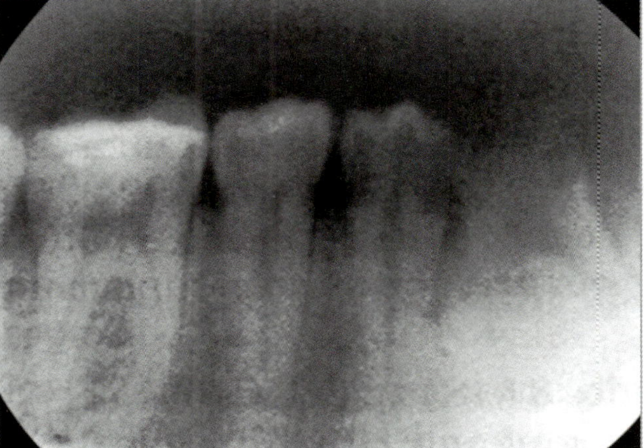

Fig. 8.5: First dental radiograph.

Roentgen presented a paper on his discovery in late December, and in January 1896, **Dr Otto Walkhoff (Fig. 8.4)**, a dentist in Brunschweig, Germany, made the first dental use of an X-ray and radiographed a lower premolar **(Fig. 8.5)**. He used a small glass photographic plate wrapped in black paper and covered with rubber with exposure time of 25 minutes.

Highlights in the History of Dental Radiology		
1895	Discovery of X-rays	WC Roentgen
1896	First dental radiograph	Otto Walkhoff
1896	First dental radiograph in USA (skull)	WJ Morton
1896	First dental radiograph in USA (Live Patient)	CE Kells
1901	First paper on dangers of X-radiation	WH Rollins
1904	Introduction of bisecting technique	WA Price
1913	First dental text (elementary and dental radiography)	HR Raper
1913	First prewrapped dental films	Eastman Kodak Company
1913	First X-ray tube	WD Coolidge
1920	Concept of paralleling technique	F McCormack
1920	First machine made film packets	Eastman Kodak Company
1923	First dental X-ray machine	Victor X-ray Corporation of Chicago
1925	Introduction of bitewing technique	HR Raper
1947	Introduction of long cone paralleling technique	FG Fitzgerald
1955	Introduction of D-speed film	
1957	First variable kilovoltage dental X-ray machine	General Electric
1960	First panoramic X-ray machine marketed	SS White and Company
1978	Introduction of dental xeroradiography	
1981	Introduction of E-speed film	
1987	Introduction of intraoral digital radiography	
2000	Introduction of F-speed film	

For his work in the discovery of X-rays, **Roentgen** was awarded the first Nobel Prize in Physics in 1901, and for years the science of imaging with the use of X-ray was called **Roentgenology**, and his name is still used today to express the units of X-ray exposure in Roentgen's.

Many of the early scientists working with dental X-rays suffered from effects of their work. Dr William Herbert **Rollins** reported burns on the skin of his hands; Dr C Edmund **Kells**, before his death, had three fingers of his hand and finally his arm amputated. He used a technique called setting the tube to adjust the X-ray beam before radiographing patients. He held his hand between the tube and a fluoroscope and adjusted the beam quality until the bones of his hand were seen clearly.

This lead to discovery of new and safer systems. In 1913, **William David Coolidge (Fig. 8.6)** invented the hot cathode X-ray tube which is the prototype of X-ray tubes today, and in 1923, the first American dental X-ray machine was manufactured by Victor X-ray Corporation which later became General Electric X-ray Corporation.

CHARACTERISTICS OF AN IDEAL RADIOGRAPH

The radiographic image should have the following characteristics to be ideal:

- **Radiographic density:** This refers to overall degree of darkening of various regions. It should not be very darker or very light.

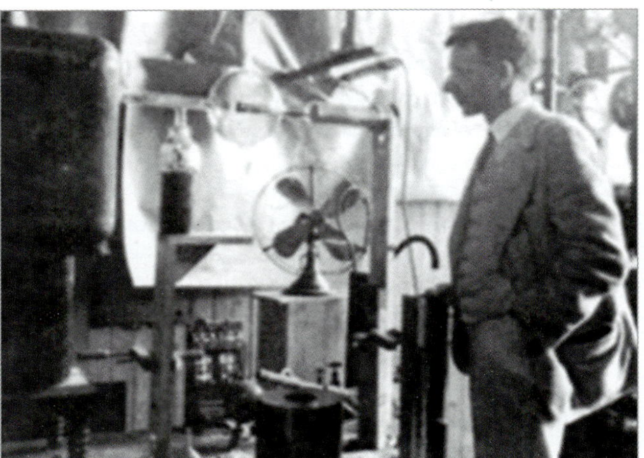

Fig. 8.6: William D Coolidge with his X-ray tube.

- **Latitude of the film:** It is the measurement of range of exposure that may be usefully recorded as a sum of distinguishable density on the film.
- **Adequate radiographic contrasts:** Difference in density of various regions, thus helping in demarcating the structures.
- **Speed of the film:** This refers to the amounts of radiation, required to produce a radiographic film of a standard density.
- **Sharpness:** It is the effectiveness of a radiograph to precisely mark the edge.
- **Resolution:** This describes the ability of radiograph to record separate structures that are close together.
- **Image quality:** Overall appearance of radiograph.

X-RAY MACHINE (FIG. 8.7)

Control panel: This consists of an on/off switch, indicator light, an exposure button, and control devices (time, kVp, mA) to regulate the X-ray beam. The control panel is plugged into an electrical outlet and appears as a panel or cabinets that are mounted.

Extension arm: The wall mounted extension arm suspends the X-ray tube head and houses the electrical wires. The purpose of the cathode is to supply the electrons necessary to generate X-rays.

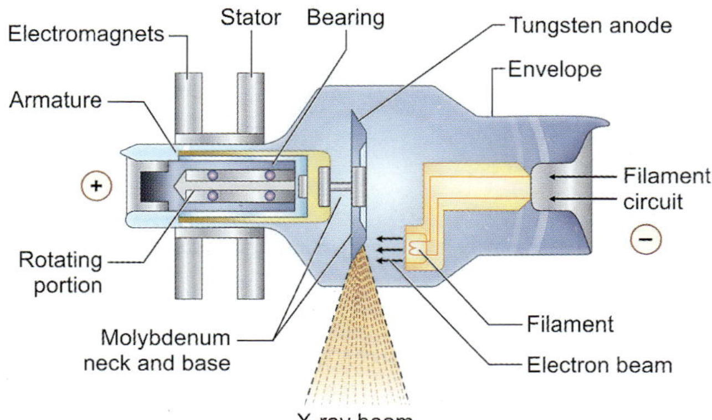

Fig. 8.7: X-ray machine.

Uses of X-ray		
General uses	***Dental uses***	***Pedodontic uses***
• X-rays are used in health sciences for diagnosis and therapeutic purposes • In industries for casting and welding • Used in preservation of food • Spectroscopy • Identification of elements, their atomic number, etc. • Photochemistry • Ionization of chemicals for oxidation and reduction purpose • Radiobiology • Crystallography • Analysis of molecules • Sterilization of instruments • Autoradiography	• To detect lesions, disease, and conditions of the teeth and surrounding structures that cannot be identified clinically • To confirm or classify suspected disease • To localize lesions or foreign objects • To provide information during dental procedures (e.g., root canal therapy) • To evaluate growth and development • To illustrate changes secondary to caries, disease, and trauma • To document the condition of a patient at a specific point of time	• Caries • Pulp pathology • Traumatic injuries • Problems of eruption • Anomalies of developments • Orthodontic evaluation • History of pain • Evidence of swelling • Unexplained tooth mobility • Unexplained bleeding • Deep periodontal pocket • Fistula formation • Unexplained sensitivity of teeth • Evaluation of sinus condition • Unusual spacing or migration of teeth • Lack of response to conventional dental treatment • Unusual tooth morphology calcification/color • Evaluation of growth abnormality • Altered occlusal relationship • Aid in diagnosis of systemic disease • Family history of dental anomalies • Postoperative evaluation

Cathode: Produced the electrons that are accelerated toward the positive anode. This includes tungsten filaments or coiled wire made of tungsten, which produces electrons when heated, and a molybdenum cup, which focuses the electrons into a narrow beam and directs the beam across the tube toward the tungsten targets of the anode.

Anode: A positive electrode consists of a wafer thin tungsten plate embedded in a solid copper rod with the purpose of converting electrons into X-ray photon. It includes a tungsten target, or plate of tungsten, which serves as a focal spot and converts bombarding electron into X-ray photons, and a copper stem, which functions to dissipate the heat away from the tungsten target.

Amperage: It is the measurement of the number of electrons moving through a conductor.

Voltage: It is the measurement of electrical force that causes electrons to move from negative pole to a positive one.

Properties of X-rays
- They are invisible.
- They travel at the same speed of light—3×10^8 m/s.
- They travel in a straight line.
- They cannot be deflected.
- They affect photographic plates.
- They produce fluorescence with some substances, for example, bario-palladium crystals.
- They can penetrate opaque objects.

INTRAORAL PERIAPICAL RADIOGRAPHIC TECHNIQUES

Two intraoral projection techniques that are used for periapical radiography are paralleling technique and bisecting angle technique.

Paralleling Technique (Fig. 8.8)

- Also called right angle technique/long cone technique/ **McCormack's** technique/**Fitzgerald** technique.

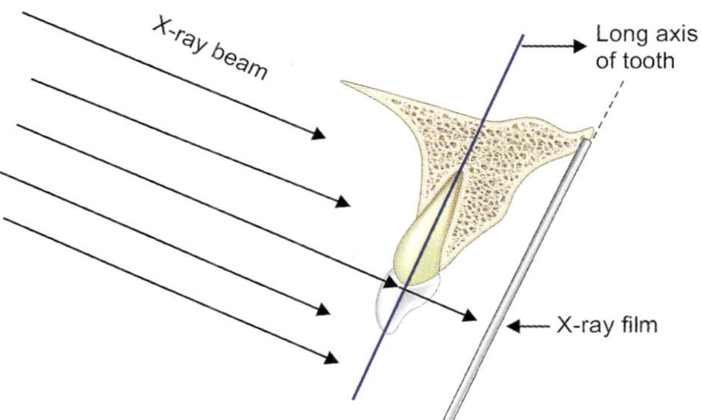

Fig. 8.8: Diagrammatical representation of paralleling technique.

- **Dr Gordon Fitzgerald** is the pioneer of this technique.
- The primary purpose of this is to obtain a true radiographic orientation of teeth and supporting structures.
- It is based on the principle that central ray should be focused perpendicular to long axis of the film with the X-ray film being parallel to long axis of tooth.
- To obtain parallelism and to reduce distortion, the film is placed away from tooth, but the use of long source to object distance reduces the size of the apparent focal spot and leads to less magnification and increased definition.
- Film holders are used to ensure proper position of the film and to maintain it in position.
- To assure that the periapical areas will be projected onto the film, it is necessary that the film be positioned away from the teeth and toward the center of the mouth, where the maximum height of the palate can be utilized.
- For maxillary projections, the superior border of the film will generally rest at the height of the palatal vault in the midline. For mandibular projections, the film will be used to displace the tongue lingually to allow the inferior border of the film to be depressed into the floor of the mouth away from the mucosa on the lingual surface of the mandible **(Fig. 8.8).**

- Also called long cone technique.
- Pioneered by **Gordon Fitzgerald**, father of modern radiology.
- Central ray should be focused perpendicular to long axis of the film with the X-ray film being parallel to long axis of tooth.
- Film holders like extended cone positioner (XCP) are used.
- More accurate.
- In case of children, film is placed within 20° of the parallel to the long axis, with the beam directed to the film.

- A variety of film holders are used for this technique. Some are XCP, precision X-ray instruments, stable bite block, and versatile intraoral positioner.
- Paralleling principle of intraoral X-ray is technique of choice, because it is more accurate and produces less distortion than bisecting angle technique.
- In case of children, there is high muscle activity in the mandible and shallow palate, thus the film cannot be placed parallel to the long axis of the teeth, but it has been demonstrated that even if the film is placed within 20° of the parallel to the long axis, with the beam directed to the film, the radiograph produced by paralleling technique will be far superior than bisecting angle technique.

Advantages

- Accurate images can be obtained with minimum magnification.
- Interdental bone levels are very well represented.
- Periapical tissue will be accurately shown with minimal foreshortening or elongation.
- Horizontal and vertical angulations are automatically determined by positioning device.
- X-ray beam is aimed correctly at the center of the film and prevents cone cut.

Disadvantages

- Positioning of the film packet is very uncomfortable for patient especially in the posterior aspect of teeth, often causing gagging.
- Positioning the holder in the mouth will be difficult for inexperienced operators.
- Anatomy of mouth sometimes makes the technique difficult.
- Positioning the holders in the lower third molar region can be very difficult.

Bisecting Angle Technique (Fig. 8.9)

- This technique was promoted by **Weston Price** in 1904.
- Also called Millers right angle technique/short cone technique/isometric triangulation technique.
- This technique is based on the principle of Cieszynski rule of isometry which states that two triangles are equal when they share one complete side and have two equal angles.
- In this technique, the film is placed close to the teeth and central ray is directed at right angles to the line bisecting the angle formed by the plane of the film and the long axis of the tooth **(Fig. 8.9)**.
- Although film holders are not used in this technique for positioning, there are some special film holders like Renn-Snap or Snap-A-Ray that can be used to prevent exposure of patient's hand, avoid slippage of film in mouth, and prevent cone cut.

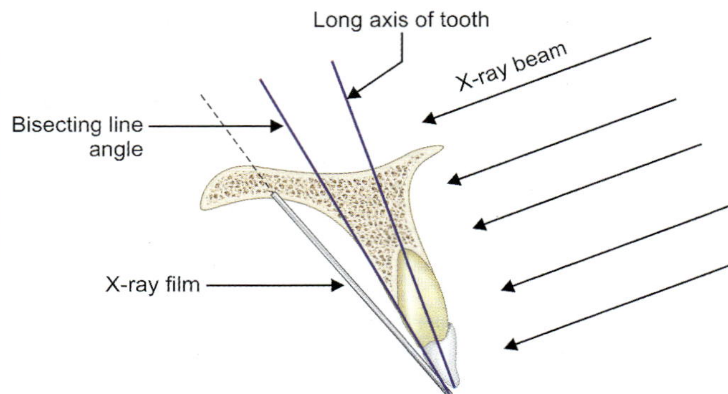

Fig. 8.9: Diagrammatical representation of bisecting angle technique.

- Angulations of tube head **(Figs. 8.10A to F)**:
  - Horizontal angulation is 0°
  - Vertical angulation is different for all teeth

Maxillary	• Incisor: +40°, Canine: +45°, Premolar: +30°, Molar: +20° • In deciduous: Anterior: +45°, Posterior: +30°
Mandibular	• Incisor: –15°, Canine: –20°, Premolar: –10°, Molar: –5° • In deciduous: Anterior: –15°, Posterior: –10°

- Also called short cone technique.
- Pioneered by **Weston Price.**
- Film is placed close to the teeth and central ray is directed at right angles to the line bisecting the angle formed by the plane of the film and the long axis of the tooth.
- More accurate.
- In case of children, film is placed within 20° of the parallel to the long axis, with the beam directed to the film.

Advantages

- Positioning of film or film packet will be reasonably comfortable for patient and for operator in all areas of mouth.
- Positioning of film is simple and quick.
- If we give proper angulation, there will not be any distortion of image.

Disadvantages

- Improper vertical angulations may lead to shortening or lengthening of image.
- Interdental bone less will be poorly demonstrated.
- Shadow of zygomatic bone frequently overlies the roots of upper molars.
- Horizontal and vertical angles have to be assessed for every exposure, considerable skill is needed.
- Cone-cut may result if improper positioning of tube is done.
- Incorrect horizontal angulation will result in horizontal overlapping of crowns and roots.

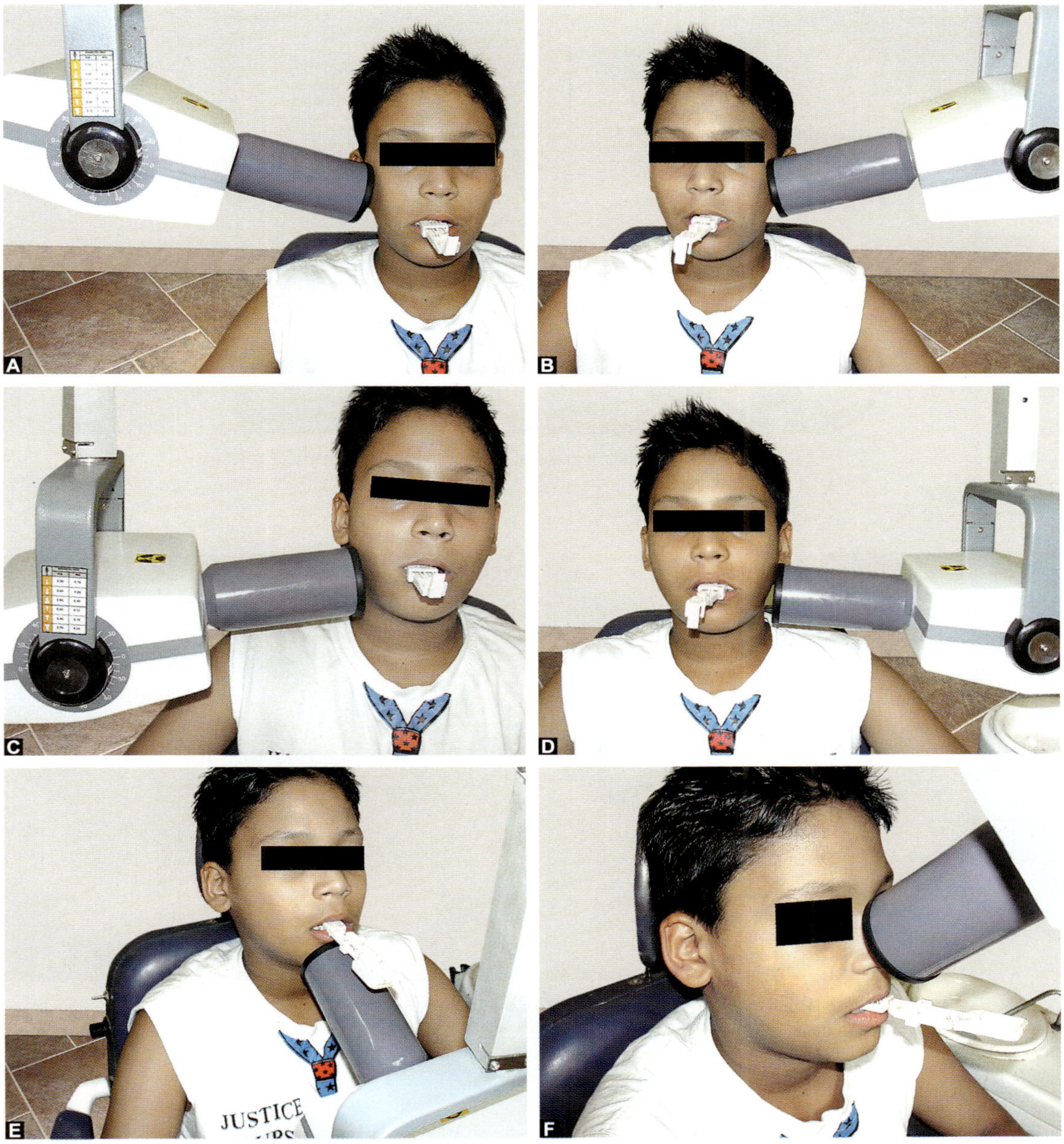

Figs. 8.10A to F: X-ray tube film placement in intraoral periapical (IOPA) radiograph: (A) Maxillary right posterior; (B) Maxillary left posterior; (C) Mandibular right posterior; (D) Mandibular left posterior; (E) Mandibular anterior; (F) Maxillary anterior.

- Crowns of teeth are often distorted, thus preventing detection of proximal caries.

SUPPLEMENTARY INTRAORAL RADIOGRAPHIC TECHNIQUE

Bitewing Radiography

- Developed by **Howard Raper** in 1925.
- Periapical films are used to record the coronal portions of both maxillary and mandibular teeth in one image **(Fig. 8.11).**
- Size 1 film is used in children and size 2 films are used in adults.
- Used mostly to detect inter-proximal caries and to check the level of bone.

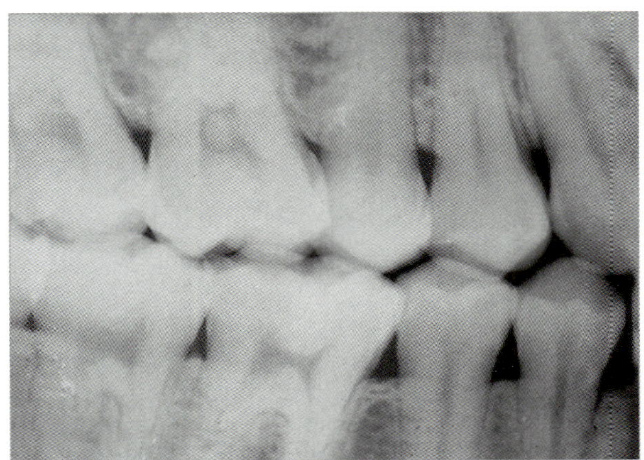

Fig. 8.11: Bitewing radiograph.

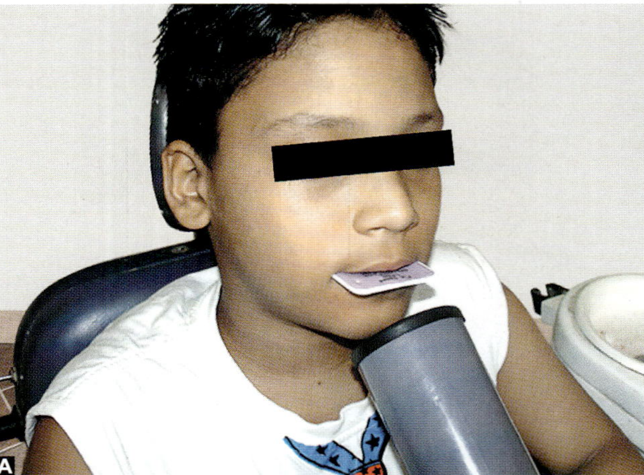

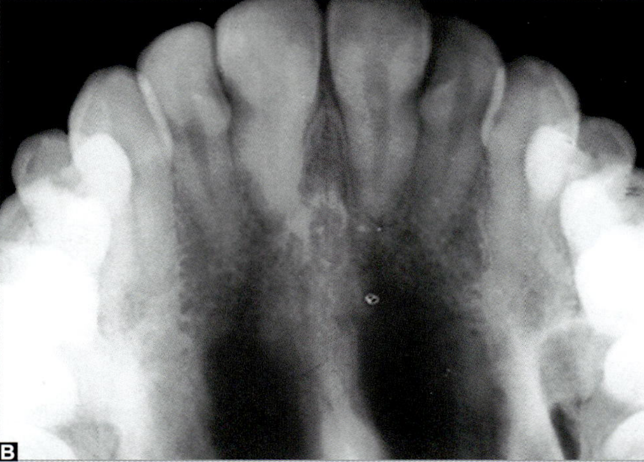

Figs. 8.12A and B: Maxillary occlusal radiograph technique and X-ray.

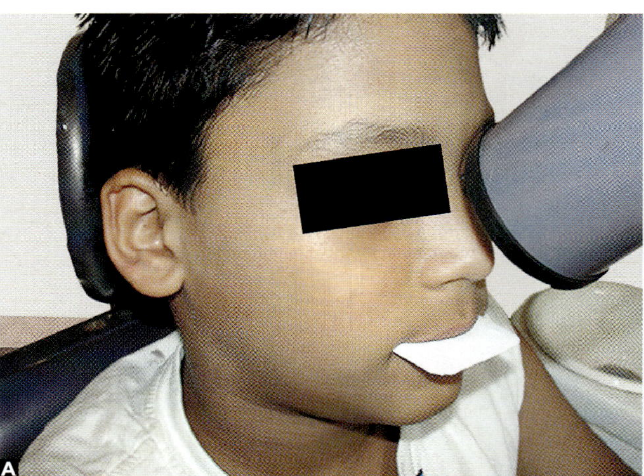

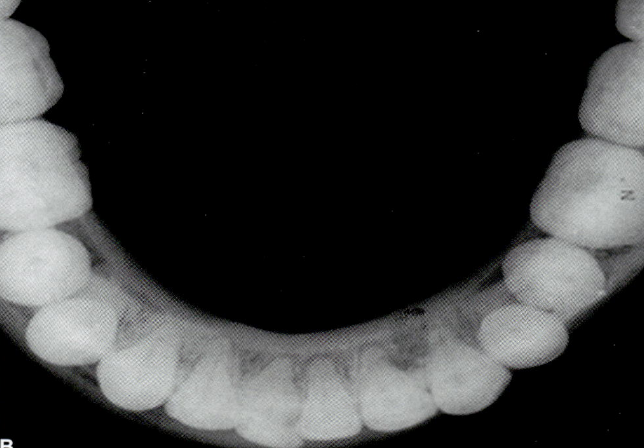

Figs. 8.13A and B: Mandibular occlusal radiograph technique and X-ray.

Occlusal Radiography

- Used to take the jaw radiographs of maxilla and mandible to detect large lesions, fractures, impactions, supernumerary teeth and to localize foreign bodies **(Figs. 8.12 and 8.13).**
- The film is partially held in between teeth and partially supported by patient.
- The vertical angulation for maxilla is +45° and for mandible is –55°.

Specialized Intraoral Radiographic Technique

- This technique is used exclusively for children and called bent film radiographic technique.
- This technique works well with young children, requires little skill as patient bites down.
- Used when young patient do not tolerate the placement of film holder inside their mouth.
- Top portion of the film is bent at right angle and this serves as a bite block to hold the film in place. Patient is instructed to bite the film slowly and radiograph is taken. Care must be taken to straighten the film before processing.
- This can be used both with paralleling cone or bisecting angle technique.
- Size 1 or 2 film should be used.

Radiographic Localization Procedure

Clark's Technique (Fig. 8.14)

- This is also called as ***S***ame Lingual-***O***pposite ***B***uccal (**SLOB**) rule, tube shift localization technique or buccal object rule.
- It was discovered by **Clark** in 1910.
- To locate or determine the buccolingual relation of an impacted tooth/foreign body within the maxilla.
- Buccal object rule states that the image of a buccally oriented object appears to move in the *opposite direction* from a moving X-ray source. And the image of any lingually oriented object appears to move in the *same direction* as a moving X-ray source.

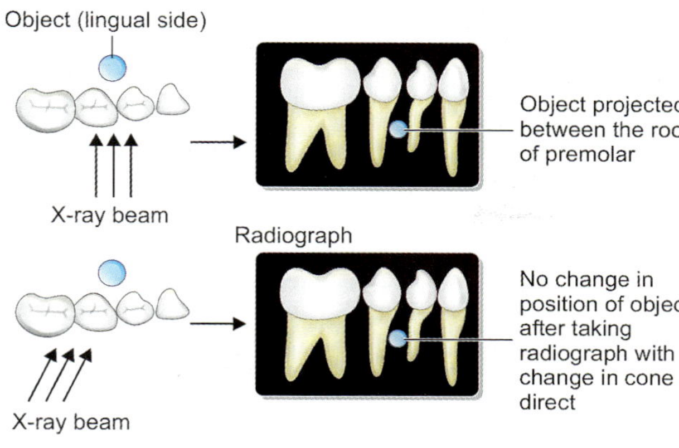

No change in position of object after taking radiograph with change in cone direct

Fig. 8.14: Clark's technique.

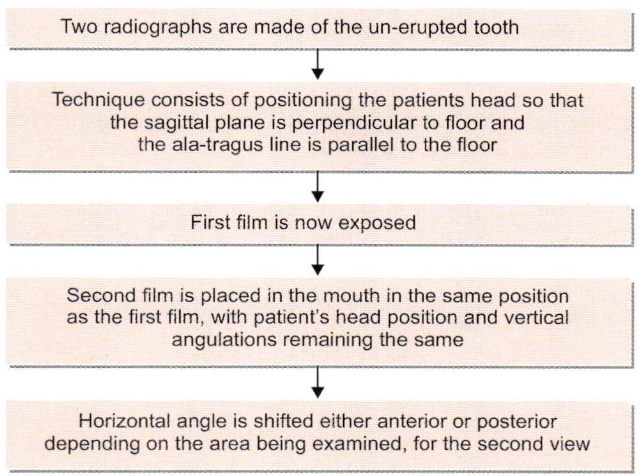

Two radiographs are made of the un-erupted tooth
Technique consists of positioning the patients head so that the sagittal plane is perpendicular to floor and the ala-tragus line is parallel to the floor
First film is now exposed
Second film is placed in the mouth in the same position as the first film, with patient's head position and vertical angulations remaining the same
Horizontal angle is shifted either anterior or posterior depending on the area being examined, for the second view

Miller's Technique

- This is also called right angle technique
- It is used to achieve the same goal as Clark's technique in mandibular arch.

Cross-sectional Occlusal Radiograph

- X-rays are taken at right angles to each other.
- Cross-sectional occlusal radiograph of maxilla with patient's sagittal plane is perpendicular and ala-tragus line is parallel to the floor.

RADIOGRAPHIC PROTOCOL

When a new patient is seen at the dental office and no previous radiographs are available, it may be necessary to obtain a base line series of radiographs. This is governed by radiographic protocol **(Table 8.1)**.

Radiographic examination/survey: To accomplish the task of radiographic protocol, specific X-rays are needed to be done at each age. These X-rays are mostly individualized for each patient and depending upon the age, and caries may be classified as 4-, 8-, 12-, or 16-film series **(Table 8.2)**. This entire set of X-ray series is called *radiographic survey* **(Fig. 8.15)**.

Table 8.1: Radiographic protocol.

Age (years)	*Considerations*	*Radiographs*
3–5	No apparent abnormalities (open contacts)	None
	No apparent abnormalities (closed contacts)	2 posterior bitewing
	Extensive caries	4-film survey
	Deep caries	2 bitewing of size 0, 1 selected periapical radiographs in addition to 4-film survey
6–7	No apparent abnormalities/extensive caries	8-film survey/selected periapical X-ray and 8-film survey
8–9	No apparent abnormalities/extensive caries	12-film survey
10–12	No apparent abnormalities/extensive caries	12- or 16-film survey

Table 8.2: Radiographic survey.

Survey	*Radiographs*
4-film series	Maxillary and mandibular anterior occlusal and two posterior bitewing radiographs
8-film series	Maxillary and mandibular anterior occlusal (or periapicals), right and left maxillary posterior occlusal (or periapical), right and left mandibular posterior periapicals and two posterior bitewing radiographs
12-film series	Two primary molar–premolar periapical radiographs, four canine periapical radiographs, two incisor periapical radiographs, two posterior bitewing radiographs
16-film series	12-film survey, four permanent molar radiographs

4-film series
8-film series
12-film series
16-film series

Fig. 8.15: X-ray film series for radiographic survey.

PANORAMIC RADIOGRAPHY

- It was developed by **Numata** (1933).
- This is also called orthopantomography (OPG)/maxillo-mandibular radiography/pantomography/rotational tomography.
- This uses a mechanism by which the X-ray film and the source of the X-rays move simultaneously in opposite direction at the same speed **(Figs. 8.16A and B)**.

Indications

- Condylar fracture.
- Traumatic cysts.
- Evaluation of tooth development (mixed dentition).
- Developmental anomalies.
- Disabled child.

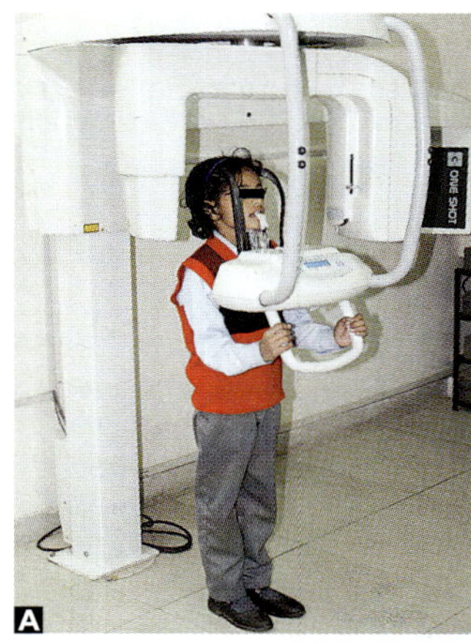

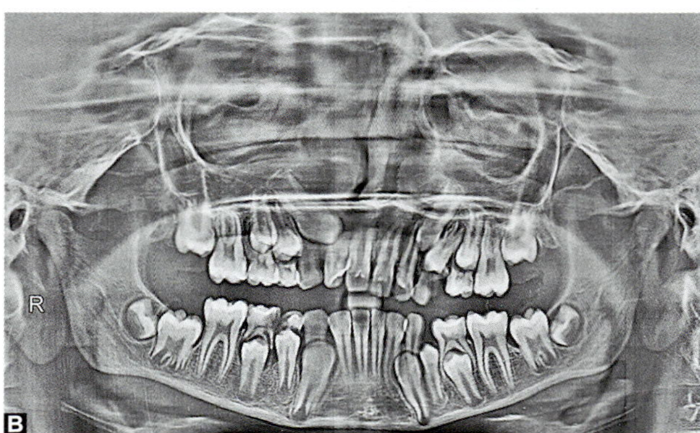

Figs. 8.16A and B: (A) Orthopantomography radiograph being taken; (B) Final OPG radiograph.

Advantages

- Broad anatomic region imaged.
- Relatively low radiation dose.
- Convenience, speed, and ease.
- Useful in patients who are unable to open mouth.

Disadvantages

- Lack of image detail for diagnosis of early carious lesion.
- Cost of X-ray machine.
- Overlaps images of teeth.
- Staying completely immobile for 15 seconds may not be possible for very young children.

Uses

- Evaluation of gross carious status.
- Assessment of advance bone heights.
- Extensive cystic and tumor cases.
- Assessment of mixed dentition.
- Overall assessment of bone pattern.
- Fractures (trauma).
- Preliminary assessment of maxillary sinus diseases.
- General assessments of condyles morphology.
- Pre- and postoperative evaluation of oral surgical procedures and orthodontic treatment.
- Changes in alveolar bone due to systemic diseases like leukemias, Paget disease.
- Evaluation of third molars
- To assess lesions in edentulous jaws.
- To assess the radiologic assessment of implant site.
- Patients who have gagging sensation to intraoral films.
- Ankylosis of temporomandibular joint (TMJ).
- Patients with restricted mouth opening.
- Evaluation of tooth development.

Extraoral radiography

This is accomplished with the film placed outside the oral cavity and it includes:

- Panoramic radiography.
- Skull projections which include Reverse-Towne, submentovertex (SMV), PA view, PNS view, and lateral cephalogram.
- Hand and wrists radiograph.
- Cephalometric radiography.

SPECIALIZED RADIOGRAPHY

Xeroradiography

- Xeroradiography which is a method of imaging uses the xeroradiographic copying process to record images produced by diagnostic X-rays.
- It differs from halide film technique; in that, it involves neither wet chemical processing nor the use of dark room
- The imaging method was discovered by an American physicist, **Chester Carlson** in 1937.
- **Pogorzelska-Stronczak** became the first to use xeroradiograph to produce dental images with extraoral dental use in cephalometry, sialography, and panoramic xeroradiography.

Principle

Xeroradiography is an electrostatic process which uses an amorphous selenium photoconductor material, vacuum deposited on an aluminum substrate, to form a plate

↓

The plate, enclosed in light tight cassette, may be likened to films used in halide-based technique

↓

The key functional steps in the process involve the sensitization of the photoconductor plate in the charging station by depositing a uniform positive charge on its surface with a corona-emitting device called scorotron

↓

The photoconductor will then conduct its electrostatic charge into the grounded base in proportion to the intensity of the exposure

↓

After charging, the cassette is inserted into a thin polyethylene bag to protect the cassette and plate from saliva

↓

The generated latent image is developed through and electrophoretic development process using liquid toner

↓

The process involves the migration to and subsequent deposition of toner particles suspended in aliquid onto subsequent deposition under the influence of electrostatic field forces

↓

That is, by applying negatively charged powder (toner) which is attracted to the residual positive charge pattern on the photoconductor, the latent image is made visible

↓

The image can be transferred to a transparent plastic sheet or to paper

↓

The toner is thereafter fixed to a receiver sheet onto which a permanent record is made

Advantages

- **Elimination of accidental film exposure:** Large light intensity is required for photoconduction and even when there is exposure, the charged area intrinsically gets erased. As a result, there is minimal need for storage for film protection during processing.
- **High resolution:** Xeroradiography has excellent characteristics of the forces around the electrostatic charges which form the latent image.
- **Simultaneous evaluation of multiple tissues:** Because the technique records tissues of differing thicknesses and densities in a xeroradiograph.
- **Ease of reviewing:** Use of reflected or transmitted light is allowed by xeroradiography, so image can be mounted either in a transparent plastic sheet or on opaque paper.
- **Better ease and speed of production:** No special skills are required, dark room requirements are unnecessary, and the entire xeroradiographic process may be completed within 60 seconds.
- **Economic benefit:** When compared with halide radiography, the expenditure is one-eighth.
- **Reduced exposure to radiation hazards:** Because there is no need to make multiple exposures as tissues of different densities and thicknesses can be recorded in one exposure, patient is at a very low risk of radiation hazards.
- **Wide applications:** Generally, xeroradiography has interesting applications in the management of neoplasm of laryngopharyngeal area, mammary and joint region, as well as an aid in cephalometric analysis.

Disadvantages

- The electrostatic charges in xeroradiographic process stand the risk of being lost in confined humid oral environment.
- Technical difficulties.
- Fragile selenium coat.
- Transient image retention.
- Slower speed.

Sialography

It is the radiographic examination of the salivary glands. It usually involves the injection of a small amount of contrast medium into the salivary duct of a single gland, followed by routine X-ray projections.

Procedure

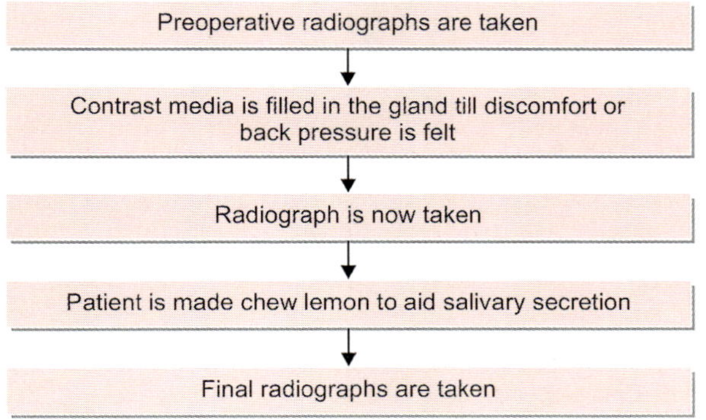
Preoperative radiographs are taken
Contrast media is filled in the gland till discomfort or back pressure is felt
Radiograph is now taken
Patient is made chew lemon to aid salivary secretion
Final radiographs are taken

Indications

- In the evaluation of the functional integrity of the salivary glands.
- In case of obstructions.
- To evaluate the ductal pattern.
- In case of facial swellings, to rule out salivary gland pathology.
- In case of intraglandular neoplasms.

Contraindications

- Persons who have allergy to iodine and/or contrast medium.
- Cases where there is acute infection.
- Patients with thyroid function tests.
- When calculi are located in anterior part of the salivary gland duct.

- Usually the radiographs taken are lateral oblique views of the face
- Used for diagnosis of foreign body, calculus, or tumor in salivary gland
- Water-soluble contrast media include Conray 480, Hypaque, Renagraffin
- Fat-soluble media are ethiodol and lipiodol

Clinical Picture

Variable clinical pictures via sialography can be seen in **Figures 8.17 to 8.21**.

Variable clinical pictures via sialography

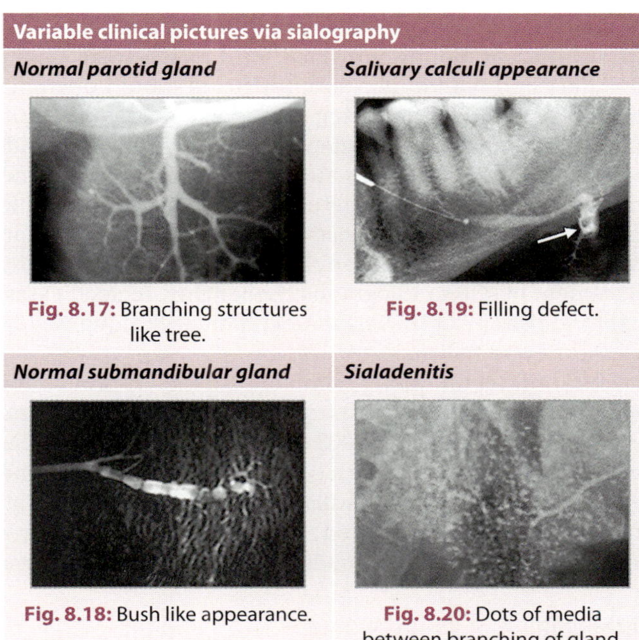

Normal parotid gland

Fig. 8.17: Branching structures like tree.

Salivary calculi appearance

Fig. 8.19: Filling defect.

Normal submandibular gland

Fig. 8.18: Bush like appearance.

Sialadenitis

Fig. 8.20: Dots of media between branching of gland.

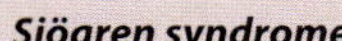

Sjögren syndrome

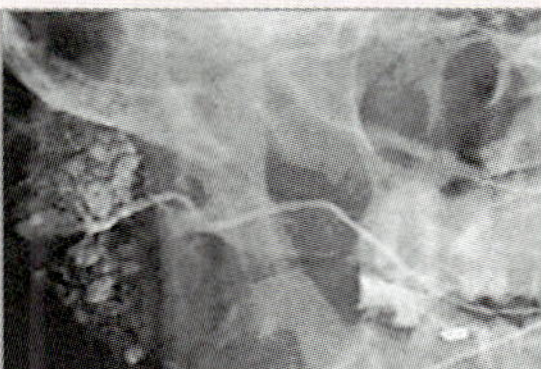

Fig. 8.21: Huge dots of media between branching of gland like cherry blossom appearance.

Hand-wrist radiograph

- The hand-wrist region is made up of numerous small bones which show a predictable and scheduled pattern of appearance, ossification, and union from birth to maturity. Thus by comparing a patients' radiograph with the standards that represent different skeletal ages, we find out the skeletal maturation status of that individual (detailed in Chapter 13).

Cephalometrics

- It is the study of the dental and skeletal relationships in the head and is used by dentists, as a treatment planning tool to evaluate facial growth abnormalities prior to treatment, in the middle of treatment to evaluate progress, or at the conclusion of treatment plan (detailed in Chapter 31).

EXTRAORAL PERIAPICAL (EOPA) RADIOGRAPHIC TECHNIQUE

A young child has little understanding of a dental disease, but during this period strong family attachments make the children experience stranger and separation anxiety when in new and unfamiliar situations especially at the dental office. Intraoral periapical radiographs are an integral part of diagnosis and the fear of unknown compels the child to become uncooperative for the same.

Periapical radiographs due to its high image resolution and excellent image contrast have always been considered for radiographic diagnosis technique by diagnostician to determine the nature and characteristics of bone, dental structures, and lesions. Due to some uncertain conditions and anatomical difficulties such as large tongue; shallow palate and/or floor of mouth; impacted third mandibular molar; maxillary and mandibular tori; restricted mouth opening; neurological difficulties; exaggerated gag reflex; pediatric patients; dental phobic patients with low pain threshold; painful mucosal conditions such as ulcers, infections, and intraoral abscesses; differently abled patients who are unable to follow the clinician's instructions; residual ridge resorption in edentulous patients; and any lingual interference make the placement of IOPA radiographs challenging. In such cases, extraoral periapical (EOPA) radiographic technique can be used as an alternative.

Extraoral technique is relatively a novel approach for periapical imaging and was introduced by Michael Newmann and Seymour Friedman in 2003 for maxillary and mandibular teeth. This technique can be a boon in pediatric patients who are generally anxious and unwilling to intraoral film placement, if the technique is mastered. This technique may play a significant role in behavior modification of pediatric patients.

Technique

- The technique involves placement of the radiographic film/sensor extraorally parallel to the teeth to be imaged, such that the tooth of interest comes in the center and the beam is directed through the opposite side buccal soft tissue without exposing the crowns of opposite side teeth **(Fig. 8.22)**.
- The X-ray equipment is set at 70 kVp and 7 mA and exposure is provided for 180 milliseconds for digital X-rays and 65 kVp, 10 mA and exposure is provided for 0.50–0.55 seconds E-speed periapical films.

Positioning of the Patient for Maxillary Teeth

For the maxillary teeth, Frankfort horizontal plane is kept parallel to the floor and X-ray beam is directed with a negative angulation from the contralateral side (around 20–35° to the horizontal plane such that it is perpendicular to the film) **(Fig. 8.22)**. The film/sensor is kept parallel to ala tragus line and centring at the point of intersection of ala tragus line and parasagittal lines.

Positioning of the Patient for Mandibular Teeth

For the mandibular teeth, occlusal plane is kept parallel to the floor and the X-ray beam is directed with a positive angulation (around 20–35° to the horizontal plane such that it is perpendicular to the film) **(Fig. 8.23)**. The film/sensor is placed parallel and 2 cm above inferior border of mandible.

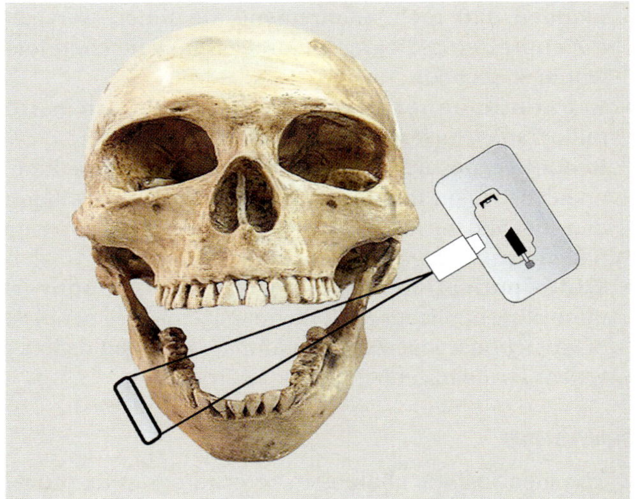

Fig. 8.22: Positioning of the film/sensor and X-ray beam for maxillary teeth. (A negative angulation: Around 20°–35° to the horizontal plane such that it is perpendicular to the film).

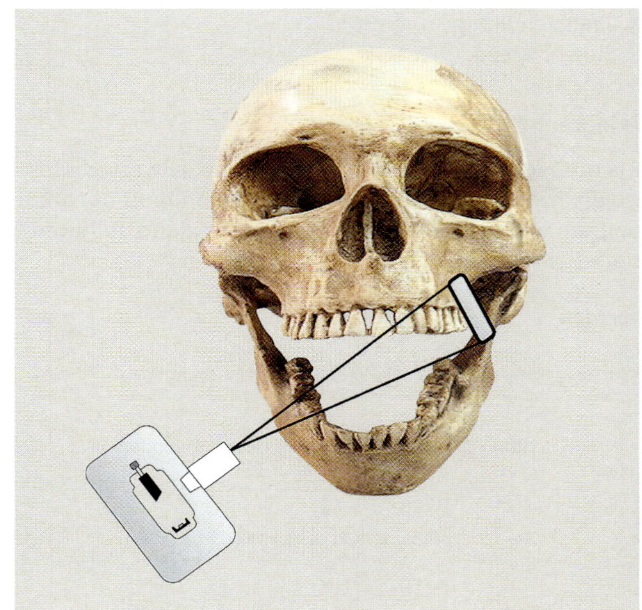

Fig. 8.23: Positioning of the film/sensor and X-ray beam for mandibular teeth. (A positive angulation: Around 20°–35° to the horizontal plane such that it is perpendicular to the film).

Direct technique: Exposing surface of the film/sensor is placed toward the cheek, overlying the tooth in question, with mouth wide open to avoid overlapping of contralateral teeth on image receptor, facing the direction of X-rays. A cotton roll may be placed between the film and the cheek to achieve parallelism **(Fig. 8.24)**.

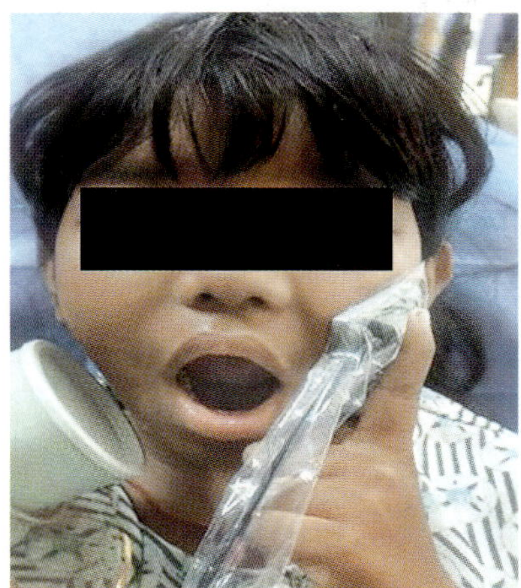

Fig. 8.24: Direct placement of sensor for maxillary right posterior teeth imaging.

PID technique: Using the modified intraoral position indicating device (PID) that is constructed as indicated by Chen et al. The X-ray beam is directed at the film/sensor with the locator ring as a guidance such that the tooth of interest comes in the center of film. The mouth is kept wide open to avoid overlapping of contralateral teeth on image receptor **(Fig. 8.25)**.

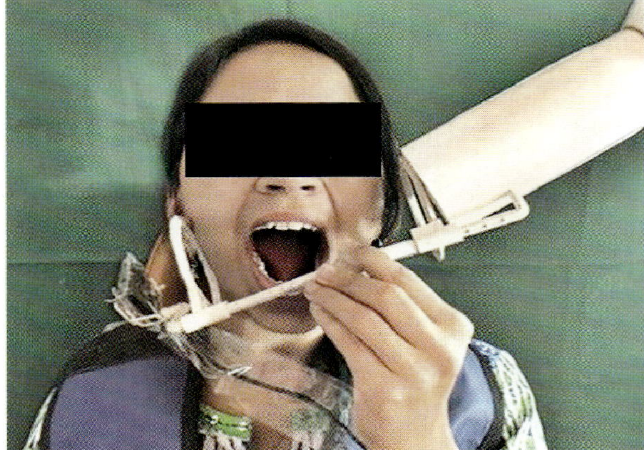

Fig. 8.25: Imaging of mandibular left posterior teeth with use of modified PID.

Advantages

- Lesser radiation exposure and cost in comparison to alternatives like panoramic radiograph.
- EOPA technique is advantageous as it reduces cross infections.

Uses

- Pediatric patients who are uncooperative
- Non-cooperative patients with exaggerated gag reflex, unable to tolerate receptor intraorally
- Low pain threshold
- Soft tissue pathology in conditions like ulcerative and vesiculobullous lesions or malignant lesions
- Reduced oral opening like cellulitis, Ludwig's angina, periapical abscess
- In cases with TMJ disorders and trismus

Disadvantages

- Though diagnostic quality of EOPA is good, it falls low when compared to image resolution and contrast of IOPA radiographs.
- Increased dose of radiations to patient to obtain diagnostic image as compared to intraoral technique. This limitation can however be overcome by digital imaging system.
- Overlapping of adjacent structures, which might decrease the image quality.

RADIATION PROTECTION

Radiograph for children should be conducted in a way that the chances for harmful effects from the diagnostic exposure are minimized as much as possible. Rigid rules have been replaced with a philosophy of radiation protection called the concept As Low As Reasonably/Diagnostically Achievable (ALARA/ALADA). The concept is one of minimum exposure without specifying a specific dose or level of exposure to radiation that is unacceptable or deemed potentially harmful. There are many effective methods of minimizing exposure to patients and dental office personnel.

- **Prescribing needed dental radiographs:** The first important step in limiting the amount of X-radiation to a patient is proper ordering of radiograph. A dentist should have professional judgment about the numbers, type, and frequency of dental radiographs as per the recommended guidelines.
- **Proper equipment**: The dental X-ray tube head must be equipped with appropriate aluminum filters, lead collimator, and position-indicating device (PID) and no leakage should be present.
- **Aluminum filtration:** The purpose of the aluminum filter in the X-ray tube head is to absorb long wavelength, poorly penetrating X-rays that are not useful in producing the radiographic image thus reducing somatic exposure by as much as 57% **(Fig. 8.26)**.

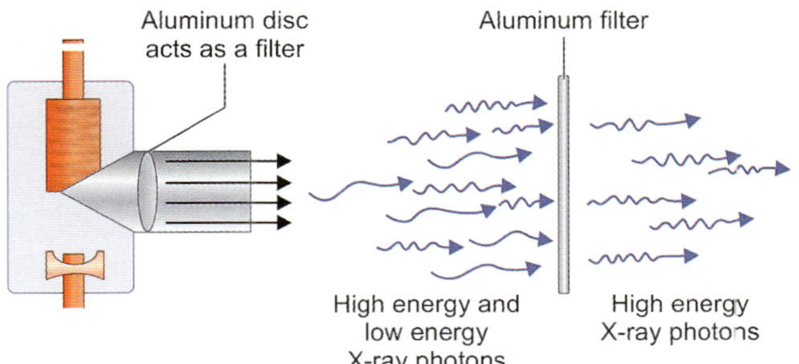

Fig. 8.26: Filtration.

- **Lead collimation (Fig. 8.27):** A collimator is a lead plate with a hole in the middle and is fitted directly over the opening of the machine housing where the X-ray beam exits the tube head. Collimation is used to restrict the size and the shape of the X-ray beam and to reduce patient exposure.

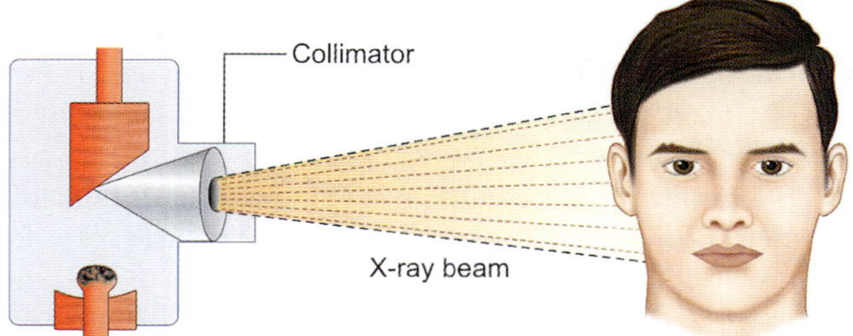

Fig. 8.27: Collimation.

- **Position indicating device (PID) (Fig. 8.28):** Appears as an extension of the X-ray tube head and is used to direct the X-ray beam. Three types of PID are conical, rectangular, and round. All these types are further available in long and short types, the former being more useful as it causes less divergence of X-ray. Rectangular cone irradiates 80–85% less tissue than short circular cones.

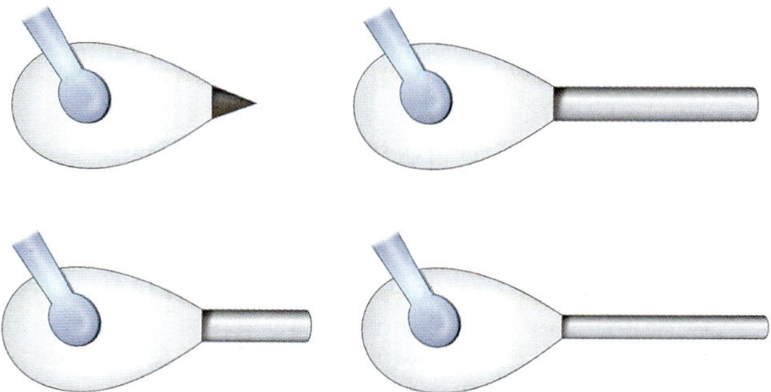

Fig. 8.28: Position indicating device.

- **Thyroid collar (Figs. 8.29A and B):** It is a flexible lead shield that is placed securely around the patient's neck to protect the thyroid gland from scattered radiation. The use of thyroid collar is recommended for all intraoral films, and it reduces thyroid gland exposure of primary beam by 50%.

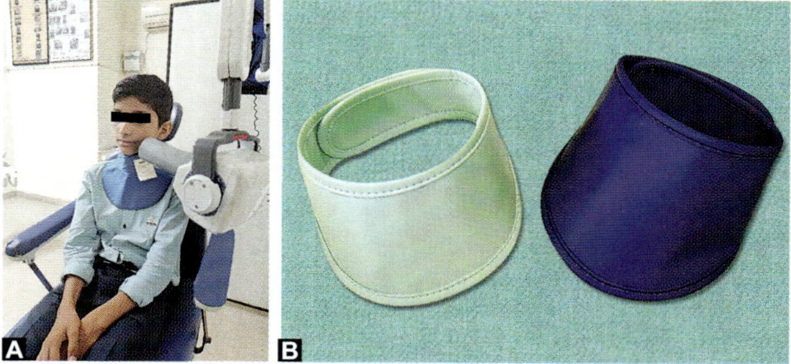

Figs. 8.29A and B: Use of thyroid collar.

- **Lead apron (Fig. 8.30):** It is a flexible shield that is placed over the patient's/radiographer's chest and lap to protect the reproductive and blood forming tissues from scattered radiation from reaching these radiosensitive organs. It is recommended for all intraoral and extraoral films. Reduces scattered radiation to 98% and minimizes exposure to chest pelvis, long bones, where major portion of hemopoietic systems are located.

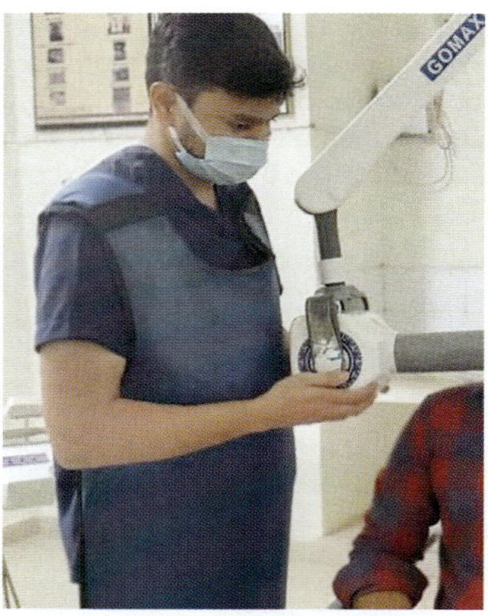

Fig. 8.30: Radiographer with lead apron.

- **Fast film:** Is the single most effective method of reducing exposure to X-radiation. E-speed is twice as fast as D-speed film and requires only one half the exposure time.
- **Film holding devices (Fig. 8.31):** Helps to stabilize the film position in the mouth and therefore, the patient's finger is not exposed to unnecessary radiation.
- **Proper film handling:** It is required to produce a diagnostic radiograph and to limit patient's exposure to radiation.
- **Correct film processing procedures:** Significantly improves the quality of radiograph. Following factors are important to assure the quality of radiograph, viz., dark room free from light leaks, adequate dark room safe lighting, and time–temperature processing.

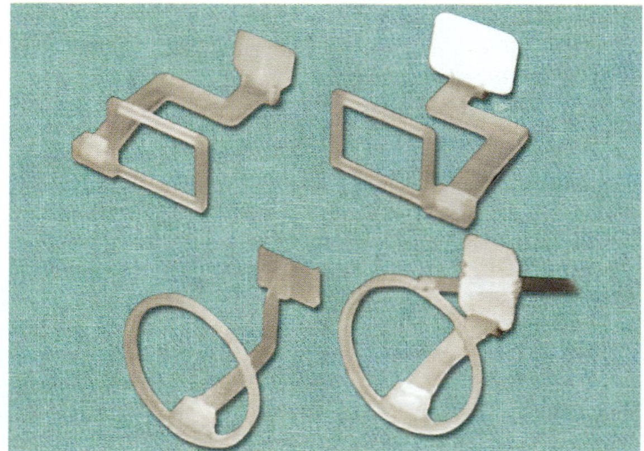

Fig. 8.31: Film holding devices.

Operator Protection Guidelines

Used to provide basic safety information that is needed when working with X-radiation. Operator protection guidelines include recommendation on distance, position, and shielding **(Fig. 8.32)**.

- Dental radiographer must avoid the primary beam.
- Stay 6 feet away from X-ray tube during X-ray procedure (distance rule).
- Use protective barriers.
- To avoid the primary beam the dental radiographer must be positioned at 90–135° angles to the beam (position rule).

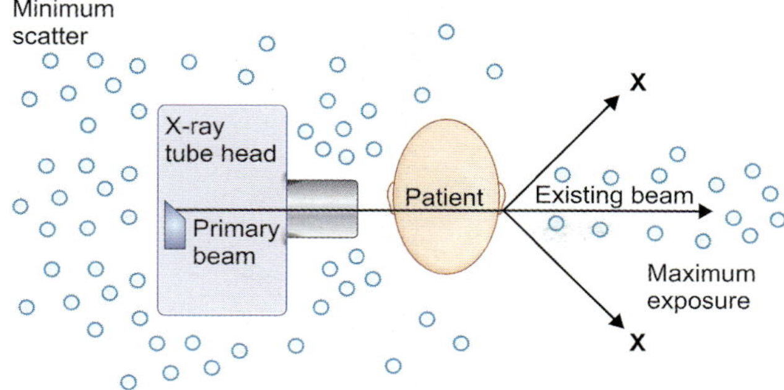

Fig. 8.32: Design for operator protection.

- ❖ The dental radiographer must never hold a film in place for a patient during X-ray exposure.
- ❖ Never hold a tube head during X-ray exposure.
- ❖ Should stand behind a protective barrier like lead screens.
- ❖ X-ray machine should be monitored for leakage radiation.
- ❖ Amount of X-radiation that reaches the body of the dental radiographer can be monitored by use of personnel monitoring device known as film badge. This should be worn at waist level. After the dental radiographer has worn the film badge for a specific time interval, it has to be returned to service company for dosage calculation.

RADIOGRAPHIC INFECTION CONTROL

In dental radiography, the main concerns arise from saliva contamination of work areas and equipment. Suitable precautions for prevention and spread of any disease are:

- ❖ Training of staff in infection control procedures.
- ❖ All clinical staff should be vaccinated in this COVID era.
- ❖ Open wounds on hands should be covered with waterproof dressings.
- ❖ Latex gloves should be worn for all radiographic procedures, but eye safety protection and masks are not usually necessary.
- ❖ Gloved hands should be washed under running water.

Common conditions that can spread due to inadequate radiographic infection control

- Infective hepatitis caused by hepatitis B or hepatitis C virus (HBV or HCV)
- HIV disease and AIDS caused by HIV
- Cold sores caused by herpes simplex virus
- Rubella (German measles)
- Tuberculosis
- Syphilis
- Diphtheria
- Mumps
- Influenza
- COVID-19 (Newest)

- ❖ Before and after X-raying every patient, using a disinfectant such as povidone iodine 7.5%, surgical scrub (Betadine) or chlorhexidine 4% (Hydrex).
- ❖ All required film packets and holders should be placed on disposable trays to avoid contamination of work surfaces.
- ❖ To prevent salivary contamination of film packets, they can be placed in small barrier envelopes before use. After use, the film packets can be emptied out of the barriers envelope into a clean surface and then handled safely.
- ❖ Film packets must only be introduced into daylight loading processors using clean hands or washed gloves.
- ❖ All film holders/bite blocks/bite pegs should be rinsed after use and then autoclaved or discarded, if disposable.
- ❖ X-ray equipment including tube head, control panel, time switch, and cassettes which have been touched should be wiped after each patient with a surface disinfectant like sodium hypochlorite, quaternary ammonium aldehyde, or peroxidase.

BEHAVIORAL CONSIDERATIONS IN PEDODONTIC RADIOGRAPHY

A radiographic appointment may be a source of anxiety or discomforts for the young patients. New surroundings, separation from parental support and intimidating machinery create an early sense of fear and apprehension. A balance should be established by the pedodontic radiographs between the child's inner resources and the demands of the appointment. It is believed that radiographs provide a pleasant and painless means of introducing a patient to dental treatment. Any subjective fears of radiography can easily be dissipated by demonstration of taking of radiographs.

- ❖ Reduce source of unnecessary anxiety.
- ❖ Motivate the child to do his best to cooperate.
- ❖ Use minimum number of films and in as short a time as possible.
- ❖ The communicating principles of tell, show and do, and modeling are effective in radiographic appointment.

Radiographic recommendations for children with disabilities

- Only radiographic investigations appropriate to the limitations imposed by the patient's age, cooperation, or disability should be attempted.
- Select intraoral films of appropriate size, modifying standard techniques as necessary.
- Utilize assistants to help hold the film.
- Avoid dental panoramic radiography because the patient will have to sit still for 18 seconds.
- Oblique lateral radiograph should be regarded as the extraoral view of choice.
- Use of paralleling technique, if possible for periapical radiography because with this technique the relative positions of film packet, teeth, and X-ray beam are maintained irrespective of position of patient's head.

- ❖ At the first appointment, the interview may be more personal and less intimidating by giving an invitation "to come in while we take pictures of your teeth." The decision to invite parent depends upon the assessment of the child patient. In the X-ray room, the operation of the chair is demonstrated by giving the child a ride to an appropriate level for filming. The radiographer introduces the protective lead apron as blankets and X-ray unit as camera **(Fig. 8.33)**. It is also helpful to demonstrate the clicking and buzzing sound associated with an exposure before filming begins.
- ❖ In the next visit, procedures of biting on the film packets may be modeled by the parent or dental assistant or a child of similar age group.
- ❖ It is sometimes wise to bring the X-ray tube into contact with your own face to dispel any fears a child may have **(Fig. 8.34)**.

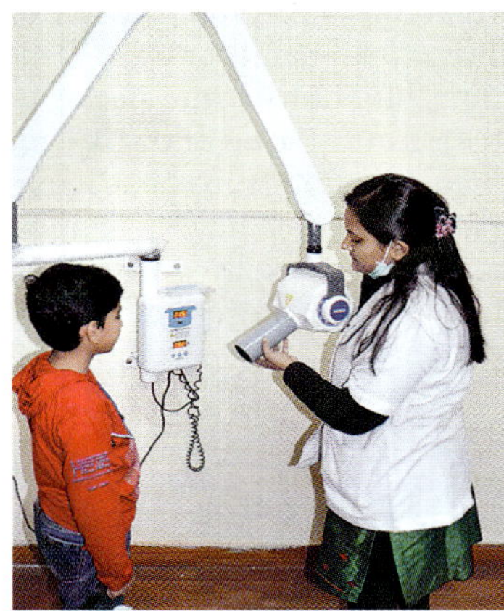

Fig. 8.33: Dentist explaining the X-ray apparatus.

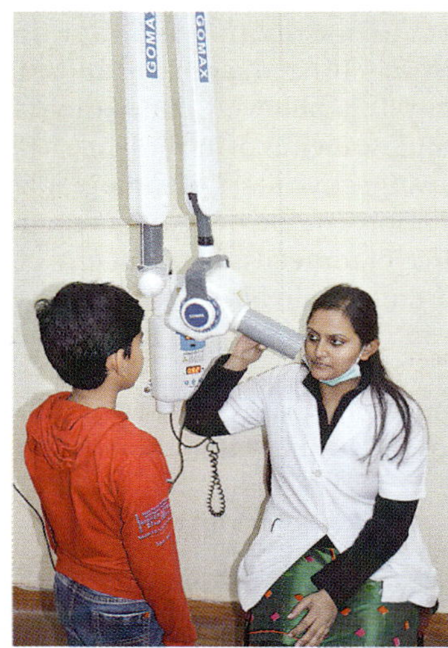

Fig. 8.34: Dentist performing tell-show-do (TSD).

- A good idea is to have the X-ray tube set at the needed angulation and placed next to child's face prior to insertion of film.
- Allow the patient to inspect and touch the film packet before it is placed in the mouth.
- If the child has a tendency to reject the film, the one should dampen the film packet. Such dampening takes away taste of the packet.
- Do not insert the packet in directly, but place the film in a horizontal plane and then gently rotate into vertical position.
- Before inverting the film, curve it slightly so as not to impinge on lingual tissue. The film should not be forced into the floor of the mouth **(Fig. 8.35)**.
- To ensure an initial success, the easiest areas are radiographed first like anterior films.
- For posterior projections, some form of film holding device is recommended.
- The observation of other children getting exposed for radiograph reduces anxiety and increases cooperation in young patients. This imitation or modeling is most effective when the model performs successfully and is reinforced for his behavior **(Fig. 8.36)**.
- Movements must be minimized and the child should be asked to focus on a wall objects so that his eyes do not follow the operator when he leaves the room. Once the film is placed, the dentist slowly counts to 10 and in the meantime the operator completes his cone-positioning moves to his safe position and exposes the film.
- If the patient is very uncooperative, it is also advisable to take the radiographs while the patient is seated in parent's lap **(Fig. 8.37)**.

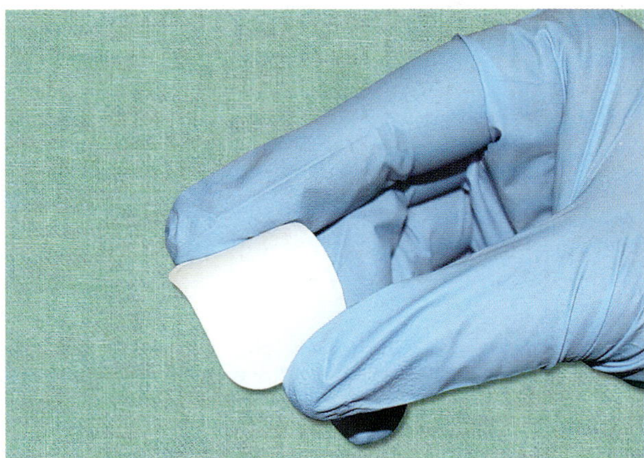

Fig. 8.35: Dampening and bending of film.

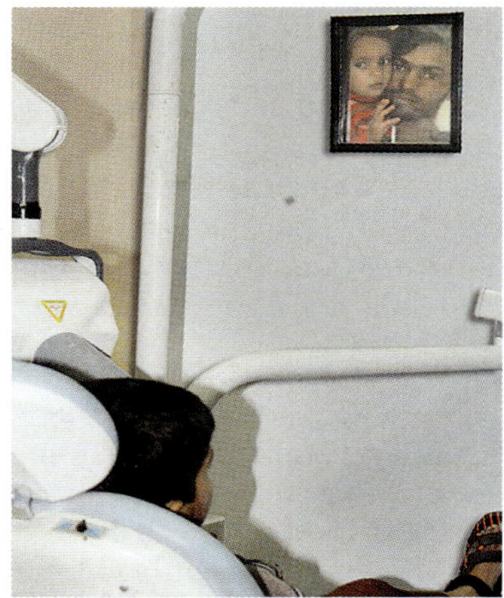

Fig. 8.36: Modeling during X-ray procedure.

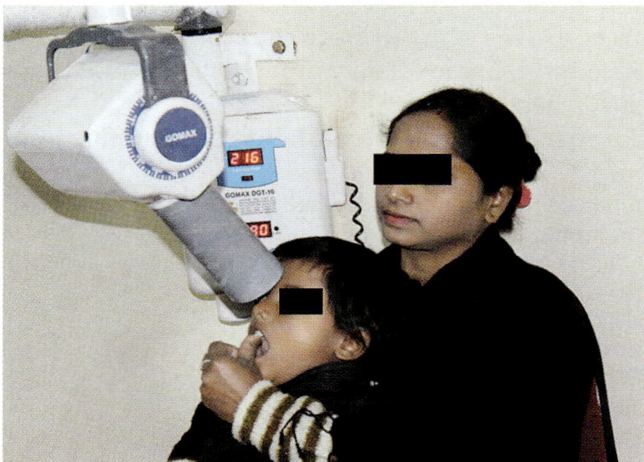

Fig. 8.37: Parent lap X-ray technique.

The importance of radiographs in dentistry needs no elaboration. It is important to realize that taking of radiographs often is a part of child's first dental experience which must be a pleasant experience so as to make him a good dental patient.

Clinical significance of radiography in pediatric dentistry

I. Pathologic evaluation
- Caries detection
- Traumatic injuries
  - Fractured roots or crowns
  - Fractured alveolar bone
  - Displaced tooth
  - Tooth or bone embedded in soft tissue
- Degree of pulpal involvement
  - Proximity of caries to pulp horn
  - Internal resorption
  - Calcific degeneration
- Periodontal diseases
  - Thickening of periodontal membrane
  - Furcation involvement
  - Periapical infection
  - Bone loss
  - External resorption

II. Developmental factors
- Stages of development
- Root formation
- Physiologic root resorption
- Bony support
- Stages of eruption and exfoliation

III. Degree of pulp maturity
- Size of pulp chamber
- Size of pulp canals
- Amount of apical closure
- Location of pulp horns

IV. Developmental anomalies
- Widely divergent roots
- Sharply curved pulp canals
- Number and length of roots
- Ectopic positioned roots
- Ankylosis
- Supernumerary teeth
- Congenitally missing teeth
- Malformed teeth
  - Microdontia and macrodontia
  - Dens in dente
  - Taurodontism
  - Gemination, fusion
  - Root dilacerations

V. Postoperative results of dental treatment
- Accuracy of restoration
- Type and success of pulp treatment
- Postsurgical healing
- Treatment failure

POINTS TO REMEMBER

- *Radiology:* The science or study of radiation as used in medicine, a branch of medical science that deals with the use of X-rays, radioactive substances, and other form of radiant energy in the diagnosis and treatment of disease.
- *Dental radiograph:* A photographic image produced on film by the passage of X-ray through teeth and related structure. The X-ray was discovered in November 1895 by Wilhelm Conrad Roentgen.
- Dr Otto Walkhoff a dentist in Germany made the first dental use of an X-ray and radiographed a lower premolar.
- *Properties of X-rays:* They are invisible, travel at the same speed of light (3×10^8 m/s), travel in a straight line, cannot be deflected, affect photographic plates, produces fluorescence with some substances.
- Paralleling cone technique was pioneered by Gordon Fitzgerald. In this central ray should be focused perpendicular to long axis ofthe film with the X-ray film being parallel to long axis of tooth.
- In bisecting angle, the film is placed close to the teeth and central ray is directed at right angles to the line bisecting the angle formed by the plane of the film and the long axis of the tooth.
- Vertical angulations of tube head in maxillary—incisor: +40°, premolar: +30°, canine: +45°, molar: +20° and in deciduous: anterior: +45°, posterior: +30°; mandibular—incisor: –15°, premolar: –10°, canine: –20°, molar: –5° and in deciduous: anterior: –15°, posterior: –10°.
- Clark's tube shift technique or localization procedure is to locate or determine the buccolingual relation of an impacted tooth/foreign body within the maxilla.
- *SLOB rule:* Buccal object rule states that the image of a buccally oriented object appears to move in the opposite direction from a moving X-ray source. And the image of any lingually oriented object appears to move in the same direction as a moving X-ray source.
- Panoramic radiography was developed by Numata (1933) and is used for diagnosis of traumatic injuries, cysts, evaluation of dentition, and anomalies.
- Xeroradiography that is a method of imaging uses the xeroradiographic copying process to record images produced by diagnostic X-rays.
- Radiographic protection can be done by prescribing needed dental radiographs, maintaining proper equipment: by aluminum filtration, by lead collimation, use of PID, thyroid collar, wearing lead apron, using fast films, and film holding devices.
- Behavioral modification for pedodontic patient is done by motivating the child: use minimum number of films; communicate using tell, show, and do; modeling and euphemisms; use the X-ray on similar age group child to show or even take in parents lap; dampen and curve the film; take anterior radiographs first.

Clinical Significance

- Radiographic examination forms a quintessential part of our path to reach the diagnosis. Although radiographic examination is necessary but one must always remember that it is a 2D image of an 3D object. Hence its corporation in clinical finding or supplementary radiographic technique is utmost necessary for conclusion.
- Radiation protection is often missed and most overlooked part in dental X-ray examination by dentist but one must realize its importance and not only wear proper protection gear himself but also provide proper radiation protection to the patient and parent with special care being taken for young children and pregnant women.
- Behavior modifications during X-ray in children holds a very important place in our treatment protocol. The dentist must take special care to use these behavior modifications in children as these are initial steps in first dental visit and any discomfort to child would lead to a negative reaction in further dental visits.

Questionnaire

1. Discuss the history and discovery of X-rays.
2. Describe the uses of X-rays.
3. What are the ideal requisites of a radiograph?
4. Describe the role of radiographs in pediatric dentistry.
5. What is 12-film survey?
6. Explain radiographic protocol.
7. Describe the diagram and working of X-ray unit.
8. Discuss paralleling and bisecting angle radiographic techniques.
9. What are radiographic localization procedures?
10. Write a note on xeroradiography.
11. What are different radiographic views visible on sialography of common pathological conditions?
12. Describe the patient and operator radiation protection guidelines.
13. Behavioral modifications for radiology in case of pediatric dentistry.

FURTHER READING

1. Arav L. Radiographic examination in pediatric dentistry. A review. NY State Dent J. 1991;57(2):36-7.
2. Browne RM, Edmondson HD, Rout PGJ. Atlas of dental and maxillofacial radiology and imaging. St. Louis: Mosby-Wolfe; 1995.
3. Espelid I, Mejàre I, Weerheijm K. EAPD guidelines for use of radiographs in children. Eur J Paediatr Dent. 2003;4(1):40-8.
4. Goaz PW, White SC, Pharoah MJ. Oral radiology; principles and interpretation, 4th ed. St. Louis: Mosby; 2000.
5. Langland OE, Langlais RP, McDavid WD, Delbal S. Panoramic radiology; 1988.
6. Mason RA, Bourne SA. Guide to dental radiography. London: Oxford Medical Publications; 1998.
7. Razmus TF, Williamson GF. Current oral and maxillofacial imaging. Philadelphia, PA: WB Saunders; 1996.
8. Richardson PS. Panoramic radiographic screening: a risk-benefit analysis. Prim Dent Care. 1997;4(2):71-7.
9. Udoye CI, Jafarzadeh H. Xeroradiography: stagnated after a promising beginning? A historical review. Eur J Dent. 2010;4(1):95-9.
10. White SC. Assessment of radiation risk from dental radiography. Dentomaxillofac Radiol. 1992;21(3):118-26.
11. Sridhara A, Konde S, Noojadi SR, et al. Comparative Evaluation of Intraoral and Extraoral Periapical Radiographic Techniques in Determination of Working Length: An *In Vivo* Study. Int J Clin Pediatr Dent. 2020;13(3):211-6.
12. Reddy SS, Kaushik A, Reddy SR, Agarwal K. Extraoral periapical radiography: A Technique Unveiled, JIAOMR. 2011;23(3):S336-9.
13. Saberi E, Hafezi L, Farhadmolashahil N, Mokhtari M. Modified Newman and Friedman Extraoral Radiographic Technique. IEJ. 2012;7(2):74-8.

CHAPTER

Digital Radiographic Diagnosis

Nikhil Marwah, Senchhema Limbu, Satyapal Yadav

Chapter Outline

- Digital Imaging
- Radiovisiography
- Digora System
- Magnetic Resonance Imaging
- Nuclear Imaging in Dentistry
- Digital Substraction Radiography
- Computed Tomography
- Spiral Computed Tomography
- Tuned Aperture Computed Tomography
- Ultrasound
- Cone Beam CT Technology
- Recent Advances of Dental Imaging
- Application of Dental Imaging in Dental Clinic

Digital or electronic imaging was first made known to dentistry in 1984 when radiovisiography (RVG) was launched in Europe by a French company **Trophy Radiologie** in 1987. **Dr Francis Mouyen**, invented and described in literature in 1989 a way to employ fiber optics to narrow down large radiographic image onto smaller size and sensed by CCD (charge-coupled device) image sensor chip that was specialized by Finnish engineer **Paul Suni**.[1,2] This type of technique has increased manifold in days and been used in dentistry. In the early days, digital radiograph was achieved by digitizing the film by camera or scanner which led to considerable loss of image properties, but today, we have digital imaging. This can be either of direct-CCD (charge-coupled device) or indirect-PSP (photo stimulable phosphor) type **(Table 9.1)**.

Terminologies of digital imaging
- *Brightness:* Digital equivalent to density or overall degree of image darkening
- *Dynamic range:* Numerical range of each pixel or shades of gray that can be represented
- *Linearity:* Direct relation between exposure and image density
- *Contrast resolution:* Ability to differentiate small differences in density as displayed on image
- *Spatial frequency:* Measure of resolution

DIGITAL IMAGING

Digital radiography is a filmless imaging system that is being stored in the computer. Digital radiographic images can be

Table 9.1: Intraoral receptor comparisons of digital imaging.

Feature	*Film*	*CCD*	*PSP*
Radiation dose	High	Low	Low
Generation of image	Chemical	Computer	Scanner, computer
Image viewing	Delayed on illuminator view box	Instant on computer	Delayed on computer
Resolution	16–20 lp/mm	8–10 lp/mm	6–8 lp/mm
Construction	Thin, flexible	Thick, rigid	Thin, flexible
Lifespan	Single	Reusable	Reusable after erasure
Infection control	Dropout	Barrier	Barrier
Image enhancement	Fixed	Multiple operation	Multiple operations
Storage	Patient record	CPU, CD	CPU, CD

(CCP: charge-coupled device; PSP: photostimulation phosphor; CPU: central processing unit; CD: compact disc)

Flowchart 9.1: Digital imaging (direct and indirect).

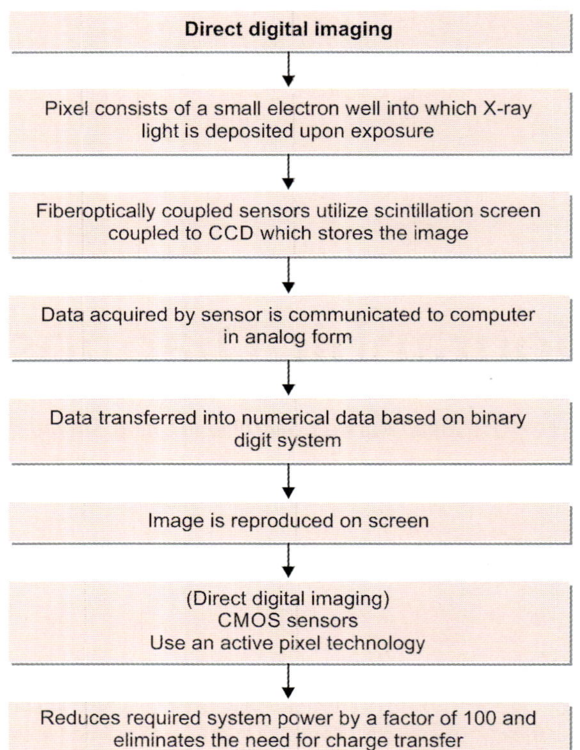

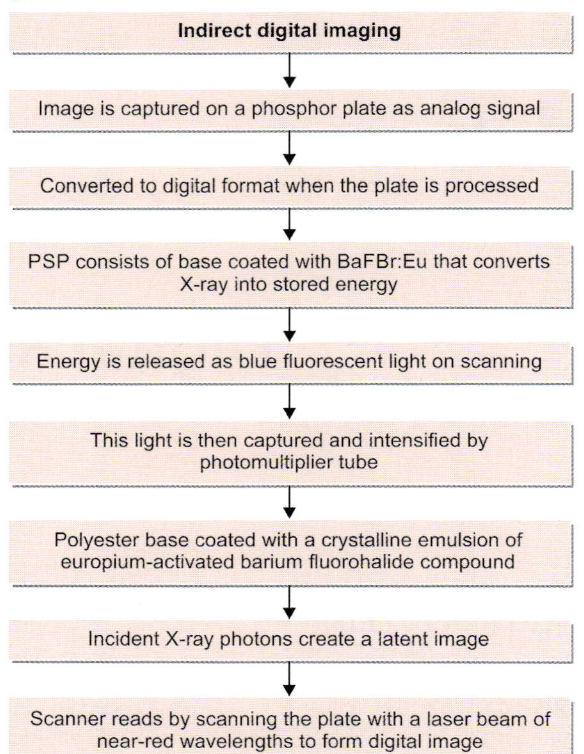

indirect, semi-direct or direct depending upon the system used. Currently there are three types used in dental imaging: (1) CCD-Charge-Coupled Device (direct system); (2) CMOS-Complementary Metal Oxide Semiconductor (direct system); and (3) PSP-photo-stimulable phosphor (indirect system) **(Flowchart 9.1).**

Radiographic produced by flatbed scanners with a transparency adapter, slide scanners, and digital cameras are referred to as indirect digital radiographs. The semi-direct images are obtained using phosphor plate system. Direct digital images are acquired using a solid-state sensor such as CCD or complementary metal-oxide-semiconductor (CMOS)-based chips.

Advantages of Digital Imaging

- Its full daylight system.
- Digital image is a dynamic image, so its contrast and density can be changed according to the diagnostic task. The digital receptors have wider latitude so in principle should reduce the number of retakes.
- Digital radiography has the reduction of radiation dose up to 80%, when compared to conventional plain film radiograph.
- PSP is more flexible and is cordless, so is easy to place
- Elimination of processing chemicals
- Working time is reduced by instant image production
- Patient education
- Easy storage
- Safest method with reduced exposure.

Disadvantages of Digital Imaging

- Increased rigidity and thickness of sensor in case of CCD
- Unknown life span of sensor
- High cost
- Care of usage, high maintenance
- Inability to perform complete infection control.
- System crash

RADIOVISIOGRAPHY

- Radiovisiography (RVG) was introduced by **Dr Francis Mouyen** in 1987 and introduced commercially by **Trophie Radiologie France** in 1984.
- Radiovisiography has less exposure time with minimal radiation exposure and within seconds image is displayed.
- It produces high quality images that can be optimized, due to the availability of preprogrammed auto-filters.
- Original system was useful in diagnosis of occlusal and approximal caries only, whereas the periodontal assessments have been made possible recently with invention of second generation system.
- RVG comprises of four basic components, viz., X-ray set with electronic timer, an intraoral sensor, a display processing unit (DPU), and a printer **(Table 9.2).**
- The original system, which was based on digital hardware without a microprocessor, will be referred to as Mark 1.
- An initial second generation (Mark 2) system, outwardly identical to the second generation system, was based on a 32-bit software-driven central processing unit but failed to achieve abilities of Mark 1 system. The first Mark 2 lacked the memory to use fully the resolving power of the sensor chip, and the number of gray levels which could be displayed on the monitor screen was only 64 compared with 256 in the Mark 1 model. Improvements to the system resulted in the second Mark 2 (available in some countries as a mobile unit).

Table 9.2: Components of RVG system.

X-ray set	*Intraoral sensor*	*Display processing unit (DPU)*	*Video printer*
• A conventional X-ray tube with generation operating at 70 kVp for use with the RVG system **(Fig. 9.1)** • It's connected to a microprocessor-controlled timer which allows very short exposure time of 0.02 second • The timer and X-ray set may also be used for conventional intraoral radiography	• The original intraoral sensor supplied with the Mark 1 system was approximately 40 × 22 × 14 mm • The sensor houses a rare-earth intensifying screen which is optically coupled to an array of CCDs • In the Mark 2 system, both normal and ZHR was available • The updated sensor supplied with the Mark 3 has a 25% larger sensitive area and less thickness by 16% **(Fig. 9.2)** • A waterproof sensor has been developed which can undergo "cold sterilization" procedures	• The analog signal obtained from the CCD after radiation exposure is stored in this unit and converted pixel by pixel into discrete gray levels • The CCD receiver (originally 256 × 256 pixels, upgraded to 480 × 380 in the Mark 3 system), together with digitizing boards and an 8-bitprocessor, allows up to 256 levels of gray to be obtained • In the Mark 2 system, more flexible digital image processing was available along with facility for storing the image data by transmission to a microcomputer • The Mark 3 model uses a 13-in color VGA monitor **(Fig. 9.3)** • The main distinction between the two Mark 3 models is that the "stand-alone" version can be used as such, or may be connected to a compatible PC and used with appropriate software	• The original video printer sold in the UK with the Mark 1 system was manufactured by Sony (Sony Corporation, Tokyo, Japan) • A dry silver imager (3M United Kingdom) was used in the Mark 2 mobile unit • The digital graphic printer used with the Mark 3 system is also manufactured by Sony **(Fig. 9.4)**

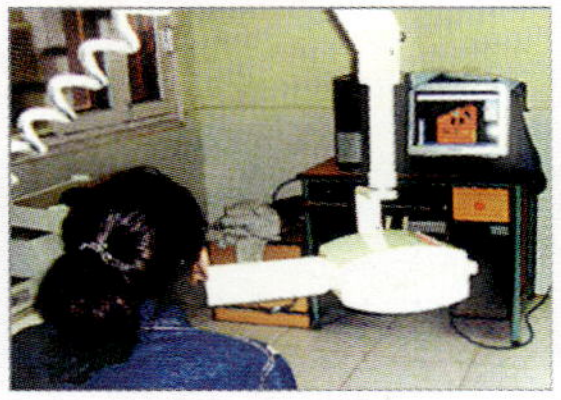
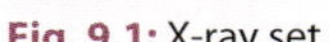

Fig. 9.1: X-ray set.

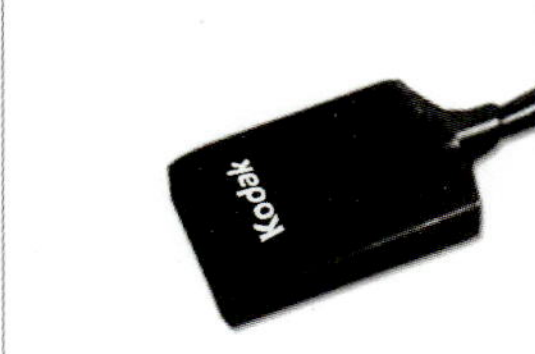

Fig. 9.2: Intraoral sensor.

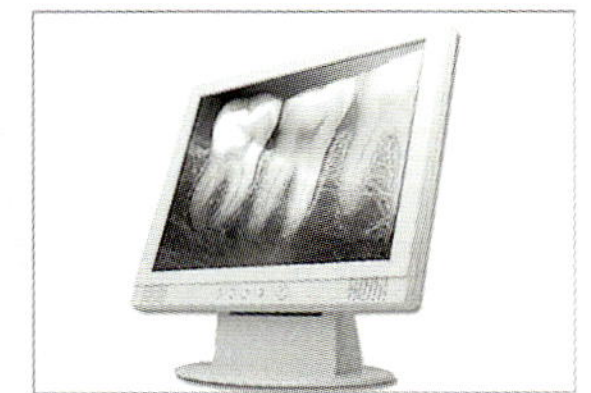

Fig. 9.3: Display processing unit.

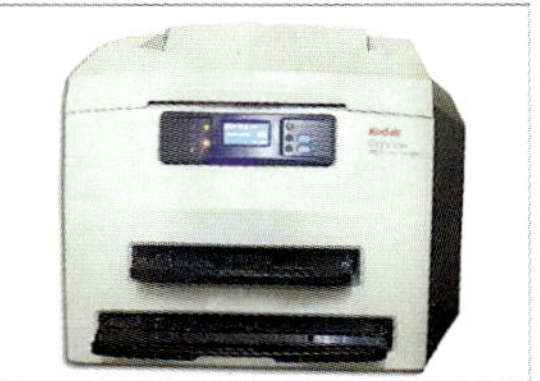

Fig. 9.4: Video printer.

(RVG: radiovisiography; CCD: charge-coupled device; ZHR: zoom high resolution)

- In RVG, upgraded softwares has made editing of the digital image possible for better understanding of the underlying conditions. Edits include changing levels of the contrast resolution, brightness, heat mapping, etc. The images on the screen can be magnified from 100% to 300% view.
- Very recent developments have resulted in two new RVG (third generation or Mark 3) systems: a "stand-alone" and a "PC" version.

Features of RVG

- **Image enhancement:** The image clarity in RVG is such, that it utilizes 256 shades of gray to give a distinct image of the dental condition. The "gray-window" effect, alternatively described as the "X-function," allows the operator to select and expand on a specific 60 levels of gray from the 256 available and may aid in diagnosis of accessory root canals. It has also been demonstrated that, using this mode, RVG is as sensitive as conventional radiography for detecting occlusal and proximal caries in-vitro in non-cavitated teeth. Improvements in the computer boards and further developments of the software available allowed an extensive range of image configurations for use with the Mark 2, which have been integrated into the third generation. The image can be electronically enhanced by smoothing, edge enhancement, and edge detection. A millimeter grid has been incorporated into the Mark 3 system and may prove to be an additional aid when positioning instruments during root canal therapy. The use of pseudo color available as part of the Mini-Julie software and integrated in the Mark 3 system. This feature assigns different colors to certain gray levels and can help to visualize particular features unclear on images and also helps in communication with patients.
- **Radiation dose:** Current radiation protection regulations recommend the use of the fastest available films consistent with satisfactory diagnostic results. **Horner** and **Walker** determined the radiation dose on the RVG setting on the Mark 1 system to be 23% of that required for D-speed film or 41% of the dose required for exposure of E-speed film.
- **Resolution:** The limiting resolution of the Mark 1 system was estimated to be 5–6 lp/mm in normal mode and 7–8.5 lp/mm in "zoom" mode 2. The introduction of the zoom high resolution (ZHR) function increased the resolution to 11 lp/mm in this mode. In the Mark 3 and the subsequent deletion of the ZHR function, the resulting resolution of the system is 9 lp/mm. In vitro and in vivo experiments suggest that although this is inferior to the resolution achieved by conventional X-ray films, it is adequate for most diagnostic tasks.
- **Collimation:** Incorporating rectangular collimation to the RVG sensor would permit a further decrease in radiation dose.

Comparatively little has been published regarding the recently developed (and rapidly developing) digital imaging dental radiographic system known as RVG. The RVG has considerable merit, although it is constrained by certain limitations. Significant improvements in the hardware have occurred and results in vitro for some applications are promising. However, full clinical evaluations across a range of dental applications are required, as are further studies.

Advantages of RVG
- Substantial dose reduction
- Production of instantaneous images
- Control of contrast
- Ability to enlarge specific areas, which may be of use in visualizing instrument location during endodontic treatment
- The potential for computer storage and subsequent transmission of the images

Disadvantages of RVG
- Sensor size and its greater thickness than conventional film
- There also appears to be a loss of resolution of the RVG image from the screen to the videoprint due to the transfer of the signal from the DPU to the printer
- Cost of equipment

DIGORA SYSTEM

- The Digora image plate system is an alternative, with fundamentally different digital image acquisition from that of CCD systems.
- Digora was introduced in 1994, and it provides two sizes of imaging plates comparable with the size 0 and 2 film.
- A single plate can be scanned for approximately 30 seconds.
- In 1997, the DenOptix system was introduced. The system has five sizes of imaging plates which are mounted in a carousel which can hold up to 29 imaging plates for scanning.
- Soredex Digora Optime latest 5th generation system is wireless, fastest and easiest visually guided system. The unit automatically without pressing any button scans imaging plates during the imaging workflow. It has intraoral imaging plates in sizes 0, 1, 2, and 3. These thin, flexible and reusable imaging plates are easy to handle, resistant to wear and replaceable.
- The durable imaging plates of Soredex Digora Optime **(Fig. 9.5)** come with patented IDOT identification system.
- The Soredex Digora Optime system's fully automatic with economical network sharing and optimized image processing leads to high-quality images (30 um super resolution, 60 um high resolution) that are displayed in just seconds (5–10 seconds depending on plate size), with display speed not dependent on image resolution.
- Comfort occlusal 4C makes occlusal projection imaging pleasant, even for pediatric patients **(Fig. 9.6)**.
- Reading out of the image plate takes less than 30 s, during which the image gradually appears on the computer monitor. The exposure range of the image plate is wide and linear. Because of the expanded exposure range, the high sensitivity of the image plate and the high quality of modern photomultiplier tubes, the image plate system can acquire data over many orders of magnitude in exposure compared to CCD or film systems.

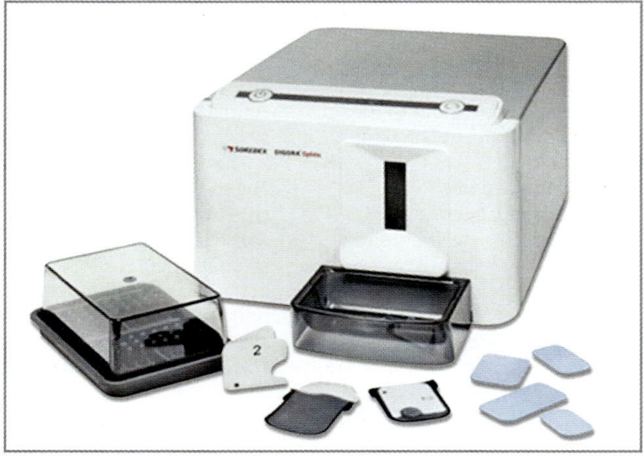

Fig. 9.5: Soredex Digora Optime.

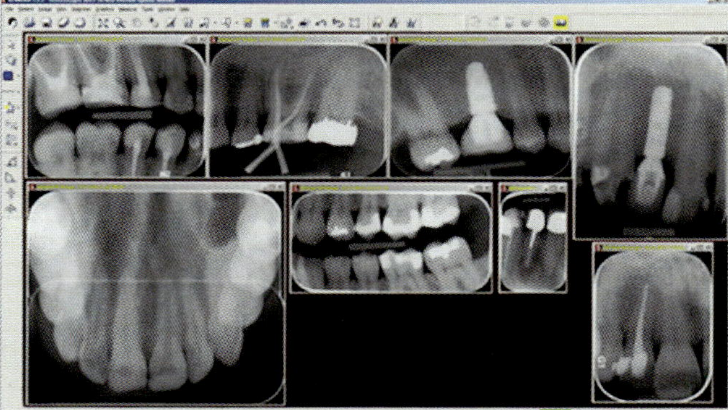

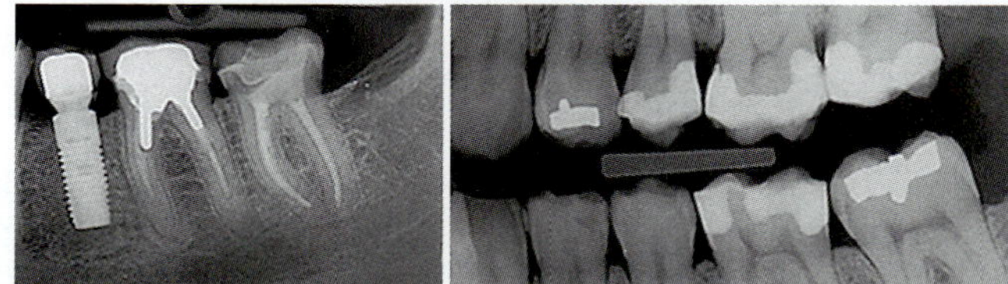

Fig. 9.6: Images displayed by Soredex Digora Optime.

- The digitized image is displayed instantly on the unit's display. The user can immediately verify image quality to the smallest clinical details and determine if a retake is needed.
- As with the other digital systems, the Digora image scan be altered after exposure to enable task-specific image characteristics. The system works in a Microsoft Windows environment, which simplifies all operating procedures. Image brightness and contrast can be changed by moving and angulating, respectively, a line displayed in a coordinate system where the gray level values in the original image are seen on the X-axis and Y-axis, respectively.
- The image-processing software allows edge enhancement and gray-scale in version.
- In addition, different types of measurements, such as measurements of linear distances (in tenths of millimeters) and angles, can be performed. All values are displayed on the screen.
- It is possible to display a histogram of the distribution of the gray levels within a chosen area, the mean gray level, and the deviation around the mean.

- It has the system guides to use correct exposure settings and does not accept improperly inserted imaging plate.
- Recently there is Digora Optime with interactive display that eliminates the need to have a dedicated PC next to it.

MAGNETIC RESONANCE IMAGING

In 1946 **Purcell and Bloch**, discovered the nuclear magnetic resonance (MR) phenomenon that are used to produce anatomic and functional information. The imaging capabilities were not commercialized until the 1980s. MRI is a noninvasive radiology technique where static magnetic field pulsed radiowaves and gradient magnetic fields are used to create an image of body structures **(Fig. 9.7)**. The images obtained are unique as no ionizing radiation from radiofrequency band of electromagnetic spectrum (10.9–10.11 nm of wavelength) is used for bringing no biological damage. It is a noninvasive imaging modality that uses electrical signals generated from response of hydrogen nuclei to strong magnetic field and radiowave/radiofrequency pulses to produce an image. The tissues appear different with different machine settings, and these images are analyzed that give diagnostic information not readily available with any other imaging modality. MRI offers the best resolution of tissues of low inherent contrast **(Fig. 9.8)**.

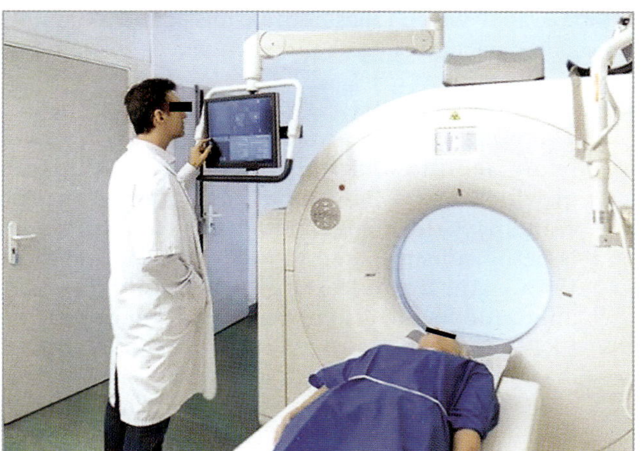

Fig. 9.7: Magnetic resonance imaging.

MR Imaging Process

Patient is placed in magnetic field and they act as magnet. Radiowave is sent in and turned off then patient emits signals that are received and used for construction of the picture.

Uses of Magnetic Resonance Imaging

- For lesions of the extracranial head and neck
- Imaging for the tumors of the skull base, paranasal sinuses, nasopharynx, parapharyngeal space.
- It identifies soft tissue diseases, especially neoplasia, involving tongue, maxilla and mandible, cheek, salivary glands, neck, vascular structures and lymph nodes.
- Superior sensitivity in detecting small lesions.
- For detection of internal derangement of TMJ.
- More accuracy in staging the lesion and narrowing the diagnostic possibilities.
- MRI also helps in 3D visualization of the carious lesion, determining its extent and its relationship with the adjacent surrounding tooth structures.[3]
- MR sialography is used in salivary gland for ductal structure, and dynamic evaluation of ducts.
- The high contrast sensitivity of MRI to soft tissue differences is the major reason MRI have replaced CT for imaging soft tissues.
- MR imaging is not considered to be hazardous to the fetus but cautionary approach should be used in pregnant

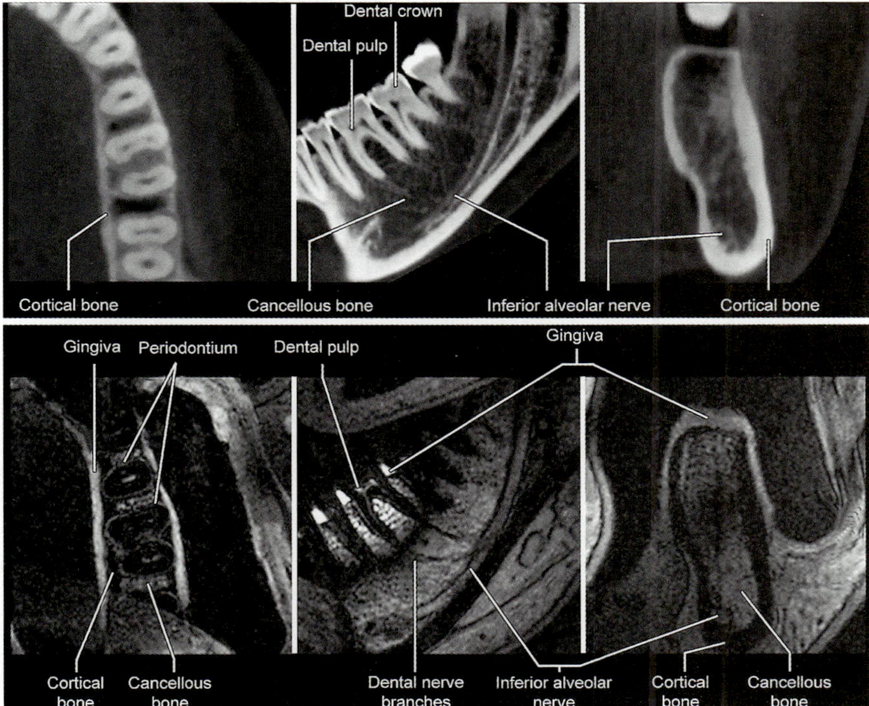

Fig. 9.8: Images displayed by magnetic resonance imaging.

women if other non-ionizing forms of diagnostic imaging are inadequate.

A recent MRI technology is called Sweep Imaging with Fourier Transform to visualize dental tissues. It can simultaneously image both hard and soft dental tissues with high resolution in short enough scanning times and hence is practical for clinical applications. It can also determine the extent of carious lesions and simultaneously assess the status of pulpal tissue, whether reversible and irreversible pulpitis, which can impact clinical decision on treatment planning.[4]

NUCLEAR IMAGING IN DENTISTRY

The advent of clinical nuclear imaging occurred in the early 1950s, when radiopharmaceuticals were first used to localize radioactive molecules in specific organs for diagnostic purposes. Nuclear imaging produces images by detecting radiation from different parts of the body after a radioactive tracer material are injected in the body that emits gamma rays which are detected by special image receptors and images are recorded on computer and on film **(Fig. 9.9)**. Bone-seeking radiopharmaceutical uptake provided a mechanism for the visualization of physiologic alterations in bone metabolism and blood-flow rate, in contrast to standard radiography, wherein imaging was based on the absorption of externally applied X-rays by the patient and the recording of the remnant beam on film.

Various nuclear imaging modalities include scintigraphy, positron emission tomography (PET) and single photon emission computed tomography (SPECT) which can assess any functional changes that occur within a diseased cell.[5]

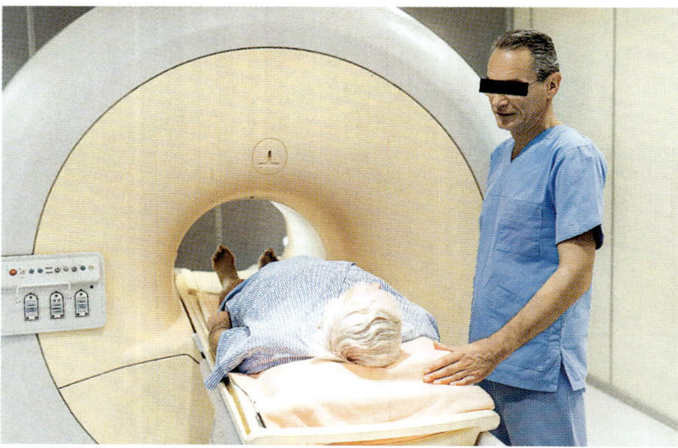

Fig. 9.9: Nuclear medicine imaging technique.

Various Nuclear Imaging Techniques

- **Scintigraphy:** Scintigraphy produces two-dimensional images due to radiation emitted from an organ, injected with a radioisotope. The radioisotope emits characteristic radiation captured by specialized external gamma cameras. It provides useful information about salivary gland function by measuring the rate and density of technetium-99m (^{99m}Tc) pertechnetate uptake in the mouth after intravenous injection. Scintigraphy is used in bone and salivary glands scanning.

  Scintigraphy of salivary glands: The procedure entails injecting of radiopharmaceutical (technetium-99m pertechnetate) and recording the resultant distribution utilizing scintillation camera. This is a means of evaluating mass lesions and functional evaluation of salivary glands. It is used in salivary glands include assessing obstructive disorders, distinguishing agenesis and aplasia, traumatic lesions, and salivary gland functioning postoperatively.[6]
- **Positron emission tomography (PET):** PET utilizes radioisotopes that emit the positron, for the biological or metabolic studies in the various organs of interest. 18F-fluorodeoxyglocose (18F-FDG) is the radiopharmaceutical most commonly used in PET scanning. PET is used for diagnostic and prognostic purposes in the region of head and neck malignancy.
- **Single photon emission computed tomography (SPECT):** SPECT is similar to PET in its use of radioactive tracer material and detection of gamma rays but it uses single photon gamma-ray emission as the source of information, in contrast with the conventional computed tomography which relies on transmission of X-rays. It is used in detection of head and neck cancer, the temporomandibular joint (TMJ).
- **Fusion imaging (PET-CT, PET-MRI, SPECT-CT):**
  - The molecular and functional imaging provided by nucleotide imaging and anatomical imaging provided by CT/MRI have been merged into so-called Hybrid/Fusion imaging.[6] Fusion imaging is being substantiated to be more accurate rather than using individually in the detection and anatomic localization of head and neck cancers.
  - PET/CT has also proved its utmost efficiency in diagnosis of head and neck carcinomas at initial stage of the disease enabling early treatment interventions for better prognosis.[3]
  - PET/MRI and its application is into the clinical settings with high accuracy in T-staging of tumor entities.
  - Integration of functional and anatomic image data via union of PET/SPECT and CT/MRI provides additional clinically relevant information. It can be the inquest of choice for imaging because it can almost eliminate the false-positive and false-negative PET findings.

Uses of Nuclear Imaging in Dentistry

- Useful in diagnosis of disease in the oral and maxillofacial region **(Fig. 9.10).**
- Used as a routine diagnostic method to evaluate the osteoblastic activity around implants and in periodontal disease.
- To identify the fractures, benign and metastatic tumors of head and neck, bone grafts and TMJ disorders at a

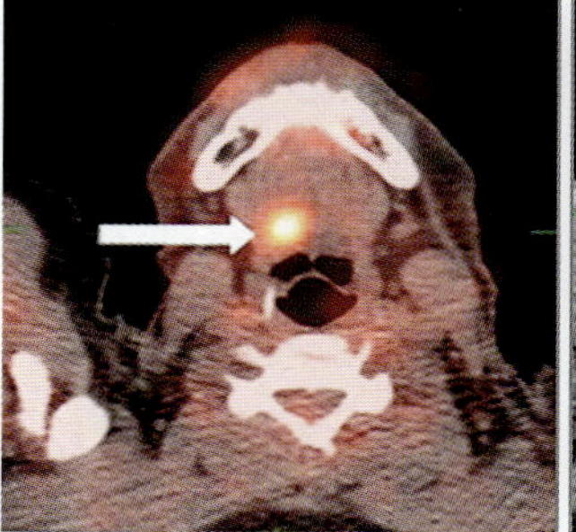

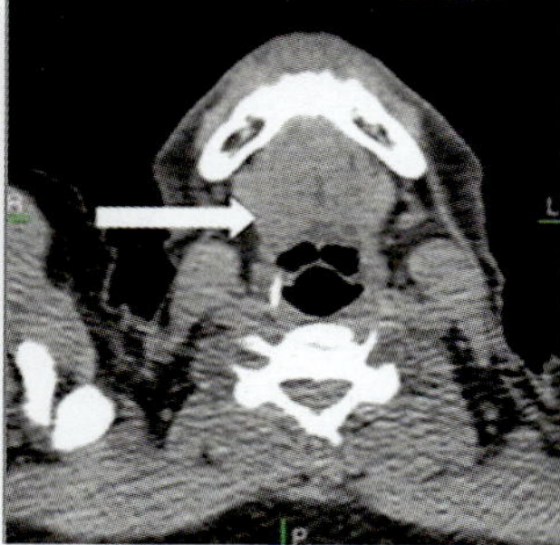

Fig. 9.10: Dental images in nuclear medicine imaging techniques.

very early stage and aids to bring about an intervention therapy.

- NM can be utilized for studies involving detection of caries, the disease of the periodontium, investigating fluorosis, microleakage of various dental materials, resorption of roots, endocrine and nutrition effects.
- Used in many metabolic and inflammatory disorders, salivary gland dysfunction and other diseases afflicting the oral and maxillofacial region.
- Positron emission tomography (PET) was a test with a good predictive value for identifying recurrent malignancies in the head and neck when used in conjunction with computed tomography (CT).
- Nuclear imaging has been reported to be useful in the evaluation of bone metabolism in bony components of the temporomandibular joint (TMJ) for assessment of facial skeletal growth.

Advantages of Nuclear Imaging

- Functional images of the diseased tissues are obtained
- Whole skeletal system can be scanned within less span of time
- Recurrence can be easily detected and sensitivity is high

Disadvantages of Nuclear Imaging

- The spatial resolution in NM imaging is reduced when compared to other imaging modalities like MRI or CT,
- It is rather expensive
- Contraindicated in pregnant and lactating women.

DIGITAL SUBTRACTION RADIOGRAPHY (DSR)

- Subtraction method was introduced by BG Zeides des Plantes in the 1920s and introduced in the year 1980s.[7]
- DSR is obtained mainly by eliminating the anatomical sturctures on the radiography and storing it digitally and combining it with the post treatment image and displaying the final subtracted image **(Fig. 9.11)**.
- It is a technique used to determine qualitative changes that occur between two images taken at different points in time. The first image is the baseline image and the second image shows the changes that have occurred since the time the first image was taken.

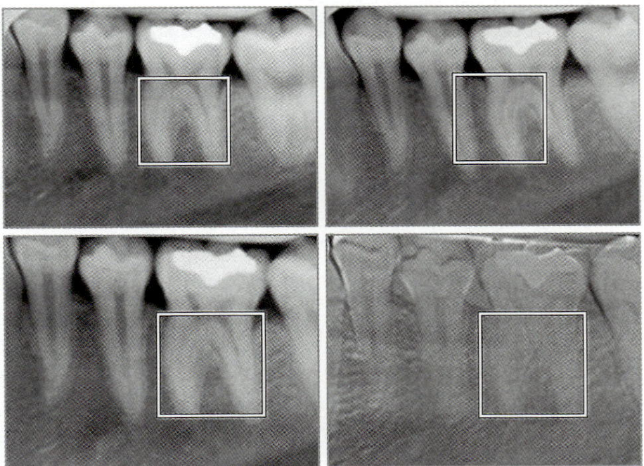

Fig. 9.11: Dental images in digital subtraction radiography.

- DSR cancels out the complex anatomic background against which this change occurs.
- For DSR to be diagnostically useful, it is crucial that the baseline projection geometry and image intensities be reproduced.

Uses of DSR

- It helps to detect the alveolar bone changes of 1–5% per unit volume and of crestal bone height change of 0.78 mm.
- DSR with or without enhancement improved the likelihood of a correct cancellous defect diagnosis when compared to other methods to detect oral cancellous bone lesions.
- In the diagnosis of periodontal bone resorption and in the analysis of level of bone in implants and in accessing the process of healing in periapical lesions.[7]
- It allows qualitative evaluation by underscoring small changes such as caries progression, periapical lesions, or even quantitative evaluation of periodontal bone loss.

COMPUTED TOMOGRAPHY

- **Radon** (1917) was the first person to lay the foundation for such an imaging, and later in 1972, the first clinical CTX-ray unit was developed by **G N Hounsfield** in England.
- CT uses X-rays to portray across sectional image of an object without superimpositions **(Fig. 9.12)**. The CT scanner makes multiple projections of an object, radiation detectors measure the object's X-ray attenuation at each of these projections, and a computer reconstructs the attenuation data to produce a cross-sectional image, or "slice" of the object.

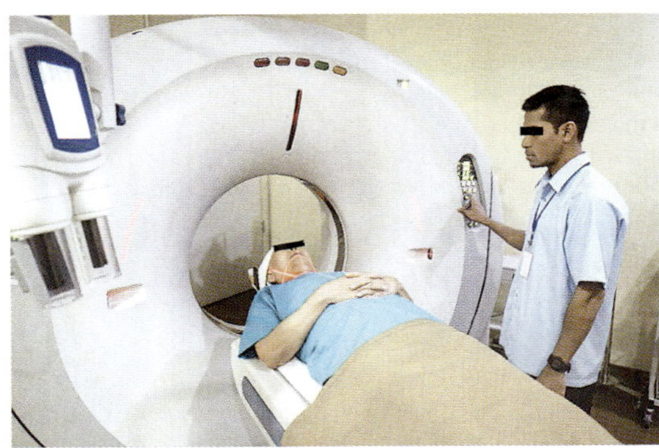

Fig. 9.12: Computed tomography.

- Current CT scanners are called multi-slice CT scanners and have a linear array of multiple detectors (up to 64 rows) that simultaneously obtain tomographic data at different slice locations.
- It provides various advantages including significant reduction in scan time, reduced artifacts, and sub-millimeter resolution (up to 0.4 mm isotropic voxel).
- CT images have less noise (i.e., they are less grainy), which results from superior collimation of the exit beam in CT machines.
- CT software programs can highlight pathologic lesions from normal anatomic structures using color-enhancement features. CT images have the ability to show slices of a given tissue, with each slice thickness (1–2 mm) and location chosen by the operator.

Applications of computed tomography[8]

- CT can be useful for the study of anatomic or pathologic structure
- It is useful for diagnosis, treatment planning, and postoperative follow-up of patients with craniofacial anomalies.
- It is used for assessing injuries of the maxillofacial skeleton region and detecting complex facial fractures involving frontal sinus, nasoethmoidal region and orbits.
- The most accurate method in the diagnosis of mandibular fractures, and also undisplaced fractures of the mandible and the condyle.
- In defining the displacements of fractures prior to surgical reduction and fixation.
- CT may be used for the noninvasive estimation of bone mass.
- It offers visualization of impacted teeth and its relation to nearby anatomic structures.
- It has been used for the study of salivary gland disease.
- Used in the assessment of traumatic injuries to the skeleton.
- Used in dental implant treatment planning **(Fig. 9.13).**
- It can be used to image the extent of pathologic conditions.
- To assess presurgical implant treatment planning.

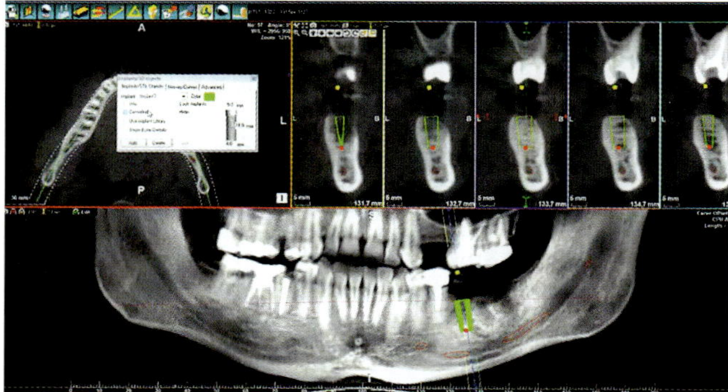

Fig. 9.13: Dental images in computed tomography.

Disadvantages of computed tomography

- High radiation dose relative to that of plain-film radiography
- High cost
- Relatively long time of image acquisition
- Poor resolution compared to conventional radiographs

SPIRAL COMPUTED TOMOGRAPHY

- Tomography had been one of the pillars of radiologic diagnostics until the 1970s when the availability of minicomputers and of transverse axial scanning method (due to the work of **Godfrey Hounsfield** and **Allan McLeod Cormack**) gradually supplanted it as the modality of CT. The technique of "Dental CT" also called as "Dentascan" was developed by **Schwartz et al.** (1987) when these investigators first used curved multi-planar reconstructions of the jaw. It is also called helical computed tomography. Existing diagnostic methods such as the computerized transverse axial scanning (CT) greatly facilitates access to the internal morphology of the soft tissue and skeletal structures.
- Recently, a newer CT technique, spiral computed tomography (SCT) **(Fig. 9.14)** or volume acquisition CT, has been developed which employs simultaneous patient translation through the X-ray source with continuous rotation of the source detector assembly; SCT acquires raw projection data with a spiral-sampling locus in a relatively short period, and without any additional scanning time, these data can be viewed as conventional transaxial

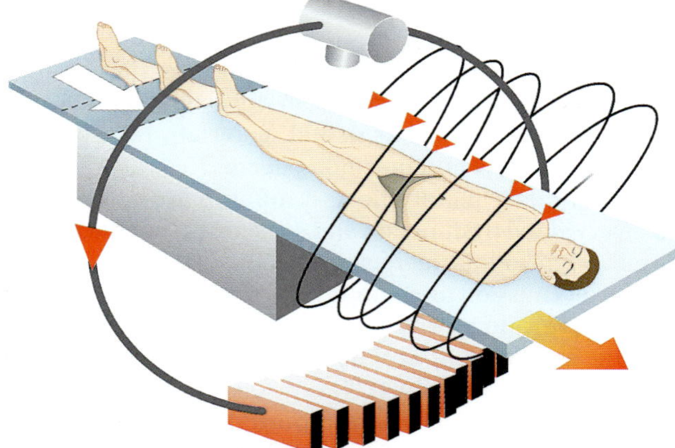

Fig. 9.14: Spiral computed tomography.

images, such as multiplanar reconstructions, or as three-dimensional (3D) reconstructions. With SCT, it is possible to reconstruct overlapping structures at arbitrary intervals and thus the ability to resolve small objects is increased.
- It is used to help diagnose disease, plan treatment, or find out how well treatment is working. 3-D images from spiral CT helped in evaluating the close relationship between maxillary sinus disease and adjacent periodontal defects and their treatment **(Fig. 9.15).**
- Advantages of spiral CT includes shortened examination times, improved visibility of vascular structures, better enhancement of parenchymal organs, capability for retrospective imaging and three-dimensional (3D) vascular studies, and potential reduction in use of contrast material.

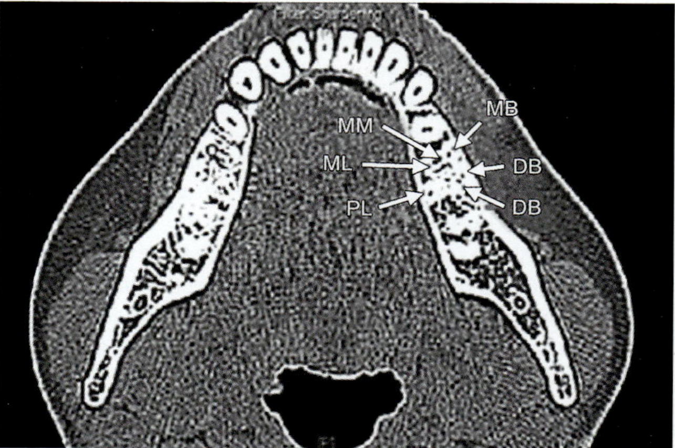

Fig. 9.15: Dental images in spiral computed tomography.

TUNED APERTURE COMPUTED TOMOGRAPHY

- Tuned aperture computed tomography (TACT) is a new imaging digital radiography, developed by **Webber** and colleagues where substraction radiographs are used based on the concept of tomosynthesis and optical aperture theory.
- TACT uses 2-D periapical radiographs acquired from different projection angles as base images and permits retrospective generation of longitudinal tomographic slices (TACT-S) lining up in the Z axis of the area of interest. It produces true 3-D data from any number of arbitrarily oriented 2-D projections.

- Its advantages are that there is decrease in superimposition of overlying anatomical structures and it is relatively simple; faster method for reconstructing tomographic images; overall radiation dose of TACT is not greater than 1 to 2 times that of a conventional periapical X-ray film; the resolution is stated to be similar with 2-D radiographs; artefacts associated with CT, such as starburst patterns seen with metallic restorations, do not exist with TACT.
- It is mainly used in external root resorption diagnosis and is considered more effective and accurate imaging modality for non-destructive quantification of osseous changes within the healing bony defects **(Fig. 9.16).**

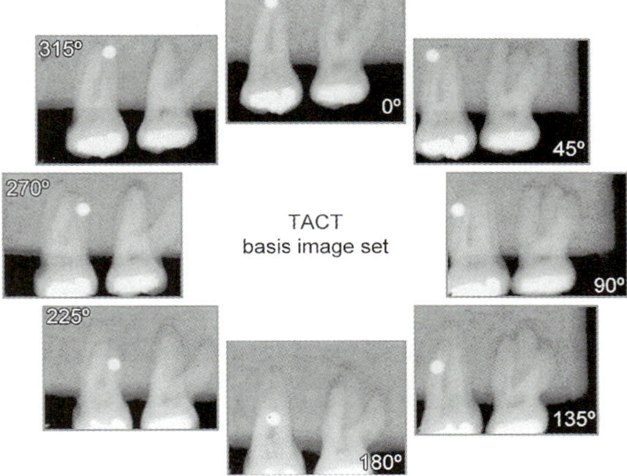

Fig. 9.16: Dental images in tuned aperture computed tomography.

ULTRASOUND

- Ultrasound (US) is a noninvasive, inexpensive and painless imaging method. Unlike X-rays, it does not cause harmful ionizing radiation.
- The first data of US diagnostic in dentistry was reported in 1963 by **Baum et al**.
- Here sound waves are used to generate an image and scanners generate electric impulses that convert to ultra-high frequency sound waves by transducer and the image is produced in sonography. They used a 15 MHz transducer to visualize the interior structures of teeth.
- It can be an important diagnostic tool for patients in whom MRI is contraindicated, such as those with cardiac pacemakers, claustrophobia and metallic prosthesis.

Uses of ultrasound (Fig. 9.17):
- Used to diagnose fractures of the orbital margin and nasal bone, zygomatic arch, and the anterior wall of the frontal sinus.
- It is also capable in the detection of extracapsular subcondylar fractures.
- It also detect sialoliths in parotid, submandibular and sublingual salivary glands.
- Ultrasound guidance can prevent injuring the facial nerve during biopsy of the parotid gland.
- It has been used in guided fine-needle aspiration, measurement of tongue cancer thickness, and diagnosis of metastasis to cervical lymph nodes.
- US can measure soft tissue thickness which could help practitioners to select the proper orthodontic mini-screw in clinical practice.

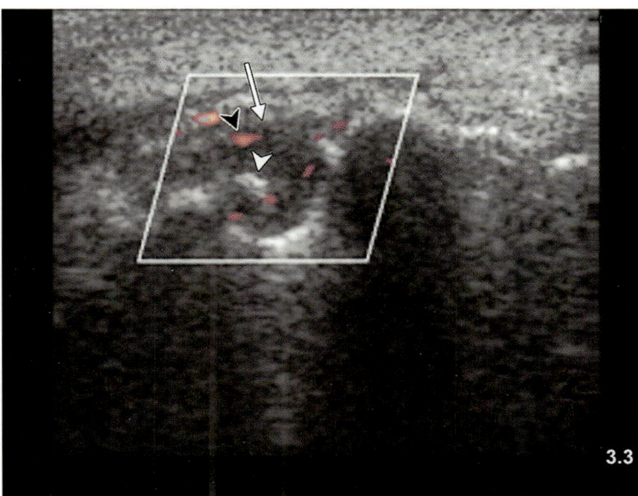

Fig. 9.17: Dental images in ultrasound.

CONE-BEAM CT TECHNOLOGY

- Cone-beam computed tomography (CBCT) is an imaging technique consisting of X-ray CT where the X-rays are divergent, forming a cone.
- **Attilio Tacconi, Piero Mozzo, Daniele Godi, and Giordano Ronca** are the pioneers of this technology.
- CBCT allows the creation in "real time" of images not only in the axial plane but also two-dimensional (2D) images in the coronal, sagittal, and even oblique or curved image planes—a process referred to as multiplanar reformation. In addition, CBCT data are amenable to reformation in a volume, rather than a slice, providing 3D information.
- CBCT scanners **(Fig. 9.18)** are based on volumetric tomography, using a 2D extended digital array providing an area detector. This is combined with a 3D X-ray beam. The cone-beam technique involves a single 360° scan in which the X-ray source and a reciprocating area detector synchronously move around the patient's head, which is stabilized with a head holder. At certain degree intervals, single projection images, known as "basis" images, are acquired. This series of basis projection images is

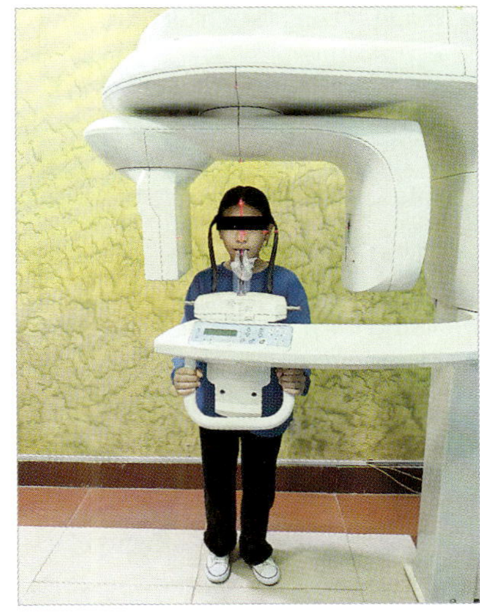

Fig. 9.18: Cone-beam computed tomography (CBCT) machine.

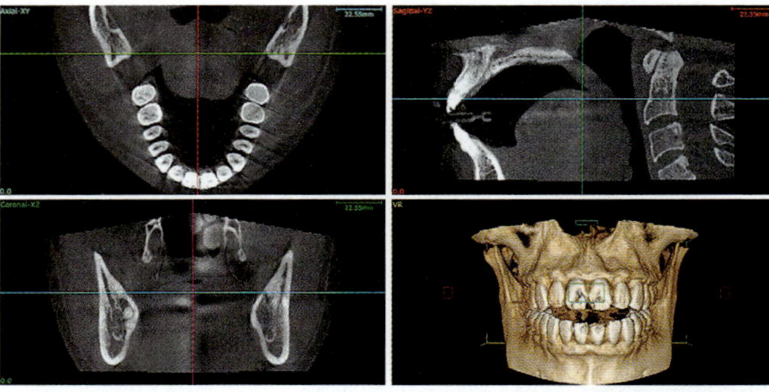

Fig. 9.19: Cone-beam computed tomography (CBCT) images.

referred to as the projection data. Software programs incorporating sophisticated algorithms including back-filtered projection are applied to these image data to generate a 3D volumetric data set, which can be used to provide primary reconstruction images in three orthogonal planes (axial, sagittal, and coronal) **(Fig. 9.19).**

- The first system introduced was NewTom QR DVT 9000 (Quantitative Radiology SRL Verona, Italy) introduced in April 2001 and the two currently used systems are 3D Accuitomo—XYZ Slice View Tomograph (J Morita Mfg Corp., Kyoto, Japan) and I-CAT (Xoran technologies, Ann Arbor, Mich., and Imaging Sciences International, Hatfield, PA).
- CBCT is categorized into large, medium, and limited volume units based on the size of their field of view (FOV). The size of the FOV depicts the scan volume of CBCT machines. It depends on various factors like the size and shape of the detector, beam projection geometry and the ability to collimate the beam. Collimation of the beam limits the X-radiation exposure to the region of interest and ensures the most favorable FOV to be selected, based on disease presentation. Smaller scan volumes produce higher resolution images and lowers the effective radiation dose to the patient. Size of the field irradiated is the principal limitation of large FOV cone beam imaging.

To Reduce the Exposure Dose in CBCT

- Collimation
- Largest voxels size in relation to Rx need
- Change in image settings such as ultra-low dose settings
- Shorter exposure time
- Lower amount of projections (resolution)
- Lower beam intensity (mA)
- Reduction of the potential (kv)
- Use of a thyroid shield and the use of AEC

Advantages of CBCT

- CBCT is well suited for imaging the craniofacial area
- It provides clear images of highly contrasted structures and is extremely useful for evaluating bone
- X-ray beam limitation as the effective patient dose to approximately that of a film-based periapical survey of the dentition
- Because CBCT acquires all basis images in a single rotation, scan time is rapid (10–70 sec)
- Reconstruction of CBCT data are performed natively by a personal computer. In addition, software can be made available which provides the clinician with the opportunity to use chair-side image display, real-time analysis.
- CBCT images can result in a low level of metal artifact, particularly in secondary reconstructions designed for viewing the teeth and jaws.

Disadvantages of CBCT

- Increased susceptibility to movement artifacts
- Lack of appropriate bone density determination
- Dental CBCT systems do not employ a standardized system for scaling the gray levels that represent the reconstructed density values and, as such, they are arbitrary and do not allow for assessment of bone quality.
- CBCT cannot be used for estimation of bone density due to distortion of Hounsfield units.
- Scan time for CBCT are lengthy at 15–20 sec thus requires patients to stay completely still during imaging.

Uses of CBCT

Large field of view (FOV) units are mainly useful in the assessment of maxillofacial trauma, orthodontic diagnosis and treatment planning, temporomandibular joint (TMJ) analysis and pathologies of the jaws. Medium FOV range from 10–15 cm and are useful for mandibulomaxillary imaging and for pre-implant planning and pathological conditions. Small FOV units (limited FOVs) of <10 cm with some as small as 4 cm × 4 cm in size are suitable for dento-alveolar imaging and are most advantageous for endodontic applications.

- Implantology
  - To assess osseointegration
  - To determine quality of bone
  - To check the relation of implant
  - During surgical guidance
- Maxillofacial surgery
  - To diagnose tumors, impacted teeth, fractures
  - To identify relation of teeth with nerve canals
  - Cystic lesions and delimitations
  - Traumatic injuries to teeth
  - Fracture or inflammation of jaws and sinuses
- Orthodontics
  - Planning of orthognathic surgery
  - Cephalometric analysis
- Endodontics
  - In diagnosing of periapical lesions
  - Identification of canals
  - Endodontic surgery
- Pediatric Dentistry
  - TMJ evaluation
  - Evaluation of growth
  - In cleft cases for volumetric assessment of defects
  - In autotransplantation of teeth, surgical guide
  - Calculating dental age
- Oral pathology
  - Developmental anomalies (impaction, supernumerary teeth, odontomes, etc.)
- Periodontology
  - Bone lesions and healing
- Forensic dentistry
  - Identification, diagnostic accuracy

RECENT ADVANCES OF DENTAL IMAGING

- **Artifical intellegence**: Image analysis using artificial intelligence in dentistry has been applied to various tasks, such as tooth segmentation or localization, bone quality (osteoporosis) assessment, bone age assessment using hand-wrist radiographs, and cephalometric landmark localization. Deep learning systems using CNN structures have been applied in the dental field, and a system that used 3D CBCT images as well as 2D images was developed.[9]

- **Tele radiography**: Teleradiology, a subset of telemedicine, involves the interpretation of diagnostic imaging examinations at a site geographically remote from that of image acquisition. In order to execute this teleradiography both user and sender must be able to produce image that is being viewed by a software system. It helps in interpretation of noninvasive imaging such as digital, MRI,CT, ultrasound and nuclear medicine. Teleradiology networks can result in fewer repeat CT examinations, decreased cumulative radiation exposure in a population, decreased time in an emergency department, and cost savings.[10]
- **Digital Imaging and Communications in Medicine (DICOM)**: It is a common method of transmission for dental radiographic images. It encompass primary and secondary diagnostic images acquired digitally that provides a basis for interoperability of digital system's output. It is a set of collection of instructions that explains format, exchange the information regarding image. DICOM standard was first adopted by medical professional to overcome the difficulty in imaging system communication and in data exchange. Presently in dentistry digital radiographic vendors had adopted it and is universally accepted. DICOM compliant system utilizes common file formats that are universally recognized. Used as contemplating digital image submission to insurance companies.[11]

APPLICATION OF DIGITAL RADIOLOGY IN DENTAL CLINIC

- Digital radiography requires 90% lesser dose compared to E-speed film and image quality can be interactively manipulated after image acquisition, i.e., contrast, blur and noise can be altered digitally.
- Digital imaging allows measuring bone loss extent using image analysis tools. High-resolution technology and/or dedicated endodontic filtering improves the visibility of small file tips as small as 0.06 mm.
- Diagnostic accuracy of the detection of carious lesions is increased by digital contrast enhancement and filtering. Measurements of length, angle, and area can be made on a digital image.
- Digora Optime is fast, automated image processing, optimized image quality, reliable and a maintenance-free design for quality patient care. Users just need to keep inserting the exposed imaging plates into the system.
- Digora Optime is fully automatic and optimized image processing and one unit serves multiple operatories.
- Soredex Digora Optime has Internal UV cleaning system that inactivates viruses and bacteria on the plate transport mechanism making it clinic friendly.
- Nuclear Medicine (NM) imaging is a noninvasive imaging modality which has a potential of detecting various pathologies in the region of head and neck with a high sensitivity, specificity rates for precise diagnosis.
- Newer imaging techniques include ultrasonography, MRI, magnetic resonance sialography, dynamic MRI and quantitative scintigraphy. Their sensitivity and specificity range from 70–95%.
- Dental MRI appears to be a safe tool for 3D imaging without ionizing radiation. However, due to high cost, its use is limited to special cases, specifically indicated for correct diagnosis.
- Ultrasonography and MRI disclose the structure, volume and pathology of the affected glands. Magnetic resonance sialography visualizes the salivary ducts and dynamic. MRI, along with scintigraphy, may provide useful information on the functional status of the salivary glands.
- The use of spiral CT instead of conventional CT for dental multiplanar reconstruction (MPR) because examination time is shorter and patient comfort is improved. Spiral CT can replace conventional CT for maxillofacial imaging.
- Newer diagnostic methods such as computed tomography (CT) and spiral (SCT) or helical CT have emerged as powerful tools for evaluation of root canal morphology.
- Spiral CT provides a better resolution as compared with other scanning methods, such as cone beam CT.
- CBCT has less scanning time, reduced dosage and is less complicated, decreasing anxiety and images obtained are highly magnified along with less distortion.
- High resolution of CBCT helps in detecting variety of cysts, tumors, infections, developmental anomalies and traumatic injuries involving the maxillofacial structures. It has been used extensively for evaluating dental and osseous disease in the jaws and temporomandibular joints and treatment planning for dental implants.

Recent advances in imaging technologies have revolutionized dental diagnostics and treatment planning. Dental imaging technology and interpretation should follow the ALARA (as low as reasonably achievable) principles and cost-effectiveness. Newer radiographic techniques help to detect pathologies in very early stages, which ultimately help to reduce morbidity and mortality and improving the quality of life of the patients.

POINTS TO REMEMBER

- Dr Francis Mouyen in 1981 invented RVG.
- Original system was useful in diagnosis of occlusal and approximal caries only whereas now they have high usage in endodontics.
- RVG comprises four basic components, viz., X-ray set with electronic timer, an intraoral sensor, a DPU, and a printer.
- The original system, which was based on digital hardware without a microprocessor, will be referred to as Mark 1. This was followed by Mark 2; recent development shave resulted in two new RVG (third generation or Mark 3) systems: a "stand-alone"and a "PC" version.
- The advantages of RVG are substantial dose reduction, production of instantaneous images, control of contrast, ability to enlarge specific areas, potential for computer storage, and subsequent transmission of the images.
- Digora was introduced in1994 and the most advantageous aspect of this is the possibility of linear measurements.

- Digora Optime is fast, automated image processing, optimized image quality, reliable and a maintenance-free design for quality patient care. Users just need to keep inserting the exposed imaging plates into the system
- CBCT has less scanning time, reduced dosage and is less complicated, decreasing anxiety and images obtained are highly magnified along with less distortion.
- Newer imaging techniques include ultrasonography, MRI, magnetic resonance sialography, dynamic MRI and quantitative scintigraphy
- Sialography visualizes the salivary ducts and dynamic. MRI, along with scintigraphy, may provide useful information on the functional status of the salivary glands.

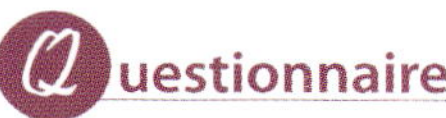

Clinical Significance

Current advancements in radiographic examination eliminate the need for processing image correction and also help in correct diagnosis by providing 3D image of our object. Hence radiographic assessment like CBCT/RVG should be part of routine protocol of treatment.

Questionnaire

1. What are the types of intraoral receptors?
2. Explain the principle of digital imaging.
3. Discuss in detail the components, functions, and uses of RVG.
4. Explain the Digora system.
5. What is nuclear imaging? Various nuclear imaging techniques in dentistry?
6. Write about CBCT and its uses.
7. Recent uses of dental imaging.

REFERENCES

1. Mouyen F, Benz C, Sonnabend E, Lodter JP. Presentation and physical evaluation of RadioVisioGraphy. Oral Surg Oral Med Oral Pathol. 1989;68(2):238-42.
2. Fidanoski B. Digital Radiography. Available from: www.fidanoski.ca/dentistry/ digital-dentalradiography.htm.
3. Madan K, Baliga S, Thosar N, Rathi N. Recent advances in dental radiography for pediatric patients: A review. J Med Radiol Pathol Surg. 2015;1:21-5.
4. Levin LG, Law AS, Holland GR, Abbott PV, Roda RS. Identify and define all diagnostic terms for pulpal health and disease states. J Endod. 2009;35:1645-57
5. Dathar S, Reddy S, Koneru J, Preethi M, Guvvala S. Nuclear Imaging in Dentistry -A novel modality to explore. International J of Health. 2015;3:38-41.
6. Buch SA, Babu SG, Castelino RL, Rao S, Madiyal A, Bhat S. Nuclear imaging in the field of dentistry: A review.
7. Shah N, Bansal N, Logani A. Recent advances in imaging technologies in dentistry. World J Radiol. 2014;6(10):794-807.
8. Heo M, Kim J, Hwang J, Han S, Kim J, Yi W, et al. Artificial intelligence in oral and maxillofacial radiology: what is currently possible?. Dentomaxillofac Radiol. 2021;50:20200375.
9. Whaites E, Brown J. An update on dental imaging. Br Dent J. 1998;185:558-9.
10. Hanna TN, Steenburg SD, Rosenkrantz AB, Pyatt Jr RS, Duszak Jr R, Friedberg EB. Emerging challenges and opportunities in the evolution of teleradiology. American Journal of Roentgenology. 2020;215(6):1411-6.
11. American Dental Association Council on Scientific Affairs. The use of dental radiographs: Update and recommendations. J Am Dent Assoc. 2006;137:1304-12.

FURTHER READING

1. Analoui M, Stookey GK. Direct digital radiography for caries detection and analysis. Monogr Oral Sci. 2000;17:1-19.
2. Borg E, Attaelmanam A, Grondahl HG. Image plate system differ in physical performance. Oral Surg Oral Med Oral Pathol Oral Radiol Endod. 2000;89:118-24.
3. Cederber RA, Tidwell E, Frederiksen NL. Endodontic working length assessment: comparison of PSP and film. Oral Surg Oral Med Oral Pathol Oral Radiol Endod. 1998;85:325-8.
4. De Vos W, et al. Cone-beam computerized tomography (CBCT) imaging of the oral and maxillofacial region: a systematic review of the literature. Int J Oral Maxillofac Surg. 2009;38:609-25.
5. Fossum ER. Active pixel sensors. SPIE. 1993;1900:2-14.
6. Freedman ML, Lurie AG, Reiskin AB (Eds). Advances in oral radiology. St Louis: Mosby-Year Book; 1980.
7. Matteson SR, Deahl ST, Alder ME, Nummikoski PV. Advanced imaging methods. Crit Rev Oral Biol Med. 1996;7:346-95.
8. Merdietio Boedi R, Shepherd S, Mânica S, Franco A. CBCT in dental age estimation: A systematic review and meta-analysis. Dentomaxillofacial Radiology. 202;51:20210335.
9. Miles DA. Imaging using solid state detectors. Dent Clin North Am. 1993;37:531-40.
10. Mouyen M, Benz C, Sonnabend E. Presentation and physical evaluation of radiovisiography. Oral Surg Oral Med Oral Pathol. 1989;68:238-42.
11. Parks ET, Williamson GF. Digital radiography: an overview. J Contemp Dent Pract. 2002;3:23-39.
12. Petrikowski CG. Introducing digital radiography in the dental office: an overview. J Can Dent Assoc. 2005;71:651.
13. Russell M, Pitts NB. Radiovisiography: an update. Dent Update. 1993. pp.141-4.
14. Sanderink GC, Miles DA. Intraoral detectors. Applications of digital imaging modalities of dentistry. Dent Clin North Am. 2000;44:249-55.
15. Swennen GRJ, Schutyser F. Three-dimensional cephalometry: spiral multislice vs cone-beam computed tomography. Am J Orthod Dentofacial Orthop. 2006;130:410-6.
16. Van der Stelt PF. Digital radiology using the Digora registration technique. Rev Belge Med Dent (1984). 1996;51:93-100.
17. Van der Stelt PF. Digital radiology: deficiency, failures and other adventures. Dentomaxillofac Radiol. 1995;24:67-8.
18. Van der Stelt PF. Improved diagnosis with digital radiography. Editorial review. Orthodnt Pedodont. 1992;2:1-6.
19. Vannier MW. Craniofacial computed tomography scanning: technology, applications and future trends. Orthod Craniofac Res. 2003:6:23-30, discussion 179-82.
20. Versteeg CH, Sanderink GC, Van der Stelt PF. Efficacy of digital intra-oral radiography in clinical dentistry. J Dent. 1997;25:215-24.
21. Wallace JA, Nair MK, Colaco MF. Comparative evaluation of diagnostic efficacy of film and digital sensors for detection of simulated periapical lesions. Oral Surg Oral Med Oral Pathol Oral Radiol Endod. 2001;92:93-7.
22. Wenzel A. Digital radiography and caries diagnosis. Dentomaxillofac Radiol. 1998;27:3-11.

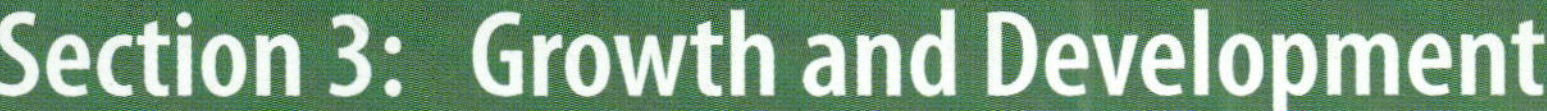

CHAPTER 10

Developmental Milestones in Children

Ravi GR, Nikhil Marwah

CHAPTER OUTLINE

Infancy and childhood are dynamic periods of growth and development wherein the neural and physical growth proceed in a sequential and predictable pattern under the influence of predetermined intrinsic factors. The skills progress from cephalic to caudal; from proximal to distal; and from generalized, stimulus-based reflexes to specific, goal-oriented reactions that become increasingly precise. By convention, these neurodevelopmental "laws" or sequences often are described in terms of the traditional developmental milestones.

The different types of developmental milestones include gross motor, fine motor, problem-solving, receptive language, expressive language, and social-emotional milestones. These milestones provide a framework for observing and monitoring a child over time. A thorough understanding of the normal or typical sequence of development in all these domains will aid the clinician to derive a correct overall impression of a child's true developmental status.

Although neurodevelopment follows a predictable course, yet each child's developmental path is unique due to the variations produced by both the intrinsic and extrinsic forces. Intrinsic influences include genetically determined attributes (e.g., physical characteristics, temperament) as well as the child's overall state of wellness. Extrinsic influences during infancy and childhood originate primarily from the family. Parent and sibling personalities, the nurturing methods used by caregivers, the cultural environment, and the family's socioeconomic status with its effect on resources of time and money all play a role in the development of children.

GROSS MOTOR MILESTONES (TABLE 10.1)

- The ultimate goal of gross motor development is to gain independent and volitional movement.
- During gestation, primitive reflexes develop and persist for several months after birth to prepare the infant for the acquisition of specific skills.

Table 10.1: Key development milestones: Gross motor.

Age (months)	*Milestone*
3	Neck holding
5	Sitting with support
8	Sitting without support
9	Standing with support
10	Walking with support
11	crawling (creeping)
12	Standing without support
13	Walking without support
18	Running
24	Walking upstairs
36	Riding tricycle

Neonatal reflexes		
Neonatal reflexes are inborn reflexes which are present at birth and occur in a predictable fashion. A normally developing newborn should respond to certain stimuli with these reflexes, which eventually become inhibited as the child matures		
Name of reflex	***Explanation***	***Appearance and exit***
Rooting reflex	Gently stroke the infant from the lips to the cheek and the normal response of the infant is to turn his head toward the stimulated side with the mouth opening	Appears at birth and is inhibited between 6 and 12 months of age
Moro reflex	This is stimulated by a sudden movement or loud noise. the neonate will respond by throwing out the arms and legs and then pulling them toward the body	Emerges in 8–9 weeks in utero, and is inhibited by 16 weeks of age
Sucking reflex	When a finger or nipple is placed in the infant's mouth, it responds by rhythmical sucking	Onset is 28 weeks of gestation
Palmer reflex	Stimulated when an object is placed into the baby's palm. A neonate responds by grasping the object	This reflex emerges 11 weeks in utero and is inhibited 2–3 months after birth
Babinski reflex	Stimulated by stroking the sole of the foot, which results in toes of the foot should fan out and the foot itself should curl in	Emerges at 18 weeks in utero and disappears by 6 months after birth
Asymmetric Tonic neck reflex	When we gently turn the infant's head to one side, a the flexion tone on the side opposite to the head turn with an increase in the extensor tone in the side to which the head is turned	This reflex is present at 18 weeks in utero and disappears by 6 months after birth
Tonic labyrinthine reflex	Arms and legs extend when head moves backward (away from spine), and will curl in when the head moves forward	Emerges in utero until 4 months postnatally
Galant reflex	When the neonates back is stimulated, their trunk and hips should move toward the side of the stimulus	This reflex emerges 20 weeks in utero and is inhibited by 9 months
Landau reflex	When neonate is placed on stomach, their back arches and head raises	Emerges at 3 months postnatally and lasts until the child is 12 months old

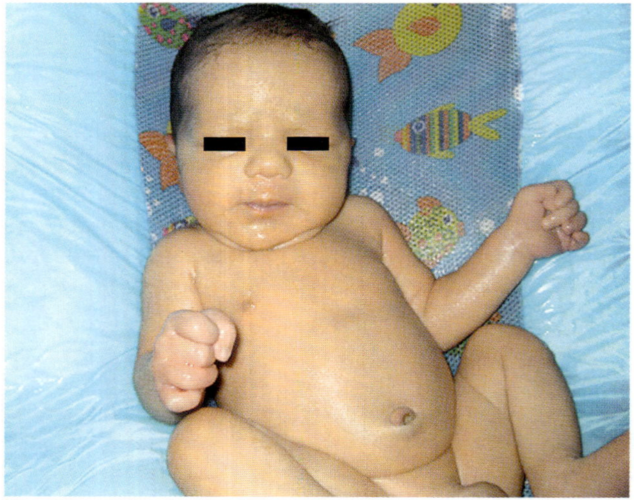

Fig. 10.1: Moro reflex: This reflex occurs spontaneously to loud noises which produces sudden extension and abduction of the upper extremities with hands open, followed by flexion of the upper extremities to midline (the "startle reflex").

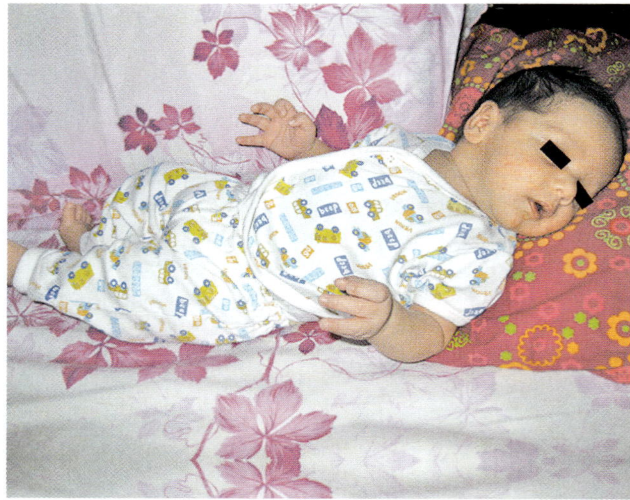

Fig. 10.2: Asymmetric tonic neck reflex (AtnR). With active or passive head rotation, the baby extends the arm and leg on the face side and flexes the extremities on the contralateral side (the "fencer posture").

- These brainstem and spinal reflexes are stereotypic movements generated in response to specific sensory stimuli. Examples include the Moro **(Fig. 10.1)**, asymmetric tonic neck **(Fig. 10.2)**, and positive support reflexes.
- As the central nervous system matures, these reflexes are inhibited which in turn enables the infant to make purposeful movements. For example, Moro reflex interferes with head control and sitting equilibrium. As this reflex lessens and disappears by 6 months of age, the infant gains progressive stability in a seated position **(Fig. 10.3).**
- Higher cortical centers mediate the development of equilibrium responses and permit the infant to pull to stand by 9 months of age **(Fig. 10.4)** and begin walking by 13 months. Additional equilibrium responses develop during the second year after birth to allow for more complex bipedal movements, such as moving backward, running, and jumping.
- By 18 months of age, a child can do a well-coordinated movement that includes rapid change of direction and speed **(Fig. 10.5)**. Simultaneous use of both arms and legs occurs after successful use of each limb independently.
- At age 2 years, a child can kick a ball, jump with two feet off the floor, and throw a big ball overhand **(Fig. 10.6).**

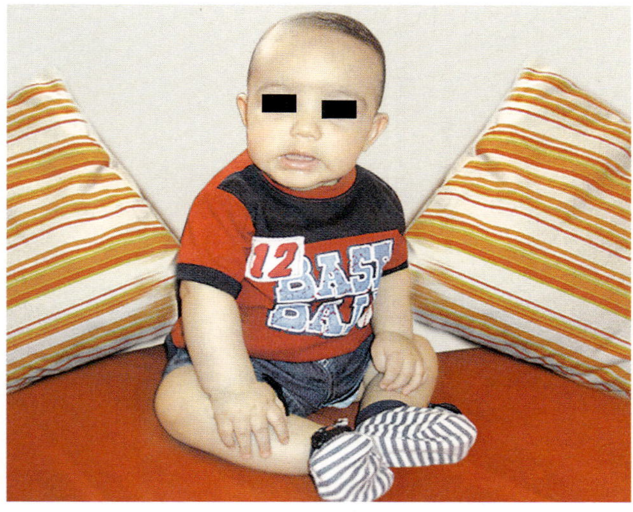

Fig. 10.3: Stable seating position (6 months).

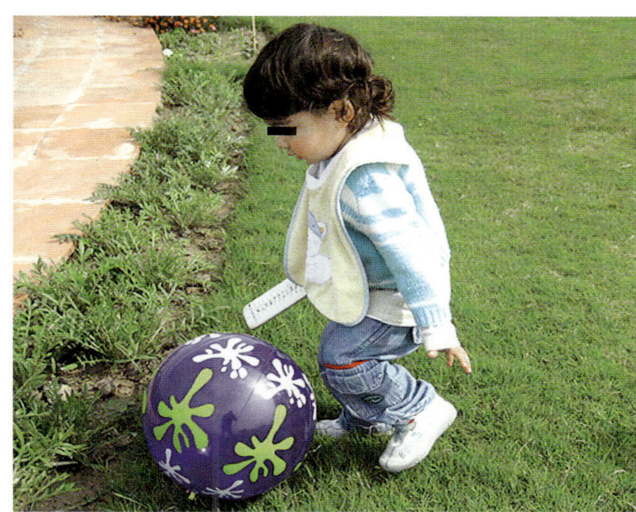

Fig. 10.6: Kick ball and play (2 years).

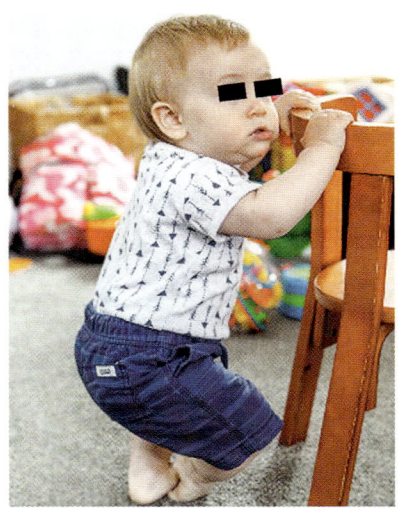

Fig. 10.4: Child takes support to stand up (9 months). *(Source:* Reprinted with permission from ©Heinz Wattie's).

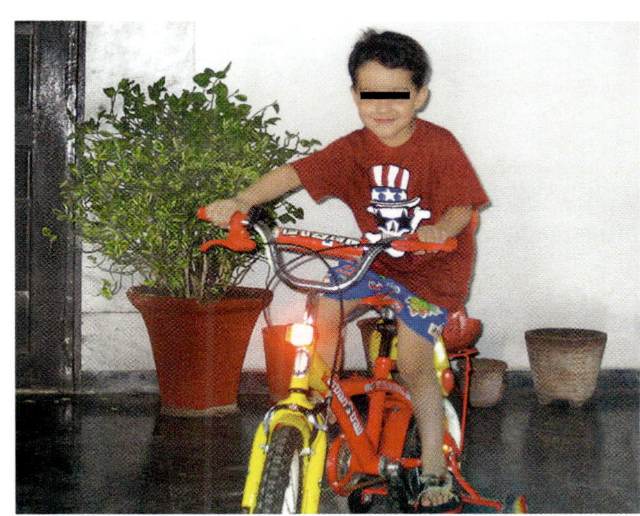

Fig. 10.7: Maintaining balance, steering on a bicycle.

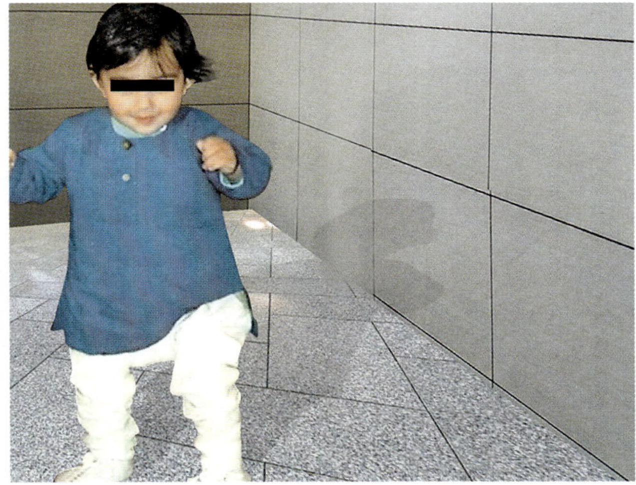

Fig. 10.5: Ability of child to do multidirectional movement (18 months).

- By the time a child starts school, he/she is able to perform multiple complex gross motor tasks simultaneously (such as pedaling, maintaining balance, and steering while on a bicycle) **(Fig. 10.7).**
- During the first postnatal year, an infant thus moves from lying prone, to rolling over, to getting to hands and knees, and ultimately to coming to a seated position or pulling to stand **(Fig. 10.8)**.

FINE MOTOR MILESTONES (TABLE 10.2)

- Fine motor skills are concerned with the use of the upper extremities to engage and manipulate the environment. These skills are necessary to perform self-help tasks, to play, and to accomplish work
- At birth, infants do not have any apparent voluntary use of their hands. They open and close them in response

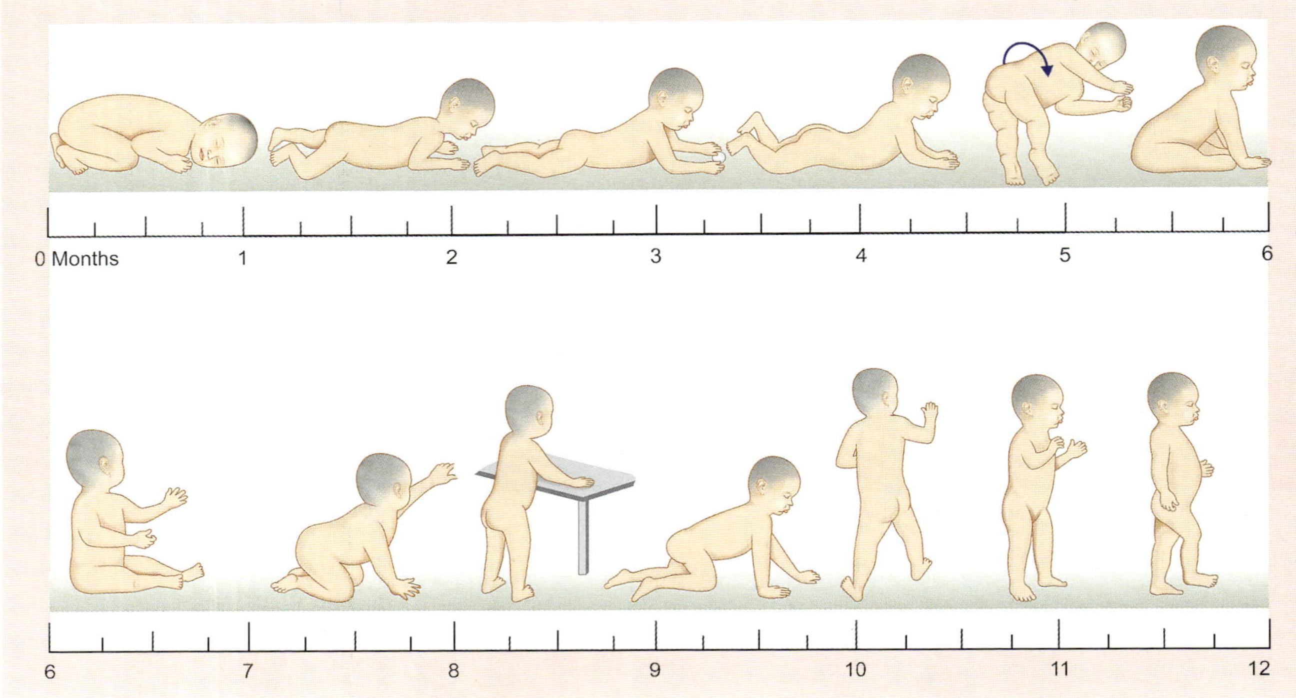

Fig. 10.8: Chronologic progression of gross motor development.

Table 10.2: Key development milestones: Fine motor.

Age (months)	*Milestone*
4	Grasps a rattle or rings when placed in hand
5	Reached out to an object and hold it with both hands (international reaching with bidextrous grasp)
7	Holding objects with crude grasp from palm (palmar grasp)
9	Holding small object, like a pellet, between index finger and thumb (pincer grasp)

to touch and other stimuli, but movement otherwise is dominated by a primitive grasp reflex **(Fig. 10.9).**

- As the primitive reflexes decrease, infants begin to prehend objects voluntarily, first using the entire palm toward the ulnar side (5 months) and then predominantly using the radial aspect of the palm (7 months) **(Fig. 10.10).**
- Infant learns to transfer objects from one hand to the other, first using the mouth as an intermediate stage (5 months) and then directly hand to hand (6 months). Between 6 and 12 months of age, the grasp evolves to allow for prehension of objects of different shapes and sizes. The thumb becomes more involved to grasp objects, using all four fingers against the thumb (a "scissors" grasp) at 7 months, and eventually to just two fingers and thumb (radial digital grasp) at 9 months. A pincer grasp emerges as the ulnar fingers are inhibited while slightly extending and supinating the wrist. By 10 months of age, infants can release a cube into a container or drop things onto the floor **(Fig. 10.11).**
- As infants move into their second year, their mastery of the reach, grasp, and release allows them to start using objects as tools. Fine motor development becomes more closely associated with cognitive and adaptive

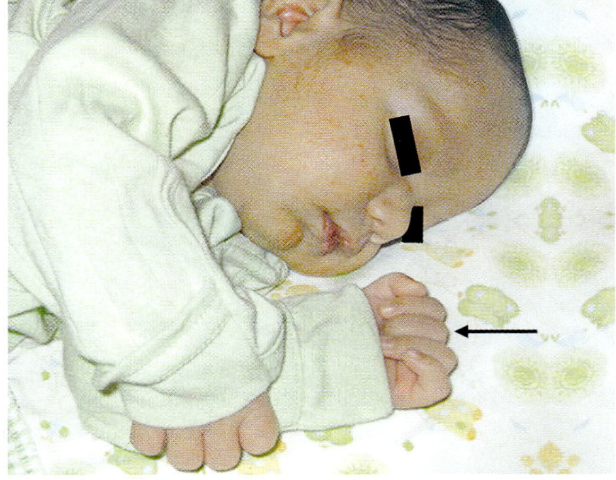

Fig. 10.9: Primitive grasp reflex.

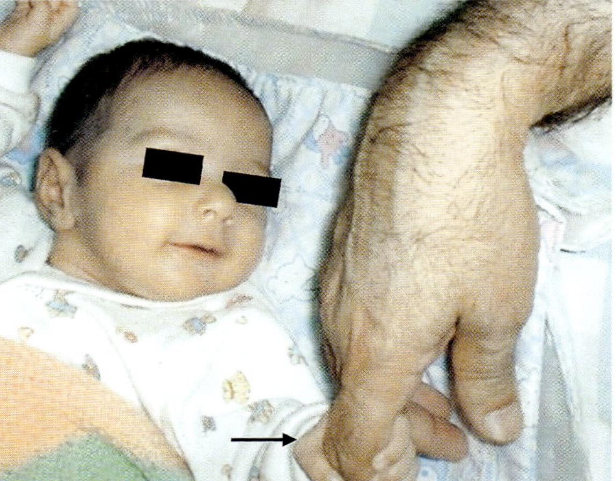

Fig. 10.10: Firm grasp (5 months).

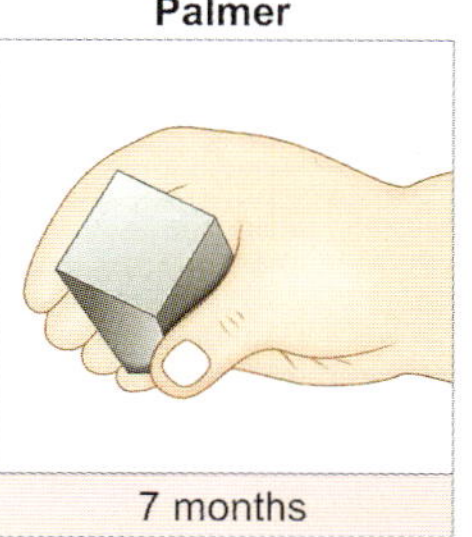

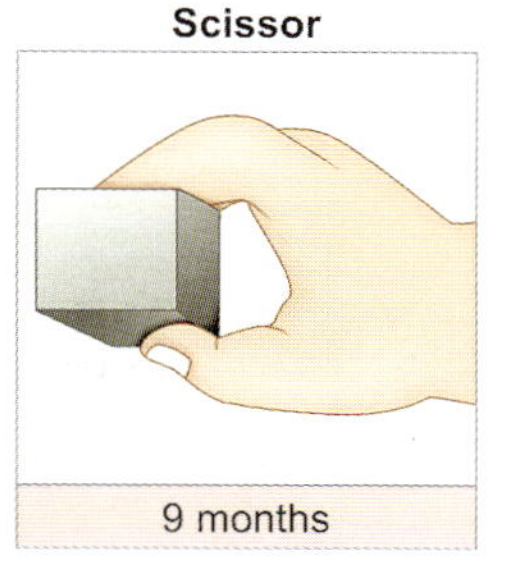

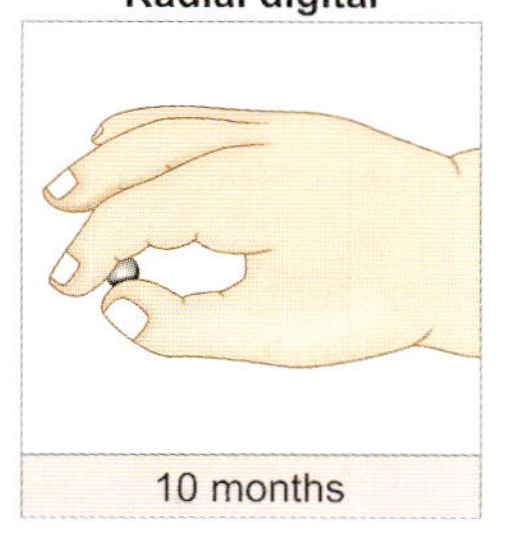

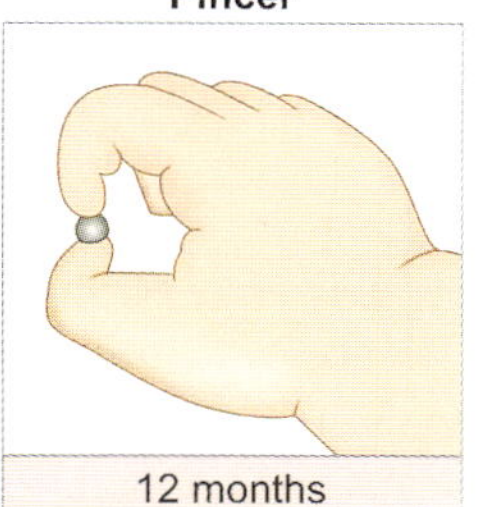

Fig. 10.11: Development of grasp.

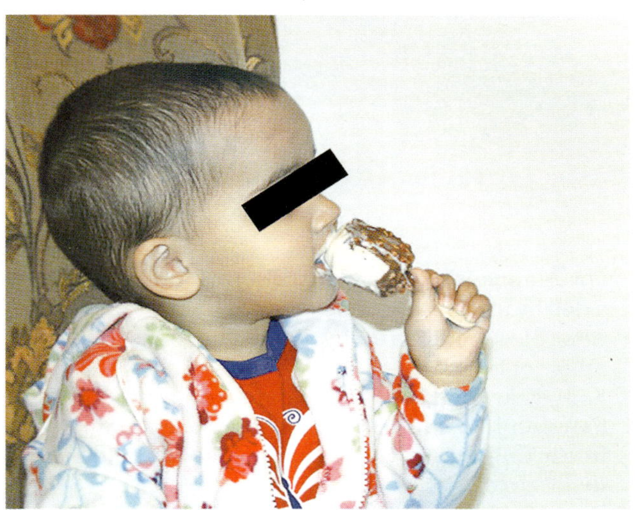

Fig. 10.12: Independent eating (20 months).

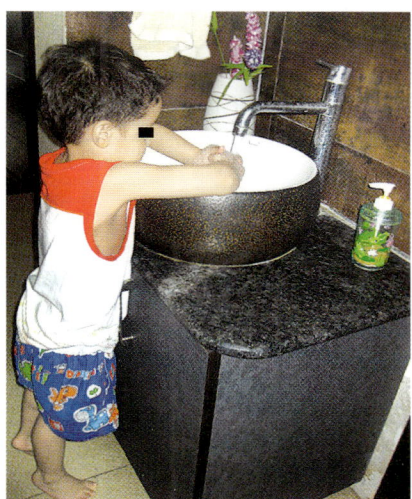

Fig. 10.13: Washing hand independently.

development, with the infant knowing both what he/she wants to do and how he/she can accomplish it. Intrinsic muscle refinement allows for holding flat objects, such as crackers or cookies. By 15 months of age, voluntary release has developed further to enable stacking of three to four blocks and releasing small objects into containers. The child starts to adjust objects after grasping to use them properly, such as picking up a crayon and adjusting it to scribble spontaneously (18 months of age) and adjusting a spoon to use it consistently for eating (20 months of age) **(Fig. 10.12).**

- By 36 months of age, they can draw a circle, put on shoes, and stack 10 blocks. They make snips with scissors by alternating between full-finger extension and flexion. Their grasp and in-hand manipulation skills allow them to string small beads and unbutton clothes and wash hands independently **(Fig. 10.13).**
- By the age of 5 years, child can dress and undress independently, brush the teeth well, and spread with a knife **(Fig. 10.14).**

LANGUAGE MILESTONES (TABLE 10.3)

- Infants communicate long before they speak their first words or phrases. At birth, crying is the primary form of communication. It is nonspecific but very effective in initiating a response from a caregiver.
- In a trial-and-error process, the infant begins making vowel and consonant sounds that she can put together into

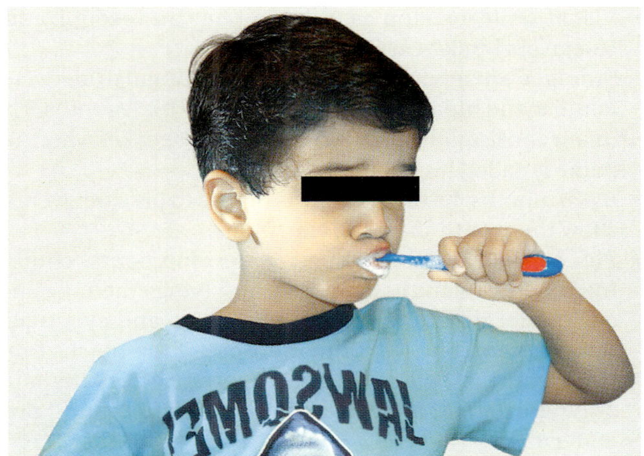

Fig. 10.14: Brushing independently (5 years).

Table 10.3: Key development milestones: Language.

Age (months)	*Milestone*
1	Turns head to sound
3	Cooing
6	Monosyllables ("ma,""ba")
9	Bisyllables ("mama,""baba")
12	Two words with meaning
18	Ten words with meaning
24	Simple sentence
36	Telling a story

"mama" and "dada" by 9 months of age. Although she is not using the words discriminately, if her caregivers respond to the sounds she makes, she will continue to use them.

- By the first birthday, the child can say her first word and can point to communicate a request.
- By 15 months, the toddler is able to give a clear "no" with a headshake. His ability to imitate sounds increases, and he can repeat an entire word and even mimic environmental sounds.
- By 18–24 months of age, he is starting to use pronouns such as "me," and his vocabulary has expanded to 50 words. New words are learnt quickly, and he begins to combine them into two-word phrases (noun–verb). He now is able to communicate basic wants ("more drink") and social interest ("bye, mama").
- Between 2 and 3 years of age, his vocabulary continues to increase, and the phrases he uses increase to three to four words in length.

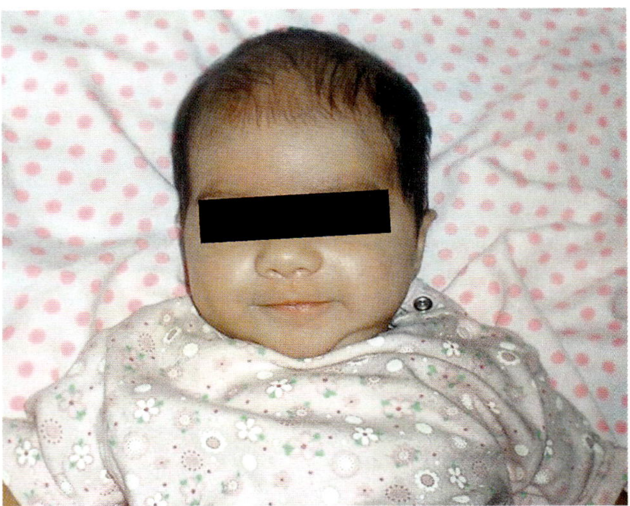

Fig. 10.15: Social smile (3 months).

SOCIAL MILESTONES (TABLE 10.4)

- Most children are born with an inherent drive to connect with others and share feelings, thoughts, and actions.
- The earliest social milestone is the bonding of a caregiver with the infant, characterized by the caregiver's feelings for the child. The infant learns to discriminate his mother's voice during the first month after birth.
- The first measurable social milestone is the smile. The infant smiles at first in response to high-pitched vocalizations ("baby talk") and a smile from his caregiver, but over time, less and less stimulation is required **(Fig. 10.15)**.
- Visual skills develop as well, and he can recognize his caregivers by sight at 5 months.
- Stranger anxiety, or the ability to distinguish between familiar and unfamiliar people, emerges by 6 months. The infant consistently turns her head to the speaker when her name is called by 10 months.
- By 18 months, he brings objects or toys to his caregivers to show them or to share the experience.
- Play skills also follow a specific developmental course. Initially, an infant holds blocks and bangs them against each other or on the table, drops them, and eventually throws them. She learns that dropping the blocks from her high chair will cause her caregiver to pick them up and return them to her; so she repeats this "game" over and over.
- By 18 months, she engages in simple pretend play, such as using miniature representative items in a correct fashion. For example, she pretends to talk on a toy phone or "feeds" a doll by using a toy spoon or bottle.
- After his second birthday, the child begins to play with others of his own age.
- Four-year olds usually have mastered the difference between real and imaginary. They become interested in tricking others and concerned about being tricked themselves.
- By age 5 years, children have learnt many adult social skills, such as giving a positive comment in response to another's good fortune, apologizing for unintentional mistakes, and relating to a group of friends.

Table 10.4: Key development milestones: Personal social.

Age	*Milestone*
2 months	Social smile
3 months	Recognizing mother
6 months	Smile at mirror image
9 months	Waves "bye-bye"
12 months (1 year)	Plays a simple ball game
36 months (3 years)	Knows gender

EMOTIONAL MILESTONES

- Coinciding with the development of social skills is a child's emotional development.
- As early as birth, all children demonstrate individual characteristics and patterns of behavior that constitute that individual child's temperament. Temperament influences how an infant responds to routine activities, such as feeding, dressing, playing, and going to sleep.
- Emotional development involves three specific elements: neural processes to relay information about the environment to the brain, mental processes that generate feelings, and motor actions that include facial expressions, speech, and purposeful movements.
- Studies have demonstrated that three distinct emotions are present from birth: anger, joy, and fear. All infants demonstrate universal facial expressions that reveal these emotions, although they do not use these expressions discriminately before the age of 3 months.
- At 15 months, a child demonstrates empathy by looking sad when she sees someone else cry. She also develops self-conscious emotions (embarrassment, shame, pride) as she evaluates her own behavior in the context of the social environment. Having once performed cute tricks on demand, she suddenly seems embarrassed and refuses to perform when she realizes that others are watching.

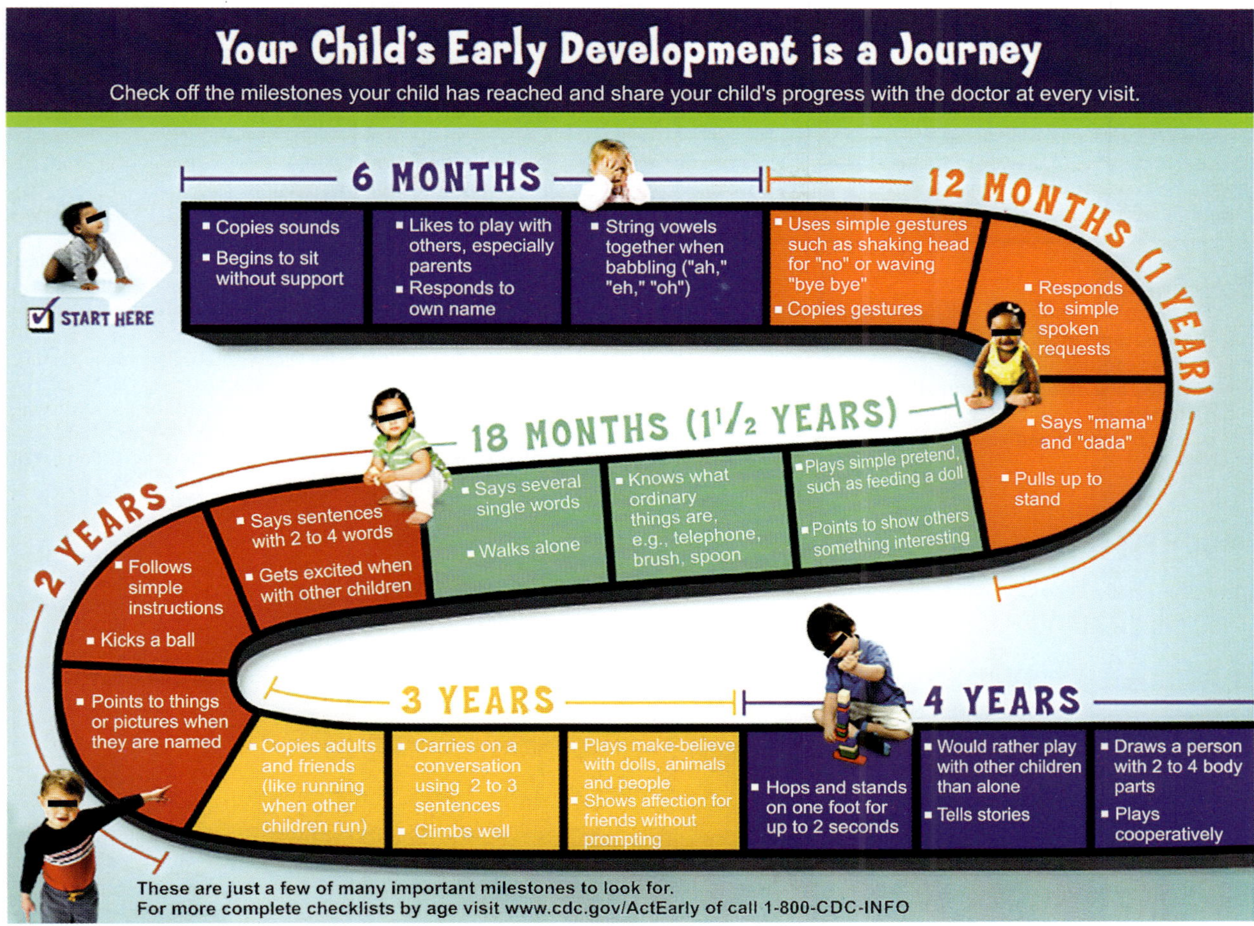

Fig. 10.16: Developmental milestones checklist of children. (*Source:* With permission from www.cdc.gov/Actearly).

- By age 2 years, he starts to mask emotions for social etiquette. During the preschool years, children learn more and more behavioral strategies to manage their emotions, depending on a given situation. They begin to understand that their expressed emotion—whether a facial, vocal, or behavioral expression—does not necessarily need to match their subjective emotional experience.
- Children learn to substitute their expressions (smile and say "thank you" even though they are disappointed in the birthday present), amplify expressions (exaggerate a painful response to get sympathy), neutralize expression (put on a "poker face" to hide true feelings), or minimize emotion (look mildly upset when feeling extremely angry).

POINTS TO REMEMBER

- Developmental milestones provide a valuable framework with which the pediatrician can appropriately evaluate and observe children over time.
- The development of motor skills is critical for a child to move independently and to interact with his/her environment meaningfully and usefully.
- Skills develop in a cephalic-to-caudal progression and from proximal to distal.
- Skills also progress from generalized responses to stimuli (primitive reflexes) to goal-oriented, purposeful actions with ever-increasing precision and dexterity.
- The development of a child from infancy to preschool years is truly remarkable. As with physical growth, neurodevelopment proceeds in a sequential and predictable fashion that can be observed, measured, and followed over time.
- As the children grow, they change from completely being dependent entirely on their caregivers to small beings with independent movement, complex language, and problem-solving skills, as well as the ability to interact in positive and productive ways with others.
- Children thus become well-suited for the next phase of development, characterized by academic achievement and more complex problem-solving and thinking skills.

Clinical Significance

- Importance of developmental milestones is crucially understood as dentist has to evaluate the mental and physical development of child in case of milestone delays.
- The uncooperative behavior of a child below 3 years of age should be considered as normal due to lack of fully developed cognitive skills.

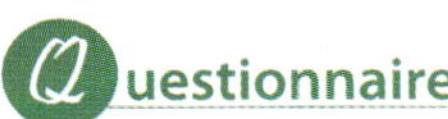

Questionnaire

1. Explain the gross motor milestone developments in a child from birth to 4 years.
2. Explain the fine motor milestone developments in a child from birth to 4 years.
3. What are the social and emotional milestones from birth to 4 years?

FURTHER READING

1. Canadian Family. Developmental milestones charts. http:// www. canadianfamily.ca/milestone0-1/http://www.cdc.gov/ actearly.
2. Developmental milestones: chart of early childhood development IMM5738.
3. Gerber RJ, Wilks T, Erdie-Lalena C. Developmental milestones: cognitive developments. Pediatr Rev. 2010;31:364.
4. Gerber RJ, Wilks T, Erdie-Lalena C. Developmental milestones: motor developments. Pediatr Rev. 2010;31:267.
5. Gerber RJ, Wilks T, Erdie-Lalena C. Developmental milestones: social-emotional developments. Pediatr Rev. 2011;32:533.
6. Lipsitt LP. Learning and emotion in infants. Pediatrics. 1998;102: 1262-7.
7. NIDCD fact sheet: speech and language developmental milestones. US Department of Health and Human Services. National Institutes of Health. National Institute on Deafness and other Communication disorders.
8. Poon JK, Larosa AC, Pai GS. Developmental delay: timely identification and assessment. Indian Pediatr. 2010;47:415-21.
9. WHO. Assessment of motor development. http://www.who. int/ childgrowth/standard/motor_milestones/en/index. html.
10. Zeman JC, Perry-Parish C, Stegall S. Emotion regulation in children and adolescents. J Dev Behav Pediatr. 2006;27: 155-68.

CHAPTER

Theories of Growth

Nikhil Marwah, Rishi Tyagi, Pallavi Pawar, Lumbini Pathivada

CHAPTER OUTLINE

- Bone Remodeling Theory
- Genetic Theory/Genetic Blueprint
- Sutural Dominance Theory/Weinmann Sicher's Hypothesis
- James Scott's Hypothesis/Cartilaginous Theory/Nasal Septum Theory
- Functional Matrix Concept/Moss Hypothesis
- Van Limborg's Concept
- Cybernetics/Servo-System Theory
- Neurotrophism
- Enlow's Expanding "V" Principle
- Functional Matrix Hypothesis Revisited

Facial growth and development is a morphogenic process working toward a composite state of aggregate structural and functional balance among the entire multiple, regional growth centers and changing hard and soft tissue body parts. The same underlying process continues to work in order to sustain ongoing equilibrium throughout adulthood in response to ever-changing internal and external conditions and relationships.

The processes commonly referred to as growth and development in multicellular organisms is an extraordinary complex and ordered program of changes that occur during the development of a mature being from the fertilized egg. Throughout the time from fertilization to maturation and subsequently to senescence, a broad range of diverse functions are simultaneously orchestrated to produce the harmonious pattern of normal development.

DEFINITIONS

Growth

It is a dynamic process with stable pattern of changes resulting in the increase in physical change of mass during the course of development. It has been defined by a number of authors as:

- **Stewart** (1982): *Defined as developmental increase in mass.*
- **Proffit** (1986): *Growth refers to increase in size or number.*
- **Moyer** (1988): *Changes in amount of living substance.*
- **Moyer:** *Quantitative aspect of biologic development per unit time.*
- **Moss:** *Change in any morphological parameter which is measurable.*
- **Todd** (1931): *Growth refers to increase in size.*
- **JS Huxley:** *Self-multiplication of living substance.*
- ***Krogman:*** Increase in size, change in proportion and progressive complexity.

Development

It is defined as:

- **Todd** (1931): *Increase in complexity.*
- **Todd** (1931): *Progress toward maturity.*
- **Moyers** (1988): *Naturally occurring unidirectional changes in the life of an individual from its existence as a single cell to its elaboration as a multifunctional unit terminating in death.*
- **Pinkham** (1994): *Development addresses the progressive development of a tissue.*
- **Enlow:** *A maturational process involving progressive differentiation at the cellular and tissue levels.*

Theory

A set of ideas formulated to explain something—an opinion; a supposition.

Concept

An idea; a general notion.

Hypothesis

A supposition put forward as a basis for reasoning or investigation.

Principle

General truth used as a basis of action.

THEORIES OF GROWTH

Initially, all the attempts to understand the concept of growth were at a simpler genetic level. It is a well-known concept that growth is strongly influenced by genetic factors, but we must not forget the role of environment on the same. Until recently, the explanations for growth control process were regarded as more or less complete, with theories underlying them secure. This has now changed and we are beginning to recognize the problems that are involved with them, and the concept of growth control has changed and has been re-evaluated. The theories of growth need to be evaluated in order to understand the etiological process of malocclusion and dentofacial deformities and to learn the influence on facial growth. Some of the major theories that have been postulated over the years are:

- Bone remodeling theory—**Brash**, 1930
- Genetic theory—**Brodie**, 1940
- Sutural dominance theory—**Sicher and Weinmann**, 1941
- Scott's cartilaginous theory—**Scott**, 1950
- Functional matrix concept—**Moss**, 1962
- Van Limborg's concept—**Von Limborg**, 1970
- Cybernetics—**Petrovic, Stutzman**, 1974

Other theories related to craniofacial growth are:

- Enlow's expanding "V" principle
- Enlow's counterpart principle
- Neurotrophic process in orofacial growth.
- Modern Composite Theory[1]
- Growth Relativity Hypothesis[1]

BONE REMODELING THEORY (BRASH, 1930)

- The research by **Brash** on bone provided the foundation for the development of the first general theory of craniofacial growth—the bone remodeling theory.
- Principle
  - Bone only grows appositionally at surfaces **(Fig. 11.1)**.
  - Growth of jaws is characterized by deposition of bone at posterior surface of maxilla and mandible. Sometimes described as "Hunterian growth of the jaws".
  - Postulated that all of craniofacial skeletal growth occurs exclusively by bone remodeling—selective addition and resorption of bone at its surfaces.
  - Failed to explain the role of unique structures such as sutures, cranial bone synchondroses, and the mandibular condylar cartilage provide in growth of craniofacial skeleton.

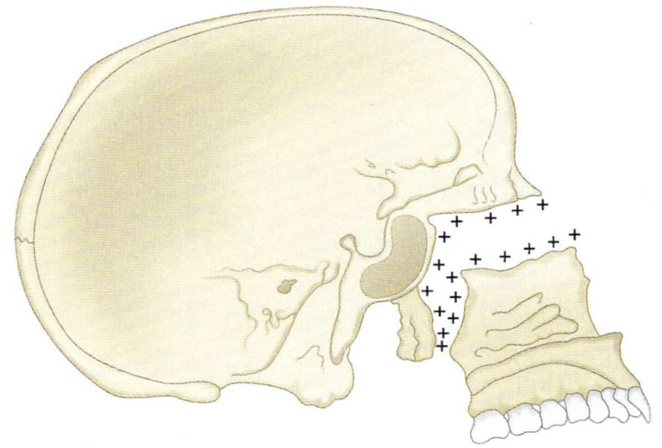

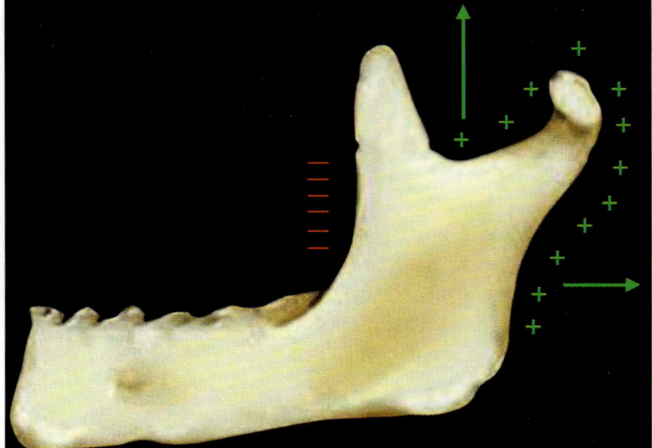

Fig. 11.1: Bone remodeling theory.

GENETIC THEORY/GENETIC BLUEPRINT (ALLAN G BRODIE, 1940)

- This theory had proposed that genes control all the functions of growth and development.
- The role of genetic programming has long been presumed by many to have a fundamental and perhaps overriding influence in establishing the basic facial pattern **(Fig. 11.2)**.
- Epigenetic regulation can determine the behavioral growth activities of certain tissues.[2]

Example to support this theory[3]

Blending of data from vertebral paleontology created the neo-darwinism synthesis which is currently accepted paradigm of phylogenetic regulation.

Examples against this theory

- It failed in understanding the mechanism by which the traits are transmitted at that time.
- It did not take into account the effects of environment in growth.

SUTURAL DOMINANCE THEORY/WEINMANN SICHER'S HYPOTHESIS (SICHER, 1941)

- **Sicher** proposed that sutures cause most of craniofacial growth, and to support his theory, he conducted some experiments using vital dyes.
- He said that primary event was proliferation of connective tissue between two bones leading to appositional growth.
- **Sicher** felt that connective tissue in sutures of vault and nasomaxillary complex produced forces that separate the bones and cause expansion.

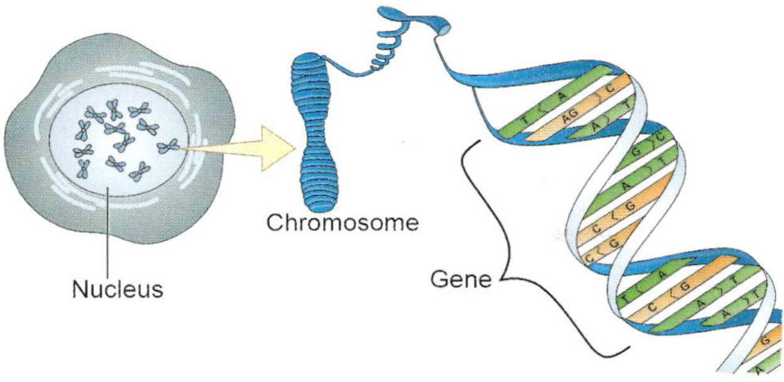

Fig. 11.2: Genetic theory.

Examples to support this theory

- If sutures are pulled apart, bone fills in, and if sutures are compressed, then there is impeded growth.

Examples against this theory

- Sutures when transplanted from face to abdominal pouch do not grow.
- Presence of forces triggers bone resorption and not deposition.
- Growth can be seen in cases of untreated cleft palate patients even in absence of sutures.
- Thus, we can conclude that sutures are not primary determinants of growth and are just the growth sites.

JAMES SCOTT'S HYPOTHESIS/CARTILAGINOUS THEORY/ NASAL SEPTUM THEORY (SCOTT, 1950)

- **James Scott** an Irish anatomist proposed that cartilaginous nasal septum has features and occupies a strategic position that might cause the midfacial region to displace rather than the sutures.
- Because the cartilage is more pressure tolerant, it has more capacity to push the nasomaxillary complex downward and forward, thus giving rise to the nasal septum theory.
- This theory states that determinant of craniofacial growth is by growth of cartilages **(Fig. 11.3).**
- The fact that cartilage does not grow while bone merely replaces it makes this theory attractive.

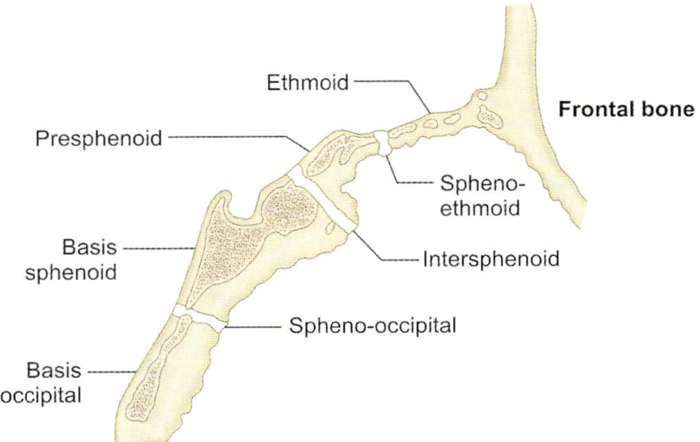

Fig. 11.3: Diagram of synchondrosis of cranial base showing growth site.

Examples to support this theory

- Although there is no cartilage in maxilla, there is a cartilage in nasal septum and this nasomaxillary complex grows as a unit.
- Nasal septum and epiphyseal cartilages continue to grow when implanted in cultures thus showing their innate growth potential.
- Removal of nasal septum leads to midfacial deformities.

Examples against this theory

- Mandibular condylar cartilage does not grow in culture showing that there are some cartilages that are not growth centers but are just sites of growth.
- In case of injury, mandibular condyle resorbs, but if it is the growth stimulator, then it should grow back after injury.

FUNCTIONAL MATRIX CONCEPT/MOSS HYPOTHESIS (MELVIN MOSS, 1962)

This theory was introduced by **Melvin Moss** *based on the functional cranial component by* **Van Der Klaaus.**

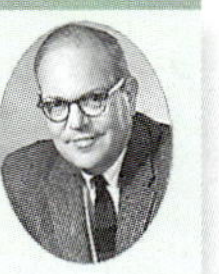

- This theory claimed that the control for growth was not in cartilage or bone but in adjacent soft tissues thus emphasizing that neither the nasal septum nor the mandibular condyle are determinants of growth. He theorizes that growth of face occurs as a response to functional needs and is mediated by the soft tissues in which jaws are embedded.
- The *functional matrix hypothesis* (FMH) claims that the origin, form, position, growth, and maintenance of all skeletal tissues and organs are always secondary, compensatory, and necessary response to chronologically and morphologically prior events or processes that occur in specifically related nonskeletal tissues, organs, or functioning spaces.
- A large number of functions are carried out independently in the craniofacial region like respiration, olfaction, hearing, chewing, etc. Each of these is carried out by a functional cranial component **(Flowchart 11.1)** which can be divided into functional matrix and skeletal unit **(Fig. 11.4).**

Flowchart 11.1: Algorithm showing functional cranial component.

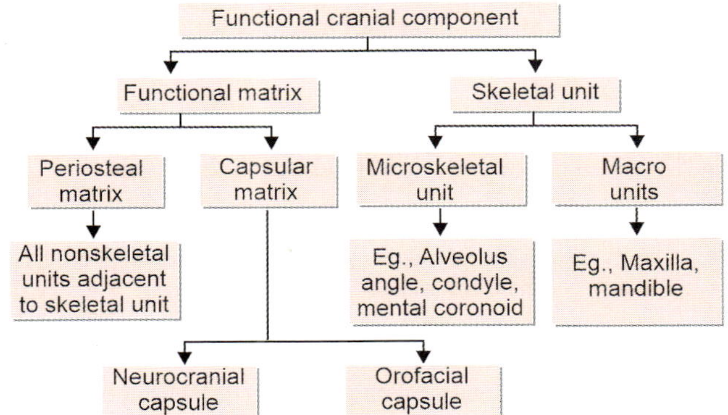

Functional Matrix

This consists of teeth, organs, glands, muscles, nerves, and vessels as well as nonskeletal cartilages. It is divided into periosteal and capsular matrix:

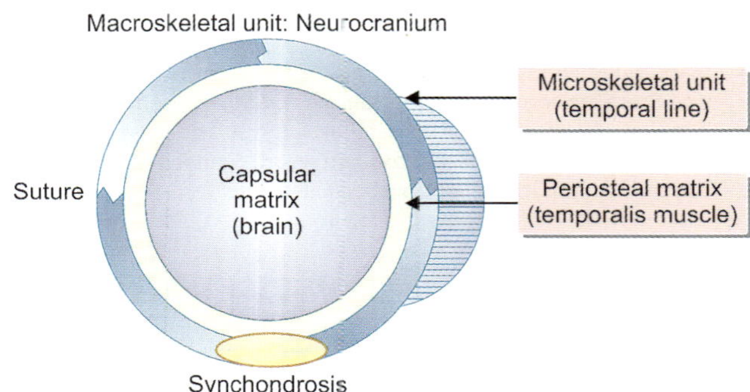

Fig. 11.4: Diagrammatic display of functional matrix theory.

Periosteal Matrix

- All nonskeletal units adjacent to skeletal units.
- Act directly and actively upon their related skeletal units producing a secondary compensatory transformation.

Capsular Matrix

- **Neurocranial capsule:**
  - Sandwiched between skin and dura mater.
  - Act indirectly and passively upon their related skeletal units producing a secondary compensatory translation.
  - Expansion of capsule takes place and the skeletal units move in the expanded capsule thus giving translative growth without deposition and resorption.
- **Orofacial capsule:**
  - Surround and protect oronasopharyngeal space.
  - Volumetric growth of these spaces is the primary morphogenic event in facial growth.

Skeletal Unit

This skeletal unit may be comprised of bone, cartilage, or tendon. All skeletal tissues are related to a specific functional matrix, that is, all skeletal tissues are associated with a single function.

Microskeletal Unit

- Bones consisting of number of small skeletal units.
- When a combination of several bones makes up this unit, it is called microskeletal unit like mandible.

Macroskeletal Unit

When there is a contribution of parts of many adjacent bones, such a unit is called macroskeletal unit like maxilla.[4]

Examples to support this theory
- Growth of cranial vault is directly a response of growth of brain.
- Enlarged or small eye will correspondingly change the size of orbit.

Example against this theory
- In hydrocephalic patients, the size of brain is small but the cranial vault is bigger.

VAN LIMBORG'S CONCEPT (VAN LIMBORG, 1970)

- According to him, all the previous theories were not complete and acceptable, but each had some elements of significance that cannot be denied.
- This made him postulate **Van Limborg's** multifactorial theory.
- This theory suggested five factors that control growth:
  1. *Intrinsic genetic factors:* Genetic control of the skeletal units themselves.
  2. *Local epigenetic factors:* Bone growth is determined by genetic control originating from adjacent factors like brains, eyes, etc.
  3. *General epigenetic factors:* Genetic factors determining growth from distant structures like growth hormones, sex hormones, etc.
  4. *Local environmental factors:* Nongenetic factors from external environment like habits, muscle forces, etc.
  5. *General environmental factors:* General nongenetic factors like nutrition, oxygen, etc.

- Chondrocranial growth is mainly controlled by intrinsic genetic factors.
- Desmocranial growth is controlled by intrinsic genetic factors.
- Cartilaginous part of skull is the growth center.
- Sutural growth is controlled by influence from skull cartilages.
- Periosteal growth depends upon growth of adjacent structures.
- Sutural and periosteal growth is governed by nongenetic environmental factors.

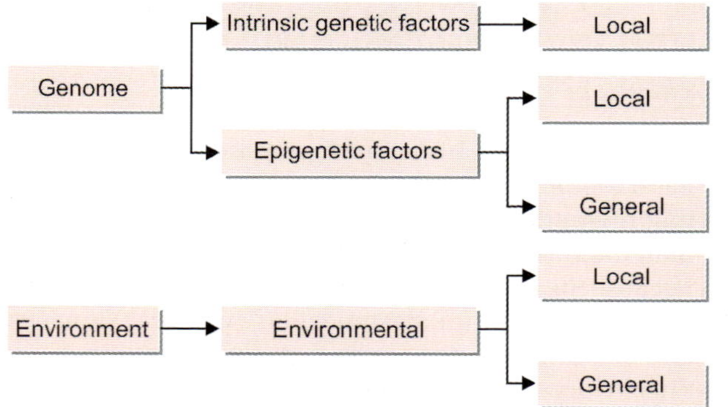

CYBERNETICS/SERVOSYSTEM THEORY (PETROVIC, STUTZMAN, 1974)

- Using the language of cybernetics, **Petrovic** reasons that it is the interaction of series of casual changes of feedback mechanisms which determine the growth of craniofacial regions.
- According to this theory, control of primary cartilage takes a cybernetics form of a command, whereas control of secondary cartilage is comprised of indirect and direct effects of cell's multiplication.

Cybernetics

Science dealing with comparative study of operations of complex computers of human nervous system.

Servosystem

Its components are **(Fig. 11.5):**

- **Command:** Signal established independent of feedback system. It affects the behavior of the control system without being affected by the consequences of the behavior, for example, secretion of growth hormone or testosterone is not modulated by variations in craniofacial growth.

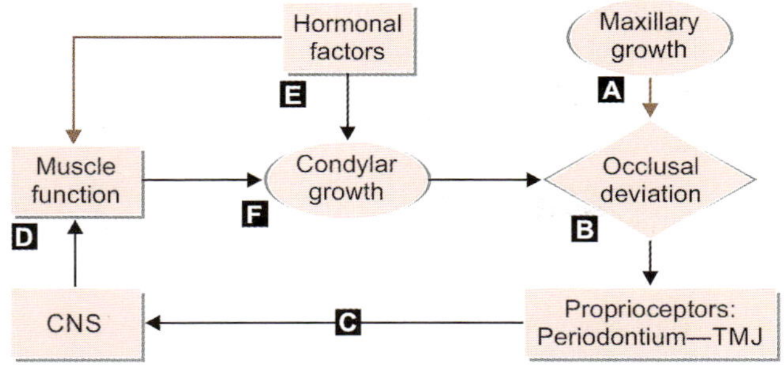

Fig. 11.5: Servosystem theory of craniofacial growth.

- **Reference input elements:** Establish relation between command (growth hormone) and reference input (sagittal position of maxillary arch). They include septal cartilage, septopremaxillary frenum, and maxillary bones.
- **Reference input:** Signal established as a standard of comparison.
- **Peripheral comparator:** Compares reference input and output, for example, position of jaws.
- **Controller:** Located between deviation and actuating signal.
- **Actuating signal:** Corresponds to output signal of controller.
- **Controlled system:** Part of control system between actuating signal and directly controlled variable.
- **Controlled variable:** Output signal of the system.
- **Gain:** Output divided by input.
- **Feedback signal:** Function of controlled variable that is comparable to reference input.
- **Disturbance:** Any input other than reference chosen to be responsible for deviation of output signal.

NEUROTROPHISM (BEHRENT, MOSS, 1976)

- The physiology of neurotrophism is based on the fact that nervous system apart from conducting efferent and afferents is also concerned with the integrity of body structures.
- Nerve control of skeletal growth by transmission of a substance through its axons is called neurotrophism **(Fig. 11.6).**

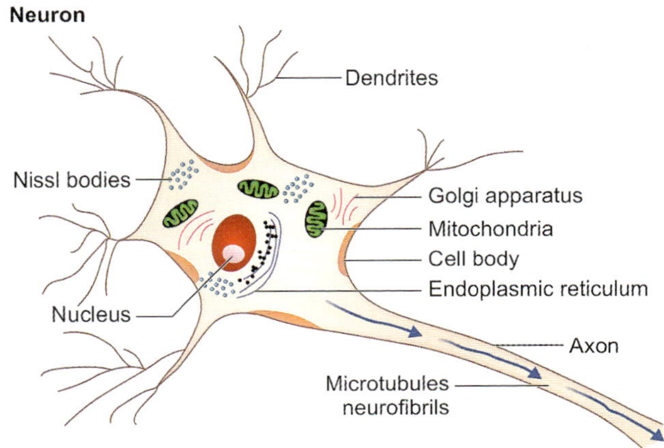

Fig. 11.6: Neurotrophic pathway.

Types of neurotrophic mechanisms

- *Neuroepithelial trophism*
  - Epithelial mitosis and synthesis is neurotrophically controlled
  - Normal epithelial growth is controlled by release of neurotrophic substances from nerve synapse.
  - Presence of taste buds is dependent on intact innervation.
- *Neurovisceral trophism*
  - Salivary glands, fat tissue are partly trophically regulated.
- *Neuromuscular trophism*
  - Innervation is required at the myoblast stage of differentiation.

ENLOW'S EXPANDING "V" PRINCIPLE

- This is the most basic and useful concept of growth.
- Many facial and cranial bones have a V-shaped pattern of growth, and the expansion of these occurs along the ends of V as a result of selective bone resorption and deposition.
- The pattern of growth is such that there is deposition along the inner side and wide ends of V and resorption on the outer aspect **(Fig. 11.7).**
- Some of the bones which grow according to this pattern are end of long bones, base of mandible, mandibular body, and palate.

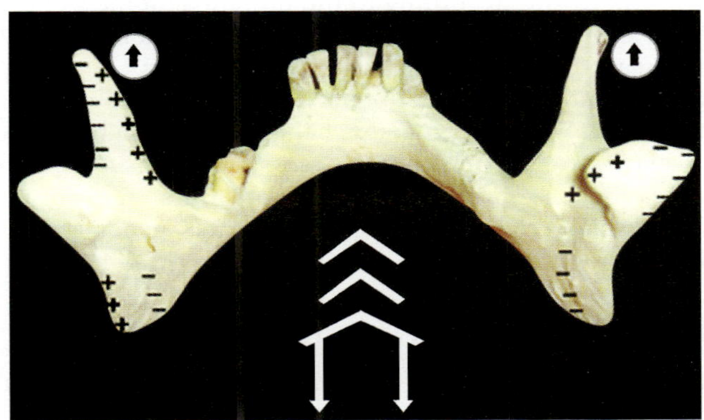

Fig. 11.7: Enlow's "V" principle.

Enlow's Counterpart Principle

This principle states that growth of any facial or cranial part relates specifically to other structural and geometric counterparts in face and cranium.

Body part and their geometric counterparts

- Nasomaxillary complex—anterior cranial fossa
- Maxillary arch—mandibular arch
- Bony maxilla—corpus of mandible
- Maxillary tuberosity—lingual tuberosity

FUNCTIONAL MATRIX HYPOTHESIS REVISITED (1997)

FMH was first put forth by **Melvin Moss** based on his study of the regulatory roles of intrinsic (genomic) and extrinsic (epigenetic) factors in cephalic growth for a decade. The initial version stressed upon epigenetic primacy and became peer accepted as one explanatory paradigm, as it was improvised. With inclusions on advances in the biomedical, bioengineering, and computer sciences, more comprehensive explanatory versions of FMH were proposed. Thus functional matrix theory was revisited and based on:

- ❖ The role of mechanotransduction
- ❖ The role of osseous connected cellular network
- ❖ The genomic thesis
- ❖ The epigenetic antithesis and the resolving synthesis.

T Melvin Moss in 1997 proposed continuation of his classical functional matrix theory with the new concept. He published series of articles in *American Journal of Orthodontics in 1997.*

According to this concept, the mechanical stimulus is pursued by the specialized cells by a process called mechanoperception. Then these signals are transmitted through the tissues by the way of mechanoconduction or mechanotransmission. Finally, these signals are transmitted to the genome of the bone where protein synthesis is taking place.

These signals alter the protein metabolism depending upon the severity and longevity of the mechanical stimulus. In short, the earlier concept of FMH theory remained same as form is determined by the function.

Moss also recognizes the important role of genetics and human genome in determining the ultimate size and shape of the craniofacial skeleton. He quotes reference of human genome project which is being carried in a mega scale all over the world. According to the human genome project, human chromosomes containing the genetic information are necessary for building up of entire human body.

Genes now beyond doubt have been proved to effect the physical growth of the person, behavior of the person, and psychology of the person. Thus Moss FMH revisited theory states that the ultimate growth controlling factor of the craniofacial skeleton depends on two factors: genetic factors and environment factors.

Modern Composite Theory[1]

- ❖ It tries to explain the growth of the maxilla and mandible.
- ❖ It separates the facial cranium into:

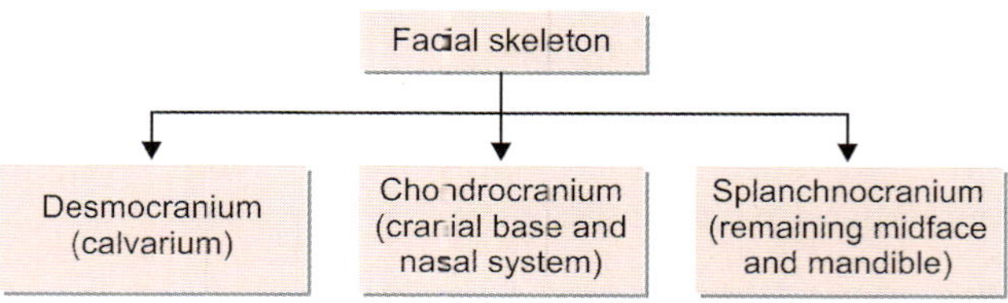

Essence of the Theory (Fig. 11.8)

- ❖ Chondrocranium is considered the dominant factor in craniofacial growth.
- ❖ Cranial basal cartilage (spheno-occipital synchondrosis predominantly) and the nasal cartilage act as growth centers.
- ❖ Local epigenetic (capsule) and local environmental (periosteal matrix) then control the calvarium.
- ❖ Sutures are considered only as growth sites.
- ❖ The growth of nasal cartilage pushes the maxilla downward and forward.
- ❖ The growth of the mandible seems to be controlled by both local epigenetic and local periosteal factors.

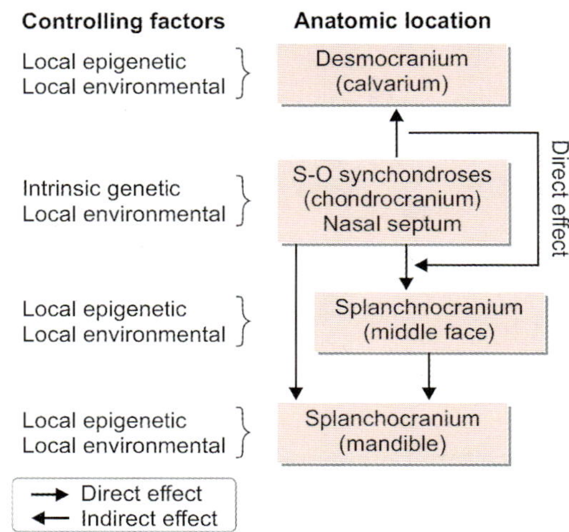

Fig. 11.8: Craniofacial growth as per composite theory.

- ❖ The position of mandible is also affected by cranial base flexion and growth by altering the posture of glenoid fossa.

Growth Relativity Hypothesis (John C Voudouris, 2000)

- ❖ Growth relativity refers to the growth that is relative to its displaced condyles from actively relocating fossa.
- ❖ **John Voudouris** introduced this concept to explain the possible effect of functional appliances on condyles and resulting growth.
- ❖ The main foundation of growth relative hypothesis are:
  - ■ ***Displacement of condyle:***
    - ◆ The displacement that takes place initially following mandibular advancement affects the fibrocartilagenous lining in the glenoid fossa to induce bone formation locally.
  - ■ ***Viscoelastic stretch:***
    - ◆ Once the condyles are displaced, it is followed by the stretch of nonmuscular viscoelastic tissues.
    - ◆ Due to viscoelastic stretch there is influx of nutrients and other biodynamic factors into the region, through engorged blood vessels of the stretched retrodiscal tissue that feed into the fibrocartilage of the condyle.
  - ■ ***Force transduction and new bone formation:***
    - ◆ This is the most interesting aspect wherein new bone formation takes place at some distance from actual retrodiscal tissue attachments in the fossa.
    - ◆ Effect of three growth stimuli (displacement + viscoelasticity + transduction of force):
      - » Modification of growth "first" occurs as a result of the action of anterior mandibular displacement.
      - » "Second", the condyle is affected by the posterior viscoelastc tissue anchored between the glenoid fossa.
      - » And "third", displacement and viscoelasticity further stimulate the normal condylar growth by transduction of forces over the fibrocartilage cap of the condylar head.

POINTS TO REMEMBER

- Growth is an increase in mass or size and development is naturally occurring unidirectional changes in the life of an individual from its existence as a single cell to its elaboration as a multifunctional unit terminating in death.
- Genetic theory by Brodie states that genes control all the functions of growth and development.
- Scott's cartilaginous theory states that the determinant of craniofacial growth is by growth of cartilages with nasal septum governing growth of nasomaxillary complex.
- Functional matrix concept given by Melvin Moss explains that the origin, form, position, growth, and maintenance of all skeletal tissues and organs are always secondary, compensatory, and necessary response to chronologically and morphologically prior events or processes that occur in specifically related nonskeletal tissues, organs, or functioning spaces.
- Van Limborg's multifactorial concept emphasizes on five factors that control growth, viz., intrinsic genetic factors, local and general epigenetic factors, and local and genetic environmental factors.

Clinical Significance

Myofunctional therapy should be initiated in the mixed dentition phase pertaining to the growth of the maxilla and mandible during that phase of life in children.

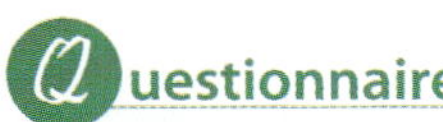

Questionnaire

1. Define growth and development.
2. Explain cartilaginous theory with experiments.
3. Describe functional matrix concept.
4. What is cybernetics?
5. Explain the growth principle of mandible.

REFERENCES

1. Wang Y, et al. Composite growth model applied to human oral and pharyngeal structures and identifying the contribution of growth types; Stat Methods Med Res; 2016.
2. Carlson DS. Growth modification from molecules to mandible. In: Mcnamara JA (Ed). Center for human growth and development. Ann Arbor, MI, University of Michigan. 1999;35:17-65.
3. Moss ML. Experimental alteration of sutural area morphology. Anat Rec. 1957;127:569-89.
4. Carlson D. Semin Orthod. 2005;11:172-83.

FURTHER READING

1. Bhalajhi SI. Orthodontics: the art and science, 3rd edition. Arya (Medi) Publishing House; 2006.
2. Dixon AD. Fundamental of craniofacial growth. CRC Press; 1997. p. 512.
3. Enlow DH. Growth and remodeling of the human maxilla. Am J Orthod. 1965;51(6):446-64.
4. Enlow DH. Handbook of facial growth. WB Saunders Co; 1982.
5. Graber TM. Orthodontics: principle and practice, 3rd edition. WB Saunders.
6. Moss M, et al. The capsular matrix. Am J Orthod. 1969;56(5).
7. Proffit WR. Contemporary orthodontics. 5th edition. Mosby; 2012. p. 768.
8. Graber TM, Rakosi T. Dentofacial orthopaedics with functional appliances, 2nd edition.
9. Scott JH. Growth of facial sutures. Am J Orthod. 1956;42:381-7.
10. Le Douarin NM. The neural crest. Cambridge University Press;1982.

CHAPTER

Prenatal and Postnatal Development of Head and Face

Rishi Tyagi, Nikhil Marwah

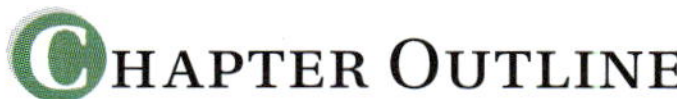

- Prenatal Growth and Development
- Postnatal Growth of Maxilla
- Postnatal Growth of Mandible

Growth and development of an individual can be divided into prenatal and postnatal periods with the former being more dynamic as the growth in prenatal period being 5,000 times more than what happens in postnatal era.

PRENATAL GROWTH AND DEVELOPMENT

Prenatal period can be divided into three periods:
1. Period of ovum.
2. Period of embryo.
3. Period of fetus.

Period of Ovum

- This is also called the preimplantation period.
- During this, the ovum extends for first 7 days after which it cleaves and attaches to intrauterine wall.

Spermatogenesis: It is the process of forming of spermatozoa in the walls of seminiferous tubules of testes **(Fig. 12.1)**.

Oogenesis: Process of formation of ovum by cells called oogonia **(Fig. 12.2)**.

Events of period of ovum
- Spermatogenesis
- Oogenesis
- Ovulation
- Fertilization
- Cleavage formation
- Blastocyst formation
- Implantation

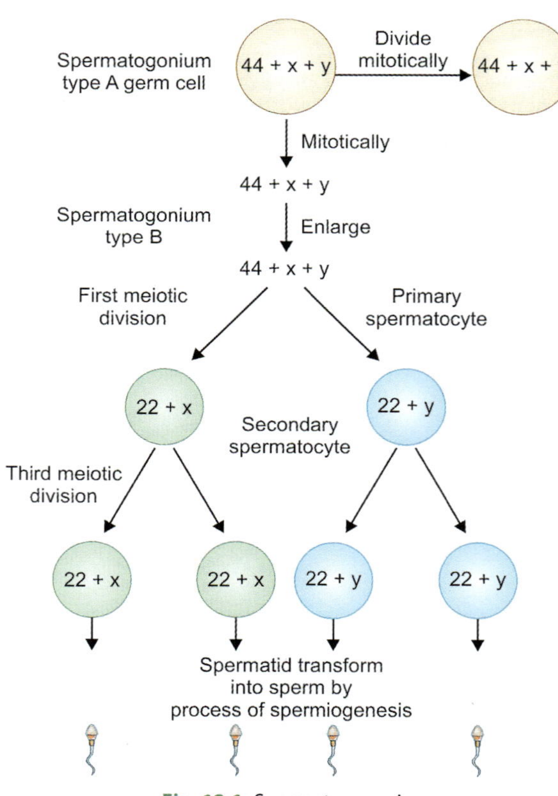

Fig. 12.1: Spermatogenesis.

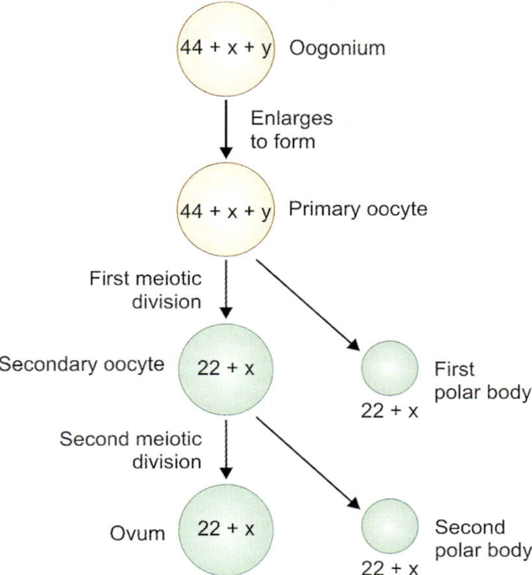

Fig. 12.2: Oogenesis.

Ovulation: Ovarian follicle is very small compared to cortex of ovary **(Fig. 12.3)**. As it enlarges, it becomes so big that it cannot reach the surface of ovary, and so it forms a bulging that ruptures to shed the ovary. This process is called the ovulation.

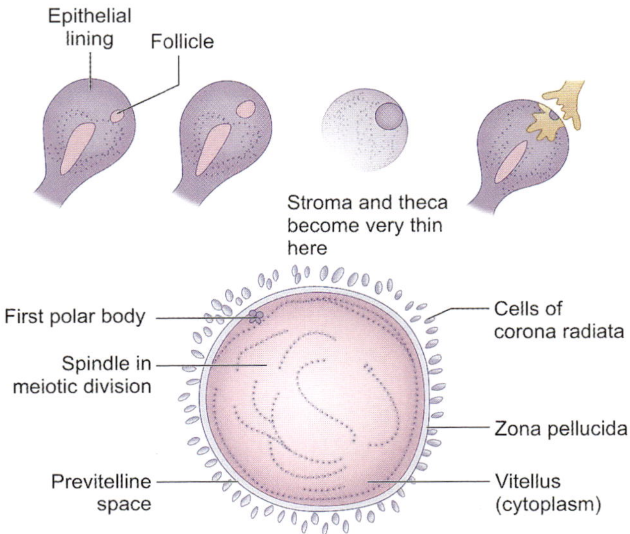

Fig. 12.3: Structure of ovum at time of ovulation.

Fertilization: It is the process in which male and female gamete fuse to form a zygote and fertilization takes place in ampulla of uterine tube **(Fig. 12.4)**.

Cleavage formation: A series of mitotic divisions decrease the size of zygote and increase the number of cells present. This stage happens 3 days after fertilization when the embryo is about to enter uterus. At this stage, zygote is called morula whose inner cell mass gives rise to embryo proper and outer cell mass contributes to placenta **(Fig. 12.5)**.

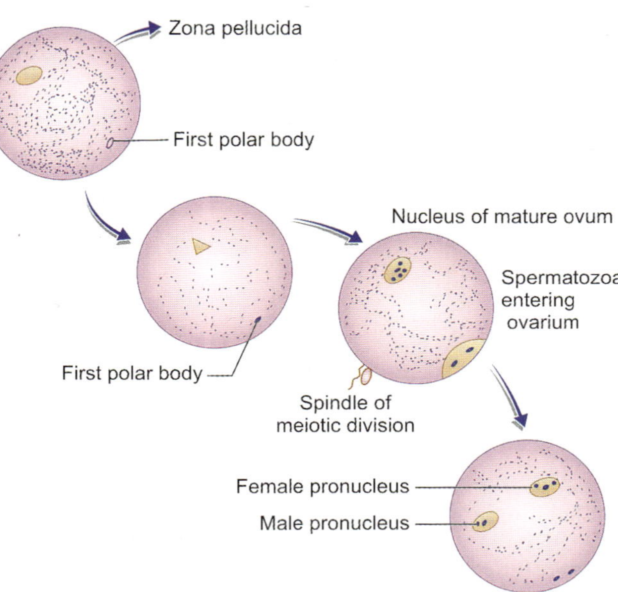

Fig. 12.4: Fertilization.

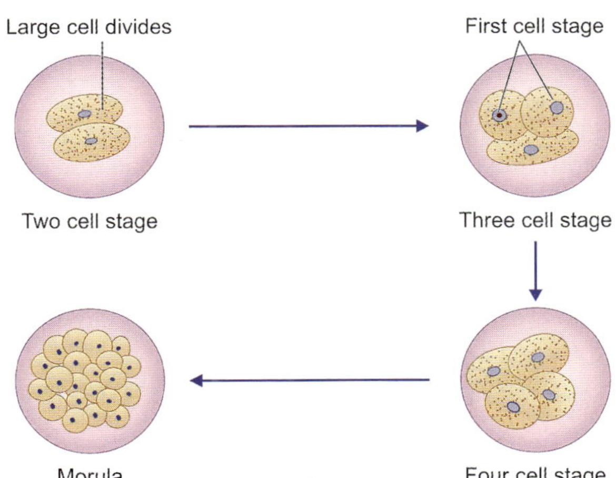

Fig. 12.5: Cleavage formation.

Blastocyst formation: As the morula enters uterine cavity, fluid penetrates it, and inner cellular space becomes one cavity called blastocyst **(Fig. 12.6)**.

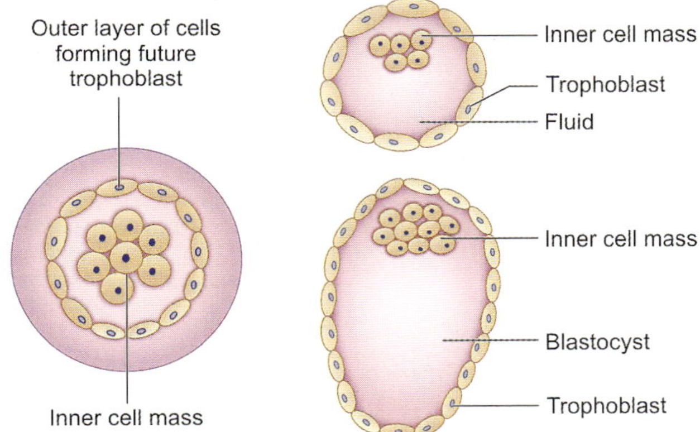

Fig. 12.6: Blastocyst formation.

Implantation: This happens at the end of first week when trophoblast cells invade epithelium **(Fig. 12.7)**.

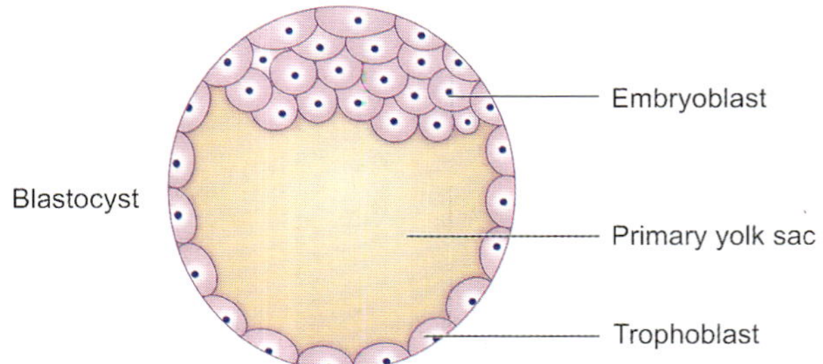

Fig. 12.7: Implantation.

Period of Embryo

It extends from the end of first week till the 8th week and is divided into presomite, somite and postsomite period.

Presomite Period (8–21 Days)

- Blastocyst now has two cell population, viz., trophoblast cells and embryoblasts.
- Embryoblast differentiates into epiblast and hypoblast which matures into two-layered germ disc (8 days).
- Primordial embryonic germ disc is composed of ectoderm and endoderm (2 weeks).
- Axis of embryo is established and enlargement of ectodermal and endodermal cells at head end occurs forming the prechordal plate which distinguishes and organizes the head **(Fig. 12.8)**.

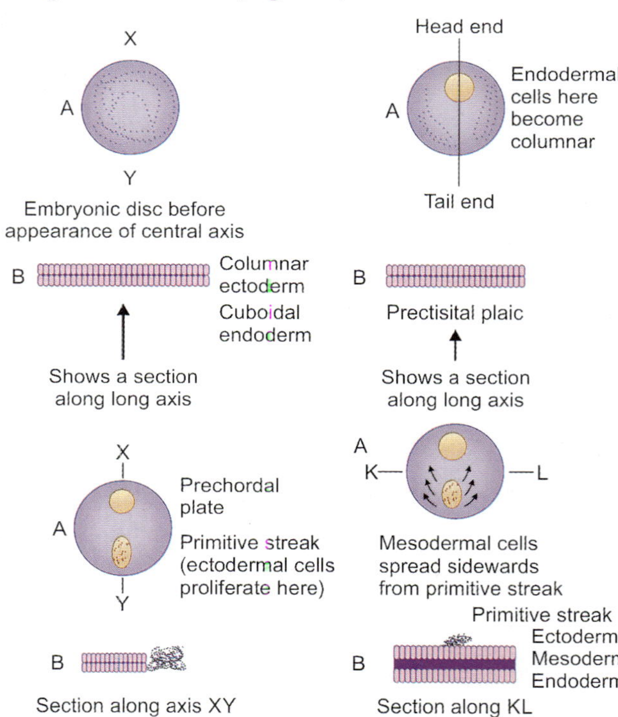

Fig. 12.8: Establishment of axis of embryo and organization of head.

- Development of primitive streak which forms the mesoderm (3 weeks) **(Fig. 12.9)**.

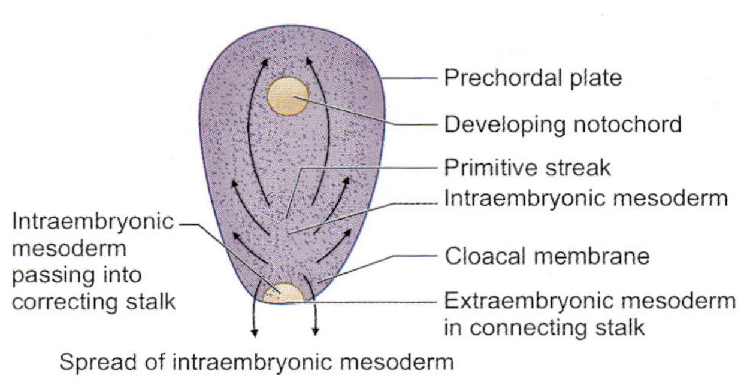

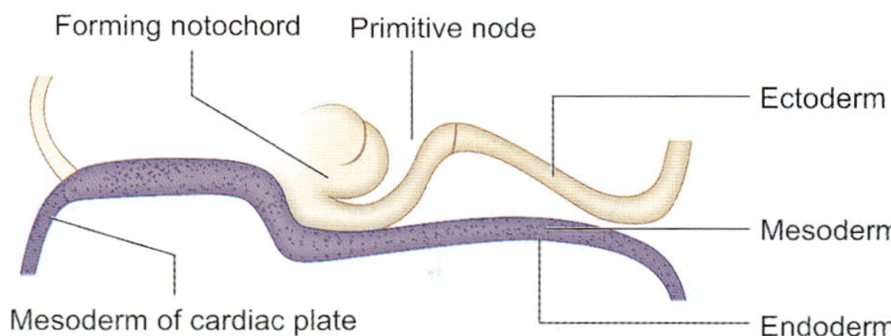

Fig. 12.9: Development of primitive streak.

Somite Period (21–31 Days)

- Ectodermal layer at the head end of embryo forms the neural plate **(Fig. 12.10)**.
- Major organs and tissues differentiate during this period, thus making it susceptible to environmental influences.

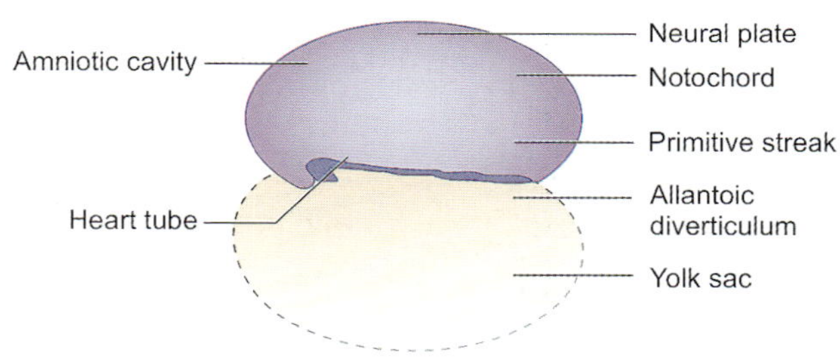

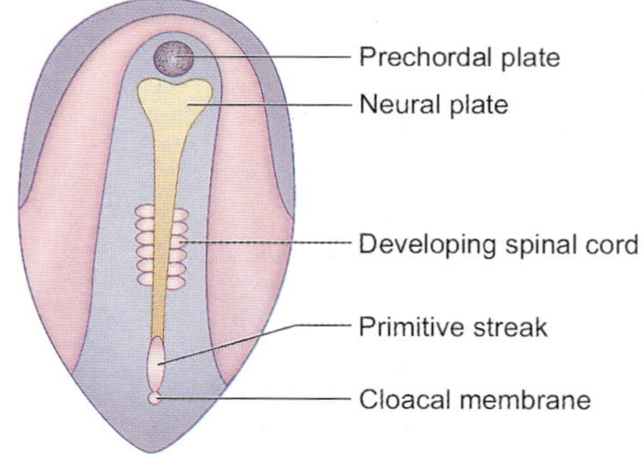

Fig. 12.10: Somite period.

Postsomite Period (32–56 Days)

- Characterized by formation of external features and branchial arches **(Fig. 12.11)**.
- Facial features become recognizable.
- Embryo is now called fetus.

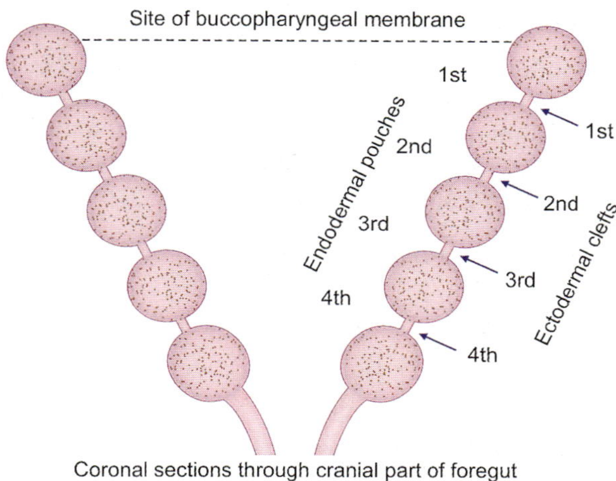

Fig. 12.11: Postsomite period.

Period of Fetus

Development of Face

- After the formation of head fold, the developing brain and the pericardium, two prominent swellings appear on the ventral aspect of embryo separated by stomatodeum **(Figs. 12.12 and 12.13)**.

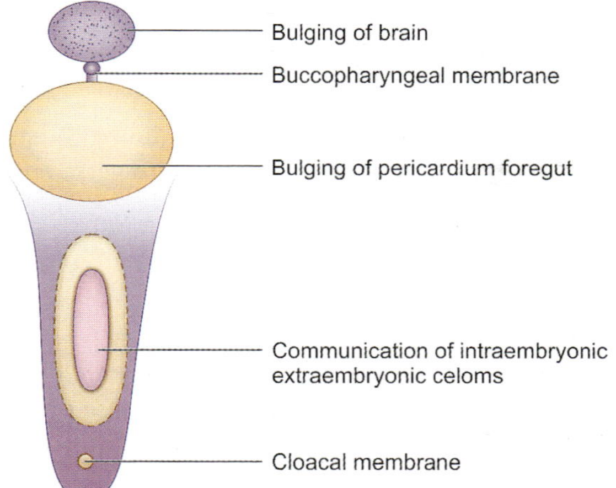

Fig. 12.12: Period of fetus.

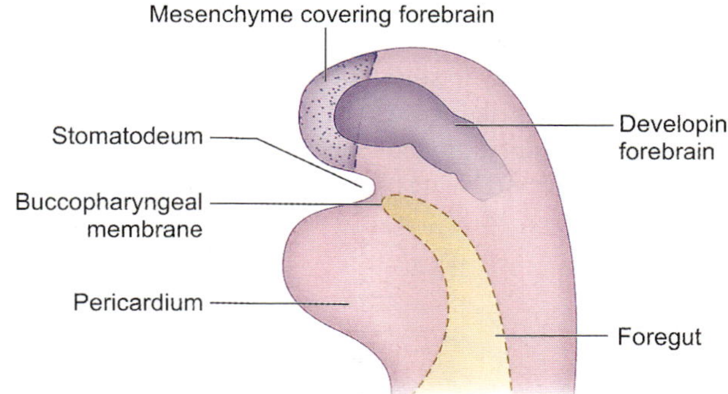

Fig. 12.13: Formation of stomatodeum.

- Mesoderm covering the developing forebrain proliferates and overlaps stomatodeum to form frontonasal process **(Figs. 12.14 and 12.15)**.

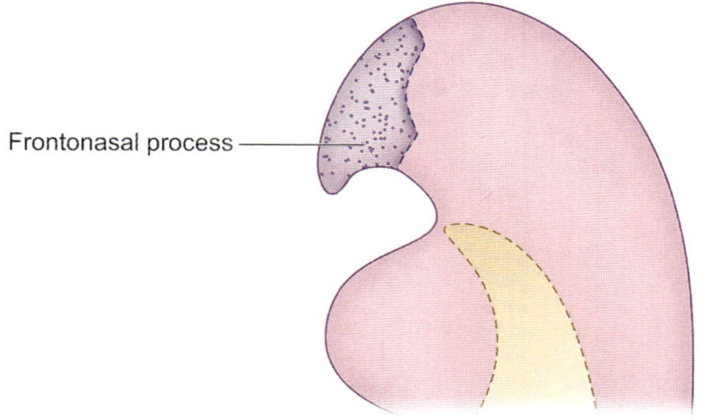

Fig. 12.14: Formation of frontonasal process.

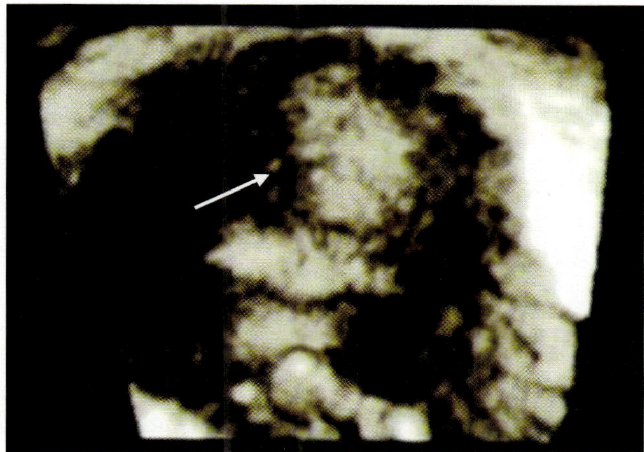

Fig. 12.15: Ultrasound of embryo showing formation of frontonasal process and stomatodeum.

- Mandibular arch which forms the lateral wall of stomatodeum gives off a bud from its dorsal end called maxillary process **(Fig. 12.16)**.
- The ventromedial growth of this process is called the mandibular process **(Fig. 12.16)**.

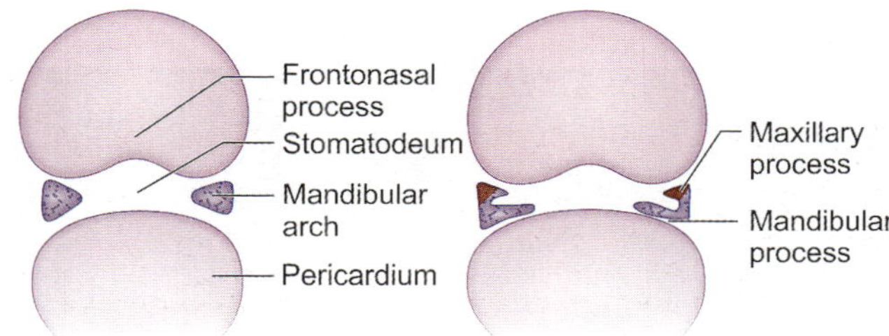

Fig. 12.16: Formation of maxillary and mandibular process.

Development of Nose

Bilateral localized thickenings appear over ectoderm overlying frontonasal process called nasal placodes **(Fig. 12.17)**.

- These placodes sink below to form the nasal pits.
- The edges of these nasal pits are raised and called medial and lateral nasal process **(Fig. 12.18)**.

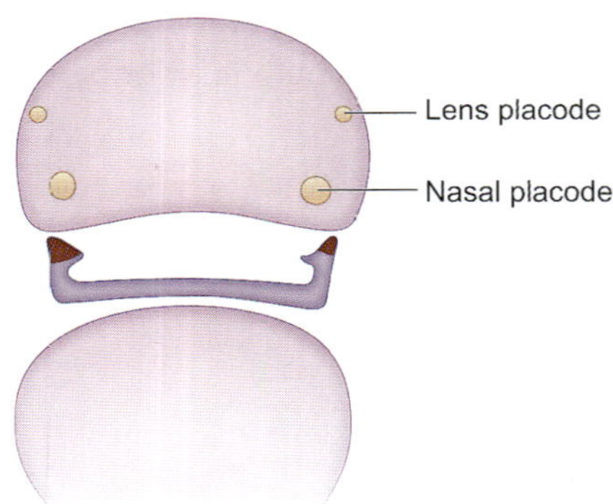

Fig. 12.17: Development of nasal placodes.

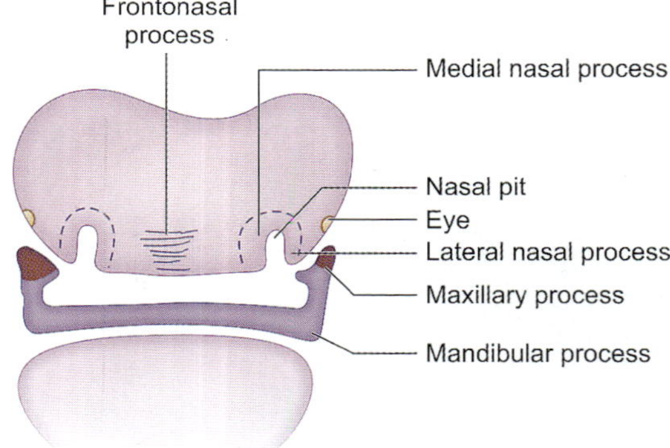

Fig. 12.18: Development of nose.

- ❖ Maxillary processes grow and fuse with lateral and medial nasal process, and both lateral and medial nasal processes also fuse with each other cutting off nasal pits from stomatodeum. These are now called external nares **(Fig. 12.19).**
- ❖ Growth of maxillary process and narrowing down of frontonasal process make the external nares to come close rapidly.
- ❖ This leads to formation of horse-shoe shaped ridge that connects nasal pits to olfactory apparatus and thus form the nose.

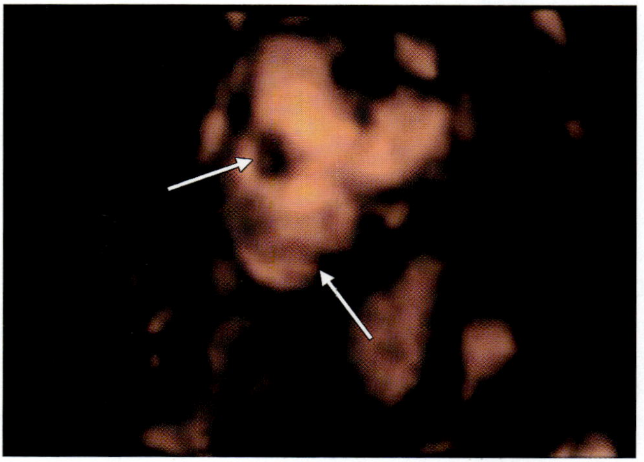

Fig. 12.19: Ultrasound of embryo showing formation of nose, eyes and maxillomandibular process.

Development of Lips

- ❖ Mandibular processes on both sides grow and fuse in midline to form lower jaw and lip **(Figs. 12.20A and B).**
- ❖ Formation of nose leads to rounding of stomatodeum to form upper part of upper lip. Lateral part of upper lip is formed by maxillary process and median part by frontonasal process **(Figs. 12.20A and B).**

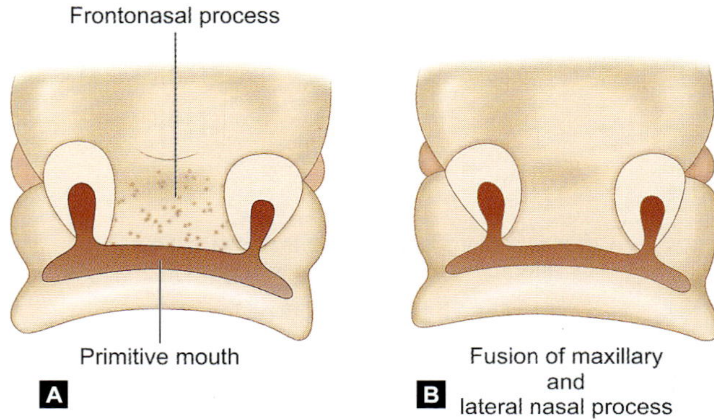

Figs. 12.20A and B: Development of lips.

Development of Maxilla

- ❖ Maxilla develops from a center of ossification in mesenchyme of maxillary process of first arch.
- ❖ From this center, bone formation spreads posteriorly below the orbit toward developing zygoma and anteriorly toward incisor region.
- ❖ Downward extension also extends to form alveolar plate for maxillary tooth germs. Medial alveolar plate which forms the body of maxilla along with lateral alveolar plate form a trough of bone around maxillary tooth germ enclosing them in bony crypt.
- ❖ Some secondary cartilages like malar cartilage also help in development of maxilla.

Development of Cheeks

After formation of upper and lower lips, the stomatodeum is called the mouth. This initially is very broad, but progressive fusion of mandibular and maxillary processes reduces it forming the cheeks.

Development of Eyes

- ❖ Eye is first seen as an ectodermal thickening called lens placode which appears on ventrolateral side of developing forebrain.
- ❖ It then sinks below to separate from surface ectoderm and appear as twin bulging that are directed laterally and lying between maxillary and lateral nasal processes. These come forward by the narrowing of frontonasal process **(Fig. 12.21).**

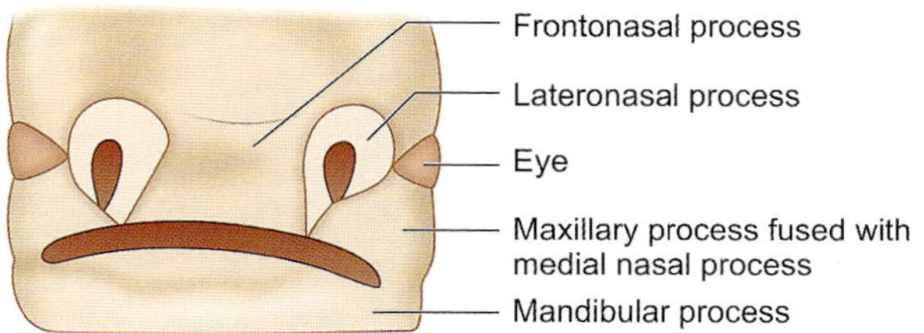

Fig. 12.21: Development of eyes.

Development of Mandible

- Mandible develops from the cartilage of first arch, that is, **Meckel's** cartilage **(Fig. 12.22)**.
- At sixth week of intrauterine life, a hyaline cartilaginous rod surrounded by fibrocellular capsule extends from otic capsule to midline of fused mandibular process from both sides
- Condensation of mesenchyme occurs

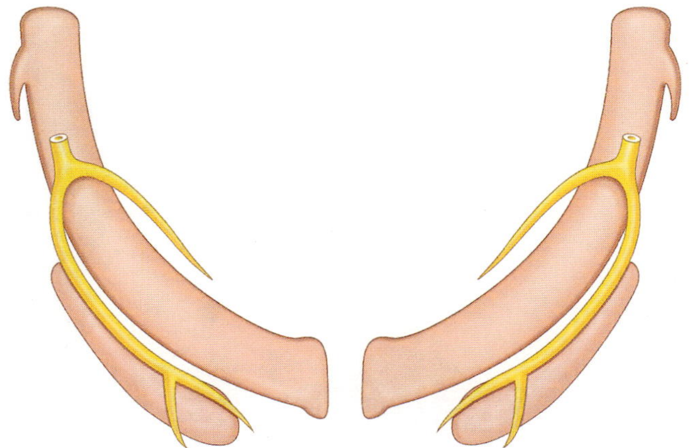

Fig. 12.22: Development of mandible from Meckel's cartilage.

- During seventh week, intramembranous ossification begins from center of mandible and spreads anteriorly and posteriorly along lateral aspect of Meckel's cartilage.
- Bone troughs from both side of mandibular process come in close approximation and remain separated in symphysis region till birth. Posteriorly, ossification proceeds till the point of division of mandibular nerve.
- Medial and lateral alveolar plates develop upward in relation to tooth germs.
- Ramus develops by rapid spread of ossification posteriorly into the mesenchyme of first arch turning away from Meckel's cartilage **(Fig. 12.23).**

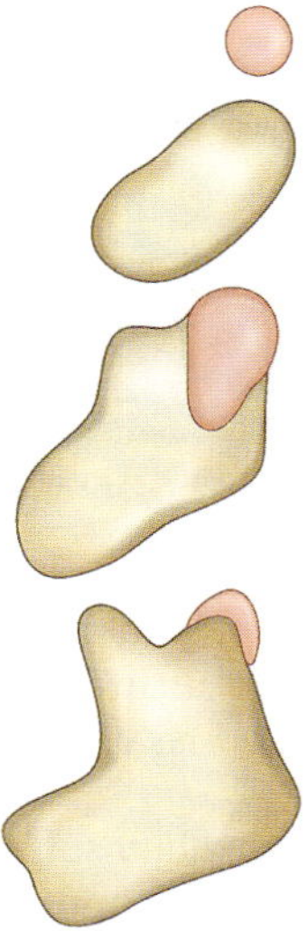

Fig. 12.23: Development of ramus.

- An area of mesenchymal condensation is seen on ventral part of developing mandible in fifth week of IUL. This cone shape cartilage starts ossification about 14 weeks and then fuses with ramus to form condylar process.

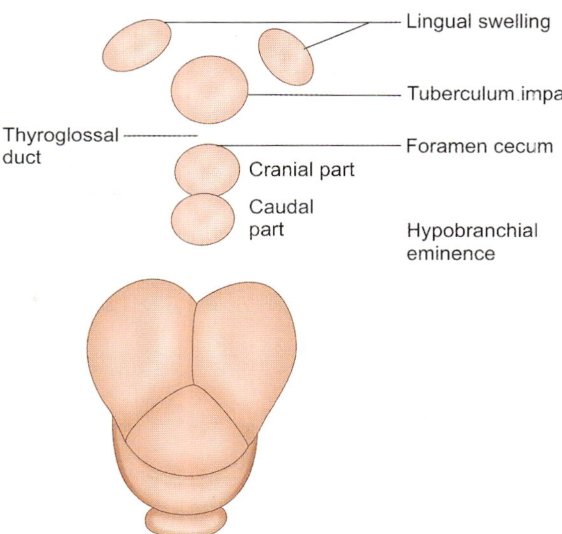

Fig. 12.24: Development of tongue.

- Accessory cartilages appear in coronoid region also, but they disappear before birth; however, when these appear in mental region, they form mental ossicles.

Development of Tongue (Fig. 12.24)

- Medial part of mandibular arch proliferates to form two lingual swellings which are separated from each other by median swelling called tuberculum impar. Epithelium from tuberculum impar grows to form a downgrowth called thyroglossal duct and is marked by a depression called foramen cecum.
- Another swelling medial to second, third, fourth arches is hypobranchial eminence which is divided into cranial and caudal parts.
- These three swellings, that is, lingual swelling, tuberculum impar and hypobranchial eminence contribute to formation of tongue.
- Anterior two-thirds of tongue is formed by two lingual swellings and tuberculum impar. Posterior one-third is derived from cranial part of hypobranchial eminence (copula).

Development of Palate

- Initially, oronasal cavity is bounded anteriorly by primary palate and occupied mainly by tongue. Distinction between oral and nasal cavity is outlined after formation of secondary palate. The palate proper however develops from contributions of both primary and secondary components.
- Medial nasal process and frontonasal process give rise to primary palate **(Fig. 12.25).**
- Formation of secondary palate starts at eighth week of IUL with fusion of palatal shelves from maxillary process and contribution of frontonasal process **(Fig. 12.26).**
- Palatal shelves from maxillary process are first directed downward on each side of tongue.
- As the tongue develops during the end of seventh week and moves to a more downward position, the palatal shelves begin to grow and move toward each other **(Fig. 12.27).**

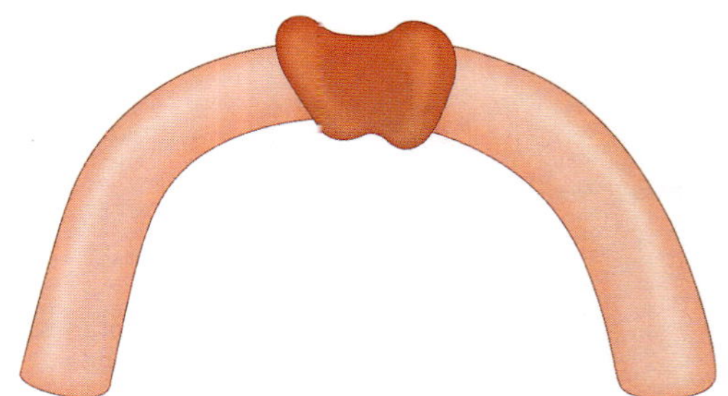

Fig. 12.25: Development of primary palate.

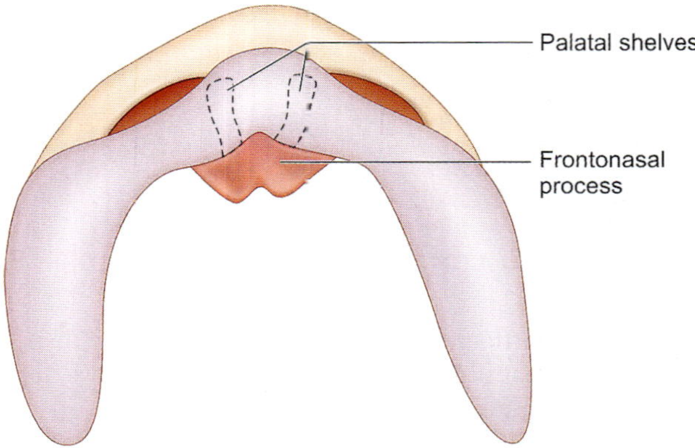

Fig. 12.26: Secondary palate initiation.

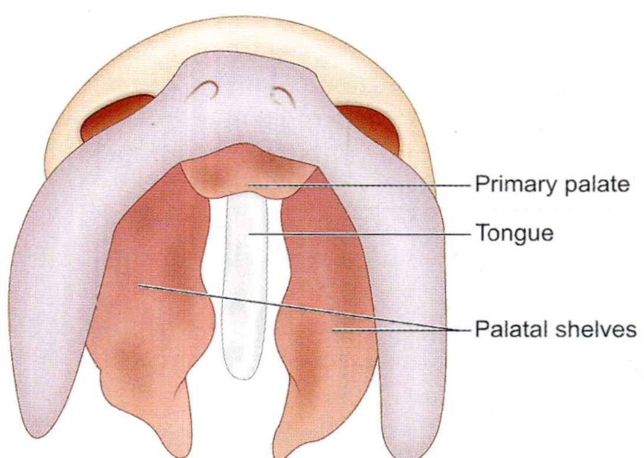

Fig. 12.27: Fusion of palatal shelf.

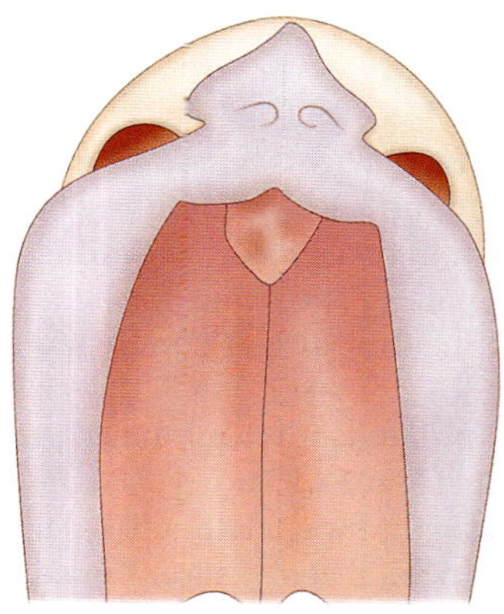

Fig. 12.28: Secondary palate formation.

- By 8.5 weeks, the shelves are in close approximation with each other and fuse with each other as well as primary palate fusing first from central region and the anterior and posterior **(Fig. 12.28)**.

POSTNATAL GROWTH OF MAXILLA

This occurs by primary and secondary displacement, growth at sutures and by surface remodeling.

Primary Displacement

Posterior directional movement due to growth in maxillary tuberosity causes maxilla to move anteriorly **(Fig. 12.29)**.

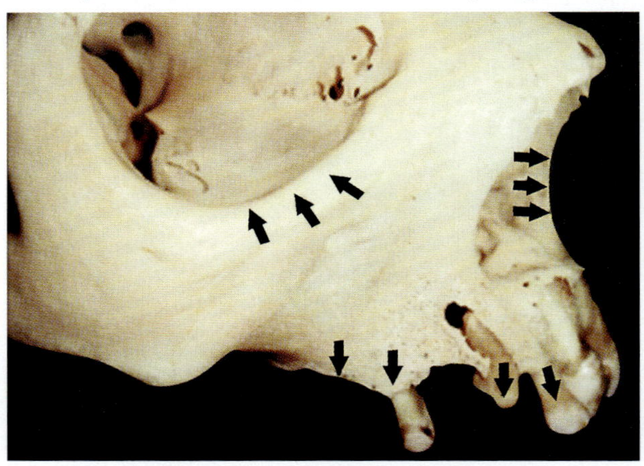

Fig. 12.29: Primary displacement.

Secondary Displacement

As the cranial base grows, it exerts pressure on the nasomaxillary complex displacing it in a downward and forward direction **(Fig. 12.30)**.

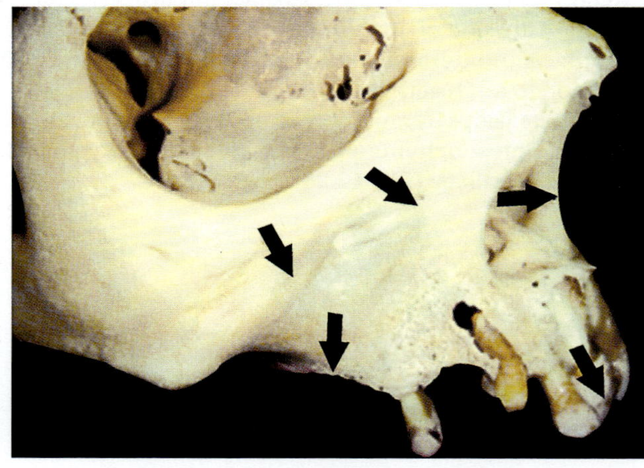

Fig. 12.30: Secondary displacement.

Growth at Sutures

- Whenever growth at sutures takes place, it leads to downward and forward displacement of maxillary complex.
- Some of the craniomaxillary sutures are frontomaxillary, frontonasal, zygomaticotemporal, zygomaticomaxillary and pterygopalatine sutures.

Remodeling (Fig. 12.31)

- Resorption on lateral surface and deposition on external surface of orbital rim—for lateral movements of eyeball.

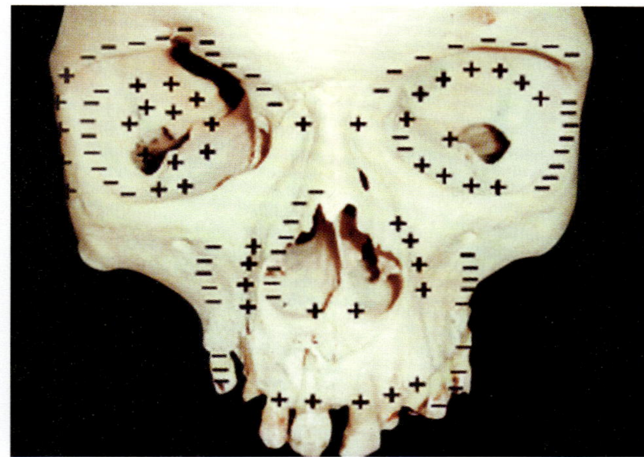

Fig. 12.31: Remodeling.

- Surface deposition on superior, lateral and anterior surface of floor of orbit.
- Deposition along posterior aspect of maxillary tuberosity—third molar accommodation.
- Resorption along lateral wall of nose—increase size of nasal cavity.
- Resorption on anterior and deposition on posterior surface of zygomatic bone.
- Bone deposition along alveolar margins— to accommodate teeth.

POSTNATAL GROWTH OF MANDIBLE

- Mandible is the most diverse bone in human craniofacial structure as it is made up of many small individual bones which on their own are miniskeletal units.
- The postnatal growth of mandible is best understood if the development of all parts of mandible is undertaken individually.

Ramus

Deposition on posterior aspect and resorption on anterior aspect to move the ramus posteriorly to accommodate for molars and to accommodate increasing muscle mass of masticatory muscles **(Fig. 12.32)**.

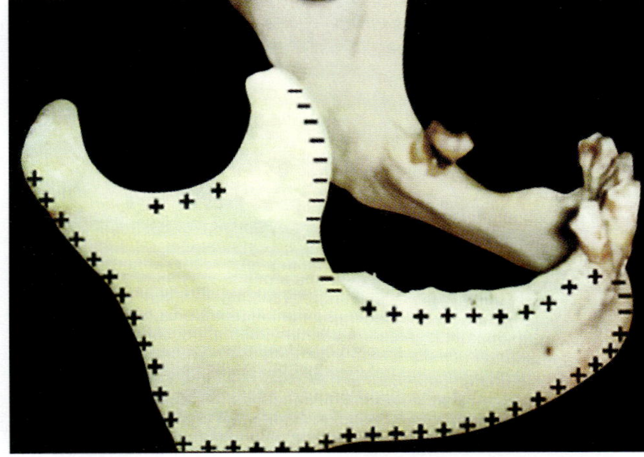

Fig. 12.32: Ramus growth pattern.

Body

Due to resorption of ramus, the old ramal bone changes to posterior body limit. Bone deposition also occurs along inferior margins of body of mandible, thus lengthening mandibular body **(Fig. 12.33)**.

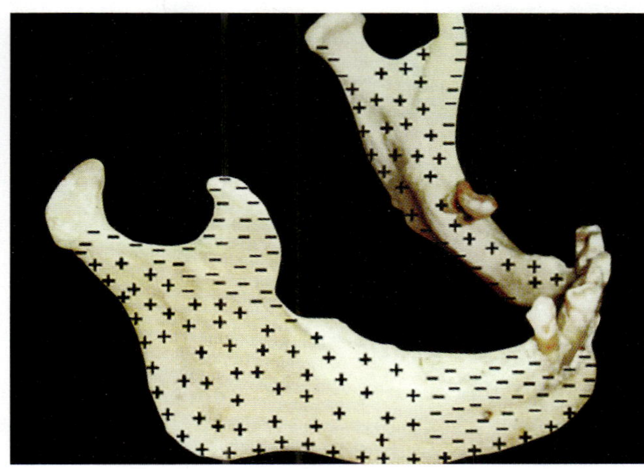

Fig. 12.33: Growth at body.

Lingual Tuberosity

This moves posteriorly by deposition along posterior surface and resorption below in lingual fossa **(Fig. 12.34)**.

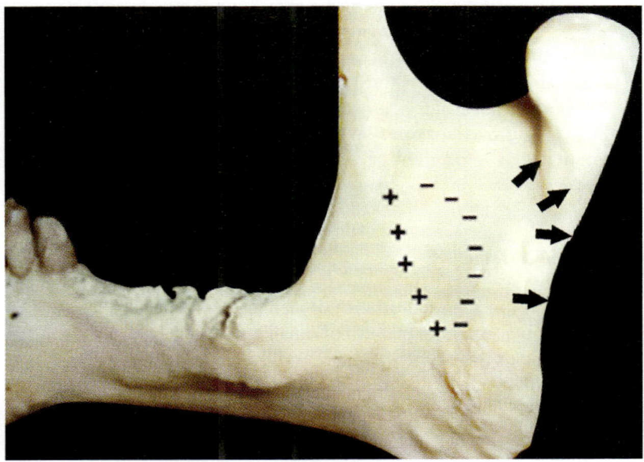

Fig. 12.34: Tuberosity growth.

Angle

Lingually, there is resorption on posterioinferior aspect and deposition on anteriosuperior aspect. Buccally, there is deposition on posteriosuperior aspect and resorption on anteriosuperior aspect. This results in flaring of angle of mandible **(Fig. 12.35)**.

Coronoid Process

Deposition occurs on lingual surface, and further growth is based on enlarging "V" principle that takes place posteriorly **(Fig. 12.35)**.

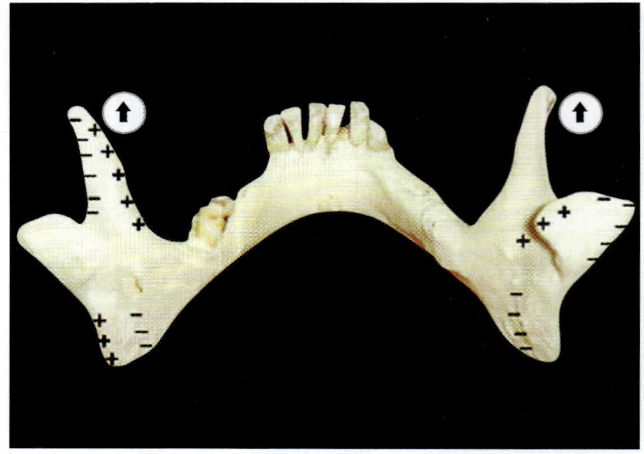

Fig. 12.35: Growth at angle and coronoid process.

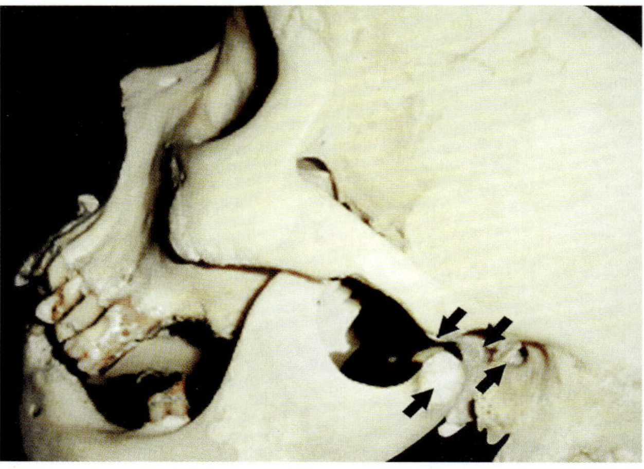

Fig. 12.36: Condylar growth.

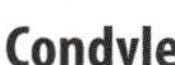

Condyle

Growth may either occur by bone deposition along condylar cartilage which then interacts with cranial base, thus displacing mandible downward and forward, or it may occur as growth of soft tissues surrounded in the region later followed by bone formation **(Fig. 12.36)**.

Alveolar Process

Develops as a response to presence of teeth by increasing in thickness and height by depositions at margins.

Chin

Bone resorption occurs in superior aspect over the concavity in mental region.

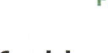

POINTS TO REMEMBER

- Prenatal period can be divided into period of ovum, period of embryo, period of fetus.
- Events of period of ovum are spermatogenesis, oogenesis, ovulation, fertilization, cleavage formation, blastocyst, implantation.
- Mandible develops from the cartilage of first arch, that is, Meckel's cartilage.
- Anterior two-thirds of tongue is formed by two lingual swellings and tuberculum impar. Posterior one-third is derived from cranial part of hypobranchial eminence.
- Postnatal growth of maxilla is by displacement, remodeling and growth at sutures.
- Postnatal development of mandible is based on remodeling and Enlow's principle.

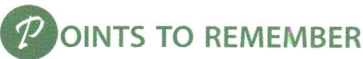

Questionnaire

1. Explain the prenatal growth of face.
2. Describe postnatal growth of maxilla.
3. Discuss postnatal growth of mandible.
4. Explain the development of palate.
5. Describe dimensional changes in maxillary arch.
6. Age changes in mandible.

FURTHER READING

1. Bhalajhi SI. Orthodontics: The Art and Science, 3rd edition. Arya (Medi) Publishing House; 2006.
2. Enlow DH. Handbook of Facial Growth. WB Saunders Co; 1982.
3. Hagg T, Attstrom H. Estimated mandibular growth. Am J Orthod. 1992:146.
4. Henneberke A, Andersen P. Cranial base growth. Am J Orthod. 1994:5014.
5. Nielsen IL, Bravo LA, Miller AJ. Normal maxillary and mandibular growth and dentoalveolar development. Am J Orthod. 1989:405.
6. Profitt WR. Contemporary Orthodontics. St Louis: CV Mosby; 1986.
7. Tencate AR. Oral Histology: Development, Structure and Function. St. Louis: CV Mosby; 1980.

CHAPTER

Principles, Assessment, and Factors Influencing Growth

Nikhil Marwah, Pallavi Pawar, Lumbini Pathivada

CHAPTER OUTLINE

- Factors Affecting Growth and Development
- Growth-pattern, Variability, and Timing Concept
- Differential Growth
- Growth Spurts
- Growth Trends
- Growth Assessment Parameters
- Dental Age
- Computerized Growth Forecasting

Growth and development are an extremely complex series of events that are best evaluated by careful examination at different stages. No one would disagree that it is more difficult to hit a moving target than a stationary one. This analogy seems appropriate to apply to pedodontists who are working with growing children. It is to be kept in mind that the child is in a dynamic, changing state and presents no static picture. The fully developed craniofacial skeleton represents the sum of its separate parts, in which the growth is highly differentiated and occurs at different states in different durations.

FACTORS AFFECTING GROWTH AND DEVELOPMENT

Factors influencing postnatal growth are so innumerable, and it is sometimes suggested that >1% of all human beings end up with their genetic final height; 99% are shorter owing to negative factors during postnatal life. The regulation of growth in terms of rate, timing, form, and character depends upon a combination and interactions of genetic and environmental factors.

Genetic Factors

- The genes contained within the nucleus of each cell are said to be necessary to produce an entire organism and are primarily responsible for orchestrating the phenomenon of normal growth.
- A genetic control influences the size of the organism to a great extent and the rate of onset of growth event.
- Polani indicated that size at birth relates about 18% to genome of fetus, 20% to maternal genome, and 30% to unknown factors.
- After birth the infant's growth rate is no longer determined by maternal factors but increasingly related to his own genetic makeup.
- **Bayley** emphasizes the resemblance of the child to the parent in stature and in performance becoming ever closer with increasing growth thus indicating the genetic background size for a newborn baby.

Summary of factors affecting growth

- Genetic factors
- Extracranial and intracranial pressure
- Maternal factors
- Socioeconomic factors
- Nutrition
- Hormones
- Muscular function
- Growth factors
- Race
- Illness
- Climate and seasonal effect
- Adult physique
- Exercise
- Family size and birth order
- Secular trend
- Psychological disturbance

Extracranial and Intracranial Pressure

- Any factor affecting physical growth is expected to be associated with effect on size and shape of cranial vault.
- For example, raised intracranial pressure during infancy results in an increased cranial circumference; if pressure is long-standing, sutural margin develop interdigitation with spiky appearance, and so when sutures are closed, it leads to excessive resorption of inner table of cranial vault.

Maternal Factors

The size of a full-term infant correlates well with the size of mother.

Socioeconomic Factors

- These factors play role as a growth factor.
- Children living in favorable socioeconomic conditions tend to be larger, display different types of growth, and show variations in timing of growth.
- **Leachtig A et al**. concluded that lower the socioeconomic status, shorter are the children.

Nutrition

- The raw materials for energy and biosynthesis are obviously essential for normal growth.
- Lack of nutrition delays growth, affects size of body part, body properties, body chemistry, quality and texture of some tissues. For example, iodine deficient diet retards craniofacial growth.
- Unless the mother's nutrition is quite poor, the fetus is able to obtain adequate nutrition for prenatal growth at the expense of the mother. In case this does not happen, the growth slows down. They wait for better time, and with return of good nutrition, growth takes place unusually fast until the genetically determined curve is neared once more. This is called catch-up growth.

Hormones

Table 13.1. shows hormones responsible for growth.

Muscular Functions

- The close relation between muscles and bone growth is seen due to the fact that the muscles influence the growth both as tissue affecting vascular supply and as a force element.
- The increased loading of jaws leads to increased sutural growth and bone apposition resulting in transverse growth of maxilla and broader base of dental arches.
- For example, wrestlers have well-developed dental arches, whereas patients of myotonic dystrophy have deteriorated craniofacial morphology.

Growth Factors

- These are peptides that transmit signals within and between cells and play a comprehensive role in modulation of tissue growth and development.
- These factors regulate a number of mechanisms like gene regulations, migration, and differentiation.

Race

- There are various factors like nutrition and environment that may lead to difference in growth in different races, but there is sufficient evidence to suggest that race alone has a role to play in the growth process.
- For example, calcification and eruption of teeth occurs around 1 year faster in blacks as compared to their white counterparts.

Illness

Any systemic disease or a prolonged debilitating disease has a profound effect on the growth process of a child.

Climate and Seasonal Effect

- A large amount of skeletal variations are associated with seasonal and climatic variations and these may affect the growth rate and weight of newborn.
- Although, there is no data to prove that there is direct effect of climate on rate of growth, those living in old climates tend to have more of adipose tissue, whereas those living hot climate are thinner.

Table 13.1: Hormones responsible for growth.

Group I	*Group II*	*Group III*	*Group IV*
Hormones influencing skeletal bone growth	Hormones responsible for ossification of long bones	Hormones responsible for pubertal growth spurt	Miscellaneous
• Growth hormone • Insulin • Thyrotropic hormone	• Parathormone	• Androgens • Progesterone • Estrogen	• Prolactin
• Stimulates production of proteins • Excess or deficiency may cause dwarfism, cretinism, acromegaly, or gigantism	• Increases bone resorption by intensifying osteoclastic activity • Facilitates conversion of vitamin D • Facilitates calcium absorption	• Development of secondary sexual characteristics • Sex differentiation • Making the muscles bulkier • Growth of female genital tract and breast • Behavioral changes in brain on puberty • Developing the secretory phase of menstrual cycle • Development of alveoli of breast	• Synthesis of milk

- Growth also varies according to seasons like it is faster in springs and summers and comparatively slower in winters.

Adult Physique

- There exists a definite relation between physique and development according to somatotypes.
- For example, tall women mature at a later age as compared to the other women of their age groups.

Exercise

It is useful for fitness and increase in muscles mass but has no relation with linear growth.

Family Size and Birth Order

- In a family, there will always exist a difference between the various members of a family with respect to their individual sizes, maturation level, and intelligence.
- Data also supports the fact that firstborns usually weigh less at birth, have less stature and higher IQ.

Secular Trend

- Size and maturational changes in a large population can be shown to occur with time.
- For example, 15-year-old boys nowadays are 5 inch taller than 15-year-old boys 50 years back.

Psychological Disturbance

- These can lead to inhibition of growth depending upon the severity of psychological disturbances.
- This is due to the fact that in stressful conditions, children will display inhibition of growth hormone.

GROWTH-PATTERN, VARIABILITY, AND TIMING CONCEPT

- A complete knowledge about the concepts of growth is necessary to understand the mechanism underlying. Pattern reflects proportionality usually of a complex set of proportions. In other words, the physical arrangement of the body at any one time is a pattern of spatially proportioned parts. It can be seen as the overall change in body proportions that occur during normal growth and development.
- *In fetal life at about one-third month of intrauterine development, the head takes up almost 50% of total body length. The cranium is large relative to face and represents more than half of total head, whereas the limbs are still rudimentary and the trunk is underdeveloped. By the time of birth, the trunk and limbs have grown faster than head and face so that the proportions of entire body devoted to head have decreased by 30% with the progressive reduction in relative size for head to about 12% the adult. At the birth, legs represent one-third of total body length, while in adult, they represent one-half. There is more growth of lower limbs than upper limbs during postnatal life. This means there is an axis of increased growth extending from head toward feet. This is called* **cephalocaudal gradient of growth (Fig. 13.1).**
- Second concept in growth and development is variability. Since everybody is not alike, it is very difficult but very important to decide whether an individual is merely at the extreme of normal variation or falls outside the normal range. Variability is thus expressed quantitatively.
- The final concept in study of growth and development is timing. Variation from timing arises because the same event happens for different individuals at different times. The timing concept can be explained by examples. For example, some children grow rapidly and mature early thereby being on the high side of developmental charts, whereas slow growers will lag behind, but with the onset of catch-up growth, they might even surpass the fast growers. Also seen in girls is the same mechanism. If a girl reaches her menarche at the age of 10–11 years she will mature faster as compared to the girl who has menarche at 13–15 years.

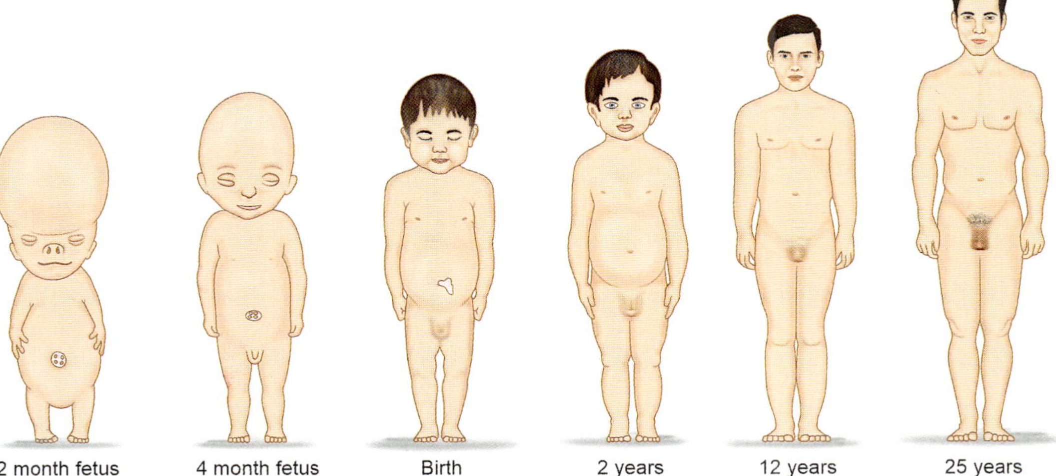

Fig. 13.1: Cephalocaudal gradient of growth.

DIFFERENTIAL GROWTH

The human body does not grow at the same rate throughout life. Different organs grow at different rates at a different amount and at different times. This is called **differential growth**.

Scammon curves for growth: The body tissues, namely, lymphoid, general, genital, and neural grow at different rates at different times. Upon analysis of the size of various parts and organs of the body, **Scammon** proposed that the growth of different tissues and systems could be summarized in four patterns (or curves) of growth. These configurations when plotted on a chart represent **Scammon** growth curves **(Fig. 13.2)**.

- **General tissue:** The general, or body, curve describes the growth of the body as a whole and of most of its parts—the growth pattern of stature, weight, and most external dimensions of the body. This consists of bones, muscles, and other organ systems. These exhibit an "S"- shaped curve with rapid growth up to 2–3 years of age followed by a slow phase till about 10 years. Then the growth again enters rapid phase in the 10th year and continues till terminating about 18–20 years.
- **Neural tissue:** The neural curve characterizes the growth of the brain, nervous system, and associated structures, such as the eyes, upper face, and parts of the skull. These tissues experience rapid growth early in postnatal life, so that about 95% of the total increment in size of the central nervous system between birth and 20 years is already attained by about 7 years of age. Grows very rapidly and reaches adult size by 6–7 years and very little growth occurs after that.
- **Genital tissue:** The genital curve characterizes the growth pattern of the primary and secondary sex characteristics. The former include the ovaries, fallopian tubes, uterus, and vagina in females, and the testes, seminal vesicles, prostate, and penis in males. Secondary sex characteristics include breast development in females, pubic and axillary hair in both sexes, and facial hair and growth of the larynx in males. This shows negligible growth until puberty, but grows rapidly on reaching puberty till adult level is achieved.

Scammon curve
- *General tissue:* These exhibit an "S"-shaped curve
- *Lymphoid tissue:* It increases rapidly in late childhood andreaches almost 200% of its adult size
- *Neural tissue:* Grows very rapidly and reaches adult size by 6–7 years
- *Genital tissue:* This shows negligible growth until puberty but grows rapidly on reaching puberty till adult level is achieved

- **Lymphoid tissue:** The lymphoid curve describes the growth of the lymph glands, thymus gland, tonsils, appendix, and lymphoid patches of tissue in the intestine. These tissues are involved in general with the child's developing immunological capacities, including resistance to infectious diseases. It increases rapidly in late childhood and reaches almost 200% of its adult size. This is due to the fact that children are more prone to infectious. By 18 years, the lymphoid tissue undergoes involution to reach adult size.

GROWTH SPURTS

- *Growth does not take place uniformly at all times. There seem to be periods when a sudden acceleration of growth occurs. This sudden increase in growth is called* **growth spurt.**
- The growth spurt in prenatal period and infantile period differs because they are more of a biological process involving division of the cells.
- On the other hand, the physiological alteration in hormonal secretion is believed to be the cause for accentuated growth associated with pubertal period.

Prediction and Clinical Applications of Growth Spurts

The prediction of direction, amount, and timing of growth spurt is very important with respect to orthodontic treatment. Growth spurt is the best time for interceptive orthodontics as growth can then be modeled according to the desired effect **(Fig. 13.3)**.

- Orthodontic treatment must be done earlier in girls as their growth spurt is early.
- The earlier the onset of puberty, the smaller is the adult.

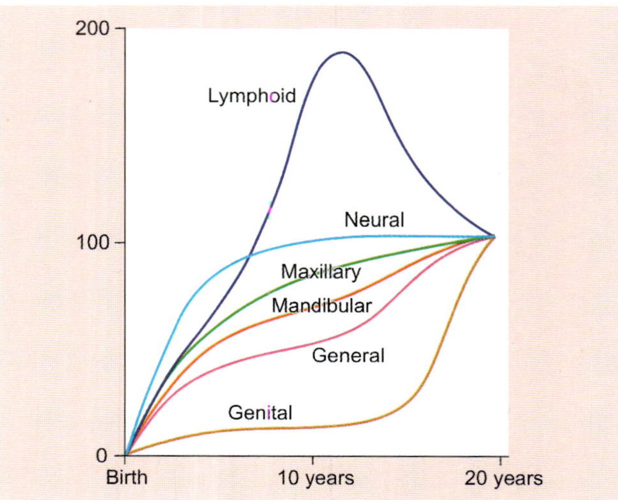

Fig. 13.2: Scammon curves.

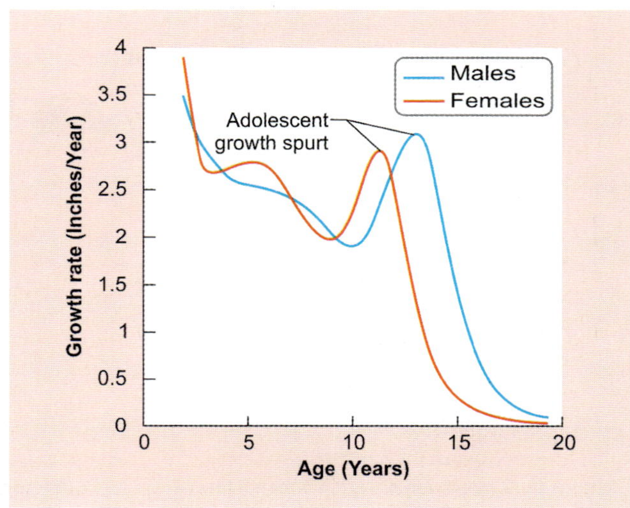

Fig. 13.3: Graphical representation of growth in children.

Table 13.2: Adolescent growth spurt.

Girls	*Boys*
First stage • Occurs about beginning of physical growth spurt • Appearance of breast buds and early stages of development of pubic hair • The peak velocity of physical growth occurs 1 year after inhibition of stage 1 *Second stage* • Secondary sexual characteristics begin to appear *Third stage* • Occurs 1–1.5 years after stage 2 and is marked by onset of menstruation • At this stage, there is more adult type of fat distribution occurring	*First stage* • Initial sign of sexual development in boys is "fat spurt" • Maturing boy gains weight and there is feminine like fat distribution due to estrogen production by Leydig cells *Second stage* • This occurs 1 year after stage 1 and coincides with beginning of increase in height • Redistribution and decrease of fat • Growth of sexual organs also takes place in this stage *Third stage* • Occurs 1–12 months after stage 2 and coincides with peak velocity of gain in height • Axillary and facial hairs appear • The sexual organs reach adult size • There is also muscular growth spurt *Fourth stage* • This occurs between 15 and 24 months after stage three • The growth in height ends • Hair appears on full face • Increase in muscular strength

- Girls mature earlier but also finish their growth sooner and that leads to the difference in adult size of men and women.
- Growth spurts are also affected by environmental variations.

The timing of growth spurts
- Just before birth
- One year after birth
- Mixed dentition growth spurt
  - Boys: 8–11 years
  - Girls: 7–9 years
- Adolescent growth spurt **(Table 13.2)**
  - Boys: 14–16 years
  - Girls: 11–13 years

- Malocclusion requiring surgical correction should only be undertaken after the growth spurt is completed.
- Arch expansion can be done during growth spurts.
- Class III tendency with mandibular prognathism should be treated before prepubertal growth spurt.
- Class II, III malocclusion should be treated during growth spurt.
- If the jaw growth has to be accelerated, it has to be done before adolescent growth spurt in girls.
- In the timing of orthodontic treatment, clinicians have a tendency to treat girls too late and boys too soon. Forgetting the disparity in physiologic maturation, if the treatment is delayed, the opportunity to utilize the growth spurt is missed. Therefore, it is very necessary to carefully assess the physiologic age while planning for orthodontic treatment.

GROWTH TRENDS

By overlapping consequent cephalograms, **Tweed** discerned a pattern of growth and termed it as growth trends.

Type A

- The maxilla and mandible grow together and thus ANB angle remains same.
- Should this be accompanied by class I relationship and ANB does not exceed 4.5°, no treatment is indicated.
- Seen in >25%.

Type A Subdivision

- Maxilla is protruding with ANB angle >4.5°.
- The treatment is to restrict the growth of maxilla while allowing mandible to catch up.
- The prognosis is good but may sometimes require extraction of premolars.

Type B

- Mandible and maxilla grow forwards and downwards with the growth of maxilla exceeding that of mandible.
- Poor prognosis and indicates that point B will not catch up with point A.
- Growth of middle and lower face is predominantly in vertical direction.

ANB angle
- According to **Sterner**, it is the angle between point A on maxilla and point B on mandible
- It is the difference between SNA and SNB and indicates the magnitude of skeletal join discrepancies
- The normal value of ANB angle is 2°
- If it is <2°, then it is indicative of class II, and if it is >2°, then indicative of class III malocclusion **(Fig. 13.4)**

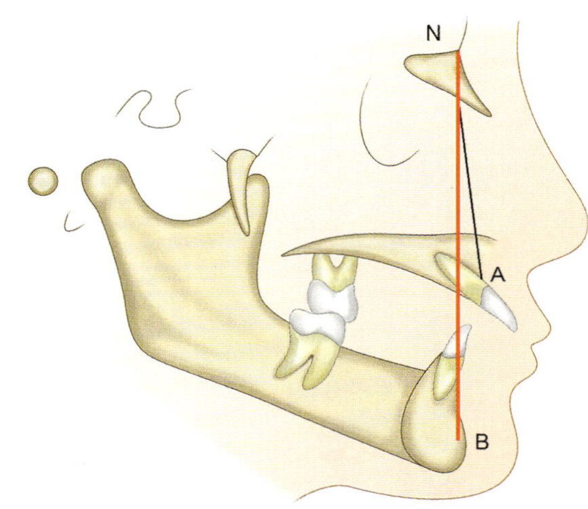

Fig. 13.4: ANB angle.

Type B Subdivision

The ANB angle is large and continues to grow indicating unfavorable growth trend.

Type C

- The maxilla and mandible grow forwards and downwards with mandible growing forward more rapidly.
- The ANB angle is seen to be decreasing with the mandible catching up with maxilla.
- This indicates favorable trend and no treatment is required until eruption of canine.

Type C Subdivision

- The mandible is found to be growing more forward when compared to maxilla; with this the mandible incisors touch the lingual surface of maxillary incisors.
- Therefore mandibular incisors are tipped lingually and maxillary incisors are tipped labially.

GROWTH ASSESSMENT PARAMETERS

The correct knowledge of facial age, developmental age, chronologic age, etc. is very necessary for formulating treatment plan. These anthropometric measurements are also useful in the interdisciplinary evaluation of patients.

Somatotypic Age

- In the overall assessment of child, a general somatotype may be appreciated.
- **Sheldon**[1] defined somatotype **(Figs. 13.5A to C)** by a series of 17 anthropometric measurements and is not related to nutritional status.
  - *Endomorph:* Stocky abundant subcutaneous fat, digestive viscera that are highly developed.
  - *Mesomorph:* Upright, sturdy, athletic, muscle bone and connective tissue is predominant.
  - *Ectomorph:* Tall, thin, and fragile with minimal subcutaneous fat and muscle tissue.
- In terms of chronologic age, ectomorph matures very late, whereas endomorph matures very early.
- Although somatotype may give gestalt about child's developmental pattern, it is not an accurate predictor of growth.

Chronologic Age

- This is the most obvious and most easily determined developmental age parameter, which is figured from child's date of birth.
- There might be difference in children of same chronologic age due to difference in thing of maturation, diseases, and various environmental factors.
- Although, it is easy to determine, chronologic age is not an accurate indicator of development nor is it a good predictor of growth.

Height and Weight Age

- Height has been commonly employed as determinant of development age.
- The standard growth curve commonly employed to characterize a child's height compared to that of children of same chronologic age is used to assess development age.
- Growth of all children up to puberty follows nearly the same curves, but the difference in adolescent growth spurts change the growth curves during and after puberty greatly.

Types of age according to Krogman[2]

- Chronologic age
- Biologic age
  - Morphologic age
  - Skeletal age
  - Dental age
  - Circumpubertal age
- Behavioral age
- Mental age
- Self-concept age

- Because height of each child is related to genetic as well as environmental factors, it is clear that a single measurement is limited as a predictor of development age.
- If at all height age has to be considered, then longitudinal height of a child which expresses the child's own growth curve is of more value.
- Weight and height age are correlated well with each other **(Fig. 13.6)**, but weight age alone is a poor indicator if

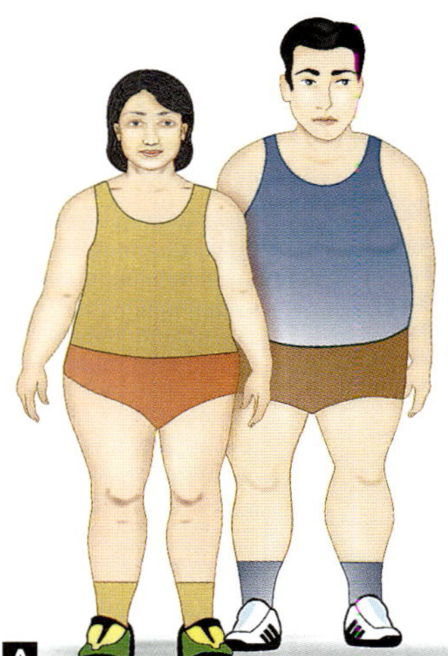

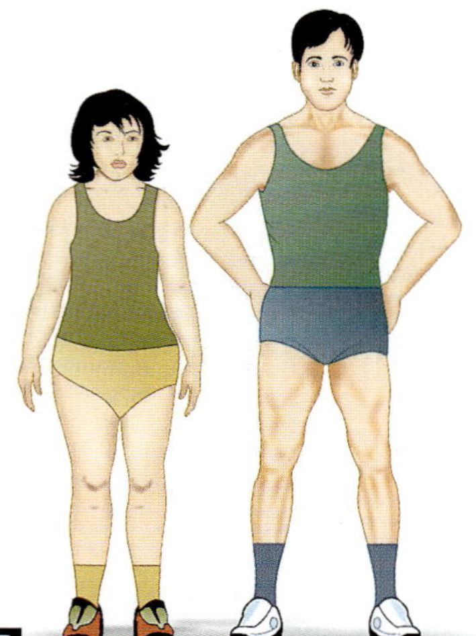

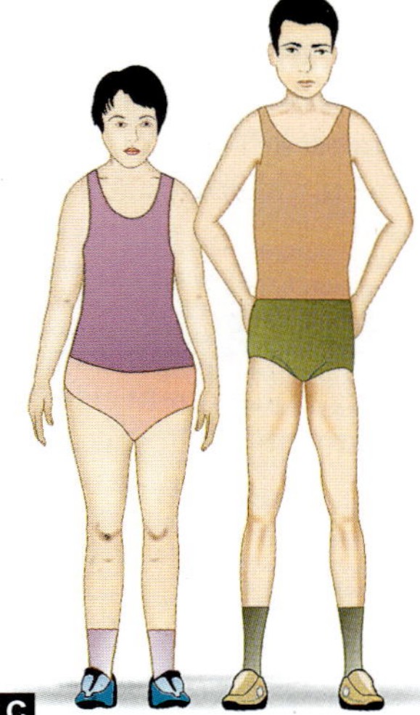

Figs. 13.5A to C: Somatotypic classification: (A) Endomorph; (B) Mesomorph; (C) Ectomorph.

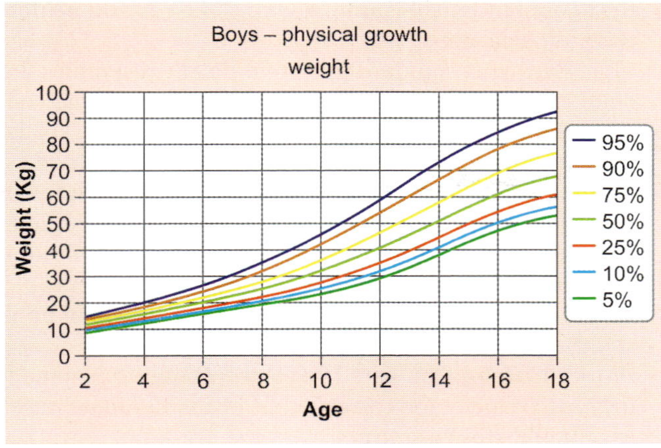

Fig. 13.6: Height/weight comparative chart for age assessment.

growth or developmental age owes to a large number of variations.

- Clinical implications of this age are that earlier the spurt occurs, shorter it is, and therefore late matures are taller which also accounts for the difference in males and females.

Sexual Age

- At puberty differential hormones actions yield characteristic body charges.
- These changes are classified into five stages according to **Reynolds, Wines,** and **Tanner**.[3]
- They outlined the stages of secondary sexual characteristics and their relation to pubertal growth spurt in height and their relation with developmental age **(Table 13.3)**.

Facial Age

- The ultimate goal of developmental growth assessment of children being evaluated for craniofacial intervention is facial age.
- The aim is to identify whether they are on their own facial growth curve and to use this as a predictor of future growth.
- Various methods used for measurement of facial age and prediction of craniofacial growth are anthropometric measurement, facial growth velocity curve, and cephalometric radiographs.

Skeletal Age

- This is a very important aspect of assessing the developmental age of child as skeletal age was found to more highly correlate with the developmental age than any other growth parameter.
- Each endochondral bone begins with a primary center of ossification which then changes shape, size, and contour till its fusion.
- Any of the skeletal growth centers can be used for skeletal age assessment but hand and wrist have been most commonly used for assessment of pubertal maturation.
- Advantages of using skeletal age are readily recognizable stage of ossification; regular sequence of developmental changes occurring from birth to adulthood; characteristic pattern of progression of ossification of epiphyseal centers can be identified.

Hand and Wrist Radiographs

The hand-wrist region is made up of numerous small bones which show a predictable and scheduled pattern of appearance, ossification, and union from birth to maturity. Thus by comparing a patients' radiograph with the standards that represent different skeletal ages, we find out the skeletal maturation status of that individual.

Anatomy of hand-wrist region: This region is made up of four groups of bones, namely, forearm, carpals, metacarpals, and phalanges **(Fig. 13.7)**.

1. **Distal ends of long bones of forearm:** The distal ends of radius and ulna form the first group of bones. These give rise to distal projections on their respective sides called radial and ulnar styloid.
2. **Carpals:** These consist of eight small irregularly shaped bones arranged in two rows:
   - *Proximal row:* Scaphoid, lunate, triquetral, pisiform.
   - *Distal row:* Trapezium, trapezoid, capitate, hamate.
3. **Metacarpals:** Five miniature long bones forming the skeletal framework of palm of hand. Each metacarpal ossifies from one primary and one secondary center.
4. **Phalanges:** These are small bones forming the fingers. These are three in number except for thumb which has two. The three bones are called as proximal, middle, and distal.
5. **Sesamoid bone:** Small nodular bone often present embedded in the tendinous region of thumb.

Table 13.3: Sexual age.

Stage	*Pubic hair ratings for girls and boys*	*Breast development ratings in girls*	*Genitalia maturity rating in boys*
Stage 1	No pubic hair	Elevation of papilla only	Testes, penis are the same size and proportion as in childhood
Stage 2	Sparse growth, straight hair	Enlargement of breast bud with increase in areolar diameter	Enlargement of testes and scrotum with change in texture of skin
Stage 3	Dark, coarse, curled hair	Further enlargement without separation of contour of areola from breast	Enlargement of penis in length with continued growth of testes and scrotum
Stage 4	Adult type hair but cover less area	Projection of areola to form a secondary mound	Increase in breadth of penis with glans development and continued enlargement of testes
Stage 5	Adult quantity and type with spread to medial surface of thigh	Further projection of papilla	Adult size and shape

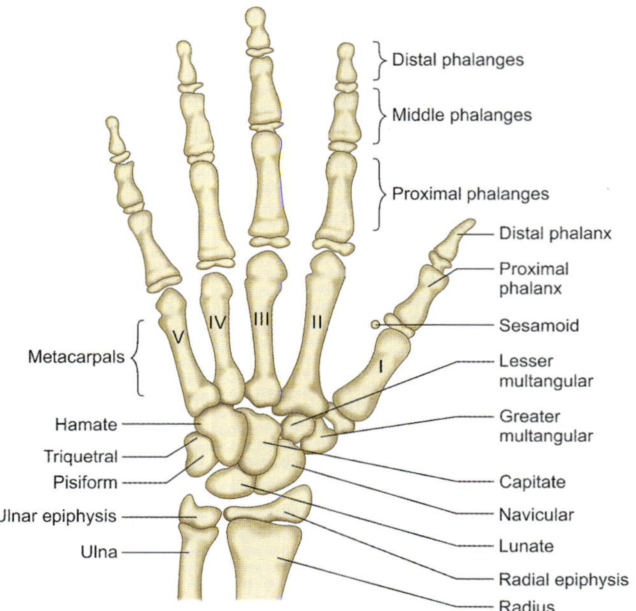

Fig. 13.7: Tracing of male standard 13 years, 6 months hand-wrist radiograph.

Indications of hand-wrist radiographs
- In patients who exhibit major difference between chronological and dental age
- Determination of skeletal maturity prior to treatment of skeletal malocclusion
- To assess skeletal age in patients whose growth is affected by neoplastic, infectious conditions
- Helps predict future skeletal maturation rate and status
- To predict pubertal growth spurt
- Studying role of heredity, environment, nutrition on the skeletal maturational pattern
- In patients with skeletal malocclusion needing orthognathic surgery to assess growth status

Determination of skeletal age:

The APA view radiograph of left hand and wrist are considered to be standard for determining skeletal age. The following are conventionally followed methods for skeletal age assessment:

- **Greulich** and **Pyle**[4] published an atlas of standard hand-wrist radiographs for males and females at various ages **(Figs. 13.8A to G).**
- For determination of skeletal age, one compares the radiograph of left hand-wrist region of the child with the atlas standards beginning with same sex and nearest chronological date.
- The hand-wrist standard that superficially resembles the child's radiograph is chosen for more detailed comparison.
- All the bones are assessed and each center is given a skeletal age of the standard. An overall age is then determined.
- **Tanner** and **Whitehouse:**[5] Suggested three methods of scoring maturity of individual bones to determine skeletal age: radius, ulna, short bone (RUS) score, carpal bone method, TW2 method (scores all the growth centers).
- **Tarranger et al.:**[6] Mean appearance time (MAT) of bone stages.
- **Bjork** and **Helm:** Compared the stages of bone development to growth velocity and correlated seven maturational stages to pubertal growth spurt.
- **Grave** and **Brown:**[7] They further corroborated the evidence of **Bjork** and **Helm** and included more ossification centers. They divided skeletal development into nine stages, each representing a level of skeletal maturity. **Schopf** in 1978 gave specific chronological ages to each of these stages **(Table 13.4).**

DENTAL AGE

- Dental age is estimated according to the last tooth erupted in oral cavity in normal sequence.
- This is the simplest but, the least accurate method.

Dental age measurement approaches[8]
- Atlas approach where we see the distinct stages of mineralization of tooth on radiographs and identify the age, for example, Massler method, Moorrees method, Anderson method
- Scoring approach where each development is divided into stages and each stage given a score, for example, Demirjian method, Nolla classification, Jhonson's method

- This involves recognizing the teeth clinically present in the oral cavity in comparison to dental eruption charts.
- The disadvantages of this technique are the wide variations in time of eruption, influence of local and environmental factors, and the fact that no or several teeth may erupt during the same time interval.
- Dental age is not well correlated with the developmental status of the child but there are a few methods which give the development quotient to a fairly accurate level thus signifying the close relation between dental and chronologic age.

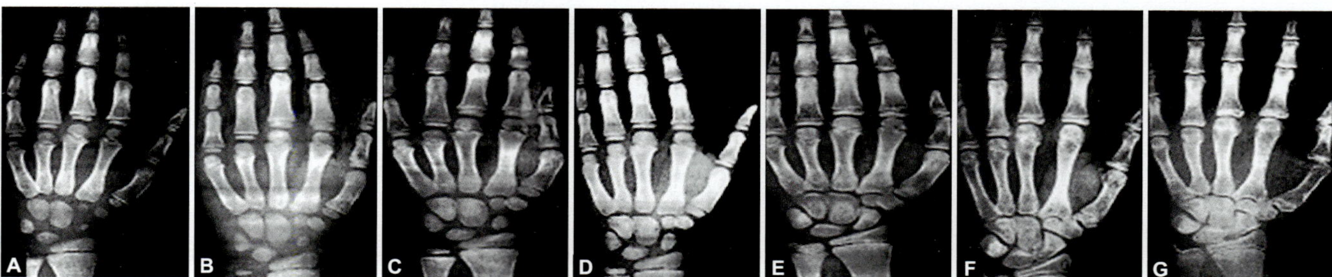

Figs. 13.8A to G: Hand-wrist radiograph of children ranging from 5 to 15 years.

Table 13.4: Stages of skeletal development.

Stage 1	***Stage 2***	***Stage 3***
• Epiphysis and diaphysis of proximal phalanx of index finger are equal • 3 years before peak velocity of pubertal growth spurt • Males—10.6 years; females—8.1 years 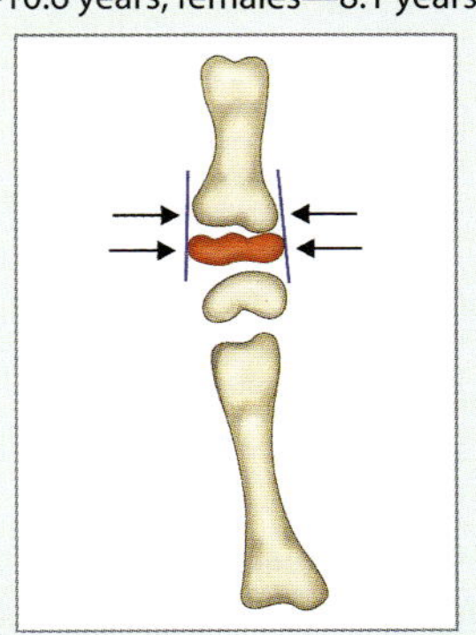	• Epiphysis and diaphysis of middle phalanx of middle finger are equal • Males—12.0 years; females—8.1 years 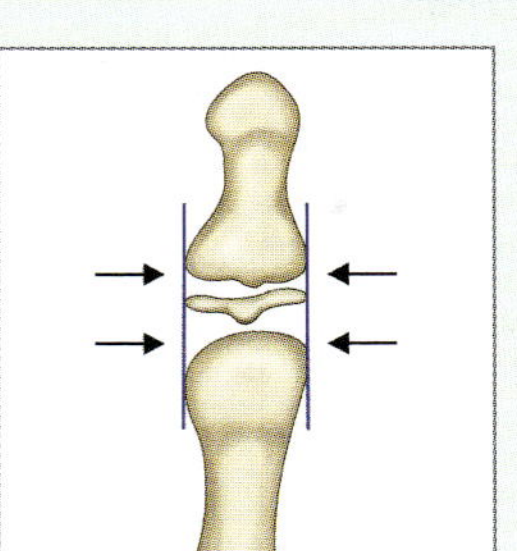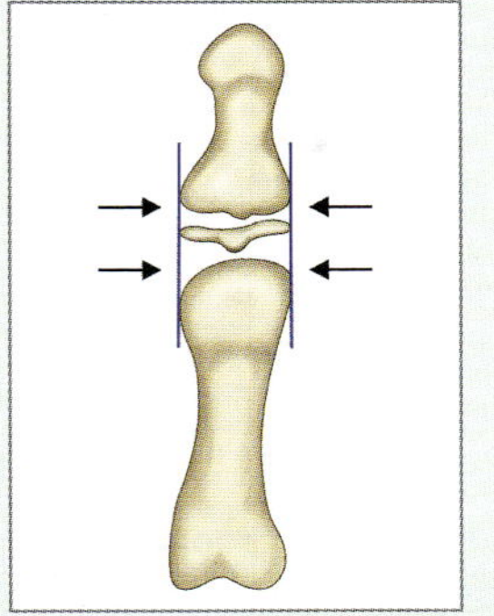	• Characterized by areas of ossification, viz., hamular process of hamate, ossification of pisiform • Males—12.6 years; females—9.6 years 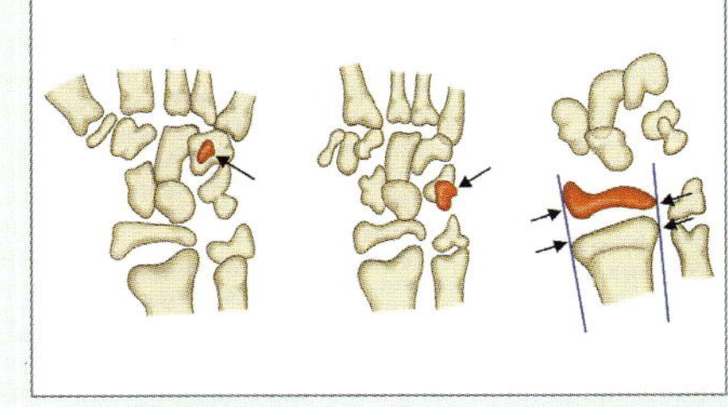
Stage 4	***Stage 5***	***Stage 6***
• Marks the beginning of pubertal growth spurt • Increase mineralization of ulnar sesamoid in thumb • Increased ossification of hamular process of hamate • Males—13.0 years; females—10.6 years 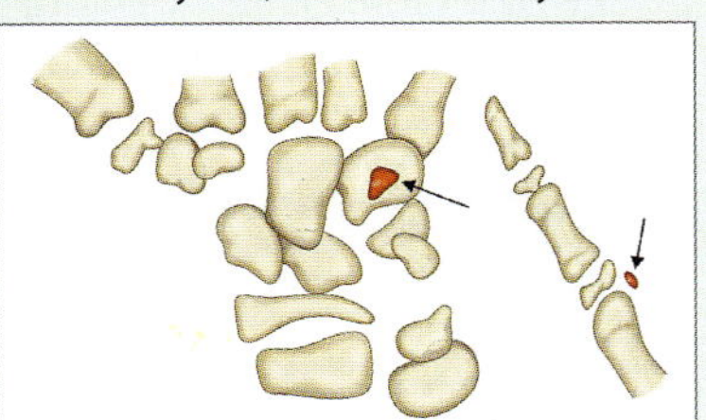	• Peak of pubertal growth spurt • Epiphysis caps diaphysis in middle phalanx of 3rd finger, proximal phalanx of thumb and radius • Males—14.0 years; females—11.0 years 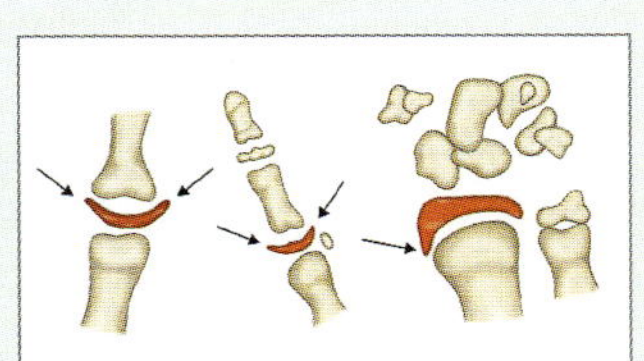	• End of pubertal growth spurt • Union of epiphysis and diaphysis of distal phalanx of middle finger • Males—15.0 years; females—13.0 years 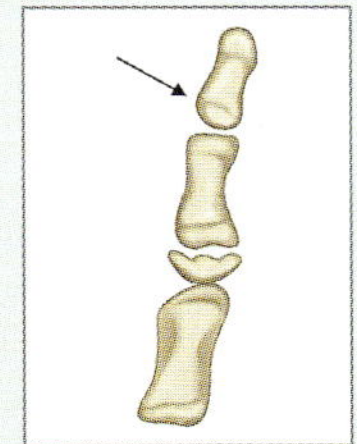
Stage 7	***Stage 8***	***Stage 9***
• Union of epiphysis and diaphysis of proximal phalanx of middle finger • Males—15.9 years; females—13.3 years 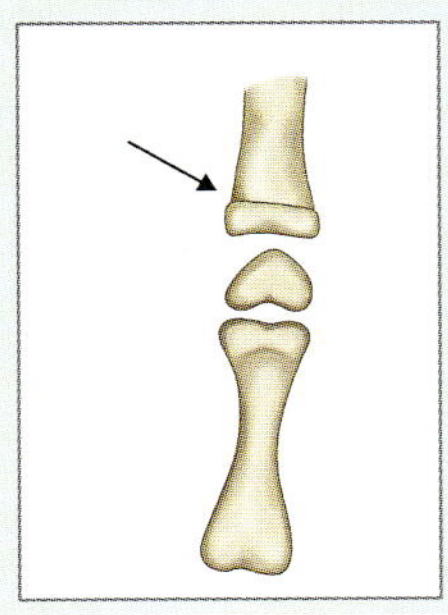	• Fusion between epiphysis and diaphysis of middle phalanx of middle finger • Males—16.9 years; females—13.9 years 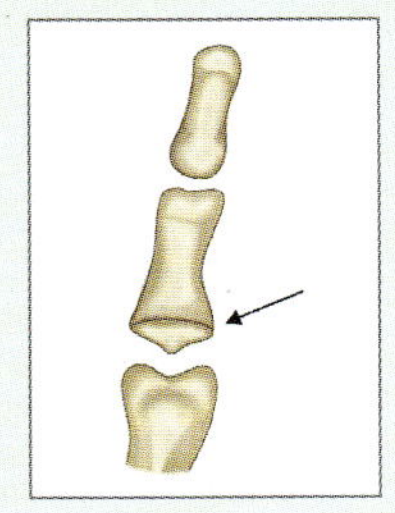	• Signifies end of skeletal growth • Fusion of epiphysis and diaphysis of radius • Males—18.5 years; females—16.0 years 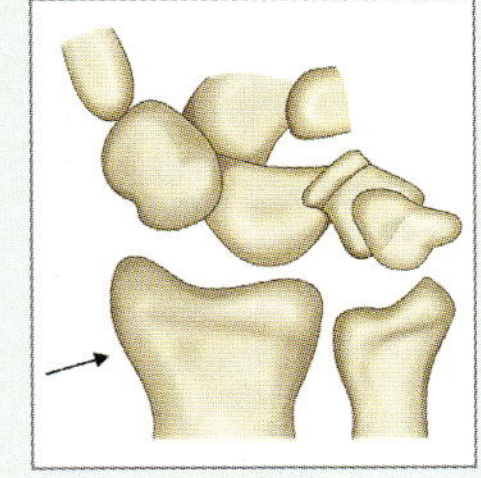

Gron and Moorrees Method[9,10]

- They helped formulate what is to date the most commonly used method of determining dental age.
- This method involved scoring of 10 permanent teeth according to crown and root formation using standard dental films **(Figs. 13.9A and B).**
- The teeth which were scored were maxillary and mandibular incisor, mandibular canine, premolars, and molars.
- Scores are plotted on a chart composed of horizontal segment for each tooth with demarcation for developmental stages and horizontal segment marked in years of age. For each tooth, appropriate stage is checked and a vertical line drawn through the corresponding checks, yielding a mean dental age.
- This was later modified by **Anderson** who added third molar also.

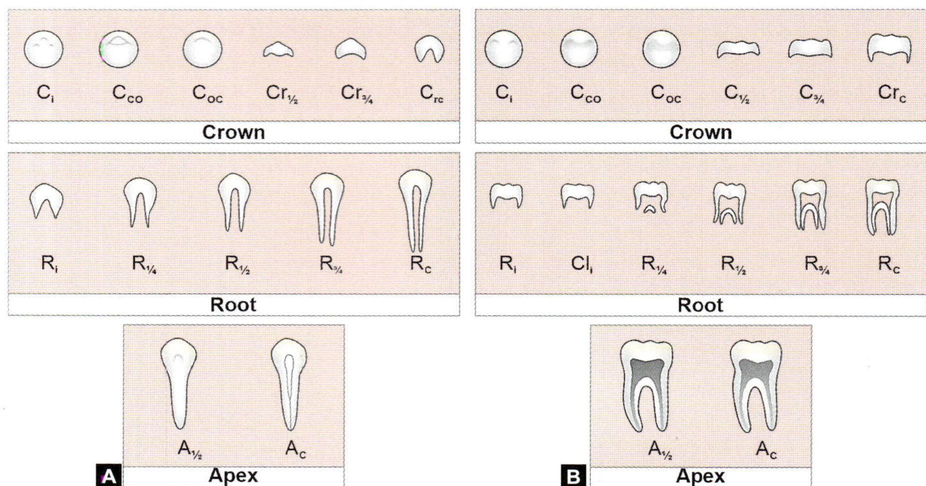

Figs. 13.9A and B: Tooth formation: (A) single-rooted; (B) multirooted. Coding symbols: C_i: initial cusp formation; C_{co}: cusp coalescence; C_{oc}: cusp outline complete; $Cr_{1/2}$: crown half complete; $Cr_{3/4}$: crown three quarters complete; Cr_c: crown complete; R_i: initial root formation; $R_{1/4}$: root length one quarter; $R_{1/2}$: root length one half; $R_{3/4}$: root length three quarters; R_c: root length complete; $A_{1/2}$: apex half closed; A_c: apex completely closed. (*Source:* Moorrees CFA, Fanning EA, Hunt EE. Age variation of formation stages of 10 permanent teeth. J Dent Res. 1963;42:1490).

Demirjian Method[11]

- **Demirjian** and **Goldstein** devised a new method for assessment of development of dental age.
- All teeth are rated on a scale of A–H **(Fig. 13.10)** and **(Table 13.5).**
- Each tooth having a stage was converted into a score using conversion table. The scores of all the teeth were then added to give the total maturity score. This score was then converted to dental age by a table given by **Demirjian** in 1973.

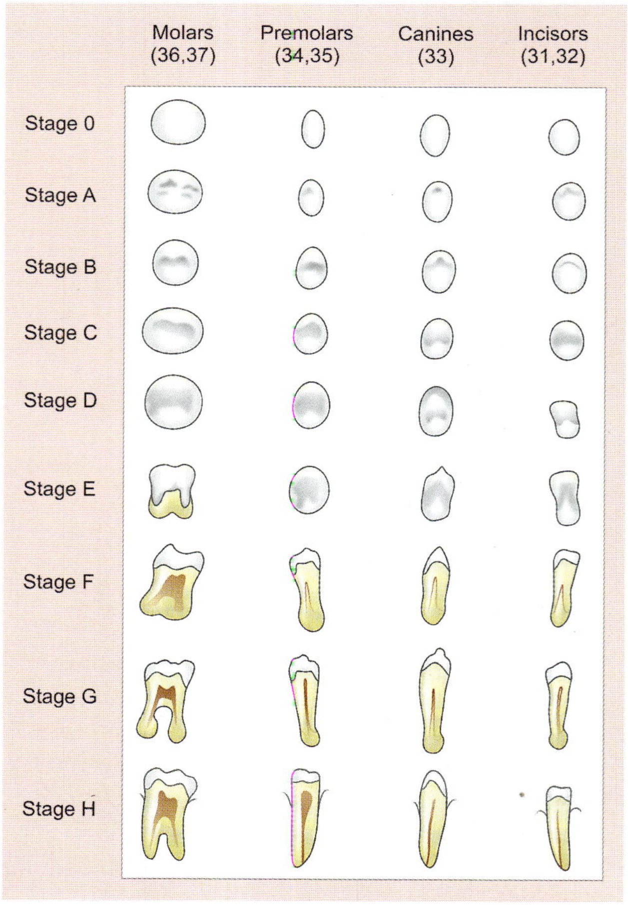

Fig. 13.10: Demirjian method for dental age assessment.

Table 13.5: Demirjian scale.

Stage	*Description*
O	No sign of calcification
A	Beginning of calcification seen at superior level of crypt
B	Fusion of calcification points in the cuspal area to form occlusal surface
C	• Enamel formation is complete with convergence toward cervical region • Beginning of dentinal deposit • Outline of pulp chamber has a curved shape at the occlusal border
D	• Crown formation is completed till CEJ • Superior border of pulp chamber in uniradicular teeth is curved and in molars is in trapezoidal form • Projection of pulp horn starts • Beginning of root formation in form of a spicule
E	• In uniradicular teeth pulp chamber forms straight line whose continuity is broken by pulp horns • Initial formation of bifurcation is seen in molars • Root length is less than crown height
F	• Walls of pulp chamber form a triangle and apex ends in funnel shape in uniradicular teeth • Calcified region of bifurcation in molars is more developed thus giving roots of the teeth a more distinctive outline • The root length is equal to or greater than crown height
G	• Walls of root canal are parallel and apical end is still open in molars
H	• Apical end of distal root in molars is closed • Periodontal membrane has uniform width around the root and apex

Cameriere Method[13]

It is a method for assessing chronological age in children based on relationship between age and measurement of open apices in teeth. This method was reported to be much more accurate than other methods. Using radiographic methods for age estimation is simple, nondestructive and reliable.

Nolla Stages[12]

They classified the developing tooth according to its radiographic status as given in **Figure 13.11**.

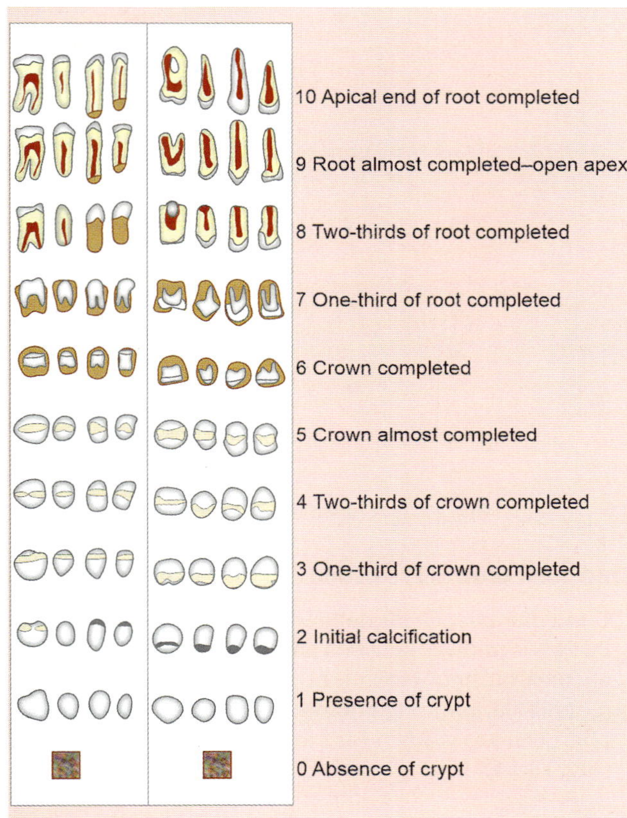

Fig. 13.11: Diagram of tooth maturation showing the progression from initial appearance of crypt through the last stage of apical root closure for the developing tooth. (*Source:* Based upon data published by Nolla C. Development of the permanent teeth. J Dent Child. 1960;27:254).

Willem's Method[14]

Dental age (DA) determination is required in various clinical and scientific disciplines such as pediatric dentistry, orthodontics, archaeology, paleontology and forensic dentistry. In certain communities, the chronological age (CA) of living people bears significant importance regarding social benefits, employment and marriage. Age of an unknown person can be assessed by correlating the physical, skeletal, and dental maturity of an individual. To be able to measure DA directly is important because it is a useful tool to estimate the CA of a child with an unknown birth date. Several methods have been proposed for assessing dental development, which is generally referred to as dental aging. Willem's method is one of the accurate method for assessment of dental age. It is the modified form of Demirjian method. In this method dental age is assessed with the help of OPGs. Digital OPGs were used as the images can be magnified to make analysis easier.

Stages	Description
A	A beginning of calcification is seen at the superior level of crypt in the form of cones. There is no fusion of these calcified points.
B	Fusion of the calcified points forms one or several cusps, giving a regularly outlined occlusal surface
C	• Enamel and dentin formation is complete at the occlusal surface and converge at cervical region. • Dentin deposition is seen. • The outline of the pulp chamber has a curved shape at the occlusal border.
D	• Crown formation is completed down to the • cementoenamel junction. • Superior border of pulp chamber in uniradicular teeth has a definite curved form; projection of pulp horns gives an umbrella top. In molars, pulp chamber has a trapezoidal form. • Beginning of root formation is seen in the form of a spicule.
E	• Uniradicular teeth • The walls of pulp chamber form straight lines, whose continuity is broken by the pulp horn. • The root length is less than the crown height. • In molars • Initiation of radicular bifurcation is seen as a calcified point or a semi-lunar shape. • Root length is less than crown height.
F	• Uniradicular teeth • The walls of pulp chamber form isosceles triangle. Apex ends in a funnel shape. • The root length is equal to or greater than the crown height. • In molars • The bifurcation has developed down to give the roots a distinct outline with funnel shaped endings • Root length is equal to or greater than crown height.
G	• The walls of root canal are now parallel and its apical end is partially open (distal root in molars).
H	• The apical end of the root canal is completely closed. • Periodontal membrane has a uniform width around the root and apex.

Cervical Spine Maturation Method (CVM)[15]

It evaluates the shape of the cervical spine obtained from lateral cephalometric radiographs. There have been numerous reports on the use of carpal bones for evaluation of bone age as they contain many bone nuclei, can be radiographed easily, and require a smaller exposure dose. The cervical spine consists of seven vertebrae, and it supports the skull. Ossification of the cervical spine continues from the embryonic stage into adulthood. CVM correlates with carpal bone age assessment and is also suitable for mandibular growth assessment **(Fig. 13.12)**. The size of the mandibular bone and timing of growth are important to achieve good intermaxillary relationships in orthodontic treatment.

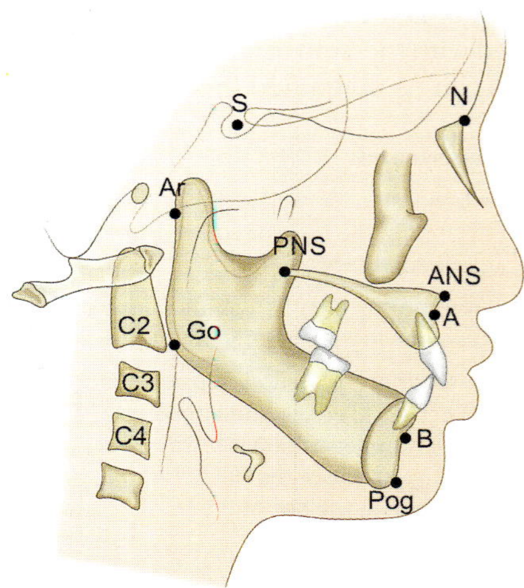

Fig. 13.12: Cephalometric landmarks used to construct the two linear measurements and angular measurements analyzed in this study. Linear parameters: ANS-PNS; Distance between ANS and PNS, Ar-Go; Distance between Articulare and Gonion, Go-Pog; Distance between Gonion and Pogonion. Angular parameters: (FMA; Mandibular plane to Frankfort-Horizontal plane, SNA; Sella-Nasion to Point A, SNB; Sella-Nasion to Point Cephalometric landmarks used to construct the two linear measurements and angular measurements analyzed in this study: Linear parameters: ANS-PNS; Distance between ANS and PNS, Ar- Go; Distance between Articulare and Gonion, Go-Pog; Distance between Gonion and Pogonion: Angular parameters: FMA; Mandibular plane to Frankfort-Horizontal plane, SNA; Sella-Nasion to Point A, SNB; Sella-Nasion to Point)

COMPUTERIZED GROWTH FORECASTING

This describes the growth of various components of craniofacial complex thus enabling the clinicians to evaluate the development of face and also to forecast the future direction of jaw growth. Ricketts was the pioneer of this concept of growth forecasting and his findings laid the foundation for future computerization of direction and magnitude of craniofacial growth. Based upon the knowledge of previous cephalometric investigations, **Schulhof** and **Bagha** utilized the science of biomathematics to computerize the growth and development of craniofacial complex. This is called computerized growth forecasting.

Growth Prediction

- **Ricketts**[13] in 1950 recognized the clinical usefulness of growth prediction.
- Prediction of growth changes requires specification of the amount of growth change at a given point in a given period and also the direction of growth.
- Several studies were done in which children who needed no orthodontic treatment were used as subjects to analyze their growth prediction. Cephalometric radiographs were taken at regular intervals and the data was grouped to provide a picture of normal growth changes.
- The major difficulty with growth prediction based on average changes is that an individual patient may have neither the average nor the amount or direction of growth and thus there is a possibility of a significant error.

Cranial-base Prediction

- The cranial base is extremely important in growth and development of entire cranium because of its relation with sphenoethmoidal and spheno-occipital synchondroses and their relationship to endochondral bone formation.
- The cranial base is designated by a line joining the most anterior point of foramen magnum (basion) with anterior point of frontonasal suture (nasion) **(Fig. 13.13).**
- In a normal child, cranial base will grow 2 mm/year. This is expressed by 1 mm forward growth of nasion and 1 mm backward growth of basion, both along the original cranial baseline.

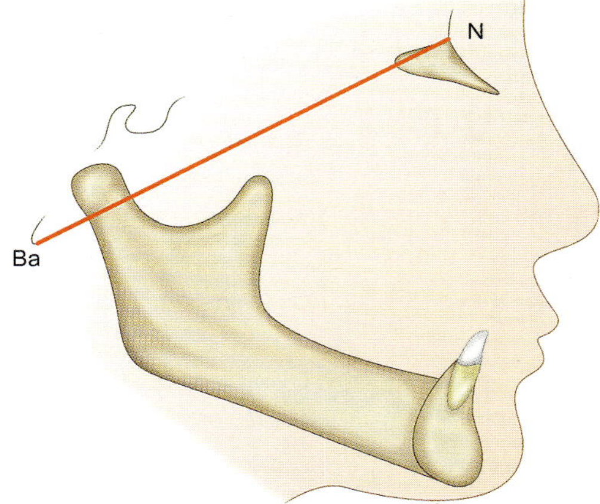

Fig. 13.13: Cranial-base prediction.

Mandibular Growth Prediction

- **Condylar axis:** This is defined as a line from a point on the Ba-N line midway between anterior and posterior borders of condylar neck (DC point), to the geometric center of mandibular ramus (Xi point). During 1 year of growth, Xi point will grow downward along condylar axis by 1 mm **(Fig. 13.14).**

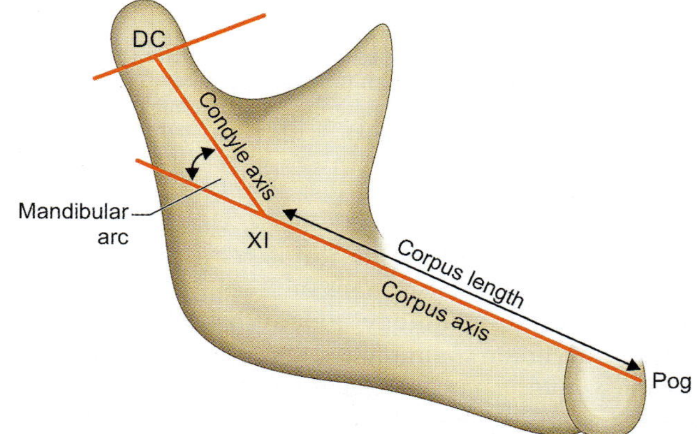

Fig. 13.14: Mandibular growth prediction.

- **Corpus axis:** The length of body of mandible is defined by a line from Xi point to the anterior point on mandibular symphysis. Each year, corpus axis grows 2 mm. The angle formed by condylar and corpus axis describes the configuration of mandible.

- **Small angle**
  - Steep mandibular plane.
  - Vertically growing mandible.
- **Large angle**
  - Square mandibular plane.
  - Forward mandibular growth.

Maxillary Growth Prediction

- Point A on maxilla grows forward same as nasion. Therefore the N-A angle or facial reference line remains the same during growth **(Fig. 13.15).**
- Skeletal convexity of a patient is determined by the relationship between point A and facial plane.
  - Point A forward (ahead of N-Pog line)—convex profile.
  - Point A backward (behind N-Pog line)—concave profile.

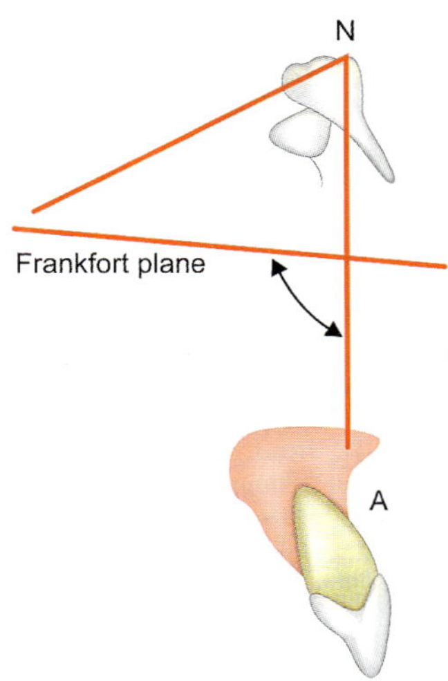

Fig. 13.15: Maxillary growth prediction.

Dentition

Related to A-Pog line

- *Lower incisor:* Stays in constant relation with A-Pog line throughout growth. Normal distance between A-Pog line and incisal edge is 1 mm.
- *Upper incisor:* Normal distance between A-Pog line and incisal edge is 3.5 mm.
- *Interincisal relation:* Normal angle is 130° with upper incisor 28° and lower incisor 22° to A-Pog line.
- *Molars:* In class I relation, distal surface of upper molar is 3 mm behind the distal surface of its lower counterpart.

Visual Treatment Objectives

- Whenever a dentist is dealing with factors that are changing, a treatment plan is more effective when those changes are anticipated and plans made.
- Bench incorporated the idea of orthodontic treatment design to computerized growth and designed visual treatment objective (VTO) for the purpose of diagnosis and treatment planning.
- The treatment design procedure outlined constructs VTO that first, changes areas due to normal growth in cranial base, chin, and maxilla; second, changes in area affected by orthopedic alteration; and third, visualize the orthodontic movement of the teeth within the jaws to a more normal relationship.
- VTO takes into consideration the changes with normal growth as well as the alteration due to treatment, and this helps the clinician to perform the treatment procedures with success.

POINTS TO REMEMBER

- Some factors affecting growth are genetic factors, maternal factors, socioeconomic factors, nutrition, hormones, race, family size and birth order, secular trend, and psychological disturbance.
- Lower the socioeconomic status, shorter are the children.
- Growth also varies according to seasons like it is faster in springs and summers and comparatively slower in winters.
- There is more growth of lower limbs than upper limbs during postnatal life. This means there is an axis of increased growth extending from head toward feet which is called cephalocaudal gradient of growth.
- The timing of growth spurts are just before birth, 1 year after birth, mixed dentition growth spurt, adolescent growth spurt.
- Orthodontic treatment must be done earlier in girls as their growth spurt is early.
- Malocclusion requiring surgical correction should only be undertaken after the growth spurt is completed.
- Arch expansion can be done during growth spurts.
- Chronological age is the most obvious and most easily determined developmental age parameter, which is figured from child's date of birth.
- Dental age is estimated according to the last tooth erupted in oral cavity in normal sequence.
- Atlas approach of dental age assessment is where we see the distinct stages of mineralization of tooth on radiographs and identify the age. For example, Massler method, Moorrees method, Anderson method, and scoring approach where each development is divided into stages and each stage is given a score. For example, Demirjian method, Nolla classification, Jhonson's method.
- Skeletal age assessment done by hand-wrist radiograph is the most reliable method of age assessment.
- Computerized growth and designed VTO for the purpose of diagnosis and treatment planning.

Clinical Significance

- Clinical significance of growth assessment parameter is of paramount importance to the dentist especially in cases of orthodontic treatment
- Correct knowledge of dental age would also help in identifying treatment plan for the child.

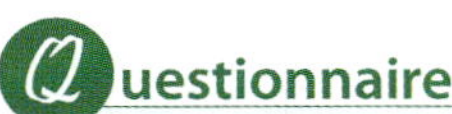

uestionnaire

1. Explain the factors affecting growth.
2. What is cephalocaudal gradient of growth?
3. Describe Scammon curve of growth.
4. What are growth spurts? Explain adolescent spurts.
5. Write a note on hand-wrist radiographs.
6. Define dental age and explain the methods to evaluate it.
7. What is Nolla classification?
8. Explain mandibular growth forecasting.

REFERENCES

1. Sheldon WH. Atlas of men a guide for somatotyping males at all ages. New York: Harper & Brothers; 1954.
2. Krogman WM. Biological timing and dentofacial complex. J Dent Child. 1968;35:176.
3. Reynolds EL, Wines JV. Physical changes associated with adolescence in boys. Am J Dis Child. 1951;82:529.
4. Greulich WW, Pyle SI. Radiographic atlas of skeletal development of hand and wrist. 2nd ed. Stanford, CA: Stanford University Press; 1959.
5. Tanner JM, Whitehouse RH, Marshall WA. Assessment of skeletal maturity and prediction of adult height. New York: Academic Press Inc.; 1975.
6. Tarranger J, Bruning B, Classon I. New method of assessment of skeletal maturity MAT. Acta Pediatr Scand Suppl. 1976; 258:121.
7. Grave KC, Brown T. Skeletal ossification and the adolescent growth spurt. Am J Orthod. 1976;69:611.
8. Willems G. A review of most commonly used age estimation techniques. J Forensic Odontostomatol. 2001;19:9-17.
9. Gron A. Prediction of tooth emergence. J Dent Res. 1962;41:573.
10. Moorrees CFA, Fanning EA, Hunt EE. Age variation of formation stages of 10 permanent teeth. J Dent Res. 1963;42:1490.
11. Demirjian A, Goldstein H. A new system of dental age assessment. Ann Hum Biol. 1976;3:411.
12. Nolla C. Development of the permanent teeth. J Dent Child 1960;27:254.
13. Nair VV, et al. Comparison of Cameriere's and Demirjian's methods of age estimation among children in Kerala: a pilot study. Clinics and Practice. 2018; 8 (991): 28-30.
14. Mohammed RB, et al et al.Dental age estimation using Willems method: A digital orthopantomographic study.Contemporary Clin Den. 2014;5(3):371-76.
15. Manabe A. Evaluation of maxillary and mandibular growth pattern based on cervical vertebral maturation in Japanese.
16. Ricketts RM. A principle of arcial growth of mandible. Angle Orthod. 1972;42:368.

FURTHER READING

1. Andrew D. Fundamental of craniofacial growth. Dixon.
2. Bhalajhi SI. Orthodontics: the art and science. 3rd edition. Arya Medi Publishing House; 2006.
3. El-Bakary AA, Hammad SM, Mohammed F. Dental age estimation in Egyptian children, comparison between two methods. J Forensic Leg Med. 2010;17:363-7.
4. Gustafson G, Koch G. Age estimation up to 16 years of age based on tooth development. Odontol Revy. 1974;25:297.
5. Helm S, Siersbaek NS, Skieller V, Bjork A. Skeletal maturation of hand in relation to pubertal growth in body height. Tandlaegebladet. 1971;75:1223.
6. Stewart RE, Barber TK, Troutman KC, Wei SHY. Pediatric dentistry: scientific foundation and clinical practice. St. Louis: CV Mosby; 1982.
7. Tanner JM, Whitehouse RH, Takaishi M. Standards from birth to maturity for height, weight, height velocity and weight velocity: British children (1965) I, II. Arch Dis Child. 1966;41:454-613.
8. Todd TW. Atlas of skeletal maturation. I. Hand. London: Henry Kimpton; 1937.

CHAPTER 14

Tooth Eruption and Shedding

Nikhil Marwah, Srinivas LS

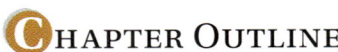

CHAPTER OUTLINE

- Pattern of Tooth Movement
- Theories of Tooth Eruption
- Shedding of Deciduous Teeth
- Chronology of Human Dentition

The word eruption properly refers to the cutting of the tooth through the gum. It is derived from the Latin word *erumpere*, meaning "to break out." It is generally understood to mean the axial or occlusal movement of the tooth from its developmental position in the occlusal plane. The emergence of the tooth through the gingiva is the first clinical sign of eruption. However, eruption is only a part of the total pattern of physiologic tooth movement, because teeth also undergo complex movements related to maintaining their position in the growing jaws and compensating for masticatory wear.

Maury Massler and **Schour** (1941) *defined eruption as a process whereby the forming tooth migrates from its intraosseous location in the jaw to its functional position within the oral cavity.*

Osborne *concluded that eruptive movement is defined as the axial movement of the tooth which brings the crown of the tooth from its developmental position within the bone of the jaw to its functional position in the occlusal plane.*

James K Avery *defined eruption as the movement of the teeth through the bone of the jaws and the overlying mucosa to appear and function in the oral cavity.*

PATTERN OF TOOTH MOVEMENT

Eruptive movements begin with the onset of the root formation, well before the teeth are seen in the oral cavity.

Movements leading to eruption of tooth can be divided into three phases:

1. Phase 1: Pre-eruptive phase.
2. Phase 2: Prefunctional eruptive or eruptive phase.
3. Phase 3: Functional eruptive or posteruptive phase.

Pre-eruptive Phase

- The pre-eruptive phase of tooth movement is preparatory to the eruptive phase.
- It consists of the movement of the developing tooth germs within the alveolar processes prior to root formation.
- During this phase, the growing tooth moves in two directions to maintain its position in the expanding jaws, viz., bodily movement and eccentric movement.
- Bodily movement, which occurs continuously as the jaw grows, is a movement of the entire tooth germ. This causes bone resorption in the direction of tooth movement and bone apposition behind it **(Fig. 14.1).**
- Eccentric growth refers to relative growth in one part of the tooth, while the rest of the tooth remains constant **(Fig. 14.2)**. For example, the root elongates, yet the crown does not increase in size. The crown maintains a constant relationship to the surrounding alveolar bone, while increase in alveolar height compensates for the root growth.
- During the early pre-eruptive phase, the successional permanent teeth develop lingual and near to occlusal level of their primary predecessor. But at the end of this phase,

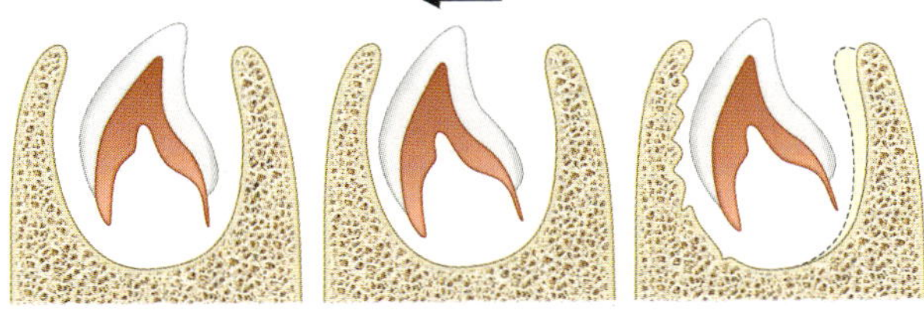

Fig. 14.1: Bodily movement of crown during eruption.

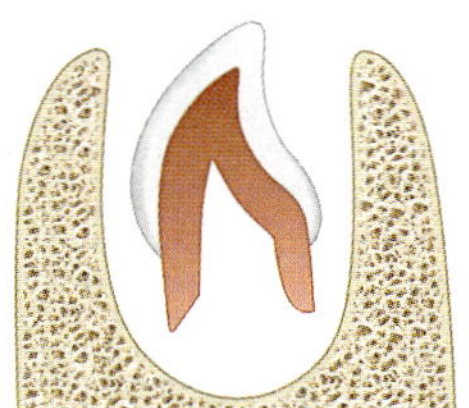
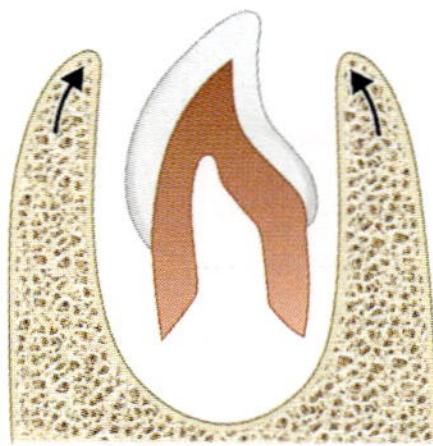

Fig. 14.2: Eccentric movement of crown during eruption.

the teeth are positioned lingually and near the apical third of the primary anterior teeth. The change in the position of the permanent tooth germ is mainly due to the eruption of the primary teeth and the coincident increase in the height of the supporting tissues. The permanent molars, having no primary predecessors, develop without this kind of relationship.

Eruptive Phase

The eruptive phase begins with the initiation of the root formation and ends when the teeth reach occlusal contact.

Anatomic stages of tooth eruption: Given by **Noyes** and **Schour (Fig. 14.3)**.

Stage I: Preparatory stage (opening of the bone crypt).
Stage II: Migration of the tooth toward the oral epithelium.
Stage III: Emergence of crown tip into the oral cavity (beginning of clinical eruption).
Stage IV: First occlusal contact.
Stage V: Full occlusal contact.
Stage VI: Continuous eruption.

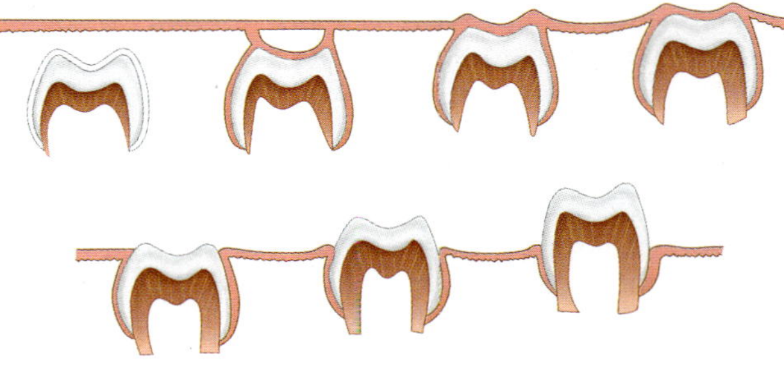

Fig. 14.3: Sequence of eruption of teeth.

Stages of tooth eruption.

Roots begin their formation as a result or proliferation of both the epithelial root sheath and the mesenchymal tissue of the dental papilla and dental follicle

↓

The erupting tooth moves through the bone of the crypt and the connective tissue of the oral mucosa

↓

The reduced enamel epithelium covering the crown comes in contact with the oral epithelium

↓

Reduced enamel epithelium of the crown proliferates and forms a thin attachment with the oral epithelium

Contd...

Contd...

↓

Tip of the crown enters the oral cavity by degenerating the membrane and breaking through the center of the double-layered epithelium

↓

Crown erupts further and the lateral border of the oral mucosa now becomes the dentogingival junction (DGJ)

↓

The reduced enamel epithelium now surrounding like a cuff, becomes known as the junctional or attachment epithelium

↓

Erupting tooth continues to move occlusally as the result of active eruption, exposing more of the clinical crown

↓

Separation of the attachment epithelium from the crown and the resulting apical shift of the attachment epithelium

Changes in Tissues Overlying Teeth

- The initial changes seen in the tissues overlying the teeth, prior to clinical emergence of the crown is the alteration of the connective tissue of the dental follicle to form pathway for the erupting teeth.
- Histologically, the future eruption pathway appears as a zone with decreased and degenerated connective tissue fibers, cells, blood vessels and terminal nerves. These changes are probably due to the loss of blood supply to this area, as well as the release of enzymes that aid in degradation of these tissues.
- An altered tissue space overlying the tooth becomes visible as an inverted funnel-shaped area with the follicle fibers directed toward the mucosa. This is called the gubernacular cord **(Fig. 14.4)**. This structure guides the tooth in its eruptive movements.

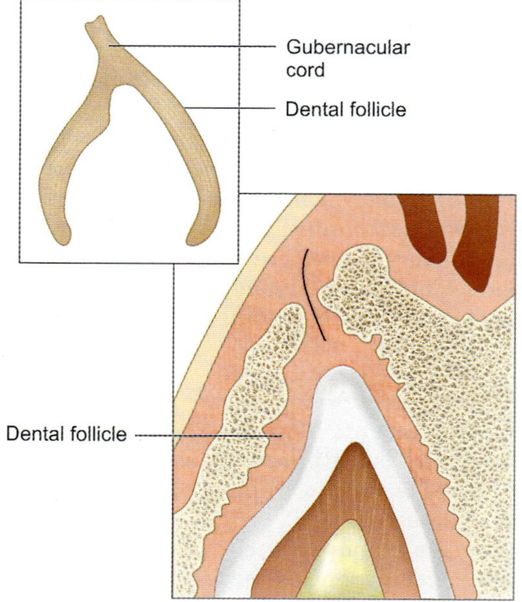

Fig. 14.4: Gubernacular cord.

- For successful tooth eruption, there must be some resorption of the overlying bony crypt so that the tooth can erupt. This can be considered as a part of remodeling growth. Osteoclasts differentiate and resorb a portion of the bony crypt overlying the erupting tooth.
- The eruption pathway, which is at first small, increases in dimension, thus allowing movement of the tooth.
- When the tooth nears the oral mucosa, the reduced enamel epithelium comes into contact with the overlying mucosa
- Simultaneously, the oral epithelial cells proliferate and fuse into one membrane.
- Further movement of the tooth stretches and thins the membrane over the crown tip. At this stage, the mucosa becomes blanched because of the lack of blood supply to the area.
- The tooth that will erupt slightly remain stationary for few days and then again erupt. In this manner, the supporting tissues are able to make adjustment to the eruptive movement.
- Each eruption movement result in more of the crown appearing in the cavity and further separation of the attachment epithelium from the enamel surface.

Changes in Tissues Around the Teeth

The tissues around the teeth also undergo changes during tooth eruption.

- Initially, the dental follicle is composed of delicate connective tissue. Gradually, as eruptive movement commences, collagen fibers become prominent, extending between the forming knot and the alveolar bone surface.
- The first noticeable periodontal fiber bundles appear at the cervical area of the root and extend at an angle coronally to the alveolar process. At the same time, the alveolar bone of the crypt is remodeled, and the bone fills into conform the smaller root diameter.
- As the eruption proceeds, other collagen fibers bundles become visible along the forming root. These are then populated with fibroblasts and myofibroblasts, with contractile capabilities.
- Very early in the eruptive process, periodontal fibers attach on the root surface and in the alveolar bone as cementogenesis proceeds. Some fibers release as the tooth moves and then reattach to stabilize the tooth. In this manner, the tooth-stabilizing process is performed by the same group of fibers throughout tooth eruption.
- Alveolar bone remodeling continues during eruption; as the tooth moves occlusally, the alveolar bone increases in height and changes shape to accommodate the crown. These actions are coordinated during the entire eruption process as well as they are throughout the life.

Changes in Tissues Underlying Teeth

- Changes also occur in the follicular tissues underlying the developing teeth.
- These changes take place in the soft tissue and fundic bone (bone surrounding the apex of the root).
- As the tooth erupts, space is provided for the root to lengthen, primarily due to the crown moving occlusally and the increase in the height of the alveolar bone. Changes in fundic regions are, thus, believed to be largely compensatory to the lengthening of the root.
- During the pre-eruptive and early eruptive phase, the follicular fibroblasts and fibers are in a plane parallel to the base of the root. The tooth moves rapidly in the socket during prefunctional eruption than at any other period. Fine bony trabeculae appear in the fundic area.
  They compensate for tooth eruption and provide some support at the apical tissues. Some authors describe this as a bony ladder. The ladder becomes denser as alternate layers of bone plates and connective tissue are laid down.
- At the end of the prefunctional eruptive phase, when the tooth comes into occlusion, about one-third of the enamel remains covered by the gingiva, and the root is incomplete. At this time, the bony ladder is gradually resorbed and one plate at a time, to make space for the developing root tip. Root completion continues for a considerable time after teeth have been in function. This process takes place from 1 to 1.5 years in deciduous teeth and from 2 to 3 years in permanent teeth.

Posteruptive Phase

- The posteruptive phase begins when the teeth reach occlusion and continues for long as each tooth remains in the oral cavity. During this phase or process, the alveolar process increases in height, and the roots continue to grow. In other words, the teeth continue to move occlusally, which accommodates the jaw and allows for root elongation.
- The most marked changes occur as the occlusion is established. Alveolar bone density increases, and the principal fibers of the periodontal ligament establish themselves into separate groups orient about the gingival third, the alveolar crest and the alveolar surface around the root **(Fig. 14.5).**
- The diameter of the fiber bundle increases also from delicate, five groups of fibers to heavy, securely stabilized bundles.
- Later in life, attrition may wear down the occlusal surfaces of the teeth. The teeth erupt slightly to compensate for loss of tooth structure and to prevent over closure. If the occlusal wear is excessive, cementum is deposited on the apical third of the root. It is deposited in the furcation region to compensate for the overeruption of teeth, and some bone apposition occurs at the alveolar crests. In

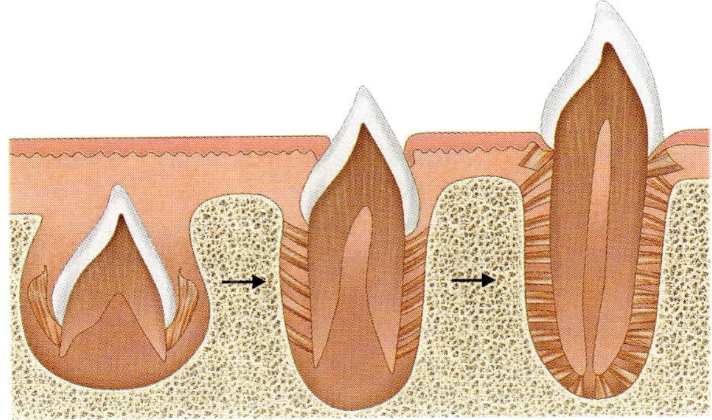

Fig. 14.5: Development of periodontal fibers.

addition to slight occlusal movement, the teeth tend to move anteriorly. This is termed mesial drift and results in bone resorption on the mesial wall of the socket and bone apposition on the distal wall. This phase is characterized by movements of the tooth after it has reached its functional position in the occlusal plane.

- These movements include those to accommodate the growing jaws, to compensate for continued occlusal wear, to accommodate interproximal wear.

THEORIES OF TOOTH ERUPTION

The mechanism of tooth eruption is an enigma which has perplexed many investigators. It is a process that has been the subject of scientific enquiry since 1778 when Hunter attributed the mechanism to root elongation. Recent reviews have concluded that there is no simple explanation for this biological phenomenon which is not surprising since most teeth erupt during periods of active craniofacial growth, and therefore eruption should be considered as a part of a multifactorial event. Recent advances in biochemistry, immunology and structural and molecular biology have renewed interest in understanding the mechanisms of bone remodeling and tooth eruption because it is now possible to determine the activity of cytokines, membrane receptors, signal transduction molecules and postactivation intercellular events.

SHEDDING OF DECIDUOUS TEETH

The human dentition like those of most mammals consists of two generations. The first generation is known as the deciduous dentition and the second as the permanent dentition. The necessity of two dentitions exists because infant jaws are small, and the size and number of teeth they can support is limited. Since teeth, once formed, cannot increase in size, a second dentition, consisting of larger and more teeth, is required for the larger jaws of the adult.

The physiologic process resulting in the elimination of the deciduous dentition is called shedding or exfoliation.

Pattern of Shedding

The shedding of deciduous teeth is the result of progressive resorption of the roots of teeth and their supporting tissues. In general, the pressure generated by the growing and erupting permanent tooth dictates the pattern of deciduous tooth resorption.

Theory	***Explanation***
Root elongation theory	According to this theory, the simplest and most obvious mechanism of eruption would be that the crowns of the teeth are pushed into the oral cavity by virtue of growth and elongation of the roots *Evidence for the theory:* Root of tooth elongates as crown erupts into the oral cavity *Evidence against the theory:* Rootless teeth often erupt without the concomitant elongation of the root, submerged teeth often continue the formation of their roots but do not erupt
Pulpal constriction theory	This theory states that the growth of the root dentin and the subsequent constriction of the pulp may cause sufficient pressure to move the tooth occlusally *Evidence for the theory:* The pulp is progressively constricted by growth of root dentin *Evidence against the theory:* Pulpless teeth erupts at the same rate as the normal teeth, premolar will often "jump" into occlusion after the premature extraction of the deciduous molar without any appreciable growth of dentine or pulpal constriction
Growth of periodontal tissues	• *Pull by surrounding connective tissue:* Underwood suggests that the connective tissue surrounding the tooth may function in pulling the tooth into the oral cavity. This theory is invalidated by histological examination of the direction of the periodontal fibers during tooth eruption, which shows that the periodontal fibers are being pulled by the tooth and not vice versa • *Alveolar bone growth:* **Herman** believed that the growth of the alveolar bone might push or squeeze the tooth out of its alveolus and into the oral cavity. However, X-ray and histological sections show that the bone does not actually touch the tooth. In addition, this mechanism can operate only upon single conical roots but not on multirooted teeth
Pressure from muscular action	**Berten** suggested that the action of the musculature of the cheeks and lips upon the alveolar process might serve to squeeze the crown of the tooth out into the oral cavity like a pumpkin seed from between the fingers. This process continues until the tooth is in occlusion, being halted by the antagonism of the teeth. the theory, however, fails to explain the teeth eruption in the cases of unilateral facial paralysis
Resorption of the alveolar crest	Resorption of the alveolar crest would serve to expose the crown of the tooth into the oral cavity. This theory is not tenable since histological examination shows that the alveolar crest is the site of the most rapid and continuous growth of bone
Hormonal theory	**Sir Arthur Keith** suggested that the hormones secreted by the thyroids and pituitary glands might govern the eruption of the teeth. This theory does not attempt to explain the mechanism of the eruption of the teeth and only points out the fact the hormones may affect the eruption of the teeth
Foreign body theory	**Gottlieb** foreign body theory states that a calcified body such as the tooth tends to be exfoliated by the tissues just as does any foreign body
Cellular proliferation theory	**Noyes** points out that the tremendous pressure, which is evolved from cellular proliferation, provides the growing plant with sufficient force to break through hard obstacles. Similarly, the osmotic pressure and forces resulting from cellular proliferation in the pulp and surrounding tissues may account for the eruption of the teeth
Vascularity theory	**Constant** (1896) points out the fact that the tissues, which lie between the developing tooth and its bony surrounding, possess a very rich vascular supply. He said that the blood pressure exerted in the vascular tissue which lies between the developing tooth and its bony surroundings is the active mechanical factor in the process known as eruption of teeth *Evidence for the theory:* Submerged teeth often erupt under the influence of hyperemia, the hyperemia in periodontitis causes a supraeruption of teeth

Contd...

Contd...

Blood vessel thrust theory	This theory proposed that eruption involves the blood supply to the tooth like the vascularity theory. The blood generates the force by hydrodynamic and hydrostatic forces within the blood vessels
Periodontal ligament contraction theory	Suggests that the contractile elements within the periodontal ligament, collagen constriction and constriction due to fibroblasts are responsible. Furthermore, there is evidence that the actual force required to move the tooth is linked to the contractility of fibroblasts. When fibroblasts are plated onto silicone rubber, they crawl about, and in doing so create wrinkles or folds in the rubber indicating that tractions forces are associated with locomotion. A model system consisting of a well, lined by a perforated mesh (mimicking the cryptal bone) and containing a gel plated with fibroblasts and a slice of root dentin has shown that not only there is three-dimensional network established but also this network generates sufficient force to raise the root slice from the bottom to the top of the well
Dental follicle theory	It is clear that the dental follicle is essential to achieve the bony remodeling required to accommodate tooth movement, for it is from this tissue that the osteoblasts differentiate
Bony remodeling theory	Bony remodeling of the jaws has been linked to tooth eruption as in the pre-eruptive phase; the inherent growth pattern of the mandible or maxilla supposedly moves teeth by the selective deposition and resorption of the bone in the immediate surroundings of the tooth. When the developing premolar is removed without disturbing the dental follicle, an eruptive pathway still forms overlying the enucleated tooth. Whereas, if the dental follicle is removed, no eruptive pathway is formed. Furthermore, if the tooth germ is replaced by a metal or silicone replica, and the dental follicle is retained, the replica will erupt, with the formation of an eruptive pathway. These observations clearly demonstrate that "programed" bony remodeling can and does occur, that is, an eruptive pathway forms in bone without a developing and growing tooth. Second, they show that the dental follicle is involved but perhaps only indirectly
Bite forces sensed by soft tissue dental follicles theory	This theory postulates that follicular soft tissues detect bite-forces and so direct bone remodeling with the effect of enabling tooth eruption. Examination of the soft tissue dental follicles, suggested broad areas of compression in overlying crowns, and wide zones of tension in follicle below root apices. So, these soft act as relevant stress sensors.[1]
Innervation-provoked pressure theory	This theory postulates that the root membrane acts as a glandular membrane. So, the innervation in this membrane causes pressure in the apical part of the tooth which results in tooth eruption.[2]
The equilibrium theory	After the functional plane is reached, the eruption of the tooth is balanced in response to the growth of the vertical growth of the mandible. As the mandible grows vertically away from the maxilla, the teeth have more room to erupt occlusally in order to maintain occlusal contact with the opposing arch. This model of tooth eruption reinforces the idea that post-emergent tooth eruption, after reaching functional occlusion, is controlled by forces impeding eruption, as opposed to encouraging forces. These balancing forces of masticatory function and the soft tissue pressures from the lips, cheeks, and tongue are the rate limiting factors of post functional occlusal eruption[3]
Neuromuscular theory or unification theory	The neuromuscular theory or unification theory of tooth eruption states that the synchronized forces of the orofacial muscles, under the control of the central nervous system, are responsible for the active movements of a tooth and the molecular events prepared a pathway under the control of these forces.[4,5]

Resorption of Anterior Teeth

- The position of the permanent anterior tooth germ is lingual to the apical third of the roots of primary tooth; hence, the resorption is in the occlusal labial direction, which corresponds to the movements of the permanent tooth germ **(Fig. 14.6)**.
- Later, the crown of the permanent tooth lies directly apical to the root of primary tooth, which causes resorption to proceed horizontally.
- This horizontal resorption allows the permanent tooth to erupt into the position of the primary tooth.

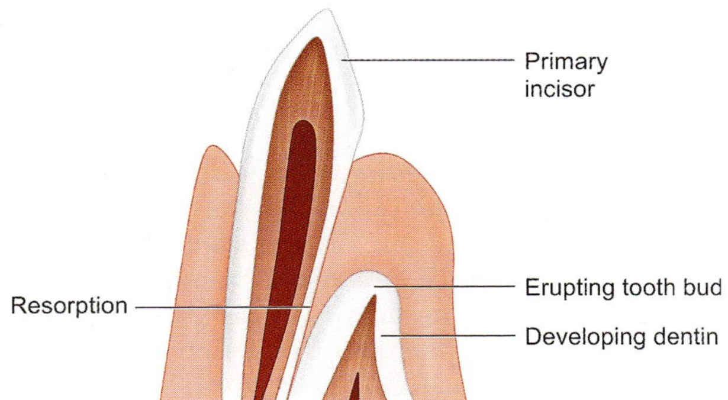

Fig. 14.6: Resorption position of anterior teeth.

Resorption of Posterior Teeth

- The growing crowns of the premolars initially are situated between the roots of the primary molars.
- The initiation is by the resorption of the inter-radicular bone followed by resorption of the adjacent surfaces of the root of primary tooth **(Fig. 14.7)**.
- Meanwhile, the alveolar process is growing to compensate for lengthening roots of the permanent tooth. As this occurs, the primary molars move occlusally; this allows the premolar crowns to be more apical.

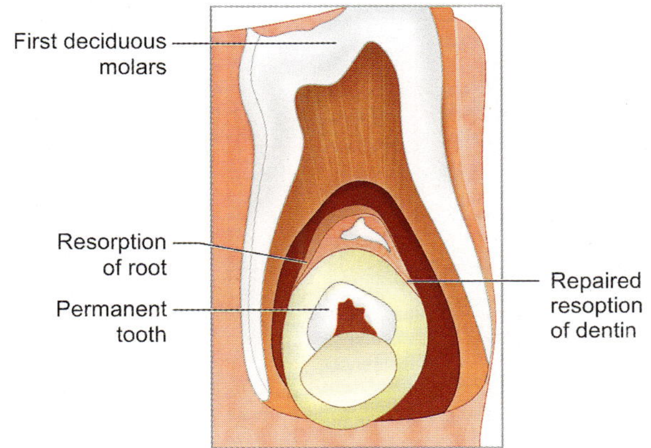

Fig. 14.7: Resorption position of posterior teeth.

- The premolars continue to erupt until the primary molars roots are entirely resorbed and the teeth exfoliate. The premolars then appear in place of the primary molars.

Mechanism of Resorption and Shedding

- The exact causes of resorption and shedding of deciduous teeth cannot be underlined; however, three main reasons have been attributed to this which are loss of root, loss of bone and increased force.
- **Kronfield** was one of the first researchers to suggest role of stellate reticulum and dental follicle in shedding mechanism.
- As permanent teeth grow, they exert pressure to induce differentiation of osteoclasts and odontoclasts, which causes resorption of hard tissues and supporting structures of root.
- Osteoclasts are bone resorbing cells derived from monocyte-macrophage lineage with giant multinuclear cells with 4–20 nuclei. Osteoclasts cells have striated border and are housed in Howship lacunae **(Fig. 14.8)** which attach to the resorbing front of hard tissue and release acid phosphatase. This disrupts collagen network and releases crystals which are digested by the vacuoles of osteoclasts. The disrupted collagen is then destroyed by fibroclasts **(Fig. 14.9)**. Resorption occurs at the ruffled border which greatly increases the surface area where the osteoclasts are in contact with bone.

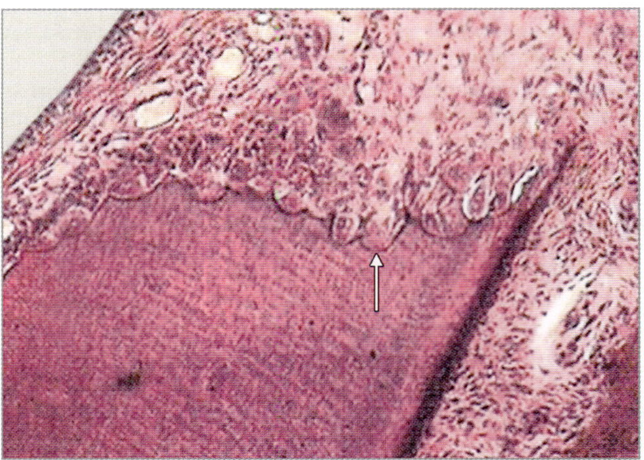

Fig. 14.8: Osteoclasts cells housed in Howship lacunae.

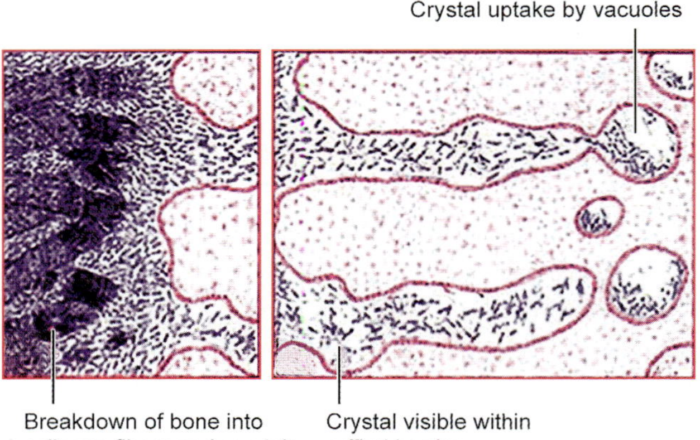

Fig. 14.9: Breakdown of collagen.

- During the process of resorption, the pressure from tooth is first directed to the bone, and following its resorption, the forces are directed to primary tooth.
- Although resorption of teeth is multifactorial, the pressure from the erupting successional tooth plays a key role because the odontoclasts differentiate at predicted sites of pressure. It must be however noted that presence of succedaneous teeth is a contributor in resorption not prerequisite.
- Forces of mastication are also synergistically involved in the mechanism of shedding. Due to growth and increased loading of jaws, these forces far exceed the limit that the deciduous tooth periodontal ligament can withstand, thereby causing trauma to the ligament and the initiation of resorption.
- Recently **Evlambia**[6] demonstrated a new concept in the shedding of primary teeth. He explained that this process is regulated in the same manner as bone remodeling involving receptor ligand system (RANK, i.e., receptor activator of nuclear factor of kappa B) which stimulates osteoclast formation.

Remnants of Deciduous Teeth

- Sometimes, parts of the roots of the deciduous teeth that are not in the path of eruption remain embedded in the jaw for a considerable time.
- They are most frequently found in association with the permanent premolars because the roots of the lower second deciduous molars are strongly curved or divergent.
- Root remnants may later be found deep in the bone, completely surrounded by and ankylosed to the bone. When they are close to the surface of the jaw, they may ultimately be exfoliated.
- Progressive resorption of the root remnants and replacement by bone may cause the disappearance of these remnants.

Retained Deciduous Teeth

- Deciduous teeth may be retained for a long time beyond their usual shedding schedule. Such teeth are usually without permanent successor, or their successors are impacted.
- Retained deciduous teeth are most often the upper lateral incisor, less frequently the mandibular second primary molars and rarely the lower central incisors.

CHRONOLOGY OF HUMAN DENTITION

The regular sequence of eruption suggests that it is under genetic control, while the same is an event highly subject to nutritional, hormonal and disease states. Disturbances of the normal sequence and ages of tooth eruption are one of the contributing factors to the development of malocclusion and consequently of significance to us as pedodontists. At birth, jaws contain the partly calcified crowns of 20 deciduous teeth and beginning of calcification of the first permanent molars. Eruption of deciduous dentition begins at an average of 7.5 months of age and terminates at about 29 months. Dental eruption is then quiescent for nearly 4 years. At the age of 6 years, the jaws contain more teeth than at any other time; 48 teeth are filling the body of mandible. After this extreme activity, there is a 2.5 years of quite period until 10.5 years of age. Then during the next 18 months, the remaining 12 deciduous teeth are lost and 16 permanent teeth erupt. The 6 years of period of the mixed dentition from 6 to 12 years is the most complicated period of dental development and the one in which malocclusion is most likely to develop. A long and valuable period of 3–7 years of quiescence follows before eruption of the lower third molars to complete the dentition. The third molars do not begin calcification until 9 years of age, and their eruption from the 16 years onward heralds the completion of dentofacial growth and development **(Figs. 14.10 and 14.11)**.

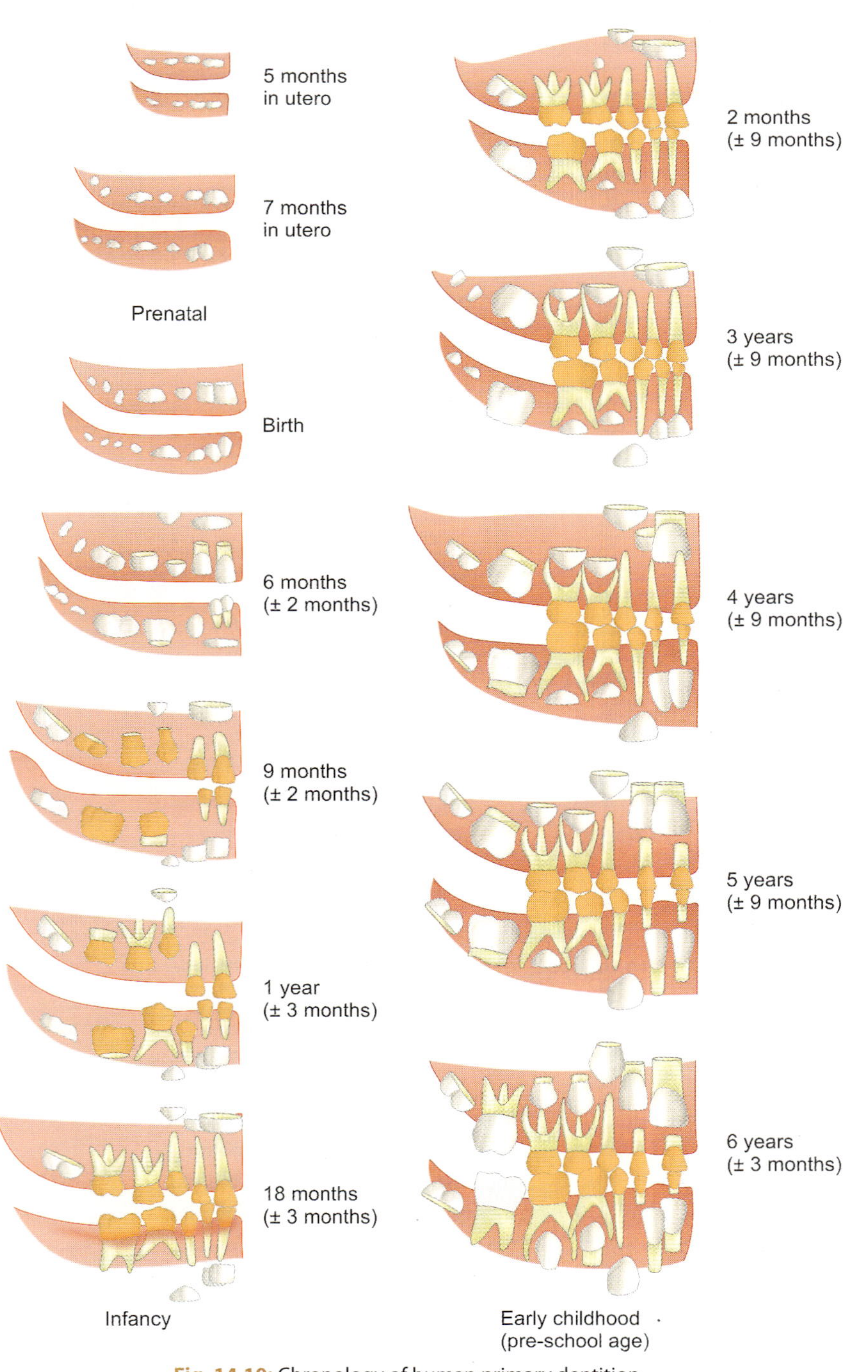

Fig. 14.10: Chronology of human primary dentition.

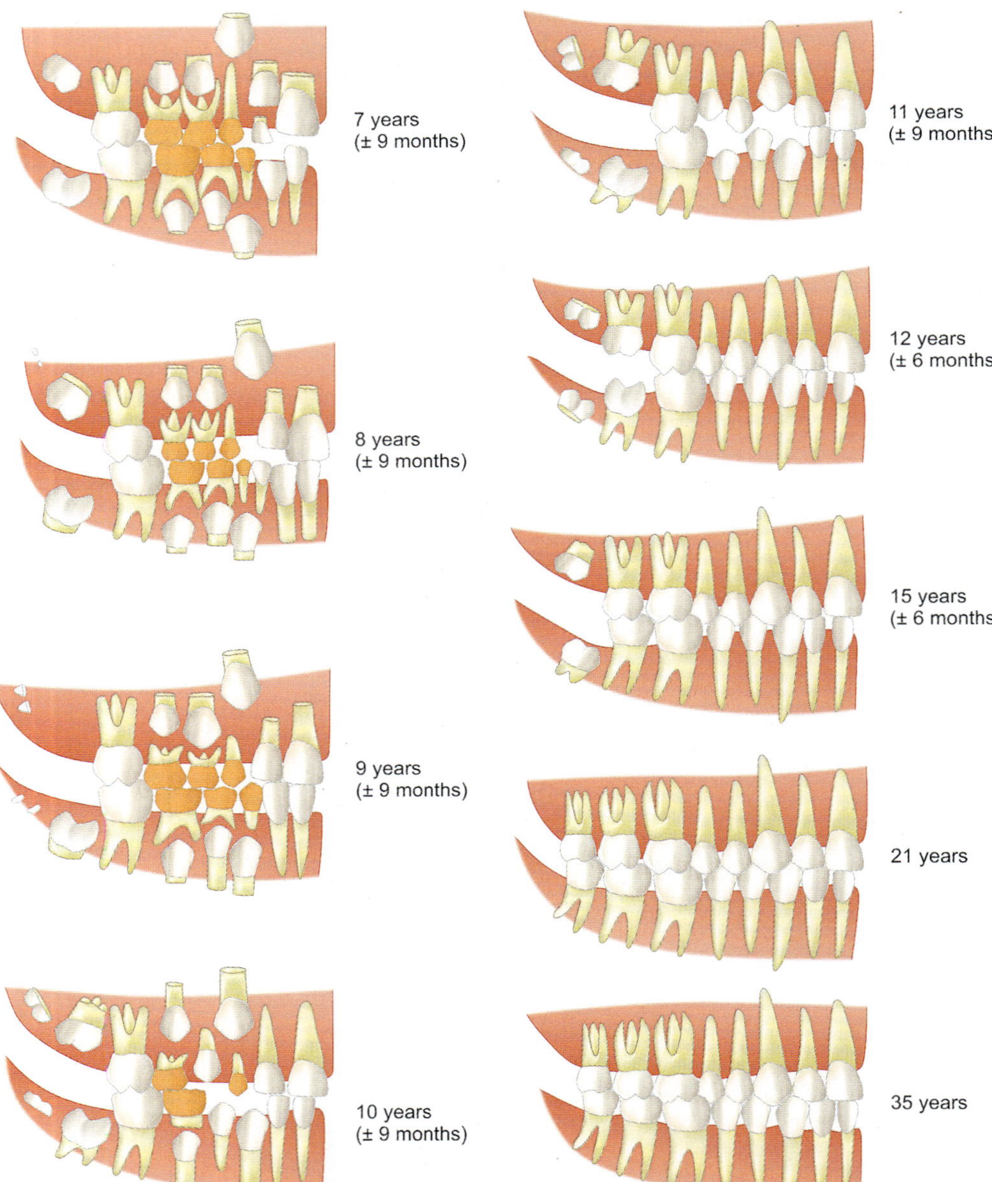

Fig. 14.11: Chronology of human mixed and permanent dentition.

Primary dentition				
Tooth	***Hard tissue formation begins***	***Crown completed***	***Eruption***	***Root completed***
Maxilla				
Central incisor	4 months in utero	4 months	7.5 months	1.5 years
Lateral incisor	4.5 months in utero	5 months	9 months	2 years
Canine	5 months in utero	9 months	18 months	3.25 years
1st molar	5 months in utero	6 months	14 months	2.5 years
2nd molar	6 months in utero	11 months	24 months	3 years
Mandible				
Central incisor	4.5 months in utero	4.5 months	6 months	1.5 years
Lateral incisor	4.5 months in utero	4 months	7 months	1.5 years
Canine	5 months in utero	9 months	16 months	3 years
1st molar	5 months in utero	5.5 months	12 months	2.25 years
2nd molar	6 months in utero	10 months	20 months	3 years

Permanent dentition				
Tooth	***Hard tissue formation begins***	***Crown completed***	***Eruption***	***Root completed***
Maxilla				
Central incisor	3–4 months	4–5 years	7–8 years	10 years
Lateral incisor	10–12 months	4–5 years	8–9 years	11 years
Canine	4–5 months	6–7 years	11–12 years	13–15 years
1st premolar	1.5–1.75 years	5–6 years	10–11 years	12–13 years
2nd premolar	2–2.25 years	6–7 years	10–12 years	12–14 years
1st molar	Birth	2.5–3 years	6–7 years	9–10 years
2nd molar	2.5–3 years	7–8 years	12–15 years	14–16 years
3rd molar	7–9 years	12–16 years	17–24 years	18–25 years
Mandible				
Central incisor	3–4 months	4–5 years	6–7 years	9 years
Lateral incisor	3–4 months	4–5 years	7–8 years	10 years
Canine	4–5 months	6–7 years	9–10 years	12–14 years
1st premolar	1.75–2 years	5–6 years	10–11 years	12–13 years
2nd premolar	2.25–2.5 years	6–7 years	11–12 years	13–14 years
1st molar	Birth	2.5–3 years	6–7 years	9–10 years
2nd molar	2.5–3 years	7–8 years	11–13 years	14–15 years
3rd molar	8–10 years	12–16 years	17–21 years	18–25 years

Guna Shekhar et al.[7] conducted a longitudinal on study chronology of eruption primary teeth among Indian children and compared the obtained data with other population. The observations of the study were **(Tables 14.1 and 14.2):**

- Indian children experienced delayed eruption of primary teeth when compared to their counterparts in other populations
- Boys showed tendency toward earlier eruption for all teeth except maxillary second molar and maxillary/mandibular first molars which erupted earlier in girls
- Comparison between maxillary and mandibular showed a tendency to earlier mandibular eruption of central incisors, lateral incisors and second molars in both genders

Table 14.1: Mean and standard deviation age (in months) of eruption of the primary teeth for boys.

	Maxilla				***Mandible***			
	Right side		***Left side***		***Right side***		***Left side***	
Tooth	***Mean***	***SD***	***Mean***	***SD***	***Mean***	***SD***	***Mean***	***SD***
Central incisor	11.88	0.74	12.05	0.84	10.86	0.73	10.50	0.41
Lateral incisor	13.35	0.88	13.36	1.03	12.55	0.92	12.66	0.79
Canine	21.04	1.28	21.15	1.35	22.18	1.37	21.89	1.14
First molar	17.28	1.05	17.50	1.11	19.00	0.85	19.13	0.79
Second molar	29.29	1.02	29.48	1.39	26.82	1.80	27.16	0.78

(SD: standard deviation)

Table 14.2: Mean and standard deviation age (in months) of eruption of the primary teeth for girls.

	Maxilla				***Mandible***			
	Right side		***Left side***		***Right side***		***Left side***	
Tooth	***Mean***	***SD***	***Mean***	***SD***	***Mean***	***SD***	***Mean***	***SD***
Central incisor	12.00	0.74	12.16	0.85	10.97	0.72	10.56	0.42
Lateral incisor	13.56	0.79	13.57	0.97	12.55	0.98	12.69	0.84
Canine	21.17	1.36	21.32	1.40	22.35	1.41	21.99	1.21
First molar	17.09	1.06	17.16	0.92	18.94	0.93	18.91	0.74
Second molar	27.81	0.78	28.14	1.25	27.53	0.98	27.19	0.85

(SD: standard deviation)

Causes for delayed eruption of permanent teeth

- Obstructions can be either soft tissue or hard tissue obstructions
- Nutritional deficiencies like prolonged malnutrition can delay tooth eruption, especially vitamin A and D[8]
- Endocrinal disturbances like hypothyroidism, hypopituitarism and hypoparathyroidism
- Preterm babies: **Seow** has reported about the delays in growth and dental development leading to delayed tooth eruption. Apart from this enamel and maxillary growth defects are noted.[9]
- HIV infection
- Anemia
- Renal failure
- Long-term drugs for intake for chemotherapy
- Drugs which inhibit prostaglandin pathway
- Genetic disorders like Apert syndrome, cleidocranial dysostosis, and Gardner syndrome.[10]
- Genetic diseases like amelogenesis imperfect and dentinogenesis imperfecta associated with osteogenesis imperfecta (type 3) are associated with delayed eruption.
- Syndromes associated with delayed eruption of permanent teeth are Down syndrome or trisomy 21, Turner syndrome (XO), Gardner syndrome, cleidocranial dysostosis, Sainton's disease, Anhidrotic ectodermal dysplasia, Hutchinson–Gilford syndrome, dentinal dysplasias, Apert syndrome[11]

Causes for early eruption of permanent teeth

- Hyperpituatrism
- Hyperthyroidism
- Premature loss of primary predecessor
- Localized hemangiomata

- **Mainali S et al.,** 2019: In a cross-sectional study found that tendency of eruption of permanent teeth was earlier in female than in males and there was no significant difference in eruption age between the right and left side of the oral cavity was observed.[12]
- **Indira MD et al.,** 2018: Conducted a study to evaluate time and sequence of eruption of primary teeth of children of Mysuru and concluded that eruption of primary tooth is delayed by 3–4 months as compared to standard eruption.[13]
- **Verma N et al** (2017): Conducted a cross sectional study and found that there is significant relation between tooth eruption and birth weight, feeding habits, socioeconomic status, and body mass index (BMI), Also Indian children experienced delayed eruption of primary teeth when compared with children of different countries and standard norms.[14]
- **Vahdat et al** (2019): Showed that no significant relationship between sex, type of diet, mother's education level and birth rank in the family, and the period of eruption of the first primary tooth. There was a significant relationship between birth weight and the time of the first deciduous tooth eruption, infants with lower or higher weight than normal at birth showed delayed deciduous tooth eruption[15]
- **Badruddin IA et al**: Conducted a cross-sectional study and concluded that children from mother with poor nutritional status during pregnancy had later timings and longer tooth eruption process duration in primary teeth.[16]

POINTS TO REMEMBER

- Eruption is defined as a process whereby the forming tooth migrates from its intraosseous location in the jaw to its functional position within the oral cavity.
- First movement of teeth is within the jaw and are eccentric and bodily movements. Gubernacular cord guides the tooth in its eruptive movements.
- Most comprehensive theories of tooth eruption are bony remodeling and periodontal ligament traction theory.
- Resorption of primary teeth is postulated due to pressure from erupting tooth, odontoclastic resorption and masticatory forces.
- At the age of 6 years, the jaws contain more teeth than at any other time; 48 teeth are filling the body of mandible. First tooth to erupt in oral cavity is mandibular primary central incisor.
- First permanent tooth to erupt in oral cavity is mandibular first molar.

Clinical Significance

Proper knowledge about the chronology of eruption of primary and permanent teeth is of utmost importance so as to evaluate any delay in dentition or formulate any treatment plan for the specified dentition.

Questionnaire

1. Explain the pattern of tooth movements.
2. What are the anatomic stages of tooth eruption?
3. Discuss the changes which take place in the tissues during eruption of tooth.
4. Enumerate the theories of tooth eruption with special reference to periodontal traction and bony remodeling theory.
5. What is the mechanism of shedding of primary tooth?
6. Write the chronology of eruption of primary teeth.

REFERENCES

1. Sarrafpour B, Swain M, Li Q, Zoellner H. Tooth eruption results from bone remodeling driven by bite forces sensed by soft tissue dental follicles: a finite element analysis. PLoS One. 2013;8(3):1-18.
2. Kjær I. Mechanism of human tooth eruption: review article including a new theory for future studies on the eruption process. Sci Tech Rep. 2014;2014:1-13.
3. Proffit WR. Contemporary orthodontics. fifth ed. Elsevier; 2013.
4. Loto AO. Tooth eruption: a neuromuscular theory, part one. J. Craniomax. Res. 2017;4(1):278-83.
5. Wise GE, King GJ. Tooth movement. J Dent Res. 2008;87:414-34.
6. Evlambia HH. Physiologic root resorption in primary teeth: molecular and histological events. J Oral Sci. 2007;49:1-12.
7. Guna SM, Tenny J. Longitudinal study of age and order of eruption of primary teeth in Indian children. J Clin Exp Dent. 2010;3:e 113-6.
8. Moulis E, Thierrens CFD, Goldsmith TM, Torres JH. Anomalies of the eruption. Http://www.em-Premiumcomdatatraitespem04-931499. http://www.em-premium.com. rproxy.sc.univ-paris-diderot.fr/ article/15429/resultatre-cherche/1Accessed August 31, 2015

9. Seow WK. Effects of Preterm Birth on Oral Growth and Development. Aust Dent J. 1997; 42(2):85-91
10. Alshukairi H. Delayed tooth eruption and its pathogenesis in paediatric patient: a review. J Dent Health Oral Disord Ther. 2019;10(3):209-212.
11. Choukroune C. Tooth eruption disorders associated with systemic and genetic diseases: clinical guide. J Dentofacial Anom Orthod. 2017;20(4):402.
12. Mainali S, Chaulagain R, Poudyal S, Pradhan A. Age and Sequence of Permanent Tooth Eruption in Children. Journal of KIST Medical College. 2019;1(2):32-7.
13. Indira MD, Bhojraj N, Narayanappa D. A cross-sectional study on eruption timing of primary teeth in children of Mysore, Karnataka. Indian J Dent Res. 2018;29:726-31.
14. Verma N, Bansal A, Tyagi P, Jain A, Tiwari U, Gupta R. Eruption Chronology in Children: A Cross-sectional Study. Int J ClinPediatr Dent 2017;10(3):278-282.
15. Vahdat G, Zarabadipour M, Fallahzadeh F, Khani R. (2019). Factors influencing the eruption period of the first primary tooth. Journal of Oral Research. 2019; 8(4):305-9.
16. Badruddin IA, Putri MR, Rahardjo A. Factors associated with primary teeth eruption pattern in children under three years old in BejiDepok, West Java. Journal of International Dental and Medical Research. 2017;10:564-8.

FURTHER READING

1. Berkovitz BK, Moxham BL. Colored Atlas of Oral Anatomy, Histology and Embryology. Mosby; 1992.
2. Bhaskar SN. Orban's Oral Histology and Embryology. 10th ed. Elsevier Publications; 2009.
3. Mc Donald RE, Avery DR, Dean JA. Dentistry for the child and adolescent. 9th edn. Elsevier Health Sciences; 2010.
4. Tencate R. Oral Histology: Development, Structure and Function, 5th edn.
5. The mechanism of tooth eruption. Br Dent J 1996.pp.181-3.

Teething

Nikhil Marwah, Srinivas LS

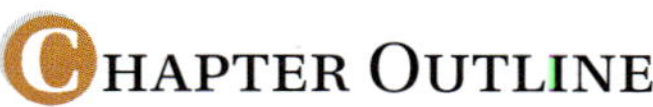

- Signs and Symptoms of Teething
- Management of Teething
- Teething Problems

The appearance of an infant's first tooth is regarded by most parents as one of the series of significant developmental landmarks. Anecdotally, however, the period associated with the eruption of the deciduous teeth in infants can be difficult and distressing for both the child and their respective parents. The enigma of teething is, at least, in part historical even though many unexplained teething myths continue to pervade contemporary child health. This chapter examines the features of teething and the historical and contemporary principles of the management of teething.

Other synonyms for teething include dentito difficilis, pathological dentition, difficult dentition, breeding teeth, teething per se.[1] Teething is a natural physiological process which consist of migration of tooth from its intraosseous position in the jaw to eruption in the oral cavity or it can simply be described as a process of tooth eruption through the gums.[2] Teething may occur without any problems or it may be associated with certain organic or systemic manifestations. Historical perspectives pertaining to teething has been given in the **Table 15.1**.

Table 15.1: Historical perspectives pertaining to teething.[3,4]

1200 BC	**Homeric hymns**	Explained the teething difficulties.
4th century BC	**Hippocrates**	Wrote a short treatise, on dentition, *Teething children suffer from itching of the gums, fevers, convulsions and diarrhea, especially when they cut their eye teeth and when they are very corpulent and costive* *Similar opinions were expressed by Pliny (1st century AD, Soranus and Galen (2nd century AD), Oreibasius (4th century), Aetius century), and Avicenna (10th century).*
117 AD	**Soranus of Ephesus**	First to suggest using hare's brain to ease teething. This remained a favored remedy until the 17th century. *If they are in pain, smear the gums with dog's milk or hare's brain; this works also if eaten. But if a tooth is coming through with difficulty, smear Cyperus with butter and oil-of-lilies over the part where it is erupting.*
6th century AD	**Aëtius of Amida**	He recommended, *Root of colocynth (a wild, poisonous vine) hung on the child in a gold or silver case, or bramble root, or the tooth of a viper, especially a male viper, set in gold or green jasper, suspended on the neck so as the hang over the stomach.*
1429	**Von Louffenberg**	Explained following for the care of a teething baby. Now when your baby's teeth appear, you must take prudent care. For teething comes with grievous pain, so to my word take heed again. When the teeth are pushing, through, to rub the gums thou thus shall do. Take fat from chicken, brain from hare, and these full of on gums shall smear. If ulcers sore thereon should come, then thou shall rub upon the gum. Honey and salt and oil thereto. But one a salve of oil of violet, for neck and throat and gums to get, and also bathe his head a while, with water boiled with chamomile.
1545	**Thomas Phaire**	His recommended charm was, *The first cast tooth of a colt set in silver and bone, or red coralle in upon the chylde should oftentimes labor his gums.* "By consent of all authors, it resists the force of lightening, help the children of the falling evil (epilepsy) and is very good to be made in powder and drunken against all manner of bleeding of the nose or fundament".

Contd...

Contd...

1575	**Ambriose Pare**	He developed the method, from the examination of a dead child. *When we diligently sought for the cause of his death, we could impute it to nothing else than the contumacious hardness of the gums ... when we cut the gums with a knife we done when we found all the teeth appearing ... if it had been done when he lived, doubtless he would have been preserved. And later, ... of which kind remedy I have with prosperous and happy success made trial in some of mine own children ... which is much better and more safe to do as some nurses do, who taught only by instinct of Nature, with their nails and scratching, break and tear and rent the gums.*
1668	**Francois Mauriceau**	Be done with a lancet rather than a knife, although a thin groat (a small coin) is as good or better either. Mauriceau challenged the effectiveness of charms, although he believed that the silver coral stick was helpful only because its hard smoothness soothed the child's gums. *There are many remedies which diverse precutting of teeth, as rubbing them with Bitches' milk, hare's or pig's brains and hanging a viper's tooth about the neck of the child and suchlike trifles: but since they are founded more on superstition, than any reason, I will not trouble myself to enlarge on what is so useless.*
1742	**Joseph Hurlock and John Hunter**	Both wrote works on teething. Hurlock in his book, *Treatise Upon Dentition*, he was convinced that many more children died from teething than was generally believed. Hurlock tried to encourage the lancing of gums ("would lance a baby's gums up to ten times") to prevent these deaths. John Hunter's view was that lancing was never attended by dangerous consequences.
1850	**Condie**	In his book, *Diseases of Children*, reported: *A curious case is related by M Robert, in his treatise on the Principal Objects of Medicine, of one of the effects of difficult dentition, as of the division of the gum. A child, having suffered greatly from difficult dentition apparently died and was laid out for internment. M Lemonnier was desirous of ascertaining the condition of the alveola. He accordingly made a free incision through the gums but on preparing to pursue further his examination, he perceived the child to open his eyes and give other indications of life. He immediately called for assistance; the shroud was removed from the body and by careful and persevering attention, the child's life was saved. In due time the teeth made their appearance and the child's health was fully restored.*
1887	**J W White**	He wrote, 'The nervous perturbation occasioned by the eruption of teeth increases the susceptibility and lessens the resistive power of the child'. It was believed that the difficulty experienced by an erupting tooth whilst penetrating gingival tissue affected trigeminal nerve endings. A 'reflex stimulation' of other cranial and spinal nerves ensued, producing 'functional derangements' and diseases in other organs. Lancing over an erupting tooth was recommended to allow bleeding and to release tissue pressure that was causing reflex stimulation of the trigeminal nerve. Any sick infant could be found to have an erupting tooth, even if the 'tooth bud' was deeply buried. This theory of reflex stimulation was reiterated as late as 1954.
1896	**Dr SS Foster**	In Dental Cosmos, explained, *The teething child becomes wakeful, restless and fretful, refuses nourishment; the alimentary canal becomes more active, diarrhea follows and if relief is not given, relaxation of the vital forces follows and we have nausea, vomiting, convulsions, paralysis and not infrequently, death.* He stated that more deaths occur in the teething period than in any similar period during the human lifespan.
1900	**Dr WC Barrett**	Addressed the First District Dental Society of New York with his paper called *The Slaughter of the Innocents* and attacked the hypocrisy of his colleagues. The child is teething is the vague explanation given to many anxious mothers by practitioners who are either incompetent to form a complete diagnosis, or too indolent and careless to seek for the hidden springs of disease... only teething. To how many pronouncing young existences in which were corrected the hopes, the ambitions, the heart affections of a family circle, have these words sounded the knell. *Only teething*, and the parents looked with but little alarm upon the symptoms of the gravest character.

SIGNS AND SYMPTOMS OF TEETHING

It is now generally accepted that the eruption of the deciduous teeth is accompanied by a number of relatively minor symptoms. **Macknin et al.**[5] identified several symptoms to be associated with teething like general irritability, disturbed sleep, gum inflammation, drooling, loss of appetite, diarrhea, circumoral rash, intraoral ulcers, increase in body temperature, increased biting, gum rubbing, sucking, wakefulness, and ear rubbing . According to them, teething can be considered as 8 day period, starting from 4 days prior to tooth emergence and extending 3 days after the event. These symptoms can be categorized as local and systemic symptoms:

Local symptoms (intra-oral and perioral region)	*Systemic symptoms*	*Behavioral changes*
• Pain • Inflammation of the mucous membrane overlying the tooth (possibly with small hemorrhages) • Facial flushing/ circumoral rash • Drooling • Gum irritation • Increased biting • Intraoral ulcers	• Malaise • Fever • Diarrhea/loose stools • Loss of appetite • Ear rubbing • Sleep disturbances • Rhinorrhea • Vomiting • Coughing • Colic • Convulsions • Croup • Malodors urine • Otitis media • Throat infection • Weight loss	• Crying • Fussiness • General irritability • Sucking of digits • Rubbing of gingiva

In a survey of parents, it was found that there is a spectrum of opinions held by parents regarding the teething-associated symptoms. Whilst only one parent in this study believed that teething is not problematical, between 70% and 85% of parents reported that teething was causally related to fever, pain, irritability, disturbed sleep, biting, drooling, and red cheeks. Furthermore, between one third and one half of these parents felt that nappy rash, ear pulling, feeding difficulties, runny nose, loose stools, and infections were related to teething, whereas a few parents related smelly urine, constipation, colic, and convulsions to eruptive difficulties.

- **Carpenter**[6] found that in 120 subjects, during the eruption of the anterior teeth, only 39% exhibited one of several symptoms (fever, vomiting, diarrhea, drooling, irritability, facial rashes, or rhinorrhea), and 78% exhibited the symptoms in case of eruption of posterior teeth. He also observed that the symptoms disappeared on either the day of or the day after eruption of the tooth.
- **Obiajuru IOC et al.**[7] conducted a study to find out the influence of microbial infection to teething problems and found that teething problems such as fever and diarrhea are not associated with teething rather caused by microbial infections such as plamodiasis, bacterial and intestinal parasitic infection.
- **Adnan M et al.**[8] conducted a study to assess parental knowledge about infant teething and concluded that most common symptoms of teething believed by parents were loose stool, fever, pain and desire to bite and the most common practice by parents to tackle teething symptoms is to allow child to bite on chilled object.

Signs and symptoms of teething
- Pain
- Inflammation of the mucous membrane overlying the tooth (possibly with small hemorrhages)
- General irritability/malaise
- Disturbed sleep/wakefulness
- Facial flushing/circumoral rash
- Drooling/sialorrhea
- Gum rubbing/biting/sucking
- Bowel upset (ranging from constipation to loose stools and diarrhea)
- Loss of appetite/alteration in volume of fluid intake
- Ear rubbing on the same side as the erupting tooth

Management of teething
- Teething rings (chilled)
- Hard sugar-free teething rusks
- Cucumber (peeled)
- Frozen items (anything from ice cubes to frozen bagels, frozen banana, sliced fruit, pretzels, vegetables)
- Pacifier (even frozen)
- Rub gums with clean finger, wet gauze
- Reassurance
- Analgesic/antipyretics
- Topic anesthetic agents
- Alternative holistic medicine

Management of teething		
Nonpharmacological methods	***Pharmacological methods***	***Alternate holistic medicines***
• Teething rings and gels for children to gnaw • Cuddle therapy • Rubbing gums • Food for chewing (>6 months old) • Placement of ice wrapped towels • Gentle massage of gums	• Topical anesthetic gels • Analgesics	• Acupressure • Aromatherapy • Homeopathic drugs • Ayurvedic and Unani medicines

MANAGEMENT OF TEETHING

The majority of investigations of "teething" have sought to confirm the presence or absence of associated features. Comparatively little research has investigated the management of teething, in particular the treatment of teething pain. The current methods of the management of teething are presented; however, infants with severe systemic upset should be promptly referred to a physician for an accurate diagnosis and appropriate treatment.

Nonpharmacological Management

- A wide range of teething rings are commercially available for infants to "gnaw;" however, parents should be advised to check the packaging carefully for any potentially harmful substances used in manufacturing.
- Solid silicone-based teething rings are superior to their liquid-filled counterparts, as the potentially irritant contents may leak, if damaged, and furthermore, usually, they cannot be sterilized.
- Temporary pain relief is provided by the pressure produced by chewing the teething ring, maximal when chilled first. Teething rings **(Fig. 15.1)** should be attached to the infants clothing, and not tied around the neck, as strangulation could result.

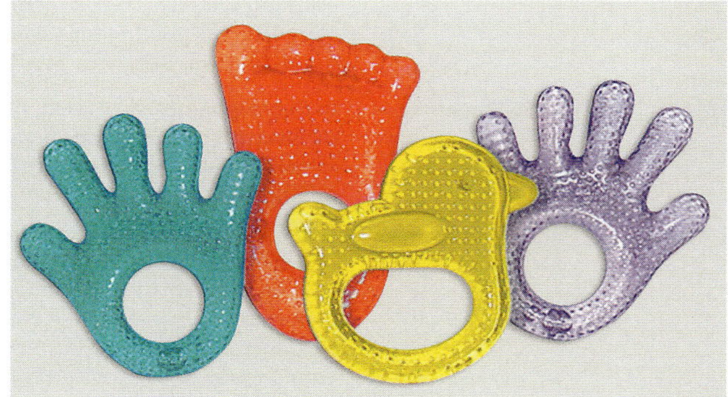

Fig. 15.1: Teething rings.

- Hard, unsweetened rusks made from flour and wheat with no sugar or sweetener can also be attached onto the infant's clothing.
- Biting or sucking cold or frozen objects including fruits, vegetables or other foods causes localized vasoconstriction and decreases inflammation; in addition, the pressure on the gums reduces pain.[9]
- Although many parents have strong views about providing infants with a pacifier at any time, many teething children are comforted by a pacifier and will chew the teat to provide temporary pain relief.
- Reassurance can often be one of the most effective methods of calming stressed teething child.

Pharmacological Management

Pharmacological methods aim to achieve analgesia, anesthesia, sedation or combination. Most parents prefer to avoid using pharmacological preparations during teething; however, a wide range of effective topical and systemic preparations are available when local measures fail to provide relief.

- **Topical anaesthetic agents:** Lignocaine 5% and benzocaine 20% are the two most frequently used anaesthetic agents in teething preparations. They act on the mucosa by decreasing the permeability of sodium ion channels in neuronal membranes leading to inhibition of depolarization and inhibition of nerve impulse propagation and conduction and provide temporary pain relief. The onset starts from 2–5 minutes and can last for 10–20 minutes. Around 7.5 mm of lignocaine gel should be placed on a clean finger or cotton bud and rubbed onto the painful area and only 6 applications per day to prevent systemic toxicity. Benzocaine being as ester, there is increased risk of hypersensitivity and methemoglobinemia.
- **Choline salicylate-based products:** Choline salicylates are synthetic NSAIDs, with mild analgesic, antipyretic and anti-inflammatory actions. It acts as a counter irritant, which when applied topically irritates sensory nerve endings and causes vasodilatation, which alters pain in the underlying tissues served by the same nerves.
- For children over 4 months old, 0.5 in. (7.5 mm) of gel to be massaged onto the painful area not more often than 3 hourly, with a maximum of six applications daily. Excessive application can lead to chemical burn and can cause Reyes syndrome in susceptible individuals, especially in those having viral or recovering from viral infection.
- **Systemic analgesics:** Both paracetamol and ibuprofen can be used as systemic analgesics. Paracetamol which is also known as acetaminophen is the medicament of choice in teething because of its action in reducing pain and pyrexia. It reduces synthesis of prostaglandins by inhibiting cycloxygenase-3 in the central nervous system. Analgesia results from the peripheral blockage of nociceptive impulses and their generation. Antipyresis results from the central inhibition of the hypothalamic heat-regulatory center. In addition, paracetamol reduces hyperalgesia by reducing production of Substance P and nitric oxide. Recommended paracetamol dosage is 3–12 months = 60–120 mg; 1–5 years = 120–250 mg. These doses are repeated at 4–6 hourly intervals, with a maximum of four doses in 24 hours. Ibuprofen is a commonly used nonsteroidal anti-inflammatory drug (NSAID) in children. It exerts analgesic, antipyretic and anti-inflammatory effects. Compared to paracetamol, ibuprofen may be more efficacious for management of pain and fever though it causes more frequent adverse reactions in children.[10,11]

Alternative Holistic Medicine

Alternative nonpharmacological holistic therapies (acupressure, aromatherapy, massage, and homeopathy) have been suggested as giving relief from the symptoms of teething.

- Acupressure requires the parent to apply pressure to certain key skin points, providing immediate, if temporary pain relief. Aromatherapy uses essential oils (clove oil, tea tree oil, olive oil, natural liquorice sticks, fennel, green onion, ginger root, and vanilla), often with massage to neutralize the inflammatory mediators produced during teething. Alternatively, chamomile oil may be placed in an aromatherapy diffuser in the infant's bedroom.
- Homeopathy treats the whole person, not solely the illness, and is becoming a more popular method of treating the symptoms of teething. The active ingredient in Ashton and Parsons Infant Powders (SSL International PLC, Knutsford) is matricaria tincture (4 mg), a carminative related to chamomile. Other homeopathic medications include Teetha (Nelson Bach USA Ltd., Wilmington, MA, USA) and Boots Homeopathic Teething Granules (The Boots Co plc, Nottingham) **(Fig. 15.2)** contain 6C potency of chamomilla, one sachet should be poured into the infant's mouth every 2 hours, up to a maximum of six doses in 24 hours. The main indications of these products are to "soothe the child, correct the motions, relieve restlessness, fretfulness and similar troubles incidental to the teething period...." all potentially useful benefits during teething.

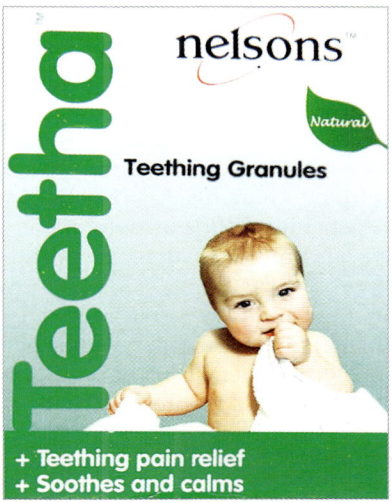

Fig. 15.2: Homeopathic teething granules.

Hellwig J (2017) described about FDA warning on teething products stating that homeopathic teething tablets and gels may pose a risk to infant and children. They are not approved by FDA for safety and efficacy, medical care should be taken immediately if child experience seizures, difficulty in breathing, lethargy, constipation, muscle weakness, difficulty in urination after using homeopathic gels or tablets.[12]

General Advice

- Parents should be advised that a number of outdated practices are potentially harmful.
- Adding or dipping sugar, honey, or jam to feeding bottles has absolutely no pain relieving effect and is highly cariogenic.
- Parents should also be advised that the repeated application of alcohol to the mucous membrane of an infant is ineffective as a topical anesthetic and due to an infant's small body weight may lead to hypoglycemia.
- Teething remedies should be kept well out of reach of all children, because of added flavorings, children can unwittingly overdose themselves.
- Medicines, including teething remedies, should never be added to food or feeding bottles, as parents cannot accurately control the dosage ingested.

Steward's approach to teething[13]

- First, give the child teething objects to bite. Cold objects bring greatest relief, so teething rings can be kept in the fridge.
- If pain is troublesome, use the appropriate dose of a paracetamol elixir, preferably sugar free. This may be given regularly, every 4–6 hours.
- If additional analgesia is required, lignocaine-based teething gels should be used.

TEETHING PROBLEMS

Eruption Hematoma (Eruption Cyst)

- A bluish purple, elevated area of tissue, commonly called eruption hematoma or eruption cyst, occasionally develops few weeks before the eruption of primary or permanent tooth **(Fig. 15.3)**.
- It is an analogue of dentigerous cyst and arise from the separation of the epithelium from the enamel of the crown of the tooth due to an accumulation of fluid or blood in a dilated follicular space following trauma.[14] Clinically it appears as dome shaped swelling in the mucosa of the alveolar ridge, whose color varies from transparent, bluish, reddish, purple to blue black. It may be asymptomatic or pain on palpation and is most frequently seen in the primary second molar or the first permanent molar regions.
- Most often, the condition is self-limited or ruptures on its own. The treatment may occasionally be justified, if it is symptomatic. Simple incision or partial excision of the overlying tissue to drain out the content.

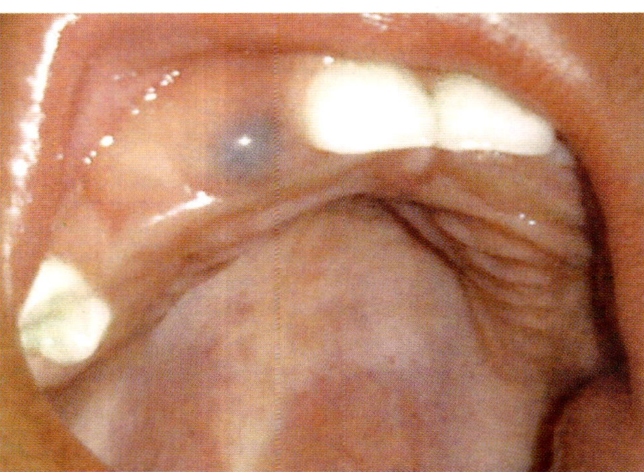

Fig. 15.3: Eruption hematoma.

Eruption Sequestrum

- The eruption sequestrum is seen occasionally in children at the time of the eruption of the first permanent molar. An eruption sequestrum is composed of fragments of calcified masses formed within the dental follicle overlying the crown of the erupting permanent molar.[15]
- Regardless of its origin, the hard tissue fragment is generally overlying the central fossa of the associated tooth embedded and contoured within the soft tissue. As the tooth erupts and the cusps emerge, the fragment sequestrates or can be resorbed completely before the tooth erupts. It is usually caused because of the apoptosis of reduced enamel epithelium, which has cells of osteoclastic potential, bringing about bone resorption mediated by dental follicle during tooth eruption.[16]
- Eruption sequestra are usually of little or no clinical significance as it may spontaneously resolve without noticeable symptoms, sometimes it may retain biofilm accumulation and lead to pericoronitis, localized swelling, discomfort during mastication, and demineralization or dental caries if it remains for a prolonged time. In such situation it has to be surgically removed.[17]

Ectopic Eruption

- It is defined as "a condition in which the permanent teeth, because of deficiency of growth in the jaw or segment of jaw, assume a path of eruption that intercepts a primary tooth, causes its premature loss and produces a consequent malposition of the permanent tooth".[18]
- Arch length inadequacy or a variety of local factors may influence a tooth to erupt in a position other than normal **(Fig. 15.4)**. Failure to treat ectopic eruption can result in loss of arch length, inadequate space for the succedaneous premolar, and malocclusion".[19]
- Some of the treatment modalities for ectopically erupting molars includes, interproximal wedging using brass ligature wires and helical orthodontic springs, distal tipping using Humphreys and Halterman appliance.

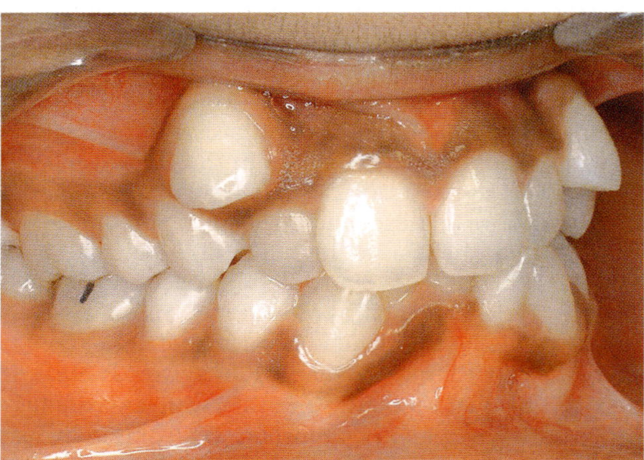

Fig. 15.4: Ectopic eruption.

Sweet[20] classified ectopic eruption on the following basis:

- Eruption of mandibular permanent lateral incisors initiating loss of the primary canines
- Eruption of the maxillary first permanent molar initiating loss of the second primary molar
- Eruption of the maxillary permanent lateral incisor initiating loss of the primary canine
- Eruption of the mandibular first permanent molar initiating loss of primary second molar

Natal and Neonatal Teeth

- Eruption of teeth at or immediately after birth is a relatively rare phenomenon. These have been defined by **Massler** and **Savara.**[21] These teeth are known as "natal" teeth if present at birth and "neonatal" teeth if they erupt during the first 30 days of life **(Fig. 15.5)**.

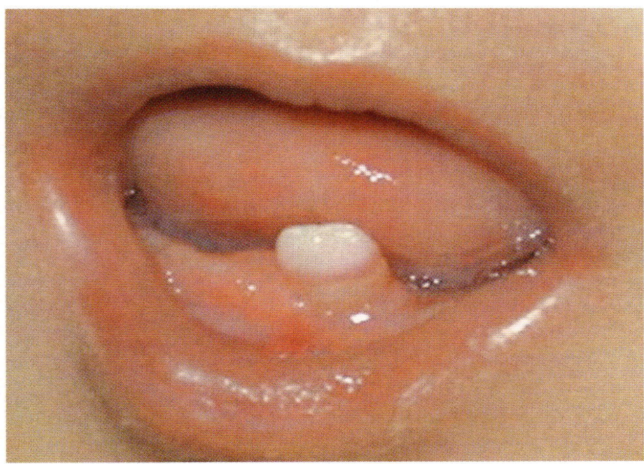

Fig. 15.5: Natal teeth.

- Prematurely erupted primary teeth present at birth have also been described in the literature as "congenital teeth," "predeciduous teeth," "fetal teeth," or "dentition praecox."
- Neonatal teeth often present with hypoplastic enamel and underdeveloped roots with resultant mobility; however, such teeth also should be further classified according to their degree of maturity. A mature natal or neonatal tooth is one that exhibits normal development, hence has a relatively good prognosis, while the term immature natal or neonatal tooth implies defective development and poor prognosis for retention.

History[22]

- Because of its rare occurrence, in the past, this anomaly of eruption was associated with superstition and folklore, being related to good or bad omens.
- This explains the many reports about this topic since 59 BC, as observed in cuneiform inscriptions detected in the 19th century as this condition has been the subject of curiosity and study since the beginning of time, being surrounded by beliefs and assumptions.
- **Titus Livius**, in 59 BC, considered natal teeth to be a prediction of disastrous events. **Caius Plinius Secundus** (the Elder), in 23 BC, believed that a splendid future awaited male infants with natal teeth, whereas the same phenomenon was a bad omen for girls.
- In Poland, India, and Africa, superstition prevailed for a long time, and in many African tribes, children born with teeth were murdered soon after birth because they were believed to bring misfortune to all they would contact.
- In England, the belief was that babies born with teeth would grow to be famous soldiers, whereas in France and Italy, the belief was that this condition would guarantee the conquest of the world. Historical figures such as **Zoroaster, Hannibal, Luis XIV, Mazarin, Richelieu, Mirabeau, Richard III**, and **Napoleon** may also have been favored by the presence of natal teeth.

Prevalence

- The reported prevalence[22] of natal and neonatal teeth has varied considerably from 1 in every 11.25–30,000 births **(Table 15.2).**

Table 15.2: Prevalence of natal and neonatal teeth reported in the literature.

Authors	*Prevalence*	*Number of children in the sample*
Magitot (1876)	1:6,000	17,578
Puech (1876)	1:30,000	60,000
Ballantyne (1897)	1:6,000	17,578
Massler and Savara (1950)	1:2,000	6,000
Allwright (1958)	1:3,408	6,817
Bodenhoff (1959)	1:3,000	–
Wong (1962)	1:3,000	–
Bodenhoff and Gorlin (1963)	1:3,000	–
Mayhall (1967)	1:1,125	90
Chow (1980)	1:2,000–3,500	–
Anderson (1982)	1:800	–
Kates et al. (1984)	1:3,667	7,155
Leung (1986)	1:3,392	50,892
Bedi and Yan (1990)	1:1,442	–
Rusmah (1991)	1:2,325	9,600
Almeida and Gomide (1996)	1:21.6	1,019

- Natal teeth are encountered more often than neonatal teeth in an approximate ratio of 3:1.
- More predilections in females.

Teeth Affected

- The teeth most often affected are lower primary central incisors.
- According to **Bodenhoff's**[23] study of natal and neonatal teeth, 85% are mandibular incisors, 11% maxillary incisors, 3% are mandibular canines and molars, and only 1% are maxillary canine or molars.

Etiology

- Over the years, there have been many postulations regarding the cause of premature eruption including dietary deficiencies, pyelitis during pregnancy, poor maternal health, hereditary factor hypovitaminosis, hormonal stimulation, trauma, febrile states, and syphilis, but a cause and effect relationship has not yet been established.
- The current concept suggests that natal and neonatal teeth are attributed to a superficial position of the developing tooth germ, which predisposes the tooth to erupt early. The tooth was not located in an alveolus but slightly below the surface of the alveolar bone, very much above the germ of the permanent successor.
- **Boyd** and **Miles** showed this clearly in both their anatomical section and radiographs of the fetal mandible. The erupted primary central incisors were located not in an alveolus but slightly below on the surface of the alveolar bone, very much above the germ of the permanent successor.
- Hereditary factors in the occurrence of these teeth are explained by **Holt** and **McIntosh** who reported a family in which natal teeth occurred in members of three successive generations.
- **Hyatt** also described a family in which five siblings had the presence of natal teeth.

- Natal and neonatal teeth are also found to be associated with multisystem syndromes and developmental abnormalities providing the evidence of genetic contribution.

Natal and neonatal teeth are associated with certain syndromes:
- Ellis-Van Creveld syndrome
- Van der Woude syndrome
- Rubinstein-Taybi syndrome
- Pierre Robin syndrome
- Down syndrome
- Cleft lip and palate
- Goltz Syndrome

Clinical Appearance

- Natal and neonatal teeth may resemble normal primary teeth, but, in many instances, they are poorly developed, small, conical, yellowish, with white hypoplastic enamel and dentin, and with poor or total failure of development of roots.
- Most affected teeth are mandibular central incisors, followed by maxillary incisors, rarely in maxillary and mandibular canine and molars.
- Natal teeth usually occur in pairs.
- The appearance of each natal tooth can be classified in one of the following categories by **Hebling:**[24]
  - **Category 1:** A shell-like crown structure loosely attached to the alveolus by a rim of oral mucosa; no root **(Fig. 15.6A).**
  - **Category 2:** A solid crown loosely attached to the alveolus by oral mucosa; little or no root **(Fig. 15.6B).**
  - **Category 3:** The incisal edge of the crown just erupted through the oral mucosa **(Fig. 15.6C).**
  - **Category 4:** A mucosal swelling with the tooth unerupted but palpable **(Fig. 15.6D).**

Histology

- Histological investigations have demonstrated that most of the crowns of natal and neonatal teeth are covered with hypoplastic enamel with varying degrees of severity, absence of root formation, ample and vascularized pulp, irregular dentin formation, and lack of cementum formation.
- **Friend et al.,**[25] in a clinical and histological report on an upper natal molar, proposed that the alteration in amelogenesis detected was due to premature exposure of the tooth to the oral cavity, which resulted in metaplastic alteration of the epithelium of the normally columnar enamel to a stratified squamous configuration.

Management

- A radiograph should be made to determine the amount of root development and the relationship of a prematurely erupted tooth to its adjacent teeth.
- **King** and **Lee**[26] recommended that inflamed gingival tissue around teeth should be controlled by applying chlorhexidine gluconate gel three times a day.
- In some cases, the sharp incisal edge of the tooth may cause laceration of the lingual surface of the tongue and selective grinding of tooth is advisable in such conditions.
- Most prematurely erupted teeth are hyper mobile because of the limited root development. Some teeth may be mobile to the extent that there is danger of aspiration, in which case, the removal of the tooth is indicated.

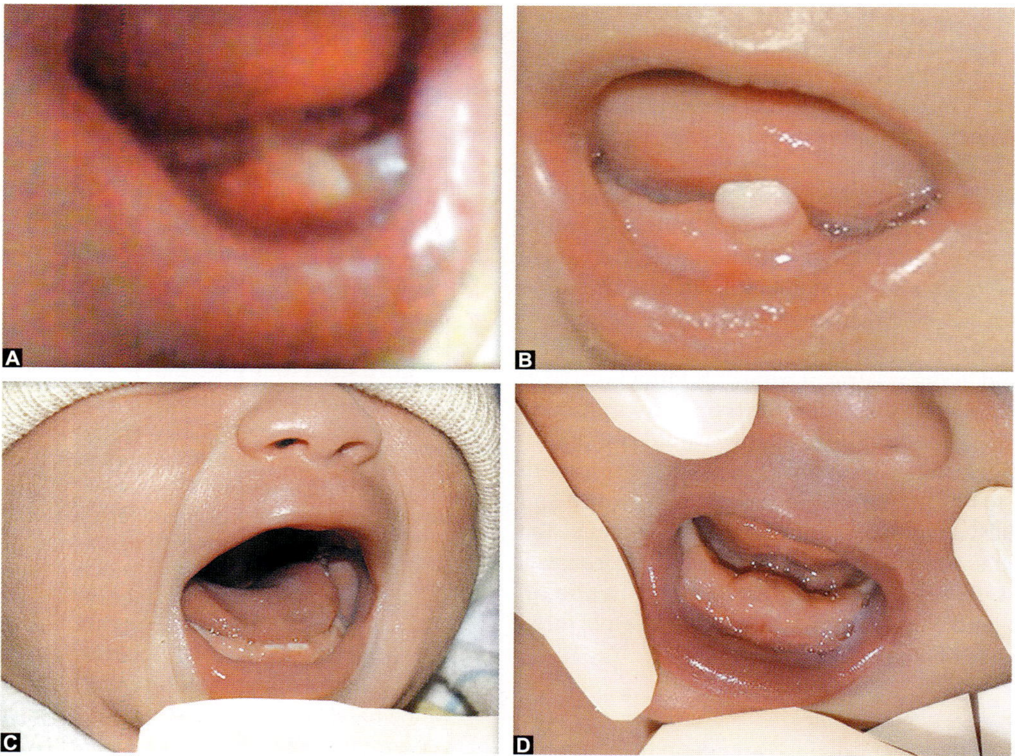

Figs. 15.6A to D: Clinical appearance of natal/neonatal teeth: (A) Shell-like crown structure loosely attached to the alveolus; (B) Solid crown loosely attached to the alveolus; (C) Incisal edge of the crown visible; (D) Mucosal swelling with the tooth unerupted. (*Source:* (A, C and D) With permission from LPCH Newborn Nursery at Stanford, Division of General Pediatrics, Stanford School of Medicine).

- If extraction of tooth is indicated, after the tooth is removed, careful curettage of the socket is indicated in an attempt to remove any odontogenic cellular remnants that may otherwise be left in the extraction site. Such retained remnant may subsequently develop a typical tooth-like structure that requires additional treatment. Earlier it was recommended to delay surgical procedures on newborns until after 10th postpartum day due to inability of clotting but nowadays, it is no longer considered because of prophylactic administration of vitamin K as a standard procedure in most hospitals.
- Eruption of neonatal teeth may cause difficulty for a mother who wishes to breastfeed her infant. If breastfeeding is too painful for mother initially, the use of a breast pump **(Fig. 15.7)** and bottling the milk are recommended. However, the infant may be conditioned not to bite during suckling in a relatively short time, if the mother persists with breastfeeding. It seems that the infant senses the mother's discomfort and learns to avoid causing it.

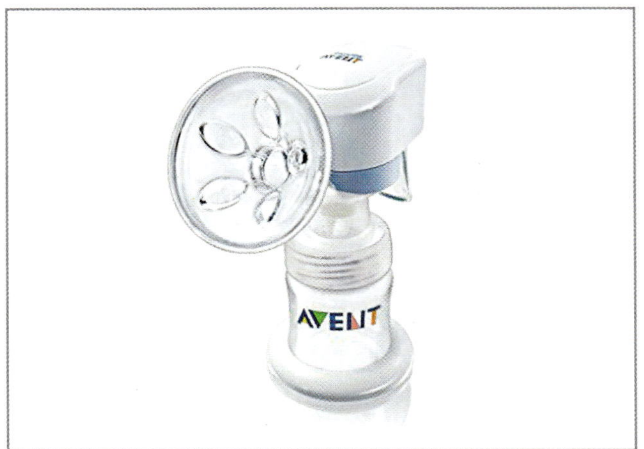

Fig. 15.7: Breast pump.

- The preferable approach is however to leave the tooth in place and to explain to the parents the desirability of maintaining this tooth in the mouth because of its importance in the growth. Adjacent teeth would erupt within a short time and the prematurely erupted tooth will become stabilized as the other teeth in the arch will erupt.

Flowchart 15.1: Management of natal or neonatal teeth.

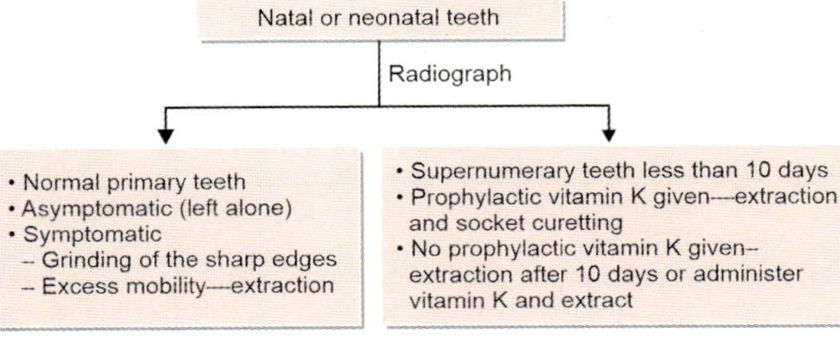

Complications

- Traumatic ulceration on the ventral surface of the tongue, frenulum, or lip is the most commonly associated complication of natal teeth

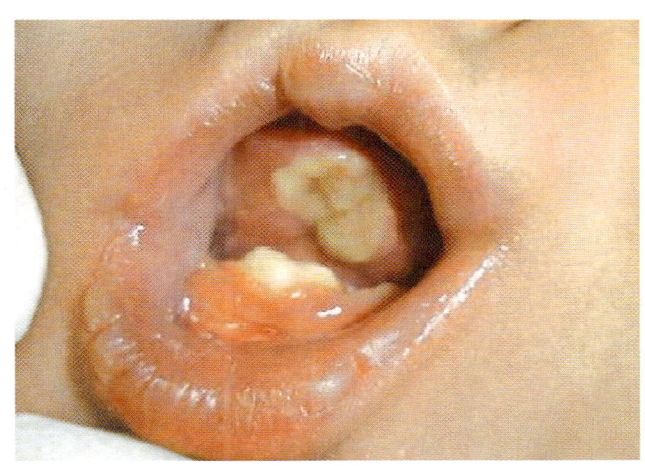

Fig. 15.8: Riga-Fede disease.

- In 1881 and 1890, **Antonio Riga** and **Fede** described this lesion histologically and it has subsequently been known as "Riga-Fede disease"[27] **(Fig. 15.8)**, although a more appropriate, descriptive term is "neonatal sublingual traumatic ulceration". Other associated terminologies are traumatic atrophic glossitis, traumatic eosonophilic ulceration of tongue and oral mucosa, sublingual fibrogranuloma.
- Ulceration of the sublingual area in infants was first described in 1857 by **Cardarelli.** It starts as a small ulcer with raised edges and with continous trauma becomes a large fibrous mass.
- Histopathologically, ulcerated mucosa with granulation tissue along with mixed inflammatory infiltrate of lymphocytes, mast cells, macrophages and eosonophills are observed.
- Lesion may cause difficulty for the child to feed thereby increasing risk of nutritional deficiency.
- First approach of managing such cases should always be conservative and focus on removal of stimuli. This can be done by trimming the edges of natal teeth or covering them with adhesive restorations. Alternatively the next step would be the extraction of the associated natal/neonatal tooth.

Non-eruption of Teeth

In case of non-eruption of teeth beyond their common eruption schedule, it is sometimes advisable to give a minor incision to facilitate their eruption if they are not associated with impactions or pathologies **(Figs. 15.9A and B)**.

The beliefs and superstitions associated with teething throughout history appear amusing and it may cause concern that the profession was so willing to go along with practices so incorrect. Yet, it is sobering to appreciate that our historic colleagues were acting on their existing knowledge and their professional and personal standing relied heavily on their reputation amongst their peers and patients. The diagnosis of teething, although historically having been applied to almost any condition whatsoever, is now reserved for a specific collection of variable signs and symptoms. The currently accepted methods of pain relief for teething infants have progressed considerably since the days leeching and

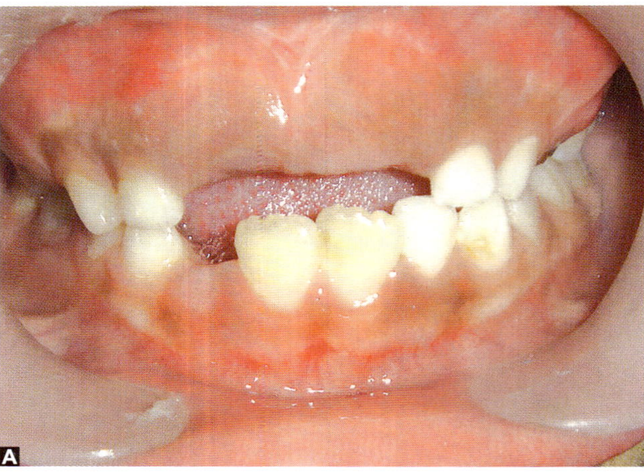

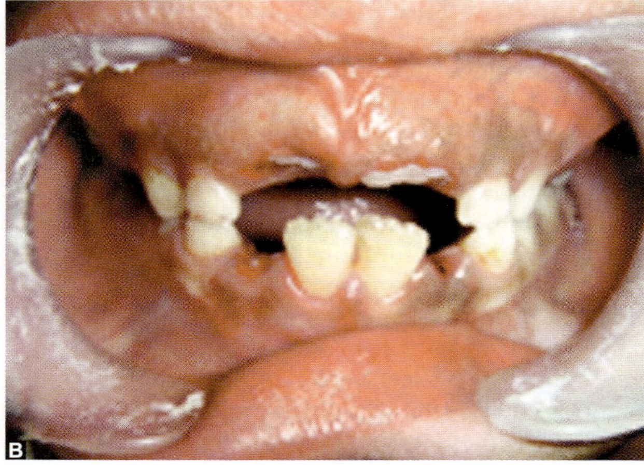

Figs. 15.9A and B: (A) Nonerupting central incisor; (B) Eruption after incision.

gum lancing and a number of supportive measures as well as topical and systemic pharmacological preparations, in addition to alternative holistic therapies can be used to relieve the pain of teething.

POINTS TO REMEMBER

- Hippocrates was the first one to advocate a treatise on teething.
- Dr WC Barrett was the first physician to change the line of treatment from lancing.
- Signs and symptoms of teething include pain, inflammation of the mucous membrane, disturbed sleep, drooling, bowel upset, loss of appetite.
- Management of teething includes teething rings, frozen items, pacifier, analgesic/antipyretics, anesthetic agents, alternative holistic medicine.
- Alternative nonpharmacological holistic therapies include acupressure, aromatherapy, massage, and homeopathy like Teetha (Nelson Bach USA Ltd., Wilmington, MA, USA) and Boots Homeopathic Teething Granules.
- Teething complications include eruption hematoma, eruption sequestrum, natal teeth, and ectopic eruption.
- Natal teeth are present at birth and neonatal teeth are seen within first 30 days of birth. They are more prevalent in females with teeth most often affected being lower primary central incisors. The current concept suggests that natal and neonatal teeth are attributed to a superficial position of the developing tooth germ, which predisposes the tooth to erupt early. Management includes selective grinding of tooth, extraction and curettage, use of breast pumps, and most prevalent complication of natal teeth is Riga-Fede disease.

Clinical Significance

- The dentist should be aware of concepts of teething and specially its management as the parent will first report to the family dentist. In such an eventuality the dentist should know the pharmacologic, holistic, alternate therapies for management.
- Natal and neonatal teeth offer a unique prospective to the dental clinician as their management is often long term and patient specific. Correct knowledge of when to modify the tooth preparation and when to extract is of utmost importance.

Questionnaire

1. Write a note on historical perspectives of teething.
2. Explain management of teething.
3. Enumerate teething complications with a note on eruption hematoma.
4. Describe history, prevalence, appearance, management, and complications of natal teeth.

REFERENCES

1. King LD. Teething revisited. Pediatric Dentistry: May/June 1994 -Volume 16, Number 179-82.
2. Wake M, Hesketh K, Lucas J. Teething and tooth eruption in infants: A cohort study. Pediatrics. 2000;106:1374-9.
3. Ingram CS. Teething: myth and reality; a review of the literature. J N Z Soc Periodontol. 1981;52:13-4.
4. Dally A. The lancet and the gum-lancet: 400 years of teething babies. Lancet. 1996;348:1710-1.
5. Macknin ML, Piedmonte M, Jacobs J, Skibinski C. Symptoms associated with infant teething: a prospective study. Pediatrics. 2000;105:747-52.
6. Carpenter JV. The relationship between teething and systemic disturbances. J Dent Child. 1978;45:381-4.
7. Obiajuru IO, Ikpeama CA, Ohalete CN, Uduchi IO. Teething Problems and the Influence of Microbial Infections. 2017;6:2.
8. Adnan M, Khan A, Ahmad W, Ahmed T, Farhat A. Parental knowledge, misconceptions and treatment practices about infant teething. Rawal Medical Journal. 2021;46(1):148.
9. Markman L. Teething: facts and fiction. Pediatr Rev. 2009;30:59-64.
10. Titchen T, Cranswick N, Beggs S. Adverse drug reactions to nonsteroidal anti-inflammatory drugs, COX-2 inhibitors, and paracetamol in a paediatric hospital. Br J Clin Pharmacol. 2005; 59:718-723.
11. Pierce CA, Voss B. Efficacy and safety of ibuprofen and acetaminophen in children and adults: a meta-analysis and qualitative review. Ann Pharmacother. 2010; 44(3): 489-506.
12. Hellwig JP. FDA Warning on Teething Products.Nursing for Women's Health. 2017;21(1):15.
13. Steward M. Infant care-teething troubles. Community Outlook. 1988; 27-8.

14. Boj JR, Garcia-Godoy F. Multiple eruption cysts: Report of case. J Dent Child. 2000;67:282-4.
15. Starkey PE, Shafer WG. Eruption sequestra in children. J Dent Child. 1963;30:80-2.
16. Park SJ, Bae HS, Cho YS, Lim SR, Kang SA, Park JC. Apoptosis of the reduced enamel epithelium and its implications for bone resorption during tooth eruption. J Mol Histol. 2012.
17. Schuler JL, Camm JH, Houston G. Bilateral eruption sequestra: report of case. ASDC J Dent Child. 1992;59:70-2.
18. Nikiforuk G. Ectopic Eruption: Discussion and clinical report. J Ont Dent Assoc. 1948;25:243-6.
19. Yaseen SM, Naik S, Uloopi KS. Ectopic eruption - A review and case report. Contemp Clin Dent. 2011;2(1):3-7.
20. Sweet CA. Ectopic eruption of permanent tooth. J Am Dent Assoc. 1939;26:574-9.
21. Massler M, Savara BS. Natal and neonatal teeth: a review of 24 cases reported in the literature. J Pediatr. 1950;36:349-59.
22. Cunha RF, Carrilho AF, Torriani DD. Natal and neonatal teeth: review of the literature. AAPD. 2001;23:158-62.
23. Bodenhoff's J. Dentitio connatalis et neonatalis. Odent Tidskr. 1959;67:645-95.
24. Hebling J, Zuanon ACC, Vianna DR. Dente natal—a case of natal teeth. Odontol Clín. 1997;7:37-40.
25. Friend GW, Mincer HH, Carruth KR, Jones JE. Natal primary molar: case report. Pediatr Dent. 1991;13:173-5.
26. King DL. Teething revisited. Pediatr Dent 1994;16:179-81.
27. Bray C. Riga's disease. W V Med J. 1927;23:249-50.

FURTHER READING

1. Ashley, M. It's only teething... A report of the myths and modern approaches to teething. Br Dent J. 2001;191: 4-8.
2. Cabate HF, Gomide MR, Costa B. Evaluation of primary dentition in cleft lip and palate children with and without natal/neonatal teeth. Cleft Palate Craniofac J. 2000; 37:406-9.
3. Kurian K, Shanmugam S, Harshvardhan T, Gupta S. Chondroectodermal dysplasia: Ellis van Creveld syndrome: A report of three cases with review of literature. Indian J Dent Res. 2007; 18:31-34.
4. Naederland R. Teething—a review. J Dent Child. 1952;19:127-32.
5. Ndiokwelu E, Adimora GN, Ibeziako N. Neonatal teeth association with Down's syndrome. A case report. Odontostomatol Trop. 2004; 27(107):4-6.
6. Swann IL. Teething complications, a persisting misconception. Postgrad Med J. 1979;55:24-5.
7. To EWH. A study of natal teeth in Hong Kong Chinese. Int J Paediatr Dent. 1991;2:73-6.
8. Vaysse F, Noirrit E, Bailleul-Forestier I, Bah A, Bandon D. Eruption and teething complications. Arch Pediatr. 2010;17:756-7.
9. Zhu J, King D. Natal and neonatal teeth. J Dent Child. 1995; 123-8.

CHAPTER 16

Development of Occlusion

Nikhil Marwah

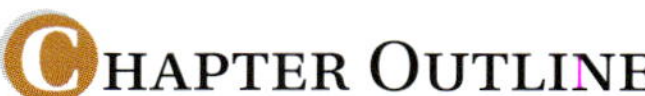

CHAPTER OUTLINE

- Predentate Period
- Deciduous Dentition Period
- Mixed Dentition Period
- Permanent Dentition
- Self-correcting Anomalies

Development of occlusion is a genetically and environmentally conditioned process, which shows a great deal of individual variations. In order to facilitate the understanding and comprehension of the developmental process, the aim of this chapter is to focus on the clinical features of developing dentition and establishment of their relationship. The term occlusion is derived from the Latin word '*occluso*' defined as the relationship between all the components of the masticator system in normal function, dysfunction, and parafunction. The various stages of occlusal development are:

- Predentate jaw relationship
- The deciduous dentition period
- The mixed (transitional) dentition period
- The permanent dentition period.

PREDENTATE PERIOD

- This is the period soon after birth. During this, the neonate has no teeth but the relation of the gum pads is of equal importance.
- The alveolar process at the time of birth is called the gum pads **(Fig. 16.1)**.
- They are horseshoe-shaped pads that are pink, firm and covered with a layer of dense periosteum **(Fig. 16.2)**.
- They are divided into two parts (labiobuccal and lingual) by dental groove. The gum pad is further divided into 10 segments by transverse groove; each segment has one developing tooth sac.
- A very important landmark in gum pads is lateral sulcus, which is the transverse groove between canine and first molar. This is helpful in predicting interarch relation at a very early stage.

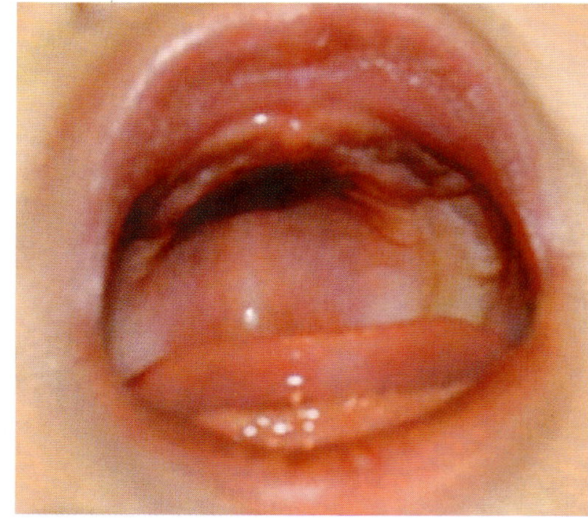

Fig. 16.1: Gum pad. (*Source:* Stanford Medicine Children Hospital, UK).

- The maxillary gum pad is wider and longer than the mandibular; thus, when they are approximated, there is a complete overjet all around. The only contact that occurs is around the molar region while space exists in anterior region. This is called infantile open bite, which is considered normal and helpful during suckling **(Fig. 16.3)**.

Mer Clinch's classification of gum pad relationship

- ***Type 1:*** 70% mandibular arch is slightly lingual to maxillary arch in incisor and molar regions.
- ***Type 2:*** 27% mandibular arch slightly distal in molar region but definitely distal in anterior region.
- ***Type 3:*** 3% mandibular arch is definitely distal in both molar and incisor region.

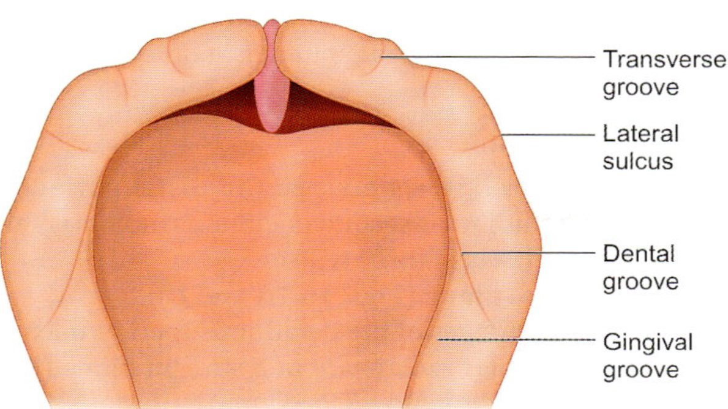

Fig. 16.2: Shape of gum pads.

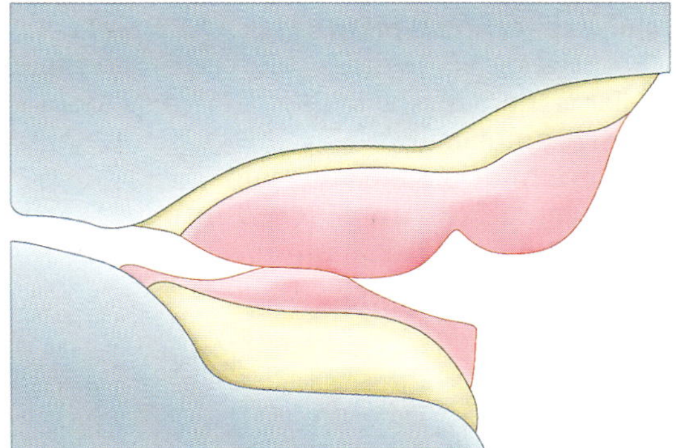

Fig. 16.3: Anterior open bite relation between upper and lower gum pads at birth.

DECIDUOUS DENTITION PERIOD

The initiation of primary teeth occurs during first 6 weeks of intrauterine life and the first primary tooth erupts at the age of 6 months. The individual variations apart, it takes around 2.5–3.5 years for all the primary teeth to establish their occlusion.

Spacing

- **Delabarre** in 1918 was the first to describe interdental spacing in primary dentition.
- **Baume** in 1950 divided the primary dentition into two parts, that is, spaced and nonspaced. He also concluded that primary spacing occurs around 70% in maxilla and 63% in mandible.
- **Foster** and **Hamilton** (1969) reported that only 1% of British children had no space.
- **White** and **Gardiner** (1976) reported that failure of incisor spacing occurs in 20% of cases before 5 years of age and usually indicated crowding in the permanent dentition.
- **Joshi** and **Makhija** (1984) found out more amount of primary teeth spacing in males than in females.

Spaced dentition: It is supposed to be good, as spaces in between the teeth can be utilized for adjustment of permanent successors, which are always larger in size compared to the deciduous teeth. The spaces present are of two types:

- **Primate spaces (Figs. 16.4A and B)**: *Exist between the maxillary lateral incisors and the canines (present mesial to maxillary deciduous canines) and mandibular canines and first deciduous molars (present distal to mandibular deciduous canines).* These spaces are also called **anthropoid or simian spaces** as they were initially found in our ancestral simian species.

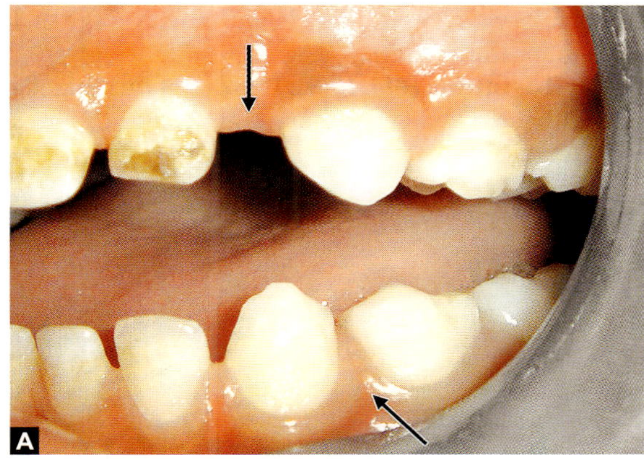

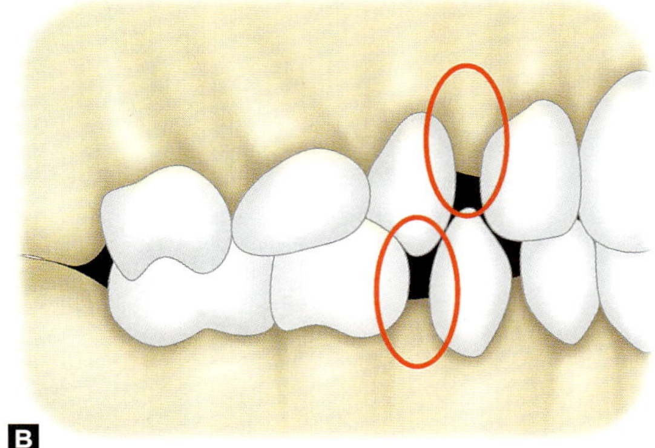

Figs. 16.4A and B: Primate spaces.

Characteristic features of deciduous dentition
- Both the dental arches are half round in shape or ovoid
- Almost no curve of Spee is present
- Shallow cuspal interdigitation
- Slight overjet
- Deep bite
- Vertical inclination of the incisors
- Spaced dentition
- Different maxillo-mandibular relations like flush, mesial, and distal terminal planes

- **Physiologic spaces (Fig. 16.5)**: *Present in between all the primary teeth and play an important role in normal development of the permanent dentition.* The total space present may vary from 0 to 8 mm with the average 4 mm in

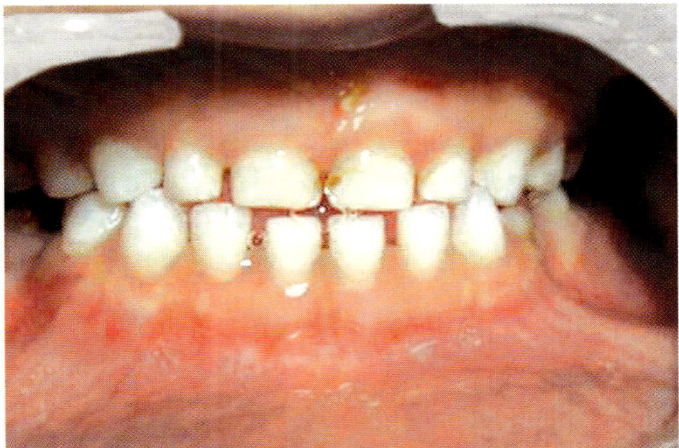

Fig. 16.5: Physiologic spaces.

the maxillary arch and 1–7 mm with the average of 3 mm in the mandibular arch.

Non-spaced dentition (Fig. 16.6): This dentition is highlighted by lack of space between primary teeth either due to small jaw or larger teeth. This type of dentition usually indicates to crowding in developing permanent dentition.

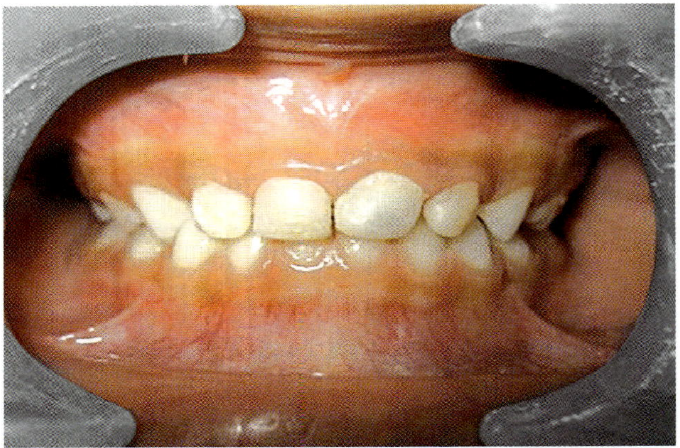

Fig. 16.6: Nonspaced dentition.

Terminal Planes

The mesiodistal relation between the distal surfaces of maxillary and mandibular second deciduous molars is called terminal plane. This is of three types:

1. **Flush terminal plane (Figs. 16.7A and B)**:
   - The distal surfaces of the deciduous second maxillary and mandibular molars are in a straight plane (flush) and therefore situated on the same vertical plane.
   - It is usually most favorable relationship to guide the permanent molars into class I. It is seen in 74%.
2. **Mesial step terminal plane (Figs. 16.8A and B)**:
   - The distal surface of the deciduous second mandibular molar is more mesial to that of the deciduous second maxillary molar. Invariably, this guides the permanent molars into a class I relationship.
   - However, a few can proceed into half cusp class III during molar transition and further into full

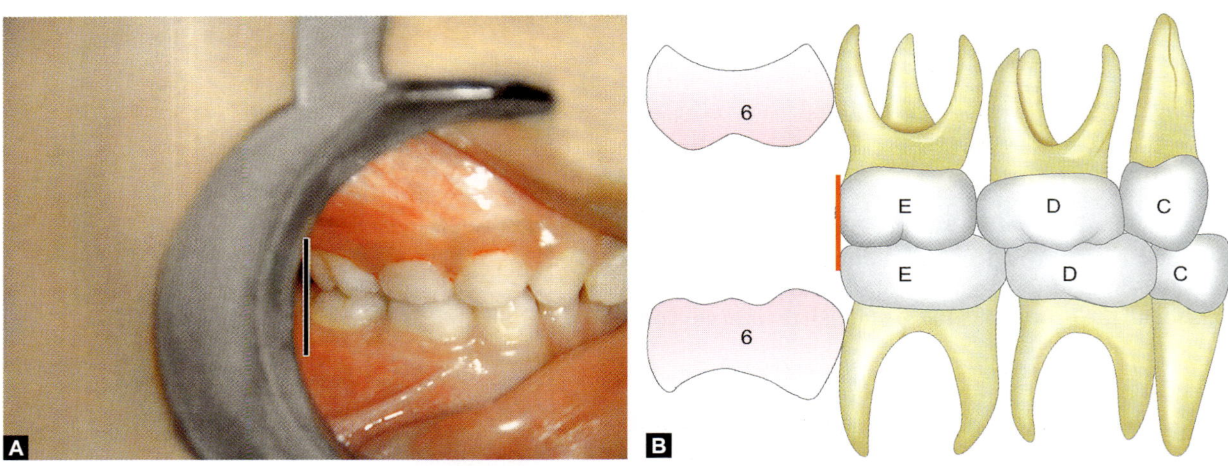

Figs. 16.7A and B: Flush terminal plane.

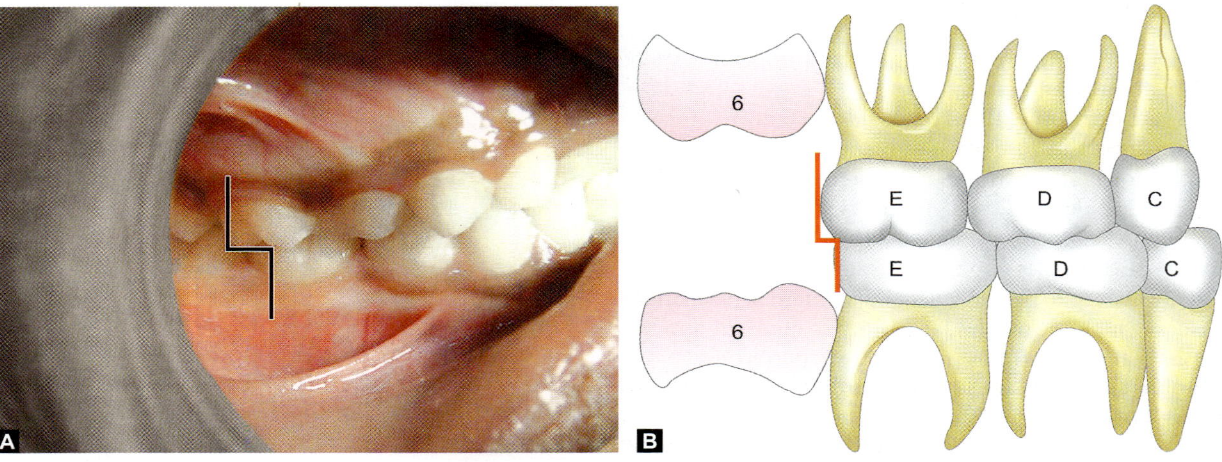

Figs. 16.8A and B: Mesial step terminal plane.

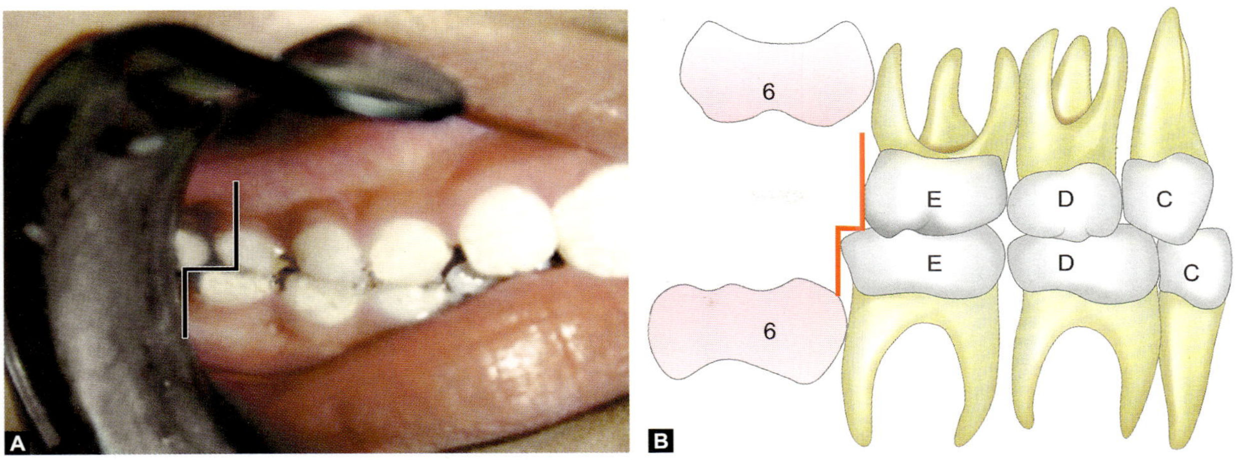

Figs. 16.9A and B: Distal step terminal plane.

class III relationship with continued mandibular growth.
- Seen in 14%.

3. **Distal step terminal plane (Figs. 16.9A and B):**
   - The distal surface of the deciduous second mandibular molar is more distal to that of the deciduous second maxillary molar. This relationship is unfavorable as it guides the permanent molars into distal occlusion.
   - Seen in 10%.

Anterior Teeth Relationship

- **Overbite:** It is the distance, which the incisal edge of the maxillary incisors overlaps vertically past the incisal edge of the mandibular incisors. The primary incisors erupt in a deep overbite which is corrected by eruption of posterior teeth around 5 years of age. The average overbite in the primary dentition is 2 mm.
- **Edge-to-edge bite:** When the incisal edges of the two incisors are in the same plane, this is also called a zero overbite. This is most common due to attrition, lengthening of ramus, and downward-forward growth of mandible.
- **Overjet:** It is the horizontal distance between the lingual aspect of the maxillary incisors and the labial aspect of the mandibular incisors when the teeth are in centric occlusion. The average in primary dentition is 1–2 mm.

Canine Relationship

The relationship of the maxillary and mandibular deciduous canines is one of the most stable in primary dentition:

- **Class I:** The mandibular canine interdigitates in embrasure between the maxillary lateral incisor and canine **(Fig. 16.10).**
- **Class II:** The mandibular canine interdigitates distal to embrasure between the maxillary lateral incisor and canine **(Fig. 16.11).**
- **Class III:** The mandibular canine interdigitates in any other relation **(Fig. 16.12).**

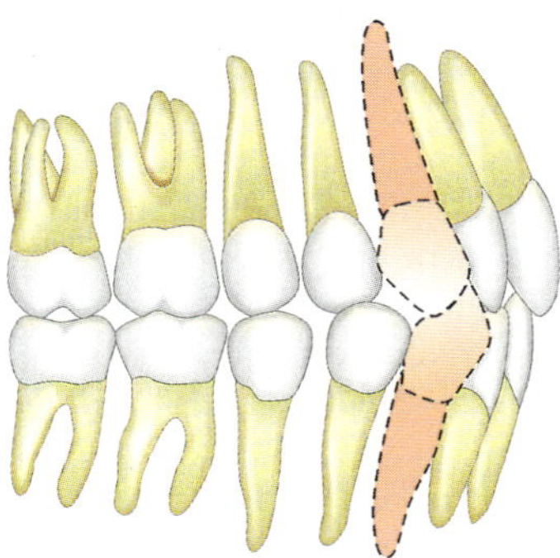

Fig. 16.10: Class I canine relation.

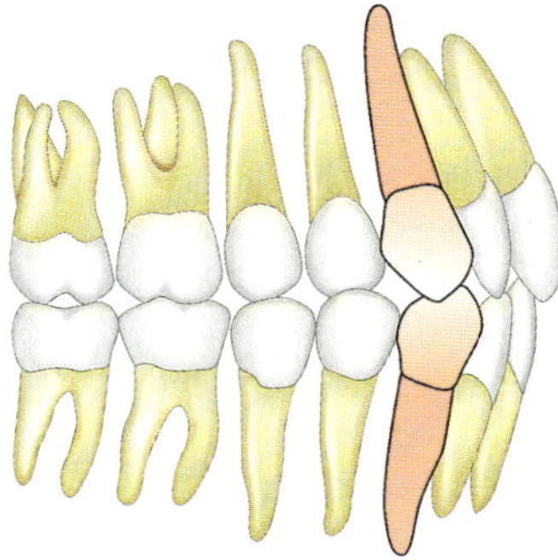

Fig. 16.11: Class II canine relation.

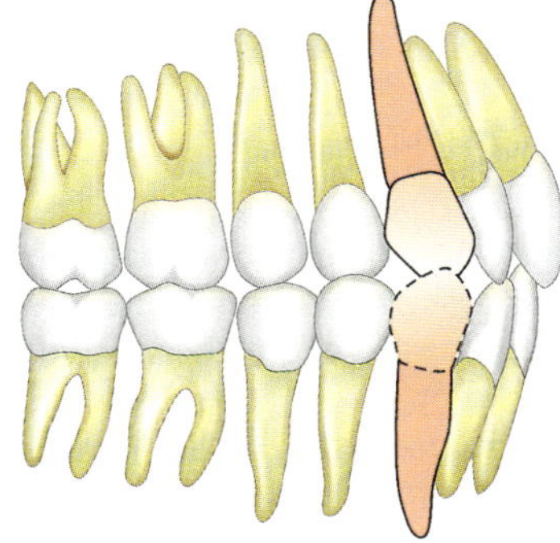

Fig. 16.12: Class III canine relation.

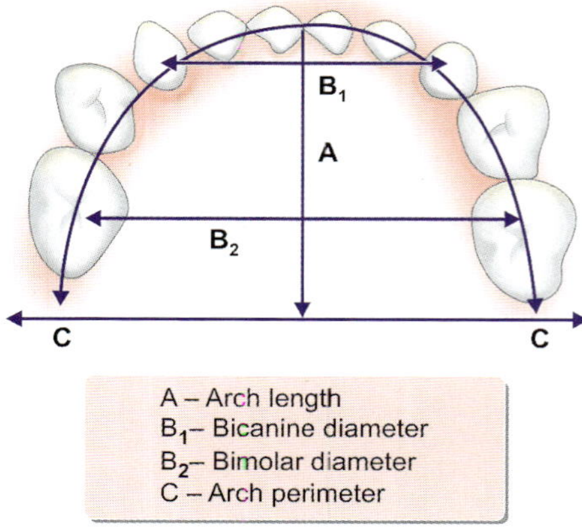

Fig. 16.13: Arch dimensions.

Arch Dimensions

- These were first measured by **Zsigmondy** in 1890.
- **Frank** and **Baume** later described the changes which can take place in arch dimensions by loss of primary teeth and during the development of occlusion **(Fig. 16.13).**
  - *Arch size:* Size of the primary dental arch is the arch width between primary canine and second molars.
  - *Arch length:* Measured from the most labial surface of primary central incisor to canine and to second primary molars.
  - *Arch circumference:* It is determined by measuring the length of curved line passing over the incisal edges and buccal cusps of teeth from the distal surfaces of primary second molar around the arch to the distal surface of second primary molar on the other side.
  - *Arch width:* Bicanine or bimolar width is called the arch width.

MIXED DENTITION PERIOD

The period during which both the primary and permanent teeth are present in the mouth together is known as mixed dentition. The permanent teeth erupting in place of previous deciduous teeth are the successional teeth, whereas those erupting posteriorly to the primary teeth are called the accessional teeth. This phase begins at around 6 years with the eruption of first permanent molars and lasts till about 12 years of age.

First Transitional Period

This is characterized by emergence of first permanent molars and exchange of deciduous incisors with permanent incisors.

- **Emergence of first permanent molars:**
  - The anteroposterior relation between the two opposing first molars after eruption depends on their positions previously occupied within the jaws, sagittal relation between the maxilla and mandible and occlusal relationship is established by the cone and funnel mechanism with the upper palatal cusp (cone) sliding into the lower occlusal fossa (funnel).
  - The mandibular molars are the first to erupt at around 6 years of age. Their position and relation is dependent on the relation of second deciduous molars as they are guided into dental arch by the distal surfaces of these teeth **(Fig. 16.14).**

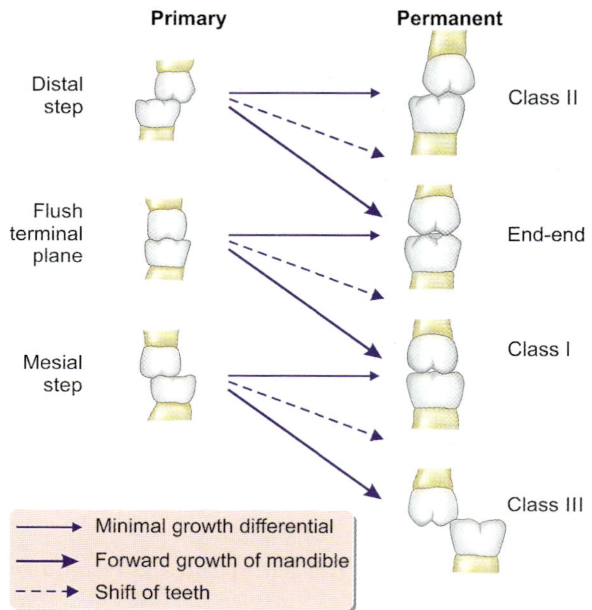

Fig. 16.14: Terminal plane prediction.

  - If the second deciduous molar is in flush terminal plane, then the erupting permanent molar will also be in the same relation. For this, to change into class I relation, the molar has to move 2–3 mm in a forward direction, this is accomplished by.

> **Terminal plane prediction**
> - *Flush terminal plane:*
>   - Class I—56%
>   - Class II—44%
> - *Mesial step:*
>   - <2 mm—80% Class I
>   - 2 mm—20% Class III
> - *Distal step:*
>   - Class II

  - *Early mesial shift:* The eruptive forces of first permanent molars are strong enough to push the deciduous molars forward in the arch, thereby utilizing the primate spaces and thus establishing class I relationship **(Fig. 16.15).**
  - *Late mesial shift:* Many children lack primate spaces and have a nonspaced dentition and thus erupting permanent molars are not able to establish Class I relation even as they erupt. In these cases, the molars establish Class I relation by drifting mesially and utilizing the Leeway space after exfoliation of deciduous molars and this is called late mesial shift **(Fig. 16.16).**
- If the second deciduous molar is in mesial step terminal plane, then the erupting permanent molar will directly erupt in Class I relation. But if further growth occurs or if there is more utilization of spaces, the relation can even change to Class III.
- If the second deciduous molar is in distal step terminal plane, then the erupting permanent molar will erupt into

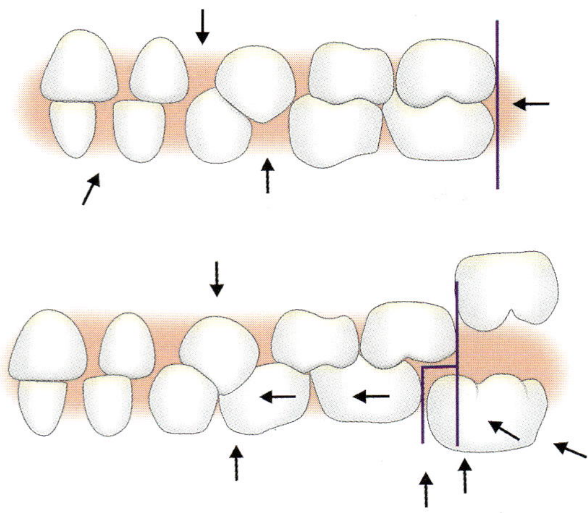

Fig. 16.15: Early mesial shift.

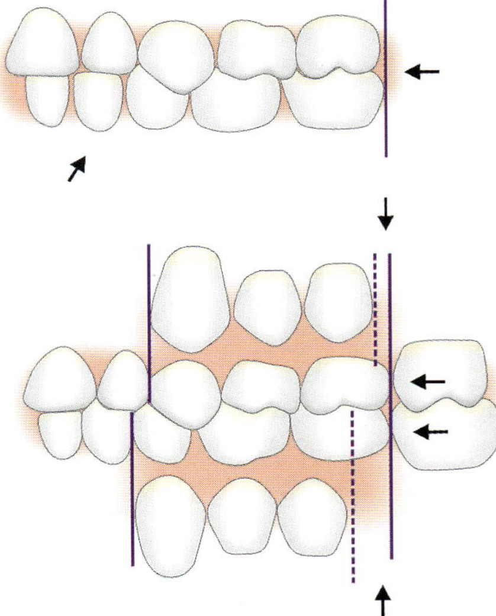

Fig. 16.16: Late mesial shift.

Class II relation. If further growth occurs or there is more utilization of spaces, then it can lead into end on molar relation.

Mixed dentition period
- First transitional period:
  - Emergence of the first permanent molars
  - Incisors transition
- Intertransitional period
- Second transitional period:
  - Emergence of cuspids, bicuspids, and the second permanent molars
  - Establishment of occlusion

❖ **Exchange of incisors:**
- The deciduous incisors are replaced by permanent incisors during this phase.
- This period of transition is from 6.5 to 8.5 years.
- The permanent incisors are larger as compared to their primary counterparts and thus require more space for their alignment. This difference between space available and space required is called the incisor liability **(Fig. 16.17).**

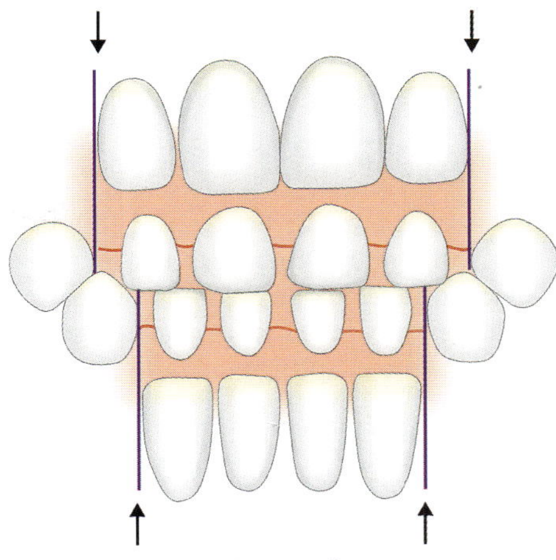

Fig. 16.17: Exchange of incisors.

- This is 7 mm for maxillary arch and 5 mm for mandibular arch.
- Some of the factors that help in alignment of incisors by gaining space are:
  - *Utilization of interdental spacing of primary incisors:* Averages 4 mm in the maxillary arch and 3 mm in the mandibular arch.
  - *Increase in intercanine arch width:* This occurs as the child grows. In males, it is 6 mm for maxilla and 4 mm for mandible whereas in females, it is 4.5 mm in maxilla and 4 mm in mandible.
  - *Increase in intercanine arch length:* This is due to growth of jaws.
  - *Change in interincisal angulations:* The angle between the maxillary and mandibular incisors is about 150° in primary dentition, whereas it is about 123° in permanent dentition, thus allowing more proclination and gaining space for incisor alignment. This is called incisor liability **(Fig. 16.18).**

Intertransitional Period

❖ In this period, the maxillary and mandibular arches consist of permanent incisors and permanent molars that sandwich the deciduous canines and molars.

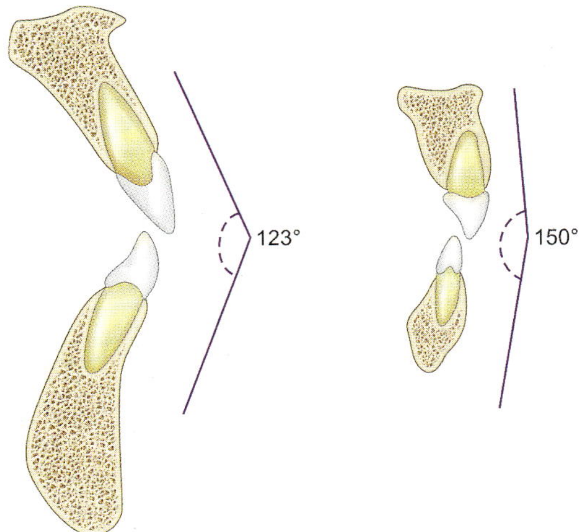

Fig. 16.18: Change in incisor angulation.

- This phase lasts for 1.5 years and is relatively stable.
- Only a few changes in the morphology of deciduous teeth are seen because they undergo attrition.

Second Transitional Period

This phase is characterized by replacement of deciduous molars and canines by premolars and permanent cuspids and the eruption of maxillary lateral incisors and canines. This takes place around 9–11 years of age and is very critical for the alignment of the erupting permanent teeth.

Replacement of Deciduous Molars and Canine

- *The combined mesiodistal width of permanent canine and premolars is less than that of deciduous canine and molars.* This extra space is called **Leeway space of Nance (Fig. 16.19)** and is utilized by mandibular molars to establish Class I relationship through late mesial shift.

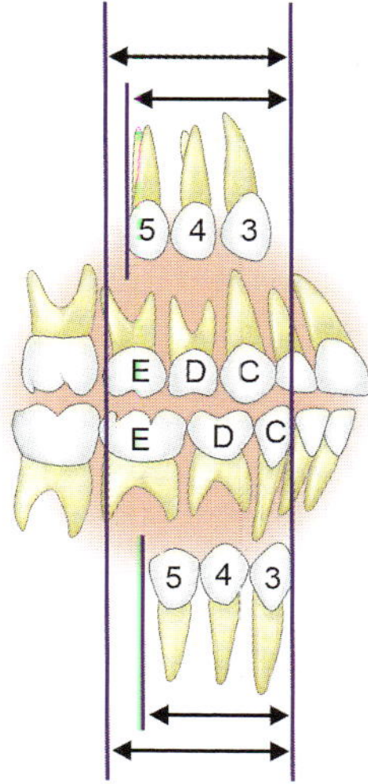

Fig. 16.19: Leeway space of Nance.

- It is 1.8 mm (0.9 mm on each side) in maxillary arch and 3.4 mm (1.7 mm on each side) in mandibular arch.
- The dimensions of deciduous second molars is more than that of second premolars, this excess space is called **E-space (Fig. 16.20)**.

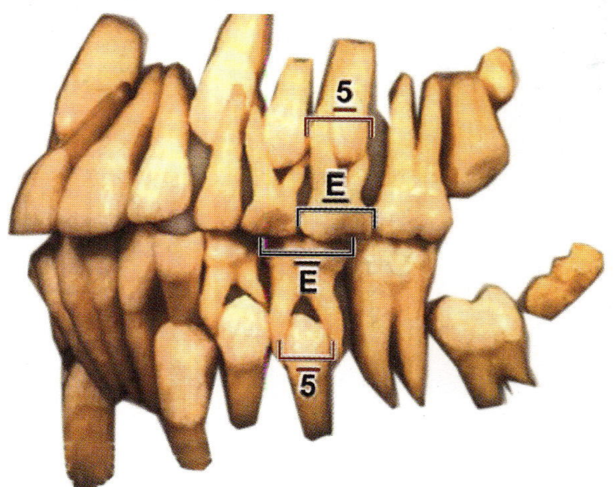

Fig. 16.20: E-space.

Eruption of Maxillary Canine

- The other event of significance in second transition period is eruption of maxillary lateral incisors and canines.
- This self-correcting malocclusion is seen around 8–11 years of age or during eruption of canines and was first described by **H Broadbent** in 1937.
- As the permanent maxillary canines erupt, they displace the roots of maxillary lateral incisors mesially. This force is transmitted to the central incisors and their roots are also displaced mesially. Thus, the resultant force causes the distal divergence of the crown in an opposite direction, leading to midline spacing **(Figs. 16.21A to E)**. This is called *Ugly Duckling Stage* or *Broadbent phenomenon*. The term ugly duckling stage indicates the unesthetic appearance of child during this stage **(Figs. 16.22 and 16.23).**
- This condition corrects itself after the canines have erupted. The canines after eruption apply pressure on the crowns of incisors, thereby causing them to shift back to original positions.
- No orthodontic treatment should be attempted at this stage as there is a danger of deflecting the canine from its normal path of eruption.

PERMANENT DENTITION

The entire permanent dentition is formed within the jaws after birth except for the cusps of first molar, which are formed before birth. Some changes that can be seen in permanent dentition are:

- Horizontal overbite decreases.
- Dental arches become shorter.
- Vertical overbite decreases up to the age of 18 years by 0.5 mm.
- Overjet decreases by 0.7 mm between 12 and 20 years of age.

Keys of Occlusion

- The permanent dentition after establishing itself is governed by various factors. These were underlined as Andrew's six keys of occlusion.
- **Andrew** in 1970 put forward these keys to occlusion after studying 120 patients with ideal occlusion. He hypothesized that the presence of the following features is necessary for an ideal occlusion:
  - Molar interarch relationship
  - Mesiodistal crown angulation
  - Labiolingual crown inclination
  - Absence of rotation
  - Tight contacts
  - Curve of Spee
  - Bolton's discrepancy.

Sequence of eruption

Maxillary arch 6-1-2-4-5-3-7-8

(First molar-central incisor-lateral incisor-first premolar-second premolar-canine-second molar-third molar)

Mandibular arch 6-1-2-3-4-5-7-8

(First molar-central incisor-lateral incisor-canine-first premolar- second premolar-second molar-third molar)

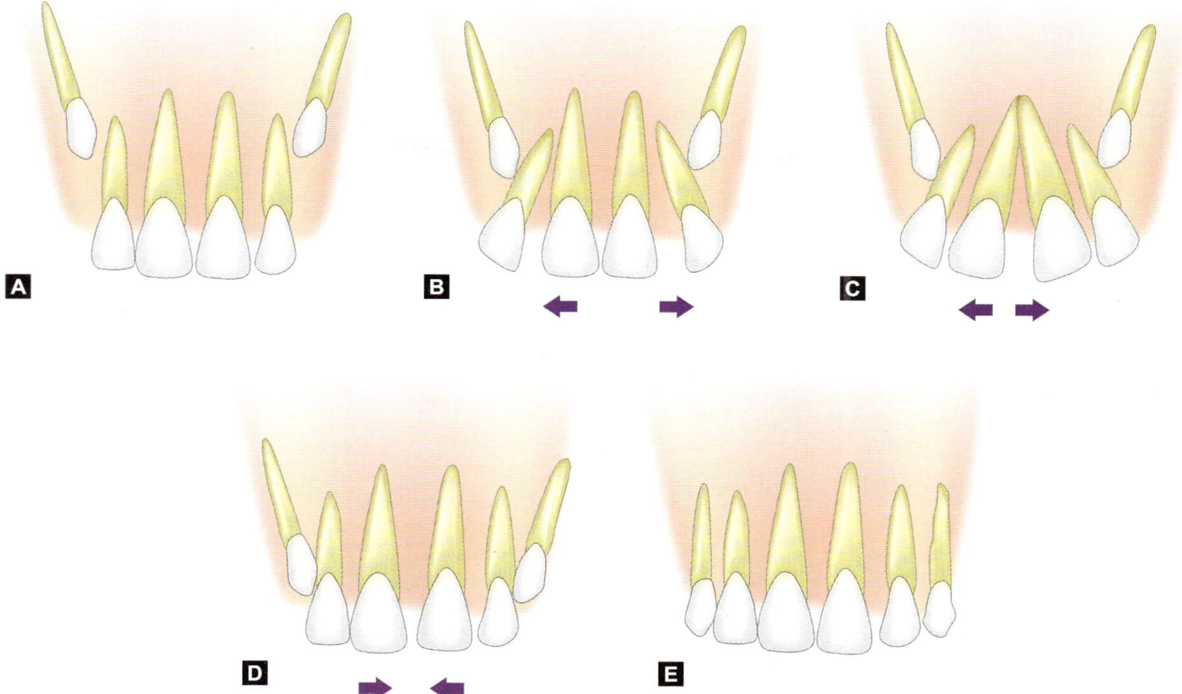

Figs. 16.21A to E: Broadbent phenomenon: (A) Erupting canine; (B) Erupting canine applying pressure on incisors; (C) Deviation of incisors due to pressure of canine; (D) Creation of midline diastema; (E) Self-correction of anomaly.

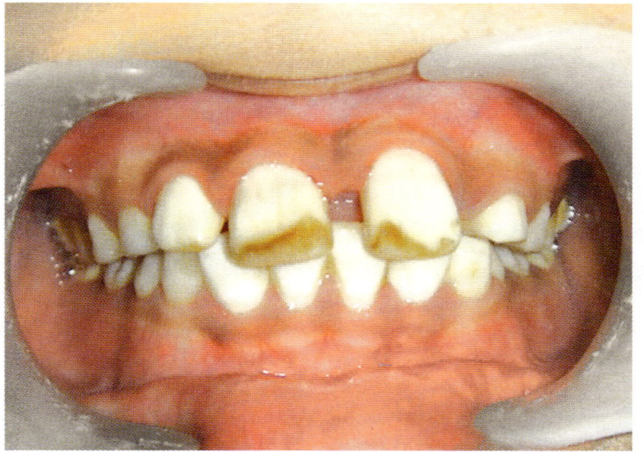

Fig. 16.22: Clinical appearance of ugly duckling stage.

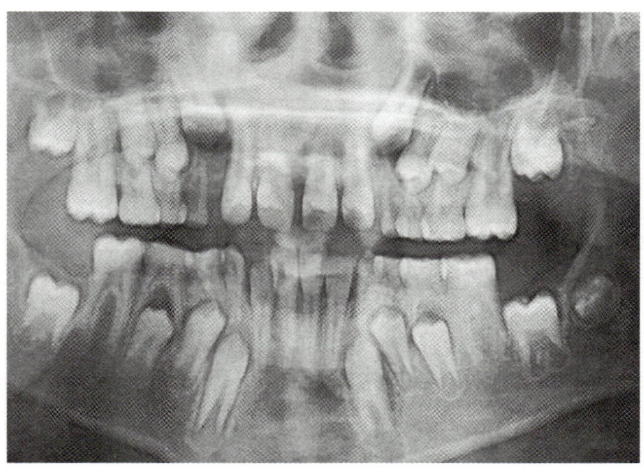

Fig. 16.23: Radiographic appearance of ugly duckling stage.

Molar Interarch Relationship (Fig. 16.24)

- The distal surface of the distobuccal cusp of the upper first permanent molar made contact and occluded with the mesial surface of the mesiobuccal cusp of the lower second molar.
- The mesiodistal cusp of the upper first permanent molar fell within the groove between the mesial and middle cusps of the lower first permanent molar.
- The canines and premolars enjoyed a cusp-embrasure relationship buccally, and a cusp fossa relationship lingually.

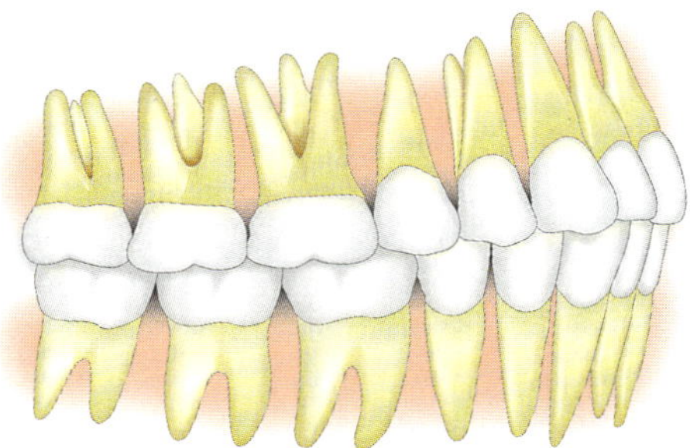

Fig. 16.24: Molar interarch relationship.

Mesiodistal Crown Angulation (Figs. 16.25 A and B)

- Crown angulation refers to angulation (or tip) of the long axis of the crown, not to angulation of the long axis of the entire tooth.
- The gingival part of the long axis of the crown must be distal to the occlusal part of the axis. The long axis of the crown for all teeth, except molars, is judged to be the mid-developmental ridge, which is the most prominent and centermost vertical portion of the labial or buccal surface of the crown. The long axis of the molar crown is identified by the dominant vertical groove on the buccal surface of the crown.

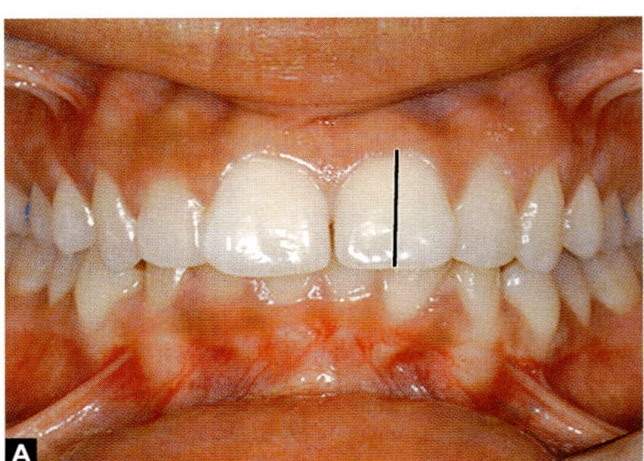

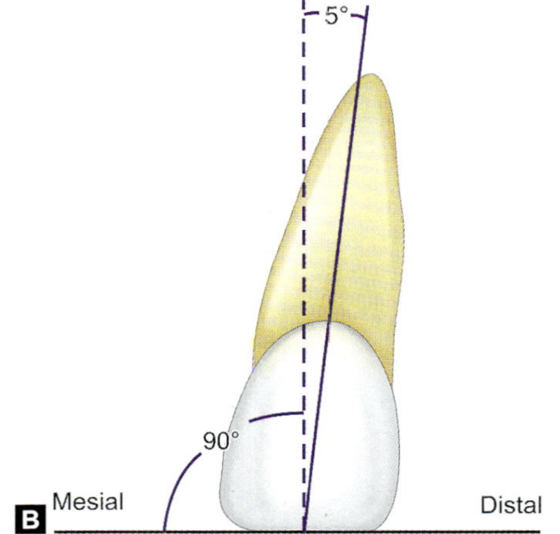

Figs. 16.25A and B: Mesiodistal crown angulation.

Crown Inclination (Fig. 16.26)

- Crown inclination refers to the labiolingual or buccolingual inclination of the long axis of the crown, not to the inclination of the long axis of the entire tooth.
- Crown inclination is determined by the resulting angle between a line 90° to the occlusal plane and a line tangent to the middle of the labial or buccal clinical crown.
- If cervical area of crown is lingually placed, then it is called positive crown inclination and if it is more bucally, then it is called negative crown inclination.
- Maxillary incisors positive, mandibular incisors negative, posteriors negative crown inclination.

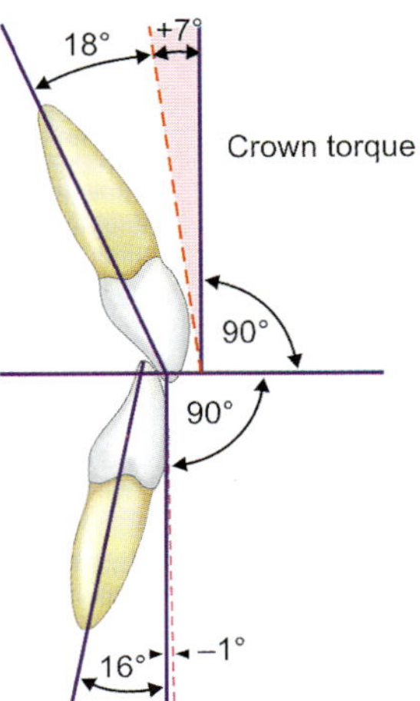

Fig. 16.26: Crown inclination.

Absence of Rotation (Fig. 16.27)

- Rotated teeth will occupy more space, hence normal occlusion should be free from rotation.
- Rotated molars and premolars occupy more space in the dental arch than normal, rotated incisors may occupy less space than those correctly aligned, and rotated canines adversely affect esthetics and may lead to occlusal interferences.

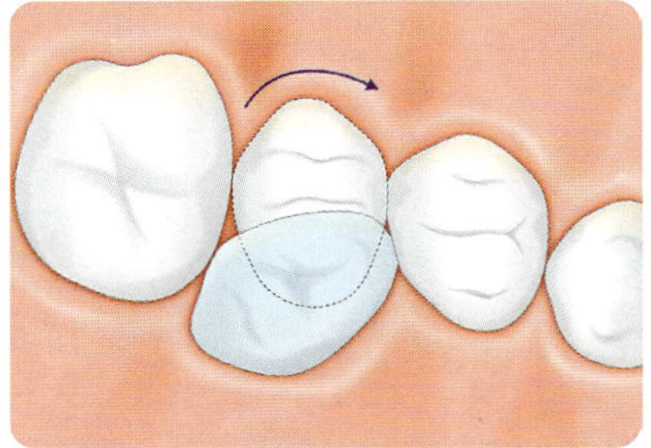

Fig. 16.27: Absence of rotation.

Tight Contacts (Fig. 16.28)

- Permanent dentition should have close contact to optimize space.
- Persons who have genuine tooth size discrepancies, pose special problems but in the absence of such abnormalities, tight contact should exist.

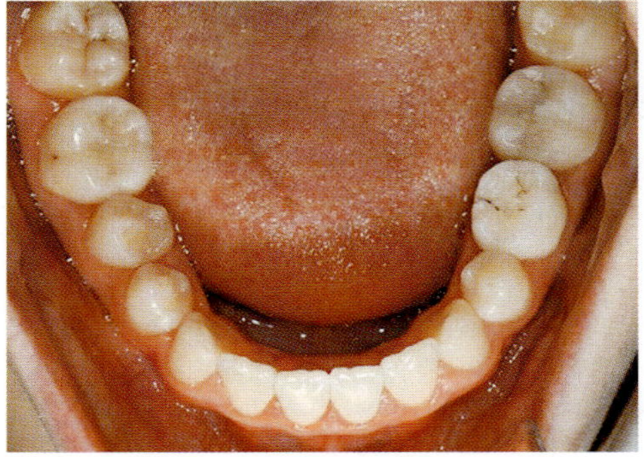

Fig. 16.28: Tight contacts.

Curve of Spee (Fig. 16.29)

- Occlusal plane should be flat with curve of Spee not exceeding 1.5 mm.

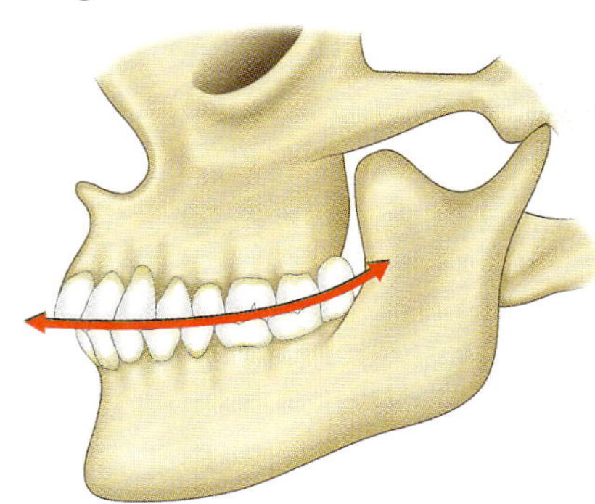

Fig. 16.29: Curve of Spee.

- There is a natural tendency for the curve of Spee to deepen with time, for the lower jaw's growth downward and forward sometimes is faster and continues longer than that of the upper jaw, and this causes the lower anterior teeth, which are confined by the upper anterior teeth and lips, to be forced back and up, resulting in crowded lower anterior teeth and/ or a deeper overbite and deeper curve of Spee **(Figs. 16.30A to C)**.

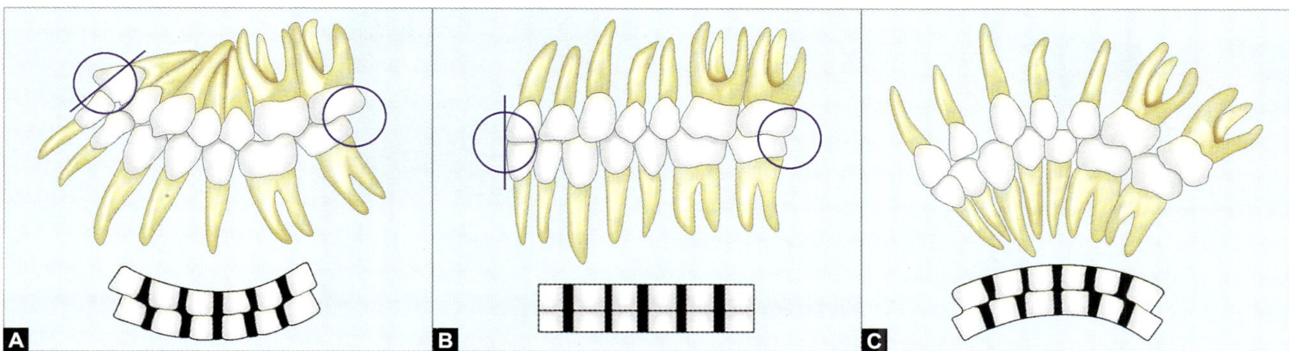

Figs. 16.30A to C: (A) A deep curve of Spee results in a more confined area for the upper teeth, creating spillage of the upper teeth progressively mesially and distally; (B) A flat plane of occlusion is most receptive to normal occlusion; (C) A reverse curve of Spee results in excessive room for the upper teeth.

SELF-CORRECTING ANOMALIES

Anomalies, which arise in the child, develop dentition during the period of transition from predentate period to permanent dentition period and get corrected on their own without any dental treatment **(Table 16.1)**.

Table 16.1: Self-correcting anomalies.

Anomaly	*Corrected by following mechanism*
Predentate period	
Retrognathic mandible	Differential and forward growth of mandible
Anterior open bite	Eruption of primary incisors
Infantile swallow pattern 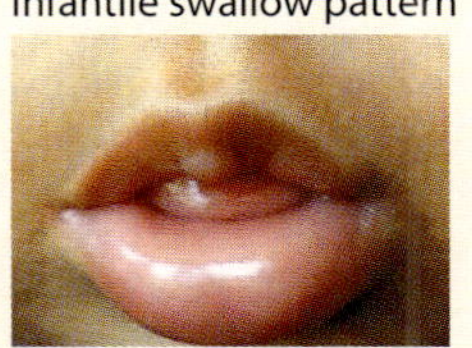	Eruption of teeth Change of diet from liquid food to solid food
Deciduous dentition	
Anterior deep bite 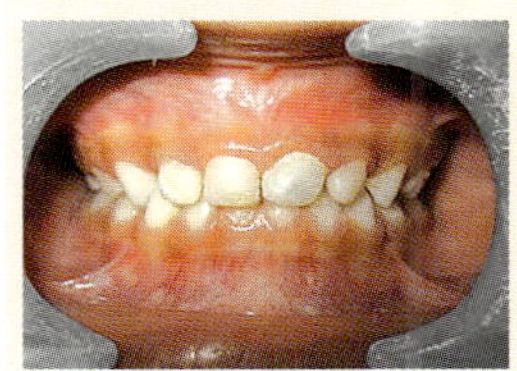	• When the attrition of incisal edges of incisors occurs • When the permanent molars erupt • When the mandible grows forward and downward
Physiologic spaces 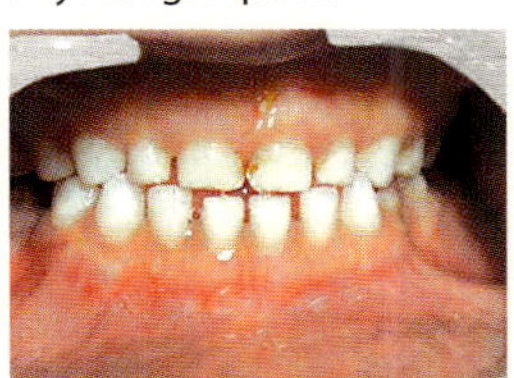	When the permanent incisors erupt, they use the spaces. In maxilla, it is around 7 mm and in mandible, it is 5 mm

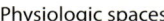

Contd...

Contd...

Anomaly	Corrected by following mechanism
Primate space 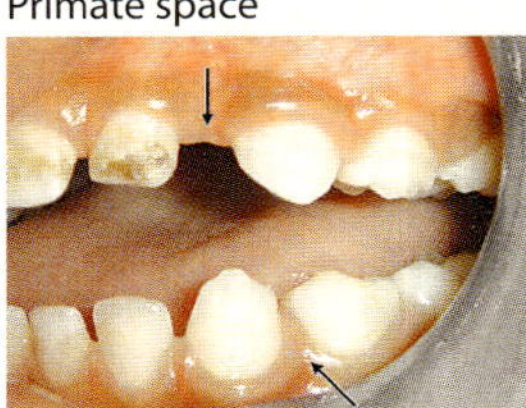	When there is early mesial shift
Flush terminal plane 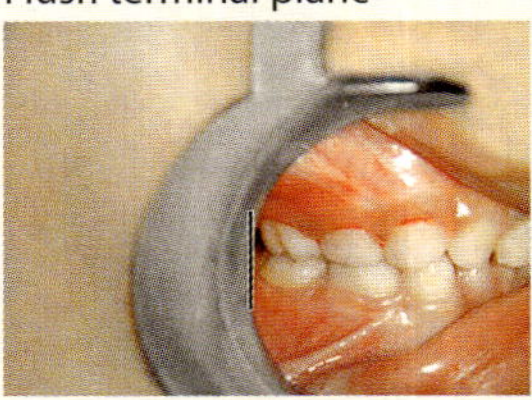	When there is early mesial shift and late mesial shift
Mixed dentition 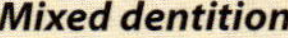	
Anterior deep bite 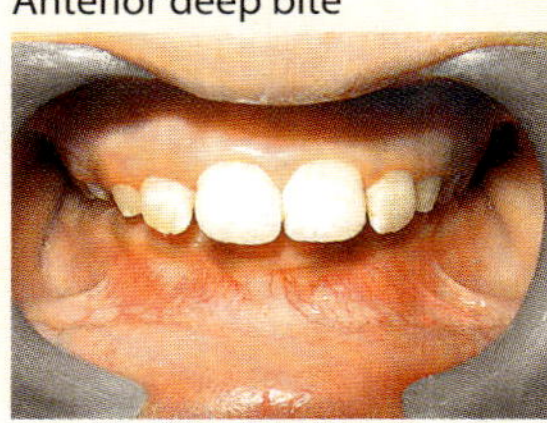	By slight supraeruption of permanent molars and premature contact of pads of tissue

Contd...

Anomaly	Corrected by following mechanism
Mandibular anterior crowding 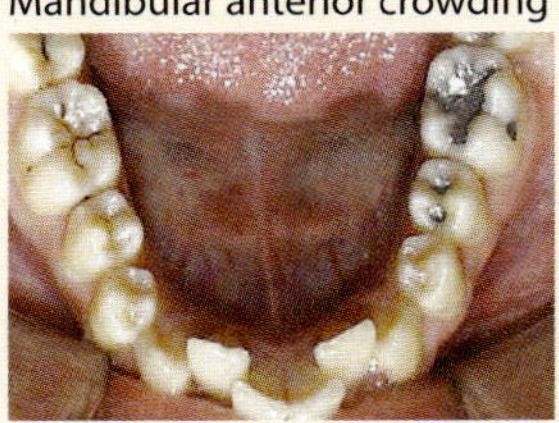	• Intercanine width gets increased • With the muscular forces from lip and tongue, there will be labial movement and incisors gets inclined
Ugly duckling stage 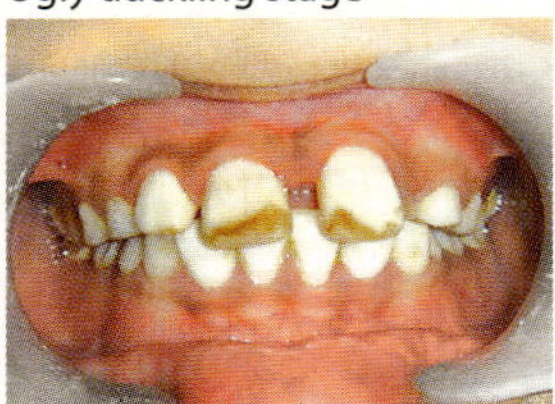	Eruption of maxillary canine
End on molar relation 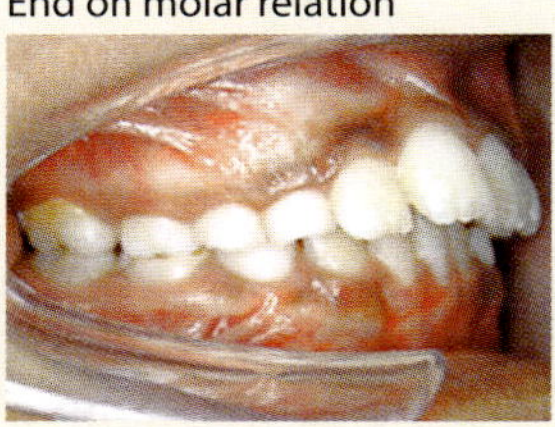	During late mesial shift by using Leeway space of Nance

Contd...

POINTS TO REMEMBER

- The alveolar process at the time of birth is called the gum pads.
- Dental groove divides gum pads into labiobuccal and lingual portions.
- Lateral sulcus is the transverse groove between canine and first molar.
- Delabarre in 1918 was the first to describe interdental spacing in primary dentition.
- Primate spaces are present mesial to maxillary deciduous canines and distal to mandibular deciduous canines.
- The total physiologic space present may vary from 0 to 8 mm with the average 4 mm in the maxillary arch and 1–7 mm with the average of 3 mm in the mandibular arch.
- Flush terminal plane is when distal surfaces of the deciduous second maxillary and mandibular molars are in a straight plane (flush) and therefore situated on the same vertical plane. It is usually most favorable relationship to guide the permanent molars into class I and is seen in 74% cases.
- The permanent incisors are larger as compared to their primary counterparts and thus require more space for their alignment. This difference between space available and space required is called the incisor liability. This is 7 mm for maxillary arch and 5 mm for mandibular arch.
- The combined mesiodistal width of permanent canine and premolars is less than that of deciduous canine and molars. This extra space is called Leeway space of Nance. It is 1.8 mm (0.9 mm on each side) in maxillary arch and 3.4 mm (1.7 mm on each side) in mandibular arch.
- As the permanent maxillary canines erupt, they displace the roots of maxillary lateral incisors mesially. This force is transmitted to the central incisors and their roots are also displaced mesially. Thus, the resultant force causes the distal divergence of the crown in an opposite direction, leading to midline spacing. This is called Ugly Duckling Stage or Broadbent phenomenon.
- Andrew's six keys of occlusion for permanent teeth are molar interarch relationship, mesiodistal crown angulation, labiolingual crown inclination, absence of rotation, tight contacts, curve of Spee, and Bolton's discrepancy.

Clinical Significance

- Early prediction of malocclusion through terminal plane relation and spaced/non-spaced dentition is to be correctly identified by the dentist.
- Myofunctional therapy should be initiated by the clinicians during the mixed dentition phase initiating from 6–12 years of age.
- Ugly duckling stage or creating of transition midline diastema due to eruption of canine (9–11) years of age is often misconceptualized as orthodontic issue. Hence, the dentist must always fully evaluate the eruption status of lateral incisors and canines before any orthodontic recommendations.

Questionnaire

1. Describe the development of dentition from birth to adolescence.
2. Describe predentate period with reference to gum pads.
3. Explain the spacing in primary teeth.
4. Define terminal planes and explain flush terminal plane.
5. What is the fate of terminal planes?
6. Describe the canine relation in primary dentition.
7. What is incisor liability?
8. What is Leeway Space of Nance?
9. What is E-space?
10. Explain Broadbent phenomenon.
11. Describe keys of occlusion.
12. What are self-correcting anomalies?

FURTHER READING

1. AAPD. Guideline on management of the developing dentition and occlusion in pediatric dentistry. Reference Manual. 2012; 34: 239-51.
2. Andrews LF. The six keys to normal occlusion. Am J Orthod Dentofacial Orthop. 1972;296-309.
3. Baume LJ. Physiological tooth migration and its significance for the development of occlusion. J Dent Res. 1950;29: 123, 331-4, 440.
4. Bishara SE, Khadivi P, Jakobsen JR. Changes in tooth size arch length relationships from the deciduous to the permanent dentition: a longitudinal study. Am J Orthod Dentofacial Orthop. 1995; 108:607-13.
5. Dean JA, Mc Donald RE, Avery DA. Management of the developing dentition. In: McDonald RE, Avery DR, Dean JA, editors. Dentistry for the Child and Adolescent. 8th edn. St. Louis, MO: Mosby, Inc; 2004. pp. 646-51.
6. Gron AM. Prediction of tooth emergence. J Dent Res 1962; 41: 573-85.
7. Moorees CFA. The dentition of the growing child. A longitudinal study of dental development between 3 and 18 years of age. Harward University Press; 1959.
8. Moorrees CFA. Growth of dental arches: a longitudinal study. J Can Dent Assoc. 1958;24:449-57.
9. Moyers RE. Development of occlusion. Dent Clin North Am. 1969;13: 523-36.
10. Proffit WR. Contemporary orthodontics. 3rd ed. St Louis: Mosby Year Book; 1999.
11. Sanin C, Savara BS. The development of an excellent occlusion. Am J Orthod. 1972; 61:345-52.
12. Williams RE, Ceen RF. Craniofacial growth and the dentition. Pediatr Clin North Am. 1982;29: 503-22.
13. Woodside DG. The significance of late developmental crowding to early treatment planning for incisor crowding. Am J Orthod Dentofacial Orthop. 2000;117:559-61.

Morphology of Primary Dentition

Nikhil Marwah, M Kirthiga, MS Muthu

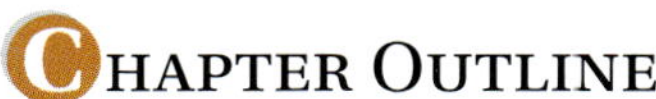

INTRODUCTION

The morphology of the primary teeth is smaller in overall size when compared with their counterparts in the permanent dentition. They have markedly more prominent cervical edges, are narrower at their "necks" are lighter in colour and have roots that are more widely flared; in addition, the buccolingual diameter of primary molar teeth is less than that of permanent teeth. The morphology of the individual teeth has been described in this chapter.

INDIVIDUAL DESCRIPTION OF PRIMARY TEETH

Table 17.1 shows the individual measurements of all the primary teeth. The detailed description of the morphology of deciduous teeth is provided below.

Maxillary Central Incisor

- The first notable difference between the maxillary central incisor and its permanent successor is the fact that it has a

Table 17.1: Measurements of all the primary teeth.

	Length overall	*Length of crown*	*Length of root*	*Mesiodistal diameter of crown*	*Mesiodistal diameter at cervix*	*Labiolingual diameter of crown*	*Labiolingual diameter at cervix*
Upper teeth							
Central incisor	16.0	6.0	10.0	6.5	4.5	5.0	4.0
Lateral incisor	15.8	5.6	11.4	5.1	3.7	4.0	3.7
Canine	19.0	6.5	13.5	7.0	5.1	7.0	5.5
First molar	15.2	5.1	10.0	7.3	5.2	8.5	6.9
Second molar	17.5	5.7	11.7	8.2	6.4	10.0	8.3
Lower teeth							
Central incisor	14.0	5.0	9.0	4.2	3.0	4.0	3.5
Lateral incisor	15.0	5.2	10.0	4.1	3.0	4.0	3.5
Canine	17.5	6.0	11.5	5.0	3.7	4.8	4.0
First molar	15.8	6.0	9.8	7.7	6.5	7.0	5.3
Second molar	18.8	5.5	11.3	9.9	7.2	8.7	6.4

mesiodistal measurement greater than the incisocervical measurement **(Fig. 17.1)**

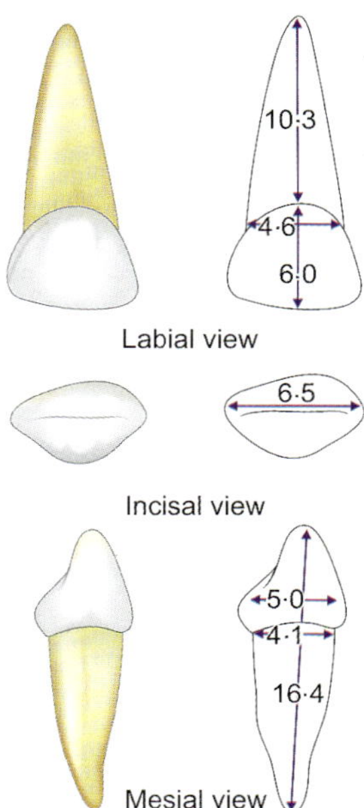

Fig. 17.1: Maxillary central incisor.

- The labial surface is slightly convex and relatively smooth, with little evidence of developmental lines or grooves. The incisal edge joins the mesial surface at an acute angle, and the distal surface at a more obtuse angle.
- The lingual surface shows a well-developed cingulum and marginal ridges, but developmental anatomic features such as pits and grooves are usually missing.
- The root of the maxillary central is conical and tapered toward the apex.

Maxillary Lateral Incisor

- The maxillary lateral incisor is essentially smaller in most dimensions than the central incisor **(Fig. 17.2).**

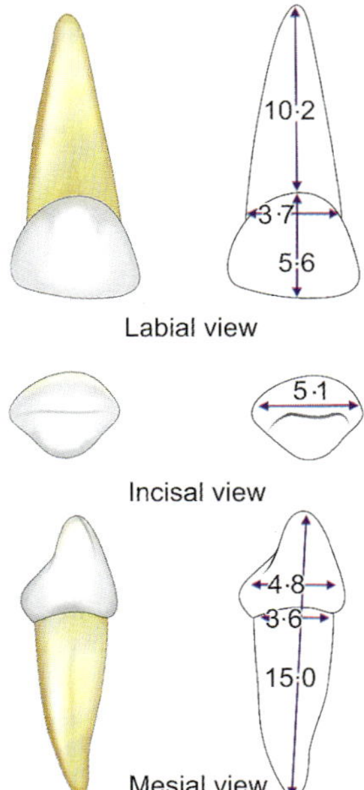

Fig. 17.2: Maxillary lateral incisor.

- The distoincisal angle is more rounded than the corresponding angle on the central incisor, and the lingual anatomy is usually less prominent.
- The morphology of the root is essentially the same as that of the central incisor, except that it is longer in proportion to the crown.

Maxillary Canine

- It is larger than maxillary incisors in all dimensions **(Fig. 17.3).**
- All surfaces of the crown are convex, creating a more pronounced constriction at the cervix than is seen in the maxillary incisors.
- It has a prominent cusp dividing the incisal aspect into a mesioincisal and a distoincisal edge, the mesioincisal edge being the longer of the two.
- The lingual surface presents a prominent lingual ridge, lingual fossae, and marginal ridges.
- The root of the maxillary canine is long and tapered toward the apex, but it shows a characteristic increase in diameter just apical to the cervical line.

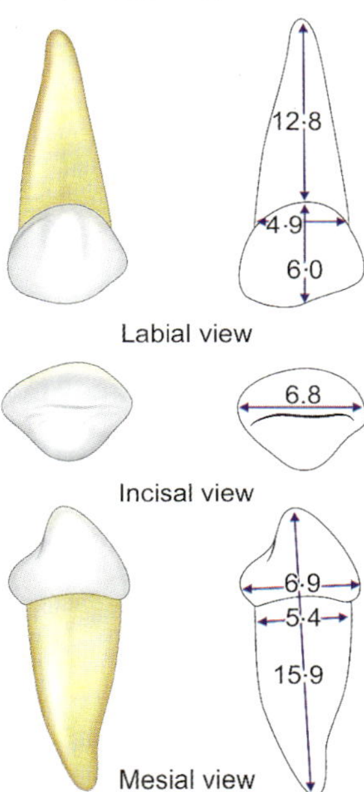

Fig. 17.3: Maxillary canine.

Mandibular Central Incisor

- The mandibular central incisor is smaller in all dimensions than the maxillary central incisor **(Fig. 17.4).**
- When viewed from the labial aspect, the tooth is symmetric with both the mesio and distoincisal angles joining the incisal edge at almost right angles.
- The incisal edge is usually perfectly straight in the horizontal plane.
- The labial surface is less convex than that of the maxillary central incisor, but it is also smooth without evidence of developmental anatomic landmarks.
- The lingual surface is usually smooth with a poorly defined fossa and marginal ridges.
- The root of the mandibular central incisor is long, evenly tapered toward the apex, and at times slightly compressed on its mesial and distal surfaces.

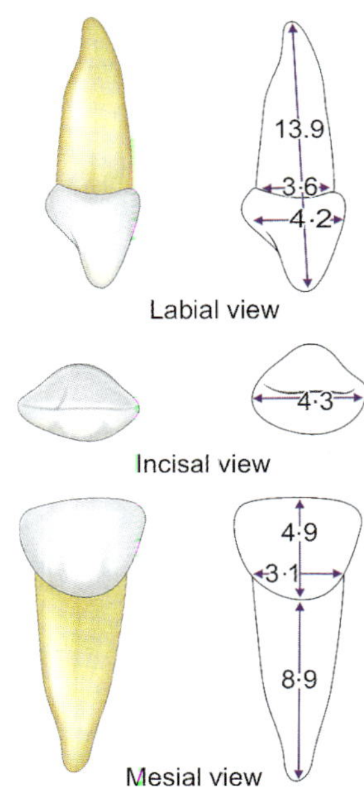

Fig. 17.4: Mandibular central incisor.

Mandibular Lateral Incisor

- The morphology of the mandibular lateral incisor is similar to that of the central incisor, except that the incisal edge slopes downward distally forming a more obtuse distoincisal angle **(Fig. 17.5)**.
- The crown is also slightly larger incisocervically and mesiodistally than that of the central incisor.
- The root is conical, longer than that of the central incisors, and shows a definite distal inclination at its apex.
- The distal surface of the root will often show a longitudinal depression or groove, separating the root into labial and lingual moieties.

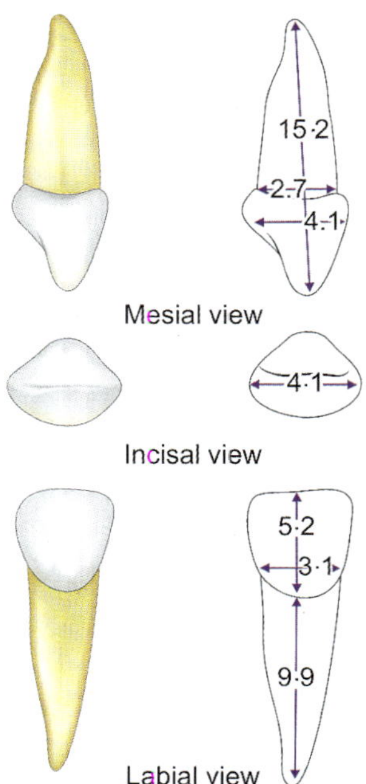

Fig. 17.5: Mandibular lateral incisor.

Mandibular Canine

- The mandibular canine appears more slender than the maxillary canine because of the smaller mesiodistal diameter in relation to crown height.
- The relative lengths of the incisal edges are reversed in the mandibular canine **(Fig. 17.6)**, making the distoincisal edge the longer of the two.
- The marginal ridges and cingulum are much less prominent, making the labiolingual diameter smaller than that of the maxillary canine.
- The root is smoothly tapered from the cervical line to the apex.

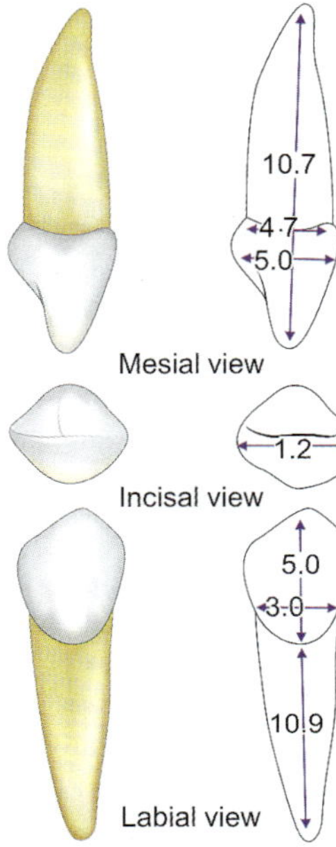

Fig. 17.6: Mandibular canine.

Maxillary First Molar

- The geometric form of the maxillary first molar when viewed from the occlusal is triangular **(Fig. 17.7)**.
- The proximal surfaces converge toward the lingual, creating a crown that is wider mesiodistally at the buccal surface. The mesiolingual cusp is the largest, followed by the mesiobuccal and the distobuccal.
- The mesiobuccal shows a greater mesiodistal development than the distobuccal cusp, occupying two-thirds of the buccal surface.
- The mesiobuccal cusp is also developed to a greater degree in an incisocervical direction, creating an increased curvature in the cervical line in the mesial half of the crown.
- A view of the crown from the mesial aspect shows the prominent buccocervical ridge which is characteristic of primary molars and, in particular, first primary molars.
- The maxillary first molar has three long and slender roots.
- The lingual root is the longest, followed by the mesiobuccal and the distobuccal.
- All three roots extend from extremely short root base in a divergent manner which is characteristic of the primary molars.

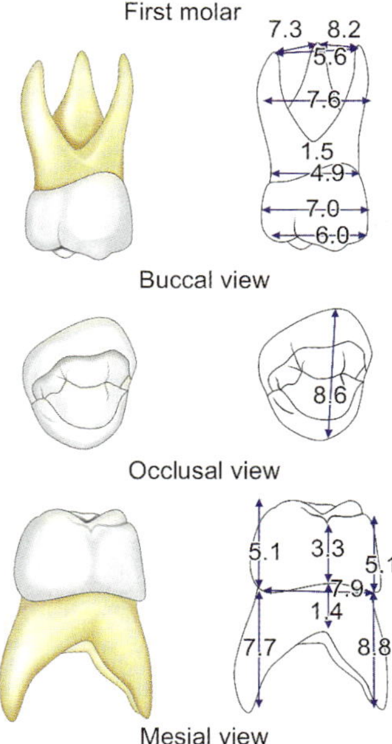

Fig. 17.7: Maxillary first molar.

Maxillary Second Molar

- The morphology of the maxillary second molar is similar to that of the maxillary first permanent molar, with a similar crown form, pit, groove, and cuspal arrangement **(Fig. 17.8).**
- There are four major cusps. The largest is the mesiolingual. The distolingual is the smallest, while the mesiobuccal and distobuccal cusps are nearly equal in size.
- The occlusal surface shows three pits—distal, central, and mesial which mark the intersection of the developmental grooves. The lingual root is the largest of the three roots; the distobuccal is the smallest.
- The root morphology is similar to that of the maxillary first permanent molar, except that the roots of the second primary molar are thinner and diverge more from the root base.

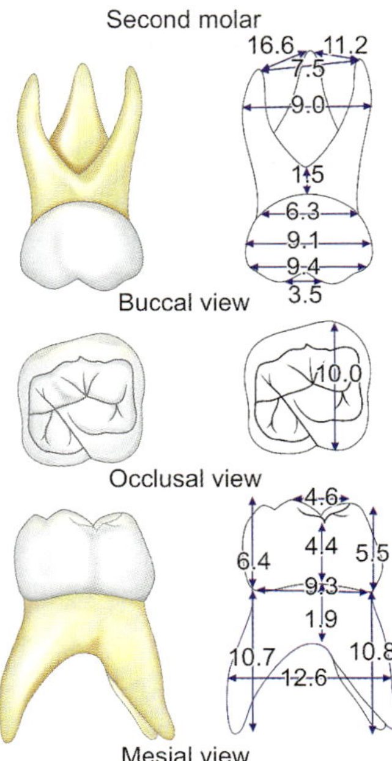

Fig. 17.8: Maxillary second molar.

Mandibular First Molar

- The general outline of the crown of the mandibular first primary molar when viewed from the occlusal is rhomboid. There are usually two buccal and two lingual cusps
- When viewed from the buccal, the greater mesiodistal and incisocervical deve-lopment of the mesiobuccal cusp is immediately noticed
- A marked apical curvature of the cervical line and a well-developed bucco-cervical ridge occur in the same area, a characteristic of the mandibular first primary molar **(Fig. 17.9).**

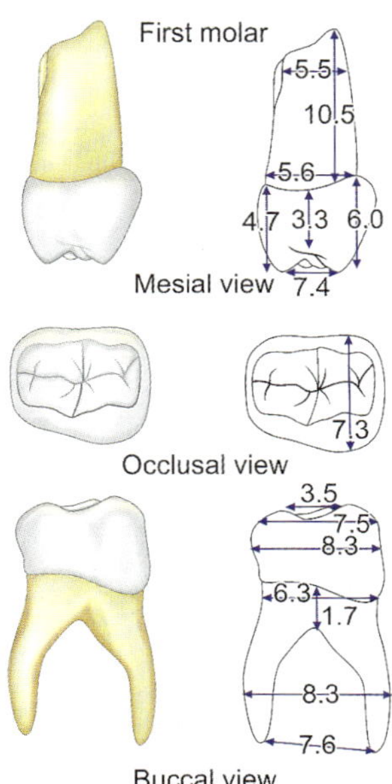

Fig. 17.9: Mandibular first molar.

- A distinguishing characteristic of this molar when viewed from the occlusal is the heavy transverse ridge connecting the mesiobuccal and mesiolingual cusps.
- There are generally three pits found on the occlusal surface central, mesial, and distal, with the first being the most prominent of the three.
- The two roots—mesial and distal show the typical flaring characteristic of primary molars; both, however, end in a sharp edge which may be slightly bifid.

Mandibular Second Molar

- Similar to its counterpart in the maxillary arch, the mandibular second primary molar is a smaller replica of the mandibular first permanent molar **(Fig. 17.10).**
- There are three buccal cusps; the distobuccal is the largest, followed by the mesiobuccal and the distal. There are two lingual cusps which are similar in size.
- There are three pits on the occlusal surface, the central pit being the deepest and the distal and mesial pits less prominent. The crown morphology shows the typical cervical constriction and buccocervical ridge seen on the other primary molars.
- As in the mandibular first primary molar, the two roots of the mandibular second molar are narrow mesiodistally, but broad buccolingually.
- The second molar shows more divergence of the roots than the first primary molar.

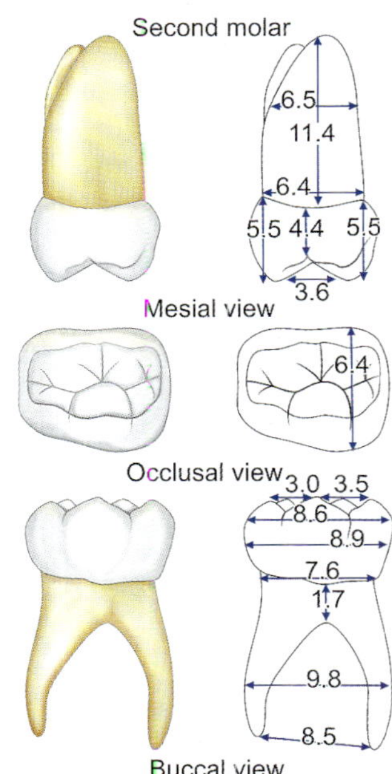

Fig. 17.10: Mandibular second molar.

CONTACTS OF PRIMARY TEETH

A contact area denotes the height of contour of the proximal surfaces of two adjacent teeth in the same arch. An ideal contact area is vital for maintenance of the stability and integrity of the dental arches and health of the supporting structures. A well-contoured, firmly established proximal contact defines the gingival embrasure and the height of the interdental papilla. Traditional literature reveals that contacts observed between primary molars are broad, flat, and situated gingivally when compared with those of permanent molars. The broad proximal contact areas observed in primary molars are likely to increase caries susceptibility, since self-cleansing action would be reduced due to the limited movement, leading to greater plaque accumulation.

OXIS Classification

In 2018, four specific types of contact areas between primary molars have been reported and hence the OXIS classification has been proposed by **Kirthiga M et al.**[1,2] The contacts areas in primary teeth have been classified as OXIS classification **(Figs. 17.11A to D)**.

- O (open contact)—When there is no contact between the primary molars.
- X (point contact)—When there is a point contact (</= 1 mm) between the primary molars.
- I (straight contact)—When there is a straight contact (> 1 mm) between the primary molars.
- S (curved contact)—When there is a curved contact (> 1 mm) between the primary molars.

Features of OXIS

- The presence of OXIS contacts have been clinically and radiographically confirmed in the studies.[3-5]
- The most common type of contact is I type and the least common type differed with different populations.
- The contact area observed at the occlusal level determined the overall type of contact based on OXIS criteria. This was in contradiction to the statement that contact areas are broad, flat, and extend further gingivally and should be revised.
- Variation in tooth contacts is known to be a risk factor for proximal caries.
- Among them, the S contact was the most susceptible type of contact among OXIS contacts, followed by the I, X, and, finally, the O contacts.

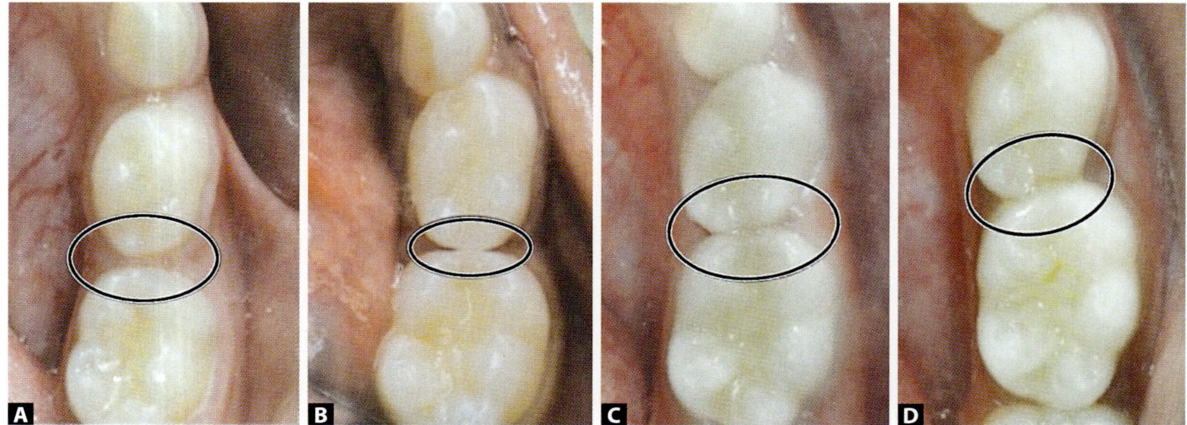

Figs. 17.11A to D: (A) Open contact; (B) Point contact; (C) Straight contact; (D) Curved contact.

Clinical Significance

It is recommended that the contacts between primary teeth are identified during the child's dental visit between the age of 3–6 years (after complete eruption of primary molars). Early identification of teeth of high-risk contacts namely S and I contacts should be followed by proper oral hygiene instructions, including regular brushing and flossing between the primary molars.

Aarthi J et al. have modified the classification to classify the primary canines.[6] The major modification was that the S contact was classified as S Type 1 and S Type II. When the canine was rotated and only one of its surfaces (either proximal or labial/lingual) was in contact with the adjacent tooth, the contact was classified as S Type I. When the canine was rotated and had two surfaces — proximal (mesial/distal) and labial or lingual — in contact with the adjacent tooth, the contact was classified as S Type II.

A thorough and basic knowledge about the morphology of primary teeth is important for an undergraduate student to perform clinical procedures like teeth identification, cavity preparation and restoration and for a postgraduate student to apply their understanding in areas of space management, operative dentistry and management of malocclusion.

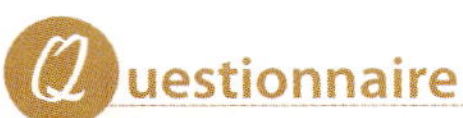

uestionnaire

1. Differences between primary and permanent teeth.
2. Unique morphological characteristics of mandibular primary first molar.
3. OXIS contacts of primary teeth.

REFERENCES

1. Kirthiga M, Muthu MS, Kayalvizhi G, Krithika C. Proposed classification for inter proximal contacts of primary molars using CBCT: a pilot study. Wellcome Open Res 2018;3:98.
2. Kirthiga M, Muthu MS, Cheuon Lee JJ, et al. Prevalence and correlation of OXIS contacts using Cone Beam Tomography images (CBCT) and photographs. Int J Paediatr Dent. 2021;31(4):520-7.
3. Muthu MS, Kirthiga M, Kayalvizhi G, Mathur VP. OXIS classification of inter proximal contacts of primary molars and its prevalence in 3–4-year-old children. Pediatr Dent. 2020;42:197-202.
4. Muthu MS, Kirthiga M, Lee JC, Kayalvizhi G, Mathur VP, Kandaswamy D, Jayakumar N. OXIS contacts as a risk factor for approximal caries: a retrospective cohort study. Pediatr Dent.2021;43(4):296-300.
5. Walia T, Kirthiga M, Brigi C, Muthu MS, Odeh R, Pakash Mathur V, Rodrigues S. Interproximal contact areas of primary molars based on OXIS classification – a two centre cross sectional study. Wellcome Open Res 2021, 5:285.
6. Aarthi J, Muthu M, Kirthiga M, Kailasam V. Modified OXIS classification for primary canines. Wellcome Open Res 2022, 7:130.

FURTHER READING

1. Kramer WS, Ireland RL. Measurements of the primary teeth. J Dent Child. 1959;26:252.
2. Kraus BS, Jordan RE, Abrams L. Dental anatomy and occlusion. Baltimore: Williams & Wilkins;1969.
3. Wheeler RC. Dental anatomy, physiology and occlusion. 5th edition, Philadelphia, PA:WB Saunders; 1971.
4. Zeisz RC, Nuckolls J. Dental anatomy. St.Louis:CVMosby;1949.

CHAPTER

Child Psychology

Nikhil Marwah, Rishi Tyagi, Divya Singh

Chapter Outline

- Theories of Child Psychology
- Approaches in Psychology
- Classical Psychoanalytical Theory/Psychosexual Theory
- Psychosocial Theory/Theory of Developmental Tasks
- Theory of Cognitive Development
- Classical Conditioning
- Operant Conditioning
- Social Learning Theory
- Hierarchy of Needs

A study of the psychology of childhood if conscientiously and intelligently pursued provides a rich background of information about children's behavior and psychological growth under a variety of environmental conditions. It provides information about psychological scales for appraising a child's developmental status; provides certain norms of growth for comparative purpose; provides understanding of basic psychological processes like learning, motivation, maturation, and socialization. It gives general principles of development with which to evaluate new trends and fads in child care and training and offers practical suggestion for guiding the psychological growth of children and other personal and natural components of their culture.

An understanding of the developmental tasks and behavior common to a certain age group will equip the dentist with the knowledge of fear and needs of child at that age. It will also enable him to detect any deviation in these patterns that may interfere with the treatment process. Therefore, the knowledge of psychological growth and development is essential to view the child's development in terms of psychologic, social, cognitive, and physical parameters.

Interest in scientific studies of children was given great importance by the work of **G Stanley Hall** (1883). He emphasized that children are not immature adults. Based on his studies many psychologists and educationalists started studying children without referring to education. Therefore, **G Stanley Hall** is known as the *"Father of the Child Study Movement"*. Psychology was born in 1879 when **Wilhelm Wundt** opened up the first psychology laboratory, at the University of Leipzig in Germany and he is now known as *"Father of Scientific Psychology"*. According to Wundt, the subject matter of the psychology was consciousness—the awareness of immediate experience. Thus, psychology became the scientific study of conscious experience and this orientation made psychology to focus mainly on the mind. Wundt's conception of psychology dominated for about two decades.

In the 19th century, the work of **Darwin**, on the principles of natural evolution, focused the scientist's interests on human development. Darwin emphasized the importance of adjustment to the continuing survival of an organism and thus laid the ground work for the concept of psychological adjustment. **Mendel's** contribution to the understanding of genetics also influenced certain movements toward the study of children. **Pavlov** contributed significantly to child psychology in developing the experimental technique of the conditioned response. This work influenced research on learning at all levels of human development. As a result of his work on emotional conditioning in infants, **Watson** prepared a treatise on the psychological care of infants that had a potent effect on earlier child care and training recommendations. **Sigmund Freud's** work was from then on a major influence in understanding of the concepts of psychology and he is called *"Father of Child Psychology"*.

- The term psychology is derived from two Greek words—psyche and logos. The root word psyche is equivalent to "soul" in Greek, and ology equivalent to "study of a subject".
- **Psychology:** It is the science dealing with human mature function and phenomenon of his soul in the main.

Flowchart 18.1: Theories of child psychology.

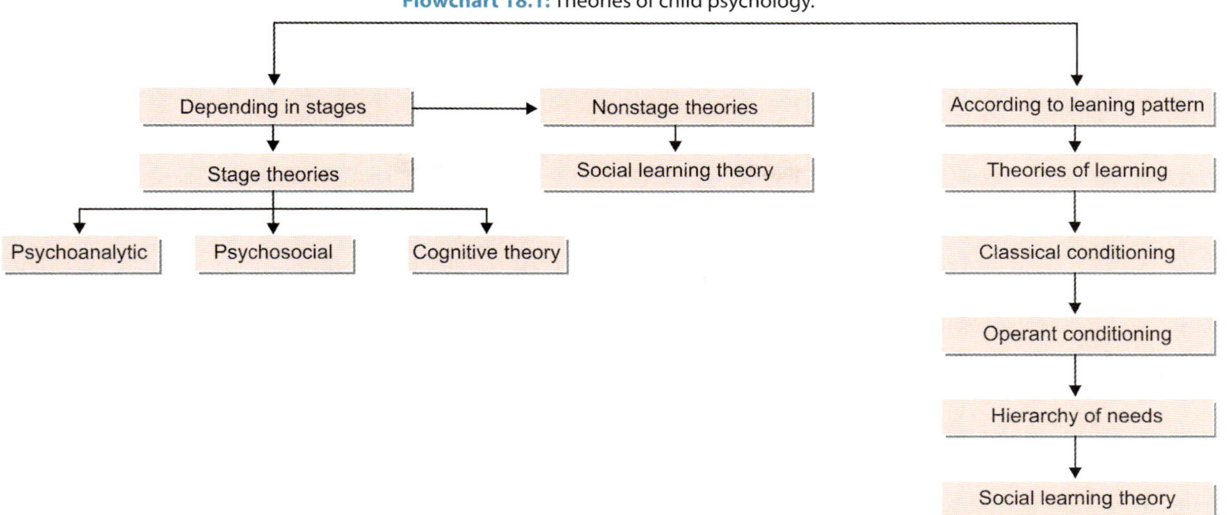

- **Child psychology:** It is the science that deals with the mental power or an interaction through the conscious and subconscious element in a child.

Aims of child psychology

Knowledge of the child psychology will help us to:

- Understand the child better and therefore deal with him more effectively and efficiently
- Better planning and interaction between treatment plan
- To identify the problems of psychosomatic origin
- To train the child so that he understands his own oral hygiene
- Helps modify child's developmental process

THEORIES OF CHILD PSYCHOLOGY

There are many theories that have been hypothesized over the centuries to understand child development. However, no one theory is able to account for the intricate matrix of psychology. But all these theories integrated together to throw some light on the child's developmental status **(Flowchart 18.1)**.

Child psychology theories can be broadly classified in two groups:

1. Psychodynamic theories:
   a. Psychosexual theory/psychoanalytic theory by **Sigmund Freud** (1905)
   b. Cognitive theory by **Jean Piaget** (1952)
   c. Psychosocial theory/ model of personality development by **Erik Erikson** (1963)
2. Theories of learning and development of behavior:
   a. Classical conditioning by **Ivan Pavlov** (1927)
   b. Operant conditioning by **BF Skinner** (1938)
   c. Hierarchy of needs by **Abraham Maslow** (1954)
   d. Social learning theory by **Albert Bandura** (1963)

SCHOOLS OF THOUGHT OF PSYCHOLOGY

- Structuralism (structure of consciousness) was based on the notion that the task of psychology is to analyze consciousness into its basic elements and to find out that how these elements are related. It was shaped by **Wundt's** ideas and his student **Edward Tetchier**, an Englishman who migrated to the United States in 1892. Structuralists wanted to identify and examine the fundamental components of conscious experience, such as sensations, feelings and images and most of their work were related with sensation and perception in vision, hearing, and touch.
- Functionalism (function of consciousness) was based on the belief that psychology should investigate the function or purpose of consciousness, rather than its structure. The chief architect of functionalism was **William James** (1842–1910), a brilliant American scholar. James was impressed by **Charles Darwin's** theory of natural selection. The cornerstone notion of Darwin's evolutionary theory suggested that "all the characteristics of a species must serve some purpose." Applying this idea to humans, James noted that consciousness is an important character of human and psychology should investigate the functions rather the structure of consciousness. He was more interested in how the people adapt their behavior to the demands of the real world around them.

APPROACHES IN PSYCHOLOGY

There are various different approaches in contemporary psychology. An approach is a perspective (i.e., view) that involves certain assumptions (i.e., beliefs) about human behavior: the way they function, which aspects of them are worthy of study and what research methods are appropriate for undertaking this study. Each perspective has its strengths and weaknesses and brings something different to our understanding of human behavior. For these reasons, it is important that psychology does have different perspectives to the understanding and study of human behavior.

- **The biological perspective:** The study of physiology played a major role in the development of psychology as a separate science. Today, this perspective is known as biological psychology, this perspective emphasizes the physical and biological bases of behavior. This perspective has grown significantly over the last few decades, especially with advances in our ability to explore and understand the human brain and nervous system.
- **The behavioral perspective:** Behavioral psychology is a perspective that focuses on learned behaviors. In 1913, radical behaviorist **John B Watson** gave the principles

of behavioral approach in his paper "*Psychology as the Behaviorist Views It*". In which he emphasized the "objective" nature of the approach, he believed that scientific methods could be applied to human behavior, and that a person's behavior could be observed, measured and quantified through experimentation. While behaviorism dominated psychology early in the 20th century, it began to lose its hold during the 1950s. Today, the behavioral perspective is still concerned with how behaviors are learned and reinforced.

- **The cognitive perspective:** In 1932, psychologist **Frederic Bartlett**, in a famous experiment known as the *War of the Ghosts* revealed the reconstructive nature of memory, with its use of schemas to recall past events. During the 1960s, a new perspective known as cognitive psychology began to take hold. This area of psychology focuses on mental processes such as memory, thinking, problem solving, language, and decision-making. Influenced by psychologists such as **Jean Piaget** and **Albert Bandura**, this perspective has grown tremendously in recent decades. As a result of prior knowledge, schemas was developed which enable us to anticipate and understand the world around us.
- **The cross-cultural perspective:** Cross-cultural psychology is a fairly new perspective that has grown significantly in recent years. These psychologists and researchers look at human behavior across different cultures. By looking at these differences, we can learn more about how our culture influences our thinking and behavior.
- **The evolutionary perspective:** Evolutionary psychology is focused on the study of how evolution explains physiological processes. Psychologists and researchers take the basic principles of evolution, including natural selection, and apply them to psychological phenomena. This perspective suggests that these mental processes exist because they serve an evolutionary purpose—they aid in survival and reproduction.
- **The humanistic perspective:** During the 1950s, a school of thought known as humanistic psychology emerged. Influenced greatly by the work of prominent humanists such as **Carl Rogers** and **Abraham Maslow**, this perspective emphasizes the role of motivation on thought and behavior. Concepts such as self-actualization are an essential part of this perspective.
- **The psychodynamic perspective:** The psychodynamic perspective originated with the work of **Sigmund Freud**. This perspective emphasizes the role of the unconscious mind, early childhood experiences, and interpersonal relationships to explain human behavior and to treat people suffering from mental illnesses.

CLASSICAL PSYCHOANALYTICAL THEORY/ PSYCHOSEXUAL THEORY

This theory was given in 1905 by **Sigmund Freud**, an Australian physician and Father of Modern-day Psychiatry.
Understanding the human mind is the core of classical psychoanalytic theory.

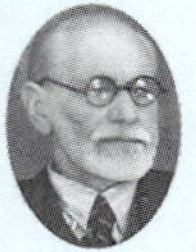

- He advocated the method of free association which means the person should say everything that comes to his mind regardless of how trivial and embarrassing it might be.
- **He said that a body has two types of neurons:** Phi neuron—concerned with condition of emotion and psi neuron—concerned with storage of emotion. When the emotions reach a certain level, a discharge is sparked off and this overdisplay of emotions is called archaic discharge.
- Freud compared the human mind to an iceberg. The small part that shown above the surface of the water represents the conscious experience, and the much larger base below water level represents the unconscious store house of impulses, passions, and inaccessible memories that affect thoughts and behaviors (**Figs. 18.1A and B**). Freud did not exactly invent the idea of the conscious versus unconscious mind, but he certainly was responsible for making it popular. The conscious mind is what you are aware of at any particular moment; your present perceptions, memories, thoughts, and fantasies. Working closely with the conscious mind is what Freud called the preconscious mind or available memory; anything that can be easily made conscious like the memories you are not at the moment thinking about but can readily bring to mind. The type of mental activity associated with the preconscious is called secondary process thinking/ realistic thinking. Such thinking is aimed at binding

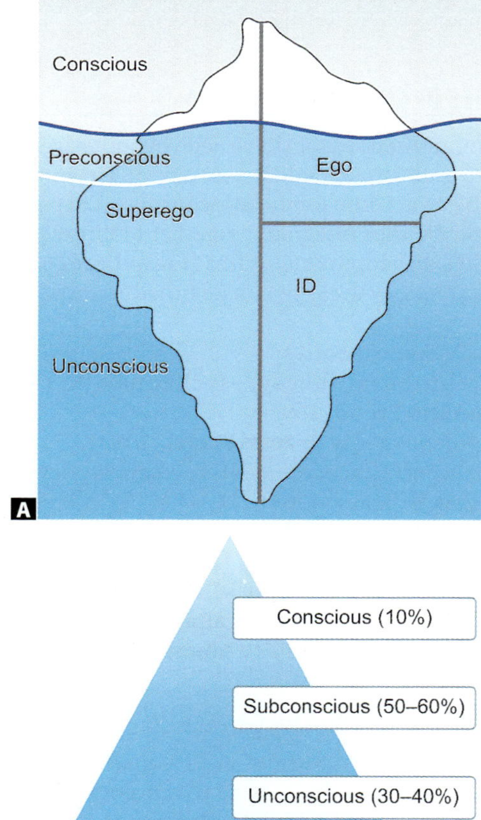

Figs. 18.1A and B: (A) Freud's conscious/unconscious concept; (B) The conscious, subconscious, and unconscious mind work together and create our reality.

person's mental energy in accordance with the demands of external reality and the person's moral values. The largest, most complex, and hidden is unconscious part. According to Freud, unconsciousness is the source of our motivations whether they may be simple desires of food or sex, neurotic compulsions, or the motives of an artist or scientist, and yet we are often driven to deny or resist becoming conscious of these motives, and they are often available to us only in disguised form. It is characteristic of very young children, who are dedicated to the immediate gratification of their desire, i.e., experience pleasure without delay.

Psychic Triad

- Freud in 1923 made the tripartite structural model of ego, ID, and superego and hypothesized three structures in this theory to understand the intrapsychic process called the psychic triad **(Fig. 18.2).**
- Freud's general notion that our behavior is influenced by biological drives (ID), social rules (superego), and mediating thought processes (ego) may not seem farfetched. However, his heavy emphasis on the primitive, sexual nature of human drives and energy (libido) helped make his theory very controversial.
- **ID:** It is the most primitive part of a personality. It is the basic structure of personality, which serves as a reservoir of instincts.

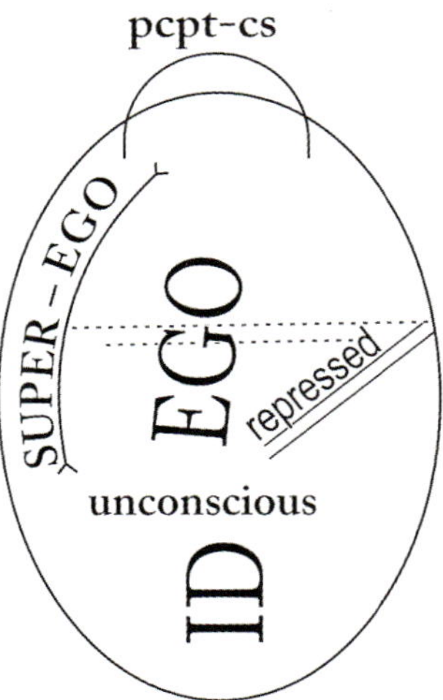

Fig. 18.2: Freud's structural model.

It is present at birth as impulse and strives for immediate pleasure and gratification. Operating under the guidance of primary process, the ID lacks the capacity to modify the drive. For example, need to eat in a young child is based on pleasure principle, that is, the child wants food irrespective of the external circumstances.

- **Superego:** That part of personality that is internalized representation of the values and morals of society as taught to the child by parents and others. It is essentially an individual conscience, and it judges whether the action is right or wrong. Superego is always trying to get you to behave in a socially appropriate way. It contains two subparts.
  a. *Conscience:* It contains moral prohibitions against certain behaviors, especially those expressing the sexual and aggressive drives of the id.
  b. *Ego ideal:* It is the image of what one ideally can be and how one ought to behave.
- **Ego:** It is the part of self, that is, concerned with overall functioning and organization of personality through its capacity to test reality and utilization of ego-defense mechanism and other functions like memory, language, and creativity. Ego is concerned with a state in which an adequate expression of ID can occur within the constraints of reality and demands and restriction of superego. For example, hunger must wait until food is given. The ego spans all three topographic dimensions of conscious, preconscious, and unconscious. The ego is the executive organ of the psyche and controls motility, perception, contact with reality, and, through the mechanisms of defense available to it, the delay, and modulation of drive expression. Freud believed that ego substitutes the reality principle for the pleasure principle. The basic dilemma of all human existence is that each element of the psychic apparatus are incompatible with the other two hence inner conflict is inevitable. For example, the superego can make a person feel guilty if rules are not followed. When there is a conflict between the goals of the id and superego, the ego must act as a referee and mediate this conflict. The ego can deploy various defense mechanisms (Freud, 1894) to prevent it from becoming overwhelmed by anxiety **(Fig. 18.3).**

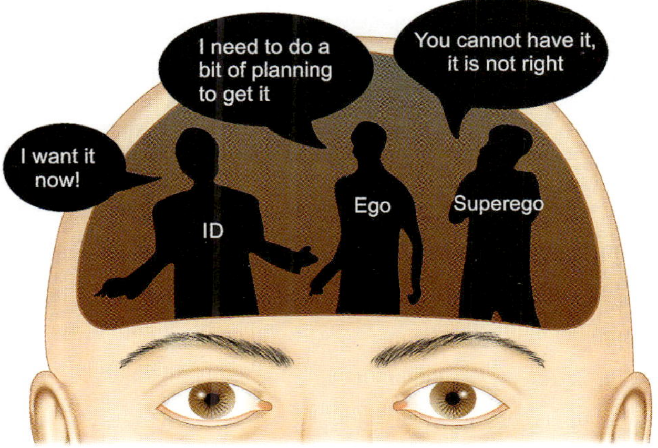

Fig. 18.3: Role-play of ID, ego, superego.

Psychosexual Stages of Development

- According to Sigmund Freud, what we do and why we do it, who we are and how we become this way are all related to our sexual drive differences in personalities originating in childhood. In the Freudian psychoanalytical model, child personality development is discussed in terms of psychosexual stages of development.

- Freud outlined five stages of manifestations of the sexual development. At each stage, different areas dominate source of sexual arousal and differences in satisfying the sexual urges at each stage will lead to differences in adult personalities. A proper resolution of the conflicts will lead the child to progress past one stage to another. Failure to achieve a proper resolution, however, will make the child fixated in the present stage, and this is believed to be the cause of many personality and behavioral disorders.

Oral Stage

Age: 0–1.5 years.

Erogenous zone in focus: Mouth.

Gratifying activities: Nursing, eating, as well as mouth movement including sucking, biting, and swallowing.

Interaction with the environment: To the infant, the mother's breast not only is the source of food and drink but also represents her love. Because the child's personality is controlled by the ID and therefore demands immediate gratification, responsive nurturing is key (both insufficient and forceful feeding can result in fixation in this stage). The id dominates, because neither the ego nor the superego is yet fully developed, and, since the infant has no personality (identity), every action is based upon the pleasure principle.

- The infantile ego is forming during the oral stage. There are two factors that contribute to its formation:
  1. In developing a body image, e.g., the child understands pain when it is applied to his/her body, thus identifying the physical boundaries between body and environment.
  2. Experiencing delayed gratification, e.g., crying gratifies certain needs
- One of the important feeling the infant experiences in oral stage of psychosexual development is weaning. It is the first feeling of losing the physical intimacy of feeding at mother's breast.
  a. It increases the infant's self-awareness that he/she does not control the environment.
  b. It help them learning delayed gratification, which leads to the formation of the capacities for independence (awareness of self) and trust (behaviors leading to gratification).

Symptoms of oral fixation: Smoking, nail biting, drinking, sarcasm.

Anal Stage

Age: 1.5–3 years.

Erogenous zone in focus: Anus.

Gratifying activities: Bowel movement and the withholding of such movement.

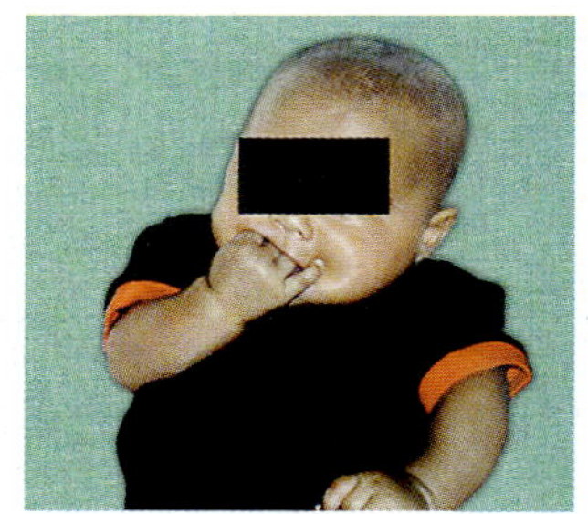

Interaction with the environment: The major event at this stage is toilet training, a process through which children are taught when, where, and how excretion is deemed appropriate by society. Children at this stage start to notice the pleasure and displeasure associated with bowel movements through toilet training. By exercising control over the retention and expulsion of feces, a child can choose to either grant or refuse parent's wishes.

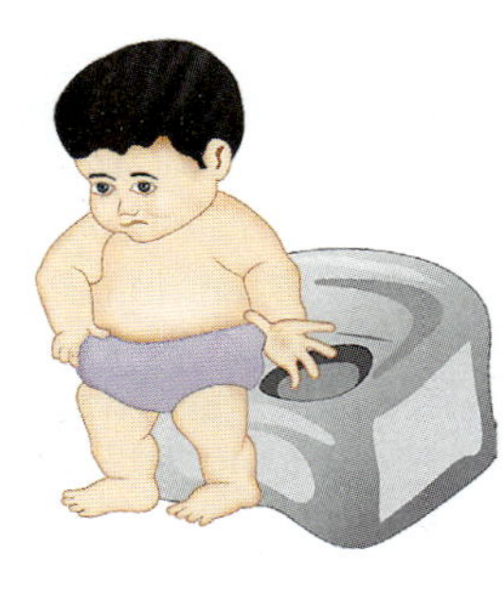

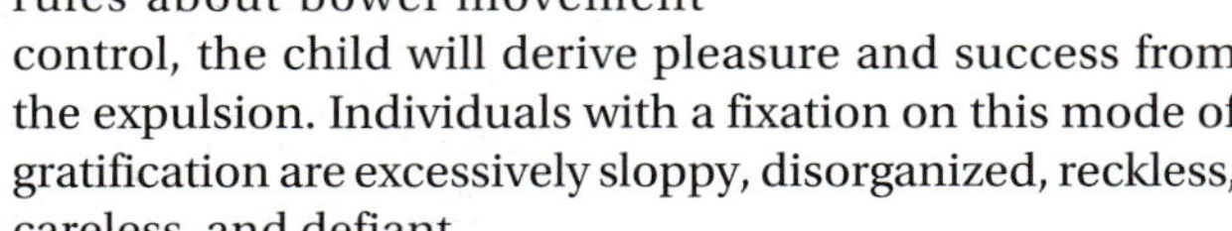

Symptoms of anal fixation

- **Anal-expulsive personality:** If the parents are too lenient and fail to instill the society's rules about bowel movement control, the child will derive pleasure and success from the expulsion. Individuals with a fixation on this mode of gratification are excessively sloppy, disorganized, reckless, careless, and defiant.
- **Anal-retentive personality:** If a child receives excessive pressure and punishment from parents during toilet training, he will experience anxiety during bowel movements and hence will withhold such functions. Individuals with such fixation are clean, orderly, and intolerant to those who are not clean.

Urethral Stage

Age: 3–4 years.

Erogenous zones: This is a transitional stage between anal and phallic stages and has characteristics of both.

Gratifying activities: Pleasure in urination.

Interaction with environment: The characteristics of the urethral stage are often subsumed under those of the phallic stage. Urethral erotism, however, is used to refer to the pleasure in urination, as well as the pleasure in urethral retention analogs to anal retention. Similar issues of performance and control are related to urethral functioning. Urethral functioning may also be invested with a sadistic quality, often reflecting the persistence of anal sadistic urges. The predominant urethral trait is that of competitiveness and ambition, probably related to the compensation for shame due to loss of urethral control. Besides the health effects, analogs to those from the anal period urethral competence provides a sense of pride and self-competence as a small boy can imitate and match his father's adult performance.

Phallic Stage

Age: 4–5 years.

Erogenous zone in focus: Genitals.

Gratifying activities: Genital fondling.

Interaction with the environment: This is probably the most challenging stage in a person's psychosexual development. The key event at this stage according to Freud is the child's feeling of attraction toward the parent of the opposite sex together with envy and fear of the same sex parent. In boys, this situation is called the **Oedipus complex** named after the young man in a Greek myth, who killed his father and married his mother unaware of their true identities. Boys in the midst of Oedipus complex often experience intense "*Castration Anxiety*," which comes from the fear of punishment from the father for their desire for the mothers. In the process

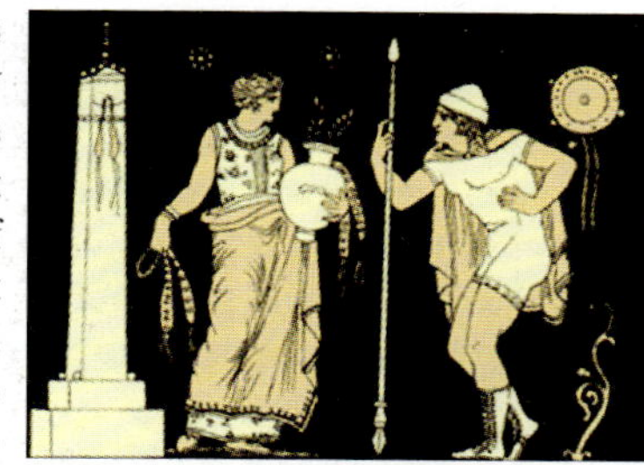

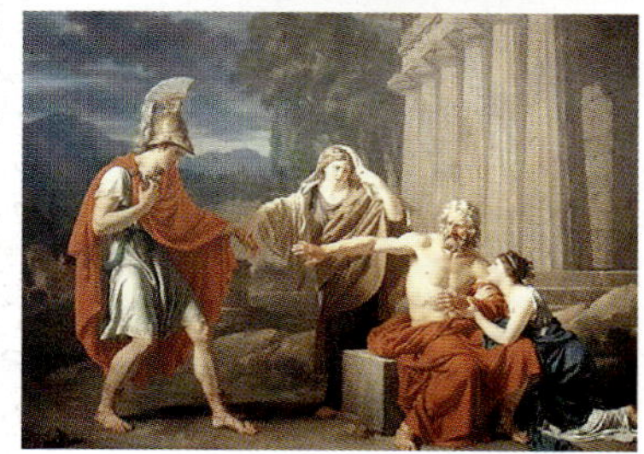

of identifying with his father, the boy not only takes on his father's behavior patterns but also his father's ideas of right and wrong. Thus, it is rough identification in the phallic stage that the boy's superego begins to form. In girls, this type of attraction is called the **Electra complex** after Agamemnon's daughter, who arranged for her mother to be murdered. For the girl, the sequence begins with an erotic focus on the father. But, in addition, the girl notices that she does not have the sexual organs of her father or brothers, and she experiences "*Penis Envy*." She suspects that she may actually have been castrated by her mother; this makes her angry, and she comes to resent and devalue her mother. Nonetheless, she eventually identifies with her mother partly because she knows if she takes on her mother's characteristics, she will stand a better chance in her own "romantic relationship" with her father. Thus, in spite of her affection for her father and her resentment of her mother, the little girl identifies with her mother, behaving like her and incorporating her values. Oedipus and Electra complexes occur in unconscious mind. The ego fears the consequences of expressing them and realizes that these drives cannot be satisfied directly. It holds the original sexual wish in the unconscious mind and derive partial satisfaction by identifying with the parent of the same sex. For example, boys try to be as much as their father and girls try to be like their mother. This process is known as "identification" through which an important part of the personality is developed.

Symptoms of phallic fixation

For men: Anxiety and guilty feelings about sex, fear of castration, and narcissistic personality (interest in one's own features).

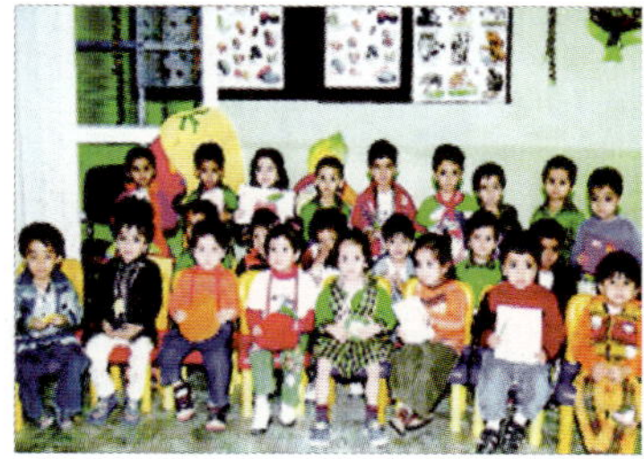

For women: It is implied that women never progress past this stage fully and will always maintain a sense of envy and inferiority, but there are no possible fixations resulting from this stage.

Latency

Age: 5 years—puberty.

Erogenous with in focus: None.

Interaction with the environment: This is a period during which sexual feelings are suppressed to allow children to focus their energy on other aspects of life. This is a time of adjusting to the social environment outside of home, absorbing the culture forming beliefs and values, developing same sex friendships, engaging in sports, etc. Much of the child's energies are channeled into developing new skills and acquiring new knowledge, and play becomes largely confined to other children of the same gender.

Genital Stage

Age: Puberty onwards.

Erogenous zone in focus: Genital.

Gratifying activities: Heterosexual relationships.

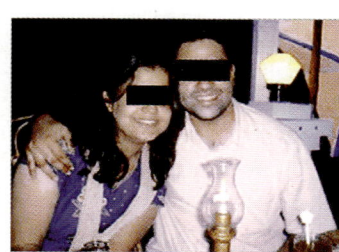

Interaction with the environment: This stage is marked by a renewed sexual interest and desire and the pursuit of relationships. There are three major sources of sexual arousal during this period: memories and sensations from earlier childhood periods, physical manipulation of genitals and other erogenous zones, and hormonal secretions. Many of the themes and anxieties of earlier stages resurface, but in new and more mature forms. In particular, the targets of sexual arousal now lie outside the tiny circle of self and family. Mature heterosexual relations emerge, with the species preserving possibility of procreation now very real.

Freud's stages of psychosexual development and associated fixations

State	*Characteristics associated with fixation*
Oral	Display many activities centered around the mouth: excessive eating, drinking; smoking, talking
Oral eroticism	Sucking and eating predominately: cheerful, dependent, and needy, expects to be taken care of by others
Oral sadism	Biting and chewing predominately; tends to be cynical and cruel
Anal—retentive	Excessively neat, clean, meticulous, and obsessive
Anal—expulsive	Moody, sarcastic, biting, and often aggressive; untidy in personal habits
Phallic	Overly preoccupied with self, often vain and arrogant, unrealistic level of self-confidence
Latency	Demonstrates sexual sublimation and repression
Genital	Traditional sex roles and heterosexual orientation

Symptoms of genital fixation: This stage does not cause any fixation. According to Freud, if people experience difficulties at this stage, the damage was done in earlier oral, anal, and phallic stages. These people come into this last stage of development with fixations from earlier stages, for example, attractions to the opposite sex can be a source of anxiety at this stage if the person has not successfully resolved the Oedipus or Electra conflict.

Summary of Freud's psychosexual theory

Basic assumptions	*Areas of application*
• The major causes of behavior have their origin in the unconscious • Psychic determinism: All behavior has a cause/reason • Different parts of the unconscious mind are in constant struggle • Our behavior and feelings as adults are rooted in our childhood experiences	• Gender role development • Therapy (psychoanalysis) • Attachment • Moral development (superego) • Aggression • Personality (Erikson, Freud)
Strengths	***Limitations***
• Made the case study method popular in psychology • Defense mechanisms • Free association • Projective tests (TAT, Rorschach) • Highlighted the importance of childhood • Highlighted the importance of the unconscious mind dream analysis	• Case studies—subjective/cannot generalize results • Unscientific (lacks empirical support) • Too deterministic (little free will) • Biased sample (e.g., middle-aged women from Vienna) • Rejects free will • Unfalsifiable (difficult to prove wrong)

PSYCHOSOCIAL THEORY/THEORY OF DEVELOPMENTAL TASKS

I have nothing to offer except a way of looking at things.
–Erik Erikson

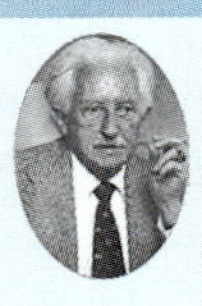

Erik H Erikson was a Danish–German–American developmental psychologist and psychoanalyst known for his theory on social development of human beings. He may be most famous for coining the phrase identity crisis.

- His interest in identity developed early on in life based upon his own experiences in school. He published a number of books on his theories and research, including "Childhood and Society" and "The Life Cycle Completed." His book "Gandhi's Truth" was awarded a Pulitzer Prize.
- The psychosocial theory was proposed by Erikson in 1950 in his book "Childhood and Society."
- Erikson was a close friend and student of Freud, and he elaborated and modified Freud theory by superimposition of psychosocial and psychosexual factors simultaneously contributing to personality development.
- Erikson stress that children are active, adaptive explorers who seek to control their environment rather than passive creatures that are slaves to their biological urges and are moulded by their parents.
- Erikson assumed that human beings are rational creatures whose thoughts, feelings and actions are controlled by the ego while Freud felt that behavior stemmed from conflicts between the id and superego.
- Erikson gave more importance on social influences rather than Freud who emphasized the sexual urges.
- This theory postulates that society responds to a child's basic needs or developmental tasks in a specific period of life and in doing so, society ensures child's healthy growth and survival in culture and traditions. According to Erikson, each individual passes through eight developmental stages. Each stage is characterized by a different psychological crisis, which must be resolved by the individual before he can move on to the next stage **(Fig. 18.4)**. If the person copes with a particular crisis in a maladaptive manner, the outcome will be more struggles with the same issue later in life.

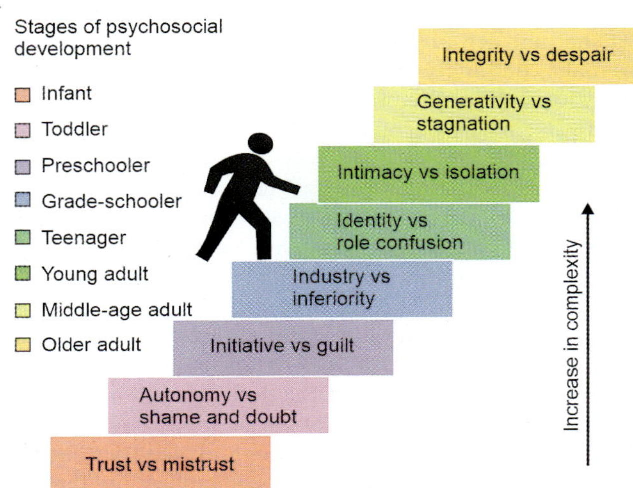

Fig. 18.4: Theory of developmental tasks by Erikson.

Stage 1: Infancy—age 0–1 year

Crisis: Trust versus Mistrust.

Description: In the first year of life, infants depend on others for food, warmth, and affection and therefore must be able to blindly trust the parents (or caregivers) for providing these.

Positive outcome: If their needs are met consistently and responsively by the parents, infants not only will develop a secure attachment with the parents but will learn to trust their environment in general as well.

Negative outcome: If no infant will develop mistrust toward people, environment, and even toward themselves.

Dental applications: This stage identifies with development of separation anxiety in the child. So, if necessary to provide dental treatment at this early age, it is preferable to do with the parent present and preferably with parent holding the child.

Stage 2: Toddler—age 1–2 years

Crisis: Autonomy versus Doubt or Shame.

Description: Toddlers learn to walk, talk, use toilets, and do things for themselves. their self-control and self-confidence begins to develop at this stage.

Positive outcome: If parents encourage their child's use of initiative and reassure him when he makes mistakes, the child will develop the confidence needed to cope with future situations that require choice, control, and independence. The parents should not discourage the child but neither should they push. A balance is required. People often advise new parents to be "firm but tolerant" at this stage. This way, the child will develop both self-control and self-esteem.

Virtue of will emerges during second stage of life. Child learns from themselves and from others what is expected and what is expectable. The elements of will are increased gradually through experiences involving awareness and attention, manipulation, verbalization and locomotion.

Erikson calls the ritualization of this stage judicious, because the child begins to judge him/her and others and to differentiate between right and wrong.

Negative outcome: If parents are over protective or disapproving of the child's acts of independence, he may begin to feel ashamed of his behavior or have too much doubt of his abilities. Another failure factor is unrestricted freedom, or if you try to help children do what they should learn to do for themselves, you will also give them the impression that they are not good for much. if you are not patient enough to wait for your child to tie his or her shoe-laces, your child will never learn to tie them and will assume that this is too difficult to learn.

Dental application: Child is moving away from mother but still will retreat to her in threatening situations. So, parent's presence is essential in dental clinic. At this stage as the child takes pleasure in doing tasks by himself, dentist must obtain cooperation from him by making him believe that the treatment is his choice and not of the dentist/parent.

Stage 3: Early childhood—age 2–6 years

Crisis: Initiative versus Guilt.

Description: Children have newfound power at this stage as they have developed motor skills and become more engaged in social interaction with people around them. They now must learn to achieve a balance between eagerness for more adventure and more responsibility and learn to control impulses and childish fantasies.

Positive outcome: If parents are encouraging but consistent in discipline, children will learn to accept without guilt that certain things are not allowed and at the same time will not feel shame when using their imagination and engaging in make believe role plays.

Negative outcome: If no children may develop a sense of guilt and may come to believe that it is wrong to be independent.

Dental application: For most children, the first visit to dentist comes during the stage of initiative. Going to the dentist can be considered a new and challenging adventure in which the child can experience success. Success is coping with the anxiety of visiting the dentist can help develop greater independence and produce a sense of accomplishment. A poorly managed, of course, dental visit can also contribute toward the guilt that accompanies failure. A child at this stage will be intensely curious about the dentist's office and eager to learn about the things out there. An exploratory visit with little work is often a good way to start the dental experience.

Stage 4: Elementary and middle school years—age 6–12 years

Crisis: Industry versus Inferiority.

Description: School is the important event at this stage. Children learn to make things, use tools, and acquire the skills to be a worker and a potential provider, and they do all these while making the transition from the world of home into the world of peers. The child who, because of his successive and successful resolutions of earlier psychosocial crisis, is trusting, autonomous, and full of initiative will learn easily enough to be industrious. In Erikson's terms, the virtue of competence emerges during this stage. Virtues of previous stages that are hope, will, and purpose will make the child become familiar with a technical way of life. Also, the child acquires industriousness and begins the preparation for entrance into a competitive world. The influence of parents as role models decreases and the influence of peer group increases.

Positive outcome: If children can discover pleasure in intellectual stimulation, being productive, seeking success, they will develop a sense of competence.

Negative outcome: If the child is allowed too little success, because of harsh teachers or rejecting peers, for example, then he or she will develop a sense of inferiority or incompetence.

Dental application: Children at this age are trying to learn the skills and rules that define success in any situation, and that includes the dental office. A key to behavioral guidance is setting attainable intermediate goals, clearly outlining for the child how to achieve those goals and positively reinforcing success in achieving these goals. Because of the child's drive for a sense of industry and accomplishment, cooperation with treatment can be obtained. Children at this stage still are not likely to be motivated by abstract concepts; rather, they can be motivated by improved acceptance or status from the peer group. This means that emphasizing how the teeth will look better as the child cooperates is more likely to be a motivating factor than emphasizing a better dental occlusion.

Stage 5: Adolescence—age 12–18 years

Crisis: Identity versus Role confusion.

Description: This is the time when we ask the question "Who am I?" to successfully answer this question, Erikson suggests the adolescent must integrate the healthy resolution of all earlier conflicts; adolescents who have successfully dealt with earlier conflicts are ready for the identity crisis which is considered by Erikson as the single most significant conflict a person must face. Adolescence, a period of intense physical development, is also the stage in psychosocial development in which a unique personal identity is acquired. This sense of identity includes both a feeling of belonging to a larger group and a realization that one can exist outside the family. It is an extremely complex stage because of the many new opportunities that arise. Emerging sexuality complicates relationships with others. At the same time, physical ability changes and academic responsibilities increase, and career possibilities begin to be defined. Members of the peer group become important role models, and the values and tastes of parents and other authority figures are likely to be rejected.

Positive outcome: If the adolescent solves this conflict successfully, he will come out of this age with a strong identity and ready to plan for the future.

Negative outcome: If not, the adolescent will sink into confusion unable to make decisions and choices especially about vocation, sexual orientation, and his role in life in general. As adolescence progresses, an inability to separate from the group indicates some failure in identity development. This in turn can lead to a poor sense of direction for the future, confusion regarding one's place in society, and low self-esteem.

Dental application: Behavior management of adolescents can be challenging. Any orthodontic treatment should be carried out if a child wants it and not parents as at this stage, parental authority is being rejected. Approval of peer group is extremely important. For example, orthodontic treatment has become so common that there may be a loss of status from being one of the few in the group who is not receiving treatment, so that treatment may even be requested in order to remain "one of the crowd." It is extremely important to realize that treatment is being done for him not to him. Abstract concepts can be grasped readily, but appeals to do something because of its impact on personal health are not likely to be heeded.

Stage 6: Young adulthood—age 19–40 years

Crisis: Intimacy versus Isolation.

Description: In this stage, the most important events are love relationships. No matter how successful you are with your work said

Erikson you are not developmentally complete until you are capable of intimacy. Successful development of intimacy depends on a willingness to compromise and even to sacrifice to maintain a relationship. An individual who has not developed a sense of identity usually will fear a committed relationship and may retreat into isolation.

Positive outcome: The adult individuals can form close relationships and share with others if they have achieved a sense of identity. Success leads to the establishment of affiliations and partnerships both with a mate and with others of the same sex in working toward the attainment of career goals.

Negative outcome: If not, they will fear commitment, feel isolated, and unable to depend on anybody in the world. Failure leads to isolation from others and is likely to be accompanied by strong prejudices and a set of attitudes that serve to keep others away rather than bringing them into closer contact.

Dental application: At this stage, external appearances are very important as it helps in attainment of intimate relation. Hence, the focus is orthodontic and esthetic treatments.

Stage 7: Middle adulthood—age 40–65 years

Crisis: Creativity versus Stagnation.

Description: By generativity Erikson refers to the adult's ability to look outside oneself and care for others through parenting. The next generation is guided in short not only by nurturing and influencing one's own children but also by supporting the network of social services needed to ensure the next generation's success. The opposite personality trait in adults is stagnation, characterized by self-indulgence and self-centered behavior.

Positive outcome: People can solve this crisis by having and nurturing children or helping the next generation in other ways.

Negative outcome: Person will remain self-centered and experience stagnation later in life.

Stage 8: Late adulthood—age 65 years–death

Crisis: Integrity versus Despair.

Description: Old age is a time for reflecting upon one's own life and seeing it filled with pleasure and satisfaction or disappointments and failures. Virtue of wisdom develops out of the encounter of integrity and despair in the last stage of life. Achieving the virtue of the stage involves the feeling of living a successful life.

Positive outcome: If the other seven psychosocial crises have been successfully resolved, the mature adult develops the peak of adjustment: integrity. If the adult has achieved a sense of fulfilment about life and a sense of unity within himself and with others, he will accept death with a sense of integrity just as healthy child will not fear life.

Negative outcome: The opposite of this is despair. This is often expressed as disgust and unhappiness on a broad scale, frequently accompanied by a fear that death will occur before a life change that might lead to integrity can be accomplished.

THEORY OF COGNITIVE DEVELOPMENT

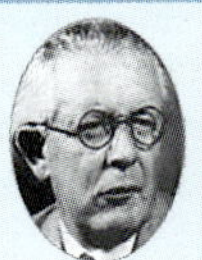

Jean Piaget world's leading theorist in the field of cognitive development proposed this theory in 1952.

Cognition refers to the mental processes by which knowledge is acquired, elaborated, stored, retrieved, and used to solve problems. This includes detecting, interpreting, classifying and remembering information, evaluating ideas, inferring principles, reducing rules, imagining possibilities, generating strategies, fantasizing and dreaming.

Cognitive theory is an approach to psychology that attempts to explain human behavior by understanding their thought processes. Based on the brain and how it learns/processes information, cognitive theories are the one that emphasize on children's conscious thoughts.

Piaget has studied every aspect of acquisition of knowledge from language skills to concept of time and space to understanding mathematical symbols. The Geneva school of psychology in which Jean Piaget is the leading figure since the early 1920s studied the child's view of the world, his acquisition of such system of knowledge as logic measurement morality, concept formation language development, and theory of physical reality.

He has written over 25 books and published over 160 articles on the psychology. His theories are concerned with practice application and understanding and were originally described to classroom teachers and specialists in child psychology. His theory of cognitive development and epistemological view is together called "Genetic epistemology." This Piaget defined as the study of acquisition, modification, and growth of abstract ideas on the basis of inherited substrate an intelligent functioning that makes growth possible. Piaget derived his theory by asking questions to children. He was less interested if the answers given were correct, he was more concerned with the way child arrived at the answer. Piaget proposed that a child's development proceeds from an egocentric position through predictable expansion and incorporation of learned

A summary of Erikson's stages

Stage	*Approximate age*	*Positive outcomes*	*Negative outcomes*
1. Trust vs mistrust	Birth–1.5 years	Feelings of trust from environmental support	Fear and concern regarding others
2. Autonomy vs shame and doubt	1.5–3 years	Self-sufficiency if exploration is encouraged	Doubts about self and lack of independence
3. Initiative vs guilt	3–6 years	Discovery of ways to initiate actions	Guilt from actions and thoughts
4. Industry vs inferiority	6–12 years	Development of sense of competence	Feelings of inferiority and no sense of mastery
5. Identity vs role confusion	Adolescence	Awareness of uniqueness of self	Inability to identify appropriate roles in life
6. Intimacy vs isolation	Early adulthood	Development of loving, sexual relationships, and same sex friendships	Fear of relationships with others
7. Generativity vs stagnation	Middle adulthood	Sense of contribution to continuity of life	Trivialization of one's activities
8. Ego integrity vs despair	Late adulthood	Sense of unity in life's accomplishments	Regret over lost opportunities of life

experiences. It deals with cognitive development beginning with primitive reflexes and motor coordination of infancy to thinking and problem solving of adolescence till adulthood. He proposes that the world is a stable environment, and the child acquires this through the knowledge of mathematics and logic as reality. Then as the child grows, he is required to adapt according to people he is living with. These all stages can be grouped as follows:

a. **Operation:** An action, which the child performs mentally and which has the added property of being reversible.
b. **Schema:** Represent a dynamic process of differentiation and reorganization of knowledge with the resultant evolution of behavior and cognitive functioning apparatus for the age of child. Schemas are categories of knowledge that help us to interpret and understand the world. According to Piaget, schema includes both a category of knowledge and the process of obtaining that knowledge. With experience, the new information is used to modify, add to, or change previously existing schemas. For example, a child who has just learned the word "bird" will tend to assimilate all flying objects into his idea of bird. When he sees a bee, he will probably say, "Look, bird!"
c. **Assimilation:** New object or idea interpreted in terms of idea or action, the child has already acquired within his age-specific skills. The process of taking in new information into previously existing schemas is known as assimilation. The process is somewhat subjective, because we tend to modify experience or information to fit in with our pre-existing beliefs.
d. **Accommodation:** Accommodation involves altering existing schemas, or ideas, as a result of new information or new experiences. New schemas may also be developed during this process. For example, the child who has just learned the word bird will tend to assimilate all flying objects in his idea of bird. When he sees a helicopter, he will probably say "Look bird." However, for intelligence to develop, the child must also have the complementary process of accommodation. Accommodation occurs when the child changes his or her cognitive structure or mental category to better represent the environment, like to distinguish between birds and helicopter. In other words, the child will accommodate the events of seeing a helicopter by creating a separate category of flying objects for helicopter.
e. **Equilibrium:** State established as a result of new knowledge to the child. Piaget believed that children try to balance between assimilation and accommodation, which is achieved through a mechanism called equilibration. As children progress through the stages of cognitive development, it is important to maintain a balance between applying previous knowledge (assimilation) and changing behavior to account for new knowledge (accommodation). Equilibration helps explain how children are able to move from one stage of thought into the next.

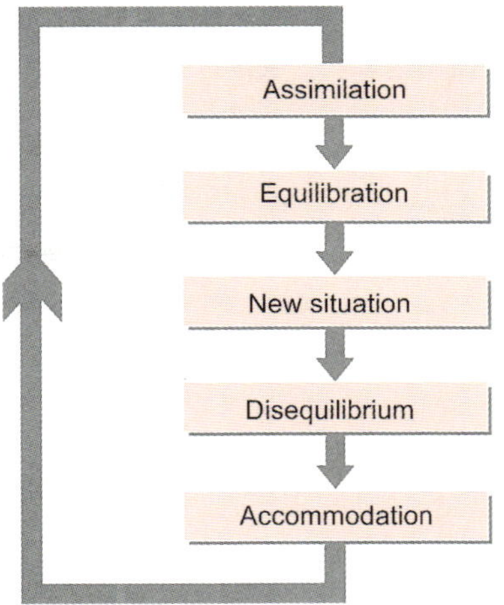

Piaget marked four stages of cognitive growth, each characterized by a different type of thinking and in each child relies more upon internal stimuli.

- Sensorimotor period (birth to 2 years of age)
- Preoperational period (2–7 years of age)
  - Preconceptual period (2–4 years of age)
  - Intuitive stage (4–7 years of age)
- Concrete operational period (7–11 years of age)
- Formal operational period (beyond 11 years).

Sensorimotor Period

- This is from birth to 2 years of age. During the first 2 years of life, a child develops from a newborn infant who is almost totally dependent on reflex activities to an individual who can develop new behavior.
- During this stage, child develops basic concept of object including the idea that object in the environment are permanent and do not disappear when the child is not looking at them.
- Simple modes of thought that are the foundation of language develop during this time, but communication between a child and adult at this stage is extremely limited because of the child's simple concepts and lack of language capabilities.
- Animism is imparting life to inanimate objects, like furniture, wall, and floor or doors, etc. And if the child gets hurt by those objects, the child will feel happy by hitting them or if the caretaker or parents hit them.
- Dental application is that the child begins to interact with the environment and can be given toys while sitting on the dental chair in his/her hand.
- This stage can be subdivided into six stages **(Table 18.1)**.

Preoperational Period

- This is from 2 to 7 years of age and is called a transition period. Manipulation of symbols or words is a characteristic feature of this stage. During this period, marked inconsistencies appear in the knowledge of a child.

Table 18.1: Sensorimotor stages.

Stage	Age	Schemata	Coordinated reflexes
1st stage Simple Reflexes	Birth to 2 months	Automatic inborn reflexes of infants	Uses inborn motor and sensory reflexes (sucking, grasping, looking) to interact and accommodate to the external world
2nd stage Primary Circular Reactions Phase	2–5 months	Coordination of reflexes improves	Primary circular reaction—coordinates activities of own body and five senses (e.g., sucking thumb); reality remains subjective— does not seek stimuli outside of its visual field; displays curiosity
3rd stage Secondary Circular Reactions Phase	5–9 months	Infants try to perceive and maintain interesting experiences	Secondary circular reaction—seeks out new stimuli in the environment; starts both to anticipate consequences of own behavior and to act purposefully to change the environment; beginning of intentional behavior
4th stage Coordination of Secondary Circular Reactions Stages	9 months to 1 year	Coordinate sensorimotor scheme	Shows preliminary signs of object permanence; has a vague concept that objects exist apart from itself; plays peekaboo; imitates novel behaviors
5th stage Tertiary Circular Reactions, Novelty and Curiosity	1 year to 18 months	New sensorimotor schemes are invented	Tertiary circular reaction—seeks out new experiences; produces novel behaviors
6th stage Internalization of Schemas	18 months to 2 years	Invent new schemes through mental exploration in which they imagine certain events and outcomes	Symbolic though—uses symbolic representations of events and object; shows signs of reasoning, e.g., uses one toy to reach for and get another; attains object permanence

- Preoperational period can be divided into two stages:
  a. Preconceptual stage (2–4 years):
     - This stage marks the start of symbolic activity
     - The child's reactions are based not simply on the physical nature of the stimulus but on its meaning
     - During this stage, a stimulus begins to take on meaning, and the child can use a stimulus to represent other objects
  b. Intuitive stage (4–7 years):
     - Prelogical reasoning appears based on preconceptual appearances unhampered by reversibility
     - Trial and error may lead to an intuitive discovery of correct relationships, but the child is unable to take more than one attribute into account at one time.
- At preoperational period capabilities for logical reasoning are limited.
- The child's thought process is dominated by the immediate sensory impressions.
- At this stage, the child is first shown two equal size glass with water in them. The child agrees that both contain the same amount of water. Then the contents of one glass are poured into a taller, narrower glass while the child watches. Now when asked which container has more water, the child will usually say that tall one. His impression is dominated by the greater height of the water in the tall glass **(Figs. 18.5A to C)**.
- **Dental application:** A preoperational child will have trouble in understanding a chain of reasoning like brushing and flossing to remove food particles which in turn prevents bacteria from forming acids which prevents tooth decay. But in this stage, he is much more likely to understand; brushing makes your teeth white, clear, and smooth. The three main areas of focus in this stage are:
  a. *Constructivism:* The child likes to explore things and make own observations. For example, child surveys the dental chair and airway syringe.
  b. *Cognitive equilibrium:* Child is explained about the equipment or instrument and allowed to deal with it
  c. *Animism:* Child correlates things with other objects which they are more used to or accustomed, for example, the handpiece can be called "Whistling Willie" who is happy when he works at polishing the child's teeth.

Concrete Operational Period

- This lasts from 7 to 11 years of age
- As the child moves into this stage typically after a year or so of preschool and first grade activity, an improved ability to reason emerges. He can use a limited number of logical processes especially those involving object that can be handled or manipulated

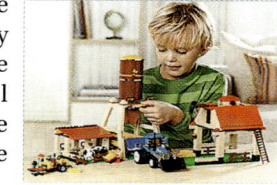

- The child is able to decenter, that is, focus attention on more than one attribute at the same time and also capable of rationale thinking so that he can classify objects according to their sizes and shapes
- The child at this stage undergoes enormous surge in intellectual development and is able to compare and tolerate different point of views. Syllogistic reasoning, in which a logical conclusion is formed from two premises, appears during this stage
- The principle of conservation and reversibility are also enhanced at this stage. At this age, the child could watch the water being poured from one glass to another; imagine the reverse of this process; and conclude that the amount of water remains the same
- Important processes during this stage are:
  - *Seriation:* The ability to sort objects in an order according to size, shape, or any other characteristic.

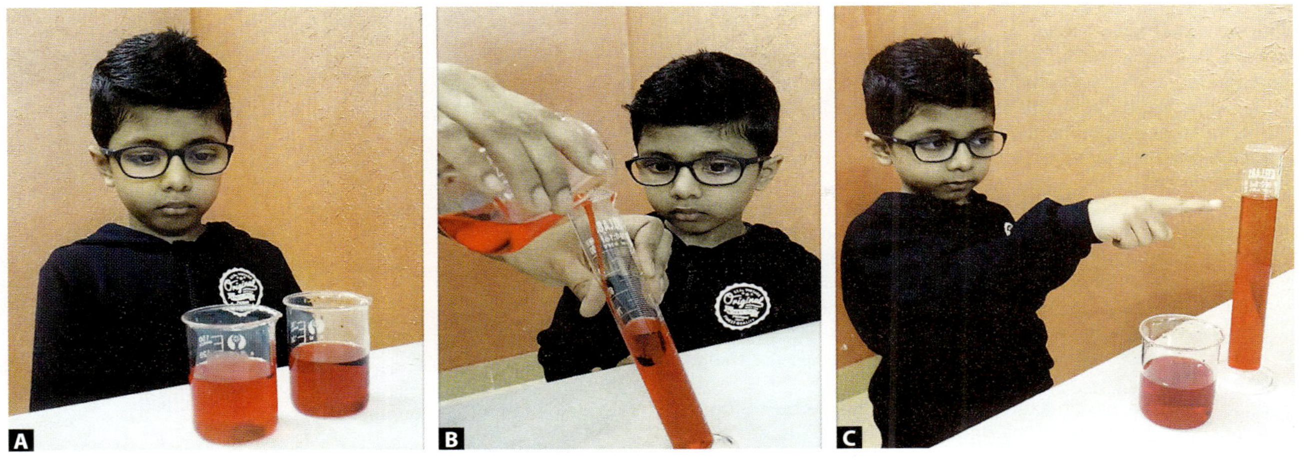

Figs. 18.5A to C: The glass water experiment to identify logical reasoning.

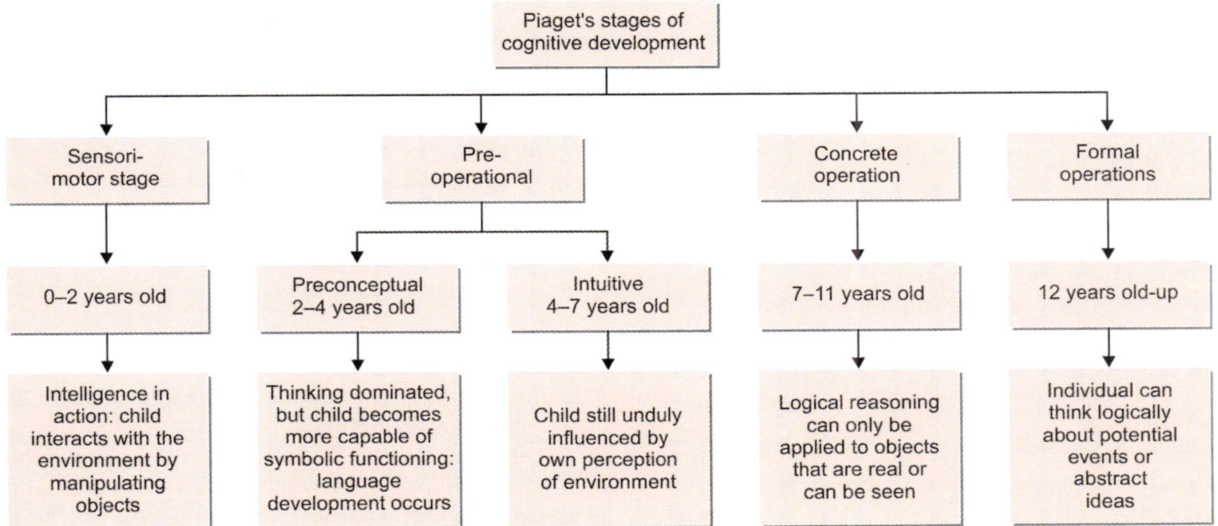

For example, if given different-shaded objects, they may make a color gradient.

- *Transitivity:* The ability to recognize logical relationships among elements in a serial order and perform "transitive inferences" (e.g., if A is taller than B and B is taller than C, then A must be taller than C).
- *Classification:* The ability to name and identify sets of objects according to appearance, size, or other characteristics, including the idea that one set of objects can include another.
- *Decentering:* Where the child takes into account multiple aspects of a problem to solve it.
- *Reversibility:* The child understands that numbers or objects can be changed then returned to their original state. For this reason, a child will be able to rapidly determine that if 4+4 equals t, t–4 will equal 4, the original quantity.
- *Elimination of Egocentrism:* The ability to view things from another's perspective.

❖ Dental application include giving concrete instructions like this is a retainer, brush like this, allowed to hold the mirror to see what is being done on his teeth, gets involved in the treatment, for example, holds the suction tip by himself.

Formal Operational Stage

❖ This is after 11 years of age

❖ Ability to deal with abstract concept and abstract reasoning develops by about 11–12 years of age. This stage is more related to experiences than age and is predictive of ability. In addition to the ability to deal with abstractions, teenagers have developed cognitively to the point where they can think about thinking. They are now aware that others think, but usually in a new expression of egocentrism, presume that they and others are thinking about the same thing

❖ At this stage, the child's thought process has become similar to that of an adult, and the child is capable of understanding concepts like health diseases and preventive treatment

❖ The child can reason a hypothetical problem and do a systematic search for solution. Dental applications include esthetic and corrective dental treatment

Limitations of Piaget theory

- First, as Piaget himself noted, development does not always progress in the smooth manner his theory seems to predict.
- Development is not sudden as a stage theory. There are subtle changes that happens gradually in child's thinking.
- Do not give adequate attention to individual variations in cognitive development.
- Issue of timing: The most frequent complaint about Piaget's theory is that children do not always display various intellectual skills or enter a particular stage of development as mentioned by Piaget. Some cognitive abilities emerge earlier than Piaget's thought; some aspects of object permanence emerge earlier than he believed, understanding of conservation of number has been demonstrated as early as age 3, although Piaget did not think it emerged until 7.
- Culture and education exert a stronger influence on children's development than Piaget believed.
- Major shortcoming of Piaget's theory is that it does not clearly indicate how children move from one stage of intellect to the next.

CLASSICAL CONDITIONING

This theory was first described by the Russian psychologist **Ivan Pavlov** in 1927. He discovered during his studies of reflexes that apparently un-associated stimuli could produce the reflexive behavior.

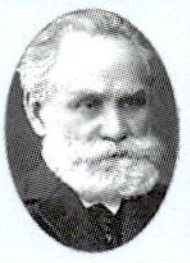

- Classical conditioning is defined as when a conditioned stimulus is paired with an unconditioned stimulus.
- Conditioned stimulus—neutral stimulus (e.g., the sound of a tuning fork or bell):
  - Unconditioned stimulus—biologically potent (e.g., the taste of food)
  - Unconditioned response—to the unconditioned stimulus unlearned reflex response (e.g., salivary secretion).
- Pavlov classical experiment involved the presentation of food to a hungry animal along with some of the other stimulus, for example, the ringing bell **(Fig. 18.6)**. In this famous experiment with dog, he showed that the sight and smell of food produced an unconditional response of salivation in the animal. He then presented the food together with ringing bell. The sound of bell is called neutral stimulus because it does not produce any response by itself. But the two events occurring together also led to the unconditioned response of salivation and later the ringing of the bell alone brought about conditional response of salivation **(Fig. 18.7)**.
- Classical conditioning thus operates by simple process of association of one stimulus with other. For this reason, this mode of learning is sometimes referred to as learning by association.

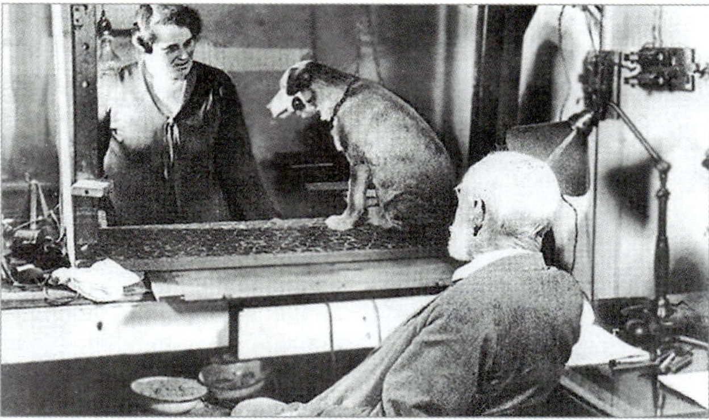

Fig. 18.6: Pavlov doing his experiment.

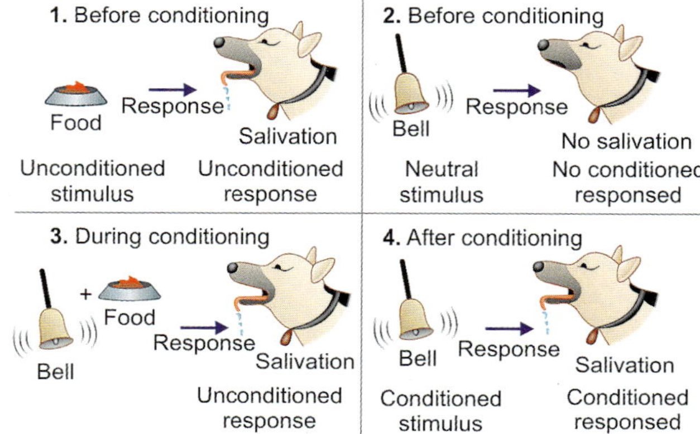

Fig. 18.7: Bell–dog experiment.

Principles of Classical Conditioning

- **Acquisition:** Learning a new response from the environment by conditioning.
- **Generalization:** Wherein the process of conditioning is evoked by a band of stimuli centered around a specific conditioned stimulus. For example, a child who had a painful experience with doctor in white coat will always associate any doctor in white coat with pain.
- **Extinction:** Removal of conditioned behavior results if the association between the conditioned and the unconditioned response is not reinforced. For example, in a fearful child, subsequent visits to the doctor without any unpleasant experience result in extinction of fear.
- **Discrimination:** It is the opposite of generalization. For example, the conditioned association of white coats with pain can easily be generalized to any office setting. If child is exposed to clinical setting which are different to those associated with painful experiences, a dental office, for instance, where painful injections are not necessary, the child learns to discriminate between two clinics and a generalized response to any office as a place where painful things occur will be extinguished.

Dental Application

- A young child is exposed to an initial stimulus like sound of the handpiece which produces anxiety. This is an unconditioned reflex. When the sound of the handpiece was coupled with dentist who was the neutral stimulus, it again produced an unconditioned reflex of anxiety. Later when dentist was presented alone, it also produced a conditioned response of anxiety.
- Classical conditioning occurs readily with young children and has considerable impact on them on first dental visit. By the time a child is brought for the first visit to a dentist,

it is highly likely that the child would have had many experiences with other doctors. When child experiences pain, reflex reaction is crying and withdrawal. In Pavlovian terms, the infliction of pain is unconditioned stimulus. For instance, it is unusual for a child to encounter people who are dressed entirely in white uniforms or long white coats. If the unconditioned stimulus of painful treatment comes to be associated with the conditioned stimulus of white coats, a child may cry and withdraw immediately at the first sight of a white coated adult. Later, the mere sight of the white coat is enough to produce the reflex behavior initially associated with pain. If individual in white coats are the ones who give painful injections that cause crying, the sight of an individual in white coat soon may provoke an outburst of crying.

Classical conditioning

First visit

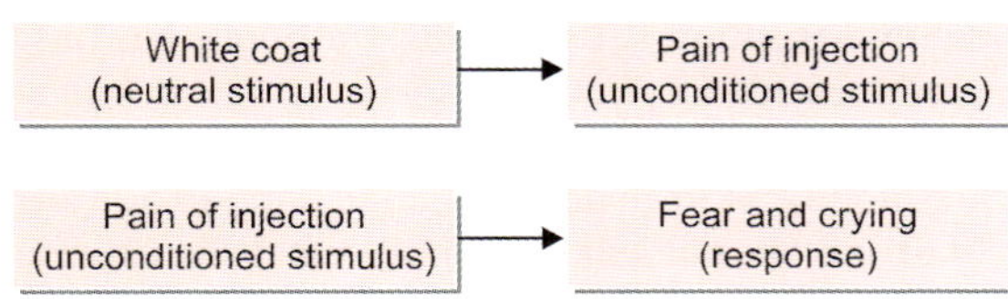

Second visit

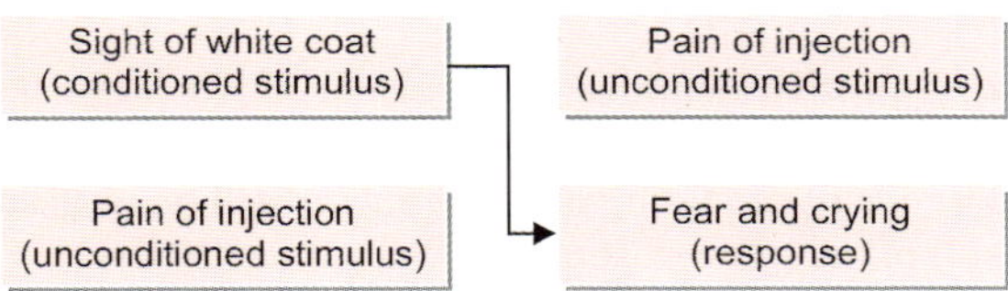

Limitations of classical conditioning

- It does not help create new behaviors.
- It only connects a naturally occurring response to a stimulus and deals with visceral responses.
- There is a lot of variables that can affect the degree to which this method would occur or not in different situations.
- It can trigger the development of phobias in humans.
- Research by John B Watson on Pavlov's work conducted on an infant child found that the child became afraid of a white rat by pairing the animal with a jarring and loud noise, though the child was not afraid when introduced to the rat alone the first time. This implies that classical conditioning can cause phobias in humans.

OPERANT CONDITIONING

This was given by **BF Skinner** in 1938.

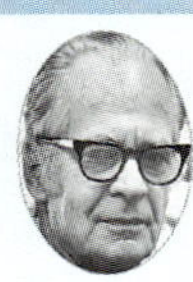

Operant conditioning can be viewed conceptually as a significant extension of classical conditioning. Skinner contended that the most complex human behaviors can be explained by operant conditioning.

- His theories, which downplay the role of the individual's conscious determination in favor of unconscious determined behavior, have met with much resistance but have been remarkably successful in explaining many aspects of social behavior far too complicated to be understood from the perspective of classical conditioning.
- Skinner concluded that the most complex human behaviors could be explained by operant conditioning. The basic principle of operant conditioning is that the consequence of a behavior itself is a stimulus that can affect future behavior response **(Fig. 18.8)**. Individual learns to produce a positive response where consequences of outcome are instrumental in bringing about recurrence of stimulus. The individual response is changed as a result of reinforcement of extension of previous experiences.
- Behavior that operates and controls the environment is called operant. It stresses that reinforcement is critical factor for learning and therefore for development of personality. The relationship between operant and consequences that follows them is called contingency.

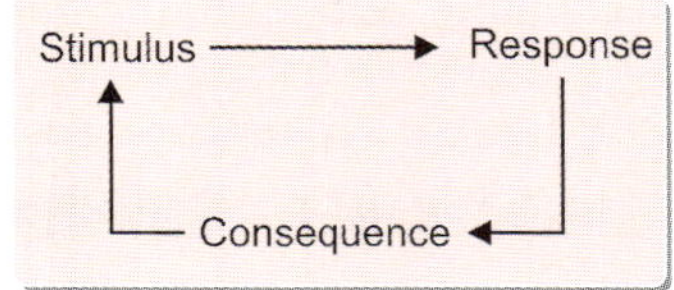

Fig. 18.8: Principle of operant conditioning.

Type of Operant Conditioning

Positive reinforcement: If a pleasant consequence follows a response, the response has been positively reinforced and the behavior that led to this pleasant consequence become more likely in the future. For example, if a child is given a reward such as a toy for behaving well during treatment, he is likely to behave well during future dental visits as his behavior was positively reinforced.

Negative reinforcement: It involves the withdrawal of an unpleasant stimulus after a response. Like positive reinforcement, negative reinforcement also increases the likelihood of a response in the future. For example, a child who visits to the dental clinic with an unpleasant experience may throw a temper tantrum to go from clinic. If this behavior (response) succeeds in allowing the child to escape, the behavior has been negatively reinforced and is more likely to occur the next time.

Omission or time out: Involves removal of a pleasant stimulus after a particular response. For example, if a child who throws a temper tantrum has his favorite toy taken away for a short time as a consequence of this behavior, the probability of similar misbehavior is decreased.

Punishment: Where an unpleasant stimulus is presented after a response. This also decreases the probability that the behavior that prompted punishment will occur in the future. Punishment is effective at all ages. Result of adding negative outcomes or removing positive ones thus weakening the response. For example, use of palatal rake or tongue crib for correction of tongue thrusting habit. One milder form of punishment that can be used in children is the "voice control." It involves speaking to child in a firm voice to gain his/her attention, telling him that his present behavior is unacceptable, and directing him as to how he should behave.

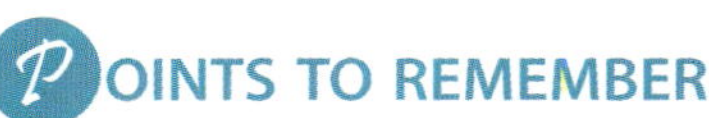

POINTS TO REMEMBER

- Reinforcement is most effective when administer immediately after the response (**Domjan Burkhard**, 1986).
- Scheduling of reinforcements is also important. New admirable habits are most easily instilled if the desirable behavior is reinforced every time it occurs—continuous reinforcement.
- These habits can be maintained for long periods with only partial reinforcement that is occasional or intermittent reinforcement.
- There is no doubt that operant conditioning can be used to modify behavior in individuals of any age, and that it forms the basis for many of the behavior patterns of life. Operant conditioning is a powerful tool for learning of behavior which influences throughout life.

Limitations of the study

- Operant conditioning fails to take into account the role of inherited and cognitive factors in learning, and thus is an incomplete explanation of the learning process in humans and animals.
- Skinners theory seems to deal strictly with distinct behavior: good, and bad. Also, a parent, or a teacher cannot keep positively reinforcing the child's good behavior after the first few times. After the reward stops being enforced, the child may be likely to stop the good behavior as well.

SOCIAL LEARNING THEORY/OBSERVATIONAL LEARNING THEORY

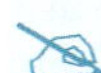

This theory was proposed by **Albert Bandura** in 1963. In social learning theory, reinforcement is considered a facilitative rather than a necessary condition for learning.

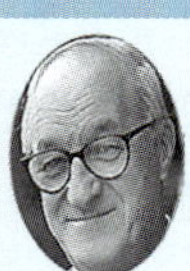

- ❖ Bandura believes that behavior is largely motivated by social needs. Reinforcement is a powerful method for regulating performance of behavior but is a relatively ineffective method for learning behavior.
- ❖ The two most essential components of this theory are the concepts of modeling and reinforcement.

Principle of Social Learning Theory

Attentional Process

- ❖ A child cannot learn by observation if the child does not attend the essential feature of the model's behavior. Simply exposing the child to the model does not assure his attention.
- ❖ Factors related to gaining his attention involve the relevancy of the model's behavior to that of the observing child. This means that the observer must be able to associate and identify with the model.
- ❖ Observational learning can be an important tool in management of dental treatment. If a young child observes an older sibling undergoing dental treatment without complaint or uncooperative behavior, he or she is likely to imitate this behavior. If the older sibling is observed being rewarded, the younger child will also expect a reward for being well.

Retention Process

- ❖ If the observer is to reproduce the model's behavior when the model is no longer present to serve as a guide, the response pattern must be memorized and coded in symbolic form
- ❖ Immediate imitation does not require much cognitive functioning; however, delayed imitation requires symbolic transformation and organization of the modeling stimuli, thus the learning requires cognitive development.

Motoric Reproduction

- ❖ The amount of observational learning that a child can exhibit depends upon the level of skills that the child has attained. These skills must be coordinated and refined through self-corrective adjustment based upon performance feedback.
- ❖ Sitting in one dental chair watching the dentist work with someone else in an adjacent chair can provide a great deal of observational learning about what the experience will be like.

Reinforcement and Motivation

When positive incentives are provided, observational learning will be promptly translated over performance. Therefore, the influence of modeling upon behavior will be weakened as a result of failure to observe the relevant activities.

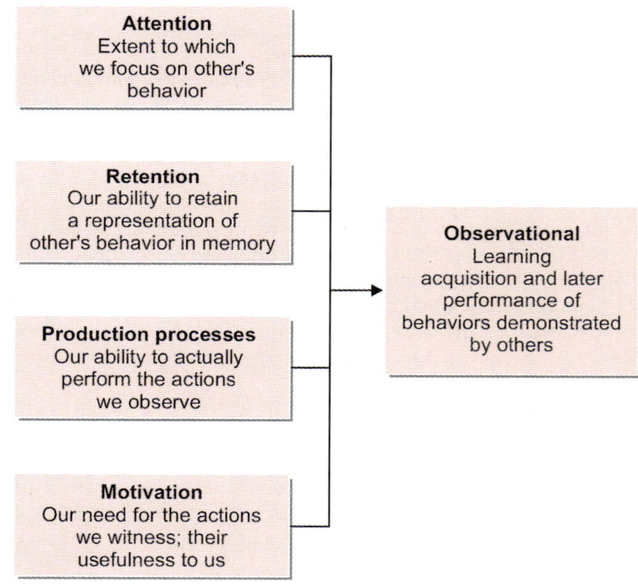

Limitations

- ❖ This theory does not take into account physical and mental changes.
- ❖ All the behaviors are not explained.
- ❖ Does not explain behavioral differences.
- ❖ Does not take in account that what one person views as punishment, another person may view as a reward.

HIERARCHY OF NEEDS OR MASLOW'S THEORY OF SELF-ACTUALIZATION

This was given in 1943 by **Abraham Maslow** in his paper "A Theory of Human Motivation".

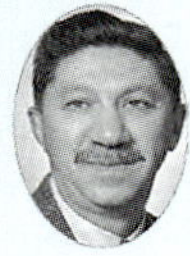

This theory developed a classification of the individual priority needs and motivations during personality development. A five-level triangular hierarchy of these needs from the most basic and important to the most elaborate shows a trend from instinctive motives to more rational intellectual ones.

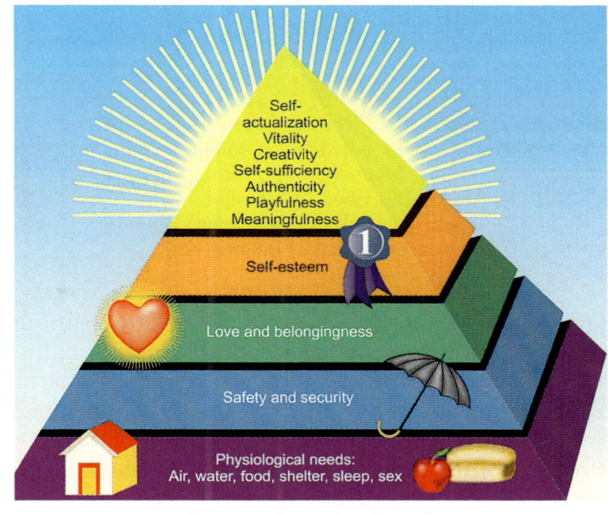

Fig. 18.9: Hierarchy of needs.

Levels of Hierarchy of Needs

Level 1: Physiologic needs: These are basic needs, such as food and water along with air, sleep, clothing, and must be satisfied before other needs. If they are not fulfilled, people will direct all their energy and resources toward satisfying them. Biological necessities such as food, water, oxygen, sleep, sex, are the important needs because a person would feel sickness, irritation, pain, discomfort, etc., or may even die if they were not fulfilled.

Level 2: Safety needs: Both physical and psychological safety is necessary to meet these needs. These are protection, stability, pain avoidance, etc. Maslow believed that children need safety more than adults when they feel afraid. Safety needs are mostly psychological in nature which can be safety and security of a home and family.

Level 3: Love and belonging needs: These needs are also termed as social needs that include affection, acceptance, and inclusion in integrated groups; the need for affection from parents, peers, and other loved ones. This is to give and receive love, and also for a feeling of belonging.

Level 4: Esteem needs: This includes self-respect and self-esteem which are the needs to be respected; to have self-respect and to respect others. Humans include the need to be competent, to achieve, to be successful, and to be open and independent. In addition, esteem needs include the desire to be acknowledged and appreciated for their achievements.

Level 5: Self-actualization needs: Maslow considered that a very small group of people reach a level called self-actualization, where all of their needs are met. And it is described as a person finding their "passion or mission" **(Fig. 18.9)**.

SEPARATION-INDIVIDUATION THEORY OF CHILD DEVELOPMENT

Margaret Mahler (1897–1986) represents a group of ego psychologists whose interest focuses on the development of psychic structures, In the field of 'Ego Psychology', Mahler is regarded as one of the main contributors.

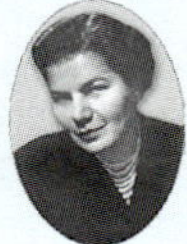

- She primarily focuses on mother-infant interactions within the first three years of life. This fills the gaps in psychodynamic stage theories, such as Freud's psychosexual stages of development, and Erikson's psychosocial stages of development.
- According to Mahler, successful completion of the developmental stages in the first few years of life results in separation and individuation. Although interrelated, it is possible for one to develop more than the other, which is largely depending on the mother's attitude towards the child.
- Separation refers to an internal process of mental separation from the mother, while individuation refers to a developing self concept.

Stages of Development

- ***Normal autistic stage (0–1 month):*** At the beginning of life, the infant is primarily focused on himself/herself. The mother is viewed as an intrinsic part of the infant, without having a separate existence. At this point the primary goal is to achieve a state of equilibrium, while lacking the understanding that the satisfaction of needs may come from an external source.
- ***Normal symbiotic stage (1–5 months):*** In this phase, the infant barely acknowledges the mother's existence as a unique entity, but as the main source of need-satisfaction. The fulfilment of the infant's physiological needs becomes intertwined with psychological desires, which serves as the basis for formation of future relationships. Availability and the ability of the mother to adapt successfully to the infant's needs are crucial to successful progression through the next stages.
- ***Separation-Individuation stage (5–24 months):*** This is the final stage in which the final stage a significant transition occurs in two overlapping realms. In separation, the infant develops an understanding of boundaries of the self, and thus the mother is increasingly viewed as an individual. Meanwhile, individuation marks the development of a sense of self.

ATTACHMENT THEORY

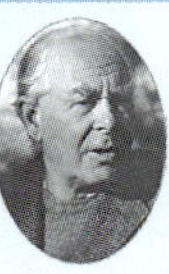

John Bowlby (1969) subsequently described attachment as a unique relationship between an infant and his caregiver that is the foundation for further healthy development. Bowlby described attachment theory as an inherent biological response and behavioral system in place to provide satisfaction of basic human needs.

Attachment theory is focused on the relationships and bonds between long-term relationships, including those between a parent and child and between romantic partner. **Schaffer** and **Emerson** outlined four distinct phases of attachment:

- **Pre-attachment stage:** From birth to 3 months, infants do not show any particular attachment to a specific caregiver. The infant's signals, such as crying and fussing, naturally attract the attention of the caregiver and the baby's positive responses encourage the caregiver to remain close.
- **Indiscriminate attachment:** Between 6 weeks to 7 months, infants begin to show preferences for primary and secondary caregivers as they develop trust towards their caregivers. They start distinguishing between familiar and unfamiliar people and responds more positively to the primary caregiver.
- **Discriminate attachment:** At this point, from about 7 to 11 months of age, infants show a strong attachment and preference for one specific individual. They started showing separation anxiety (on separation from primary figure), and stranger anxiety (around strangers).
- **Multiple attachments:** After approximately 9 months of age, children begin to form strong emotional bonds with other caregivers beyond the primary attachment figure, including the father, older siblings, and grandparents.

Factors that influence attachment

- **Opportunity for attachment:** Children who do not have a primary care figure may fail to develop the sense of trust needed to form an attachment like those in orphanages.
- **Quality caregiving:** This is a vital factor in which children learn that they can depend on the people who are responsible for their care when caregivers respond quickly and consistently.

Patterns of attachment

- **Ambivalent attachment:** It is an uncommon style affecting an estimated 7–15% of US children. As a result of poor parental availability, these children cannot depend on their primary caregiver to be there when they need them. These children become very distressed when a parent leaves.
- **Avoidant attachment:** This attachment style might be a result of abusive or neglectful caregivers, in which children who are punished for relying on a caregiver will learn to avoid seeking help in the future. Children tend to avoid parents or caregivers, showing no preference between a caregiver and a complete stranger.
- **Disorganized attachment:** These children seems disoriented, dazed, or confused and avoid or resist the parent. Lack of a clear attachment pattern is likely linked to inconsistent caregiver behavior. In such cases, parents may serve as both a source of comfort and fear, leading to disorganized behavior.
- **Secure attachment:** Children shows distress when separated and joy when reunited as they are dependent on their caregivers. Although the child may be upset, they feel assured that the caregiver will return and when frightened, securely attached children are comfortable seeking reassurance from caregivers.

Stage	*Related stages*	*Emotional development*	*Cognitive development*	*Social development*	*Dental intervention*
1. Infancy (15 months)	Corresponds to oral stage of Freud's psychoanalytical theory and the stage of trust vs mistrust in Erikson's theory.	Emotions like anger, fear, curiosity, joy and affection between 4–10 months of age. Stranger and separation anxiety starts at 6 months and peaks between 13–18 months. Anxiety occurs due to the concept of trust versus mistrust	From first day of life cognitive changes occur Mussen and co-workers (1948) described four major areas of cognitive development: 1. Area of perception—infant has the ability to perceive movements, facial reactions and color. 2. Recognition of information—infants can recognize face. They can encounter crucial event in their consciousness. 3. Ability to categorize—by the age of 1 year infants can group things by their shape, color etc. 4. Enhancement of memory—even very young infants have some memory and by the age of 6 months they can recall any past experience.	Infant is totally dependent on their parents. Non-reflexive smiling occurs at 2–3 months and signifies the first major social behavior of the infant other than crying.	Dental intervention for infant is minimal. The dental treatment may be best achieved in the hospital setting using a general anesthesia. Minor treatments may be carried out in dental office.

Contd...

Contd...

Stage	***Related stages***	***Emotional development***	***Cognitive development***	***Social development***	***Dental intervention***
2. Toddler (15 months to 2 years)	Corresponds to anal stage of Freud's psychoanalytical theory and stage of autonomy vs shame or doubt in Erikson's theory.	Toddlers progress emotionally by end of 2 years. Rocky emotional behavior is seen. By the end of 15–18 months separation anxiety is exchanged by object permanence.	Object permanence seen. They become symbol oriented. Around age 21 months, toddlers learn scripts, or routines, about how certain things are done. Around age 24 months, they cultivate the ability to pretend and imagine things that aren't there in front of them.	Toddlers start participating in family routines. They also begin "to and fro" play with caregivers and other peers. They start realizing they can include other people in their fun and play.	Dental examination-should be done with the child in parent's lap. Radiographs to be taken with the help of parents or assistant by using protection. Caries should be excavated using spoon excavator or bur using slow speed handpiece. Major procedures may require oral sedation or general anesthesia. Dietary counseling and oral hygiene maintenance advised.
3. Preschooler (2–6 years)	Corresponds to genital stage of Freud's psychoanalytical theory and stage of initiative vs guilt in Erikson's theory.	The emotions such as frustration, fear, jealousy, envy, grief develops dramatically between the age 3 and 6 years. At the 6th birthday they become emotionally complex with friendship and hostility, acting out aggression and experiencing guilt and anxiety.	The child acquires the capacity to think symbolically with mental imagery. The period of intuitive thought develops around the age of four and lasts until age of seven or eight. Late in this period the child will begin to acquire writing and reading skills	The period between the 2nd and 3rd birth days has been considered as "terrible twos". Resist by saying No. They do not hesitate to state their opinions in front of everyone. They become conscious of things due to more social indulgence.	Dentist should use communication methods if the child likes to verbalize. Usage of euphemistic descriptions of dental procedures. Modelling is effective.
4. Middle school child (6–11 years)	Corresponds to latency stage of Freud's psychoanalytical theory and the stage of industry vs inferiority in Erikson's theory.	By 6-12 years, emotional satisfaction occurs when they are accepted socially by their peers. Lack of acceptance, isolation, teasing can be very damaging for the child emotionally.	During the years 6 to 12, mental ability of a child grows extensively. They remain attentive to any problem, produce sophisticated oral and written communication.	There is an increasing importance of peers, and the massive expansion of the child's social environment. School is very important for this age group as it signifies an extra familial world.	For dentist and staff, middle school age represent minimum behavior entanglement. Anxiety can be dealt with in a sensible way by staff personnel and the dentist.
5. Adolescent (11–18 years)	Corresponds to adolescence stage of Freud's psychoanalytical theory and stage of Identity vs role confusion in Erikson's theory.	The confidence and personal identity of an adolescent may be compromised if their feelings about body image are negative. The advent of puberty and the hormones associated with puberty lead to sexual feelings and urges.	Intellectual tasks and ability at abstract thinking allows the adolescent to deal with complex and vocational and educational challenges. Kiell 1967 stated that adolescents are "passionate, irascible and apt to be carried away by the impulses".	Importance of peers escalates. Popularity is an essential desire in adolescence.	Dentist and staff will find working for the adolescent a pleasant experience. There may be a period of time during pubescence when the individual may be sensitive and irritable, requiring thorough attention and patience on the part of the dental staff.

POINTS TO REMEMBER

- Child psychology: It is the science that deals with the mental power or an interaction through the conscious and subconscious element in a child.
- Psychodynamic theories are psychosexual theory/psychoanalytic theory by Sigmund Freud (1905), cognitive theory by Jean Piaget (1952), psychosocial theory/model of personality development by Erik Erikson (1963).
- Theories of learning and development of behavior include classical conditioning by Pavlov (1927), operant conditioning by Skinner (1938), hierarchy of needs by Maslow (1954), social learning theory by Bandura (1963).
- Freud explained that psychic triad is governed by biological drives (iD), social rules (superego), and mediating thought processes (ego).
- Stages of Freud's psychosexual theory include oral, anal, urethral, phallic, latency, genital.
- According to Erikson, each individual passes through eight developmental stages. Each stage is characterized by a different psychological crisis, which must be resolved by the individual before he can move on to the next stage.
- Piaget marked four stages of cognitive growth each characterized by a different type of thinking namely sensorimotor period, preoperational period, concrete operational period, formal operational period.

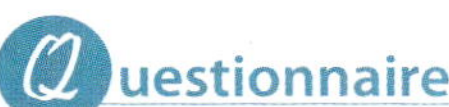

Questionnaire

1. Define child psychology and give its aims.
2. Classify theories of child psychology.
3. Explain psychosexual theory by Freud.
4. What is Erikson's psychosocial theory?
5. Describe Piaget's cognitive development.
6. Explain the behavior learning theories.

FURTHER READING

1. Agras WS. Learning theory. In: Kaplan HL, Sadock BJ (Eds). Comprehensive textbook of psychiatry, 5th edition. Baltimore: Williams and Wilkins; 1989. p. 262.
2. Atkinson RC, Shiffrin RM. Chapter: Human memory: A proposed system and its control processes. In: Spence KW, Spence JT (Eds). The psychology of learning and motivation (Volume 2). New York: Academic Press; 1968.pp. 89-195.
3. Baddeley AD, Hitch G. Working memory. In: Bower GH (Ed). The psychology of learning and motivation: Advances in research and theory. New York: Academic Press. 1974;8:47-89.
4. Bartlett FC. Remembering A study in experimental and social psychology. Cambridge University Press; 1932.
5. Byrnes JP. Categorizing and combining theories of cognitive development and learning. Educ Psychol Rev. 1992;4:309.
6. Erikson E. Childhood and society. New York: Norton; 1950.
7. Erikson E. Freud's "The Origin of Psychoanalysis". Int J Psychoanal. 1995;36:1.
8. Erikson, Encyclopedia 1959/1980, p. 97.
9. Feldman RS. Understanding psychology. 4th edition.
10. Freud S. An outline of psycho-analysis. New York: Norton; 1969.
11. Freud S. Beyond the pleasure principle. New York: Norton; 1961.
12. Freud S. Ego and the Id. New York: Norton; 1960.
13. Freud S. The interpretation of dreams. In: Standard edition, 1900:4 & 5:1-627.
14. Jean Piaget a Swiss psychologist: Encyclopedia Britannica.
15. King M. Introduction to psychology. 7th edition. Tata Mc Graw Hill Publishing Ltd.
16. Mahler M, Furer M. Certain aspects of the separation-individuation phase. Psychoanalytic quarterly. 1963;32:1-14.
17. Mahler M. On child psychosis and schizophrenia: autistic and symbiotic infantile psychoses. Psychoanalytic study of the child. 1952;7:286-305.
18. Maslow's Need Hierarchy Theory: Applications and Criticisms Avneet Kaur.
19. McLeod M, Saul E. "Erik Erikson"Simply Psychology; 2017.
20. Miller PH. Theories of developmental psychology. 2nd edition. WH Freeman & Company.
21. Pavlov IP. Conditioned reflexes. London: Oxford University Press; 1927.
22. Santrock JW. Cognitive Developmental Approaches, Child development, 11th edition. 210-32.
23. Sarles RM, Forester DJ, Wagner ML. Psychological growth and development; 2017. pp. 27-30.
24. Skinner BF. Science and human and behavior. New York: Macmillan; 1953.
25. Sternberg RJ. The biological basis of learning. In: Psychology-in search of human mind. 3rd edition.
26. Walker S. Learning theory and behavior modification. London: Methuen; 1984.
27. Watson JB. Psychology as the behaviorist views it. Psychological Review. 1913;20(2):158-77.

CHAPTER

Dental Fear, Anxiety and Phobia

N Sivakumar, Anant Nigam, Nikhil Marwah, Kunal Gupta

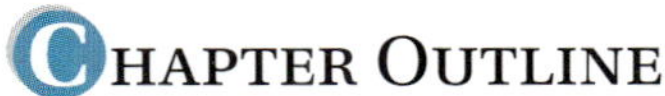

Chapter Outline

Children experience mild fears that appear or disappear spontaneously and follow a predictable path. These developmentally appropriate or "normal" fears should be differentiated from phobias and anxiety disorders, which are out of proportion to the demands of the situation that elicits them, cannot be rationalized, are involuntary, leading to avoidance of the situation, and interfere with daily functioning (American Psychiatric Association, 2000). Modern dentistry has made much progress in providing a patient-friendly environment, but despite revolutionary new dental techniques, anxiety and fear toward dentistry has stayed relatively constant over the past many years. Dental fear is a normal emotional reaction to one or more specific threatening stimuli in a dental situation and is said to be ranked fourth among common fears and ninth among intense fears. The normative fear literature now spans over one century with the first investigation into normal fear having been published by **Hall** in 1897.

DEFINITIONS

Fear: *The unpleasant emotional state consisting of psychological and psychophysiological responses to a real external threat or danger including agitation, alertness, tension, and mobilization of the alarmed reaction.* — *Dorland Medical Dictionary*

It is defined as a painful feeling of impending danger, evil, trouble, etc. — *Delbridge*

Defined as a reaction to a known danger. — *Rubin*

Emotion: *It is defined as an expression of readiness to establish, maintain, or change one's relation to the environment on a matter of personal importance.* It is a conscious mental reaction subjectively experienced as a strong feeling usually directed toward a specific object and typically accompanied by physiological and behavioral changes in the body.

- Fear is a reaction to known danger
- Anxiety is reaction to unknown or anticipated stimuli
- Worry is thinking about a known stimulus
- Phobia is anxiety about a specific thing

Dental anxiety: *Denotes a state of apprehension that something dreadful is going to happen in relation to dental treatment and it is coupled with a sense of losing control.*

Dental phobia: *It is an irrational fear resulting in conscious avoidance of specific feared object, activity or situation related to dentistry. It represents a severe type of dental anxiety and is characterized by marked and persistent anxiety in relation either to clearly discernible situations/objects (e.g., drilling, injections) or to the dental situation in general. Dental phobia is an extreme form of dental anxiety.*

FEAR-RELATED EMOTIONAL PATTERNS

Shyness

- It is a form of fear characterized by shrinking from contact with others who are strange and unfamiliar. It is always aroused by people never by objects, animals, or situations.
- Shyness in the presence of strangers is so common at this age level that it is often labeled the "strange age" or the "period of infantile fearfulness." The reason for this period of fearfulness is that, at 6 months, babies are intellectually mature enough to recognize the difference

between familiar and unfamiliar people, but they are not mature enough to recognize that their unfamiliarity poses no threat.

- If, however, shyness is extremely intense and frequent, it may lead to a generalized timidity that affects children's social relationships long after babyhood is over. They then become "shy children".
- In babies, the usual response in shyness is crying, turning the head away from the stranger, and clinging to a familiar person for protection. Later, when babies are able to creep or walk, they run away and hide as they do when they are frightened. Older children show their shyness by blushing, by stuttering, by talking as little as possible, by nervous mannerisms, such as pulling at the ears or clothing, shifting from one foot to the other, and bending the head to one side and then raising it coyly to look at the stranger.

Embarrassment

- Like shyness, embarrassment is a fear reaction to people, not to objects or situations.
- It differs from shyness in that it is not aroused by strangers or by familiar people in unfamiliar clothes or roles, but rather by uncertainty about how people will judge one and one's behavior.
- It is, therefore, a state of self-conscious distress.
- It is usually not present in a child <5 or 6 years of age. As children grow older, embarrassment is heightened by memories of experiences in which their behavior fell below social expectations. This tends to exaggerate their fear of how others will judge them in the future.

Distress

- *Distress was defined as the stress behavior displayed by a child which might not be the result of pain.*
- It is an occurrence of emotions felt or behavior displayed during (dental) treatment caused by factors other than pain (e.g., fear, anxiety, and anticipatory or situational stress).

Worry

- Worry is usually described as "imaginary fear" or "borrowing trouble".
- Unlike real fear, it is not aroused directly by a stimulus in the environment but is a product of the child's own mind. It comes from imagining dangerous situations which could arise.
- The most common worries center around the home, family, and peer relationships and school problems, with the latter becoming more prominent as children progress in school.
- Children who feel inferior and inadequate tend to internalize their worries, thinking about them and exaggerating them out of all proportion. Better adjusted children, by contrast, are more likely to discuss their worries with people who they think will be sympathetic. Children who feel both insecure and rejected often verbalize their worries in the hopes of winning sympathy and through it, improving their social acceptance. Extroverts at all ages verbalize their worries more than introverts.

Effect of emotions on children

- Emotions add pleasure to everyday experiences. Emotions prepare the body for action
- Emotional tension disrupts motor skills. Emotions serve as a form of communication. Emotions interfere with mental activities
- Emotions act as sources of social evaluation. Emotions color children's outlooks on life
- Emotions affect social interactions
- Emotions leave their mark on facial expressions. Emotions affect the psychological climate
- Emotional responses if repeated develop as habits
- All children express their worries by their facial expression. Only as children grow older and realize that worry is not a particularly acceptable emotional pattern, will they try to conceal their facial expressions. Some children, however, deliberately try to look worried in order to win attention and sympathy.

Anxiety

- Anxiety is an uneasy mental state concerning impending or anticipated danger.
- It is marked by apprehension, uneasiness, and foreboding from which the individual cannot escape; it is accompanied by a feeling of helplessness because the anxious person feels blocked, unable to find a solution for problems. The uneasy mental state characteristic of anxiety may in time become a generalized "free-floating" anxiety in which children experience a mild state of fear in any situation which is perceived as a potential threat.
- Though anxiety develops from fear and worry, it is distinguished from them in several respects. It is vaguer than fear. Unlike fear, it does not come from an existing situation, but from an anticipated one.
- Like worry, anxiety is due to imaginary rather than real causes. Anxiety differs from worry, however, in two respects. First, worry is related to specific situations, such as parties, examinations, or money problems, whereas anxiety is a generalized emotional state. Second, worry comes from an objective problem, whereas anxiety comes from a subjective problem.

TYPES OF FEAR

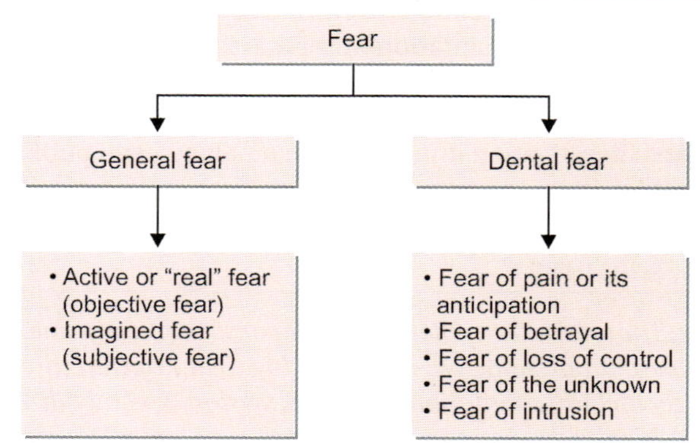

Objective Fear or "Real" Fear

- Objective fears are those produced by direct physical stimulation of the sense organs and are generally not of parental origin. Objective fears are responses to stimuli that are felt, seen, heard, smelled, or tasted by the child and are of a disagreeable or unpleasant nature.

- A child who has had previous contact with a dentist and has been managed so poorly that undue and unnecessary pain has been inflicted necessarily develops a fear of future dental treatment. It is difficult to get a child is hurt previously, to return to the dentist of his own volition. When he is induced to return, the dentist must realize his emotional state and proceed slowly to re-establish the child's confidence in the dentist and in dental treatment.
- A child who has been improperly handled or subjected to intense pain in a hospital by persons in white uniforms may develop an intense fear of similar uniforms on dentists or dental hygienists.
- Even the characteristic smell of certain drugs, chemicals or dental materials previously associated with unpleasantness may arouse unwarranted fear.
- Fear also lowers the pain threshold so that any pain produced during dental treatment becomes magnified and leads to even greater apprehension.

Subjective Fear or "Imagined Fear" or "Suggested Fear" or "Imitative Fear"

- Subjective fears are those based on feelings and attitudes that have been suggested to the child by others about their experiences without the child's having had the experience personally.
- The young inexperienced child, hearing of some unpleasant or pain-producing situation undergone by apparent or others, soon develops a fear of that experience. The mental picture producing the fear is retained in the child's mind and with the vivid imagination of childhood, becomes magnified and formidable. A child hearing from parents or playmates of the supposed terror of the dental office soon accepts it as real and to be avoided if at all possible.
- **Shoben** and **Borland** reported that fear of dentistry in adults was based more on what they heard about dentistry from their parents than on anything else. In children as in adults, the greatest producer of fear is hearing unpleasant experiences in the dental office from parents or friends.
- The influence of parents is one of the most important in the child's attitude toward dentistry. It is imperative that parents inform their children of what to expect in the dental office. The child should be familiarized in a general way with the procedures that will be encountered and the appearance and description of the office equipment before the first dental appointment.
- Suggestive fears may be acquired by imitation. A child observing fear in others may soon acquire a fear for the same object or event as real and genuine as that observed by the child in others. This is especially true if the fear is observed in parents. Children frequently identify themselves with parents. If the parent displays fear, the child is fearful.
- Imitative fears may be transmitted subtly and may be displayed by the parent and acquired by the child without either being aware of it. They are generally recurrent fears and therefore are more deep seated and difficult to eradicate.

Dental Fear

There are five factors which are important in the etiology and perpetuation of dental fear:

1. **Fear of pain or its anticipation**
   - The link between actual or misinterpreted pain, or the anticipation of pain, and dental fear is well established. Unfortunately, discomfort and sometimes pain can still be a feature of dental treatment today no matter how careful we are about trying to ensure adequate analgesia.
   - The other problem is that individuals, especially children, have their feelings of pain denied. We frequently see children who report that they said that they were experiencing pain, but the dentist ignored them and carried on. So, it is very important as dentists to recognize and address the pain symptoms of the children.
   - A very basic explanation which is suitable for children as young as five is as follows. You have lots of different types of telephone wires called nerves going from your mouth to your brain (touch appropriate body parts). Some of them carry "ouch!" messages and the others carry messages about touch (demonstrate) and hot and cold. The sleeping potion stops the ouch messages being sent, but not the touch and the hot and cold messages. So you will still know that I am touching the tooth and you will still feel the cold of the water. If you are convinced that it will hurt, it will. This is because if I make the ouch nerves go off to sleep and I touch you, a touch message gets sent. But your brain is looking for ouch messages and it says to itself. There is a message coming. It must be an ouch message: So you go "ouch" and it hurts, but all I did was to touch you.
2. **Fear of betrayal**
   - Trust may also be learned either directly from the behavior of parents, peers, and so on or indirectly from statements from others or observation of behavior.
   - It is therefore theoretically possible that children learn to trust or distrust dental personnel from their parents before they have any direct contact with such person (vicarious learning).

Determinants of fear (Flowchart 19.1)

- Dental behavior management problem (DBMP)
- Mother–child relation
- Temperament
- Pain and anxiety
- Predictability and controllability
- Gender and age
- Communication
- Age of onset
- Culture, ethnicity, and socioeconomic status
- Physical disability
- Genetics
- Determinants related to dentist
- Psychological and emotional determinants

- The research evidence that is available in adults, suggests that trust of the dentist is an important factor in dental fear.

Flowchart 19.1: Determinants of fear.

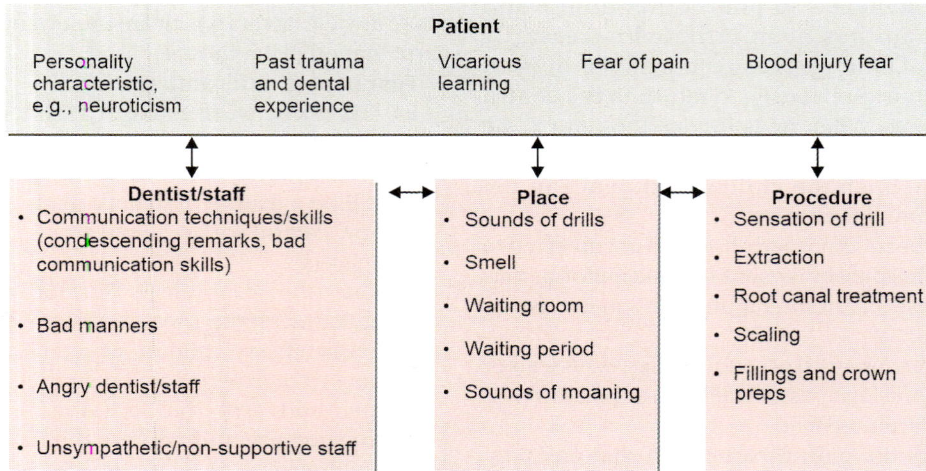

3. **Fear of loss of control**
   - Children are used to being cared for or controlled by parents. They have an innate sense though, of the boundary that defines social from personal control. Overtly offering children the opportunity to ask questions enhances their control over information gained, thus offering decisional control (by providing reasonable choices).
   - Letting a 4-year-old child choose which tooth to be polished first (not whether they wish to get teeth polished or not, which is an unreasonable choice) gives them an appropriate degree of feeling at control. Six-year olds are capable of deciding whether or not to have a local anesthetic for a particular restoration, but not whether or not to have the restoration. Ten-year-olds may request that easy treatment is completed at a particular appointment because they have examinations afterwards or they are not feeling well, thus offering control over the noxious stimulus.
4. **Fear of the unknown**
   - In anyone's eyes, a visit to the dentist may be classified as a potentially threatening situation.
   - "Helpful" comments from the mother such as, "It would not hurt;" even before an examination, will raise the possibility in the child's mind of being hurt.
   - However, it is important to provide accurate information about possible discomfort immediately before the event. One must be very cautious not to provide such information a long time in advance as it may only serve to increase fear of the unknown and the anticipation of pain. The poorer the quality and quantity of information provided by the dentist about the situation, the more important such misinformation from others becomes.
   - The provision of a developmentally appropriate level of information will not only reduce fear of the unknown, but also foster a sense of control as described above. The most usual way in which a dentist provides information is the "tell-show-do" technique.
5. **Fear of intrusion**
   - Most if not all the dental procedures are invasive
   - Intrusion involves impinging on the patient's personal space and into a bodily cavity, the mouth. Impinging on a patient's personal space is something that is taken for granted by professionals. They perceive this as part of their caring role, even if the patients dislike the procedure intensely. Some children find this invasion of personal space very threatening
   - It may evoke withdrawal by younger children and comments, usually from older children, such as "I do not like the thought of that thing squirting up inside my tooth"
   - Intrusion may also involve a threat to the persona. For example, the child who refuses to attend because every visit involves perceived criticism from the dentist about his poor diet and cleaning which becomes demoralizing for the child.

DEVELOPMENT AND PHYSIOLOGY OF FEAR

The development of fear is an innate function of the sub cortical and the amygdale which is considered to be the focus zone of this episode **(Fig. 19.1)**. Fear in children is seldom linked to their emotional status but most frequently is a conditioned response through learning experiences via friends, family and peers.

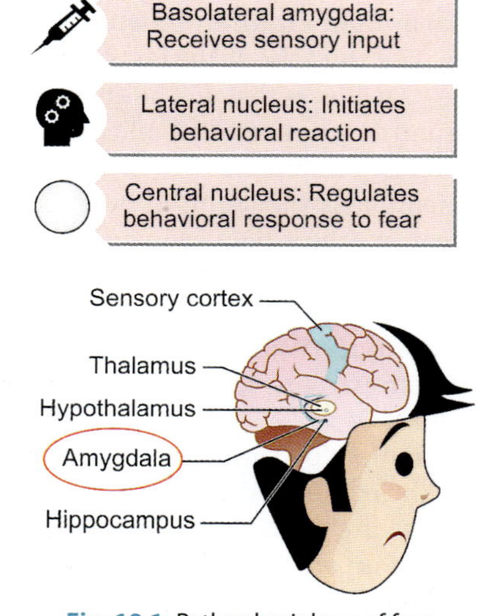

Fig. 19.1: Pathophysiology of fear.

Table 19.1: Different types of fears corresponding to age.

Age groups (years)	0–2	2–4	4–7	8–10	11–13
• Fears	• Strangers • Loud noises • Loss of support • Strange objects	• Being alone • Darkness • Animals	• Environmental threats • Imaginary creatures • Animals • Frightening movies	• Animals • Burglar • Personal harm/ harm others	• Animals • Personal harm/harm others • Separation from parents

PREVALENCE OF DENTAL FEAR AND ANXIETY

- The prevalence of dental fear among children has been reported to range between 5% and 20% across the countries **(Table 19.1).**
- In the Indian scenario, there are only a few epidemiological studies available regarding prevalence of dental anxiety and fear.
- In 1997, **Rao et al.,** reported that about 51% of the students aged between 17 and 22 reported some fear of dentistry with females and dental students being more fearful than males and medical students.
- **Pramila M** and **Murthy AK** (2010) reported a 23.4% prevalence of high dental fear among 12–15-year-old school children.
- **Ekta AM** and **Ajithkrishnan CG** (2011), reported that around 41% of patients waiting in the OPD for dental treatment were dentally anxious with females and subjects living in villages showing increased dental anxiety than males and city dwellers.
- **Marya CM et al.,** reported that prevalence of dental anxiety was high (50.2%) as compared to phobia (4.38%) and most of the anxious patients were in the age group 20–30 years.

Responses to Fear

Fear is a complex entity in itself and hence the response to fear is also one of multidimensional type with the individual exhibiting inner feeling/cognitive response, outer behavioral expression, and accompanying physiological changes **(Fig. 19.2)**.

Cognitive
The child expresses fear, e.g., I am scared

Behavioral
Child's behavior suggests threatening environment

Physiological
Body responds to fear

Fig. 19.2: Response to fear.

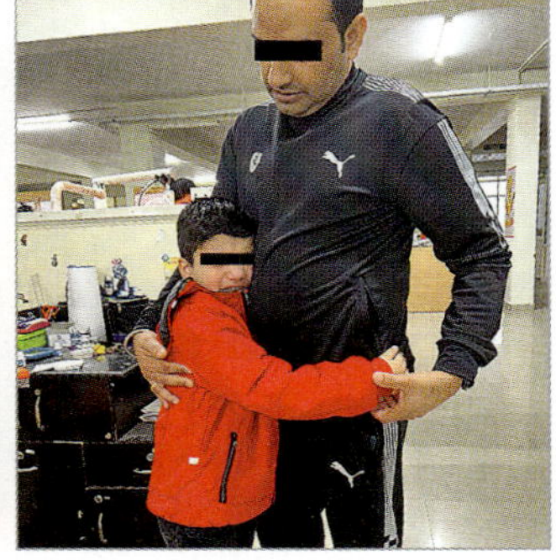

Fig. 19.3: Behavioral response of child to fear.

- **Inner feeling/cognitive response:** Negative statements such as "I am scared of the dentist" or "The injection will hurt me".
- **Behavioral response:** Forceful crying, holding on to parents tightly or trying to pull parents towards exit **(Fig. 19.3)**
- **Physiological response:** This varies from person to person but is usually associated with high speed of breathing, sweating and change of facial expressions.

MANAGEMENT OF FEAR AND ANXIETY

Various approaches outline the behavior management treatment strategies for pediatric dental patient, viz., informative, psychotherapeutic, modeling, behavioral, cognitive, and hypnotic approaches. Many of these titles are descriptive and some have psychologic definitions. Procedures that enhance a feeling of control include giving the child choices, helping within treatment or otherwise manipulating dental objects, and acknowledging the child's experience. When a child is given a multitude of small choices, he or she comes to believe that his or her thoughts and judgment are important. As a result, the child's ability to cope is enhanced. Various behavior management strategies (detailed in Chapter 21, Nonpharmacologic Behavior Management) are summarized in **Table 19.2**.

Important points to remember for combating fear in children
- Never make fun of a child's fear.
- Positive reinforcement for a child's good behavior.
- Try to be supportive and empathetic
- Explore strategies to overcome their fears like imagery, music, hypnosis.

The reality approaches for managing a fearful and anxious child in dental clinic.

- **The patient is granted the reality of his symptoms or complaints:** By so doing, the patient's discomfort or pain is confirmed and he is made to feel that this is a real problem being brought to the dentist. This must be apparent in the

Table 19.2: Various behavior management strategies.

Primary prevention	*Secondary prevention*	*Tertiary behavioral treatment strategies*	*Pharmacologic management strategies*
Environment based approaches	*Behavioral treatment of fearfulchildren*	*Behavioral treatment of anxious children*	*Behavioral treatment of uncooperative/handicapped children*
• Home and child-rearing • Preappointment approaches • A safe, controlled environment • Sense of control to the child • Introduction of the child to the dental office	• Communication • Euphemisms • The guidance-cooperation model • Time-structuring • Distraction • Guided imagery • Behavior modification • Parent in the operatory	• Desensitization • Modeling • Tell–show–do • Combined behavioral treatments	• Nitrous oxide sedation • Oral sedation • Rectal sedation • Parenteral sedation • Aversive techniques • General anesthesia

attitude and demeanor of the examining doctor. It is not a principle that can be mechanically applied but must be internally motivated.

- **The patient's anxiety or fear requires a thorough exploration of the symptoms and complaints:** The examination should not be cursory. We cannot underestimate the patient's need for a procedure that will assure him that everything possible is being done to understand the problem and its solution.
- **A positive statement of assurance at some stage is mandatory:** Examinations conducted in silence or with wise expressions and grunts are in themselves anxiety producing. Therefore, it is important to reassure the patient that the problem is understandable and that he is not alone in his difficulty. We attempt to overcome the sense of isolation, and constantly seek to establish during the examination a warm human relationship.
- **The dentist states that he/she does not know all the answers to the patient's problems:** (Anxiety, fears, and so forth) to remove the aura of omnipotence that the preceding statement might cause. The patient might attempt to manipulate this omnipotence, as a form of magic, to cure all ills. It is, therefore, necessary to qualify this by saying that we do not know all the answers.
- **The search for effective psychological treatment of anxiety and phobia:** At the present time, research is in an active period in two areas—the behavioral and the pharmacologic. These two methods take a different approach, although there is much evidence that in the more severe multiphobias, a joint approach may work best.

Being a good dentist in today's world means along with producing a fine, accurate restoration; the dentist must have the knowledge of the dynamics of child development and an understanding that a patient's behavior which is crucial to the outcome of treatment. It is essential to employ dental fear and behavior management techniques which are considered "as much an art form as it is a science." It is not an application of individual techniques created to "deal" with children but rather a comprehensive methodology meant to build a relationship between patient and doctor which ultimately builds trust and allays fear and anxiety. The dentist must primarily aim in prevention of dental fear by creating safe atmosphere for children in the dental environment starting from the first call made to the clinic, parent education, and a friendly dental team. By integrating the sound knowledge of dental fear and management skills, treatment of children will be rewarding and satisfying to the dentist and positively reinforcing and less stressful to patients.

POINTS TO REMEMBER

- Fear is defined as the unpleasant emotional state consisting of psychological and psychophysiological responses to a real external threat or danger including agitation, alertness, tension and mobilization of the alarmed reaction.
- Dental anxiety denotes a state of apprehension that something dreadful is going to happen in relation to dental treatment and it is coupled with a sense of losing control.
- Fear is a reaction to known danger; anxiety is reaction to unknown anticipated stimuli; worry is thinking about a known stimulus; phobia is anxiety about a specific thing.
- Fear-related patterns include shyness, embarrassment, worry, and anxiety.
- Objective fears are real fears which are produced by direct physical stimulation of the sense organs and are generally not of parental origin. These are responses to stimuli that are felt, seen, heard, smelled or tasted and are of a disagreeable or unpleasant nature.
- Subjective fears are imagined fears and are based on feelings and attitudes that have been suggested to the child by others without the child having had the experience personally.
- Dental fear includes fear of pain or its anticipation, fear of betrayal, fear of loss of control, fear of the unknown, and fear of intrusion.

Questionnaire

1. Define dental fear, anxiety and phobia.
2. What are the different types of fears?
3. Enumerate the determinants of fear.
4. Outline the approach for management of dental fear and anxiety.

FURTHER READING

1. Agras S, Sylvester D, Oliveau D. The epidemiology of common fears and phobia. Compr Psychiatry. 1969;10:151-6.
2. Agras S. Panic: facing fears, phobias and anxiety. In: The portable stanford, Chapter 1, 1985. pp. 2.
3. Armfield JM, Heaton LJ. Management of fear and anxiety in the dental clinic: a review. Aust Dent J. 2013;58(4):390-407.

4. American Psychiatric Association. Diagnostic and Statistical Manual of Mental Disorders, 4th edition, text revision (DSM-IV-TR). Washington, DC: American Psychiatric Association. 2000
5. Chapman HR, Kirby-Turner NC. Dental fear in children--a proposed model. Br Dent J. 1999;187(8):408-12.
6. Delbridge A, Bernard JRL, Blair D, Peters P, Butler S (Eds). Macquarie dictionary. NSW, Australia: The Macquarie Library, Macquarie University; 1991.
7. Klingberg G, Broberg AG. Dental fear, anxiety and dental behaviour management problems in children and adolescents: a review of prevalence and concomitant psychological factors. Int J Paediatr Dent. 2007;17:391-406.
8. Malvania EA, Ajithkrishnan CG. Prevalence and socio- demographic correlates of dental anxiety among a group of adult patients attending a dental institution in Vadodara city, Gujarat, India. Indian J Dent Res. 2011;22:179-80.
9. Marya CM, Grover S, Jnaneshwar A, Pruthi N. Dental anxiety among patients visiting a dental institute in Faridabad, India. West Indian Med J. 2012;61:187-90.
10. Pramila M, Murthy AK, Chandrakala B, Ranganath S. Dental fear in children and its relation to dental caries and gingival condition: a cross-sectional study in Bangalore City, India. Int J Clin Dent Sci. 2010;1:1-5.
11. Rao A, Sequeire PS, Peter S. Characteristics of dental fear amongst dental and medical students. Indian J Dent Res. 1997;8:111-14.
12. Rubin GJ, Slovin M, Krochak M. The psychodynamics of dental anxiety and dental phobia. Dent Clin North Am. 1988;32:647-56.
13. Slovin M, Wasserman JF. Special needs of anxious and phobic dental patients. Dent Clin North Am. 2009;53:207-19.
14. Versloot J, Veerkamp JS, Hoogstraten J. Assessment of pain by the child, dentist, and independent observers. Pediatr Dent. 2004;26(5):445-9.
15. Weiner AA. The basic principles of fear, anxiety and phobia: past and present. In: Weiner AA (Eds). The fearful dental patient: a guide to understanding and managing. Iowa: Wiley Blackwell; 2011. pp. 4.
16. Winer G. A review and analysis of children's fearful behaviour in dental settings. Child Dev. 1982;53:1111-33.

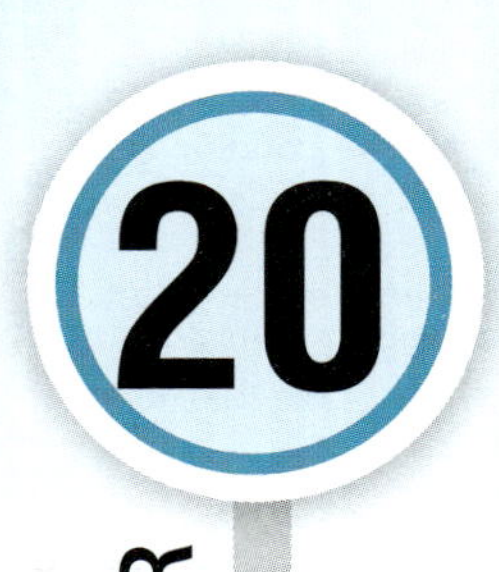

CHAPTER

Psychometric Assessment of Dental Fear and Anxiety

Nikhil Marwah, N Sivakumar, Mili Meghpara

Chapter Outline

Contemporary pediatric dentistry has made much progress in providing a child-friendly environment. However, despite revolutionary new dental techniques, anxiety toward dentistry has stayed relatively constant over the past 50 years. Dental fear, anxiety, and phobia create a challenging environment for both the child and the dentist to work together. The behavioral sciences have become an increasingly important component of dental education and research. One component of this has been the application of psychological methods to the study of behavior and attitudes relevant to health, illness, and health care. This chapter focuses on measurement techniques to assess dental fear and anxiety, in particular, fear of dentists and dentistry as well as of dental pain. There are many tests for anxiety and fear evaluation about they are primarily divided into two types:

1. Observation of child's reaction/behavior by dentist or other person during dental treatment.
2. Reports of anxiety made by the child himself or herself or by the accompanying parent (most often the mother) using psychometric scales. Self-reports are most often used for older children who can understand and comprehend the concept, whereas parental reports are for young children.

Commonly used fear and anxiety scales

Used in adults and children	*General scales used to measure dental anxiety*	*Child-specific dental anxiety scales*
• Corah DAS	• STAI-S	• CFSS-DS
• MDAS	• HADS-anxiety subscale	• MCDAS
• Kleinknecht's DFS		• FBRS
• DFAS		• VPS
• Gatchel's 10-point FS		• VAS
• Stouthard's DAI		• FIS
• DAI-S		• SFP
• Gale's RQ		• Anxiety thermometer
• PAQ		• Morin's AFDTCI
• HAQ		
• FDP questionnaire		
• Single-item measures		

(DAS: dental anxiety scale; STAI-S: Spielberger state-trait anxiety inventory; CFSS-DS: children's fear survey schedule-dental subscale; MDAS: modified dental anxiety scale; HADS: hospital anxiety and depression scale; MCDAS: modified child dental anxiety scale; DFS: dental fear survey; FBRS: Frankl behavior rating scale; DFAS: dental fear assessment scale; VPS; Venham picture scale; FS: fear scale; VAS: Venham anxiety scale; DAI: dental anxiety inventory; FIS: facial image scale; DAI-S: dental anxiety inventory short version; SFP: Smiley Faces Program; RQ: ranking questionnaire; PAQ: photo anxiety questionnaire; AFDTCI: adolescent's fear of dental treatment cognitive inventory; HAQ: hierarchical anxiety questionnaire; FDP: fear of dental pain)

CORAH DENTAL ANXIETY SCALE (TABLE 20.1)

- The most widely used measure of dental anxiety, the dental anxiety scale (DAS), was originally based on a single-item question that was developed to measure "psychologic stress" (**Corah NL** 1969).[1]
- The four questions in the DAS relate to scenarios varying in temporal and distal proximity from the dental experience. Presumably, increased physical and temporal proximity to the dental encounter was believed to be related to increases in anxiety, and this has formed the basis of other scales, such as the dental anxiety inventory (DAI).[2]
- This is a four-item measure, where respondents are asked about four dentally related situations and are asked to indicate which option is closest to their likely response to that situation.

Table 20.1: Corah's dental anxiety scale, revised (DAS-R).

***Name*______________________ *Date*______________**

Norman Corah's dental questionnaire

1. If you had to go to the dentist tomorrow for a check-up, how would you feel about it?
   a. I would look forward to it as a reasonably enjoyable experience
   b. I would not care one way or the other
   c. I would be a little uneasy about it
   d. I would be afraid that it would be unpleasant and painful
   e. I would be very frightened of what the dentist would do
2. When you are waiting in the dentist's office for your turn in the chair, how do you feel?
   a. Relaxed
   b. A little uneasy
   c. Tense
   d. Anxious
   e. So anxious that I sometimes break out in a sweat or almost feel physically sick
3. When you are in the dentist's chair waiting while the dentist gets the drill ready to begin working on your teeth, how do you feel?
   a. Relaxed
   b. A little uneasy
   c. Tense
   d. Anxious
   e. So anxious that I sometimes break out in a sweat or almost feel physically sick
4. Imagine you are in the dentist's chair to have your teeth cleaned. While you are waiting and the dentist or hygienist is getting out the instruments which will be used to scrape your teeth around the gums, how do you feel?
   a. Relaxed
   b. A little uneasy
   c. Tense
   d. Anxious
   e. So anxious that I sometimes break out in a sweat or almost feel physically sick

Scoring the DAS-R (this information is not printed on the form that patients see)

a = 1, b = 2, c = 3, d = 4, e = 5 Total possible = 20

Anxiety rating

- 9–12 = Moderate anxiety but have specific stressors that should be discussed and managed
- 13–14 = High anxiety
- 15–20 = Severe anxiety (or phobia). May be manageable with the dental concerns assessment but might require the help of a mental health therapist

(DAS-R: dental anxiety scale, revised)

- However, the four questions also vary in what they measure, with the first two questions relating to anxiety generally and the second two questions seeming to relate to anticipated fear of specific stimuli—the drill and cleaning instruments.
- The advantages of DAS are that first, it can aid the dentist to be aware of what to expect from patients and take measures to help alleviate the anxiety of the patient and second, it can be self-administered in the waiting room in 2 min.
- The DAS is widely used but has been criticized for exhibiting a range of scores too narrow to be used effectively in clinical studies.

KLEINKNECHT'S DENTAL FEAR SURVEY (TABLE 20.2)

- The second most commonly used measure of dental anxiety and fear is the dental fear scale (DFS).
- Originally developed as a 27-item scale (**Kleinknecht et al.,** 1973) and subsequently reduced to 20 items as a result of a later factor analytic study.[3]
- The original 27-item scale had 2 items on the avoidance of dentistry, 6 items related to felt physiological arousal, 14 items assessing fear of specific stimuli, a single item concerning overall fear, and 4 items on the reaction to dentistry among family and friends.
- The subsequent 20-item scale retained the 2 items focused on avoidance and the single item tapping overall fear but reduced the number of questions that were related to physiological arousal from 6 to 5, of specific dental items from 14 to 12, and eliminated the items related to dental reactions of friends and family.
- Lacking any explicit direction or rationale for combining the items, researchers have almost universally summed the 20 items to create a single score ranging from 20 to 100.

Table 20.2: Kleinknecht's dental fear survey.

1. Has fear of dental work ever caused you to put off making an appointment?				
1	2	3	4	5
Never	Once or twice	A few times	Often	Nearly every time
2. Has fear of dental work ever caused you to cancel or not appear for an appointment?				
1	2	3	4	5
Never	Once or twice	A few times	Often	Nearly every time
When having dental work done				
3. My muscles become tense....				
1	2	3	4	5
Never	Once or twice	A few times	Often	Nearly every time
4. My breathing rate increases....				
1	2	3	4	5
Never	Once or twice	A few times	Often	Nearly every time
5. I perspire				
1	2	3	4	5
Never	Once or twice	A few times	Often	Nearly every time
6. I feel nauseated and sick to my stomach....				
1	2	3	4	5
Never	Once or twice	A few times	Often	Nearly every time
7. My heart beats faster....				
1	2	3	4	5
Never	Once or twice	A few times	Often	Nearly every time

Contd...

Contd...

	1 None of all	2 A little	3 Some what	4 Much	5 Very much
8. Making an appointment for dentistry....					
9. Approaching the dentist's office....					
10. Sitting in the waiting room...					
11. Being seated in the dental chair....					
12. The smell of the dentist's office...					
13. Seeing the dentist walk in....					
14. Seeing the anesthetic needle...					
15. Feeling the needle injected...					
16. Seeing the drill....					
17. Hearing the drill....					
18. Feeling the vibrations of the drill....					
19. Having your teeth cleaned....					
20. All things considered, how fearful are you of having dental work done?					

(*Source:* © 1978, Kleinknecht, Klepac, Alexander).

- Despite the DFS being widely used as a measure of dental fear, the scale was not developed to produce a single fear score but rather to provide information on the variety of specific stimuli that might elicit fear or avoidance responses as well as the patient's specific and unique response to those stimuli.

CHILDREN'S FEAR SURVEY SCHEDULE

Children's fear survey schedule was developed by **Scherer** and **Nakamura**.[4] It consists of 80 items on a 5-point Likert's scale.

- It has been demonstrated to have high reliability and validity for measuring dental fear in children.
- The cumbersome nature of the questionnaire designed to be filled by the child patient has limited its use despite established validity report.
- The dental subscale of children's fear survey schedule (CFSS-DS) developed by **Cuthbert** and **Melamed**[5] consists of 15 items and each item can be given 5 different scores ranging from "not afraid at all (1)" to "very much afraid (5)".
- The CFSS-DS has a total score range of 15–75 and a score of 38 or more has been associated with clinical dental fear.
- Its reliability and validity have been aptly demonstrated but the dental-specific items comprising the CFSS-DS do not even reflect aspects or components of dental fear *per se*. Rather, they present specific moments of treatment, much as the fear-specific stimuli used in the DFS.
- The cognitive, physiological, behavioral, and emotional aspects of dental fear are not measured, which undermines any claim that the CFSS-DS is a theoretically sound measure of dental fear.

Items:
- Dentists
- Doctors
- Injections (shots)
- Having somebody examine your mouth
- Having to open your mouth
- Having a stranger touch you
- Having somebody look at you
- The dentist drilling
- The sight of the dentist drilling
- The noise of the dentist drilling
- Having somebody put instruments in your mouth
- Choking
- Having to go to the hospital
- People in white uniforms
- Having the nurse clean your teeth

MODIFIED DENTAL ANXIETY SCALE (TABLE 20.3)

- In 1995, Corah's DAS was modified by **Humphris et al.,**[6] to overcome its shortcomings by adding a fifth question relating to local anesthetics as it is a major cause of anxiety for many individuals.

Table 20.3: Modified dental anxiety scale (MDAS).

Can you tell us how anxious you get, if at all, with your dental visit? Please indicate by inserting "X" in the appropriate box

1. If you went to your dentist for treatment tomorrow, how would you feel?
   Not anxious ☐ Slightly anxious ☐ Fairly anxious ☐ Very anxious ☐ Extremely anxious ☐
2. If you were sitting in the waiting room (waiting for treatment), how would you feel?
   Not anxious ☐ Slightly anxious ☐ Fairly anxious ☐ Very anxious ☐ Extremely anxious ☐
3. If you were about to have a tooth drilled, how would you feel?
   Not anxious ☐ Slightly anxious ☐ Fairly anxious ☐ Very anxious ☐ Extremely anxious ☐
4. If you were about to have your teeth scaled and polished, how would you feel?
   Not anxious ☐ Slightly anxious¨ Fairly anxious ☐ Very anxious¨ Extremely anxious¨
5. If you were about to have a local anesthetic injection in your gum, above an upper back tooth, how would you feel?
   Not anxious ☐ Slightly anxious ☐ Fairly anxious ☐ Very anxious ☐ Extremely anxious ☐

Each item scored as follows

Not anxious = 1 Slightly anxious = 2 Fairly anxious = 3

Very anxious = 4 Extremely anxious = 5

Total score is a sum of all 5 items, range 5–25

Cutoff is 19 or above which indicates a highly dentally anxious patient, possibly dentally phobic

- The answer options were also modified ("not anxious," "slightly anxious," "fairly anxious," "very anxious," and "extremely anxious") so that the same options were available for all five questions, and they were rephrased to be in a clearer order of anxiety.

DENTAL ANXIETY QUESTION

- The dental anxiety question (DAQ) is a single-item construct.
- "Are you afraid of going to the dentist?" It has four possible responses: "no," "a little," "yes, quite," and "yes, very." These responses are scored from 1 to 4 in the direction of increasing anxiety.
- This question also has been used with a 5-point response scale.
- The DAQ correlates well with Corah's DAS in studies of adult and child populations.
- Single item inventories have been regarded with scepticism by scale developers because they do not provide opportunities to control for response-set bias (such as the tendency to give responses that the participant believes are "correct"), and because they do not allow for the isolation of components of multidimensional constructs.
- However, for some purposes, such as screening people who are likely to be highly anxious about dental treatment, it is a useful and brief tool, although it has a tendency to overestimate the prevalence of severe dental anxiety.

STATE-TRAIT ANXIETY INVENTORY

- In 1983, **Spielberger** developed the state-trait anxiety inventory (STAI), which comprises 40 questions divided into 2 sections to distinguish between 2 different types of anxiety.
- State anxiety is defined as the anxiety state we experience when something causes us to feel appropriately and temporarily anxious and this anxiety then retreats until we feel "normal" again.
- Trait anxiety is defined as the "pre-set" level of anxiety experienced by an individual who has a tendency to be more anxious, to react less appropriately to anxiety provoking stimuli.
- The two sections differ in the item wording, the response format, and the instructions on how to respond. To control the response sets, half of the questions are formulated in terms of positive emotions and the others state negative emotions. The scaling of the positively formulated questions is then reversed when computing the total score.
- Although the STAI was not specifically designed for use in dentistry, it is commonly used and has been proven to significant have positive correlation with CDAS.

State-trait anxiety inventory—state

How do you feel right now, at this moment?

Answers: 1—not at all; 2—somewhat; 3—moderate; 4—very much

1. I feel calm
2. I feel secure
3. I am tense
4. I feel strained
5. I feel at ease
6. I feel upset
7. I am presently worrying over misfortunes
8. I feel satisfied
9. I feel frightened
10. I feel comfortable
11. I feel self-confident
12. I feel nervous
13. I am jittery
14. I feel indecisive
15. I am relaxed
16. I feel content
17. I am worried
18. I feel confused
19. I feel steady
20. I feel pleasant

State-trait anxiety inventory—trait

How do you generally feel?

Answers: 1—not at all; 2—somewhat; 3—moderate; 4—very much

21. I feel pleasant
22. I feel nervous and restless
23. I feel satisfied with myself
24. I wish I could be as happy as others seem to be
25. I feel like a failure
26. I feel rested
27. I am *calm, cool, and collected*
28. I feel that difficulties are piling up so that I cannot overcome them
29. I worry too much over something that really does not matter
30. I am happy
31. I have disturbing thoughts
32. I lack self-confidence
33. I feel secure
34. I make decisions easily
35. I feel inadequate
36. I am content
37. Some unimportant thought runs through my mind and bothers me
38. I take disappointments so keenly that I cannot put them out of my mind
39. I am a steady person
40. I get in a state of tension or turmoil over my recent concerns and interests

VENHAM PICTURE TEST

- This scale consists of a series of eight paired drawings of a child **(Fig. 20.1)**.
- Each pair consists of a child in a nonfearful pose and a fearful pose (e.g., running away).

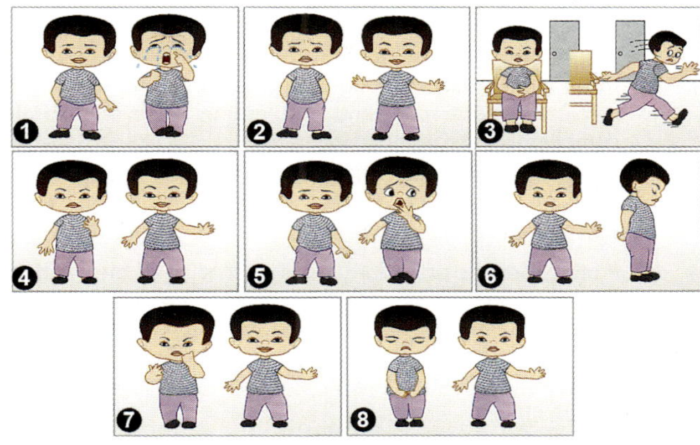

Fig. 20.1: Venham picture test.

- The respondent is asked to indicate, for each pair, which picture more accurately reflects his or her feelings at the time.
- Scores are determined by summing the number of instances in which the child selects the high-fear stimulus.

VENHAM'S ANXIETY SCALE (TABLE 20.4)

- **Venham et al.**,[7] developed two scales to evaluate the child's response to dental treatment, an anxiety rating scale and an uncooperative behavior rating scale.
- Each is a 6-point scale, with scale points anchored in objective, specific, and readily observable behavior.

Table 20.4: Venham's anxiety scale.

Anxiety rating scale	
0.	Relaxed, smiling, willing, and able to converse
1.	Uneasy, concerned. During stressful procedure may protest briefly and quietly to indicate discomfort. Hands remain down or partially raised to signal discomfort. Child willing and able to interpret experience as requested. Tense facial expression may have tears in eyes
2.	Child appears scared. Tone of voice, question, and answers reflect anxiety. During stressful procedure, verbal protest, (quiet) crying, hands tense and raised (not interfering much—may touch dentist's hand or instrument, but not pull of it). Child interprets situation with reasonable accuracy and continues to work to cope with his/her anxiety
3.	Shows reluctance to enter situation, difficulty in correctly assessing situational threat. Pronounced verbal protest, crying. Using hands to try to stop procedure. Protest out of proportion to threat. Copes with situation with great reluctance
4.	Anxiety interferes with ability to assess situation. General crying not related to treatment. More prominent body movement. Child can be reached through verbal communication, and eventually with reluctance and great effort, he or she begins the work of coping with the threat
5.	Child out of contact with the reality of the threat. General loud crying, unable to listen to verbal communication, makes no effort to cope with threat. Actively involved in escape behavior. Physical restraint required
Behavior rating scale	
0.	Total cooperation, best possible work conditions, no crying or physical protest
1.	Mild, soft verbal protest or (quiet) crying as a signal of discomfort but does not obstruct progress. Appropriate behavior for procedure, i.e., slight start at injection, "ow" during drilling if hurting etc.
2.	Protest more prominent. Both crying and hand signals. May move head around making it hard to administer treatment. Protest more distracting and troublesome. However, child still complies with request to cooperate
3.	Protest presents real problem to dentist. Complies with demands reluctantly, requiring extra effort by dentist. Body movement
4.	Protest disrupts procedure, requires that all of the dentist's attention be directed toward the child's behavior. Compliance eventually achieved after considerable effort by dentist, but without much actual physical restraint (may require holding child's hands or the like to start). More prominent body movement
5.	General protest, no compliance or cooperation. Physical restraint is required

- This is one of the most reliable indicators of observed anxiety and has been used predominantly in anxiety assessment protocols.

FACIAL IMAGE SCALE (FIG. 20.2)

- Facial image scale (FIS) has a row of five faces ranging from very happy to very unhappy.
- Original nine face facial affective scale was designed by **McGrath et al.**, (1996) to evaluate pain and discomfort (emotional distress) in children.
- Children are asked to point at which face they felt most like at the moment.
- The face is scored by giving a value of one for the most positive face and five for the most negative face.
- Faces four and five indicate high dental anxiety.

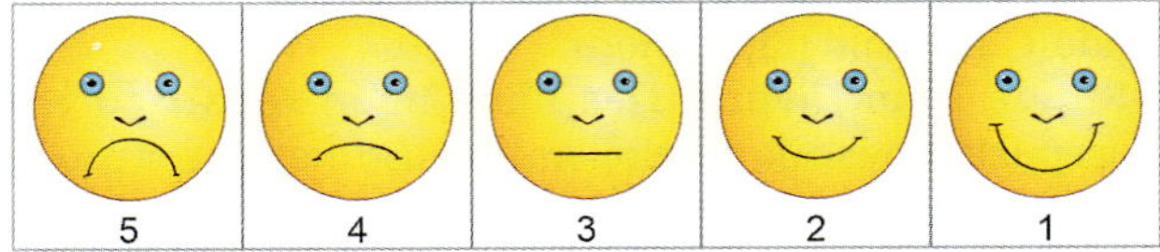

Fig. 20.2: Facial image scale with image scores.

SMILEY FACES PROGRAM

- **Buchanan**,[8] using multimedia tool book, developed an interactive computerized version of the FIS and this windows program was entitled Smiley Faces.
- This is a fully computerized scale where the child must select from a range of seven facial expressions indicating how they feel. It is based on the modified dental anxiety scale (MDAS) and consists of five questions relevant to a child's experience in the dental practice environment.
- The Smiley Faces Program (SFP) is a four-item computerized DAS.
- The faces describe the child's response to a range of dental stimuli ranging from going to the dentist to having an injection.
- The questions appear on the computer screen for a matter of seconds and then the child is asked to replace the neutral face with one of seven faces which describes how they feel about the dental item. The SFP has the psychometric properties as well as the potential to engage dentally anxious children in a novel and innovative way while assessing their dental anxiety.

ANXIETY THERMOMETER

This is an image of a thermometer where the respondent selects a point on the thermometer to rate anxiety, where no anxiety and 10 = extreme anxiety **(Fig. 20.3)**.

The treatment of the dentally anxious or phobic individual can turn out to be most gratifying to a dental staff. These patients desperately need comprehensive dental care with an emphasis on their special needs and become most appreciative of the treatment provided by sensitive caregivers. A wide range of methodological approaches and techniques, especially the use of questionnaires and behavioral measures, are available to assess the fear and anxiety of individuals related to dental treatment. It is important that such psychometric measures are reliable, valid, and applicable to the population toward which they are aimed. These techniques can be used by the

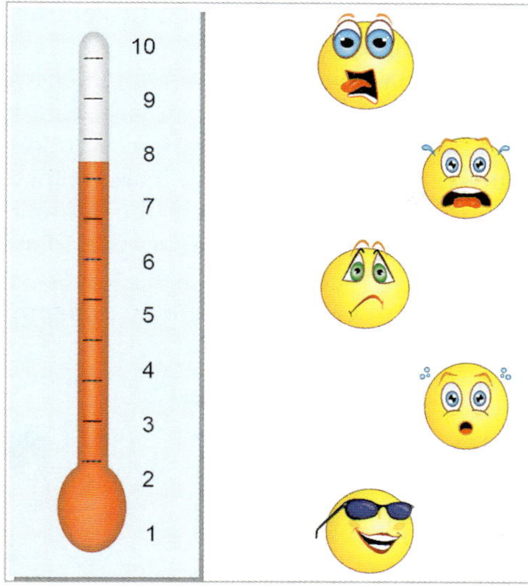

Fig. 20.3: My fear thermometer.

dentist in an individual setting to assess the level of dental anxiety and fear and also to analyze the effectiveness of any counseling program directed toward behavior modification.

RMS-PICTURE SCALE

Raghavendra, Madhuri, and Sujata Pictorial Scale (RMS-PS) is an innovative scale for the of child's dental anxiety assessment given in 2015 by **Raghvendra Shetty** et al.[9] It comprises a row of five faces from very happy to unhappy faces. Two separate sets of photographs were used for boys and girls, to maximize its acceptability among both the genders **(Fig. 20.4)**. The children will be asked to choose the face they can identify themselves at that moment. The scale will be scored by giving a value of one to very happy and five to the very unhappy face. The RMS-PS has many advantages such as:

- Attractive and colorful for children with ease of understanding.
- Needs a short time to complete the scale.
- Provides immediate feedback about the child's anxiety to the dental team, in the waiting room and post-treatment. It can also be used to get the feedback in subsequent visits, so that the appropriate behavior guidance can be used.

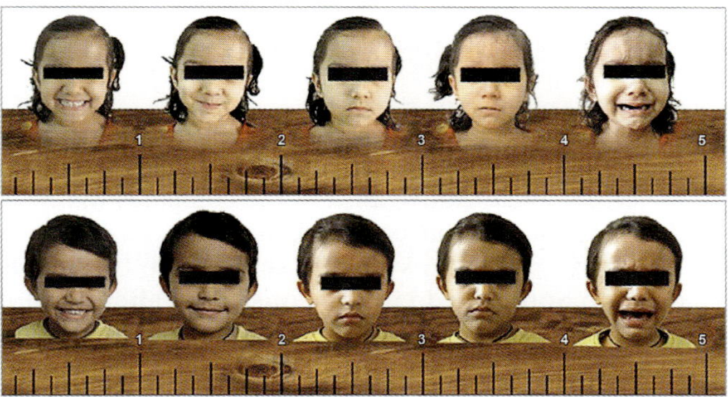

Fig. 20.4: RMS Pictorial Scale (RMS-PS) for girls (top) and boys (bottom). (*Source:* Shetty R M, Khandelwal M, Rath S. RMS Pictorial Scale (RMS-PS): An innovative scale for the assessment of child's dental anxiety. J Indian Soc Pedod Prev Dent. 2015;33:48-52).

- With the original color photographs in RMS-PS, the children can identify themselves better compared to black and white and cartoon figures used in other scales.

ANIMATED EMOJI SCALE

- Animated emoji scale (AES), was designed by **Jyothsna V Setty** (2017) using motion emoticons/animojis.[10]
- This was based on the interest and attraction of today's generation towards multimedia, and their preference of motion pictures on electronic devices rather than still cartoons on paper.
- The AES has five graphic interchange formats of animated emoji faces showing different feelings ranging from very happy/laughing to very unhappy/sad and crying (most positive to most negative feelings). The child can be asked to choose one of these animated emojis on the electronic display (mobile screens, tabs, laptops, computer screens, television screens, etc) that best matched their feelings at that moment.
- The scale has scores from 1 (very happy emoji) to 5 (very unhappy emoji) as shown in **Figure 20.5**.

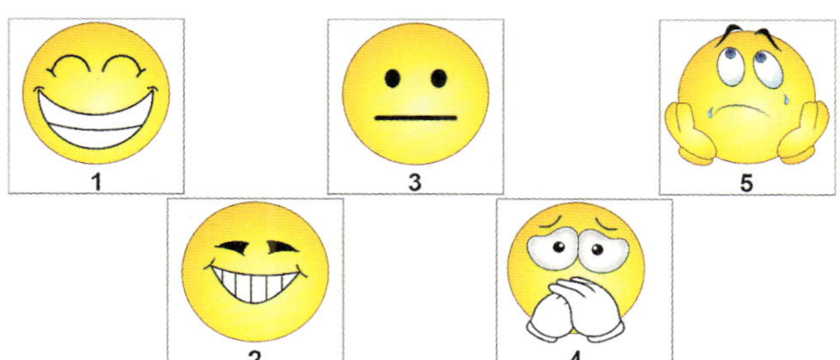

Fig. 20.5: Five animated emoji faces in AES.

Advantages of AES

- It is very attractive.
- Easy for children to relate with feelings.
- Less time consuming.
- Universal (no languages or questionnaires are used)
- Common to both sexes, and offers immediate scoring of dental anxiety, thus helping the dental team to use appropriate behavior management modalities for efficient and effective dental treatment.

FEAR OF DENTAL PAIN QUESTIONNAIRE

- The original questionnaire consists of 18 items and assesses fear of pain associated with a variety of dental procedures.
- Each item is answered on a rating of 1 (no fear) to 5 (extreme fear), resulting in a possible total score of 18–90.

Item number	Translation item
1.	Receiving an anesthetic in the mouth
2.	Having some gum burned away
3.	The dentist's hook tugging at a filling
4.	Having a lump in the mouth
5.	The filling of a molar
6.	Receiving root canal treatment

7.	Having a tooth pulled
8.	A cold sensation in the mouth close to a cavity
9.	An incision in the gums
10.	An old filling that's being removed
11.	Being drilled in the jawbone
12.	Being drilled in a tooth
13.	A cavity that's being explored with the dentist's hook
14.	Receiving an injection in the roof of the mouth
15.	Braces that are being tightened
16.	Having a wisdom tooth extracted
17.	A severe toothache
18.	A cavity that's being excavated with a rough drill

FEAR ASSESSMENT PICTURE SCALE

- This is used in 6-8 year old children.
- The FAPS was designed by taking a part of Klingberg's children dental fear picture test (CDFP) pointing picture. The FAPS was designed by taking a part of Klingberg's CDFP pointing picture and the images were drawn in frontal aspects so that the expressions can be seen. A girl or a boy cartoon in the dental chair was drawn both these figures were paired with "not fearful" and "fearful" facial expression **(Fig. 20.6)**. In "not fearful" cartoon the expressions were calm, and relaxed while in "fearful" there was change in expressions such as increased eye white area and facial grimace. [11]

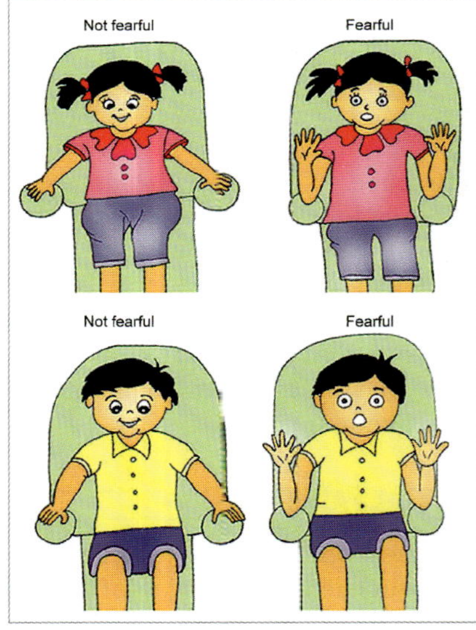

Fig. 20.6: Figures of FAPS. (*Source:* Tiwari N, Tiwari S, Thakur R, Agrawal N, Shashikiran ND, Singla S. Evaluation of treatment related fear using a newly developed fear scale for children: "Fear assessment picture scale" and its association with physiological response. Contemp Clin Dent. 2015;6:327-31).

CHOTTA BHEEM–CHUTKI SCALE

- This is a newly designed scale developed in the Department of Pedodontics, Sri Guru Ram Das Institute of Dental Sciences and Research, Amritsar.[12]
- This scale comprises two separate cards; one for boys and the other for girls.
- For boys, Chotta Bheem cartoon character was chosen to depict various emotions, and for girls, Chutki cartoon character was chosen to depict various emotions.
- Each card consists of a series of six figures depicting happy to unhappy and running emotion by the cartoon character. Children were asked to choose the face they identified with at that instant. To record on the scale, a score of one was assigned to a happy face and six to an unhappy face and running **(Fig. 20.7)**.

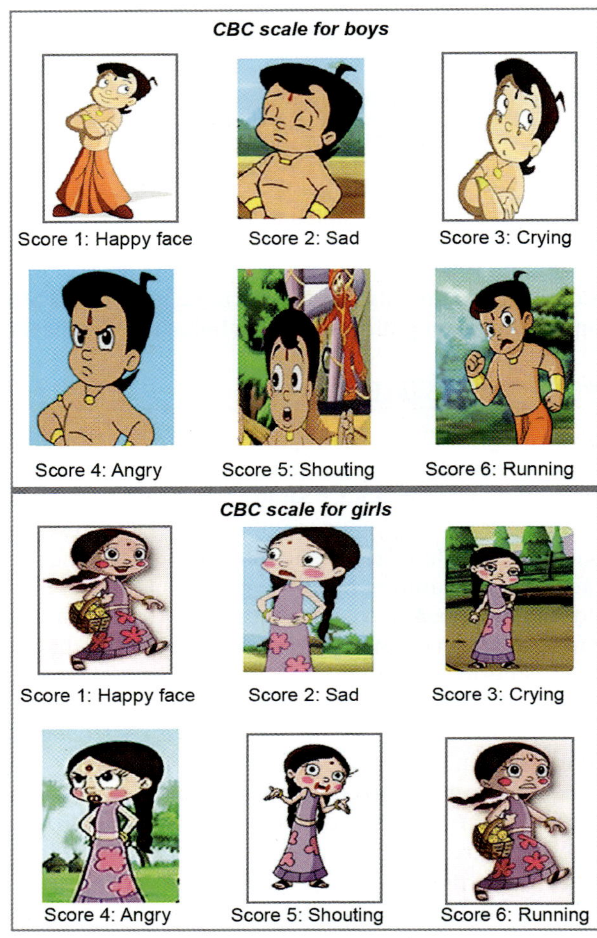

Fig. 20.7: Depictive figures of CBC scale. (*Source:* Sadana G, Grover R, Mehra M, Gupta S, Kaur J, Sadana S. A novel Chotta Bheem–Chutki scale for dental anxiety determination in children. Journal of International Society of Preventive and Community Dentistry; 2016).

DAVE'S HAND GESTURE SCALE

- Dave's hand gesture scale is a useful and valid method for measuring preoperative anxiety and compares well with the visual analog scale for anxiety.[13]
- The main objectives of this scale were to define, develop and provide initial construct validation for an updated and more refined measure of anxiety in children.
- Dave's hand gesture scale for anxiety measurement appears to hold promise as a reliable and potentially valid measure for use in children of all age groups **(Fig. 20.8)**.

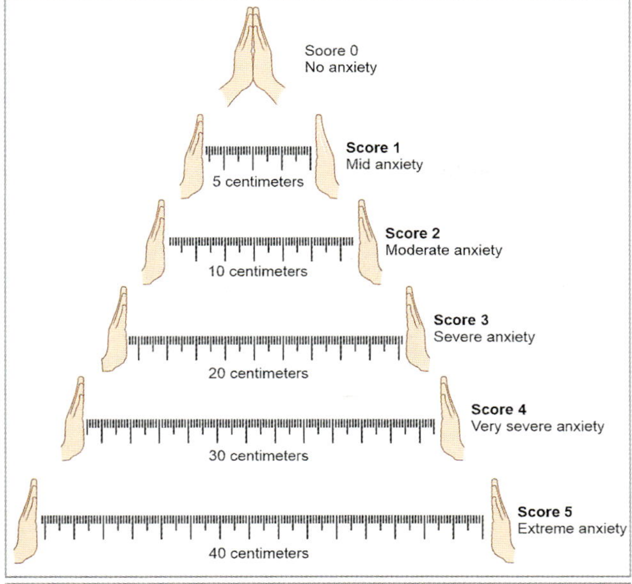

Hand gesture	DHG scale score	VAS score	Scoring criteria
Hand are joined	0	0	No anxiety
Hands 5 cm apart	1	2	Mild anxiety
Hands 10 cm apart	2	4	Moderate anxiety
Hands 20 cm apart	3	6	Severe anxiety
Hands 30 cm apart	4	8	Very severe anxiety
Hands 40 cm apart	5	10	Extreme anxiety

VAS: Visual Analog Scale

Fig. 20.8: Depicitve figures of DHG scale. (*Source:* Dave BH, Thaker BA, Inderchand B. Dental anxiety among 4-7-year-old children measured by hand gestures: A new modified visual analog scale (Dave's hand gesture scale). J Integr Health Sci. 2021;9:65-9).

POINTS TO REMEMBER

- Anxiety is evaluated by two means, either observation of the behavior or self-report.
- Commonly used anxiety scales are Corah's DAS, MDAS, Kleinknecht's dental fear survey (DFS), dental fear assessment scale (DFAS), CFSS-DS, modified child dental anxiety scale (MCDAS), Frankl behavior rating scale (FBRS), Venham picture scale (VPS), Venham anxiety scale (VAS), and FIS.
- Corah's DAS is the most frequent used scale.
- The CFSS-DS developed by Cuthbert and Melamed is best for usage in children.
- VAS is most effective in observational anxiety assessment.
- Venham picture test and FIS are two reliable picture tests for anxiety measurement in children.
- Newer methods for anxiety assessment include SFP and anxiety thermometer.

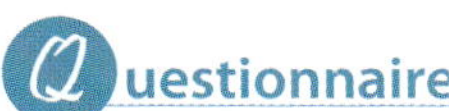

Questionnaire

1. Enumerate the fear and anxiety scales used in children.
2. Discuss Corah's dental anxiety scale.
3. Explain children's fear survey schedule.
4. What is facial image scale?
5. Explain the anxiety assessment parameters proposed by Venham.
6. What is Smiley Faces Program?

REFERENCES

1. Corah NL. Development of a dental anxiety scale. J Dent Res. 1969;48:596.
2. Stouthard MEA, Mellenbergh GJ, Hoogstraten J. Assessment of dental anxiety: a facet approach. Anxiety Stress Coping. 1993;6:89-105.
3. Kleinknecht R, Thorndike RM, McGlynn FD, et al. Factor analysis of the dental fear survey with cross-validation. JADA. 1984;108:59-61.
4. Scherer MW, Nakamura CY. A fear survey schedule for children. Behav Res Ther. 1968;6:173-82.
5. Cuthbert ML, Melamed BG. A screening device: children at risk of dental fear and management problems. ASDC J Dent Child. 1982;49:432-6.
6. Humphris GM, Morrisson T, Lindsay S. The modified dental anxiety scale: validation and United Kingdom norms. Community Dent Health. 1995;12:143-50.
7. Venham, et al. Interval ratings scales for children's dental anxiety and uncooperative behavior. Pediatr Dent. 1980;2:195-202.
8. Buchanan H. Assessing dental anxiety in children: the Revised Smiley Faces Program. Child Care Health Dev. 2010;36:534-8.
9. Shetty R M, Khandelwal M, Rath S. RMS Pictorial Scale (RMS-PS): An innovative scale for the assessment of child's dental anxiety. J Indian Soc Pedod Prev Dent. 2015;33:48-52.
10. Jyothsna V Setty, Ila Srinivasan, Sreeraksha Radhakrishna, Anjana M Melwani, Murali Krishna DR. Use of an animated emoji scale as a novel tool for anxiety assessment in children.J Dent Anesth Pain Med. 2019;19(4):227-33.
11. Tiwari N, Tiwari S, Thakur R, Agrawal N, Shashikiran ND, Singla S. Evaluation of treatment related fear using a newly developed fear scale for children: "Fear assessment picture scale" and its association with physiological response. Contemp Clin Dent. 2015;6:327-31.
12. Sadana G, Grover R, Mehra M, Gupta S, Kaur J, Sadana S. A novel Chotta Bheem-Chutki scale for dental anxiety determination in children. Journal of International Society of Preventive and Community Dentistry; 2016.
13. Dave BH, Thaker BA, Inderchand B. Dental anxiety among 4-7-year-old children measured by hand gestures: A new modified visual analog scale (Dave's hand gesture scale). J Integr Health Sci 2021;9:65-9.

FURTHER READING

1. Newton JT. Anxiety and pain measures in dentistry: a guide to their quality and application. JADA. 2000;131:1449-57.
2. Tiwari S, Kulkarni P, Agrawal N, Mali S, Kale S, Jaiswal N. Dental Anxiety Scales Used in Pediatric Dentistry: A Systematic Review and Meta-analysis. The Journal of Contemporary Dental Practice. 2022;22(11):1338-45.

CHAPTER

Nonpharmacologic Behavior Management

Nikhil Marwah, Ravi GR, Sharath Asokan, Priyanka Lekhwani

Chapter Outline

Although the operative dentistry may be perfect, the appointment is a failure, if the child departs in tears.

—Mc Elroy (1895)

Behavior is the manner in which a person acts, behaves or performs. Behavior management is not just the application of individual technique formulated to deal with individuals but rather is a comprehensive methodology meant to build a relationship between patient and dental professional. Since childhood experience plays an important role in forming the adult behavior, proper behavior management from the early stages will help in the development of a proper oral health attitude among individuals throughout life. Most children willingly accept dental treatment when approached in a positive, supportive manner, but for those who exhibit considerable anxiety or problematic behaviors, child behavior management requires skills in expressive communication, empathetic listening, and coaching. Treatment of the fearful and anxious or physically resistive child is a formidable task. Successful and efficient management of those children requires considerable time, effort, and expertise from the dental practitioner. Thus, behavioral management of children in clinics is an integral part of pediatric dentistry.

Although the aim of behavior management is to instill a positive dental attitude and create a long-term interest on the patient's part so as to facilitate ongoing prevention and improved dental health in the future, none of the methods discussed in this chapter are applicable in all situations. The appropriate management technique(s) should be chosen based on the individual child's requirements and the individual dentist's experience and expertise.

DEFINITIONS

- **Behavior** *is any activity that can be observed, recorded, and measured. It is an observable act or any change in the functioning of an organism.*
- **Behavior management** *is the means by which the dental health team effectively and efficiently performs dental treatment for a child and thereby, instills a positive dental attitude.* ***—Wright (1975)***
- **Behavior modification** *is defined as the attempt to alter human behavior and emotion in a beneficial manner and in accordance with the laws of learning.* ***—Eysenck (1964)***
- **Behavior shaping** *is the procedure, which slowly develops behavior by reinforcing a successive approximation of the*

desired behavior until the desired behavior comes into being. For example, desensitization, tell-show-do (TSD), modeling, distraction, contingency management.

- **Behavior guidance** *is a continuum of individualized interaction involving the dentist, and patient directed toward communication and education "which ultimately builds trust and allays fear and anxiety".*
- **Behavioral pedodontics** *is the study of science that helps to understand development of fear, anxiety, and associated acts as it applies to the child in the dental situation.*

"Behavior management" has been the conventional term that states the effort by families, caregivers, therapists, and also dentists to control troublesome behaviors of people with special needs during daily activities or clinical treatment. But it has been understood that no one likes to be managed and that such terminology degrades the individual. Every human grows, learns, and benefits from many sources of support and guidance throughout the life in order to function in social and family settings. Thus, the American Academy of Pediatric Dentistry (AAPD) has recently changed its terminology from "behavior management" to "behavioral guidance".

Objectives of behavior management
Snowder (1980)

- To establish effective communication with child and parent
- Gain child and parent confidence for dental treatment
- Teach child positive aspect of preventive dental care
- Provide a comfortable, relaxing environment to the child

BEHAVIORAL CHARACTERISTICS

University of Washington Nursing School and Forrester have developed a series of word picture of various ages, which help us determine the different behavioral patterns of children at different ages **(Tables 21.1 to 21.4)**.

Table 21.1: Word picture of a 2-year old.

Emotional development	*Mental development*	*Motor development*
• Self-centered	• Investigative—touch, taste	• Whole body action
• Cannot share	• One thing at a time	• Marks time
• Gives up readily	• Cannot recognize	• Climbs onto stairs
• Clings to familiar people	• Remembers order of routine	• Push-pull, pokes
• People are as inanimate objects	• Attention span 1–5 min	• Awkward with small objects
• Watches others	• Irresponsible	• Rotates, fits object
• Dependent on routines	• Concepts of family only	• Unsteady
• Contacts by pushing and shoving	• Needs own name used	• Wide stance, body forward
• Easily distracted	• Matches words with objects	• Depends on adult for dressing
• Easily frustrated	• One/two word sentences	• Hugs, topples
• Complete dependence on adults	• May stutter	
	• Wide vocabulary range 5–200 words	

Table 21.2: Word picture of a 3-year old.

Emotional development	*Mental development*	*Motor development*
• Highly imitative of adults	• Lively imagination	• Well-balanced body
• Jealous	• Makes simple choice	• Rides a tricycle
• Asserts independence often	• Very talkative regardless of a listener	• Walks erect
• Exuberant—very talkative	• Alert, excited, curious	• Alternates feet in stair climbing
• Beginning parallel play	• Moves and talks at the same time	• Enjoys rhythm
• Lively humor (mixed identities, incongruities)	• Puts words into action	• Nimble on feet
• Beginning to share	• Tries new words	• Some finger control in handling of small objects
• Often gets frustrated	• Talks about imaginary situations	• Can carry liquids
• Enjoys contacts	• Attention span 4–8 min	
• Wants to please adults	• Vocabulary 800–900 words	
• Goes after what he wants	• Names and matches simple colors	
	• Difficulty in combining two activities	

Table 21.3: Word picture of a 4-year old.

Emotional development	*Mental development*	*Motor development*
• Dominates—bossy, boastful	• Can do two things at once	• A longer, leaner body built
• Hits, grabs for what he wants	• Likes variety of materials	• Throws large ball, kicks with some accuracy
• Explosive; destructive	• Accepts changes with preparation	• Vigorous, dynamic
• Loyalties shift frequently	• Judges which of two is bigger	• Dresses self-except for back buttons, bow ties
• Cooperative play (with 2 or 3)	• Confuses fact and fancy	• Cannot set limits—active until exhausted
• Easily over stimulated, excitable, goes out of bounds	• Concepts of life and death	• Accurate, but rash in body movements
• Assertive	• *Attention span:* 8–12 min	• Sureness and control in finger hand activities
• Impatient and intolerant in large groups	• Produces recognizable forms	• Can jump about own height
• A show-off, cocky, noisy	• Calls people names	• Lands upright
• Insists on what he wants	• Constructive	
• Can jump about own height	• Enjoys silly words, rhymed without meaning	
• Loves to tease, to outwit	• Dynamic intellectual drive	
• Terrific humor, nonsense loving, silly	• Understands simple reasons for thing	
	• Able to talk to solve conflicts	
	• Age conscious and birthday conscious	
	• Comments, criticizes, compares	
	• Vocabulary about 1,500 words	

Table 21.4: Word picture of a 5-year old.

Emotional development	*Mental development*	*Motor development*
• Becoming poised, self-confident • Harbors wounded feelings • Copies adult behavior—acts grown up • Likes companionship with adults • Plays in groups of 2–5 children • Has to be right • Enjoys group play, circle games • Talks about home, reveals family secrets • Sensitive of ridicule • Conscious of sex differences of playmates, sex play • Accepts and respects authority, will ask permission • Growing competitiveness • Silly, giggling • May get high, wide, wild • Enjoys pointless riddles and jokes	• Curious about everything • *Attention span:* 12–28 minutes • Seeks information on how and why • Ready for short trips into community • Defines familiar objects in terms of their use • Knows name and address • Enjoys making up songs, dictating own stories • Self-centered in thinking • Uses complete sentences readily • Counts ten objects • Likes to display his new knowledge and skills • Uses big words • Makes a plan before starting project • Vocabulary—about 2,200 words	• Enjoys activities requiring hand skills • Adult like posture in throwing and catching ball • Draws a recognizable man • Able to skip on both feet • Learning how to tie a bowknot • Skill and accuracy with simple tools • Surging physical drives • Can sit still for brief periods • Likes dancing—rhythmic, graceful • Enjoys jumping, running, stunting

FACTORS INFLUENCING CHILD'S BEHAVIOR IN DENTAL OFFICE

Wright[1] summarized the following factors:
- Medical history
- Maternal anxiety
- Family and peer influence
- Dental office environment
- Growth and development
- Personal factors
- Environmental factors
- Other variables.

Medical History

When studying a child's medical experience, it is the emotional quality of past visits rather than the number of visits to the physician that is significant. If the patient views a physician favorably, then the child is likely to have less apprehension when visiting the dentist. Fears can thus be transferred from one situation to another; hence preformed attitude concerning health care can be of prime importance.

Maternal Anxiety

In past years, it has been customary for mothers more often than fathers to accompany children on a visit to the dentist; therefore, maternal anxiety was considered important. Highly anxious mother had a negative influence on the child.

Family and Peer Influence

Socioeconomic status of the family directly affects child's attitude toward the values of the dental health process. Those of low socioeconomic class, below average education, have a tendency to attend dental needs when symptom dictates. These families harbor anxiety from dental treatment and these children take on these fear and tend to be less cooperative. On the other hand if financial and educational means are ample, families value good dental health easily established in preventive program.

Dental Office Environment

Bohuslov (1970) stated that psychological preparation of the child is based on the physical environment. Since the child may enter the dental office with some fear, the first objective of the dentist should be to put the child at his ease and make him realize that his experience is not unusual. Finn summarized the following factors related to the dental office which influence child's behavior:
- Waiting room should be made in respect to home environment
- Make the reception room comfortable, so that the room is not foreign to them
- Have library with books for children of all ages
- Simple but sturdy toys must be kept to amuse very small children
- A handy record player with well-chosen records will provide comfort for a frightened child
- Appointment cards and announcements should be made attractive to children
- A sketch of some cartoon on card helps
- Operating room may be made more appealing to the child if a few pictures on the wall are suggestive of child at play. A portrait of a carefree and laughing child is good
- Have an assistant skilled in making animals object out of cotton rolls
- Try to avoid the child patient, seeing anybody expressing in pain or sight of blood on others.

Growth and Development

A child's chronological age plays a significant role in growth and developmental patterns. Younger the child, more atypical will be the response. The intellectual age of 3 years signifies a maturational readiness to accept dental treatment. Different age groups will show different behavior patterns as explained in the word picture charts.

Fundamentals of behavior management
- Team attitude
- Organization
- Positive approach
- Truthfulness
- Tolerance
- Flexibility

Personal Factors

Temperament and general fearfulness are some of the personal characters which are known to influence the behavior of the child. Although these are to influence the child's behavior the most, personal characters are also affected by the environmental factors.

Environmental Factors

Various environmental factors like age of the child, socioeconomic status, family situation, frequent exposure to invasive medical care, past experience of operative dental care, etc., have been identified to influence the child's behavior. However, parental dental fear has been noted to be the most influencing factor amongst all environmental factors.

Other Variables

Stephen Wei explained that many other variables affect the child in dental office like socioeconomic status, culture, sex, sibling relation, number of children, presence of parent, and attitude of dentist.

Scientific research pertaining to child behavior in dental office

- According to **Klingberg L** and **Raadal M**, dental fear and behavior are multifactorial and can be broadly classified into personal characters, environmental factors, or situational factors
- **Locker** (1996), **Tenberge** (2001), and **Versloot** (2009) concluded that past medical and dental experiences are the most prominent ofall the factors
- **Milgrom** (1997) found out that fear of injections (belonephobia) is the major cause for fear and uncooperative behavior in children
- **Lee** (2008) found out that younger children exhibit more dental fear than elder. In addition, invasive and painful experience during first dental visit contributed significantly for the disruptive behavior in children
- According to **Davey** (1989), traumatic experiences during first dental visit are more likely to cause to dental anxiety in children
- **Rachman S** (1977) in his conditioning theory of fear suggested that objective experiences like previous visit to pediatrician or experience during first dental visit play a greater role than subjective experiences due to siblings and child rearing practices in the family
- **Klingberg**[2] (2007) observed cooperative children were fearful and uncooperative children were nonfearful. This indicated that the children with behavior management issues need not always be fearful
- **Kyritsi** (2009) studied the behavior of Greek children and suggested that behavior of the child was not related to gender of the child but related to age of child. Children with siblings or in joint families are known to learn patience, tolerance and tend to be cooperative. However, in nuclear families, parents play a major role in shaping the behavior
- **Gao**[3] (2013) studied dental fear and anxiety in children and adolescents and concluded that DFA has multifaceted manifestations, impacts, and origins; some of the themes only become apparent when using internet social media like YouTube
- **Sharath Asokan**[4] (2014) used a ten-point scale to observe the overt and subtle behavioral characteristics of a child in the waiting room to predict the behavior during dental treatment.

ROLE OF DENTIST IN CHILD'S BEHAVIOR

- **Appearance of dental office:**
  - Make one corner of waiting room for the child only where he can play, sit, and read.
  - Record player playing soothing music to ease fear.
  - Appointment cards to be appealing to the child.
  - Try to avoid children during adult treatment and vice versa.
  - Operating room should be appealing to the child having cartoon and pictures on walls.
- **Personality of dentist:** Should be impressive.
- **Time and length of appointment:** Better to have morning appointments and also prevent appointments during the child's sleeping, playing, or eating time. Duration should be short and can last for a maximum of 20–30 minutes.
- **Dentist's skill and speed:** Dentist should be skilled or he will lose the child's confidence.
- **Dentist's conversation:** Keep talking to the child to gain his confidence. Use simple words and answer all questions.
- **Attention to patient:** Treat the patient as he is the only one seen during that day. Never leave him alone in chair and do not change rooms as all this increases anxiety.
- **Use of simple words:** Do not use fear promoting words like needle, injection.
- **Reasonableness of dentist:** Be realistic and reasonable. Try to put yourself in the child's place and see why he behaves in this particular way. Give the child an opportunity to participate in procedure.
- **Use of admiration, subtle flattering, praise, and reward:** Enforces the behavior for future.
- **Self-control of dentist:** Dentist should never lose his temper. It is a mark of defeat and indication to child that he has succeeded in undermining your dignity.

MATERNAL INFLUENCE ON CHILDREN'S BEHAVIOR IN DENTAL SITUATION

The parent-child relationship was termed as "one-tailed" by **Bell** because parental characteristics have a unilateral influence on the developing child. Most of the characters of the child like behavior, personality, anxiety, and reaction to stress are directly influenced by the parent's characters. Both mother and the father play an important role in child's psychologic development, but more emphasis is placed on mother. This is because mother generally has intimate contact with the child since prenatal period. The mother-child relationship falls into two broad categories: (1) autonomy vs control, (2) hostility vs love. Mothers either have control over the child's behavior or they give the child freedom/autonomy. The other category includes loving/caring or hostile mothers.

Maternal attitude summarized by Bayley and Schaefer

Maternal attitude	*Features*	*Child's behavior*
Overprotective	• Mother gives excessive care for child in terms of feeding, dressing, bathing and these conditions continue past the usual age • Constantly involved with child's daily social activities and may not allow him to participate in risk-involving games • Excessive concern about routine dental condition • Infantilizes the child, retards normal psychological maturation • Submissive child, shy • Aggressive child, demanding and expects constant attention and service • Displays temper tantrums • He will not be anxious of new environment *Factors for this attitude:* » Miscarriages » Long delay in conception may be due to family financial condition/sterility » Death of other sibling » Serious illness/handicapped child	Submissive, shy, anxious
Overindulgence	• May be associated with overprotective or dominant natural trait • These parents give child whatever he might want, as far as financially possible including toys, candy, and clothes • Relative such as grandparents are also overindulgent • Such child is spoiled and is accustomed to getting his own way • His emotional development is impeded, keeping him in infantile dependent state in which crying and temper tantrums will produce the behavior from his parents that he demands • He is usually incapable of amusing himself and he keeps the adults around him busy devising diversion for him	Aggressive, spoilt, demanding, displays temper tantrums
Under affectionate	• May vary from mild detachment to indifference to neglect • Mother becomes less emotionally supportive of her child due to her outside interests, employment, or because the child is unwanted • Child is well behaved and appears to be well adjusted • They are unsure of decision-making capacity • Since they have not experienced love and affection at home, emotional contact with them is difficult • Dentist may find that they cry easily and are shy and unable or unwilling to cooperate • They respond well to a dentist who gives them emotional support and affection	Usually well behaved but may be unable to cooperate, may cry easily
Rejecting	• Acceptance vs. rejection is one of the most significant of family influences • Maternal rejection may arrive under any circumstance in which a child is unwanted • Rejection is usually overt • Mother's behavior is characterized by neglect of the child, severe punishment, nagging, and resistance to spending time and money on the child • He may show extreme anxiety and be aggressive, overactive, and disobedient • He will usually resort to any behavior to gain attention • Abuse and neglect can be both physical and emotional	Aggressive, overactive, disobedient
Authoritarian	• The authoritarian parent chooses technique for controlling child's behavior that may be termed non-love oriented • Discipline often takes the form of physical punishment or verbal ridicule • The authoritarian mother will insist that the child conform to her set of norms and will expend much effort to train child along those lines • The authoritarian mother is usually the product of an authoritarian upbringing • Child to authoritarian control is submissive coupled with resentment and evasion • Where the child will not directly disobey a command, he has heightened avoidance gradient	Evasive

Research regarding maternal influence on behavior

- **Hane**[5] (2008) suggested that the function of maternal behavior was different across the two general trajectories—maternal positivity and negativity—and these influenced the development of social withdrawal in childhood. Maternal negativity is associated with poor social functioning in children who have an established history of social withdrawal, whereas maternal positivity is associated with better social outcome for preschoolers who are viewed as temperamentally shy
- **Hane** and **Fox** (2006): The quality of maternal interactive behavior with infants influences the physiological and behavioral response to stress, including expression of fearfulness and positive sociability with novel partners
- **Landry**[6] (2000) observed that the mother's maintaining of children's interests and child characteristics of 2–3.5 years children indirectly influenced on their 4.5 years old independent cognitive and social functioning

Effect of the Parental Presence in the Operatory

- It is quite probable that dentists generally prefer to have parents absent from the operating room while children are being treated because most children behave satisfactorily without parental presence. In fact, as children get older and develop emotional independence, they themselves prefer they have their parent remain in the waiting room.
- If a child exhibits uncooperative behavior, the presence of the parent will sometimes lend support to this type of behavior and it can also limit the range of behavior control techniques of the dentist **(Fig. 21.1)**. Parent should not, however, be routinely excluded from the operatory as there are certain occasions when their presence is desirable and actually enhances positive behavior on the part of child **(Fig. 21.2)**.

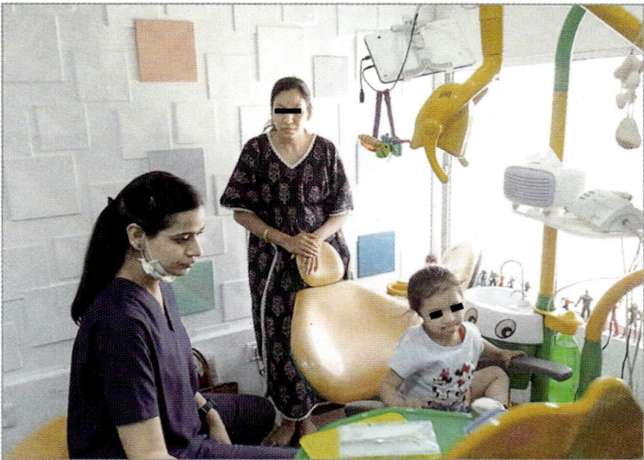

Fig. 21.1: Parental presence. (*Pic Courtsey:* 4 Kids Dental Clinic).

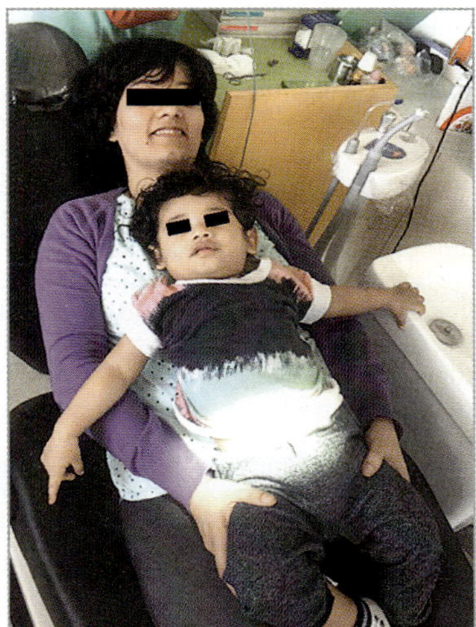

Fig. 21.2: Treatment of child in mother's lap. (*Pic Courtsey:* Abhinav Palekar).

- **Frankl** found that children in age group of 42–49 months are benefited from mother's presence.
- Young children are more prone to a number of fears, like fear of unknown, and hence exhibit anxiety during short-term separation and the degree of response is affected by length of separations.

Parental Behavior in the Dental Office

Parental behavior in the dental office also plays an important role in child management. Parents must understand that once the child is in the office, the dentist knows how to prepare the child emotionally for the necessary treatment. If a parent is invited into the treatment room, he must assume the role of a passive guest and either sit or stand away from the chair. Some instructions that should be told to the parents are:

- Tell the parents not to voice their own personal fears in front of the child.
- Tell the parents never to use dentistry as a threat of punishment.
- Parents should familiarize their children with dentistry by taking the child to the dentist to become accustomed to the dental office and the dentist.
- Explain to the parent that an occasional display of courage on his part in dental matters will build courage in the child.
- Consult the parent about the home environment and the importance of moderate parental attitudes in building well-adjusted child.
- Parents should stress the value of regular dental care, not only in preserving the teeth but also in formation of good dental patients.
- Discourage parents from bribing their child to go to the dentist.
- The parent should be instructed never to shame or ridicule to overcome the fear.
- The parent should not promise the child what the dentist is or is not going to do.
- Several days before the appointment, the parent should be instructed to convey to the child in a casual manner that they have been invited to visit the dentist.

Parent–Child Separation

Wright noted that excluding the parent from the operating room could contribute in controlling the child's positive behavior. Most dentists probably are more relaxed and comfortable when parent remains in the reception area and their action has positive effect on children's behavior. Some factors which influence the dentist not to include parent in the operatory are:

- Parents often repeat orders, creating an annoyance for both dentist and child patient
- Parents impose orders, becoming a barrier to the development of rapport between the dentist and child
- Dentist is unable to use voice intonation in the presence of the parent because he may be offended
- Child divides attention between parent and dentist
- Dentist's attention is divided between parent and child.

CLASSIFICATION OF CHILD BEHAVIOR IN DENTAL OFFICE

Classification of behavior management techniques	
Psychological approach	• Preappointment behavior modification • Communication • Use of second language • Tell–show–do • Tender love care • Desensitization • Contingency management • Visual imagery • Modeling • Behavior shaping • Assimilation and coping • Hypnosis • Retraining • Distraction • Externalization • Parental presence or absence • Reframing • Voice control
Physical approach	• Hand over mouth • Physical restraints
Pharmacological	• Premedication • Conscious sedation • General anesthesia

Frankl's classification

- **Frankl** in 1962 introduced a behavior-rating scale, which is one of the most reliable tools developed for behavior measurement
- This consists of a ratings of determination numbered from 1 to 4, each defining a specific behavior
- **Wright** in 1975 suggested that a symbol be added to this rating scale, permitting the dentist to record a behavior base at the inception of dental treatment and to keep a progressive record of the child's behavior
- **Wright** (1975) gave the symbols to **Frankl's** four types of behavior. They also gave a right sided arrow mark (→) indicating the change in behavior in the dental operatory (due to fear or behavior guidance)

Behavior	*Rating*	*Symbol*	*Features*
Definitely negative	Rating No. 1	(– –)s	◆ *Refuses treatment:* » *Immature behavior:* Cannot reason or cope with the situation, e.g., babies, special child » *Uncontrolled behavior:* Temper tantrum suggestive of extreme anxiety, e.g., preschooler » *Defiant behavior:* Exhibits resistance, e.g., spoiled, stubborn child, middle school years ◆ *Cries forcefully:* Uncontrollable behavior, e.g., late preschooler or middle years child ◆ *Extreme negative behavior associated with fear:* » *Uncontrollable behavior:* Exhibited in the older children possessing deep-rooted emotional problems » *Defiant behavior:* Includes passive resistance in the individual approaching adolescence
Negative	Rating No. 2	(–)	◆ *Reluctant to accept treatment:* » *Immature behavior:* Babies or preschooler » *Timid behavior:* Seen in children, who are » overprotected, exposed to few people or dominated by strange environment » *Influenced behavior:* Includes family and peer pressure ◆ *Displays evidence of slight negativism:* » Timid behavior » Whining behavior
Positive	Rating No. 3	(+)	*Accepts treatment:* ◆ *Tense cooperative behavior:* Observed in all stages, follows dentists' directions but may be resistant and cautious ◆ *Conservative behavior:* Responds harmoniously ◆ *Timid behavior:* Follows dentist direction in a shy, quiet manner. Can become uncooperative due to any bad experience during treatment
Definitely positive	Rating No. 4	(++)	*Unique behavior:* Looks forward to understand the importance of good preventive care and establishes a good rapport

Wright classification (1975)

- Cooperative behavior
- Lacking cooperative behavior
- Potentially cooperative behavior (five subtypes):
    1. *Incorrigible/uncontrolled behavior:* This is typically presented by 3–4 years old children at their first dental visit or by older children at the time of injection. There is loud crying, kicking, and temper tantrums. These children fall under the hypermotive category of Lampshire
    2. *Defiant/obstinate behavior:* This child has been termed as "spoiled kid" by Lampshire in 1970. He controls his behavior in a sense by challenging the authority of the dentist. Typical responses are "I do not want my teeth fixed" or "you cannot make me open my mouth." These children have potentially severe emotional problems that are manifested at home, school, and other areas of life
    3. *Timid behavior:* Often expressed by young children, particularly at the initial dental appointment. It is a result of child's anxiety about the dental experience and how he is expected to perform in the office. The child's anxiety may prevent him from listening attentively to the dentist, so instruction must be given slowly, quietly, and repeated when necessary. Once the child gains confidence in the dentist, he can become excellent patient
    4. *Tense cooperative—borderline behavior:* They are extremely tensed; body language is different; tremor in voice; sweating palms, hands. They can be cooperative if behavior managed well
    5. *Whining behavior:* The child with this type of behavior can be extremely frustrating to treat. He allows treatment, but he whines throughout the entire procedure
- Stoic behavior is a type of behavior commonly mistaken to be a part of potentially cooperative group. The child is generally cooperative, sits quietly, and accepts all dental treatment including the injection without protest or any sign of discomfort. This behavior is characteristic of children who have been physically abused.

Pinkham's classification

Category I	Emotionally compromised child
Category II	Shy, introvert child
Category III	Frightened child
Category IV	Child who is adverse to authority

Lampshire classification

Cooperative	Children who remain physically and emotionally relaxed and cooperative throughout the entire visit, regardless of treatment undertaken
Tense cooperative	Children who are tense but nevertheless cooperative
Outwardly apprehensive	Child, who hides behind the mother in the waiting room, uses stalling techniques and avoids talking to the dentist. These children will eventually accept dental treatment
Fearful	Children who require considerable support in order to overcome their fear of dental situation. Modeling is useful for them
Stubborn/defiant	Children who passively resist or try to avoid treatment by using techniques that have been successful for them in other situations
Hypermotive	Children who are agitated and who adopt procedures such as screaming or kicking as their coping defense mechanism
Handicapped	Children who are physically, mentally, or emotionally handicapped
Emotionally immature	This category includes the young children who have not yet achieved sufficient emotional maturity to rationalize the need for dental treatment and to cope with it

PREAPPOINTMENT BEHAVIOR MODIFICATION

Audiovisual Modeling

- The goal is for the patient to reproduce the behavior exhibited by model.
- Child sees the video cassette before proceeding to dental clinic, on day of appointment. Type of model used can be siblings, other children, or parents **(Fig. 21.3).**
- It is best recommended to use the model of the same age as that of the child patient so that he can easily relate himself with the model.

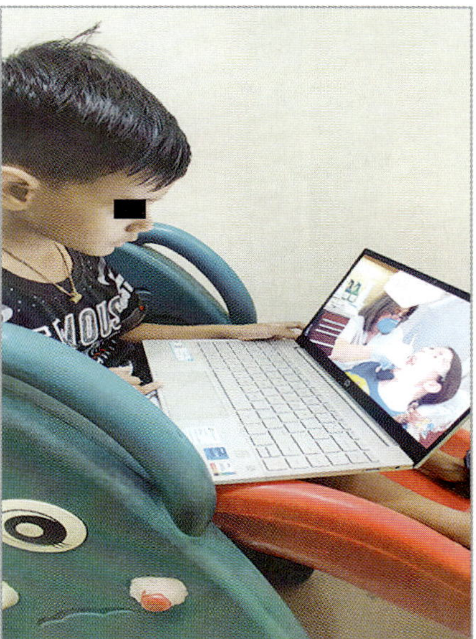

Fig. 21.3: Child watching dental video on counseling visit in play area.

- **Advantages:**
  - Stimulation of new behavior
  - Facilitation of behavior in more appropriate manner
  - Elimination of inappropriate behavior because of fear
  - Extinction of fear
- **Disadvantages:**
  - Expensive
  - Time-consuming process.

Preappointment Mailing

- Contact with the child's parents before the first dental visit can alienate some concerns
- It increases the likelihood of a success as it prepares the patient for first dental visit
- Parent can be contacted by telephone as a reminder the day before the dental appointment, it may serve in establishing good relationship **(Fig. 21.4)**.

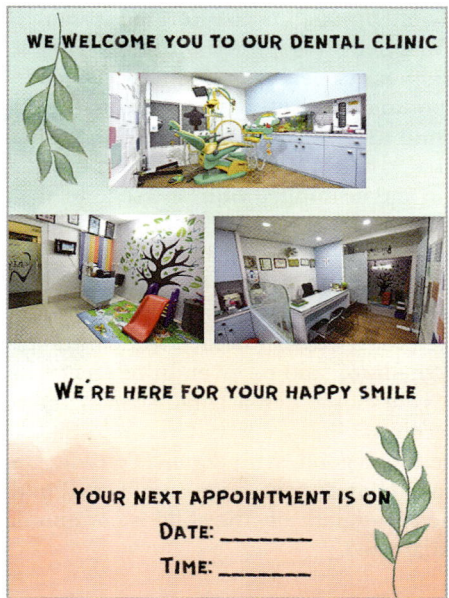

Fig. 21.4: Sample of pre-appointment mailing card.

COMMUNICATION

- First objective in successful management of the young child is to establish communication **(Fig. 21.5).**
- By involving the child in conversation, the dentist not only learns about the patient but also may relax the youngster.

The fears and natural innate curiosity of the child demand that explanations be given for each and every step of dental treatment.

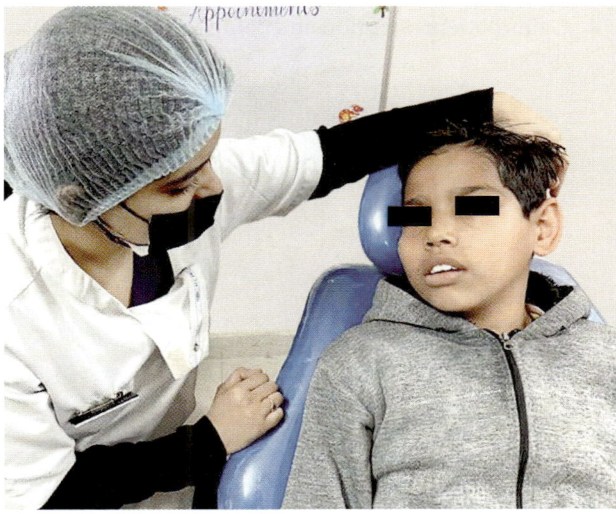

Fig. 21.5: Dentist-child communication.

- There are two ways of establishing communication:
  1. *Verbal:* Spoken language to gain confidence.
  2. *Nonverbal:* Expression without words like welcome handshake, patting, eye contact.
- Effective vocabulary is important aspect as the dentist must only use the words that are understandable by the child. Communication with children aged 2–7 years should be based on Piagetian concept (*Animism*—giving life to an inanimate object) which involves giving life like names to dental instruments like handpiece is called whistling Charlie.

- Honesty of approach is also very important, if the child knows that dentist is honest with his words, it will bring out a cooperative behavior in him.
- The important aspect of communication is getting the child to respond to dentist's commands. Two things must be remembered here. First, the command may take some time to sink in and be implied with, and second, the command should be within the ability of child. It is imperative to use positive language like *please can you move your hand* rather than use negative aspect like *do not get your hand here.*
- The three most important facets of communication are source, medium, and receiver. In reference to dentistry, dentist is the source, dental clinic is the medium, and child is the receiver.
- If the dentist is good, sympathetic, confident, and honest and dental clinic is neat, quiet, familiar to children, full of toys, then automatically the child is communicating and is well managed.

NONVERBAL COMMUNICATION

Nonverbal communication is the reinforcement and guidance of behavior through appropriate contacts, posture, facial expression and body language **(Fig. 21.6).**

- **Objectives:**
  - Enhances the effectiveness of other communicative management techniques
  - Gains patient attention and compliance and motivates him.

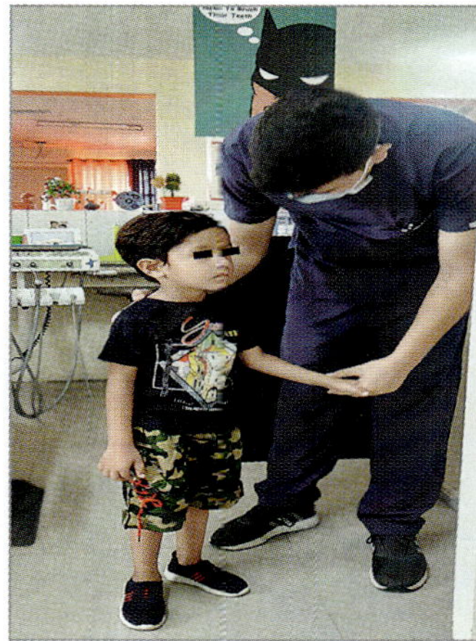

Fig. 21.6: Motivation by nonverbal method.

DESCRIPTIVE PRAISE

This praise emphasizes specific cooperative behaviors (e.g., "Thank you for sitting still", "you are doing a great job keeping your hands in your lap") rather than a generalized praise (e.g., "good job").

SIGNALING

Armfield[7] 2013 stated the relationship of trust is greatly improved by the clinician responding promptly and appropriately to the young patient's signal.

Signaling allows the patient to communicate with the dental team during any phase of treatment by means of previously established signal with specific meanings **(Fig. 21.7)**. The patient, by raising a hand or a finger can communicate their wish to stop the treatment (for rest breaks, or notify dentists of any unpleasant feelings).

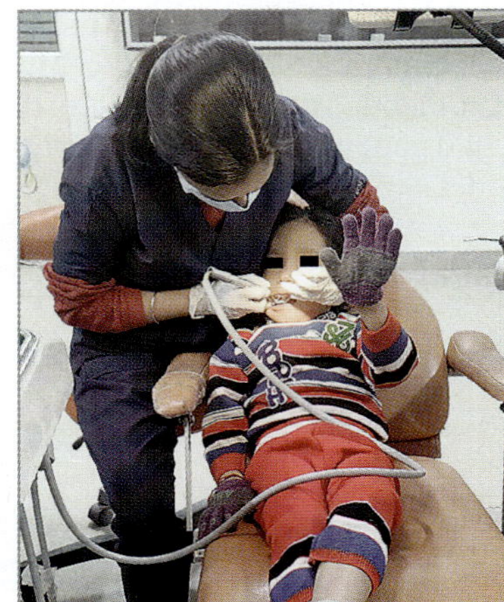

Fig. 21.7: Patient using signaling as communication.

USE OF SECOND LANGUAGE (EUPHEMISMS)

- Address the child at his or her level of comprehension. This does not suggest the use of baby talk but rather employing words that have meaning for that child **(Fig. 21.8)**. This means not speaking to an 8-year old as if he or she were 3 and vice versa. Does a 3-year old understand what it means to "evacuate" or "vacuum" the mouth or what is meant by a "rubber dam clamp"? The use of inoffensive or mild expressions may be substituted for those that suggest unpleasantness or are fear promoting. "Spraying sleepy water on the tooth" is much less offensive and fear promoting than "I am going to give you a shot on your gum!".
- The dental staff as well as the dentist should be oriented to the use of a "second language." The different expressions that can be employed are limited only by the creativity of the dentist. It should be emphasized that word substitutes are most effectively used with preschool children. Use with older children may be perceived by the child as "talking down".

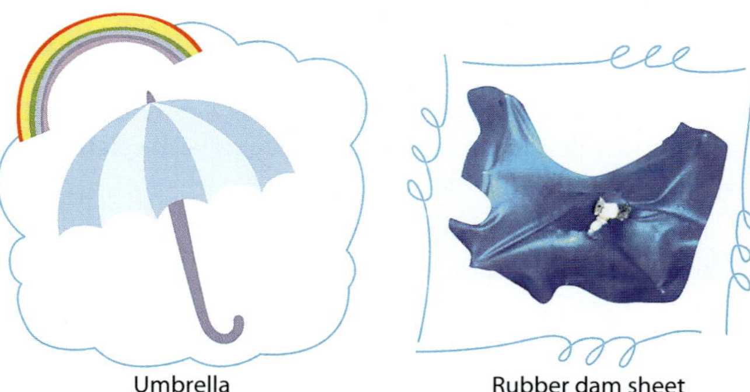

Fig. 21.8: Euphemisms depiction. (*Source:* Deshpande A, Shah Y. AY DentalPictionary, L-92022/2020; Literary work, copyright date 2020).

- The tone of the voice can also be very effective in altering the child's behavior. A change of tone or volume can be used to communicate a feeling or sense to the child. A kind, firm, or a soft or a loud voice says a lot to the child. It is not what you say, but it is how you say it.
- **Aboulenain am** et al[8] (2017): The use of second language plays a major role in the interaction between the pediatric dentist and the child patient and the easier the word substitute, the better is the behavior of children in the dental clinic.

Dental terminology	*Word substitute*
• Air	• Wind
• Impression material	• Pudding, mashed potatoes
• Anesthetic	• Sleepy medicine or sleepy water
• Bur	• Brush or pencil
• Caries	• Brown spot: sugar bugs
• Explorer	• Tooth counter
• Evacuator	• Vacuum cleaner
• Matrix	• Fence for filling
• Rubber dam	• Raincoat
• Stainless steel band	• Ring for the tooth
• Stainless steel crown	• Hat for the tooth
• X-ray	• Camera
• Radiograph	• Picture
• Handpiece	• Whistling train

POSITIVE PREVISIT IMAGERY

Patients are shown positive photographs and images of dentistry and dental treatment in the waiting area before the dental appointment.

- **Objectives:**
  - To provide children and parents with visual information on what to expect during the dental visit.
  - To provide children with context, to be able to ask the provider relevant questions, before dental procedures are initiated.

TELL-SHOW-DO

- Tell-show-do (TSD), the cornerstone of behavior management, was given by Harold **Addleston** in 1959.
- The classic model for communicating with children and favorably conditioning them to the dental experience is "Tell, Show, and Do".
- Specifically, the dentist tells the child what is going to be done in words the child can understand. Second, the dentist demonstrates to the child exactly how the procedure will be conducted. Finally, the practitioner performs the procedure exactly as it was described and demonstrated.[9]
- **Objectives:**
  - To teach the patient aspects of dental visit and to familiarize him with the dental setting
  - To shape patients response to various procedures.
- **Tell:**
  - Verbal explanations of procedures in phrases appropriate to the developmental level of the child **(Fig. 21.9A).** In telling, explain to the child exactly what you are going to do.
  - Tell the child before you do it, while you are doing it, and after you have done it.
  - Your voice should be soft, yet firm, confident, and continuous.
  - You should be truthful with the child, and if the procedure is going to be painful or uncomfortable, say so.
  - Talk about the dental situation. Sometimes talking about other things (distraction) is indicated, but not at the expense of the child being properly informed as to what you are doing.

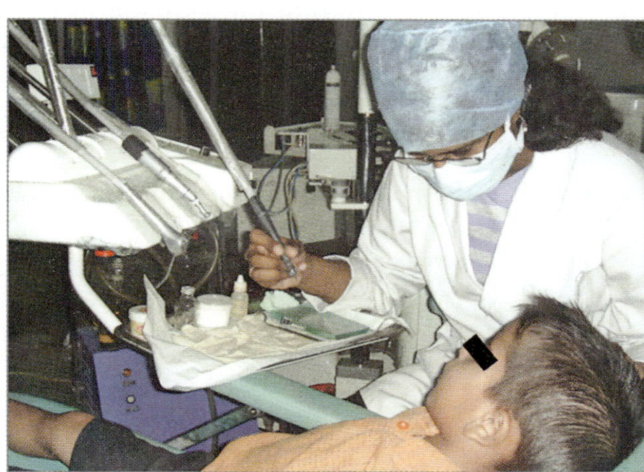

Fig. 21.9A: Verbal explanations of procedures.

- **Show:**
  - Demonstration of the visual, auditory, olfactory, and tactile aspects of the procedure in a carefully defined, nonthreatening setting **(Fig. 21.9B).**
  - The dentist can either demonstrate on himself or on an inanimate object. In showing, demonstrate to the child what will happen, how and with what equipment. Remember, you can use all the senses to show a child.

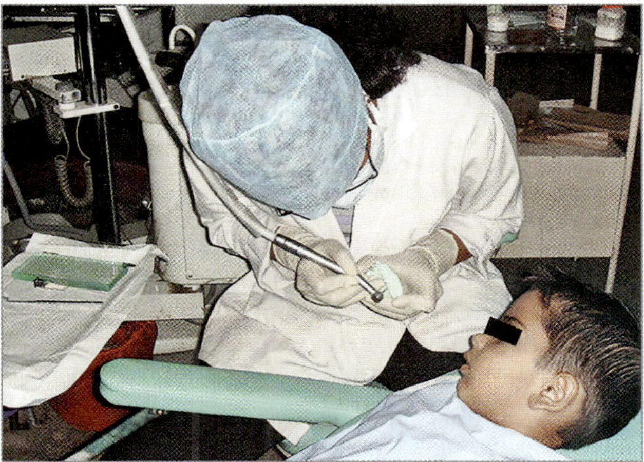

Fig. 21.9B: Demonstration for the patient.

  - "The noise" of a running handpiece shows the child through the hearing medium. A pinch on the arm before anesthesia administration demonstrates to the child how the pinch of the injection in the mouth might feel.
  - Although showing the child is a basic guideline, it is wise to avoid showing fear promoting instruments such as the anesthesia syringe.

- Consequently, bringing equipment from behind the child or below the visual level is preferred. In selected situations, the child can be shown the anesthetic syringe with the sleeve over the needle, an explanation that this is the instrument used to "spray the sleepy medicine on your tooth".
- Always remember the multisensory approach. The child can see, touch, smell, and hear.

❖ **Do:**
- Without deviating from the explanation and demonstration, the dentist proceeds directly to perform the previewed operation **(Fig. 21.9C).**
- In doing, do what you said you would do.
- Use the same tone of voice in telling what you are doing as you do it.
- Do not perform the task until the child has a clear awareness of what it is you are going to do.

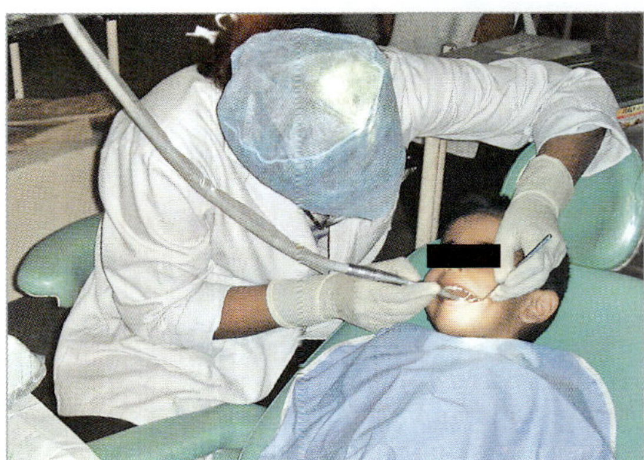

Fig. 21.9C: Perform the previewed operation.

Research pertaining to use of Tell–Show–Do technique in behavior management
- **Levy and Domoto** (1979) observed TSD as one of the most highly employed behavior management technique.
- **Carr et al.**[10] in a survey of pediatric dentists in South-Eastern states of the USA found that only 62% of them used TSD with all children
- **Crossley and Joshi**[11] (2002) reported that TSD was the most popular technique for managing children, which was listed by 87% of pediatric dentists
- **Grewal**[12] mentioned that 70% of respondents use this technique, but normal conversation was listed as the first strategy when dealing with children
- **Peretz** et al.[13] (2003) found that 97% of pediatric dentists use this technique
- **Sharma and Tyagi**[14] from their retrospective study concluded that TSD modifies the behavior of child and aids in achieving the treatment goals effectively in all age groups
- **Al Daghanin S and Balharith M**[15] (2017) revealed that the most accepted technique by parents was TSD, and the second preferred was nitrous oxide inhalation sedation followed by general anesthesia and the least preferred was passive restraint followed by HOM technique. Male parents preferred general anesthesia while female parents preferred nitrous oxide inhalation sedation.

Sayed Azhar[16] (2016) used live visual output of the dental operating microscope (DOM) as an adjunct to the TSD technique and found reduction in anxiety from the first visit to the second visit for restorative treatment when the DOM was used.
- **Tiwari et al**[17] concluded that Tell-Show-Do technique is very effective in achieving treatment goals in all age groups.
- **Samara et al**[18] demonstrated a reduction in physiological signs of anxiety in children aged 6- to 15-years-old when Tell-Show-Do was applied.

ASK-TELL-ASK

❖ Ask-Tell-Ask technique is given by Clinical Affairs Committee—Behavior Management Subcommittee and Council on Clinical Affairs in 2015.

❖ When clinicians tell the child about the dental treatment, too much information regarding the treatment sometimes may alarm the patient. By using this technique it is possible to improve the child's knowledge regarding the dental procedure.

❖ This technique involves inquiring about the patient's visit and feelings towards or about any planned procedure (Ask): explaining the procedures through demonstrations in a nonthreatening language appropriate to the cognitive level of the patient (Tell): and again inquiring if the patient understands and how he/she feels about the impending treatment (Ask).

❖ The dentist can ask the child or the parent to 'Teach-Back' what they have learned.

TELL-PLAY-DO

❖ Given by **Viswakarma AP**[19] in 2017

❖ This technique is based on the learning theory where interchange of thought and two-way interchange of information takes place. This is done by performing dental treatment on dental imitating toys, where child understands the dentist's frame of reference and feels more comfortable and develops cooperative behavior **(Fig. 21.10).**

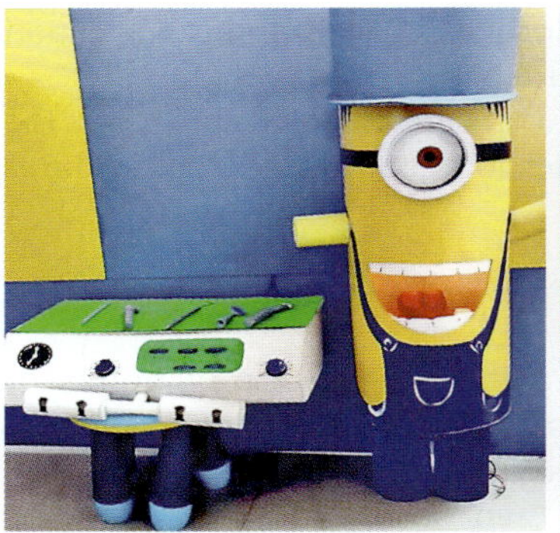

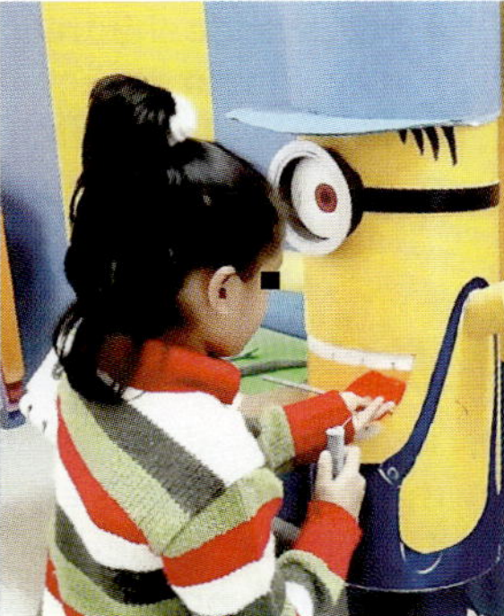

Fig. 21.10: Child performing the Tell-Play-Do game.

❖ **Kevadia et al**[20] compared Tell-Play-Do technique with Live Modelling for managing the behavior of child during dental treatment and found that Tell-Play-Do technique is more effective in reducing the child's fear and anxiety about dental treatment than live modelling.

❖ **Shah and Bhatia**[21] compared the effectiveness of Tell-Play-Do with AV distraction and found that Tell-Play-Do is equally effective as AV distraction for reducing anxiety during dental treatment.

TELL SHOW PLAY DOH

❖ Given by **Radhakrishna S et al.**[22] in 2019.

❖ A reusable modelling compound known as Play-Doh is generally used by children for arts and craft projects. Play-Doh dentist Drill N Fill set consists of head which contains slot into which moulded teeth are inserted and a battery operated drill. The child is allowed to play with the battery operated toy drill **(Fig. 21.11)**.

- The main aim is to familiarize the child with the dental equipment and to reduce the anxiety thereby preparing the child for the treatment. Radhakrishna S et al compared the techniques of Tell-Show-Play-Doh, a smartphone dentist game, and a conventional Tell-Show-Do method in the behavior modification of anxious children in the dental operatory and found that Tell-Show-Play-Doh and smartphone dentist game techniques are effective tools to reduce dental anxiety in pediatric patients.

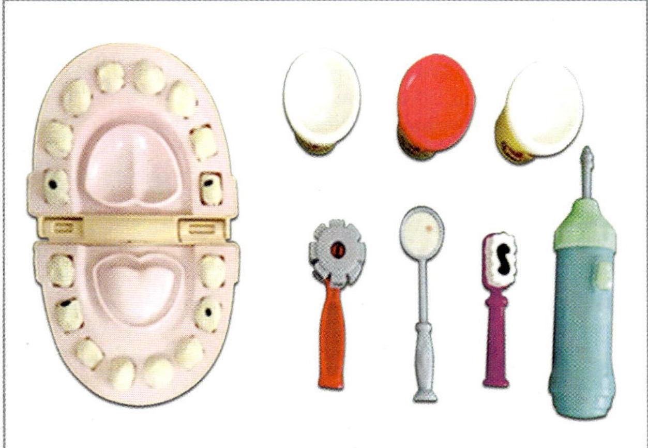

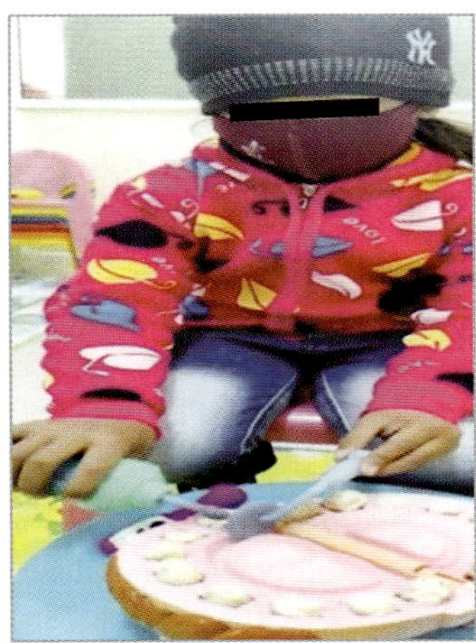

Fig. 21.11: Child playing with Play-Doh set.

TELL-PLAY-DO WITH SMART PHONE DENTIST GAME

- **Patil et al.,**[23] in 2017 and **Meshki et al.,**[24] in 2018 introduced the Android application dentist games to reduce dental fear and to make comfortable and aware of the dental procedures and idea of the performance of treatment.
- This modification helps the children to get first-hand experience of the dental treatment and they can easily relate their experience of dental treatment with the simulation game, thereby reducing the anxiety during the treatment **(Fig. 21.12)**.
- **Shah et al.,**[25] stated that smartphone application intervention reduce anxiety in pediatric patients in a better way when compared to conventional behavior modification techniques.
- **Lee et al.,**[26] stated that engaging a child with smartphone applications can be a distraction in the behavior guidance technique and concluded that smartphones were most effective in reducing preoperative anxiety in children.

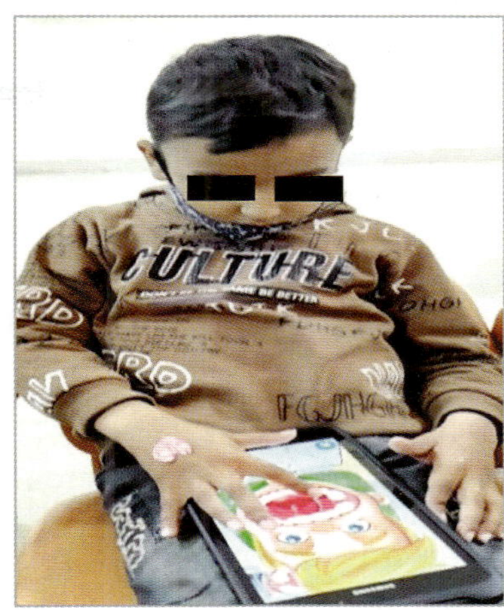

Fig. 21.12: Child engaged in the act of playing dentist game.

DESENSITIZATION

- This technique was demonstrated by **James** and popularized by **Wolpe.**
- It means to take away ones sensitivity to a type of behavior.
- This is used in children having pre-established fears and uncooperative behavior.
- Desensitization is a therapeutic technique that pairs an anxiety-evoking stimulus with a response inhibitory to anxiety. In such situations, the perceived link between the stimulus and the anxiety response is weakened.
- **Wolpe** used relaxation as the inhibitor of anxiety-visual imagery of anxiety-provoking stimuli with the patient maintaining profound muscle relaxation. The technique calls for a hierarchy of fear stimuli, whereby the patient conquers fear or anxiety toward low-anxiety or moderate-anxiety stimuli before approaching the more dramatic stimuli.
- **Gale** and **Ayer** have written a description of this technique as used with dental phobia. Technique usually involves teaching the patient to induce a state of deep muscle relaxation, and while the patient is in relaxation state, tell him to imagine scenes that are relevant to his fears. Imaginary scenes are presented to the patient in a graduated fashion so that scenes provoking only minimal anxiety are initially described and gradually more stressful situations are presented.
- Preventive desensitization is philosophically possible for the child dental patient approaching the first dental appointment. A graded introduction of the child to dentistry, TSD approaches, and accomplishment of easy procedures (examination, prophylaxis, fluoride treatment, brushing instruction) are aspects of preventive desensitization.
- The conflict in the term preventive desensitization is due to the fact that logically nothing can be desensitized unless previously sensitized. However, because of mass media and fears acquired from siblings, peers, and parents, it is reasonable to believe that most children aged 30 months

or older are to a degree sensitized to dentistry before their first appointment. Additionally, medical appointments may have sensitized the child to any clinical setting.

- **Howitt** and **Stricker** addressed the hierarchy of anxiety-evolving stimuli in the dental experience in children as injection → exposure to dental environment → dental drill → rubber dam → hand instruments > prophylaxis.

MODELING

- It is based on **Bandura's** social learning theory, which states that one's learning or behavior acquisition occurs through observation of suitable model performing a specific behavior **(Fig. 21.13).**
- Modeling is based on the psychologic principle that much of one's learning or behavior acquisition occurs through observation of a suitable model performing a specific behavior.
- Modeling and/or learning by observation of a model have many synonymous terms: imitation, observational learning, identification, internalization, introjections, coping, social facilitation, contagion, and role taking.

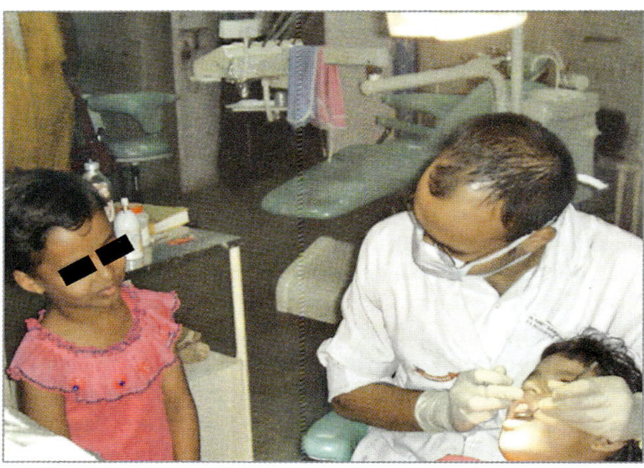

Fig. 21.13: Model performing a specific behavior.

Objectives of modeling
- Stimulates acquisition of new behavior
- Facilitating the behavior already in the patients in a more appropriate manner
- Elimination of avoidance behavior
- Extinction of fear

- The efficacy of modeling as a learning technique has been demonstrated by producing behavioral changes in situations requiring cooperation, aggressive behavior, language development, and moral judgments.
- Modeling has been used as a technique to eliminate or minimize fear of dentistry in children by allowing the child to observe an older sibling undergoing dental treatment.
- **Types of modeling:**
  - Audiovisual
  - Live modeling by sibling or parent
- **Types of models:**
  - Mastery (cooperative patient who enjoys dental treatment)
  - Coping (just manages to cope up with the treatment)

Advantages of modeling (Rim and Masters, 1974)
- Patient's attention is obtained
- Designed behavior is modeled
- Physical guidance of the desired behavior
- Reinforcement of the guided behavior

Research pertaining to use of modeling
- **Sharma Karan** and **Malik Manvi**[27] (2016) found that mother as a live model can be a highly effective regimen for concrete delivery of oral health care in a child patient. They also found that live model is a tangible technique in the list of nonpharmacological techniques of behavior management and can be safely incorporated in routine clinical practice.
- **Nada Farhat Mchayleh**[28] (2009) compared efficiency of TSD and live modeling on children's heart rates during dental treatment and found children who received live modeling with the mother as model had lower heart rates than those who received treatment with the father as model and those with TSD method ($p<0.01$). The model used for live modeling (father or mother) and the child's age are determining factors for the results.
- **Roberts**[29] (2010) and **Shapiro** (2007) stated modeling based on the principle that a patient can be conditioned to exhibit positive behavior after observing the behavior of another patient, and older sibling, or a family member in the similar situation (e.g., in dental chair).
- **Johnson** and **Machen**[30] have found that children who viewed a 12-min videotape presentation of a child undergoing an examination, radiographs, local anesthetic administration, and restorative treatment similar to their own upcoming experiences exhibited more positive behavior than did a control group with no modeling experience. It is also a proven fact that if the model is of the same age group as the patient, the effect is even more pronounced.
- **Chambers**[31] **(1970):** Both live and filmed modeling are effective in reducing child's fear and anxiety about dental treatments and promoting adaptive behavior.
- **Karekar P et al**[32]**:** Conducted a study to assess the effect of live modelling, filmed modelling and tell show do technique and concluded that modelling is more effective when compared to TSD technique.

DIRECT OBSERVATION

Patients are shown a video or are permitted to directly observe a young cooperative patient undergoing dental treatment **(Fig. 21.14).**

- **Objectives:**
  - Familiarize the patient with dental sitting and specific steps involved in a dental procedure.
  - Give the patient and parents an opportunity to ask questions about the dental procedure in a safe environment.

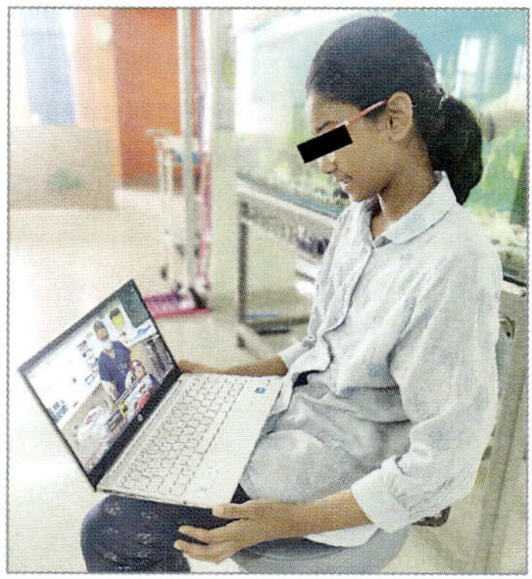

Fig. 21.14: Child watching a dental treatment video.

BEHAVIOR SHAPING

- *It is defined as a process which slowly develops a behavior by reinforcing successive approximations of the desired behavior until the desired behavior is expressed.*
- It is based on the established principles of social learning.
- Proponents of the theory hold that most behavior is learned and that learning is the establishment of a connection between a stimulus and a response. For this reason, it is sometimes called stimulus–response (S–R) theory.
- When shaping behavior, the dental assistant or dentist is teaching a child how to behave. Young children are led through these procedures step by step. They have to be communicative and cooperative to absorb information that may be complex for them. The following is an outline for a behavior shaping model:
  - State the general goal or task to the child at the outset
  - Explain the necessity for the procedure
  - Divide the explanation for the procedure slowly
  - Make all explanations at a child's level of understanding with use of euphemisms
  - Use successive approximations
  - Reinforce appropriate behavior
  - Disregard minor inappropriate behavior.

CONTINGENCY MANAGEMENT

- This behavior management technique is based on **BF Skinner's** operant conditioning
- The presentation of positive reinforcers or withdrawal of negative reinforcers is termed contingency management. It includes:
  - Positive reinforcement
  - Negative reinforcement
  - Omission or time out
  - Punishment
- **Levy** and **Domoto** (1979) found out that positive reinforcement was one of the highly preferred techniques in the pedodontic dental practices in the state of Washington.

Types of Reinforcers

- **Positive reinforcers:** It is the one whose presentation increases the frequency of desired behavior.
- **Negative reinforcers:** It is the one whose contingent withdrawal increases the frequency of a behavior.
- **Material:** Stickers, pencils, small toys (preferably not candies and sweets). Rewards are given after the dental procedure and bribes are given before. Bribes should not be given in pediatric dental practice. The reward in one visit will act like a bribe for the next visit and the child will behave properly to receive his gift.
- **Social:** Praise, positive facial expression, handshake, smile, hug, pat on the shoulder. This is the best kind of positive reinforcer which works well with children.
- **Activity:** Opportunity of participating in a preferred activity like a cartoon show, visit to the park. Before patient can accomplish this activity he has to behave accordingly in the dental office.
- **Positive reinforcement:** It is the presentation of the pleasant stimulus and is done to appreciate the child for the good behavior. Either of the above reinforcers can be used.
- **Negative reinforcement:** Withdrawal of the unpleasant stimulus like high-speed handpiece. Care should be taken not to confuse this punishment. The unpleasant stimulus is withdrawn and not given to the child. It is similar to de-emphasis or substitution type of retraining.
- **Time-out (or) omission:** It is the withdrawal of the pleasant stimulus to reinforce good behavior. Asking the mother (pleasant stimulus for the child) to stay out of the dental operatory to make the child cooperative is an example of time-out.
- **Punishment:** It is the presentation of the unpleasant stimulus to the child, for example, voice control, hand-over-mouth exercise (HOME).

EXTERNALIZATION (FIG. 21.15)

- It is a process by which child's attention is focused away from the sensation associated with dental treatment by involving in verbal or dental activity.
- **Objectives:**
  - To decrease perception of unpleasantness
  - To interest and involve children.

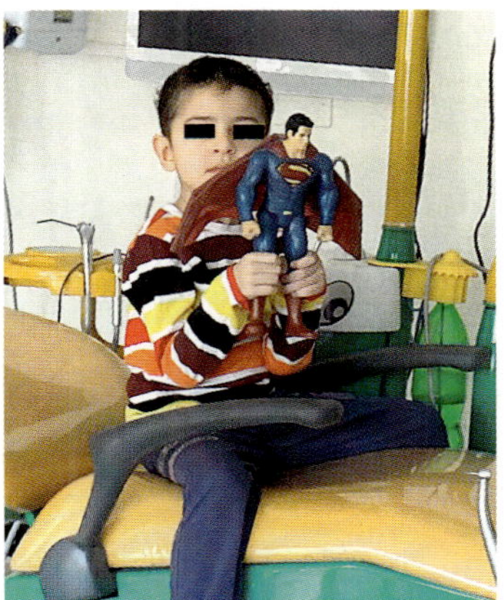

Fig. 21.15: Externalization.

DISTRACTION

- This is a newer method of behavior management in which the patient is distracted from the sounds and/or sight of dental treatment thereby reducing the anxiety.
- Objective is to relax the patient and to reduce anxiety during treatment
- Use stories and fairy tales
- Use slow instrumental music
- Relaxation effect of music and the sound of music will eliminate unpleasant dental sounds like the sound of handpiece.
- Choice of distraction is chosen by the patient; this will help child gain control over the unpleasant stimulus and give them a feeling of being in a familiar environment.
- Child seeing the audiovisual presentation will have multisensory distraction as he will tend to concentrate on the TV screen thereby screening out the sight of dental treatment, and the sound of the program will help eliminate the unpleasant dental sounds like the sound of handpiece.
- Placebo effect

❖ **Types:**

- *Audio distraction:* Patient listens to audio presentation through headphones throughout the course of the treatment **(Fig. 21.16)**.

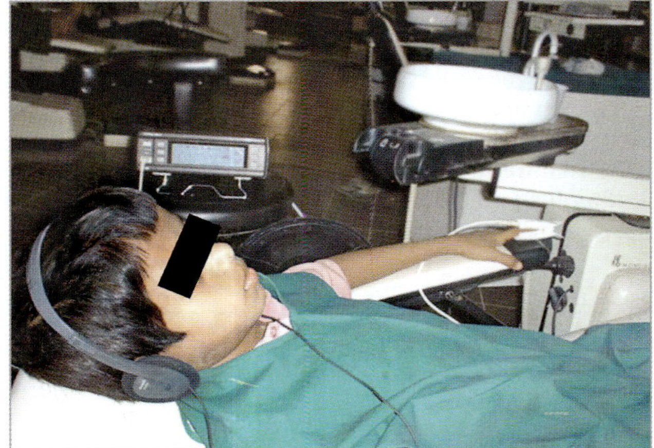

Fig. 21.16: Audio distraction.

- *Audiovisual distraction:* Patient is shown audiovisual presentation through television during the entire treatment **(Fig. 21.17A)**. The same can also be accomplished by either video games **(Fig. 21.17B)** or by the use of audiovisual glasses **(Fig. 21.17C)**.

Types of distraction:
1. *Active: Active distraction promotes child participation which involves several sensory components such as toys, virtual reality, relaxation.*
2. *Passive: Distraction through child observation of an activity or stimulus rather than active participation, e.g., listening to music, watching television or videos.*

Videogame distraction: The use of videogame as a distraction tool is based on the principles of cognitive—behavioral therapy and neuro-feedback mechanism for children with anxiety disorders.Videogames are very effective distractors for children as they engage multiple sensory systems. They provide vivid visual and auditory stimulation and typically require close attention to visual cues in order to execute various tasks. They also engage tactile and kinesthetic senses as the individual plays the game.

- **Virtual reality based distraction**
  - In 1968, **Ivan Sutherland and Bob Sproull** invented virtual reality with a head mounted device that was connected to a computer and in 1998, **Heim** described virtual reality as an interactive computer based software that can be used to immerse children in the virtual environment which completely obstructs the present situation.
  - VR even combines the audio, visual, and kinesthetic sensory modalities. Depending on how immersive the presented stimuli are, the person's attention will be more or less drained from the real world, leaving less attention to the real world processes, including painful stimuli.
  - The application of VR distraction is based on assumption that pain perception has a large psychological component and the pain attracts a strong attentive response because of the potential threat of damaged tissue associate with sensation. The redirection of this attention manipulates the pain perception. Recently it has also been established that VR changes the way people intercept incoming pain signals and it reduces amount of pain related activity.
  - However, it should be emphasized that virtual reality goggles are effective if young patients watch pictures they already know, such as cartoons. Using new, previously unknown pictures might cause discomfort and stress.

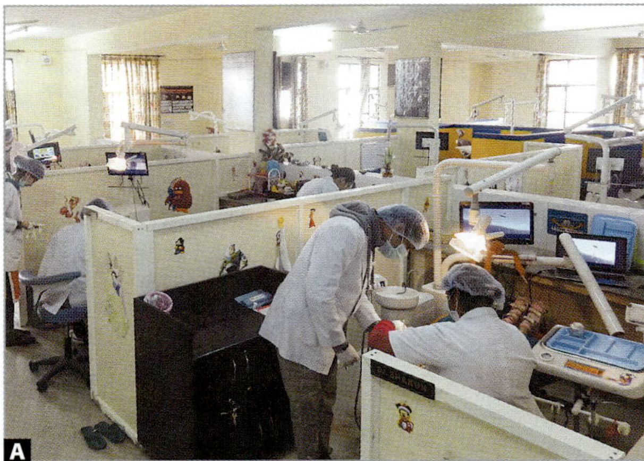

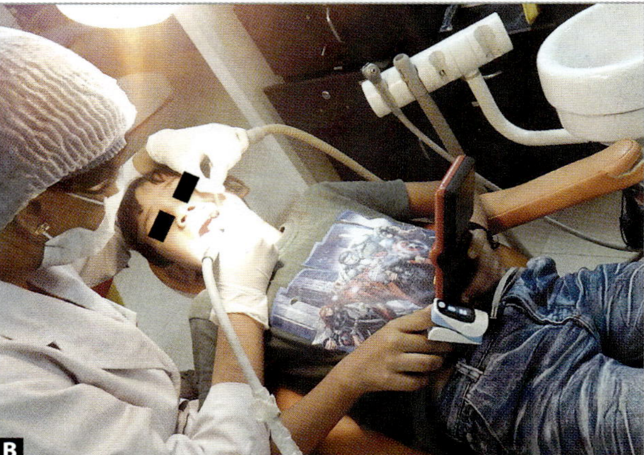

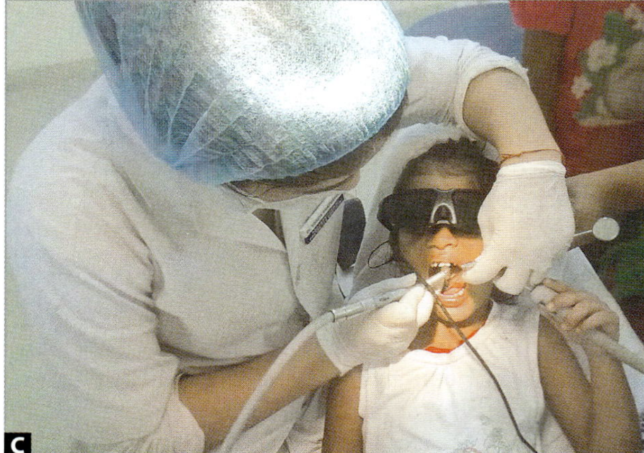

Figs. 21.17A to C: Audiovisual distraction using: (A) Audiovisual; (B) Video games; (C) AV glasses.

Theories of distraction:
1. *Gate Control Theory: Part of brain processing painful stimuli are less active when patient is under distraction.*
2. *Limited Attention Capacity Theory: Human's capacity to pay attention is limited, therefore, an individual should concentrate on painful stimuli in order to perceive pain.*
3. *Masking: Music is able to mask unpleasant sounds such as noise of dental drill thereby reducing the anxiety.*

Research on distraction technique
- **Levy and Domoto** (1979) found out that distraction was one of the highly preferred techniques in the pedodontic dental practices in the state of Washington
- **Magora** (2010) observed audiovisual wireless eyeglasses method of distraction [audiovisual distraction (AVD)] was able to replace the visual and auditory signals from the environment by a pleasant movie. As, this method offered the possibility of nonpharmacological sedation in patients undergoing dental treatment AVD may be of benefit especially to uncooperative, very anxious children and prevent pharmacologic means of sedation by offering a pleasurable method without adverse effects
- **Frere** (2001), **Bensten** (2001), **Prabhakar**[33] (2007), and **Ram** (2010) in their studies observed AVD as a promising technique that offers an additional nonpharmacological mode of sedation conceived to diminish the unpleasantness often associated with dental procedures in children and adults
- **Abdelmonien Soad** and **Mahmoud Sara**[34] (2015) found both passive, active and passive–active distraction techniques effective in reducing pain perception during local anesthesia administration.
- **Agarwal Nidhi** and **Dhawan Jayata et al**[35] (2017) found eutectic mixture of local anesthetic (EMLA) cream with AV aids was better when compared with EMLA without AV aids followed by Benzocain with AV aids.
- **Sivakumar et al**[36] (2014) evaluated the effect of 3D glasses for AVD in children during local anesthesia administration and concluded that this technique is helpful in reducing anxiety of child patients and has better effect as compared to music
- **Attar RH et al**[37]**:** Compared active and passive distraction and concluded that active distraction enhance visual, mental and motor participation of child which provides anxiolysis and analgesia
- **Dahlquist LM et al**[38] 2010 evaluated videogame and virtual reality with and without head mounted display and found virtual reality with head mounted display could reduce pain tolerance during cold pressor trials.
- **Fakhruddin et al**[39] have observed that using goggles along with behavioral methods in the treatment of children with hearing problems increases the levels of dental anxiety. Using behavioral methods and visual distractions is therefore recommended for such children. However, the operating field should remain fully visible, although in the case of patients with no hearing issues, watching pictures on a screen is less effective than using VR goggles. This may be due to the fact that children with impaired hearing have no control over their surroundings and experience anxiety whenever they are unable to maintain visual contact.

ASSIMILATION AND COPING

- Stress can act to increase pain perception while coping decrease it by a process called as assimilation.
- Coping refers to cognitive and behavioral efforts made by individuals to master, tolerate, or reduce stressful situations.
- **Behavioral coping:** Efforts include physical or verbal activities in which the child engages to deal with stress. These are readily visible to dentist, for example, inquisitive question about the procedure.
- **Cognitive coping:** Efforts which involve manipulation of emotions. These are not visible to dentist, but these play a crucial role in child's ability to deal with the treatment as well as forming a positive outlook for future.
- Children taught coping skills like imagery, relaxation, self-talk demonstrated less stress during treatment.
- **Kasimoglu Y et al:**[40] Robotic technology can successfully help in coping the dental anxiety and stress and help children to behave better.

Coping strategies and dentist's behavior

Sl. No.	*Coping strategy*	*Dentist's behavior*
1.	Distraction/ displacement	Talk to patient about hobbies, or just babble
2.	Expressive communication (verbalization fear)	Ask what the patient is feeling, or describe what you think they feel
3.	Relinquishing control to authority figure	Display confidence
4.	Gaining manipulative control over source	Tell patient what if something bothers them to put up their hand like this (demonstrate a safe way). Tell patient to count to 10 with you as you go through the procedure, finishing at the end of the count. Give patient a mirror to watch with structure choices, for example, "Would you like orange or strawberry flavor?" "Would you like to play with my chair?"
5.	Affiliation	Be empathetic
6.	Conscious instruction to oneself	Tell patient to count to "Breath deep", or "Relax"
7.	Mental rehearsal	Inform patient of the steps to be performed prior to the procedure, and use Tell-Show-Do

PARENTAL PRESENCE OR ABSENCE

- **Objectives:**
  - To gain patient's attention and compliance
  - To avert avoidance behavior
  - To establish authority
- **Advantages of parental presence:**
  - Supporting and communicating with the child
  - Very young patients

Research on parental presence or absence from operatory
- **Ajlouni** (2010) observed that 82% of pediatric dentists allow parents to be present during dental treatment
- **Adair**[41] (2004): Parents may prefer or insist on being with their children during treatment, or they would like to assist the pediatric dentist if any behavioral problem arises
- **Crossley**[11](2002) found high percentage of pediatric dentists allowing presence of parents during treatment
- **Grewal**[12] showed that only 61% of respondents allow parents to be in the clinic during treatment, and there is a significant relationship between the length of experience and the allowance of parents in the operatory
- **Carr et al**[10] reported that 84% of practitioners allow parent to be in clinic with their children during treatment

- **Advantages of parental absence:**
  - Overcoming parental conditioning
  - Avoiding communication interference
  - Avoiding parental interference

RETRAINING

- A technique similar to behavior shaping, designed to fabricate positive values and to replace the negative behavior.
- Children who require retraining approach the dental office displaying considerable apprehension or negative behavior. This may be due to previous eventful dental visit or the effect of improper parental or peer orientation or even due to the child's experience in medical setting.
- The essence here is to locate the problem that it can either be avoided or distracted. The dentist should try to build up a new relation with the child so that the child is able to forget his previous thought process of dental clinic.
- If the child has had a previous eventful dental experience with some other dentist in another operatory, he will always have a fear and associate this clinic and dentist with the same; so it is up to the dental team to make his experience different so that he is retrained.
- **Approaches:**
  - Avoidance (e.g., avoid extensive pulp therapy with pulp capping)
  - De-emphasis and substitution (e.g., substitute high-speed handpiece with spoon excavator)
  - Distraction (e.g., distract the child with stories/activities/audiovisual aids).

MEMORY RESTRUCTURING

It is a behavioral approach in which memories associated with a negative or difficult event (e.g., first dental visit, LA, restorative procedures, extraction) are restructured into the positive memories using information suggested after the event has taken place **(Kenath 2013)**. Restructuring involves four components:

1. Visual reminder
2. Positive reinforcement through visualization
3. Concrete example to encode sensory details
4. Sense of accomplishment.

- A visual reminder could be a photograph of the child smiling at the initial visit (i.e., prior to the difficult experience).
- **Objective:** Restructures difficult or negative past dental experience and improves patient behavior at subsequent dental visits.

Reframing

- Proposed by **Watzlawick et al. 1974**
- It refers taking a situation outside the frame up to the moment the individual is in different state and visualize in a way acceptable to the person. When using this technique of reframing, it is not the fact that changes, rather meaning attributed to them that changes.
- Ultimate achievement is the second order change. (Different reality)
- It is especially useful in younger children 3–4 years, more so in a 4-year old child because of their lively mind.
- Successful reframing converts the notion of unpleasantness to notion acceptance and approval by the patients.

MAGIC TRICK

- The use of a magic trick has been shown to be an effective alternative behavioral management strategy in strong-willed young children. The technique is useful for all patients who can verbally communicate. There are no contraindications.
- The magic trick is used to encourage children who on a previous visit to the dental surgery had refused to enter the dental surgery, to sit in the dental chair and have a radiograph. The simple use of the trick increased cooperation when compared to no intervention **(Fig. 21.18)**. It is unclear the mechanism of action for this technique but one element may be the rapport building involved.

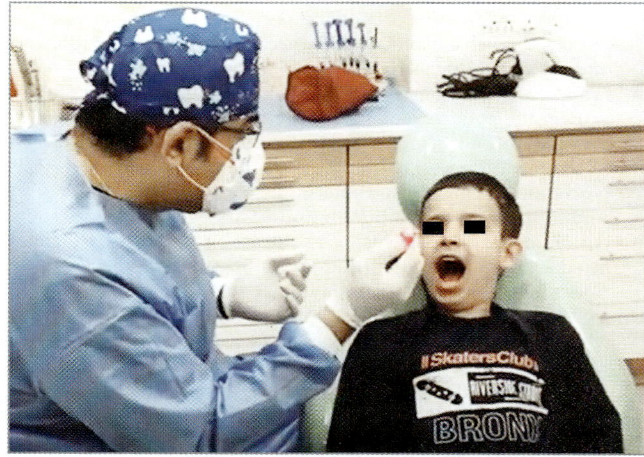

Fig. 21.18: Magic trick by dentist. (*Pic courtesy:* Dr Nikhil Grover).

RELAXATION BREATHING

- This exercise is believed to benefit almost every fearful patient in relaxation through paced breathing.
- The physiologic changes accompanying relaxation breathing, or diaphragmatic breathing, effectively forms a counterpart to the emergency "fight or flight reaction" characterizing an anxious individual.
- It is difficult to be tense and to breathe from your abdomen at the same time.

Research on relaxation breathing
- **Armfield**[7] (2013) stated breathing relaxation is easy to perform and can be adopted by anxious patients in the dental chair immediately before treatment or at home
- **Milgran**[42](2009) revealed breathing relaxation provides more oxygen to the body, thus reducing the heart rate.

- It is believed that relaxation breathing can also be effective in reducing perceived pain.
- While a systematic review involving the period 1996–2005 found no association between rhythmic breathing relaxation and pain relief in a single identified study, one recent study has shown that relaxation breathing does appear to lower both anxiety and perceived pain.

PROGRESSIVE MUSCLE RELAXATION

- The process of progressive muscle relaxation is based on the principle of muscle physiology that even if the muscle is tensed, releasing the tension causes relaxation in the muscle.
- The basic process of progressive muscle relaxation requires the patient to focus on specific voluntary muscles and in sequence, tense and then relax the tension in that muscle.

As the tensing and relaxing sequence progresses, other aspects of the relaxation response also actively occur: breathing becomes slower and deeper, heart rate and BP decreases and vasodilation in the small capillaries of the extreme may occur, meeting a subjective sense of calmness and ease.

BUBBLE BREATH PLAY THERAPY

It is simple, inexpensive, exceptionally engaging and non-threatening technique in which children are encouraged to blow big bubbles and exhale slowly **(Azher U et al,[43] 2020)**. To blow bubbles, children take deep breaths which help to train them in controlled breathing enhancing relaxation **(Fig. 21.19)**.

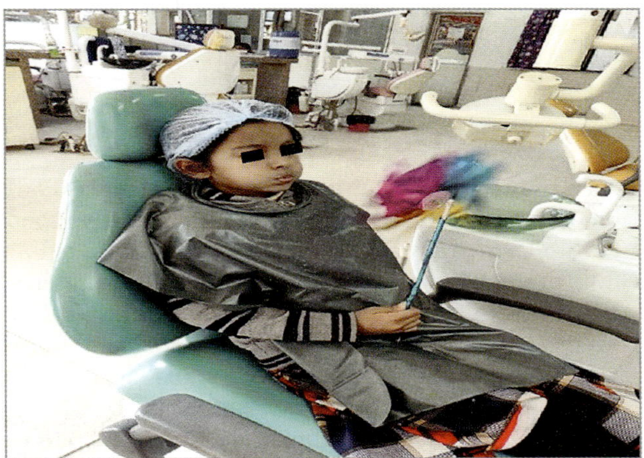

Fig. 21.19: Bubble breath play therapy.

VISUAL IMAGERY

- Controlled day dreaming
- Subject is asked to imagine being in his favorite place/ performing his favorite activity and this can act as a fantasy during his dental treatment.

AROMATHERAPY

- It is noninvasive, inexpensive therapy which uses essential oils extracted from flowers, barks, stem, leaves, roots, flowers and other parts of plant.
- Term aromatherapy was coined by **Rene Gattefosse.**
- It involves inhalation of scented oil which reaches the lungs and rapidly diffuse into blood causing brain activation through systemic circulation. Essential oils contain neroli as main component. Inhaling the neroli essential oil is thought to transmit messages to part of brain (limbic system) that controls emotions, which in turn influences the nervous system thereby casing stress reduction and enhancement of mood.
- **Nirmala K et al:[44]** Aromatherapy with levander oil or sweet orange using nebulizer or inhaler decreases dental anxiety of children.

VOICE CONTROL

- Given by **Pinkham** in 1985
- Sudden and firm commands that are used to get the child's attention and stop the child from his current activity
- Soft, monotonous soothing conversation can also be used as it is supposed to function like music to set the mood
- In both cases what is heard is more important because the dentist is attempting to influence behavior directly and not through understanding
- The tone of voice and the facial expression of the dentist are also important as they function like a mirror
- **Objectives:**
  - To gain the patient attention and compliance
  - To avoid negative or avoidance behavior
  - To establish authority
- **Indications:** Uncooperative and inattentive patients
- **Contraindications:** Children who due to age, disability, mental or emotional immaturity are unable to understand.

USE OF POETRY AND DRAWINGS

Use of Poetry

- This technique is employed in children above 7 years of age.
- The poem is written as a collective effort, the dentist contributing one line and the child next, for example, teeth are white, when they are bright; teeth do shine, when you clean; teeth are happy, when they are healthy; teeth stay long, when they are strong.
- By selecting words like shine, happy, and long, it was easy to make the child discover clean, healthy, and strong. By doing this, it allows the child to discover information about his teeth and their well-being.

Use of Drawings

- This technique was developed when it was discovered that with a little manipulation, the forms of the familiar teeth could be altered to look like common animals, birds, and insects.
- This is useful for children of 3–5 years of age.
- Child is given a paper and pencil or a crayon and asked to draw some picture. Then slowly the child is asked to draw teeth and showed how teeth can be made to look like his pets. He is then told that like his pets, the tooth also have to be looked after and kept clean.

Advantages

- It allows repetition without monotony.
- The rhyme and rhythm can be used to guide the child toward the information to be implied.
- It gives the child a sense of achievement and increases self-esteem.
- Above all, it will destroy the preconception the child has formed about dentistry, the dentist, and the dental clinic.

HYPNOSIS

It was first suggested by **Franz A Mesmer**, a Viennese physician, in 1773. It is defined as a state of mental relaxation and restricted awareness in which subjects are usually engrossed in their inner experiences such as imagery, are less analytical and logical in their thinking, and have enhanced capacity to respond to suggestions in an automatic and dissociated manner. This is explained in detail in Chapter 87.

Uses

Hennon outlined the following uses:
- To reduce nervousness and apprehension
- To eliminate defense mechanisms that patients use to postpone dental work
- To control functional or psychosomatic gapping
- To prevent thumb sucking and bruxism
- To induce anesthesia.

ROLE-PLAY

- Effective communication with the child is the backbone of all behavior management techniques, role-play is perceived as gratifying in terms of developing effective communication and appropriate behavioral and attitudinal skills.
- In role-play, the learner develops and practices newly acquired skills by simulating a scenario. It involves a minimum of two or a group of students, who communicate both as dentists and as patients as they switch between these roles. Role-play can be recommended by educators as a new teaching modality, as it offers the opportunity for active student engagement and the integration of learned concepts into practice **(Fig. 21.20)**.
- **Khubchandani et al.**[45] in 2022 conducted a study among undergraduates. To compare role play with group discussion and found that role-play as a teaching tool was highly effective in instilling behavior management skills among students to deal with young patients in clinical situations as compared to the group discussion method.

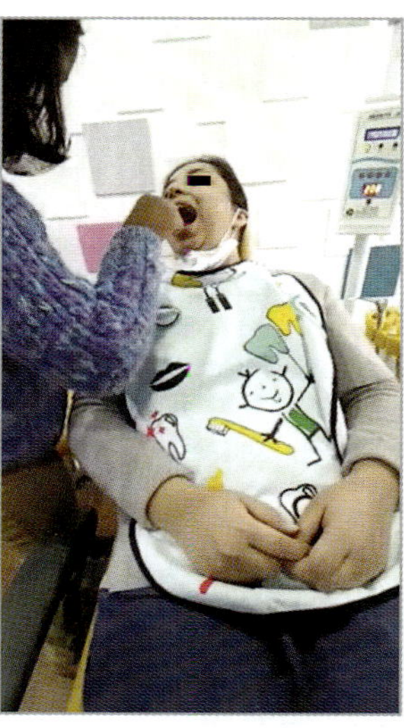

Fig. 21.20: Role-play.

HUMANOID ROBOTICS

- Robots have captured the interest, curiosity, and attention of children.
- Medical robots have only been in use for a few decades, and humanoid robots are started to be used to implement technopsychological distraction for children in order to reduce their pain as a result of stress and anxiety during a medical procedure **(Fig. 21.21)**.

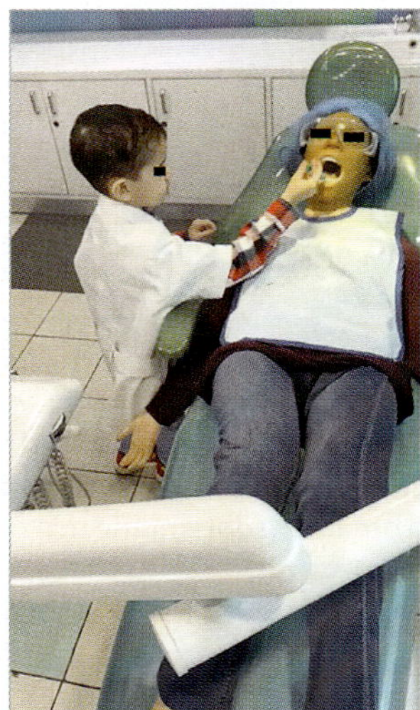

Fig. 21.21: Humanoid robotics.

- Human-robot interaction design, the clinical application of robot technologies to dental services might be good option for modern dentistry. iRobiQ is a small, autonomous, humanoid robot manufactured by Yujin Robot. It has a touch-screen LCD display on its body, multicolor LEDs on its face and hands allow further communication of emotions by colored light. Programming facilitates the robot show different facial expressions such as happy, sad, surprise, or angry. In this study, iRobiQ was chosen for human facial expressions contents.
- **Yelda Kasimoglu et al.,**[46] in 2020 conducted a study in 4–10 year old children to reduce their anxiety and improve their behavior during dental treatment and concluded that robotic technology can successfully help in coping with dental anxiety and stress, and helps children to behave better in dental office.

FLOODING TECHNIQUE

Described as behavior modification technique that eliminates a child's attempts to avoid experiences that he perceives to be undesirable, for example, HOM, physical restraints.

HAND-OVER-MOUTH TECHNIQUE

This technique was first described in 1920 by **Dr Evangeline Jordan** who wrote "If a normal child will not listen but continues to cry and struggle—hold a folded napkin over the child's mouth and gently but firmly hold the mouth shut. His scream increases his condition of hysteria, but if the mouth is held closed, there is little sound, and he soon begins to reason **(Fig. 21.22)**."

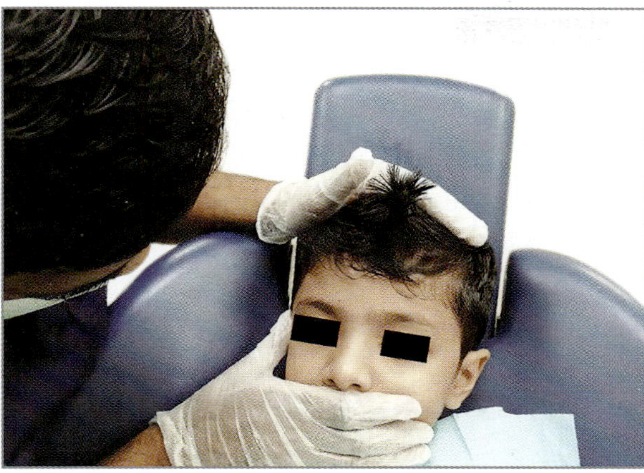

Fig. 21.22: Hand-over-mouth exercise.

Other terminologies

- Aversive conditioning by **Lenchner** and **Wright**
- Emotional surprise therapy by **Lampshire**
- HOM airway restricted (HOMAR) by **Levitas** (1947)
- Aversion by **Crammer** (1973).

Objectives

- To gain child's attention enabling communication with dentist so that appropriate behavioral expectation can be explained.
- To eliminate inappropriate avoidance behavior to dental treatment and to establish appropriate learned response.
- To increase child's confidence in coping with anxiety provoking dental stimuli.
- To assure child safety in delivery of quality dental care.

Indication

A healthy child who is able to understand and cooperate but who exhibits defiant, obstreperous, or hysterical behavior to dental treatment.

Contraindications

- Immature child
- When it prevents child from breathing
- When the dentist is emotionally involved with the child.

Technique

When indicated, a hand is placed over child's mouth and behavioral expectations are calmly explained. Child is told that the hand will be removed as soon as the appropriate behavior begins. When child responds, the hand is removed and child's appropriate behavior is reinforced. If the child shows negative behavior, again the procedure is repeated.

Research regarding Hand-Over-Mouth Exercise (HOME)

- Association of Pedodontic Diplomates in 1970 found out that 80% used HOME technique frequently
- **Carr et al.**[10] found out the number of clinicians who did not practice HOME was around 57%
- **Adair et al.,**[41] observed that 79% of the clinicians did not use HOME.
- **Newton** and **Patel H et al.,**[47] (2004): determined the attitudes of UK specialist pediatric dentists towards the HOM technique and the use of physical restraints and found very small number of specialist dentists endorse HOM as a technique for the control of un-cooperative children. Approximately 60% of the respondents reported that HOM should never be used. Those who used and suggested it, said that it should be used with cases of hysterical, tantrum behavior (57 respondents, 32%). The most commonly anticipated psychological sequel which may accompany the use of these techniques was subsequent fear of dental treatment.
- **Sharath et al.,**[48] have shown that the usage of aversive techniques like voice control and HOME reduced over the subsequent visits in an Indian structured postgraduate dental program.

Variations of the Techniques

Airway uninstructed, hand-over both nose and mouth, HOMAR, towel held over mouth only, dry towel over nose and mouth, wet towel over nose and mouth **(Figs. 21.23A to C).**

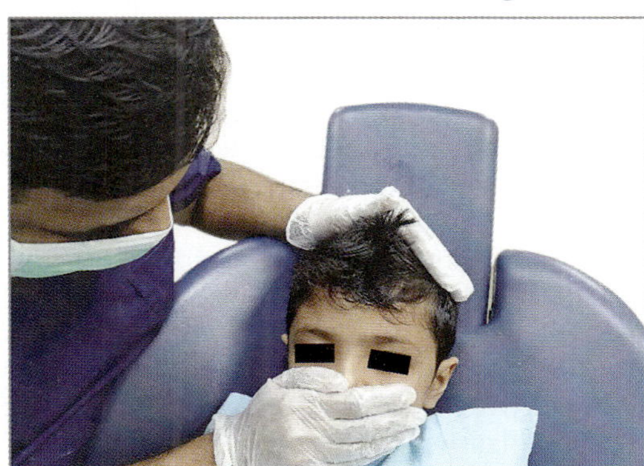

Fig. 21.23A: Hand-over-mouth airway restricted.

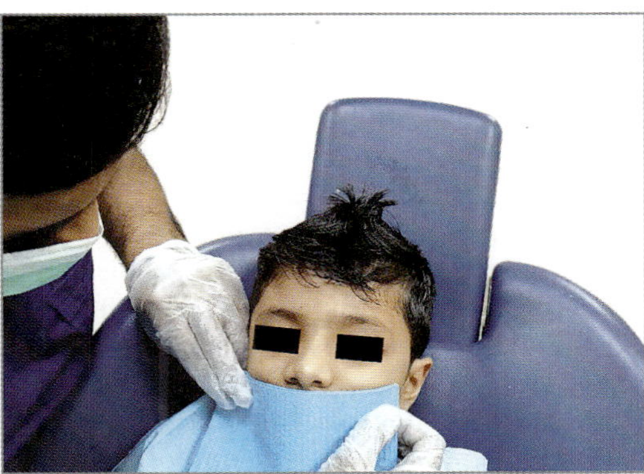

Fig. 21.23B: Towel held over mouth only.

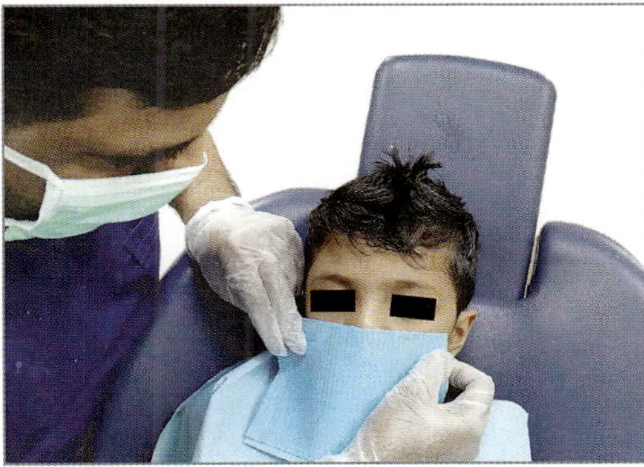

Fig. 21.23C: Towel held over mouth and nose.

Legality of Use of HOME

- It has been pointed out that the use of HOME will not subject the dentist to liability by the patient when it is used properly with parental consent.
- Use of HOMAR is more nearly objectionable legally and may result in liability of the dentist.

PROTECTIVE STABILIZATION

Partial or complete immobilization of the patient is sometimes a necessary and effective way to diagnose and deliver dental care to patients who need help in controlling their extremities. Immobilization is also useful for managing combative, resistant patients, so that the patient, practitioner, or dental staff may be protected from injury while care is being provided. The parents must be informed and the consent must be documented, before immobilization is used, they should have a clear understanding of the type of immobilization to be used, the rationale, and duration of use.

The American Academy of Pediatric Dentistry's Standard of Care for Behavior Management, revised in May 1996, indicates that the need to diagnose and treat, as well as protect the safety of the patient and practitioner, must justify the use of immobilization. This decision should take into consideration the patient's emotional development, physical and medical considerations, dental need, other alternative behavioral modalities, and the quality of dental care. The older terminology of physical restraints has been replaced with the term medical immobilization or protective stabilization because we are not just strapping the child to the chair minimizing his movement. The idea is to immobilize the child benefiting and protecting both the child and the dentist.

Indications for Using Immobilization

- A patient who requires diagnosis or treatment and cannot cooperate because of lack of maturity.
- A patient who requires diagnosis or treatment and cannot cooperate because of mental or physical disabilities.
- A patient who requires diagnosis or treatment and does not cooperate after other behavior management techniques have failed.
- When the safety of the patient or practitioner would be at risk without the protective use of immobilization.

Contraindications

- A cooperative patient
- A patient who cannot be safely immobilized because of underlying medical or systemic conditions
- As punishment
- It should not be used solely for the convenience of the staff.

Research regarding protective stabilization

- Association of Pedodontic Diplomats in 1972 conducted a survey and found out that 84% of the pedodontists used physical restraints in selected patients
- **Nathan** (1989) observed that only 4% of the pedodontists employed immobilization technique

Types of Restraints

1. **Active:** Restraining performed by dentist, staff or parent without aid of any restraining device.
2. **Passive:** Restraining performed with aid of restraining device.

Types of mechanical aids for protective stabilization

Part	Aid	Features
Mouth	Tongue blades Open wide mouth prop 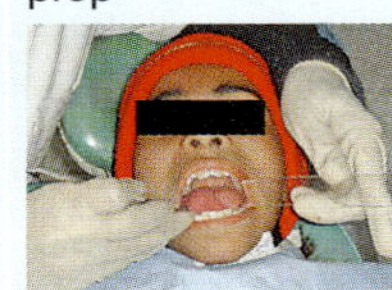	• These can be used directly to open mouth • It has a durable foam core on the outside of a tongue depressor • It is also easy to use, durable, and available in two sizes
	Molt mouth prop 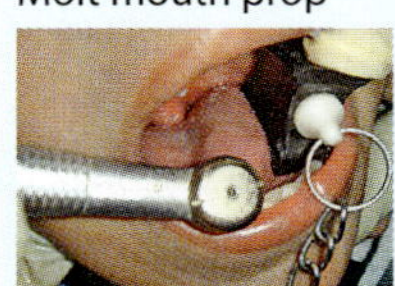	• It can be very helpful in the management of a difficult patient for a prolonged period. It is made in both adult and child sizes, allows accessibility to the opposite side of the mouth • Its disadvantages include the possibility of lip and palatal lacerations and luxation of teeth if it is not used correctly • The patient's mouth should not be forced beyond its natural limits because patient's • Discomfort and panic will result, causing further resistance and perhaps airway compromise
	Rubber bite blocks 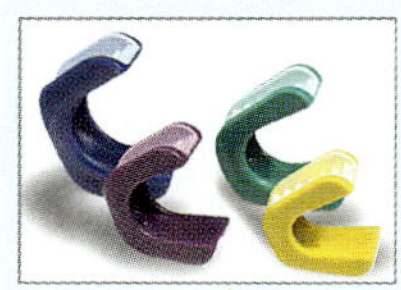	• Available in various sizes to fit on the occlusal surfaces of the teeth and stabilize the mouth in an open position. The bite blocks should have floss attached for easy retrieval if they become dislodged in the mouth
	Finger guards 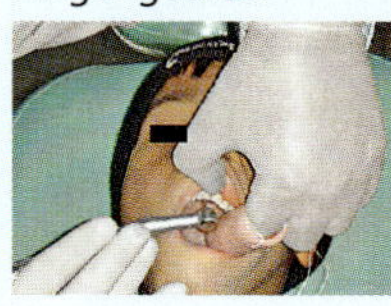	• Used directly to open mouth
Extremities	Posey straps Velcro straps Towel and tape Extra assistant 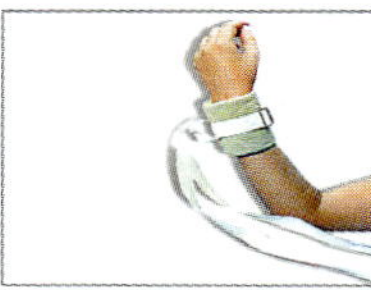	• Fasten to the arms of the dental chair and allow limited movement frequently preventing overreaction by resistant or combative patients • Helpful for an athetoid-spastic cerebral palsy patient who tries desperately, but without success, to control body movements

Part	Aid	Features
Body	Papoose board	• Simple to store and use • It is available in areas to hold both large and small children • It has attached head stabilizers • It is reusable • Necessary to monitor respiration if it is used in combination with sedation • An extremely resistant patient may develop hyperthermia if immobilized too long • Any restrained patient requires constant attendance and supervision
	Triangular sheet	• Mink described this technique using a triangular sheet to control an extremely resistant child • It allows the patient to upright during radiographic examinations • Its disadvantages include the frequent need for straps to maintain the patient's position in the chair, the difficulty of its use on small patients, and the possibility of airway impingement • Hyperthermia may be another problem during long periods of immobilization • The need for constant supervision is emphasized so that these problems may be avoided
	Pedi-Wrap	• Comes in various sizes and allows some movement while still confining the patient • Its mesh fabric prevents developing hyperthermia • Requires straps to maintain body position in the dental chair • Constant supervision to prevent the patient from rolling out of the chair
	Bean bag Dental chair Insert	• Developed to help comfortably accommodate hypnotic and severely spastic persons who need more support and less immobilization in a dental environment • It is reusable and washable, and one size fits most people • Many patients with physical disabilities relax more in this setting
	Safety belt and extra assistant	• Useful in controlling movements
Head	Head positioner Plastic bowl Extra assistant	• Used to stabilize head

POINTS TO REMEMBER

- Behavior management is the means by which the dental health team effectively and efficiently performs treatment for a child and at the same time instills a positive dental attitude.
- Factors influencing child's behavior in dental office are history, maternal anxiety, family and peer influence, dental office environment, growth and development, environmental factors.
- Objectives of behavior management are to establish effective communication with child and parent; gain child and parent confidence for dental treatment; teach child positive aspect of preventive dental care and provide a comfortable, relaxing environment to the child.
- *Role of dentist in child's behavior:* Appearance of dental office should be pleasing; personality of dentist should be impressive; time and length of appointment should be short; dentist should be skilled; dentist should use simple words; dentist should treat the patient with importance; dentist should be realistic and reasonable; dentist should exercise self-control.
- Frankl found that children in age group of 42–49 months are benefited from mother's presence in operatory.
- Frankl in 1962 introduced a behavior-rating scale, which is one of the most reliable tools developed for behavior measurement. It consists of a ratings of determination numbered from 1 to 4, each defining a specific behavior.
- Wright in 1975 suggested that a symbol be added to this rating scale, permitting the dentist to record a behavior base at the inception of dental treatment and to keep a progressive record of the child's behavior.
- Psychological approach of behavior management are preappointment behavior modification, communication, use of second language, TSD, tender love care, desensitization, contingency management, visual imagery, modeling, behavior shaping, assimilation and coping, hypnosis, retraining, distraction, externalization, parental presence or absence, reframing and voice control.
- Physical approach of behavior management are HOME and physical restraints.
- Communication acts as a means for the dentist to know the child and his fears and can be of verbal or nonverbal type.
- Euphemism is use of second language like camera for X-ray.
- Animatopia is giving animated sounds to objects like handpiece is called whistling train.
- TSD is the cornerstone of behavior management was given by Addleston in 1959. Specifically, the dentist tells the child what is going to be done in words the child can understand. Second, the dentist demonstrates to the child exactly how the procedure will be conducted. Finally, the practitioner performs the procedure exactly as it was described and demonstrated.

- Objectives of modeling are to stimulate acquisition of new behavior, facilitating the behavior already in the patients in a more appropriate manner, elimination of avoidance behavior, and extinction of fear.
- Live modeling by the same age group peer is one of the best methods of behavior management of a child.
- Distraction is a newer method of behavior management in which the child seeing the audiovisual presentation will have multisensory distraction as he will tend to concentrate on the TV screen thereby, screening out the sight of dental treatment and the sound of the program will help eliminate the unpleasant dental sounds like the sound of handpiece.
- Voice control was given by Pinkham in 1985. It is sudden and firm commands are used to get the child's attention and stop the child from his current activity.
- HOM technique is also called aversive conditioning, emotional surprise therapy, HOME, and aversion by Crammer. Objective is to gain child's attention enabling communication with dentist so that appropriate behavioral expectation can be explained, to eliminate inappropriate avoidance behavior to dental treatment and to establish appropriate learned response. It is indicated in a healthy child who is able to understand and cooperate but who exhibits defiant, obstreperous, or hysterical behavior to dental treatment.
- Immobilization is indicated in patient who requires diagnosis or treatment and cannot cooperate because of lack of maturity or because of mental or physical disabilities and in patients in whom all other behavior management techniques have failed. Restraints for mouth—mouth props, tongue blade, rubber bite blocks, finger guard; body—Papoose board, triangular sheet, Pedi-Wraps, beanbag dental chair insert; extremities—straps, tapes; head—head positioner.

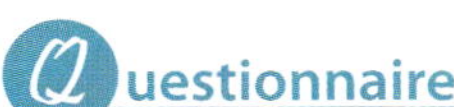

Questionnaire

1. Define behavior and behavior management and enumerate the techniques for child management.
2. What are the factors influencing child behavior in dental office?
3. What are the objectives of behavior management?
4. Describe the role of dentist in child management.
5. Write a note on maternal influence in dental operatory.
6. Classify child behavior and give details about Frankl's classification.
7. Describe preappointment behavior modifications.
8. Differentiate between communication and euphemisms.
9. Explain TSD technique.
10. Write a note on distraction.
11. Describe the indications and procedure of modeling.
12. Give the indications, procedure, modifications of HOME.
13. Explain the different types of mechanical restraints used for immobilization.

REFERENCES

1. Wright GZ, Starkey PE, Gardner DE. Child management in dentistry, 2nd edition. Oxford: John Wright and Sons; 1991. pp. 58-75.
2. Lenchner V, Wright GZ. Non-pharmacologic therapeutic approaches to behavior management. In: Wright GZ (Ed). Behavior management in dentistry for children. Philadelphia, PA: WB Saunders Co.; 1975. pp. 91-114.
3. Gao X, Hamzah SH, Yiu CKY, et al. Dental fear and anxiety in children and adolescents: qualitative study using YouTube. J Med Internet Res. 2013;15:e29.
4. Asokan S, Surendran S, Punugoti D, Nuvvula S, GeethaPriya PR. Validation of a novel behavior prediction scale: A two-center trial. Contemp Clin Dent. 2014;5(4):514-7.
5. Hane AA, Cheah C, Rubin KH, et al. The role of maternal behavior in the relation between shyness and social reticence in early childhood and social withdrawal in middle childhood. Soc Dev. 2008; doi: 10.1111/j.1467-9507.2008.00481.x.
6. Landry SH, Smith KE, Swank PR, et al. Early maternal and child influences on children's later independent cognitive and social functioning. Child Dev. 2000;71:358-75.
7. Armfield JM, Heaton LJ. Management of fear and anxiety in the dental clinic: a review. Australian Dental Journal. 2013;58:390-407.
8. Aboulenain AM, Abdellatif AM, El-agamy RA. Effects of different modifications of second language on child's behavior in the dental office. Dental journal. 2017;63:563-8.
9. Adelson R, Goldfried MR. Modeling and the fearful child patient. J Dent Child. 1970;37:476.
10. Carr KR, Wilson S, Nimer S, et al. Behavior management techniques among pediatric dentists practicing in the southeastern United States. Pediatr Dent. 1999;21:347-53.
11. Crossley ML, Joshi G. An investigation of pediatric dentists' attitude toward parental accompaniment and behavioral management techniques. BR Dent. 2002;11,192(9)517-21.
12. Grewal N. Implementation of behavioral management technique—how well accepted they are today. J Indian Soc Pedo Prev Dent. 2003;21:70-4.
13. Peretz B, Glaicher H, Ram D. Child management technique. Are there differences in the way female male pediatric dentists in Israel practice? Braz Dent J. 2003;14:82-6.
14. Sharma A, Tyagi R. Behavior assessment of children in dental settings: a retrospective study. Int J Clin Pediatr Dent. 2011;4:35-9.
15. Al Daghanin S, Balharith M, Alhaznis, et al. Behavior management techniques in pediatric dentistry: how well they are accepted? A Cal J Ped Neonatal. 2017;5:1-6.
16. Sayed A, Ranna V, Padawe D, et al. Effect of the video output of the dental operating microscope on anxiety levels in a pediatric population during restrictive procedures. J Indian Soc Pedod Prev Dent. 2016;34:604.
17. Tiwari S, Arora R. Behaviour Management Techniques in Paediatric Dentistry; Comparative study based on heart rate Between Live Modelling and Tell-Show-Do. 2016;3(6):160-3.
18. Samara-Quintero PA, Bernardoni-Socorro C, Borjas AM, Fuenmayor NR, Estevez J, Arteaga-Vizcaino M. Changes in blood pressure in children undergoing psychological treatment before dental procedures. Acta Odontol Latinoam. 2006;19(1):9-12.
19. Vishwakarma AP, Bandarde PA, Patil SB, et al. Effectiveness of two different behavioral modification techniques among 5-7 year old children. A randomized controlled trial. J India Soc Ped Prev Dent. 2017;35:143-5.
20. Kevadia MV, B Sandhyarani, Patil AT, et al. Comparative Evaluation of Effectiveness of Tell-Play-Do, Film Modeling and Use of Smartphone Dental Application in the Management of Child Behavior. Int J Clin Pediatr Dent. 2020;13(6):682-7.
21. Shah U, Bhatia R. Effectiveness of Audiovisual Eyeglass method compared to Tell-Play-Do technique among 4–7 year old children: A randomized control trial. International Journal of Oral Care and Research. 2018;6(2):1-7.
22. Radhakrishna S, Srinivasan I, Shetty J, Krishna M, Melwani A, Hegde K. Comparison of three behavior modification technique for management of anxious children aged 4-8 years. J Dent Anesth Pain Med. 2019;19(1):29-36.
23. Patil VH, Vaid K, Gokhale NS, Shah P, Mundada M, Hugar SM. Evaluation of effectiveness of dental apps in management of child behaviour: A pilot study. Int J Pedod Rehabil. 2017;2:14-8.
24. Meshki, et al. Effects of Pretreatment Exposure to Dental Practice Using a Smartphone Dental Simulation Game on Children's Pain and Anxiety: A Preliminary Double-Blind Randomized Clinical Trial. Journal of Dentistry, Tehran University of Medical Sciences, Tehran, Iran. 2018;15(4):250-8.
25. Shah HA, Nanjunda Swamy KV, Kulkarni S and Choubey S. Evaluation of dental anxiety and hemodynamic changes (Sympatho-Adrenal Response) during various dental procedures using smartphone

applications v/s traditional behaviour management techniques in pediatric patients. International Journal of Applied Research 2017; 3(5): 429-433.
26. Lee JH, Jung HK, Lee GG, Kim HY, Park SG, Woo SC. Effect of behavioral intervention using smartphone application for preoperative anxiety in pediatric patients. Korean J Anesthesiol. 2013;65:508-18.
27. Karan S, Manvi M, Vinod S. Relative efficacy of Tell-Show-Do and the modeling techniques on suburban Indian children during dental treatment based on heart rate valves: a clinical study. J Dent Specialties. 2016;4:178-82.
28. Farhet N, Mc Mayley, Harfouche A, et al. Techniques for managing behavior in pediatric dentistry: comparative study of live modeling and tell-show-do based on children's heart rates during restraint. JCDA. 2009;75:283a-283f.
29. Roberts JF, Curean ME, Koch G, et al. Newton: behavior management technique in pediatric dentistry. Eur Arch Pedia Dent. 2010;11:166-74.
30. Johnson DC. Managing the patient and parent in dental practice. In: Wei SHY (Ed). Pediatric dentistry. Total patient care. Philadelphia, PA: Lea & Febiger; 1988. p. 140.
31. Chambers DW. Behavior management techniques for pediatric dentists: an embarrassments of riches. ASDC J Dent Child. 1977:30-4.
32. Karekar P, Bijle MN, Walimbe H. Effect of three behavior guidance techniques on anxiety indicators of children undergoing diagnosis and preventive dental care. Journal of Clinical Pediatric Dentistry. 2019;43(3):167-72.
33. Prabhakar AR, Marwah N, Raju OS. Comparison between audio and audio-visual distraction technique in managing anxious pediatric dental patients. JISPPD. 2007:177-82.
34. Mahmoud SA. Comparative evaluation of passive, active and passive active distraction techniques on pain perception during local anesthesia administration in children. J Advan Res. 2016;7:551-6.
35. Agarwal N, Dhawan J, Kumar D, et al. Effectiveness of two topical ansesthetic agents used along with audiovisual aids in pediatric Dental Patients. J Clin Diag Res. 2017;11: ZC80-3.
36. Nuvvula S, Alahari S, Kamatham R, et al. Effect of audiovisual distraction with 3D video glasses on dental anxiety of children experiencing administration of local analgesia: a randomised clinical trial. Eur Arch Paediatr Dent. 2014;16:43-50.
37. Attar RH, Baghdadi ZD. Comparative efficacy of active and passive distraction during restorative treatment in children using an iPad versus audiovisual eyeglasses: a randomised controlled trial. European Archives of Paediatric Dentistry. 2015;16(1):1-8.
38. Dahlquist LM, Weiss KE, Law EF, Sil S, Herbert LJ, Horn SB, et al. Effects of videogame distraction and a virtual reality type head-mounted display helmet on cold pressor pain in young elementary school-aged children. J Pediatr Psychol. 2010;35(6):617-25.
39. Fakhruddin KS, Gorduysus MO, El Batawi H. Effectiveness of behavioral modification techniques with visual distraction using intrasulcular local anesthesia in hearing disabled children during pulp therapy. Eur J Dent. 2016;10(4):551-5.
40. Kasimoglu Y, Kocaaydin S, Karsli E, Esen M, Bektas I, Ince G, Tuna EB. Robotic approach to the reduction of dental anxiety in children. Acta Odontologica Scandinavica. 2020;78(6):474-80.
41. Adair SM, Waller JL, Schafer TE, et al. A survey of members of American Academy of Pediatric Dentistry on their use of behavior management techniques. Pediatr Dent. 2004;26:159-66.
42. Milgran, Weinstein P, Newton LJ. Treating fearful dental patients: a patient management handbook, 3rd edition. Seattle (WA). Dental Behavior Research; 2009.
43. Azher U, Srinath SK, Nayak M. Effectiveness of bubble breath play therapy in the dental management of anxious children: a pilot study. The Journal of Contemporary Dental Practice. 2020;21(1):17-21.
44. Nirmala K, Kamatham R. Effect of Aromatherapy on Dental Anxiety and Pain in Children Undergoing Local Anesthetic Administrations: A Randomized Clinical Trial. Journal of Caring Sciences. 2021;10(3):111.
45. Monika MK, Srivastava T, Vagha S, Baliga S, Thosar N, Rathi N. Comparative evaluation of role play and group discussion as teaching-learning method for behavior management in pediatric dentistry. International Journal of Health Sciences. 2022; 870-81.
46. Kasimoglu Y, Kocaaydin S, Karsli E, Esen M, Bektas I, Ince G, et al. Robotic approach to the reduction of dental anxiety in children. Acta Odontol Scand. 2020;78(6):474-480. doi: 10.1080/00016357.2020.1800084. Epub 2020 Jul 30. PMID: 32730719.
47. JT Newton, Patel H, Shah S, et al. Attitudes towards the use of hand-over-mouth (HOM) and physical restraint amongst pediatric specialist practitioners in the UK. Int J Pediat Dent. 2004;14):111-7.
48. Sharath A, Rekka P, Muthu MS, RathnaPrabhu V, Sivakumar N. Children's behavior pattern and behavior management techniques used in a structured postgraduate dental program. J Indian Soc Pedod Prev Dent. 2009;27(1):22-26.

FURTHER READING

1. Ajlouni O, Al-Moherat F, Habahbeh R, et al. Behavior management techniques among Jordanian pediatric dentists. J R Med Serv. 2010;17(Suppl 2):62-6.
2. Allen KD, Stonely RTM. Evaluation of behavioral management technology dissemination in pediatric dentistry. Pediatr Dent. 1990;12(2):79-82.
3. American Academy of Pediatric Dentistry. Clinical guidelines on behavioral management. Pediatr Dent Reference Manual. 2003;25(7 suppl):69-74.
4. Chambers DW. Communicating with the young patient. J Am Dent Assoc. 1976;93:793-9.
5. Choate BB, Seale NS, Parker WA, et al. Current trends in behavior management techniques as they relate to new standards concerning informed consent. Pediatr Dent. 1990;12:83-6.
6. Christen A. Pjagetian psychology: some principles as helpful in treating the child dental patient. J Dent Child. 1971:44.
7. Connick C, Palat M, Pugliese S. Appropriate use of physical restraints. ASDC J Dent Child. 2000. pp.256-62.
8. Craig W. Hand over mouth technique. J Dent Child. 1971;38:387.
9. Crall JJ. Behavior management conference panel 2 report- third-party payer issues. Pediatr Dent. 2004;26:171-4.
10. Curry SL. The role of coping in children's adjustment to dental visit. ASDC J Dent Child. 1988. pp.231-46.
11. Florella M, Sarale C, Ram RD. Audiovisual iatrosedation with video eyeglasses distraction method in pediatric dentistry: case history. J Int Dent Med Res. 2010;3:133-6.
12. Greenbaum PE, et al. Dentist's voice control: effects on children's disruptive behaviors. Health Psychol. 1990;9:46-58.
13. Hagan PP. The legal status of informed consent for behavior management techniques in dentistry. Pediatr Dent. 1984;6:204-8.
14. Kuhn BR, Allen KD. Expanding child behavior management technology in pediatric dentistry: a behavior science perspective. Pediatr Dent. 1994;16:13-7.
15. Lawrence SM. Parental attitudes toward behavior management techniques in pediatric dentistry. Pediatr Dent. 1991;13:151-5.
16. Levitas TC. HOME—hand over mouth exercise. J Dent Child. 1974;41:178-82.
17. Machen JB, Johnson R. Desensitization, model learning and dental behavior in children. J Dent Res. 1974:83-7.
18. Maruyama S, Koyazu T. Effect of dental drawings and coloring on attitudes of child dental patients. ASDC J Dent Child. 1988:129-32.
19. McKnight-Hanes C, Myers DR, Dushku JC, Davis HC. The use of behavioral management techniques by dentists across practitioner type, age and geographic region. Pediatr Dent. 1993;15:267-71.
20. Peretz B, Bimstein E. Use of imagery suggestions during administration of LA in pediatric dental patients. ASDC J Dent Child. 2000:263-7.
21. Peretz B, Gluck GM. Reframing—reappraising an old behavioral technique. J Clin Pediatr Dent. 1999;23:103-6.
22. Shaw AJ, Welbury R. The use of hypnosis in sedation clinic for dental extraction in children. ASDC J Dent Child. 1996: pp. 418-20.
23. Suprabha BS, Rao A, Choudhary S, et al. Child dental fear and behavior: the role of environmental factors in a hospital cohort. J Ind Soc Pedod Prev Dent. 2011;29:95-101.
24. Wepman BJ, Sonnenberg EM. Effective communication with the pedodontic patient. J Pedod. 1979;2:316-21.

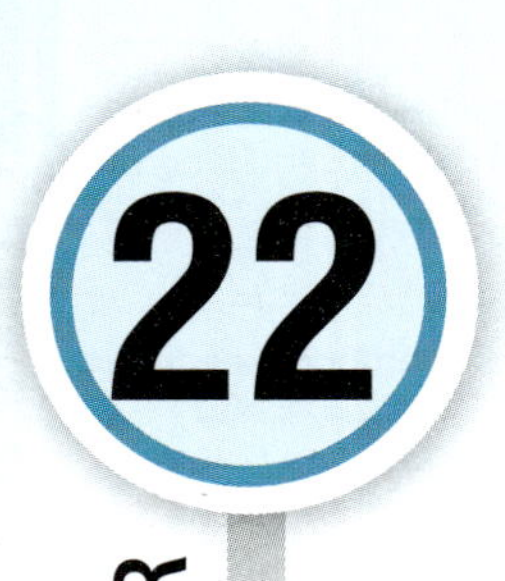

CHAPTER

Nitrous Oxide—Oxygen Anxiolysis and Conscious Sedation

Kunal Gupta, Ashwin Rao, Nikhil Marwah, Abhilasha Agarwal, Akash Patodia

Chapter Outline

Most children can be managed effectively using the techniques outlined in basic behavior guidance. These basic behavior guidance techniques should form the foundation for all of the management activities provided by the dentist. Children, however, occasionally present with behavioral considerations that require more advanced techniques. These children often cannot cooperate due to lack of psychological or emotional maturity and/or mental, physical, or medical disability. The advanced behavior guidance techniques commonly used include protective stabilization and sedation.

Objectives of sedation in Pediatric Dentistry

- For the child:
  - Reduce anxiety and modify perception of pain during the treatment
  - Facilitate coping with the treatment
  - Prevent development of dental fear and anxiety
  - Minimize physical discomfort and pain
  - Control behavior and/or movement so as to allow the safe completion of the procedure
  - Minimize psychological trauma, and maximize the potential for amnesia
- For the dentist:
  - Facilitate accomplishment of dental procedures
  - Reduce stress and unpleasant emotions
  - Prevent "burn-out" syndrome

Ideal objectives for pediatric oral health include absence of dental fear and anxiety as well as healthy oral structures. The ultimate aim is to lay strong foundations for good oral health throughout life. This implies two main dimensions in pediatric oral care: (1) to keep the oral environment healthy, and (2) to keep the patient capable of, and willing to utilize the dental service. In recognition of the expanding need for both the elective and emergency use of sedative agents and the importance of delivering painless treatment to children, guidelines for the use of sedative agents among children are important. Pediatric dentists should be aware that sedation represents a continuum. Thus, a patient may move easily from a light level of sedation to a deeper level, which may result in the loss of the patient's protective reflexes. The distinction between conscious (minimal to moderate) sedation and deep sedation is made for the purpose of describing the level of monitoring needed, as well as the responsibility of the dentist.

DEFINITIONS

Moderate sedation:[1] *"Moderate sedation (old terminology, "conscious sedation") is a drug-induced depression of consciousness during which patients respond purposefully to verbal commands or after light tactile stimulation. No interventions are required to maintain a patent airway, and spontaneous ventilation is adequate. Cardiovascular function is usually maintained. The caveat that loss of consciousness should be unlikely is a particularly important aspect of the definition of moderate sedation; drugs and techniques used should carry a margin of safety wide enough to render unintended loss of consciousness unlikely".*

Deep sedation:[1] *A drug-induced depression of consciousness during which patients cannot be easily aroused but respond*

Objectives of conscious sedation[2,3]

- Reduce or eliminate anxiety
- Reduce untoward movement and reaction to dental treatment
- Enhance communication and patient cooperation
- Raise the pain reaction threshold
- Increase tolerance for longer appointments
- Aid in treatment of the mentally/physically disabled or medically compromised patient
- Reduce gagging

Goals of conscious sedation

- To provide the most comfortable, efficient, and high-quality dental service for the patient
- To control inappropriate behavior that interferes with such provision of care
- To produce in the patient a positive psychological attitude toward future care
- To promote patient welfare and safety
- To return the patient to a physiologic state in which safe discharge is possible

Indications[2,3]

- Lack of psychological or emotional maturity
- Medical, physical, cognitive disability
- Fearful, highly anxious, or obstreperous patient
- A patient whose gag reflex interferes with dental care
- A cooperative child undergoing a lengthy dental procedure
- Certain patients with special healthcare needs
- A patient for whom profound local anesthesia cannot be obtained

purposefully following repeated or painful stimulation. The ability to independently maintain ventilatory function may be impaired. Patients may require assistance in maintaining a patent airway, and spontaneous ventilation may be inadequate. Cardiovascular function is usually maintained.

General anesthesia:[1] *A drug-induced loss of consciousness during which patients are not arousable, even by painful stimulation. The ability to independently maintain ventilatory function is often impaired. Patients often require assistance in maintaining a patent airway, and positive pressure ventilation may be required because of depressed spontaneous ventilation or drug-induced depression of neuromuscular function. Cardiovascular function may be impaired.*

Minimal sedation (old terminology "Anxiolysis"):[1] *A drug-induced state during which patients respond normally to verbal commands. Although cognitive function and coordination may be impaired, ventilatory and cardiovascular functions are unaffected.*

CLINICAL GUIDELINES FOR USE OF CONSCIOUS SEDATION BY DENTISTS[1]

Patient Evaluation

- Patients considered for minimal to moderate sedation must be suitably evaluated prior to the start of any sedative procedure.
- In healthy or medically stable individuals (American Society of Anaesthesiologists [(ASA) I, II], this may consist of a review of their current medical history and medication use.
- However, patients with significant medical considerations (ASA III, IV) may require consultation with their primary care physician or consulting medical specialist.

Documentation before Sedation

Documentation shall include, but not be limited to, the guidelines that follow:

- **Informed consent:** The patient's record shall document that appropriate informed consent was obtained according to local, state, and institutional requirements.
- Instructions and information should be provided to a responsible person.
- The practitioner shall provide verbal and/or written instructions to the responsible person. Information shall include objectives of the sedation and anticipated changes in behavior during and after sedation.
- Special instructions shall be given to the adult responsible for the child patients who will be transported home in a car safety seat regarding the need to carefully observe the child's head position so as to avoid airway obstruction.
- A 24-hour telephone number for the practitioner or his or her associates shall be provided to all patients and their families.
- An appropriate sedative record must be maintained, including the names of all drugs administered, time administered and route of administration, including local anesthetics, dosages, and monitored physiological parameters.
- Instructions shall include limitations of activities and appropriate dietary precautions.

Classification of patient selection (according to American Society of Anesthesiologists)[4]	
ASA physical status I	A normal healthy patient
ASA physical status II	A patient with mild systemic disease
ASA physical status III	A patient with severe systemic disease
ASA physical status IV	A patient with severe systemic disease that is a constant threat to life
ASA physical status V	A moribund patient who is not expected to survive without the operation
ASA physical status VI	A declared brain-dead patient whose organs are being removed for donor purposes
E	Emergency operation of any variety (used to modify one of the above classifications)

Preoperative Preparation

- The patient, parent, guardian, or care giver must be advised regarding the procedure associated with the delivery of any sedative agent and informed consent for the proposed sedation must be obtained.
- Determination of adequate oxygen supply and equipment necessary to deliver oxygen under positive pressure must be completed.
- Baseline vital signs must be obtained unless the patient's behaviour prohibits such determination.
- A focused physical evaluation must be performed as deemed appropriate.
- Preoperative dietary restrictions must be considered based on the sedative technique prescribed **(Table 22.1).**
- Preoperative verbal and written instructions must be given to the patient, parent, escort, guardian, or caregiver.

Table 22.1: Appropriate intake of food and liquids before elective sedation.*

Ingested material	*Minimum fasting period (h)*
Clear liquids, water, fruit juices without pulp, carbonated beverages, clear tea, black coffee	2
Breast milk	4
Infant formula	6
Nonhuman milk; because nonhuman milk is similar to solids in gastric emptying time, the amount ingested must be considered when determining an appropriate fasting period	6
Light meal: A light meal typically consists of toast and clear liquids. Meals that include fried or fatty foods or meat may prolong gastric emptying time. Both the amount and type of foods ingested must be considered when determining an appropriate fasting period	6

*American Society of Anesthesiologists. Practice guidelines for preoperative fasting and the use of pharmacologic agents to reduce the risk of pulmonary aspiration: Application to healthy patients undergoing elective procedures. A report of the American Society of Anesthesiologists. Available at "http://www.asahq.org/publicationsAndServices/npoguide.html".

Personnel and Equipment Requirements

- At least one additional person trained in basic life support for healthcare providers must be present in addition to the dentist.
- A positive-pressure oxygen delivery system suitable for the patient being treated must be immediately available.
- When inhalation equipment is used, it must have a fail-safe system that is appropriately checked and calibrated.
- The inhalation sedation equipment must also have either (1) a functioning device that prohibits the delivery of <30% oxygen or (2) an appropriately calibrated and functioning in-line oxygen analyzer with audible alarm An appropriate scavenging system must be available if gases other than oxygen or air are used.

Preparation and Setting-up for Sedation Procedures

- Part of the safety net of sedation is to use a systematic approach so as to not overlook having an important drug, piece of equipment, or monitor that should be immediately available at the time of a developing emergency.
- To avoid this problem, it is helpful to use an acronym that allows the same setup and checklist for every procedure. A commonly used acronym useful in planning and preparation for a procedure is SOAPME:

S	Size-appropriate suction catheters and a functioning suction apparatus
O	An adequate oxygen supply and functioning flow meters/other devices to allow its delivery
A	Airway: Size-appropriate airway equipment
P	Pharmacy: All the basic drugs needed to support life during an emergency, including antagonists
M	Monitors: Functioning pulse oximeter and other monitors as appropriate like capnograph
E	Special equipment or drugs for a particular case

Monitoring during Sedation

- A dentist, or at the dentist's direction, an appropriately trained individual, must remain in the operatory during active dental treatment to monitor the patient continuously until the patient meets the criteria for discharge to the recovery area.

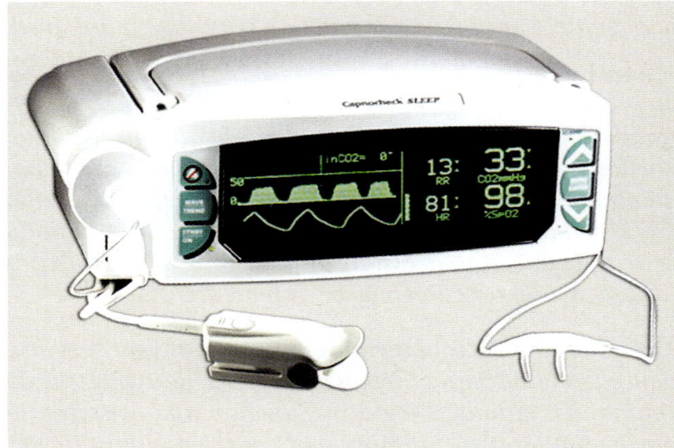

Fig. 22.1: Capnography machine with pulse oximeter.

- The appropriately trained individual must be familiar with monitoring techniques and equipment. Monitoring must include oxygenation, circulation, and ventilation.

Oxygenation

- Color of mucosa, skin, or blood must be evaluated continuously.
- Oxygen saturation is measured by pulse oximetry.
- Pulse oximetry **(Fig. 22.1)** measures the amount of oxygen carried on hemoglobin in the arterial blood. It can measure multiple parameters like SpO_2, perfusion, and heart rate. Its advantages are continuous monitoring, multiple sites of usage, noninvasive, and user friendly.

Ventilation

- The dentist and/or appropriately trained individual must verify respirations continuously.
- Capnography **(Fig. 22.1)** usually includes capnometry to provide the digital display of a numeric value along with the waveform and it gives a digital display of the CO_2 on inspiration and expiration. Capnography measures end tidal carbon dioxide ($ETCO_2$).

Circulation

Blood pressure and heart rate should be evaluated preoperatively, postoperatively, and intraoperatively as necessary (unless the patient is unable to tolerate such monitoring).

Recovery and Discharge

- Oxygen and suction equipment must be immediately available if a separate recovery area is utilized.
- The qualified dentist or appropriately trained clinical staff must monitor and document that level of consciousness, oxygenation, ventilation and circulation are satisfactory prior to discharge and during recovery until the patient is ready for discharge by the dentist.
- Postoperative verbal and written instructions must be given to the patient, parent, escort, guardian, or caregiver.

Discharge criteria
- Cardiovascular function and airway patency are satisfactory and stable.
- The patient is easily arousable.
- The patient can talk (if age appropriate).
- The patient can sit up unaided (if age appropriate).
- Presedation level of responsiveness achieved.
- The state of hydration is adequate.

Emergency Management

- If a patient enters a deeper level of sedation, the dentist must stop the dental procedure until the patient returns to the intended level of sedation.
- The reversal agents and emergency drugs must be available at all times to the dentist for usage.
- The qualified dentist is responsible for the sedative management, adequacy of the facility and staff, diagnosis and treatment of emergencies related to the administration of sedation, and providing the equipment and protocols for patient rescue.
- Emergency management of sedation is described in more detail below in the chapter. **Flowchart 22.1** shows summary of conscious sedation.

Flowchart 22.1: Summary of conscious sedation.

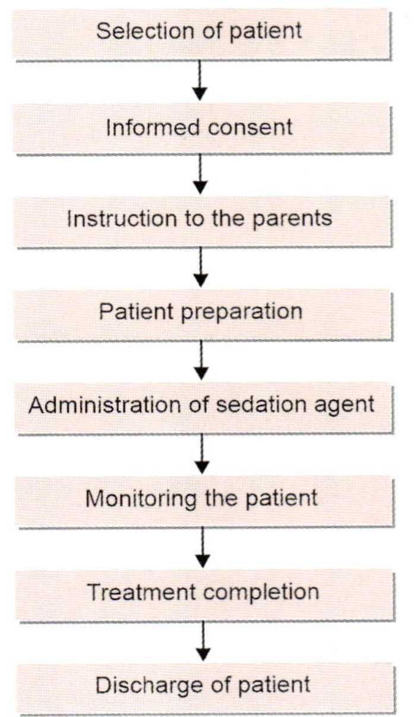

INSTRUCTIONS TO THE PARENTS FOR CONSCIOUS SEDATION

Eating and drinking	To avoid vomiting and complications during treatment with sedation, do not allow your child any food or drink (even water) unless directed by your doctor. The following schedule should be followed (*Refer* **Table 22.1**)
Change in health	Any change in the child's health, especially the development of a cold or fever, within 7 days before the day of treatment is very important. For the child's safety, a new appointment may be made for another day
Arriving	A responsible adult must accompany the patient to the dental office and must remain until treatment is completed. Plan to arrive early for your appointment
Medications	Give your child only those medications that he or she takes routinely, such as seizure medications or prophylactic antibiotics, and those prescribed by your child's physician. Do not give your child any other medicines, before or after treatment, without checking with dental office
Activities	Do not plan to permit activities for the child after treatment. Allow the child to rest closely supervise any activity for the remainder of the day
Getting home	The patient must be accompanied by a responsible adult. Someone should be available to drive the patient home. The child should be closely watched for signs of breathing difficulty and carefully secured in a car seat or seat belt during transportation
After treatment	After treatment, the first drink should be plain water. Sweet drinks can be given next. Small drinks taken repeatedly are preferable to taking single with large amounts
Temperature	The child's temperature may be elevated for the first 24 hours after treatment. Acetaminophen every 3-4 hours and fluids will help alleviate this condition
Seek advice	• If vomiting persists beyond 4 hours • If the temperature remains elevated, beyond 24 hours, or goes above 101°F • If there is any difficulty in breathing • If any other matter causes your concern

SEDATION TECHNIQUES

There are a variety of methods for producing sedation or alteration of mood in the pediatric patient. These systemic procedures are based on thoughtful utilization of various drugs that produce sedation as one of their principal effects. Sedative drugs may be administered by inhalation, oral, intramuscular (IM), intravenous (IV), submucosal (SM) and rectal routes. The primary objective of these techniques is to produce a quiescent patient to ensure the best quality of care and to help train a child to willingly accept dental care. Another objective might be to accomplish a more complex or lengthy treatment plan in a shorter period by lengthening appointment times, thereby reducing the number of repeat visits required. Various routes of conscious sedation are:

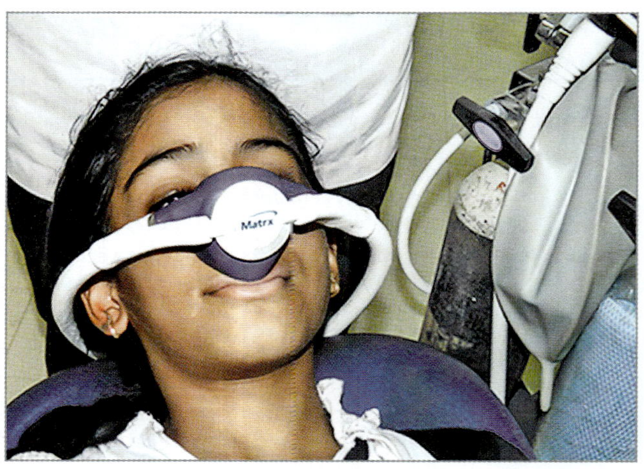

Fig. 22.2: Inhalational sedation.

Inhalation Sedation

- This is the most popular route for conscious sedation in Pediatric Dentistry.
- The inhalational route (**Fig. 22.2**) is the most reliable in terms of onset and recovery.
- Efficacy is reduced when children object to the nasal hood or have difficulty breathing through the nose.
- The use of a rubber dam improves the effect of the sedation and reduces atmospheric pollution.

Oral Sedation

- It is the most universally accepted and easiest route of drug administration.
- The advantages of oral sedation are ease of administration, relatively safe, easy acceptance by the patient, low cost, low side effects, and no need for needles, syringes or equipment.
- Disadvantages associated with this are objectionable taste, variable results, variable consistency, difficult reversal of unwanted effect, and slow recovery time.
- This route is mostly recommended for premedication.
- The oral sedative agent should only be prescribed and administered by the operating dentist within the facility where the dental procedure is to take place. Children who are given an oral sedative should be placed in a quiet room together with their escort and a competent member of staff and should be monitored clinically and electronically.

Intramuscular Sedation

- Anatomic consideration of the injection site and additional training of the operator is required. In children, anterior thigh (vastus lateralis muscle) is the preferred site for intramuscular drug administration **(Figs. 22.3A to E)**.
- In children displaying disruptive behavior, this route is useful and helps the operator reliably deliver the entire drug dose to the child.

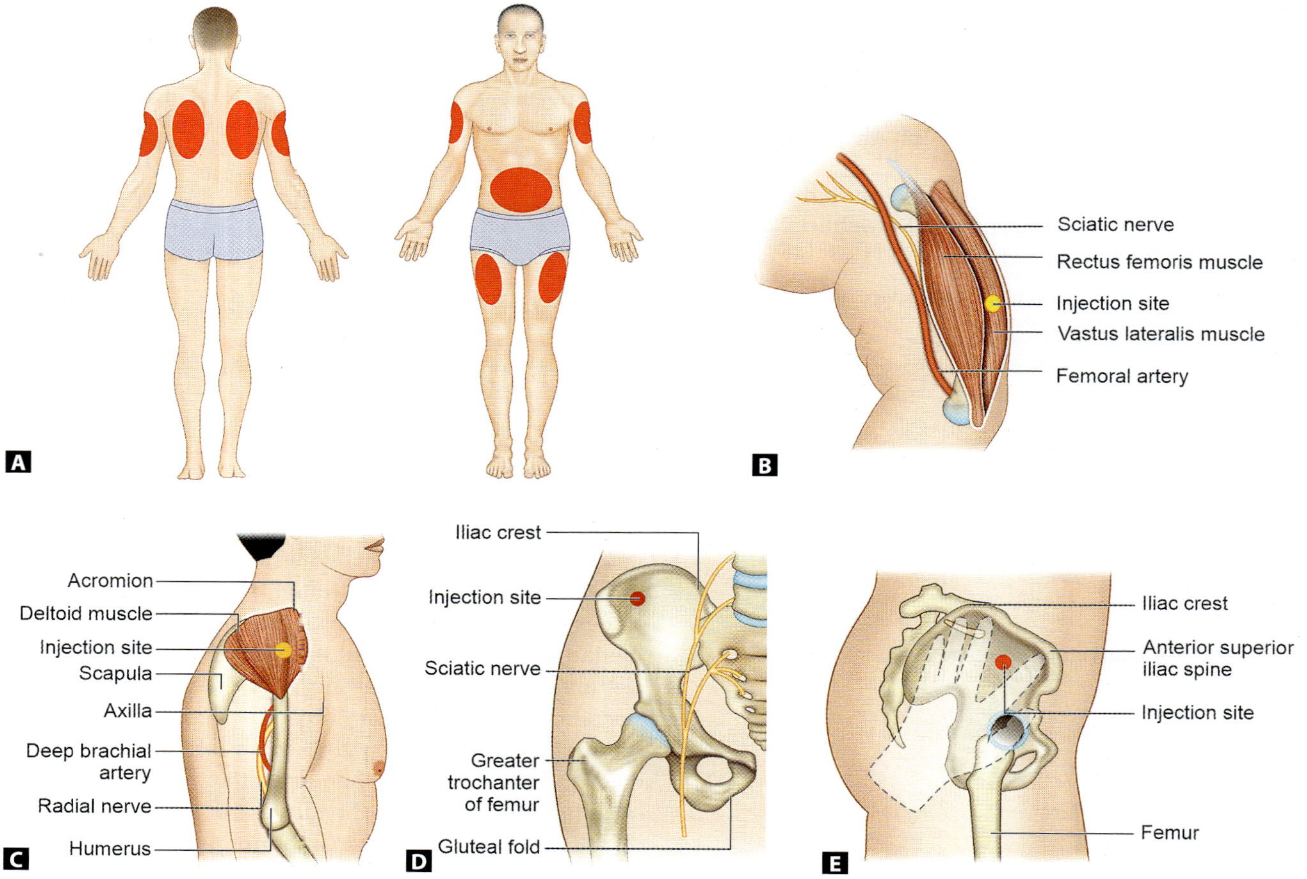

A

B

Sciatic nerve
Rectus femoris muscle
Injection site
Vastus lateralis muscle
Femoral artery

C

Acromion
Deltoid muscle
Injection site
Scapula
Axilla
Deep brachial artery
Radial nerve
Humerus

D

Iliac crest
Injection site
Sciatic nerve
Greater trochanter of femur
Gluteal fold

E

Iliac crest
Anterior superior iliac spine
Injection site
Femur

Figs. 22.3A to E: Site of intramuscular sedation.

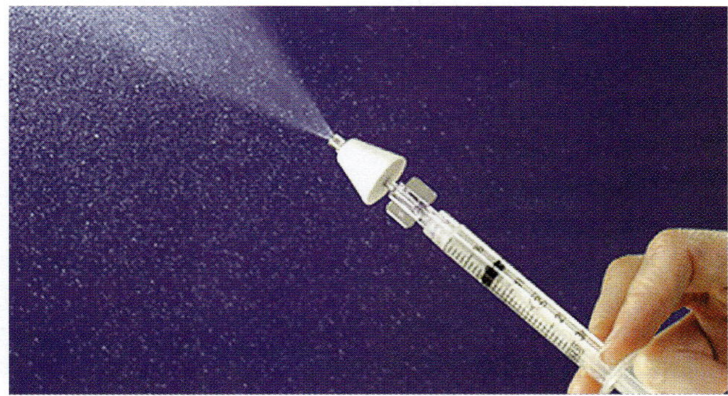

Fig. 22.4: Mucosal atomizer device (MAD).

Submucosal Sedation

- This involves deposition of the drug beneath the mucosa (i.e., sublingual, intranasal).
- Best method is intranasal.
- The oral site usually chosen is the buccal vestibule.
- Intranasal administration is used as an alternative to sedation by oral or injection, especially in pediatric patients. Intranasal administration is a painless, inexpensive and easy to apply method. The duration of onset of action in intranasal administration is close to intravenous administration.
- There are two ways to administer IN medications: by dripping or atomization. The first doesn't require other equipment in addition to a syringe but a compliant child is necessary. In the last years, the mucosal atomizer device (MAD) **(Fig. 22.4)** is the most used IN delivery device that breaks medications into smaller, easily absorbed particles and administers them in a relatively rapid fashion **(Figs. 22.5A and B).**
- The necessity of patient compliance for application limits the use of the method in younger and non-compliant patients.

Intravenous Sedation

- This is the most efficient, and safest method of parenteral sedation next to inhalation. This is because the drug can be titrated to clinical effect. The onset of action of the drug is within 30 seconds.
- Few disadvantages include frequent monitoring, incidence of phlebitis, and hematoma at the site.
- Intravenous sedation is not recommended in precooperative children. Dentists should consider whether the provision of an elective general anesthetic might be preferable in such circumstances.
- Single-drug IV sedation, for example, midazolam, is recommended for adolescents who are psychologically and emotionally suitable.
- Intravenous sedation should only be administered by an experienced dental sedationist with a trained dental nurse in an appropriate facility.
- A pulse oximeter, at least, should be used to augment alert clinical observation.
- Intravenous sedation for dental treatment in children below the16 years is not recommended for conscious sedation, except in special cases, and should be performed in a hospital facility.
- Controlled sedation may be of value for anxious adolescents.

Rectal Sedation

- Rectal administration is not socially acceptable.
- It is currently not recommended without a hospital facility and requires the assistance of a qualified anesthetist.

NITROUS OXIDE—OXYGEN ANXIOLYSIS

Nitrous oxide—oxygen anxiolysis is also known as relative analgesia or inhalation sedation. This technique is considered as a basic behavior guidance technique because the objective of this technique is to build trust and faith in a child patient needing dental treatment, develop a positive dental attitude and allay dental fear and anxiety. Nitrous oxide—oxygen anxiolysis is based on psychological reassurance and hence other basic guidance techniques must be used in conjunction with nitrous oxide inhalation. If other basic behavior guidance techniques such as audiovisual distraction, tender love care, positive reinforcement are not used, then the effectiveness of nitrous oxide inhalation is compromised.

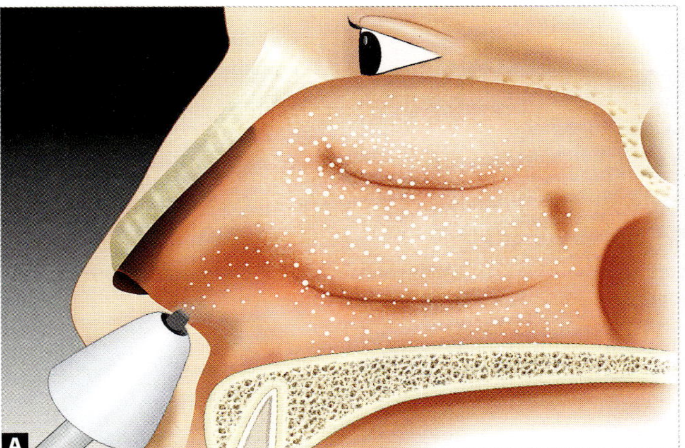

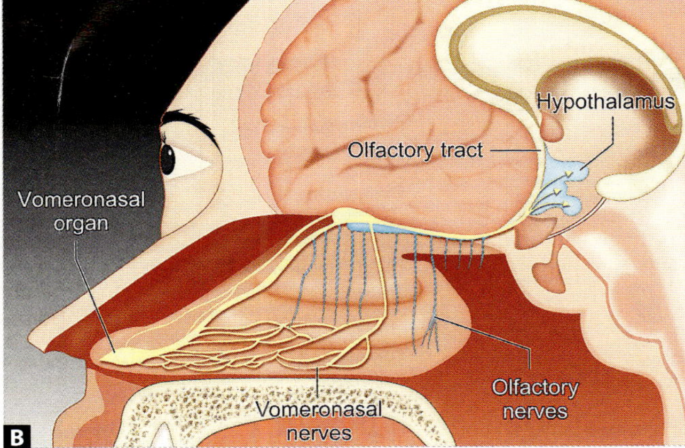

Figs. 22.5A and B: Intranasal medication administration (mechanism of action).

Objectives of using nitrous oxide—oxygen anxiolysis in Pediatric Dentistry

- Reduce fear and anxiety for dental treatment and dental visit
- Enhances communication
- Reduces gag reflex
- Instills a positive dental treatment
- Improves the quality of dental treatment being provided to the children
- Increases efficiency of the operator
- Reduces fatigue of the dentist
- Reduce stressful environment in the clinic

Sedation Continuum

The American Society of Anesthesiologists has divided the sedation spectrum into four depths with minimal sedation or anxiolysis at one end and general anesthesia at the other end **(Table 22.2)**. There is no clear demarcation between various planes of sedation and that is why it is known as a continuum **(Fig. 22.6)**. The depth of sedation is not governed by the choice of medication, meaning that a medication will not help in achieving a specific depth of sedation but may produce a depth greater than intended.

Because sedation is a continuum, it is not always possible to predict how an individual patient will respond. Hence, practitioners intending to produce a given level of sedation should be able to rescue patients whose level of sedation becomes deeper than initially intended. Individuals administering moderate sedation/analgesia ("Conscious Sedation") should be able to rescue patients who enter a state of deep sedation/analgesia, while those administering deep sedation/analgesia should be able to rescue patients who enter a state of general anesthesia (GA).

While administering nitrous oxide/oxygen gases, the desirable level of sedation is minimal sedation or anxiolysis.

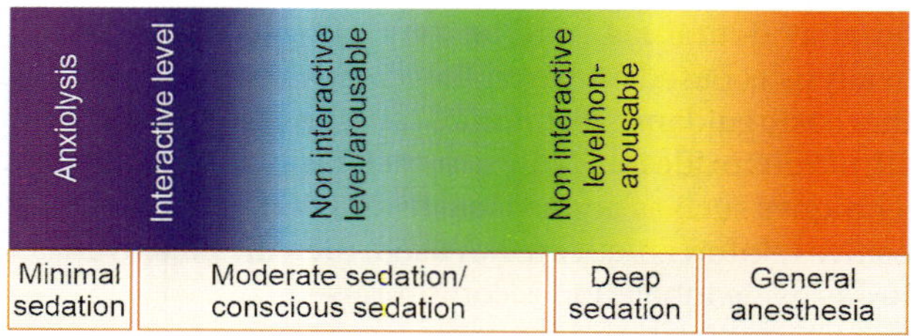

Fig. 22.6: Sedation continuum.

Since sedation is a continuum, there could be periods of moderate sedation.

Minimal sedation (old terminology "Anxiolysis"):[5] *A drug-induced state during which patients respond normally to verbal commands. Although cognitive function and coordination maybe impaired, ventilatory and cardiovascular functions are unaffected.*

Moderate sedation:[5] *"Moderate sedation (old terminology, "conscious sedation") is a drug-induced depression of consciousness during which patients respond purposefully to verbal commands or after light tactile stimulation. No interventions are required to maintain a patent airway, and spontaneous ventilation is adequate. Cardiovascular function is usually maintained. The caveat that loss of consciousness should be unlikely is a particularly important aspect of the definition of moderate sedation; drugs and techniques used should carry a margin of safety wide enough to render unintended loss of consciousness unlikely".*

Deep sedation:[5] *A drug-induced depression of consciousness during which patients cannot be easily aroused but respond purposefully following repeated or painful stimulation. The ability to independently maintain ventilatory function may be impaired. Patients may require assistance in maintaining a patent airway, and spontaneous ventilation maybe inadequate. Cardiovascular function is usually maintained.*

General anesthesia:[5] *A drug-induced loss of consciousness during which patients are not arousable, even by painful stimulation. The ability to independently maintain ventilatory function is often impaired. Patients often require assistance in maintaining a patent airway, and positive pressure ventilation may be required because of depressed spontaneous ventilation or drug-induced depression of neuromuscular function. Cardiovascular function maybe impaired.*

Indications[6]

- *Child is fearful and apprehensive.* The child should be willing to communicate with the dentist otherwise the dentist will not be able to explain the process of using the nasal hood to the child.
- *Child with previous negative dental experience:* The child who had negative experience earlier would be quite fearful and associate the dental visit with previous dental visit.

Table 22.2: Continuum of depth of sedation[1]

	Minimal sedation (anxiolysis)	***Moderate sedation (conscious sedation)***	***Deep sedation***	***General anesthesia***
	Drug-induced state	Drug-induced depression of consciousness	Drug-induced depression of consciousness	Drug-induced loss of consciousness
Responsiveness	Normal response to verbal stimulation	Purposeful response to verbal or tactile stimulation	Purposeful response to repeated tactile or painful stimulation	Unarousable with painful stimulus
Airway	Unaffected	No intervention required	Intervention may be required	Intervention often required
Spontaneous ventilation	Unaffected	Adequate	May be adequate	Frequently inadequate
Cardiovascular function	Unaffected	Usually maintained	Usually maintained	May be impaired

Hence, for these children nitrous oxide should be used even for doing an examination.

- *Children with special needs :* Since these children are more anxious, hence nitrous oxide inhalation may be useful for managing these children.
- *Reduce fatigue in children:* Children may get fatigued keeping their mouth open for a long duration during the dental procedure, and hence may interrupt frequently. Using nitrous oxide facilitates practice of quadrant dentistry.
- *Children who gag even during examination*: Nitrous oxide would help to reduce gagging thereby making it easier to do examination and take radiographs.
- *To improve analgesia:* Since nitrous oxide is an analgesic, it may help in managing inflamed tooth.

Contraindications[6] (Table 22.3)

- Extremely fearful and anxious children
- Children with COPD (although rare)
- Abdominal pain
- Middle ear infection/recent middle ear or eye surgery
- Children with psychiatric disorders
- Children undergoing treatment with bleomycin sulfate
- Children with immunosuppressive therapy
- Children with cobalamin deficiency
- Children in precooperative age
- Children with multiple sclerosis
- Children needing surgical intervention in anterior part of maxilla
- Children who are mouth breathers
- Children with upper respiratory tract infection

Special indications nitrous oxide–oxygen inhalation sedation[8]	
Cardiovascular disease	N_2O–O_2 inhalation sedation can minimize the risk of myocardial infarction
Cerebrovascular disease	Patient who has cerebrovascular disease can receive N_2O–O_2 for stress/anxiety reduction
Respiratory disease	Patients with bronchial asthma can receive nitrous oxide because it is non-irritating to the bronchial and pulmonary tissues
Hepatic disease	N_2O–O_2 is not biotransformed anywhere in the body; it can be used in patients with hepatic disease
Epilepsy and other seizure	N_2O–O_2 can be useful in these patients to avoid stress

(*Source:* Bowen DM. Aiding in administration of nitrous oxide analgesia. Idaho: Idaho State Board of Dentistry;2005).

Advantages

- Rapid onset and rapid recovery due to its property of low blood gas partition coefficient
- Ease of administration as it has to be inhaled from a nasal hood and does not involve any injection prick or ingestion of bitter tasting drugs
- Ability to communicate during procedure as child does not lose consciousness
- Depth of sedation can be controlled by the operator based on clinical monitoring
- Safe compared to other agents
- No impact on daily duties

Table 22.3: Contraindications of nitrous oxide—oxygen inhalation.[7]

No contraindications	Possible contraindications	Absolute contraindications
Cardiovascular system Heart murmur, congenital conditions, rheumatic fever, transplant	Sinus infection/congestion—may need postponement of appointment	Recent eye surgery
Central nervous system Seizure disorders	Tuberculosis or upper respiratory infection	Recent ear surgery
Respiratory system Asthma: N_2O is not contraindicated as it reduces the stress provoking stimuli which usually precipitate asthma	Ear infection—may require postponement of appointment	Latex allergy
Hematological disorders Anemias, methemoglobinemia, sickle cell anemia, leukemia, hemophilia, polycythemia vera	Mental illness, autism, psychiatric disorders	Bleomycin therapy
Hepatic diseases Hepatitis, jaundice	Stomach pain May require postponement	COPD/emphysema
Endocrine system Thyroid/adrenal dysfunction, diabetes	Claustrophobia	
Kidney diseases No effects of nitrous oxide		
Neuromuscular system Multiple sclerosis, muscular dystrophy, cerebral palsy, myasthenia gravis		
Cancer N_2O creates sense of well being and relaxation		

Disadvantages

- Poor acceptance of the nasal mask by a child
- Space requirement in the operatory for placing the delivery system
- Initial cost of delivery system
- Possibility of occupational hazard for the dental staff

Disadvantages of other modes of sedation over nitrous oxide.[6]	
Route of administration	**_Disadvantages over nitrous oxide sedation_**
Oral	• Cannot titrate the drug • Delay in onset • Varying response due to difference in gastric absorption • No oral reversal drug present • Longer preprocedural fasting required
Intramuscular	• Difficult for patients who are needle phobic • Can cause muscular pain • Over sedation possible • Longer preprocedural fasting required
Intravenous	• Difficult for patients who are needle phobic • Over sedation possible • Longer preprocedural fasting required
Intranasal	• Difficult to administer • Can cause burning sensation in nasal mucosa • Over sedation possible

Nitrous Oxide Delivery System

The nitrous oxide delivery system consists of the following parts **(Figs. 22.7 to 22.9)**:

- *Flowmeter*—these are two glass tubes which indicates the flow rate of nitrous oxide and oxygen. These tubes are color coded with green or white color for oxygen and blue color for nitrous oxide
- *Pressure gauges*—monitors the pressure of the gases in cylinders
- *Flow control knob*—controls the combined flow of oxygen and nitrous oxide gases
- *Concentration control knob*—controls the concentration of oxygen or nitrous oxide gases
- *Oxygen flush*—provides extra delivery of oxygen to the reservoir bag
- *Emergency air inlet*—automatically provides the patient with ambient air if gas flow is interrupted

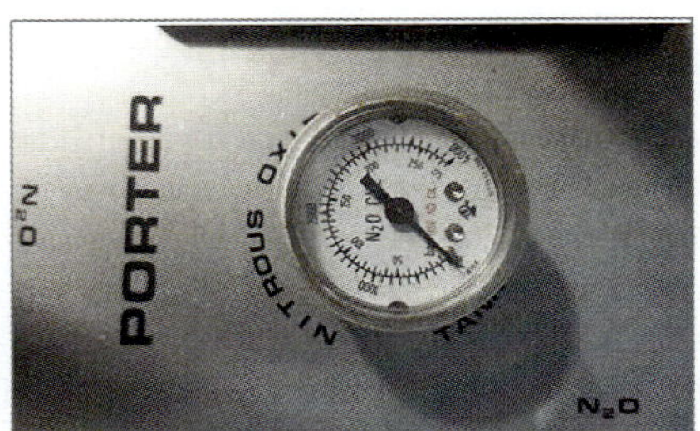

Fig. 22.8: Pressure gauge.

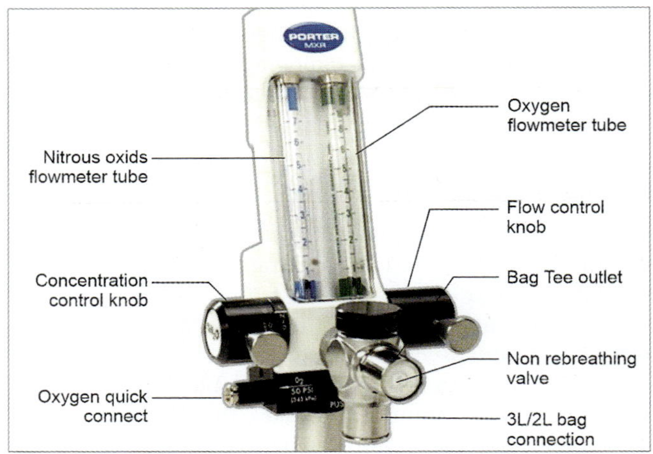

Fig. 22.9: Parts of flowmeter assembly.

- *Reservoir bag*—provides the pool of gases which are inhaled by the child. It also helps in monitoring the ventilation of the child.
- *Fail safe mechanism*—it is a dual seal oxygen piloted valve system that automatically prevents flow of nitrous oxide gas if the oxygen flow is reduced to zero. It hence, ensures that in any situation, nitrous oxide is not delivered to the child without mixing with oxygen.
- *Bag tee*—supports reservoir bag
- *Scavenging breathing circuit*—one end of breathing circuit is connected to the bagtee and other end is connected to a vacuum unit for flushing out exhaled gases from the breathing circuit preventing their leakage into the ambient air **(Fig. 22.10)**
- *Nonrebreathing valve*—guards against carbon dioxide build up and rebreathing of gases.

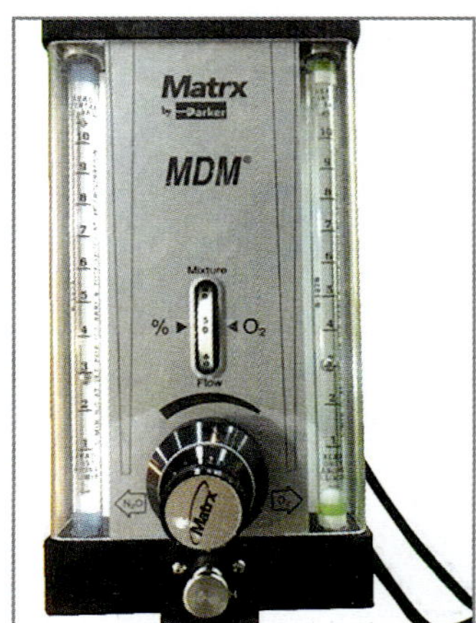

Fig. 22.7: Flowmeter.

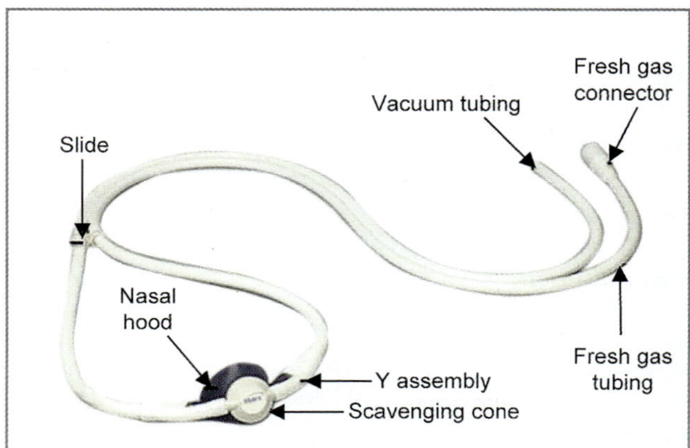

Fig. 22.10: Scavenging breathing circuit.

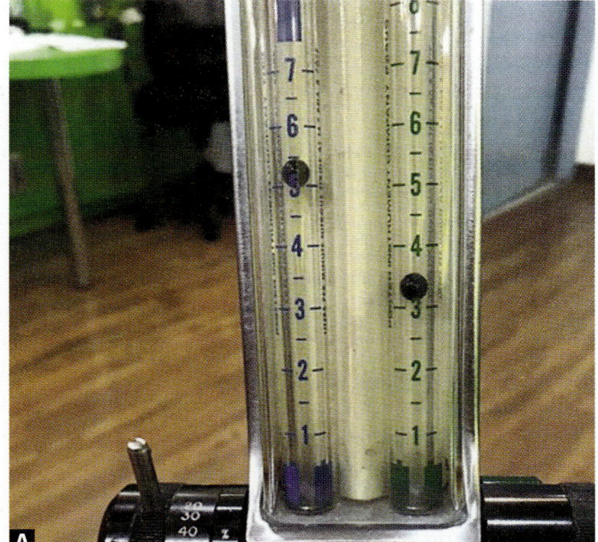

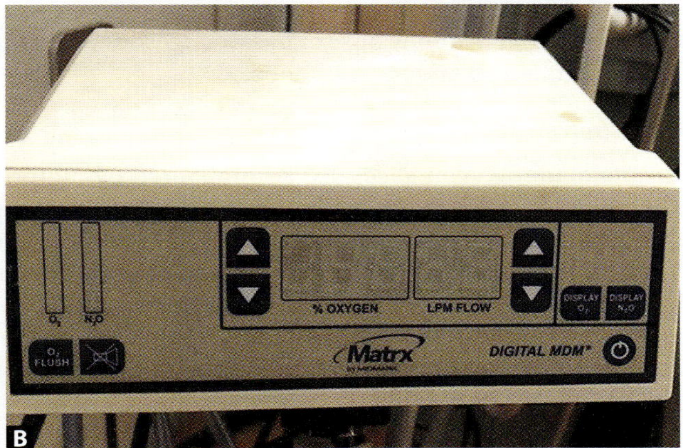

Figs. 22.11A and B: Types of flowmeter: (A) Analog flowmeter; (B) Digital flowmeter.

Nitrous Oxide Flowmeters

Analog Type (Fig. 22.11A)

Analogue type has flowmeters with glass indicator tubes and single motion controls. It consists of flow control knob and a concentration knob (which could be indicating oxygen or nitrous oxide based on the manufacturer).

Digital Type (Fig. 22.11B)

Digital type flowmeter has digital display with simple push button operation.

Scavenging

Scavenging should be carried out to prevent build up nitrous oxide gas in ambient air as this gas is an occupational hazard for the dentist. Since nitrous oxide gas is heavier than air, it settles down inside the dental clinic in an unscavenged setting, thereby increasing its concentration in ambient air. As per US occupational safety and health administration guidelines, ambient nitrous oxide concentration should be less than 25 ppm in the dental operatories.[9] Usually in an unscavanged operatory concentration of ambient nitrous oxide would be 3500 ppm.[10]

Recommendations for controlling nitrous oxide exposure in the dental office.

Equipment	• Properly installed nitrous oxide delivery system • Appropriate scavenging equipment with a readily visible and accurate flowmeter • Vacuum pump with capacity up to 45 L of air per minute per workstation • Variety of mask sizes to ensure proper fit
Ventilation	• Vacuum exhaust and ventilation exhaust vented outside • Outside venting not in close proximity to fresh air vents • Good room air mixing for general ventilation
Inspections	• With each use and when gas cylinder is changed, pressure connections tested for leaks using a soap solution or a portable infrared spectrophotometer • Daily, price to first use, inspected for worn parts, cracks, holes or tears, and replaced as necessary • Appropriate flow rates (up to 45 L/minor per manufacturer's recommendations) verified
Patients	Before administration • Use properly sized masks to ensure a good, comfortable fit • Check for over-or under inflation of reservoir (breathing) bag while the patient is breathing oxygen (before nitrous oxide administration)
	During administration • Minimize talking and mouth breathing by patient while mask is in place • Reservoir bag periodically inspected for changes in tidal volume • Vacuum flow rate verified
	After administration • 100% oxygen delivered to patient for 5 minutes before removing mask to purge patient and system of residual nitrous oxide • System oxygen flush should not be used
Dental personnel	• Periodic (i.e., semi-annual) sampling of dental personnel, especially chair-side personnel exposed to nitrous oxide (e.g., with a diffusive sampler, such as a dosimeter or infrared spectrophotometer)

(*Source:* ADA Council on Scientific Affairs and the ADA Council on Dental Practice).[11]

In active scavenging, loose end of the breathing circuit is connected to a vacuum pump (having 45 L/min vacuum pressure) which actively removes exhaled gases having higher concentration of nitrous oxide.

Nitrous Oxide Breathing Mask

- *Single mask system*: There is a single mask which has a scavenging cone attached on the top of the mask **(Fig. 22.12A)**
- *Double mask system:* This consists of two masks—an outer mask which completely covers an inner liner. The space between the outer and inner masks is connected to the scavenging tubing **(Fig. 22.12B)**.
- *Silhouette mask:* It is an anatomic shaped nasal mask with adhesive strips on the sides to prevent leakage of nitrous oxide gas around the mask, thereby enhancing the effect of nitrous oxide. This mask is considered to have the best scavenging efficiency **(Fig. 22.12C)**.

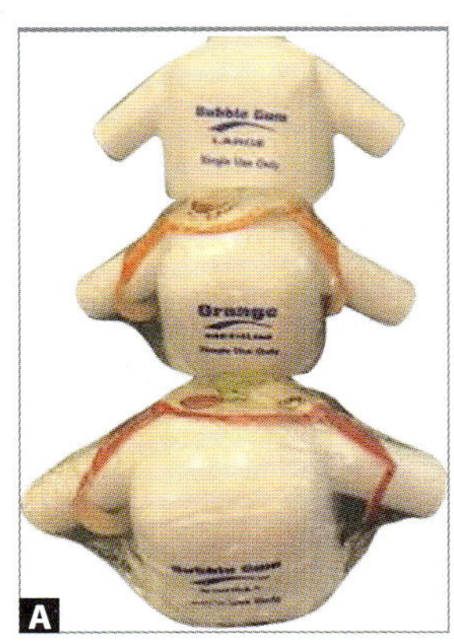

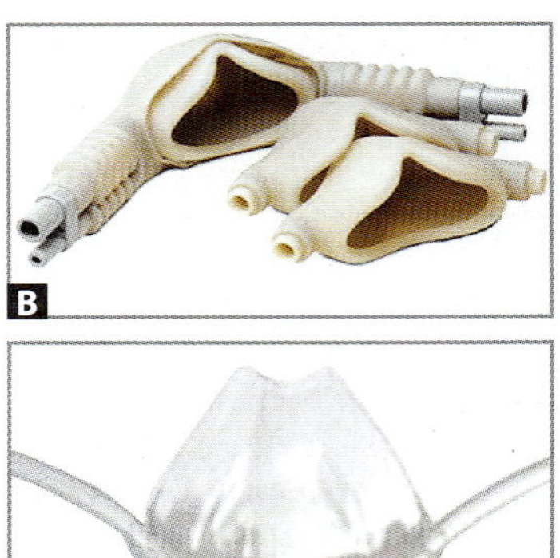

Figs. 22.12A to C: Nitrous oxide breathing masks: (A) Matrx breathing mask; (B) Porter double mask system; (C) Silhouette mask.

Common nitrous oxide equipment providers are:
- Matrx by Porter
- Accutron
- Baldus
- Smartsed
- Consed

Physical properties of nitrous oxide gas
- Colorless, sweet smelling gas
- Heavier than air (1.53 times heavier than air)
- Nonflammable but it supports combustion
- It is influenced by atmospheric pressure. More amount of nitrous oxide has to be administered at higher altitudes as less atmospheric pressure reduces pressure to deliver into lungs. The cylinders have a filling ratio of 0.75 in temperate countries and 0.67 in tropical countries.
- Nitrous oxide is eliminated unchanged from the body. Major part of the inhaled gas is excreted through lungs and small part diffuses through the skin.

Planes of Nitrous Oxide/Oxygen Anxiolysis or Relative Analgesia

Langa (1968)[12] has described three planes of relative analgesia.

Plane 1: Slight Analgesia and Amnesia

In this phase the child will have reduced fear or anxiety. He/she will feel warm and tingling in extremities or in circumoral region.

Plane 2: Moderate Analgesia and Amnesia

In this phase the child can keep mouth open, hands may drop down (hand drop phenomenon), there is a feeling of relaxation, voice changes can be appreciated and there is decreased motor coordination.

Plane 3: Complete Analgesia and Amnesia

In this phase the mandible becomes more rigid and child tends to close mouth, the eyes will have dazed look, child will not follow directions and may begin to hallucinate.

The most desired plane of nitrous oxide sedation is Plane 2.

Technique of Administration[13]

The objectives of using nitrous oxide should be explained to the parents as well as child patient to make it successful and effective. Parents should be told that it has a role in reducing fear/anxiety, bringing about relaxation of child and reduce pain or sensitivity during the dental procedures.

Children should be introduced to the nasal mask using the tell-show-do technique. The child should be trained to breathe in and out into the mask with the mouth open to minimize incidences of mouth breathing during the dental procedures. Positive reinforcement through verbal praises should be done during the process of introducing nasal mask. Modeling and audiovisual distraction may also be used for children who have higher anxiety.

Presedation Instructions

- Avoid milk and other solid foods for two hours prior to appointment.
- If the child has running nose or nasal congestion, then the appointment should be postponed.

Administration of Gases

Nitrous oxide/oxygen gases are administered by method of titration. Titration is the method of administering a drug based on desirable clinical effects, with no fixed dosage based on body weight, etc. Therefore, clinical effects govern the concentration of the gases to be delivered and is not dependent on the age or weight of the child. Each patient may need a different concentration to achieve the desirable clinical effects.

There are two methods of titration for administering nitrous oxide gas.

1. Standard titration
2. Rapid titration

Standard Titration/Slow Titration

In this technique concentration of nitrous oxide gas is administered in increments of 10% every minute. The phases of administration are:

- **Oxygenation phase:** Initially 100% oxygen is delivered for a period of 3–5 minutes.
- **Induction phase:** In this phase nitrous oxide is increased in increments of 10% every minute till the desired clinical effects are achieved.
- **Maintenance phase:** Once the desired clinical effects are achieved, the nitrous oxide and oxygen concentrations are maintained until the completion of procedure.
- **Injection phase:** If administration of local anesthesia is needed, the nitrous oxide concentration is raised to 50–60% to achieve better analgesic properties. After local anesthesia has been administered, the concentration is reduced to the level decided during the maintenance phase.
- **Recovery phase:** After the treatment is completed, nitrous oxide concentration is reduced to zero and oxygen

concentration increased to 100% for 5 minutes to prevent diffusion hypoxia.

Rapid Titration

This technique is usually used for children who have higher anxiety. In this technique the nitrous oxide concentration is directly increased to 50–60% so that the clinical effects may be achieved quickly. After reduction of initial anxiety, the concentration of nitrous oxide gas is then gradually reduced to a level where the clinical effects may be maintained.

Clinical Signs and Symptoms

- Dull and lazy eyes
- Reduced eyeball movement
- Dazed look or trance-like appearance
- Voice changes
- Smile on face or laughter
- Relaxed hands and feet in abduction
- Indifference to surroundings
- Lesser awareness of pain
- Floating sensation

End of Titration

Once the dental procedure ends, the child may be allowed to leave after a verbal check is done to ensure that there is no dizziness, headache or nausea.

Procedure of Administration (Figs. 22.13A to F)

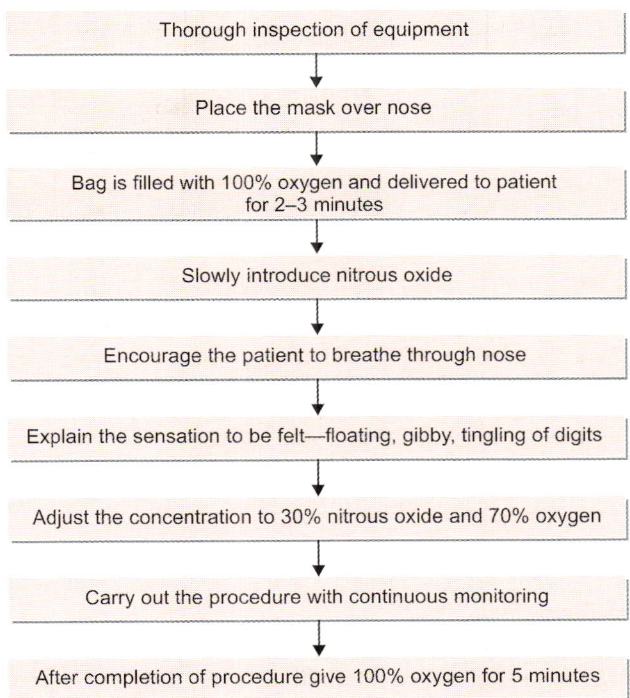

Thorough inspection of equipment
Place the mask over nose
Bag is filled with 100% oxygen and delivered to patient for 2–3 minutes
Slowly introduce nitrous oxide
Encourage the patient to breathe through nose
Explain the sensation to be felt—floating, gibby, tingling of digits
Adjust the concentration to 30% nitrous oxide and 70% oxygen
Carry out the procedure with continuous monitoring
After completion of procedure give 100% oxygen for 5 minutes

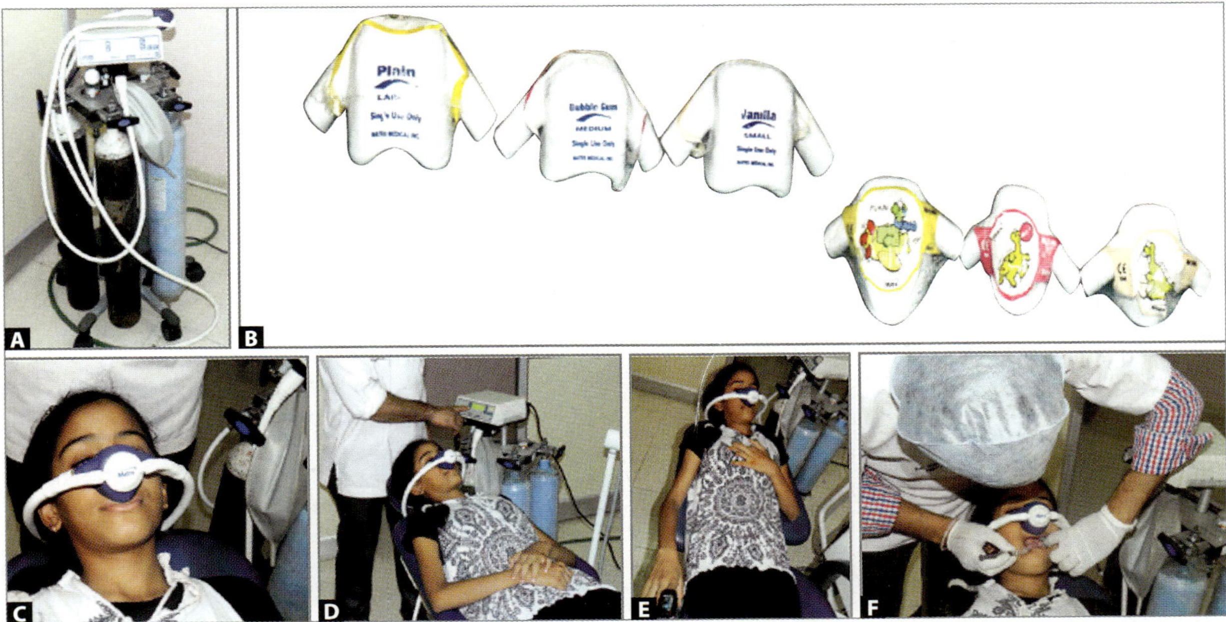

Figs. 22.13A to F: Nitrous oxide sedation equipment and procedure: (A) Nitrous oxide and oxygen cylinder; (B) Different sizes of mask and odor; (C) Application of nasal hood on the child; (D) Final adjustment of nitrous oxide and oxygen ratio; (E) Sedated child under observation; (F) Dentist performing dental treatment.

Flowchart 22.2: Steps of clinical monitoring.

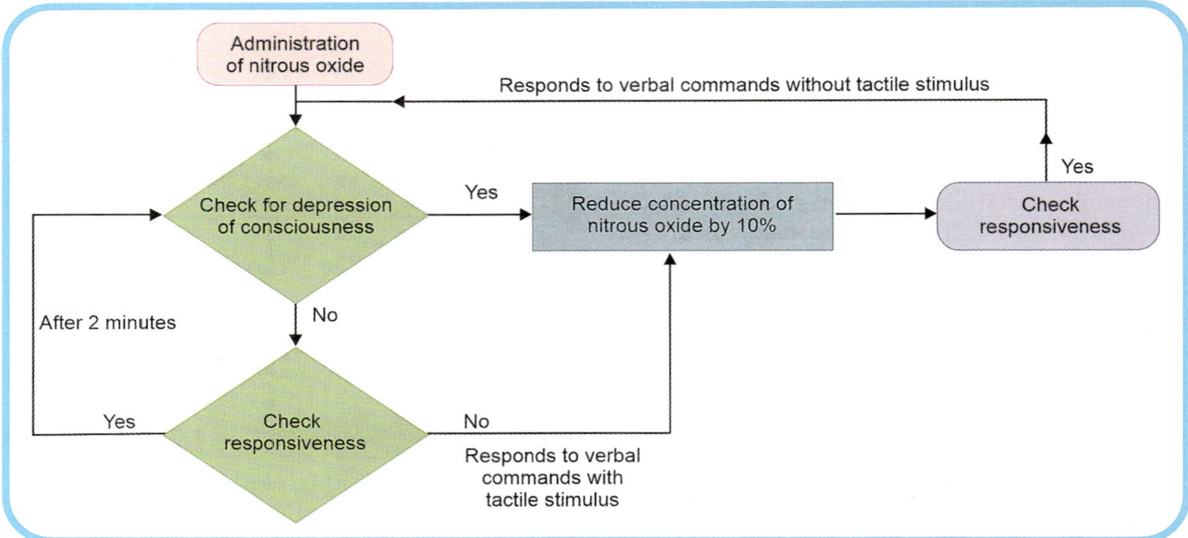

Monitoring

Monitoring is an important aspect of nitrous oxide sedation to ensure that the child is maintained in the "minimal level of sedation" **(Flowchart 22.2)**. This is achieved by alert clinical monitoring and technological monitoring (use of electronic devices like pulse monitors). Clinical monitoring involves determining the level of consciousness and establishing responsiveness which helps in deciphering the depth of sedation.

If the child appears to be in moderate level of sedation (with depression of consciousness) based on clinical signs **(Figs. 22.14)**, then the nitrous oxide concentration should be reduced by 5–10%. The clinical signs should be checked again in 2 minutes and if the child seems to be in minimal level of sedation (with no depression of consciousness), the concentration of nitrous oxide is then maintained at that level. However, if the child still seems to be in moderate level of sedation (with continued depression of consciousness), then the concentration of nitrous oxide should be further reduced till alertness is achieved **(Fig. 22.15)**.

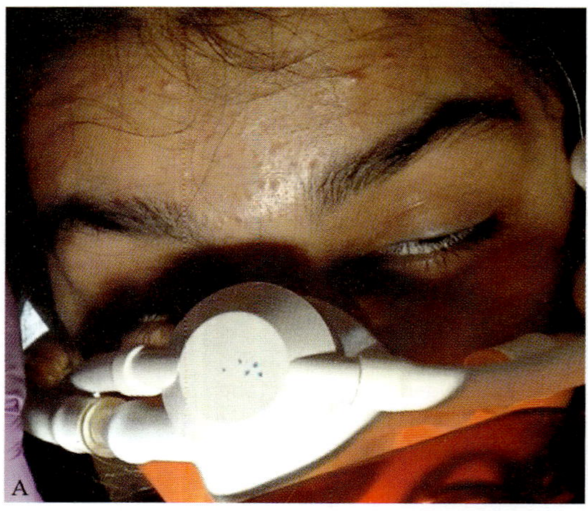

Fig. 22.14: Shows depression of consciousness (moderate sedation).

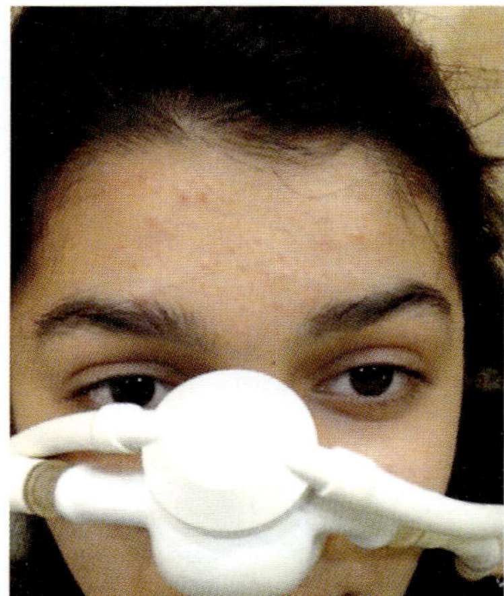

Fig. 22.15: Shows no depression of consciousness (minimal sedation).

Various authors have expressed different views regarding use of pulse oximeter.

- Its use in children is not advocated because movement of hands or feet which may displace the sensor leading to inaccurate readings.
- Its use in children may create a negative impact on minds of parents and they may develop anxiety for the minimal sedation procedure.

American Academy of Pediatric Dentistry "recommends" use of pulse oximetry though it is "not mandatory".[14]

Adverse Events

Nitrous oxide/oxygen anxiolysis may be associated with minor adverse events which include headache, dizziness, nausea, vomiting, stomach pain and flatulence. The incidence of minor side defects varies from 4–10%.[15] It has also been reported that the incidence of minor side effects may increase if nitrous oxide is administered at a concentration of 50% for more than two hours.

Diffusion hypoxia may occur as the sedation is reversed at the termination of the procedure. The nitrous oxide escapes into the alveoli with such rapidity that the oxygen present becomes diluted; thus, the oxygen– carbon dioxide exchange is disrupted and a period of hypoxia is created. However, this phenomenon is clinically insignificant in healthy pediatric patients. Nonetheless, to minimize this effect, the patient should be oxygenated for 3–5 minutes after a sedation procedure.

DRUGS USED FOR MINIMAL TO MODERATE (CONSCIOUS) SEDATION

Other than nitrous oxide oxygen drugs intended to produce minimal to moderate sedation primarily come under three groups:

1. Opoids.
2. Antianxiety agents.
3. Sedative hypnotics.

Opioids

- Opioids are primarily intended for analgesia. Sedation is their secondary action.
- They are usually used for their analgesic actions along with a drug that produces sedation as its primary effect.
- They have the propensity to cause respiratory depression in high doses.
- They act on the opioid receptors in the CNS.
- Commonly used opioid for its analgesic properties and as an adjunct in moderate sedation/analgesia is meperidine.
- Naloxone is an opioid reversal drug to reverse any complications like respiratory depression.

Meperidine (Demerol)

- Meperidine is about one-tenth as potent as morphine.
- It is a synthetic opioid with atropine-like properties.
- The onset of meperidine is 3-4 minutes (IV) and 10-15 minutes (IM).
- The peak effect of meperidine is 15 minutes (IV) and 45 minutes (IM).
- The duration of action is 2-4 hours.
- It can also be administered orally.
- In large dosages, it can produce tachycardia, tremors, muscle twitching, and seizures.

Fentanyl (Sublimaze)

- Fentanyl is not intended for moderate sedation. It is indicated for deep sedation/general anesthesia.
- Fentanyl has more rapid onset and shorter duration than morphine.
- It is 100 times more potent than morphine.
- The onset of fentanyl is 30 seconds (IV) and 5–10 minutes (IM).
- The peak effect of fentanyl is 10 minutes (IV) and 30–45 minutes (IM).
- The duration of action is 30–60 minutes.
- Fentanyl in moderate doses of 2–10 µg/kg or higher doses when given rapidly IV can produce skeletal muscle rigidity called "stiff chest syndrome".
- Fentanyl lacks histamine release and suppresses the stress response associated with surgery or invasive procedures and also depresses the respiratory center in the brainstem so that normal response to hypoxia and hypercarbia is reduced.

Anti-anxiety Agents

- The primary action of these drugs is to produce anxiolysis and not sedation (drowsiness) or hypnosis (sleep).
- They act on the limbic system in the CNS which is the "Seat of Emotions".
- Benzodiazepines like midazolam are the most popular drugs in this group for use in Pediatric Dentistry. Diazepam and lorazepam are other benzodiazepines used in adults commonly in oral form.
- Antihistamines like hydroxyzine and diphenhydramine are other drugs that fall into this category. But, it should be noted that anxiolysis, sedation and hypnosis are not their intended primary pharmacological actions. Hence they are not useful individually for minimal to moderate sedation in Pediatric Dentistry.

Midazolam (Versed)

- Midazolam is the most commonly used sedative in Pediatric Dentistry after nitrous oxide oxygen.
- It is an excellent anxiolytic and sedative.
- It can be administered through multiple routes including the oral, intravenous, intranasal, intramuscular or rectal route.
- Midazolam has also been shown to enhance anterograde amnesia when used preoperatively in pediatric patients.
- Midazolam is a short-acting anxiolytic agent, with short duration of action that makes its use limited to short dental procedures only.
- High lipophilicity at physiological pH and very high clearance and elimination allow rapidity of onset and speedy recovery.
- After 45 minutes, the sedative effect wears off. The elimination half time is 2 hours, which facilitates a fast recovery.
- Midazolam should be used only in anxious children. It should be used in children displaying combative or disruptive behavior. If used in these children, it can lead to a paradoxical reaction which is known by many as "Angry Child Syndrome".
- Flumazenil[2] can be used to reverse the effects of benzodiazepines. A dose of 0.01 mg/kg may be repeated four times as needed.

Intravenous Midazolam

- Intravenous midazolam is useful in anxious adolescent children.
- Midazolam can be safely titrated to the ideal level of sedation which is the major advantage of the intravenous route.
- The intravenous route can also provide an emergency intravenous access in case of an emergency.
- The dose is 0.1 mg/kg body weight.

Oral Midazolam[16,17]

- Oral midazolam can be administered as a sweetened mixture for delivery either via a drinking cup or drawn into a needleless syringe and deposited in the retromolar area.
- Though tablets and syrups are commercially manufactured, they are not easily available.

- Oral mixtures given approximately 20-30 minutes before treatment.
- It reaches the systemic circulation via the portal circulation; this decreases the drug's bioavailability, necessitating a higher oral dosage compared to IV administration.
- Midazolam is rapidly absorbed in the gastrointestinal tract and produces its peak effect in 30 minutes.[3] It has a short half-life of about 1.75 hours.
- When given in doses between 0.5 and 0.75 mg/kg of body weight, oral midazolam has been found to be a useful sedative agent for pediatric dental outpatients.
- A disadvantage through the oral route is the possibility of the child spitting out the drug.

Intranasal Midazolam[18]

- It produces a sedative effect within 10 minutes of administration.
- The administered dose is limited by the volume of the solution, as large volumes can cause coughing, sneezing, and expulsion of part of the drug.
- There have been reports of transient burning and discomfort affecting the nasal mucosa.
- It is not recommended in children who have copious nasal secretions or who suffer from an upper respiratory tract infection.
- Midazolam may be given by the intranasal route at doses of 0.2–0.4 mg/kg.
- Onset time is intermediate between the oral and IV routes of administration (10–15 minutes).
- The effectiveness of this route of administration is well established as a premedication for anesthesia.
- Adverse effects possibly include respiratory depression especially if dosages have been grossly violated.
- Best administered through the Mucosal Atomization Device (MAD) is shown in **Figure 22.4**.

Rectal Midazolam

- It is an ethical/human right concern in some countries.[19]
- Children under 25 kg of weight shall have 0.3–0.4 mg midazolam per kilogram bodyweight with maximum dose 10 mg midazolam.
- Rectal solution is administered approximately 10 minutes before treatment starts.

Sedative Hypnotics[20]

- The principle action of these drugs is to activate sleep.
- Inadequate dosages may only leady to a drowsy (sedated), but irritated child. This group of drugs usually do not possess anxiolytic properties.
- They mainly act on the reticular activating system which is the area of the brain controlling consciousness.
- The most common drugs in this category are barbiturates and non barbiturates.
- Examples of non-barbiturates are chloral hydrate and dexmedetomidine.
- Barbiturates are no longer used for moderate sedation in Pediatric Dentistry because of their narrow therapeutic index or a steep dose-response curve. This means that there is a very small difference in the dosage of a barbiturate which causes moderate sedation to the dosage that will lead to general anesthesia.
- Other drugs like Propofol cannot be classified in this category because it is primarily a general anesthetic and not recommended for moderate sedation in Pediatric Dentistry.

Chloral Hydrate

- Chloral hydrate is a chlorinated derivative of ethyl alcohol that is easy to administer and has a low incidence of adverse effects.
- The normal oral dose is 50 mg/kg of body weight with a suggested range of 40–60 mg/kg.
- Following oral administration, the onset of action of chloral hydrate is rapid, drowsiness or arousable sleep usually developing within 30–45 minutes.
- Duration of action is 2–5 hours.[3]
- It is a weak analgesic with an elimination half-life of approximately 8 hours.
- In small doses, mild sedation occurs and, in intermediate doses, natural sleep is produced.
- Common complications include nausea and vomiting. It also irritates the gastrointestinal tract in the vast majority of patients. Gastric discomfort can be reduced by diluting the drug or by drinking a glass of water or milk after the drug.
- The combination of chloral hydrate with alcohol is thought to produce a potentiation drug interaction through an alteration of alcohol metabolism. This combination, known colloquially as a "Mickey Finn" or "knock-out drops," can induce severe alcohol intoxication with stupor, coma, or death.
- Chloral hydrate is contraindicated in children with heart disease as well as those with renal or hepatic impairment.

Dexmedetomidine (Precedex)

- Dexmedetomidine is the *S*-enantiomer of medetomidine
- It is a highly selective, potent $\alpha 2$-adrenergic agonist, with a short duration of action.
- It has the ability to provide rapid and stable hypnosis (sleep) and provide analgesia while still maintaining patient arousability and respiratory function.
- The IV dose is 0.2–0.7 μg/kg/h.
- The unique mechanism of action of dexmedetomidine allows the patient to be awakened and respond to verbal commands, take neurological tests, and be interactive while remaining calm and comfortable. When the awakening stimulus is removed, the patient returns to sleep.
- Can also be administered orally and intranasally.

Ketamine[21]

- Ketamine was first synthesized by **Parke-Davis** scientist **Calvin Stevens** and got Food and Drug Administration (FDA) approval in 1970.
- Though ketamine has been used to obtain moderate sedation, it should be noted that it is primarily a general anesthetic and should be used only by medical personnel

trained to handle general anesthesia. It is not a moderate sedation drug and is mentioned here only to emphasize this point.

- Ketamine is a NMDA antagonist and phencyclidine derivative that results in dissociation between the cortical and limbic systems of the brain called dissociative anesthesia.
- It is a dissociative agent, which makes a state of catalepsy that gives sedation, control of pain and amnesia.
- Ketamine prevents the higher cortical centers from perceiving visual, auditory, and painful stimuli.
- An IV dose of 1 mg/kg induces dissociative anesthesia in 2 minutes, and effects last 15–30 minutes.
- Patients demonstrate nystagmus and display a blank stare that is characteristic of dissociative anesthesia.
- Ketamine maintains cardiovascular stability as well as muscle tone and airway reflexes.
- Disadvantages of ketamine may include increased intracranial and intraocular pressures, hypertension, tachycardia, and postemergence delirium (i.e., vivid nightmares).
- Chronic use of ketamine may lead to cognitive impairments, including memory problems.
- It is one of the most prevalent drugs for recreational use owing to its dissociative properties.

COMPLICATIONS ASSOCIATED WITH MODERATE SEDATION[22,23]

Every practitioner administering moderate sedation should be able to recognize sedation related complications and be able to rescue that patient. Some of the major complications are:

- Airway obstruction.
- Ineffective ventilation resulting from respiratory depression causing hypoxia and hypercarbia.
- Problems with the cardiovascular system including hypotension.
- Drug overdose or reaction (anaphylaxis or anaphylactoid reactions).
- Aspiration associated with loss of protective airway reflexes
- Nausea and vomiting.
- Problems with equipment compromising patient safety.

Airway Obstruction

- Airway obstruction is the most common complication associated with moderate sedation.
- The obstruction of the airway commonly occurs secondary to loss of the muscle tone especially in an obese child with a flabby soft palate. Other reasons could be:
  - Improper positioning of the child's head on the dental chair.
  - Pooling of saliva in the throat.
  - Working on the mandibular arch thereby applying pressure and pushing it back.
  - Tongue falling back and physically obstructing the airway.
- Signs of airway obstruction include inspiratory stridor or snoring, rocking chest movements, absence of breath sounds, hypoxemia, and hypercarbia.
- The signs are similar in respiratory depression. But, hypoventilation or respiratory depression is characterized by a shallow depth and rate of chest and abdominal movements.
- Hypercarbia is defined as a $PaCO_2$ >44 mm Hg and is the result of hypoventilation.
- Hypoxemia is present when PaO_2 is <60 mm Hg or SpO_2 by pulse oximeter is <90%.
- *If airway obstruction is suspected consider:* Repositioning the patient's head providing a head tilt, applying a chin lift or jaw thrust and providing 100% oxygen.
- Persistent airway obstruction may require the use of airway adjuncts and suspend further drug administration.
- For respiratory depression, positive pressure ventilation (PPV) that includes a 100% oxygen source and a bag valve mask (BVM) device should be used.

Anaphylaxis and Anaphylactoid Reactions

- Anaphylaxis and anaphylactoid reactions are acute and are characterized by wheezing, dyspnea, syncope, hypotension, and upper airway obstruction.
- Can be caused by histamine release or latex allergy.
- Treatment of anaphylactic or anaphylactoid reactions: prompt recognition of the clinical situation and stopping the administration of the suspected offending drug, ventilation with 100% oxygen, securing the airway with endotracheal intubation, prompt use of fluids and intramuscular epinephrine (1:1000).

Aspiration

- Risk factors for aspiration are inadequate fasting or recent oral intake, diabetes, pregnancy, obesity, altered consciousness.
- Suspect aspiration in patient with the above risk factors having respiratory difficulty, tachypnea, tachycardia, cyanosis, and oxygen desaturation.
- Blood gases may reveal hypoxemia with mixed metabolic and variable respiratory acidosis.
- In severe cases of aspiration, systemic hypotension, pulmonary hypertension, and pulmonary edema may occur.

Nausea and Vomiting

- Nausea and vomiting can cause hypertension or hypotension, tachycardia, bradycardia, and aspiration.
- Nausea and vomiting is the leading cause of unexpected hospital admission.
- Predisposing factors of nausea and vomiting are age (younger patient more susceptible), female gender, history of postoperative emesis, presence of hypoglycemia, pain, hypotension, or hypoxia.
- When intra operative vomiting is encountered, the priority is to clear the airway to enable oxygen to reach the lungs. This is made possible by immediately rolling the child to the side and suctioning the mouth and the pharynx.

Research regarding conscious sedation

- **Beirne** concluded that conscious sedation when used with local anesthesia for pain control can be an effective method for treatment of anxious patients without making them unconscious.[24]
- **Damle et al.** observed oral midazolam to be better tolerated and accepted by both the child and parents and was associated with negligible side effects when compared with oral ketamine.[25]
- **Barbosa et al.** suggested that sedation with N_2O-O_2 is recommended along with behavior control techniques that can provide more safety and comfort for children during the dental treatment.[26]
- **Al-Zahrani et al.** stated that the use of nitrous oxide-oxygen along with midazolam is a safe and synergistic combination.[27]
- **Silva et al.** founded conscious sedation can be recommended to anxious patients who have dental and needle phobia, to patients that present an increased vomiting reflex and also to patients with special needs but capable of communicating.[28]
- **Krishna Priya et al.** concluded that conscious sedation is a safe method with a wide safety margin that can be used effectively in managing dental fear and anxiety in children and can reduce the need for general anesthesia.[29]
- **Galeotti et al.** observed that inhalation conscious sedation represented an effective and safe method to obtain cooperation, even in very young patients, and it could reduce the number of pediatric patients referred to hospitals for general anesthesia.[30]
- **Attri et al.** studied that safe and adequate administration of sedative and analgesic medications can make painful and anxiety provoking situations tolerable.[31]
- **Ashlay PF et al.** in a recent systematic review evaluating the efficacy of conscious sedation agents used for behavior management in Pediatric Dentistry showed oral midazolam to be an effective agent.[32]
- **Fantacci C et al.** investigated the type of administration of IN drugs: drop instillation or by a Mucosal Atomizer Device (MAD) and the results showed that the use of MAD even gives a better bioavailability of drugs. They concluded that in sedation via MAD is effective and safe and should be one of the first choices for procedural sedation in children.[33]
- **Sado-Filho J et al.** concluded that all the three regimens intranasal ketamine and midazolam, oral ketamine and midazolam, or oral midazolam provided moderate dental sedation with minor adverse events and the combination of ketamine with midazolam proved to be more effective in comparison to midazolam alone.[34]
- **Funda AR.** concluded that hypnosedative anaesthetic medications have been used for various indications and purposes outside the operating room by different specialists other than anaesthesiologists. Midazolam, propofol, ketamine, fentanyl, and dexmedetomidine were the most common hypnosedative agents that were used either alone or in various combinations. The most common route of administrations were oral and intravenous routes.[35]

POINTS TO REMEMBER

- Sedation and general anesthesia can prove to be valuable adjuncts to regular dental treatment. Use of sedation is advocated in children lacking the ability to cooperate because of their age and anxious children.
- Conscious sedation is defined as a minimally depressed level of consciousness that retains the patient's ability to independently and continuously maintain an airway and respond appropriately to physical stimulation or verbal command and that is produced by a pharmacological or nonpharmacological method or a combination thereof.
- Objectives of conscious sedation are to reduce or eliminate anxiety, reduce untoward movement and reaction to dental treatment, enhance communication and patient cooperation, raise the pain reaction threshold, aid in treatment of the mentally/physically disabled or medically compromised patient.
- Indications of conscious sedation are lack of psychological or emotional maturity, medical, physical, cognitive disability, fearful, highly anxious or obstreperous patient, a patient whose gag reflex interferes with dental care, a patient for whom profound local anaesthesia cannot be obtained.
- There is only one inhalation agent that meets the requirement of conscious sedation and that is nitrous oxide ideal concentration for nitrous oxide sedation is 30% N_2O and 70% O_2.
- Diffusion hypoxia may occur as the nitrous oxide sedation is reversed; this can be checked by administrating oxygen for 3–5 minutes.
- Reversal agents used for benzodiazepines sedation are flumazenil and that for opioids sedation is naloxone.
- Midazolam is the best drug of choice for sedation in children with oral route being most preferred.
- Ketamine is the drug most often used for recreational abuse due to induction of dissociative anesthesia.
- Day care/ambulatory anesthesia is indicated in healthy ASA I and ASA II patients specifically.

Questionnaire

1. Define conscious sedation, deep sedation, and general anesthesia.
2. Write about importance of nitrous oxide in Pediatric Dentistry.
3. Which drugs are used in premedication?
4. Enumerate the indications and objectives of conscious sedation.
5. Classification of patient selection according to American Society of Anesthesiologists.
6. Write a note on ketamine.
7. Write about reversal agents for benzodiazepines and opioids.
8. What is diffusion hypoxia?
9. Describe midazolam sedation.
10. What are the complications of sedation?
11. Describe the drugs used for conscious sedation.

REFERENCES

1. Coté CJ, Wilson S. Guidelines for Monitoring and Management of Pediatric Patients Before, During, and After Sedation for Diagnostic and Therapeutic Procedures. Pediatr Dent. 2019 Jul 15;41(4):259-260.
2. Wilson S. Management of child patient behavior: quality of care, fear and anxiety, and the child patient. Pediatr Dent. 2013;35:170-4.
3. American Academy of Pediatric Dentistry. Clinical guideline on the elective use of minimal, moderate, and deep sedation and general anesthesia in pediatric dental patients. Pediatr Dent. 2004;26:95-103.
4. American Society of Anesthesiologists. Pediatric anesthesia practice recommendations: task force on pediatric anesthesia of the ASA Committee on Pediatric Anesthesia. Park Ridge, IL: ASA; 2002.
5. American Society of Anesthesiologists, Position on Monitored Anesthesia Care, Last Amended on October 17, 2018.
6. Gupta K., Ritwik P. Rationale for Using Nitrous Oxide in Pediatric Dentistry. In: Gupta K, Emmanouil D, Sethi A (Eds), Nitrous

Oxide in Pediatric Dentistry. Springer, Cham. 2020. https://doi.org/10.1007/978-3-030-29618-6_1

7. Paarmann C, Royer R. Pain control for dental practitioners: an interactive approach, 1st edn. Wolters Kluwer; 2008.
8. Bowen DM. Aiding in administration of nitrous oxide analgesia. Idaho: Idaho State Board of Dentistry;2005.
9. Alert request for assistance in controlling exposure to Nitrous oxide during anesthesia administration. Cincinnati. US Dept of Health and Human Services. Public Health Service. Centre of Disease Control, National Institutes of Occupational Safety and Health. 1994; DHHS/NIOSH Publication number 94–100. Accessed 15 Jan 2019.
10. Hillman KM, Saloojee Y, Brett I, Cole PV. Nitrous oxide concentrations in the dental surgery. Anaesthesia. 1981;36:257.
11. Nitrous oxide in the dental office. ADA Council on Scientific Affairs; ADA Council on Dental Practice. J Am Dent Assoc. 1997;128(3):364-5. PMID: 9066223.
12. Langa H. Relative analgesia in dental practice—inhalation analgesia and sedation with nitrous oxide. Philadelphia: Saunders; 1976.
13. Gupta K, Ritwik P. Clinical Application of Nitrous Oxide in Pediatric Dentistry. In: Gupta K, Emmanouil D, Sethi A (Eds), Nitrous Oxide in Pediatric Dentistry. Springer, Cham. 2020. https://doi.org/10.1007/978-3-030-29618-65.
14. American Academy of Pediatric Dentistry. Use of nitrous oxide for pediatric dental patients. The Reference Manual of Pediatric Dentistry. Chicago, Ill.: American Academy of Pediatric Dentistry; 2021:338-43.
15. Pedersen RS, Bayat A, Steen NP, Jacobsson ML. Nitrous oxide provides safe and effective analgesia for minor paediatric procedures--a systematic review. Dan Med J. 2013 ;60(6):A4627. PMID: 23743110.
16. Bhatnagar S, Das UM, Bhatnagar G. Comparison of oral midazolam with oral tramadol, triclofos and zolpidem in the sedation of pediatric dental patients: an in vivo study. J Indian Soc Pedod Prev Dent. 2012;30:109-14.
17. Alzahrani AM, Wyne AH. Use of oral midazolam sedation in pediatric dentistry: a review. Pak Oral Dent J. 2012;32:444-55.
18. Karl HW, Keifer AJ, Rosenberger JL, et al. Comparison of the safety and efficacy of intranasal midazolam or sufentanil for pre-induction of anesthesia in pediatric patients. Anesthesiology. 1992;76:109.
19. Lejus C, Renaudin M, Testa S, Malinovsky JM, Vigier T, Souron R. Midazolam for premedication in children: nasal vs. rectal administration. Eur J Anaesthesiol. 1997 May;14(3):244-9. doi: 10.1046/j.1365-2346.1997.00013.x.
20. Thikkurissy S, Gosnell ES. Pain reaction control: Sedation. In: Nowak AJ, Christensen JR, Mabry TR Townsend JA, Wells MH (eds). Pediatric Dentistry infancy through adolescence, 6th edition. Philadelphia, Elsevier,2019;116-127.
21. Kaviani N, et al. The effect of orally administered ketamine on requirement for anesthetics and postoperative pain in mandibular molar teeth with irreversible pulpitis. J Oral Sci. 2011;53:461-5.
22. Simmons D. Sedation and patient safety. Crit Care Nurs Clin North Am. 2005;17:279-85.
23. Malviya S, Voepel-Lewis T, Tait AR. Adverse events and risk factors associated with the sedation of children by non- anesthesiologists. Anesth Analg. 1997;85:1207-13.
24. Beirne OR. Current and future research in dental sedation and anesthesia. Anesth Prog. 1986;33:193-6.
25. Damle SG, Gandhi M, Laheri V. Comparison of oral ketamine and oral midazolam as sedative agents in pediatric dentistry. J Indian Soc Pedod Prevent Dent. 2008;26:97-101.
26. Barbosa ACBM, Mourão J, Milagre V, Andrade DC, Areias C. Inhalation conscious sedation with nitrous oxide/oxygen in pediatric dentistry. Med Express. 2014;1:102-4.
27. Al-Zahrani AM, Wyne AH, Sheta SA. Comparison of oral midazolam with a combination of oral midazolam and nitrous oxide-oxygen inhalation in the effectiveness of dental sedation for young children. J Indian Soc Pedod Prev Dent. 2009;27(1):9-16. doi: 10.4103/0970-4388.50810.
28. Silva CC, Lavado C, Areias C, Mourão J, Andrade D. Conscious sedation vs general anesthesia in pediatric dentistry—a review. Med Express. 2015;2:15-8.
29. Krishna Priya V, Gaur D, Ganesh M, Kumar CS. Conscious sedation in pediatric dentistry: a review. Int J Contemp Med Res. 2016;3:1577-80.
30. Galeotti A, Garret Bernardin A, D'Antò V, et al. Inhalation conscious sedation with nitrous oxide and oxygen as alternative to general anesthesia in precooperative, fearful, and disabled pediatric dental patients: a large survey on 688 working sessions. Biomed Res Int. 2016;2016:1-6.
31. Attri JP, Sharan R, Makkar V, et al. Conscious sedation: emerging trends in pediatric dentistry. Anesth Essays Res. 2017;11:277-81.
32. Ashley PF, Chaudhary M, Lourenço-Matharu L. Sedation of children undergoing dental treatment. Cochrane Database Syst Rev. 2018;12(12):CD003877. doi: 10.1002/14651858.CD003877.
33. Fantacci C, Fabrizio GC, Ferrara P, Franceschi F, Chiaretti A. Intranasal drug administration for procedural sedation in children admitted to pediatric Emergency Room. Eur Rev Med Pharmacol Sci. 2018;22(1):217-22.
34. Sado-Filho J, Viana KA, Corrêa-Faria P, Costa LR, Costa PS. Randomized clinical trial on the efficacy of intranasal or oral ketamine-midazolam combinations compared to oral midazolam for outpatient pediatric sedation. PloS One. 2019;14 (3): e0213074.
35. Funda AR. Hypnosedative and Analgesic Drug Choice for Pediatric Procedural Sedation: a Review of Recent Literature. Pediatric Practice and Research.7(Ek): 644-8.

FURTHER READING

1. American Academy of Pediatric Dentistry pediatric dent Pediatric Dentistry Pediatric Dentistry. Use of nitrous oxide for al patients. The Reference Manual of. Chicago, Ill.: American Academy of ; 2020:324–329. https://www.aapd.org/media/Policies_Guidelines/BP_UseofNitrous.pdf. Last accessed on 9Feb 2022.
2. American Society of Anesthesiologists. Continuum of Depth of Sedation: Definition of General Anesthesia and Levels of Sedation/Analgesia. October 23, 2019. https://www.asahq.org/standards-and-guidelines/continuum-of-depth-of-sedation-definition-of-general-anesthesia-and-levels-of-sedation analgesia. Last accessed on 9Feb 2022.
3. An Updated Report by the American Society of Anesthesiologists Task Force on Sedation and Analgesia by Non-Anesthesiologists; Practice Guidelines for Sedation and Analgesia by Non-Anesthesiologists. Anesthesiology 2002;96:1004–1017. https://pubs.asahq.org/anesthesiology/article/96/4/1004/39315/Practice-Guidelines-for-Sedation-and-Analgesia-by. Last accessed on 9Feb 2022.
4. Australian Dental Association. Policy statement 6.33. Relative analgesia in Dentistry. https://www.ada.org.au/Dental-Professionals/Policies/Dental-Practice/Relative-Analgesia/PS6-33-Relative-Analgesia11-12Apr19_Approved.aspx. Last accessed on 9 Feb 2022.
5. Bauman BH, McManus Jr. JG. Pediatric pain management in the emergency department. Emerg Med Clin North Am. 2005;23:393-414.
6. Berge TI. Nitrous oxide in dental surgery. Best Practice & Research. Clinical Anaesthesiology. 2001;15(3):477-89.
7. Chiaretti A, Barone G, Rigante D, et al. Intranasal lidocaine and midazolam for procedural sedation in children. Arch Dis Child 2011;96:160-3.
8. Dummett CO, Adair SM. Workshop on practical and cost effective issues of behavior management. Pediatr Dent. 1999;21:470-1.
9. Gupta K, Chopra R, Kulkarni P. Use of pulse oximetry during nitrous oxide- oxygen inhalation sedation: mandatory or recommended? Eur Arch Paediatr Dent. 2022;23(4):647-652. doi: 10.1007/s40368-022-00717-7. Epub 2022 Jun 2. PMID: 35655051.
10. Gupta K, Ritwik P. Nitrous Oxide-oxygen Inhalation in Dental Practice: Sedation or Behavior Guidance? Journal of South Asian Association of Pediatric Dentistry. 2022;5(1):54. doi: 10.5005/jp-journals-10077-3213
11. Gupta K, Ritwik P. Rationale and pre-requisites for use of nitrous oxide in pediatric dentistry. Clin Dent Rev. 2021; 5:2. https://doi.org/10.1007/s41894-020-00090-y

12. Gupta K, Ritwik P. The "First Nitrous Oxide Visit" in a pediatric dental practice. Clin Dent Rev. 2021; 5:14. https://doi.org/10.1007/s41894-021-00101-6
13. Hosey MT. UK National Clinical Guidelines in Paediatric Dentistry. Managing anxious children: the use of conscious sedation in paediatric dentistry. Int J Paediatr Dent. 2002;12:359-72.
14. Mistry RB, Nahata MC. Ketamine for conscious sedation in pediatric emergency care. Pharmacotherapy. 2005;25:1104-11.
15. Oznurhan F, Derdiyok C. The drugs and application methods in dental sedation. J Dent Res Pract. 2020;4:1-6.
16. Piira T, Sugiura T, Champion GD, Donnelly N, Cole AS. The role of parental presence in the context of children's medical procedures: a systematic review. Child Care Health Dev. 2005;31:233-43.
17. Report of the intercollegiate advisory committee for sedation in dentistry. Standards for conscious sedation in the provision of dental care of dentistry. 2015. https://www.rcseng.ac.uk/-/media/files/rcs/fds/publications/dental-sedation-report-2015-web-v2.pd. Last accessed on 9Feb 2022.
18. Spitalnic S, Blazes C, Anderson A. Conscious sedation: a primer for outpatient procedures. Hosp Physician. 2000:22-32.

CHAPTER

Behavior Management of Differently-abled Child

Priya Verma Gupta, Nikhil Marwah

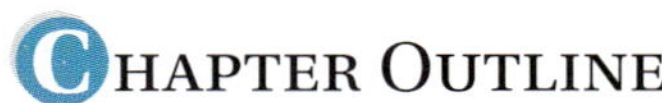

Dental professionals and parental groups alike agree that individuals with a disability, whether developmental or acquired, are entitled to the opportunity to achieve appropriate rehabilitation to enable them to realize their maximal level of functioning and to assist them in "normalizing" their lives. Historically, five basic reasons have been given to account for the inadequacy of dental care for this group by *Plummer:*

1. On the part of the profession, there has been lack of knowledge, understanding, and actual experience in treating the differently-abled patient.
2. There has been inadequate information on the oral hygiene status and dental needs of the differently-abled population.
3. The importance of dental care for the differently-abled has been overlooked by health planners and administrators in establishing programs for the noninstitutionalized population.
4. Parents and guardians of differently-abled children have not been made aware of the importance of oral health and may lack knowledge of the healthcare system and financial resources available to them.
5. Home care has been so neglected that most differently-abled patients need extensive dental treatment.

MENTAL RETARDATION

Mental retardation has been defined by the American Association of Mental Deficiency (AAMD) as "Sub-average general intellectual functioning which originates during the developmental period and is associated with impairment in adaptive behavior."

American Academy of Pediatric Dentistry (1996)

A person should be considered dentally handicapped if he has pain, infection, or lack of functional dentition which affects the following:

- Restricts consumption of diet adequate to support normal growth and developmental needs
- Delays or alters growth and development
- Inhibits performance of any major life activity including work, learning communication, and recreation

Dental treatment of a person with mental retardation: Providing dental treatment for a person with mental retardation requires adjusting to social, intellectual, and emotional delays. A short attention span, restlessness, hyperactivity, and erratic emotional behavior may be encountered while treating patients with mental retardation undergoing dental care. The following procedures have proved beneficial in establishing dentist–patient rapport and reducing the patient's anxiety about dental care.

- Give the family a brief tour of the office before attempting treatment.
- Introduce the patient and family to the office staff. This will familiarize the patient with the personnel and reduce the patient's fear of the unknown.
- Allow the patient to bring a favorite item (stuffed animal, blanket, or toy) to hold for the visit.
- Be repetitive; speak slowly and in simple terms.
- If the individual has an alternative communication system, such as a picture board or electronic device, be sure it is available to assist with dental explanations and instructions.

- Give only one instruction at a time.
- Reward the patient with compliments after the successful completion of each procedure.
- Actively listen to the patient. People with mental retardation often have trouble with communication, and the dentist should be particularly sensitive to gestures and verbal requests.
- Invite the parent into the operatory for assistance and to aid in communication with the patient.
- Keep appointment short.
- Gradually progress to more difficult procedures (e.g., anesthesia and restorative dentistry) after the patient has become accustomed to the dental environment.
- Schedule the patient early in the day, when the dentist, the staff, and the patient will not be fatigued

Note: There is no mention of general anesthesia.

CEREBRAL PALSY

Nelson used the term cerebral palsy to describe a group of nonprogressive disorders resulting from malfunctioning of the motor centers and pathways of the brain.

Dental treatment of a person with cerebral palsy: To an uninformed dentist, a person with cerebral palsy might be perceived as an uncooperative and unmanageable patient. A clinician who lacks knowledge about physically and mentally disabling conditions may not be comfortable in treating such patients and may refuse to do so. The following suggestions are offered to the clinician as being of practical significance in treating a patient with cerebral palsy.

- Consider treating a patient who uses a wheelchair in the same itself.
- If a patient is to be transferred to the dental chair, ask about a preference for the mode of transfer. If the patient has no preference, the two person lift is recommended.
- Make an effort to stabilize the patient's head through all phases of dental treatment.
- Try to place and maintain the patient in the midline of the dental chair with arms and legs as close to the body as feasible. Keep the patient's back slightly elevated, to minimize swallowing (supine position).
- On placing the patient in the dental chair, determine the patient's degree of comfort and assess the position of the extremities. Do not force the limbs into unnatural positions.
- Use immobilization judiciously for controlling movements of the extremities.
- For control of involuntary jaw movements, choose from a variety of mouth props and finger splint. Patient preference should weigh heavily, since a patient with cerebral palsy may be very apprehensive about the ability to control swallowing. Such appliances may also trigger the strong gag reflex.
- To minimize startle reflex reactions, avoid stimuli, such as abrupt movements, noises, and lights, without forewarning the patient.
- Introduce intraoral stimuli slowly to avoid eliciting a gag reflex or to make it less severe. Consider the use of the rubber dam, a highly recommended technique, for restorative procedures. Work efficiently and minimize patient's time in the chair to decrease fatigue of the involved muscles.

CHILDHOOD AUTISM

Kanmer (1944) described a clinical syndrome in children with inability to relate appropriately to people and situations.

Dental treatment of a person with autism

- A prominent symptom of infantile autism is an intense desire to maintain consistency in the environment.
- Minor changes in the environment may elicit extreme anxiety in autistic children.
- They often exhibit an extreme resistance on being held and show an inappropriate reaction to fearful situations.
- Eye contact is difficult to achieve, and the children are prone to tantrums and aggressive or destructive behavior.
- Oral hygiene is often very poor because of finicky dietary habits.
- Behavior modification techniques by **Lovaas** have proved to be effective in producing behavioral changes in autistic children.
- The key to all behavior modification programs lies in the use of positive reinforcement to promote desirable behavior.
- An appropriate reward is often difficult to find for autistic children. In the early stages of the program, sweet foods can serve as desirable rewards. In the latter stages of modifying behavior, such oral rewards should be changed to social rewards, such as a pat on the back or a hug.

Source: Kaur K, Suneja B, Jodhka S, Kaur J, Singh A, Singh SR, Metallic insignia in primary teeth: A biomarker for Autism Spectrum Disorders. J indian Soc Pedod Prev Dent 2021; 39:61-6.

It has been estimated worldwide, that one in 160 children have ASD. There is a dramatic rise in the prevalence of autistic spectrum disorders in India in the past few decades, affecting almost 0.15–1.00% of the children (one in 400–500). The diagnosis of autistic spectrum disorders is multifactorial and depends on its etiology, which itself is poorly understood. Previously, it had been the school of thought, that all such disorders are the result of genetic inheritance. Prenatal and environmental exposures have been implicated in the occurrence of developmental disabilities in children, but the research relating to the roles of metals or chemicals in the causation of these disorders has been slow. It has been hypothesized that exposure to environmental factors such as metals like zinc and manganese can be a causative factor for autistic spectrum disorders. The maximum susceptibility is prominent during the prenatal period when the placenta is permeable and the fetal blood–brain barrier and the neuronal growth is immature. Children, in their early childhood also are particularly vulnerable to the neurotoxic effects of exposures to heavy metals because their brains are still in the developing stage.

The contributions of multiple metal exposures and the occurrence of ASDs are unclear, although dysregulation of the metals like zinc and manganese has been implicated because of their potential roles in the central nervous system. These elements play an important role in the synaptic transmission of impulses across the central nervous system. Their toxicity or deficiency can lead to neurological or psychological disorders. Zinc is a trace element in human body and is involved in the regulation of neurogenesis, neuronal migration, and differentiation, consequently maintaining healthy brain function and shaping cognitive development. Manganese (Mn) is also a naturally occurring trace element which is an essential cofactor for metalloenzyme-superoxide dismutase, which protects cells against antioxidant processes. Dysregulation of manganese results in the enhanced formation of oxygen reactive species in the areas of the brain which can lead to oxidative stress and cause impaired propagation of impulses.

To assess the effects of metals on the neurological development of children, there is a need of a biomarker or a parameter. The commonly used biological matrices to assess the exposure of the child, such as blood and urine, provide access to single point serum concentrations only, the values of which show diurnal variations. Hair and nails are other biomarkers which can be used to provide information about exposures in this period, but these can be contaminated by shampoos, nail paints, etc., and do not provide access to the prenatal period. These markers cannot retrospectively assess the prenatal and early postnatal exposure. Therefore, using these biomarkers to aid in the diagnosis of ASD is not feasible. Consequently, the children suspected to have ASD are subjected to psychological interventions and multiple behavior screening tests which are also not very definitive of diagnosing autism and can be very exhausting for the child and the parent.

A primary tooth can suffice as a reliable biomarker to assess the environmental exposure of both the mother and the child in early childhood years. The mineralization of these teeth proceeds in an incremental pattern, akin to growth rings of trees, spanning the entire prenatal and early postnatal phases. Enamel formation in primary teeth begins in utero and completes by approximately 3 months to 1-year postbirth as according to the particular tooth period of mineralization. The metals are accessible through the placental barrier which go into the fetal bloodstream and deposit these metals in the teeth while they are mineralizing. Data on the fine incremental microstructure of teeth can be used to uncover the cumulative chemical exposures which the mother might have had during her gestation period. In this study, the primary incisors were analyzed for concentrations of metals by a method called Inductively Coupled Plasma Optical Emission Spectrometry (ICP-OES). And it was found that much higher concentrations of zinc and manganese were found in ASD children' teeth as compared to the teeth of typically developing children.

The results of the current study supported the fact that there are associations between metal exposures to a pregnant mother and a child during his early years of childhood. This study could be a surpassing contribution by Pediatric Dentistry to the world of medicine to aid in the diagnosis of ASD, where genomics can sometimes fail to unfold the jumble, especially for the diagnosis of a disorder in a country like India where parents are in the greatest denial for accepting their child's disability.

VISUAL IMPAIRMENT

A person is considered to be affected by blindness if the visual acuity does not exceed 20/200 in the better eye, with correcting lenses, or if the acuity is >20/200 but accompanied by a visual field of no >20°.

Dental treatment of a person with blindness

- Determine the degree of visual impairment (e.g., can the patient tell light from dark).
- If a companion accompanies the patient, find out if the companion is an interpreter. If he or she is not, address the patient.
- Establish rapport; offer verbal and physical reassurance. Avoid expressions of pity of references to visual impairment as an affliction.
- In guiding the patient to the operatory, ask if the patient desires assistance. Do not grab, move, or stop the patient without verbal warning. Encourage the parent to accompany the child.
- Paint a picture in the mind of the visually impaired child, describing the office setting and treatment. Always give the patient adequate descriptions before performing treatment procedures. It is important to use the same office setting for each dental visit to ally the patient's anxiety.
- Introduce other office personnel very informally.
- When making physical contact, do so reassuringly. Holding the patient's hand often promotes relaxation.
- Allow the patient to ask questions about the course of treatment and answer them keeping in mind that the patient is highly individual, sensitive, and responsive.
- Allow a patient who wears eyeglasses to keep them on for protection and security.
- Rather than using the tell-show-feel-do approach, invite the patient to touch, taste, or smell, recognizing that these senses are acute. Avoid sight references.
- Describe in detail instruments and objects to be placed in the patient's mouth. Demonstrate a rubber cup on the patient's fingernail.
- Because strong tastes may be rejected, use smaller quantities of dental materials with such characteristics.
- Some patients may be photophobic. Ask parents about light sensitivity and allow them to wear sunglasses.
- Explain the procedures of oral hygiene, and then place the patient's hand over yours as you slowly but deliberately guide the toothbrush.
- Use audiocassette tapes and Braille dental pamphlets explaining specific dental procedures to supplement information and decrease chair time.
- Announce exits from the entrances to the dental operatory cheerfully. Keep distractions minimal, and avoid unexpected loud noises.
- Limit the patient's dental care to one dentist whenever possible.
- Maintain a relaxed atmosphere. Remember that your patient cannot see your smile.

HEARING LOSS

Dental treatment of a person with hearing loss

- Prepare the patient and parent before the first visit with a welcome letter that states what is to be done and include a medical history form.
- Let the patient and parent determine the initial appointment how the patient desires to communicate (i.e., interpreter, lip reading, sign language, writing notes, or a combination of these).
- Look for ways to improve communication. It is useful to learn some basic sign language.
- Face the patient and speak slowly at a natural pace and directly to the patient without shouting.
- Assess speech, language ability, and degree of hearing impairment when taking the patient's complete medical history.
- Identify the age of onset, type, degree, and cause of hearing loss, whether any other family members are affected.
- Enhance visibility for communication.
- Watch the patient's expression.
- Have the patient use hand gestures if a problem arises.
- Write out and display information.
- Reassure the patient with physical contact; hold the patient's hand initially, or place a hand reassuringly on the patient's shoulder while the patient maintains visual contact.

- The child may be startled without visual contact, so explain to the patient if you must leave the room.
- Use visual aids and allow the patient to see the instruments, and demonstrate how they work.
- Display confidence; use smiles and reassuring gestures to build up confidence and reduce anxiety.
- Adjust the hearing aid (if the patient has one) before the handpiece is in operation, since a hearing aid will amplify all sounds.

RECOMMENDATIONS OF AAPD

This guideline by American Academy of Pediatric Dentistry (AAPD) for individuals with special healthcare needs (SHCN) is intended to educate healthcare providers, parents, and ancillary organizations about the management of oral health care needs particular to individuals with SHCN.

Scheduling Appointments

- The parent's/patient's initial contact with the dental practice allows both parties an opportunity to address the child's primary oral health needs and to confirm the appropriateness of scheduling an appointment with that particular practitioner.
- Along with the child's name, age, and chief complaint, the receptionist should determine the presence and nature of any SHCN and, when appropriate, the name(s) of the child's medical care provider(s).
- The office staff, under the guidance of the dentist, should determine the need for an increased length of appointment and/or additional auxiliary staff in order to accommodate the patient in an effective and efficient manner.

Dental Home

- Patients with SHCN who have a dental home are more likely to receive appropriate preventive and routine care.
- The dental home provides an opportunity to implement individualized preventive oral health practices and reduces the child's risk of preventable dental/oral disease.

Patient Assessment

- Familiarity with the patient's medical history is essential to decreasing the risk of aggravating a medical condition while rendering dental care.
- An accurate, comprehensive, and up-to-date medical history is necessary for correct diagnosis and effective treatment planning.
- Information regarding the chief complaint, history of present illness, medical conditions and/or illnesses, medical care providers, hospitalizations/surgeries, anesthetic experiences, current medications, allergies/ sensitivities, immunization status, review of systems, family and social histories, and thorough dental history should be obtained.
- At each patient visit, the history should be consulted and updated. Recent medical attention for illness or injury, newly diagnosed medical conditions, and changes in medications should be documented. A written update should be obtained at each recall visit. Significant medical conditions should be identified in a conspicuous yet confidential manner in the patient's record.
- A caries-risk assessment should be performed. An individualized preventive program, including a dental recall schedule, should be recommended after evaluation of the patient's caries risk, oral health needs, and abilities.
- A summary of the oral findings and specific treatment recommendations should be provided to the patient and parent/caregiver.

Medical Consultations

The dentist should coordinate care via consultation with the patient's other care providers. When appropriate, the physician should be consulted regarding medications, sedation, general anesthesia, and special restrictions or preparations that may be required to ensure the safe delivery of oral health care.

Patient Communication

- When treating patients with SHCN, similar to any other child, developmentally appropriate communication is critical.
- An attempt should be made to communicate directly with the patient during the provision of dental care. A patient who does not communicate verbally may communicate in a variety of nontraditional ways.

Informed Consent

All patients must be able to provide signed informed consent for dental treatment or have someone present who legally can provide this service for them. Informed consent should be well documented in the dental record through a signed and witnessed form.

Behavior Guidance

- Behavior guidance of the patient with SHCN can be challenging because of dental anxiety or a lack of understanding of dental care; children with disabilities may exhibit resistant behaviors. These behaviors can interfere with the safe delivery of dental treatment.
- With the parent/caregiver's assistance, most patients with physical and mental disabilities can be managed in the dental office.
- Protective stabilization can be helpful in patients for whom traditional behavior guidance techniques are not adequate.
- When protective stabilization is not feasible or effective, sedation or general anesthesia is the behavioral guidance armamentarium of choice.

Preventive Strategies

- Individuals with SHCN may be at increased risk for oral diseases; these diseases further jeopardize the patient's health.
- Education of parents/caregivers is critical for ensuring appropriate and regular supervision of daily oral hygiene.

- Toothbrushes can be modified to enable individuals with physical disabilities to brush their own teeth. Electric toothbrushes and floss holders may improve patient compliance. Caregivers should provide the appropriate oral care when the patient is unable to do so adequately.
- A noncariogenic diet should be discussed for long-term prevention of dental disease.
- Patients with SHCN benefit from sealants and fluoride programs.
- Preventive strategies for patients with SHCN should address anticipatory guidance about risk of trauma and what to do if dentoalveolar trauma occurs.

Barriers

- Dentists should be familiar with community-based resources for patients with SHCN and encourage such assistance when appropriate.
- While local hospitals, public health facilities, rehabilitation services, or groups that advocate for those with SHCN can be valuable contacts to help the dentist/patient address language and cultural barriers, other community-based resources may offer support with financial or transportation considerations that prevent access to care.

POINTS TO REMEMBER

- A person should be considered dentally handicapped if pain, infection, or lack of functional dentition which affects the following: restricts consumption of diet adequate to support normal growth and developmental needs; delays or alters growth and development; inhibits performance of any major life activity including work, learning communication, and recreation.
- Tell-show-do technique, short appointment time, and allowing child his favorite toy in operatory are best approaches in dental management of children with mental retardation.
- Treatment in wheelchair and immobilization for extremities are best used for managing children with cerebral palsy.
- In case of autism, the main precaution is to avoid sudden movements and the focus is to maintain consistency in the environment.
- During treatment of patient with hearing loss, lip reading and sign language are good tools to be used.
- While managing a blind child for dental treatment, the use of Braille signs and feel-show-do technique is the most effective.

Questionnaire

1. Enumerate the reasons for lack of dental care in differently-abled children.
2. Describe the management of a child with mental retardation.
3. How will you manage a child with cerebral palsy in dental operatory?
4. Explain dental management of autistic child.
5. What are the dental management strategies in case of a child with vision or hearing loss?

FURTHER READING

1. American Academy of Pediatric Dentistry. Definition of special health care needs. Pediatr Dent. 2012;34(special issue):16.
2. American Academy of Pediatric Dentistry. Symposium on lifetime oral health care for patients with special needs. Pediatr Dent. 2007;29:92-152.
3. Anders PL, Davis EL. Oral health of patients with intellectual disabilities: A systematic review. Spec Care Dentist. 2010;30:110-7.
4. Charles JM. Dental care in children with developmental disabilities: attention deficit disorder, intellectual disabilities, and autism. J Dent Child. 2010;77(2):84-91.
5. Glassman P, Subar P. Planning dental treatment for people with special needs. Dent Clin North Am. 2009;53:195-205, vii-viii.
6. Kaur K, Suneja B, Jodhka S, Kaur J, Singh A, Singh SR. Metallic insignia in primary teeth: A biomarker for Autism Spectrum Disorders. J Indian Soc Pedod Prev Dent. 2021;39:61-6.
7. Mink JR. Dental care for the differently-abled child. In: Goldman HM, et al., editors. Current therapy in dentistry (vol. 2). St. Louis: Mosby; 1966.
8. Nowak AJ, Casamassimo PS, Slayton RL. Facilitating the transition of patients with special health care needs from pediatric to adult oral health care. J Am Dent Assoc. 2010;141:1351-6.
9. Nowak AJ. Patients with special health care needs in pediatric dental practices. Pediatr Dent. 2002;24:227-8.
10. Nunn JH. The dental health of mentally and physically handicapped children: a review of the literature. Community Dent Health. 1987;4:157-68.
11. Ohmori I, Awaya S, Ishikawa F. Dental care for severely handicapped children. Int Dent J. 1981;31:177-84.
12. Shenkin JD, Davis MJ, Corbin SB. The oral health of special needs children: dentistry's challenge to provide care. J Dent Child. 2001;86:201-5.

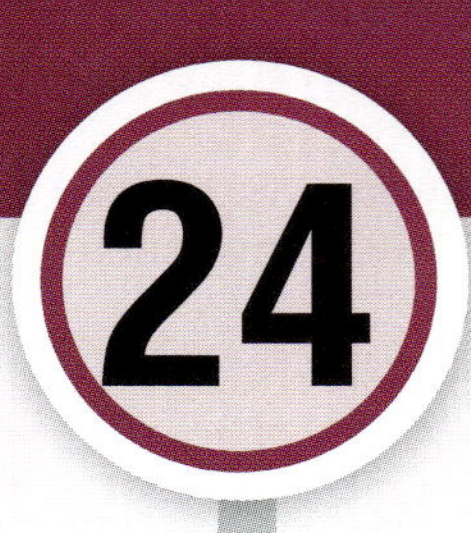

CHAPTER

Diet and Nutrition

Nikhil Marwah, Ambika Joshi

Chapter Outline

- Basal Metabolism and Basal Metabolic Rate
- Energy for Physical Activity
- Specific Dynamic Action of Food
- Recommended Dietary Allowance
- Food Group Guides
- Food Guide Pyramid
- Dietary Goals

A balanced diet is one in which nutrients from each food group in recommended servings is present for the optimal functioning of the human. Since energy is of prime importance in the life process, the study of nutrition is concerned with the basic question of how the human body metabolizes and transforms the elements of food into energy. In fact, our need for energy has such a high priority that a nutrient such as protein, whose primary function is to build tissue, can be used to provide energy when adequate amounts of carbohydrates and fats—the usual nutrient energy sources are not eaten. The energy from food is made available to the body in four basic forms: chemical, for synthesis of new compounds; mechanical, for muscle contraction; electrical, for brain and nerve activity; and thermal, for regulation of body temperature.

The overall energy needs of the body are calculated to be the sum of three factors: basal metabolism, energy for physical activity, and the specific dynamic action (SDA).

BASAL METABOLISM AND BASAL METABOLIC RATE

- Basal metabolism is the minimum amount of energy needed to regulate and maintain the involuntary essential life processes, such as breathing, circulation of the blood, cellular activity, keeping muscles in good tone, and maintaining body temperature.
- The basal metabolic rate (BMR) is defined as the number of kilocalories expanded by the organism per square meter of body surface per hour (kcal/m^2/h).
- The basal metabolism of healthy men requires about 1,600–1,800 kcal daily; basal expenditure of women is about 1,200–1,450 kcal.

ENERGY FOR PHYSICAL ACTIVITY

- Muscular activity affects both energy expenditure and heat production.
- Energy expenditure increases with muscular activity.

Various types of dietary activities	
Maintenance activity	Sitting most of the day, about 2 h of moving about slowly or standing
Light activity	Typing teaching, shop-work, laboratory work; some walking
Moderate activity	Walking, housework, gardening, carpentry, cycling, tennis
Strenuous activity	Picking and shovel work, swimming, basketball, football, running

SPECIFIC DYNAMIC ACTION OF FOOD

- Specific dynamic action (SDA) is the term used to describe the expenditure of calories during the digestion and absorption of food.
- It is 2% for fats, 6% for carbohydrates, and 12% for protein-rich foods.

RECOMMENDED DIETARY ALLOWANCE

- Since 1943, the Food and Nutrition Board, a group of nutrition scientists, has published at approximately 5-year intervals revised and updated editions of the recommended dietary allowances (RDAs).
- The RDAs are sets of values for levels of intake of the nutrients currently considered essential and which meet the physiological needs of nearly all individuals **(Tables 24.1 to 24.4).**

Table 24.1: Vitamins.

Vitamin	Name	Functions	Deficiency	RDA	Food sources	Oral manifestations
B_1	Thiamine	• Coenzyme • Helps in DNA, RNA formation • Metabolism of fats, proteins • Role in neurophysiology	Wet, dry, and infantile beriberi	1 mg/day	Cereals, meat, liver, peas, beef, nuts, milk, leafy legumes, pork, vegetable	No oral manifestations
B_2	Riboflavin	• Coenzyme • ATP generation • Metabolism	Dermatitis, glossitis, angular stomatitis	1.5 mg/day	Milk, liver, cheese, eggs, cereals, whole grains, vegetables	Angular cheilosis, atrophy of filiform papillae, enlarged fungiform papillae, shiny red lips, magenta tongue, sore tongue
B_4	Niacin	• Coenzyme • Tissue respiration • CNS functioning	Pellagra	16–33 mg/day niacin equivalents	Liver, yeast, meat, legumes, cereals	Angular cheilosis, mucositis, stomatitis, oral pain, ulceration, ulcerative gingivitis, denuded tongue, glossitis, glossodynia, tip of tongue is red and swollen, dorsum is dry and smooth
B_5	Pantothenic acid	• Involved in Kreb's cycle • Component of sterols	Paresthesia, fatigue, abdominal stress	4–7 mg/day	Eggs, cereals, legumes, milk, potatoes	–
B_7	Biotin	• Stimulates growth of yeast • Constituent of DNA	Dermatitis, paresthesia, glossitis	100–200 µg/day	Liver, milk, egg yolk, yeast	–
B_6	Pyridoxine	• Cofactor for enzymes • Synthesis of amino acids	Dermatitis, glossitis, convulsions	0.3–2 mg/day	Meat, liver, yeast, legumes, wheat bran, cereals	Angular cheilosis, sore or burning mouth, glossitis, glossodynia
B_{12}	Cyanocobalamin	• Coenzyme • Maintenance of myelin sheath	Atrophic glossitis, combined system disease	3 µg/day	Meat, egg, milk, cheese, fish	Angular cheilosis, mucositis, stomatitis, sore or burning mouth, hemorrhage gingiva, halitosis, epithelial dysplasia of oral mucosa, loss or distortion of taste, ulceration, denuded tongue, glossitis, "beefy" red, smooth and glossy, delayed wound healing, xerostomia, bone loss, aphthous ulcers
B_9	Folic acid	• Maturation of blood cells • Coenzyme • DNA synthesis	Malabsorption, anemia, angular cheilosis	0.4 mg/day	Liver, dark green leafy vegetables, nuts, orange asparagus, soya	–
C	Ascorbic acid	• Formation of collagen • Wound healing • Role in hematology • Role in phagocytosis • Metabolism of amino acids	Scurvy, hemorrhagic skin, follicles, swollen, and bleeding gums	60 mg/day	Pepper, turnip, citrus fruits, cabbage, beans, tomatoes, carrot, tamarind	Scurvy-red swollen gingivae, gingival friability, periodontal destruction, sore burning mouth, soft tissue ulceration, increased risk of candidiasis, malformed teeth (inadequate dentine)
A	Retinol	• Formation of visual purple • Differentiation of epithelium • Promotion of bone remodeling • Activation of cell membrane	Night blindness, keratomalacia, xerophthalmia, hyperkeratosis, hypoplasia	5,000 iu	Yellow and vegetables, carrot, cabbage, spinach, potatoes	Inadequate cell differentiation—impaired healing and tissue regeneration, desquamation of oral mucosa, keratosis, increased risk of candidiasis, gingival hypertrophy and inflammation, xerostomia, disturbed or arrested enamel development, irregular tubular dentine formation and increased caries risk
D	Cholecalciferol	• Calcium and phosphorus absorption	Rickets and osteomalacia	400 iu	Fish, egg, liver, butter, milk	Incomplete mineralization of teeth and alveolar bone excess pulp calcification, enamel hypoplasia
E	Tocopherol	• Antioxidant • Stabilizes cell membrane • Prevents fats from decay	Anemia	10–20 iu	Cereals, soybean, corn, meat, milk, egg	No oral manifestation
K	Menadione	• Synthesis of prothrombin and other clotting factors	Clotting disorders	70–140 µg/day	Lettuce, spinach, cauliflower, cabbage	Increased risk of bleeding and candidiasis

(RDA: recommended dietary allowance)

Table 24.2: Minerals.

Mineral	*Functions*	*Sources*	*Deficiency*
Calcium	• Gives rigidity to bones and teeth • Aids in transmission of impulses across neuromuscular junction • Acts as a chemical trigger in the contraction of muscles • Essential factor in the clotting of blood	• Milk and milk products • Leafy green vegetables—kale, mustard greens, broccoli (spinach contains oxalic acid which binds calcium so that it cannot be absorbed)	Hypocalcemia tetany
Phosphorus	• Development and maintenance of skeletal structure • Involved in the storage and release of energy in carbohydrate metabolism • Component of RNA and DNA • Component of cell membranes	• Meat, poultry, fish, eggs • Milk, dried peas, and beans • Whole grain breads and cereals are rich sources, but much of the phosphorus is bound by phytic acid	Irritability, weakness, blood cell disorders, gait dysfunction
Sodium and chlorine	• Major components of extracellular fluid—helps maintain osmotic pressure • Helps regulate acid–base balance	• Salt used in processing food, cooking, and at the table	• Sodium—hyponatremia, coma, confusion chlorine—alkalosis, failure to thrive
Potassium	• Helps to maintain osmotic pressure and acid–base balance	• Bran, Brewer's yeast, dried peas and beans, oranges	• Hypokalemia, paralysis, cardiac problems
Magnesium	• Role in the body's anabolic and catabolic processes	• Leafy green vegetables, nuts, soybeans, snails	• Neuromuscular irritability
Sulfur	• Component of sulfur-containing amino acids, the vitamins thiamine and biotin, enzymes (coenzyme A) and hormones (insulin)	• Wheat germ, lentils, peanuts, cheese • Major source is the amino acid cystine	
Iron	• Component of hemoglobin (carries oxygen from lungs to tissues) • Component of myoglobin (stores oxygen temporarily in muscle) • Component of catalysts in the metabolism of glucose	• Meat, organ meats, egg yolks, clams, oysters, leafy green vegetables	• Anemia, enteropathy, decreased work performance, impaired learning ability
Iodine	• Essential component of thyroxin and triiodothyronine (regulates the rate of oxidation-reduction reactions)	• Iodized salt • Seafood • Seaweed	• Cretinism, deaf/mutism, impaired fetal growth, retarded brain development
Manganese	• Cofactor in enzyme systems	• Dry tea, instant coffee, whole grains, peanut butter	• Arthralgia, neuralgia
Copper	• Present in several enzymes essential for development of young red blood cells	• Cocoa powder, dry tea, beef and pork liver, peanut butter	• Anemia, Menkes syndrome
Zinc	• Component of several metalloenzymes	• Meat, poultry, seafood, eggs	• Growth retardation, hypogonadism
Cobalt	• Constituent of vitamin $B1_2$		–
Molybdenum	• Not established in man	• Legumes, cereal grains, liver	• Tachycardia, nausea, headache
Fluorine	• Incorporated into tooth structure, aids in resistance to caries	• Fluoridated water, seafood, dry tea	• Osteoporosis, dental caries
Chromium	• Role in glucose tolerance in humans	• American cheese, dry beans, meat, whole grains	• Impaired glucose tolerance
Selenium	• Nonspecific antioxidant catalyst	• Meat, eggs, milk, seafood, whole grains	• Muscle weakness

- The RDAs are primarily designed for planning and procuring nutritionally adequate food supplies for population groups rather than for individuals.
- If the foods consumed contain the amounts of nutrients that meet the RDA, the probability of developing nutritional deficiencies is negligible.
- These are recommendations for the average daily amounts of nutrients that will meet nutritional requirements of most people.
- In addition to providing standards for the USRDA nutritional labeling, the RDA also serves as the basis for:
  - The food guides.
  - The development of diets and products for therapeutic uses.
  - The formulation of new food products.
  - A guide for food provided by community resources such as senior centers, home-delivered meals, and food stamps.

Table 24.3: Summary of RDA for Indians – 2020.

Age group	Category of work	Body Wt	Protein	CHO	Cal cium	Magne sium	Iron	Zinc	Iodine	Thiamine	Ribo flavin	Niacin	Vit B6	Folate	Vit B12	Vit C	Vit A	Vit D
		(kg)	(g/d)	(g/d)	(mg/d)	(mg/d)	(mg/d)	(mg/d)	(μg/day)	(mg/d)	(mg/d)	(mg/d)	(mg/d)	(μg/d)	(μg/d)	(mg/d)	(μg/d)	(IU/d)
Men	Sedentary Moderate Heavy	65	54.0	130	1000	385	19	17	150	1.4 1.8 2.3	2.0 2.5 3.2	14 18 23	1.9 2.4 3.1	300	2.5	80	1000	600
Women	Sedentary Moderate Heavy	55	45.7	130	1000	325	29	13.2	150	1.4 1.7 2.2	1.9 2.4 3.1	11 14 18	1.9 1.9 2.4	220	2.5	65	840	600
	Pregnant woman	55 + 10	+9.5 (2nd trimester) +22.0 (3rd trimester)	175	1000	385	40	14.5	250	2.0	2.7	+2.5	2.3	570	+0.25	+15	900	600
	Lactation 0–6 m 7–12 m		+16.9 +13.2	200 200	1200	325	23	14	280	2.1 2.1	3.0 2.9	+5 +5	+0.26 +0.17	330 330	+1.0	+50	950	600
Infants	0–6 m*	5.8	8.1	55	300	30	-	-	100	0.2	0.4	2	0.1	25	1.2	20	350	400
	6–12 m	8.5	10.5	95	300	75	3	2.5	130	0.4	0.6	5	0.6	85	1.2	27	350	400
Children	1–3 y 4–6 y 7–9 y	11.7 18.3 25.3	11.3 15.9 23.3	130 130 130	500 550 650	135 155 215	8 11 15	3.0 4.5 5.9	90 120 120	0.7 0.9 1.1	0.9 1.3 1.6	7 9 11	0.9 1.2 1.5	110 135 170	1.2 1.2 2.5	27 32 43	390 510 630	600
Boys	10–12 y	34.9	31.8	130	850	270	16	8.5	150	1.5	2.1	15	2.0	220	2.5	54	770	600
Girls	10–12 y	36.4	32.8	130	850	255	28	8.5	150	1.4	1.9	14	1.9	225	2.5	52	790	600
Boys	13–15 y	50.5	44.9	130	1000	355	22	14.3	150	1.9	2.7	19	2.6	285	2.5	72	930	600
Girls	13–15 y	49.6	43.2	130	1000	325	30	12.8	150	1.6	2.2	16	2.2	245	2.5	66	890	600
Boys	16–18 y	64.4	55.4	130	1050	405	26	17.6	150	2.2	3.1	22	3.0	340	2.5	82	1000	600
Girls	16–18 y	55.7	46.2	130	1050	335	32	14.2	150	1.7	2.3	17	2.3	270	2.5	68	860	600

Table 24.4: Summary of recommended intakes for other minerals and trace elements.

Sl. No.	Minerals/trace element	Recommended intake
1.	Phosphorous	1,000 mg/day
2.	Sodium	2,000 mg/day
3.	Potassium	3,500 mg/day
4.	Copper	2 mg/day
5.	Manganese	4 mg/day
6.	Chromium	50 µg/day
7.	Selenium	40 µg/day

FOOD GROUP GUIDES

The objective of national food guides has been to translate dietary standards into simple and reliable devices for the nutrition education of the layperson. The factors that were taken into consideration in the development of food guides were the customary food patterns, the availability of food, food economics, and the nutritive value of foods in a particular locale. The food group guides serve as a practical and workable plan for helping the homemaker select the type and amount of food that needs to be included in each day's meals in order to provide a balanced diet. The USDA daily food guide divides commonly eaten foods into five groups according to their respective nutritional contributions—(1) vegetable-fruit, (2) bread-cereal, (3) milk-cheese, (4) meat, poultry, fish, and beans, and (5) fats, sweets, and alcohol.

Vegetable–Fruit Group

- Vegetables and fruits are important because they contribute vitamins A and C and fiber as well as trace amounts of other nutrients.
- In general, the color of the vegetable or fruit is a guide to its food value.
- Dark green and deep yellow vegetables are good sources of vitamin A.
- Most dark green vegetables, if not overcooked, are also reliable sources of vitamin C as well as riboflavin, folic acid, iron, and magnesium.
- The food guide recommends four basic servings daily from this group. This includes one good vitamin C source each day and a dark green and a deep yellow vegetable at least every other day and more frequently if possible.
- To ensure adequate fiber, unpeeled raw fruits and vegetables and edible seeds should be eaten when possible.
- A serving is one-half cup of a vegetable or fruit, or a portion as ordinarily served, such as one medium-size apple, or potato; one bowl of salad; or half of a medium-size grapefruit.

Bread–Cereal Group

- The bread and cereal group is the most economical source of nutrients in our daily diets.
- A wide variety of cereal grain is available, including wheat, rice, corn, rye, oats, and barley.
- Whole-grain or enriched bread and cereals contain substantial amounts of the B vitamins and iron.
- Bread and cereals also provide protein and are a major source of this nutrient in vegetarian diets.
- Whole-grain products also contribute magnesium and fiber.
- Many breakfast cereals are enriched at nutrient levels higher than those that occur in natural whole grain. In some cases, fortification adds vitamins, such as A, B, C, and D, not normally found in cereals (which is not desirable or recommended, especially the addition of vitamins A and D).
- However, fiber and other still unidentified vitamins and trace minerals that may normally be present in whole grain are not replaced in the usual restoration process of the refined cereals.
- Therefore, it is strongly recommended that natural whole-grain products be included in the diet whenever possible.
- Four servings daily of breads and cereals, especially of whole-grain products, are recommended.
- Counted as one serving are 1 oz of ready-to-eat cereal, one-half to three-fourth cup of cooked cereal, corn meal, grits, macaroni, noodles, spaghetti, or rice, and one slice of bread.

Milk–Cheese Group

- Milk products are an important part of the diet as they provide about two-thirds of the calcium, one half of the riboflavin, and one-fourth of the protein in the foods normally eaten.
- Milk is low in vitamin C and iron, but it supplies more of the other essential nutrients in significant amount than any other single food.
- An average serving is one 8-oz cup of milk or about a 1-inch cube of cheddar cheese.
- Children and adolescents should have the equivalent of 3–4 serving daily.

Meat, Poultry, Fish, and Beans Group

- The choices within this group are many: Beef, lamb, veal, pork, fish, poultry, eggs, dried beans or peas, and nuts.
- These foods are valued for protein, phosphorus, niacin, vitamin B_{12}, and iron. Only foods of animal origin provide vitamin B_{12}. Foods in this group are usually the most expensive items in the diet.
- In this group, the organ meats (liver, heart, and kidneys) deserve special mention for their high nutritional value in relation to cost. There is relatively little difference in the protein and iron content of beef, veal, lamb, and pork, although pork is richer in thiamine.
- Fish, poultry, and eggs are complete protein foods and can be used as meat equivalents. Nuts and their products, such as peanut butter, can be included in the diet for variety.
- It is strongly recommended that the choices among the above-mentioned food be varied, because each has distinct nutritional advantages. For example, red meats and oysters are good sources of zinc. Liver and egg yolks are valuable sources of vitamin A. Dry beans, dry peas, soybeans, and nuts are worthwhile sources of magnesium. Fish and poultry are low in saturated fat. Sunflower and sesame seeds contribute polyunsaturated fatty acids. Cholesterol is

found in high concentration in organ meats and egg yolks, whereas fish and shellfish except shrimp are relatively low in cholesterol.

- To obtain full advantage of the protein from the foods in this group, it is preferable to have an occasional egg for breakfast, a fish or meat sandwich at noon, and some meat, fish, poultry, or beans at night rather than to have a large serving at only one meal and no food from this group at other meals.
- Suggested daily amounts from this group of foods are two or more servings.
- Count 3–4 oz of lean cooked meat, or fish filet as a serving. One-half to three-fourth cooked beans, dry peas (split peas), soybeans, or lentils; two tablespoons peanut butter, and one-fourth to one-half cup nuts, sesame seeds, or sunflower seeds count as 1 oz of meat, poultry, or fish.

Fats, Sweets, and Alcohol Group

- This group of foods provides mostly calories.
- Included in the group are butter, margarine, mayonnaise, other salad dressings, other fats and oils; candy, sugar, jams, jellies, syrups, sweet toppings, soft drinks and other highly sugared beverages; wine, beer, and liquor.
- Refined flour products that are not restored or enriched used as ingredients in prepared foods are also included in this group.
- The most desirable food in this group are vegetable oils which supply vitamin E and essential fatty acids and margarine and butter which provide some vitamin A.
- In general, with the exception of the fats just mentioned, these foods provide practically no essential nutrients such as vitamins, minerals, and protein; therefore, no serving sizes are defined.

FOOD GUIDE PYRAMID

- A food guide pyramid is a pyramid-shaped guide of healthy foods divided into sections to show the recommended intake for each food group.
- The USDAs first dietary guidelines were published in 1894 by **Dr Wilbur Olin Atwater**. In Atwater's 1904 publication titled *Principles of Nutrition and Nutritive Value of Food,* he advocated variety, proportionality, and moderation; measuring calories; and an efficient, affordable diet that focused on nutrient-rich foods and less fat, sugar, and starch.
- The historical perspective of food guides was explained by **Welsh** and **Shaw** in 1992.

Basic Seven

- The first food guide proposed in 1943 was basic seven **(Fig. 24.1)**.
- In 1943, during World War II, the USDA introduced a nutrition guide promoting the "Basic seven" food groups to help maintain nutritional standards under wartime food rationing. The basic seven food groups were:
  1. Green and yellow vegetables (some raw; some cooked, frozen or canned).
  2. Oranges, tomatoes, grapefruit (or raw cabbage or salad greens).
  3. Potatoes and other vegetables and fruits (raw, dried, cooked, frozen, or canned).
  4. Milk and milk products (fluid, evaporated, dried milk, or cheese).
  5. Meat, poultry, fish, or eggs (or dried beans, peas, nuts, or peanut butter).
  6. Bread, flour, and cereals (natural whole grain, or enriched or restored).
  7. Butter and fortified margarine (with added vitamin A).

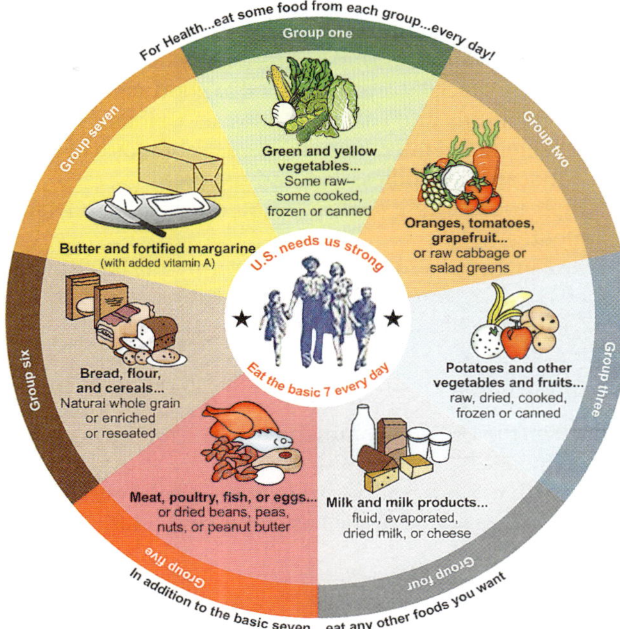

Fig. 24.1: Basic seven food guide. (*Source:* Reprinted with permission from USDA's Center for Nutrition Policy and Promotion).

Basic Four

- Basic seven was then upgraded in 1957 to the four food groups, the basic four (1956–1992) **(Fig. 24.2)**.
- These food groups were:
  1. *Vegetables and fruits:* Recommended as excellent sources of vitamins C and A, and a good source of fiber.

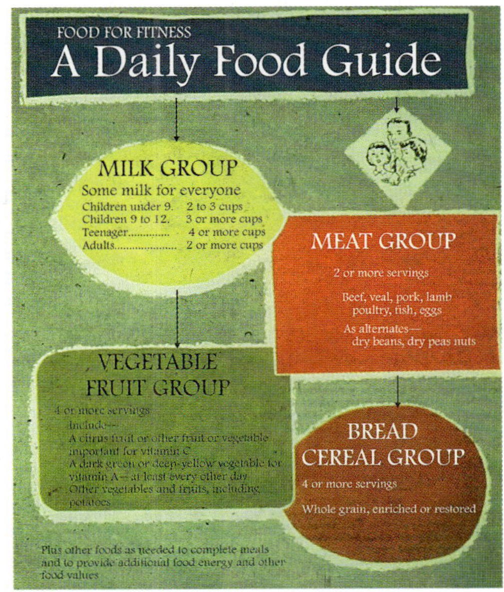

Fig. 24.2: Basic four-group guide. (*Source:* Reprinted with permission from USDA's Center for Nutrition Policy and Promotion).

A dark-green or deep-yellow vegetable or fruit was recommended every other day.

2. *Milk:* Recommended as a good source of calcium, phosphorus, protein, riboflavin, and sometimes vitamins A and D. Cheese, ice cream, and ice milk could sometimes replace milk.
3. *Meat:* Recommended for protein, iron, and certain B vitamins. Includes meat, poultry, fish, eggs, dry beans, dry peas, and peanut butter.
4. *Cereals and breads:* Whole grain and enriched breads were especially recommended as good sources of iron, B vitamins and carbohydrates, as well as sources of protein and fiber. Includes cereals, breads, cornmeal, macaroni, noodles, rice, and spaghetti.

- "Other foods" were said to round out meals and satisfy appetites.
- These included additional servings from the basic four, or foods such as butter, margarine, salad dressing and cooking oil, sauces, jellies, and syrups.

Five-Group Guide

- In 1979, the USDA recommended a five-food groups daily food guide.
- In the five-food groups guide fats, sweets, and alcohol groups were added to the basic four **(Fig. 24.3)**.

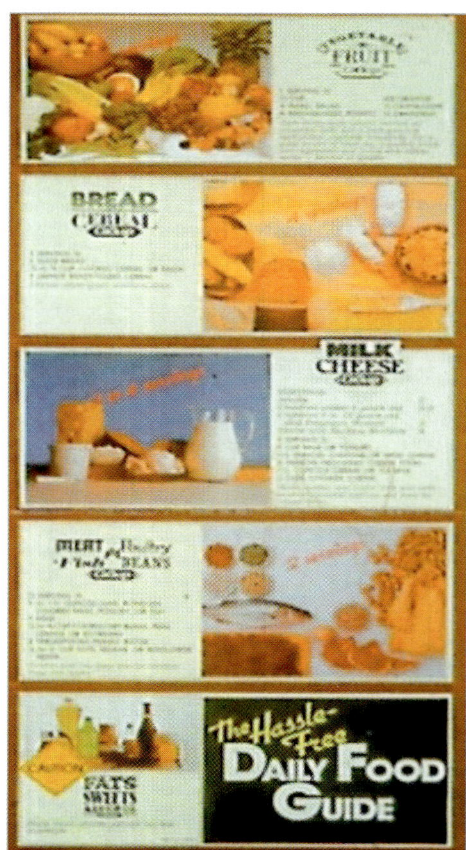

Fig. 24.3: Five-group guide. (*Source:* Reprinted with permission from USDA's Center for Nutrition Policy and Promotion).

Food Wheel Approach

- Total diet approach included goals for both nutrient adequacy and moderation.
- Five-food groups and amounts formed the basis for the food guide pyramid.
- Daily amounts of food provided at three calorie levels.
- First illustrated for a red-cross nutrition course as a food wheel **(Fig. 24.4)**.

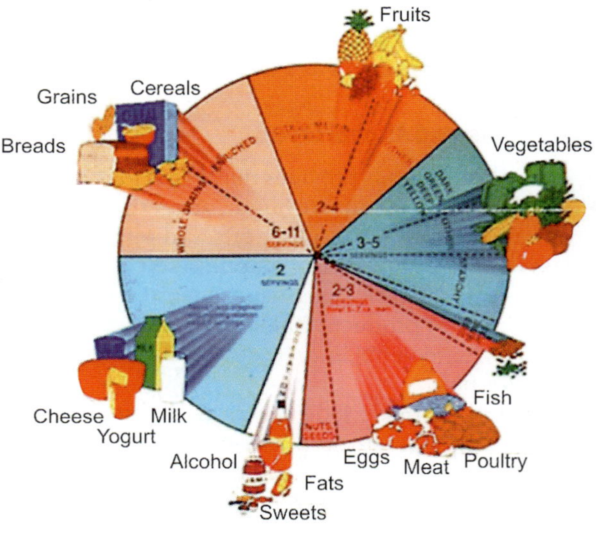

Fig. 24.4: Food wheel approach. (*Source:* Reprinted with permission from USDA's Center for Nutrition Policy and Promotion).

Food Guide Pyramid

- The first food pyramid was published in Sweden in 1974.
- But the popular food guide pyramid was proposed in 1992 **(Fig. 24.5)** which was again modified in March 1999.
- The introduction of the USDAs food guide pyramid in 1992 attempted to express the recommended servings of each food group.

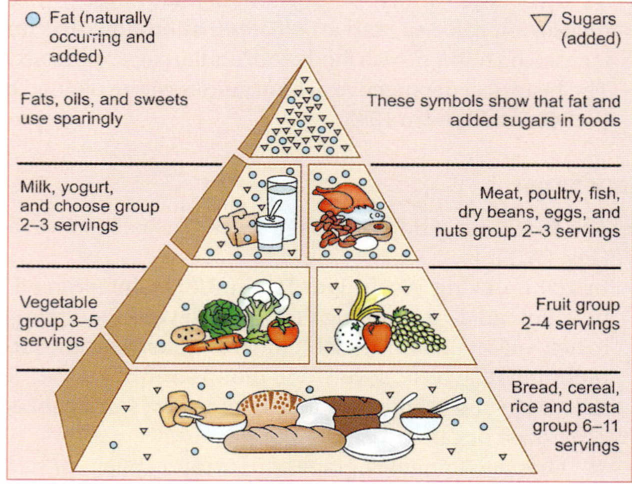

Fig. 24.5: USDA first food guide pyramid. (*Source:* Reprinted with permission from USDA's Center for Nutrition Policy and Promotion).

- On April 15, 2005, the USDA updated its guide with my pyramid [for adults **(Fig. 24.6)**, for children **(Fig. 24.7)**, and for vegetarians **(Fig. 24.8)**], which replaced the hierarchical levels of the food guide pyramid with colorful vertical wedges, often displayed without images of foods, creating a more abstract design. Stairs were added up the left side of the pyramid with an image of someone climbing them to represent exercise. The share of the pyramid allotted to grains now only narrowly edged out vegetables and milk, which were of equal proportions. Fruits were next in size, followed by a narrower wedge for protein and a small sliver for oils. An unmarked white tip represented discretionary calories for items such as candy, alcohol, or additional food from any other group.

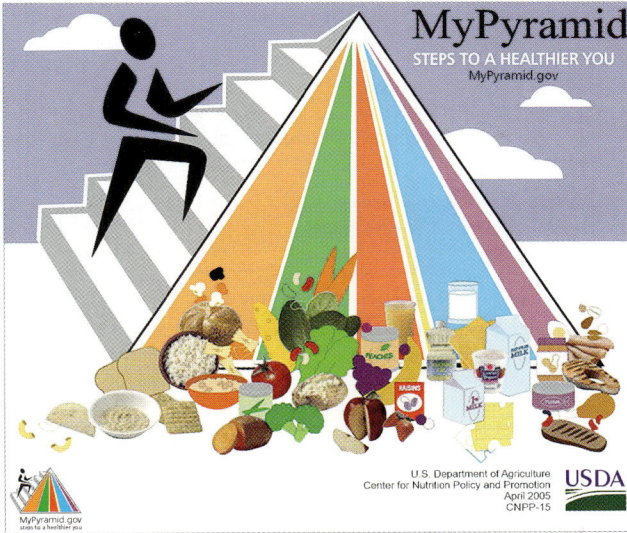

Fig. 24.6: Food guide pyramid for adults based on basal metabolic rate (BMR) (modified 2005). (*Source:* Reprinted with permission from USDA's Center for Nutrition Policy and Promotion).

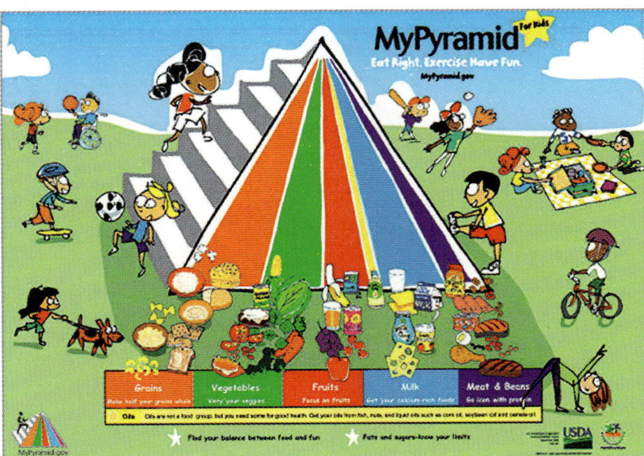

Fig. 24.7: Food guide pyramid for children (modified 2005). (*Source:* Reprinted with permission from USDA's Center for Nutrition Policy and Promotion).

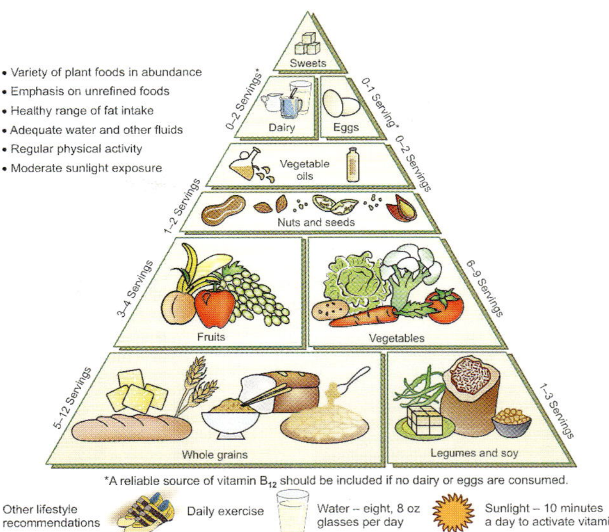

Fig. 24.8: Food guide pyramid for vegetarians. (*Source:* Department of Nutrition, Loma Linda University, USA 2008).

My Plate

- The food guide pyramids were discontinued and a new alternative program named my plate **(Fig. 24.9)** was initiated in June 2, 2011.
- My plate is divided into four slightly different sized quadrants, with fruits and vegetables taking up half the space, and grains and protein making up the other half.
- The vegetables and grains portions are the largest of the four (30% grains, 30% vegetables, 20% fruits, and 20% protein), accompanied by a smaller circle representing dairy, such as a glass of low-fat/nonfat milk or a yogurt cup. Some of the additional recommendations are "make half your plate fruits and vegetables," "switch to 1% or skim milk," "make at least half your grains whole," and "vary your protein food choices".
- The guidelines also recommend portion control while still enjoying food, as well as reductions in sodium and sugar intakes.

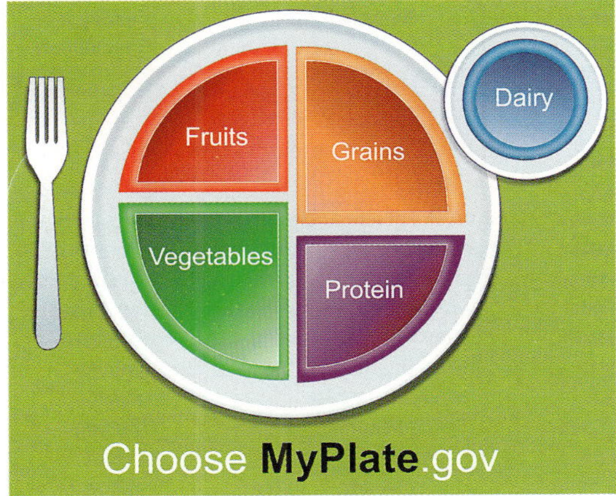

Fig. 24.9: My Plate Program 2011. (*Source:* Reprinted with permission from USDA's Center for Nutrition Policy and Promotion).

My Vegetarian Plate

- Loma Linda University developed a vegetarian food pyramid which included recommended servings of relevant food groups based on energy needs for vegans.
- The General Conference of Seventh-Day Adventists has now brought upon the vegetarian MyPlate **(Fig. 24.10).**

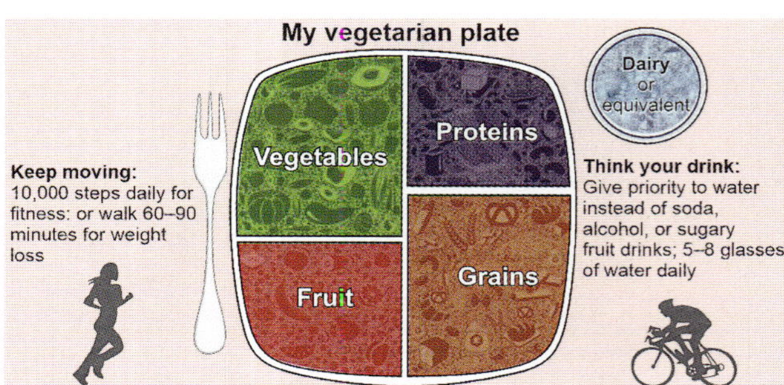

Fig. 24.10: My vegetarian plate program.

Food Guide Pyramid in India—ICMR (Fig. 24.11)

Guideline 1: Eat variety of foods to ensure a balanced diet

Rationale: Nutritionally adequate diet should be consumed through a wise choice from a variety of foods

- Nutrition is a basic prerequisite to sustain life.
- Variety in food is not only the spice of life but also the essence of nutrition and health.
- A diet consisting of foods from several food groups provides all the required nutrients in proper amounts.
- Cereals, millets and pulses are major sources of most nutrients.
- Milk which provides good quality proteins and calcium must be an essential item of the diet, particularly for infants, children and women.
- Oils and nuts are calorie-rich foods, and are useful for increasing the energy density and quality of food.
- Inclusion of eggs, flesh foods and fish enhances the quality of diet. However, vegetarians can derive almost all the nutrients from diets consisting of cereals, pulses, vegetables, fruits and milk-based diets.
- Vegetables and fruits provide protective substances such as vitamins/minerals/phytonutrients.
- Diversified diets with a judicious choice from a variety food groups provide the necessary nutrients.

Guideline 2: Ensure provision of extra food and healthcare to pregnant and lactating women

Rationale: Additional food and extra care are required during pregnancy and lactation

- Pregnancy is physiologically and nutritionally a highly demanding, period. Extra food is required to meet the requirements of the fetus.
- A woman prepares herself to meet the nutritional demands by increasing her own body fat deposits during pregnancy.
- A lactating mother requires extra food to secrete adequate quantity/quality of milk and to safeguard her own health.

Guideline 3: Promote exclusive breastfeeding for six months and encourage breastfeeding till two years or more, if possible

Rationale: Exclusive breastfeeding ensures safe nutrition to the infant and all round development of health

- Breast milk is the mast natural and perfect food for normal growth and healthy development of infants.
- Colostrum is rich in nutrients and anti-infective factors and should be fed to infants.
- Breast-fee ding reduces risk of infections.
- It establishes mother-infant contact and promotes mother-child bonding.
- It prolongs birth interval by fertility control (delayed return of menstruation).
- Breastfeeding helps in retraction of the uterus.
- Incidence of breast cancer is lower in mothers who breast feed their children.
- Breastfeeding is associated with better cognitive development of children and may provide some long-term health benefits.

Guideline 4: Feed home based semi-solid foods to the infant after six months

Rationale: Easy to cook homemade preparations are hygienic and healthy foods for the growing baby

- Breast milk alone is not adequate for the infant beyond 6 months of age.
- Introduction of food supplements (semi-solid complementary foods) along with breastfeeding is necessary for infants after 6 months of age.
- Provision of adequate and appropriate supplements to young children prevents malnutrition.
- Hygienic practices should be observed while preparing and feeding the complementary food to the child; otherwise, it will lead to diarrhea.

Guideline 5: Ensure adequate and appropriate diets for children and adolescents both in health and sickness

Rationale: Well-formulated balanced diets for children and adolescents help optimum growth and boosts their immunity

- A nutritionally adequate and balanced diet is essential for optimal growth and development.
- Appropriate diet and physical activity during childhood is essential for optimum body composition, BMI and to reduce the risk of diet-related chronic diseases in later life and prevent vitamin deficiency.
- Common infections and malnutrition contribute significantly to child morbidity and mortality.
- A child needs to eat more during and after episodes of infections to maintain good nutritional status.

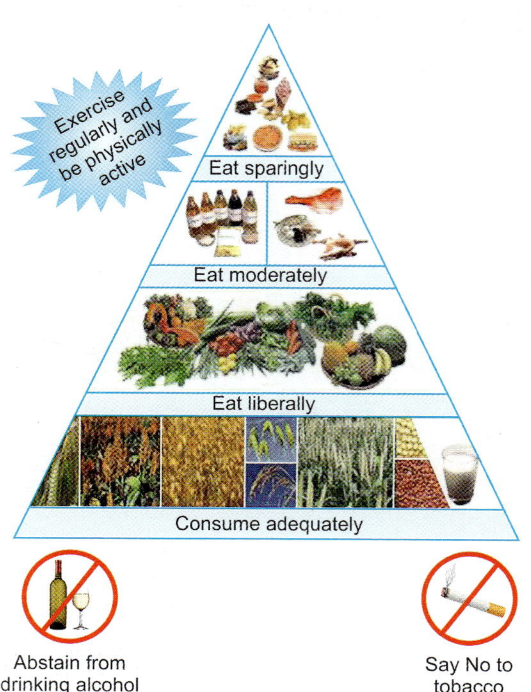

Fig. 24.11: Food Guide Pyramid in India.

DIETARY GOALS

The following dietary goals and changes in food selection and preparation are recommended so as to provide adequate nutrition:

- Increase the consumption of complex carbohydrates and naturally occurring sugars from about 28% to about 48%.
- Reduce the consumption of refined and processed sugars by about 45%.
- Reduce overall fat consumption from approximately 40% to about 30%.
- Reduce saturated fat consumption.
- Reduce cholesterol consumption to about 300 mg/day.
- Limit sodium intake by reducing salt to about 5 g/day.

Changes in Food Selection and Preparation Suggested by the Dietary Goals

- Increase consumption of fruits, vegetables, and whole grains.
- Decrease consumption of refined sugars.
- Decrease consumption of food high in total fat and replace saturated fats with polyunsaturated fats.
- Decrease consumption of animal fat, choosing meats such as poultry to reduce saturated fat intake.
- Decrease consumption of butterfat, eggs, and other sources high in cholesterol.
- Decrease consumption of salt and foods high in salt content.

Implementation of Dietary Goals

- Eat a variety of foods.
- Eat foods with adequate starch and fiber, such as whole-grain bread, cereals, raw vegetables, and fruits.
- Eat a minimum to moderate amount of sugar.
- Eat a minimum to moderate amount of salt.
- Consume alcohol only in moderation.
- Achieve and maintain ideal weight.

POINTS TO REMEMBER

- A balanced diet is one in which nutrients from each food group in recommended servings is present for the optimal functioning of the human.
- The RDAs are sets of values for levels of intake of the nutrients currently considered essential and which meet the physiological needs of nearly all individuals.
- The food group guides serve as a practical and workable plan for helping the homemaker select the type and amount of food that needs to be included in each day's meals in order to provide a balanced diet.
- The USDA daily food guide divides commonly eaten foods into five groups according to their respective nutritional contributions: (1) vegetable–fruit, (2) bread–cereal, (3) milk–cheese, (4) meat, poultry, fish, and beans, and (5) fats, sweets, and alcohol.
- Vegetables and fruits are important because they contribute vitamins A and C and fiber as well as trace amounts of other nutrients.
- Bread and cereal group is the most economical source of nutrients in our daily diets.
- Milk products are an important part of the diet as they provide about two-thirds of the calcium, one-half of the riboflavin, and one-fourth of the protein in the foods normally eaten.
- Meats are valued for protein, phosphorus, niacin, vitamin B_{12}, and iron.
- The USDA's first dietary guidelines were published in 1894 by Dr Wilbur Olin Atwater. The first food pyramid was published in Sweden in 1974.
- First food guide proposed in 1943 was basic seven, changed to basic four in 1957, upgraded in five-group guide in 1979, changed to food guide pyramid in 1992, modified with component of BMR in 2005, and a new alternative program named My Plate was initiated on June 2, 2011.

Questionnaire

1. What is specific dynamic action?
2. Explain RDA.
3. Describe the food group guides.
4. Explain the historical evolution of food guide pyramid.
5. What is My Plate concept?

FURTHER READING

1. Burkholder N, Sabaté J. Encyclopedia of Food and Health, 2016.
2. Burt BA. Diet, nutrition and oral health; a rational approach for the dental practice. J Am Dent Assoc. 1984;109:21.
3. Committee on Dietary Allowances, Food and Nutrition Board, National Academy of Sciences, National Research Council. Recommended dietary allowances. 9th rev. edition. Washington, DC: National Academy Press; 1980.
4. Forrester DJ, Wagner ML, Flemming J. Pediatric dental medicine. Philadelphia, PA: Lea & Febiger; 1981.
5. Hertzler AA, Anderson HL. Food guides in the United States. J Am Assoc. 1974;64:19.
6. McDonald RE, Avery DR. Dentistry for Child and Adolescent, 7th edition. St. Louis: Mosby; 2000.
7. Nizel AE. Nutrition in Preventive Dentistry: Science and Practice. Philadelphia, PA: WB Saunders; 1972.
8. USDA–DHHS Nutrition and Your Health: Dietary Guidelines for Americans, 2nd edition. Washington, DC: GPO; 1985.
9. Welsh S, Davis C, Shaw A. A brief history of food guides in the United States. Nutrition Today November/December 1992. pp.6–11.
10. Wilson ED, Fisher KIL, Fuqua MD. Principles of Nutrition, 3rd edition. New York: John Wiley; 1975.
11. "USDAs My Plate". United States Department of Agriculture. Retrieved 2 June 2011.

CHAPTER 25

Diet Counseling for the Prevention of Dental Caries

Nikhil Marwah, Ambika Joshi

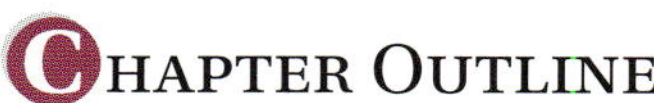

CHAPTER OUTLINE

- Principles of Diet Management
- Diet Counseling

During the pre-eruptive period, foods exert nutritional effect on the formation of dental matrix and mineralization. However, during the posteruptive periods foods exert a dietary and topical effect. Therefore, when giving dietary counseling, some food choices and eating habits merit attention. These include frequency of between-meal snacking, physical form and retentiveness of sugar- sweetened snacks, and the amount of sugar added to food or beverages for sweetening.

A basic prerequisite for accomplishing dietary change is the advice that the patient, not the counselor, bears the responsibility for making the change. Minimal requirements for a successful dietary counseling service include enrolling, active patient involvement in planning, implementing, and evaluating the diet before and after counseling and insisting on a series of follow-up visits to tailor the diet to the patient's needs and likes without jeopardizing the dental-health status.

PRINCIPLES OF DIET MANAGEMENT

A rational nutrition program for dental caries prevention based on the effects of various nutrients and food practices on the production or inhibition of dental caries coupled with some basic dietetics principles can be formulated. Therefore, these four rules should be adopted when making dietary modifications:

1. Maintain overall nutritional adequacy by conforming to the United States Department of Agriculture (USDA) daily food guide for at least the recommended number of servings from each of the food groups.
2. The prescribed diet should vary from the normal diet pattern as little as possible.
3. The diet should meet the body's requirements for the essential nutrients.
4. The prescribed diet should take into consideration and accommodate the patient's likes and dislikes, food habits, and other environmental factors as long as they do not interfere with the objectives.

Effective diet counseling can thus help us formulate the following conclusion:

- The dietary guidance advocated here can improve general as well as dental health.
- Personalized dietary counseling added to other caries-preventive measures should reduce caries recurrence significantly.
- The daily ingestion of a balanced and varied selection of foods from the different food groups, avoidance of sweets that are retained next to tooth enamel, and discontinuance of between-meal snacking are the basic elements in achieving a diet that produces few caries.
- To realize maximum patient acceptance and cooperation with the diet prescription, determine and manage the reasons for the original diet, and suit the new diet to the patient's daily routine and lifestyle.
- The objectivity, personalization of the diet, and the time spent in counseling are rewarded both financially and by the satisfaction of performing a useful health care and preventive dentistry service.

Calculation of dental-health diet score

Dental-health diet score = [Food score (adequate intake of foods from each of the food groups) + nutrient score (consuming foods from especially recommended groups of 10 nutrients)] – sweet score (ingestion of foods that are overtly sweet sugars)

Food group score table (highest possible score is 96)

Food	*RDA*	*Number of servings*	*Points*
Milk	3	× 8	
Meat	2	× 12	
Fruits and vegetables	1	× 6	
Vitamin C	1	× 6	
Others	2	× 6	
Breads and cereals	4	× 6	

Nutrient score table

Mark one score for each nutrient consumed

Protein and vitamin A	*Iron*	*Folic acid*	*Riboflavin*	*Vitamin C*
Cheese, dried peas, dried beans, eggs, fish, meat, milk, apricot, butter, carrot, liver, milk, and spinach	Beef, eggs, liver, green leafy vegetables	Cereals, spinach, yeasts	Broccoli, chicken breasts, eggs, milk, mushrooms	Grapefruit, green peppers, oranges, strawberries, tomatoes, calcium and phosphorus—cheese, eggs, green leafy vegetables, milk

Sweet score table

Classify the sweet by its nature and multiply according to severity

Liquid: (×5)	*Solid and sticky: (×10)*	*Slowly dissolving: (×15)*
Soft drinks, fruit drinks, cocoa, sugar and honey in beverages, ice cream, flavored yogurt, pudding, custard	Cake, doughnuts, sweet rolls, pastry, canned fruit in syrup, bananas, cookies, chocolate candy, caramel, chewing gum, dried fruit, marshmallows, jelly, jam	Hard candies, breathe mints, antacid tablets, cough drops

Assessment of dental-health diet score

Score	*Result*	*Interpretation*
72–96	Excellent	Counseling not required
64–72	Adequate	Educate the patient
56–64	Barely adequate	Counseling required
56 or less	Not adequate	Counseling with diet modifications

DIET COUNSELING

Patient Selection

- Diet counseling will not succeed with every dental patient.
- Potential candidates for counseling should give high priority to preventive dentistry and should be willing to expend long-term efforts to maintain their natural dentition good health for a lifetime.
- In addition to a positive attitude, they should have a demonstrable need for dietary improvement, based on their current food intake regimen.

Food Diary

- A food diary is, as the name implies, a record of all food and beverages consumed during a specific period **(Fig. 25.1)**.
- If the child is young, the mother usually completes the food diary at home, writing in foods after they are eaten. The patient is instructed to be as accurate as possible in determining quantities and to record in detail everything eaten or drunk during or between meals, the size serving in household measures, the addition of sugar, milk, syrups, to anything consumed.
- A food or diet diary can be either of 24 hours or 1 week. The 24-hours recall is a valuable tool for obtaining a sketchy picture of a patient's food intake.

Assessment of Sweet Score

- < 5: Excellent
- 5–10: Fair
- >15: Watch out zone

Diet Workbook

Date: ***Name:***

What are dental caries?
The plaque that forms on your teeth every day contains bacteria (germs).
These bacteria change the sugar in your food into acid.
Sugar (in food) + Bacteria (germs) = Acid
These acids begin the breakdown of the tooth .... dental caries.

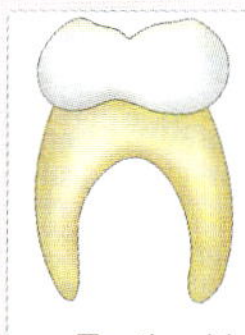
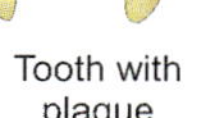
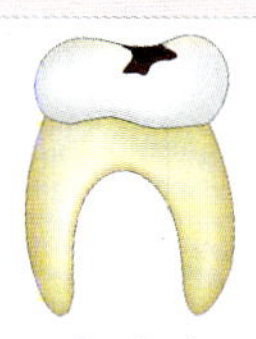
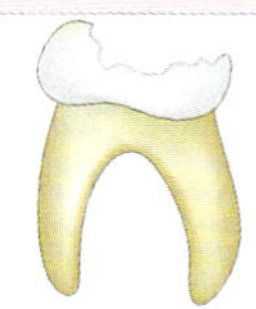

Note: Sticky foods that are sweet are much worse than liquid sweet foods. The longer the sugar is on the tooth, the more acid is made by the bacteria. Very bad: candy, cookies, chocolate-covered ice cream, cake, pie, jam. Not so bad: plain ice cream, pudding, jell-O, soft drinks.
How many circles are on your food diary? _______________
There are 20 minutes of acid forming on your teeth for each circle .....
____ × 20 – _____ minutes (or _____ hours)
What foods can you eliminate to reduce the number of circles?

How many servings are you having from the four food groups?

	Now having	***Should have***	***Difference***
Milk group			
Milk—fluid whole evaporated, skim, dry, buttermilk	3	2–3 or more servings	OK
Cheese—American, natural, cottage			
Meat group			
Beef, veal, pork, lamb, poultry, fish, eggs, dry peas and beans, peanuts	$1^4/_5$	2 or more servings	–1/5
Vegetable-fruit group include a source of:			
Vitamin C (citrus fruits, green pepper, cantaloupe, strawberries)	3	4 or more servings	–1
Vitamin A (dark green or deep yellow vegetables)			
Read-cereal group			
Whole gain, enriched or restored. Includes rice, pasta, crackers, and rolls	4	4 or more servings	OK

Food group	***Day 1***	***Day 2***	***Day 3***	***Day 4***	***Day 5***	***Calculate***	***Average (per day) intake***
Milk	√√√	√√	√√√√	√√√√	√√	15/5 = 3	3
Meat	√√	√	√√√	√√	√	9/5 = $1^4/_5$	$1^4/_5$
Fruit-vegetable	√√√	√√√√√	√√	√√√	√√	15/5 = 3	3
Bread-cereal	√√√√√	√√√√	√√	√√√√√	√√√√	20/5 = 4	4

Diet prescription

Continue eating:
Milk group
Bread-cereal group

Eat more of:
Meat group—eggs, cheeseburger, bologna, tuna fish
Vegetable-fruit group—apples, peaches, tomato juice, raw carrot

A suggested menu for you

Breakfast:
Orange juice
Cereal with fruit and milk

Lunch:
Bologna sandwich
Fruit
Milk

After school:
Juice
Crackers and cheese

Supper:
Meat, fish or poultry
Vegetables
Rice, milk
Jell-O

Before bed:
Toast with cream cheese
Milk

Snack suggestions

Raw vegetables:

Celery sticks	Lettuce wedges	Keep in water in refrigerator all ready to eat
Carrot sticks	Cucumber sticks	Fill celery stalk with cream cheese, meat or cheese spread or peanut butter
Cauliflower bits	Radishes	
Green pepper rings	Tomatoes	

Fruits:

Oranges	Melon	Have a plate of fruit chunks on toothpicks fixed in the refrigerator
Plums	Grapes	
Peaches	Apples	Add to milk and blenderize to make a fruit shake
Pears	Grapefruit	
Pineapple	Tangerines	
Strawberries		

Drinks: Milk, unsweetened fruit and vegetable juices, sugar-free carbonated beverages

Other snacks: Slices of—turkey, chicken, beef, bologna, salami or cheese, served by itself or as a sandwich, on bread or crackers unsweetened dry cereal, with milk, nuts, chips, popcorn pretzels

Popsicles: Put unsweetened juices (or mix yogurt or buttermilk with juices) into popsicle molds and freeze

Fig. 25.1: Sample food diary.

Calculation of Dental Health Diet Score

It is a simple scoring procedure that can disclose a potential dietary problem that is likely to adversely affect a patient's dental health.

Communication Techniques

- Communication is a basic tool in the practice of preventive dentistry.
- Communication is the giving and receiving of information; it involves the knowledge, thoughts, and opinions of the counselor and patient.
- Both the dentist and the dental hygienist, by virtue of their education and training, should recognize that they render a vital dental-health service when they advise patients on diet and nutrition.
- Because diet and inadequate nutrition can be major etiological factors in dental–oral health problems, it is necessary that the dentist or dental hygienist give diet counseling when indicated.
- During a face-to-face interview, keeping eye contact with the patient is a persuasive and powerful device for motivating behavioral change.
- Communications can be both verbal and nonverbal. Words transmit information. The interviewer's tone of voice, facial expression, and gestures convey sincerity, enthusiasm, and empathy. These nonverbal actions can be influential in helping the patient to change his or her behavior.
- The message must be adapted to the patient's needs and level of understanding. Personalization of the message is more likely to result in a sustained change in behavior.
- To communicate with a patient, a combination of interviewing, teaching, counseling, and motivation is used.

Interviewing

- **Purpose:** The basic goal in interviewing is to understand the problem, the factors that contribute to it, and the personality of the patient.
- **Advantages of a dietary interview:** It can serve as a valuable diagnostic aid to provide knowledge of a person's daily routine for adapting a caries-preventive diet.
- **Physical setting:** Privacy, comfortable and relaxed atmosphere are important requisites for an interview. The interview should not take place on chair side in the dental operatory, as it can be a threatening atmosphere that may lead to fear and withdrawal. Rather, it should take place in a separate counseling room that contains a small conference table, few chairs, a blackboard, and visual aids.
- **Diet interviewer:** Good dietary interviewing requires skill, time, and some background knowledge of the science and practice of nutrition, including familiarity with ways in which food habits are formed.
- **Procedure for interviewing the patient:** Start with a brief introductory statement about the purpose of the interview. Ask questions that will encourage the patient's expression of feelings about his or her current dental- health condition and the importance of preserving the natural dentition. An important advantage is listening before speaking as the patient himself may reveal answers to his problems and provide a direction for the course of action. In general, the interviewer should be encouraging and sympathetic and should not assume an adversary position. Allow the patient to make choices based on what has been learned and with which the patient can cooperate. When closing an interview, it is usually a good plan to end by recapitulating what the patient has learned and the future action that you have agreed on.

Teaching and Learning

- Patient education is more than simply giving information: It requires the presentation of information with sufficient impact to stimulate action by the learner.
- A number of teaching aids may be used, including booklets on nutrition and dental health, which can be purchased at little cost.

Counseling

- Approaches to counseling may be directive or non-directive.
- In directive counseling, the role of the patient is passive and the decisions are made by the counselor.
- In nondirective counseling, the counselor's role is merely to aid the patient in clarifying and understanding his or her own situation and to provide guidance so that the patient can make his or her own final decision as to the type of action that should be taken.
- The nondirective counseling approach is recommended for diet counseling.

Guidelines for Counseling

- A prerequisite for successful nutrition counseling is a realistic and honest statement that the patient, not the counselor, bears the responsibility for making changes in food selections and eating habits
- The guidelines for counseling are:
  - **Gather information:** Personal identifying data, likes and dislikes, and the patient's perception.
  - **Evaluate and interpret information:** Relative adequacy of the diet and eating habits.
  - **Develop and implement a plan of action:** Qualitative modifications of the diet.
  - Seek active participation of the patient's family in all aspects of dietary change.
  - Follow-up to assess the progress made.

Prerequirements of Counseling

- **Elicit a true response:** If the counselor is hoping for truthful responses to his questions, he must follow some simple rules which will relax the patient. It is important to give neither positive nor negative feedback when the patient is recalling his food intake. Since people tend to avoid negative reinforcement and seek positive reinforcement, they may alter their responses in pursuit of these goals.

Example

Counselor (C): What did you eat for breakfast?

Patient (P): An ice cream

C: An ice cream? (registers shock, displeasure, ridicule)

P: (shyly) Yes

C: What did you eat for dinner last night?

P: Meat, potatoes, spinach, and salad
(patient really did not eat dinner last night but wants to avoid another negative response from the counselor so she fabricates a dinner)

C: That's great (positive reinforcement)

Patient then continues to give answers which elicit positive responses only

- **Phrase the questions correctly:** Do not put words in the patient's mouth. If information is sought, it is best to ask an open-ended question, one that will allow the patient to answer with a response other than yes or no.

Example

Right		*Wrong*	
Q:	What did you put inyour cereal?	Q:	Did you put milk in your cereal?
A:	Milk and sugar	A:	Yes
Q:	How much milk?	Q:	Did you put 1/2 cup of milk?
A:	About 2/3 cups	A:	Yes

It is easy for the patient to say "Yes" rather than to go to the trouble of explaining a different response. This can give a false picture of food intake.

- **Listen and wait for an answer:** When you ask a question, give the patient time to think of his answer.

Example

Right		*Wrong*	
Q:	What did you eat for breakfast?	Q:	What did you eat for breakfast?
A:	(Silence)	A:	(Silence)
Q:	(Silence)	Q:	Was it cereal?
A:	I had eggs	A:	(Silence)

Do not let the silence make you uncomfortable so that you rush in with an answer for him.

Counseling Visit

Step 1: *Pursue diary for completion:* Remember that diaries are often inaccurate, so keep an educated ear open to clues about eating behavior. For example, the patient enters the office chewing gum. You check the food diary and find no gum mentioned on it. it is a good idea to ask "How often do you chew gum?" rather than ignore it because it was not entered.

Step 2: *Determine daily routine:* It is important to have an understanding of not only what the patient is eating but also why he is eating it. This is best accomplished by examining the daily routine

Step 3: *Explain cause of decay:* Explain that the bacteria living on our teeth rely on the sugar in our diets for their supply of energy. In the process of breaking down the sugar, an acid is formed which can "dissolve" the tooth.

Step 4: *Isolate sugar factor:* All the food consumed is scanned and the number of sugar exposures is circled. This includes sugar or syrups added to cookies, cakes, cereals, fruit, and beverages. Dried fruits are also included.

Step 5: *Analyze sweets intake:* Examine the foods that are circled. Explain that it is not the amount of sugar as much as it is the form and the frequency of intake that determines cariogenicity of the diet. Count the circles in the diet workbook and ask the patient which circled foods on the diary can be eliminated.

Step 6: *Determine adequacy of diet:* This is done by dental-health diet score.

Step 7: *Diet prescription and suggested menu:* It is now time to put together a personalized diet for the patient based on what we have learned about his usual dietary pattern and daily routine.
Commend the patient.
Allow the patient to suggest improvements and write his or her own diet prescription.
Allow the patient to delete sugar from the plaque-forming foods.
Allow the patient to select nonplaque promoting snack substitutes.
Allow the patient to select menus starting with the existing.
menu as a nucleus

Step 8: *Reinforcement by follow-up re-evaluation:* Schedule a follow-up visit for 2 weeks later. The patient is asked to complete a second 5-day food diary in the same manner first just before returning. evaluate the new food diary and compare the results with the original plan to note whether recommendations have been followed. repetition, clarification, and encouragement are the keys to success in long-term maintenance of the new, acceptable, less cariogenic, and more nutritious diet.

No dentistry should be done on the day when diet counseling occurs, so that the counseling is given due importance and use-of-diet workbook is emphasized.

Motivation

- It is an incentive for action.
- The counselor's positive attitude and conviction as to the necessity and effectiveness of nutrition counseling can stimulate the patient to initiate an improved dietary pattern.
- A person passes through five preliminary decision stages in changing a dietary pattern-awareness, interest, involvement, action, and forming a new habit:
    - Awareness is recognition that a problem exists, but without an inclination to solve it, for example, "Hard candies produce acid, which can cause my teeth to decay."
    - Interest is greater degree of awareness but still with no inclination to act, for example, "May be I should give up the hard candies; I do not want any more sensitive or painful teeth".
    - Involvement is a definite intention to act, for example, "I definitely will give up hard candy".
    - Action is a trial performance, for example, "I have given up hard candies and chew sugarless gum instead to prevent the dry feeling in my mouth".
    - Habit is a commitment to perform this action regularly over a sustained period of time, for example, "I have not consumed a hard candy in 6 months".

The pedodontist is in a unique position to promote good nutrition in his patients and their families as he is treating a disease to which diet contributes dramatically to both etiology and treatment. It is our hope that the dentist who looks into a child's mouth and thinks "What is this child eating?" will use this chapter to help him evaluate and improve the diets of his patients.

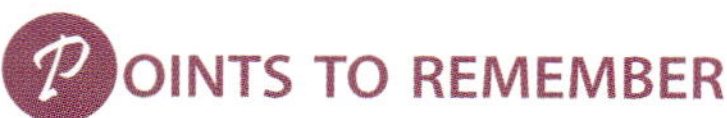

POINTS TO REMEMBER

- Diet is important requisite for healthy dentition both in prenatal and postnatal period of life.
- A food diary is, as the name implies, a record of all food and beverages consumed during a specific period.
- Dental-health diet score = [Food score (adequate intake of foods from each of the food groups) + nutrient score (consuming foods from especially recommended groups of ten nutrients)] – sweet score (ingestion of foods that are overtly sweet sugars).
- In nondirective counseling, the counselor's role is merely to aid the patient in clarifying and understanding his or her own situation and to provide guidance so this approach is recommended for diet counseling.
- Diet counseling involves the following: Pursue diary for completion, determine daily routine, explain cause of decay, isolate sugar factor, analyze sweets intake, determine adequacy of diet, diet prescription, reinforcement by follow-up.

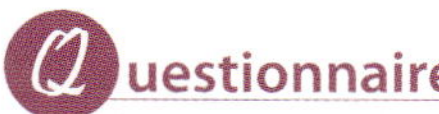

Questionnaire

1. What are the principles of diet management?
2. Explain the concept of food diary.
3. Describe counseling of a dental patient.
4. What is dental-health score?
5. Explain the diet counseling of a child for caries prevention.

FURTHER READING

1. Burt BA. What recommendations should dentists make to their patients regarding the effect of diet and nutrition on their oral health? What kind of diet and consumption patterns promotes better oral health and what kinds are less consistent with good oral health? Diet, nutrition and oral health. A rational approach for the dental practice. J Am Dent Assoc. 1984;109:21.
2. Committee on Dietary Allowances, Food and Nutrition Board, National Academy of Sciences, National Research Council. Recommended Dietary Allowances. 9th rev. edition. Washington, DC: National Academy Press; 1980.
3. Nizel AE, Shulman JS. The science and art of inhibiting caries in adolescents via personalized nutritional counseling. Dent Clin North Am. 1969;13:387.
4. Nizel AE. Nutrition in Preventive Dentistry: Science and Practice. Philadelphia, PA: WB Saunders; 1972.
5. Palmer C, Rounds M. Nutrition counseling. Clinical Preventive Dentistry Student Manual. Boston: Tufts University School of Dental Medicine; 1986.
6. Wilson ED, Fisher KIL, Fuqua MD. Principles of Nutrition. 3rd eedition. New York: John Wiley; 1975.

CHAPTER 26

Pit and Fissure Sealants

Nikhil Marwah, Divya Reddy

Chapter Outline

- Morphology of Pits and Fissures
- Types of Pit and Fissures
- Histopathology of Fissure Caries
- Types of Pit and Fissure Sealants
- Requisites of an Efficient Sealant
- Fissure Sealant Cycle
- Clinical Technique for Placement of Pit and Fissure Sealant
- Critical Issues Regarding Pit and Fissure Sealant Usage
- Current Status of Pit and Fissure Sealant

The prevalence of caries has decreased in the past two decades and contributing to this decline are water fluoridation, dentifrices, improved oral hygiene, and changes in diet and awareness. These caries preventive strategies were found to have greater effects in reduction of smooth surface caries rather than the pits and fissures caries. The plaque retentive nature of pits and fissures makes them difficult to clean, and therefore are more susceptible to caries when compared to smooth surfaces. Pit and fissure sealant application is a preventive, conservative approach involving the sealing of pits and fissures of caries prone teeth providing a physical barrier that inhibits the ingress of bacteria and nutrients.

Pit (**Ash**, 1993): *It is defined as a small pinpoint depression located at the junction of developmental grooves or at terminals of those grooves.*

Fissure (**Orbans**, 1954): *Fissure is defined as deep clefts between adjoining cusps.*

Pit and fissure sealant: *This term is used to describe a material that is introduced into the occlusal pits and fissures of caries-susceptible teeth, thus forming a micromechanically bonded, protective layer cutting access of caries-producing bacteria from their source of nutrients.*[1]

Fissure sealant: *It is a material that is placed in the pits and fissures of teeth in order to prevent or arrest the development of dental caries.*[2]

HISTORY

1867	**Arthur**	Stated that decay was inevitable, and that obliteration of the fissures could prevent its occurrence
1905	**Miller W**	First attempt to prevent occlusal caries by applying silver nitrate on the tooth surfaces
1923	**Hyatt**	In his famous paper "Prophylactic odontomy," he advocated filling the fissures of teeth with silver or copper oxyphosphate cement as soon as the teeth erupted and then later, when they erupted fully into the oral cavity, class I cavity was prepared involving all deep pits and fissures and were prophylactically restored with amalgam.
1929	**Bodecker**	Introduced an alternative method of caries prevention with mechanical widening of fissures so as to transform deep, retentive fissures to cleansable ones.
1939	**Gore**[3]	The use of polymers as fissure sealants and to a lesser extent as coatings owes its origin to him as he used solutions of cellulose nitrate inorganic solvents to fill the surface enamel made porous by the action of acids in the saliva
1955	**Buonocore**[4]	Published his classic study introducing the acid etch and bonding technique of resin-based materials. He used 85% phosphoric acid for 30 seconds to increase the adhesion of methyl methacrylate material to enamel.
1965	**Gwinnett and Buonocore**	Showed that approximately 50% phosphoric acid solution etched enamel and the porosity resulted—was penetrated by the cyanoacrylate, with production of a strong bond

Contd...

Contd...

1965	**Cueto and Buonocore**	Developed first sealant material; they used 50% phosphoric acid with 7% zinc oxide and a mixture of methyl cyanoacrylate with silicone cement, as sealant material. A retention rate of 71% was observed after 1 year, while reduction of caries reached 87%. However, this material was prone to bacterial disintegration over time.
1965	**Bowen**	Bis-GMA was developed at the National Bureau of Standards from the adduct of bisphenol A and glycidyl methacrylate
1968	**Rodyhouse[5]**	Reported on the use of Bis-GMA monomer using methyl methacrylate as diluents together with a peroxideamine polymerization system. Over a 3-year period, he demonstrated a 30% reduction in caries in the 130 children studied. However, he did not employ acid etching before application to the teeth
1970	**Buonocore**	Utilized Bis-GMA system but employed an ultraviolet-sensitive polymerization initiator (benzoinmethylether), which allowed more flexibility in the clinical application of the material to the teeth and more complete filling of the fissures
1971	**Nuva-Seal**	First pit and fissure sealant developed and commercially introduced by LD Caulk Company
1974	**McLean and Wilson**	Introduced glass ionomer pit and fissure sealants

MORPHOLOGY OF PITS AND FISSURES

The fissure contains organic plug composed of reduced enamel epithelium, microorganism forming dental plaque, and oral debris. The increased susceptibility of this surface to caries is due to the fact that fissure provides a protected niche for plaque accumulation (**Rohr et al.,** 1991; **Hicks,** 1986). Recently erupted teeth have a porous enamel lining and the fissures are rich in cellular and organic debris. Theoretically, this porous zone of enamel bordering the fissures offers a three-dimensional honeycombed structure into which fissure sealants could be locked. Any procedure must be carried out at the earliest possible time after eruption to make effective preventive use of fissure sealants.[6] The penetration of liquids into cracks and crevices is given by the equation of Bikerman.

$$1.50z^2 = \frac{S \cdot \gamma Cos\theta}{6\eta} t$$

Where z = is the depth of the crevice

S = is the width of the crevice

γ = is the surface tension of the liquid

θ = is the advancing contact angle of the liquid

η = the viscosity

t = the time.

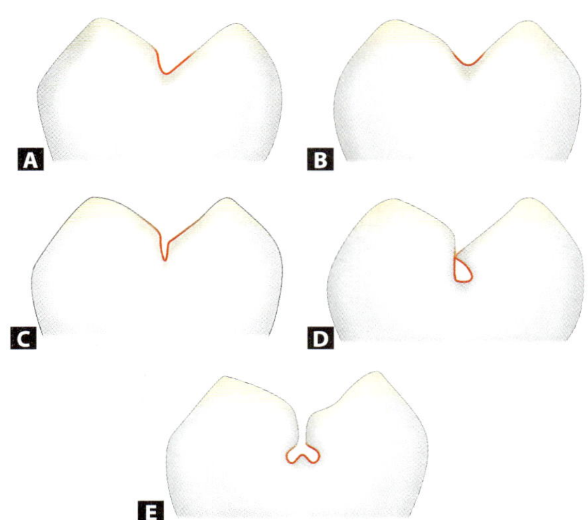

Figs.26.1AtoE: Morphology of pits and fissures: (A) U type—almost the same width from top to bottom; (B) V type—wide at the top and gradually narrowing towards the bottom; (C) I type—extremely narrow slit; (D) IK type—extremely narrow slit with a larger space at bottom; (E) Inverted Y type.

TYPES OF PITS AND FISSURES

Nagano,[7] 1961classified the shapes of occlusal fissures based on anatomical form into following types **(Figs. 26.1A to E)**: Nagano established the close relationship of form and depth of pits and fissures with V type being shallow, the U-type with medium depth and most of the remaining types deep. He also observed the relationship between form and depth of pits and fissures and the localization of primary carious lesion. Caries was observed to start at the bottom in V-type; starts halfway down in U-type, while in I-type and IK-type, starts from the top.

1. V-type (34%)
2. U-type (14%)
3. I-type (19%)
4. IK-type (26%)
5. Inverted Y-type (7%)

HISTOPATHOLOGY OF FISSURE CARIES

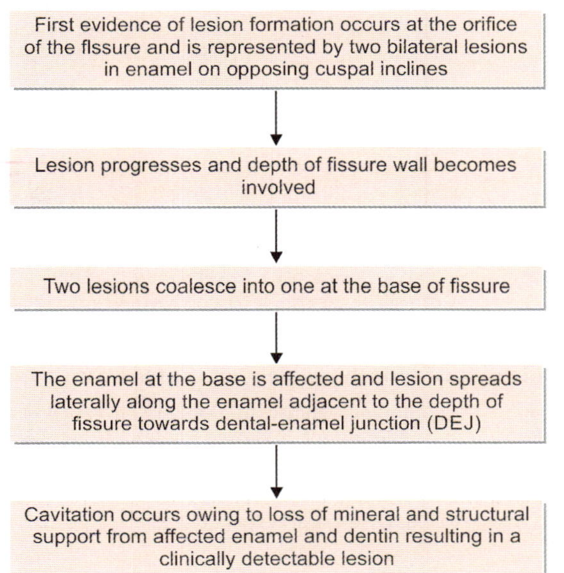

First evidence of lesion formation occurs at the orifice of the fissure and is represented by two bilateral lesions in enamel on opposing cuspal inclines
Lesion progresses and depth of fissure wall becomes involved
Two lesions coalesce into one at the base of fissure
The enamel at the base is affected and lesion spreads laterally along the enamel adjacent to the depth of fissure towards dental-enamel junction (DEJ)
Cavitation occurs owing to loss of mineral and structural support from affected enamel and dentin resulting in a clinically detectable lesion

TYPES OF PIT AND FISSURE SEALANTS

As per 'evidence-based clinical practice guideline for the use of pit and fissure sealants' (AAPD, 2016)[8] sealants are broadly classified into three categories:

1. Resin-based Sealants

These are further classified based on:

A. Method of polymerization
B. Viscosity
C. Translucency

Resin-based sealants classification based on the method of polymerization

1st generation	UV light polymerizing sealants	Polymerized by the action of UV rays on the initiator present in the material which initiates the process; however, is no longer used, e.g., Nuva-Seal® (First sealant introduced in the market)
2nd generation	Autopolymerizing resin-based sealants or chemically cured sealants	The activator, a tertiary amine, is added to one component and mixed with another one. The reaction between these two components produces free radicals that initiate the polymerization of the resin sealant material (1–2 min setting time), e.g., Delton (Dentsply)
3rd generation	Visible light-polymerising resin-based sealants	Photoinitiators present in sealant material are activated by visible light in the wavelength of around 470 nm (blue); longer working time and shorter setting time (10–20 seconds) compared to previous generation, e.g., Dyract Seal (Dentsply), Prime Pit and Fissure Sealant, etc
4th generation	Fluoride-releasing resin-based sealants	Fluoride-releasing particles are added to light-polymerizing resin-based sealants, in an attempt to inhibit caries, e.g., 3M Clinpro Sealant, SDI Conceal F Pit and Fissure Sealant, etc.

Classification of resin-based sealants based on viscosity

Filled	Possesses higher wear resistance; but their penetration ability into fissures is low. Therefore, filled sealants usually require occlusal adjustments, which lengthens the procedure, e.g., PF Seal SC, Premier Biocoat, etc.
Unfilled	Exhibits lower viscosity, better penetration into fissures. Also, it allows a better retention and lower microleakage rates, e.g., 3M Clinipro, Ultradent Ultraseal, etc.

Classification of resin-based sealants based on translucency

Opaque	Opaque white fissure sealants are easier to see during application and easier to detect clinically during recall examination, e.g., Delton (Dentsply)
Transparent	Transparent sealants can be clear, pink, or amber, eg., Helioseal® Clinpro®

2. Glass Ionomer Sealant Materials

- Glass ionomer cement has also been used as a pit and fissure sealant.
- It is easy to place, is moisture friendly compared to the hydrophobic resin-based sealants.
- Glass ionomer cements can be used as 'transitional sealants' when the resin-based sealants cannot be placed due to difficulty in moisture control in cases of partially erupted permanent teeth requiring sealants, especially when the operculum is covering the distal part of the occlusal surface. It can also be used in deep fissures on primary molars that are difficult to isolate due to uncooperative behavior of the child.
- The fluoride releasing property and the fluoride recharging ability are invariably the most advantageous features of these type of sealants.

3. Polyacid-modified Resin Sealants

- Polyacid-modified resin sealants, also referred to as compomers, combines traditional visible-light polymerizing resin-based sealants with GI sealants with fluoride-releasing property.
- As resin-based, they do not contain water, are hydrophobic and can be polymerized after positioning the bonding agents; similar to the GIs, they release fluoride, but in much smaller amounts.
- Therefore, the polyacid modified resin sealants have better adhesion property, are less water-soluble compared to GI sealants, and are less technique sensitive compared to resin-based sealants.

REQUISITES OF AN EFFICIENT SEALANT

Brauer[9] in1978 suggested the following pre-requisites for a sealant to be effective **(Table 26.1)**:

- Viscosity allowing penetration into deep and narrow fissures even in maxillary teeth.
- Adequate working time.
- Rapid cure.
- Good and prolonged adhesion to enamel.

Table 26.1: Properties of an ideal sealant.

Property	*Ideal sealant*	*Self-cured*	*Light cured (unfilled)*	*Light cured (filled)*
Penetration	High	Medium	Low–high	Low–medium
Working time	Medium	Short–medium	Medium–long	Medium–long
Setting time	Short	Medium	On demand	On demand
Water sorption	Low	High	High	Medium
Thermal expansion	Low	High	High	Medium
Wear resistance	High	Low	Low	Medium
Ratings	100%	53%	62%	75%

- Low sorption and solubility.
- Resistance to wear.
- Minimum irritation to tissues.
- Cariostatic action.

Indications of Pit and Fissure Sealant

- Deep, retentive pits and fissures, which may cause wedging of an explorer.
- Pits and fissures of permanent teeth of children and adolescents with high caries risk.
- Stained pits and fissures with minimum appearance of decalcification.
- No radiographic or clinical evidence of proximal caries.
- Possibility of adequate isolation.
- Questionable enamel caries in pit and fissures.
- Caries free pit and fissures.
- If the patient desires.
- Caries pattern indicative of more than one lesion per year.
- Morphology of pit at risk of caries.
- Routine dental care with active preventive dentistry program.
- Community-based sealant program.

Contraindications for Sealant Usage

- Wide, self-cleansing pits and fissures.
- Radiographic or clinical evidence of interproximal caries
- Teeth that cannot be isolated.
- Life expectancy of tooth is limited.
- Occlusal surfaces that are already carious requiring restoration.
- Individuals with no previous carious experience with well-coalesced pits and fissures.

CLINICAL TECHNIQUE FOR PLACEMENT OF PIT AND FISSURE SEALANT

Step 1: Tray Set-up

- Prior to the start of the procedure, a tray with all necessary instruments, supplies, and equipment should be prepared.
- Each operator needs to determine what should be included on the tray based on personal preferences and the sealant material being used.
- The items included in the sample tray set-up are mouth mirror, slow speed handpiece, explorer (No. 5), applicator brush, cotton pliers, sealant material, isolation device like saliva ejector, curing light, syringe tip, and articulating tape.

Step 2: Cleaning of Tooth Surface or Tooth Preparation

- The tooth surface must be cleaned thoroughly to remove adherent plaque and debris prior to sealant placement.
- Cleaning the tooth with pumice and a prophylaxis cup or a bristle brush is advised **(Fig. 26.2A)**. Debris can also be removed using an explorer through the fissure and forceful washing with water spray or by using a dry bristle toothbrush.
- More aggressive methods such as mechanical preparation of fissures prior to etching (enameloplasty) have been followed such as, air abrasion, eliminating fissures with dental burs (fissurotomy burs), sand blasting **(Fig. 26.2B)**. However, enameloplasty with these methods removes

Pit and fissure treatment alternatives

Diagnosis	*Treatment*
Caries-free surface: No explorer wedging • No explorer wedging • Well coalesced, self-cleansing shallow pits and fissures • Stained pits and fissures	Observation only and re-evaluation at 6-month recall examinations
Caries-free surface: No explorer wedging • Stained or minimal decalcified or opacified appearance of pits and fissures • No radiographic or clinical evidence of interproximal caries	Sealant placement • Adequate isolation from saliva—place sealant • Isolation not possible allow further eruption and place sealant within 1–3 months
Caries-free surface: Explorer wedging • Explorer wedging due to pit and fissure anatomy • Stained or decalcified appearance of pits and fissures • No radiographic or clinical evidence of interproximal caries	Sealant placement • Adequate isolation from saliva-place sealant • Isolation not possible allow further eruption and place sealant within 1–3 months • Remove overlying tissues and place sealant or allow further • Eruption and place sealant within 1–3months
Incipient caries: Minimal involvement • Explorer catch due to incipient or minimal caries involving limited areas of pits and fissures • Decalcified appearance of fissures enamel with involvement of adjacent pit and fissures • No radiographic or clinical evidence of interproximal caries • Possible radiographic evidence of occlusal caries	Preventive restoration • Preventive restoration placement (restoration of isolated pits and fissures) • Preventive resin restoration placement • Glass ionomer-preventive restoration • Sealant—amalgam-preventive restoration (amalgam in isolated pits and fissures without extension for prevention and sealant) • Glass ionomer resin-preventive restoration
Carious surface obvious clinical caries • Explorer catch with obvious clinical caries • Loss of enamel lining the pits and fissures • Generalized involvement of pits and fissures by caries with undermining of enamel • Probable radiographic evidence of occlusal caries	Restoration • Posterior composite restoration • Amalgam restoration • Glass ionomer restoration • Glass ionomer resin restoration • Glass ionomer/posterior composite restoration

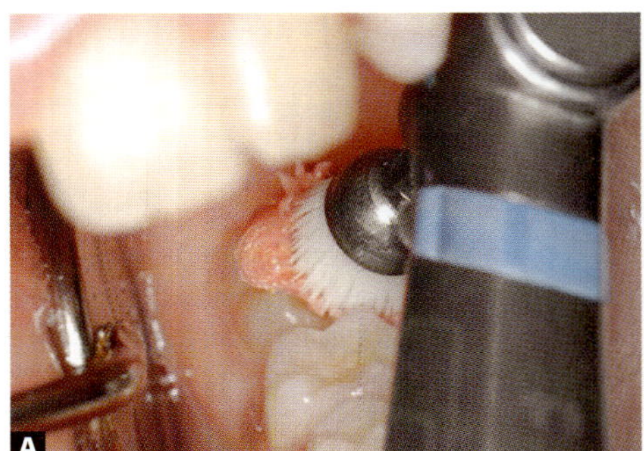

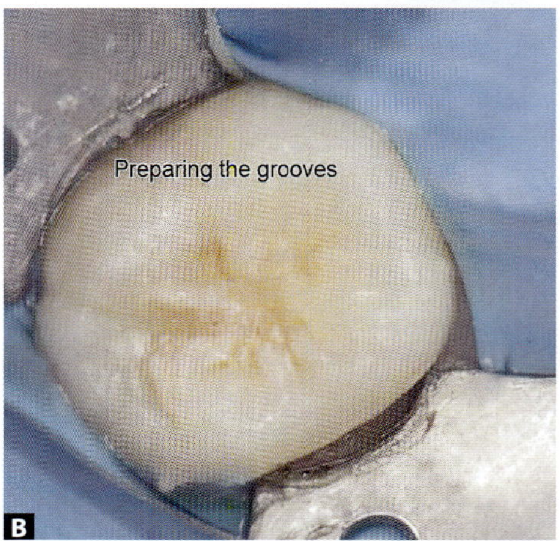

Figs. 26.2A and B: (A) Cleaning of fissures; (B) Preparation of tooth.

enamel overlying dentin at the bottom of the fissure, making the tooth more susceptible to caries if sealant is lost.

- Some manufacturers advise against use of fluoride containing prophylactic pastes or topical fluoride application on the tooth prior to sealant placement as fluoride decreases enamel solubility and thereby interferes with proper etching of enamel. However, several authors have proved that the use of fluoride containing prophylactic pastes or topical fluoride prior to sealant application does not adversely affect the retention of sealants.

> - **Brockleherst** (1992), suggested that air abrasion with aluminium oxide particles is the best method of cleaning as it results in an improved surface for resin wetting, more number of resin tag formation, and more depth of sealant penetration
> - **Sol et al.** (2000) found out that use of sodium bicarbonate air polishing system resulted in higher retention of cement
> - **Garcia Godoy et al.,** (1994) and **Zervou et al.**,[10] recommended enameloplasty as it increases the surface area and decreases microleakage. It can be concluded that type of prophylaxis medium is unimportant and unless plaque, debris, or stains are present on the tooth surface obscuring diagnosis, a prophylaxis before sealing is not essential, although tooth preparation can be useful.

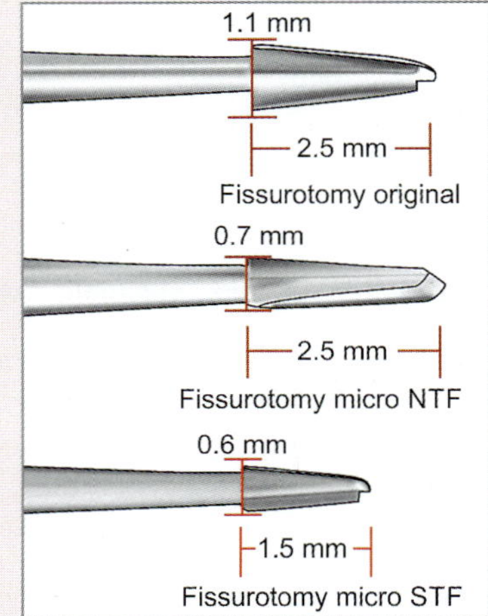

> **Fissurotomy burs**
> The fissurotomy system gives you a viable alternative to be conservative and protect as much healthy tooth structure as possible. The fissurotomy bur tip is extremely small (just 0.33 mm) and fast. It cuts a smooth, minimally invasive groove in suspicious fissures to allow for explorer access. Advantages of these burs include exact drilling depth, pain-free use, ideal cavity form and ability to explore, and restore in just 3–5 minutes. Fissurotomy burs are available in three different configurations: Fissurotomy original (1.1 mm wide/2.5 mm long), fissurotomy micro NTF (0.7 mm wide/2.5 mm long), and fissurotomy micro STF (0.6 mm wide/1.5 mm long).[11]

Step 3: Isolation

- Isolation is the most critical factor during the placement of sealants; loss of sealants and immediate failure of retention are most often due to salivary or moisture contamination.
- **Silverstone** (1984) concluded that salivary contamination allows rapid precipitation of glycoproteins onto the etched surface, greatly decreasing the bond strength. Even 1 second of exposure to saliva can form a protein layer resistant to 30 seconds of vigorous irrigation.
- Rubber dam provides most ideal and controllable isolation **(Fig. 26.3A)**. However, in young children or for newly erupted teeth, it may not be always possible to position rubber dam. In such cases, use of cotton rolls with effective suction, dry field pads, dry field kits or single tooth isolation can be done **(Fig. 26.3B)**.
- The use of moisture control system such as Isolite® system (Innerlite Incorporation, Santa Barbara, CA, USA) has also been reported in the literature for the effective isolation of teeth receiving pit and fissure sealants **(Fig. 26.3C)**.[11]

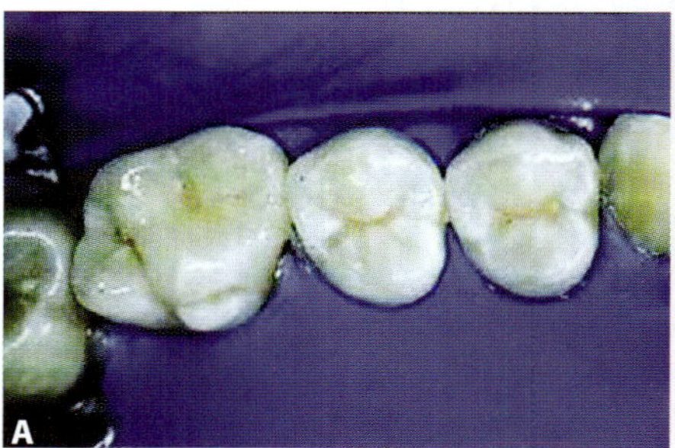

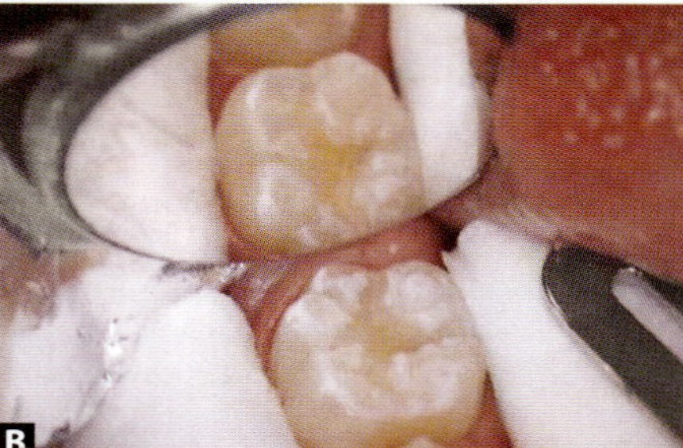

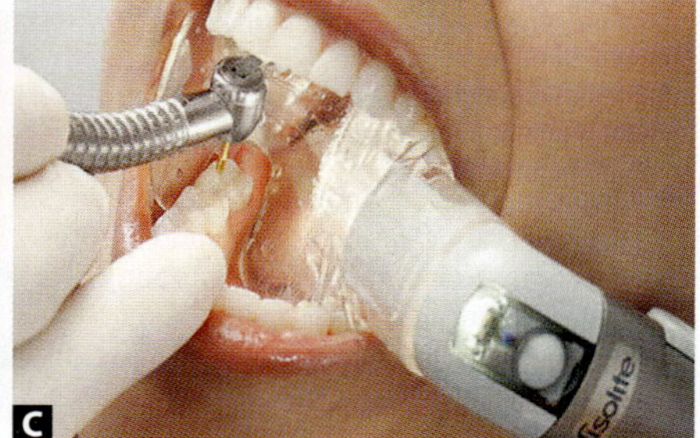

Figs. 26.3A to C: Methods of Isolation of teeth: (A) Rubber dam isolation; (B) Cotton roll isolation; (C) Isolation with Isolite® system.

Step 4: Acid Etching

- Prior to the sealant application, the enamel must be prepared by acid etching with 35-37% phosphoric acid followed by rinsing and drying **(Fig. 26.4).**

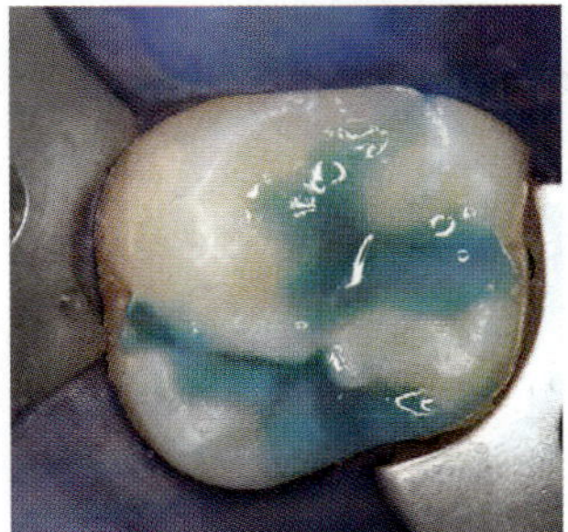

Fig. 26.4: Acid etching with 37% phosphoric acid.

- Acid-etching times have been reduced from 60s to 15s or 20s owing to the findings of several studies investigating if shorter etching times are acceptable in conditioning of enamel prior to sealant placement. Earlier recommendation for primary teeth etching was double the recommended time for permanent teeth, i.e., 60s for permanent teeth and 120s for primary teeth. The longer etching times in primary teeth were advocated due to the presence of thicker aprismatic enamel layer. However, this finding was found not to be clinically significant for sealant retention. A rinsing time of 30s followed by drying for 15s has been recommended by most of the manufacturers.
- The etchant (either in liquid or gel form) should be liberally applied to flow into all the susceptible fissures. Following this, the etchant should be rinsed off with air-water spray and high-volume suction and dried to obtain chalky white enamel appearance.
- Acid-etching facilitates removal of organic pellicle, removes the uppermost aprismatic layer of enamel, partially dissolving the mineral crystallites to create irregular topographical micro-retentive patterns for the infiltration of resinous material.
- After completion of etching process, it is extremely important to maintain isolation. Any contamination at his point would require repetition of etching process.

> - **Duggal et al.,**[12] (1997) have used different etching timing of 15, 30, 45 and 60 seconds and concluded that there is no difference in retention of sealant using different etching time.
> - **Tandon et al.,**[13] (1989) proposed an etching time of 15 seconds to be sufficient for primary teeth.

> - The most accepted times and the currently applicable times were given in **International Association for Dental Research** (IADR) sealant symposium in 1991.

Step	*Primary tooth*	*Permanent tooth*
Acid etch	30 seconds	20 seconds
Wash	30 seconds	30 seconds
Dry	15 seconds	15 seconds

- **Scientific basis for acid etching:**
  - It was given by **Silverstone.**[14] Acid etching on the surface enamel has shown to produce a degree of porosity **(Fig. 26.5).**

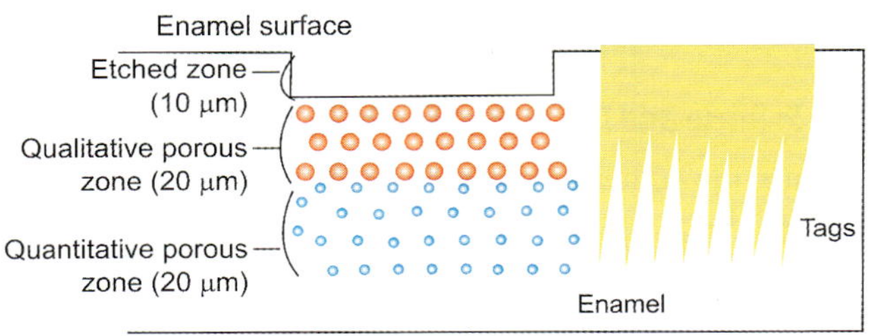

Fig. 26.5: Zones of etching.

  - First, a narrow zone of enamel is removed by etching. In this, plaque and pellicles are dissolved. Fully reacted inert mineral crystals in the surface enamel are also removed, resulting in a more reactive surface, with increase in surface area, and decrease in surface tension that allows the resin to wet the enamel surface more readily. This zone is 10 μm in depth.
  - The second zone is a qualitative porous zone, which is 20μm in depth. Because of the porosities created, this zone may be distinguished qualitatively from enamel by polarized light microscopy.
  - The third zone is quantitative porous zone with small porosities and is 20 μm deep.
- **Types of etching pattern:**
  - **Silverstone**[15] in 1975 identified three basic patterns of etching:
    - **Type1 (Fig. 26.6A):** Preferential dissolution of prism cores, resulting in honeycomb like appearance.
    - **Type 2 (Fig. 26.6B):** Preferential dissolution of prism peripheries, giving a cobblestone-like appearance.
    - **Type 3 (Fig. 26.6C):** A more random pattern, with areas corresponding to both type 1 and type 2 patterns together.

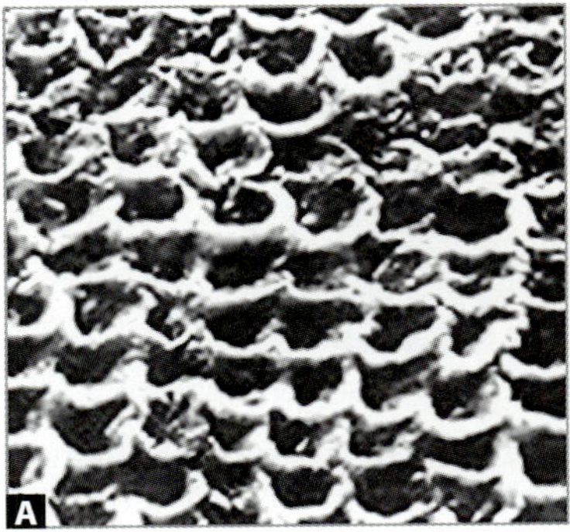

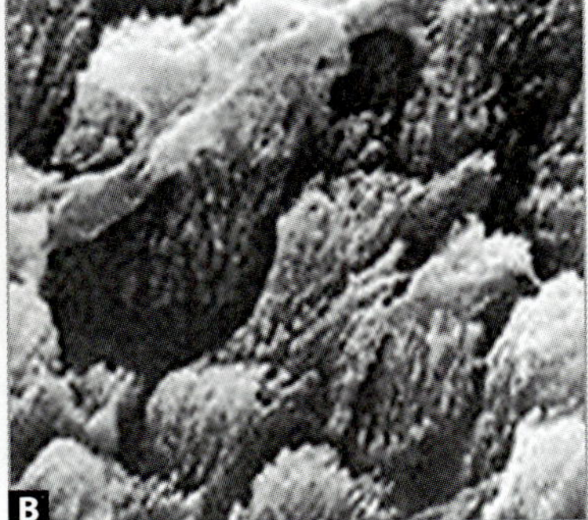

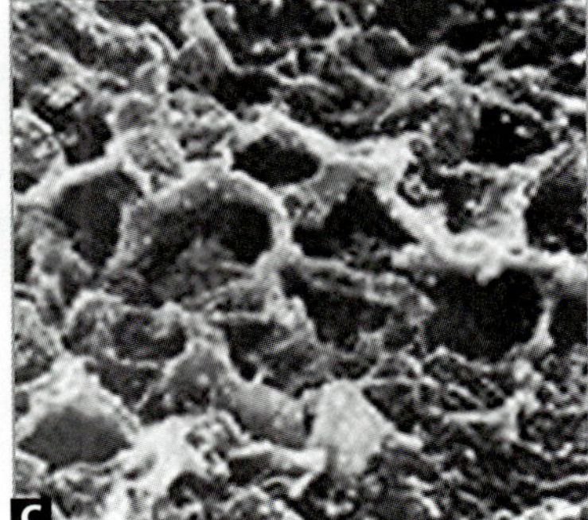

Figs. 26.6A to C: Patterns of etching.

Galil KA (1975)[16] observed type 4, type 5, which were less well-defined patterns mostly in the cervical regions of the buccal surfaces.

- **Type 4:** Pitted enamel surfaces as well as structures that looked like unfinished maps or networks.
- **Type 5:** Flat smooth surfaces, lacking micro irregularities for penetration and retention of resins.

Functions of resin tags
- Provide mechanical means for retention
- Surround the enamel crystals and provide resistance to demineralization by acid products from plaque
- Bis-GMA sealants are resistant to acid dissolution and provide protection against caries along enamel resin interface
- Creates a protective barrier against bacterial colonization of sealed fissure.

Step 5: Rinse and Dry Etched Tooth Surface

- Rinse the etched tooth surface with air water spray for 30 seconds.
- This removes the etching agent and reaction products from etched enamel surface.
- Dry the tooth for 15 seconds with uncontaminated compressed air.
- The dried etched enamel should have a frosted white appearance **(Fig. 26.7)**.
- If salivary contamination has occurred, re-etch for 10 seconds, and repeat the procedure.

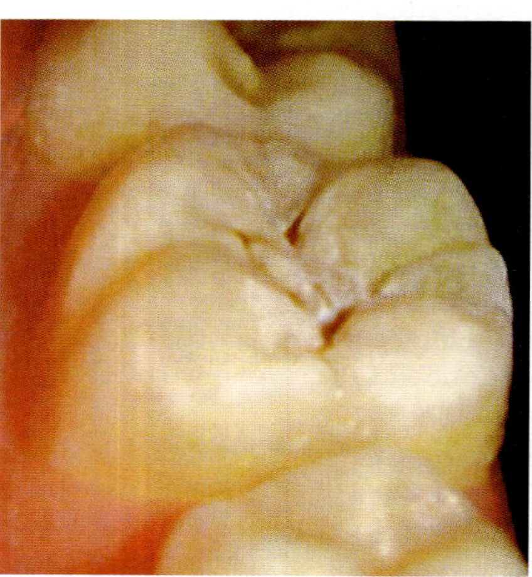

Fig. 26.7: White frosted appearance of etched surface.

Step 6: Application of Bonding Agent

- An additional step of application of bonding agent between etched enamel and sealant was recommended by various authors. Hitt and Feigal (1992) were the first to use hydrophilic bonding materials as a way of optimizing bond strength when the sealant is applied in a moist environment.
- **Hitt** (1992) and **Feigal**,[17] postulated that applying halogenated bonding agent after etching can increase bond strength in saliva-contaminated enamel (0.0005–17.8 MPa) and in uncontaminated enamel (16.7–20.5 MPa) because bonding agent displaces saliva from enamel, improving sealant wetting of surface.
- The use of dentin bonding agents prior to sealant application has also been found to improve long-term sealant retention in mildly hypomineralized permanent molars **(Fig. 26.8)**.

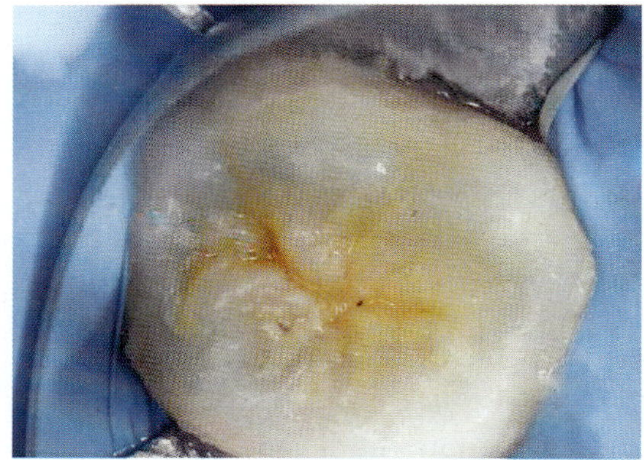

Fig. 26.8: Application of bonding agent.

- However, this step can increase the working time and cost of sealant placement and is usually followed at clinician's discretion.
- Most of the sealants today are provided with single step etching and bonding agents combined into one (e.g., Xeno Bond).

Step 7: Application of Sealant

- Use of minimum amount of sealant to adequately cover all the susceptible pits & fissures is the followed recommendation.
- Sealant may be applied using a variety of instruments: an explorer tip, a small brush, or the dispenser system consisting of a preloaded syringe with a small tip that allows direct application of sealant material on to the tooth.
- In mandibular teeth, apply the sealant distally and allow it to flow mesially with the converse being true for the maxillary teeth. Allow the sealant to flow in the etched pits and fissures to avoid incorporating air into material and creating voids **(Fig. 26.9)**. Then using a fine brush or applicator, carry a thin layer up the cuspal inclines to seal secondary and supplemental fissures.

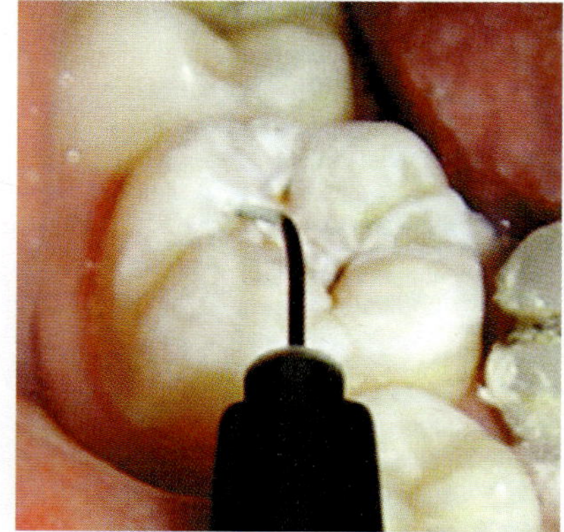

Fig. 26.9: Application of sealant.

- Overfilling must be avoided as excess sealant material can alter the patient's occlusion. In case of overfilling, excess material is removed with a small brush before curing.

Historical development of dentin bonding agents

Generation	*Steps*	*Description*	*Examples*
First generation (mid-1950s and early 1960s)	2-steps	Etching enamel only adhesive application	Cervident (SS White, Lakewood, NJ, USA) No longer used
Second generation (late 1970s)	2-steps	Etching enamel only followed by adhesive application, slightly improved bond strength due to modifications in the coupling agent	Clearfil™ Bond system F (Kuraray, Tokyo, Japan) Scotchbond™ (3M ESPE, Saint Paul, MN, USA) Bondlite (Kerr, Orange, CA, USA) No longer used
Third generation (1980s)	3-steps	Partial removal of smear layer acid etching, primer, then unfilled adhesive resin application	Scotchbond™ 2 (3M ESPE, Saint Paul, MN, USA) Clearfil™ New Bond (Kuraray, Tokyo, Japan)
Fourth generation (1990s)	3-step etch-and-rinse adhesive	Complete removal of the smear layer and the formation of a hybrid layer. Total etch technique (etching enamel and dentin, rinsing, primer, adhesive)	Scotchbond™ Multi-Purpose (3M ESPE, Saint Paul, MN, USA) All-Bond 2® (BISCO, Schaumburg, IL, USA)
Fifth generation (mid-1990s)	3-step etch-and-rinse adhesive	Separate etching step, rinsing enamel and dentin, followed by application of combined primer-adhesive solution	OptiBond® Solo (Kerr, Orange, CA,USA) Adpcr™ Sinile Bond (3M ESPE, Saint Paul, MN, USA) Primc & Bond (DENTSPLY, York, PA, USA)
Sixth generation (late 1990s and early 2000s)	2-step self-etching adhesive	Alter the smear layer forming a thin hybrid layer. It is composed of an acidic primer (etchant + primer in one bottle) followed by bonding resin—no rinsing step	Clearfil™ SE Bond (Kuraray, Tokyo, Japan) OptiBond® Solo Plus Self-Etch (Kerr, Orange, CA, USA)
	1-step 2 component self-etching adhesive	It combines etchant, primer and adhesive in one step but requires pre-mixing before application	Adper™ Prompt™ L-Pop™ (3M ESPE, Saint Paul, MN, USA) Xeno® ID (DENTSPLY, York, PA, USA)
Seventh generation (2002)	1-step self-etching adhesive	It combines etchant, primer and adhesive in a single bottle	Clearfil™ S3 Bond (Kuraray, Tokyo, Japan) G-Bond™ (GC America, Alsip, IL, USA) iBond® (Heraeus Kulzer, Hanau, Germany)
Eighth generation (2010)	1-step self-etching adhesive	Acidic hydrophilic adhesive in a single bottle	Futurabond DC (Voco, Cuxhavcn, Germany) Nanobonding agent
Multimode or universal (2011)	Self-etching adhesive or etch and rinse adhesive or selective enamel etching	Phosphoric acid pre-etching in total or selective etching	Scotchbond™ Universal (3M ESPE, Saint Paul, MN, USA) Futurabond U (Voco, Cuxhaven, Germany)

Additionally, if an excessive amount of sealant is applied such that it extends beyond the etched area of the occlusal surface, the margins will leak and stain over subsequent months.

Step 8: Curing/Polymerization of Sealant

- Once the sealant material is satisfactorily placed on all the susceptible areas, curing of the material should be carried out by placing the tip of light curing unit as close as possible to the tooth surface for as long as recommended by the manufacturer. **(Fig. 26.10).**

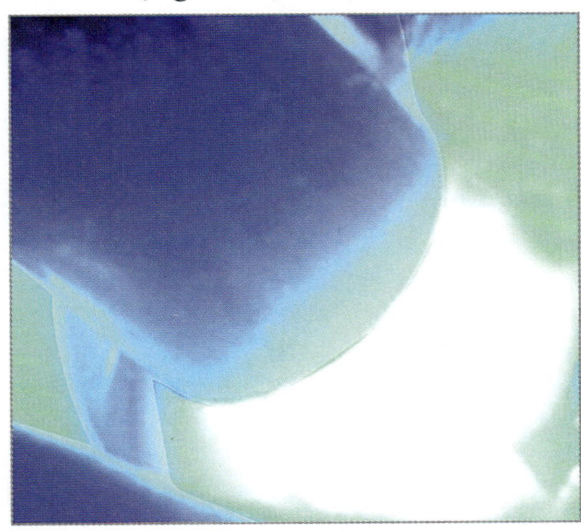

Fig. 26.10: Curing of sealant.

- **Chosak** and **Eidelman**[18] found that the longer sealants were allowed to sit on the etched surface before being polymerized, the more the sealant penetrated the microporosities, creating longer resin tags, which are critical for micromechanical retention
- **Hicks et al.** (2000) found that argon laser curing of sealant material may enhance caries resistance

Step 9: Evaluation of Sealant

- After polymerization and before the removal of isolation material, visual and tactile examination of sealant must be done to check for any voids, air bubbles or deficient material. In that case, sealant material can be directly applied on these defects as the oxygen-inhibited layer has not been disturbed.
- Sealant retention should also be evaluated with a probe by attempting to remove the sealant. If the sealant is dislodged, the tooth should be re-etched, and a new sealant material should be applied.
- The operator should also remove excess sealant material over the distal margin of the tooth that may create a ledge **(Fig. 26.11).**

Step 10: Occlusal Adjustment

- Evaluation of occlusion of sealed tooth surface with articulating paper should be done to determine if any excessive sealant is present and necessary adjustments are to be made to ensure patient's comfort.

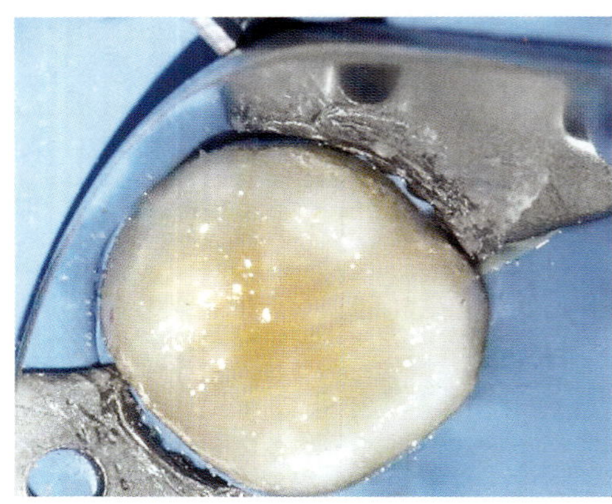

Fig. 26.11: Evaluation of sealant.

- A small discrepancy in occlusion in case of unfilled sealant is easily tolerated as the cement abrades away but in case of filled-resin sealant, occlusal adjustment is a must to avoid discomfort.

Step 11: Recall and Re-evaluation

- Sealants needs evaluation for retention during the routine recall examinations.
- It is necessary to re-evaluate sealed tooth surface for loss of material, exposure of voids, and caries development, and sealants are to be reapplied if any defect or less is detected.
- When sealants are partially lost and require repair, the clinician should vigorously attempt to dislodge the remaining sealant material with an explorer. If it remains intact on probing, there is no need to completely remove the old material before placing the new.
- Although, a single application of resin fissure sealant has been shown to be beneficial in reducing caries of a population, on an individual basis, there is general agreement that the caries-preventive effect of resin fissure sealant relies on the maintenance of integrity of the fissure sealants.

CRITICAL ISSUES REGARDING PIT AND FISSURE SEALANT USAGE

Sealant Retention

- Retention of sealant is critical for long-term effectiveness of pit and fissure sealants in preventing dental caries.
- The first report that discussed on the retention of pit and fissure sealants was Horowitz's landmark Kalispell study.[19] In the 5-year report of this study, the authors reported 42% complete retention at 5 years. Horowitz also noted that teeth with sealant partially missing had a lower incidence of caries (7%) than paired unsealed control teeth that were not sealed (41% caries). Thus, from the results of this pioneering clinical trial, one can conclude that even partially sealed teeth are considerably less susceptible to caries than unsealed teeth. Horowitz concluded, "The findings of this study clearly show that when this pit and fissure sealant is retained, it is effective in preventing caries in sealed tooth surfaces."
- **Simonsen**[20] reported 15-year retention rates for single application of sealants on permanent molars. Around 27.6% showed complete retention, 35% showed partial retention, 68.8% remained caries free but only 17% of unsealed teeth were caries free. None of the teeth that either completely or partially retained sealants developed caries.
- Clinical evidence suggests that sealant loss (retention failure) occurs in two phases: there is an initial loss due to faulty technique (such as moisture contamination), followed by a second loss associated with material wear under the forces of occlusion.
- Various factors associated with sealant retention includes Initial cleaning of tooth before sealant placement, isolation of the tooth, enamel surface preparation, adhesive application, type of the sealant material used and the type of tooth on which sealant is placed.
- A meta-analysis investigated the clinical retention rates of pit and fissure sealants with regard to different types of materials at different observation-times. The resin-based sealants showed the best retention rates: the five-year retention rates for light-polymerizing, auto-polymerizing, and fluoride-releasing resin-based sealants were 83.8%, 64.7%, and 69.9%, respectively. The GI-based fissure sealants, on the other hand, had a 5.2% retention rate at the five-year observation-time. Polyacid modified resin sealants also showed low retention rates.[21]
- **Corona SAM et al.,**[22] stated that the flowable restorative system yielded optimal retention on primary molars. Its retention rate was significantly higher than that of the conventional pit-and-fissure sealant on primary teeth.
- **Maher MM et al.,**[23] stated that replacing phosphoric acid-etching with self-etching adhesive Adper Prompt L-Pop does not compromise sealant retention in primary teeth after a 1-year period.
- **Unal M et al.,**[24] stated that resin-based sealants containing ACP or fluoride are more retentive than conventional resin-based sealants.
- **Joshi S et al.,**[25] stated that retention by high-viscosity GIC sealant applied with or without additional light curing was found to be similar.

Success of sealant restorations

Study	*Duration (years)*	*Success (%)*
Simonsen and Stallard	1.0	100
Azhadri et al.	1.0	86
Walker et al.	1.25	82
Houpt et al.	1.5	91
Gray	2.0	67–97
Walls et al.	2.0	97
Simonsen and Jensen	2.5	96
Raadal	2.5	84
Simonsen	3.0	99
Houpt et al.	3.0	77
Houpt et al.	4.0	64
Welbury et al.	5.0	26
Houpt et al.	6.5	65
Simonsen and Landy	7.0	90
Houpt et al.	9.0	54
Merzt-Fairhurst	9.0	28

Postulated reasons for lack of sealant usage	
Reasons for limited use of sealants	***Rankings***
Dentist users	
Lack of insurance reimbursement	1
Concern of sealing over caries	2
Concern of sealant retention	3
Cost effectiveness	4
Dentist non-users	
Concern of sealing of decay	1
Occlusal filling preferred	2
Sealants do not last long	3

Cost Effectiveness of a Sealant

- Although it is evident that sealants provide significant caries protection for pits and fissures, the use of sealants has been limited in the past owing to questions about their cost effectiveness.
- The total expense incurred with sealant placement must be compared with the cost of restoration of the teeth in which sealants are not placed and caries eventually developed. **Simonson** (1987) over a 10-year period, observed that it is 1.6 times as costly to restore the carious lesions in the first permanent molars in an unsealed group of 5–10-year-old children living in a fluoridated area than it is to prevent, with a single application of pit and fissure sealant, the greater number of lesions observed if pit and fissure sealant is not utilized.
- **Burt**[27] noted that cost effectiveness of sealants would be enhanced by: (1) using trained auxiliaries to apply sealant to the fullest extent allowed by law, (2) applying the most recently developed sealants in which retention rates appear to be most favorable and (3) their application in areas where proximal caries is low.

Estrogenicity Issue

- Bisphenol-A (BPA) is the precursor chemical of the most commonly used monomers such as bisphenol-a dimethacrylate (Bis-DMA) and bisphenol-a glycidyl dimethacrylate (Bis-GMA) in resin composites and resin-based sealants.
- BPA is known for its estrogenic potential with potential reproductive and developmental human toxicity owing to its ability to bind to and activate human estrogen receptors. Although it is not a direct ingredient of dental sealants; it is a chemical that appears in the final product only when the raw materials fail to fully react.
- **Olea et al.**, (1996) reported that 89.8 to 93.1 µg of BPA was identified in the saliva of patients treated with a commercially available dental sealant and confirmed the estrogenicity of this resinous material by proliferation tests of human breast cancer and implicated bisphenol-A dimethacrylate (bis-DMA) as an estrogenic factor. A systematic review reported high levels of BPA in saliva samples collected immediately and one hour after placement of resin-based sealants. Urine samples also showed high levels of BPA.[28]
- However, it should also be remembered that none of the dental sealants that carry the American Dental Association (ADA) seal release detectable BPA to place patients at risk,[29] A report by ADA and American Academy of Pediatric Dentistry did not support the occurrence of adverse effects after sealant placement and described BPA effect as a small transient effect.

CURRENT STATUS OF PIT AND FISSURE SEALANTS

Fluoride Releasing Sealants

- Fluoride releasing resin-based sealant is a product manufactured by adding fluoride releasing particles to resin-based sealants in an attempt to prevent caries. The fluoride releasing sealants available in the market, contain either a soluble-fluoride salt such as sodium fluoride or fluoride releasing glass filler or both.
- **Garcia Godoy** (1997) found out that all the fluoridated sealants exhibited greatest amount of fluoride release during the first 24 hours after sealant application and the fluoride release gradually decreased thereafter.
- **Cooley et al**. (1990) and **Hicks et al**. (1992) conducted laboratory studies on a fluoride releasing sealant material composed of a modified urethane Bis-GMA resin. They also concluded that fluoride release dips considerably as the days go by. But they reported 60% reduction in secondary caries and enhanced degree of caries resistance.
- The researchers who worked with fluoride releasing sealants named the phenomenon of higher fluoride release during the first days as **"burst effect."**
- Examples of fluoride fissure sealants are Seal-Rite® (Pulpdent), FluoroShield® (Dentsply), Conceal F®(SDI), Helioseal-F (Ivoclar vivadent), Delton Plus® (Dentsply).

Colored Pit and Fissure Sealant

- The colored pit and fissure sealants change their color during curing phase or polymerization which facilitates easier and proper application of sealant on the tooth.
- Examples are Clinpro (3M ESPE), Helioseal Clear Chroma (Ivoclar Vivadent).
- Helioseal changes color from clear to green during polymerization. The degree of color change is also an indicator of its setting and adequate polymerization.
- Clinpro changes color from pink to opaque white after being exposed to visible light.
- It is much faster to assess retention with a white sealant than with a clear sealant at later time intervals. Also, documentation of retention is much easier over long time periods with a colored sealant.

Fluorescing Pit and Fissure Sealant

- This sealant eliminates the guess work involved with placing sealants and confirming placement during recall appointments.
- Through the use of a UV penlight, this sealant fluoresces a blue/white color.
- The fluorescent glow provides clinicians with a visual verification of the sealant margins at the time of placement and offers the easiest way to verify retention and inspect margins during patient recall appointments.
- For example, DeltonSeal-N-Glo (Dentsply).

Moist Bonding Pit and Fissure Sealant

- Placement of resin-based sealant is very technique sensitive, as they are Bis GMA based materials that are primarily hydrophobic in nature and require a dry field. In recent years, resin-based sealant technology has been developed that incorporates moisture-tolerant resin chemistry and behaves favorably in the moist oral environment.
- "Embrace Wet Bond™" is one of the recent advances which is a unique moisture tolerant resin-based sealant that contains no bis-GMA and no bisphenol A (BPA) and uses hydrophilic resin chemistry. Embrace incorporates di-tri and multifunctional acrylate monomers into an advanced acid integrating chemistry that is activated by moisture. It forms a unique resin acid-integrating network (RAIN) that improves penetration into pits and fissures and provides superior sealing of the margins. It bonds chemically and micromechanically to the moist tooth, integrating with the tooth structure to create a strong, margin-free bond that virtually eliminates microleakage.
- The use of moisture-tolerant resin-based sealant could be encouraged in situations difficult to attain moisture control as it incorporates a hydrophilic chemistry. Application of moisture tolerant resin-based sealant is highly beneficial in treating children because it is often difficult to maintain a dry field, and the fact that the material works well in a slightly moist field is a great benefit to the practitioner. The ability to bond in the presence of moisture simplifies the sealant procedure and makes it less technique sensitive.
- For example: Embrace Wet Bond™ (Pulpdent Corporation).

Hydrophilic, Fluorescent, BPA Free Pit and Fissure Sealant

- This is a new sealant developed which combines the best properties of nearly all sealants. Some of its major properties are hydrophilic chemistry, advanced adhesive technology, fluorescent properties, thixotropic viscosity, and BPA-free formula.
- Thus, not only can it be used in wet environment but also is easy to place owing to thixotropic viscosity and is easy to follow up due to fluorescence.
- For example, UltraSeal XT® hydro.

Pit and Fissure Sealant with ACP

- It is a light-cured sealant that contains the "smart material" amorphous calcium phosphate (ACP) which has an ability to release calcium and phosphate ions and remineralize tooth structure by enhancing tooth's natural repair mechanism.
- ACP is referred to as a "smart material" because it only releases calcium and phosphate ions when the pH drops to 5.5 and ceases when the pH rises. Once the calcium phosphate is released, it will act to neutralize the acid and buffer the pH. It causes supersaturation of calcium and phosphate ions locally, thereby promoting the formation of hydroxyapatite.
- It has a controlled flowability that keeps the sealant on the tooth structure while completely filling occlusal surfaces and it forms a chemical and thermal barrier protecting the tooth enamel on the occlusal surface from carious attacks.
- For example: Aegis® Pit and fissure sealant.

Sealants with S-PRG Filler

- This is a sealant that was developed incorporating newly developed technology involving a pre-reacted glass ionomer (Ikemura et al., 2008). This technology enables the formation of a stable glass-ionomer phase in fillers by pre-reacting acid-reactive glass containing fluoride with polyacrylic acid in the presence of water.
- These S-PRG filler uniquely releases 6 ions: fluoride, sodium, strontium, aluminum, silicate and borate, all with known bioactive properties. Strontium and fluoride improve the acid resistance of teeth by acting on hydroxyapatite to convert it to strontium apatite and fluorapatite.
- Beauti sealant is a resin-based fissure sealant containing 40% S-PRG fillers developed by Shofu Co., Kyoto, Japan. It is a tooth colored, fluoride recharging pit and fissure sealant with a self-etching primer that reduces the treatment time by eliminating the need for phosphoric acid etching.

Glass Carbomer as Pit and Fissure Sealant

- A novel glass-ionomer-based material—"the glass-carbomer", with powder particles reduced to nano size is an additional option as a sealant material apart from glass ionomer and rein-based sealants.
- Glass carbomer is a glass-based material with an additional carbon chain and contains nano sized powder particles and fluorapatite as a secondary filler. The liquid of glass carbomer is polyacrylic acid.
- The major advantage of this material in Pediatric Dentistry is that it is moisture tolerant making it easy to place in children.

POINTS TO REMEMBER

- Pit and fissure sealant is a term used to describe a material that is introduced into the occlusal pits and fissures of caries-susceptible teeth, thus forming a micro mechanically bonded, protective layer cutting access of caries-producing bacteria from their source of nutrients.[1]
- Buonocore (1955) observed that, after treatment of the enamel with concentrated phosphoric acid solution, attachment of acrylics into tooth surfaces was greatly increased.
- First pit and fissure sealant Nuva-seal developed and commercially introduced by LD Caulk Company in 1971.
- Fissure types include V, U, I, IK, inverted Y; most prone to caries being inverted Y.
- Procedure for sealant placement is tray set up, isolation, tooth preparation, acid etching, washing and drying, application of bonding agent, application of sealant, curing and evaluating.
- Etching time is 30 seconds for primary teeth and 20 seconds for permanent teeth.

- Main functions of resin tags include retention, caries protection, and prevention of bacterial colonization.
- Fluoride releasing sealants—Seal-Rite®(Pulpdent), FluoroShield®(Dentsply), ConcealF®(SDI).
- Clear pit and fissure sealant—Helioseal®.
- Colored pit and fissure sealant—Clinpro®.
- Fluorescing pit and fissure sealant—DeltonSeal-N-Glo®.
- Moist bonding pit and fissure sealant—Embrace WetBond®.
- Pit and fissure sealant with ACP—AegisPit®and fissure sealant.
- Hydrophilic fluorescent BPA-free pit and fissure sealant—UltraSealXT® hydro.

Questionnaire

1. Define pit and fissure sealant and discuss the method of its placement.
2. Explain the classification, indications, and ideal properties of sealants.
3. Write a note on history of pit and fissure sealants.
4. Explain acid etching.
5. What are the new developments in the field of sealants?

REFERENCES

1. Simonsen RJ. Pit and fissure sealants. In: Clinical applications of the acid etch technique.1st edition. Chicago,IL: Quintessence Publishing Co. Inc.;1978. pp. 19-42.
2. Welbury R, Raadal M, Lygidakis NA. EAPD guidelines for the use of pit and fissure sealants. Eur J Paediat rDent. 2004;5:179-84.
3. GoreJT. Etiology of dental caries enamel immunization experiments. J Dent Res. 1939; 26:958.
4. Buonocore MG. Simple method of increasing the adhesion of acrylic filling materials to enamel surfaces. J Dent Res.1955;34:849.
5. Rodyhouse RH. Prevention of occlusal fissure caries by use of a sealant: a pilot study. ASDC J Dent Child. 1968; 35:253-62.
6. Grewal N, Chopra R. The effect of fissure morphology and eruption time on penetration and adaptation of pit and fissure sealants: an SEM study. J Indian Soc Pedod Prevent Dent. 2008;26:59-63.
7. NaganoT. Forms of pits and fissures. Dent Abst. 1961;6:426.
8. Wright JT, Crall JJ, Fontana M, et al. Evidence-based Clinical Practice Guideline for the Use of Pit-and-Fissure Sealants. American Academy of Pediatric Dentistry, American Dental Association. Pediatr Dent. 2016;38(5): E120-E36.
9. Subramanian EMG, Muthu MS, Sivakumar N. Pit and fissure sealants and preventive resin restorations. Chapter 21. In: Muthu MS,SivakumarN(Eds). Pediatric dentistry: principles and practice. 2nd edition. Elsevier; 2011. pp. 241-8.
10. ZervouC, Doherty EH, et al. An in vitro study of microleakage of pit and fissure sealants in the presence of occlusal forces. J Clin Pediatr Dent. 2000;24:273-8.
11. Alhareky MS, Mermelstein D, Finkelman M, Alhumaid J, Loo C. Efficiency and Patient Satisfaction with the Isolite System Versus Rubber Dam for Sealant Placement in Pediatric Patients. Pediatr. Dent. 2014;36:400-4.
12. Duggal MS, Tahmassebi JF, Toumba KJ, Mavromati C. The effect of different etching times on the retention of fissure sealants in second primary and first permanent molars. Int J Pediatr Dent. 1997;7(2):81-6.
13. Tandon S, Mathew TA. Effect of acid-etching on fluoride-treated caries-like lesions of enamel: a SEM study. ASDC J Dent Child. 1997;64(5):344-8.
14. Silverstone LM, Dogon IL. The effect of phosphoric acid on human deciduous enamel surfaces in vitro. J Int Assoc Dent Child. 1976;7:11.
15. Silverstone LM. Invitro studies with special reference to enamel surface and the enamel-resin interface. In: Silverstone LM, DogonIL, (Eds). Proceedings of an international symposium on the acid etch technique. St.Paul: Central Publishing Co; 1975.
16. Galil KA, Wright GZ. Acid etching patterns on buccal surfaces of permanent teeth. Pediatr Dent. 1979;1(4):230-4.
17. Feigal RJ. The use of pit and fissure sealants. Pediatr Dent. 2002;24:415-22.
18. ChosakA, EidelmanE. Effect of time from application until exposure to light on the tag lengths of a visible light-polymerized sealant. Dent Mater. 1988;4:302-6.
19. Horowitz HS, Heifetz SB, Poulsen S. Retention and effectiveness of a single application of an adhesive sealant in preventing occlusal caries: final report after five years of a study in Kalispell, Montana. J Am Dent Assoc. 1977;95:1133-9.
20. Simonsen RJ. Pit and fissure sealant: review of the literature. Pediatr Dent. 2002;24:393-414.
21. Kühnisch J, Mansmann U, Heinrich-Weltzien R, Hickel R. Longevity of materials for pit and fissure sealing --Results from a meta-analysis. Dent Mater. 2012;28:298-303.
22. Corona SAM, Borsatto MC, Garcia L, Ramos RP, Palma-Dibb RG. Randomized, controlled trial comparing the retention of a flowable restorative system with a conventional resin sealant: one-year follow up. Int J Paediatr Dent. 2005;15:44-50.
23. Maher MM, Elkashlan HI , El-Housseiny AA. Effectiveness of a Self-etching Adhesive on Sealant Retention in Primary Teeth. Pediatric Dentistry 2013;35(4):351-4.
24. Ünal M, Oznurhan F, Kapdan A, Dürer A. A Comparative Clinical Study of Three Fissure Sealants on Primary Teeth: 24-Month Results. The Journal of Clinical Pediatric Dentistry. 2015;39:2.
25. Joshi S, Sandhu M, Suma SHP, Garg S, Dhindsa A. Split-mouth Randomised Clinical Trial on the Efficacy of GIC Sealant on Occlusal Surfaces of Primary Second Molar. Oral Health Prev Dent. 2019;17: 17-24.
26. Burt BA. Fissure sealants: clinical and economic factors. J Dent Educ.1984;48:96-102.
27. Olea N, Pulgar R, Perez P, Orea-Serrano F, Rivas A, Novillo-Fertrell A. Estrogenicity of resin-based composites and sealants used in dentistry. Environ Health Perspect. 1996;104:298-305.
28. Kloukas D, Pandis N, Eliades T. In vivo bisphenol-A release from dental pit and fissure sealants: A systematic review. J Dent. 2013;41:659-67.
29. Association AD. Estrogenic effects of bisphenol A lacking in dental sealants. Available at: http://www.ada.org/prof/prac/issues/statements/sealest.html(accessed1998).

FURTHER READING

1. Ahovuo-Saloranta A, Hiiri A, Nordblad A, Worthington H, MakelaM. Pit and fissure sealants for preventing dental decay in the permanent teeth of children and adolescents. Cochrane Database Syst Rev. 2004:CD001830.
2. Ahovuo-Saloranta A, Hiiri A. Nordblad A, Mäkelä M, Worthington HV. Sealants for preventing dental decay in the permanent teeth --A review. Cochrane Database Syst Rev; 2013.
3. BravonLJ, et al. Dental caries and sealant usage in US children. J Am Dent Assoc. 1996;127:335-43.
4. Donly KJ. Sealants: where we have been, where we are going. Gen Dent. 2002;50:438-40.
5. Gilpin JL. Pit and fissure sealants: a review of the literature. J Dent Hyg Summer. 1997;71:150-8.
6. Gwinnett AJ, Buonocore MG. Adhesives and caries prevention. Br Dent J. 1965;119:77.
7. Hassall DC, Mellor AC. The sealant restoration: indications, success and clinical technique. Br Dent J. 2001;191:358-62.
8. Locker D, Jokovic A. Series Editor Kay EJ. Prevention Part 8: The use of pit and fissure sealants in preventing caries in the permanent dentition of children. Brit Dent J. 2003;195:375-8.
9. Rethman J. Trends in preventive care: caries risk assessment and indications for sealants. J Am Dent Assoc. 2000;131:8S-12S.
10. Strassler HE. Incisal edge: clinical update: flowable composite resins. 2013;7:61-70.
11. Waggoner WF, Seigal M. Pit and fissure sealant application: updating the technique. J Am Dent Assoc.1996;1:351-61.

CHAPTER

Plaque Control in Children

Nikhil Marwah, Koya Srikanth, Ayushi Bansal

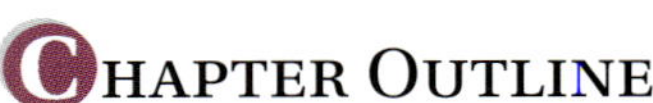

CHAPTER OUTLINE

- Disclosing Solution
- Dentifrice
- Toothbrush
- Toothbrush Modifications and Current Concepts
- Techniques of Toothbrushing
- Tongue Cleansing
- Interdental Cleaning Aids
- Chemotherapeutic Plaque Removal
- Guidelines for Home Oral Hygiene

The emergence of a new philosophy and dentistry based on prevention rather than repair and replacement has been one of the most significant developments in the history of dentistry. Despite these substantial improvements in health, dental disease, however, remains a chronic health problem. Two main oral disease, dental caries and periodontal disease, frequently begin in childhood and often have long sequelae; therefore, to prevent these problems, primary preventive dentistry must begin early in life before the insidious onset of these diseases.

WHO (1961) *defines plaque is a specific but highly variable structural entity resulting from colonization of microorganism consisting of various species and strains embedded on an extracellular matrix on tooth surfaces, restorations and other parts of oral cavity and consists of salivary components like mucin, desquamated epithelial cells, debris and microorganims all embedded in a gelatinous extracellular matrix.*

Dental plaque (Bowen) *is defined as a structured, resilient, yellow-grayish substance that adheres tenaciously to the intraoral hard surfaces, including removable and fixed restorations.*

Dental plaque is broadly classified as supragingival or subgingival based on its position on the tooth surfaces.

The different regions of plaque are significant to different processes associated with diseases of the teeth and periodontium. For example, marginal plaque is of prime importance in the development of gingivitis; supragingival plaque and tooth associated with subgingival plaque are critical in calculus formation; fissure associated with subgingival plaque is important in the soft tissue destruction.

Methods of plaque control

Mechanical plaque control	***Chemical plaque control***
• Dentifrice	• Mouthwash
• Toothbrush	• Chlorhexidine
• Dental floss	• Other compounds
• Oral irrigation	
• Interdental cleaning aids	

Plaque control *is the removal of plaque and the prevention of its accumulation on the teeth and adjacent gingival surfaces.* Plaque control is the key to prevention and successful treatment of periodontal disease. Removal of microbial plaque leads to resolution of gingival inflammation in its early stages, and cessation of plaque control measures leads to its recurrence. Plaque control is accomplished by professional plaque removal and by patient performing oral hygiene practices or both.

DISCLOSING SOLUTION

According to Wilkins (1959) a disclosing agent is a selective dye in solution, tablet or lozenge form used to visualize and identify dental biofilm on the surfaces of the teeth.

Uses

- ❖ Effective motivation tool for patient education
- ❖ Instructions to patient about plaque control
- ❖ Self-assessment by the patient
- ❖ Evaluation of effectiveness of long term plaque control measures
- ❖ Assessment of the clinician
- ❖ Preparation of plaque indices.
- ❖ Caries risk assessment
- ❖ Photodynamic therapy

Formulations

Name	***Preparation***	
Skinner solution	Diluted (21 mL of tincture Iodine in 15 mL of water) tincture of iodine water—15.0 mL	
Iodine preparations	Iodine crystals—3.3 g Tincture of iodine—21.0 mL Potassium iodide—1.0 g Zinc iodide—1.0 g Water (distilled)—16.0 mL Glycerin—16.0 mL	
Mercurochrome preparations	Mercurochrome (Merbromin: Disodium salt of 2,7-dibromo-4 hydroxymercurifluorescein)—1.5 g Water—30 mL Oil of peppermint—three drops Artificial noncalorigenic sweetener	
Bismarck brown (Easlick's disclosing solution)	Bismark brown—3.0 g Ethyl alcohol—10 mL Glycerin—120 mL Flavoring agent—one drop	
	Topical application	***Tablet***
Erythrosin (most widely used) 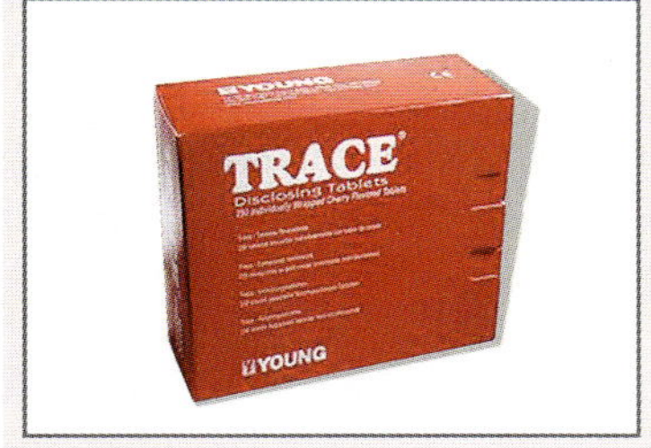 	Erythrosine—0.8 g, Water—100 mL Alcohol (95%)—10.0 mL Oil of peppermint—two drops	FD and C Red No. 3—15.0 mg Sodium chloride—0.747% Sodium sucaryl—0.747% Calcium stearate—0.975% Soluble saccharin—0.186% White oil—0.124%, flavoring—2.239%
2-tone solution **(Block et al.,** 1975**)** 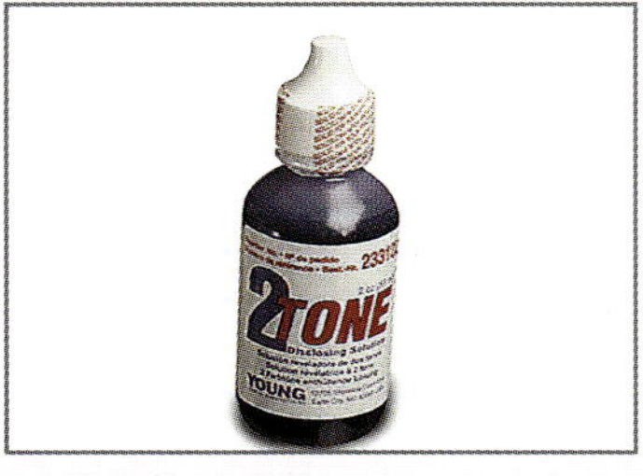 	Combination of erythrosin with FD and C Green No. 3, FD and C blue No. 1 or Hercules green shade 3 Thicker (older) plaque stains blue Thinner (newer) plaque stains red	
Plak light system **(Squillaro et al.)** 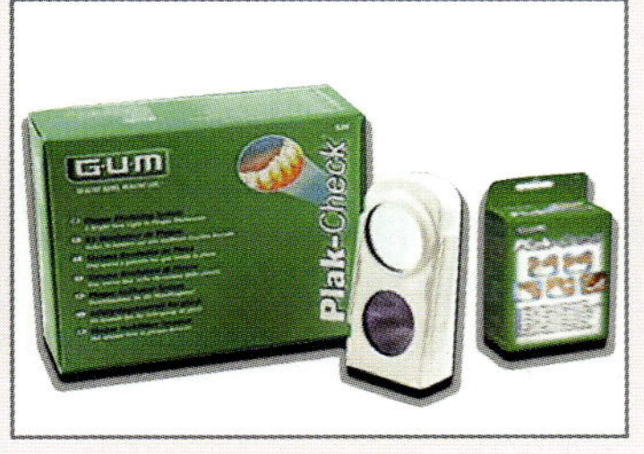 	Sodium fluorescein Glycerin—75%, FD and C Yellow No. 8 Fluorescence is affected by pH When excited with blue light, fluorescence is yellow-green.	

DENTIFRICE

According to ADA "A dentifrice is a substance used with a toothbrush for the purpose of cleaning the accessible surface of the teeth" **(Fig. 27.1)**. Egyptian medical manual the Ebers Papyrus written about 1500 BC mentions the use of dentifrice for cleaning the mouth, and Hippocrates was the first to recommend the use of dentifrices.

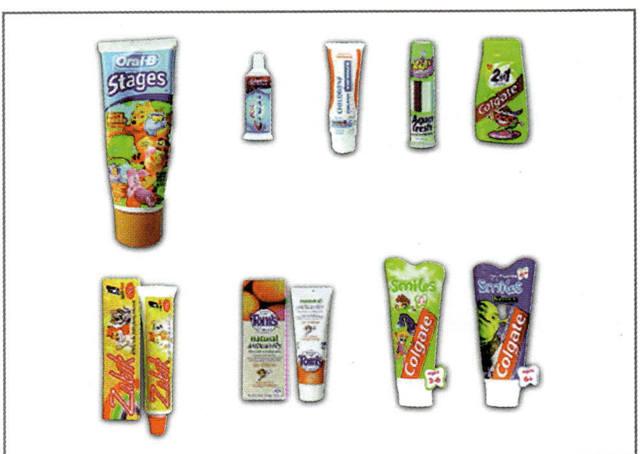

Fig. 27.1: Dentifrices for children.

Therapeutic dentifrices

- A toothpaste is an excellent delivery system and has been widely used to deliver fluorides(stannous fluoride, sodium fluoride (NaF) 0.24% (1,100 ppm), sodium monofluorophosphate ($Na_2PO_4F_2$) 0.76% (1,000 ppm), antibiotics, enzymes and to inhibit dental caries
- Reduction of tooth sensitivity, calculus promotion, bacterial plaque formation, and gingivitis
- Used for tooth whitening for cosmetic effect

Mechanical Plaque Control Aids

1. Toothbrushes
   a. Manual
   b. Electrical
2. Interdental aids
   a. Dental floss
   b. Triangular toothpicks (hand held, proxapic)
   c. Interdental brushes (proxabrush, bottle brushes, single tufted brushes)
   d. Yarn
   e. Superfloss
   f. Perio-aid
3. Aids for gingival stimulation
   a. Rubber tip stimulator
   b. Balsa wood edge
4. Others
   a. Gauze strips
   b. Pipe cleaners
   c. Water irrigation device
5. Aids for edentulous or partially edentulous patients
   a. Denture and partial clasp brushes
   b. Cleansing solutions

TOOTHBRUSH

History

- The mechanical cleaning of teeth can be traced back to ancient times. Toothbrushes were probably developed from the ancient custom of chewing twigs of lentsik wood or similar aromatic twigs.
- Evidence says that oral hygiene was practiced by Egyptians 5,000 years ago; Romans used toothpick made up of bone and metals **(Fig. 27.2)**.

Composition of dentifrices

Component	*% Added*	*Use*	*Example*
Detergent	1.2%	• To lower surface tension • Penetrate and loosen surface deposits and strains • Emulsify debris for easy removal by the toothbrush • Contribute to the foaming action	Sodium lauryl sulfate
Cleaning and polishing	20–40%	• A dentifrice may have a combination of agents in an abrasive system to accommodate both cleaning and polishing objectives • Abrasive is used to clean • A polishing agent is used to produce a smooth, shining tooth surface that resists discoloration, bacterial accumulation, and retention	Calcium carbonate, calcium pyrophosphate, bicalcium phosphate
Binders	1–2%	• To prevent separation of the solid and liquid ingredients during storage • Contribute to the stability and consistency of the toothpaste	Organic hydrophilic colloids, alginates, magnesium aluminum silicate, colloidal silica
Humectants	20–40%	• These are added to retain moisture • Prevent hardening on exposure to air • To stabilize the preparation	Glycerin, sorbitol
Preservatives		• To prevent bacterial growth and to prolong shelf life	Alcohols, formaldehyde, and dichlorinated phenols
Sweetener	2–3%	• To impart a pleasant flavor for patient's acceptance	Sorbitol and glycerin
Flavoring agent	1–15%	• To make the dentifrices desirable • To mask other ingredients that may have less pleasant flavor	Peppermint, cinnamon, menthol
Therapeutic agent	1–2%	• For medicinal value	Fluoride
Coloring agent	2–3%	• Added for attractiveness	
Water	20–40%	• Main transport medium	

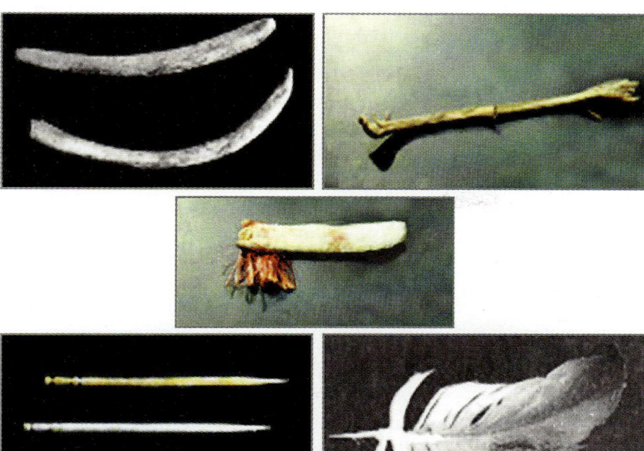

Fig. 27.2: Ancient toothbrushes.

- The first bristle toothbrush was found in China during the Tang dynasty.
- In 1223, Japanese Zen master **DÅ Gen Kigen** recorded that he saw monks in China clean their teeth with brushes made of horse-tail hairs attached to an ox bone handle.
- Toothbrush in Europe during the 17th century and the earliest identified use of the word toothbrush in English was in the autobiography of **Anthony Wood**, who wrote in 1690 that he had bought a toothbrush from **J Barret.**
- In Europe, **William Addis** of England is believed to have produced the first mass-produced toothbrush in 1780. William was basically a rag picker and in 1770, he had been jailed for causing a riot; while in prison, he decided that the method used to clean teeth by rubbing a rag with soot and salt on the teeth was ineffective and could be improved. To that end, he saved a small animal bone left over from the meal he had eaten the previous night, into which he drilled small holes. He then obtained some bristles from one of his guards, which he tied in tufts that he then passed through the holes in the bone, and which he finally sealed with glue. After his release, he started a business that would manufacture the toothbrushes he had built under the name of Wisdom Toothbrushes **(Fig. 27.3).**
- The first patent for a toothbrush was by **HN Wadsworth** in 1857 (US Patent No. 18,653) in the United States, but mass production in the United States only started in 1885. The rather advanced design had a bone handle with holes bored into it for the Siberian boar hair bristles.
- **During** the 1900s, celluloid handles gradually replaced bone handles in toothbrushes. Natural animal bristles were also replaced by synthetic fibers, usually nylon, by **DuPont** in 1938.

Toothbrush development timeline

3000 BC	Egyptians use small branches to clean teeth
1223	Chinese invent bristle toothbrush
1690	First reference to word toothbrush in Europe
1780	**William Addis** invents toothbrush
1857	First patent for a toothbrush by **HN Wadsworth**
1938	First nylon bristles introduced by **DuPont**
1954	Electric toothbrush invented by **Philippe-Guy Woog**
1960	First electric toothbrush in the US—**Broxodent**
1980	First modified angulation of toothbrush—**Reach**
1987	First rotary action electric toothbrush for home use
2000	Low-price power toothbrushes become popular

- The first nylon bristle toothbrush, made with nylon yarn, went on sale on February 24, 1938 **(Fig. 27.4)**. The first electric toothbrush was invented in Switzerland in 1954 by **Dr Philippe-Guy Woog.**
- The first American electrical toothbrush in the United States called the **Broxodent** was released in 1960 by **Squibb**. General Electric introduced a rechargeable cordless toothbrush in 1961.
- In 1987, **Interplak** was the first rotary action electrical toothbrush for home use.
- **Johnson** and **Johnson** (1980), developed Reach toothbrush as the first to have a specialized design intended to increase its effectiveness.
- In January 2003, the toothbrush was selected as the number one invention (Lemelson-MIT survey).

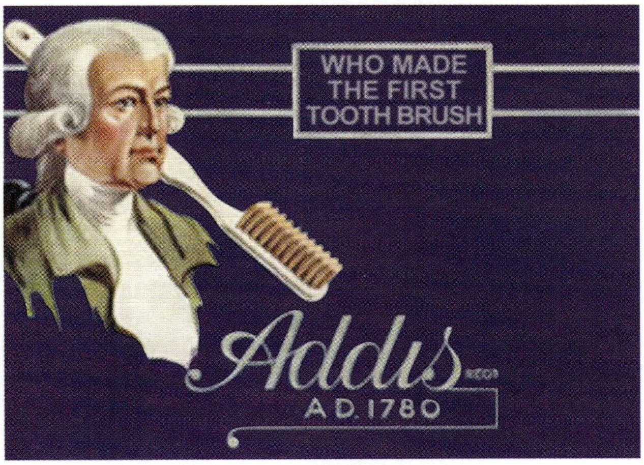

Fig. 27.3: First toothbrush by Addis.

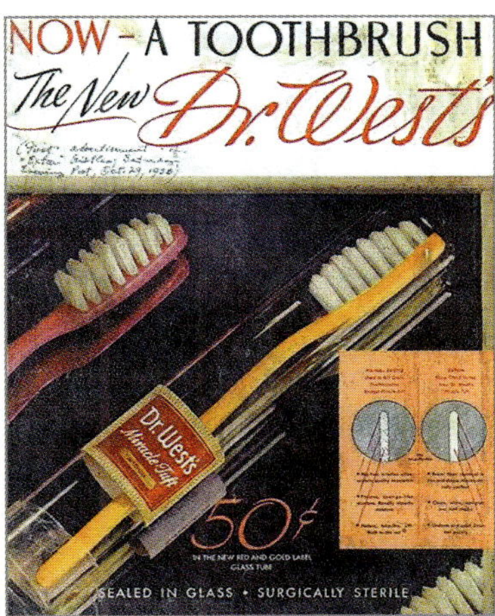

Fig. 27.4: First nylon toothbrush by DuPont.

Parts of Toothbrush

Toothbrushes should be able to reach and effectively clean most areas of the teeth. The type of brush is a matter of individual preferences. Parts of manual toothbrush include **(Fig. 27.5)**:

- **Handle**—grasped in the hand during tooth brushing.
- **Head**—the working part that consists of tufts of bristles or filaments.
- **Shank**—the location that connects the head and the handle.

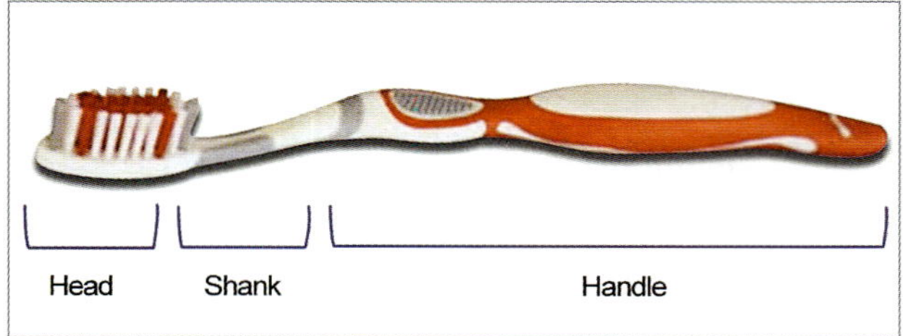

Fig. 27.5: Parts of manual toothbrush.

ADA specifications
- Length—1–1.25 in.
- Width—5/16–3/8 in.
- Surface area—2.54–3.2 cm
- No. of rows—2–4 rows of brushes
- No. of tufts—5–12 per row
- No. of bristles—80–85 per tuft
- Diameter for soft brushes—0.007 in., for medium brushes—0.12 in., and for hard brushes—0.014 in.

Types of Toothbrush Bristles

- There are two kinds of bristle material used in toothbrushes.
- Natural bristles from logs and artificial filaments made predominantly of nylon.
- Both types remove plaque; however, in homogenecity of the material, uniformity of bristle size, elasticity, resistances to fracture, and repulsion of water and debris, nylon filament is clearly superior **(Fig. 27.6).**
- Research has found out that soft nylon, multitufted bristles remove more plaque than hard bristles even when applying more pressure. It is also noted that brushes that have end-rounded filaments produce less gingival abrasion then filaments cut across.
- The recently introduced rippled bristle pattern may increase the efficiency of plaque removal especially in the proximal areas.

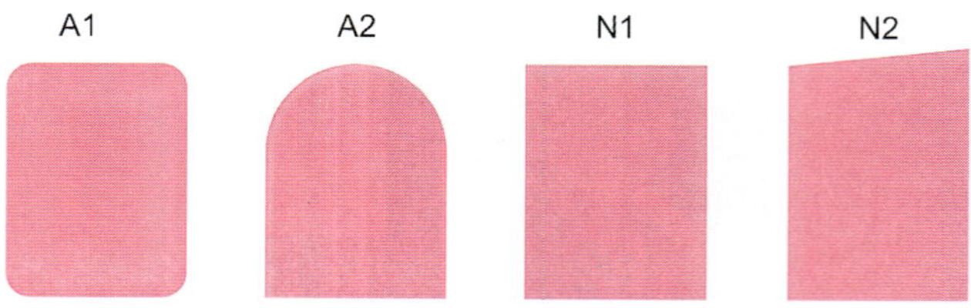

Fig. 27.6: Geometrical design of bristles.

Different types of toothbrush bristle patterns

Toothbrush	*Bristle pattern*
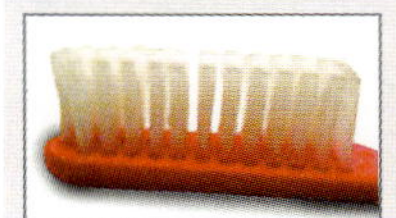	*Block pattern* The bristles are of the same length and are arranged neatly like a block
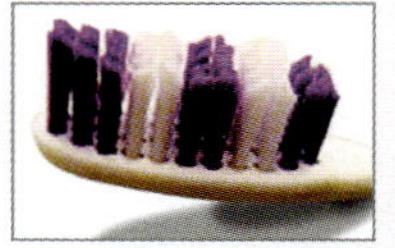	*Wavy or V-shape pattern* The bristles form a V-shape or wavy pattern. According to the manufacturer, this is intended to give the bristles a better contact with the areas around the adjacent tooth surfaces
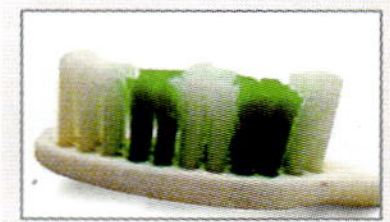	*Multilevel trim pattern* The manufacturer claimed that it enables the brush to reach difficult-to-clean areas
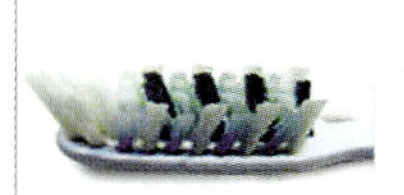	*Criss-cross pattern* According to the manufacturer, this design can lift up plaque effectively
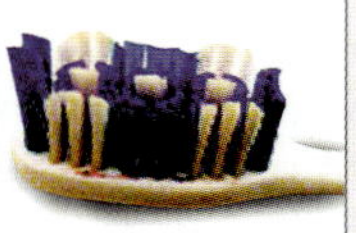	*Cross-action with gum stimulator* Removes plaque more efficiently and also stimulates gingiva
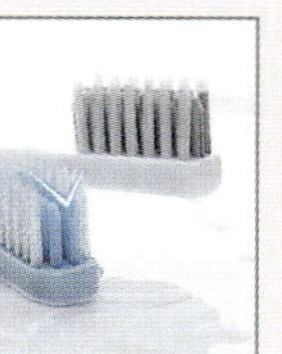	V or U groove brush are used in orthodontic patients for proper cleaning

Size of Toothbrush According to Age

A toothbrush with any kind of brush head cleans teeth effectively. However, the size of the brush head should be considered according to the size of the oral cavity.

Age	*Description*
0–2 years	Brush head size should be approximately the diameter of 15 mm
2–6 years	Brush head size should be approximately the diameter of 19 mm
6–12 years	Brush head size should be approximately the diameter of 22 mm
Above 12 years	Brush head size should be approximately the diameter of 25 mm

Types of Toothbrush Handles

Type of handle	*Feature*
Straight handle	All conventional toothbrushes have straight handles that are easier to control
Contra- angle handle	This handle design is similar to a dental instrument, intending to access to the difficult-to-clean areas
Flexible handle	This kind of handle intends to reduce gum injury caused by excessive brushing force
Grip handle	This handle intends to prevent the toothbrush from slipping away during toothbrushing

Frequency and Duration of Brushing

- ❖ **Jenkins** suggested that toothbrushing before meal is optimal.
- ❖ He says that saliva is a good remineralizing agent that will neutralize and buffer the lowered pH of oral fluids caused by acidic foods and fermentable carbohydrates.
- ❖ So, if toothbrushing is done after meals, it may remove saliva and decrease the remineralizing action **(Fig. 27.7)**.

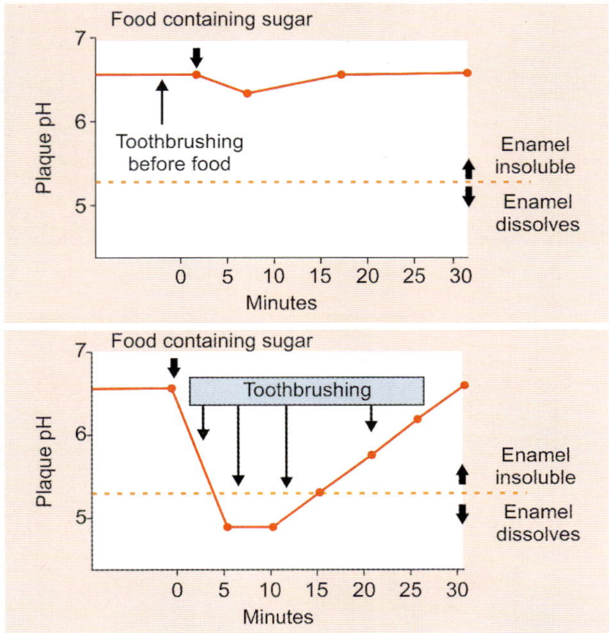

Fig. 27.7: Jenkins concept.

TOOTHBRUSH MODIFICATIONS AND CURRENT CONCEPTS

Powered Toothbrush

- ❖ The level of oral hygiene achieved by an individual is dependent on technique, motivations, dexterity, and perseverance. Since the behavioral practices cannot be modified, the greatest potential for improving oral hygiene will come from advancements of brush design that enhance plaque removal.
- ❖ First electric toothbrush **(Fig. 27.8)** was conceived in Switzerland in 1954 by **Dr Philippe-Guy Woog.**

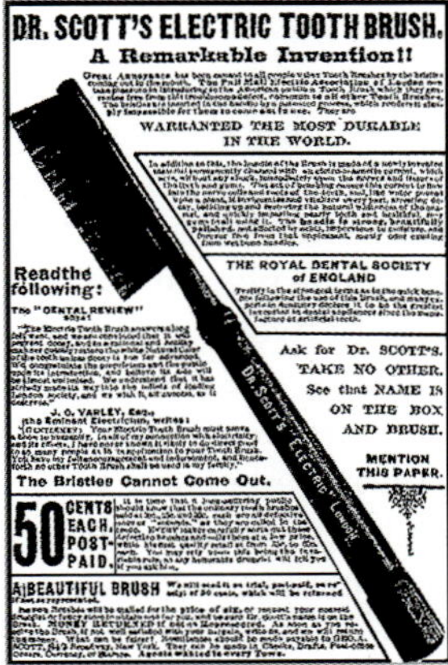

Fig. 27.8: First electrical toothbrush.

- ❖ The Broxo Electric Toothbrush was introduced in the USA by ER Squibb and Sons Pharmaceuticals 1959. After introduction, it was marketed in the USA by Squibb under the names Broxodent **(Fig. 27.9)**. In the 1980s, Squibb transferred distribution of the Broxodent line to the Somerset Labs division of Bristol Myers/Squibb.

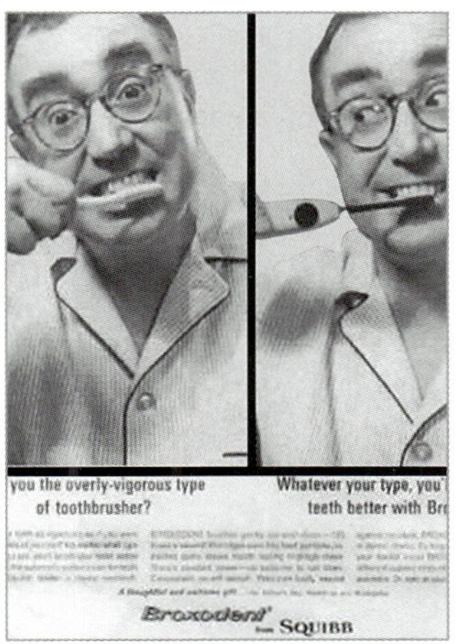

Fig. 27.9: Broxodent toothbrush.

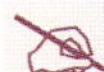

The first electric toothbrush was conceived in Switzerland *in 1954* by **Dr Philippe-Guy Woog** and was manufactured in Switzerland and later in France for Broxo SA. The device plugged into a standard wall outlet and run on AC line voltage. Electric toothbrushes were initially created for patients with limited motor skills, as well as orthodontic patients.

- ❖ The GE Automatic Toothbrush was introduced in the early 1960s; it was cordless with rechargeable NiCad batteries, and although portable, was rather bulky. The GE Automatic Toothbrush came with a charging stand which held the handpiece upright. Also, early NiCad batteries tended to have a short life span. The batteries were sealed inside the GE device, and the whole unit had to be discarded when the batteries failed.
- ❖ In 1987, Interplak was the first rotary action electrical toothbrush for home use.
- ❖ **Braun-Oral-B kids power toothbrush D10** is most effective in removing plaque in children. It has an oscillatory round brush head, so causes no soft tissue damage. It appeals to children as it plays music at 1-min interval thereby monitoring brushing time **(Fig. 27.10)**.

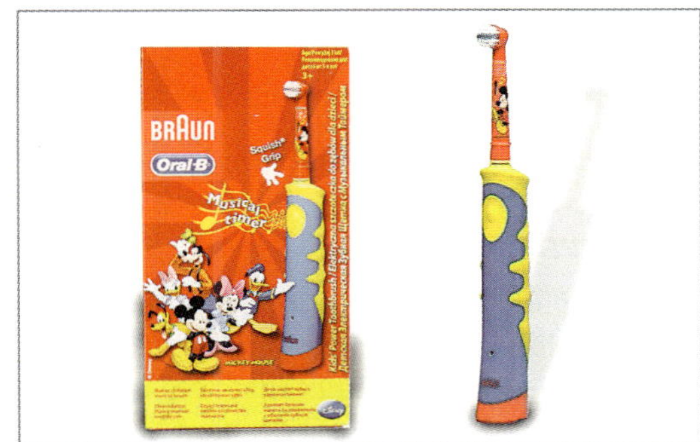

Fig. 27.10: Braun Oral-B kids power toothbrush D10.

- Current modifications of powered brushes have three motions:
  1. Back and forth
  2. Circular
  3. Elliptical.

Indications of powered toothbrush
- Individual lacking motor skill
- Handicapped patients
- Patients who have orthodontic appliances
- Whosoever wants to use.

Contraindication of powered toothbrush
- Hypersensitivity
- Patient with cardiac pacemaker

Advantages
- Better patient compliance
- Better accessibility in interproximal and lingual tooth surface
- Less brushing force
- Brushing time incorporated in some brushes

Disadvantages
- Cost and maintenance
- Noise and discomfort due to vibration

Difference between manual and powered toothbrushes

Characteristic	*Manual*	*Powered*
Brushing duration	20–40 s	1–3 min
Teeth brushed at a time	Multiple	One/multiple
Brush head motion	Cross and multiple	Minimal
Brush head speed	Zero	1,000 s/min
Brush head strokes	40–100/min	10–40/min
Brush head load	150–1,000 g	50–250 g

Generation of powered tooth brush

Generation	*Description*	*Example*
First	Powered by electricity, battery operated	Broxodent
Second	Vibrating, reciprocal, rotating head, rechargeable	Braun Oral-B, Interplak
Third	Sonic, rechargeable	Sonic care

ALTERNATIVE NEWER CONCEPTS IN TOOTHBRUSHES

Superbrush

- It is designed to simultaneously clean the outer, inner, and chewing surfaces of teeth.
- Three brush heads are combined together in the superbrush. When the brush is placed on the chewing surface, all the three surfaces of the tooth are cleaned simultaneously **(Fig. 27.11).**
- It shortens the brushing time.
- Mostly indicated in disable children.

Pulsar Toothbrush

- New concept in toothbrush technology where a pulsating chip is embedded on the base of bristles.
- Pulsar has soft vibrating bristles that help breakup plaque between teeth and facilitate easy removal.
- Oral-B Pulsar is first to incorporate this technology in manual toothbrushes **(Fig. 27.12).**

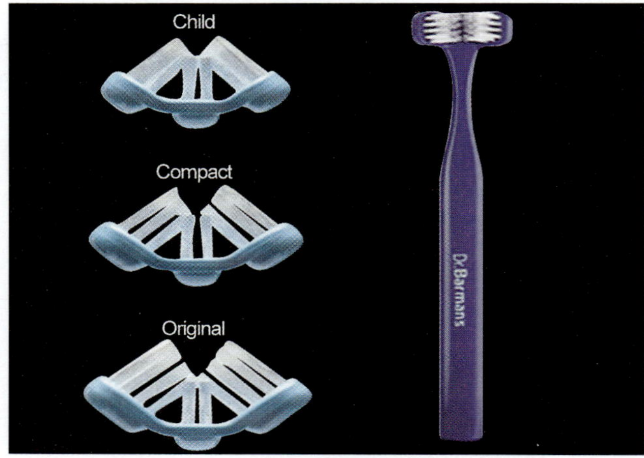

Fig. 27.11: Superbrush.

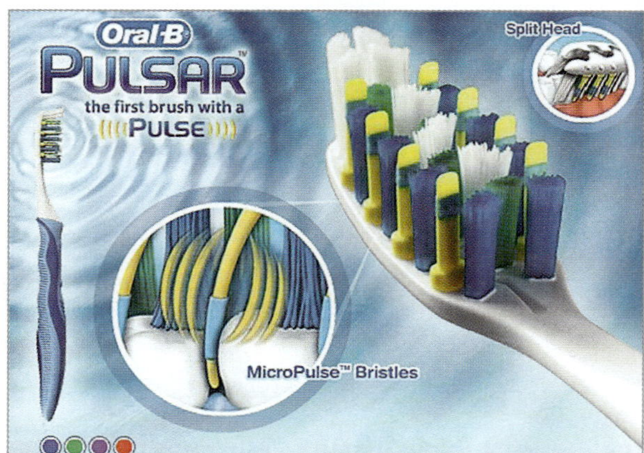

Fig. 27.12: Oral-B Pulsar.

Ultrasonic Toothbrush

- The newest development in this field is the ultrasonic toothbrushes, or simply sonic toothbrushes using ultrasonic waves to clear the teeth.
- In order for a toothbrush to be considered "ultrasonic," it has to emit a wave at a minimum frequency of 20,000 Hz or 2,400,000 movements per minute. Typically, ultrasonic toothbrushes approved by the FDA operate at a frequency of 1.6 MHz, which translates to 192,000,000 movements per minute.
- Any toothbrush operating at a frequency or vibration less than 2,400,000 movements per minute (20,000 Hz) is a "sonic" toothbrush. It is called sonic because its operating frequency (movements per minute) falls into the human hearing range of between roughly 20 Hz and about 20,000 Hz.
- Emmi-dent® is the first ultrasonic toothbrush that generates ultrasound with its patented ultrasonic microchip, which is embedded inside the brush head. This chip creates up to 96 million ultrasonic (air oscillations) impulses per minute, and transmits them via the bristles together

with the specially formulated Nano Bubble toothpaste onto the teeth and gums. This popular and revolutionary beyond sonic toothbrush is a unique method of cleaning your teeth and removing harmful bacteria even in hard to reach areas, and beats other toothbrushes in many ways **(Fig. 27.13)**.

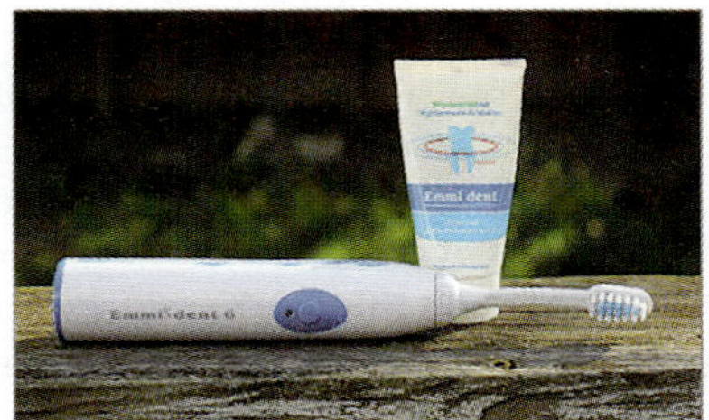

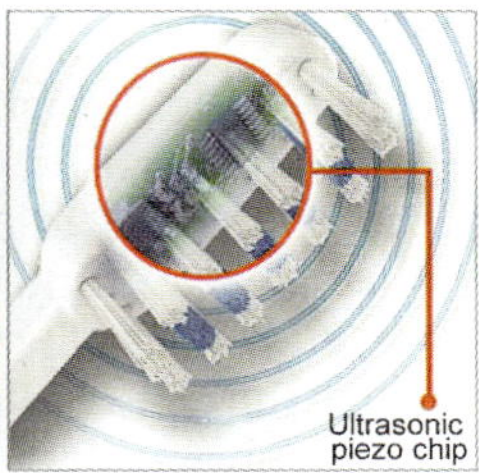

Fig. 27.13: Emmi-dent ultrasonic toothbrush.

Chewable Toothbrush

- A chewable toothbrush is a miniature plastic molded toothbrush that can be used when no water is available **(Fig. 27.14).**

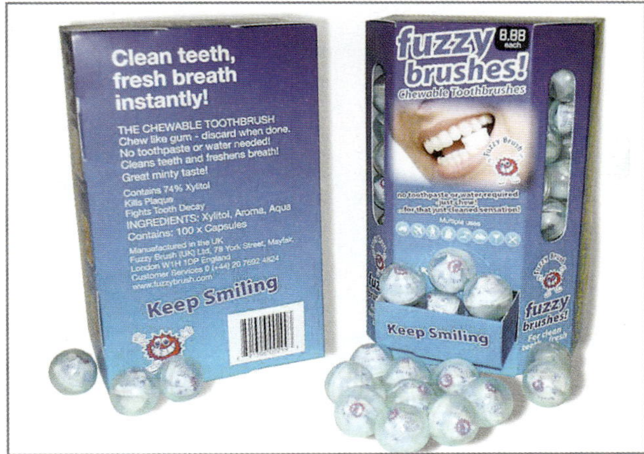

Fig. 27.14: Chewable toothbrush.

- They tend to be very small, but should not be swallowed.
- They are available in different flavors such as mint or bubblegum and should be disposed of after use.
- Other types of disposable toothbrushes include those that are a small breakable plastic ball of toothpaste on the bristles, can be used without water, and prove to be quite handy to travelers.
- **Bezgin et al**. in 2015 also conducted a pilot study on the effectiveness of chewable brush in removing plaque in children and found no adverse clinical signs or symptoms caused by the toothbrushes.

Possi Toothbrush for Kids

- Developed by Kyocera and Lion to make tooth brushing enjoyable for children.
- It has a ceramic piezoelectric element inside the head which turns electric signals into pulsation to transmit music directly without the use of external speakers **(Fig. 27.15)**.

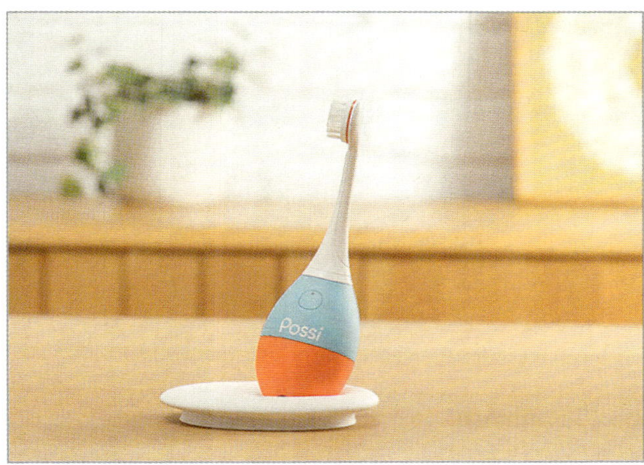

Fig. 27.15: Possi toothbrush for kids.

U shaped Toothbrush

- It is available for both children and adults. It is useful in patients with psychomotor difficulties.
- Available in manual, ultrasound and electric forms.
- Bristles are at 45° which promotes the Bass technique of brushing, yet till now they have not proved to be as effective as manual toothbrushing **(Fig. 27.16)**.

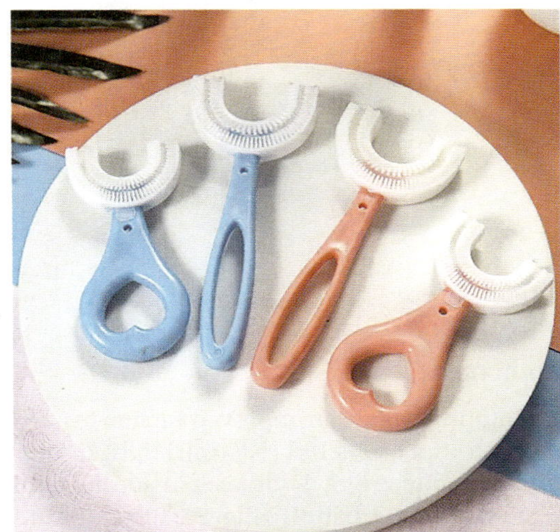

Fig. 27.16: U-shaped toothbrush for kids.

Ionic/Proton Toothbrush

- Ionic brushes work on the principle of polarity. They remove plaque through deposition of positive charged ions on the surface of the tooth. Plaque having the same charge, is repelled from the tooth surface and deposited on negatively charged bristles of the brush **(Fig. 27.17)**.
- The bonding between the pellicles and bacteria is mediated by Ca^{2+} bridge formation. The anions supplied by the lithium battery inhibits the bonding between the bacteria and Ca^{2+} and prevents the bacteria from adsorbing to the pellicles. Hence, the plaque accumulation is reduced because the abovementioned anions continuously supplied from the tips of the bristles of the ionic toothbrushes prevent the mild electrostatic bonding between the bacteria itself.

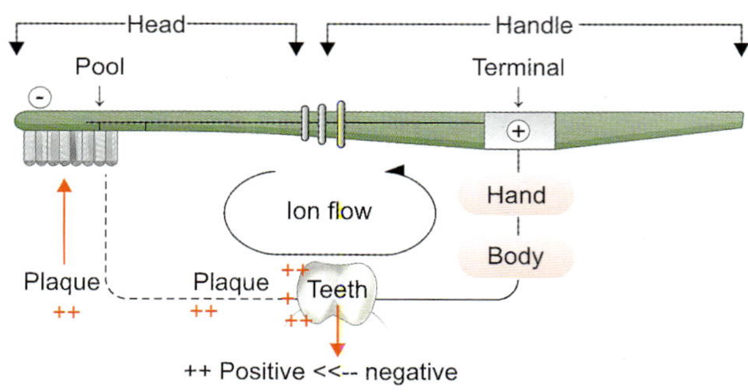

Fig. 27.17: Mechanism of ionic toothbrush.

Smart Toothbrush

- These advanced toothbrushes do not just restrict their functions of scrubbing teeth with a plastic handle; they also promote better oral health with less effort using their additional cleaning mechanisms **(Fig. 27.18).**

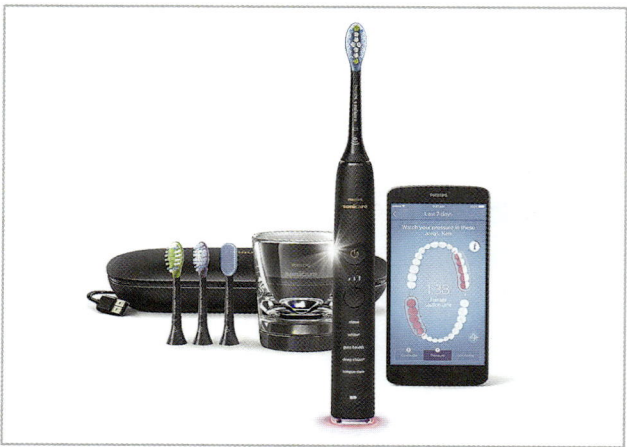

Fig. 27.18: Smart toothbrush.

Laser Toothbrush

- Laser toothbrushes are an improved version of the modern toothbrush that emits red (635 nm) light in the visible spectrum produced by a diode laser inside the toothbrush powered with an AA battery **(Fig. 27.19).**

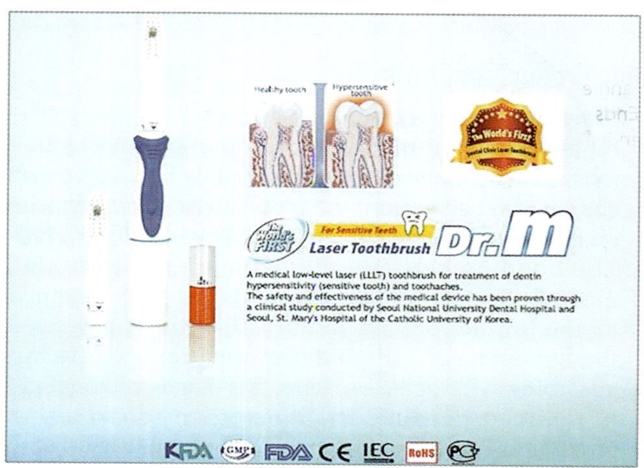

Fig. 27.19: Laser toothbrush.

- The LLLT with the help of such toothbrushes help to reduce dentinal hypersensitivity. Another advantage of using laser in toothbrush is that the patient can use it at home, which is cost effective, less time consuming and easily used by patients.

Tooth Towelettes

- These are being marketed as a method of plaque removal when tooth brushing is not possible.
- Finger brushes are mounted on the index finger of the brushing hand, and the agility and sensitivity of the finger are used to clean the teeth. Consequently, the pressure with which they are applied can be well controlled because the finger can actually feel the tooth and gingival surfaces and helps in positioning the brush for more effective scrubbing. **(Fig. 27.20).**
- However, the plaque removal efficacy of such brushes, in particular proximal plaque reduction is less than a regular manual toothbrush.

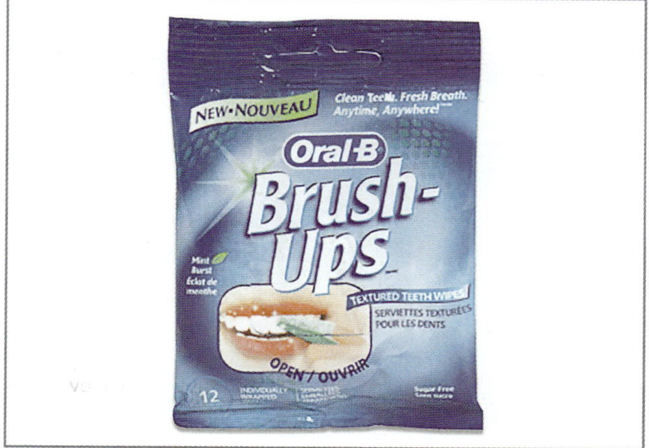

Fig. 27.20: Tooth wipes.

TECHNIQUES OF TOOTHBRUSHING

- There are six major techniques of toothbrushing **(Table 27.1)**, viz., scrub, bass, charters, fones, roll, and Stillmans.
- The most recommended technique for brushing in small children is scrub, followed by bass as they grow up after they achieve full manual dexterity.

TONGUE CLEANSING

- Tongue is one such structure which retains plaque and requires brushing.
- The tongue is anatomically perfect for harboring bacteria. The fungiform papillae create elevation and depressions in the tongue, which can house debris and microorganisms.
- The brushing of the tongue helps reduce the debris, plaque, and number of microorganisms.
- Place the head of the tongue cleaning brush **(Fig. 27.21)** near the middle of the tongue, with bristles pointed toward the throat, then the tongue is extruded, and the brush is

Table 27.1: Techniques of toothbrushing.

Method	*Bristle placement*	*Motion*	*Advantage/disadvantage*
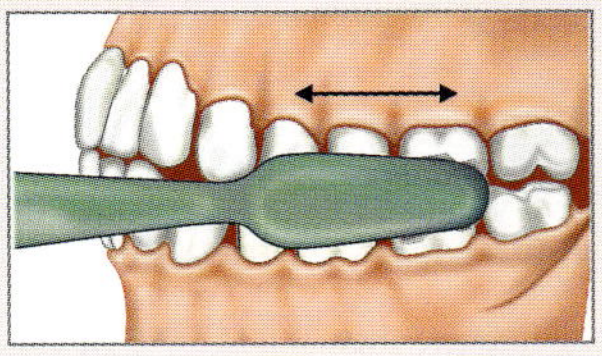 Scrub	Horizontal, on gingival margin	Scrub in anterior–posterior direction keeping brush horizontal	• Easy to learn • Best suited for children
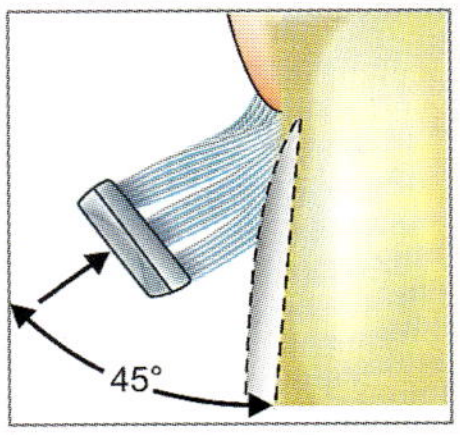 Bass	Apical, toward gingival into sulcus at 45°, to tooth surface	Short back and forth vibratory motion while bristles remain in sulcus	• Remove plaque from cervical area and sulcus • Easily learned • Good gingival stimulation
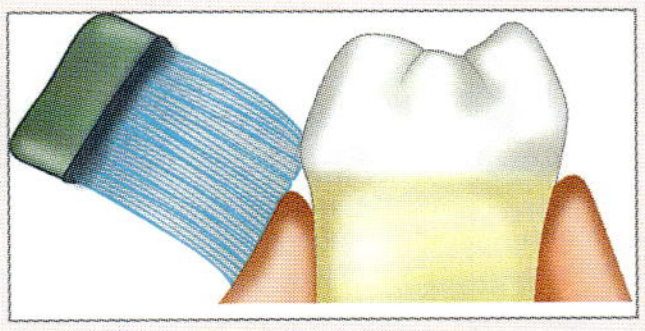 Charters	Coronally, 45°, sides of bristles half on teeth and half on gingiva	Small circular motions with apical movement toward gingival margin	• Hard to learn and position brush • Clears interproximal • Gingival stimulation
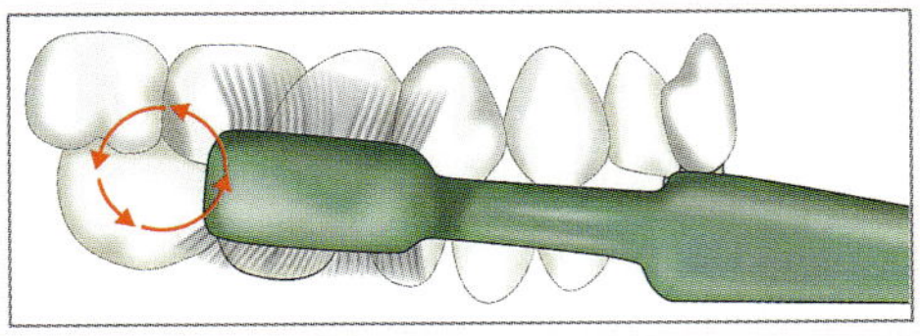 Fones	Perpendicular to the tooth	With teeth in occlusion, move brush in rotary motion over both arches and gingival margin	• Easy to learn Interproximal areas not cleaned • May cause trauma
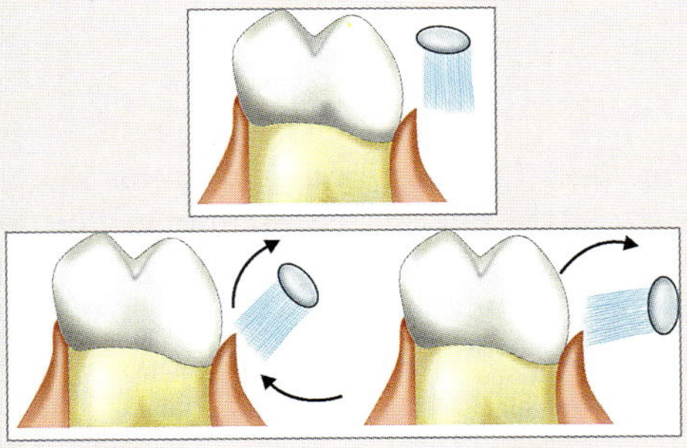 Roll	Apically, parallel to tooth and then over tooth surface	On buccal and lingual inward pressure, then rolling of head to sweep bristle over gingiva and tooth	• Does not clean sulcus area • Easy to learn • Good gingival stimulation
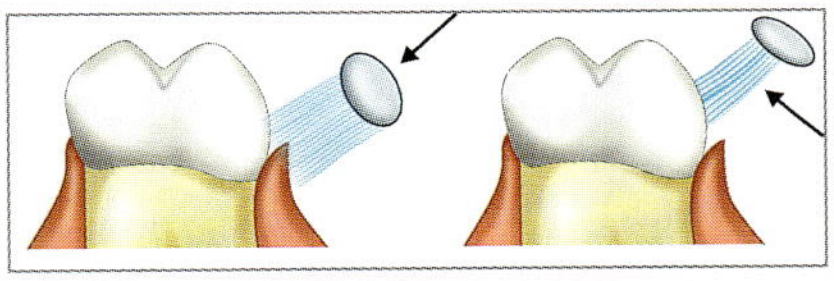 Stillman	On buccal and lingual, apically at an oblique angle to long axis of tooth. Ends rest on gingiva and cervical part	On buccal and lingual slight, rotary motions with bristle ends stationary	• Excellent gingival stimulation Moderate dexterity required Moderate cleaning of interproximal area
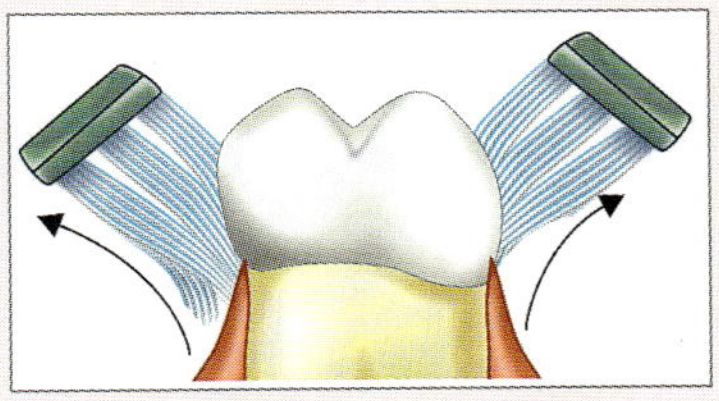 Modified Stillman	Pointing apically at an angle of 45° to tooth surface	Apply pressure as in Stillman method but vibrate brush and also move occlusally	• Good gingival stimulation Cleaning of interproximal area Easy to master

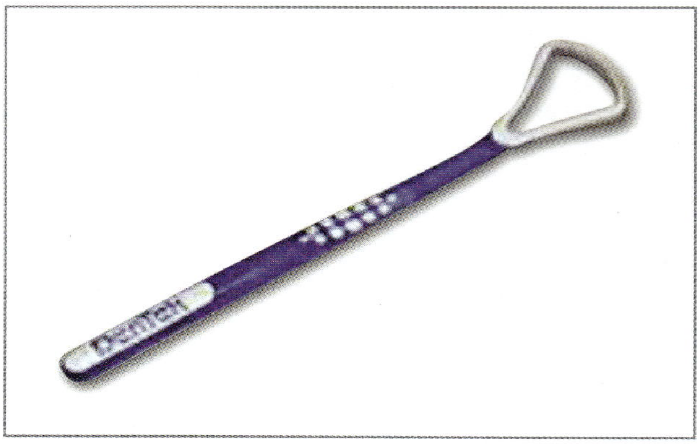

Fig. 27.21: Tongue cleaning brush.

swept forward, and this motion is repeated six to eight times.

- The patient is advised to use firm, overlapping scrub-type strokes starting at the back of the tongue and moving toward the tip.

INTERDENTAL CLEANING AIDS

Anatomy of the interdental area is a major factor in the selection of interdental aids. The most frequent interdental aids include dental floss, interproximal brush, wooden tips, oral irrigation devices, dental tapes, and end-tufted brushes.

Dental Floss

- First paper on dental floss was published by **Parmly** in 1819, and he is credited as the inventor of floss.
- Later in 1882, **Codman** and **Shurtuff** made first commercial floss made of silk. A lot of research had been going on about the different types of flosses and their benefits, but it was **Dr Charles C Bass** who in 1948, recommended that nylon floss is superior to silk.
- The Johnson and Johnson Company of New Brunswick; New Jersey was the first to patent dental floss in 1898.
- Size of dental floss can vary from 300 to 1,500 denier (D). Floss is constructed with the help of individual filaments 2–3-D thick.
- Floss is dispensed in boxes and can be readily used and disposed off from there **(Fig. 27.22)**. For additional ease of flossing, various floss holders are available throughout which vary in designs **(Fig. 27.23)**.

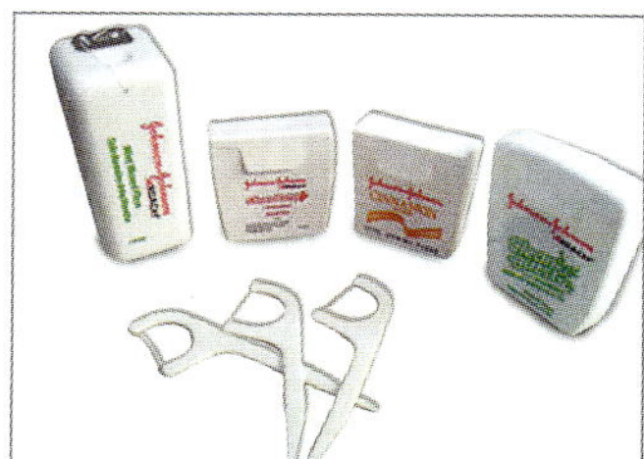
Fig. 27.22: Dental floss.

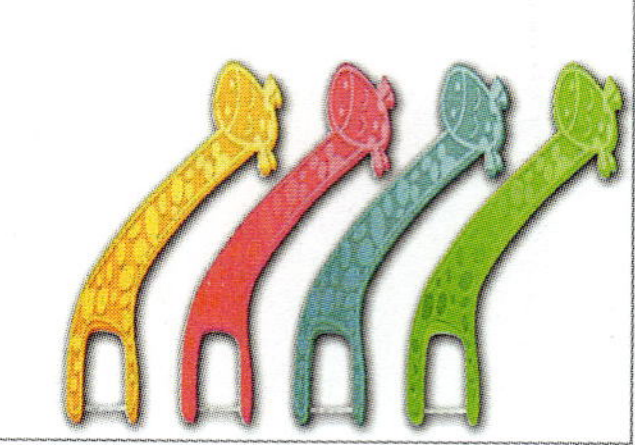
Fig. 27.23: Dental floss with holders.

Types of Floss

- Twisted and nontwisted
- Banded and nonbanded
- Thin and thick
- Microfilament and multifilament
- According to ADA specification
    - *Type I:* Unbonded dental floss composed of yarn having no additives.
    - *Type II:* Bonded dental floss composed of yarn having no additives other than binding agent or agent for cosmetic performance.
    - *Type III:* Bonded or unbonded loss having drug for therapeutic usage.

Method of Holding Floss

- *String floss method:* Use 18 in. of floss. Wrap 2–3 in. of floss around middle finger of left hand and similarly to the right hand **(Fig. 27.24).**

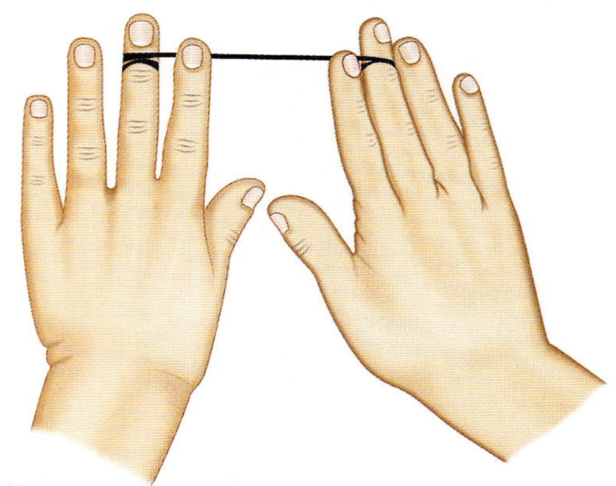
Fig. 27.24: String floss method.

- *Circle of floss method:* Take floss and tie a double knot to secure it. The size of the circle is like an orange. Position the knot to the left side of working area and place middle, little, and ring fingers of both hands on the inside of circle to keep it taut. Rotate counterclockwise for fresh segments **(Fig. 27.25)**.

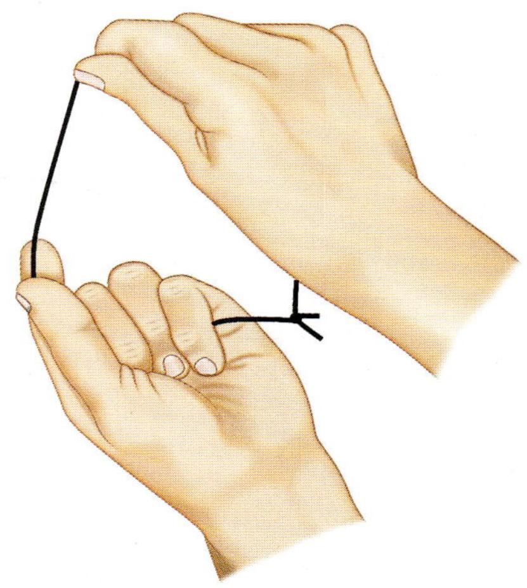
Fig. 27.25: Circle of floss method.

Techniques of Flossing (Figs. 27.26 and 27.27)

In a healthy properly contoured interproximal gingival tissue, the dental floss can be correctly inserted 2 to 3 mm below the tip of the papillae without causing damage to the gingiva

↓

Hold floss firmly in a diagonal or oblique position

↓

Guide the floss past contact area with a gentle motion

↓

Control floss to prevent snapping through the contact area onto the gingival tissue

↓

Maxillary teeth: Direct the floss by holding the floss over two thumbs or a thumb and an index finger. Rest a side of a finger on teeth of opposite side of the arch to provide balance and a fulcrum
Mandibular teeth: Direct the floss down by holding the two index fingers on top of the stand. One index finger holds the floss on the lingual aspect and the other on the facial aspect. The side of thefinger on the lingual side is held on the teeth of the opposite side of the mouth to serve as a fulcrum or rest

↓

Pass the floss between the gingival margin, curve to adapt the floss around the tooth, press, and side up and down over the tooth surface. Loop the floss over the distal surfaces of the mostposterior teeth in each quadrant and teeth next to edentulous areas.
Hold finely against the tooth and move the floss in both up and down motion

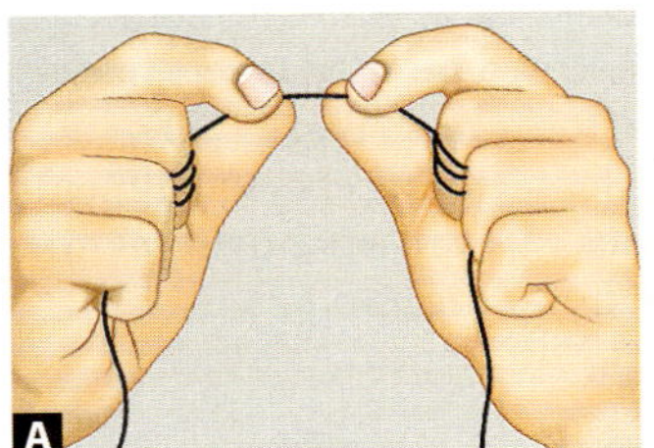

A

Step-1: Wind 18" of floss around middle fingers of each hand.
Pinch floss between thumbs and index fingers, leaving 1"–2" length in between.
Use thumbs to direct floss between upper teeth

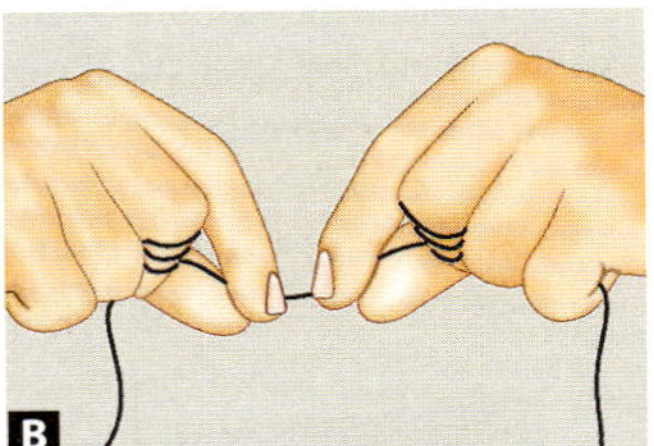

B

Step-2: Keep a 1"– 2" length of floss taut between fingers.
Use index fingers to guide floss between contacts of the lower teeth

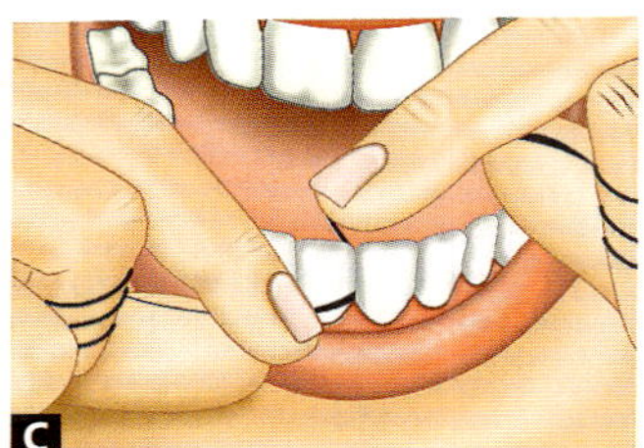

C

Step-3: Gently guide floss between the teeth by using a zig-gag motion. Do not snap floss between your teeth.
Contour floss around the side of the tooth

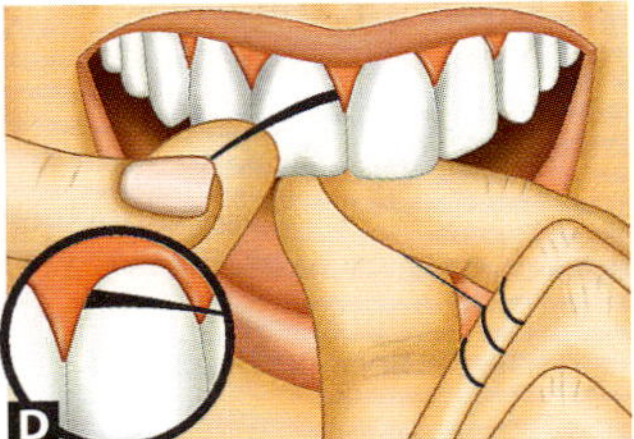

D

Step-4: Slide floss up and down against the tooth surface and under the gumline.
Floss each tooth thoroughly with a clean section of floss

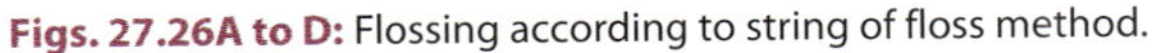

Figs. 27.26A to D: Flossing according to string of floss method.

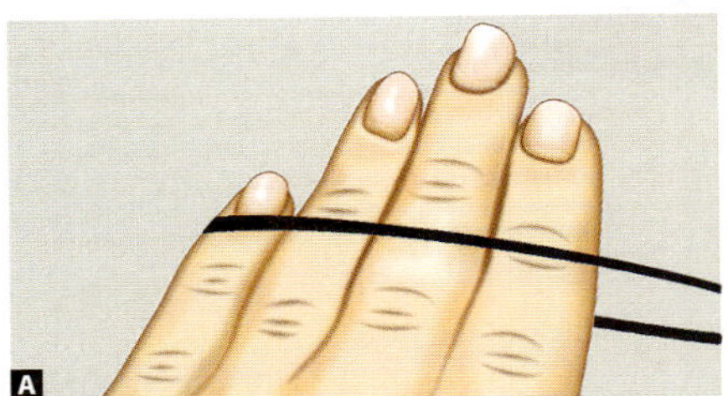

A

Step 1: Take a length of floss (waxed, up-waxed tape, etc.) about 10-12 inches.
Make the floss into a circle figners to just fit within it

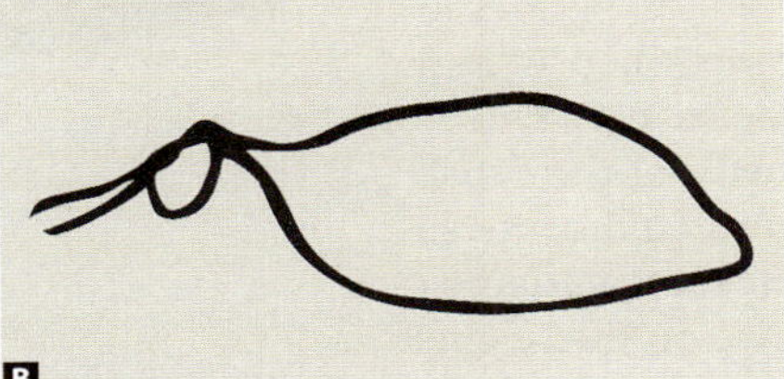

B

Step 2: Double knot the floss in a circle.
The knots must be in the same place–an old seamstress technique

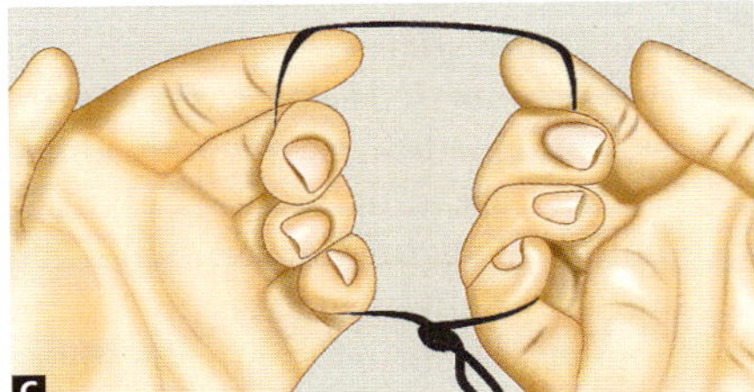

C

Step 3: This technique makes flossing much easier–no more fingers turning blue

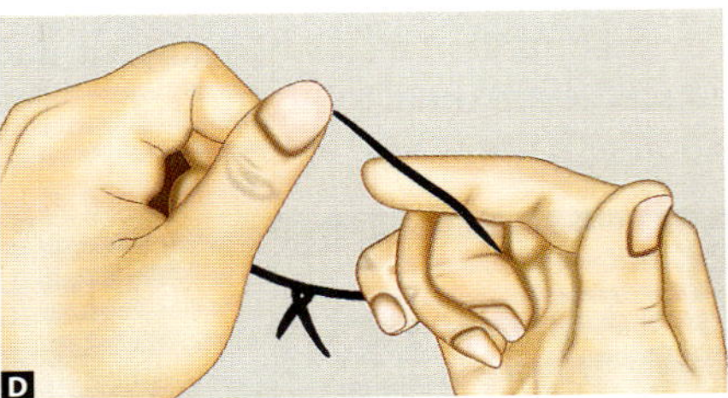

D

Step 4: To floss your upper teeth–place all fingers in the ring with floss over the left thumb and right index finger–floss upper left teeth

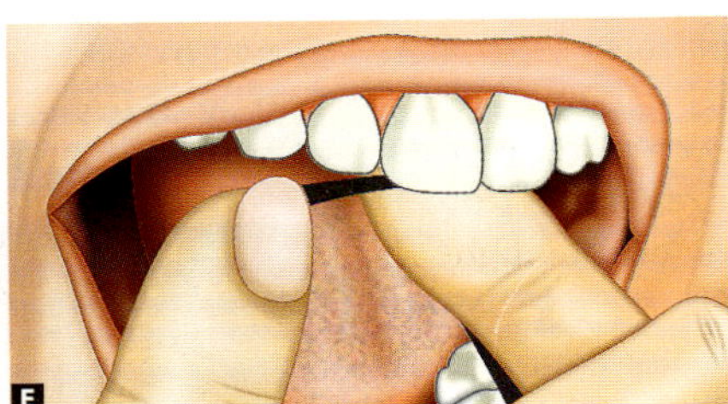

E

Step 5: Keep the floss taut at all times, no more than 1 inch between the thumb and index fingers

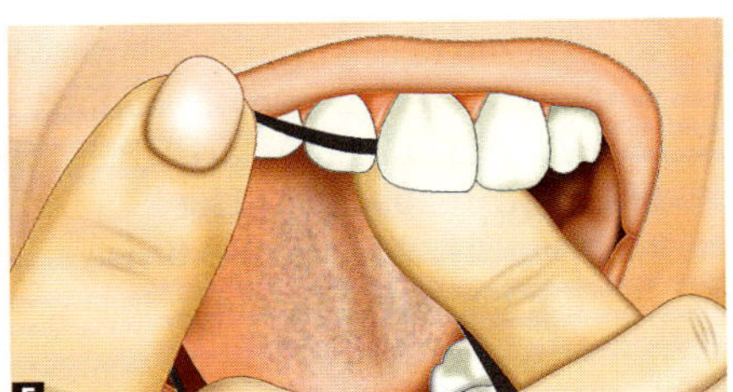

F

Step 6: Move the floss vertically; curving it gently up and down 3-6 times until the tooth feels "squeaky" clean

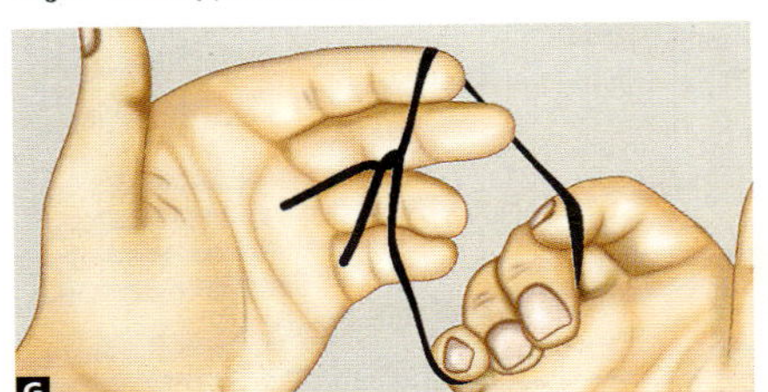

G

Step 7: Move around the cross-circle using a clean area of it for each tooth

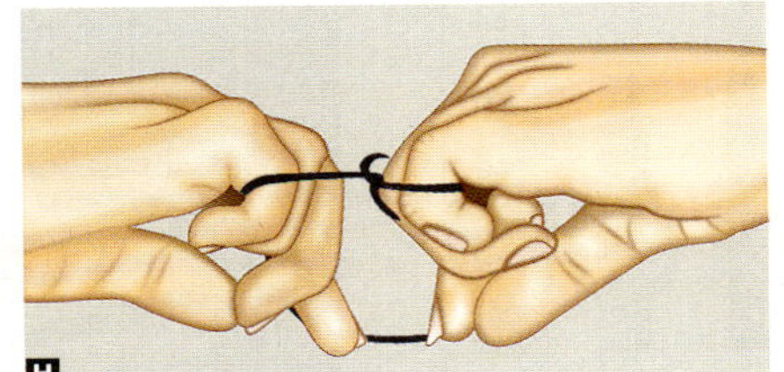

H

Step 8: Using both index fingers–floss all lower teeth

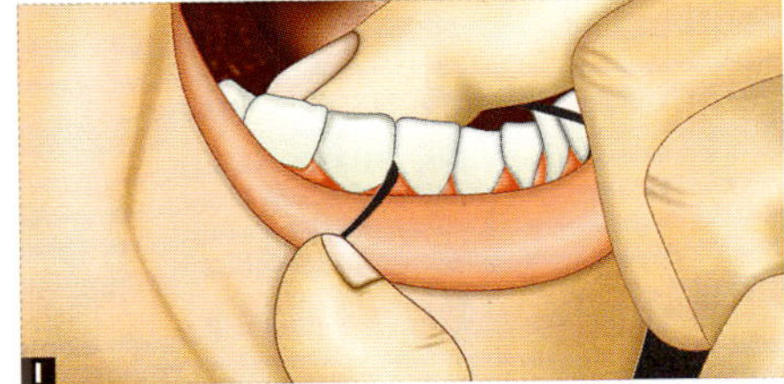

I

Step 9: Flossing thoroughly once a day before or after brushing should be enough to keep your gums healthy

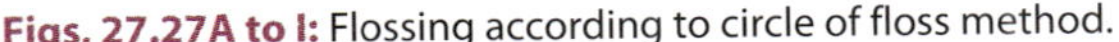

Figs. 27.27A to I: Flossing according to circle of floss method.

Additional Suggestions

- Slide the floss to a new, unused portion for succeeding proximal tooth surfaces.
- Floss may be doubled to provide a wide rubbing surface.

Precaution

- The col area is non-keratinized and is vulnerable to bacterial innervation. Too great a pressure with floss one or more times a day, particularly by fine floss that tends to tear more easily than the thicker floss, can be destructive to the attachment and is particularly significant in children in whom teeth are in the process of eruption, and the functional epithelium in less firmly attached.
- Do not use long piece of floss between the fingers when held for insertion.
- Snapping the floss through the contact area should be avoided.

Flossing for children
- Not all children can floss effectively.
- The ability to use floss is a function of age and manual dexterity.
- The ability to manipulate floss and remove plaque is highly dependent on hand and eye coordination and age.

Interproximal Brushes

- These are cone-shaped brushes made of bristles mounted on handle, single-tufted brushes, or small conical brushes.
- Interdental brushes are particularly suitable for cleaning large irregular or concave tooth surface adjacent to wide interdental spaces.
- They are inserted interproximally and are activated in short back and forth strokes in between the teeth.
- For best cleaning efficiency, the diameter of the brush should be slightly larger than the gingival embrasure so that the bristles can exert pressure on the tooth surfaces.
- Single tufted brushes are slightly effective on the lingual surface of mandibular molar and premolar, whereas a regular toothbrush is often impeded by the tongue.
- These brushes are classified as:
  - Tapered (Christmas tree appearance)
  - Nontapered (bottle neck appearance)
- Interdental brushes are classified according to ISO standard 16409:2006. The ISO brush sizes range from 1 to 7 **(Fig. 27.28)**. The ISO brush size is determined by the PHD or passage hole diameter in mm.

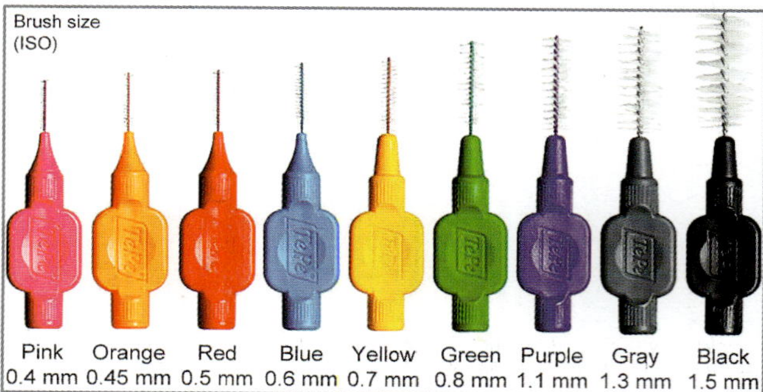

Fig. 27.28: Interproximal brushes.

Brush color	*Brush size*	*Wire size (mm)*	*PHD (mm)*
Pink	0	0.4	
Orange	1	0.45	≤0.8
Red	2	0.5	0.9–1.0
Blue	3	0.6	1.1–1.2
Yellow	4	0.7	1.3–1.5
Green	5	0.8	1.6–1.8
Purple	6	1.1	>1.9
Gray	7	1.3	
Black	7	1.5	

(PHD: passage hole diameter)

End-tufted Brush

- An end-tufted brush is a type of toothbrush used specifically for cleaning along the gumline adjacent to the teeth.
- The bristles are usually shaped in a pointed arrow pattern to allow closer adaptation to the gums **(Fig. 27.29)**.
- An end-tufted brush is ideal for cleaning specific difficult-to-reach areas such as between crowns, bridgework, crowded teeth, and fixed orthodontic appliances.

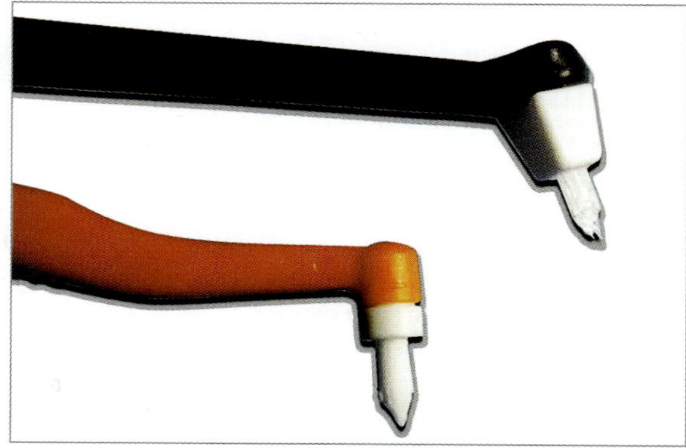

Fig. 27.29: End-tufted brush.

Wooden Tips

- Soft-triangular wooden tips such as a Stim-U-Dent **(Fig. 27.30)** are placed in the interdental space in gingiva, and they slide with contact the proximal tooth surface.
- Made up of bass wood or balsa wood.

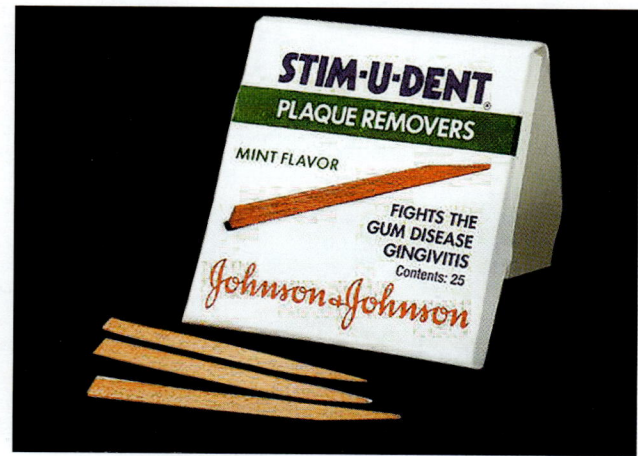

Fig. 27.30: Stim-U-Dent wooden tips.

- ❖ Repeatedly moved in and out of the embrasures, removing soft deposit for the teeth, and mechanically stimulating the gingiva.
- ❖ Use is limited to the facial surfaces.

Rubber Interdental Brush

It was found to be more efficient and comfortable than traditional interdental brushes by **NL Hennequin-Hoenderdos et al (Fig. 27.31).**

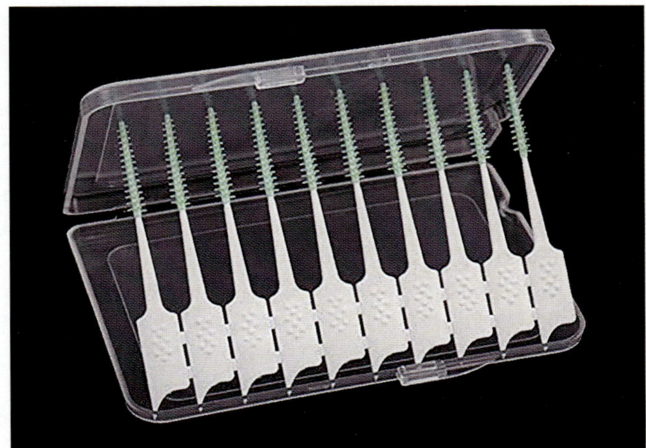

Fig. 27.31: Rubber interdental brushes.

Oral Irrigation

- ❖ Irrigation is the targeted application of a pulsated or steady stream of water or other irrigant for a cleansing and therapeutic purpose which can be done by the patient or the clinician.
- ❖ Oral irrigation cleans adherent bacteria and debris from the oral cavity more effectively than toothbrush and mouth rinse. They are particularly helpful for removing debris from inaccessible areas around orthodontic appliance and fixed prosthesis.
- ❖ When used as adjuncts to toothbrushing, these devices can have a beneficial effect on periodontal health by retarding the accumulation of plaque and calculus and by reducing gingival inflammation.
- ❖ Contraindicated in patients with advanced periodontitis and medically compromised patients like leukemia, AIDS, diabetes, bleeding disorders.
- ❖ It is delivered by:
  - ■ Power driven device **(Fig. 27.32)**
    - ◆ Generates an intermittent or pulsating jet of fluid.
    - ◆ An adjustable dial for regulation of pressure is provided along with a hand-held interchangeable tip that rotates 360° for application at the gingival margin.
  - ■ Nonpower driven device **(Fig. 27.33)**
    - ◆ It is attached to a household water supply and delivered through a hand-held interchangeable tip that can be used for application at the gingival margin.
    - ◆ Its disadvantages are uncontrolled water pressure and nonpulsatile water jet, thereby limiting its subgingival effect.

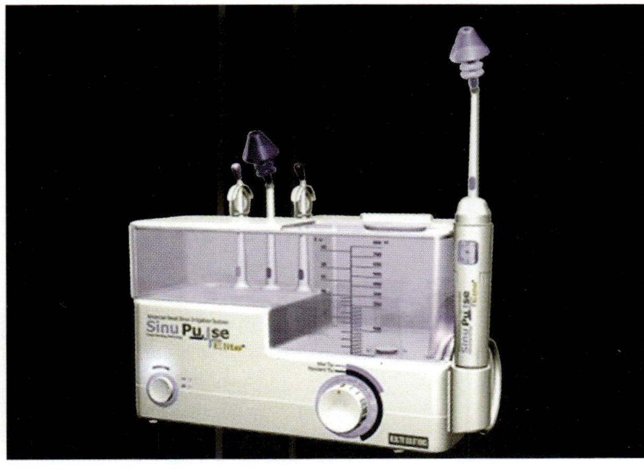

Fig. 27.32: Power driven oral irrigation device.

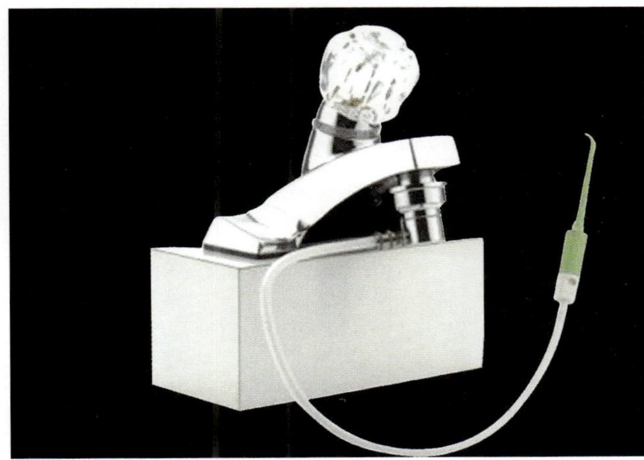

Fig. 27.33: Nonpower driven oral irrigation device.

Procedure of Irrigation

- ❖ The target of the oral irrigation in the loosely attached subgingival bacterial plaque.
- ❖ Some tips that are used to deliver the oral irrigants may be classified as:
  - ■ According to composition of tip—metal, rubber
  - ■ According to angulation—straight, angulated
  - ■ According to use—standard specialized

Pulsated irrigant is directed perpendicular to the long axis of the tooth

↓

Hydrokinetic activity is started

↓

Direct the jet tip towards the interdental area almost touching the tooth surfaces, hold tip at a right angle to the long axis of the tooth

↓

Start on the low pressure setting and increase gradually depending on the condition of the gingival tissue comfort

↓

The first is the impact zone when the irrigant makes an initial contact, and the second is the flashing, when the irrigant is deflected from the tooth surface and third action is lavage of irrigant in the subgingival region

↓

Follow a define pattern across the mouth, maxillary arch first then the mandibular arch applying for 5 to 8 sec at each interdental area

CHEMOTHERAPEUTIC PLAQUE REMOVAL

Classification of chemotherapeutic plaque removal agents	
Biguanides and related compounds • Chlorhexidine • Alhexidine	Fluoride and inorganic ions • Stannous fluoride • Hydrogen peroxide
Quaternary ammonium compounds • Cetylpyridinium	Antibiotics • Penicillin • Metronidazole
Enzymes • Dextranase • Glucose–amyloglucosidase	Organic compound • Sanguinarine • Menthol/thymol
First generation	Capable of reducing plaque scores by about 20%-50%. They exhibit poor retention within the mouth, e.g., antibiotics, phenols, quaternary ammonium compounds, sanguanarine
Second generation	Overall plaque reduction by 70%-90% and are better retained by the oral tissues. Exhibit slow release properties, e.g., chlorhexidine
Third generation	They block the binding of microorganisms to the tooth or to each other. As compared to chlorhexidine, they do not exhibit good retention properties, e.g., delmopinol

Chlorhexidine

- The dental profession has used chlorhexidine for over two decades. It is recognized as the primary agent for chemical plaque control, and its clinical efficacy is well known to the profession.
- In addition to having gained the acceptance of dental profession, chlorhexidine has also been recognized by the pharmaceutical industry as the positive control against which the efficacy of alternate antiplaque agent should be measured.
- It is a cationic bisbiguanide with broad-spectrum antibacterial activity, low mammalian toxicity, and strong affinity for binding to skin and mucous membranes.

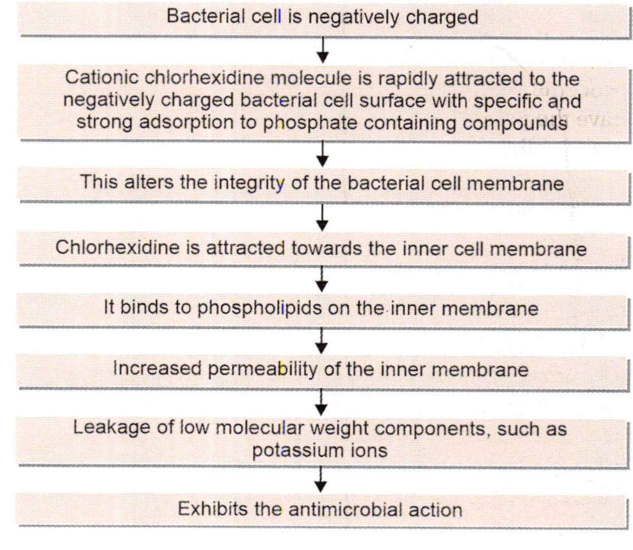

- Chlorhexidine has a wide spectrum of activity encompassing Gram-positive and Gram-negative bacteria, yeasts, dermatophytes, and some lipophylic viruses.
- Chlorhexidine shows different effects at different concentration. At low concentration, the agent is bacteriostatic, and at high concentration, it is bactericidal.
- Antiplaque mode of action: Chlorhexidine (0.12– 0.2%) binds to the different surfaces within the mouth (teeth and mucosa) and also to the pellicle and saliva. After a single rinse with chlorhexidine, the saliva itself exhibits antibacterial activity for up to 5 hours, whereas persistence at the oral surfaces has been shown for over 12 hours. The following are the mechanism of plaque inhibition:
  - An influence on pellicle by blocking the acidic groups on the salivary glycoprotein, thus reducing the protein adsorption to the tooth surface.
  - An influence on the adsorption of plaque onto the tooth surface by binding to the bacterial surface in sublethal amounts.
  - The key feature of chlorhexidine is its substantivity. Substantivity is the ability of an agent to be retained in the oral cavity and slowly released in its active form over an extended period of time.
  - An influence on the formation of plaque by precipitating the agglutination factors in saliva and displacing calcium from the plaque matrix.
- Disadvantages
  - Brownish reversible staining of teeth on restorations which may be associated with precipitation of "melanoids" from saliva. This may be enhanced by high lipid/carbohydrate diet.
  - Alteration in taste.
  - Rarely hypersensitivity has been reported.
  - Stenosis of parotid duct has also been reported.

Essential Oils

- These are the oldest form of mouthwashes. The most popular one being Listerine.
- It is a combination of the phenol-related essential oils, thymol, and eucalyptol mixed with menthol and methyl salicylate.
- Mechanism of action is by cell-wall disruption and inhibition of bacterial enzymes.
- **Goodson** (1985) has pointed out that most phenolic compounds have anti-inflammatory and prostaglandine synthetase inhibitor activity. Phenolic compounds are also known to act as scavengers of oxygen-free radicals (**Kuehl et al.,** 1977) and should have an effect on leukocyte activity.
- It has shown effectiveness in plaque reduction in the range of 20–34% and gingivitis reduction about 28–34%.
- Adverse effects include initial burning sensation and bitter taste in the mouth.

Quaternary Ammonium Compounds

- The agent most commonly used in this category is cetylpyridinium chloride at a concentration of 0.05%.
- This group of chemical agents is cationic and binds to the oral tissues, but not as strongly bisbiguanide. When used orally, they bind strongly to plaque and tooth surfaces but

are released from these binding sites more rapidly than chlorhexidine. This rapid release is one of the reasons why they are not as effective as chlorhexidine.
- Mechanism of action is related to their ability to rupture the cell wall and alter the cytoplasmic contents.
  - Adverse effects include a yellow brownish discoloration of the tongue and around gingival margin of the tooth, burning sensation, and occasional desquamation.
  - Commercial names are Cepacol (0.05%) and Scope (0.45%).

Triclosan

- Trichloro—2-hydroxydiphenyl ether.
- Triclosan is available in dentifrices and mouth rinses. It is more effective with zinc citrate or a copolymer of methoxy ethylene.
- Triclosan is both a Bisphenol and a nonionic germicide with low toxicity. It has broad spectrum of antibacterial activity and lack the staining effects of cationic agents.
- Since it does not bind well to oral sites due to its lack of a strong positive charge ions, therefore, it is used in combination with zinc citrate to take advantage of its potential antiplaque property; copolymer of methoxyethylene and maleic acid to increase its retention time, and combination with pyrophosphates to enhance its calculus-reducing properties.
- Triclosan also acts as an anti-inflammatory agent in mouth rinses. It has been shown to inhibit both cyclooxygenase and lipoxygenase and thus decrease synthesis of prostaglandin and leukotriene, which are key mediators in inflammation.

Sanguinarine

- It is currently used in both mouth rinse and toothpaste.
- It is an alkaloid extract from the bloodroot plant—*Sanguinaria canadensis.*
- It contains the extract at 0.03% (equivalent to 0.01% sanguinarine and 0.2% zinc chloride).
- 17–40% plaque reduction and 18–57% reduction in gingivitis is seen.
- The only adverse effect reported with this agent has been a burning sensation when used initially.

Propoile

- Naturally occurring bee product used by bees to seal opening on their hives.
- Consists of wax, plant extracts and contains flavones, flavanones, and flavonols.
- It has been shown that it had very low level of clinical effectiveness but significant plaque inhibitory action.

Stannous Fluoride

- In addition to decreasing the solubility of enamel to bacterial acids and enhance mineralization, stannous fluoride has shown a secondary benefit of inhibiting microbial plaque accumulation.
- Mechanism of action is that its interference with bacterial biochemical synthesis, metabolism, and aggregation.
- 0.04% concentration is the most effective.
- Available as an aqueous gel and suggested usage is one or two times daily.

Prebrushing Rinse

- PLAX is the only available agent.
- The chemical composition is sodium benzoate when combined with a soapy agent, it may have a surfactant action on plaque.
- Nonapproved by the ADA.
- Chemical plaque control has been shown to be effective for both plaque reduction and improved wound healing after periodontal surgery.

GUIDELINES FOR HOME ORAL HYGIENE

Prenatal Counseling

The goal of prenatal dental counseling is one counseling of education. Even before the baby is born, parents should be counseled on how to provide an environment that will nurture good oral health habits that contribute to life-long dental health for their child. Prenatal counseling can be quite effective because during this period, the parents are more open to health information for their children than during any other time.

The Infant

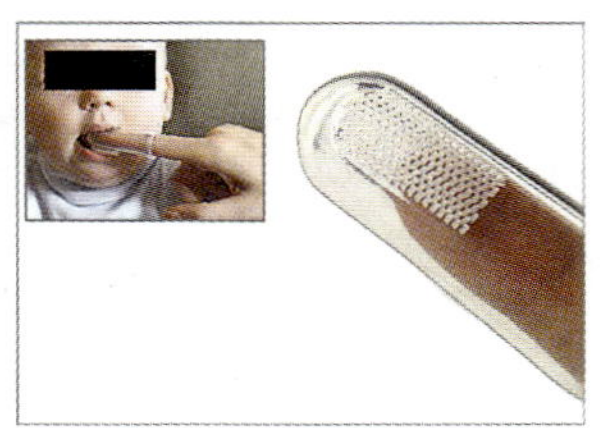

It is generally recommended that parents begin clearing the infant's mouth by the time first tooth erupts. It is suggested that secure and consistent physical support with slow, careful movement is to be employed at all time. Most have suggested that the parent wraps a damp washcloth or a piece of gauze around the index finger and clean the teeth and gum pads once a day. As more teeth erupt, the parent can begin using a small soft toothbrush. At this age, toothpaste is not necessary and may interfere with visibility for the parent. Additionally, the infant will be unable to effectively expectorate, causing unwanted toothpaste ingestion. Several methods of positioning the infants for daily oral hygiene procedures have been suggested. One effective method is to have the parent cuddle the infant in his or her arm with one of the child arms gently slipped around the parents back. In this way, the parent can stabilize the child with one hand and work with the other.

The Toddler

The parent should be totally responsible for oral hygiene of the baby, as for the infant. Establishing a specific routine is generally most convenient for parents and encourages the young child to develop good dental habits. As more teeth begin to erupt, parents should approach brushing systematically by beginning in one area of the mouth and progressing up in an orderly fashion. This is best accomplished by the use of a dampened, soft bristled toothbrush. If adjacent teeth are

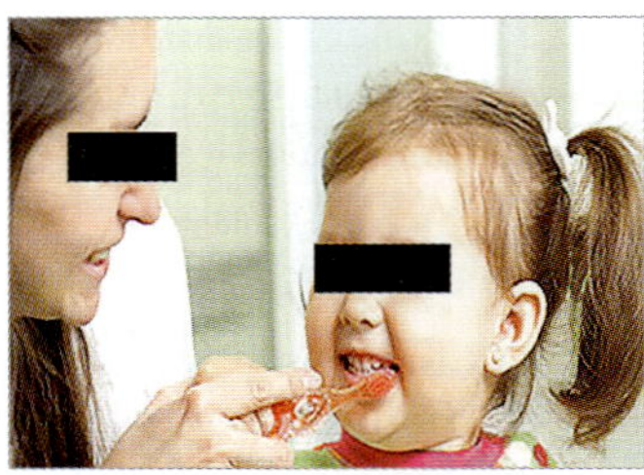

in contact, parents should also begin to floss these areas. Although parents still have the responsibility of performing a thorough, daily plaque removal for their babies, children at the age begin to demonstrate an interest in the procedure and a desire to take part. Parents should encourage this behavior and allow the child to attempt brushing procedures. Parents should, however, be advised that the child's efforts will be inadequate in thoroughly removing plaque. Therefore, the parent must perform a thorough plaque removal for the child at least once a day. As for the infant, it is important to the parent's methods of positioning and stabilizing the child so that the parents will have maximum visibility as well as control over the child's movements. The position selected for home plaque removal procedures will depend on the cooperation of the child. Many of the techniques employed with the infants may also be applied to the baby. One of the most effective positions is to have the parents face each other while the child is supine on the parent's knees. In this position, one parent assumes the role of brusher, while the other parent stabilizes the child. The preschool child is usually unable to expectorate effectively, and to any dentifrice that is placed on the toothbrush is generally ingested. Repeated ingestion of large amount of dentifrice may increase the systemic fluoride intake to undesirable levels. Thus, until the child can expectorate effectively, the parent should be responsible for dispensing the toothpaste and should place only a small pea-sized portion of dentifrice on the brush for the child.

The Early School Age Child

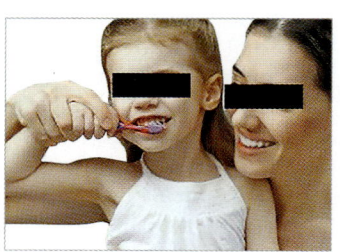

Because they are beginning to develop the necessary skill, early school aged children should be encouraged to routinely attempt brushing and flossing. However, the parent must continue to maintain the major responsibility by providing a thorough plaque removal for the child each evening before bed.

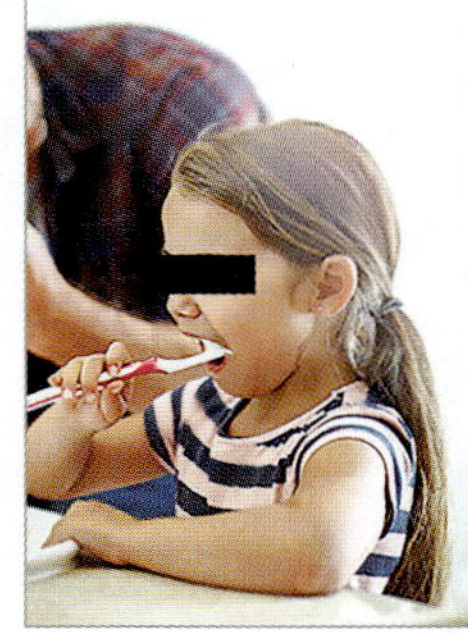

Disclosing agents may be particularly useful in this age group when one is teaching brushing and flossing techniques. The key to the success of an oral hygiene program for the preadolescent child is to encourage parents to reinforce the instructions given in the dental office. After the child attempts plaque removal procedures, the parent can promote learning by staining the teeth with disclosing solution and showing where the improvement is needed. The child should also be praised for his or her efforts when plaque has been successfully removed. Children in this age group, generally, demonstrate the ability to expectorate and should use a fluoridated dentifrice each time they brush.

The Preadolescent

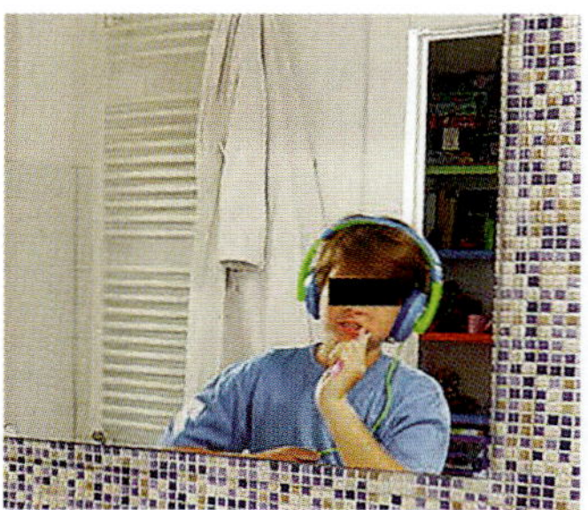

During preadolescence, the child will gradually assume more responsibility for his or her own hygiene. By 10 or 11 years of age, the child has often achieved the coordination necessary for effective brushing and flossing. The children in this age group require instruction on proper brushing and flossing techniques.

The Adolescent

The adolescent has generally attained the manual dexterity needed to properly brush and floss without direct help from an adult. Although children in this age group probably have the ability to adequately perform thorough oral hygiene procedure, they may lack the motivation to do so on a routine basis.

POINTS TO REMEMBER

- WHO defined bacterial dental plaque as a specific but highly variable structural entity resulting from colonization and growth of microorganism consisting of various species and strains embedded on an extracellular matrix.
- Plaque control is the removal of plaque and the prevention of its accumulation on the teeth and adjacent gingival surfaces. Mechanical plaque control is done by dentifrice, toothbrush, dental floss, oral irrigation, and interdental cleaning aids.
- Chemical plaque control is done mostly by mouthwash of chlorhexidine or other compounds.
- Two-tone disclosing solution was discovered by Block (1975) and has FD and C Green No. 3 and FD and C Red No. 3. It stains thicker (older) plaque stains blue and thinner (newer) plaque stains red.
- William Addis of England discovered toothbrush.
- The first nylon bristle toothbrush, made with nylon yarn, went on sale on February 24, 1938 by DuPont. The first electric toothbrush was invented in Switzerland in 1954 by Dr Philippe-Guy Woog.
- *ADA specifications of toothbrush:* Length—1–1.25 in., width—5/16–3/8 in., surface area—2.54–3.2 cm, No. of rows—2–4 rows of brushes, No. of tufts—5–12 per row, No. of bristles—80–85 per tuft.

- Jenkins concept states that toothbrushing before meal is optimal. He postulates that saliva is a good remineralizing agent that will neutralize and buffer the lowered pH of oral fluids caused by acidic foods and fermentable carbohydrates. So, if toothbrushing is done after meals, it may remove saliva and decrease the remineralizing action.
- Indications of powered toothbrush are individual lacking motor skill, handicapped patients, patients who have orthodontic appliances.
- The newest development in plaque control is the ultrasonic toothbrushes, using ultrasonic waves to clear the teeth.
- New concept in manual toothbrush technology is where a pulsating chip is embedded on the base of bristles that help breakup plaque by vibrations (Oral-B Pulsar).
- There are six major techniques of toothbrushing, viz., scrub, bass, charters, fones, roll, and Stillman technique. Scrub is the best method for brushing in small children, and bass is the best for older children.
- Flossing for children is difficult as the ability to use floss is a function of age and manual dexterity.
- Home oral hygiene guideline suggests that care of teeth must start as soon as they erupt by cleaning with warm gauze, later we can shift to use of finger brush. For infants, best is to position them in lap and do their oral cleaning; preschool children can usually accomplish brushing with parental help; preadolescent children can do the brushing on their own but under adult supervision, whereas older children can take care of their oral need like brushing and mouthwash on their own.

Questionnaire

1. Define dental plaque and enumerate the methods of plaque control.
2. Write a note on disclosing solutions.
3. What is the composition of dentifrices?
4. Explain the evolution of toothbrush.
5. What is Jenkins concept?
6. Write a note on powered toothbrush.
7. What are the newer modifications of toothbrush?
8. Explain various techniques of toothbrushing with special reference on the technique used in children.
9. What are interdental cleaning aids?
10. Write a note on chlorhexidine.
11. What are the guidelines of home oral hygiene for children from infancy to adolescence?

FURTHER READING

1. Addy M, Moran J, Davies RM, et al. The effect of single morning and evening rinses of chlorhexidine on the development of tooth staining and plaque accumulation. J Periodontal Res. 2000;134-40.
2. Biesbrock AR, Bayuk LM, Santana MV, et al. The clinical effectiveness of a novel power toothbrush and its impact on oral health. J Contemp Dent Pract. 2002;3:1-10.
3. Cochran DL, Kalkwarf KL, Brunsvold MA. Plaque and calculus removal: considerations for the professional. 2nd ed. China: Quintessence Publishing Co, Inc; 1994.
4. Deery C. The effectiveness of manual versus powered toothbrushes for dental health: a systematic review. J Dent 1999;32:197-211.
5. Gibson TA, Nash DN. Practice patterns of board-certified pediatric dentists: frequency and method of cleaning children's teeth. J Pediat Dent. 2004;26:97-9.
6. Grossman E, Proskin H. A comparison of the efficacy and safety of an electric and a manual children's toothbrush. J Am Dent Assoc. 1997;128:469-74.
7. Kimmelman BB, Tassman GL. Research in design of children's toothbrushes. J Dent Child. 1960;27:60-4.
8. McClure DB. A comparison of toothbrushing techniques for the preschool child. J Dent Child. 1966;33:205-10.
9. Mentes A, Atukeren J. A study of manual toothbrushing skills in children aged 3 to 11 years. J Clin Pediatr Dent. 2002;27:91-4.
10. Schonfeld SE, Farnoush A, Wilson SG. In vivo antiplaque activity of a sanguinarine-containing dentifrice: comparison with conventional toothpastes. J Periodontal Res. 2004;21:298-303.
11. Wright GZ, Banting DW, Feasby WH. Effect of interdental flossing on the incidence of proximal caries in children. J Dent Res. 1977;56: 574-8.
12. Wojtyla C, Ciebiera M, Kowalczyk D, Panek G. Cervical cancer mortality in East-Central European Countries. Int J Environ Res. Public Health. 2020; 17(13): 4639.
13. Chandra S, Jain N, Garg R, et al. Ionic vs manual toothbrushes: Effect on plaque and oral hygiene status in children. Int J Clin Pediatr Dent. 2019;12(5):375-8.)
14. NL Hennequin-Hoenderdos, et al. Efficacy of a rubber bristles interdental cleaner compared to an interdental brush on dental plaque, gingival bleeding and gingival abrasion: A randomized clinical trial. Int J of Dental Hygiene. 16 (3); 2018, 380-88.
15. Mandal A, Singh DK, Siddiqui H, Das D, Dey AK. New dimensions in mechanical plaque control: An overview. Indian J Dent Sci. 2017;9:133-9.

CHAPTER 28

Plaque Control for the Differently-abled Child

Nikhil Marwah, Koya Srikanth, Jyoti S Isaac

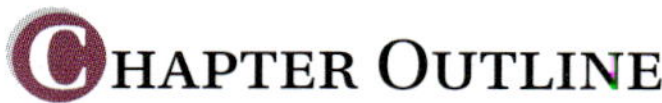

Chapter Outline

The aim of plaque removal procedures is to disrupt the bacterial plaque that accumulates on the teeth and to remove food debris from tooth surfaces. These procedures result in better periodontal health and to some extent a reduction in caries. The most effective approach is still frequent mechanical disruption of the plaque material by means of tooth brushing and flossing. It is important to begin cleansing procedures as soon as primary teeth erupt. When a parent or another adult performs the cleansing procedure for a small child, proper positioning of the child is crucial. The position chosen must provide support for the child's head and body, provide adequate visibility and must be near a good source of light. The dental professional who is teaching the procedure should evaluate the abilities of each person involved and recommend an appropriate position.

Home dental care should begin in infancy; the dentist should instruct the parents to gently cleanse the teeth daily with a soft cloth or an infant toothbrush. For older children who are unwilling or physically unable to cooperate, the dentist should teach the parent or guardian correct toothbrushing techniques to safely restrain the child when necessary. The goals and purpose of preventive dental services for persons with severe disabilities, including personal oral hygiene (POH) procedures, are no different than those for the general population. However, the physical, cognitive, and behavioral limitations presented by severely differently-abled individuals require modification of usual preventive practices including the choice of materials and techniques utilized. Although the dentist maintains overall responsibility for preventive as well as restorative services, the dental hygienist together with other auxiliaries usually are the dental professionals most involved with these programs.

DEVELOPMENT OF A PERSONAL ORAL HYGIENE PROGRAM

- The dental hygienist usually leads the dental team in the development and monitoring of an individual's POH program.
- This program is developed utilizing information obtained at the first dental examination, discussions with appropriate direct care staff, consultations with other professionals from the program team, and occasionally from visits to the residential area where oral hygiene procedures will be carried out.
- Pertinent information including the person's cognitive and physical limitations and abilities, the ability to cooperate with POH procedures, the level of periodontal health and caries risk, the level and rate of plaque, and calculus accumulation, significant drugs used (including sugar content) and type, and consistency of diet will impact the selection and prescription of specific POH techniques.
- The procedures prescribed include toothbrush selection and use, flossing techniques and materials (e.g., floss holder) needed, antimicrobial agents prescribed, mouth props or restraints required, and positioning techniques indicated.
- One of the vital components of a successful POH program is monitoring to determine if the procedures are being performed as prescribed. This will allow the dental practitioner to evaluate the program's effectiveness and make modifications as needed. Monitoring is often accomplished using a "checklist" or other measurements of staff compliance with prescribed procedures.

Evaluation of effectiveness is often made at the time of recall.

LEVEL OF CAREGIVER SUPPORT

The level of mental functioning and the individual's capacity for interaction with others dictates the level of home care that can be performed by the individual and his/her degree of dependency on the caregiver. There are numerous strategies for categorizing the level of caregiver support necessary for adequate oral hygiene. One of these includes the following categories:

- Independent toothbrushing—no assistance.
- Partial independent toothbrushing—with staff assistance including prompting by verbal instructions or by physical manipulation (staff's hand over person's hand).
- Complete staff dependence requiring no significant behavior management.
- Complete staff dependence requiring head stabilization, lip retraction, and mandibular pressure to maintain oral access; or
- Complete staff dependence requiring more than one staff person. The additional staff person(s) would provide physical stabilization of the person necessary for adequate oral hygiene procedures to be safely completed.

ORAL HYGIENE AIDS

Devices used in the mouth to control plaque should be selected on an individual basis and training in their use is necessary to prevent damage to oral tissues. There are a wide variety of oral care products available for use. When deciding on the appropriate devices to be tried, the following issues should be considered:

- Ability of the individual or caregiver performing daily oral hygiene.
- Time constraints placed on staff or caregiver.
- Level of person's cooperation.
- Physical and environmental conditions where oral care is provided.
- Degree of parent involvement.
- A plaque control program is essential in monitoring oral hygiene in the special child and determining the level of success achieved by each patient. The brushing technique for these patients, who have fine or gross motor deficiencies limiting their ability to brush should be effective as well as simple for the person performing the brushing. Often recommended technique is the horizontal scrub method because it is easy to perform and yields good results. This technique consists of performing gentle horizontal strokes on cheek, tongue and biting surfaces of all teeth and gums. Other patients with special health care needs without such motor problems can use age-appropriate techniques.

Toothbrush

- The choice of a toothbrush for persons with disabilities is often the same as for the general population.
- Usually a soft nylon bristle, rounded end, multitufted brush with a long strong neck is the preferred choice. Brushes with longer handles facilitate reaching the posterior teeth. The size of the brush head is determined by the size of the oral cavity and the person's ability to open.
- As with any individual, the proper application of the toothbrush is far more important than toothbrush choice.
- There are numerous commercially available modified toothbrushes that have been designed for special patients. This usually entails the modification of the handle and special designs for bristle placement. A list including description and source of some modified brushes and other materials currently available are presented in **Table 28.1.**
- Several studies have found the automatic toothbrush to be superior to manual brushes for some individuals.
- However, most studies that compare the effectiveness of toothbrush choices, whether manual, adapted, commercially modified, or automatic, have found that improvement in oral hygiene levels occurs regardless of which toothbrush is used, indicating that toothbrush choice is far less important than conscientious use and follow-up.

Toothbrush Modifications

- The most common tool for effective mechanical control of dental plaque is a toothbrush, but the presence of physical and/or cognitive disabilities can create difficulties both in holding and manipulating a toothbrush.
- For patients whose main deterrent to personal self-care is related to grasp, manipulation, or control of the brush, adaptations have been devised which include enlarged handles, hand attachments, and elongated handles.
- The aim of the toothbrush adaptation is to provide a handle with a stable grip, whilst its shape enables the person to feel how to manipulate the brush in the mouth adequately during cleaning.
- **Grasp:** For people who cannot grasp and hold, the objective is to fasten the brush handle to the hand. This can be achieved by using a Velcro strap with a pocket on the palm side into which the toothbrush can be inserted **(Fig. 28.1).**
- **Fixed fingers:** For a patient with fingers permanently flexed or fixed in a fist, toothbrushes with variation in the grip and handle width in all shapes and sizes are available commercially, and a suitable brush that inserts directly into the patient's grasp can be selected **(Fig. 28.2).**

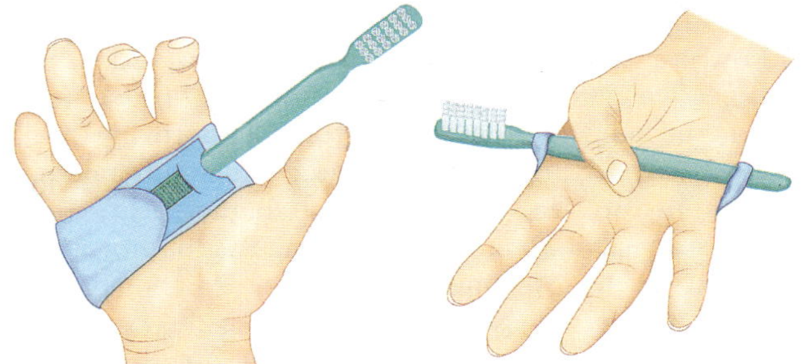

Fig. 28.1: Velcro strapped brush. (*Source:* Picture from https://www.nidcr.nih.gov/imagegallery/oralhealth/ ToothbrushAdaptations.htm).

Table 28.1: Commercially available modified toothbrushes.

Brush name	Description	Findings
Collis Curve®	Three rows of bristles, outer two rows are curved inward with a single short straight row running down the center	The Collis Curve brush is a popular, commercially available adapted brush. It has the advantage of being able to cover buccal, occlusal, and lingual surfaces simultaneously
Improve®	Standard-shaped head with the bristles arranged in a deep "V" groove design	Position over teeth to do simultaneous lingual–buccal brushing. However, when one side is at 45° angle, then other side no longer makes contact with the corresponding gingiva and cervical surface
Action 2®	Double-headed brush with sides angled at 45°	This brush is very difficult to insert correctly, and when in the mouth, the heads are too small to cover the crowns and reach the gingiva
Twinbrush®	Twin heads angled at 45° with outside rows softer than inside rows	Easy to use and insert and seems to work best with a small amount of toothpaste. It is most effective for brushing the lingual posteriors. Brush by placing over the anterior teeth and moving backward
Omniadent®	A six-sided brush with very small heads to allow brushing of all surfaces (both arches) at the same time	This brush is very impractical. The double side is not as useful as the size of the brush makes it uncomfortable to use and interproximal tips are too large to clean as they are intended
Vac-U-Brush®	A suction brush designed for bedside use on patients who may be at risk of aspiration while receiving mouth care. It has a moderate length, wide handle with a suction attachment on the end	The brush fits easily on all the bedside suction units tested. The head is small enough for a child-size mouth. The handle is able to be maneuvered comfortably by the operator. The head is small with a row of soft bristles set in a horseshoe pattern with a suction groove in the center for fluid removal
Colgate Plus®	Diamond-shaped head with a long-curved handle. The outer bristles are very soft while the inner bristles are more firm	The tapered head may help in insertion when the patient remains clenched. The long handle is comfortable and helps to reach the posteriors
Flex (Aquafresh)®	Large, tapered head with soft bristles. The handle is long with section that is bent into a fan-like arrangement	Except for the textured handle which offered a more secure grip, this brush did not offer any benefit over a standard tapered head brush. The flexed section did not seem to serve any real purpose
Radius®	Brush has a larger than average head with soft nylon bristles and large built-up handle shaped for left or right hands	The larger head allows for all sides to be brushed at the same time. Also available in child size

- **Limited hand closure or reduced manual dexterity:** Objective is to enlarge the diameter of the brush handle to fit the hand. The simplest method of improving the grip involves inserting the brush handle into another material to improve its size, shape, or surface characteristics. Simple and successful methods of adapting the toothbrush grip include the use of sponges, tubing, bicycle handlebar grips, or pushing it into a soft rubber ball **(Fig. 28.3).**
- **Manipulation:** For those patients who can position a toothbrush but cannot manipulate it sufficiently to clean all the surfaces of the teeth, double-headed brushes are useful and commercially available. **Kaschke et al.** in his trial to evaluate the effectiveness of different toothbrushes showed that a three-headed brush (such as the "Superbrush") performed best for adults who otherwise required help with their toothbrushing **(Fig. 28.4)**. Use of powered toothbrush is also best indicated in these individuals.
- **Limited shoulder or arm movement:** For this group of people, where there is limited arm and hand movement, the objective is to lengthen the handle of the brush with a material strong enough to maintain the brush in contact

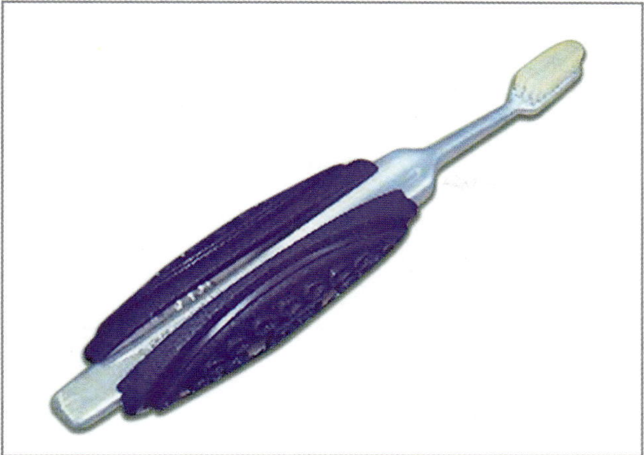

Fig. 28.2: Gripped toothbrush.

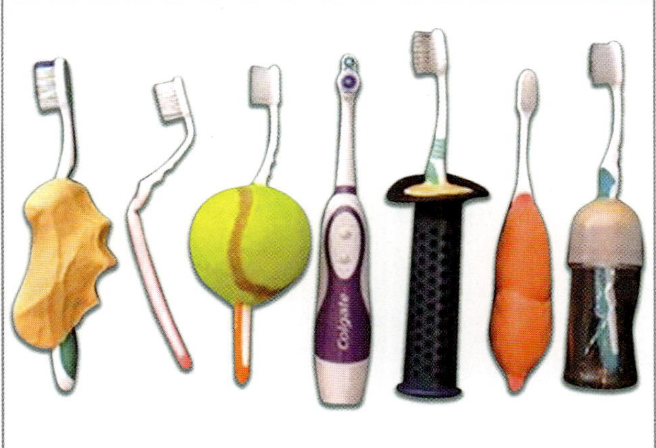

Fig. 28.3: Toothbrush grip modifications. (*Source:* Picture fromhttps://dentistryofthecarolinas.com/2017/02/23/hand-pain-dental-care/).

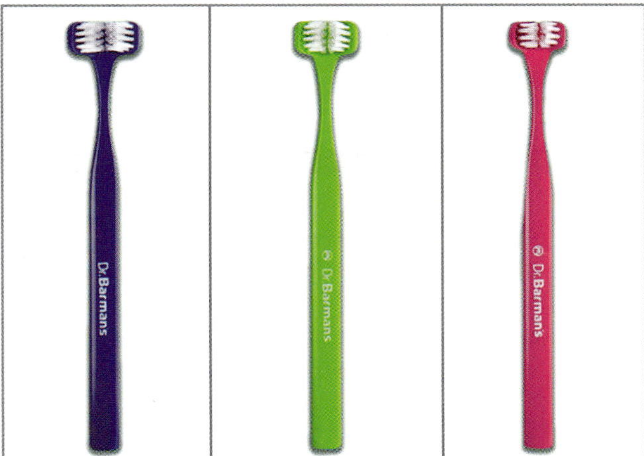

Fig. 28.4: Superbrush.

with tooth surfaces so as to apply sufficient lateral pressure to remove plaque effectively **(Fig. 28.5)**.

- Electric tooth brushes have also been used effectively with special children. The vibration and noise tend to

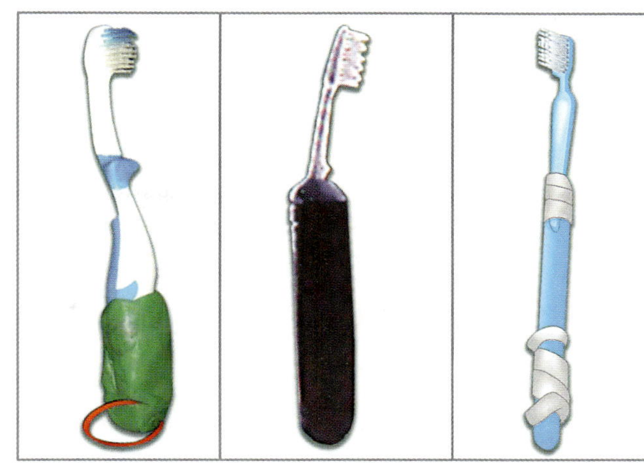

Fig. 28.5: Long handle modification.

desensitize the patient for future dental appointments if followed by positive reinforcement while the design and color is motivational for the child.

Dentifrices

- For many severely differently-abled patients, the foaming caused by toothpaste together with copious amounts of saliva stimulated by toothbrushing obstructs visualization of the areas to be brushed and can stimulate gagging.
- Some individuals may ingest excessive amounts of toothpaste.
- An alternative for these persons is the elimination of toothpaste during brushing. The toothbrush can simply be moistened with water or a flavorful mouthwash.
- A commercially available dentifrice that is non-foaming, safe for ingestion, and has a pleasant taste (NASA Dent®) is available, but the need for such toothpaste with this population is questionable.

Mouthwash

- The use of antimicrobial agents, especially chlorhexidine mouth rinse, has been proven effective in reducing the severity of plaque accumulation and gingivitis. There has been an increased interest in use of these agents with the differently-abled population since adequate mechanical plaque removal remains a problem.
- Since the usual method of rinsing and expectorating is difficult for the person with severe disabilities, alternative methods such as a spray or application by swab (e.g., Toothette®) is often indicated.
- The use of other antimicrobial agents may also be indicated. These include Listerine® mouthwash, stannous fluoride gels and mouthwashes, povidone iodine (Betadine®) mouthwashes, sanguinarine products (e.g., Viadent®) and similar mouthwashes have proven effective antiplaque agents, are cheaper than chlorhexidine and do not cause problems with staining and taste alteration. They do, however, contain alcohol and should be used with caution in patients who may swallow them.

Fluoride Application

- Professionally prescribed stannous fluoride gels are generally more effective antiplaque agents than commercially available fluoride mouthwashes, but their application is more difficult with this population.
- Foam or plastic trays are usually contraindicated due to lack of patient cooperation and frequent bruxism. Professionally constructed acrylic mouthguard- type trays are difficult to fabricate for uncooperative individuals, difficult for direct care staff to use, and are frequently misplaced.
- The application of fluoride gels by toothbrush after normal brushing has been completed is often the method of choice.

GUIDELINES FOR HOME ORAL CARE OF DIFFERENTLY-ABLED CHILDREN (FIG. 28.6)

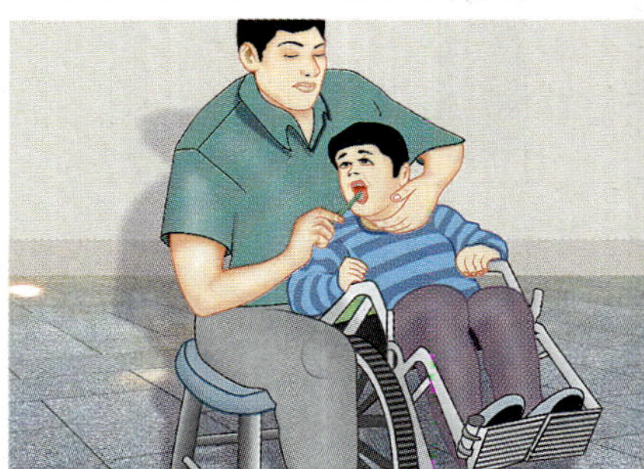

Wheelchair:
Or sit behind wheelchair. Remember to lock chair wheels first, then tilt chair back into your lap.

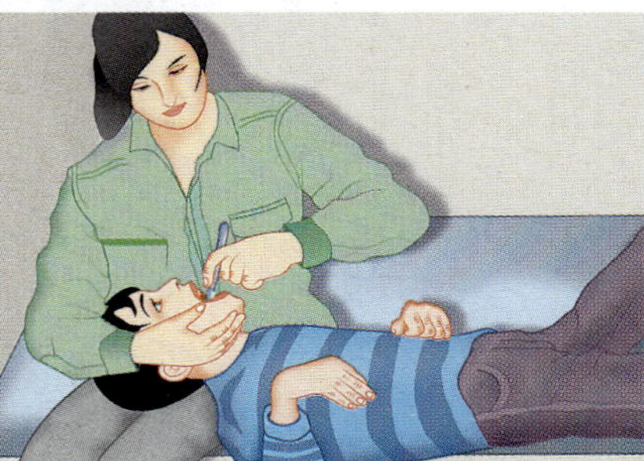

Bed or sofa:
Patient lies on bed or sofa with head in your lap. Support individual's head and shoulder with your arm.

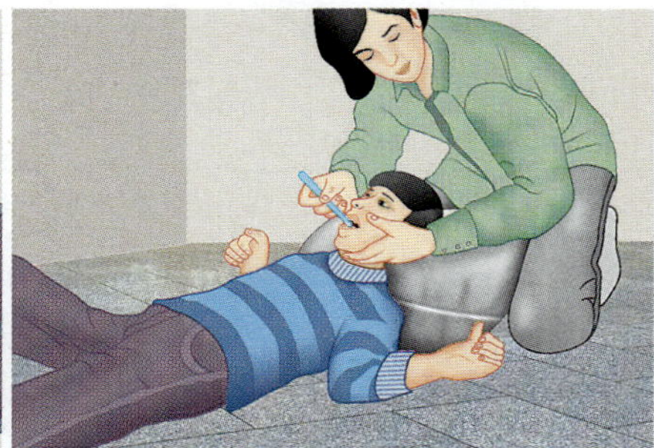

Lying on floor:
Patient lies on floor with head on pillow. You kneel behind his/her head. You can use your arm to hold person still.

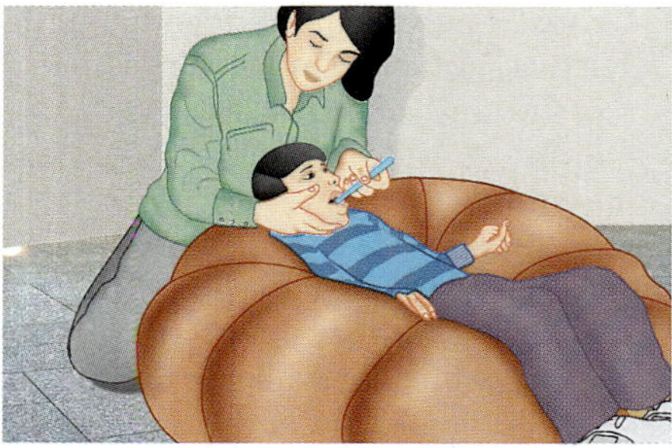

Beanbag chair:
For people who have difficulty sitting-up straight, a beanbag chair lets them relax without fear of falling.
Use same position as for bed or sofa.

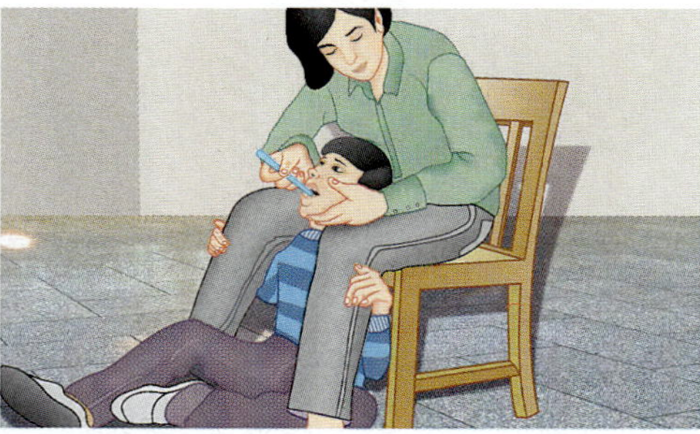

Sitting on floor:
Patient sits on floor; you sit behind person on chair. Individual leans head against your knees. If individual is uncooperative or uncontrollable, you can place your legs over his/her arms to keep them still.

Fig. 28.6: Guidelines for home oral care of differently-abled children.

POINTS TO REMEMBER

- Home dental care should begin in infancy.
- For older children who are unwilling or physically unable to cooperate, the dentist should teach the parent or guardian correct toothbrushing techniques to safely restrain the child, when necessary.
- Usually a soft nylon bristle, rounded end, multitufted brush with a long strong neck is the preferred choice.
- Powered brushes are preferred choice in differently-abled children.
- For people who cannot grasp and hold brush handle is attached to Velcro strap on the palm.
- In case of limited hand closure or reduced manual, simplest method of improving the grip involves inserting the brush handle into another material to improve its size, shape, or surface characteristics, like bicycle handlebar grips or pushing it into a soft rubber ball.
- For those patients who can position a toothbrush but cannot manipulate it sufficiently to clean all the surfaces of the teeth, double-headed brushes and powered toothbrush are best indicated.
- When there is limited arm and hand movement, the objective is to lengthen the handle of the brush with a material strong enough to maintain the brush in contact with tooth surfaces so as to apply sufficient lateral pressure to remove plaque effectively.
- Use of dentifrices has a limited role, whereas the mouthwashes form an important component of maintenance control of oral hygiene in differently-abled children.

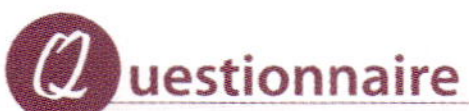

1. Explain plaque control for a differently-abled child.
2. What are the modifications of toothbrush for a differently-abled child?
3. Explain the guidelines for home care of oral hygiene in differently-abled children.

FURTHER READING

1. Albertson D, Johnson R. Plaque control for the institutionalized child. J Am Dent Assoc. 1973;87:1389-94.
2. Bay LM, et al. Effect of chlorhexidine on dental plaque and gingivitis in mentally retarded children. Comm Dent Oral Epid. 1975;3:267-70.
3. Bratel J, et al. Electric or manual toothbrush? A comparison of effects on the oral health of mentally handicapped adults. Clin Prevent Dent. 1988;10:23-6.
4. Crawford PJ, et al. The effect of modifying toothbrush handles on plaque control in handicapped children: preliminary report. Proc Br Paedod Soc. 1977;7:11-3.
5. Dickinson C, Millwood J. Toothbrush handle adaptation using silicone impression putty. Dent Update. 1999;26:288-98.
6. Dougall A, Fiske J. Access to special care dentistry, Part 4. Education. Br Dent J. 2008;205:119-30.
7. Ettinger RL, et al. Oral hygiene and the handicapped child. J Int Asso Dent Child. 1978;9:3-11.
8. Ettinger RL, et al. Toothbrush modifications and the assessment of hand function in children with hand disabilities. J Dent Handi. 1980;5:7-12.
9. Johnson R, et al. Plaque control for handicapped children. J Am Dent Assoc. 1972;84:824-8.
10. Kaschke I, Klaus-Roland J, Zeller A. The effectiveness of different toothbrushes for patients with special needs. J Disabil Oral Health. 2005;6:65-71.
11. Loesche WJ. Plaque control in the handicapped: the treatment of specific plaque infections. Can Dent Assoc J. 1981;47: 649-56.
12. Nowak AJ. Dentistry for the Handicapped Patient. St Louis: CV Mosby Co.; 1976. p. 3.
13. Scully C, Dios PD, Kumar N. Special Care in Dentistry. Chapter 2. London: Churchill Livingstone; 2007.
14. Soncini JA, et al. Individually modified toothbrushes and improvement of oral hygiene and gingival health in cerebral palsy children. J Pedod. 1989;13:331-4.
15. Southern Association of Institutional Dentists: Self-Study Course Module 11. Preventive Dentistry for Persons with Severe Disabilities.
16. Williams NJ, et al. The curved bristle toothbrush: an aid for the handicapped population. J Dent Child. 1988;55:291-3.
17. Wells JE, Reed MW, Coury VM. Review of Basic Science and Clinical Dentistry (Vol-II).
18. McDonald's Dentistry for the Child and Adolescent, 9th edition.

Fluorides

Puneet Goenka, Nikhil Marwah, Suruchi Juneja

Chapter Outline

- Fluoride in the Environment
- Fluoride Content in Some Commonly Used Foods
- Metabolism of Fluoride
- History of Fluorides
- Shoe Leather Survey
- Mechanism of Action of Fluoride
- Water Fluoridation
- School Water Fluoridation
- Salt Fluoridation
- Milk Fluoridation
- Dietary Fluoride Supplements
- Topical Fluorides
- Sodium Fluoride
- Stannous Fluoride
- Acidulated Phosphate Fluoride
- Newer Topical Fluorides
- Fluoride Varnish
- Fluoride Dentifrices
- Fluoride Toxicity
- Dental Fluorosis Indices
- Defluoridation
- Recent Advances in Fluoride

The greatest contribution of last century to the improvement of oral health is perhaps the discovery and utilization of fluoride as a caries preventive measure. Extensive research has been carried out about the utility of this salt in variety of ways to draw maximum systemic and topical benefits of its cariostatic properties. Fluoride is one of those remarkable elements, which have not only notable chemical qualities but also physiological properties of great interest and importance for human health. Fluoride has been described as an essential nutrient in the Federal Register of United States Food and Drug Administration (1973) and World Health Organization (WHO) expert committee on trace elements and human health. They have also included fluoride in the list of 14 elements recognized to be physiologically essential for the normal development and growth of human beings. The term fluoride is derived from a Latin word Fluore, which means to flow. Its atomic weight is 19 and atomic number is 9. Fluoride is never encountered in nature in the elemental form, as it is the most electronegative and reactive of all elements, and thus it is found in salt form.

FLUORIDE IN THE ENVIRONMENT

Lithosphere

- In the lithosphere, fluoride is present as a wide variety of minerals like fluorspar, cryolite, apatite mica, and hornblende.
- High concentrations of fluoride are also present in certain pegmatite like topaz and tourmaline, as well as volcanic and hypabyssal rocks. Salt deposits of marine origin also contain abundance of fluoride.

Facts file

Concentration of fluoride in:
- Rain water: Negligible
- Lake Nakuru (Kenya) water: 2,800 ppm
- Tea leaves: 82–371 ppm [Wei SH, et al. Nutrition. 1989;5(4):237-40]
- Coconut water: Negligible

- In spite of being in abundance, very little fluoride is biologically available. This is mainly because of its reactive nature thus rendering it to be bound firmly to minerals and other chemical compounds. The availability of free fluoride ions in the soil is governed by the natural solubility of the fluoride compound considered, the acidity of the soil, the presence of other minerals or chemical compounds, and the amount of water present.
- The concentration of fluoride in soil also increases with depth.

Hydrosphere

- Due to universal presence of fluorides in Earth's crust, all water contains fluoride in various concentrations.

- For example, negligible in rain water, high in lakes and wells like fluoride in sea water—0.8–1.4 mg/L and in river—0.5 mg/L.
- Highest content of fluoride in water is in Lake Nakuru (Kenya)—2,800 ppm.

Atmosphere

- Fluoride mainly enters the atmosphere through the dusts of fluoride-containing soil, from gaseous industrial waste, from burning of coal fires, and from gases emitted in areas of volcanic activity.
- The fluoride content in the air in some factories can reach levels as high as 1.4 mg/m.

FLUORIDE CONTENT IN SOME COMMONLY USED FOODS

The mean value of fluoride content, in ppm, of commonly used food items in India as given by **Lakdawala** and **Punekar**[1] are tabulated below:

Type of food	*Fluoride content (ppm)*
Cereals	
Whole wheat	2.920
Wheat flour milled	5.402
Rice	7.720
Bajra	1.885
Pulses and legumes	
Bengal gram flour, milled	8.065
Bengal whole gram	4.215
Green gram dal	2.965
Green gram whole	5.882
Red gram dal	3.590
Leafy vegetables	
Spinach	2.113
Fenugreek leaves	3.011
Cabbage	1.880
Colocasia leaves	4.959
Amaranth leaves	6.154
Roots and tubers	
Potatoes	1.856
Onions	2.088
Carrots	3.425
Other vegetables	
Cucumber	2.457
French beans	1.530
Tomato	1.366
Brinjal	2.024
Ladies finger	2.730
Fruits	
Banana	1.096
Chikoo	1.238
Grapes	1.360
Oranges	1.745
Mango	1.320
Water melon	0.739
Apple	1.744
Guava	0.392
Animal foods	
Milk	0.499
Eggs	1.531
Mutton	3.083
Beef	4.416
Pork	3.533
Fish	0.933–3.149
Prawns	2.749
Beverages	
Tea	56.640
Coca cola	10.393
Sugarcane juice	1.198
Coconut water	0.508
Miscellaneous	
Groundnuts	2.088
Coconut fresh	2.148
Sugar	0.420
Betel leaves	2.680–9.320

Fluoride Distribution (Figs. 29.1 and 29.2)

Fluorosis is worldwide in distribution and endemic at least in 25 countries. It has been reported from fluoride belts: one that stretches from Syria through Jordan, Egypt, Libya, Algeria, Sudan and Kenya, and another that stretches from Turkey through Iraq, Iran, Afghanistan, India, northern Thailand and China. There are similar belts in the America and Japan.

High levels of Fluoride were reported in 230 districts of 20 States of India (after bifurcation of Andhra Pradesh in 2014). The population at risk as per population in habitations with high fluoride is 11.7 million (as on 1.4.2014). Rajasthan, Gujarat and Andhra Pradesh are worst affected states. Punjab, Haryana, Madhya Pradesh and Maharashtra are moderately affected states while Tamil Nadu, West Bengal, Uttar Pradesh, Bihar and Assam are mildly affected states.

In India fluorosis is mainly due to excessive fluoride in water except in parts of Gujarat and Uttar Pradesh where industrial fluorosis is also seen.

METABOLISM OF FLUORIDE

Absorption

Fluoride is primarily absorbed from stomach. This process occurs by passive diffusion and is also inversely related to pH so that factors which promote the secretion of gastric acid increase the rate of fluoride absorption, which leads to earlier and high peak plasma levels and vice versa.

Transportation

- **In plasma, fluoride exists in two forms:** Ionic fluoride (inorganic or free fluoride) and nonionic or bound fluoride.
- Almost all fluoride in plasma is in ionic form and is not bound to any macromolecules. The plasma half-life of fluoride is reported to be ~10 hours. Studies have indicated that the fluoride is not bound to the plasma proteins or

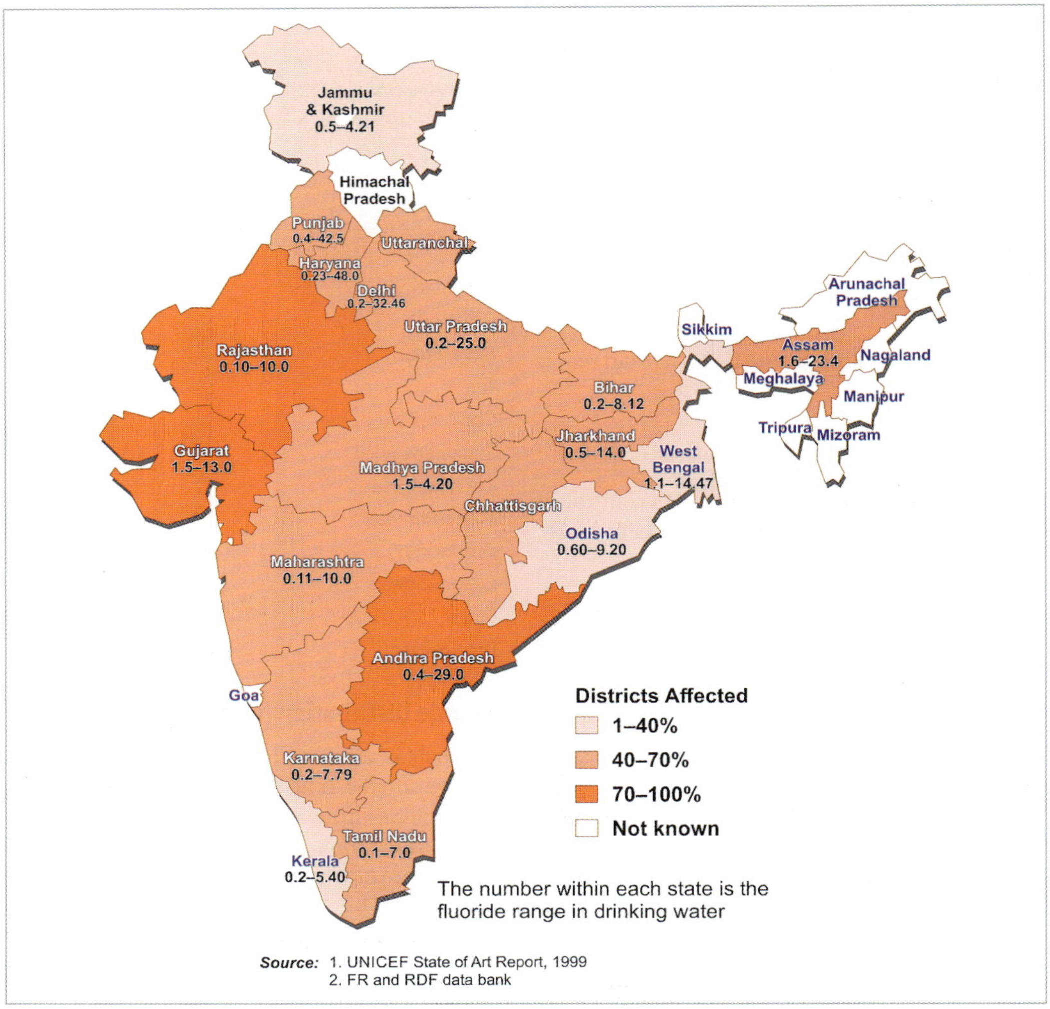

Jammu
& Kashmir
0.5–4.21
Himachal
Pradesh
Punjab
0.4–42.5
Uttaranchal
Haryana
0.23–48.0
Delhi
0.2–32.46
Rajasthan
0.10–10.0
Uttar Pradesh
0.2–25.0
Sikkim
Arunachal
Pradesh
Assam
1.6–23.4
Nagaland
Meghalaya
Manipur
Tripura
Mizoram
Bihar
0.2–8.12
Jharkhand
0.5–14.0
West
Bengal
1.1–14.47
Gujarat
1.5–13.0
Madhya Pradesh
1.5–4.20
Chhattisgarh
Odisha
0.60–9.20
Maharashtra
0.11–10.0
Andhra Pradesh
0.4–29.0
Goa
Karnataka
0.2–7.79
Tamil Nadu
0.1–7.0
Kerala
0.2–5.40
Districts Affected
1–40%
40–70%
70–100%
Not known
The number within each state is the
fluoride range in drinking water
Source: 1. UNICEF State of Art Report, 1999
2. FR and RDF data bank

Fig. 29.1: Fluorosis distribution in India according to Susheela.[2]

Iraq
Turkey
Syria
Jorden
Palestine
Morocco
Algeria
Libya
Egypt
Senegal
Mexico
United Arab
Emirates
Argentina
Japan
China
Bangladesh
Thailand
Iran
Pakistan
India
Ethiopia
Uganda
Kenya
Tanzania
Sri Lanka
Australia
New Zealand

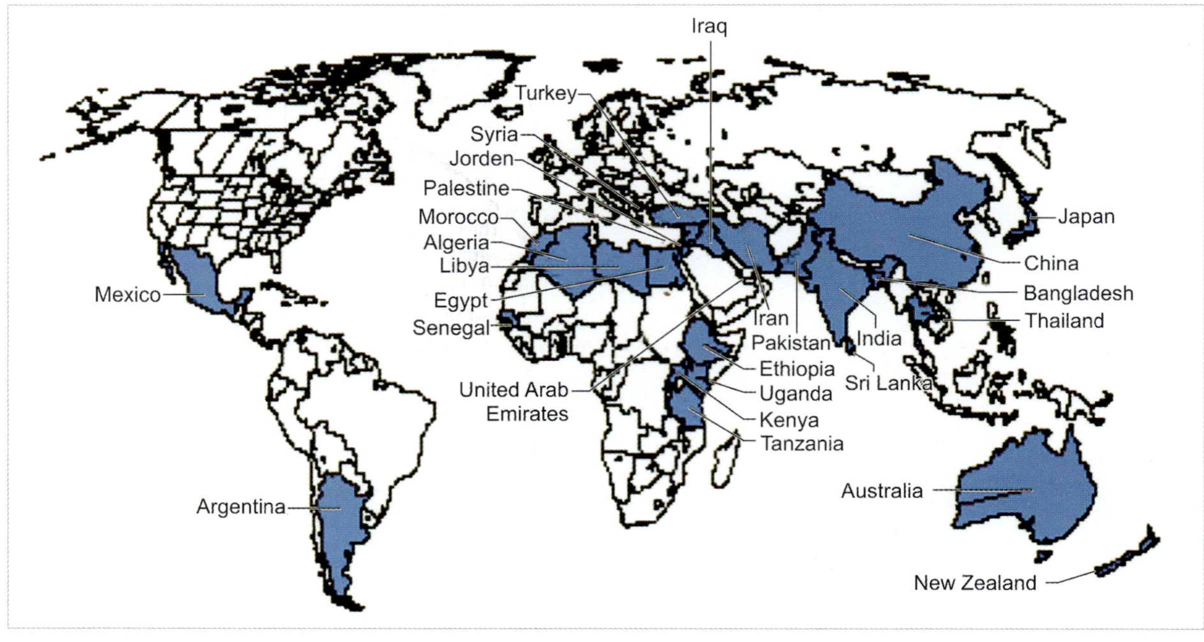

Fig. 29.2: Countries with endemic fluorosis (according to UNICEF).[3]

to any other constituent of plasma. Therefore, it may be assumed that the interstitial fluid and the plasma have virtually the same composition.
- The plasma concentration of fluoride is variable, being dependent on the level of intake and several physiological factors.
- Considering the above facts, the height of plasma peak is proportional to the fluoride dose ingested, the rate of absorption, and the body weight (volume of distribution) of the subject, that is, the larger the body weight, the lower is the plasma peak and vice versa.

Soft Tissue Distribution

- Once absorbed, fluoride is distributed within minutes through the extracellular fluid to most organs and tissues.
- The fluoride concentration in most soft tissues is lower than the plasma level except in the healthy kidney where, because of urine production, an occasional fluoride accumulation may result.
- Fluoride passes through the placenta, and studies have shown that the fetal fluoride level is about 75% of that of the maternal blood. Gedalia has described that when the fluoride intake is low, fluoride freely passes through the placenta, but when the fluoride intake is high, the placenta plays a regulatory role and protects the fetus from excess.
- The fluoride concentration of human breast milk is lower than that of maternal plasma. Thus, the fluoride intake of infants who are solely or mainly breastfed is unusually low.
- In subjects with a normal diet, the fluoride concentration in the saliva is about 1 μm/L.

Excretion

- The main route of fluoride excretion is via the kidneys.
- Because ionic fluoride is not bound to plasma proteins, its concentration in the glomerular filtrate is undoubtedly the same as in plasma. Also, there exists a "steady state" between the concentrations of fluoride in the plasma and the urine, that is, the fluoride concentrations in plasma and urine tend to parallel each other very closely.
- The kidneys are very efficient in removing fluoride from the body. The renal clearance of fluoride in the adult typically is 30–50 mL/min. Compared to the other halogens whose clearance rates are normally about ≤1.0 mL/min.
- Excretion of fluorides.
  - *Renal:* 30% within 3 hours and 40–60% in 24 hours.
  - *Gut:* 10% in feces.
  - *Breast milk:* 0.01–0.05 ppm.
  - *Sweat:* 10–25% in 1 hours.

Distribution of Fluoride in the Body

It depends upon physical form of dose, presence of food in stomach, gastric pH, gastric motility, and concurrent oral administration.
- *Plasma concentration:* 0.7–2.4 μm.
- *Kidney:* 4.16 ppm.
- *Bone:* 99%.
- *Enamel:* 2,200–3,200 ppm.
- *Dentin:* 200–300 ppm.
- *Cementum:* 4,500 ppm.
- *Pulp:* 100–650 ppm.

HISTORY OF FLUORIDES

1901	**Dr Fredrick McKay** of Colorado, USA observed apparently permanent stain on the teeth of many of his patients: commonly known as "Colorado stains" by the local inhabitants. **McKay** at this stage failed to relate this stain with any factor and named it as "mottled enamel"
1908	**Dr McKay** presented a case at the annual meeting of State Dental Association in Boulder and found that the condition was not confined to Colorado but extended to other towns as well
1912	**Dr McKay** came across an article written by **Dr JM Eager** (1902), a US Marine Hospital surgeon who reported that a high proportion of Italian residents in Naples had brown stains on their teeth known as "denti di Chiaie"
1916	**McKay** and **Black** conducted a survey over 6,873 individuals in 26 communities in USA reporting that an unknown factor possibly present in domestic water during the period of tooth calcification may be the cause of mottled enamel
1918	**McKay** observed that individuals reared up in Britton since 1898 had mottling, whereas all those who had passed through childhood before had normal teeth. It was also observed that prior to 1898, Britton had changed its water supply from individual shallow wells to deep drilled artesian wells. Thus, it was concluded by **McKay** that some mysterious element in water supply was the causative agent for mottled enamel
1925	The inhabitants of Oakley, Idaho were so much convinced by the water supply hypothesis that they switched their water supply from deep artesian wells to shallow water supply following concerns about discoloration to teeth. **McKay** found no brown stains in the permanent teeth of 24 children born in Oakley, seven and half years later following the change in water supply
1931	**Churchill** developed a method for determining concentrations of fluoride in drinking water. He found 13.7 ppm of fluoride in Bauxite. In addition, the level of fluoride was very high in the water from other endemic areas for mottled teeth. Thus, this was finally established that "Fluoride" was the culprit behind this ugly condition. Further supported by the experimental production of dental lesions similar to human fluorosed enamel, in experimental animals by water from endemic areas and water to which fluoride had been added (**Smith**, 1931)
1934	**Dean** conducted the famous "Shoe Leather Survey" and established that concentration of fluoride in drinking water was directly correlated to the severity of fluorosed enamel. Dean also developed a standard classification of mottling and an index to quantify it mottling index
1939	To test the correlation of fluoride in water and dental caries, a survey of four Illinois cities was planned by Dean. The cities were **Galesburg** and **Monmouth** (1.8 and 1.7-ppm fluoride, respectively) and **Macomb** and **Quincy** (0.2-ppm fluoride). The results showed that caries experience in low fluoride areas with 0.2-ppm fluoride was more than twice as high as that in the areas with 1.7 and 1.8-ppm
1942	**Dean** finally concluded that at 1-ppm of fluoride in drinking water near maximal reduction of caries experience, i.e. 60% was achieved and only "sporadic instances" of the mildest form of dental fluorosis of no practical or esthetic significance were observed
1945	First community level water fluoridation program started in Grand Rapids, USA
1950s	Water fluoridation started in the United States in the states of Florida, Illinois, California (1952), Ohio (1955), and Missouri (1957)
1964	The WHO and the Pan American Health Organization endorsed the practice of water fluoridation

(WHO: World Health Organization)

SHOE LEATHER SURVEY

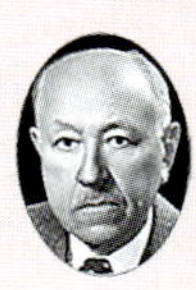

The study of relationship between fluoride concentration in drinking water, mottled enamel, and dental caries was given an impetus by the decision of ***Dr Clinton T Messner****, Head of US Public Health service in 1931, to assign a young Dental Officer* ***Dr H Trendley Dean*** *to pursue full time research on mottled enamel.*

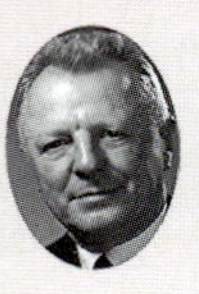

- His first task was to continue McKay's work and to find the extent and geographical distribution of mottled enamel in USA.
- He sent a questionnaire to the secretary of every local and state dental society in the country and asked if mottled enamel existed in their areas, if so, how extensive and also enquired about the water source. Out of 1197 questionnaires, 632 replies were received. Dean reported that 97 localities in the country where mottling had occurred.
- His aim was to find out the minimal threshold of fluoride—The level at which fluorine began to blemish the teeth. He showed conclusively that the severity of mottling increased with increasing fluoride concentrations in the drinking water.
- He gave the following observations:
  - Water concentration was 4 ppm or more—signs of discrete pitting.
  - Water concentration was 3 ppm or more—mottling was widespread.
  - Water concentration was 2–3 ppm—teeth had dull chalky appearance.
  - Water concentration was ≤1 ppm—no mottling of any esthetic significance.
  - He also reported that the incidence of caries in these teeth was less as compared to nonfluoridated teeth.

MECHANISM OF ACTION OF FLUORIDE

The mechanism of action of fluoride or the methods by which fluoride exhibits its anticariogenic or antimicrobial effect are improved crystallinity, void theory, acid solubility, enzyme inhibition, suppressing the flora, antibacterial action, lowering free surface energy, desorption of protein and bacteria, and alteration in tooth morphology **(Table 29.1)**. To understand these phenomena's, it is most ideal to first understand the structure of hydroxyapatite **(Fig. 29.3)**.[4]

Table 29.1: Mechanism of action of fluoride.

Improved crystallinity	Fluoride increases the crystal size and produces less strain in crystal lattice. This takes place through conversion of amorphous calcium phosphate into crystalline hydroxyphosphate
Void theory	Incorporation of fluoride results into formation of larger and more stable crystals. Fluoride replaces OH^- from the center of the Ca^{++} triangle. It forms strong coulomb interaction forces with Ca^{++}, thereby decreasing the dimension of this axis. Hydroxyapatite crystals are known to have inherent voids due to missing hydroxyl groups which makes it unstable. In hydroxyapatite crystal OH^- group is present slightly above or below the plane formed by Ca^{++} ion. To maintain symmetry, equal number of OH^- ions should be present on both the sides of the Ca^{++} plane. At times when hydrogen of adjacent OH^- groups points towards each other, this results into stearic interference resulting into the elimination of one OH^- group, thereby forming a void in the place. Voids in the crystal decreases the stability and increases chemical reactivity. When these voids are filled by Fl^-, the stability of the crystal increases, and the reactivity decreases greater stability of the crystal impart lower solubility and greater resistance to dissolution in acids. Incorporation of a small amount of Fl^- in the apatite crystal improves its properties considerably. Fl^- ions also form hydrogen bonds with neighboring OH^- ions which further helps in the stabilization of the crystal
Acid solubility	(FAP vs HAP) Fluorapatite or fluoridated hydroxyapatite (solubility constant of 10.60) is less soluble than hydroxyapatite (10.55) therefore has greater stability
Enzyme inhibition	Fluoride has enolase inhibition effect, and it also inhibits glucose transport. Enolase is a metalloenzyme that requires a divalent cation for its activity; fluoride due to its increased reactivity forms a complex with this cation, thus inhibiting the enzyme. It also inhibits nonmetalloenzymes like phosphatases, thus leading to reduced acid production
Suppressing the flora	Stannous fluoride is a potent suppressor of the bacterial growth because it oxidizes the thiol group present in bacteria, thus inhibiting bacterial metabolism
Antibacterial action	The concentration of fluoride above 2 ppm in solution progressively decreases the transport of uptake of glucose into cells of oral streptococci and also reduces ATP synthesis
Lowering free surface energy	Fluoride incorporated in enamel by substitution of hydroxyl ions reduces the free surface energy and thus indirectly reduces the deposition of pellicle and subsequent plaque formation
Desorption of protein and bacteria	Hydroxyapatite crystals are amphoteric with both positive and negative receptor sites. Acidic protein group binds to calcium site and basic to phosphate site. Fluoride inhibits the binding of acidic protein to hydroxyapatite, thereby displaying its beneficial effects
Alteration in tooth morphology	Dentition in fluoridated communities showed a tendency toward rounded cusps, shallow fissures due to selective inhibition of ameloblasts

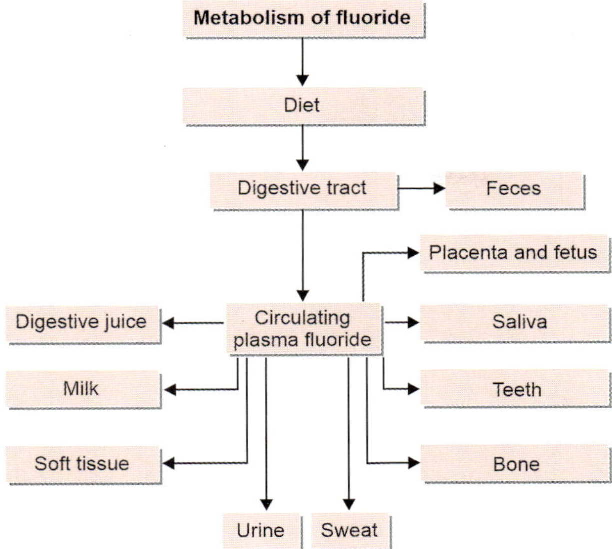

Structure of Hydroxyapatite

The hard tissues of the body, viz., bone and teeth are made of an organic part and an inorganic part. The primary chemical constituents of enamel are Ca^{++}, PO^{-3}_4, OH^-, and carbonate (CO^{-2}_3). The spatial arrangement of these ions forms microcrystals in enamel and dentin called as hydroxyapatite [$Ca_{10}(PO_4)_6(OH)_2$]. Carbonate ion [CO^{-2}_3] is an integral part of the relatively large apatite crystals of enamel. Along with these, the inorganic phase of teeth contains a large number of trace elements like F^-, Mg, Mo, Sr, Cl, Na, etc. The most significant among these is the Fl^-. The hydroxyapatite is formed by the spatial arrangement of a large number of repeating units called crystal. The smallest space unit of the HA crystal is called unit cell which is formed by 10 Ca^{++}, 6 PO^{-3}_4, and OH^-. Individual or isolated unit cell cannot exist.

Thus, $Ca_{10}(PO_4)_6(OH)_2$ does not represent the molecular formula of unit cell; rather, it is the minimum number of atoms necessary to form an unit cell through their spatial interaction. Each unit forms a rhomboid with a- and b-axes lying in the same plane, forming the floor and the roof of the rhomboid. Each side measure 9.42 A° and with two angles each of 60° and 120°. The height of the unit cell, the *C*-axis, at right angle to the a–b plane and parallel to the long axis of the crystal, measures 6.88 A°. **Figure 29.3** represents the location of the OH^- and Ca^{2+} in a repeating unit cell.

The OH^- are arranged in columns parallel to the *C*-axis at distances of 1/4th and 3/4th the height of the *C*-axis. Surrounding this column, Ca^{++} forms an equilateral triangle lying parallel to the a–b plane. Successive Ca^{++} triangles are rotated 180° with respect to each other, thereby forming a screw axis symmetry. This stacking of two such triangles shows that they do not superimpose each other but are out of phase by 60°. In addition, Ca^{++} ions are also located in vertical columns, parallel to the *C*-axis. One of it is situated just above or below the halfway point between ends of the cell and the other just above or below the a–b plane. The phosphate ions occupy the bulk of the space within each unit call. They have a tetrahedral structure with the phosphorus of the center and oxygen at each apex.

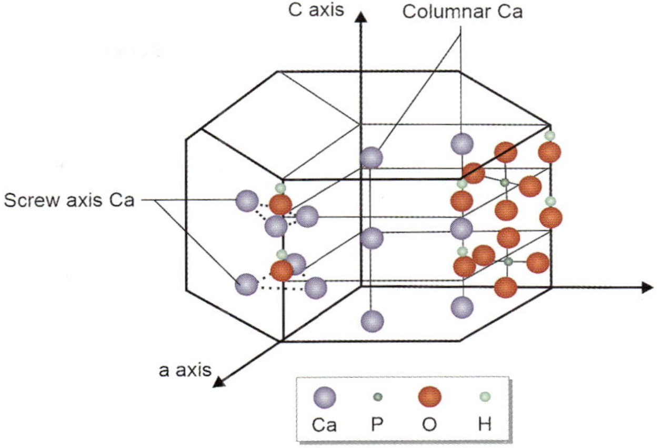

Fig. 29.3: Hydroxyapatite structure.

WATER FLUORIDATION

It is defined as the upward adjustment of the concentration of fluoride ion in public water supply in such way that the concentration of fluoride ion in the water may be consistently maintained at one part per million (ppm) by weight.

History of Water Fluoridation

- History of water fluoridation dates back many years when **Fredrick McKay** and **Trendley Dean** began their initial research, but the most significant change took place in 1942 during Grand Rapids–Muskegon study.[5]
- During many previous researches, it was noted that fluoride decreased the incidence of caries, crucial step was to see if dental caries would be reduced in a community by adding fluoride at 1 ppm to water supply.
- US public health service in December 1942 began this study in two cities Grand Rapids and Muskegon. They came to a conclusion that 1-ppm fluoride was not only best for caries control but was also well within limits of safety.
- On January 25, 1945, it was the moment of truth sodium fluoride (NaF) was added to water supply. It was for the first time that permissible quantity of a beneficial dietary nutrient was added to communal drinking water **(Fig. 29.4)**.

Countries using water fluoridation

- Argentina, Australia, Brazil, Brunei, Canada, Chile, Fiji, Guatemala, Guyana, Hong Kong, Irish Republic, Israel, Libya, Malaysia, New Zealand, Panama, Papa New Guinea, Peru, Serbia, Singapore, South Korea, Spain, United Kingdom, United States, Vietnam.

Countries which refused water fluoridation

- Portugal, Romania, Denmark, Austria, China, The Netherlands, Belgium, Hungary, Switzerland, Luxembourg, Sweden, Norway, Finland, Japan, France, Czech Republic, India, Germany.

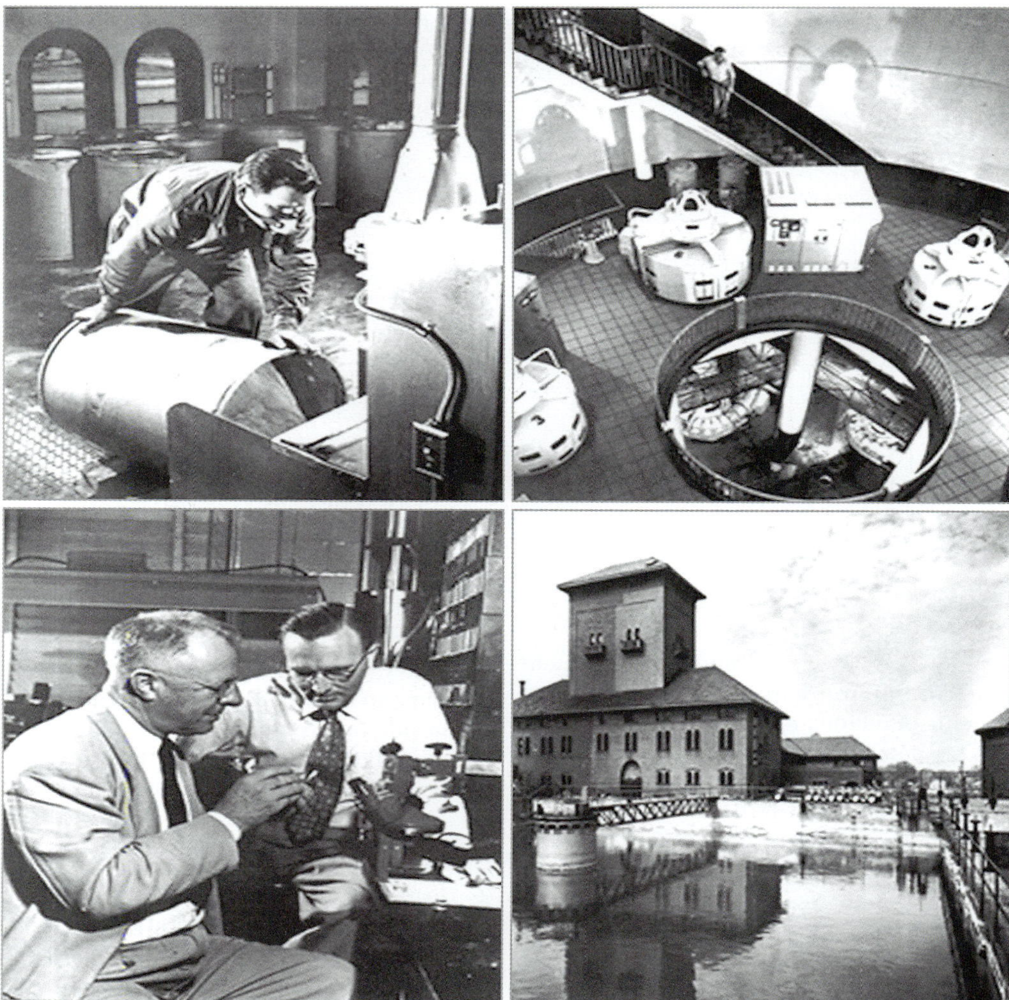

Fig. 29.4: Timeline photos of Grand Rapids—Muskegon study of water fluoridation.

Fluoride Compounds used in Water Fluoridation

- Fluorspar
- Sodium fluoride
- Silicofluorides
- Sodium silicofluoride
- Hydrofluosilicic acid
- Ammonium silicofluoride.

Optimum Level of Fluoride

- Based on extensive research, the United States Public Health Service (USPH) (1986) established the optimum concentration for fluoride in the water in the range of 0.7–1.2 parts per million. This range effectively reduces tooth decay, with minimal chances to cause dental fluorosis.
- The water intake of individuals varies widely and is influenced significantly by climate.
- Children living in a 1-ppm fluoridated area are assumed to receive an optimal intake of fluoride from water and food of 1 mg fluoride daily.
- The US Public Health Service Drinking Water Standards has recommended optimal fluoride concentration as a function of temperature.
- **Galagan** and **Vermillion**[6] developed an empiric formula for estimating the amount of daily fluid intake based on body weight and climatic conditions, using the mean annual maximum daily air temperature as follows:

Galagan and Vermillion formula

$$\textbf{ppm } F = \mathbf{0.34}/E$$

$$E = -0.038 + 0.0062 \times T$$

E—Estimated daily water intake of children in oz/lb of body weight

T—Mean maximum daily air temperature in degree Fahrenheit of the area

In 1967, **Richards et al.** made a comprehensive study of temperature and recommended water fluoridation

Temperature in °C	*Recommended ppm*
<18.3	1.1–1.3
18.9–26.6	0.8–1.0
>26.7	0.5–0.7

Advantage of Water Fluoridation

- Large number of people are benefited.
- Consumption is regular.

- ❖ Fluoridated drinking water not only acts systemically during tooth formation to make dental enamel more resistant to dental decay but also has topical effect through the release in saliva after ingestion.
- ❖ Fluoridation of community water is the least expensive and most effective way to provide fluoride to a large group of people.

Disadvantages of Water Fluoridation

- ❖ Interfere with human rights.
- ❖ Other-sources of fluoride such as fluoridated oral hygiene products, food, and beverages processed with fluoridated water, tea are not considered.
- ❖ Common source of water supply may not be present.

Equipment for Water Fluoridation

There are three systems for water fluoridation:

1. Saturator system.
2. Dry feeder system.
3. Solution feeder system.

System	*Procedure*	*Factors limiting usage*	*Recommendation*
Saturator system	4% saturated solution of NaF is produced and injected at the desired concentration in the water distribution source with aid of a pump	Need to clean gravel bed used for filtration	Suitable for medium-sized townsrequiring <3.8 million lit/day
Dry feeder	NaF or silicofluoride in the form of powder is introduced into a dissolving basin	Care in handling fluoride, obstruction of pipes, and compacting of fluoride while storage	Suitable for medium-sized townsrequiring 3.8–19 million lit/ day
Solution feeder	Volumetric pump permitting the addition of a given quantity of hydrofluosilicic acid inproportion to the amount of water treated	The equip-ment must be resistantto at-tack by hydro-fluosilicic acid, necessitating construction in polyvinyl chlorides or another plastic	Suitable for medium sized and large towns with a capacity of >7.6 million lit/day

Landmark studies of water fluoridation

- **1931**: **HV Churchill** devised method to measure the level of fluoride in water.
- **1938: Klein H** and several branches of the US Public Health Service conducted studies jointly in Texas, in Amarillo and in Wichita Falls and confirmed that fluorosis was associated with low levels of tooth decay.
- **1939**: **TH Dean** conducted study to test the correlation of fluoride in water and dental caries, in a survey of four Illinois cities Galesburg, Monmouth, MaComb, and Quincy.
- **1943**: **David Ast** made a monograph to determine the benefits of adding fluoride to drinking water.
- **1943**: **David Ast, Smith DJ, Wachs B, Cantwell KT** did Newburgh-Kingston caries-fluorine study XIV: combined clinical and roentgenographic dental findings after 10 years of fluoride experience.
- **1961**: **Backer Dirks O, Houwink B, Kwant GW** conducted a study on artificial fluoridation of drinking water in the Netherlands called The Tiel-Culemborg experiment.
- **1965**: **Brown** and **Poplove** carried out study on water fluoridation in Canada.

According to British Fluoridation Society, 2012

- Most developed nations do not fluoridate their water. In western Europe, for example, only 3% of the population consumes fluoridated water.
- While 25 countries have water fluoridation programs, 11 of these countries have less than 20% of their population consuming fluoridated water: Argentina (19%), Guatemala (13%), Panama (15%), Papa New Guinea (6%), Peru (2%), Serbia (3%), Spain (11%), South Korea (6%), the United Kingdom (11%), and Vietnam (4%).
- Only 11 countries in the world have more than 50% of their population drinking fluoridated water: Australia (80%), Brunei (95%); Chile (70%), Guyana (62%), Hong Kong (100%), the Irish Republic (73%), Israel (70% –started in 1981 and stopped in 2014), Malaysia (75%), New Zealand (62%), Singapore (100%), and the United States (64%).
- In total, 377,655,000 million people worldwide drink artificially fluoridated water. This represents 5% of the world's population.

SCHOOL WATER FLUORIDATION

- ❖ This program helps in limiting caries in school children who are our prime concern. School water fluoridation is a suitable alternative where community water fluoridation is not feasible.
- ❖ The amount of fluoride added in school drinking water should be greater than normal because children have to stay in school for a short time of the day and to compensate for holidays and vacations.
- ❖ This procedure was first started in 1954 in St Thomas US Virgin Islands by US Public Health Service Division.
- ❖ The current recommended regimen for school water fluoridation is adding 4.5 times more fluoride.
- ❖ There has been around 25–40% decrease in dental caries with this program. Simple fluoridators particularly that employ the Venturi system are most suitable, because they require almost no maintenance and can be utilized effectively in small installations of small- or medium-sized schools.

Advantages

- ❖ Good results in reducing caries.
- ❖ Minimal equipment.
- ❖ Not expensive.

Disadvantages

- ❖ Children do not receive the benefit until they go to school
- ❖ Not all children go to school in poor countries like India
- ❖ Amount of water drunk cannot be regulated.

SALT FLUORIDATION

- ❖ As a dietary vehicle for ensuring adequate ingestion of fluoride, domestic salt comes second to drinking water.

- ❖ **Wespi** in 1955 introduced salt fluoridation in Switzerland.
- ❖ Initially, the concentration of fluoride was 90 mg F/kg but has been recently made 200–350 mg F/kg.
- ❖ Antioquia, Colombia was the first American country to follow salt fluoridation in 1967.
- ❖ In 1982, WHO and FDI recommended that salt fluoridation starts as soon as possible in all countries.
- ❖ The procedure of salt fluoridation can be either by spraying concentrated solutions of NaF or KF on salt on a conveyor belt or by mixing with PO_4 carrier salt and then adding to the main bulk. Till now, salt fluoridation has been tried in Columbia, Hungary, Mexico, and Switzerland, with Switzerland being the oldest.
- ❖ A study conducted by **Toth**, in Hungary after 8 years of use of fluoridated salt, showed a reduction of 39% in deft in 6-year-old children.

Advantages

- ❖ Fluoridated salt is safe.
- ❖ Theoretically fluoridated salt prevents dental caries by both systemic as well topical action.
- ❖ No supervision of set up or distribution system.
- ❖ Low cost.
- ❖ Depends on individual acceptance and rejection.

Disadvantages

- ❖ No precise control over-indicated consumption, since salt intake varies greatly among people.
- ❖ International efforts to reduce sodium uptake.
- ❖ Fluoridated salt consumption is lowest when the need for fluorides is greatest: in the early years of life.

MILK FLUORIDATION

- ❖ **Ziegler** in 1956 was the first person to mention milk fluoridation as a method of systemic fluoridation.
- ❖ The concentration of fluoride in 250-mL milk bottle was 0.625 mg.
- ❖ It targets the fluoride directly to the children, and this could be less expensive than water fluoridation. But considerable number of children in most countries will not drink milk for one or another reason.
- ❖ The mode of action of fluoride is both systemic as well as topical.
- ❖ The amount of fluoride to be added depends upon the age of the child and the fluoride concentration in water. This is further complicated by the fact that different children consume varying quantities of milk per day.
- ❖ Countries using milk fluoridation on a regular basis are Russia, United Kingdom, China, Bulgaria.

Compounds used for Milk Fluoridation

- ❖ Calcium fluoride.
- ❖ Sodium fluoride.
- ❖ Disodium monofluorophosphate (MFP).
- ❖ Disodium silicofluoride.

Feasibly of Milk Fluoridation in India

- ❖ In spite of the controversy concerning the binding and complexing of fluoride with calcium and protein of the milk and thus making it unavailable for its anticariogenic action, **Ericsson** (1985) using radioactive isotope technique proved that availability of fluoride from milk is the same as from water 4 hours after consumption.
- ❖ Though theoretically milk fluoridation is advantageous, in addition to being the staple food for children, its consumption can be confined to groups who need it most, that practically speaking, this method does not seem to be viable and feasible because of the following facts:
  - ▪ In India, majority of the children population living in rural and urban areas cannot afford milk daily, and moreover there does not exists a central milk supply system in these areas.
  - ▪ Variation of intake and quantity of milk is another factor which cannot be controlled since it depends upon the socioeconomic, religious, and ethnic factors.

DIETARY FLUORIDE SUPPLEMENTS

- ❖ When introduced, dietary fluoride supplements were perceived to be a reasonable alternative where water fluoridation was not possible. But supplements need cooperation to a high degree and so these should be directed only to needy population for whom caries or its treatment may be difficult.
- ❖ Some examples of supplements are fluoride drops, fluoritab liquid, Vi-Daylin/F ADC drops, pediaflor*drops, etc.
- ❖ The dosage will depend upon the age of the child and the concentration of fluoride in the area. American Academy of Pediatrics recommends that fluoride supplements can be started 2 weeks after birth and continue till 16 years of age.

Dietary fluoride supplementation schedule.[7]

Age	*<0.3 ppm F*	*0.3–0.6 ppm F*	*>0.6 ppm F*
Birth–6 months	0	0	0
6 months–3 years	0.25 mg	0	0
3–6 years	0.50 mg	0.25 mg	0
6 years up to ≥16 years	1.00 mg	0.50 mg	0

- ❖ Prior to 1969, fluoride was prescribed in prenatal supplements for potential caries prevention in teeth whose development began before birth. It was assumed that fluoride would cross the placental barrier and that it would be acquired by the developing teeth sufficiently to provide caries protection. The United States Food and Drug Administration (USFDA) concluded that sufficient evidence did not exist to support claims of efficacy of prenatal fluoride supplements; therefore, in 1966, the Food and Drug Administration (FDA) banned advertising claiming that prenatal fluoride supplements provided a dental benefit, but it did not ban their sale by prescription.
- ❖ Fluoride supplements extend its cariogenic effect by acting both locally and systemically. For its local or topical effect,

fluoride must either contact the tooth surface before it is swallowed or pass through the circulation and be secreted in saliva.

- It is recommended that a child consume no >1 mg of fluoride per day from fluoride supplements and from the drinking water.
- According to Ripa, the appropriate marketed dosage forms may be given full strength of half strength, depending upon the patient's age and level of fluoride in the drinking water. The American Academy of Pediatrics has subsequently adopted this approach.

TOPICAL FLUORIDES

Fluoride has been proved to be the single most effective weapon in our limited arsenal of anticaries agents. Dean proved that individuals continuously living in a fluoride-rich area had less caries as compared to the individuals who had lived in the same fluoride rich areas during calcification of teeth but had shifted to nonfluoride areas thereafter. Simultaneously, in early 1940s, it was demonstrated that extracted teeth when exposed to dilute solutions of fluoride on for a few seconds were found to have completely bound fluoride on the enamel surface which subsequently was less soluble than the original enamel surface. These two facts brought forth the idea of topical application of fluoride solution of dental caries prevention. In 1941, began the era of topical fluorides when the first clinical study of NaF was carried out by Bibby using a 0.1% NaF solution. Subsequently, over the years, various other topical fluoride agents have been evolved which in sequential order are SnF_2 (1947), APF (1963), Na MPP (1963), amine fluoride (1965), and varnish-containing fluoride (1968). Topical fluorides can be divided into:

Professionally applied fluorides	***Self-applied fluorides***
Neutral NaF	Tooth brushing dentifrices
Stannous fluoride	Tooth brushing solutions
Acidulated phosphate fluoride	Tooth brushing prophylaxis pastes
Amine fluoride	Mouth rinses
Fluoride varnishes	
Fluoride gels	

SODIUM FLUORIDE

*Milestone studies were conducted by **Bibby**[8] in 1941 and Knutson in 1942, which varied not only in concentration of NaF used but also in number of applications per year.*

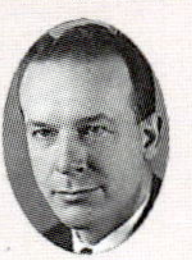

- **Knutson** and **Feldman**[9] (1948) recommended a technique of four applications of 2% NaF at weekly intervals in a year at 3, 7, 11, and 13 years.
- NaF has neutral pH, 9,200 ppm of F.
- Caries reduction in first year was 45% and in 2nd year was 36%.

Method of Preparation

- About 20% NaF solution can be prepared by dissolving 20 g of NaF powder in 1 L of distilled water in a plastic bottle.
- It is essential to store fluoride in plastic bottles because if stored in glass containers, the fluoride ion of solution can react with silica of glass forming SiF_2, thus reducing the availability of free active fluoride for anticaries action.

Method of Application (Knutson Technique)

Cleaning and polishing of the teeth
↓
Quadrants are isolated with cotton rolls and the teeth are dried thoroughly
↓
NaF is then applied with cotton applicators on one quadrant
↓
Permitted to dry on the teeth for about 4 minutes
↓
The procedure is repeated for the remaining quadrants
↓
Patient is instructed to avoid eating, drinking or rinsing for 30 minutes so as to prolong the availability of fluoride ion to react with the tooth surfaces
↓
Second, third and fourth applications are given at weekly intervals at ages 3,7,11 and 13 years

Mechanism of Action

When NaF is applied topically, it reacts with hydroxyapatite crystals to form CaF_2, which is the dominant product of reaction
↓
Choking off effect: This occurs because once a thick layer of CaF_2 gets formed it interferes with the further diffusion of fluoride from the topical fluoride solution to react with hydroxyapatite (It is because of this reason that NaF is once applied and is left to dry for 4 minutes)
↓
CaF_2 reacts with hydroxyapatite to form fluoridated hydroxyapatite which increases the concentration of surface fluoride.

- Making the tooth structure more stable
- Less susceptible to dissolution by acids
- Interferes with plaque metabolism through antienzymatic action
- Helps in remineralization of the initial decalcified areas

$$Ca\,(PO_4)\,6\,(OH)_2 + 20\,F = 10\,CaF_2 + 6\,PO_4 + 2\,OH$$
$$CaF_2 + 2\,Ca_5(PO_4)_3OH = 2\,Ca_5(PO_4)\,3F + Ca\,(OH)_2$$

Advantages

- Chemically stable.
- Acceptable taste.
- Nonirritating to gingival tissues.
- Does not discolor the teeth.
- Cheap and inexpensive.

Disadvantages

- Continuous application for 4 minutes.
- Patient has to make four visits in a short time.
- Follow-up is difficult.

STANNOUS FLUORIDE

- Stannous fluoride in the early 1950s occupied a central role in the saga of preventive dentistry. After the discovery of NaF, a wide variety of other fluoride compounds were tried like potassium, lead, silicon, tin, and zirconium.
- All yielded some cariostatic benefit, but SnF_2 was found to be three times more effective than NaF.
- **Dudding** and **Muhler** in 1957 tried single annual application of 8% SnF_2 and reported 32% caries reduction.

Method of Preparation

- Stannous fluoride solution has to be freshly prepared before use each time (stannous form of tin gets oxidized to stannic form, thus making the SnF_2 inactive for anticaries action), as it has no shelf life.
- For convenient preparation number "o", gelatin capsules are priorly filled with 0.8 g powdered SnF_2 and are stored in airtight plastic containers. Just before application, the content of one capsule is dissolved in 10 mL of distilled water in a plastic container, and the solution thus prepared is shaken briefly. The solution is then applied immediately.

Method of Application

- The recommended procedure for application of SnF_2 begins with thorough prophylaxis followed by isolation with cotton rolls and drying preferably with compressed air.
- Either a quadrant or half of the mouth can be treated at one time.
- A freshly prepared 8% solution of SnF_2 is applied continuously to the teeth with cotton applicator and reapplication of the solution to a particular tooth is done every 15–30 second so that the teeth are kept wet for 4 minutes.
- The recommended frequency of application is once per year.

Mechanism of Action

SnF_2 reacts with hydroxyapatite in addition to fluoride and forms a new crystalline product—stannous trifluorophosphate

↓

Rapid penetration of tin and fluoride in 30 seconds therefore continuous reapplication after 15–30 seconds is needed

↓

In addition to stannous trifluorophosphate three more additional products are formed, viz. stannous hydroxyphosphate, calcium fluoride and calcium trifluorostannate

Low conc. – $Ca_5(PO_4)\ 3OH + 2\ SnF_2 = 2\ CaF_2 + Sn_2(OH)\ PO_4 + Ca_3(PO_4)_2$

High conc. – $Ca_5(PO_4)\ 3OH + 16\ SnF_2 = 2\ CaF_2 + 2\ SnF_3PO_4 + Sn_2(OH)\ PO_4 + 4\ CaF_2(SnF_3)_2$

– $2\ Ca_5(PO_4)\ 3OH + CaF_2 = 2\ Ca_5(PO_4)\ 3F + Ca\ (OH)_2$

Disadvantages

- Should be prepared freshly.
- Low pH.
- Metallic taste due to stannous hydroxyl phosphate.
- Causes gingival irritation.
- Produces discoloration of teeth.
- Causes staining on margins of restorations.

ACIDULATED PHOSPHATE FLUORIDE

*The idea of acidulated phosphate fluoride as a topical agent in the prevention of dental caries emerged with the in vitro investigation by **Bibby** in 1947, which reported that as the pH of the NaF solution was lowered, fluoride was absorbed into enamel more effectively.*

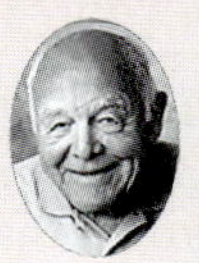

- **Brudevold et al.**[10] did systematic investigation to find out an optimal fluoride acid solution which would provide maximal fluoride deposition, while causing minimal demineralization.
- They concluded that semiannual application of 1.23% APF for 4 minutes is helpful in reducing caries by 28%.
- One of the practical difficulties of doing the topical application is that the teeth must be kept wet with solution for 4 minutes and, moreover, APF solution is acidic and sour and bitter in taste, so repeated applications are often difficult.

Method of Preparation

- It is prepared by dissolving 20 g of NaF in 1 L of 0.1 M phosphoric acid. To this, 50% hydrofluoride acid is added to adjust the pH at 3.0 and F concentrations at 1.23%.
- For the preparation of APF gel, a gelling agent like Methylcellulose or Hydroxyethyl cellulose is to be added to the solution and the pH is to be adjusted between 4 and 5.

Method of Application

After thorough prophylaxis, the teeth are isolated with cotton rolls on both lingual and buccal sides

↓

For the application of gel, position the patient upright and provide saliva ejector

↓

Place enough gel to fill one-third of the trough area of tray so that it is sufficient to cover dental arches

↓

Place loaded tray over the arch and squeeze the buccal and lingual surfaces forcing gel between them and allow tray to remain in mouth for 4 minutes

↓

Instruct the patient to expectorate immediately and avoid drinking and eating for the next 30 minutes

↓

Recommended frequency of APF topical application is semiannual

Mechanism of Action

When APF is applied on the teeth, it initially leads to dehydration and shrinkage in the volume of hydroxyapatite crystals

↓

Hydrolysis and formation of intermediate product

↓

Dicalcium phosphate dihydrate (DCPD)

↓

This DCPD is highly reactive with fluoride leading to formation of fluorapatite. The amount and depth of fluoride deposited as fluorapatite would be dependent on the amount and depth at which DCPD gets formed

↓

Since the conversion of whole DCPD so formed into fluorapatite, deeper penetration and continuous supply of fluoride is required, so APF has to be applied every 30 seconds and the teeth be kept wet for 4 minutes

$Ca_5(PO_4)$ 3OH + 4 H = 5 Ca + 3 HPO_4 + H_2O Ca + HPO_4 = Ca· HPO_4·$2H_2O$ (DCPD)

5 Ca·HPO_4·$2H_2O$ + F = $Ca_5(PO_4)$ 3F + 2 HPO_4 + 3 H + $2H_2O$

Advantages

- Has acceptable taste.
- No staining.
- No gingival irritation.
- Stable with long shelf life.
- Cheap.

Disadvantages

- Teeth have to be kept wet for 4 minutes.
- Solution is acidic.

NEWER TOPICAL FLUORIDES

Amine Fluoride

- In 1945, **Muhlemann** of the University of Zurich first studied effects of AMF.
- Amine fluoride is superior to inorganic fluorides in reducing enamel solubility because of chemical protection by fluoride and physicochemical protection by organic portion.
- They are also surface active because they hold fluoride on enamel surface for longer time.

Stannous Hexafluorozirconate

Researchers at Indiana University have developed $SnZrF_6$ effective in reducing the solubility of enamel and in preventing dental caries.

FLUORIDE VARNISH

The cariostatic effect of topical fluoride agents has generally been related to their ability to deposit fluoride in the enamel and also their depth of penetration. The topical fluoride solutions that are currently in use have a major disadvantage that they remain in contact with teeth for a very short time, that is, 5–10 minutes before getting diluted by saliva and consequently can exert relatively a superficial effect on the dental enamel. A second drawback with topical fluoride solutions is that soon after application, much of the acquired fluoride, probably representing unreacted F and CaF_2, leaches away. To enhance the caries inhibitory property of topical fluorides, experiments were carried out aiming at overcoming above mentioned drawbacks by developing methods for prolonging the contact of fluoride solutions with tooth enamel leading not only to deeper penetration but also a more permanently bound form of fluoride. To achieve prolonged fluoride action in mouth, **Schmidt** in 1964 developed a new coating method in which the teeth were coated with a lacquer containing fluoride called F-lacquer, which released fluoride ions to the dental enamel in high concentrations for several hours in the moist atmosphere of the mouth. Consequently, the use of fluoride containing varnishes in caries prevention has become the treatment of choice. The two most commonly used varnishes are Duraphat (NaF varnish containing 2.26% F) in organic lacquer and Fluor protector (silane fluoride with 0.7% F).

Composition of Duraphat and Fluor Protector

- Fluor protector is a colorless, polyurethane lacquer dissolved in chloroform and dispensed in 1-mL ampules. The fluoride compound is a difluorosilane. The fluoride content in fluor protector is 0.7% by weight, and the active fluoride available is 7,000 ppm **(Fig. 29.5).**
- Duraphat is NaF in varnish form containing 22.6 mg F/mL (2.26%) suspended in an alcoholic solution of natural organic varnishes. It is available in bottles of 30 mL suspension containing 50 mg NaF/mg. The active fluoride available is 22,600 ppm **(Fig. 29.6)**.

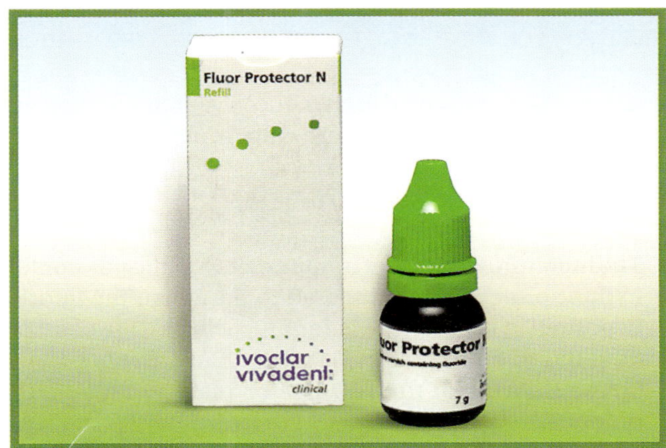

Fig. 29.5: Fluor protector varnish.

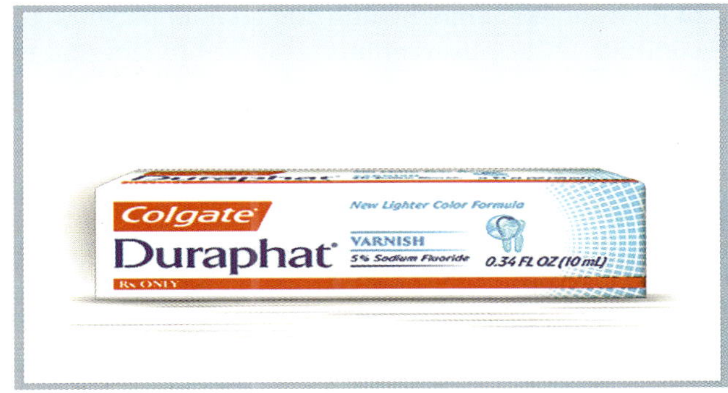

Fig. 29.6: Duraphat varnish.

Technique of Varnish Application

After prophylaxis, teeth are dried

↓

Do not isolate with cotton rolls as varnish being sticky has tendency to stick to cotton

↓

A total of 0.3 – 0.5 mL(6.9 –1.5 mg F) of varnish is required to cover the full dentition

↓

The application is done first on lower arch (as saliva collects more rapidly around it) and then on upper arch with the help of single tufted small brush starting with the proximal sufaces

↓

After application the patient is made to sit with mouth open for four minutes before spitting

↓

The patients should be clearly instructed not to rinse or drink any thing at all for one hour and not to eat anything solid but take liquids and semisolids only till next morning. A special emphasis on instructions is needed to maintain the contact between varnish and tooth surfaces for about 18 hours for prolonging interaction between varnish and enamel

Mechanism of Action

- Duraphat is NaF in varnish form with neutral pH. When applied topically under clinically controlled conditions, a reservoir of fluoride ions gets built up around the enamel of teeth. From this, fluoride keeps on slowly releasing and continuously reacting with the hydroxyapatite crystals of enamel over a long period of time leading to deeper penetration of fluoride and more formation of fluorapatite.

$$10\ Ca_5(PO_4)\ 3\ OH + 10\ F = 6\ Ca_5(PO_4)\ 3F + 2\ CaF_2 + 6\ Ca_3(PO_4)_2 + 10\ OH$$

- A part of CaF_2 so formed in low concentrations further reacts with crystals of hydroxyapatite and forms fluorapatite.

$$2\ Ca_5(PO_4)\ 3OH + CaF_2 = 2\ Ca_5(PO_4)\ 3\ F + Ca\ (OH)_2$$

- The literature shows that in spite of lower fluoride content in fluor protector as compared to duraphat, the fluoride deposited in enamel is twice as much, but on the contrary, its ability to inhibit caries is far less than duraphat.
- Silane fluoride of fluor protector reacts with water to produce considerable amount of hydrofluoric acid (HF), which penetrates into enamel more readily than fluoride. Fluorosilanes also enhance retention and penetration of fluoride in enamel by utilizing enamel network as a conduit. These observations support the fact that the fluoride deposited in enamel is more in the case of fluor protector as compared to duraphat.

$$R\text{-}SiF_2\ OH + H_2O = R\text{-}Si\ (OH)_3 + 2\ HF$$

Safety Aspect of Fluoride Varnish

- Due to the increasing use of caries prevention of fluoride varnishes with high concentrations of fluoride, it is necessary to evaluate the risk of possible side effects by examining plasma levels following such applications.
- The recommended dose of 0.5 mL of duraphat for single application contains 11.3 mg F, and 0.5 mL of fluor protector contains 3.1 mg F. The highest plasma fluoride concentration varied between 60 and 120 mg/mL and was seen within 2 hours of application. These values are far below the toxic doses and hence adjudged to be safe.

> - A review by **Marinho et al.** showed that the clinical efficacy of fluoride varnish showed decrease in caries by 35% (Primary teeth) and by 45% (Permanent teeth).
> - In terms of efficacy of Varnish
> - Acccording to **Seppa et al.** Duraphat >> Fluorprotector; **Green et al**: Duraphat = Fluorprotector; **Levy et al**: Duraphat < Fluorprotector

FLUORIDE DENTIFRICES

Fluoride dentifrices have been proven to be effective anticaries agents since 1955. Today, in industrialized countries, their sales have dominated the major part of the market of dentifrices. In most of the western countries, viz., Norway, Sweden, Denmark, United Kingdom, USA, Netherlands, and Australia, almost 95% of the available toothpastes in the market are fluoridated. The most commonly evaluated fluoride dentifrices are NaF and stannous fluoride, and more recently the sodium MFP and amine fluoride, are also being used.

Sodium Fluoride and Stannous Fluoride Dentifrices

- Sodium fluoride was the first fluoride compound to be added as an active ingredient, but its efficacy was very limited **(Fig. 29.7)**. OTC dentifrices usually contain 900-1100 ppm of fluoride. High-concentration dentifrices (5000 ppm) are available only by prescription and can be recommended for children 6 years and older and adolescents who are at high risk of caries and who are able to expectorate after brushing. Indications include history of dental caries and new lesions, xerostomia, and those with gastroesophageal reflux causing dental erosion and those undergoing orthodontic treatment.[11]

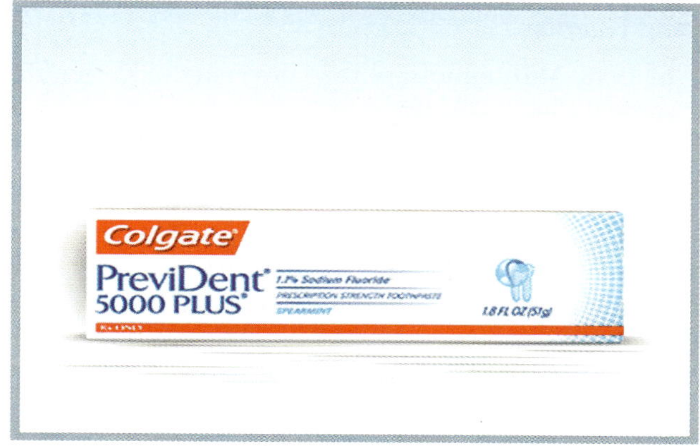

Fig. 29.7: Sodium fluoride toothpaste.

- In 1955, another milestone development in history of dentifrices was the introduction of divalent tin fluoride compound (SnF_2) in dentifrices containing 0.4% SnF_2 in a calcium pyrophosphate abrasive system **(Fig. 29.8)**.
- However, this also failed to get the desired results because of its compatibility with abrasives, staining of anterior restorations of composites resins, and a metallic astringent taste, which was not acceptable.

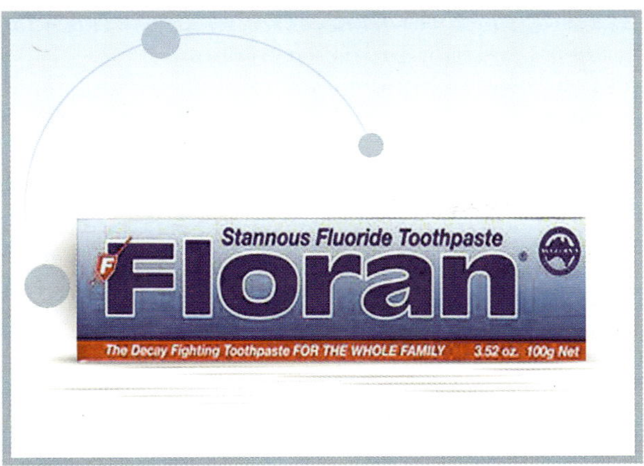

Fig. 29.8: Stannous fluoride toothpaste.

Amine Fluoride Dentifrices

- This was first tested for its cariostatic potential in Zurich, Switzerland.
- This showed organic fluorides to have antibacterial and anticariogenic properties, which were superior to inorganic fluorides and demonstrated significant reduction in caries rate.
- These dentifrices are marketed only in Europe **(Fig. 29.9)**.

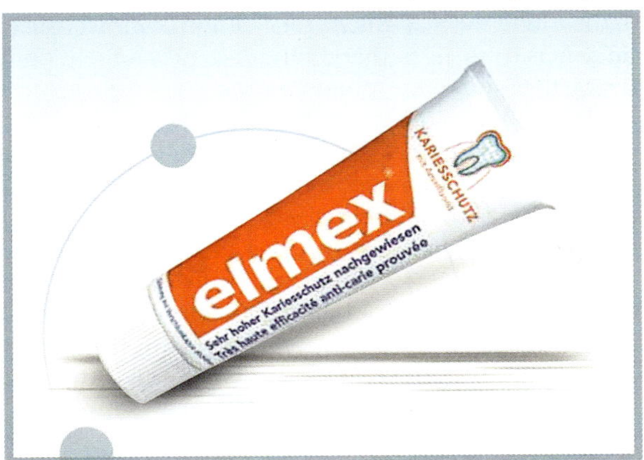

Fig. 29.9: Amine fluoride toothpaste.

Monofluorophosphate

- Monofluorophosphate (MFP) is the basic incompatibility of the NaF and SnF_2 compounds with calcium abrasives leading to decrease available fluoride has been overcome with the introduction of MFP, which has become the preferred chemical form of fluoride in most of the major commercial fluoridated tooth pastes used throughout the world ever since 1969 **(Fig. 29.10).**
- Dentifrices containing MFP at a concentration of 0.76%, 0.1% with sodium metaphosphate as abrasive, have led to variable reductions in caries rates ranging from 17% for unsupervised brushing and about 34% for supervised brushing in nonfluoridated areas.
- At present, there are two possible modes of action regarding caries inhibitory mechanism of MFP. The first mode is essentially a fluoride effect given by **Ericsson** (1963), MFP is deposited in the crystalline lattice and in subsequent intracrystalline transposition, and fluoride is released and replaces the hydroxyl group to form fluorapatite. The second mode of action according to **Ingram** (1972) attributes to the anticariogenic activity. MFP differs from other agents, in the aspect that its F-atom is covalently bonded to phosphorous atom. The mechanisms include direct incorporation into hydroxyapatite or hydrolysis to phosphate and fluoride ions, followed by reaction to form fluoroapatite.

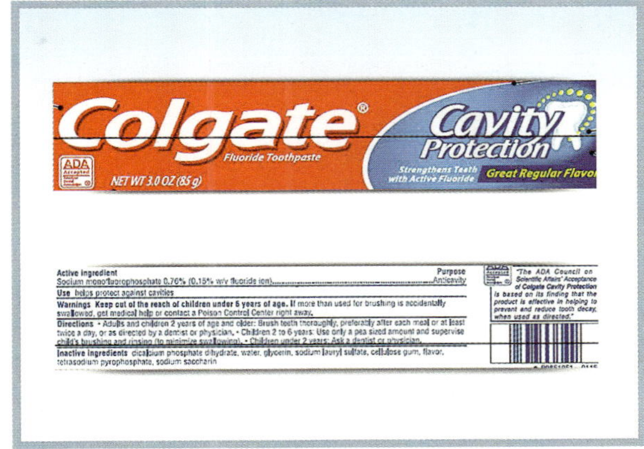

Fig. 29.10: Monofluorophosphate toothpaste.

$$PO_3F + H_2O = H_2PO_4 + FPO_3F + OH = PO_4 + F + H$$

- Advantages include neutral pH, greater stability to oxidation and hydrolysis, longer shelf life, increased availability of fluoride, and no staining of teeth.

Recommendations for use of fluoride dentifrice

Age (years)	*Recommendation*
Below 4	Not recommended
4–6	Once daily with fluoride paste and twice without paste
6–10	Twice daily with fluoride paste and once without paste
Above 10	Thrice daily with fluoride paste

FLUORIDE TOXICITY

During the latter half of 19th century and the first half of the 20th century, NaF was used as a pesticide. It was often stored in places where the residents had access to the compound. Because of this, many cases of accidental and intentional acute fluoride poisoning occurred. **Lidbech et al.** (1943) described one of the mass poisonings that occurred during that period. At the Oregon State Hospital, an evening meal of scrambled eggs was prepared with NaF which had been mistaken for powdered milk. Approximately 17 lb of NaF was added to 10 gallons of eggs. There were 263 cases of acute poisoning, of which 47 terminated fatally. Fluoride can be very harmful if large amounts are ingested in a single dose or over a period of time. This may be followed by rapidly developing signs and symptoms. It is divided into acute toxicity and chronic toxicity.[12]

Probably toxic dose (PTD): Defined as the threshold dose that could cause serious or life-threatening systemic signs and symptoms.
Safely tolerated dose: 8–16 mg/kg body weight
Toxic dose: 16–32 mg/kg body weight
Lethal dose: 32–64 mg/kg body weight

Acute Toxicity

Ingestion of large doses of fluoride at one time.

Factors Affecting Acute Toxicity

- ❖ Bioavailability.
- ❖ Route of administration.
- ❖ Age.
- ❖ Rate of absorption.
- ❖ Acid base status.

Signs and Symptoms

- ❖ Nausea, vomiting.
- ❖ Abdominal pain, diarrhea.
- ❖ Excess salivation and mucosal discharge.
- ❖ Generalized weakness and carpopedal spasms.
- ❖ Weak thready pulse, fall in blood pressure.
- ❖ Depression of respiratory center.
- ❖ Decreased plasma calcium level, increased potassium level.
- ❖ Cardiac arrhythmia.
- ❖ Coma and death.

Methods to Reduce Intake of Nondietary Fluorides

- ❖ Parental supervision.
- ❖ Small amount of paste to be used.
- ❖ Products with low fluoride level to be used.
- ❖ Teaching children not to swallow the paste.
- ❖ Strict adherence to professional advice.
- ❖ Should not be used by young children without supervision.
- ❖ Should be kept out of the reach of children.

Management of Acute Toxicity

Immediate	• Aimed at reducing fluoride absorption • Induce vomiting • Fluid replacement • Monitoring levels of plasma calcium and potassium
<5 mg/kg fluoride ingested	• Give milk • Induce vomiting
>5 mg/kg fluoride ingested	• Give milk • Induce vomiting • 5% calcium gluconate • Hospitalization
>15-mg/kg fluoride ingested	• Induce vomiting • Hospitalization • Cardiac monitoring (peaking of T-wave or prolonged Q–T interval) • Slow administration of 10% calcium gluconate • Maintain urinary output—supportive measures for shock

Chronic Toxicity

It is defined as ingestion of variant doses of fluoride over a prolonged period of time. It is of two types: (1) dental and (2) skeletal fluoroses:

Dental Fluorosis

Dental fluorosis is a developmental disturbance of dental enamel, caused by successive exposures to high concentrations of fluoride during tooth development, leading to enamel with lower mineral content and increased porosity.[12]

- ❖ It can be hypoplasia or hypomaturation of tooth enamel or dentin.
- ❖ Both primary and permanent teeth will be affected, but greater fluorosis in permanent teeth is seen because much of the mineralization of primary teeth occurs before birth and also because the placenta serves as the barrier to the transfer of high concentrations of plasma fluoride from a pregnant mother to her developing fetus.

Etiopathogenesis

There is direct inhibitory effect on enzymatic action of ameloblasts leading to defective matrix formation and subsequent hypomineralization.

Causes for Dental Fluorosis

- ❖ Excessive fluoride in water.
- ❖ Nonprescribed use of fluoride supplements.
- ❖ Ingestion of topical fluoride.

Clinical Features (Figs. 29.11A to F)

- ❖ The first signs of dental fluorosis are thin white striae across the enamel surface. These fine lines follow the perikymata pattern and can best be distinguished by drying the surface of the tooth. Even at this stage of dental fluorosis, the cusp tips, incisal edges, or marginal ridges may appear opaque white, the "snow cap" phenomenon.
- ❖ In slightly more affected teeth, the white lines are broader and more pronounced. Occasional merging of several lines occurs to produce smaller, irregular, cloudy, or paper-white areas scattered over the surface.
- ❖ With increasing severity, the entire tooth surface exhibits distinct, irregular, opaque, or cloudy white areas. Frequently, the cervical enamel appears more homogenously opaque, and the mesioincisal part of the maxillary incisors may exhibit varying degrees of brownish discoloration. Such brown stains are a result of posteruptive staining.
- ❖ The next degree of severity manifests as irregular opaque areas which merge so that the entire tooth surface appears chalky white. When such surfaces are probed vigorously, part of the surface enamel may flake off.
- ❖ In even more severe stages, the tooth surface is entirely opaque with focal loss of the outermost enamel. Such small enamel defects are usually designated "pits." With increased severity, these pits merge to form horizontal bands.
- ❖ Ultimately, the most severely fluorotic teeth exhibited an almost total loss of surface enamel whereby the normal tooth morphology is severely affected. The loss of surface enamel may be so extensive that only a cervical rim of intact, markedly opaque enamel is left. The remaining part of the tooth often exhibits a dark brownish discoloration. The discoloration is entirely dependent on such posteruptive environmental conditions as dietary habits, and the degree of discoloration should, therefore, not be used as an indication of severity of fluorosis as such.

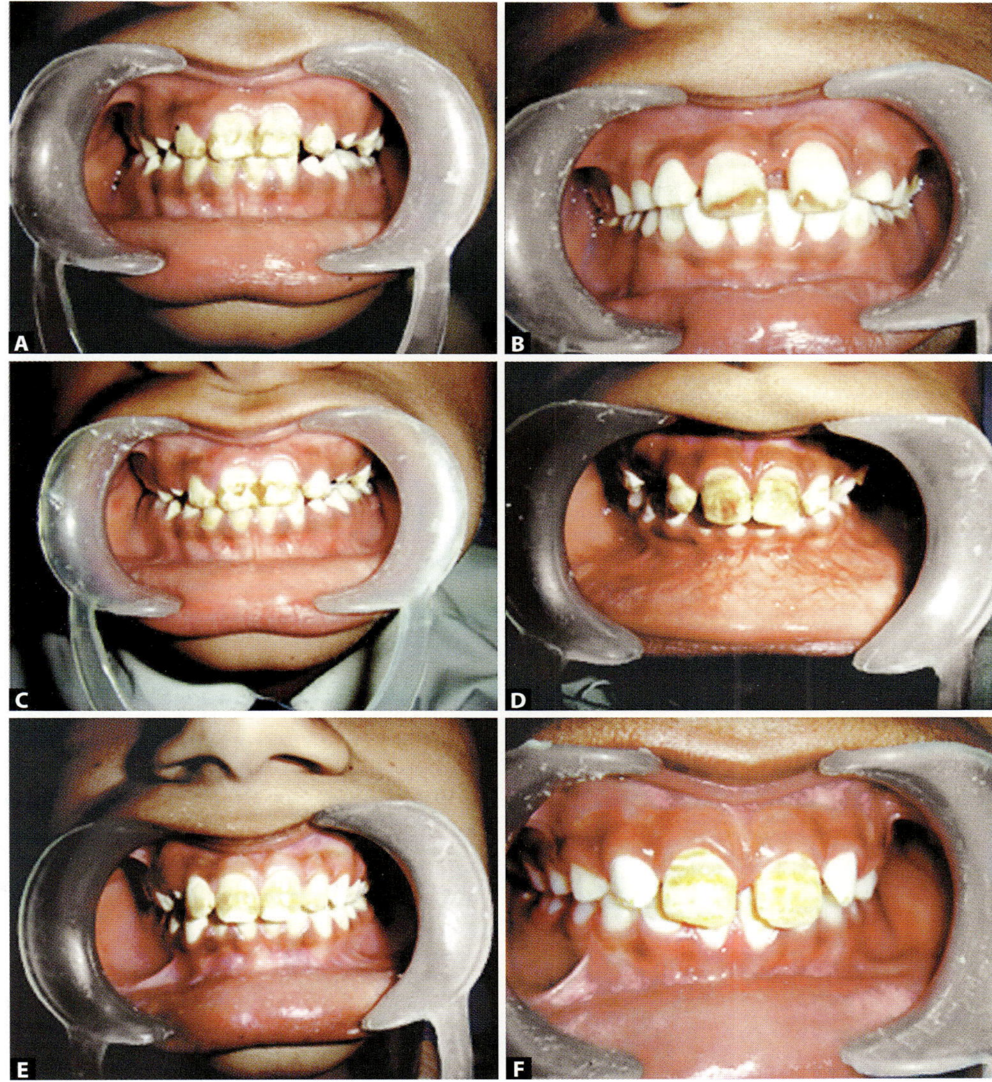

Figs. 29.11A to F: Different grades of dental fluorosis.

Skeletal Fluorosis

This is also called osteofluorosis.

Etiology

Water fluoride levels over 4 ppm causes a mild variant but levels over 8 ppm cause severe skeletal fluorosis.

Clinical Features

- Increase in bone density.
- Change in bone contours.
- Irregular periosteal growth.
- Spinal column and the pelvis show roughening and blurring of the trabeculae.
- Bone appears as marble white shadows and the configuration is wooly. The cortex of long bone is thick and dense, and the medullary cavity is diminished.
- Ligamental and tendon calcification with vague pain in joints.
- Stiffness and limitation of joint movements, immobilizing the patient—crippling fluorosis.
- Arthritic changes, cataract, thyroid problems, fractures, urinary, and gallstones may also be seen.

Classification

According to the severity, **Teotia et al.** classified skeletal fluorosis:

- Clinical
  - *Mild:* Generalized bone and joint pains.
  - *Moderate:* Mild symptoms with stiffness, rigidity, and restricted movement of spine and joints.
  - *Severe:* Symptoms of moderate fluorosis along with flexion deformities of spine, hips, and knees, genu valgum, genu varum, bowing and rotational deformities of legs, neurological complications, crippling, and bedridden stage.
- Radiological
  - *Mild:* Osteosclerosis only.
  - *Moderate:* Signs of mild fluorosis along with periosteal bone formation, calcifications of interosseous membrane, ligaments, muscular attachments, capsules, and tendons.
  - *Severe:* Signs of moderate fluorosis with associated metabolic bone disease (rickets neo-osseousmalacia, osteoporosis), exostosis, osteophytosis.

Systemic effects of chronic exposure to fluorides[13-15]

Gastrointestinal tract (GIT): Nonulcer dyspepsia, drying of goblet cells and fissure in the gastric mucosa, delayed emptying of stomach, nausea, bloated abdomen, loss of appetite.

Skeletal muscles: Destruction of the actin and myosin filaments, weakness, loss of muscle energy, inability to stand in erect position.

Red blood cells (RBCs): Erythrocyte membrane becomes pliable and is thrown into folds due to loss of calcium content. RBCs attain a shape similar to amoeba with pseudopodia-like folds projecting into different directions and are termed echinocytes.

Reproductive system: Male infertility with abnormality in sperm morphology, low testosterone levels, and testicular oxidative stress. Repeated abortions and still births due to fetal blood vessels calcification.

Neurological system: Adversely affects brain leading to nervousness, depression/tingling sensation in fingers and toes, excessive thirst and tendency to urinate more frequently. **Li et al.**[16] from China also reported low IQ among children exposed to high fluoride as compared to nonexposed children.

DENTAL FLUOROSIS INDICES

The extent of dental fluorosis can be evaluated by various indices, like Dean index, Thylstrup and Fejerskov index, Horowitz index, Moller index, FDI index, etc.

Thylstrup and Fejerskov index

Score	*Criteria*
0	Normal enamel
1	Narrow wide lines corresponding to perikymata
2	More pronounced lines
3	Merging and irregular cloudy areas
4	Entire surface is chalky white
5	Surface has opacity with pits
6	Regularly arranged pits and horizontal bands
7	Loss of outer enamel but less than half surface
8	Loss of enamel in more than half surface
9	Loss of tooth structure leading to change in anatomic appearance of tooth

FDI index

Dental developmental index modified in 1989

Score	*Criteria*
1	Normal
2	Demarcated opacities • White/cream • Yellow/brown
3	Diffuse opacities • Diffuse—lines • Diffuse—patchy • Diffuse—confluent • Confluent/patchy/staining/loss of enamel
4	Hypoplasia • Pits • Missing enamel
5	Any other defects

Dean index

Given by Trendly H Dean in 1934. Examination of all tooth surfaces was done in good natural light with the child seated facing window.

Rating	*Public health significance*	*Characteristics*
0	Normal	The enamel shows the usual translucency. The surface is smooth, shiny, and usually of a pale, creamy white to gray white color
0.5	Questionable	The enamel shows slight aberrations ranging from a few white flecks to occasional white spots
1	Very mild	Small, opaque, paper white areas scattered irregularly over tooth but not involving >25%
2	Mild	Opaque, paper white areas that is more extensive, involving >25% but <50%
3	Moderate	All enamel surfaces are affected and also show attrition
4	Severe	All enamel surfaces are affected and hypoplasia is so marked that general form of tooth is affected. Discrete or confluent pitting with brown stains is a characteristic feature

DEFLUORIDATION

It is the process of removing excess, naturally occurring fluorides from drinking water in order to reduce the prevalence and severity of dental fluorosis. WHO in 1963 has recommended that optimum limit of fluoride in drinking water for the prevention of dental caries is 0.7–1.2 ppm. In India, the work on defluoridation was taken up by National Environmental Engineering Research Institute **(NEERI)** at Nagpur, Maharashtra, India in 1961 where various methods for removal of fluoride from potable waters have been tried.

Defluoridation techniques can be broadly classified into four categories:[17]

1. Adsorption technique.
2. Ion-exchange technique.
3. Precipitation technique.
4. Other techniques, which include electrochemical defluoridation and reverse osmosis.

Adsorption Technique of Defluoridation

- This technique functions on the adsorption of fluoride ions onto the surface of an active agent. Activated alumina, activated carbon, and bone char were among the highly tested adsorbing agents.
- **Activated alumina**
    - Application of domestic defluoridation plant, based on activated alumina, was launched by UNICEF in rural India.
    - **Horowitz** and **Helfetz**, in 1972 discussed about a successfully functioning, activated alumina community defluoridation plant, which was commissioned in Bartlett, Texas, USA in the year 1952.
    - The disadvantages with activated alumina are adsorption of fluoride is possible only at specific pH range, needing pre- and post-pH adjustment of water.
    - Frequent activation of alumina is needed, which make the technique expensive.

- **Bone char**
  - **Nutthamon Fangsrekam** described the process of defluoridation by bone char as the ion exchange and adsorption between fluoride in the solution and carbonate of the apatite comprising bone char.
  - The efficacy of the plant depends upon temperature and pH of raw water; duration for which the bone char is in contact with raw water. The maximum amounts of fluoride adsorbed per gram of bone char surface at 25, 35, and 45°C are about 21.1, 22.4, and 25.7 μmol, respectively. The optimum time for the adsorption to reach saturation is 9 hours, and optimum pH of fluoride solution is between 7.00 and 7.50.
  - Disadvantages of this technique are the bone char harbors bacteria and hence unhygienic. Without a regular fluoride analysis, nothing indicates when the material is exhausted and the fluoride uptake is ceased.
- **Brick pieces column**
  - The basic principle of functioning of brick piece column is the same as that of activated alumina.
  - The soil used for brick manufacturing contains aluminum oxide. During burning operation in the kiln, it gets activated and adsorbs excess fluoride when raw water is passed through.
- **Mud pot**
  - The raw pots are subjected to heat treatment as in the case of brick production. Hence, the mud pot also will act as an adsorbent media.
  - The major advantages of mud pots are they are economic and readily acceptable for the rural communities.
- **Natural adsorbents**
  - Seeds of the drumstick tree, roots of vetiver grass, and tamarind seeds were tried as defluoridation agents.

Ion-exchange Technique

- **Anion exchange resins**
  - These include polystyrene anion exchange resins and basic quaternary ammonium type resins.
  - **Bhakuni** found that although these resins did remove fluoride, but they had some disadvantages like ionizing fluoride removal capacity on prolonged use, cost, and alteration of taste of water.
- **Cation exchange resins**
  - *Defluoron-1:* Bhakuni developed this combination of sulphonated saw dust impregnated with 2% alum solution. The disadvantages of this were poor hydraulic properties and heavy attritional losses.
  - *Carbion:* It is a cation exchange resin of good durability and can be used both on sodium and hydrogen cycles.
  - *Magnesia:* Investigations conducted by **Thergaonkar** (1971) established that magnesia removed the excess fluorides, but pH of treated water was beyond 10, and its correction by acidification or recarbonation was necessary.
  - *Defluoron-2:* To overcome the problems faced with previous methods, defluoron-2 was developed in 1968. Defluoron-2 is a sulphonated coal and works on the aluminum cycles. This type of defluoridation gave excellent results, had a good shelf life of 2–4 years, and was very cost-effective.

Defluoridation by Precipitation Technique

- Precipitation methods are based on the addition of chemicals (coagulants and coagulant aids) and the subsequent precipitation of a sparingly soluble fluoride salt as insoluble fluorapatite.
- Aluminum salts (e.g. alum), lime, polyaluminum chloride (PAC), polyaluminum hydroxyl sulfate, and brushite are some of the frequently used materials in defluoridation by precipitation technique.

Other Techniques of Defluoridation

- **Reverse osmosis**
  - In reverse osmosis, the hydraulic pressure is exerted on one side of the semipermeable membrane which forces the water across the membrane leaving the salts behind
  - The removal of fluoride in the reverse osmosis process had been reported to vary from 45 to 90% as the pH of the water was raised from 5.5 to 7.
- **Defluoridation by electrolysis**
  - The basic principle of the process is the adsorption of fluoride with freshly precipitated aluminum hydroxide, which is generated by the anodic dissolution of aluminum or its alloys in an electrochemical cell.
  - The driving force is an electric current which carries the ions through the membranes (**Hall and Crow**, 1993).
  - Advantages are it does not require addition of chemicals, low volume of sludge, units can be designed for any capacity, electrochemical reactor occupies less floor space, operator friendly, and requires less electric energy.

Nalgonda Technique[18]

Although defluoron-2 was successful in removing fluorides, the regeneration and maintenance of the plant required skilled operation, which may not be readily available. In order to overcome this problem, a method was evolved by **WG Nawalakhe** in 1974, which is so simple and adaptable that even illiterate persons can make use of it.

Working Principle

- This involved the addition of three readily available chemicals, i.e., sodium aluminate or lime, bleaching powder, and filter alum to the fluoride water in the same sequence which leads to flocculation, sedimentation, and filtration. Sodium aluminate or lime hastens settlement of precipitate and bleaching powder ensures disinfection. This technique can be used both for domestic as well as for community water supplies.
- For domestic treatment, any container of 20–25 L capacity is suitable. A tap 3–5 cm above the bottom of the container is useful to withdraw treated water but is not essential. Adequate amount of lime water and bleaching powder are sprinkled into water first and mixed well with it. Alum solution is then poured, and the water is stirred for 10 minutes. The contents are settled for 1 hour, and the clear water is withdrawn either through the tap or decanted slowly without disturbing the sediment **(Fig. 29.12)**.

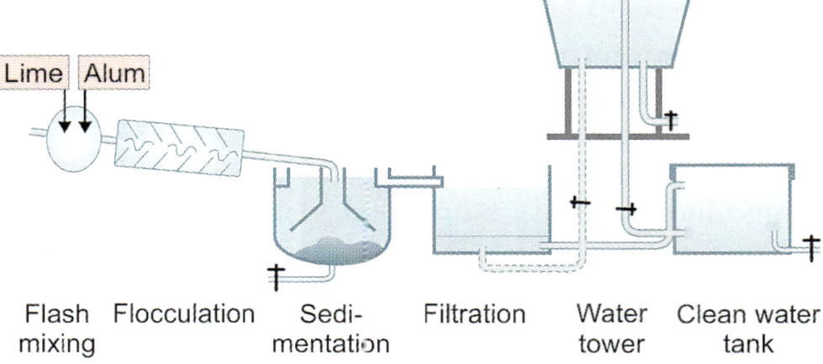

Fig. 29.12: Nalgonda technique.

Advantages

- No regeneration of media.
- No handling of caustic acids and alkalies.
- Readily available chemicals are used.
- Adaptable to domestic usage.
- Simplicity in design, construction, and maintenance.
- Little wastage of water.
- Needs minimal mechanical and electrical equipment.

Disadvantages

- Desalination may be necessary.
- Hardness of the raw water in the range of 200–600 mg/L requires precipitation softening.
- Generation of higher quantity of sludge compared to electrochemical defluoridation.
- Large amount of alum needed to remove fluoride.

Modifications for Nalgonda Technique

- **Polyaluminum chloride (PAC):** It is evident that for higher concentrations of fluoride, the removal efficiency of fluoride is higher with PAC when compared with alum.
- **Polyaluminum hydroxy sulfate (PAHS):** It is found to require less flocculation time and settling time.

Two bucket technique in Tanzania

The designed defluoridator consists of two buckets equipped with taps and a sieve on which a cotton cloth is placed. Alum and lime are added simultaneously to the raw water bucket where it is dissolved/suspended by stirring with a wooden paddle. The villagers are trained to stir fast while counting to 60 (1 min) and then slowly while counting to 300 (5 min). The flocs formed are left to settle for about 1 hour. The treated technique. water is then tapped through the cloth into the treated water bucket from where it is collected as needed for drinking and cooking.

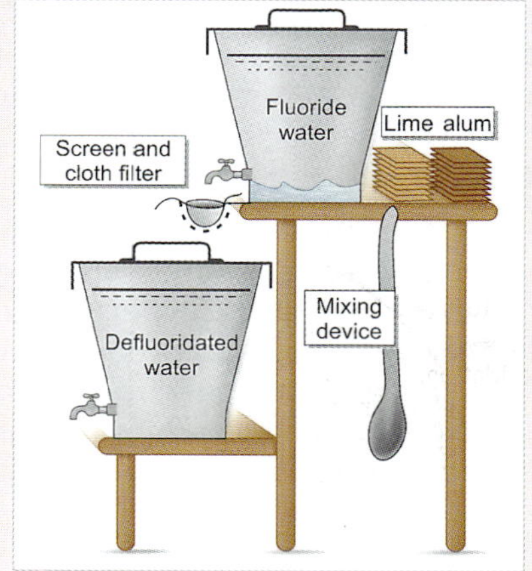

Prashanthi Technique

The Prashanthi technology for fluoride removal using activated alumina, originated as a result of research and development activities carried out at the Bio-science Department at Satya Sai University for Higher Learning at Prasanti Nilayam at Anantpur District in Andhra Pradesh.

RECENT ADVANCES IN FLUORIDE[19]

Sustained Released Intraoral Devices

Copolymer Membrane Device

- Developed by **Cowsar** (1976) in USA.
- This system was designed as a membrane-controlled reservoir-type and has an inner core of hydroxyethyl methacrylate (HEMA)/methyl methacrylate (MMA) copolymer (50:50 mixture), containing a precise amount of NaF. This core is surrounded by a 30:70 HEMA/MMA copolymer membrane which controls the rate of fluoride release from the device.
- When the matrix becomes hydrated, small quantities of granulated NaF are diluted until the matrix itself becomes saturated. The precise water absorption rates by the inner and the outer cores enables the devices to act accurately and reliably as a release controlling mechanism.
- The device is approximately 8 mm in length, 3 mm in width, and 2 mm in thickness **(Fig. 29.13)** and is usually attached to the buccal surface of the first permanent molar by means of stainless steel retainers that are spot welded to plain, standard orthodontic bands, or are bonded to the tooth surfaces using adhesive resins.
- Depending on the amount of F in the inner core, the rate of F release of these devices can be between 0.02 and 1.0 mg F/day for up to 180 days.

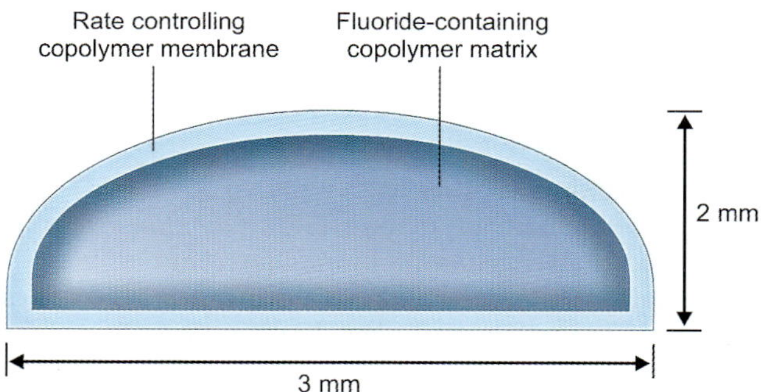

Fig. 29.13: Copolymer device.

Fluoride Glass Device

- Developed in Leeds, United Kingdom.
- The F glass device dissolves slowly when moist in saliva, releasing F without significantly affecting the device's integrity.
- The original device was dome shape, with a diameter of 4 mm and about 2 mm thick, being usually attached to the buccal surface of the first permanent molar using adhesive resins **(Fig. 29.14)**. Due to the low retention rates of the original device, it was further substantially changed to a kidney-shaped device, being 6 mm long 2.5 mm in width, and 2.3 mm in depth **(Fig. 29.15)**, and it was proven to be effective regarding both F release and retention rate.
- A new modification was introduced more recently in order to facilitate device handling, attachment, and replacement. This new device has been shaped in the form of a disk that is placed within a plastic bracket **(Fig. 29.16)**.

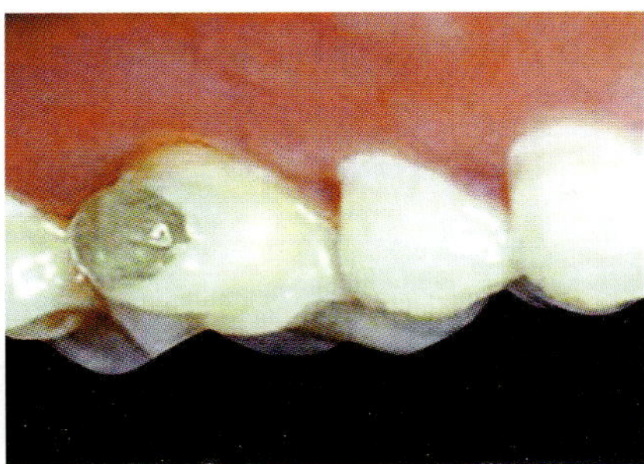
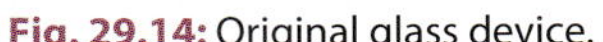
Fig. 29.14: Original glass device.

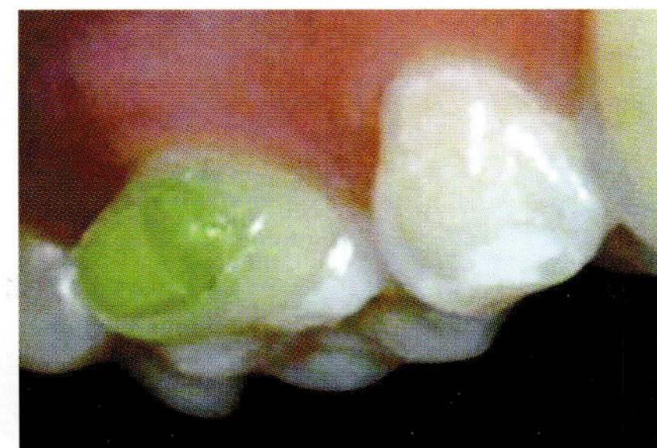
Fig. 29.15: Modified glass device.

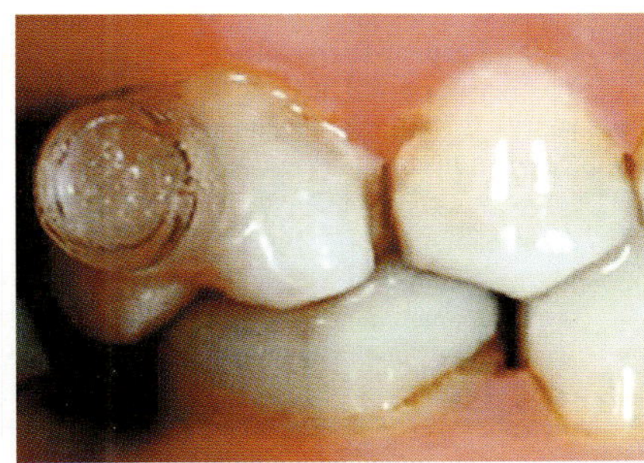
Fig. 29.16: New modification of glass device.

- Concentration of fluoride in glass: 13.3–21.9%.
- Longer shelf life with continuous release up to 2 years.

Hydroxyapatite-Eudragit RS100 Diffusion Controlled F System

- This is the newest type of slow-release F device, which consists of a mixture of hydroxyapatite, NaF, and Eudragit RS100.
- Eudragit RS100 is a copolymer of ethyl acrylate, MMA, and a low content of methacrylic acid ester with quaternary ammonium groups. The ammonium groups are present as salts and make the polymers permeable.
- It contains 18 mg of NaF and is intended to release 0.15 mg F/day.
- It was demonstrated that the use of this device is able to significantly increase salivary and urinary F concentrations for ≥1 month.
- Placed on labial aspect of maxillary incisors, buccal aspect of molars, and lingual aspect of mandibular incisors.

Silver Diamine Fluoride

- Silver diamine fluoride (SDF) is a basic solution (pH of 10-12) with a 38% w/v $Ag(NH_3)_2F$. The silver acts as an antimicrobial and fluoride promotes remineralization; the ammonia (NH_3) present stabilizes the solution.
- When SDF is applied to tooth surface, the diamine-silver ion complexes react with hydroxyapatite forming silver phosphate (Ag_3PO_4) and silver oxide (Ag_2O).
- SDF is indicated for children with high caries risk who have active cavitated caries lesions and children who present with behavioral or medical management challenges which precludes the conventional restorative treatment. (This has been dealt in detail in Chapter 46).

Researches on fluoride release

- Use of fluoride complexes—**Mc Cann et al.**[20] showed Al^{3+} and Ti^{+} ions showed increased uptake of fluoride in enamel.
- **Gron et al.**[21] evaluated that cetyl pyridinium chloride, zonyl FSC, zonyl FSN, iodyne showed increased uptake of fluoride in enamel.
- Light activated fluoride—**Zezell et al.**[22] (Nd:YAG Laser + Topical APF)
- NaF containing mucosa adhesive paste—**Gabre et al.**[23]
- Orthodontic brackets as fluoride reservoir—**Song Li et al.**[24]
- Laser activated fluoride with remineralizing agent—**Aminabadi et al.**[25] (Nd:YAG + CPP-ACP)
- Fluoridated hydroxyapatite coated preformed metal crowns—**Clark et al.**[26]

POINTS TO REMEMBER

- Fluoride has been described as an essential nutrient in the Federal Register of United States Food and Drug Administration (1973).
- The term fluoride is derived from a Latin word Fluore, which means to flow.
- Lake Nakuru (Kenya) has most concentration of fluoride, that is, 2,800 ppm.
- Tea leaves have most fluoride content among common food items: 56,640 ppm.
- In the case of teeth, maximum concentration of fluoride is found in cementum (4,500 ppm).
- Fluoride can cross the placental barrier.
- Shoe Leather Survey by Dean was done to continue McKay work on fluoridation.
- First community level water fluoridation program started in Grand Rapids, USA on January 25, 1945.
- Mechanism of action of fluoride is by improved crystallinity, filling of voids of hydroxyapatite, less acid solubility, enzyme inhibition, suppressing the flora, antibacterial action, lowering free surface energy, desorption of protein and bacteria, and alteration in tooth morphology.
- Galagan and Vermillion formula is ppm $F = 0.34/E$.
- The current recommended regimen for school water fluoridation is adding 4.5 times more fluoride.
- Salt and milk fluoridation was done by Wespi and Zieglar, respectively.
- Knutson and Feldman recommended a technique of four applications of 2% NaF at weekly intervals in a year at 3, 7, 11, and 13 years.
- Brudevold did the study on APF and concluded that semiannual application of 1.23% APF for 4 minutes is helpful in reducing caries by 28%.
- Duraphat is the most effective varnish in caries reduction.
- MFP is the most commonly used active ingredient of toothpastes today.
- *Acute toxicity:* Ingestion of large doses of fluoride at one time. Its signs and symptoms include nausea, vomiting, diarrhea, excess salivation and mucosal discharge, weakness and carpopedal spasms, fall in blood pressure, cardiac arrhythmia, and may be even death.
- Chronic toxicity includes dental and skeletal fluorosis.
- The extent of dental fluorosis can be evaluated by various indices, like Dean index, Thylstrup and Fejerskov index, Horowitz index, Moller index, FDI index, etc.

- Defluoridation is the process of removing excess, naturally occurring fluorides from drinking water in order to reduce the prevalence and severity of dental fluorosis.
- First defluoridation project was taken up by National Environmental Engineering Research Institute (NEERI) at Nagpur in 1961.
- Defluoridation techniques are adsorption technique, ion-exchange technique, precipitation technique, and electrochemical/reverse osmosis.
- Nalgonda technique was given by WG Nawalakhe in 1974, and it involves addition of three readily available chemicals, that is, sodium aluminate or lime, bleaching powder, and filter alum to the fluoride water in the same sequence which leads to flocculation, sedimentation, and filtration. Sodium aluminate or lime hastens settlement of precipitate and bleaching powder ensures disinfection. This technique can be used both for domestic as well as for community water supplies.
- The newer fluoride developments include copolymer membrane device, fluoride glass device, and Hydroxyapatite—Eudragit RS100 diffusion controlled F system.

Questionnaire

1. Discuss the distribution of fluoride in environment.
2. Describe the metabolism of fluoride.
3. Give a brief description on history of fluoride.
4. What is shoe leather survey?
5. Explain the mechanism of action of fluoride.
6. Write a note on water fluoridation.
7. What is Galagan and Vermillion formula?
8. Discuss school water fluoridation.
9. What are topical fluorides? Write a note on Knutson technique.
10. Write a short note on APF.
11. Explain choking off mechanism.
12. What are fluoride varnishes?
13. Discuss acute toxicity with its clinical features and management.
14. Explain dental fluorosis.
15. Note on fluorosis indices.
16. Discuss defluoridation with special reference to Nalgonda technique.
17. What are the recent advancements in intraoral fluoride?

REFERENCES

1. Punekar BD, Lakdawala DR. Fluoride content of water and commonly consumed foods in Bombay and a study of the dietary fluoride intake. Indian J Med Res. 1973;61:1679-87.
2. Susheela AK. Epidemiology and control of fluorosis in India. J Nutr Found India; 1984.
3. UNICEF. Fluoride in water: an overview. Available from: http://www.unicef.org/programme/wes/info/fluor.htm (accessed on 29-09-2007).
4. Tewari A, Jalili VP. Fluorides and dental caries. Indian Dental Association; 1986.
5. Dean HT, Arnold FA, Jay P, Knutson JW. Studies on mass control of dental caries through fluoridation of the public water supply. Public Health Rep. 1950;65:1403-8.
6. Galagan DJ, Vermillion JR. Determining optimum fluoride concentrations. Public Health Rep. 1957;72:491-3.
7. Clinical guidelines by AAPD revised in 2012 reference manual V 34/ NO 6 12/13.
8. Bibby BG. A new approach to caries prophylaxis. Tufts Dent Outlook. 1942;15:4-8.
9. Knutson JW, Armstrong WD, Feldman FM. Effect of topically applied sodium fluoride on dental caries experience. iv. Report of findings with two, four and six applications. Publ Health Rep. 1947;62:425.
10. Brudevold F, Savory A, Gardner DE, Spinelli M, Speirs R. A study of acidulated fluoride solutions I: In vitro effects on enamel. Arch Oral Biol. 1963;8:167-77.
11. Melinda B. Clark, Martha Ann Keels, Rebecca L. Slayton, SECTION ON ORAL HEALTH, Patricia A. Braun, Susan A. Fisher-Owens, Qadira Ali Huff, Jeffrey M. Karp, Anupama Rao Tate, John H. Unkel, David Krol; Fluoride Use in Caries Prevention in the Primary Care Setting. Pediatrics December 2020; 146 (6): e2020034637. 10.1542/ peds.2020-034637.
12. Whitford GM. Acute and chronic fluoride toxicity. J Dent Res. 1992;71:1249-54.
13. Fejerskov O, Manji F, Baelum V. The nature and mechanisms of dental fluorosis in man. J Dent Res. 1990;69 spec Iss: 692-700.
14. Susheela AK, Das TK, Gupta IP, et al. Fluoride ingestion and its correlation with gastrointestinal discomfort. Fluoride. 1992;25:5-22.
15. Susheela AK. A Treatise on Fluorosis, 2nd edition. New Delhi: Fluorosis Research and Rural Development Foundation; 2003.
16. Li XS, Zhi JL, Gao RO. Effect of fluoride exposure on intelligence in children. Fluoride. 1995;28:189-92.
17. Renuka P, Pushpanjali K. Review on defluoridation techniques of water. Int J Eng Sci. 2013;2:86-94.
18. Nawalakhe WG, Paramasivam R. Defluoridation of potable water by Nalgonda technique. Curr Sci. 1993;65.
19. Pessan JP, Al-Ibrahim NS, Buzalaf MAR, Toumba JK. Slow- release fluoride devices: a literature review. J Appl Oral Sci. 2008;16:238-44.
20. McCann HG. The effect of fluoride complex formation on fluoride uptake and retention in human enamel. Archives of Oral Biology. 1969;14(5):521-531.
21. Gron, P & Caslavska, Vera. Effect of Surface-Active Agents on Fluoride Enamel Interactions. II. Caries research.1983:17;304-309.
22. Zezell DM, Boari HG, Ana PA, Eduardo Cde P, Powell GL. Nd:YAG laser in caries prevention: a clinical trial. Lasers Surg Med. 2009;41(1):31-35.
23. Gabre P, Birkhed D, Gahnberg L. Fluoride retention of a mucosa adhesive paste compared with other home-care fluoride products. Caries Res. 2008;42(4):240-6.
24. Li S, Hobson RS, Bai Y, Yan Z, Carrick TE, McCabe JF. A method for producing controlled fluoride release from an orthodontic bracket. European Journal of Orthodontics. 2007:29(6);550-54.
25. Asl-Aminabadi N, et al. Laser-casein phosphopeptide effect on remineralization of early enamel lesions in primary teeth. Journal of Clinical and Experimental Dentistry. 2015: 7(2) e261-e267.
26. Clark DR, Czajka-Jakubowska A, Rick C, Liu J, Chang S, Clarkson BH. In vitro anti-caries effect of fluoridated hydroxyapatite-coated preformed metal crowns. Eur Arch Paediatr Dent. 2013;14(4):253-8.

FURTHER READING

1. Bali RK, Mathur VB, Talwar PP, Chanana HB. National Oral Health Survey and fluoride mapping 2002–2003. India. Available from: http://www.docstoc.com/docs/83028952/ summary-PDF.
2. British Fluoridation Society (2012). One in a Million: The facts about water fluoridation. Available online at: http://www.bfsweb.org/ onemillion/onemillion2012.html
3. Ekstrand J, Zeigler EE, Nelson SE, Formon SJ. Absorption and retention of dietary and supplemental fluoride. Adv Dent Res. 1994;8:175-80.
4. Fejerskov O, Richards A, DenBesten P. In: Fejerskov O, Ekstrand J, Burt BA (Eds). Fluoride in Dentistry, 2nd edition. Copenhagen: Munksgaard; 1996. pp. 112-52.
5. Finn SB. Clinical Pedodontics, 2nd edition. Philadelphia, PA: Saunders; 1965.
6. Koch G, Petersson LG. Caries Preventive effect of a fluoride containing varnish (Duraphat) after 1 year's study. Comm Dent Oral Epidemiol. 1975;3:262-6.

7. McCann HG. The effect of fluoride complex formation on fluoride uptake and retention in human enamel. Archs Oral Biol. 1969;14: 521-31.
8. Moller IJ, Holst JJ, Sorensen E. Caries reducing effect of a sodium monofluorophosphate dentifrice. Br Dent J. 1968;124:209-13.
9. Muhler JC, Radhike AW, Nebergall WH, Day HG. A comparison between the anticariogenic effect of dentifrices containing stannous fluoride and sodium fluoride. J Amer Dent Assoc. 1955;51:556-9.
10. Muhler JC, Stookey GK, Bixler D. Evaluation of the anticariogenic effect of mixtures of stannous fluoride and soluble phosphates. J Dent Child. 1965;32:154-69.
11. Murray JJ, Winter GB, Hurst CP. Duraphat fluoride varnish—a 2 year clinical trial in 5 years old children. Br Dent J. 1977; 143:11-7.
12. National Health Portal India. https://www.nhp.gov.in/disease/non-communicable-disease/fluorosis
13. Pollick H. Salt fluoridation–A review. Journal of the California Dental Association. 2013;41(6):395-7, 400-4
14. Susheela AK, Koacher J, Jain SK, Sharma K, Jha M. Fluroide toxicity: a molecular approach. In: Highlights of the 13th conference of the international society for fluoride research, organized by Dr Susheela AK, in New Delhi (India); 1993. pp. 13-7.
15. US Department of Health and Human Services, Centers for Disease Control, Dental Disease Prevention Activity. Water fluoridation: a manual for engineers and technicians. Atlanta; 1986.
16. Whitford GM. The metabolism and toxicity of fluoride. In: Myers HM (Ed). Monographs in Oral Science. No. 13. Basel (Switzerland): Karger; 1989.
17. Whitford GM. The physiological and toxicological Characteristics of fluoride. J Dent Res. 1990;69 (Spec Iss):539-49.
18. World Health Organisation. Fluorides and human health, Geneva. In: WHO Monograph Series No. 59. 1970.

CHAPTER 30

Oral Habits

Nikhil Marwah, Manojit Mahato

CHAPTER OUTLINE

- Definition of Habits
- Classification of Habits
- Thumb Sucking
- Pacifier Habit
- Tongue Thrusting
- Mouth Breathing
- Bruxism
- Lip Biting
- Nail Biting
- Self-Injurious Habits

Oral habits may be a part of normal development; a symptom with a deep-rooted psychological basis that may be the result of abnormal facial growth. Digit sucking, lip and nail biting, bruxism, mouth breathing, tongue thrusting may be considered as normal habits seen in children. These habits bring about harmful unbalanced pressures to bear upon the immature, highly malleable alveolar ridges, the potential changes in position of teeth and occlusion, which may become decidedly abnormal if these habits are continued for a long time.

DEFINITION OF HABITS

Boucheor OC *defined habit as a tendency toward an actor an act that has become a repeated performance, relatively fixed, consistent, easy to perform, and almost automatic.*

Dorland *(1957) defined habit as a fixed or constant practice established by frequent repetition.*

Buttersworth *(1961) defined habit as frequent or constant practice or acquired tendency which has been fixed by frequent repetitions.*

Mathewson *(1982): Oral habits are learned patterns of muscular contractions.*

CLASSIFICATION OF HABITS

Useful and Harmful Habits (James, 1923)

Useful habits	*Harmful habits*
Should include all those habits of normal function such as correct tongue position, proper respiration, and deglutition.	All those that exert perverted stress against the teeth and dental arches, for example, mouth breathing, tongue thrusting.

Compulsive and Noncompulsive Habits (Finn, 1987)

Compulsive habits	*Non compulsive habit*
Acquired as a fixation in the child to the extent that he retreats to the practice whenever his security is threatened.	Children appear to undergo continuing behavior modification, which permit them to release certain undesirable habit patterns and form new ones which are socially accepted.

Primary habit	*Secondary habits*
Habit acquired as an act	Secondary habit is a habit that is due to a supplemental problem, for example, large tongue causes tongue thrusting habit.

Meaningful and Empty Habits (Klein, 1971)

Meaningful habit	*Empty habit*
Habit with a deep-rooted psychological problem.	Meaningless habit that can be treated easily by a dentist using reminder therapy.

Normal and Abnormal Habits

Normal habits	*Abnormal habits*
Those habits that are deemed normal by children of a particular age group.	Those habits that are pursued after their physiological period of cessation.

Physiologic and Pathologic Habits

Physiologic habits	*Pathological habits*
Physiologic habits are those that are required for normal physiologic fractioning, for example, nasal respiration, sucking during infancy.	Habits that are pursued due to pathological reasons such as adenoids and nasal septal defects that may lead to mouth breathing.

Retained and Cultivated Habits	
Retained habit	***Cultivated habit***
Those that are carried over from childhood into adulthood.	Those cultivated during the socioactive life of an individual.

Morris and Bohanna Classification, 1969	
Habit	***Example***
Non-pressure habits	Mouth breathing
Pressure habits	a. Sucking habit
	» Lip sucking
	» Thumb and digit sucking
	b. Biting habit
	» Nail biting/needle holding
	» Pillow rest
Postural habit	» Chin rest
Miscellaneous	» Bruxism

Graber (1972)

- Thumb/fingers sucking
- Tongue thrusting/sucking
- Lip/nail biting
- Speech defects
- Mouth breathing
- Bruxism
- Postural defects
- Defective occlusal habits

Kingsley (1958)

- Functional–mouth breathing
- Muscular–lip sucking, pencil biting
- Combined.

THUMB SUCKING

Thumb sucking: *It is defined as the placement of the thumb in varying depths into the mouth* **(Fig. 30.1)**.

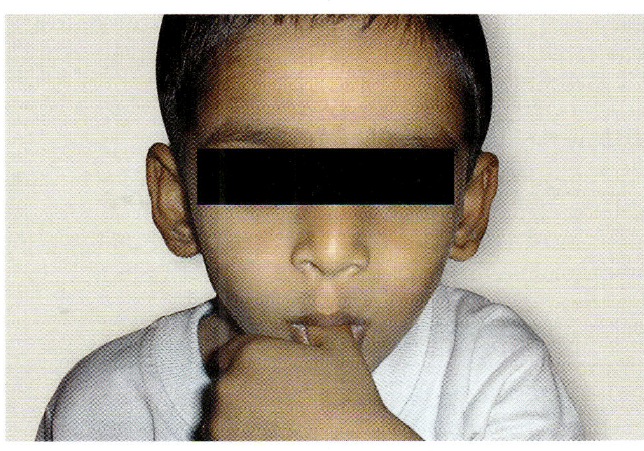

Fig. 30.1: Child performing the act of thumb sucking.

Classification

Normal Thumb Sucking

The thumb-sucking habit is considered normal during the first one and half years of life. Such a habit is usually seen to disappear as the child matures.

Abnormal Thumb Sucking

When thumb-sucking habit persists beyond the preschool period, then it could be considered as an abnormal habit. If the habit is not controlled and treated during this stage, it may cause deleterious effects on the dentofacial structures.

Psychological

The habit may have a deep-rooted emotional factor involved and may be associated with neglect and loneliness experienced by the child.

- **Habitual:** The habit does not have a psychological bearing; however, the child performs the act.
- **Nutritive sucking habits:** Breastfeeding, bottle feeding.
- **Non-nutritive sucking habit:** Thumb or finger sucking, pacifier sucking.

According to Subtelny (1973) (Figs. 30.2A toD)

Type A: This type is seen in almost 50% of the children wherein whole digit is placed inside the mouth with the pad of the thumb pressing over the palate, while at the same time, maxillary and mandibular oral contact is present.

Type B: This type is seen in almost 13–24% of the children wherein the thumb is placed into the oral cavity, and at the same time, maxillary and mandibular contact is maintained.

Type C: This type is seen in almost 18% of the children wherein the thumb is placed into the mouth just beyond the first joint and contacts hard palate and the maxillary incisors, but there is no contact with mandibular incisors.

Type D: This type is seen in almost 6% of the children wherein only a little portion of the thumb is placed into the mouth.

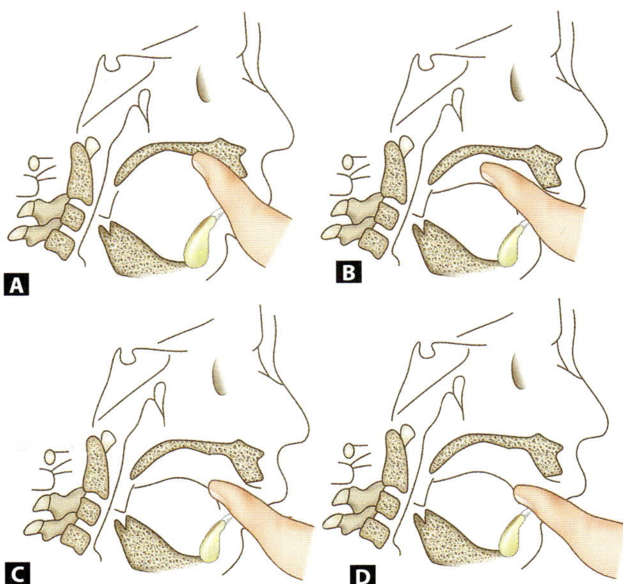

Figs. 30.2A toD: Pathophysiology of thumb sucking.

Theories and Concepts of Thumb Sucking

Classical Freudian Theory (Sigmund Freud, 1919)

The psychoanalytic theory has proposed that a child goes through various distinct phases of psychological development. In oral phase, it is believed that the mouth is the erogenous zone. During this phase, the child takes anything and everything to the oral cavity. It is believed that any kind of the deprivation of this activity will probably cause an emotionally insecure individual.

Oral Drive Theory (Sears and Wise, 1982)

They suggest that the strength of the oral drive is in part a function of how long a child continues to feed by sucking. It is not the frustration of weaning that produces thumb sucking, but in fact, it is the prolonged nursing that causes it.

Rooting Reflex (Benjamin, 1962)

The rooting reflex is movement of the infant's head and tongue toward an object touching its cheeks. He suggested that thumb-sucking arises from the rooting and placing reflexes common to all mammalian infants during the first 3 months of life.

Sucking Reflex (Ergel, 1962)

The process of sucking is a reflex occurring in the oral stage of development and is seen even at 29 weeks of intrauterine life and may disappear during normal growth between the ages of 1 and 3.5 years. It is the first coordinated muscular activity of the infant. Babies who are restricted from sucking due to disease or other factors become restless and irritable. This deprivation may motivate the infant to suck the thumb and finger for additional gratification.

Learning Theory (Davidson, 1967)

This theory advocates that non-nutritive sucking stems from an adaptive response. The infant associates sucking with feelings like pleasure and hunger and recalls these events by sucking the suitable objects available, which is mainly thumb or finger.

Etiological Factors Associated with Thumb Sucking

Socioeconomic Status

In high socioeconomic status, the mother is in a better position to feed the baby and in a short time the baby's hunger is satisfied, whereas in the low socioeconomic group, mother is unable to provide sufficient breast milk to the infants; hence, in the process, the infant suckles intensively for a long time, thereby exhausting the sucking urge. This theory explains the increased incidence of thumb sucking in industrialized areas when compared to rural areas.

Working Mother

The sucking habit is commonly observed to be present in children with working parents because such children are brought up in the hands of caretaker and develop feelings of insecurity.

Number of Siblings

The development of the habit can be related to the number of siblings because more the number increases, the attention meted out by the parents to the child gets divided. A child who feels neglected by the parents may attempt to compensate his feelings of insecurity by means of this habit.

Order of Birth of the Child

Later the sibling ranks in the family, greater is the chance of having an oral habit.

Social Adjustment and Stress

Digit sucking has also been proposed as an emotionally based behavior.

Age of the Child

The time of appearance of digit-sucking habit has significance.

- **In the neonate:** Insecurities are related to primitive demands as hunger.
- **During the first weeks of life:** Related to feeding problems
- **During the eruption of the primary teeth:** It may be used to relieve teething.

Diagnosis of thumb-sucking habit

History

Once the positive history of habit is determined, the question regarding the frequency, intensity, and duration of the habit is determined. The remedies that have been tried at home, the feeding patterns, parental care of the child are also ascertained.

Emotional status

It is essential to determine if the habit is meaningful or empty. This requires an insight into the emotional security and familial wellbeing of the child.

***Extraoral examination* (Figs. 30.3 and 30.4)**

Digits that are involved in the habit will appear reddened, exceptionally clear, chapped, and a short fingernail, that is, a clean dishpan thumb.

Lips: The position of the lips at rest or during swallowing should be observed. A short, hypotonic upper lip frequently characterizes chronic thumb suckers. Lower lip is hyperactive, and this leads to further proclination of upper anterior teeth.

Profile: Usually convex profile

Other features: Active thumb sucking also have a higher incidence of middle ear infections and frequently have enlarged tonsils accompanied by mouth breathing.

Intraoral examination

The type of malocclusion produced by digit sucking is dependent on a number of variables like position of the digit, associated or of facial muscle contractions, mandibular position during sucking, facial skeletal pattern, intensity, frequency, and duration of habit.

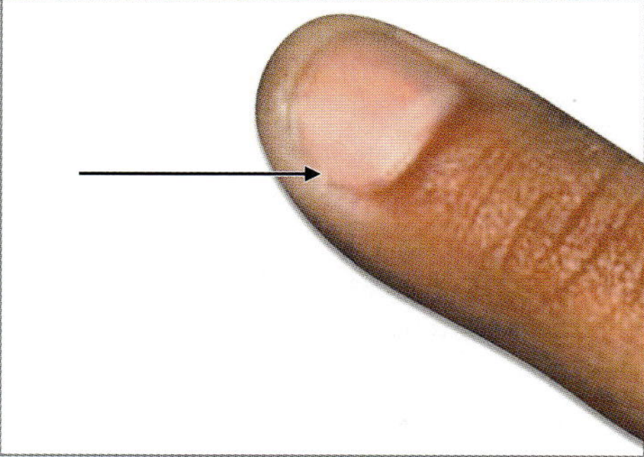

Fig. 30.3: Callus formation on nails.

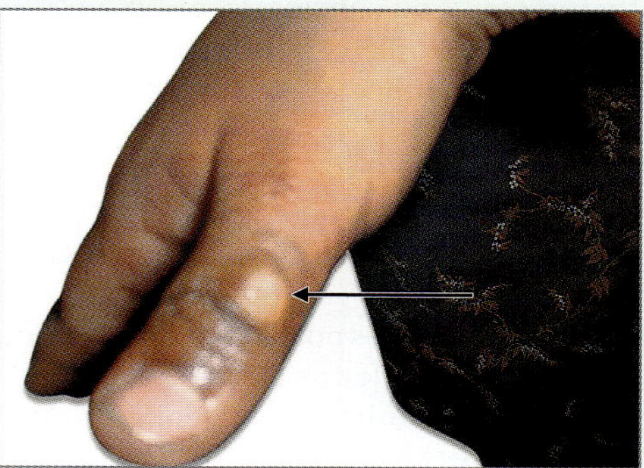

Fig. 30.4: Skin keratotic lesions.

Dentofacial Changes Associated with Thumb Sucking (Figs. 30.5 to 30.7)

Effects on maxilla

↓

- Proclination of the maxillary incisiors
- Increased maxillary arch length
- Anterior placement of the apical base of the maxilla
- Increased clinical crown length of maxillary incisor
- High palatal arch
- Atypical root resorption in primary central incisor
- Increased trauma to maxillary incisors

↓

- Retroclination of mandibular incisors
- Retrusion of mandible

↓

Effects on interarch relationship

↓

- Increased overjet
- Decreased overbite
- Posterior crossbite
- Anterior open bite

↓

Effects on lip placement and function

↓

- Development of tongue thrust
- Lower tongue position
- Hypotonic upper lip
- Hyperactive lower lip

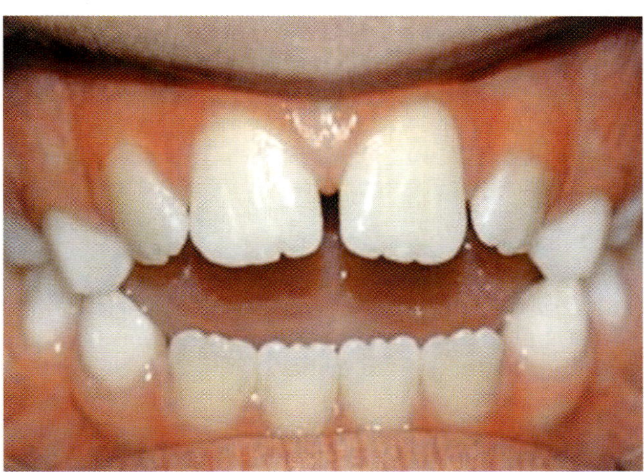

Fig. 30.5: Open bite. (*Source:* Nancyl Wehner www.omahamyology.com).

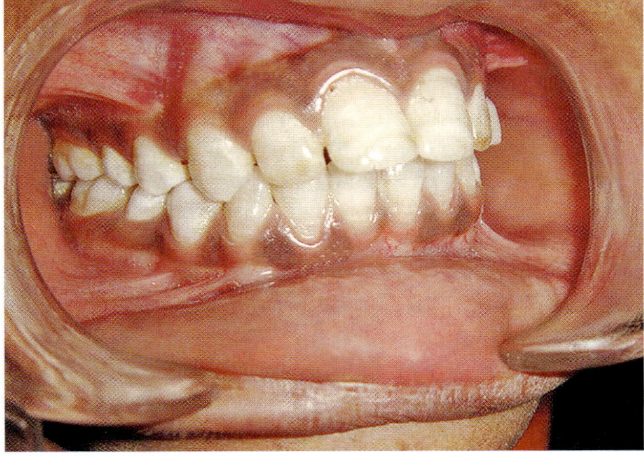

Fig. 30.6: Proclination of incisors.

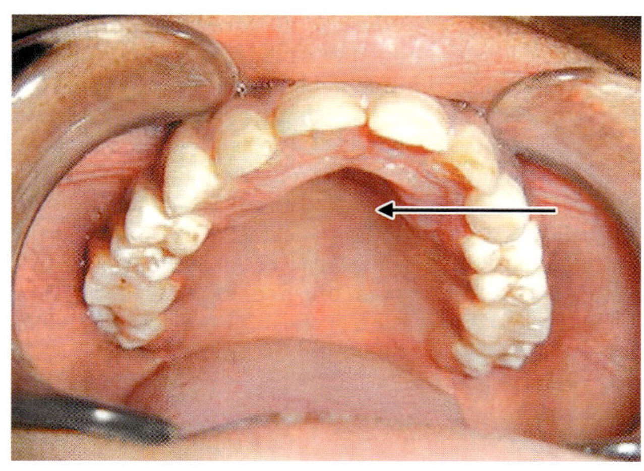

Fig. 30.7: Deep palate.

Management

The strategy for management of thumb sucking should be started when the child shows any signs of the habit or whenever a familial tendency of the habit is discovered.

Preventive Treatment

- First, feed the child whenever he is hungry and let him eat as much as he wants. Second, feed the child the natural way; importance of breastfeeding is primarily psychological and secondarily nutritive. Third, never let the habit to start, the practice must be discontinued at its inception (**Hughes**, 1941).
- **Use of a dummy/pacifier:** Encouraging the baby to suck a dummy instead of his thumb can prevent him from acquiring the habit.

Psychological Therapy

- Nagging, scolding, or frightening the child should be avoided since this could cause negativism and tend to make him resort to the habit.
- **β-hypothesis or Dunlop hypothesis:** He believed that if a subject can be forced to concentrate on the performance of the act at the time he practices it, he could learn to stop performing the act. Forced purposeful repetition of habit eventually associates with unpleasant reactions and the habit is abandoned. The child should be asked to sit in front of the mirror and asked to observe himself as he indulges in the habit.

Six Steps in Cessation of Habit (Larson and Johnson)

Step 1: Screening for psychological component
Step 2: Habit awareness
Step 3: Habit reversal with a competing response
Step 4: Response attention
Step 5: Escalated DRO (differential reinforcement of other behaviors)
Step 6: Escalated DRO with reprimands (consists of holding the child, establishing eye contact, and firmly admonishing the child to stop the habit)

- **Three-alarm system (Norton and Gellin–1968):** A chart is designed with days of the week and blank spaces. When the child engages in his habit, he is told to wrap the digit he sucks with coarse adhesive tapes. The child feels the tape in his mouth; it is the first alarm, and this reminds him to stop the habit. The elbow of the arm with the offending thumb is firmly wrapped in 2-inch elastic bandage; safety pins are placed at proximal and distal ends of bandage, and one safety pin is placed length wise at the mesial end of the elbow, and when the child sucks the thumb again, the closed pin on the medial end of elbow, mildly jabbing the elbow, indicates second alarm. If the habit persists, the bandage is tightened; this is the final or third alarm, which will definitely remind the child of the habit.

- **Reframing and symptom prescription for thumb sucking habit cessation (Yogesh Kumar TD et al., 2014)**
  - Applicable to a child from 7 to 11 years of age.
  - Step 1: Assessing the child's habit and assuring the child that no harm will be done.
  - Step 2: Symptom prescription (child to continue the habits but note down the timing).
  - Step 3: Parents are informed about the treatment plan.
  - Step 4: 2 weeks after initial conversation the child is recalled back and allowed to suck the finger in front of a mirror (Dunlop beta hypothesis).
  - Step 5: Child is shown photographs of children who continued the habit and children who stopped the habit (reframing).
  - Step 6: Photographs were given to parents and asked to stick to child room.
  - Step 7: Parents are asked to praise the child when she reduces the frequency (social reinforcement).

Chemical Treatment

It is the least effective method. Bitter and sour chemicals have been used over the thumb to terminate the practice but with very minimal success, for example, quinine, asafoetida, pepper, castor oil, etc. Nowadays, new anti-thumb sucking solutions like femite, thumb-up, anti-thumb are also being marketed, but they have also had a very moderate success **(Fig. 30.8)**.

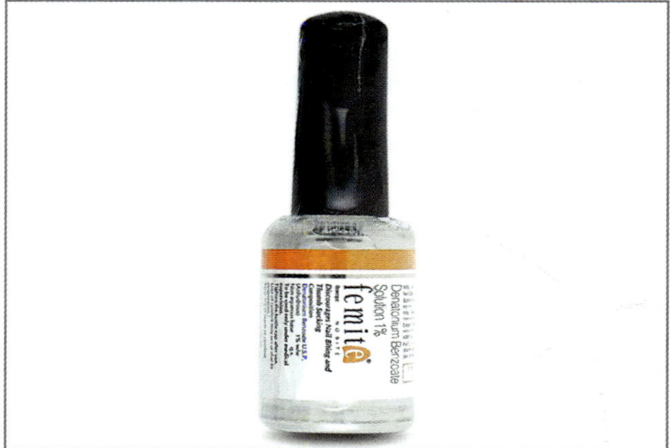

Fig. 30.8: Anti-thumb sucking solution.

Mechanical Therapy or Reminder Therapy or Response Prevention Therapy

Extraoral approach: Mechanical restraints applied to the hand and digits like splints, adhesive tapes. Thumb guard is the most effective extraoral appliance for control of the habit **(Fig. 30.9)**.

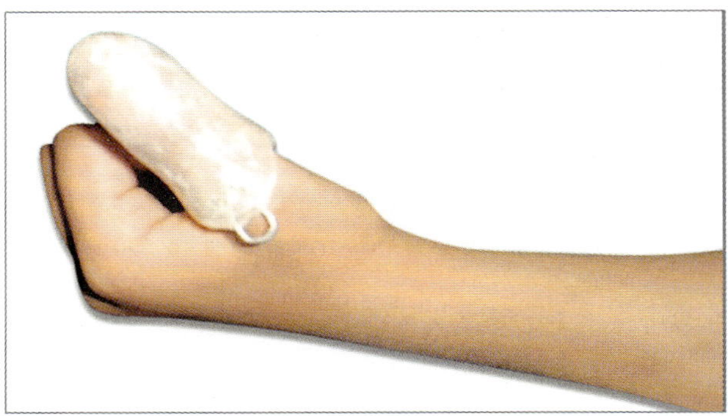

Fig. 30.9: Thumb guard.

Intraoral approach: The early years of life culminating in the oedipal period at the age of 5 years are in appropriate psychologically for this approach; therefore, the optimal time for appliance placement is between the ages of 3 and 4.5 years preferably during spring or summer, when the child's health is at its peak and the sucking desires can be sublimated in outdoor play and social activity. The following appliances are recommended:

- **Removable or fixed palatal crib (Figs. 30.10A to D)**: It breaks the suction force of the digit on the anterior segment, reminds the patient of his habit, and makes the habit a non-pleasurable one.
- **Oral screen:** Oral screen is a functional appliance introduced by **Newell** in 1912. It produces its effects by redirecting the pressure of the muscular and soft tissue curtain of the cheeks and lips. It prevents the child from placing the thumb or finger into the oral cavity during sleeping hours.
- **Hay rakes (Fig. 30.11)**: **Mack** (1951) advocated the use of dental appliance in children over 3.5 years of age who are persistent thumb suckers. The device was called hay rake as it was designed with a series of fence like lines that prevented sucking.
- **Bluegrass appliance:** Developed by **Haskell** (1991). It is a fixed appliance using a Teflon roller, together with positive reinforcement. Used to manage thumb-sucking habit in children between 7 and 13 years of age. The patient believes that he has acquired a new toy to play with. Instructions are given to them to roll the roller instead of sucking the digit.
- **Quad helix:** The quad helix is fixed appliance used to expand the constricted maxillary arch. The helixes of the appliance serve to remind the child not to place the finger in the mouth.
- **Modified bluegrass appliance (Fig. 30.12)**: This is a modification of the original appliance with the difference being that this has two rollers of different colors and material instead of one. If the patient tries to suck on his thumb, the suction will not be created, and his thumb will slip from the rollers thus breaking the act.

Current Strategies

- **Increasing the arm length of the night suit:** This is useful in children who sincerely want to discontinue the habit and only perform during their sleep. The arms of their night suit are lengthened so that they cannot reach the thumb during night.

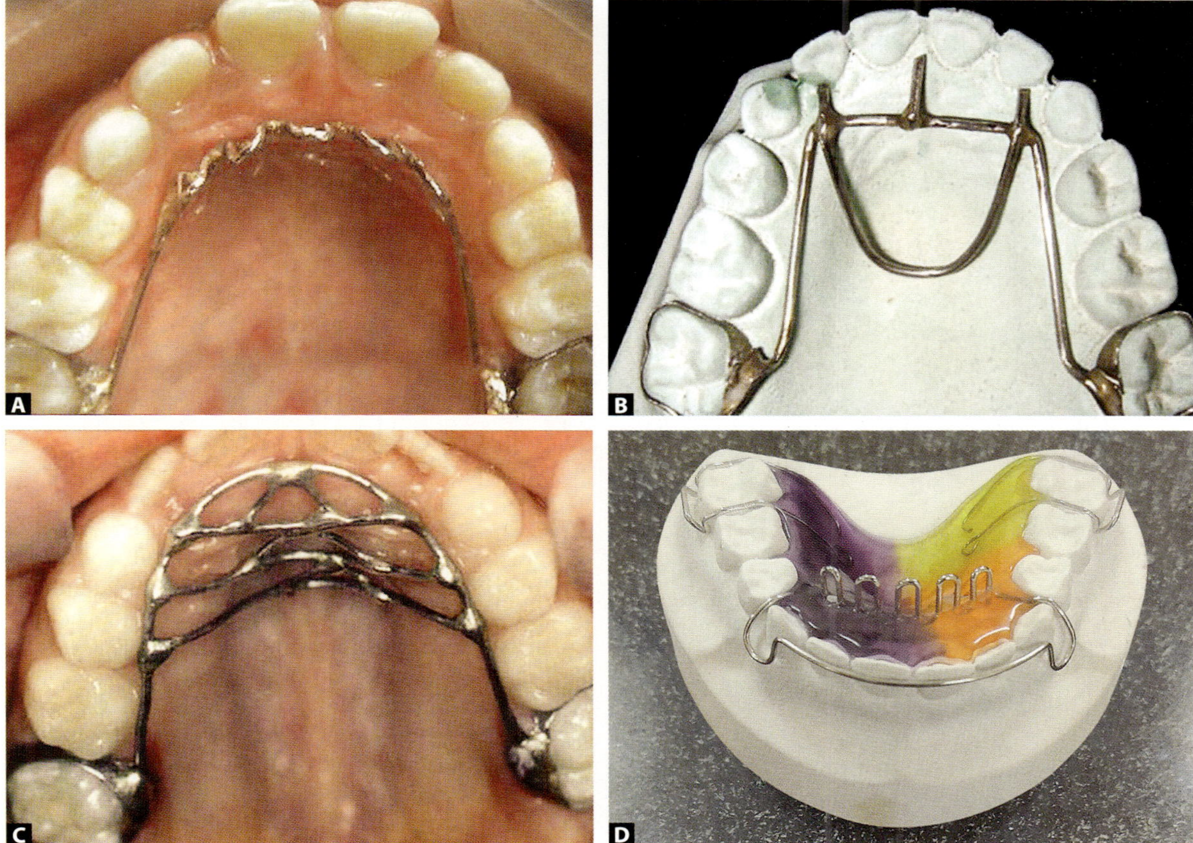

Figs. 30.10A to D: Different designs of palatal crib.

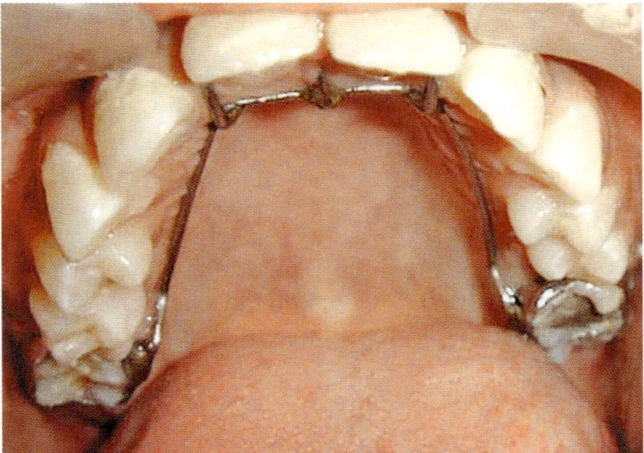

Fig. 30.11: Hay rakes.

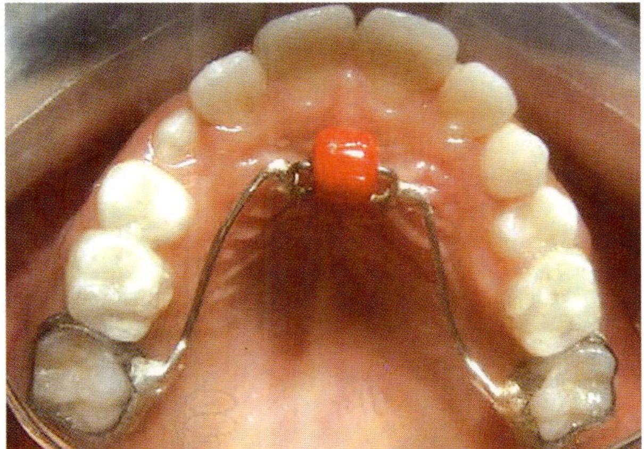

Fig. 30.12: Modified bluegrass appliance.

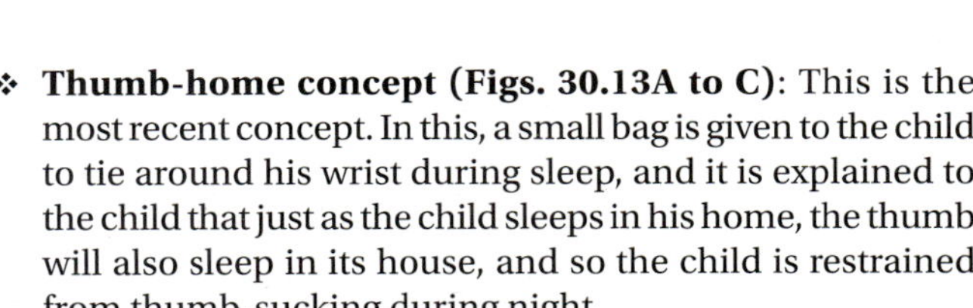

- **Thumb-home concept (Figs. 30.13A to C)**: This is the most recent concept. In this, a small bag is given to the child to tie around his wrist during sleep, and it is explained to the child that just as the child sleeps in his home, the thumb will also sleep in its house, and so the child is restrained from thumb-sucking during night.
- **Currently the use of hand puppets is gaining popularity (Fig. 30.14A):**
  - Fill toe sock with stuffing. Pack very tightly.
  - Cut tag board approximately 2 inch wide and 4 inch long.
  - Roll tag board loosely around index finger and then wrap thread around it to make a tube.

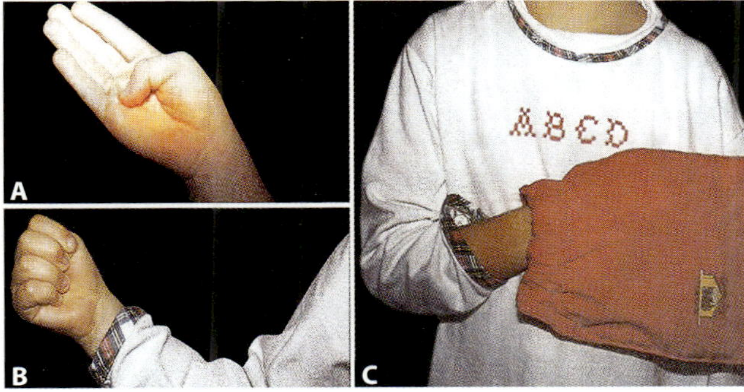

Figs. 30.13A to C: Thumb-home concept.

- Make hole in filling with index finger.
- Insert tag board tube in filling.
- Cut sock off about 1 inch below heel
- Wrap thread around sock at exposed end of tube and sew sock to end of tube.
- Dress your puppet with cloth and trimmings.
- Paint face on puppet with marking pen, crayons, of a brick paints or stitch on with colored thread.

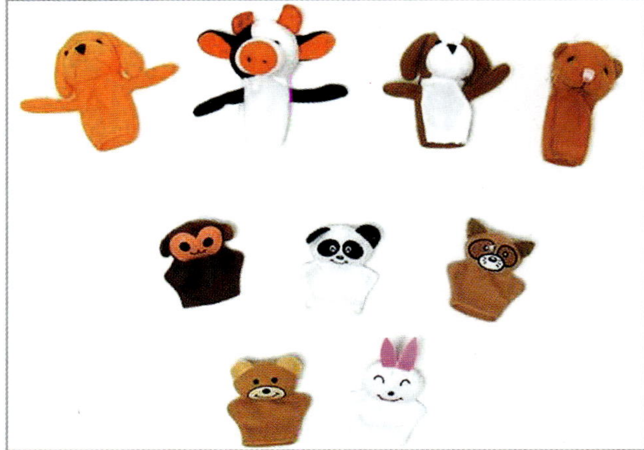

Fig. 30.14A: Hand puppets.

- **Thumb-sucking book (Fig. 30.14B)**: *"The Little Bear who Sucked his Thumb"* is a book directed at children, for children. The book has been written and illustrated by **Dr Dragan Antolos**, an experienced dentist with a special interest in thumb-sucking habits in children. He deals first hand in management of dental, social, and functional problems which can arise with persistent thumb sucking. The book and chart are a noninvasive and effective strategy for stopping thumb sucking and have received positive support from psychiatrists, speech pathologists, and pedodontic societies. He is very mindful that parents and practitioners should not place pressure on children to stop as this is only met with resistance and can entrench the problem.

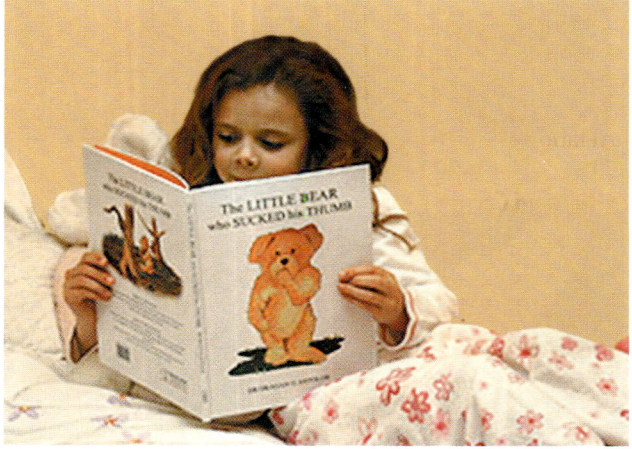

Fig. 30.14B: Child reading thumb-sucking book.

The book is beautifully illustrated, with characters that will appeal to both boys and girls. As well as a stand-alone story,

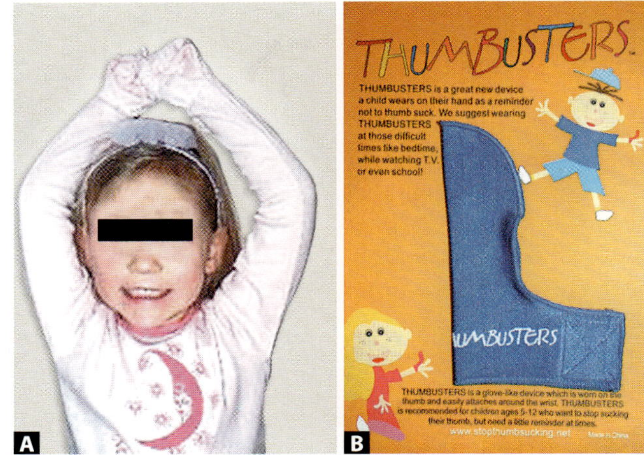

Figs. 30.15A and B: (A) Special shirt;(B) Special gloves.

The Little Bear who Sucked his Thumb is especially useful to parents with children that have a thumb-sucking habit. It addresses the problem in a fun and non-threatening way. The wall chart can be personalized with your child's name, helping to further motivate them, and in conjunction with the book, find the desire to stop sucking their thumb.

- **My special shirt (Fig. 30.15A)**: This helps in minimizing the damage of finger sucking by providing a number of tools to address the habit in a phased manner. This shirt keeps the child busy; thereby, avoiding the habit. By working as a team, your child will gain confidence, balance emotions, and stop their dependence on need to suck.
- **Thumbusters (Fig. 30.15B)**: It is a glove like device, which is worn around the thumb with support at the wrist, which provides the child with repeated reminders at all times.
- **Elbow guard and three-alarm system (Fig. 30.16)**: **RURS' elbow guard** is an innovative and unique appliance to prevent thumb/finger sucking habit in children, which was developed by **Shetty et al.**, in 2003 **(Table 30.1)**. RURS' elbow guard will allow some movement of the elbow but will not allow the thumb to reach the mouth. Children usually accept the appliance easily. They perceive it something like a wristband and thought themselves to be fashionable, so they would not try to take it off.

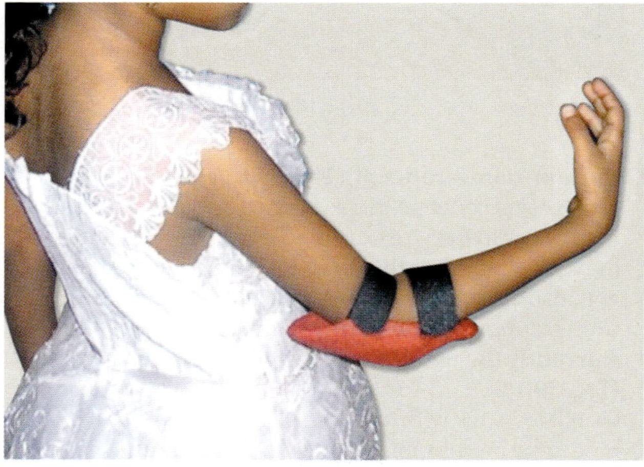

Fig. 30.16: RURS' elbow guard.

Table 30.1: Difference between the previous and revised three-alarm system.

Alarm	Previous three-alarm system (Norton and Gellin, 1968)	Revised three-alarm system (Shetty et al., 2015)
First	The child feels the tape in his mouth	The child wearing the elbow guard
Second	The closed pin mildly jabbing the elbow	The music/vibration/siren/ recorded voice played when tried to bend the elbow
Third/final	The bandage is tightened	The elbow guard restricting thumb/finger reaching the mouth

Advantages of RURS'elbow guard:

- Easy parent supervision and follow-up
- Convenience and comfort to the patient
- Easier to make impression of the elbow
- Patient acceptance is better
- Loose enough to allow sufficient blood flow
- Can be given in any age group
- Can be worn under full sleeve shirt
- Very economical.

Three-alarm system: RURS' elbow guard was modified along with the incorporation of revised three-alarm system. A musical chip with speaker was incorporated on the outer side of the acrylic elbow guard during acrylization. So, whenever, the child tries to suck the thumb or digit, the switch button will be pressed by the elbow joint, and music would play reminding the child to stop the habit.

Alarming wristwatch: **Krishnappa et al.,** 2016, reported a case of an 8-year-old male with persistent thumb sucking habit. They came up with a new device with an alarm that was activated when the child placed the finger into the mouth. The alarm was placed in a wristwatch and making it attractive for the child to accept and wear them **(Fig. 30.17)**. The child was followed for 5 months, and they found that there is decreased frequency of thumb sucking followed by discontinuing the habit totally by 5 months.

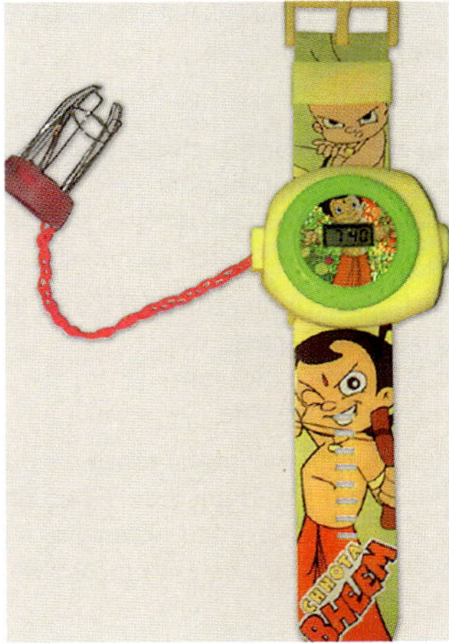

Fig. 30.17: Alarming wristwatch.

Light emitting diode habit-breaking appliance: **Sahu et al** (2017) designed a new innovative light emitting diode habit-breaking appliance. The appliance is a regular Hawley's appliance with the addition of the light-emitting diode bulb and the switch. When the child's tongue or the finger touches the appliance, the light bulb gets illuminated, thus reminding the child to quit the habit **(Fig. 30.18)**. The said appliance utilizes easily available electrical gadgets that will function by disturbing the subconsciously built vicious cycle. The reminders send by its activation will break the pleasure perception obtained during the habit. Habit breaking through this appliance is effective as it is superior to other appliances in the mode of action as well as the design itself is attractive to the children.

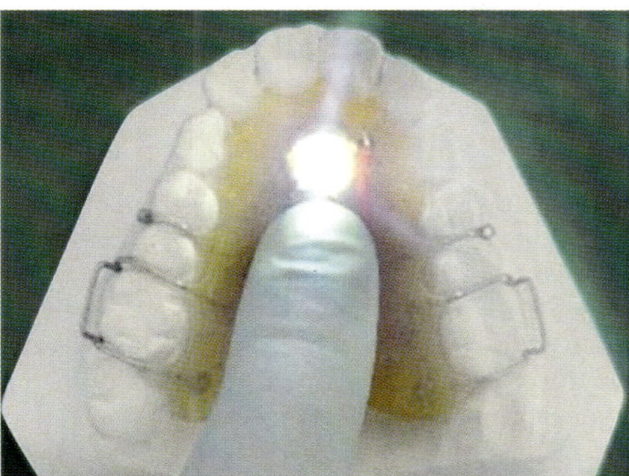

Fig. 30.18: Light emitting diode habit-breaking appliance.

PACIFIER HABIT

Pacifiers have been used by mankind for more than thousands of years. They have been identified to help children in transitioning to sleep, to soothe infants, to provide comfort while teething. The effects of pacifier sucking are the same as NNS or thumb sucking, but some other associated risks with pacifier sucking are explained here.

Effect of Pacifier Use on Breastfeeding

New man hypothesized that the use of pacifier causes "nipple confusion" in the infant and a faulty technique of breastfeeding which eventually leads to early weaning. This was also supported by Mitchell who found out that infants given pacifiers in hospitals are less likely to breastfeed mothers on discharge as compared to those who were not given pacifiers. Although there are a variety of authors like Schubiger, Franco, Fleming who feel that pacifier and breastfeeding have no correlation.

Pacifier and Caries

Prolonged use of pacifiers in children and especially those used with sugar syrups or sweetened liquids have a positive relation with caries.

Safety Issues

- **Physical safety:** Materials and designs of pacifiers that have been associated with asphyxia, infection, and death.
- **Chemical safety:** Due to presence of *N*-nitrosamines in pacifiers which are proven to be carcinogenic.
- **Immunologic safety:** Latex allergy and early sensitization.

Recommendations

- Educate parents and caregivers about the safe use of pacifiers.
- With hold the use of pacifiers until breastfeeding is established. After that point, limit their use for soothing breastfeeding infants.
- Advise parents and caregivers to exercise judgment and restraint regarding pacifier use.
- Clean pacifiers routinely and avoid sharing between siblings.
- Suggest to parents that pacifier use be curtailed beginning at 2 years of age.

TONGUE THRUSTING

Tongue thrusting is the most controversial of all oral habits. There is a wide range of attitudes and opinions among various authors regarding diagnosis and effect of tongue thrusting.

Tulley (1969) defined tongue thrust as the forward movement of the tongue tip between the teeth to meet the lower lip during deglutition and in sounds of speech, so that the tongue lies interdentally **(Fig. 30.19)**.

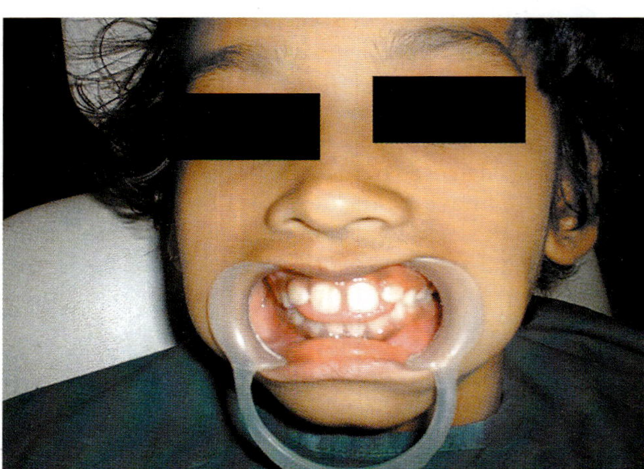

Fig. 30.19: Tongue thrusting.

Classification of Tongue Thrusting

Profitt (1990)

- **Physiologic:** This comprises of the normal tongue thrust swallow of infancy.
- **Habitual:** The tongue thrust swallow is present as a habit even after the correction of the malocclusion.
- **Functional:** The tongue thrust mechanism is an adaptive behavior developed to achieve oral seal.
- **Anatomic:** Persons having enlarged tongue can have an anterior tongue posture.

Tulley WJ (1969 classified tongue thrusting according to its etiology)

- **Tongue thrust as a habit**
  - Usually seen before 11 years of age
  - Class I or class II pattern with slight overjet or open bite
  - Gets autocorrected with appliance therapy
  - No need for speech re-education therapy
- **Tongue thrusting which is endogenous or innate**
  - Familial tendency
  - Sibilant sounds
  - If facial pattern is optimum, then we need only speech education therapy
  - If facial pattern is not optimum, then we need appliance therapy followed by speech therapy.
- **Tongue thrust as an adaptive behavior**
  - Majority of the cases fall into this category
  - Adaptive behavior of the tongue forward between the teeth
  - Anterior open bite is evident
  - Good response to appliance therapy
- **Tongue thrust due to pathologic or grossly abnormal problems**
  - Tongue size like macroglossia

Etiology of Tongue Thrusting

- **Genetic influence:** There is a complexity of factors that might predispose a child toward this habit like an extremely high narrow palatal arch, an imbalance between the number and size of teeth, and the size of the oral cavity.
- **Thumb sucking:** This act depresses the tongue and keeps the teeth apart so one can suspect that it also induces malfunctions of the tongue during deglutition.

Development of tongue thrusting habit (Mihiri Silva and David Manton, 2013)

- During breastfeeding there is no continuous flow of milk, and this places the infants orofacial muscles work more, encouraging muscle development and growth of the mandible. The action of the infant's mouth during breastfeeding has been described more as a squeezing of the mother's nipple, compared to a pistol like action of the tongue during sucking of the nursing bottle teat.
- During feeding, the nipple of the mother's breast is positioned more anteriorly in the child's mouth, compared to the teat of a nursing bottle which is directed farther back toward the pharyngeal wall, thus displacing the tongue anteriorly. These factors may lead to the development of irregular swallowing patterns, such as tongue thrust, which may, in turn, contribute to malocclusion.

Classification of tongue thrusting (James S Brauer and Townsend V Holt)

Type	*Clinical presentation*
Type 1	Non-deforming tongue thrust
Type 2	Deforming anterior tongue thrust **(Fig. 30.20A)** *Subgroup 1:* Anterior open bite *Subgroup 2:* Associated procumbency of anterior teeth *Subgroup 3:* Associated posterior crossbite
Type 3	Deforming lateral tongue thrust **(Fig. 30.20B)** *Subgroup 1:* Posterior open bite *Subgroup 2:* Posterior crossbite *Subgroup 3:* Deep overbite
Type 4	Deforming anterior and lateral tongue thrust *Subgroup 1:* Anterior and posterior open bite *Subgroup 2:* Associated procumbency of anterior teeth *Subgroup 3:* Associated posterior crossbite

- **Mixed dentition:** When a child loses deciduous teeth especially a canine or an incisor, the tongue frequently protrudes into the space at rest, during speech and swallowing activity.

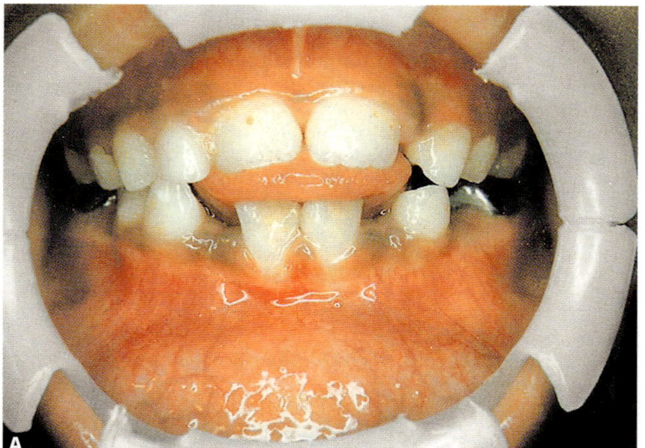

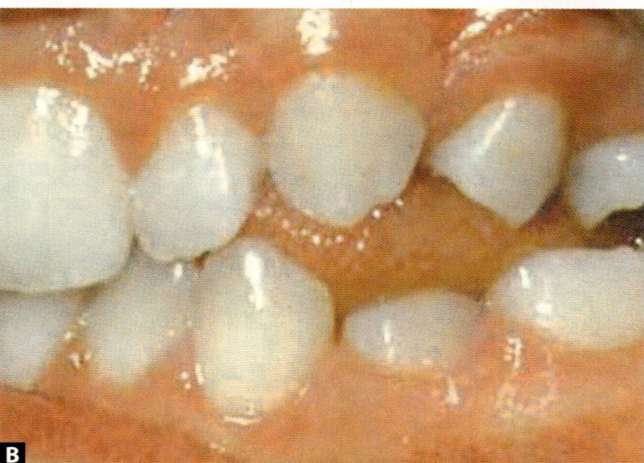

Figs. 30.20A and B: (A) Anterior tongue thrust; (B) Lateral tongue thrust.

- **Gap filling tendency:** Any space around the dental arches not occupied by teeth will tend to be filled by the tongue partly due to exploratory excursions and partly for preventing the escape of food during deglutition.
- **Allergies:** Allergies affecting the upper respiratory tract cause their effects on tonsils and adenoid leading to mouth breathing and tongue thrusting.
- **Macroglossia and microglossia:** In these situations, tongue is inadequate to fill the oral space resulting in a forward thrusting.
- **Soft diet:** Oral laxity is encouraged with resulting underdevelopment of orofacial muscles.
- **Oral trauma:** When a traumatic condition persists for a sufficient time, its effects can cause changes in deglutition pattern.
- **Sleeping habits:** Some patients who sleep on their back on a low pillow or with open mouth, the tongue rests in the mandibular arch and moves forward against the teeth during swallowing.

Role of lingual frenum in tongue thrusting habit

A force exerting on the dentition up to 6 hours per day can produce significant changes in the developing dentition. According to **Coza**, 1992, average no of swallowing by an individual is about 900–1000 times per day and per swallow last for 1 second (1000 second) which does not cause a significant effect on the dental arch. But the resting position of the tongue may be more likely to lead to malocclusion rather than the transient forces exerted during deglutition. The anterior positioning of the tongue during swallowing in the setting of an anterior open bite may be a functional adaption to form an anterior oral seal to facilitate swallowing. A high lingual frenum attachment can restrict the tongue high into palate to get a proper seal for swallowing. Also, it pulls the tongue to lower position at rest. Assessment of lingual frenum should be done before planning for any myo-exercises or appliance therapy for tongue thrusting habit.

Anterior Tongue Thrust

Extraoral Features

- Usually, dolichocephalic face.
- Increased lower anterior facial height.
- Incompetent lips.
- Expressionless face as the mandible is stabilized by facial muscles instead of masticatory muscles during deglutition.
- Speech problems like sibilant distortions and lisping, etc.
- Abnormal mentalis muscle activity is seen.

Moyer's classification of swallowing patterns

Type	*Inference*
Normal infantile swallow	During this swallow, the tongue lies between the gum pads and mandible is stabilized by contraction of facial muscles especially buccinator. This type of pattern disappears on eruption of the buccal teeth of primary dentition
Transitional swallow	intermixing of normal infantile swallow and mature swallow during the primary dentition and early mixed dentition period
Normal mature swallow	During this swallow, there is very little lip and cheek activity. Mainly there is contraction of mandibular elevators
Simple tongue thrust swallow	During this swallow, there is contraction of lips, mentalis muscle, and mandibular elevators. Tongue protrudes into an open bite that has a definite beginning and ending
Complex tongue thrust swallow	This is characteristically known as teeth apart swallow. There are marked contractions of the lip, facial, and mentalis muscles but absence of temporal muscle contraction during swallow. Anterior open bite is also present

Intraoral Features

- Proclined, spaced, and sometimes flared upper anteriors resulting in increased overjet.
- Retroclined or proclined lower anteriors depending upon the type of tongue thrust.
- Presence of an anterior open bite.
- Presence of posterior crossbites.
- The simple tongue thrust is characterized by a normal tooth contact during the swallowing act. They exhibit good intercuspation of posterior teeth in contrast to complex tongue thrust.
- The tongue is thrust forward during swallowing to help establish an anterior lip seal. At rest the tongue tip lies at a lower level.

Diagnosis of tongue thrusting

Careful differentiation must be made among a simple, complex, and retained infantile swallow. The prognosis is usually excellent for correction of simple tongue thrust, good for complex tongue thrust, and very poor for retained infantile swallowing pattern.

Examination of the tongue thrusting: Check for size, shape, and movements.

Functional examination:

- Observe the tongue position, while the mandible is in the rest position
- Observe the tongue during various swallows:
  - Conscious swallow
  - *Command swallow of saliva*
  - *Command swallow of water*
  - *Conscious swallow during mastication*

Palpatory examination:

- Place water beneath the patient's tongue tip and ask him to swallow
  - Normal: Mandible rises, and teeth are brought together, but no contraction of lips or facial muscles
  - Tongue thrusting: Marked contraction of lips and facial muscles
- Place hand over temporalis muscle and ask to swallow
  - Normal: Temporalis contracts and mandible is elevated
  - Tongue thrusting: No temporalis contraction
- Hold the lower lip and ask the patient to swallow
  - Normal: Swallow can be completed
  - Tongue thrusting: Patient cannot complete swallow

Role of cephalometry:

- To assess the tongue posture at rest
- Low tongue posture leading into open bite and proclination of anterior teeth.

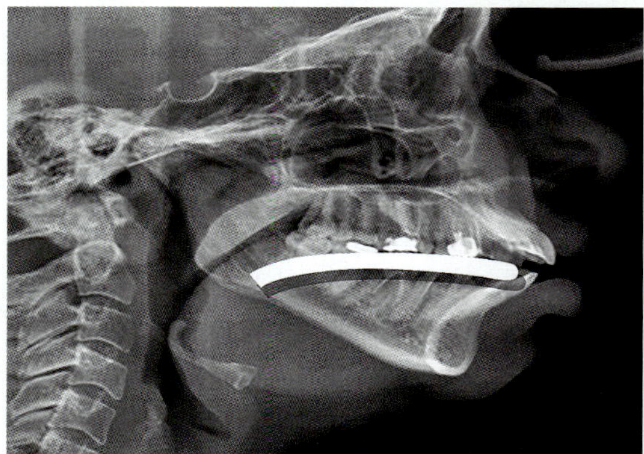

Complex Tongue Thrust

Features

- Proclination of anterior teeth, bimaxillary protrusion.
- This kind of tongue thrust is characterized by a teeth apart swallow.
- The anterior open bite can be diffused or absent.
- **Proffit and Mason** measured the data of the force, duration, intensity, and frequency of tongue thrust and concluded that the tongue thrust habit may sustain an open bite instead of creating the habit.
- Absence of temporal muscle constriction during swallowing.
- Patients with a complex tongue thrust combine contractions of the lip, facial, and mentalis muscle. The occlusion of teeth may be poor.
- Poor occlusal fit, no firm intercuspation.
- Posterior open bite in case of lateral tongue thrust.
- Posterior crossbite.

Clinical Features

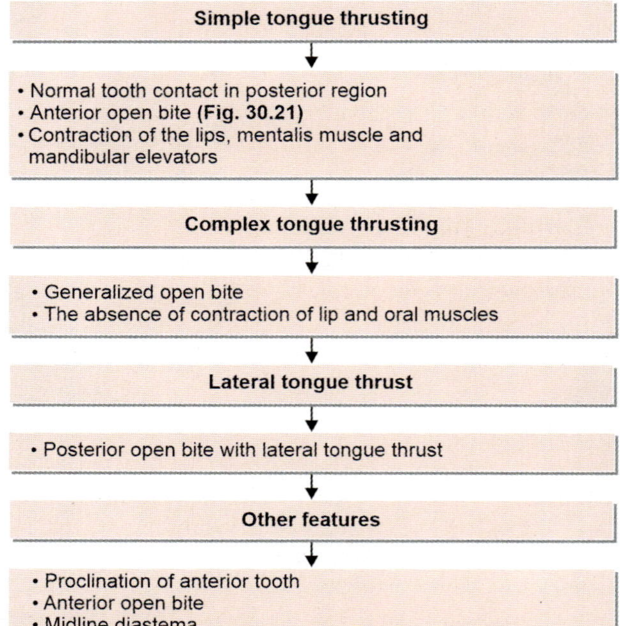

Simple tongue thrusting
• Normal tooth contact in posterior region
• Anterior open bite (Fig. 30.21)
• Contraction of the lips, mentalis muscle and mandibular elevators
Complex tongue thrusting
• Generalized open bite
• The absence of contraction of lip and oral muscles
Lateral tongue thrust
• Posterior open bite with lateral tongue thrust
Other features
• Proclination of anterior tooth
• Anterior open bite
• Midline diastema
• Posterior crossbite

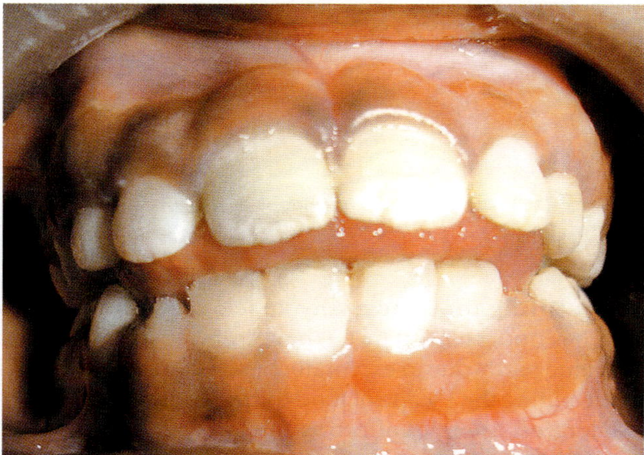

Fig. 30.21: Anterior open bite with proclination.

Treatment Considerations

Tongue thrusting often self-corrects by 8–9 years of age by the time permanent teeth erupt. If tongue thrusting is associated with other habits, then the associated habit must be treated first. **Cayley et al.,** performed a prospective clinical study and assessed the effect of tongue-education therapy on tongue function and dentofacial form in anterior open bite patients using electropalatography and lateral head cephalometric radiographs. She concluded that there was some evidence of a trend for eruption of upper and lower incisors with concomitant reduction of the anterior open bite and implied that the therapy was partially successful in improving tongue function during swallowing and in reducing anterior open bite.

Myofunctional Therapy

Garliader proposed this method in which the patient can be guided regarding the correct posture of the tongue during swallowing by various exercises like asking the child to place the tip of the tongue in the rugae area for 5 min and then asking him to swallow.

The Spot Exercises

1. Keep the tip of the tongue at the spot (5 mm behind the meeting point of upper central incisors in the midline: incisive papilla), squeeze against the palate and make a click sound and swallow. Repeat this exercise 20 times three times a day.
2. **Orthodontic elastics:** The tongue tip is held against the palate using orthodontic elastic of 5/16 and sugarless fruit drop.
3. **Lemon candy exercise:** Instead of the elastic, a lemon candy is put on the tongue tip. Patient is asked to hold the candy against the palate by the tongue tip and then asking the child to swallow.
4. **2S exercise:** This includes identifying the spot and the squeezing the spot keeping the tongue at same position.
5. **4S exercise:** This includes identifying the spot, salivating, squeezing the spot, and swallowing. Using the tongue, the spot is identified, the tongue tip is pressed against this spot, and the child is asked to swallow keeping the tongue at the same spot.

Other Exercises

The child is asked to perform a series of exercise such as whistling, reciting the count from 60 to 69, gargling, yawning, etc., to tone the respective muscles.

Lip Exercises

Tug-of-war and button pull exercise: A string is tied to two buttons; one of the buttons is placed between the lips of the patient while the other is held by the patient outside. The outer button is pulled outwards, and at the same time, the inside button is resisting the forces, thereby strengthening the lips on both aspects.

Subconscious Therapy

Once the voluntary swallowing pattern is acquired, the patient proceeds to subconscious therapy, viz., subliminal therapy, in which the patient is asked to place a reminder sign or autosuggestion which requires the patient to give self-instructions like repeating six times "I will swallow correctly all night long"—for 10 nights.

Speech/Articulation Therapy

Ask the patient to recite words with '*S*' sound like Sixty to Sixty-Nine, Mississippi, Race, Loose, Mysore, Dice, Saraswati, Place.

Mechanotherapy

Both fixed and removable appliances can be fabricated. The appliance re-educates tongue so that the dorsum of tongue approximates the palatal vault, and the tip of the tongue contacts palatal rugae during deglutition. Some of the appliances that can be used to prevent tongue thrusting are:

- Preorthodontic trainer.
- Modifications of Hawley appliance.
- Tongue crib **(Figs. 30.22A and B).**
- Oral screen.
- Galella habit appliance.
- Habit corrector.
- Froggy mouth device.

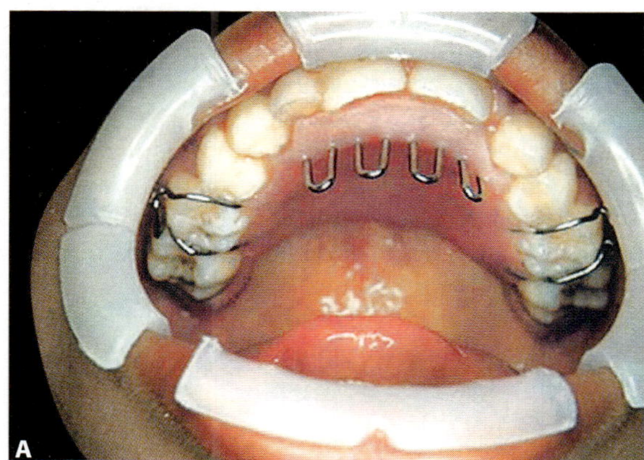

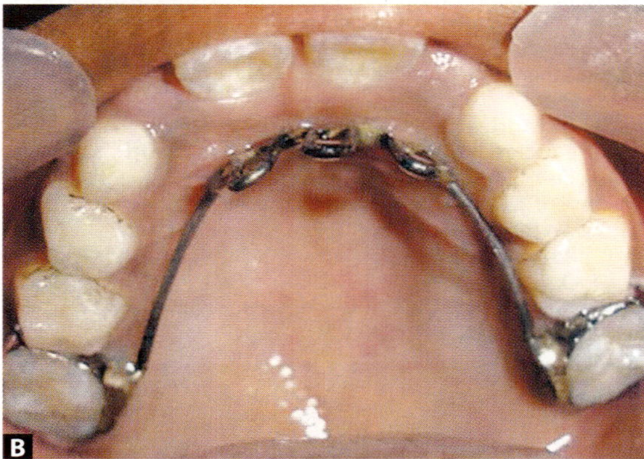

Figs. 30.22A and B: Tongue crib.

Galella Habit Appliance

It is primarily used to correct aberrant tongue habits; however, a secondary function of the appliance is to deter thumb sucking. The appliance is designed to be physiologically congruent with normal tongue function and is a simple appliance consisting only of a large coffin loop and a lingual arch wire that supports a habit bead. It is built on bands placed on the first permanent molars. The appliance is inserted into horizontal tubes (Mia tubes) that are placed on the lingual of the bands, and it is in the family of "fixed-removable" appliances. It is the design, position, and function of these components that make this appliance unique and highly effective **(Fig. 30.23).**

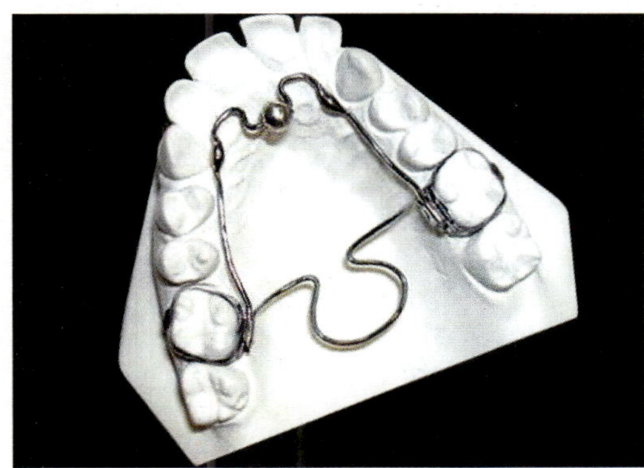

Fig. 30.23: Gallela habit appliance.

Coffin loop is large, about a third the width of the entire palate, and is positioned approximately 8–10 mm away from the palate. The lingual arch wire supports a habit bead that is positioned over the posterior third of the incisive papilla. When the patient swallows, they are instructed to wedge their tongue in between the bead and the roof of the mouth. They are also instructed to "pull" the bead toward the back of the mouth throughout the day. The coffin loop not only functions to remind the heel of the tongue of aberrant tongue swallows but also, because of its position away from the roof of the mouth, helps to intrude the molars thus aiding in the closing of the bite. The anterior position of the bead, combined with the patient's exercise of "pulling" the bead toward the back of the mouth, functions both to retrain the tip of the tongue and as a deterrent to aberrant tongue thrusting.

Habit Corrector™

- **Bergersen EO** in 1987 introduced a removable myofunctional appliance called habit corrector to intercept the atypical swallowing pattern in pediatric age groups.
- It's a preformed, patented appliance made of inert flexible plastic material that adapts to the occlusal anatomy.
- **Indication**
  - Tongue thrust habit.
  - Re-educate habits like habitual mouth breathing, thumb or pacifier sucking, low rest position of tongue.
  - Prevent or reduce open bites, crossbites and increased overjet due to functional problems like abnormal habits.
  - It is available in two forms: HC-C (CLOSE) or closed type: a single block and HC-O (OPEN) or open type in which the front part is open and is joined in the posterior region which useful for habitual mouth breathers.

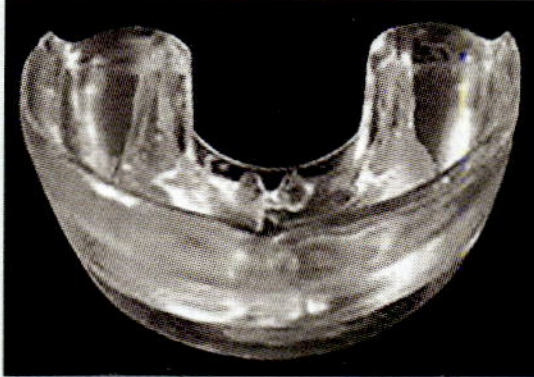
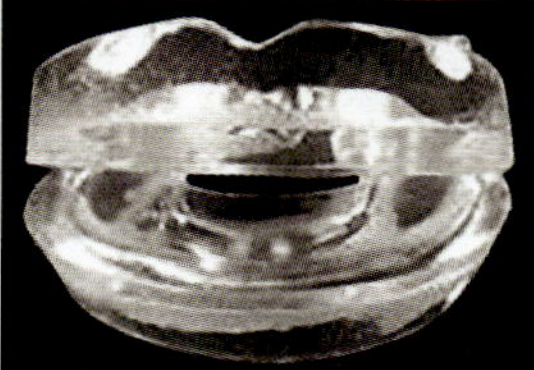

Anoetic swallowing rehabilitation device

- Froggy Mouth (FM) (Micerium, Genoa, Italy) device is a myofunctional device designed by **Dr Patrick Fellus**, Italy for swallowing re-education in atypical swallowing patients.
- Anoetic rehabilitation is a non-restrictive technique (15 minutes per day, associated with pleasure and during a few weeks only) that does not require cerebral participation.
- The FM appliance is available in 3 sizes (small, medium, large): small for children between 3 and 7 years old, medium for children between 7 and 12 years old, large for children over 12 years old.
- **Instructions for use:** The patients should wear FM for 15 min a day for a period of 6 months, while sitting in an upright position, watching television (positioned at a minimum distance of 2 m) or during recreational activity.
- **Vincenzo Quinzi et al.,** in an observational study evaluated the effect of FM appliance on 40 children of age between 5 to 13 years with atypical swallowing pattern. They observed a significant improvement in the lip strength and reduction in lip activity during swallowing. They also recommended a minimum wear of 15 min/day for maximum effect.

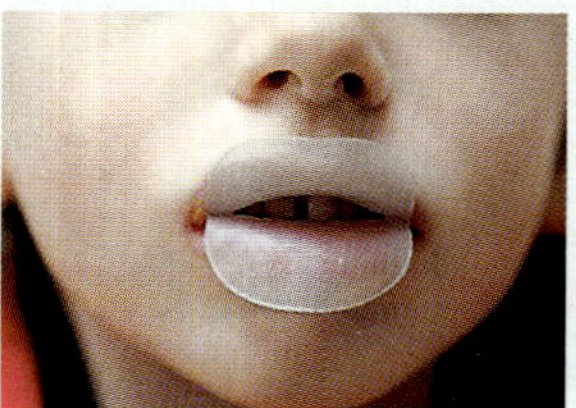

MOUTH BREATHING

Sassouni (1971) *defined mouth breathing as habitual respiration through the mouth instead of nose.* **Merle** *(1980) used the term oronasal breathing instead of mouth breathing.*

Classification of Mouth Breathing

Finn in 1987:

- **Obstructive:** Increased resistance to or complete obstruction of normal airflow through nasal passage.
- **Habitual:** As a matter of habit or persistence of the habit even after elimination of the obstructive cause.
- **Anatomical:** Short upper lip leads to incompetence of lips and hence mouth breathing.

Diagnosis of Mouth Breathing

- **Observe the patient**
  - *Mouth breathers:* Lips will be apart
  - *Nasal breathers:* Lips will be touching
- **Ask the patient to take a deep breath through nose**
  - *Mouth breathers:* No change in shape or size of external nares
  - *Nasal breathers:* Demonstrates good control of alar muscles
- **Mirror test:** it is also called Fog test. Two-surfaced mirror is placed on the patient's upper lip. If air condenses on upper side of mirror, the patient is nasal breather, and if it does so on the opposite side, then he is a mouth breather, e.g., Modified Glatzel mirror used for Fog test for mouth breathers **(Fig. 30.24)**

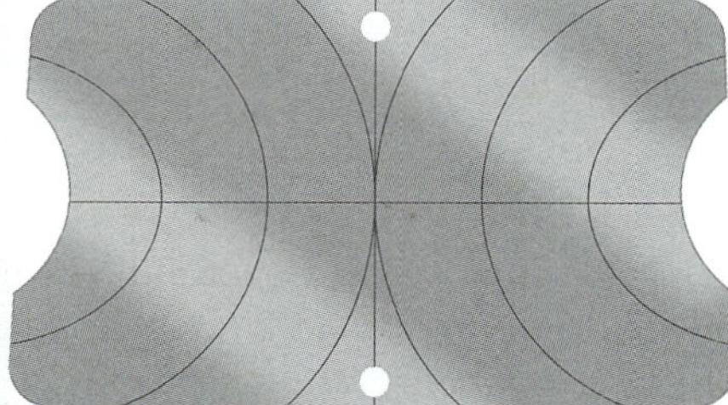
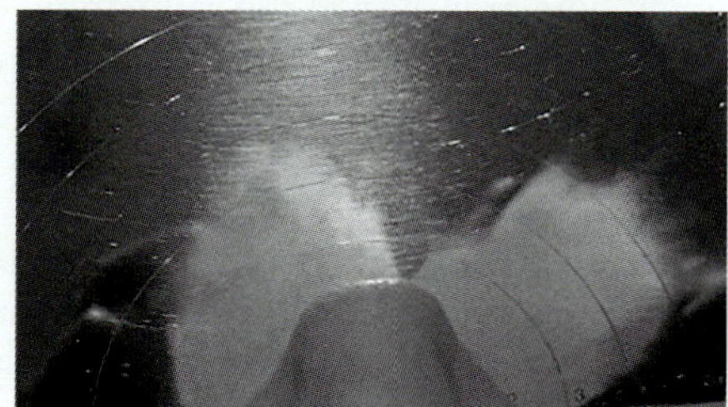

Fig. 30.24: Modified Glatzel mirror used for Fog test for mouth breathers.

- **Massler water holding test:** Patient is asked to hold the mouth full of water. Mouth breathers cannot retain the water for a long time **(Fig. 30.25)**

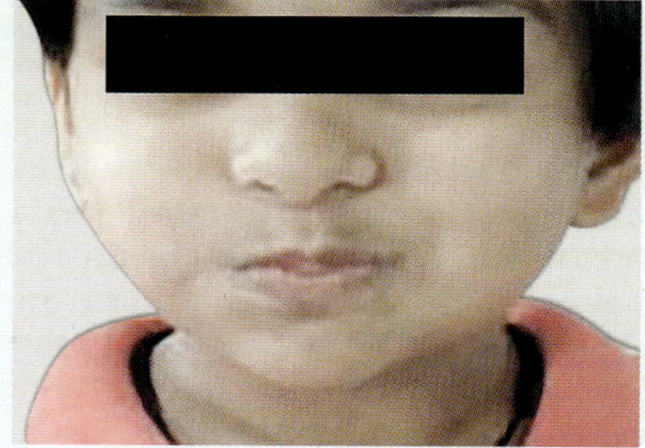

Fig. 30.25: Massler water holding test.

- **Zwemmer's butterfly test:** Take a few fibers of cotton and place it just below the nasal opening. On exhalation, if the fibers of the cotton flutter downwards patient is nasal breather, and if fibers flutter upward he is a mouth breather **(Fig. 30.26)**

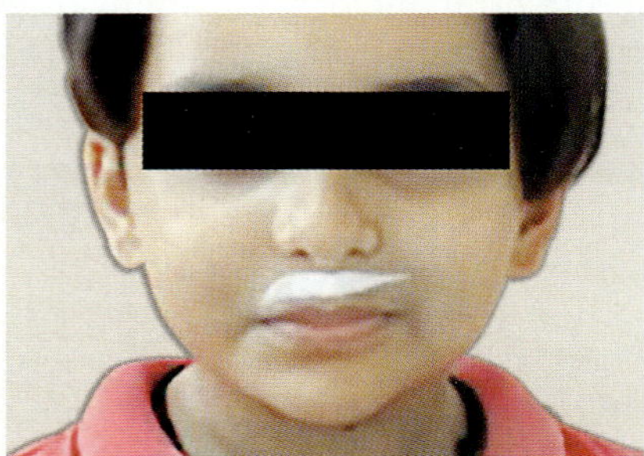

Fig. 30.26: Zwemmer's butterfly test.

- ***Lip seal test for mouth breathers:*** A micropore paper tape is used to seal the lip and observed the child for the pattern of breathing. If the child feels tight in the chest or throat under one minute is an indication of prolonged mouth breathing which can be habitual or obstructive in nature. **(Fig. 30.27)**

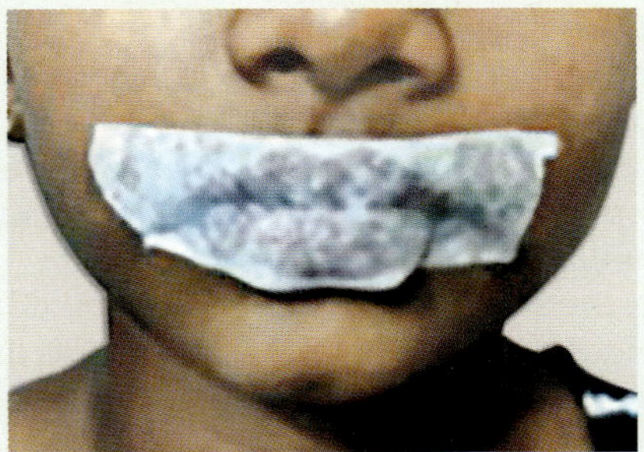

Fig. 30.27: Lip seal test for mouth breathers.

- ***Rhinometry (inductive plethysmography):*** The total air flow through the nose and mouth can be quantified using inductive plethysmography
- ***Cephalometrics:*** It can be used to calculate amount of nasopharyngeal space
- *General features to observe for a mouth breather*
  - Note the respiratory rate per minute of the child according to the age.
  - Breathing movement is observed for diaphragmatic breathing or upper chest breathing
  - Nares should increase in size while inspiration and reduce in size during expiration
  - Head posture should be noted as there is forward head posture for mouth breathers
  - Dorsal nasal hump due to unequal growth of nasal cartilage in mouth breathers

Etiology

- Developmental and morphologic anomalies like abnormal development of nasal cavity, nasal turbinates, and short upper lip.
- Partial obstruction due to deviated nasal septum, localized benign tumors.
- Infection and inflammation of nasal mucosa, chronic allergic stomatitis, chronic atrophic rhinitis, enlarged adenoids and tonsils, nasal polyps.
- Traumatic injuries to the nasal cavity.
- Genetic pattern—ectomorphic children having a genetic type of tapering face and nasopharynx are prone to nasal obstruction.

Clinical Features

General features

↓

- In order to breathe, the child bends the neck forward straightening the oro-naso-pharyngeal path
- This gives the appearance of a pigeon chest
- In mouth breathers the oropharynx is dry and can produce a low-grade esophagitis
- Maxillary sinus and nasal cavity frequently becomes narrowed
- Turbinates become swollen and engorged
- Speech acquires a nasal tone
- Sleep apnea syndrome—due to the loss of cleansing action of saliva there is generally an enlargement of the lingual tonsil at the base of the tongue this leads to partial or complete obstruction of the oropharynx during sleep

↓

Blood gas constituents

↓

- Blood gas studies reveal that mouth breathers have 20% more CO_2 and less O_2

↓

Appearance (Figs. 30.28A and B)
(Given by CV Tomes)

↓

- Adenoid facies is the characteristic feature of mouth breathers
- Lips are held wide apart
- There is lack of tone of oral musculature
- Upper lip is short
- The chin is receded and the face has typical pigeon face appearance
- The nose is tipped superiorly
- Long narrow face
- The face is expression loss
- The bridge of the nose is flat

↓

Dental and skeletal

↓

- Rolled margins and enlarged papilla
- Low tongue position
- Narrow maxillary area
- Protrusion of maxillary and mandibular incisors
- The palatal vault is high
- Mandible hangs open in a slack manner
- Anterior open bite
- Increased incidence of caries
- Mucus and plaque become more tenacious
- Chronic keratinized marginal gingivitis

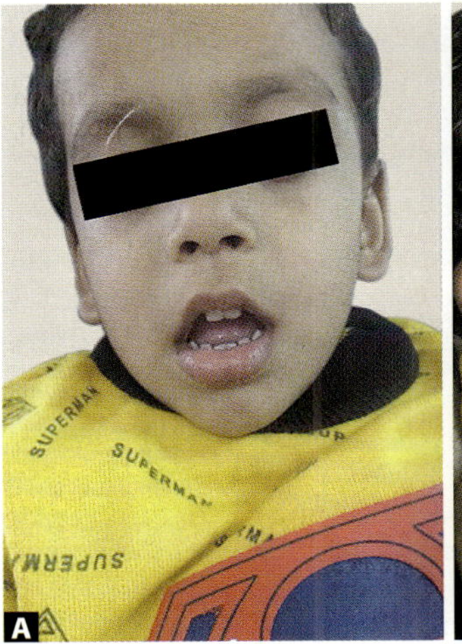

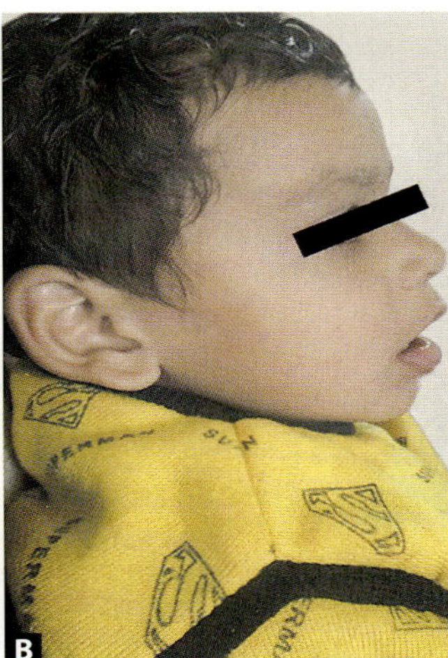

Figs. 30.28A and B: Appearance of mouth breather.

Treatment

The main aspect of management of a mouth-breathing patient is to treat and eliminate the underlying cause or pathology that has created the habit. This should be followed by symptomatic treatment. Other procedures and appliances that can be used are:

- Lip exercises15–30 min/day for 4–5 months **(Fig. 30.29)**
- Oral screen
- Habit corrector appliance (explained earlier in tongue thrusting)
- Maxillothorax myotherapy
- Deep breathing exercises

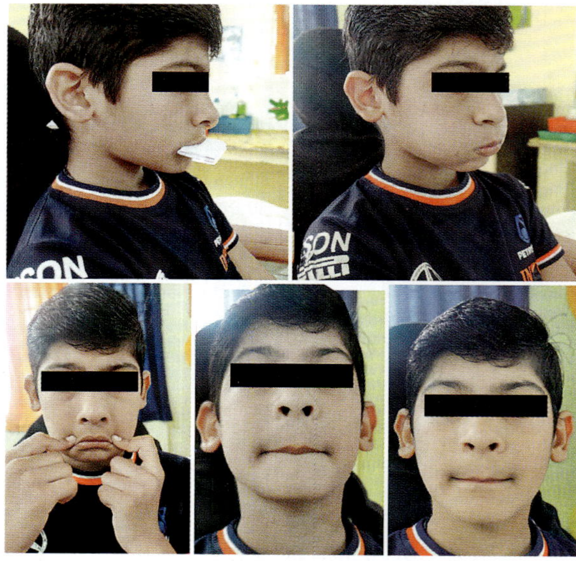

Fig. 30.29: Lip exercises.

Lip exercise for the lips (circumoral muscles) (Fig. 30.29)

- If the upper lip is hypotonic and flaccid, the child is instructed to extend the upper lip as far as possible curving the vermilion border under and behind the maxillary incisors. This exercise should be done15–20 min a day for a period of 4–5 months
- *Stretching of the upper lip to maintain lip seal:* The patient is asked to hold a thin piece of paper between the lips
- If the maxillary incisors are protruded, the lower lip can be used to augment the upper lip exercise. The upper lip is first extended under and behind the maxillary incisors. The vermilion border of the lower lip is then placed against the outside of the extended upper lip and pressed as hard as possible against the upper lip. This type of exercise exerts a strong retracting influence on the maxillary incisors while increasing the tonicity of both upper and lower lips. This exercise is particularly valuable for mouth breathers and should be done for ≥30 min a day
- Massaging of the lips
- *Button pull exercise:* A button of 1.5-inch diameter is taken and a thread is passed through the buttonholes. Then, the patient is asked to place the button behind the lips and pull the thread, while restricting it from being pulled out by lip pressure
- *Tug-of-war exercise:* This involves use of two buttons, with one placed behind the lips while the other button is held by another person to pull the thread
- *Holding and pumping of water back and forth behind the lips:* Patient is asked to hold and pump water back and forth behind the lips until they get tired
- For a developing class II division 1 malocclusion, the playing of a wind instrument may be an interceptive procedure

Oral Screen

- First introduced by **Newell** in 1912 and later advocated by **Hotz** (1980).
- Works on the principle of force application and force elimination of circumoral musculature **(Figs. 30.30A and B)**.

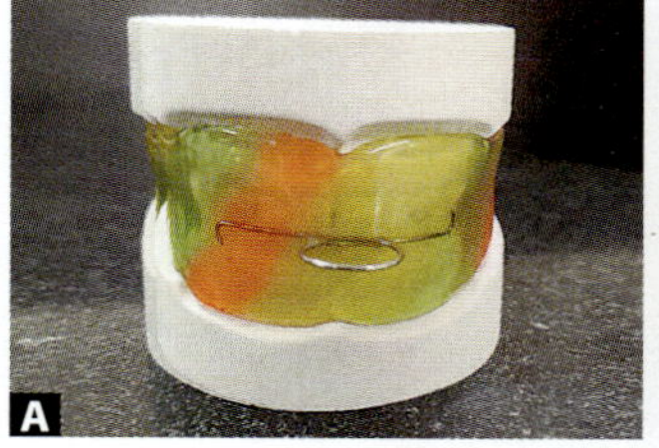

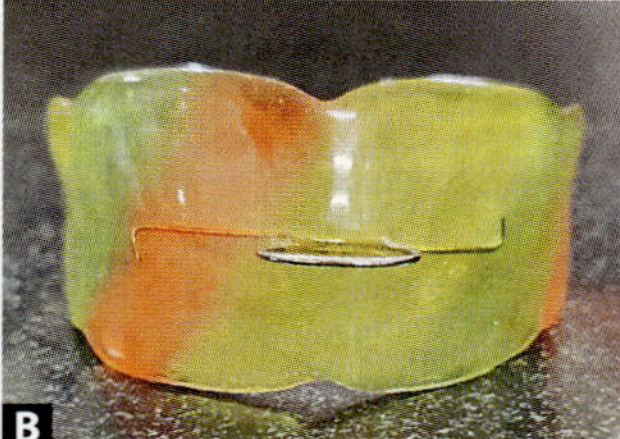

Figs. 30.30A and B: Oral screen.

- **Indications:**
  - Habit-correcting appliance.
  - It helps retrain and strengthen lip action.
  - Improves the tonicity of the lips.
  - To correct simple labio version of the maxillary anterior teeth.
- **Contraindication:** Should not be used if the child has naso-respiratory distress or a nasal obstruction.
- **Modifications:**
  - **Hotz** modification: Anterior loop made of SS wire was added to the appliance. Patient pulls the loop and resists the displacement of the appliance with lips simultaneously.
  - **Kraus** (1956), **Fingeroth** (1958) modification with breathing holes.
  - Double oral screen by **Kraus** 1956, **Selmer-Olsen** 1975.
  - **Rehak's** modification: Pacifier attached with screen.
- **Methodology of working:** After correction of the nasal obstruction this appliance can be given to enhance and promote nasal breathing. To begin with small holes are made at the inter incisal level in the anterior portion of the shield. These holes are periodically closed over the next few weeks in a phased manner such that the child is comfortable with nasal breathing.

Maxillothorax Myotherapy

This was advocated by **Macaray** 1960. These expanding exercises are used in conjunction with the Macaray activator. Macaray constructed an activator out of aluminium with which development of the dental arches and dental base relationship could be corrected at the same time as encouraging mouth breathing. The mouth breather holds the activator in the mouth and at the same time with the left and right arms alternately carries out 10 exercises.

Studies for mouth breathing and dental malocclusion

- ROMA index—risk of malocclusion assessment index: **Grippaudo et al.,** 2016 used ROMA index to assess the ratio of mouth breathing and malocclusion. They screened 3017 children using the ROMA index and found that that an increase in the degree of the index increases the prevalence of bad habits and mouth breathing, meaning that these factors are associated with more severe malocclusions. They also reported a significant association of bad habits with increased overjet and open bite and mouth breathing is closely related to increased overjet, reduced overjet, anterior or posterior crossbite, open bite. Therefore, it is necessary to intervene early on these etiological factors of malocclusion to prevent its development or worsening and, if already developed, correct it by early orthodontic treatment to promote good skeletal growth.

- **Miho Nagaiwa et al.,** did an EMG (electromyography) study of masticatory muscles for the chewing efficiency in mouth breathers and found that it takes a longer amount of time to complete chewing to obtain higher masticatory efficiency when breathing through the mouth. Therefore, mouth breathing will decrease the masticatory efficiency if the duration of chewing is restricted in everyday life.
- **Fernanda et al.,** had done a cephalometric study of changes in the dentofacial complex among nasal versus oral breathers. They observed that the inclination of the mandibular plane (**SN-Go-Gn**) in mouth breathing children are higher than those in nasal breathing children. The posterior facial height are smaller than the anterior one in mouth breathing children and also the upper anterior facial height are smaller than the lower facial height. Thus, mouth breathing children have higher mandibular plane angle with more vertical growth compared to nasal breathers.
- **Ziyi et al.,** in their meta-analysis observed the significant effect of mouth breathing in the overall facial development.
  1. *Effect of mouth breathing in the sagittal (A-P direction):* SNA and SNB angle in mouth breathers is lower when compared to nasal breathing children. The AND angle, anterior inclination of upper and lower incisor are higher in children with mouth breathing. This shows a more retrognathic mandibular development with proclined incisors in mouth breathing children.
  2. *Effect of mouth breathing in the vertical direction*: When they compared Inclination of the occlusal plane in relation to the skull base, the degree of the maxillary inclination in relation to the anterior cranial base and the inclination of the mandibular plane in relation to the skull base, there was a higher value for mouth breathing children showing an increased vertical growth.
  3. *Effect of mouth breathing on airway*: The backward and downward rotation of maxilla and mandible resulted in airway stenosis in children with mouth breathing.

Difference between oral screen and vestibular screen

- **Krauss** limited the term "oral screen" to those appliances with the objective of controlling tongue function.
- In his version of the vestibular screen, the material extended into the vestibule in contact with the alveolar process but did not touch the teeth at all.
- Other variation of Krauss is the combine oral and vestibular screen to form "double oral screen" for eliminating mouth breathing and tongue thrusting.

BRUXISM

Ramfjord in1966 defined bruxism as the habitual grinding of teeth when an individual is not chewing or swallowing.

Classification

- **Daytime:** Diurnal bruxism/bruxomania. It can be conscious or subconscious and may occur along with parafunctional habits.
- **Nighttime bruxism:** Nocturnal bruxism. Subconscious grinding of teeth characterized by rhythmic patterns of masseter.

Etiology

- **Central nervous system:** It could be a manifestation of cortical lesions, for example, in children cerebral palsy.
- **Psychological factors:** A tendency to gnash and grind the teeth has been associated with feeling of anger and aggression or is a manifestation of the inability to express emotions such as anxiety and hate.
- Occlusal discrepancies.
- Genetics.
- **Systemic factors:** Magnesium deficiency, chronic abdominal distress, intestinal parasites.
- **Occupational factors:** An overenthusiastic student and compulsive overachievers may also develop the habit.

Clinical Manifestations

The signs and symptoms of bruxism depend on frequency intensity, and age of patient. The forces of bruxism are transmitted to the structures of masticatory apparatus, and depending on the resistance of the individual, certain amount of the forces is absorbed, and the rest are passed to other structures.

- **Occlusal trauma:** This includes toothache, mobility mainly in morning.
- **Tooth structure:** Extreme sensitivity due to loss of enamel, a typical wear facets, pulp may be exposed, and many fractured teeth can also occur.
- **Muscular:** Tenderness of the jaw muscles on palpation, muscular fatigue on waking up in the morning, hypertrophy of masseter.
- **Temporomandibular joint:** Pain, crepitation, clicking in joint, restriction of mandibular movements.
- **Associated features:** Headache.

Treatment

- **Occlusal adjustments:** Premature contacts or occlusal interferences have been associated with the development of bruxism in some studies in the past and hence their corrections are a must.
- **Equilibration therapy:** The proposed idea that bruxism may be due to malocclusion makes orthodontic treatments viable options in managing the condition.
- **Occlusal splints:** These are worn at night to guide the occlusal movement so that the periodontal damage is minimal. The appliance covers all the maxillary or mandibular teeth, but it is mostly worn in the upper maxilla. Occlusal splints are generally appreciated to prevent tooth wear, injuries and reduce night-time clenching. Splints should cover the occlusal surfaces of all the teeth. With the use of a splint, there will be some reduction in muscle tone. The appliance that helps manage the consequences of nocturnal bruxism is the flat-planed stabilization splint, also called occlusal bite guard, bruxism appliance, biteplate, or nightguard **(Fig. 30.31)**.
- **Psychotherapy:** Patient counseling can lead to a decrease in tension and create awareness of the habit. This will increase voluntary control and thus reducing parafunctional movements.

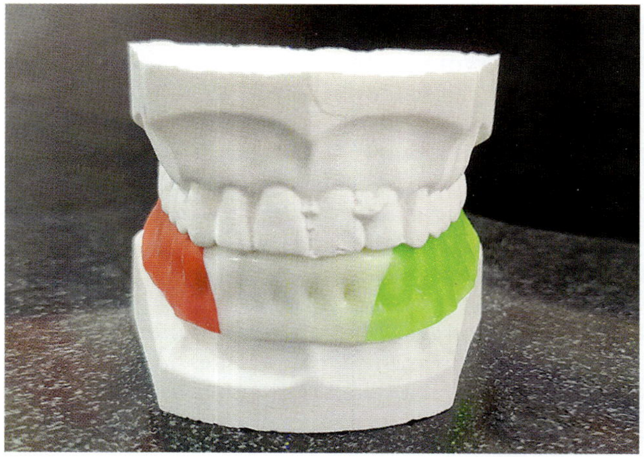

Fig. 30.31: Mouthguard for prevention of bruxism.

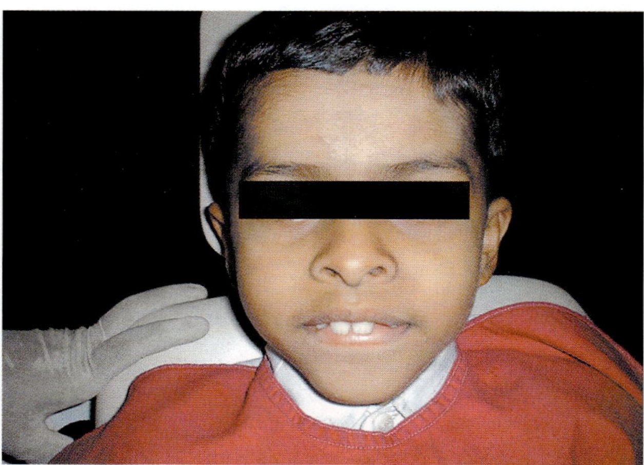

Fig. 30.32: Lip habit.

- **Physical therapy:** It may be recommended if bruxism is associated with muscle pain and stiffness.
- **Relaxation training:** In this method, the patient is trained to relax the muscle group voluntarily.
- **Medication:** The use of drugs in treating bruxism should be limited to short periods and severe cases where occlusal devices and psychological approaches were ineffective. Pharmacological management includes the use of antianxiety agents, tranquilizers, sedatives, and muscle relaxants.
- **Biofeedback:** This technique utilizes positive feedback to enable the patient to learn tension reduction. It is based on the idea that bruxers can unlearn their behavior. It is accomplished by allowing the patient to view an electromyography (EMG) monitor while the mandible is postured with minimum activity. For nocturnal bruxism, auditory, vibratory, or taste stimuli may be used.
- **Electrical method:** Electrogalvanic stimulation for muscle relaxation is currently used for the treatment of bruxism.
- **Botulin toxin:** A neurotoxin synthesized by *Clostridium botulinum*, is currently used to treat various medical conditions, including bruxism. It works by impeding acetylcholine production and blocking calcium channels in nerve endings, temporarily inhibiting muscle contraction. Botulin toxin A injections in the masseter and temporal muscles have been demonstrated to improve the quality of life of patients with bruxism.

LIP BITING

Normal lip anatomy and function is important for speaking, eating, and maintaining the balanced occlusion. The lip habit may involve either of the lips, higher predominance toward the lower lip. This is defined as a habit that involves manipulation of lips and perioral structures **(Fig. 30.32)**.

Classification

- Lip licking/wetting of lips by the tongue
- *Lip sucking habit:* Pulling the lips in to the mouth between the teeth.

Etiology

- Malocclusion
- In conjunction with other habits
- Emotional stress.

Clinical Manifestations

- Protrusion of upper incisors
- Retrusion of lower incisors
- Lip trap **(Fig. 30.33)**
- Muscular imbalance
- Lower incisor collapse with lingual crowding
- Lip has reddened and chapped area below the vermilion border **(Fig. 30.34)**
- Mento labial sulcus becomes accentuated.

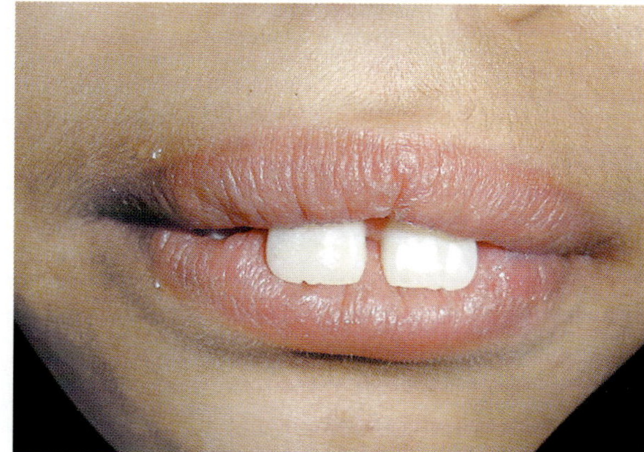

Fig. 30.33: Lip trap.

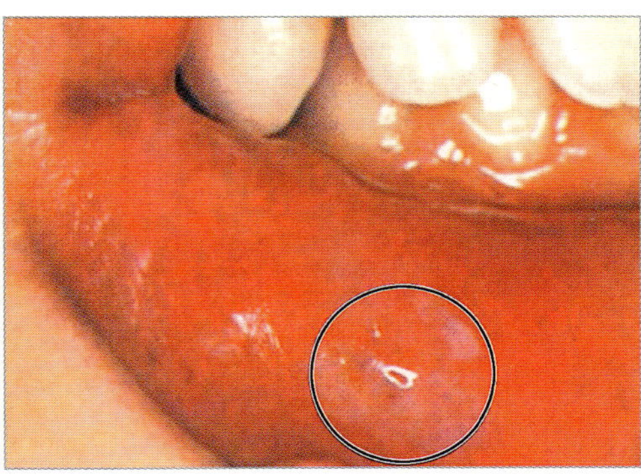

Fig. 30.34: Reddened and chapped area below the vermilion border.

Treatment

Lip habit is not self-correcting and may be come more deleterious with age because of the muscular force interacting with child's growth. Treatment of lip sucking habit should be directed initially toward the etiology followed by appliance therapy like lip protector **(Fig. 30.35)**, oral screen, and lip bumper **(Figs. 30.36A and B)**. **Gopalakrishna S et al** (2021) used clear aligner for management of lip biting and found that clear aligner/retainer was efficient and acceptable to patients.

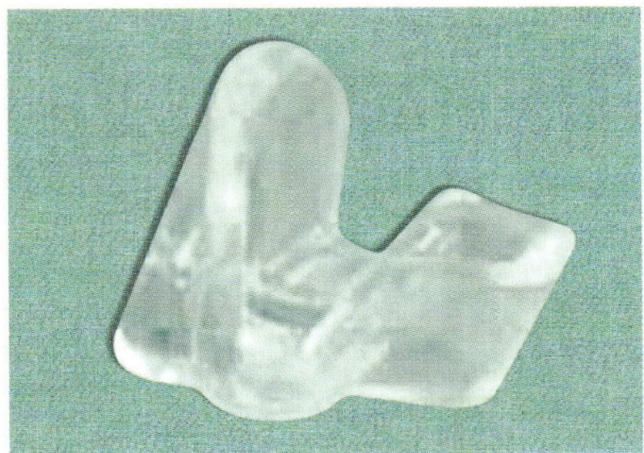

Fig. 30.35: Lip protector.

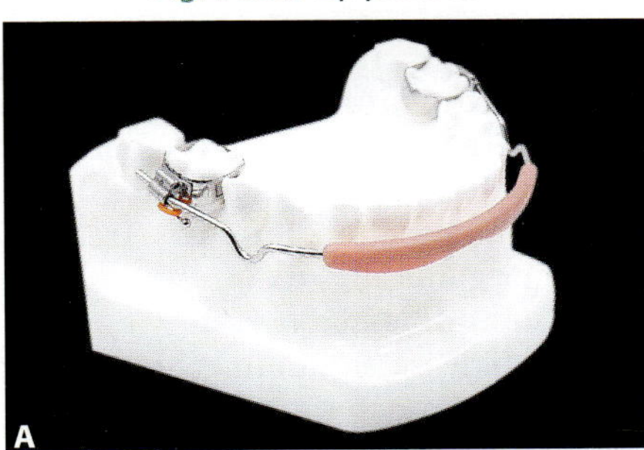

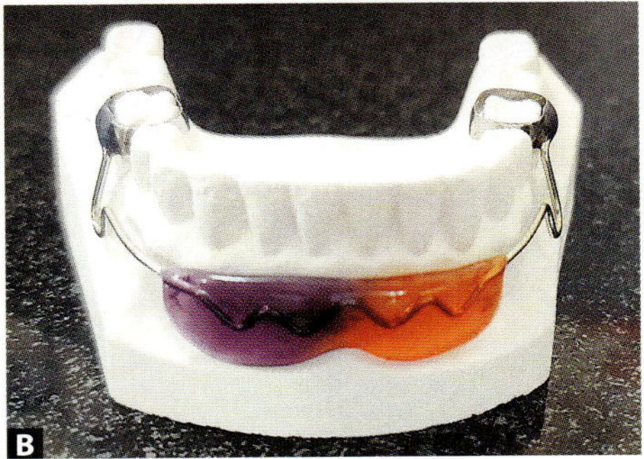

Figs. 30.36A and B: Lip bumper. (*Pic courtesy:* ODI Orthodontic lab in Buffalo, NY, USA).

NAIL BITING

Nail biting is one of the most common habits in children and adults. It is the sign of internal tension. Incidence as reported by **Weschsher** (1931) is 43% in adolescents and 25% in college students. Onychophagia also called nail biting (NB), is a common but unresolved problem. It is a pathological oral habit in which a person puts as well as bites one's nails and fingertips. Onychophagia is a Greek word, *onycho* means fingernail or toenail and *phagia* is to eat or consume. It is often neglected as a condition in clinical practice, and it may lead to negative effects on quality of life and results in physical as well as psychosocial damage. It is also considered as a self-mutilative automatic behavior.

Etiology

- **Nervousness:** When an individual is tensed, they resort to nail biting which has a calming effect on the individual.
- **Imitation:** Role models of children are their elders such as parents, and they are used to copying their adults whether it is a good or bad habit.
- **Emotions:** Shyness or low self-esteem also often leads to nail biting.
- **Boredom:** If persons feel bored, are not doing anything in particular, are inactive—these could be some common reasons to bite their nails.
- **Perfectionism:** If children find they are imperfect in specific goal, they automatically try to fix them by nail biting.
- **Psychosomatic:** Particularly seen in aggressive families.

Effects

- Crowding, rotation, and alteration of incisal edges of incisors
- Inflammation of the nail bed.
- Malformed nails,
- Infection of the nail and surrounding soft tissue
- Increased risk of parasitic infections
- Stomach infections due to swallowing nail particles and dirt
- Social and psychological complications like humiliation, emotional suffering, and social impairment.

Management

- The main goal of management of nail biting is to motivate the child and provide emotional support and to relieve stress that may help to defeat the nail biting. In mild cases, nail biting is not a distressing condition and always improve on its own, even though it needs more attention, love, affection, and comprehension; these are suitable to stop the bad habit. The best way to manage a nail biting is to make good habits, educate them, to develop awareness, to give emotional support and encouragement.
- **Aversion stimulus:** In this psychotherapy, irritant is used over the finger. This type of psychotherapy is based on reinforcement learning. An aversive stimulus such as a bitter substance on the nail biter's nail so nail biter thinks twice to put nail in mouth.
- **Stimulus control:** The main principle of this is to identify and then eliminate the stimulus, because it always triggers

biting urges. This therapy helps to identify, to get rid from environment and situation or emotions that trigger nail biting.

- **Competing response:** In this behavioral method, child performs a competing response whenever he/she has the urge to bite or finds his/hers biting nails. For example, a behavior to stop or avoid moving upper limbs towards face or lips, or a behavior to stop or inhibit entering fingers into mouth is employed. This method has been shown to be more effective than not using it.

SELF-INJURIOUS HABITS

(Masochistic habits, sadomasochistic habits, self-mutilating habits.) Repetitive acts that result in physical damage to the individual **(Fig. 30.37)**. These habits show an increased incidence in the mentally retarded population. Seen in 10–20% in mentally retarded children and in children with psychological abnormalities.

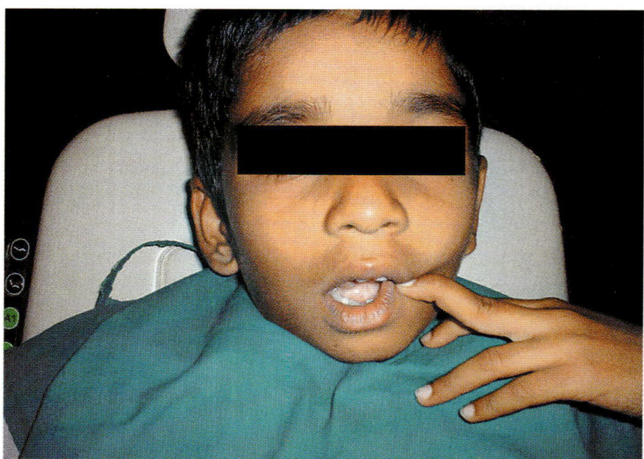

Fig. 30.37: Child with cheek biting.

Etiology

- **Organic:** Associated with Lesch-Nyhan disease and De Lange syndrome.
- **Functional:** Given by **Stewart** and **Kernohan** in 1972.

Type A: Injuries superimposed on a pre-existing lesion, for example, 3.5-year-old child who was treated for herpetic stomatitis, all but one of the numerous lesions responded well to treatment. This single ulcer was found to be perpetuated by a fingernail habit occurred mainly at night.

Type B: Injuries secondary to another established habit, for example, rotation of thumb while thumb sucking can harm soft tissues.

Type C: Injuries of the unknown or complex etiology. This type of behavior has a greater psychogenic component.

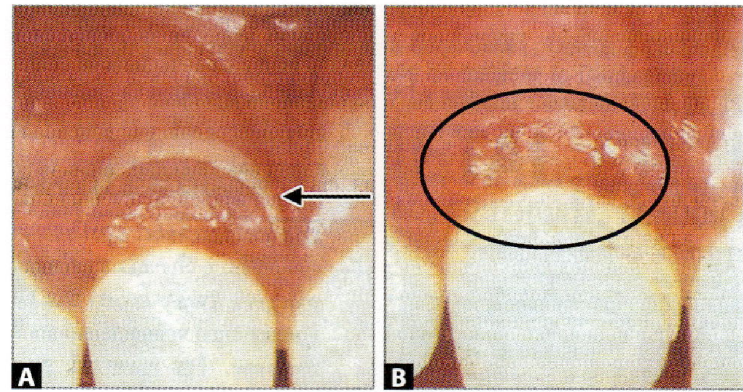

Figs. 30.38A and B: Dislodged nail by picking of gingiva, ulcer due to picking of gingiva.

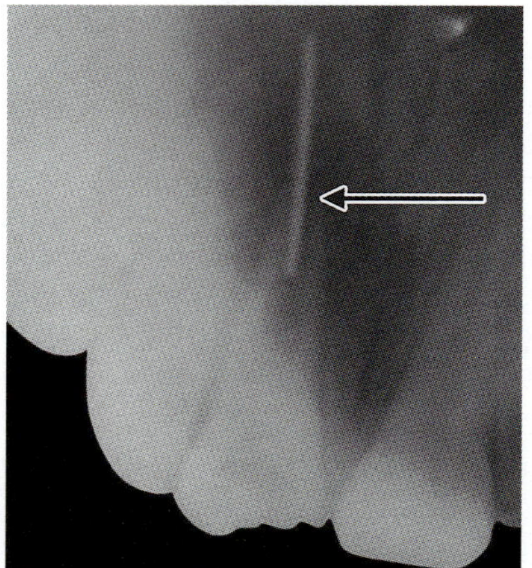

Fig. 30.39: Pin insertion inside endodontic cavity.

Clinical Features

- Biting of fingers, knees, shoulders
- Frenum thrusting
- Picking of gingiva **(Figs. 30.38A and B)**
- Insertion of sharp objects into the oral cavity **(Fig. 30.39)**.

Treatment

The initial treatment is initiated toward psychotherapy because some children experience a feeling of neglect, abandonment, and loneliness and thus use this behavior in an attempt to solicit attention and love. Treatment of self-injurious behavior generally re quires a multidisciplinary approval. Care should be taken in dealing with this form of behavior of underlying emotional component. Palliative therapy followed by mechanotherapy using protective padding and mouth guards has also been advocated.

Many oral habits may be considered normal for a certain stage of a child's development, but it is the duty of the pedodontist to work with the parents and children toward resolution of habit before it causes any deleterious effects because he is most often the first to see the patient.

INTERRELATION AMONG ORAL HABITS

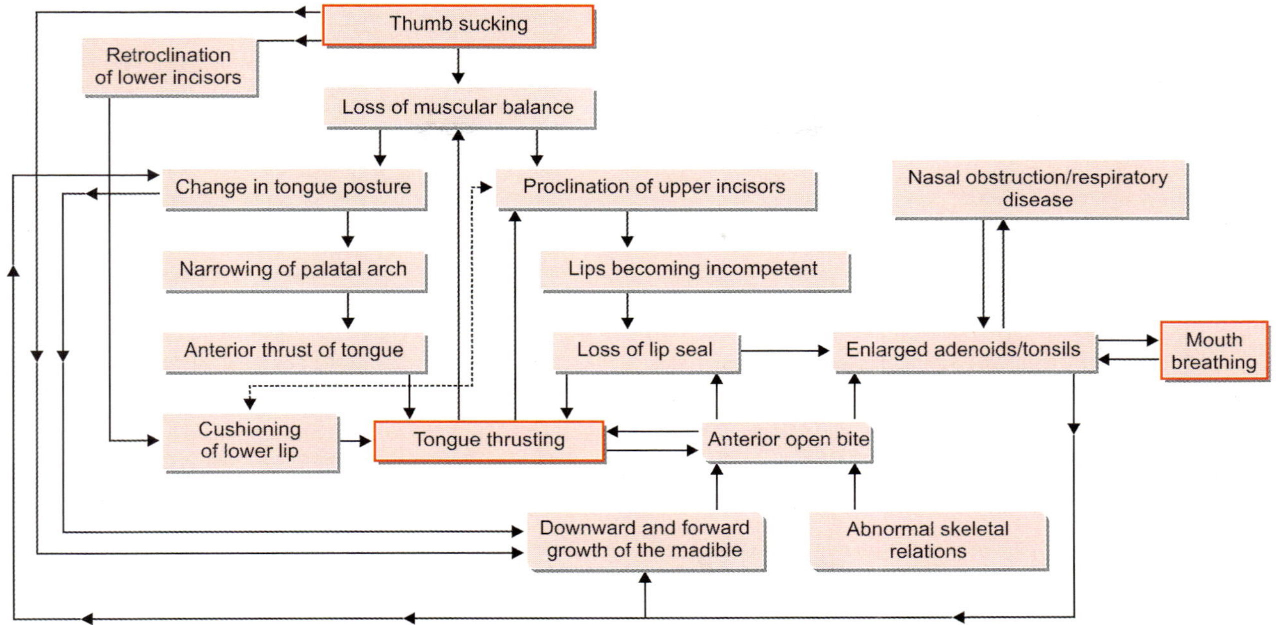

POINTS TO REMEMBER

- Boucher OC defined habit as a tendency toward an actor an act that has become a repeated performance, relatively fixed, consistent, easy to perform, and almost automatic.
- Thumb sucking is defined as the placement of the thumb in varying depths into the mouth. Its etiology varies from oral theory, rooting reflex, working mother, low socioeconomic status, stress, and age of child. The classical features include dishpan thumb with keratotic lesions, proclination of maxillary incisors, open bite, high palate. The management strategies include psychological approach, chemical approach, reminder therapy, mechanotherapy using rakes, and new reminder advancements like thumb-home concept, book reading, long sleeves, etc.
- Tongue thrust as the forward movement of the tongue tip between the teeth to meet the lower lip during deglutition and in sounds of speech, so that the tongue lies interdentally. It can be physiologic, anatomic, functional, or habitual. The classical features are open bite, crossbite, bimaxillary protrusion, and incompetent lips. Diagnosis is made by asking the patient to swallow water while observing musculature. Treatment is by mechanotherapy, subconscious therapy, myofunctional exercises, lip and elastic exercises.
- Mouth breathing as habitual respiration through the mouth instead of nose. It may be obstructive, habitual, or anatomic. The most common diagnostic tests are rhinometry, Massler water holding test, Jwemen's butterfly test. The main clinical features include adenoid facies, gingivitis, and anterior maxillary caries. Treatment is by removal of obstruction, lip exercises, and oral screen.
- Bruxism is the habitual grinding of teeth when an individual is not chewing or swallowing.
- Self-injurious habits are also called masochistic habits, sadomasochistic habits, self-mutilating habits. They are repetitive acts that result in physical damage to the individual. Its etiology is either organic which is associated with Lesch-Nyhan disease and De Lange syndrome or functional. Clinical features include biting of fingers, knees, shoulders, frenum thrusting, and picking of gingiva.

Questionnaire

1. Define and classify oral habits.
2. Describe the etiology, clinical features, and management of thumb-sucking habit.
3. Classify tongue thrusting and explain its clinical features.
4. Write a note on management of thrusting habit by exercise.
5. What are the diagnostic test and clinical features of mouth breathers?
6. What is bruxism?
7. Explain self-injurious habits.

FURTHER READING

1. Andrews RG. Tongue thrusting. J South Calif Dent Assoc. 1960;28:47-53.
2. Campos F, Lessa R, Enoki C, Fernandes M, Feres N, Cardoso F, et al. Breathing mode influence in craniofacial development. Rev Bras Otorrinolaringol. 2005:71(2):156-60.
3. Cayley AS, et al. Electropalatographic and cephalometric assessment of myofunctional therapy in open bite subjects. Aust Orthod J. 2000;16:23-33.
4. Fernández-Núñez T, Amghar-Maach S, Gay-Escoda C. Efficacy of botulinum toxin in the treatment of bruxism: Systematic review. Med Oral Patol Oral Cir Bucal. 2019;24(4):e416-24.

5. Gopalakrishnan S, Chacko T, Jacob J. Management of Lip Biting Using Clear Aligner/Clear Retainer. Journal of Indian Orthodontic Society. 2021;55(1):94-95.
6. Grippaudo C, Paolantonio EG, Antonini G, Saulle R, La Torre G, Deli R. Association between oral habits, mouth breathing and malocclusion. Acta Otorhinolaryngol Ital. 2016;36:386-94.
7. Gulati MS, Grewal N, Kaur A. A comparative study of effects of mouth breathing and normal breathing on gingival health in children. J Indian Soc Pedo Prev Dent. 1998;16:72-83.
8. Gupta T, et al. Mouth breathing—its consequences, diagnosis and treatment. Acta Scientific Dental Sciences. 2020;4(5):32-41.
9. Haas M. The different sucking habits and their influence on the development of dentition. DRecord. 1937;57:633-53.
10. Haskell BS, Munk JR. An aid to stop thumb sucking: the 'Bluegrass appliance'. Pediatr Dent.1991;13:83-5.
11. Johnson LR. Habits and their control during childhood. J Am Dent Assoc. 1937;24:1409-21.
12. Josell SD. Medical Dental Science: habits affecting dental and maxillofacial growth and development. Dent Clin North Am. 2000;44:659-69.
13. Josell SO. Habits affecting dental and maxillofacial growth and development. Dent Clin North Am. 1995;39:851-60.
14. Krishnappa S, Rani MS, Aariz S. New electronic habit reminder for the management of thumb-sucking habit. J Indian Soc Pedod Prev Dent. 2016;34:294-7.
15. Lal SJ, Weber, DDS KK. Bruxism Management. [Updated 2021 Sep 15]. In: Stat Pearls [Internet]. Treasure Island (FL): Stat Pearls Publishing; 2022. Available from: https://www.ncbi.nlm.nih.gov/books/NBK482466/
16. Lewis SJ. Thumb-sucking; a cause of malocclusion in the deciduous teeth. J Am Dent Assoc. 1930;17:1060-72.
17. Lobbezoo F, van der Zaag J, van Selms MK, Hamburger HL, Naeije M. Principles for the management of bruxism. J Oral Rehabil. 2008;35(7):509-23.
18. Nagaiwa M, Gunjigake K, Yamaguchi K. The effect of mouth breathing on chewing efficiency. Angle Orthod. 2016;86:227-34.
19. Norton LA, Gellin ME. Management of digital sucking and tongue thrusting in children. Dent Clin North Am. 1968. pp. 363-82.
20. Nowak AJ, Warren JJ. Infant oral health and oral habits. Pediatr Clin North Am. 2000;47:1034-66.
21. Nowak AJ, Warren JJ. Infant oral health and oral habits. Pediatr Clin North Am. 2000;47:1043-66.
22. Popovich F, Thompson GW. Thumb and finger sucking: its relation to malocclusion. Am J Orthod. 1973;63:148-55.
23. Proffit WR, Mason RM. Myofunctional therapy for tongue thrusting: background and recommendations. Jam Dent Assoc. 1975;90:403-11.
24. Pullen HA. Abnormal habits in the irrelation to malocclusion and facial deformity, Internat. J Orthod. 1927;13:233-52.
25. Quinzi V, Nota A, Caggiati E, Saccomanno S, Marzo G, Tecco S. Short-Term Effects of a Myofunctional Appliance on Atypical Swallowing and Lip Strength: A Prospective Study. J Clin Med. 2020;9:2652.
26. Ramfjord SP. Bruxism: a clinical and electromyographic study. J Am Dent Assoc. 1961;62:21-44.
27. Sahu A, Shyagali TR. A new innovative light-emitting diode habit-breaking appliance. Indian J Multidiscip Dent. 2017;7:149-51.
28. Shetty RM, Dixit U, Hegde RJ, Shivaprakash PK. RURS' elbow guard: an innovative treatment of the thumb-sucking habit in a child with Hurler's syndrome. J Indian Soc Pedod Prev Dent. 2010;28:227-33.
29. Shetty RM, Shetty M, Shetty NS, Deoghare A. Three-alarm system: revisited to treat thumb-sucking Habit. Int J Clin Pediatr Dent. 2015;8:82-6.
30. Siddiqui JA, Qureshi SF, Marei WM, Mahfouz TA. Onychophagia (Nail biting): A body focused repetitive behaviour due to psychiatric co-morbidity. J Mood Disord. 2017;7(1):47.
31. Tulley WJ. A critical appraisal of tongue thrusting. Am J Orthod. 1969;55:640-50.
32. Umberger FG, Van Reenen JS. Thumb sucking management are view. Int J Orofacial Myology. 1995;21:41-7.
33. Van Norman RA. Digit-sucking: a review of the literature, clinical observations and treatment recommendations. Int J Orofacial Myology. 1997;23:14-34.
34. Williams TI, Rose R, Chisholm S. What is the function of nail biting: an analog assessment study. Behav Res Ther 2007; 45: 989-995.
35. Zhao Z, Zheng L, Huang X, Li C, Liu J, Hu Zhao Y, et al. Effects of mouth breathing on facial skeletal development in children: a systematic review and meta-analysis. BMC Oral Health. 2021:21:108.

CHAPTER

Cephalometric Diagnosis

Siddharth Mehta, Nikhil Marwah

CHAPTER OUTLINE

- Cephalometric Technique
- Reference Points
- Reference Planes
- Analysis of the Cephalogram
- Down's Analysis
- Steiner's Analysis
- Tweed's Analysis
- Wit's Appraisal

The primary aim of cephalometrics is to assess the dental, skeletal and facial relationships as seen on radiograph. Cephalometric has long been studied and researched by all scientists and is an integral part of orthodontics as well as pedodontics. The development of craniofacial morphology has evolved a great deal over 50 years. The earliest reference to the shape and morphology of face was in 4th century BC by Greeks. In 1922, **Simon** introduced a photographic technique to evaluate facial morphology. **Rancini** and **Carrera** in 1926 performed first lateral view of skull. It was in 1931 that **B Holly Broadbent** recognized the need of assessment of craniofacial morphology and later **TW Todd** went on to develop first cephalometer based on anthropometer used at case Western Reserve University.

CEPHALOMETRIC TECHNIQUE

For the radiograph, the patient is positioned next to the X-ray apparatus and positioned by adjusting the ear rods and nasal piece so that the Frankfort horizontal (FH) plane is parallel to floor. The film cassette is positioned as close as possible to the patient, and the X-ray beam should be at the level of ear rods, perpendicular to film **(Figs. 31.1A and B)**.

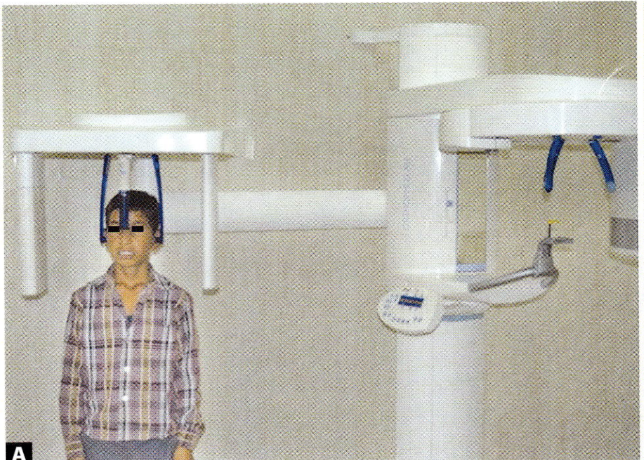

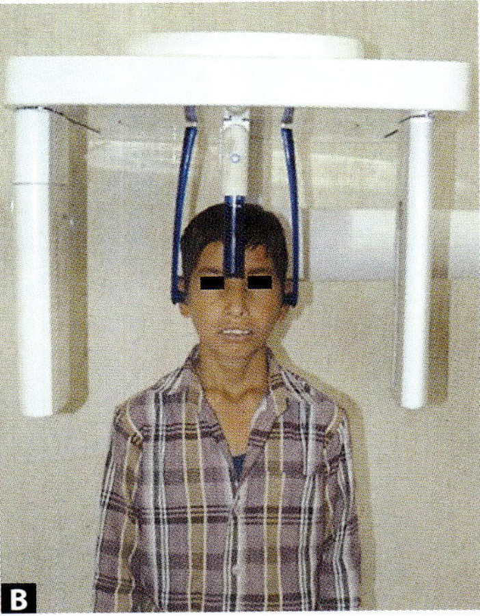

Figs. 31.1A and B: Technique for lateral cephalostat.

Table 31.1: Lateral reference points.

Symbol	Point	Details
A	Subspinale	Deepest point on maxilla
ANS	Anterior nasal spine	Tip of anterior nasal spine
Ar	Articulare	Point of intersection of dorsal contour of mandibular process and temporal bone
B	Supramentale	Most posterior point between infradentale and pogonion, anterior point of mandible
Ba	Basion	Lowest point on anterior aspect of foramen magnum
Bo	Bolton point	Highest point of retrocondylar fossa
Cd	Condylion	Most superior point on articular head of condyle
CF	Center of face	Intersection of FH plane and a line perpendicular to Pt point
Gn	Gnathion	Inferior-most point on contour of chin
Go	Gonion	Point on jaw angle that is inferiorly, posteriorly, and outwardly directed
Me	Menton	Inferior-most point on mandibular symphysis
N	Nasion	Intersection of internasal suture with nasofrontal suture
Or	Orbitale	Lowermost point on lower border of orbit
PNS	Posterior nasal spine	Tip of posterior spine of palatine bone in hard palate. Denotes posterior limit of maxilla
Po	Porion	Most superior point on external auditory meatus
Pog	Pogonion	Anterior-most point on contour of chin
Ptm	Pterygomaxillary fissure	Projected teardrop-shaped fissure created by anterior border of pterygoid plate and posterior border of maxilla
Pt	Pt point	Intersection of inferior border of foramen rotundum with posterior wall of Ptm
R	Broadbent registration point	Midpoint of perpendicular from center of sella turcica to Bolton plane
S	Sella turcica	Midpoint of hypophyseal fossa
SO	Spheno-occipital synchondrosis	Upper-most point of suture

Table 31.2: Frontal reference points.

Symbol	Point	Details
LZF/RZF	Zygomaticofrontal	Bilateral points on medial aspect of zygomaticofrontal sutures at the intersection of orbit
ANS	Anterior nasal spine	Tip of anterior nasal spine
LJ/RJ	Jugal process	Bilateral points on jugal processes at the junction of maxillary tuberosity and zygomatic buttress
LAG/RAG	Antegonial points	Points at inferior margin of antegonial protuberances
M	Menton	Inferior point of mental protuberance
I	I point	Point at the junction of crown and gingiva in maxillary and mandibular region

Table 31.3: Soft tissue reference points.

- Glabella
- Nasal tip
- Upper lip point
- Lower lip point
- Infradentale
- Soft tissue nasion
- Subnasale
- Stomion
- Supradentale
- Soft tissue pogonion

Cephalometric Landmarks

Cephalometric landmarks are of two types:

1. **Anatomic landmarks:** They are representative of actual anatomic structures, e.g., nasion.
2. **Derived Landmarks:** They are obtained from actual anatomic structures and should be easily identifiable, reproducible and allow angular and linear measurement, e.g., gnathion.

REFERENCE POINTS

Critical knowledge of anatomical landmarks is of paramount importance in cephalometrics as multiple structures sometimes make it difficult to assess the relationship on radiograph alone.

The radiograph is placed on a view-box and traced using a tracing paper and drawing pencil to demarcate all the reference points and planes. There are 18 main reference points on face; in addition to these anthropologic landmarks, there are certain arbitrary points that are also helpful in cephalometric analysis **(Tables 31.1 to 31.3)**. Reference points can be divided into **(Fig. 31.2)** lateral and frontal **(Fig. 31.3)**.

REFERENCE PLANES

Linear assessment is by joining two lines, and angular assessment is by joining three lines. By combining various linear and angular cephalometric measurements, joining various landmarks, cephalometrics offers valuable information on facial types, growth, case diagnosis, functional analysis and progress reports and all other treatment aspects of patients **(Figs. 31.4A to J)**.

- **A-Pog line:** Line from point A to pogonion.
- **Basion-nasion plane (BN plane):** From nasion (N) to basion (Ba) representing the cranial base.

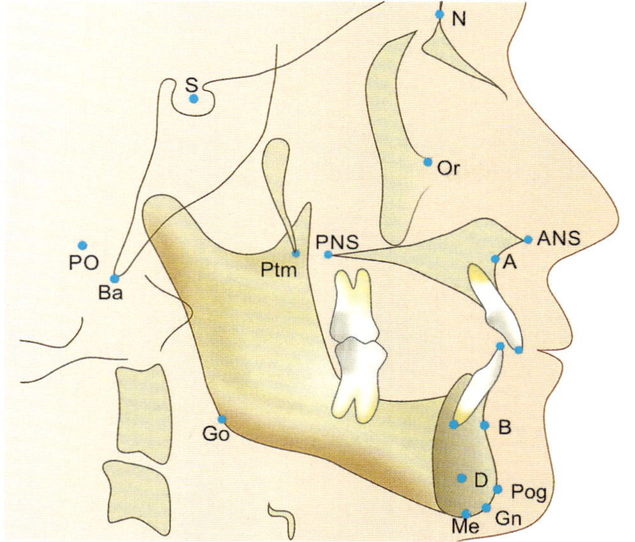

Fig. 31.2: Lateral cephalometric landmarks.

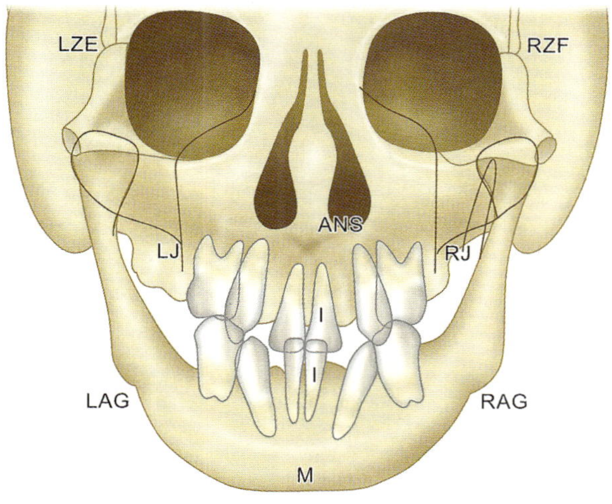

Fig. 31.3: Frontal cephalometric landmarks.

A Pogonion plane

B Basion–nasion plane

C Esthetic plane

D Facial axis

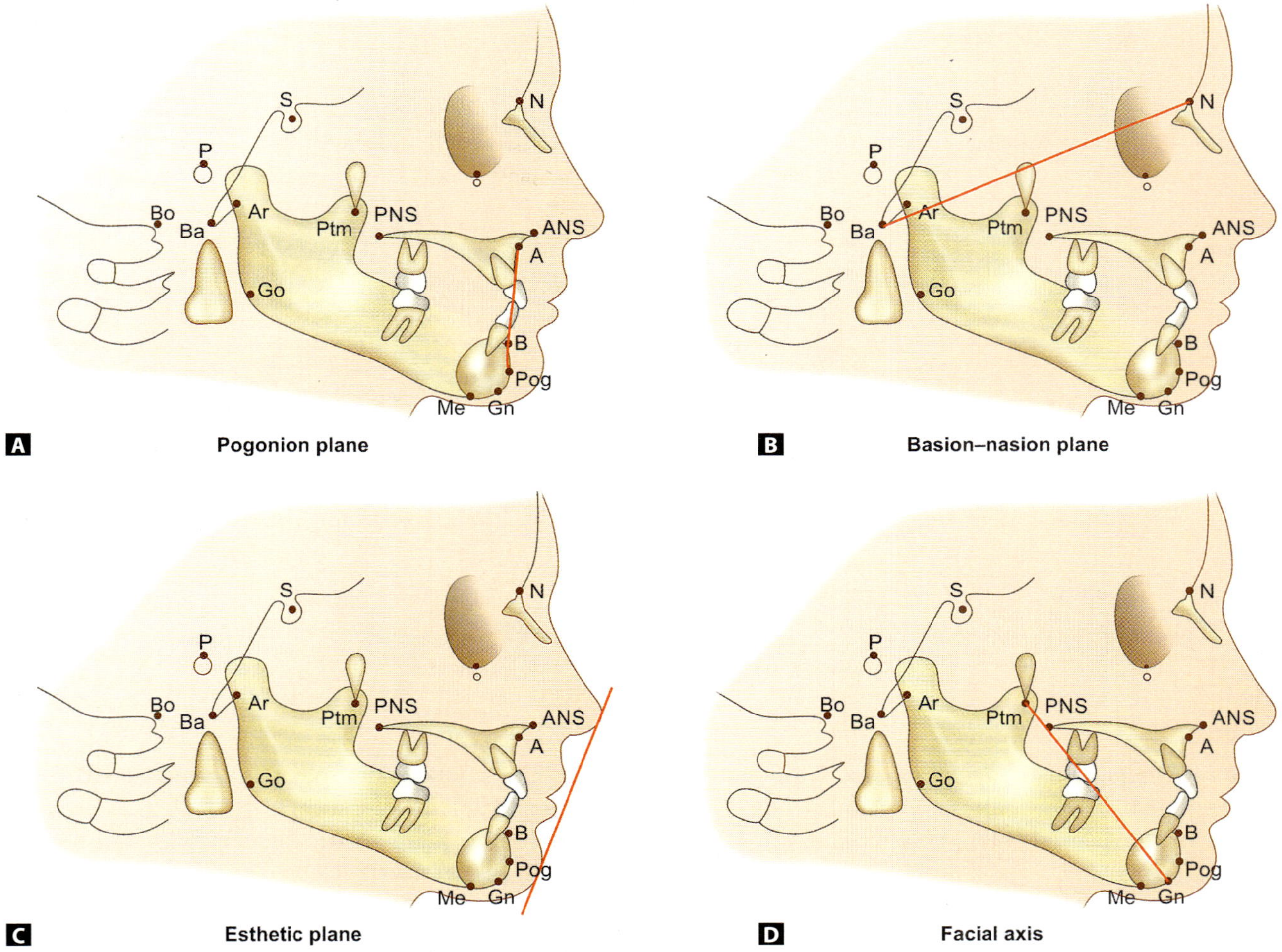

Figs. 31.4A to D: Cephalometric reference planes.

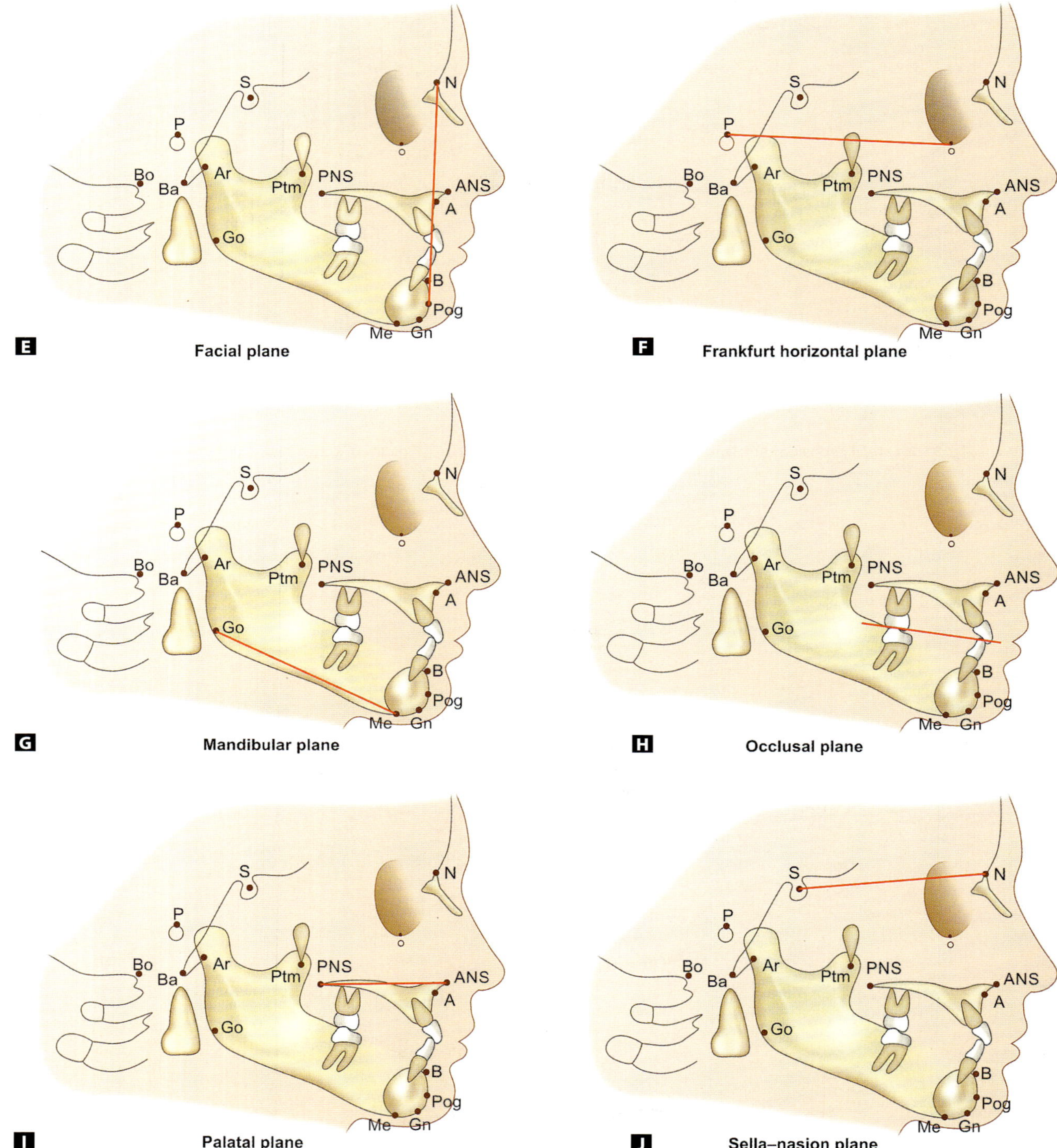

Figs. 31.4E to J: Cephalometric reference planes.

- **E-plane:** Esthetic plane is denoted by a line between anterior point on nose and anterior point on chin.
- **Frankfort horizontal (FH) plane:** From porion (Po) to orbitale (O).
- **Facial plane (FP):** Line through nasion (N) perpendicular to FH plane.
- **Facial axis (FX):** From Pt point (Pt) to gnathion (Gn) which crosses BN plane at right angle.
- **Mandibular plane (MP):** Tangent to inferior border of mandible.
- **Occlusal plane (OP):** Separates the maxillary and mandibular teeth.

- **Palatal plane (PP):** Extends from ANS to PNS.
- **Pterygoid vertical (PTV) plane:** Line perpendicular to FH plane through Pt point.
- **Sella-nasion plane (SN plane):** From sella (S) to nasion (N).

ANALYSIS OF THE CEPHALOGRAM

- The methods currently available to evaluate craniofacial form include anthropometry, cephalometry, ultrasound, computed tomographic (CT) scanning, magnetic resonance imaging (MRI) and optical surface scanning.
- Arguably, cephalometry continues to be the most versatile technique in the investigation of the craniofacial skeleton because of its validity and practicality. Despite the inherent cephalometric distortion and differential magnification of the craniofacial complex, in comparison with newer imaging techniques, the cephalogram produces a high diagnostic yield at a low physiological cost.
- Nevertheless, there are problems in deriving a numerical representation of craniofacial form using cephalometry. This is because "form" is the combination of "size" and "shape," and separating shape from size is complex. Perhaps the most important limitation of cephalometry relates to the errors inherent with the identification and recording of the structures therein.
- The traditional method of analyzing cephalograms [conventional cephalometric analysis (CCA)] has, in recent years, been supplemented with a variety of sophisticated morphometric methods. Although these newer methods possess mathematical and statistical advantages, each has limitations. There are two distinct groups of scientifically valid analytical methods used in cephalometry—landmark-based techniques and boundary outline methods.
  - Landmark-based techniques are dependent on cephalometric landmarks—discrete points defined intrinsically in terms of the surrounding anatomy to represent the craniofacial form. Landmarks convey information relating only to their location, providing no information either about the interlandmark or surrounding anatomy. In particular, landmarks cannot represent curving anatomy and all are not equally valid and reproducible. Landmark-based techniques include CCA, Procrustes superimposition techniques, Euclidean distance matrix analysis (EDMA), thin-plate spline analysis (TPS), biorthogonal grids (BOG) and finite element morphometry/finite element scaling analysis (FEM/FESA).
  - Boundary outline techniques do not require cephalometric landmarks to represent the craniofacial form. As their generic term suggests, they only investigate the shape of the perimeter of a structure. Medial axis analysis (MAA), resistant—fit theta RHO analysis, Eigen shape analysis, and elliptical Fourier functions (EFF) are considered under the boundary outline technique umbrella.

DOWN'S ANALYSIS

- One of the most frequently used cephalometric analysis.
- He did study on 20 Caucasian individuals of 12–17-year age group belonging to both sexes.
- **Consists of 10 parameters:**
  - Five skeletal
  - Five dental

Skeletal Parameters

- Facial angle.
- Angle of convexity.
- A–B plane angle.
- MP angle.
- Y-axis.

Facial Angle

- The inferior posterior angle formed by the intersection of the FH and the FP (N–Pog) **(Fig. 31.5A).**
- Average value—87.8°.
- Range—82–95°.
- Indication of anterior-posterior positioning of mandible in relation to upper face. It is used to measure degree of protrusion or retrusion of lower jaw.
- Magnitude increase in case of Class III malocclusion with prominent chin.
- Decrease in case of Class II malocclusion.

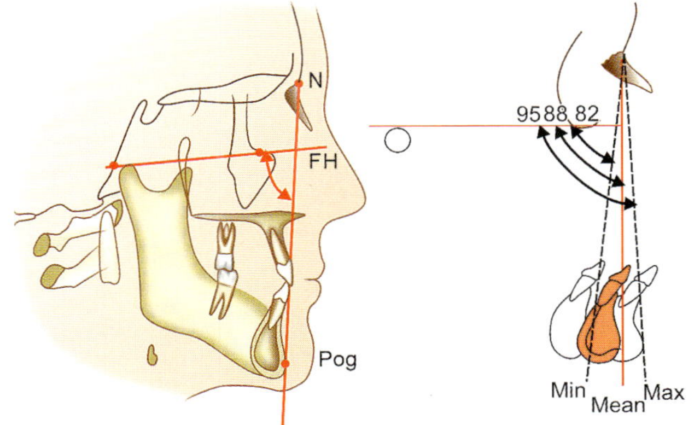

Fig. 31.5A: Facial angle.

Angle of Convexity (Fig. 31.5B)

- The angle is formed by the intersection of lines N–A and A–Pog.

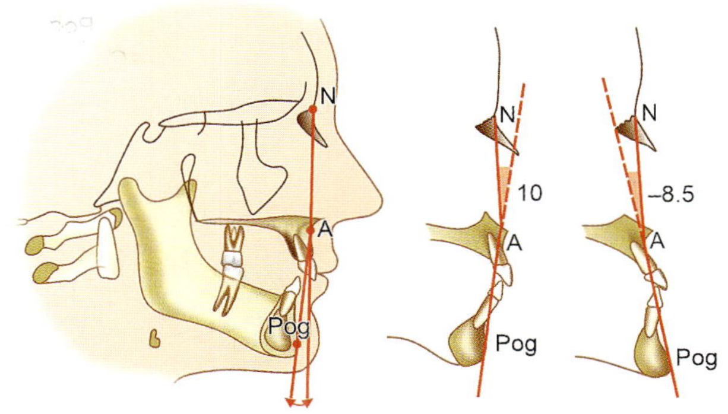

Fig. 31.5B: Angle of convexity.

- Reveals convexity or concavity of skeletal profile.
- Average value—0°
- Range—8.5-10°
- A positive value in convex profile suggesting prominent maxilla relative to mandible
- Negative value in concave profiles.

A–B Plane Angle (Fig. 31.5C)

- Line connecting points A and B and a line joining N–Pog
- Average value –4.6°.
- Range –9 to 0°.
- Indicative of maxillomandibular relationship in relation to facial plane.
- Usually negative as point B is behind point A.
- Positive angle found in Class III malocclusion.

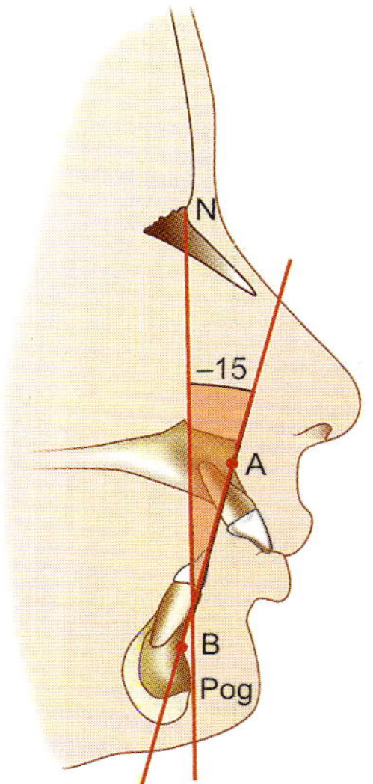

Fig. 31.5C: A–B plane angle.

Mandibular Plane Angle (Fig. 31.5D)

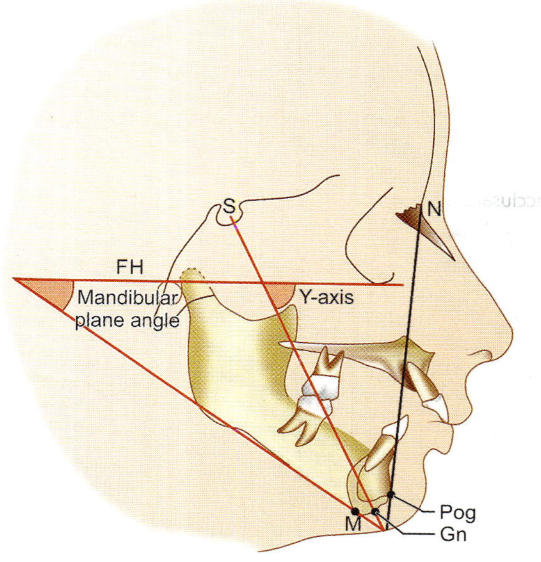

Fig. 31.5D: Mandibular plane angle.

- The anterior angle formed by the intersection of the FH plane and a tangent to the lower border of the mandible and symphysis.
- Average value—21.9°.
- Range—17-28°.
- Increased angle suggestive of vertical grower with hyperdivergent facial pattern.

Y-Axis (Growth Axis) (Fig. 31.5E)

- Angle formed by joining S-Gn line with FH plane.
- Average value—59°.
- Range—53-66°.
- Angle-larger—Class II facial pattern and vertical growth of mandible.
- Smaller angle—Class III pattern and horizontal growth of mandible.

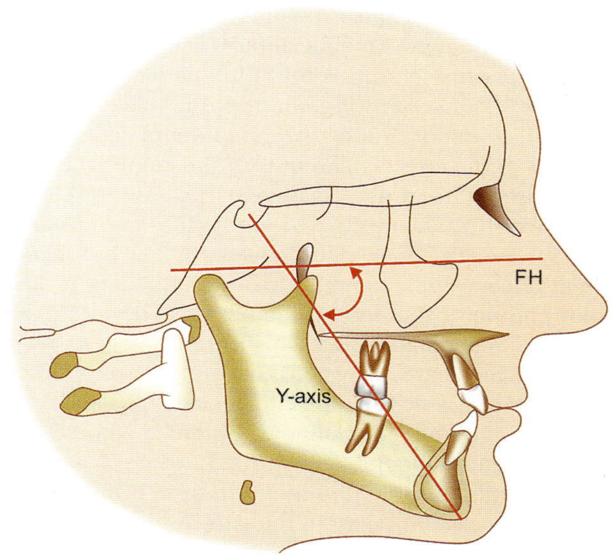

Fig. 31.5E: Y-axis (growth axis).

Dental Parameters

- Cant of OP
- Interincisal angle
- Incisor OP angle
- Incisor MP angle
- Upper incisor to A-Pog line.

Cant of Occlusal Plane (Fig. 31.6A)

- Angle between OP and FH plane
- Down's described OP as a line passing through the cusp tips of the maxillary and mandibular first permanent molars and midway between the incisal edges of the maxillary and mandibular central incisors (bisecting the overbite).
- Average value—9.3°.
- Range—1.5-14°.
- It gives us slope of OP relative to FH plane.

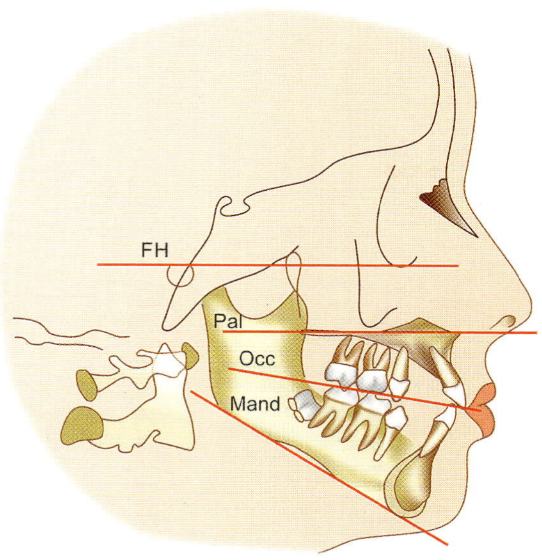

Fig. 31.6A: Cant of occlusal plane.

Interincisal Angle (Fig. 31.6B)

- A measurement of the degree of procumbency of the incisor teeth, introduced by WB Down's as the (posterior) angle formed by the intersection of the long axes of the maxillary and mandibular central incisors.
- Average—135.4°.
- Range—130-150.5°.
- Angle decrease in Class II division 1 and bimax cases.
- Increase in Class II division 2 cases.

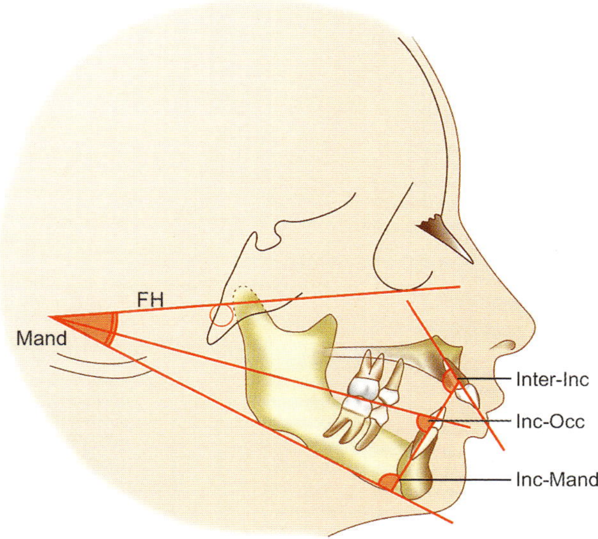

Fig. 31.6B: Interincisal angle, incisor occlusal plane angle, incisor mandibular plane angle.

Incisor Occlusal Plane Angle

- Inside inferior angle formed by intersection between the long axis of lower central incisor and OP.
- Read as + or - from right angle.
- Average—14.5°.
- Range—3.5-20°.
- Increase in angle shows lower incisor proclination.

Incisor Mandibular Plane Angle

- Angle formed by intersection of long axis of LI and MP.
- Average—1.4°.
- Range—8.5-7°.
- Increase in angle—LI proclination.

Upper Incisor to A–Pog Line (Fig. 31.6C)

- Linear measurement between incisal edge of maxillary central incisor and the line joining point A to Pog.
- Average—2.7 mm.
- Range—1-5 mm.
- More value—upper incisor proclination.

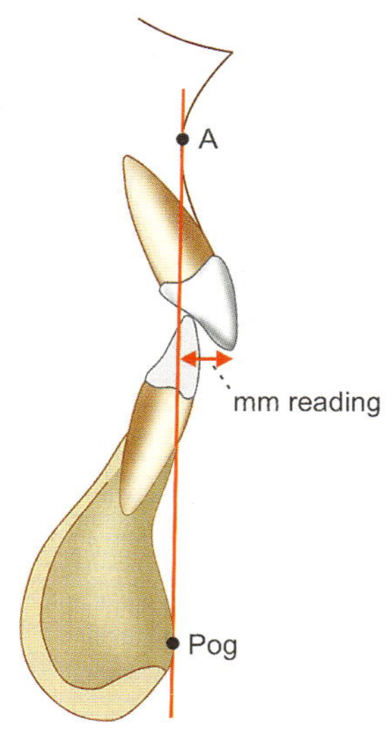

Fig. 31.6C: Upper incisor to A–Pog line.

Parameter	*Minimal (degrees)*	*Maximal (degrees)*	*Mean (degrees)*
			Skeletal pattern
Facial angle	82	95	87.0
Angle of convexity	–8.5	+10	0
A–B plane angle	–9	0	–4.6
Mandibular plane angle	17	28	21.9
Y-axis	53	66	59.4
			Dental pattern
Cant of occlusal plane	+1.5	+14	+9.3
I to I	130	150.5	135.4
I to occlusal plane	+3.5	+20	+14.5
I to mandibular plane	–8.5	+7	+1.4
I to A–P plane	–1 mm	+5 mm	+2.7 mm

STEINER'S ANALYSIS

Skeletal analysis	*Dental parameters*	*Soft tissue analysis*
• SNA angle	• Upper incisor to N–A (angle)	• S-line
• SNB angle	• Upper incisor to N–A (linear)	
• ANB angle	• Lower incisor to N–B (angle)	
• Mandibular plane angle	• Lower incisor to N–B (linear)	
• Occlusal plane angle	• Interincisal angle	

Skeletal Parameters

SNA Angle (Fig. 31.7A)

- A commonly used measurement for assessment of the anteroposterior position of the maxilla with regards to the cranial base.
- The inferior posterior angle formed by the intersection of lines SN and NA is measured.
- Mean—82°.
- Larger value—prognathic maxilla (Class II).

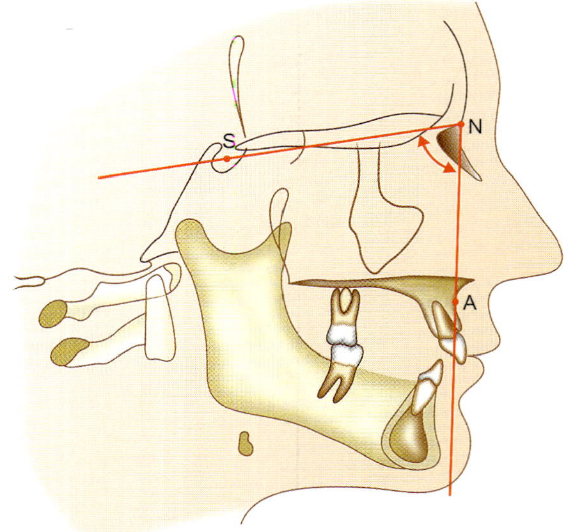

Fig. 31.7A: SNA angle.

SNB Angle (Fig. 31.7B)

- Evaluate the anteroposterior position of the mandible in relation to the cranial base.
- The inferior posterior angle formed by the intersection of lines NA and NB is measured.
- Mean—80°.
- Larger angle—prognathic mandible (Class III).

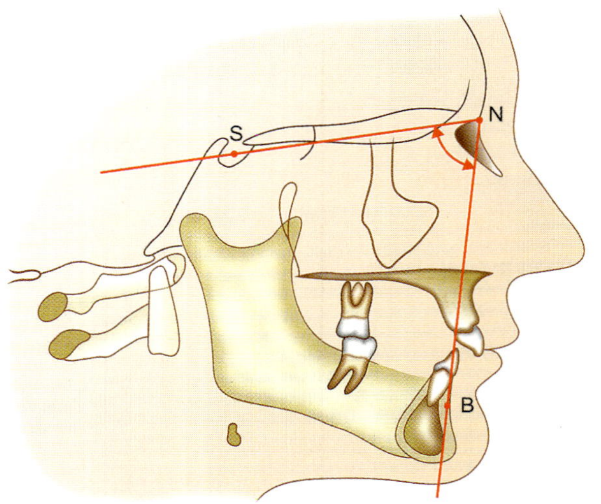

Fig. 31.7B: SNB angle.

ANB Angle (Fig. 31.7C)

- The difference between angles SNA and SNB aims at providing an evaluation of the anteroposterior relationship between the maxillary and mandibular apical bases.
- Formed by N-point A and N-point B.
- Mean—2°.
- Increase in angle—Class II skeletal tendency.

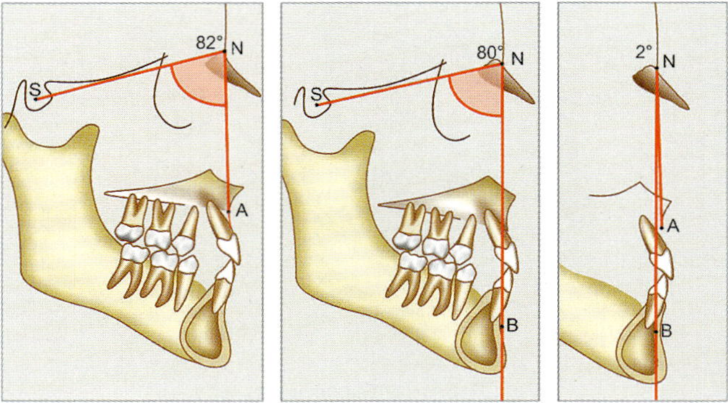

Fig. 31.7C: ANB angle.

Mandibular Plane Angle (Fig. 31.7D)

- A measurement introduced by CC Steiner's for assessment of the steepness of the MP in relation to the cranial base.
- The anterior angle formed by the intersection of SN and Go-Gn is measured.
- Mean—32°.
- Lower angle—horizontal GP.

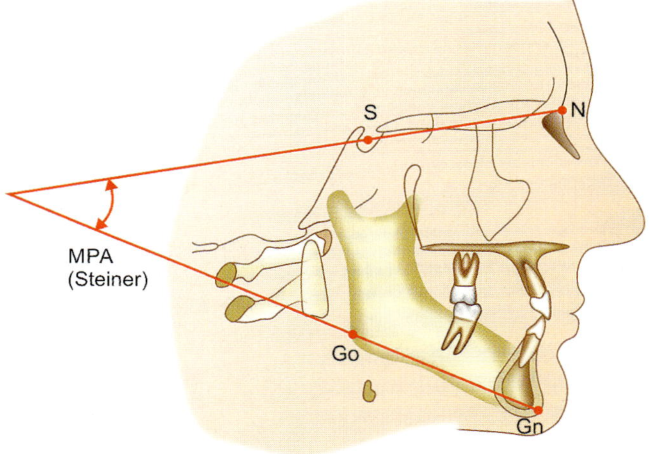

Fig. 31.7D: Mandibular plane angle.

Occlusal Plane Angle

- A line drawn through the occlusal surfaces of the maxillary and mandibular first permanent molars and first premolars.
- Formed between OP and SN plane.
- Mean—14.5°.
- Represent relation of the OP to cranial base and face.
- Indicate growth pattern.

Dental Parameters

Upper Incisor to N–A (Angle) (Fig. 31.8A)

- Formed by intersection of the long axis of upper central incisor and line joining N-point A.
- Average—22°.
- Indicate relative inclination of the upper incisors.
- Increased angle—proclination.

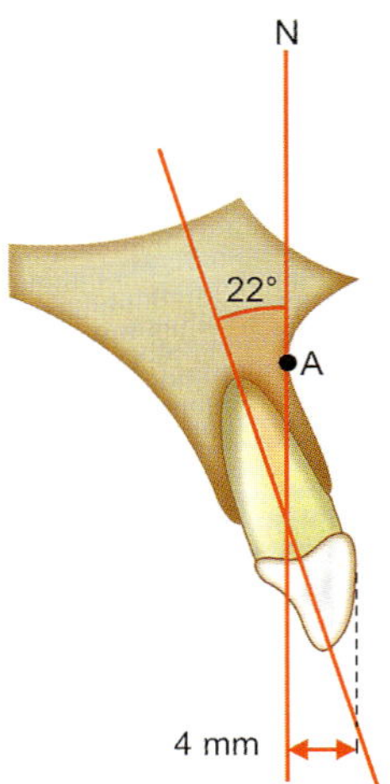

Fig. 31.8A: Upper incisor to N–A (angle and linear).

Upper Incisor to N–A (Linear)

- Linear measurement between the labial surface of upper central incisor and the line joining N-point A.
- Average—4 mm.
- Determine upper incisor position.
- Increase in case of proclination.

Lower Incisor to N–B (Angle)

- Formed by intersection of the long axis of lower central incisor and line joining N-point B.
- Average—25°.
- Indicate relative inclination of the lower incisors.
- Increased angle—proclination.

Lower Incisor to N–B (Linear) (Fig. 31.8B)

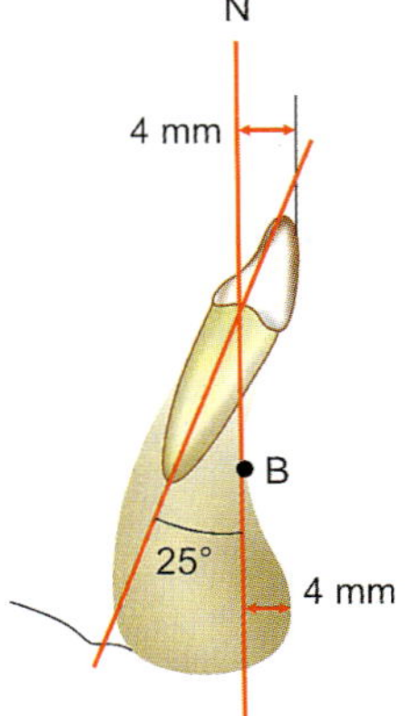

Fig. 31.8B: Lower incisor to N–B (angle and linear).

- Linear measurement between the labial surface of lower central incisor and the line joining N-point B.
- Average—4 mm.
- Determine lower incisor position.
- Increase in case of proclination.

Interincisal Angle (Fig. 31.8C)

- Interincisal angle relates the relative position of upper incisor to that of the lower incisor.
- Mean—130°.

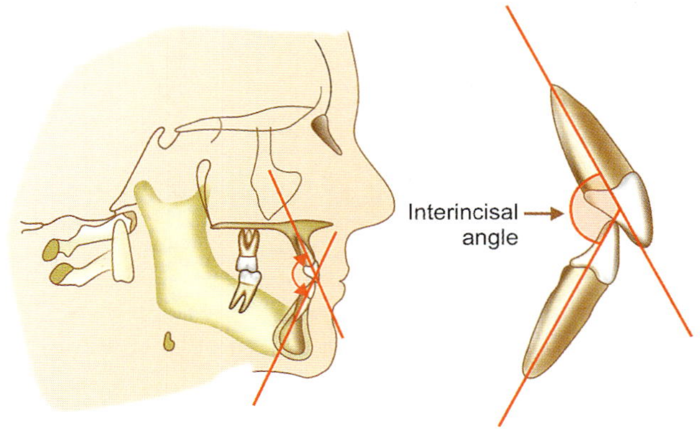

Fig. 31.8C: Interincisal angle.

Soft Tissue Analysis

S-line (Esthetic Plane of Steiner) (Fig. 31.9)

- Formed by a line extending from soft tissue contour of chin to the middle of "S" formed by lower border of nose.
- The lips should fall on this line and any deviation shows prominence or flatness of the lips.
- If lips beyond this line, then protrusive lips/convex profile.

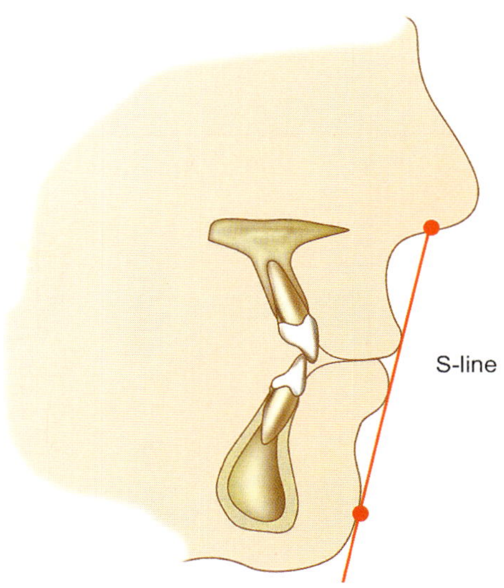

Fig. 31.9: S-line (esthetic plane of Steiner).

Parameter	Reference measurements
SNA (angle)	82°
SNB (angle)	80°
ANB (angle)	2°
I to N–A (mm)	4 mm
I to N–A (angle)	22°
I to N–B (mm)	4 mm
I to N–B (angle)	25°
Po to N–B (mm)	Not established
Po and I to N–B (difference)	–
I to I (angle)	131°
Occl to S–N (angle)	14°
GoGn to S–N (angle)	32°

TWEED'S ANALYSIS (FIG. 31.10A)

- A set of three angular measurements (which constitute what has come to be known as the Tweed's triangle), introduced by CH Tweed's in 1946.
- The three angles that were originally described are the FMA (Frankfort-MP angle—mean 25°) **(Fig. 31.10B)**, the IMPA (incisor-MP angle—mean 90°) **(Fig. 31.10C)**, and the FMIA (Frankfort-mandibular incisor angle—mean 65°) **(Fig. 31.10D)**.
- Wit's appraisal **(Figs. 31.11A and B)**
- Measure of extent to which maxilla and mandible are related to each other in anteroposterior or sagittal plane.
- Used in cases where ANB not reliable.
- In Class II—BO behind AO.
- In Class III—BO ahead of AO.

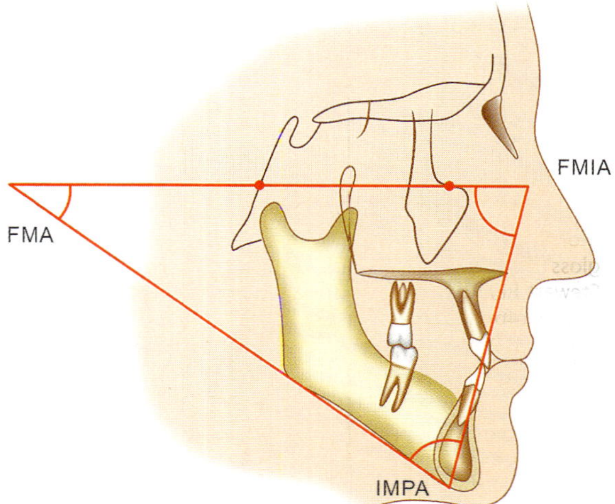

Fig. 31.10A: The Tweed's triangle.

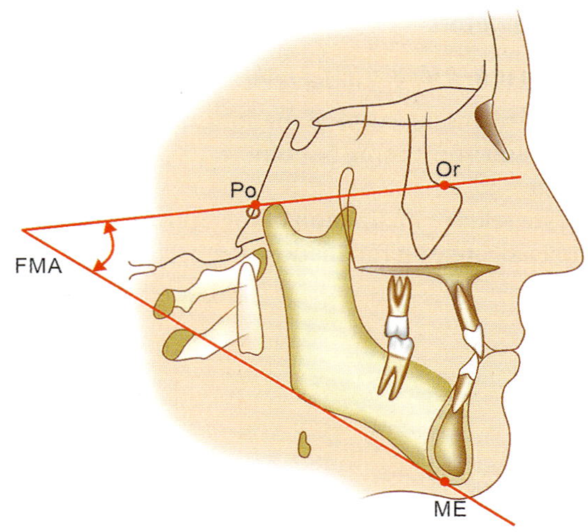

Fig. 31.10B: Frankfort-mandibular plane angle.

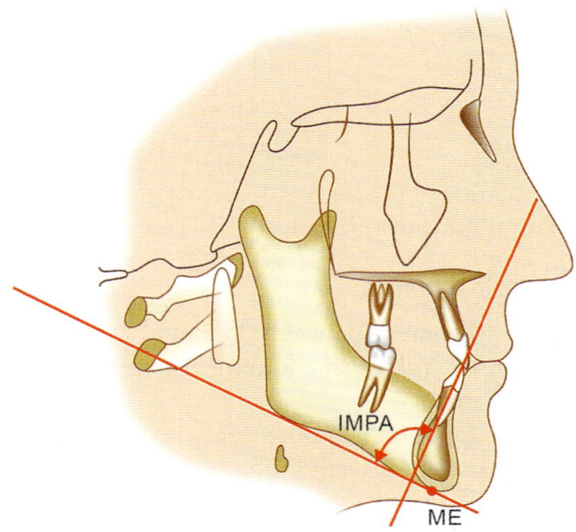

Fig. 31.10C: Incisor mandibular plane angle.

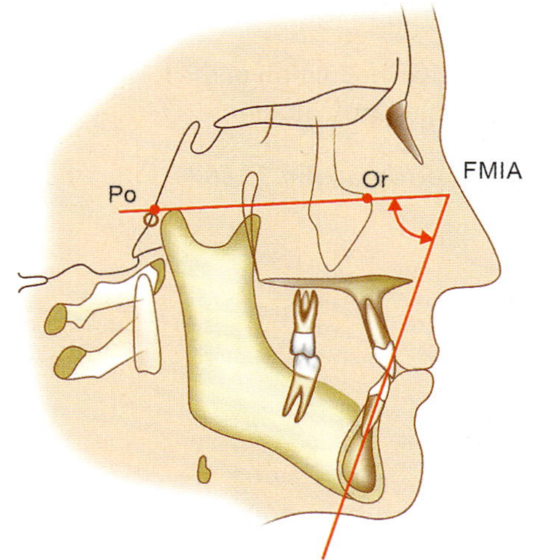

Fig. 31.10D: Frankfort-mandibular incisor angle.

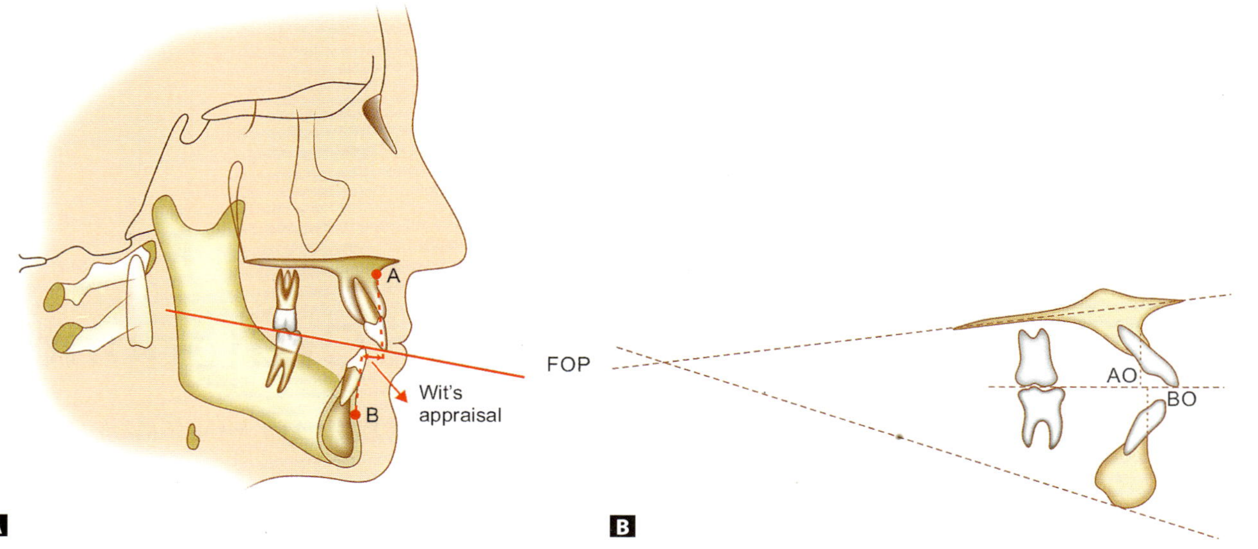

Figs. 31.11A and B: Wit's appraisal.

POINTS TO REMEMBER

- Pioneer of cephalometrics is B Holly Broadbent.
- TW Todd went on to develop first cephalometer at Western Reserve University.
- There are 18 main reference points on face and 12 reference planes.
- E-plane: Esthetic plane is denoted by a line between anterior point on nose and anterior point on chin.
- FH plane: From Po to orbitale (O).
- The two major techniques for cephalometric assessment are landmark-based techniques and boundary outline techniques.
- Down's analysis includes skeletal assessment by facial angle, angle of convexity, AB plane angle, mandibular plane angle, Y-axis and dental assessment by cant of OP, interincisal angle, incisor OP angle, incisor mandibular plane angle, upper incisor to A–Pog line.

Questionnaire

1. What are lateral reference points?
2. Explain lateral cephalometric assessment.
3. Write a note on soft tissue assessment.
4. SNA and SNB angle.
5. What is Down's analysis?
6. Explain Steiner's analysis.

FURTHER READING

1. Bhalajhi SI. Orthodontics: the art and science, 3rd edition. Arya (Medi) Publishing House; 2006.
2. Bookstein FL. On the cephalometrics of skeletal changes. 1982.
3. Broadbent BH. A new X-ray technique and its application to orthodontia. Angle Orthod. 1931;7:183.
4. Krull JT, Krull GE, Lapp TH, Bussard A. Cephalometrics and facial esthetocs: The key to complete treatment planning. In: McDonald RE, Avery DR (Eds). Dentistry for the child and adolescent, 9th edition. Mosby, St. Louis; 2011. pp. 525-49.
5. Lele S, Richtsmeier JT. Euclidean distance matrix analysis: a coordinate-free approach for comparing biological shapes using landmark data. Am J Phys Anthropol. 1991;86:415-27.
6. Lestrel PE. Method for analyzing complex two-dimensional forms: elliptical Fourier functions. Am J Hum Biol. 1989;1:149-64.
7. McIntyre GT, Mossey PA. Size and shape measurements in contemporary cephalometrics. Eur J Orthod. 2003;25:231-52.
8. Moyers RE, Bookstein FL. The inappropriateness of conventional cephalometrics. Am J Orthod. 1979;75:599-617.
9. Profitt WR. Contemporary orthodontics. St. Louis: CV Mosby; 1986.
10. Slice DE, Bookstein FL, Marcus LF, Rohlf FJ. A glossary for geometric morphometrics: Part 1. http://129.49.19.42/morph/ glossary/ gloss1html; 1998.
11. Stewart RE, Barber TK, Troutman KC, Wei SHY. Pediatric dentistry: scientific foundation and clinical practice. St. Louis: CV Mosby; 1982.
12. Straney DO. Median axis methods in morphometrics. In: Rohlf FJ, Bookstein FL (Eds). Proceedings of the michigan morphometrics workshop. Ann Arbor: University of Michigan Museum of Zoology; 1990. pp.180-200.

Preventive Orthodontics

Mridula Trehan, Deepesh Prajapati, Priya Nagar, Nikhil Marwah, Shantanu Jain

Chapter Outline

A number of procedures can be carried out by the pediatric dentist, so as to prevent or intercept a malocclusion that may develop or is developing. The terms preventive and interceptive orthodontics are sometimes used synonymously. Preventive orthodontic procedures are undertaken when the dentition and occlusion are perfectly normal, while interceptive procedures are carried out when the signs and symptoms of a malocclusion have appeared. Some of the procedures carried out in preventive orthodontics can also be carried out in interceptive orthodontics, but the timings are different. For example, extraction of supernumerary teeth before they cause displacement of other teeth is a preventive procedure, while their extraction after the signs of malocclusion have appeared is an interceptive procedure.

Preventive orthodontic procedures are aimed at elimination of factors that may lead to malocclusion, while interceptive orthodontics is undertaken at a time when the malocclusion has already developed or is developing.

Procedures undertaken in preventive orthodontics

- Parent education
- Caries control
- Care of deciduous dentition
- Extraction of supernumerary teeth
- Occlusal equilibration
- Maintenance of quadrant wise tooth shedding timetable
- Management of ankylosed tooth
- Management of abnormal frenal attachments
- Checkup for oral habits
- Prevention of damage to occlusion, for example, Milwaukee braces
- Management of deeply locked first permanent molar
- Space maintenance

- Preventive orthodontics according to **Graber** (1966) *can be defined as the action taken to preserve the integrity of what appears to be normal occlusion at a specific time.*
- **Proffit** and **Ackerman** (1980) *defined preventive orthodontics as the prevention of potential interference with occlusal development.*

PARENT EDUCATION

Knowledge of preventive dentistry for the parents especially mothers should ideally begin during the prenatal period as this is the time they are most encouraged about the well being of the unborn child and should continue even after the birth for the entire lifetime of an individual.

Prenatal Education

- The expecting mother should be educated on matters such as nutrition to provide an ideal environment for the developing fetus.
- The importance of oral hygiene maintenance by the mother is important as recent studies have indicated a possible co-relationship between the mothers' poor oral hygiene and premature births.

- ❖ The mother should be advised to have natural foods containing calcium and phosphorus, e.g., milk, milk products, egg, etc. especially during the third trimester as they would allow proper formation of deciduous teeth crowns.

Postnatal Education

This is more age specific and can be divided into four types:

1. **Birth to 1 year of age:**
   - This is the most important period of counseling.
   - Stress on breastfeeding.
   - Bottle feeding with high sugar exposures should be avoided.
   - In case the child is being bottle fed, the mother is advised on the use of physiologic nipple and not the conventional nipple. The physiologic nipple is designed to permit suckling of the milk which more or less resembles the normal functional activity as in breastfeeding.
   - Gum pads and newly erupted teeth should be cleaned with a clean, soft cotton cloth dipped in warm saline.
   - Gradual progression should be made from cloth cleaning to finger brush **(Fig. 32.1)** without the use of dentifrices.
   - Make parents aware about right use of pacifiers.

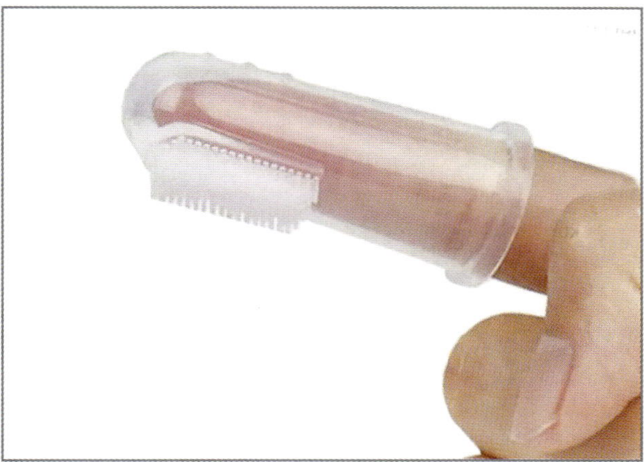

Fig. 32.1: Finger brush.

2. **One to three years of age:**
   - Importance of weaning.
   - Bottle feeding should be withdrawn completely by 18–24 months of age.
   - Brushing should be initiated twice in a day.
   - Parents should be taught the correct method brushing the teeth as at this age, they have to brush their children's teeth. Along with correct method of brushing, flossing should also be taught.
3. **Three to six years of age:**
   - The parents should be informed about the effects of oral habits on the development of occlusion **(Fig. 32.2)**
   - The parents should encourage the child to begin brushing on his own at least once a day.
4. **Six years onwards of age:**
   - The parents should be informed about the initiation of exfoliation of deciduous teeth and the eruptive pattern of permanent teeth **(Fig. 32.3)**.

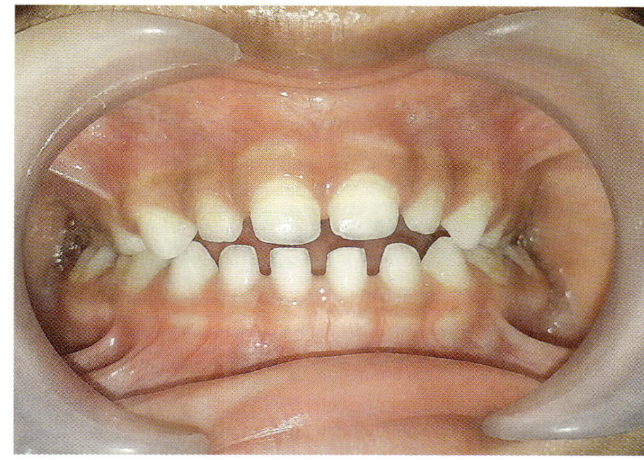

Fig. 32.2: Developing open bite.

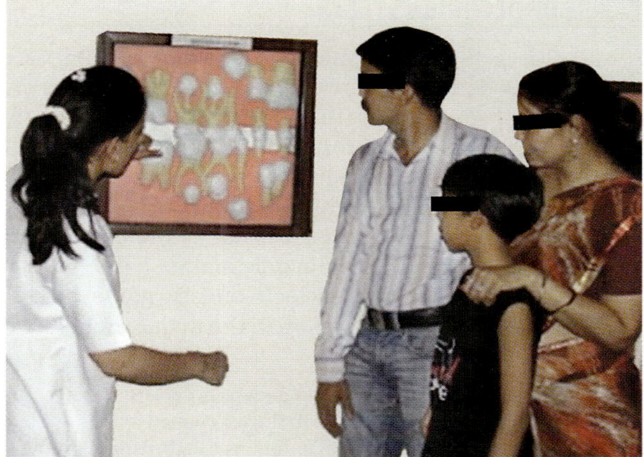

Fig. 32.3: Parents being informed about eruptive pattern.

   - Parents should be educated about the need for constant review and recall on a regular basis.
   - In case of extraction of deciduous teeth due to decay, etc. the need, advantages and importance of space maintainers should be explained to the parents.
   - Till the child cannot tie his own show laces, parents are advised to at least supervise the child's brushing and flossing.

CARIES CONTROL

- ❖ Caries involving the proximal surface of deciduous teeth if not restored at the earliest may lead to loss of arch length by movement of adjacent teeth into that space **(Fig. 32.4)**.
- ❖ The most effective tool in detecting proximal caries is the bitewing radiograph.
- ❖ Once detected, the affected teeth should be restored immediately to their proper mesiodistal dimension so as to prevent loss of arch length. Importance of flossing and avoiding soft diet should be reinforced.
- ❖ Caries initiation can also be prevented by diet counselling, topical fluoride application, and pit and fissure sealants.

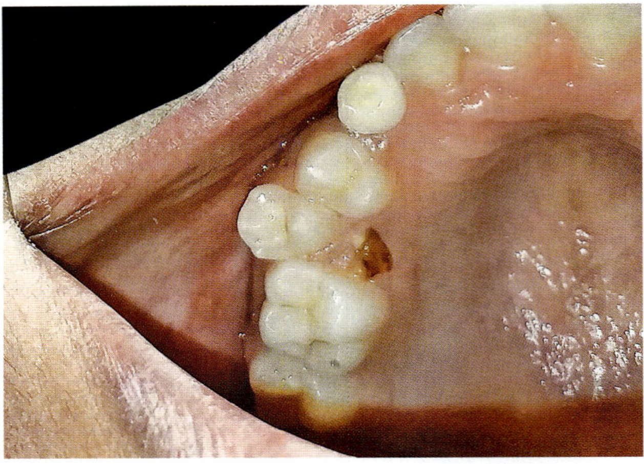

Fig. 32.4: No treatment of a grossly decayed primary molar led to space loss and hence ectopic eruption of the premolar.

CARE OF DECIDUOUS TEETH

- All efforts should be made to prevent early loss of deciduous dentition by way of prevention of caries and timely restoration of carious teeth. Simple preventive procedures such as proper diet counselling, timely application of topical fluoride or pit and fissure sealant application help in preventing caries.
- Deciduous teeth by themselves act as the best natural space maintainers, which not only maintain the space for their succeeding permanent teeth but also guide the latter teeth into their proper position in the dental arches.

Consequences of premature loss of deciduous teeth
- Migration of adjacent teeth into the space created
- Non eruption or altered path of eruption of succedaneous tooth
- Tongue thrusting may develop
- Hampered phonation in the case of anterior tooth loss
- Unesthetic appearance when there is an anterior tooth loss which leads to psychological effect on the child

EXTRACTION OF SUPERNUMERARY TEETH

- Supernumerary teeth are an additional entity to the normal series and are seen in any region of the dental arch **(Figs. 32.5A and B).**
- Their reported prevalence ranges between 0.3% and 0.8% in the primary dentition and 0.1–3.8% in the permanent dentition with more predilections for males and the anterior region.
- Some of the orthodontic complications caused by supernumerary teeth include delay of eruption, ectopic eruption, crowding, incomplete space closure during orthodontic treatment, root resorption of adjacent teeth, pathology like cyst formations, can cause complications in alveolar bone grafting and may also cause issues during implants.
- Thus supernumerary teeth should be identified and extracted before they cause any of these complications.

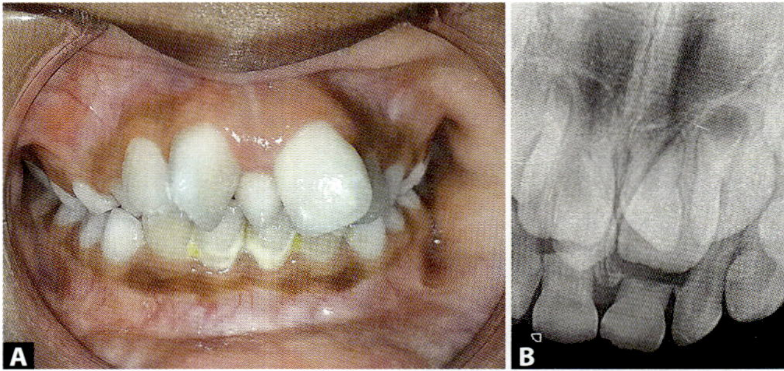

Figs. 32.5A and B: (A) Clinical presentation of supernumerary teeth; (B) Radiographic presentation of supernumerary teeth.

CLASSIFICATION OF SUPERNUMERARY TEETH

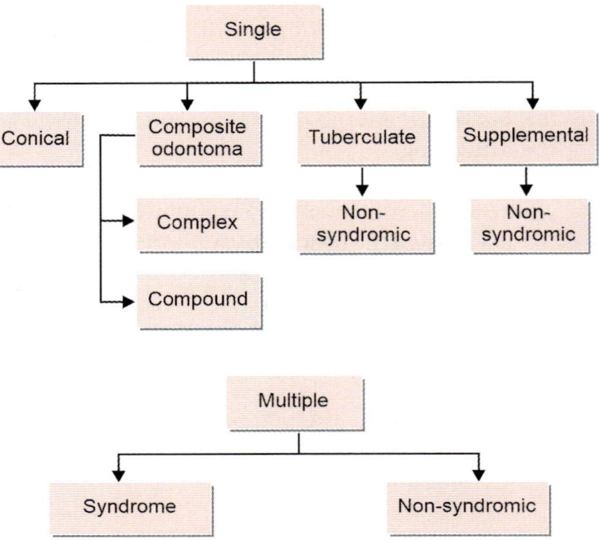

- Supernumerary teeth are classified according to the location and morphology in four types:
  1. *Conical:* It's a small peg shaped conical tooth, found high and inverted into the palate or placed horizontally, mostly in permanent dentition as a mesiodens. Formed during root formation usually earlier or at the same juncture as the permanent incisors **(Fig. 32.6).**

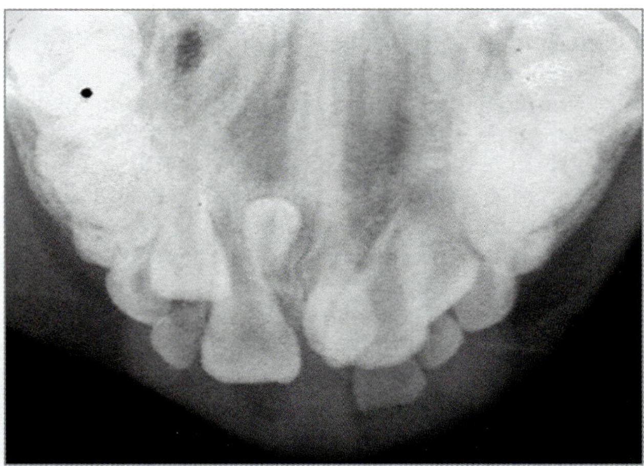

Fig. 32.6: Conical supernumerary tooth. (*Source:* Garvey MT, Barry HJ, Blake M. Supernumerary teeth--an overview of classification, diagnosis and management. J Can Dent Assoc. 1999;65(11): 612-6).

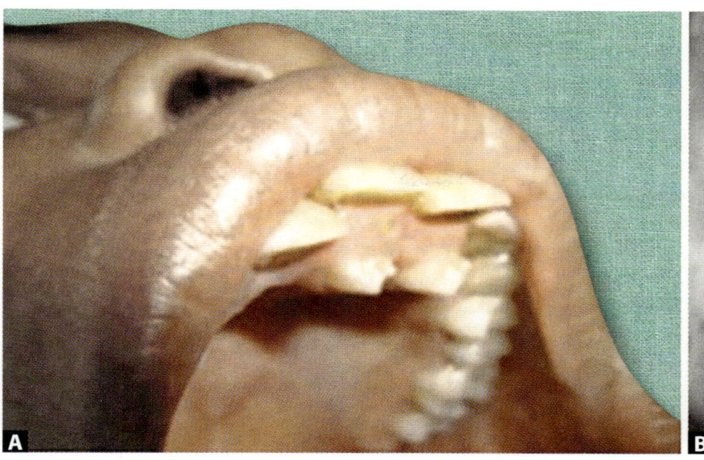

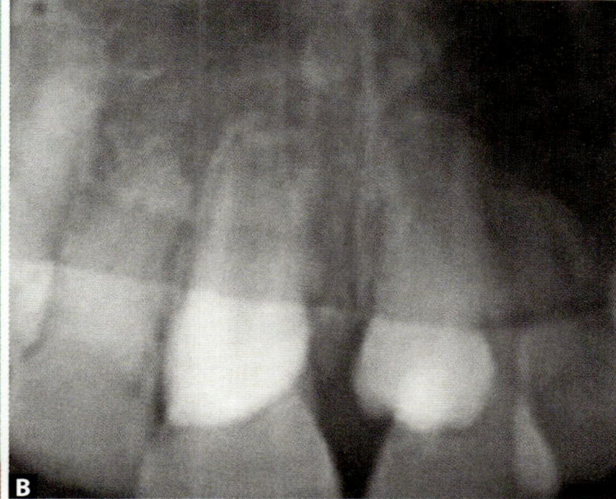

Figs. 32.7A and B: Tuberculate supernumerary tooth. (*Source:* Eigbobo JO, Osagbemiro BB. Bilateral tuberculate supernumerary teeth. Clinics and Practice. 2011; 1(2):e30).

2. *Tuberculate:* This type of supernumerary teeth has more than one cusp or tubercle, its usually cylindrical in shape and may be folded inwards. They are located generally on the palatal face of the central incisor and usually occur in pairs. Eruption of Tuberculate Supernumerary is uncommon, as its root formation is also delayed **(Figs. 32.7A and B)**.
3. *Supplemental:* When in the normal series of teeth, there is a replication of teeth occurs, its called a Supplemental type of supernumerary teeth. In the primary dentition, there is high prevalence of non-impacted supplemental type of supernumerary teeth. It has been observed that maxillary permanent lateral incisor is most prevalent supplemental supernumerary, though molars and premolars are also replicated **(Fig. 32.8)**.
4. *Composite odontoma:* Not a commonly acknowledged classification, but still can be considered a type of supernumerary tooth. The lesion is composed of more than one type of tissue, as it is not a neoplasm, but hamartomatous abnormality.

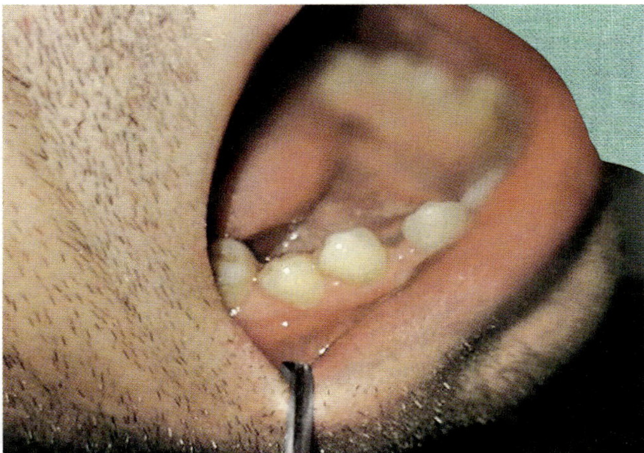

Fig. 32.8: Supplemental tooth. (*Source:* Suljkanovic N, Balic D, Begic N. Supernumerary and supplementary teeth in a non-syndromic patients. Med Arch. 2021;75(1):78-81).

OCCLUSAL EQUILIBRATION

- Occlusal equilibration may be carried out not only in the preventive phase but also in the interceptive phase as well as during the corrective orthodontic treatment.
- It is the systematic reshaping of the occlusal anatomy of teeth to minimize or eliminate the role of occlusal interferences in reflexly determined mandibular positions.
- Occlusal equilibration is done more during active growth.

Occlusal prematurities if present, can lead to deviation in the mandibular path of closure

↓

These functional shifts may lead to anterior crossbite or pseudo Class III malocclusion

↓

Using an articulating paper, it is essential to check for interferences in the retruded position, intercuspal position, protrusive and lateral occlusal contacts

↓

The premature contacts are then eliminated by selective grinding

↓

Entire grounded tooth surface should be coated with topical fluoride

MAINTENANCE OF QUADRANT-WISE TOOTH SHEDDING TIMETABLE

- There should not be >3 months difference between the shedding of deciduous teeth and eruption of permanent teeth in one quadrant as compared to other quadrants.
- Delay in eruption may be due to any one of the following reasons:
  - Presence of over retained deciduous teeth/roots.
  - Presence of supernumerary tooth.
  - Cysts and tumors of the jaw.

- Overhanging restoration in deciduous teeth.
- Fibrosis of gingiva.
- Ankylosis of deciduous teeth.
- Absence of permanent tooth bud.

- As a rule of thumb, the shedding of the deciduous dentition should be kept on schedule by extracting the tooth or teeth on one side of the arch, when they have been lost through natural process on the other side.
- Space maintainers should be given until the eruption of succedaneous teeth.

MANAGEMENT OF ANKYLOSED TEETH

- Ankylosis is a condition characterized by absence of the periodontal membrane in a small area or the whole of the root surface.
- Ankylosed deciduous teeth do not get resorbed and therefore either prevent the permanent teeth from erupting or deflect them to erupt in abnormal locations **(Fig. 32.9)**.
- These ankylosed teeth should be diagnosed and surgically removed at an appropriate time to permit the permanent teeth to erupt.

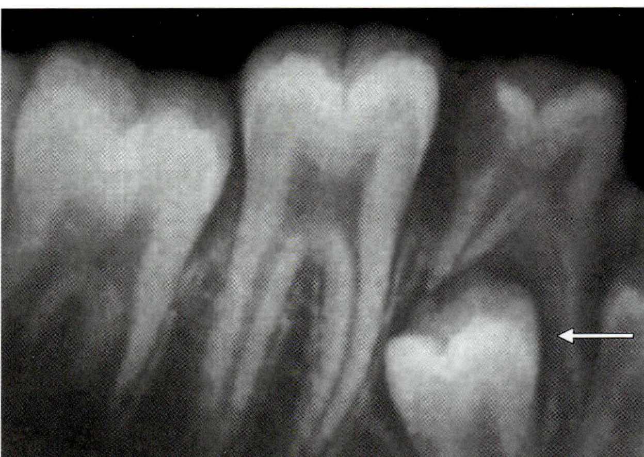

Fig. 32.9: Ankylosed primary second molar preventing eruption of premolar.

MANAGEMENT OF ABNORMAL FRENAL ATTACHMENT

- The presence of a thick and fleshy maxillary labial frenum that is attached relatively low prevents the maxillary central incisors from approximating each other **(Figs. 32.10A and B)**. This causes the development of diastema or excess spacing between the teeth, which in turn may not allow the eruption of succedaneous teeth.
- The procedure for frenectomy is usually done along with orthodontic treatment and not before it. The space should be closed at least partially, so that orthodontic movement to bring the teeth together should be resumed immediately after the frenectomy, so that the teeth are brought together quickly after the procedure. When this is done, healing occurs with the teeth together and the inevitable postsurgical scar tissue stabilizes the teeth instead of creating obstacles to final closure of the space.

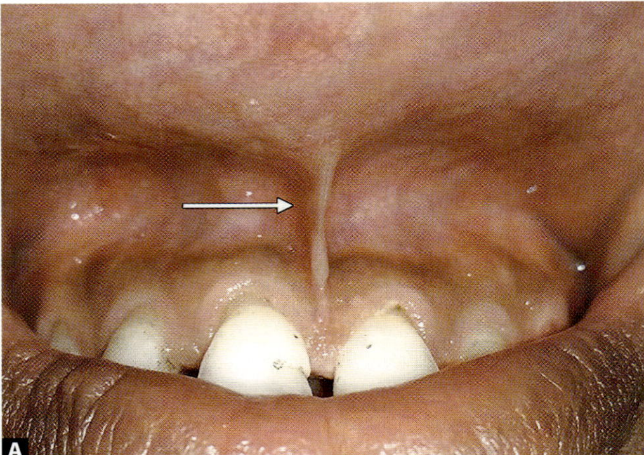

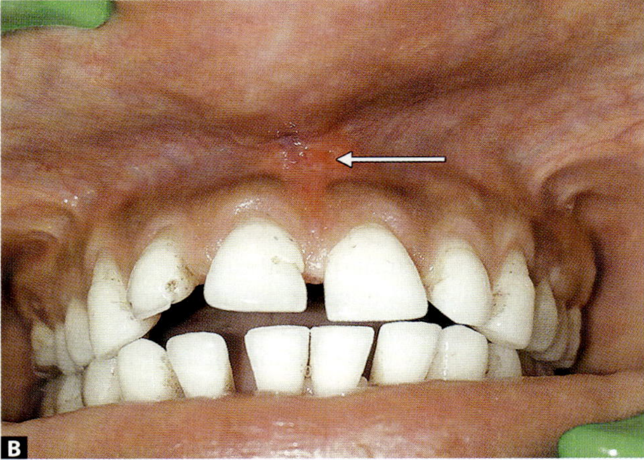

Figs. 32.10A and B: Lased high frenal attachment: (A) Preoperative; (B) Postoperative.

- Presence of ankyloglossia or tongue tie prevents functional development due to lowered position of tongue and abnormalities in speech and swallowing and hence should be surgically corrected **(Fig. 32.11)**.
- Decision whether to treat any of tethered oral tissue (TOTs) like lingual or labial frenum should based on functional issues it is causing not just the anatomy of the frenum.

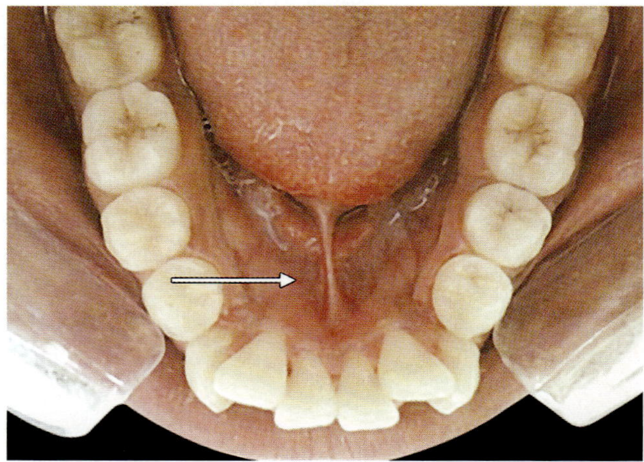

Fig. 32.11: Tongue tie.

Key to successful frenectomy

The key to successful surgery is removal of the interdental fibrous tissue. It is unnecessary, and in fact undesirable, to excise a large portion of the frenum itself. Instead, the fibrous connection to the bone is removed, and the frenum is then sutured at a higher level.

ORAL HABITS CHECK-UP AND EDUCATION

- Habits such as finger and thumb sucking, nail biting, tongue thrusting and lip biting should be identified, and the patient/parents should be educated on the ill effects of these habits and should be motivated to stop the habit by age 36 months or younger.
- If the resting tongue posture is forward of the normal position, incisor displacement is likely, but if resting tongue posture is normal, a tongue thrust swallow has no clinical significance.
- Obstructive sleep apnea syndrome (OSAS) may be associated with narrow maxilla, crossbite, low tongue position, vertical growth, and open bite. History associated with OSAS may include snoring, observed apnea, restless sleep, daytime neurobehavioral abnormalities or sleepiness, and bedwetting. Physical findings may include growth abnormalities, signs of nasal obstruction, adenoidal facies, and/or enlarged tonsils.
- Patients and their parents should be provided with information regarding consequences of a habit. Parents may play a negative role in the correction of an oral habit as nagging or punishment may result in an increase in habit behaviors; change in the home environment may be necessary before a habit can be overcome.
- Use of an appliance to manage oral habits is indicated only when the child wants to stop the habit and would benefit from a reminder.

PREVENTING MILWAUKEE BRACE DAMAGE

- Milwaukee brace is an orthopedic appliance used for the correction of scoliosis.
- This appliance exerts tremendous force on the mandible and the developing occlusion leading to retardation of mandibular growth and possible deformities.
- Specially designed intraoral splints, activators, positioners, and dentofacial orthopedic appliances may prevent malocclusion or at least reduce the deleterious effects.

MANAGEMENT OF DEEPLY LOCKED PERMANENT FIRST MOLARS

- Occasionally, the first permanent molar may get deeply locked under the crest of contour of the distal surface of deciduous second molar.
- Slicing the distal surface of the second deciduous molars helps in guiding the eruption of first permanent molars.
- Sometimes, locked permanent first molars may resorb the second deciduous molar at the cervical part of the tooth. If root resorption is severe, deciduous second molar has to be extracted and space maintained for the second premolars.
- Slightly locked permanent first molar usually erupts without treatment. Passing a ligature wire or separators interdentally frees the slight lock.

SPACE MAINTAINERS

- Premature loss of deciduous teeth can cause drifting of the adjacent teeth into the space. It can result in abnormal axial inclination of teeth, spacing between teeth and shift in the dental midline. This prevents the normal eruption path of permanent teeth leading to malocclusion.
- So corrective procedure may require some type of passive space maintainers, active tooth guidance, or a combination of both, depending on the present problem.
- Space maintainer is a device used to maintain the space created by the loss of a deciduous tooth (Detailed in Chapter 35).
- An important part of preventive orthodontics is the correct handling of spaces created by the untimely loss of deciduous teeth.

Prerequisites for space maintainers

- They should maintain the mesiodistal dimension of the space created by the lost tooth
- They should be functional, if possible, at least to the extent of preventing the overeruption of the opposing tooth
- They should be simple in construction
- They should be strong enough to withstand occlusal forces
- They must not endanger the remaining teeth by imposing excessive stresses on them
- They should not interfere with normal vertical eruption of the adjacent teeth
- They should be easily adjustable
- Their construction should be such that they do not restrict normal growth and developmental processes
- They should not interfere with functions such as mastication, speech or deglutition
- They must be easily cleansable and not serve as traps for food debris, etc. which might enhance dental caries and soft tissue pathology
- Durable and corrosion resistant
- Reasonable in cost.

Factors affecting planning for space maintenance

- Time elapsed since tooth loss
- Dental age of the patient
- Thickness of bone covering the unerupted teeth
- Sequence of eruption of teeth
- Delayed eruption of permanent teeth
- Congenital absence of permanent tooth.

Consequences of space loss

Premature loss of primary anterior tooth	***Premature loss of primary posterior tooth***
• Causes » Due to increases susceptibility to dental trauma » Early childhood caries • Premature loss of primary incisor may not have a major impact on space loss. Movement of the permanent incisor erupting may show some movement in the resulting space. *In such a situation, space maintainer is not recommended unless for esthetic purposes.* • Premature loss of unilateral primary canine may show a significant effect on midline shift, so a balancing extraction may be considered as a preventive action. *Patients with spaced dentition, may not show any movement but a regular and a careful monitoring is recommended.* • Premature loss of bilateral mandibular primary canines show that the mandibular incisors may have some lingual movement causing anterior arch length to decrease. *In such cases maintenance of the arch should be done with a lingual arch holding appliance.*	• Cause » Dental caries • Loss of primary first molar prematurely may result in 1.5 mm of space loss in mandible and about 1 mm in maxilla, which is not of much concern. *So in such cases space maintainer may not be routinely recommended.* • Premature loss of unilateral primary first molar may have an effect on the midline shift. *So careful monitoring is required and concurrent balancing extractions may be recommended.* • Premature loss of primary second molar is of critical importance as it is an important factor in maintenance of leeway space: which signifies difference in total M-D width of primary canines and molars and permanent premolars and canines. M-D width of C+D+E should be more than 3+4+5 *Primary second molar and second premolar have shown the major difference in their M-D widths and are a point of concern. This discrepancy is referred to as 'E-space'. This space available helps in easy mesial movement of first permanent molar which is of greater significance in maxilla than mandible.* *In case of a missing primary second molar, the actively erupting permanent molar may migrate mesially causing space loss, crowding and loss of arch length. This is of prime importance in Class II malocclusions.*

POINTS TO REMEMBER

- Preventive orthodontics can be defined as the action taken to preserve the integrity of what appears to be normal occlusion at a specific time.
- Procedures undertaken in preventive orthodontics are parent education, caries control, care of deciduous dentition, extraction of supernumerary teeth, occlusal equilibration, maintenance of quadrant wise tooth shedding timetable, management of ankylosed tooth, management of abnormal frenal attachments, checkup for oral habits, prevention of damage to occlusion, management of deeply locked first permanent molar and space maintenance.
- Space maintainer is a device used to maintain the space created by the loss of a deciduous tooth.
- Factors affecting planning for space maintenance are time elapsed since tooth loss, dental age of the patient, thickness of bone covering the unerupted teeth, sequence of eruption of teeth, delayed eruption of permanent teeth, congenital absence of permanent tooth.

Questionnaire

1. Define preventive orthodontics and enumerate the procedures involved.
2. Explain postnatal dental education for parents.
3. Explain the consequences of premature loss of deciduous teeth.
4. What are the treatment options for anterior tooth crossbite?
5. Describe the procedure of frenectomy.
6. Enumerate the factors affecting planning for space maintainers.

FURTHER READING

1. Garvey MT, Barry HJ, Blake M. Supernumerary teeth--an overview of classification, diagnosis and management. J Can Dent Assoc. 1999 Dec;65(11):612-6.
2. Gianelly AA. Leeway space and the resolution of crowding in the mixed dentition. Semin Orthod 1995; 1:188-194.
3. Gowri Shankar S. Textbook of Orthodontics, 1st edition. 2011.
4. Graber TM. Orthodontics: Principles and Practice, 3rd edition. Philadelphia, PA; 1972.
5. Guideline on Management of the Developing Dentition and Occlusion in Pediatric Dentistry. American Academy of Pediatric Dentistry. Reference Manual v 32 / no 6.
6. Kharbanda OP. Diagnosis and Management of Malocclusion, 2nd edition; 2013.
7. Peter S. Essentials of Preventive and Community Dentistry, 3rd edition; 2006.
8. Proffit WR. Contemporary Orthodontics, 4th edition. Elsevier Publications.
9. Ramirez-Yañez G. Treatment of anterior crossbite in the primary dentition with esthetic crowns: report of 3 cases. Pediatr Dent. 2011;33:339-42.
10. Tondon S. Textbook of Pedodontics, 2nd edition. Paras Medical Publisher; 2009.

CHAPTER

Myofunctional Therapy

Anshula Deshpande, Sonali Saha, Nikhil Marwah, Siddharth Mehta

CHAPTER OUTLINE

An early article in American orthodontic literature, "The 'three Ms': Muscles, Malformation, and Malocclusion," by **Graber** (1963) described the effects of function and malfunction. Functional appliances are considered to be primarily orthopedic tools to influence the facial skeleton of the growing child in the condylar and sutural areas. However, these appliances also exert orthodontic effects at the dentoalveolar area. The influences of natural forces and functional stimulation on form were first reported by **Roux** in 1883 as results of studies he performed on tail fins of dolphins. **Häupl** (1938) saw the potential of the Roux hypothesis and applied his concepts to correction of jaw and dental arch deformities using functional stimuli. Häupl explained the way functional appliance worked through the activity of orofacial muscle; function is inherent in all cells, tissue and organs and influences these media as a functional stimulus. A functional appliance changes the posture of the mandible or maxilla in order to generate all or a portion of its effect. These appliances, also referred to as dentofacial orthopedic appliances, use the patient's muscle movement to produce orthodontic or orthopedic forces. Loose-fitting or passive appliances, which utilize the orofacial musculature's inherent forces; and transmit them through the appliance to the teeth and alveolar bone. **A myofunctional appliance** *is defined as an appliance that harnesses the natural forces of the orofacial musculature and transmits it to the teeth and alveolar bone in a predetermined direction.*

- ***Moyer's:*** *Functional appliances are loose removable appliances designed to alter the neuromuscular environment of the orofacial region to improve occlusal development and/or craniofacial skeletal growth.*
- ***Proffit:*** *Functional appliances are appliances which alter the posture of the mandible, holding it open or open and forward or backwards.*
- ***Glossary of orthodontic terms – (2012):*** *Functional appliance is a term used to describe a class of appliances which utilize the muscle action of the patient to produce orthodontic or orthopedic forces.*

HISTORY

1879: Norman Kingsley	Forward positioning of mandible in orthodontics–Bite plane/Bite-jumping appliance (vulcanite). Drawback-tendency to relapse even with bite guide
1883: Wilhelm Roux	The influences of natural forces and functional stimulation on form-foundation of both general and dental orthopedic principles (Wolff's Law).
1906: Alfred P Rogers	Father of Myofunctional Therapy; The first to implicate the facial muscles for the growth, development, and form of the stomatognathic system.

Contd...

Contd...

1905/09: Prof Emil Herbst	Founder of Herbst appliance
1909: Viggo Andresen	Modified bite jumping appliance—inspired from Benno Lisher's theory.
1936: Karl Häupl	Saw the potential of Roux's hypothesis and explained how functional appliances work through the activity of the orofacial muscles.
1950: Prof. Dr Wilhelm Balters	Modified activator by reducing bulk from palate and substituted with a coffin spring → Bionator
1956: Dr Martin Schwarz	Double Plates → combined the advantages of the activator and the active plate by constructing mandibular and maxillary acrylic plates that occluded with the mandible in a protrusive position.
1957: Rolf Fränkel	Function regulator
1977: Dr William J Clarks	Twin block
1989: Blechman et al.	Magnetic appliances

CLASSIFICATION OF MYOFUNCTIONAL APPLIANCES

Proffit Classification

- **Tooth-borne passive appliances:** They have no intrinsic force generating components such as springs or screws and depend on the soft tissue stretch and muscular activity to produce the derived treatment results, for example, Activator, Bionator, Herbst appliance.
- **Tooth-borne active appliances:** These include modifications of activator and bionator that include springs and screws to provide force for transverse or anteroposterior changes.
- **Tissue-borne passive appliances:** These are mostly located in the vestibule and have little or no contact with the dentition, for example, oral screen.
- **Tissue-borne active appliances:** These are mostly located in the vestibule and have significant contact with the dentition, e.g. functional regulator of Frankel, functional orthopedic magnetic appliances (FOMA).

Tom Graber Classification

- **Group A:** Teeth supported.
- **Group B:** Teeth/Tissue supported.
- **Group C:** Vestibular positioned appliances.

Erdogan E Classification

- Classification of functional appliance according to the force they apply:
  - Pure functional appliance
    - Activators.
    - Regulators.
  - Mechano-functional appliance
    - Fixed.
    - Removable.
- Classification of functional appliances according to their effect mechanism:
  - Activators can be subdivided into:
    - Pure functional
    - Mechano-functional, and these are divided into subdivisions.
  - Regulators are subdivided into:
    - Oral screens
    - Lip bumpers
    - Frankel appliance (Type 4)

Other Classifications

- **Myotonic appliances:** They are functional appliances that depend on the muscle mass for their action.
- **Myodynamic appliances:** They are functional appliances that depend on the muscle activity for their function.
- **Removable functional appliances:** These can be removed and inserted by the patient.
- **Fixed functional appliances:** These are fitted to the teeth by the operator and cannot be removed by the patient at will.
- **Group I appliances:** They transmit muscle forces directly to the teeth for the correction of malocclusion, e.g. oral screen, inclined planes.
- **Group II appliances:** These appliances reposition the mandible and the resultant force is transmitted to the teeth and other structures, e.g. activator, bionator.
- **Group III appliances:** These also reposition the mandible but their area of operation is the vestibule outside the dental arch, e.g. Frankel appliance, vestibular screen.

Action of myofunctional appliances

Orthopedic changes

- Accelerate the growth in the condylar region
- Bring about remodeling of glenoid fossa
- Designed to have restrictive influence on growth
- Change the direction of growth of jaws

Dentoalveolar changes

It can bring about changes in sagittal, transverse and vertical directions

Muscular changes

Improve the tonicity of orofacial muscles

DIAGNOSIS AND CASE SELECTION

Diagnosis and case selection is important in appliance selection. Following diagnostic aids should be evaluated before finalizing the choice of myofunctional appliance.

- Age of the patient.
- Evaluation of growth spurts
- Orthodontic records
- Study models
- Radiographs: Preoperative OPG
- Photographs
- Cephalometric analysis
- Functional analysis
- Clinical inspection—fundamental guideline for a proper case selection
- Visual treatment objective of the patient

ADVANTAGES OF MYOFUNCTIONAL APPLIANCES

- Enables elimination of abnormal muscle function thereby aiding in normal development.
- Treatment can be initiated at mixed dentition.
- As it is started at an early age, psychological disturbances associated with malocclusion can be avoided.
- Less chairside time as these appliances are mostly fabricated in laboratory.
- Do not interfere with oral hygiene.
- Frequency of patients' visit to orthodontist is less.
- Most FA are worn during night.

LIMITATIONS OF MYOFUNCTIONAL APPLIANCES

- They cannot be used in adult patients when growth has ceased.
- They cannot be used to bring about individual tooth movement.
- Most functional appliances are dependent on the patient for timely wear. Thus, patient cooperation is essential for the success of the treatment.
- They may require prefunctional tooth movement for correction of minor tooth irregularities that may interfere with functional therapy.
- Fixed appliance therapy may be required at the termination of treatment for detailing of the occlusion.

VESTIBULAR SCREEN

The basic appliance for screening therapy is the vestibular screen **(Fig. 33.1)**. Common modifications include lower lip shield, tongue crib, combination of vestibular screen and tongue crib, and vestibular screen with breathing holes. The appliance is effective in eliminating abnormal sucking habits and lip dysfunction if it is properly made and worn. It helps establish a proper lip seal and indirectly influences the posture of tongue. The shield interrupts contact between the tip of the tongue and lower lip, a vestige of the infantile suckling pattern, leading to maintenance of deglutitional cycle and creates a somatic swallowing pattern.

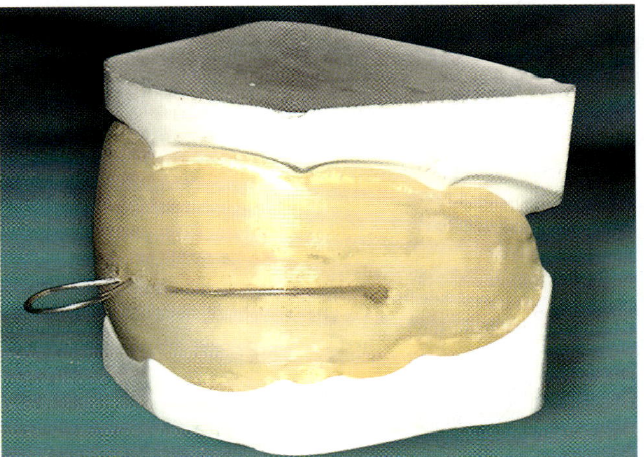

Fig. 33.1: Vestibular screen.

Indications

Deciduous Dentition

- Screening appliances intercept and eliminate all abnormal perioral muscle function in acquired malocclusions resulting from abnormal habits.
- It can also be used in the deciduous dentition as pretreatment devices, if an activator is going to be placed later, to help in reducing the severity of malocclusion.
- For hyperkinetic children or those with potential behavior problems who exhibit persistent finger sucking and concomitant tongue thrust, the use of vestibular shield first is more likely to be successful and produce less psychological trauma.
- It can be used in patients with nasorespiratory problems. The use of vestibular screen with breathing holes can help reestablish normal nasal breathing.

Mixed Dentition

- It can be used with other appliances if correction cannot be achieved by screens alone.
- It is used in pretreatment to eliminate the influence of abnormal perioral muscles function.
- Retention adjunct in dentofacial orthopedic therapy.

Fabrication

Plaster models are made after taking impression of upper and lower arch

↓

Articulated models are covered with 2 to 3 mm of wax over the labial surfaces of the teeth

↓

Shield is fabricated in self-curing acrylic over the wax relief

↓

The completed vestibular should be in contact only with the upper and lower labial folds during the anterior positioning of the mandible

↓

The shield is fabricated without a holding ring, which might interfere with desired lip seal

ACTIVATOR

In 1880, **Kinsley** introduced the concept of "Jumping the bite" for patients with mandibular retrusion. He inserted a vulcanite palatal plate consisting of an anterior incline that guided the mandible to a forward position when patient closed on it.

This maneuver corrected the sagittal relationship without tipping the lower incisors forward.

- **Hotz** used the appliance in cases of deep bite retrognathism.
- Some years before Anderson started experimenting with his working retainer; Robin created an appliance quite similar in its objectives, called the monoblock appliance and positioned the mandible forward in patients with glossoptosis and severe mandible retrognathism.

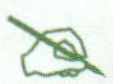

*Activator was first used by **Viggo Andresen** (1908) with vertical extensions to contact contiguous lingual surfaces of the mandibular teeth. He used modified Kinsley plate as a retainer over summer vacation for his daughter after he removed fixed appliances to correct a disto-occlusion. Seeing the continued improvement with this retainer, he called it a biomechanical working retainer.*

- When Andresen moved from Denmark to Norway, he became associated with Karl Häupl at University of Oslo. Andresen and Häupl teamed up to write about their appliance, they called it an activator, because of its ability to activate the muscle forces.

Mode of Action of Activator

According to **Andresen** and **Häupl**, the activator **(Figs. 33.2A to C)** induces musculoskeletal adaptation by introducing a new pattern of mandibular closure. The appliance loosely fits into the mouth. The patient has to move the mandible forward to engage the appliance. This results in stretching of elevator muscles of mastication. This generates kinetic energy that causes the following:

- Prevention of further forward growth of maxillary dentoalveolar process.
- Movement of maxillary dentoalveolar process distally.
- A reciprocal forward force on mandible.
- Condylar adaptation by backward and upward growth.

Construction Bite

- The construction bite is an intermaxillary wax record used to relate the mandible to the maxilla in three dimensions of space.
- The bite registration involves repositioning the mandible in a forward direction as well as opening the bite vertically.
- In most cases, the mandible is advanced by 4–5 mm and the bite opened to the extent of 2–3 mm beyond the freeway space.

Parts of Activator

- *Wire elements:* Upper labial bow (0.8–0.9 mm wire).
- *Acrylic portion:* Maxillary part; mandibular part, interocclusal part.

Management of Appliance

- Patient should be sufficiently convinced about the benefits of the appliance.
- Patient should be taught how to use, place, and remove the appliance.
- Patient should be asked to wear 2–3 h during daytime in the first week. During the second week, increase use up to 3 h a day as well as while sleeping.

Trimming

- *For vertical control:* This can be done to extrude or intrude the teeth.
- *For sagittal control:* This can be done to protrude or retrude the anterior teeth. Teeth in buccal segment can be moved mesially and distally.
- *For transverse plane:* This is done by allowing the contact of acrylic on the lingual surfaces of the teeth to be moved transversely.

Indications

- Class II div 1, Class II div 2, Class III.
- Class I open bite, deep bite.
- Preliminary treatment before fixed appliance therapy to improve skeletal jaw relationship.
- Post-treatment retention.
- Children with lack of vertical development.

Contraindications

- The appliance is not used in correction of Class I problems with crowding.
- Excess lower facial height and extreme vertical mandibular growth.
- Severely proclined lower incisor.

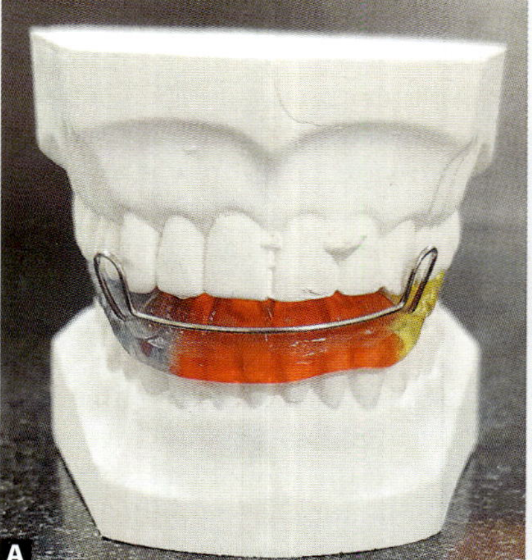

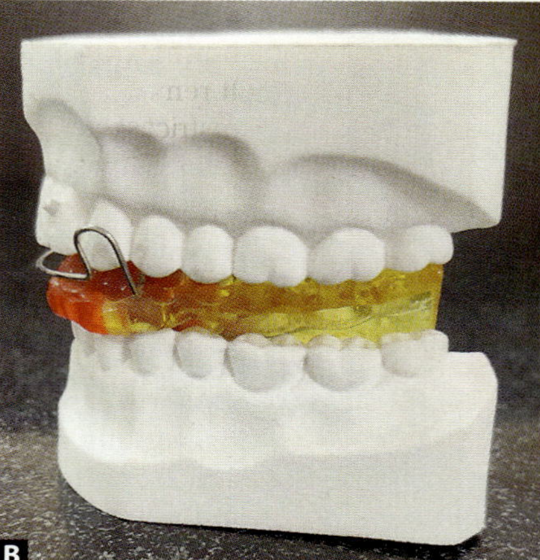

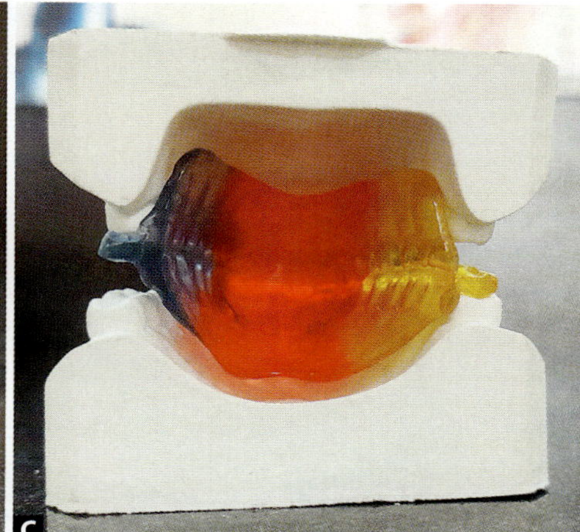

Figs. 33.2 A to C: Activator.

- Children with nasal stenosis caused by structural problems.
- Limited application in nongrowing children.

Advantages

- Uses existing growth of jaws.
- Minimal oral hygiene problems.
- Interval between appointments is long.
- Short appointment duration.
- It is economical.

Disadvantages

- Requires good patient cooperation.
- Cannot produce precise detailing and finishing.
- May produce moderate mandibular rotation.

Modifications of Activator

- **One bow activator of AM Schwarz:** Maxillary and mandibular portions are connected together by an elastic bow; this allows stepwise sagittal advancement of the mandible by adjustment of the bow.
- **Wunderer's modification:** It is used in treatment of Class III malocclusion. It is characterized by maxillary and mandibular portions connected by the anterior screw. By opening the screw the maxillary portion is moved anteriorly, with a reciprocal backward thrust in the mandibular portion.
- **The reduced activator:** This appliance resembles a bionator with acrylic portion of activator reduced from the maxillary anterior area leaving a small flange of acrylic on palatal slopes. The two halves may be connected by palatal wire.
- **Palate-free activator:** Palate is free of acrylic.
- **Karwetzky modification:** Maxillary and mandibular plates are joined by a U-loop in region of first permanent molar.
- **Heraeus modification:** Over compensating the neutral position of mandible in construction wax bite by sealing the appliance firmly against the maxillary dental arch.
- ***Teuscher activator:*** A modification that eliminates palatal acrylic with a large omega loop. It has a set of lip pads that facilitate forward growth of mandible. Torquing springs are present for each maxillary incisor on labial side. Head gear tubes are included in the molar acrylic region.

Recent Advances in Functional Appliances

- **Paolone-Kaitsas appliance (PK appliance):** This is a removable functional appliance first described in 2017. It has two acrylic plates, upper and lower joined by 2 lateral 3 loop springs. It has complete coverage of occlusal surfaces to control occlusal plane. Lateral springs facilitate progressive activation to give vertical control. An expansion screw may be added to correct maxillary transverse dimensions.
- **Dynamax appliance:** It has two parts—upper is removable, lower may be removable or fixed as a lingual arch with bands on first molars. Fixed one is more useful in mixed dentition (late). Maxillary component has Adams clasp for retention, palatal spring for expansion. Mandibular advancement is produced by vertical spring projections in first molar area that engage on shoulders present on lingual aspect of mandibular component. Springs are 14 mm long that allow protrusive action.
- In this appliance, advancement is kept minimum (3–4 mm). Upper posterior teeth have occlusal coverage of 1 mm.
- Torquing springs are present on the anterior teeth in upper arch. This appliance helps in vertical control with head gear tubes in molar region.

FUNCTION REGULATOR

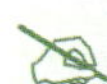

Developed by **Professor Rolf Frankel** *of Germany. It is also called Frankel appliance,vestibular appliance, and oral gymnastic appliance.*

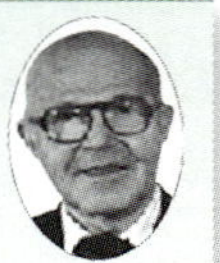

Fränkel had used the activator functional appliance and experienced mixed results with this appliance. He believed that a treatment outcome is more stable if the functional deviations of muscles are also corrected along with dentition.

Through his work he developed an approach which allowed the maxillary and mandibular muscles to play an important part in an orthodontic treatment. He achieved that through development of functional regulator appliances. These appliances allowed him to train and reprogram the musculature around the mouth. He first introduced his functional orthopedic approach in 1966 at a meeting for European Orthodontic Society.

Fränkel's Philosophy

1. Functional performance of the muscular portions of the oral capsule influences the developing functional spaces, as believed by Melvin Moss.
2. He believed that the perioral muscles had restraining effect on the dental arches and that the insertion of appliance expands the capsule and allows new functional adaptation of the muscle.

It has two main treatment effects:

1. Serves as a template against which the craniofacial muscles function. The framework of appliance provides an artificial balancing of environment thereby promoting normal pattern of muscle activity.
2. It removes muscle forces in labial and buccal areas that restrict skeletal growth thereby providing an environment that enables skeletal growth.

Mode of Action of Frankel Appliance

- Increase in transverse and sagittal directions—by use of buccal shields and lip pads.
- Increase in vertical direction—by allowing the lower molar to erupt freely because appliance is fixed to the upper arch.
- Muscle adaptation—development of new patterns of motor function by buccal shields and lip pads of FR can be achieved by:
  - Massaging the soft tissues.
  - Loosening the tight muscles.

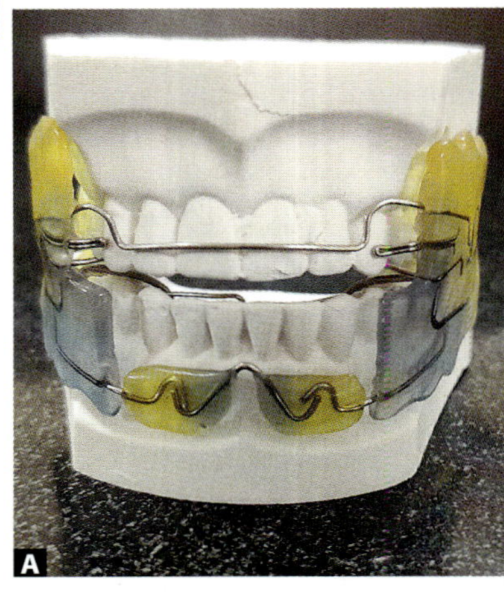
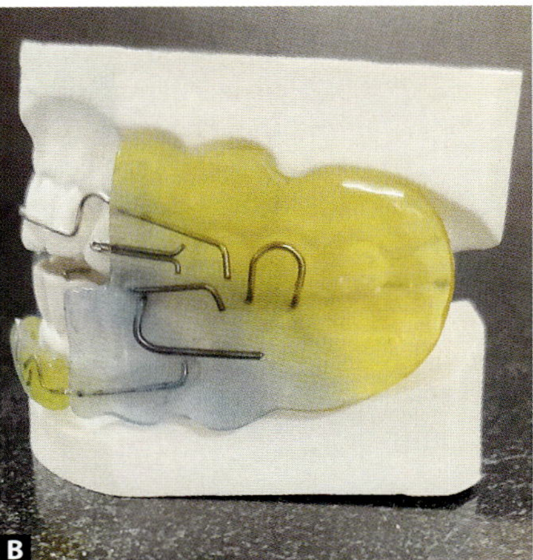
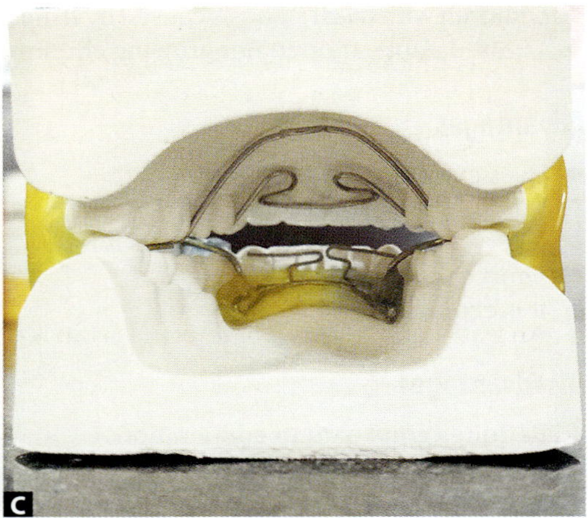

Figs. 33.3A to C: Frankel appliance.

- Improving the blood circulation.
- Improving muscle tonicity.
- Providing new functional matrix for perioral muscle to act upon it–'ought- to- be matrix'.

❖ Mandibular forward positioning—position of mandible can be changed by gradual training of the protractor and retractor muscles followed by condylar adaptation.

Components of Frankel Appliance (Figs. 33.3A to C)

❖ **Acrylic components**
- Buccal shield: They were about 2.5 mm thick and their goal was to expand the soft tissue capsule in the back.
- Lip pads: They are tear drop-shaped acrylic pads which were placed in the vestibule of the lower arch.
- Lingual shield: This allows mandibular muscles to overcome their poor posture.

❖ **Wire components**
- Palatal bow: This rests on maxillary molar and has a stabilizing action for the appliance.
- Cross-over wire: They run between 1st and 2nd premolars and are responsible for movement of the buccal segments.
- Lower lingual wires: They prevent the lingual movement of lower incisors.
- Labial bow
- Canine loop: Used for guided eruption of canine and also for intermaxillary anchorage.

Indications

- ❖ Mixed dentition. Within growth spurts.
- ❖ Schedule class two malocclusion with prognathic maxilla retrognathic mandible. (Positive VTO).
- ❖ Functional Class II malocclusion.
- ❖ In a horizontal or neural growth vector case.
- ❖ Class III malocclusions.
- ❖ Bimaxillary protrusion and open bite problems.

Contraindications

- ❖ Class I malocclusion crowding.
- ❖ Thumb sucking habit.
- ❖ Severe dentoalveolar problems in permanent dentition.
- ❖ Uncooperative patients.

Classification/Types of Frankel Appliance

Sl. No.	Classification	Indication
1.	FR I	Class I and Class II, divlsion 1 malocclusion
2.	FR Ia	Class I with deep bite, Class I with minor to moderate crowding or arrested development of basal arches.
3.	FR Ib	Class II, division 1- Overjet >5 mm
4.	FR Ic	Class II, division 1- Overjet >7mm
5.	FR II	Class II, division 1 and division 2
6.	FR III	Class III
7.	FR IV	Open bite
8.	FR V	Vertical maxillary excess + high mandibular plane angle in long face patients (along with headgear)

Advantages

- ❖ It enables elimination of abnormal muscle function thereby aiding in normal development.
- ❖ Treatment can be initiated at early age.
- ❖ Less chairside time is spent.
- ❖ The frequency of the patients visit is less.
- ❖ They do not interfere with the oral hygiene status.
- ❖ Duration of treatment is comparatively less they deal with skeletal as well as dentoalveolar problems.

Disadvantages

- ❖ The appliance is bulky and the cooperation of the patient is essential.
- ❖ They cannot be used in adult patients where the growth has ceased.
- ❖ Cannot be used to bring about individual tooth movement in case of crowding.
- ❖ Fixed appliance therapy may be required at the termination of treatment for final detailing of the treatment.

Clinical Management

- ❖ Stabilizing the appliance at the delivery is absolutely essential.
- ❖ Prior to placement, all margins are checked for smoothness.
- ❖ Check vertical dimension.
- ❖ Overextension of the labial, lingual, lip and buccal pads cause tissue irritation, so the extensions should be correct.

Wearing Time

- For the first two weeks the appliance should be worn for two to four hours during the day.
- During the next three weeks that time is extended to four to six hours.
- It usually takes two months before the appliance is worn at night.
- The appliance and treatment progress should be checked at four weeks interval.
- An initial end to end molar relationship is corrected in six months

Treatment Timing

Optimum time to start the treatment is the mixed dentition period (8 to 10 years age).

BIONATOR—A MODIFIED ACTIVATOR

- The bulkiness of the activator and its limitation to night-time wear have deterred clinician as interested in attaining the greatest potential of functional growth guidance. The bionator is a less bulky appliance, tooth-borne appliance developed in Germany by **Wilhelm Balter** in the early 1950s.
- Bionator's lower portion is narrow and its upper has only lateral extensions with a cross-palatal stabilizing bar. The palate is free for proprioceptive contact with the tongue; the buccinator wire loop holds away potentially deforming muscular action; the appliance may be worn all the time, except during meals **(Figs. 33.4A to C)**.
- According to Balters, the equilibrium between the tongue and circumoral muscles is responsible for the shape of the dental arches and intercuspation. The tongue was the most important factor in treatment. A dis-coordination of its function could lead to abnormal growth and actual deformation. The purpose of the bionator was to establish good function coordination and eliminate these forming growth restriction aberrations.

Principles of Bionator

- Not to activate the muscles but to modulate muscle activity thereby enhancing normal development of the inherent growth pattern.
- Eliminating abnormal and potentially deforming environmental factors.

Types of Bionator

1. **Standard appliance**
   - This is used for the treatment of Class II div 1 and Class I malocclusions having narrow dental arches.
   - It consists of a slender acrylic body fitted to the lingual aspects of mandibular arch and a part of maxillary arch. The acrylic extends up to the distal of the first permanent molars. The maxillary plate covers only the molars and premolars with the anterior region remaining uncovered. The acrylic extends 2 mm below the gingival margin. The interocclusal space of some of the buccal teeth is filled with acrylic extending one half of the occlusal surface of the teeth to stabilize the appliance.
   - The wire components of the bionator are the palatal arch and the vestibular wire. The palatal arch is made of 1.2 mm diameter wire. It emerges opposite the middle of the first premolars and follows the contour of the palate forming a curve that reaches the distal surface of first permanent molars. The palatal arch is kept 1 mm away from mucosa.
   - The vestibular wire is made up of 0.9 mm stainless steel wire. It emerges from the acrylic below the contact point between the upper canines and premolars. It rises vertically and is bent at right angles to go distally along the middle of the upper premolar crowns. Mesial to the molar, a round bend is made so that the wire runs at the level of the lower papilla up to mandibular canine where it is bent to reach the upper canine. It forms a mirror image on the opposite side. The vestibular wire is kept away from the surface of incisors by the thickness of a sheet of paper. The lateral portions of the wire are sufficiently away from the teeth to allow expansion of the arch.
2. **Class III appliance**
   - This is used in mandibular prognathism.
   - The acrylic parts are similar to the standard appliance.
   - The palatal arch is placed in the opposite direction so that the rounded arch is placed anteriorly. The

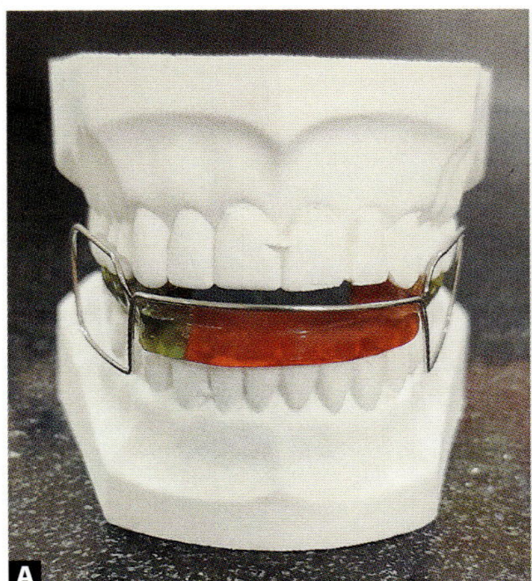

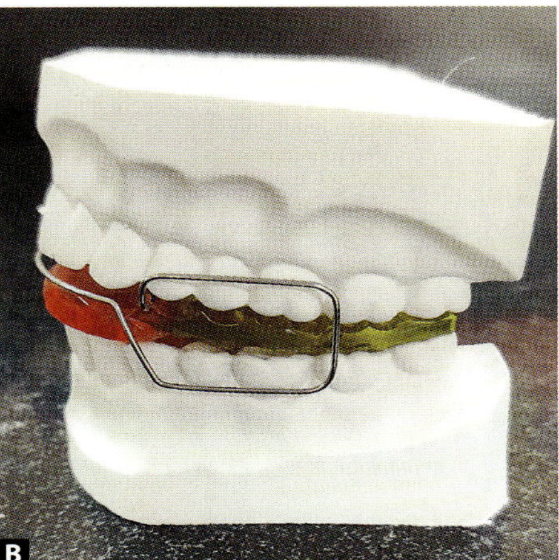

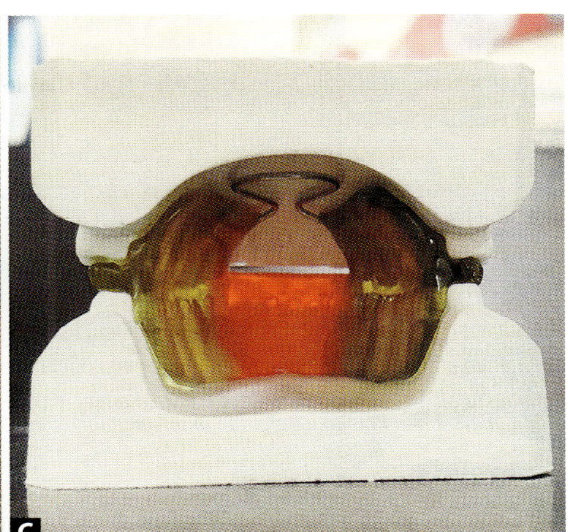

Figs. 33.4A to C: Bionator.

vestibular wire runs in front of the lower incisors instead of terminating at the lower canines.

3. **Open bite appliance**
   - The maxillary acrylic portion is modified so that even the anterior area is covered.
   - Its purpose is to prevent the tongue from thrusting between the teeth as the tongue is responsible in most cases for the open bite.

Indications of Bionator

Types of bionator	*Malocclusion treated*
Standard bionator	Class II division 1 malocclusion • Mixed dentition phase • Well-aligned dental arches • Mandible is in a posterior position • Skeletal discrepancy is not too severe • Labial tipping of the upper incisor is evident
	Deep overbite malocclusion • Trimming of acrylic is performed to permit uninhibited eruption of the buccal segment teeth
Open bite bionator	Open bite malocclusion • Buccal segment teeth are loaded with acrylic for all possible intrusive stimulus • Treat open bite cases that result from abnormal habits such as finger sucking, retained infantile deglutitional patterns and aberrant tongue function.
Reverse type bionator	Class III type malocclusion • Designed to load the mandibular teeth and unload the upper anterior alveolar portion, where growth stimulation is desired, especially during eruption of the incisors.

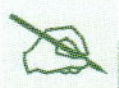

Contraindications of Bionator

- The Class II relationship caused by maxillary prognathism.
- Presence of a vertical growth pattern.
- Labial tipping of the lower incisors. Anterior posturing of the mandible with simultaneous uprighting of the lower incisors cannot be performed with the bionator.

Advantages

- Reduced in size as compared to activator.
- A constant influence on the tongue and perioral muscles because of the screening effect of the labial bow and its lateral extension.
- Bionators action is faster than that of classic activator because unfavorable external and internal muscle forces are prevented from exerting undesirable and restrictive effects on the dentition and supporting structures for a longer time.
- Constant wear results in more rapid sagittal adjustment of the musculature to the forward mandibular posture because the mandible retracts only during eating.

Disadvantages

- Simultaneous requirements of stabilization of the appliance plus selective grinding of eruption guidance.
- In the case of skeletal disturbances, the effectiveness of Balters bionator is very limited, as it is for any functional appliance.
- The vulnerability to distortion, which occurs because far less acrylic support exists in the alveolar and incisal region.

Clinical Management

- For maximal beneficial effect the bionator must be worn day and night.
- The time interval between office visits is three to five weeks, depending on the state of eruption of the teeth.
- During the first phase of the treatment the occurrence of rapid horizontal or vertical changes in mandibular position is common.
- The labial bow should be checked to ensure it touches the teeth only lightly, if at all.
- In the final stages, minor spaces can be closed by active retraction of the bow.
- The buccinator loops should be away from the deciduous first and second molar areas but should not irritate the cheek mucosa.
- Loops can be activated if expansion is required.
- The loading and unloading off acrylic areas or planes should depend on whether tooth movement is to be stimulated or retarded.

HERBST APPLIANCE

It is a fixed functional appliance that was developed by **Emil Herbst** *in the early 1900s.*

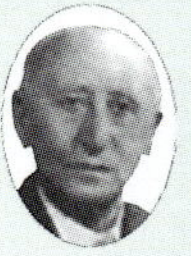

- **Hans Pancherz** again popularized its use in 1979.
- The appliance can be compared to an artificial joint working between the maxilla and mandible, keeping mandible in anterior position. The device consists of a tube into which the plunger fits. The tube is fixed to the distal end of the maxillary molars, while the rod is fixed to the lower first premolar **(Fig. 33.5).**
- It can be either of bonded type or banded type.

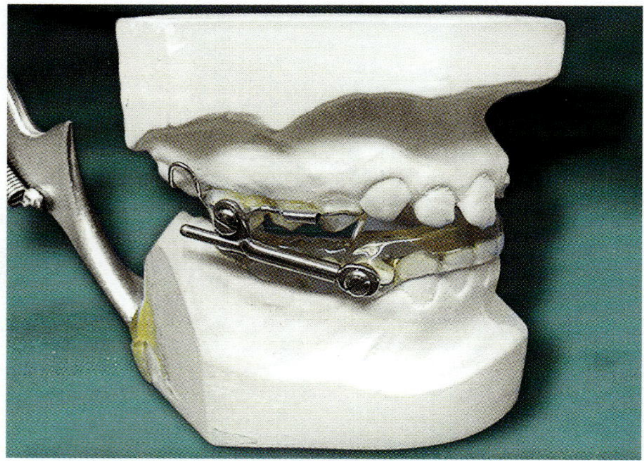

Fig. 33.5: Herbst appliance.

Indications

- Correction of skeletal Class II malocclusion due to retrognathic mandible.
- It can be used as anterior repositioning splints in patients having temporomandibular joint disorders.
- Postadolescent patients
- Mouth breathing
- Uncooperative patients

Advantages

- Fixed appliance cannot be removed by the patients, action it produces is continuous.
- The treatment duration is short due to continuous nature of action.
- Less patient cooperation is needed.
- It can be used successfully in patients who are at the end of their growth.
- It can be used in patients who have mouth-breathing habit due to nasal airway obstruction.

Disadvantages

- Initial discomfort is usually present.
- It can cause minor functional disturbances in masticatory system which are temporary.
- Repeated breakage and loosening of the appliance occurs.
- Plaque accumulation and enamel decalcification.
- Tendency for posterior open bite at the termination of therapy.

JASPER JUMPER

- It is a relatively new type of flexible, fixed, tooth-borne functional appliance that was introduced by **JJ Jasper** in 1980.
- Its actions are similar to Herbst appliance but it lacks rigidity.
- It uses a modular system commonly known as Jasper Jumper, which can be attached to fixed appliance that is placed on the upper and lower arches **(Fig. 33.6).**
- It is analogous to the tube and the plunger of Herbst appliance, but it is more flexible. It is made up of a stainless steel coil that is attached at both the ends to stainless steel end caps. The module is given an opaque covering of polyurethane for hygiene and comfort. It is available in seven sizes ranging from 26 to 38 mm in length.

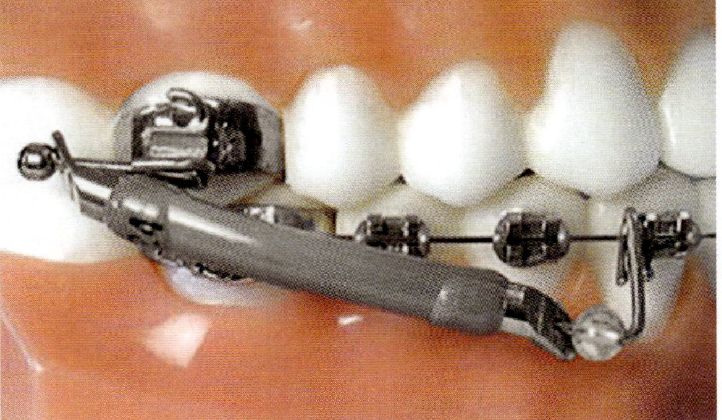

Fig. 33.6: Jasper Jumper appliance.

Indications

Indicated in skeletal Class II malocclusion with maxillary excess and mandibular deficiency.

Effects of Jasper Jumper

- According to **Rankin, Parker** and **Blockwood**, the Jasper Jumper brings about both skeletal and dentoalveolar changes in the ratio of 40:60.
- **Skeletal effects:**
  - Holds and displaces the maxilla distally.
  - A small shift of point A distally.
  - Clockwise rotation of mandible.
  - Condyle moves forward.
- **Dental changes:**
  - Posterior tipping and intrusion of upper molar.
  - Backward tipping of maxillary incisors.
  - Anterior translation and tipping of mandibular teeth.
  - Intrusion of mandibular incisor.

Advantages

- Continuous force.
- Increased patient compliance.
- Greater degree of freedom as compared to Herbst appliance.
- Oral hygiene is easier to maintain.

LIP BUMPER

- The lip bumper or lip plumber as it is sometimes called is a combined removable fixed appliance.
- The lip bumper can be called a modified vestibular screen that is used for muscular force application or for elimination.
- The appliance can be used in both the maxilla and the mandible to shield the lips away from the teeth.
- It is made up of thick stainless steel wire extending from one molar to the opposite molar. The wire is made to lie away from the anterior teeth. The lip bumper is inserted into round molar tubes of 0.93 mm diameter soldered to bands on first molars. The anterior portion of the wire from canine to canine can be reinforced with acrylic **(Figs. 33.7A and B).**
- Although lip bumpers are mostly used in the mandibular arches, they can also be used in the maxillary arch. Such an appliance is similar in design and is called **Denholtz** appliance.

Uses

- They are used in patients exhibiting lower lip habits such as lip sucking. The lip bumper shields the lower lip away.
- They are also used in patients exhibiting hyperactive mentalis activity that causes flattening or crowding of the lower anteriors.
- Lip bumpers can be used to augment anchorage.
- Distalization of first molar can be achieved by use of lip bumpers.

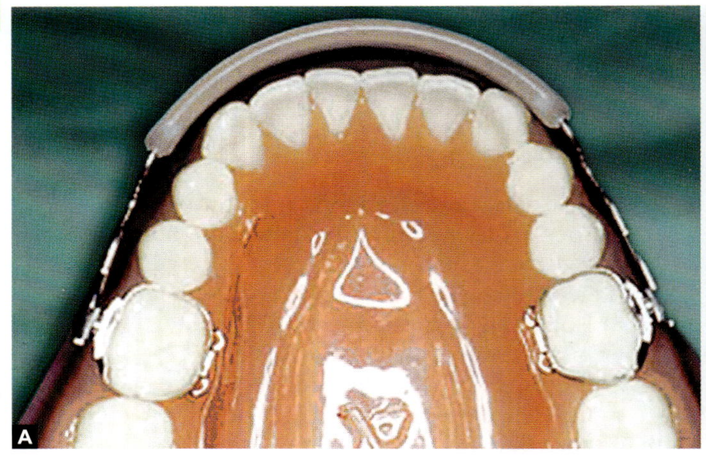
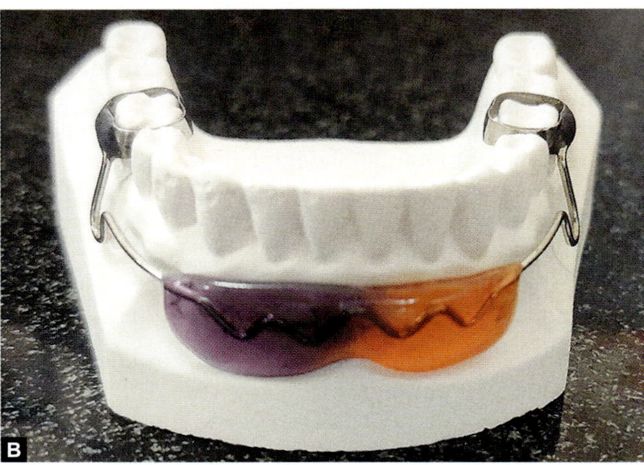

Figs. 33.7A and B: Lip bumper.

- These can be used as space regainers, if the lower molar has drifted mesially due to early loss of deciduous molars.

TWIN BLOCK APPLIANCE

The twin block appliance was developed by ***William Clark*** *in 1977 as a two-piece appliance resembling a Schwartz double plate and a split activator.*

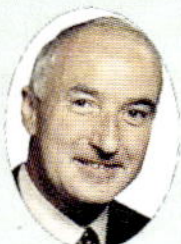

- These are simple bite blocks that effectively modify the occlusal inclined plane. These devices use upper and lower bite blocks that engage on occlusal inclined planes.
- Twin blocks are designed for full-time wear and they correct the maxillomandibular relationship through functional mandibular displacement. Achieve rapid functional correction of malocclusion by modifying occlusal inclined plane, guiding the mandible forward into correct occlusion. Upper and lower bite blocks interlock at a 70° angle; they are designed for full- time wear to take full advantage of all functional forces applied to the dentition, including the forces of mastication and patient can eat comfortably with appliance in place **(Figs. 33.8A to E)**.

Features

- Twin blocks are constructed in a protrusive bite that effectively modifies the occlusal inclined plane by means of acrylic inclined planes on occlusal bite blocks.

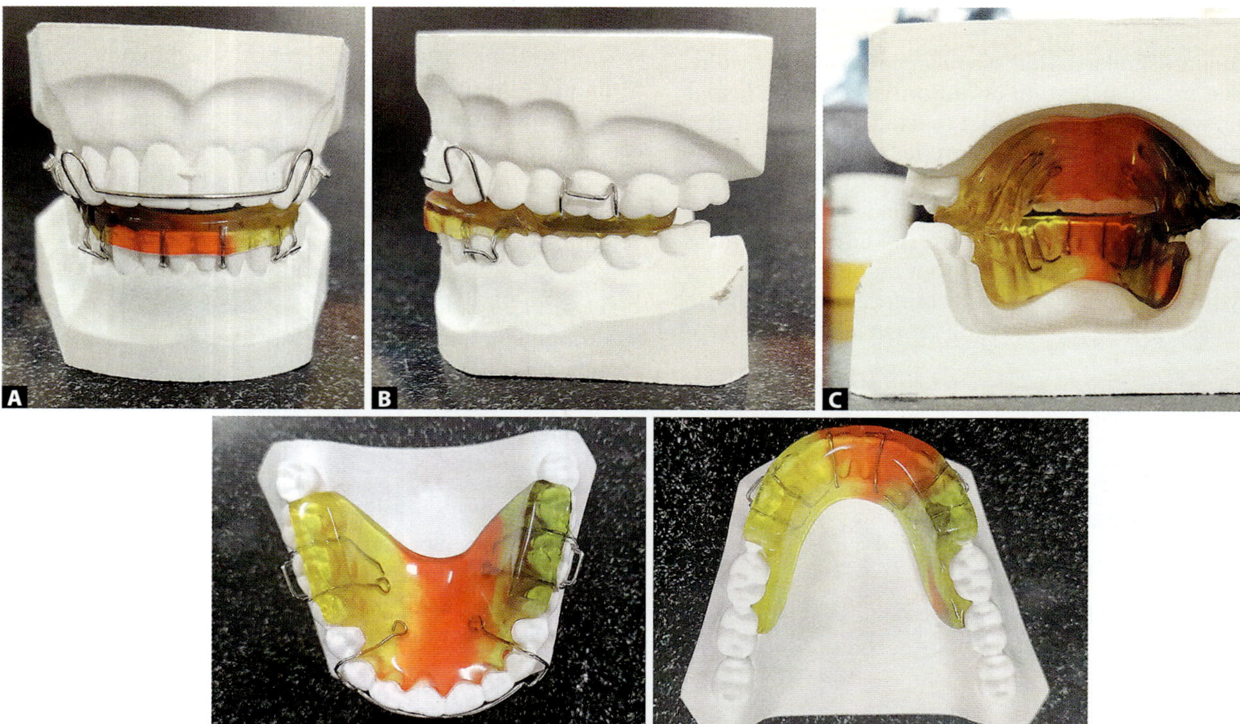

Figs. 33.8A to E: Construction design of twin block.

- The unfavorable cuspal contacts of distal exclusion are replaced by favorable proprioceptive contacts of inclined planes of the twin blocks.
- The bite blocks interlock at a 70° angle usually covering the upper and lower teeth in the buccal segment.
- Muscle behavior is immediately influenced through the placement of inclined planes between the teeth.
- Bony changes are gradual and take several months to become established. Favorably directed occlusal forces transmitted through the dentition provide constant proprioceptive stimuli to influence the growth rate and architecture of trabecular structure of supporting bone.

Mechanism of Action

- Inclined planes
- Muscles of mastication
- Force transmission
- Bone remodeling

Indications

- The primary indication for twin blocks in early mixed dentition is in Class II div 1 in which prominent upper incisors rest outside the lower lip and is vulnerable to fracture.
- Twin blocks can fulfill three objectives at this stage of development:
  - They can reduce overjet and correct distal occlusion
  - They can control overbite if overbite is deep or anterior open bite is present.
  - They can improve arch form by transverse or sagittal development.

Bite Registration

- According to **Woodside**—mandible should be positioned protruded approximately 3 mm distal to the most protrusive position that the patient can achieve, while vertically the bite is registered within the limit of the freeway space.
- According to **Roccabado**—normal physiologic TMJ movement quantifies as 70% of the total joint space. Overjet up to 10 mm—a single activation edge-to-edge incisor relation with 2 mm interincisal clearance. Overjet greater than 10 mm—initial activation of 7–8 mm followed by further activation.
- Vertical dimension—blocks should be thick enough to open the bite slightly beyond the freeway space.
- Appliances for bite registration.
  - George bite gauge.
  - Exactobite bite registration device.

Components of Twin Block

- Occlusal bite block—lower and upper
- U/L clasps - Adams clasp {delta clasp (Graber)}
- Interdental clasps on lower incisors
- Labial bow
- Midline screw
- Springs to move individual teeth
- Provision of extraoral traction

Stages of Treatment (Figs. 33.9 and 33.10)

Stage 1: Active phase—twin blocks: During the active phase of treatment, twin blocks are worn full time. The objective is to correct arch relationships in anteroposterior, vertical, and

Clark cephalometric analysis

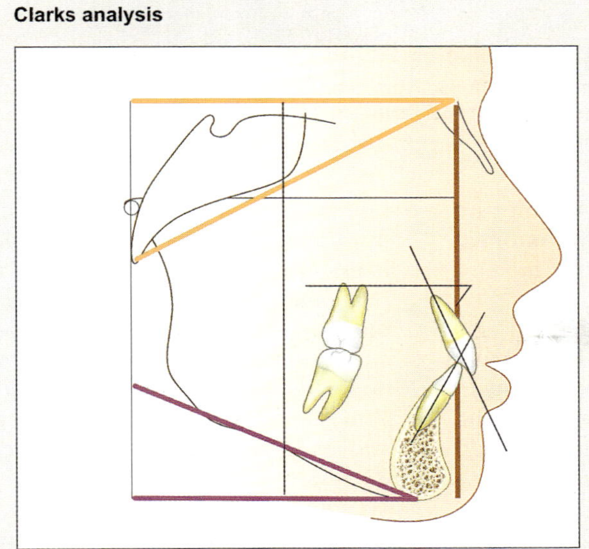

NORMS:

Angular
Cranial base – 27°
Mandibular – 26°
Craniomandibular – 53°
Facial plane - (–) 3°
Facial axis – 27°
Condyle axis –27°
Mandibular arc – 26°
Craniomaxillary – 27°
Maxillary deflection –0°

Dental
Upper 1–25°
Lower 1–25°
1 to 1 –128°
Distal 6 to PTV-age +3
Lower 1 to APo–1

Convexity –2.5 at 8 yrs
N vert to A –0 mm
N vert to pog- –10 at 8 yrs
Nasal angle
Lower lip to E plane= –2

Coben (1955) observed that superimposition of tracings in the anterior cranial base has the major disadvantage of ignoring growth at the primary growth site in the base of the skull, the spheno-occipital synchondrosis, which has the fundamental influence on facial growth. Growth of the head is observed more accurately by superimposition at basion. The same method of superimposition has been selected to demonstrate facial growth changes with twin block treatment, using basion as a fulcrum point for analysis of growth changes in the facial rectangle, with the Frankfort plane horizontal. A facial rectangle helps one to define the relative position and angulation of cranial, maxillary, mandibular, and dentoalveolar structures. The rectangular framework makes it easier to identify areas where growth departs from normal in the facial pattern.

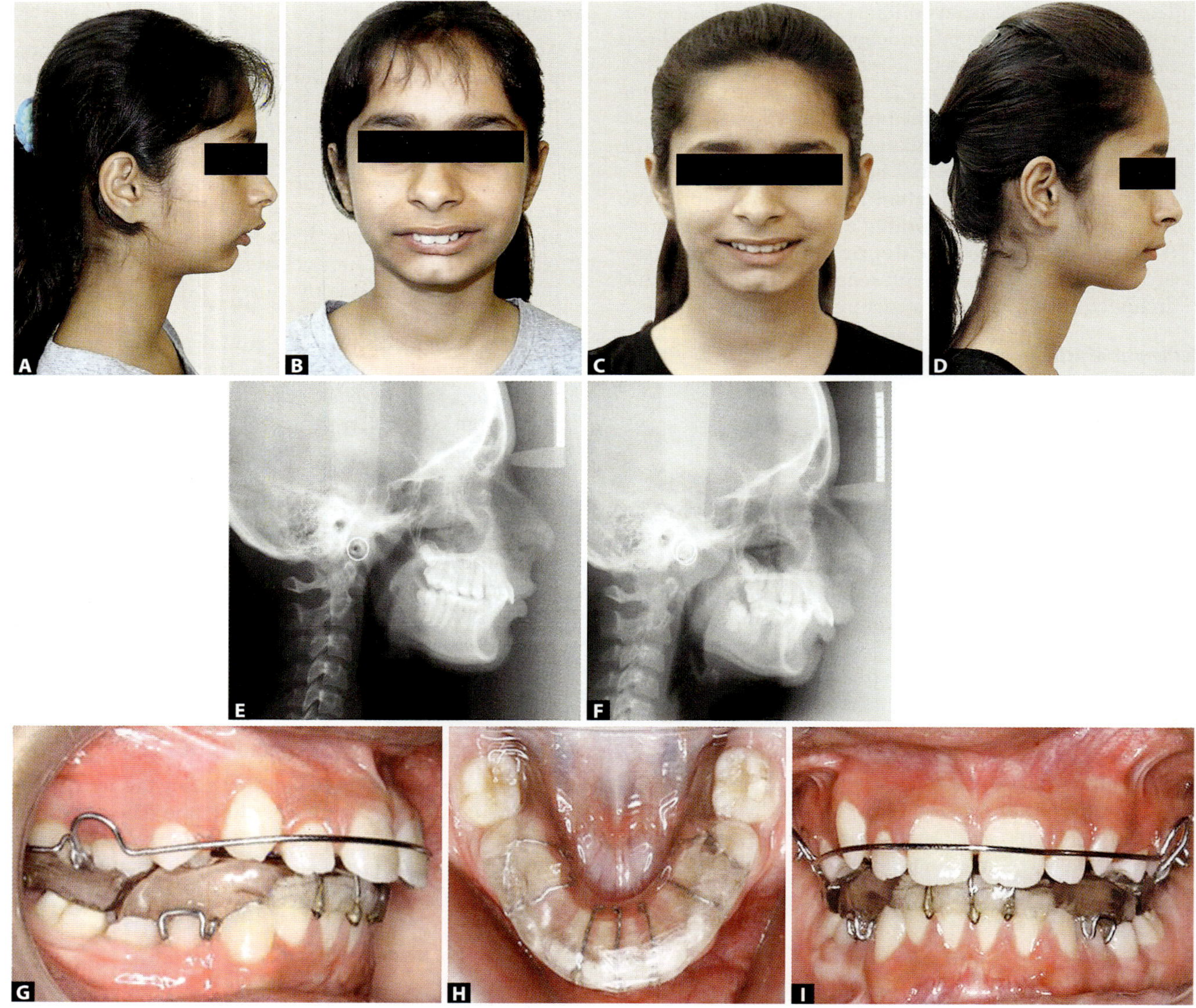

Figs. 33.9A to I: Stages of twin block appliance treatment therapy: (A) Pretreatment profile view; (B) Pretreatment frontal view; (C) Post-treatment profile view; (D) Posttreatment frontal view; (E) Pretreatment X-ray; (F) Post-treatment X-ray; (G to I) View of appliance therapy. *(Pic courtesy:* Dr Ravi Mahto,Kathmandu University School of Medical Sciences (KUSMS), Nepal).

transverse dimensions. Normally, overjet and overbite are corrected within 6 months, and the lower molars have erupted into occlusion within 9 months. The average wear time for twin blocks is 6–9 months.

- *First visit:* On fitting twin block appliances, the overjet is measured for future reference. The lingual flange must be relieved slightly lingual to the lower incisors to avoid gingival irritation as the appliance is driven in by the occlusion during the first few days. The clinician should check that the patient bites in a comfortable position in a protrusive bite.
- *Second visit:* After 10 days, the patient should be wearing the appliances comfortably and eating with them in position after 10 days. In cases of deep overbite, the upper block should be slightly trimmed occlusodistally to leave the lower molars 1 mm clear of the occlusion to allow eruption and reduce the overbite by increasing lower facial height.
- *Third visit:* After 4 weeks at each visit, progress is reviewed by measuring the overjet. At the same time, the occlusion is checked for the correction of the buccal segment relationship. Minor adjustment is necessary only to keep the labial bow out of contact with the upper incisor and to ensure that the lower molars are not in contact with the upper block in cases of deep overbite.
- *Fourth visit:* After 6 weeks, a similar pattern of adjustment and checking of occlusion and overjet should occur after 6 weeks.
- The clinician should trim the blocks in the recommended sequence to reduce the deep overbite.
- *Progress:* An overjet as large as 10 mm can be corrected without reactivating the bite block if the rate and direction of mandibular growth are favorable. Full correction of sagittal arch relationship can be achieved in as little as 2–6 months, thus producing a normal incisor relationship. At this stage, the overjet is fully corrected and the buccal

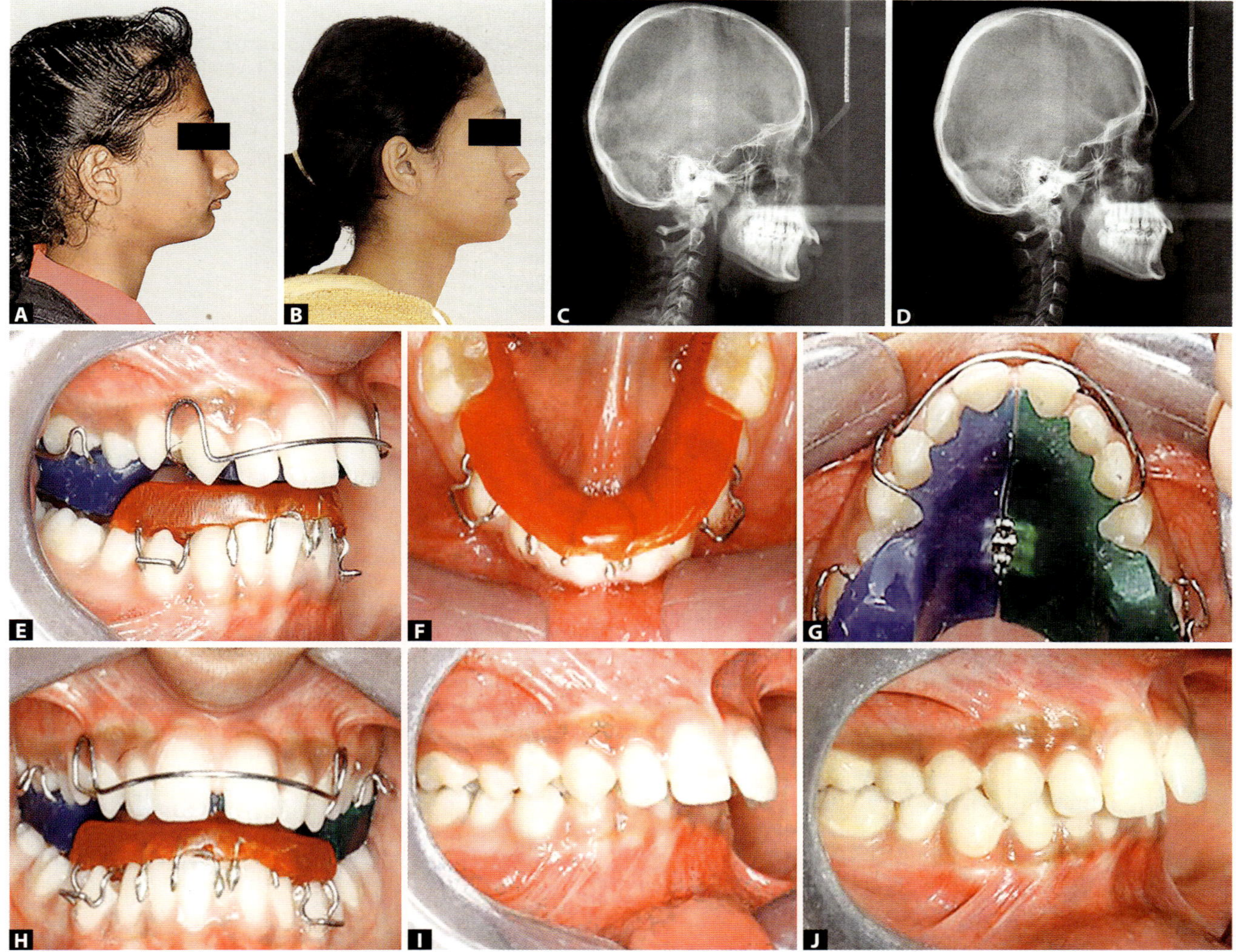

Figs. 33.10A to J: Stages of twin block appliance treatment therapy: (A) Pretreatment profile view; (B) Post-treatment profile view; (C) Pre treatment X-ray; (D) Posttreatment X-ray; (E to H) View of appliance therapy; (I) Pretherapy occlusion; (J) Post-therapy occlusion. (*Pic courtesy:* Dr Ravi Mahto,Kathmandu University School of Medical Sciences (KUSMS), Nepal).

segments are still out of occlusion because of presence of the bite block.

Stage 2: Support phase—anterior inclined plane: The objective of the second stage of treatment is to retain the corrected incisor relationship until buccal segment occlusion is fully established.

- To achieve this objective, an upper removable appliance is fitted with an anterior inclined plane to engage the lower incisors and canines. This appliance is worn full time initially to allow the buccal segment occlusion to settle; it is then used as a retainer.
- The upper and lower buccal teeth are usually in occlusion within 4–6 months. Full-time appliance wear is continued during the support phase for another 3–6 months to allow functional reorientation of trabecular system before any reduction of appliance wear occurs during the retention period.
- Stability is excellent after twin block treatment; this can be attributed partly to the support phase, during which a functional retainer is used to stabilize the corrected incisor relationship while the buccal teeth settle fully into occlusion.

Modifications of Twin Block

- Twin block for transverse development
- Twin block for sagittal development
- Twin block for transverse and sagittal appliance
- Twin block Crozat appliance
- Magnetic twin block appliance
- Twin block with a spinner
- Fixed twin block
- Reverse twin block
- Twin block hybrid appliance

Reverse Twin Block Appliance

Traditional twin block appliances by **Clark** is widely accepted and commonly used for the treatment of Class II malocclusions. Another variation of twin block, reverse twin block is used for correction of developing Class III malocclusion. In this, the occlusal inclined planes are reversed. Inclined planes are set at 70° such that upper arch receives forward component of force and distal and downward force to the lower molar region. Lower bite blocks cover lower molars and upper block covers upper deciduous molars and canines.

Invisalign Mandibular Advancement

- Invisalign treatment with mandibular advancement is meant for tweens and teens presenting with retrognathic Class II malocclusions in permanent dentition or stable late mixed dentition. The special feature of enhanced precision wings for Invisalign treatment with mandibular advancement are integrated into the Invisalign aligners.
- The benefits of Invisalign treatment with mandibular advancement with enhanced precision wings
  - Efficient treatment: Simultaneously moves the jaw forward while moving the patients' teeth.
  - Patient comfort: Patients report satisfaction and increased comfort when compared to traditional, fixed appliances.
- Clinical protocol
  - Record submission
  - Premandibular advancement (MA) phase (optional)
  - Mandibular advancement (MA) phase
  - Transitional phase
  - Standard Invisalign treatment
  - Retention

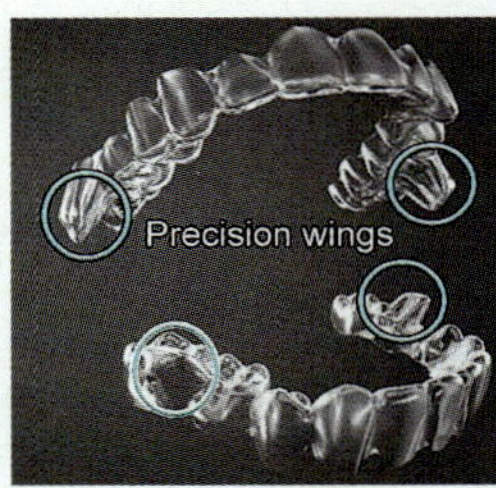

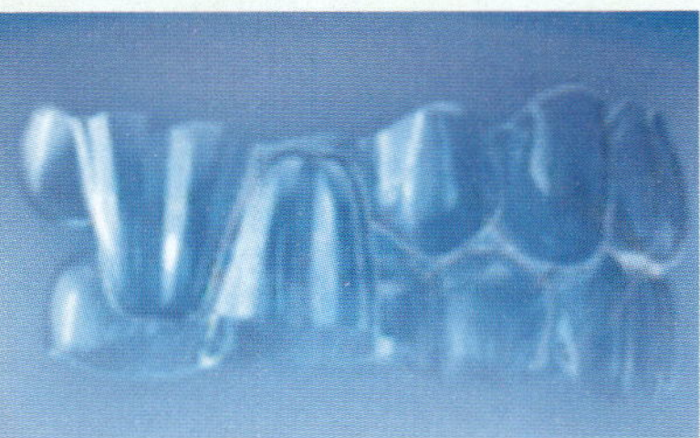

Graber Modification

- Maxilla: Modified by placing two expansion screws in the midline patients in whom significant expansion is desired during twin block treatment, the appliance becomes unstable and too flexible if only one midline screw is used. Each screw is activated once per week (≈0.2 mm) until adequate expansion is attained. Clasps are used to secure the appliance to the first molars
- Mandible: Clark recommendation using series of ball clasps lie in the interproximal areas between the canines and lower incisors. Modified by placing a labial bow anterior to the lower incisors that has labial acrylic similar to that of a lower spring retainer.

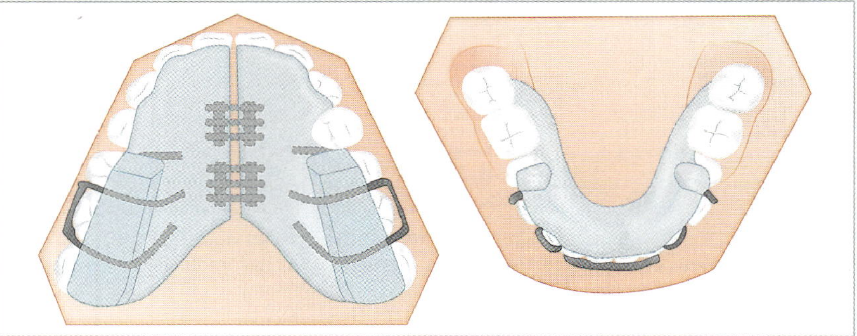

POINTS TO REMEMBER

- Tooth-borne passive myofunctional appliances have no intrinsic force-generating components such as springs or screws and depend on the soft tissue stretch and muscular activity to produce the desired treatment results, e.g. activator, bionator, Herbst appliance.
- Tissue-borne passive myofunctional appliances are mostly located in the vestibule and have little or no contact with the dentition, e.g., functional regulator of Frankel.
- Advantages of myofunctional appliances are that it enables elimination of abnormal muscle function thereby aiding is normal development, treatment can be initiated at mixed dentition, less chair side time as these appliances are mostly fabricated in laboratory, and patient acceptance is good.
- Limitations of myofunctional appliances are that they cannot be used in adult patients when growth has ceased, they cannot be used to bring abort individual tooth movement and these appliances are dependent on the patient for timely wear.
- Andresen and Häupl developed activator that induces musculoskeletal adaptation by introducing a new pattern of mandibular closure. Indicated in Class II div 1 and div 2, Class III and Class I open bite and deep bite.
- Frankel appliance was developed by Professor Rolf Frankel, and it helps in overcoming the abnormal perioral muscle activity and rehabilitates the muscles that are causing the problem.
- Bionator is used for the treatment of Class II div 1 and Class I malocclusions having narrow dental arches.
- Herbst appliance is a fixed functional appliance that was developed by Emil Herbst and is indicated in corrections of Class II malocclusion.
- The lip bumper can be called a modified vestibular screen that is used for muscular force application or for elimination. The appliance can be used in both the maxilla and the mandible to shield the lips away from the teeth.
- The twin block appliance was developed by Clark in 1977 as a two-piece appliance resembling a Schwartz double plate and a split activator that has simple bite blocks that effectively modify the occlusal inclined plane. The primary indication for twin blocks in early mixed dentition is in Class II div 1 in which prominent upper incisors rest outside the lower lip.

Questionnaire

1. Define myofunctional appliance and give its classification.
2. Write a note on vestibular screen.
3. Discuss the indications, contraindications, mode of action and modifications of activator.
4. Explain the bionator.
5. What is Frankel appliance and what are its various types?
6. Write a note on Herbst appliance.
7. What are the uses of lip bumper?
8. Describe the features, construction and treatment with twin block appliance.

FURTHER READING

1. Ackerman JL, Proffit WR. Preventive and interceptive orthodontics: a strong theory proves weak in practice. Angle Orthod. 1980;50:75-87.
2. Blomgren GA, Moshiri F. Bionator treatment in Class II, division 1. Angle Orthod. 1986;56:255-62.
3. Bogue EA. Orthodontia of the deciduous teeth. D Digest. 1913;19:79-88.
4. Chadwich SM, Banks P, Wright JL. Use of myofunctional appliances in the UK: a survey of British orthodontists. Dent Update. 1998;25:302-8.
5. Cheney EA. Aims and methods of treatment in the deciduous dentition. Am J Orthod. 1957;43:721-42.
6. Chen JY, Will LA, Niederman R. Analysis of efficacy of functional appliances on mandibular growth. Am J Orthod Dentofacial Orthop. 2002;122:470-6.
7. Frankel R. The role of Class II division 1 malocclusion with functional correctors. Am J Orthod. 1969;55:265-75.
8. Freeman JD. Preventive and interceptive orthodontics: a critical review and the results of a clinical study. J Prev Dent. 1977;4:7-23.
9. Harvold EP, Vargervik K. Morphogenetic response to activator treatment. Am J Orthod. 1971;60:478-90.
10. Hasler R, Ingervall B. The effect of a maxillary lip bumper on tooth positions. Eur J Orthod. 2000;22:25-32.
11. Houston WJB, Stephen CD, Tulley WJ. A textbook of orthodontics. 2nd edn. 1992. pp. 1-12.
12. Kloehn SJ. Mixed dentition treatment. Angle Orthod. 1950;20:75-96.
13. McNamara JA, Bookstein FL, Shaughnessy TG. Skeletal and dental changes following functional regulator therapy on Class II patients. Am J Orthod. 1985;88:91-110.
14. Moshe D, McInnis D, Lindauer J. The effects of lip bumper therapy in the mixed dentition. Am J Orthod Dentofac Orthop. 1997;111:52-8.
15. Moyers RE. Handbook of orthodontics for the student and general practitioner. 3rd edn. Chicago: Year Book Medical Publishers; 1973.
16. Nance HN. The limitation of orthodontic treatment: I. Mixed dentition diagnosis and treatment. Am J Orthod Oral Surg. 1947;33:177-233.
17. Popovich F, Thompson GW. Evaluation of preventive and interceptive orthodontic treatment between three and eighteen years of age. In: Tr Third Intern Orthod Congress; 1973. pp. 260-81.
18. Proffit WR, Fields HW. Contemporary orthodontics. 2nd edn. The development of orthodontic problems. 1993. pp.128-33.
19. Quadrelli C, Gheorgiu M, Margchetti C, Ghiglione V. Early myofunctional approach to skeletal Class II. Mondo Ortod. 2002;2:109-22.
20. West EE. Treatment objectives in the deciduous dentition. Am J Orthod. 1969;55:617-32.
21. Woodside DG, Metaxas A, Altuna G. The influence of functional appliance therapy on glenoid fossa remodeling. Am J Orthod. 1987;92:181-98.
22. Woodside DG, Reed RT, Doucet JD, Thompson GW. Some effects of activator treatment on the growth rate of the mandible and position of the midface. In: Tr. third Intern Orthod Congress; 1973. pp. 459-80.

Model Analysis

Nikhil Marwah, Vinola Duraisamy

CHAPTER OUTLINE

Model analysis is one of the most essential diagnostic aids to visualize the patient's occlusion from all aspects and also helps in making necessary measurements of teeth, dental arches, basal bone to carry out space analysis. The main advantage of this over other aids is that model analysis offers a three-dimensional view of the same.

Model analysis can be defined as the study of maxillary and mandibular arches in all the three planes of space (sagittal, vertical, transverse) and is a valuable tool in orthodontic diagnosis and treatment planning.

FUNDAMENTALS OF MODEL ANALYSIS

Study model analysis compares the space available and space required in a dentition.

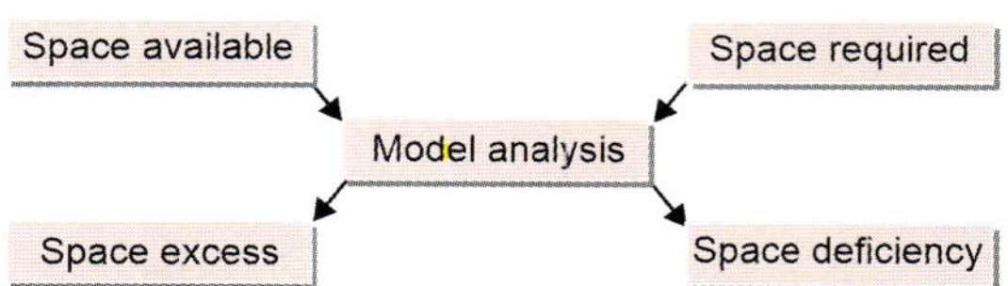

OBJECTIVES OF IDEAL STUDY MODELS

- Models should accurately reproduce the teeth and their surrounding soft tissue.
- Soft tissue should not be altered.
- Models should be well finished.

ADVANTAGES OF MODEL ANALYSIS

- They are three-dimensional records of the patient's dentition.
- Occlusion can be visualized from the lingual aspect.
- They provide a permanent record of interarch relationship.
- Helps to motivate patients as they can visualize the treatment progress.
- They are needed for comparison purposes at the end of treatment and act as a reference for post-treatment changes.

TYPES OF MODEL ANALYSIS

Permanent dentition	*Mixed dentition*	*Primary dentition*
• Pont's index	*Radiographic*	• Boston University approach
• Korkhaus analysis	• Nance Carey's analysis • Hay Nance mixed dentition analysis	• Boston University approach using Tanaka-Johnston analysis
• Linder Harth analysis	• Huckaba analysis	
• Arch perimeter analysis	*Non-radiographic*	
• Carey's analysis	• Moyer's mixed dentition analysis	
• Bolton's analysis	• Tanaka-Johnston analysis	

Contd...

Contd...

Permanent dentition	Mixed dentition	Primary dentition
• Ashley Howe's analysis	• Ballard and white	
• Peck and Peck index	*Combination*	
• Sanin-Savara tooth size analysis	• Hixon and Oldfather method	
• Schwarz analysis	• Staley Kerber • Total Space analysis	

PONT'S INDEX

Pont in 1909 presented a system whereby the measurement of the four maxillary incisors automatically established the width of the arch in the premolar and molar region **(Fig. 34.1)**.

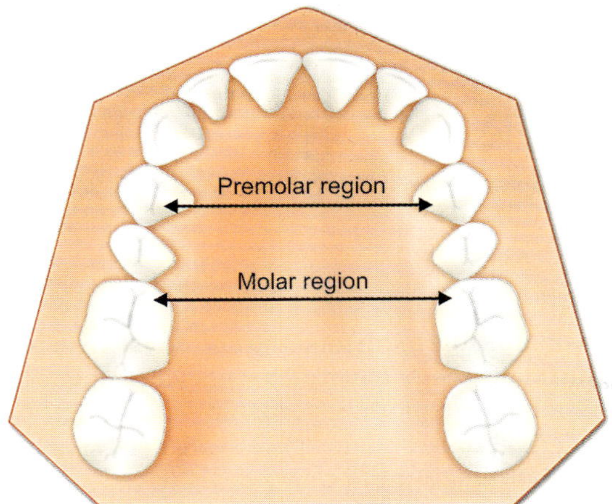

Fig. 34.1: Pont's index.

Uses

- Determining whether the dental arch is narrow or is normal.
- Determining the need for lateral arch expansion.
- Determining how much expansion is possible at the premolar and molar region.

Procedure

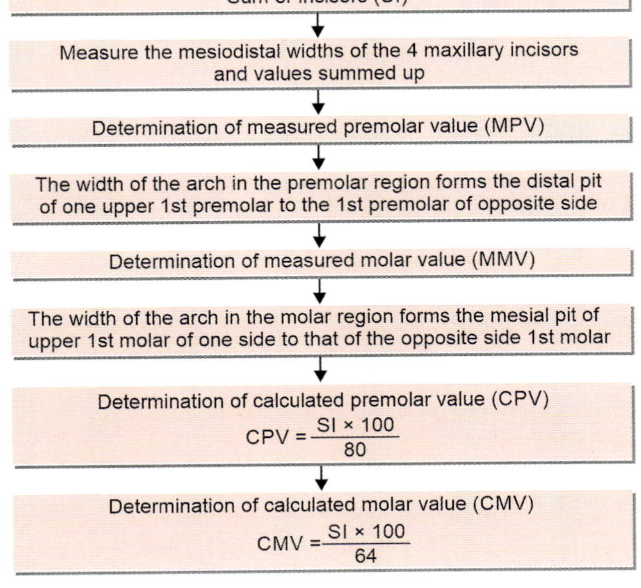

Inference

If the measured value is less than calculated value, it indicates the need for expansion. Thus, it is possible to know how much expansion is needed in the premolar and molar regions, respectively.

Drawbacks

- This is based on the study of French population and hence its universal validity is questionable.
- This analysis does not take into consideration the alignment of teeth.
- The analysis does not take into account the skeletal malocciusion.
- This analysis does not consider malformation of the teeth like peg laterals.

LINDER HARTH INDEX

This analysis is similar to Pont's analysis except that a new formula was used to determine the calculated premolar and molar values.

$$\text{Premolar value was calculated by} = \frac{(SI \times 100)}{85}$$

$$\text{Molar value was calculated by} = \frac{(SI \times 100)}{64}$$

KORKHAUS ANALYSIS

- This analysis is also similar to Pont's analysis, but he used Linder Harth's formula to determine the ideal arch width in the premolar and molar region **(Fig. 34.2)**. In addition, he also uses the measurements made from the midpoint of the interpremolar line to a point between the two maxillary incisors.
- According to Korkhaus, for a given width of upper incisors, a specific value of the distance between the midpoint of interpremolar line to the point between the two central incisors should exist.

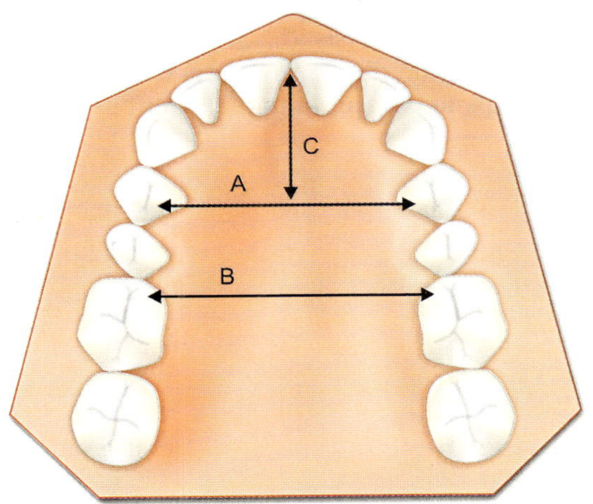

A. Arch width in premolar region
B. Arch width in molar region
C. 1st distance from midpoint of interpremolar line to point of incisor

Fig. 34.2: Korkhaus analysis.

- Korkhaus devised an instrument "the orthometer" which helps to measure the ideal arch width in premolar and molar region and also to know the perpendicular distance from the interpremolar line to the region in between the two incisors for a given sum of mesiodistal widths of the maxillary incisors.

Inference

If there is an increase in the perpendicular measurement, then ideally the anterior are proclined, and if it is less than this value, they are retroclined.

Advantages

This analysis not only tells about the ideal arch width but also about the ideal positioning of the anterior teeth.

S.No	Sum of incisors (in mm)	Arch width in premolar region (in mm)	Arch width in molar region (in mm)	Perpendicular distance from incision to interpremolar line (in mm)
1	27	32	41.5	16
2	27.5	32.5	42.3	16.3
3	28	33	43	16.5
4	28.5	33.5	43.8	16.8
5	29	34	44.5	17
6	29.5	34.7	45.3	17.3
7	30	35.5	46	17.5
8	30.5	36	46.8	17.8
9	31	36.5	47.5	18
10	31.5	37	48.5	18.3
11	32	37.5	49	18.5
12	32.5	38.2	50	18.8
13	33	39	51	19
14	33.5	39.5	51.5	19.3
15	34	40	52.5	19.5
16	34.5	40.5	53	19.8
17	35	41.2	54	20
18	35.5	42	54.5	20.5
19	36	42.5	55.5	21

ARCH PERIMETER ANALYSIS

This is an upper arch analysis. This analysis helps us to find out the difference between the basal bone and the tooth material, that is, it helps in determining the extent of discrepancy **(Fig. 34.3)**.

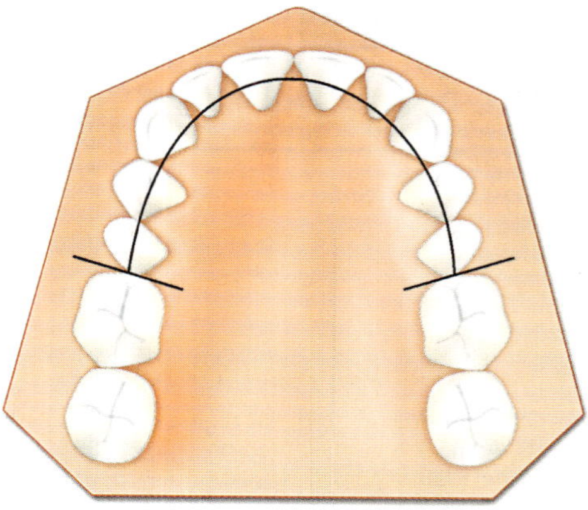

Fig. 34.3: Arch perimeter analysis.

Procedure

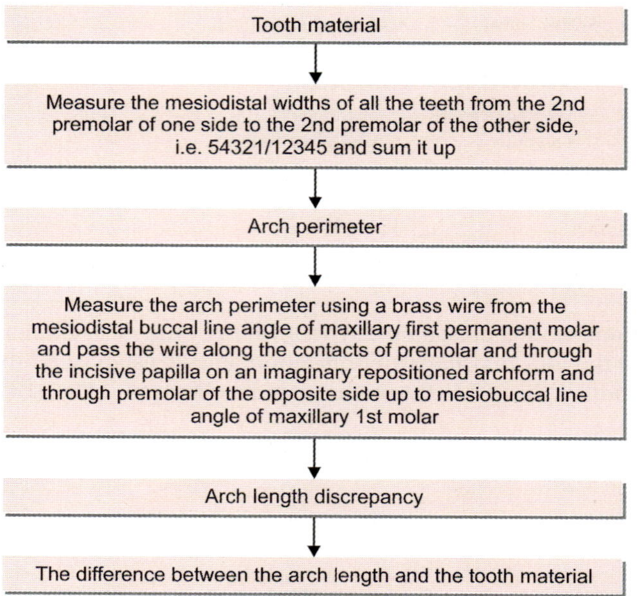

Tooth material
Measure the mesiodistal widths of all the teeth from the 2nd premolar of one side to the 2nd premolar of the other side, i.e. 54321/12345 and sum it up
Arch perimeter
Measure the arch perimeter using a brass wire from the mesiodistal buccal line angle of maxillary first permanent molar and pass the wire along the contacts of premolar and through the incisive papilla on an imaginary repositioned archform and through premolar of the opposite side up to mesiobuccal line angle of maxillary 1st molar
Arch length discrepancy
The difference between the arch length and the tooth material

Inference

- By comparing the tooth material and arch length required, we can obtain the extent of arch length discrepancy if tooth material more than space available—crowding.
- If tooth material less than space available—spacing if it is between 0 and 2.5 mm—non-extraction.
- If it is between 2.5 and 5 mm—second premolars extraction.
- If it is >5 mm—first premolar extraction.

NANCE AND CAREY'S ANALYSIS

This is same as arch perimeter analysis done for maxillary arch except that this is done on mandibular arch **(Fig. 34.4)**. The same steps as in arch perimeter analysis must be followed to determine:

- Tooth material (space required).
- Arch perimeter (space available).
- Arch length discrepancy.

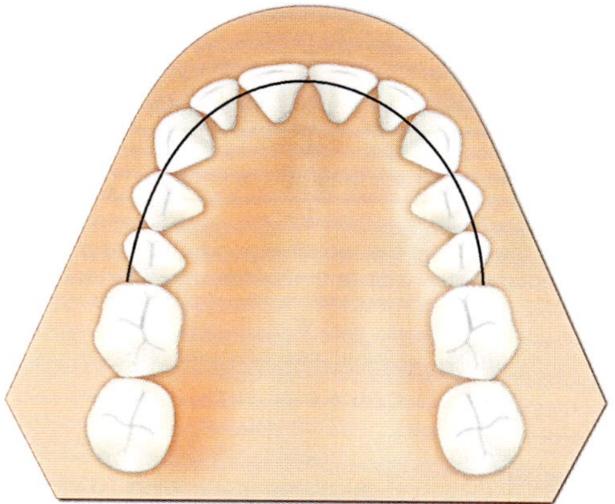

Fig. 34.4: Nance and Carey's analysis.

Procedure

- The arch length is measured anterior to the first permanent molar using a soft brass wire.
- Wire should be extended from mesial aspect of lower first permanent molar to buccal cusps of premolars and incisal edges of the anterior to continue up to mesial of the first molar of the contralateral side.
- If anteriors are proclined, brass wire should be passed along the cingulum of anterior teeth.
- If anteriors are retroclined, pass along the labial surface.
- The mesiodistal width of teeth anterior to first molar are measured and summed up as total tooth material.
- The difference between the arch length and the actual measured tooth material gives the discrepancy.

Treatment Plan

- If the discrepancy is 0–2.5 mm, it indicates minimal tooth material excess where proximal stripping is carried out to reduce the tooth material.
- If the discrepancy is between 2.5 and 5 mm, it indicates the need to extract the second premolars.
- A discrepancy of >5 mm indicates the need to extract the first premolars.

BOLTON'S ANALYSIS

- Also called Bolton's tooth size ratio analysis.
- It was introduced in the year 1952 by Wayne A Bolton.
- Bolton pointed out that the extraction of one tooth or several teeth should be done according to the ratio of tooth material between the maxillary and mandibular arch to get ideal interdigitation, overjet, overbite and alignment of teeth to attain an optimum interarch relationship.
- According to Bolton, a ratio exists between the mesiodistal widths of maxillary and mandibular teeth. He studied the interarch effects of discrepancies intooth size to devise a procedure for determining the ratio of total mandibular versus total maxillary tooth size versus maxillary anterior teeth size (**Fig. 34.5**).
- Average proportion between upper and lower teeth in overall and anterior region helps to create a normal overjet and overbite.

Procedure

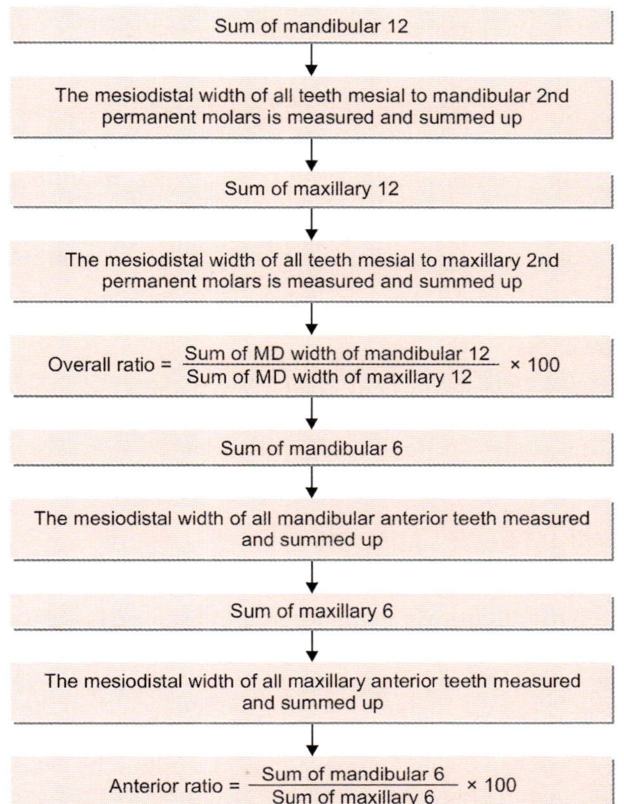

Sum of mandibular 12
The mesiodistal width of all teeth mesial to mandibular 2nd permanent molars is measured and summed up
Sum of maxillary 12
The mesiodistal width of all teeth mesial to maxillary 2nd permanent molars is measured and summed up
Overall ratio = $\frac{\text{Sum of MD width of mandibular 12}}{\text{Sum of MD width of maxillary 12}} \times 100$
Sum of mandibular 6
The mesiodistal width of all mandibular anterior teeth measured and summed up
Sum of maxillary 6
The mesiodistal width of all maxillary anterior teeth measured and summed up
Anterior ratio = $\frac{\text{Sum of mandibular 6}}{\text{Sum of maxillary 6}} \times 100$

Inference

- If overall ratio is <91.5%, it indicates maxillary tooth material excess which can be determined by:

$$\text{Sum of maxillary 12} = \frac{\text{Sum of maxillary 12}}{100} \times 91.3$$

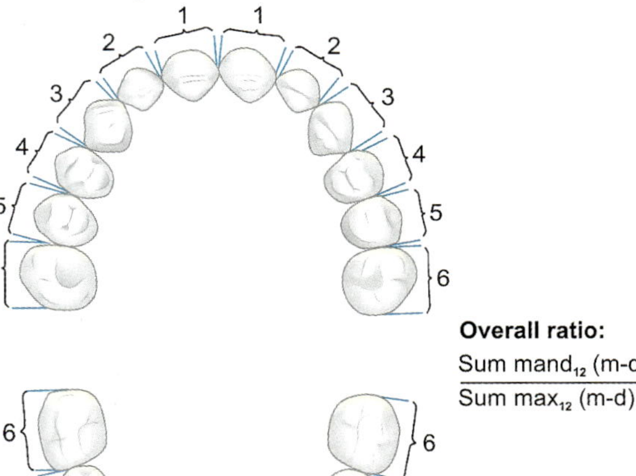

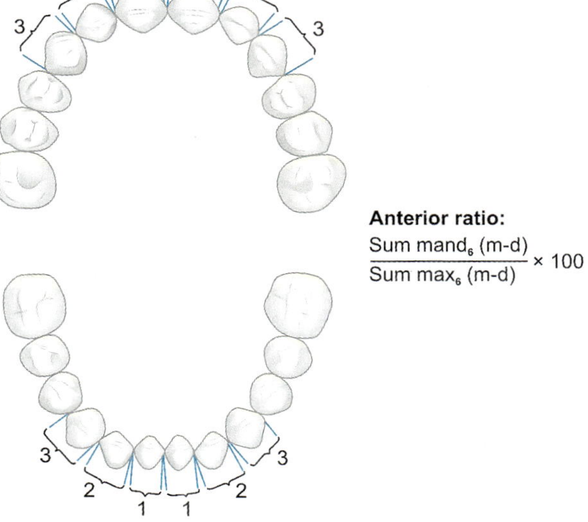

Fig. 34.5: Bolton's analysis.

- If overall ratio is >91.5%, it indicates maxillary tooth material lack which is determined by:

$$\text{Sum of mandibular 12} = \frac{\text{Sum of maxillary 12}}{91.3} \times 100$$

- If the anterior ratio is <77.2%, it indicates maxillary anterior excess which is determined by:

$$\text{Sum of mandibular 6} = \frac{\text{Sum of maxillary 6}}{100} \times 77.2$$

- If the anterior ratio is >77.2%, it indicates mandibular anterior excess which is determined by:

$$\text{Sum of maxillary 6} = \frac{\text{Sum of mandibular 6}}{77.2} \times 100$$

Drawbacks

- The study does not consider the sexual dimorphism in the maxillary canine width.
- The study was done on specific population; hence the values may change in other populations.

ASHLEY HOWE'S ANALYSIS

According to **Ashley Howe**, crowding is not only due to tooth size, but it can also result when there is inadequate apical base, that is, crowding is due to deficiency in arch width rather than arch length **(Fig. 34.6)**.

He found the relation between the total width of the 12 teeth anterior to the second molars and the width of the dental arch in the first premolar region. For this, he devised a formula to determine whether apical base of the patient could accommodate the teeth. It is done in both upper and lower arches.

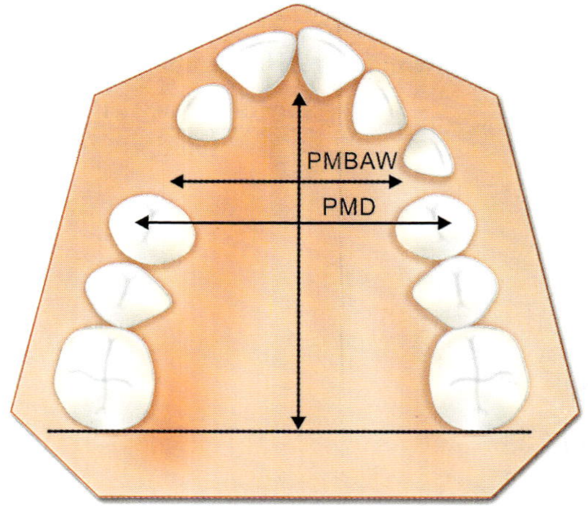

Fig. 34.6: Ashley Howe's analysis.

Inference

- If PMD > PMBAW, expansion is contraindicated.
- If PMBAW > PMD, expansion is possible.
- If PMBAW percent is–
  - Less than 37% → basal arch deficiency case, which requires extraction of teeth to manage the case.
  - 44% → ideal case and extraction not required.
  - Between 37% and 44% → borderline case.

Procedure

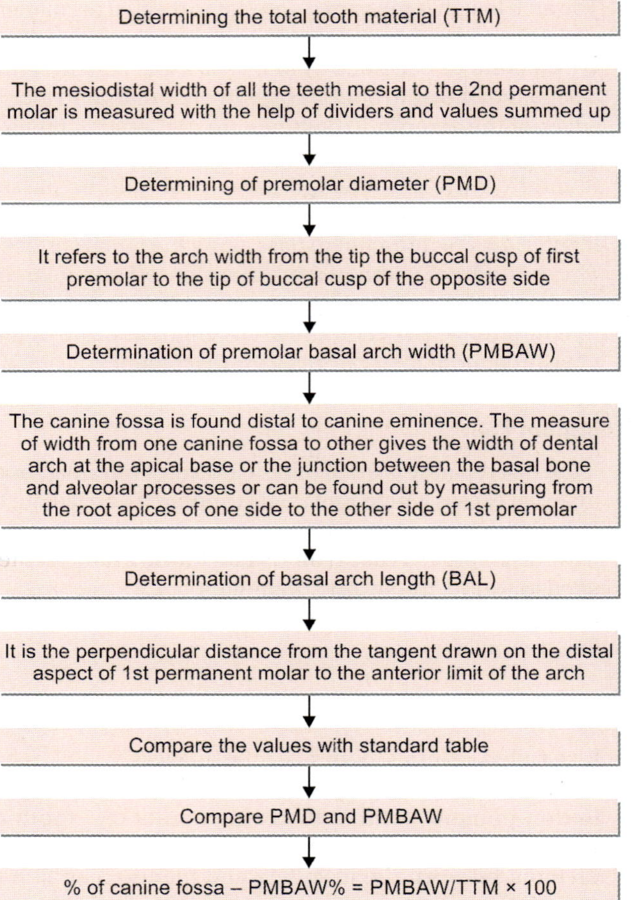

SANIN-SAVARA TOOTH SIZE ANALYSIS

- **Devised** by **Sanin** and **Savara** and colleagues (scholars of the University of Oregon).
- This is a simple and ingenious procedure to identify individual and group tooth size disharmonies.
- It makes use of precise mesiodistal measurements of crown size of each tooth, appropriate tables of tooth size distribution in the population and a chart for plotting the patients measurements. The teeth are measured with Boley gauge and tabulated.
- Mesiodistal crown-size relationship are decisive variables in search for factors associated with the development of occlusal and facial irregularities.
- The possible effects of discrepancies upon interdigitation during and after orthodontic treatment.
- The isolation of discrepant teeth of minor tooth malocclusions that may be treated in part by selective mesiodistal grinding and minor tooth movement.

PECK AND PECK INDEX

- Developed by **Harvey Peck** and **Sheldon Peck**.
- To determine the presence or absence of lower incisor crowding and related to shape (mesiodistal and facio-lingual) of the lower anterior teeth.

- This is done on the lower arch.
- Persons with ideal incisal arrangement have smaller mesiodistal width and comparatively larger labiolingual width than in persons with incisal crowding.

Procedure

Take the mesiodistal width of mandibular incisors individually (MD)

↓

Take the labiolingual width/faciolingual width of mandibular incisors individually (LL/FL)

↓

Calculate the proportion of MD of each tooth to the LL thickness of the tooth using formula

$$\frac{MD}{LL/FL} \times 100$$

- Mean value for mandibular central incisor = 88–92%
- Mean value for mandibular lateral incisor = 90–95%.

Inference

If the value for a given case is more than the mean value, then mesiodistal width of the tooth is more than the labiolingual width, and hence proximal stripping is indicated in such cases.

HIXON AND OLDFATHER METHOD

- It was given in the year 1956. It is the prediction method for the mandibular arch. It is mainly used for estimating the size of newly erupted canine and premolar.
- It's a combined form of mixed dentition space analysis.
- The original analysis which was given stated the measurement of the incisors on the left side of the arch. But modified **Hixon** and **Oldfather** method was given by **Staley** and **Kerber**. They revised this in a study they conducted in Iowa in 1980 called the Iowa facial growth study in which both the sides of the arch were used. They said that by using both sides of the midline the revised equation had a significantly reduced standard error.

Procedure

Mesiodistal width of the mandibular central incisor and lateral incisor are obtained from the cast

↓

Determine the width of the premolars from the intraoral periapical radiographs with paralleling technique

↓

Sum up the width of the central and lateral incisor along with the width of unerupted premolars of that particular side

↓

Estimated sum total width of the cuspids and bicuspids of that particular side can be obtained from the standard chart

↓

Measured sum width of incisors and bicuspids has a corresponding sum width of the cuspids and premolars in the chart

Using the measured value, the estimated value can be interpreted. The following values help in predicting the estimated tooth size.

Measured value	*Estimated tooth size*
23 mm	18.4 mm
24 mm	19.0 mm
25 mm	19.7 mm
26 mm	20.3 mm
27 mm	21.0 mm
28 mm	21.6 mm
29 mm	22.3 mm
30 mm	22.9 mm

Disadvantages

- Error is caused due to distortion of radiographic image.
- Can be used only in mandibular arch.

HUCKABA ANALYSIS

- It is also called as Proportional Equation Prediction Method and was given by **Huckaba GW**. He used both study casts and radiographs for determining the width of unerupted tooth.
- To compensate for enlargement of radiographic images, measure an object that can be seen both in radiograph and on the cast such as primary molar tooth. Accuracy of this method of determining the width of the unerupted tooth is fair to good, depending upon the quality of the radiographs and their position in the arch.
- This technique can be used both in maxillary and mandibular arches in all ethnic groups.
- Then a simple proportional relationship can be established as follows:

$$Y_1 = \frac{X_1 \times Y_2}{X_2}$$

Actual width of primary molar (X_1)
Apparent width of primary molar (X_2)
Actual width of unerupted premolar (Y_1)
Apparent width of unerupted premolar (Y_2)

Advantages

- Very easy, practical and relatively accurate method.
- Does not require any prediction table.
- Can be used in both maxillary and mandibular arches.

HAY NANCE'S MIXED DENTITION ANALYSIS

- It is similar to Carey's arch perimeter analysis in permanent dentition.
- It's a radiographic mixed dentition space analysis.

Procedure (Nanda 1993)

Measure the width of the unerupted tooth (cuspids and bicuspids) by using the IOPA
This can be called as the space required

↓

The total mesiodistal width of all the teeth in each quadrant indicates space required to accommodate permanent teeth

↓

Measure the arch perimeter from the mesial side of the first permanent molar to the contralateral side first permanent molar. This can be called as the space available

↓

The difference between the space required and available can be called as the arch length discrepancy

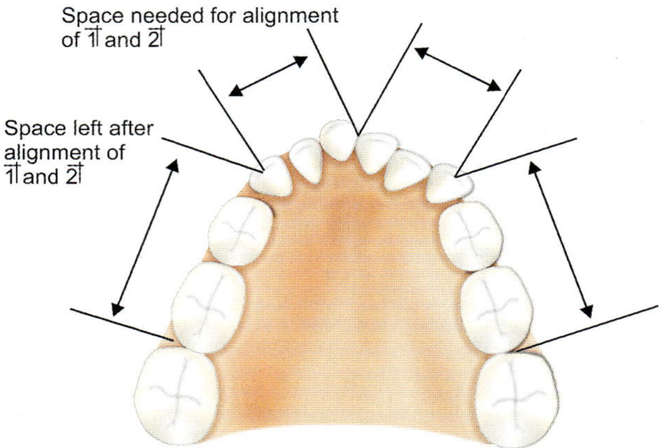

Fig. 34.7: Moyer's mixed dentition analysis.

Advantages

- Results in minimal errors.
- It can be performed with reliability.
- Allows analysis of both arches.

Limitations

- Requires cephalometric radiograph.
- Requires knowledge of Tweed's analysis and accurate tracing.
- Time-consuming.
- Needs whole mouth radiograph.

MOYER'S MIXED DENTITION ANALYSIS

- There is high correlation between sizes of different teeth in same individual, thus making it possible to predict the size of unerupted tooth by looking at the teeth present in oral cavity **(Fig. 34.7)**.
- Introduced by **Moyer**, in 1967.

Procedure (Table 34.1)

Measure the mesiodistal width of mandibular incisors

↓

Measure the space for mandibular cuspids and bicuspids from the distal of aligned lateral incisor to mesial aspect of 1st permanent molar

↓

Measure the space for maxillary cuspids and bicuspids from the distal aspect of aligned lateral incisor to mesial aspect of 1st permanent molar

↓

Using Moyer's probability chart find out sum total mesiodistal width of upper and lower cuspids and bicuspids for the given sum width of lower central and lateral incisors at 75% probability

↓

Compare the space available and space required in all four quadrants to determine arch length discrepancy

Inference

If the predicted value is greater than available arch length, crowding of teeth can be expected.

Advantages

- It has minimal error, and the range of possible error is precisely known.
- It can be done with equal reliability either by a beginner or by an expert.
- It is not time-consuming.
- It requires no special equipment.
- It can be done in the mouth as well on the cast.
- It may be used on both the arches.

Limitations

- It is a probability analysis.
- Does not account for tipping or rotation of mandibular incisors.
- Maxillary teeth size is predicted by mandibular teeth.
- It does not mention the population group from which they were calculated.
- Cannot be universally applied due to population variations.

TOTAL SPACE ANALYSIS

- This analysis was developed by **Leven Merrifield.**
- Here the lower arch is divided into three areas—anterior, middle and posterior to analyze the space required in the lower arch.
- Measurements from the study models and cephalograms are used in this analysis. This discrepancy for each area has to be calculated, and the resultant value is added together to yield the discrepancy of the arch.

Anterior Area

Space Required

- Measure the width of the mandibular incisors on the cast and the width of the cuspids from the radiographs.
- Cephalometric correction for the incisor positioning is calculated according to Tweed's method; TMIA is taken into consideration instead of IMPA of Tweed. The incisors are repositioned, and the difference in the actual and proposed TMIA is determined. The difference in angulation is multiplied by 0.8 to get the difference in mm.
- *Soft tissue modification:* Upper lip thickness is measured from the vermilion border of the upper lip to the greatest

Table 34.1: Probability tables for predicting the sizes of unerupted cuspids and bicuspids.

A. Mandibular bicuspids and cuspids

Males

21/12 =	19.5	20.0	20.5	21.0	21.5	22.0	22.5	23.0	23.5	24.0	24.5	25.0	25.5
%													
95	21.6	21.8	22.0	22.2	22.4	22.6	22.8	23.0	23.2	23.5	23.7	23.9	24.2
85	20.8	21.0	21.2	21.4	21.6	21.9	22.1	22.3	22.5	22.7	23.0	23.2	23.4
75	20.4	20.6	20.8	21.0	21.2	21.4	21.6	21.9	22.1	22.3	22.5	22.8	23.0
65	20.0	20.2	20.4	20.6	20.9	21.1	21.3	21.5	21.8	22.0	22.2	22.4	22.7
50	19.5	19.7	20.0	20.2	20.4	20.6	20.9	21.1	21.3	21.5	21.7	22.0	22.2
35	19.0	19.3	19.5	19.7	20.0	20.2	20.4	20.67	20.9	21.1	21.3	21.5	21.7
25	18.7	18.9	19.1	19.4	19.6	19.8	20.1	20.3	20.5	20.7	21.0	21.2	21.4
15	18.2	18.5	18.7	18.9	19.2	19.4	19.6	19.9	20.1	20.3	20.5	20.7	20.9
5	17.5	17.7	18.0	18.2	18.5	18.7	18.9	19.2	19.4	19.6	19.8	20.0	20.2
Females													
95	20.8	21.0	21.2	21.5	21.7	22.0	22.2	22.5	22.7	23.0	23.3	23.6	23.9
85	20.0	20.3	20.5	20.7	21.0	21.2	21.5	21.8	22.0	22.3	22.6	22.8	23.1
75	19.6	19.8	20.7	20.3	20.6	20.8	21.1	21.3	21.6	2.9	22.1	22.4	22.7
65	19.2	19.5	19.7	20.0	20.2	20.5	20.7	21.0	21.3	21.5	21.8	22.1	22.3
50	18.7	19.0	19.2	19.5	19.8	20.0	20.3	20.5	20.8	21.1	21.3	21.6	21.8
35	18.2	18.5	18.8	19.0	19.3	19.6	19.8	20.1	20.3	20.6	20.9	21.1	21.4
25	17.9	18.1	18.4	18.7	19.0	19.2	19.5	19.7	20.0	20.3	20.5	20.8	21.0
15	17.4	17.7	18.0	18.3	18.5	18.8	19.1	19.3	19.6	19.8	20.1	20.3	20.6
5	16.7	17.0	17.2	17.5	17.8	18.1	18.3	18.6	18.9	19.1	19.3	19.6	19.8

B. Maxillary bicuspids and cuspids

Males

21/12 =	19.5	20.0	20.5	21.0	21.5	22.0	22.5	23.0	23.5	24.0	24.5	25.0	25.5
(%)													
95	21.2	21.4	21.6	21.9	22.1	22.3	22.6	22.8	23.1	23.4	23.6	23.9	24.1
85	20.6	20.9	21.1	21.3	21.6	21.8	22.1	22.3	22.6	22.8	23.1	23.3	23.6
75	20.3	20.5	20.8	21.0	21.3	21.5	21.8	22.0	22.3	22.5	22.8	23.0	23.3
65	20.0	20.3	20.5	20.8	21.0	21.3	21.5	21.8	22.0	22.3	22.5	22.8	23.0
50	19.7	19.9	20.2	20.4	20.7	20.9	21.2	21.5	21.7	22.0	22.2	22.5	22.7
35	19.3	19.5	19.9	20.1	20.4	20.6	20.9	21.1	21.4	21.6	21.9	22.1	22.4
25	19.1	19.3	19.6	19.9	20.1	20.4	20.6	20.9	21.1	21.4	21.6	21.9	22.1
15	18.8	19.0	19.3	19.6	19.8	20.1	20.3	20.6	20.8	21.1	21.3	21.6	21.8
5	18.2	18.5	18.8	19.0	19.3	19.6	19.8	20.1	20.3	20.6	20.8	21.0	21.3
Females													
95	21.4	21.6	21.7	21.8	21.9	22.0	22.2	22.3	22.5	22.6	22.8	22.9	23.1
85	20.8	20.9	21.0	21.1	21.3	21.4	21.5	21.7	21.8	22.0	22.1	22.3	22.4
75	20.4	20.5	20.6	20.8	20.9	21.0	21.2	21.3	21.5	21.6	21.8	21.9	22.1
65	20.1	20.2	20.3	20.5	20.6	20.7	20.9	21.0	21.2	21.3	21.4	21.6	21.7
50	19.6	19.3	19.9	20.1	20.2	20.3	20.5	20.6	20.8	20.9	21.0	21.2	21.3
35	19.2	19.4	19.5	19.7	19.8	19.9	20.1	20.2	20.4	20.5	20.6	20.8	20.9
25	18.9	19.1	19.2	19.4	19.5	19.6	19.8	19.9	20.1	20.2	20.3	20.5	20.6
15	18.5	18.7	18.8	19.0	19.1	19.3	19.4	19.6	19.7	19.8	20.0	20.1	20.2
5	17.8	18.0	18.2	18.3	18.5	18.6	18.8	18.9	19.1	19.2	19.3	19.4	19.5

Measure and obtain the mesial–distal widths of the four permanent mandibular incisors and find that value in the horizontal row of the appropriate male or female table. Reading downward in the appropriate vertical column obtains the values for expected width of the cuspids and premolars corresponding to the level of probability you wish to choose.

Ordinarily, I use the 75% of probability rather than the mean of 50% since, although the values distribute normally toward crowding and spacing, crowding is a much more serious clinical problem, and the 75% predictive values thus protects the clinician on the safe side.

Note: That the mandibular incisors are used for the prediction of both the mandibular and maxillary cuspid and bicuspid widths.

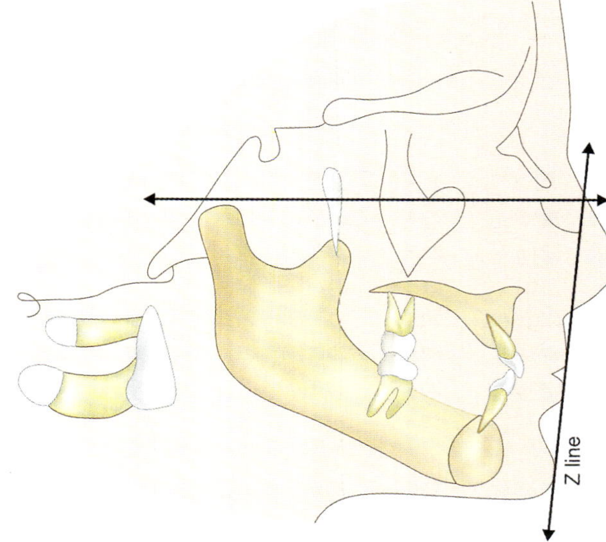

Fig. 34.8: "Z" angle of Merrifield.

curvature of the labial, surface of the central incisors. The total chin thickness is measured from the soft tissue chinto the NB line. If the lip thickness is greater than chin thickness, the difference is determined and multiplied by 2 and added to the space required.

- If it is less than or equal to chin thickness, no soft tissue modification is necessary.
- Measure the "Z" angle of Merrifield **(Fig. 34.8)** and add the cephalometric correction to it. If the correction "Z" angle is >80°, the mandibular incisor angulation was modified as necessary (up to IMPA of approximate 92°). If the corrected angle is <75°, additional uprighting of the mandibular incisor is necessary.

Space available: Measure the space available by using a brass wire from the mesiobuccal line angle of first primary molar of one side to the other.

Middle Area

Space required: MD width of the first permanent molars on the cast and measure the width of the unerupted premolar from the radiographs.

Curve of occlusion: A flat object is placed on the occlusal surface of mandibular teeth contacting the incisors and the first permanent molars. The deepest point between this flat surface and the occlusal surface of primary molars is measured on both the sides. This formula is applied to know the space required for leveling the curve of occlusion.

$$= \frac{\text{Depth on right side} + \text{depth of left side} + 0.5\,\text{mm}}{2}$$

Space available: It is measured using a brass wire from the mesiobuccal line angle of first primary molar to the distobuccal line angle of first permanent molar on either side.

Posterior Area

Space required: MD width of second and third molars is obtained from the radiographs as they might be unerupted. If these molars are not visible on the radiographs, Wheeler method is used for calculation, i.e.

$$X = \frac{Y - X^1}{Y^1}$$

where X is the estimated value of third molar in the individual patient, Y is the actual size of permanent mandibular first molar, X' is the Wheeler's value of third molar and Y' is the Wheeler's value of first molar.

Space available: The amount of space available consisted of space presently available on the casts and the estimated increase.

Inference

- *Space presently available:* This was obtained by measuring the distance on the occlusal plane tangent to distal surface of first permanent molars to the anterior border of ramus on a lateral cephalogram.
- *Estimated increase or prediction:* The estimated increase is 3 mm/year, i.e., 1.5 mm on either side until 14 years of age in girls and 16 years of age in boys. The age of the patient is subtracted from 14 or 16 according to the sex of the patient and is multiplied by 3 to obtain the estimated increase.
- *Total space deficit/discrepancy:* The total space deficit is arrived at by comparing the space required and space available in anterior, middle and posterior areas. Thus, this analysis tells us precisely where the discrepancy is present, i.e., in the anterior, middle or the posterior areas.

SCHWARZ MODEL ANALYSIS

- **Dr AM Schwarz** developed a simple analysis to determine the proper size of the arches for each patient.
- The Schwarz Model Analysis is used to determine the amount of expansion needed.

Indications

- Posterior crossbites.
- Constricted airway.
- Lack of space for all the permanent teeth to erupt properly.
- Narrow arches.
- Crowding.
- Improper space for the tongue to function normally.

Method

- To start the analysis first determine the Schwarz Index or SI by measuring the widest mesial-distal portion of the upper laterals and centrals **(Fig. 34.9).**
- If the laterals are not fully erupted or in case of peg laterals, you can estimate their size by subtracting 2 mm from the width of the centrals.
- To personalize this analysis, instead of adding 8 mm for the premolars and 16 mm for the molars, add the following amounts to compensate for the patient's facial type: Euryprosopic–8 mm/16 mm, mesoprosopic—7 mm/14 mm, leptoproscopic–6 mm/12 mm.

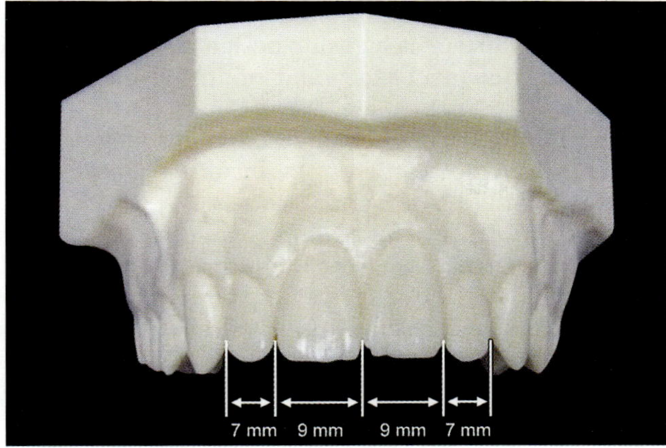

Fig. 34.9: Measurements of index.

- ❖ "Should be" measurement for premolar: After determining the SI, use that number to determine the ideal arch width in the 1st premolar area. To find the proper width, add 8 mm to the SI number. This will determine how wide the arch should be in the 1st premolar area for both arches.
- ❖ "Should be" measurement for the molars: To find the ideal arch width for the 1st molars add 16 mm to the SI number. It will determine how wide the arch should be in the 1st molar area for both arches.
- ❖ "Actual" measurement for premolars: The next step is to determine the "ACTUAL" measurement. Measure from the distal pit to the distal pit of the upper 1st premolars. On the lower arch, measure from the interproximal contact point to the interproximal contact point on the distal of the 1st premolar.
- ❖ "Actual" measurement for the molars: The next step is to determine the actual measurement for the molars. By measuring from the central fossa to the central fossa of the upper 1st molars the measurement is given under the actual column. On the lower arch measurement from the distal buccal cusp to the distal buccal cusp on the 1st molars is record.

Inference

- ❖ Determine the 'should be' and 'actual' measurements by subtracting the actual measurement from the should be measurement.
- ❖ If the actual measurement is greater than the should be measurement, the arches are wider than ideal.
- ❖ If the should be is greater than the actual measurement, then the arches are too narrow in either the premolar or molar area or both.

TANAKA-JOHNSTON ANALYSIS (1974)

- ❖ It was done as a study to check the repeatability of Moyer's analysis in a different population.
- ❖ It's a non-radiographic method of mixed dentition analysis suggested by **Tanaka** and **Johnston** in 1974.
- ❖ This method uses the width of the lower incisors to predict the widths of the unerupted cuspids and bicuspids of the upper and lower arch.
- ❖ They had conducted their study on 506 orthodontics patients in Cleveland.

Procedure

From permanent 1st molar on one side, mark the distances on casts in segments to the permanent 1st molar on the opposite side. Measure these segments over the contact points

↓

Add the measurements from step 1 to determine the total arch circumference

↓

Measure the mesiodistal widths of the mandibular central and lateral incisors

↓

Divide the sum of the widths of the mandibular incisors by 2 and add 10.5 mm for the mandibular arch

↓

This total gives the estimated size of the mandibular canine and the two premolars on one quadrant

↓

Double the total in step 6 for the canines and four premolars in the mandibular arch

↓

Subtract this dimension from the remaining space available in the arch to give a positive or negative total arch space

Available arch length = total arch length–sum of incisors + predicted width

+ Value: space surplus

– Value: space deficit

Tanaka and Johnston prediction values

- One half of the mesiodistal width of four lower incisors + 10.5 mm = estimated width of mandibular canine and premolar in one quadrant
- One half of the mesiodistal width of four lower incisors + 11.0 mm = estimated width of maxillary canine and premolar in one quadrant

Inference

- ❖ If the result is positive, there is more space available in the arch than is needed for the unerupted teeth.
- ❖ If the result is negative, the unerupted teeth require more space than is available to erupt into ideal alignment.

Advantages

- ❖ Improving on the Moyer's analysis, it is relatively accurate for children of European ancestry. The technique involves simple, easily repeated procedures and minimal material needs.
- ❖ It does not use prediction charts.
- ❖ No additional radiographs required.
- ❖ Reasonable accuracy.
- ❖ Can be applied to both the arches.

Limitations

There may be error in the predicted size of the unerupted teeth if patients are not of Northwestern European descent.

BOSTON UNIVERSITY APPROACH

- ❖ **Gianelly** proposed a prediction method, i.e., based on the mesiodistal widths (MDW) of primary mandibular canine and first molars with an idea for early prediction of unerupted permanent mandibular teeth widths.

- This was prepared in Boston University (BU) and hence named as the Boston University approach.
- This approach requires the presence of deciduous canines and first molars, which is as follows:

MD width of permanent mandibular canines and premolars	=	MDW of primary mandibular canine +2 (MDW of primary mandibular first molar)

Limitations

- Due to changes in arch dimension as well as position and inclination of primary dentition.
- The balance among the various functional and structural demands of the face and dentition are difficult to predict in an early age.

BOSTON UNIVERSITY APPROACH USING TANAKA-JOHNSTON VALUES[1]

In a new approach for primary dentition analysis, accurate prediction of canine and premolar dimension was made using the BU approach and comparing the obtained values using Tanaka-Johnston (T/J) method. It was observed that BU approach cannot be suggested in boys according to this method, although not much difference was found. However, the comparison of the mean values obtained through BU and T/J approaches showed an encouraging point.

Digital dental analysis[2]

Digital revolution that is transforming every human aspect is also affecting dentistry in a variety of ways; from electronic record keeping to newer diagnostic tools, technological advancement has helped to broaden access of dental facilities. On similar grounds, dental model analysis facilitates direct dental measurement model analysis is one of the orthodontic analyses to assess dental alignment and dental space whether the teeth are at appropriate positions and space for orthodontic treatment or dental extraction is in need. Traditional method is tedious and time-consuming with the help of software, we can perform dental width, dental arch measurement etc. Commercially available digital models can be produced by a direct or an indirect method. Indirect methods begin with dental impressions. Digital model scan then be obtained by laser scanning of plaster models or computed tomography imaging of the impressions or plaster models. The direct method uses an intraoral scanner to scan directly in the patient's mouth, making dental impressions redundant. This can be advantageous for patients with a gag reflex or with cleft lip and palate, who are at risk of aspiration and respiratory distress during taking of the dental impressions. Recently, the validity of digital models produced with an indirect method was evaluated in a systematic review by assessing the agreement of measurements on digital and plaster models. It was concluded that digital models offer a high degree of validity, and measurement differences are likely to be clinically acceptable.

CAST SCAN ANALYSIS

- **Yamamoto et al**, described an optical method for creating 3D computerized models using a laser beam on a cast. These computerized models are the platform for calculating distances by using designated software and estimating treatment effects and tooth movements in this way.
- OrthoCAD is such a system that is commercially available and provides the possibility of transforming impressions or plaster casts into 3D virtual models.
- **Tomassetti et al.** evaluated different measuring methods, including OrthoCAD, to calculate the Bolton tooth size analysis. OrthoCAD's values were found to be less correlated to the baseline values established by the average of three repeated measurements using Vernier calipers, than the values of the computerized digital calipers method (Hamilton Arch Tooth System).

Procedure

- The tooth size, intercanine and intermolar arch width are examined.
- On the computerized models, using the OrthoCAD measurement tools (version 1.17) with accuracy of 0.1 mm (method C).
- Measurements of arch width were performed on six of the setups, on the plaster, and on the computerized models. The upper and lower intercanine and intermolar widths were measured (**Fig. 34.10**). Using these measurements analysis can be carried out.

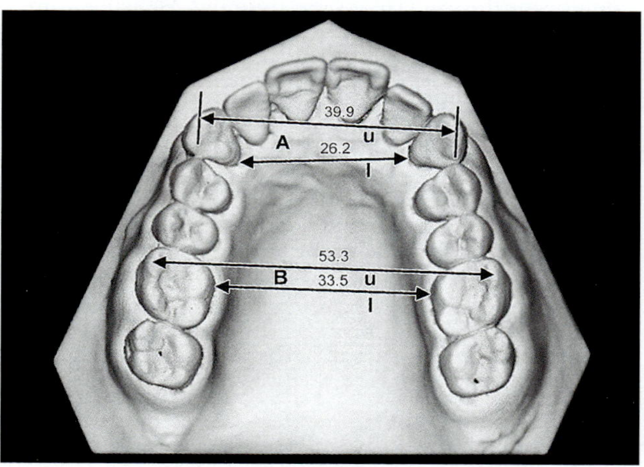

Fig. 34.10: Measurements in cast scan analysis.

Advantages

- Digital scan of the models provide a more reliable and stable configuration as hand-to-eye errors are eliminated.
- Storage of data is simpler and more concise.
- Reproducibility is very accurate.

Disadvantages

- Even though OrthoCAD is a real 3D model, the image viewed is only two-dimensional. Thus, identification of points, axes and planes becomes more difficult.
- It is very important for the observers to get familiar with the methods.

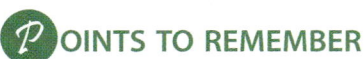

POINTS TO REMEMBER

- Model analysis can be defined as the study of maxillary and mandibular arches in all the three planes of space (sagittal, vertical, transverse) and is a valuable tool in orthodontic diagnosis and treatment planning.
- Permanent dentition analyses are Pont's index, Korkhaus analysis, Linder Harth analysis, Arch perimeter analysis, Carey's analysis, Bolton's analysis, Ashley Howe's analysis, Peck and Peck index, Sanin-Savara tooth size analysis.
- Mixed dentition analysis is Huckaba analysis, Hixon and Oldfather method, Moyer's mixed dentition analysis, Nance analysis, total space analysis.
- Korkhaus analysis is used to measure arch width in premolar and molar region. Carey's analysis is most frequently used for assessment of minor space issues. Bolton's analysis is used for tooth size ratio analysis.
- Huckaba analysis is used for determining the width of unerupted tooth. Moyer's analysis is the most reliable and comprehensive tool for space analysis.

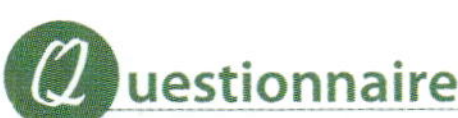

Questionnaire

1. Define model analysis and enumerate the mixed dentition analysis.
2. What is Carey's analysis?
3. Describe Huckaba model analysis.
4. Write a note on Bolton's analysis.
5. Describe Moyer's mixed dentition analysis.

REFERENCES

1. Nuvvula S, Vanjari K, Kamatham R, Gaddam KR. Primary dentition analysis: exploring a hidden approach. Int J Clin Pediatr Dent. 2016;9(1):1-4.
2. Bholsithi W, Sinthanayothin C. Digital dental model analysis. 13th International conference on biomedical engineering. pp. 472-5.

FURTHER READING

1. Adams CP, W John S Kerr. The design, construction and use of removable orthodontic appliances. 6th ed. Oxford 1995.
2. Bhalajhi SI. (2006) Orthodontics: The Art and Science. 3rd Edition, Arya (Medi) Publishing House, New Delhi.
3. Bolton WA. Disharmony intooth size and its relations to the analysis and treatment of malocclusion. Angle Orthod 1958;28:113-30.
4. Bolton WA. The clinical applications of a tooth size analysis. Am J Orthod. 1962;48:504-29.
5. Graber TM. Orthodontics: principles and practice. 3rd edn. 1972.
6. Joondeph DR, Riedel RA, Moore AW. Pont's index: a clinical evaluation. Angle Orthod. 1970;40:112-8.
7. Proffit WR. (2000) Contemporary orthodontics. 3rd edn, Mosby, St Louis.
8. Tanaka MM, Johnston LE. The prediction of the size of unerupted canines and premolars in a contemporary orthodontic population. J Am Dent Assoc. 1974;88:798-801.

CHAPTER

Pediatric Space Management

Nikhil Marwah, Ravi GR, Sharath Asokan, Joby Peter

CHAPTER OUTLINE

- Changes Seen after Premature Loss of Teeth
- Determinants of Appliance Selection
- Factors Contributing for Space Closure
- Classification of Space Maintainer
- Factors Affecting Planning for Space Maintainers
- Fixed Space Maintainers
- Band and Loop Space Maintainer
- Lingual Arch Space Maintainer
- Nance Palatal Arch Space Maintainer
- Transpalatal Arch
- Distal Shoe Space Maintainer
- Newer Modification of Space Maintainer
- Functional Space Maintainer
- Space Maintenance in Primary Anterior Region
- Anterior Esthetic Functional Space Maintainer
- Removable Space Maintainers
- Space Regainers

Pediatric Dentistry has increasingly shifted from a conservative restorative approach toward a concept of total pediatric patient care. Thus, all aspects of oral health care including diagnosis, prevention, oral medicine, restoration, and correction of malocclusion have increasingly become the responsibility of the pediatric dentist. Guidance of the eruption and development of the primary and permanent dentitions is an integral part of Pediatric Dentistry, and it should contribute to the development of a permanent dentition that is in harmonious, functional, and esthetically acceptable occlusion.

In the quest for providing optimal dental care, the age old saying "prevention is better than cure" holds true. In this endeavor, the pedodontist is most evenly poised to carry the mantle of providing the required services. For the preventive approach to be truly effective, it needs to apply at its earliest, that is, at the primary prevention level. This key difference between prevention and interception lies primarily in the matter of timing. Unlike preventive orthodontic procedures that are aimed at elimination of factors that may lead to malocclusion, interceptive orthodontics is undertaken at a time when malocclusion is developing. Thus, interceptive orthodontics basically refers to measure undertaken to prevent a potential malocclusion from progressing into a more severe one.

DEFINITIONS

Preventive Orthodontics

Graber *(1966) has defined preventive orthodontics as the action taken to preserve the integrity of what appears to be normal occlusion at a specific time.*

Interceptive Orthodontics

American Association of Orthodontists (1969) *defined it as that phase of science and art of orthodontics employed to recognize and eliminate the potential irregularities and malpositions in the developing dentofacial complex.*

Space Maintenance

This term was coined by **JC Brauer** *in 1941. It is defined as the process of maintaining a space in a given arch previously occupied by a tooth or a group of teeth.*

Space Control

Gainsforth *in 1955 defined it as careful supervision of the developing dentition; it reflects an understanding of the dynamic nature of occlusal development.*

Space Supervision

Moyers *defines, "when the judgment of the dentist determines that the individual patient's occlusion will have a better chance of obtaining optimum development through supervised intervention of the transitional dentition than without clinician directed supervision."*

Space Maintainer

According to ***Boucher****, it is a fixed or removable appliance designed to preserve the space created by the premature loss of a primary tooth or a group of teeth.*

Objectives of space maintenance
- Preservation of primate space
- Preservation of the integrity of the dental arches
- Preservation of normal occlusal planes
- In the case of anterior space maintenance, it should aid in esthetics and phonetics

CHANGES SEEN AFTER PREMATURE LOSS OF TEETH

The dentition is designed to function as a single unit, retained spatially by the sum of forces exerted upon each individual member. Three district forces, that is, occlusal, muscular, and eruptive forces contribute to space closure. The effort on each segment of the arch is different.

Buccal Segment

- **First primary molar area:** The loss of first primary molar may be maxillary, mandibular, or both; unilateral or bilateral space maintainers should always be placed. An abnormally high tongue position coupled with a strong mentalis and buccinators muscle may be damaging to the occlusion after the loss of a mandibular primary molar. A collapse of the lower dental arch and distal drifting of anterior segment will be the result. The potential for space loss is greater during eruption of first permanent molars since this is the time when the permanent molar exerts a strong eruptive force against the distal crown surface of second primary molar. A space maintainer should be in place at this time to prevent second primary molar from being displaced by first permanent molar. The maxillary first permanent molar usually erupts distally and begins a rotation to swing forward once the cusp tips appear through the tissue at the eruption site. The permanent molar then contacts the second primary molar in a less direct eruptive force. However, at the time of contact, there should be a space maintainer in place to resist the potential for mesial displacement of second primary molar.
- **Second primary molar area:** The potential for space loss is even greater when second primary molars are lost because they normally serve as a buttress for permanent molar eruption. The earlier the tooth is lost, the greater is the space management problem because of the influence these primary molar have on first permanent molar eruption. Maxillary permanent molar erupts distally and then swings forward to contact the second primary molar. If the latter is missing and no space appliance is placed, it is common for the maxillary first permanent molar crown to continue to swing mesially, until it come in contact with first molar thus blocking out the second premolar. The mandibular first permanent molar strongly depends on the presence of second primary molar distal crown surface for eruptive guidance. Thus, if the primary tooth is lost during permanent molar eruption, the latter will continue its mesial eruption pathway to produce a severe space loss and tipped position.

Anterior Segment

- **Primary canine area:** Early loss of primary canines is more common due to erupting lateral incisors rather than caries. If the loss is unilateral, there will be midline shift due to the migration of larger permanent incisor segment into the space during the process of adjustment. The midline will deviate to the side of space loss. Loss of primary cuspid could contribute to an additional decrease in circumference of arch by permitting lingual tipping of permanent incisors from the force of orbicularis oris and its associated muscles. When early loss of a primary cuspid has occurred as a result of insufficient length of the arch, it is best to remove the opposite primary cuspid to permit the permanent incisors to tip toward a symmetrical alignment and reinforce with a space maintainer.
- **Primary incisor area:** Primary incisors may be lost prematurely through early childhood caries or by traumatic injuries at any age. When loss of teeth occurs at ages close to normal exfoliation, space maintenance is not needed. But if there is still time for the permanent incisors to erupt, a space maintainer must be given for speech development, esthetics, and prevention of social trauma for child.

Ronnerman (1974) study:
- Most common to least common prematurely lost primary molar
- Maxillary second molar (72%) > mandibular second molar (61%) > mandibular first molar (38%) > maxillary first molar (30%)

SS Ahmed (2012):
- Prevalence of early loss of primary teeth was higher in boys (9.28%) than girls (7.22%)
- Prevalence of early loss of primary teeth was higher at 8 years of age
- Lower first primary molars were most commonly affected by early loss followed by upper first primary molars
- More number of teeth was lost in the right side when compared with the left

Loss of Individual Teeth

No other factor plays a more significant role in preventive and interceptive orthodontics than the preservation of primary dentition till its normal time of exfoliation. The primary teeth provide a mold for the proper growth of the jaws, so that the permanent teeth may have an adequate space for aligning themselves. Premature loss of a primary tooth or a group of teeth will lead to a wide range of implications **(Tables 35.1 to 35.3)**.

Cavalcantal AL[1] studied the prevalence of early loss of primary molars in schoolchildren in the city of Campina Grande, PB, Brazil. The results showed that 24.9% of the sample had loss of primary molars, but no differences were observed between genders ($P > 0.05$). There was larger loss prevalence among the 9-year olds (27.2%) and the most commonly missing teeth were the lower primary molars (74.3%).

Table 35.1: Loss of individual tooth.

Loss of maxillary primary 1st molar	• The primary cuspid shifts distally in the first year only, if at all • The 1st permanent molar and second primary molar shift mesially, with the amount depending on the duration of absence and age at loss • An erupting first bicuspid is guided along the mesial surface of the mesially migrating second primary molars, eventually lying close to the lateral incisor
Loss of maxillary primary 2nd molar	• If the maxillary second primary molar is lost early, the second bicuspid is generally impacted • The permanent molar shifts mesially • The cuspid and first primary molar shift distally • As the first bicuspid generally has an eruption timing advantage over the second bicuspid, will erupt earlier into the site, maintained by the first primary molar, often with distal drift • The resultant lack of space between the permanent molar and first bicuspid causes impaction of the second bicuspid
Loss of mandibular primary molar	• The effect of mandibular extractions tends to be similar for all three situations, i.e., loss of primary 1st molar, 2nd molar, or both • Timing differentials between the cuspid, first bicuspid, and second bicuspid in the mandible appear to account most for the similarity among groups • In case of loss of first primary mandibular molar, the permanent molar and second primary molar both tips forward • In case of loss of second primary mandibular molar, the permanent molar tips forward • In case of loss of first and second primary mandibular molars, the permanent molar will tip forward and primary canine will tip distally leading to impaction of bicuspids and also causing midline shift

Table 35.2: Space maintenance in the primary dentition.

Missing primary tooth	*Suggested treatment*	*Reason*
Maxillary incisor	No space maintenance required	No consequence. Exception: If incisor(s) is (are) lost prior to primary canine eruption, space closure may be observed
Maxillary canine	Band and loop space maintainer	Decrease possibility of midline shift
Maxillary 1st molar	Band/crown loop space maintainer	Prevents loss in arch dimension
Maxillary 2nd molar	Distal shoe space maintainer*	• Guides 1st permanent molar into proper position • Prevents loss in arch dimension
Mandibular incisor	No space maintenance required	No consequence. Exceptions: • If incisor(s) is (are) lost prior to primary canine eruption, space closure may be observed • Pre-existing incisor crowding (tendency of incisors to tip lingually)
Mandibular canine	Band and loop space maintainer	Decreases possibility of midline shift
Mandibular 1st molar	Band/crown loop space maintainer	Prevents loss in arch dimension
Mandibular 2nd molar	Distal shoe space maintainer*	• Guides 1st permanent molar into proper position • Prevents loss in arch dimension

*If second primary molar extraction site has healed, space maintenance may be deferred until bony eruption of the first permanent molar. At that time, a reverse band and loop space maintainer or space-regaining procedure can be employed to guide or reposition the first permanent molar into proper position.

Table 35.3: Space maintenance in the mixed dentition.

Missing primary tooth	*Suggested treatment*	*Reason*
Maxillary lateral incisor Maxillary canine	Extract antimere Prior to eruption of permanent lateral incisor(s): Removable space maintainer After eruption of permanent lateral incisor(s): Extract antimere	Decrease possibility of midline shift • Guides permanent lateral incisor into proper position • Decreases possibility of midline shift
Maxillary 1st molar	Prior to eruption of permanent lateral incisor(s): Nance appliance	• Prevents loss in arch dimension • Does not interfere with eruption of permanent laterals
	After eruption of permanent lateral incisor(s): Band/crown loop space maintainer	Prevents loss in arch dimension
Maxillary 2nd molar Mandibular lateral incisor Mandibular canine	Nance appliance Extract antimere Prior to eruption of permanent lateral incisor(s): Removable space maintainer	Prevents loss in arch dimension Decreases possibility of midline shift • Requires only minor adjustment to afford normal positioning of permanent incisors. • Decreases possibility of midline shift
	After eruption of permanent lateral incisor(s): Stopped lingual arch space maintainer	• Decreases possibility of midline shift • Prevents lingual tipping of permanent incisors
Mandibular 1st molar	Prior to eruption of permanent lateral incisor(s): Band/crown loop space maintainer	• Prevents loss in arch dimension • Does not interfere with eruption of permanent incisors
	After eruption of permanent lateral incisor(s): Lingual arch space maintainer	• Prevents loss in arch dimension • Permits distolateral repositioning of primary canine
Mandibular 2nd molar	Prior to eruption of permanent lateral incisor(s): Band/crown loop space maintainer	• Prevents loss in arch dimension • Does not interfere with eruption of permanent incisors
	After eruption of permanent lateral incisor(s): Lingual arch space maintainer	• Prevents mesial tipping of 1st permanent molar • Prevents loss in arch dimension

Indications of space maintainers

- If the space after premature loss of primary teeth shows signs of closing.
- If the use of space maintainer will aid in or make the future orthodontic treatment less complicated.
- If the need for treatment of mal occlusion at a later date is not indicated.
- When the space for a permanent tooth should be maintained for 2 years or longer.
- To avoid supraeruption of a tooth from the opposing arch.
- To improve the physiology of a child's masticatory system and restore dental health optimally.

Contraindications of space maintainers

- If the radiograph of extraction region shows that the succedaneous tooth will erupt soon.
- If the radiograph of extraction region shows one third of the root of succedaneous tooth is already calcified.
- When the space left by prematurely lost primary tooth is greater than the space needed for the permanent successor as indicated radiographically.
- If the space shows no signs of closing.
- When succedaneous tooth is absent.

Requirements of space maintainers

- It should maintain the entire space created by the lost tooth It must restore function.
- Prevent supraeruption of opposing tooth It should be simple in construction.
- Should be strong enough to withstand occlusal forces.
- Should permit maintenance of oral hygiene.
- Must not restrict the growth of jaws.
- It should not exert undue forces of its own.

DETERMINANTS OF APPLIANCE SELECTION

There are some factors that govern the selection of space maintaining appliance (according to DCNA 1978):

- **Patient cooperation:** Greater patient cooperation is needed for removable appliance. Unlike fixed appliance patients, removable appliance wearers should wear the appliance for a given time.
- **Integrity of the appliance:** When considering long- term wear, the frequency with which the appliance breaks or is lost must be considered.
- **Maintenance:** With normal usage, the clasps or the acrylic or removable appliances may require minor adjustments. The cement on the abutment areas of fixed appliances often disintegrates with time and loose bands will lead to decalcification of the underlying enamel due to food stagnation and acid production. Thus, periodic removal of appliance, checking for decalcification, polishing of tooth and cementation is necessary.
- **Modifiability:** If a successor tooth erupts out of alignment the wire of a fixed appliance may be difficult to adjust. Anticipating future modifications owing to occlusal development can reduce the number of appliances required.
- **Limitations:** The clinician should project the number of appliances needs for the patient whenever possible.
- **Time:** Usually the time required to construct removable acrylic appliances is greater than for fixed appliance.
- **Oral hygiene status and caries risk of the patient**: When selecting a space maintainer we should assess the oral hygiene status and caries risk of the patient especially for a fixed space maintainer.

FACTORS CONTRIBUTING FOR SPACE CLOSURE

- Inclination of long axis of permanent molars—tendency of molar to shift mesially because their long axis is mesially inclined.
- Premature loss of primary teeth.
- Influence of buccal musculature—buccinators exerts forces that can derange occlusion.
- Path of least resistance—this is created following loss of support because of extraction or missing tooth.
- Effect of position of center of rotation of mandible: **Smyd** pointed out that more the axis of mandibular rotation is lowered in respect to occlusal plane, less is the amount of horizontal thrust transmitted to teeth in occlusion.

CLASSIFICATION OF SPACE MAINTAINERS

According to Hitchcock	*According to Raymond C Thourow*	*According to Hinrichsen*
• Removable or fixed or semifixed	• Removable	• Fixed space maintainers *Class I*
• With bands or without bands	• Complete arch—Lingual arch and extraoral anchorage	• Nonfunctional types—bar type, loop type
• Functional or nonfunctional	• Individual tooth	• Functional types—pontic type, lingual arch type *Class II*
• Active or passive		• Cantilever type (distal shoe, band, and loop)
• Certain combinations of the above		• Removable space maintainers—acrylic partial dentures

Classification of Removable Space Maintainers

Brauer classified removable dentures for children as follows:

- **Class 1:** Unilateral maxillary posterior.
- **Class 2:** Unilateral mandibular posterior.
- **Class 3:** Bilateral maxillary posterior.
- **Class 4:** Bilateral mandibular posterior.
- **Class 5:** Bilateral maxillary anterior posterior.
- **Class 6:** Bilateral mandibular anterior posterior.
- **Class 7:** One or more primary of permanent anterior.
- **Class 8:** Complete primary.

FACTORS AFFECTING PLANNING FOR SPACE MAINTAINERS

Time Elapsed Since Tooth Loss

- It was stated by **McDonald** and **Avery**[2] that if space closure is going to occur, it will usually take place within 6 months after the loss of tooth. Therefore, the appliance must be placed as soon as possible, following the extraction of tooth.
- Incidence of closure appears to be related to the length of time since extraction; the longer the time, the greater the incidence.

Seipel (1946) reported 98% closure for spaces present >14 months.
Weber's (1949) 87% closure figure was based on an average 6 months closure.
Seward (1965) and **Breakspear** (1961) reported 99% and 98% for incidence of closure in spaces present for more than a year.

Amount of Space Loss

Maxillary spaces close faster as compared to mandibular spaces.

Research studies regarding space loss

- **Pederson et al.** (1978) documented a frequency of 50% population who underwent changes owing to premature extractions.
- **Olsen** (1959) stated that greater loss occurs in mandible owing to a mesial axial orientation of first molar.
- **Cohen** (1941), **Seipel** (1949), **Richardson** (1965)[3] stated that loss of second primary molar will cause greater space loss.
- **Stewart**:[4] More severe space loss in terms of mm is in maxillary arch, but more severe space loss in terms of clinical management is in lower arch because molar space is more difficult to regain in this arch.
- **MacGregor** reviewed the dental literature, and based on his review of the literature, he recommended the following: Maintain space of maxillary and mandibular incisors only if lost prior to eruption of the primary canines because the canines "may push the primary laterals mesially" causing space loss in the quadrant; maintain the space if a primary canine is prematurely lost to prevent midline shift; and it is not necessary to maintain space for prematurely lost mandibular primary incisors after the eruption of the canines "because the lower arch is inside the upper arch space loss ensues; space reopens when the permanent teeth erupt."
- **Tunison et al** (2008)[5] explained that immediate space loss of 1.5 mm per arch side in the mandible and 1 mm in the maxilla was found. The magnitude, however, is not likely to be of clinical significance in most cases. Nevertheless, in cases with a severe predisposition to arch length deficiency prior to any tooth loss, this amount of loss could have treatment implications.
- **Kisling** determined that after the age of 7.5–8 years (and thus after eruption of the permanent first molars), space maintainers need not be inserted when a primary first molar loss occurs.
- **Padma Kumari** and **Retnakumari** (2006)[6] conducted a study of 46–49-year old in which extraction space (D space), intermolar arch width, length, and perimeter were measured on the casts in cases of unilateral extractions. Maximum space loss occurred in first 4 months. D space decreased 0.64, 1.3, 1.64, and 1.75 mm at the 2-, 4-, 6-, and 8-month time points.
- **Laing et al** (2009)[7] and **Northway** (2000) concluded that following the premature loss of the maxillary first primary molar, the permanent canine will become impacted. Thus, while there was more space loss associated with the loss of a second primary molar than with a first primary molar, the space loss caused by the latter led to the impaction of the permanent maxillary canines.

	Maxilla		*Mandible*	
	D (mm)	*E (mm)*	*D (mm)*	*E (mm)*
First year	1.3	2.8	1.8	2.4
Second year	1.8	4.5	2.7	3.1
Third year	3.2	8.0	3.3	4.5

Rate of Space Closure

- Younger the patient, more is the space loss.
- Maximum space is lost during first 6 months of extraction and most immediate loss is within 76 hours with maximum impact being in first 24 hours due to collapse of bony trabeculae thus allowing of ease of movement of adjacent teeth.

- According to **Breakspear**:[8,9]
  - Space loss after loss of first maxillary molar is 0.8 mm
  - Space loss after loss of first mandibular molar is 0.9 mm
  - Space loss after loss of second maxillary molar is 2.2 mm
  - Space loss after loss of second mandibular molar is 1.7 mm.
- According to **Clinch**[10] and **Healy**:
  - Space loss before eruption of permanent molar is 6.1 mm
  - Space loss after eruption of permanent molar is 3.7 mm.
- **Helm** (1970) supported that space closure is more common in the mandibular segments.
- **Ronnerman** and **Thilander** (1978) said that space closure is more common in the maxillary segment.

Direction of Space Closure

- **Stewartes**[4] (1965) noted that in maxilla, all except one of 12 extraction spaces closed by mesial migration of teeth distal to the extraction space. In mandible, all space losses >2 mm were brought about mainly by a distal movement of the teeth mesial to the space.
- **Rose** (1966) states that space closure can occur in two ways either through forward migration or rotation of teeth distal to the site of extraction.

Eruption Status of the Adjacent Teeth

It helps us ascertain mesial shift for molars and distal tipping for canines.

Amount of Bone Coverage Over the Tooth

According to **McDonald**[2] 1 mm of bone resorbs in 4–5 months. If 1 mm or more bone is overlying the succedaneous tooth, it is an indication for space maintainer. If the space is >2 mm, fixed appliance, and if <2 mm, removable appliance.

Eruption Status of the Succedaneous Tooth

- It is estimated by the amount of root completion (tooth erupts in oral cavity after two-third root formation).
- According to **Sleichter CG** (1962) a faster eruption of the succedaneous tooth is anticipated if it has penetrated the cortical plate. In such condition need for a space maintainer depends on the clinical condition.
- According to **Mickey Mantle** Rule (Rule of 7 for Primary Molars) eruption delays before exfoliation age of 7 and accelerates after exfoliation age of 7. i.e., the effect decreases with increasing age.

Dental Age of Patient

It is the age calculated according to the last tooth erupted in oral cavity in normal eruption sequence. This involves recognizing the teeth clinically present in the oral cavity in comparison to dental eruption charts. It can also be calculated according to the methods of **Gustafson** and **Koch** or **Gron** and **Moorrees.**

Sequence of Eruption

Knowledge of usual eruption sequence is important. For example, if the mandibular primary second molar is prematurely lost and mandibular second permanent molar is erupting before the second premolar, arch length loss secondary to mesial forces generated on first permanent molar as the second permanent molar erupts can occur with subsequent space loss.

Delayed Eruption of Permanent Teeth

Over-retained or ankylosed primary teeth, or impacted permanent teeth, can result in a delay of the eruption process. With the removal of these types of primary teeth, an appliance may be needed to hold the space until the permanent tooth erupts into a normal position.

Available Space

An evaluation of the available space should be performed to determine whether the deficiency is developmental or a result of the pre-existing condition. A space analysis conducted in the mixed dentition, will aid the practitioner in a prediction of the amount of available space for the unerupted permanent teeth. A decision may be made at this point on the type of space maintenance that is appropriate.

Arch Length Adequacy

This will be estimated by position of incisors, leeway space, and incisor liability.

Curve of Spee

According to **Andrews**, ideal occlusion will have a near flat curve of Spee, thus additional space can be gained (1 mm of space is gained per 1 mm of depth of curve of Spee).

Abnormal Oral Habits

- They will exert abnormal pressure on dental arches and so may influence the type and planning of space maintainer.
- Strong mentalis muscle patterns may have a negative effect after loss of mandibular molars or canines with collapse of the arch and distal drifting of the anterior segment.
- Thumb or digit sucking habits may also produce abnormal forces initiating collapse of the dental arches after premature loss of primary teeth.
- Tongue thrusting habit is associated with hyperactive mentalis and inferior orbicularis oris.

Interdigitation

- It is another variable influencing space control. Cuspal height is believed to contribute to the stability of the dentition.
- **Gould** (1965) and **Devey** (1967) stressed about importance of cuspal interlocking and cuspal height, respectively. **Gould** states that cuspal interlocking will act as a physical barrier for the migration of the teeth after extraction, whereas **Davey** suggested that high cusps inhibit drifting. Hence the assessment of the type of interdigitation and its stability is extremely important when projecting the need for appliance therapy.

Miscellaneous Factors

These factors influence planning because they may be associated with either space gain or space loss. Some of these factors are:

- **Growth of jaws:** during the eruption of permanent lateral incisors, inter canine space increases to accommodate permanent lateral incisors. During this time a space maintainer that doesn't interfere with the arch development should be given.
- **Proximal caries:** MOD caries especially in second primary molar causes loss of E space due to the mesial migration of permanent first molars. An appropriate space maintainer should be designed to prevent this.
- Length of the edentulous area and the number of teeth lost.
- Space loss and early loss of primary teeth: according to **Sleichter CG** (1962) a faster eruption of the succedaneous tooth is anticipated if it has penetrated the cortical plate. In such condition need for a space maintainer deepens on the clinical condition.

FIXED SPACE MAINTAINERS

Fixed space maintainers are the appliances, which are fixed onto the teeth and utilize bands or crowns for their construction.

Advantages of Fixed Space Maintainers

- Bands require no tooth preparation.
- Do not interfere with eruption of abutment teeth.
- Jaw growth is not hampered.
- Succedaneous tooth is free to erupt.
- Can be used in uncooperative patients.

Disadvantages of Fixed Space Maintainers

- Elaborate instrumentation and skills required.
- Banded tooth is more prone to caries and decalcification.
- Supraeruption of opposing tooth.

Fabrication of Fixed Space Maintainers

- Band construction.
- Taking the impression and cast preparation.
- Loop fabrication.
- Soldering.
- Polishing.
- Cementation.

Armamentarium (Figs. 35.1A to C)

- Stainless steel band material or preformed bands.
- Pliers—contouring pliers, band forming pliers, band seater or pusher, band adapter, hoe pliers straight and curved, band cutting scissors, bird beak pliers, crimping pliers, three-pronged pliers, universal pliers.
- Stainless steel wires (round).
- Spot welding unit, soldering unit, silver solder, flux.
- Wire cutter.
- Finishing burs, polishing stones.

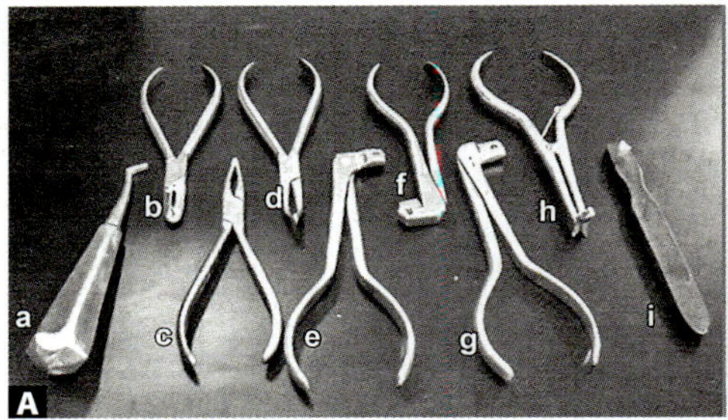

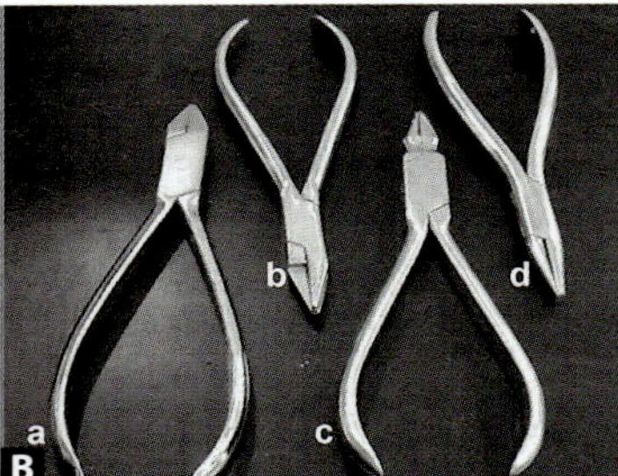

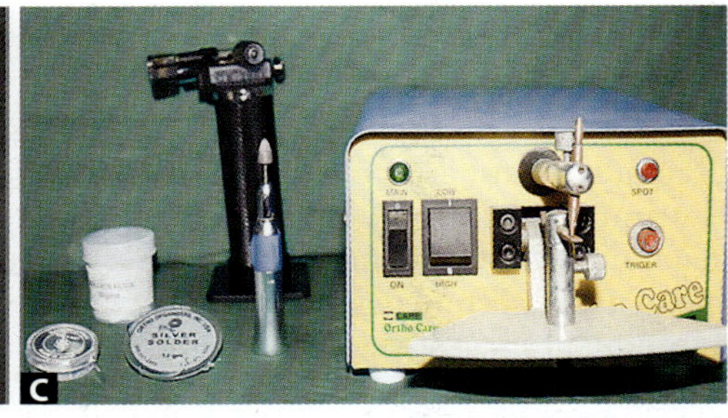

Figs. 35.1A to C: (A) Band forming armamentarium: a—Band pusher/adapter, b—Contouring plier, c—Straight hoe plier, d— Curved hoe plier, e and f—Peak pliers (rt/lt side), g—Peak plier (universal), h—Bird beak plier (universal), i—Band seater; (B) Loop forming armamentarium: a—Adams plier, b—Three-pronged plier, c—Universal plier, d—Optic plier; (C) Armamentarium for band pinching.

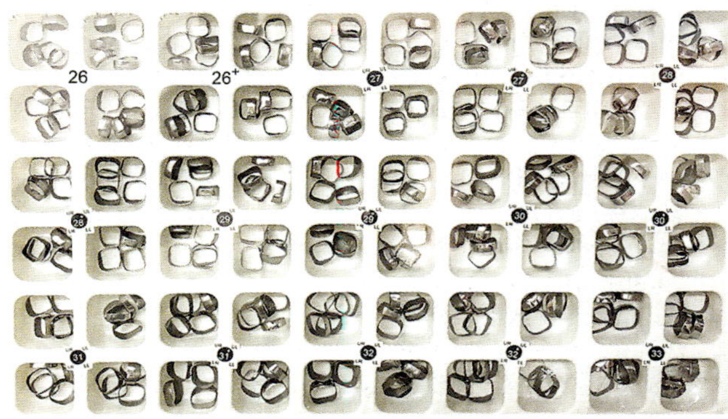

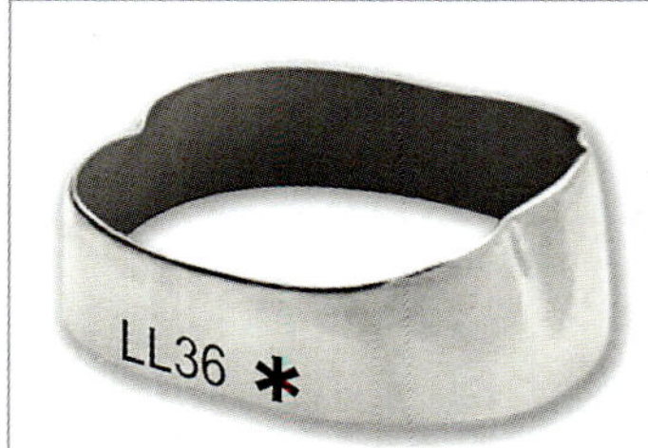

Fig. 35.1D: Preformed seamless bands.

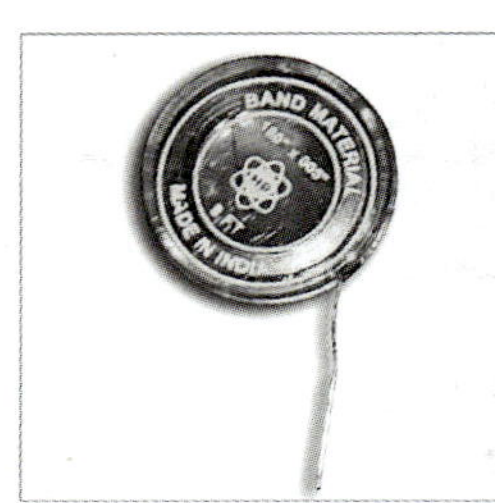

Fig. 35.1E: Band material.

Band Construction

The making of a properly fitting, contoured, strong band is a very important undertaking for fixed appliances or space maintainers. The band forms can be classified as:

According to Fabrication

Loop bands

- Precious metal (first introduced by Johnson).
- Chrome alloy bands.

Tailored bands

- Precious metal.
- Chrome alloy.

Preformed seamless bands **(Fig. 35.1D)**

Chrome alloy or precious metal, which are adapted, festooned, and stretched to fit. A range of preformed bands from 1 to 32 depending on the mesiodistal width of the tooth for the maxillary and mandibular arch are available commercially.

According to Band Material (Fig. 35.1E)

- Anterior teeth: 0.003 × 0.125 × 2 in.
- Bicuspids: 0.004 × 0.150 × 2 in.
- Primary molars: 0.005 × 0.180 × 2 in.
- Permanent molars: 0.006 × 0.180 × 2 in.

Band Fabrication

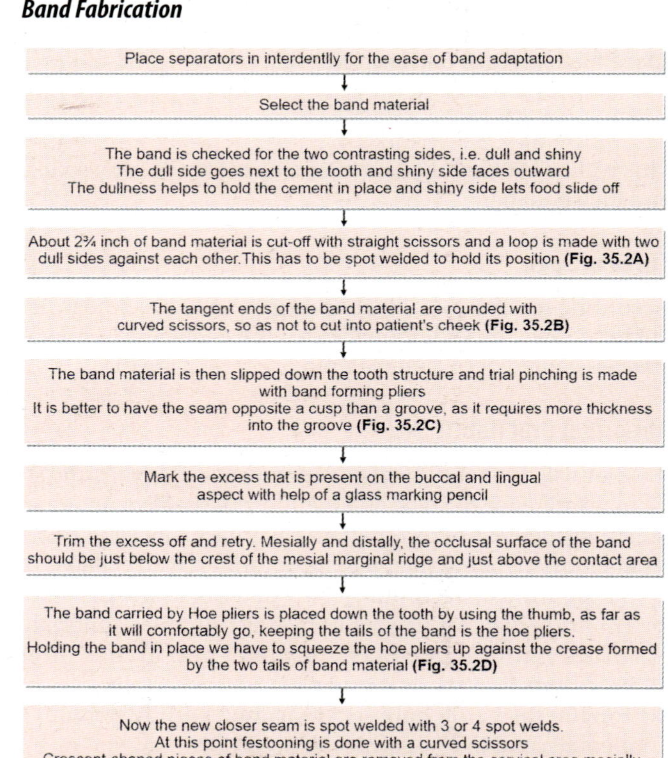

Place separators in interdentlly for the ease of band adaptation
↓
Select the band material
↓
The band is checked for the two contrasting sides, i.e. dull and shiny
The dull side goes next to the tooth and shiny side faces outward
The dullness helps to hold the cement in place and shiny side lets food slide off
↓
About 2¾ inch of band material is cut-off with straight scissors and a loop is made with two dull sides against each other.This has to be spot welded to hold its position **(Fig. 35.2A)**
↓
The tangent ends of the band material are rounded with curved scissors, so as not to cut into patient's cheek **(Fig. 35.2B)**
↓
The band material is then slipped down the tooth structure and trial pinching is made with band forming pliers
It is better to have the seam opposite a cusp than a groove, as it requires more thickness into the groove **(Fig. 35.2C)**
↓
Mark the excess that is present on the buccal and lingual aspect with help of a glass marking pencil
↓
Trim the excess off and retry. Mesially and distally, the occlusal surface of the band should be just below the crest of the mesial marginal ridge and just above the contact area
↓
The band carried by Hoe pliers is placed down the tooth by using the thumb, as far as it will comfortably go, keeping the tails of the band is the hoe pliers.
Holding the band in place we have to squeeze the hoe pliers up against the crease formed by the two tails of band material **(Fig. 35.2D)**
↓
Now the new closer seam is spot welded with 3 or 4 spot welds.
At this point festooning is done with a curved scissors
Crescent-shaped pieces of band material are removed from the cervical area mesially and distally. These concave cuts are blended into the buccal and lingual cervical portions of the band by trimming burs **(Fig. 35.2E)**
↓
Band is now ready for final seating. After placing the band pull the band from lingual aspect squeezing the excess out. Hold the band firmly in this position with the help of finger pressure from buccal aspect and pinch the band with peak pliers **(Fig. 35.2F)**
↓
Remove the band and spot weld at the new contact, cutting the excess off **(Figs. 35.2G and H)**
↓
Now refit the band and fold the seam in distal direction **(Figs. 35.2I and J)**
↓
Remove it and solder the seam. Trim any sharp points and polish the band before refitting **(Figs. 35.2K and L)**

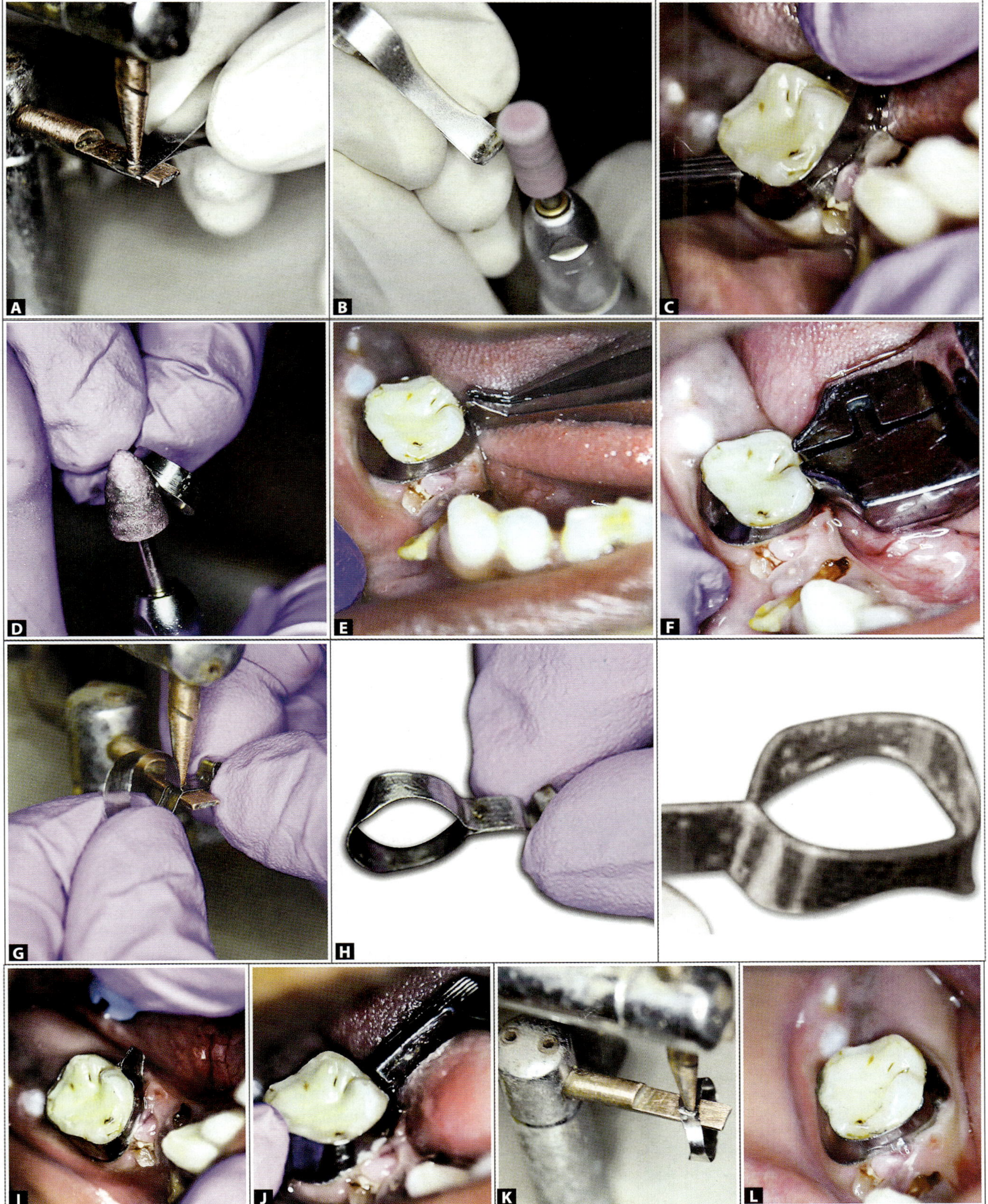

Figs. 35.2A to L: Band pinching procedure: (A) Initial spot weld; (B) Rounding off margins; (C) Buccal groove adaptation; (D) Initial trimming of band to adapt to gingival margins; (E) Pinching with hoe pliers; (F) Final pinching with peak pliers; (G) Spot welding as close as possible to the joint after pinching; (H)Presentation of band; (I)Seating of band; (J) Infolding of seam; (K) Final spot welding of band seam; (L) Completely adapted band.

Impression Making and Cast Preparation

An alginate impression of the banded tooth and appropriate abutment is made. Full arch impression is taken for lingual arch and Nance appliance, whereas a sectioned impression can be taken when planning a Band and Loop space maintainer. After taking the impression band, remover pliers is used to remove the band and place it into the impression in the same position that it occupied on the tooth. Stabilize and pour the cast.

Band Stabilization

After band pinching, the bands will be transferred to the impression. In the impression tray, their position can be reinforced by using different materials in order to avoid displacement of the band during casting process.

Sticky wax

- It is heated over the flame and dripped over the mesial and distal surfaces of the molar bands seated in the alginate impression. This hot sticky wax is known to capture and hold the band without displacement, while pouring the cast.
- **Limitation:** It does not really adhere well to alginate, besides any slight over vibration during pouring the stone, the band tend to move out of position.

Orthodontic wires

- Short sections of stainless steel wires (0.020) can be placed and dental stone poured. On the retrieved cast, the protruding wires at the base of the band needs to be trimmed before appliance fabrication.
- **Limitation:** If the wire segment is not positioned passively, it can push the band deeper into the impression thereby affecting the fit of the finished appliance.

L-shape wire

- 0.032" wires can be inserted from buccal to lingual across the banded molars. Instead of pouring the stone, it should be painted over the impression with a brush and the final fill has to be done with a spatula. A disc can be used to cut the protruding ends of the wires to flush with the model in the set cast.

Stapler pins

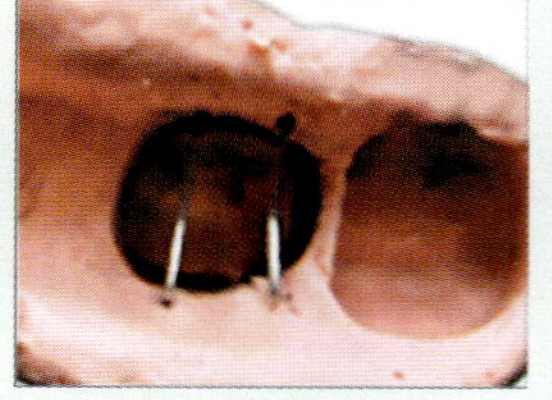

- Two stapler pins per band can be inserted into the alginate impression buccolingually with the help of tweezers over the exposed edges of the band. After casting, the exposed ends of stapler pins have to be trimmed.
- **Limitation:** These pins are non-sturdy; there could be chances of its displacement due to the vibration produced during casting, resulting in an inaccurate model.

Bobby pins

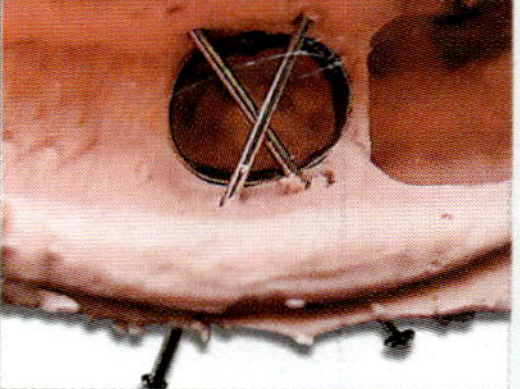

- Two bobby pins can be placed diagonally to stabilize the band. The pins should pass through the perforations in the tray running from buccal to lingual side through the set alginate impression material, bisecting the band to form an "X." They should be removed before the final set of the stone.
- **Limitation:** They should be placed passively as it would tend to push the band gingivally if active. Besides, failure to remove pins before final set of stone would result in fracture of the final cast.

Cyanoacrylate

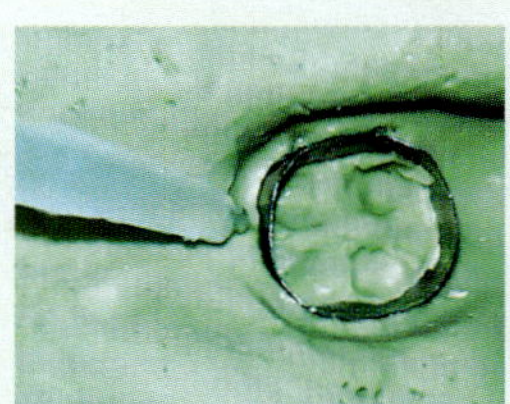

- A drop of this glue can be added at the mesial and distal margins of the orthodontic band where it contacts the impression material. It sets rapidly when it comes in contact with moisture. It is the easiest and lesser time-consuming method.
- **Limitation:** If more of cyanoacrylate glue is added to stabilize band and not cleaned from the final model, it could contaminate the solder joint area as the metal is heated.

Green stick compound

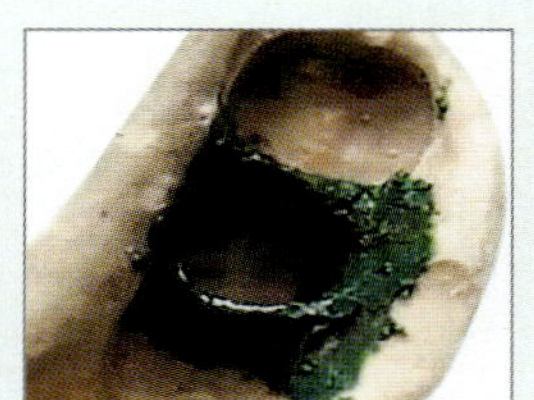

- It is softened and flown over the circumference of the band. Wax spatula is heated over the flame and is used to spread the compound over the flanges of the impression; the heated spatula is run through the inner surface of the band to merge the compound with the band. Blow torch is used to glisten the surface of the compound. The impression is then washed in running tap water so that the compound hardens, dental stone is poured once the cast has set, it is then immersed in hot water such that the green stick compound surrounding the band softens and is easily pried away with a Lecron Carver. It is very efficient, as it provides added retention to the band.
- **Limitation:** It is an elaborate and time-consuming procedure.

(*Source:* Balaji S, Gurusamy K, Sangeeta P, Neerja R. Different techniques of bank stabilization in the impression for space maintainer: clinical aid in pediatric dentistry. Eur J Pharm Med Res. 2016;3(7):157-60).

Loop Fabrication (Figs. 35.3A to G)

This is formed using round stainless steel wire. The thickness and the design of loop are different for all space maintainers and are discussed individually.

Soldering (Figs. 35.4A and B)

Quick set plaster is used to position the adapted wire on the working model. Reducing zone of the solder torch is used for soldering. A generous amount of flux should be applied above and below the point where wire contacts band. A piece of solder is transferred to solder joint with a pair of utility pliers. The flame is redirected toward the cast and the joint is heated till it is red hot and the solder flows evenly. Immediately dip this in water and remove appliance.

Finishing and Polishing (Figs. 35.5A to C)

A finished solder joint should be smooth and free of porosity. A green stone is used to contour the soldered joint to a smooth transition with the band. Rubber wheels are relied upon to reduce surface roughness, and gold rouge or rag wheel is used for final polishing.

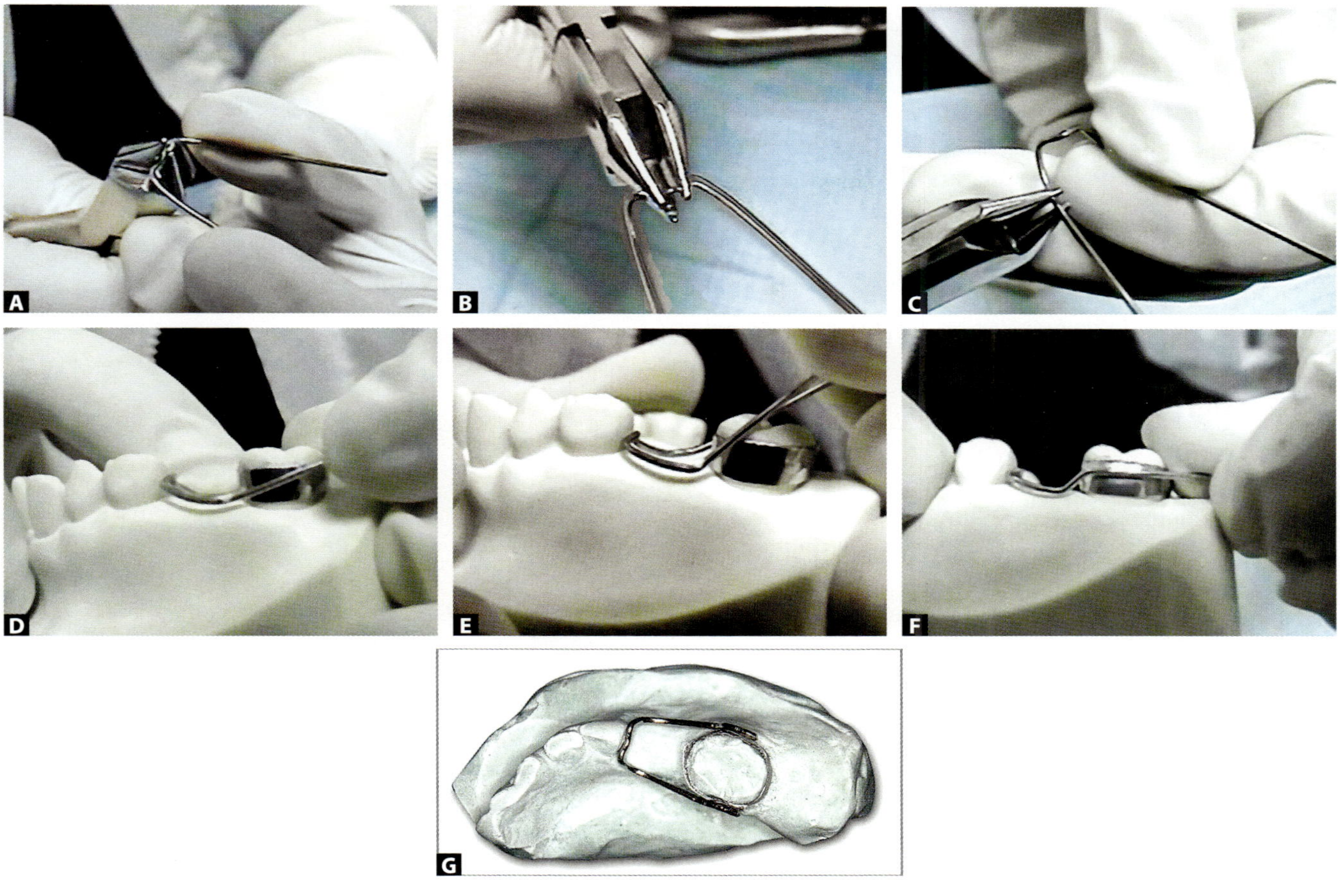

Figs. 35.3A to G: (A) Initial loop fabrication; (B) Curve formation with three prong plier; (C) Adaption according to mucosa; (D) Marginal adaption of loop; (E) Retentive band of loop; (F) Complete loop placement; (G) Final loop presentation.

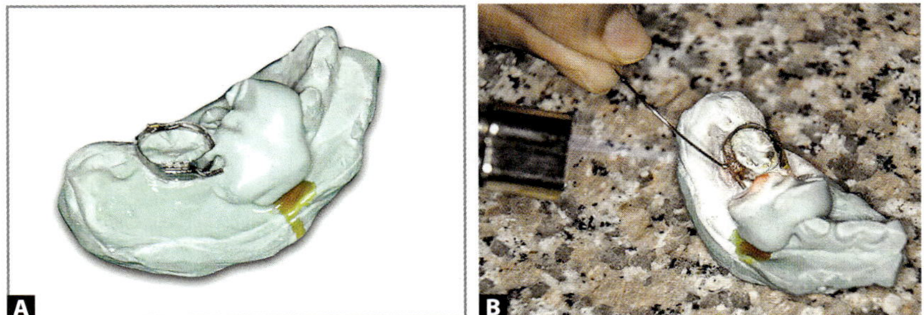

Figs. 35.4A and B: (A) Stabilization; (B) Soldering.

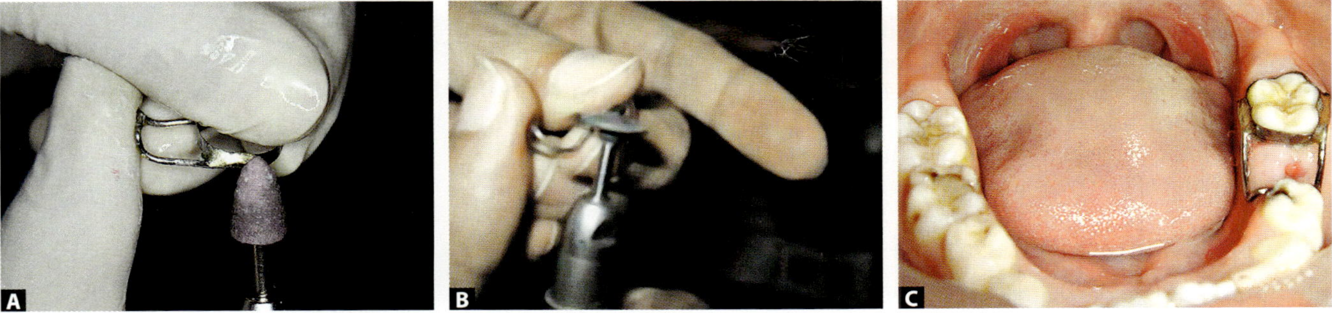

Figs. 35.5A to C: (A) Finishing; (B) Polishing; (C) Final presentation of polished space maintainer.

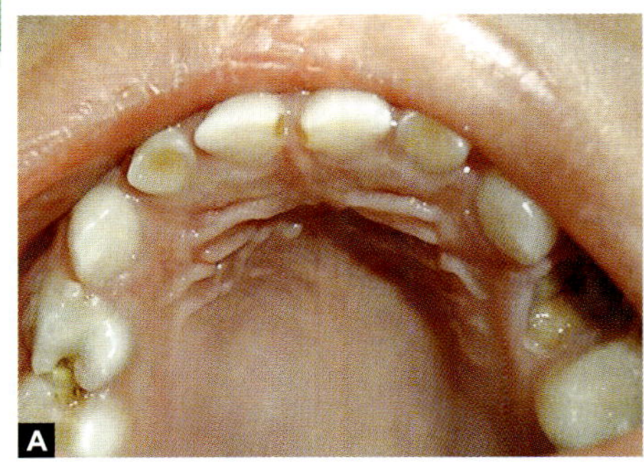
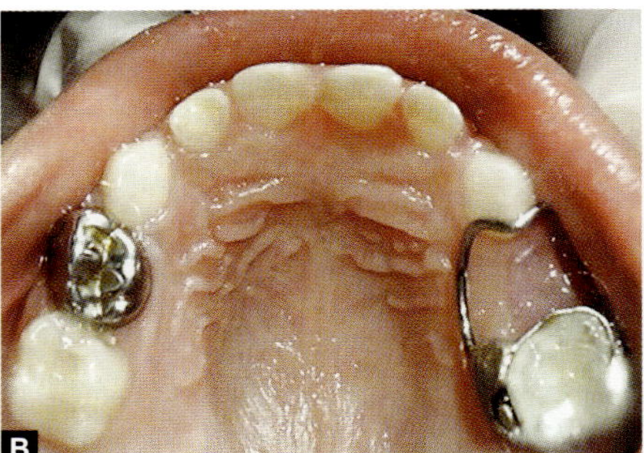
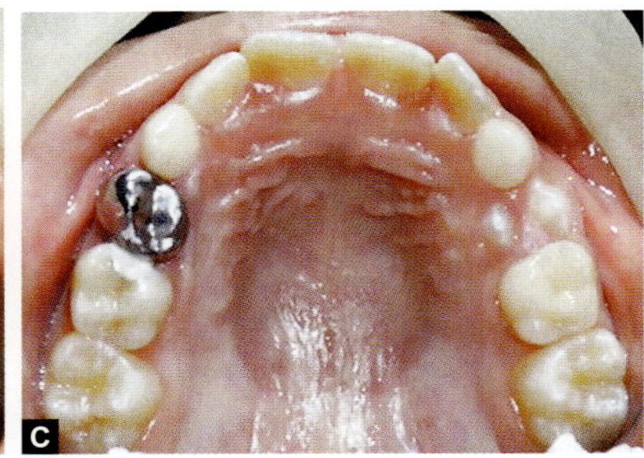

Figs. 35.6A to C: Band and loop space maintainer: (A) Preoperative extraction space; (B) Band and loop SM cemented; (C) Postoperative eruption status of teeth in exact location.

BAND AND LOOP SPACE MAINTAINER

It is a unilateral, nonfunctional, passive, fixed appliance indicated for space maintenance in the posterior segments when single tooth is lost **(Figs. 35.6A to C)**.

Indication (Moyers 1988)[11]	*Contraindication (Mathewson)*
In case of premature loss of any primary molar in primary dentition or primary maxillary molar in transitional dentition with permanent successor not erupting clinically for the next 2 years and its root length is less than one third mature	An occlusion that is extremely crowded or already exhibits marked space loss
Premature loss of a primary second molar as the permanent first molar is erupted clinically	High dental caries activity
Bilateral loss of single primary molar before eruption of permanent incisors	Replacement of primary anterior teeth
Sometimes it is given in cases of premature loss of primary canine	Replacement of primary second molar in the primary dentition without partial clinical eruption of permanent first molar
When the period of space maintenance is short and abutment tooth is intact	Replacement of primary second molars in transitional dentition with the permanent molar banded Cases that need guidance of eruption

Indications

- It is usually indicated for preserving the space created by the premature loss of single primary molar.
- Bilateral loss of single primary molar before eruption of permanent incisors. This is because the developing succedaneous tooth buds are placed lingually to permanent incisors so other space maintainers like lingual arch can lead to obstruction of these teeth.
- It is also indicated when second primary molar is lost after the eruption of first permanent molar.

Design of the Wire Loop (Figs. 35.7A and B)

- The arms of the loop should be placed in the junction of middle and cervical third, at the same time not interfering with occlusion.
- The contour of the loop should be similar and as close as possible to the gingival contour.

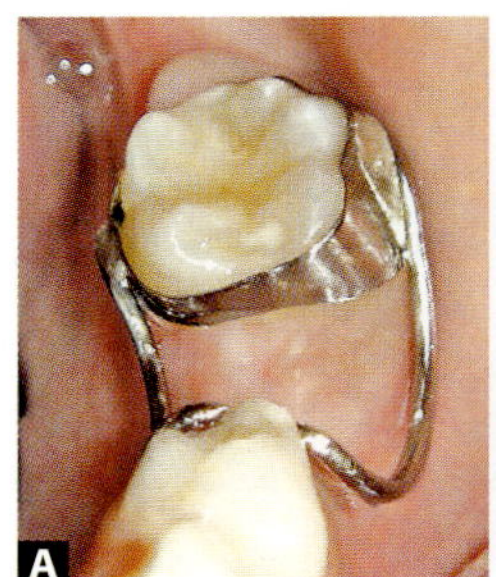
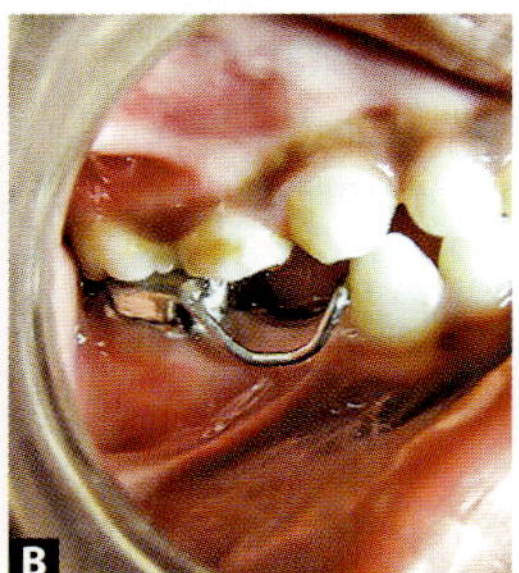

Figs. 35.7A and B: Design of the wire loop.

- The final width of the loop should be wide enough to allow eruption of premolar inside the loop.
- The loop should be placed just above the contact area of the supporting tooth in a passive manner so as not to slip down.

Advantages

- Construction is easy and faster.
- Few appointments by patient.
- Many modifications are possible.

Disadvantages

- Cannot stabilize the arch.
- Nonfunctional.
- Slippage of loop by masticatory forces.
- Cannot be used for multiple loss of teeth.
- Most of the time primary second molar (E) is lost before eruption of premolar.

Modifications in Designs of Band and Loop Space Maintainer

- **Rapp** and **Demiroz:**[12] Stoppers can be used to prevent gingival as well as buccal movements of loop **(Fig. 35.8)**.

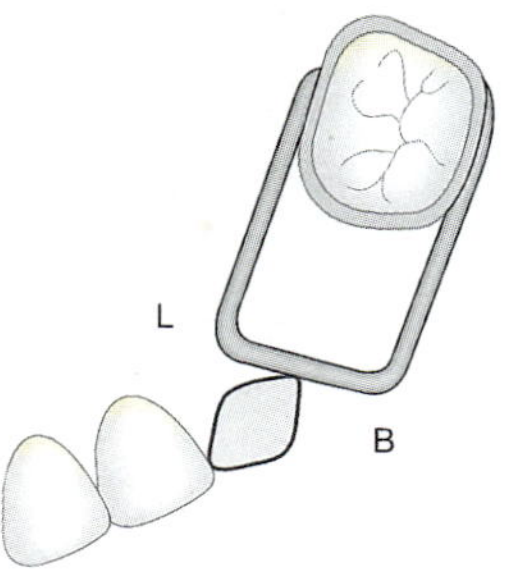

Fig. 35.8: Rapp modification with stoppers.

- **Crown and loop (Fig. 35.9)**: Same as band and loop but a stainless steel crown is used on abutment tooth instead of a band.

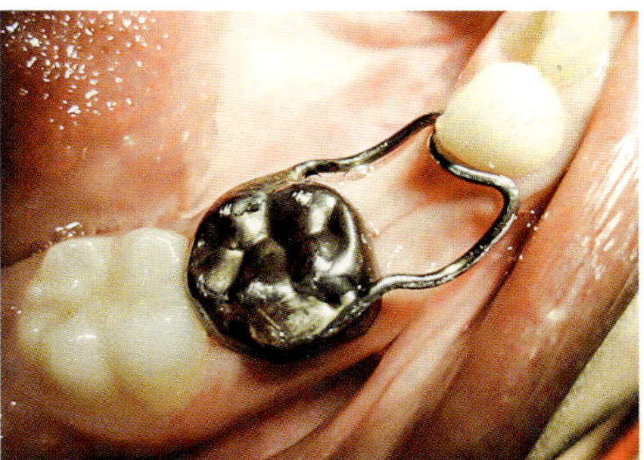

Fig. 35.9: Crown and loop. (*Source:* Dentgama.com).

- **Crown-band and loop (Fig. 35.10)**: Stainless steel crown is first placed on abutment tooth and then it is banded.

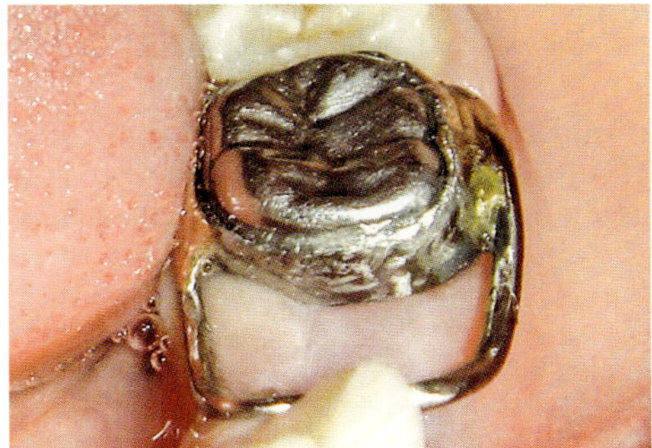

Fig. 35.10: Crown band and loop.

- **Mayne's space maintainer (Figs. 35.11A to E)**: Band and loop but the loop is halved with buccal loop eliminated and only the lingual extension given.[13] According to **Moses J** et al., lingual loop is eliminated and only buccal extension given. It can also be modified by crown-band and Mayne's loop.
- **Reverse band and loop (Fig. 35.12):** Given when there is premature loss of primary second molar and the permanent molars have not erupted fully to support a band. In such cases, primary first molar is banded and a loop is made that touches just below the marginal ridge of permanent molars.

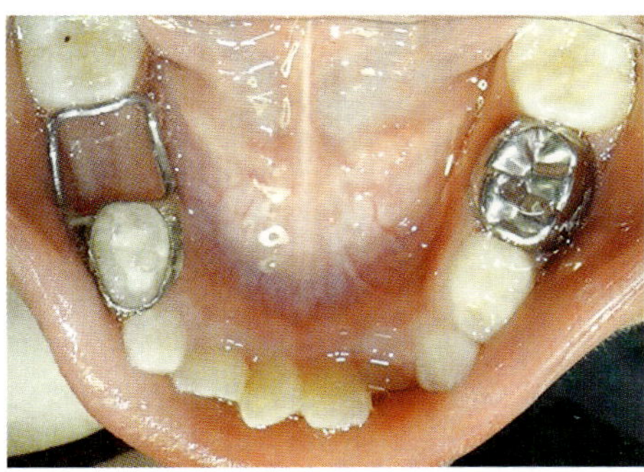

Fig. 35.12: Reverse band and loop. (*Pic courtesy:* Dr Amita Rai, PDC, Nepal).

- **Band and bar**: Prevents eruption of premolar **(Fig. 35.13)** and was used in earlier times.

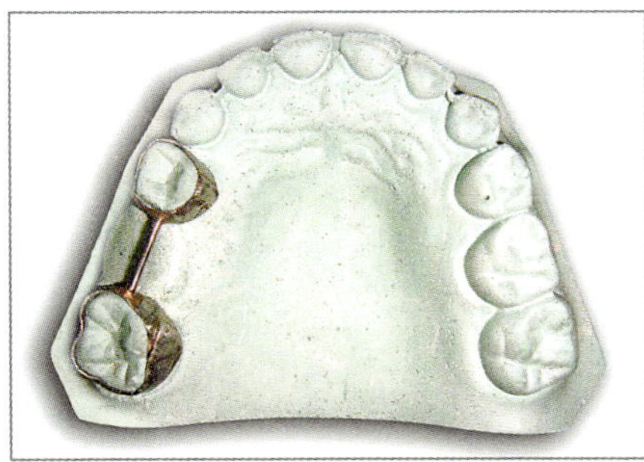

Fig. 35.13: Band and bar.

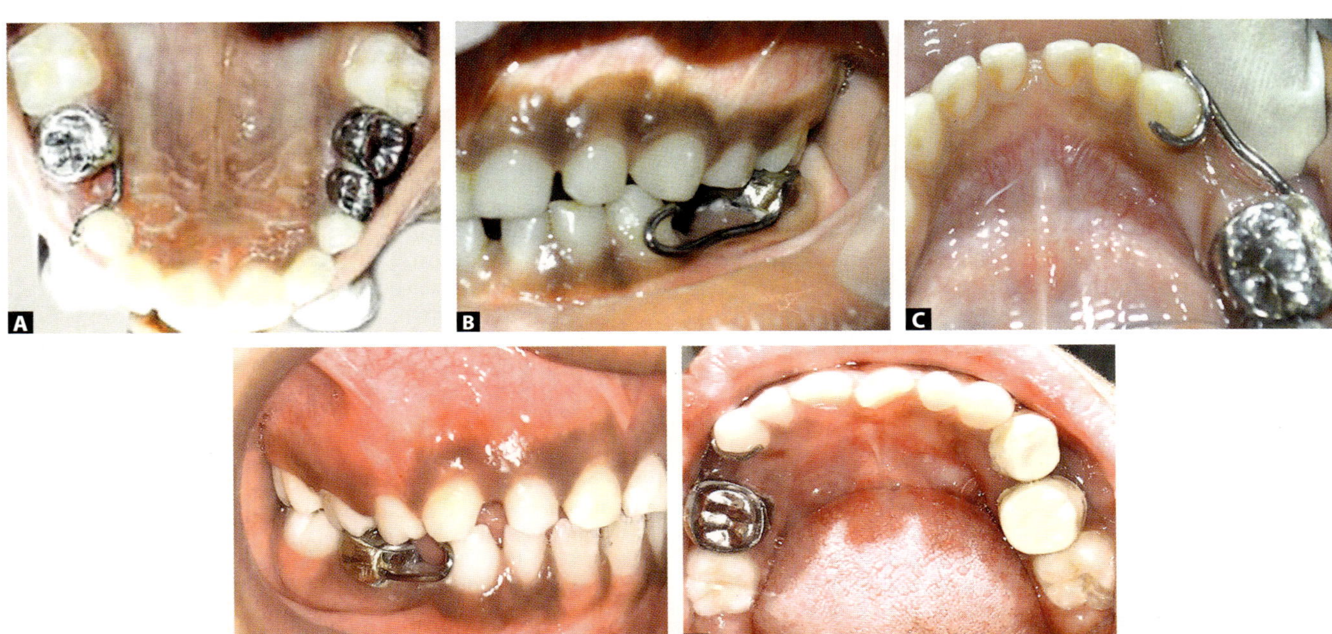

Figs. 35.11A to E: Mayne's space maintainer. [*Source (Fig. A):* Savitri et al. IJMDCR, *(Figs. B and C):* Moses J et al. IJPR (2018)], *(Figs. D and E):* Tahririan D, Safaripour M, Eshghi A, Bonyadian AH. Dent Res J. 2019).

- **Long band and loop (Fig. 35.14):** Used in case there is multiple loss of teeth in one segment and an arch stabilizing space maintainer like lingual arch cannot be given due to eruption status or if removable appliance is contraindicated.

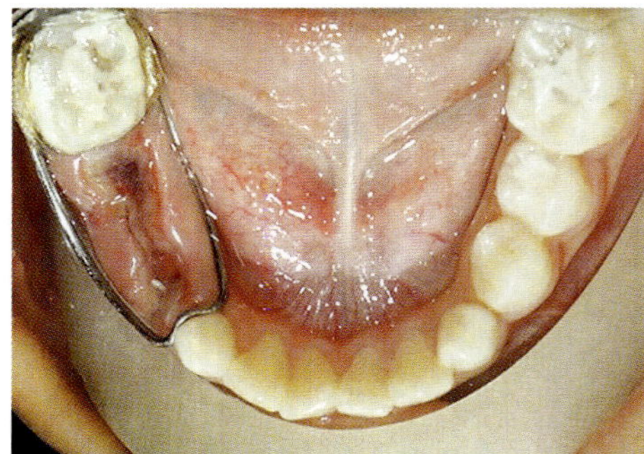

Fig. 35.14: Long band and loop.

- **Bonded band and loop space maintainer (Fig. 35.15):** With the use of acid-etch technique light curing composite systems, simple space maintainers can be more readily made. Its advantage includes ease of adhesion to the dental contours, fast technique of application, good strength.[14]
    - **Gerald Z Wright** (1976) preformed loop of 0.81 mm wire designed.
    - **Simsonsen RJ** (1978) used a metal bar (3M company).

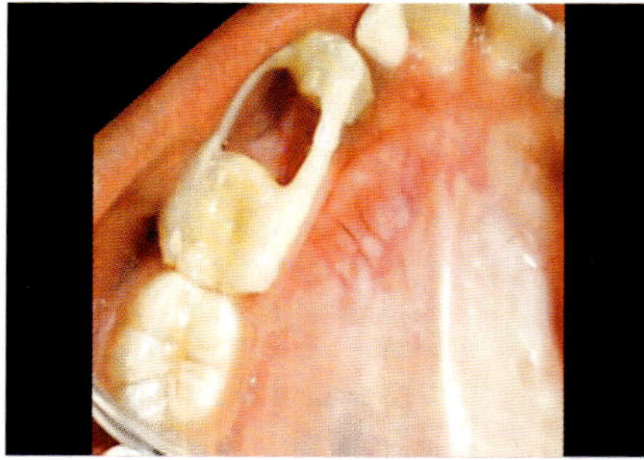

Fig. 35.15: Bonded space maintainer. (*Source:* Garg A et al.[14] JISPPD, 2008).

- **Band and loop space maintainer with NIMS modification (Fig. 35.16): Prajapati et al.**[15] 2013 proposed that in some case like long-standing loss of upper first primary molars, the primary canine occludes with primary molar of opposite arch such that cusps of molar impede in the space created by loss of tooth. In such cases, the loop has to be modified and one arm has to be removed to create space and allow proper occlusion.

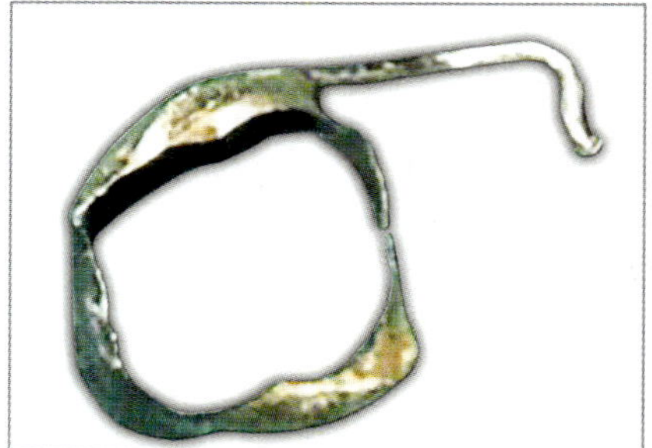

Fig. 35.16: Band and loop space maintainer with NIMS modification. (*Source:* Prajapati et al. JMDS, 2013).

- **Band and loop space maintainer** with unilateral band and bent wire design **(Fig. 35.17)** was presented by **Pushpalatha et al.**[16] 2016 in cases with space loss.

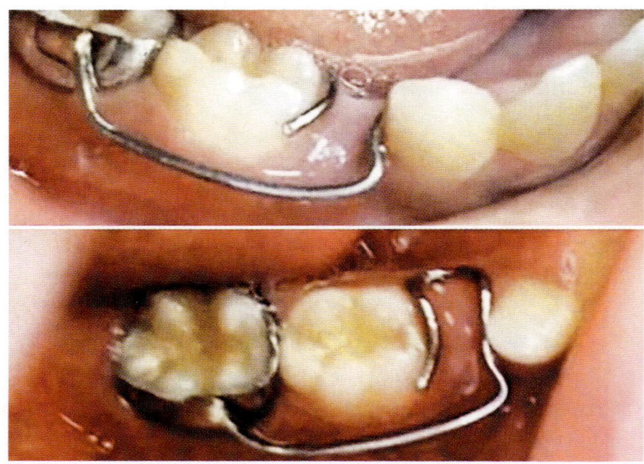

Fig. 35.17: Band and loop space maintainer with unilateral band and bent wire design. (*Source:* Pushpalatha,[16] JDCFR)

- **Functional band and loop space maintainers (Fig. 35.18): V Vinothini et al.,** in 2019 modified conventional band and loop space maintainer to make it functional.

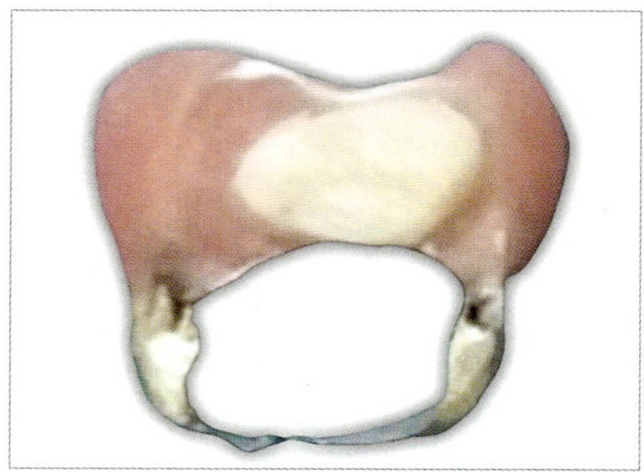

Fig. 35.18: Functional band and loop space maintainers.

Research studies regarding band and loop space maintainers (Fig. 35.17)

- **Christensen** and **Fields** advise that the crown and loop is not a recommend technique. Fields states that it is no longer considered advisable to use the crown-loop appliance because it precludes simple appliance removal and replacement. He recommends that teeth with SSC should be banded like natural teeth.
- **McDonald et al.**[2] stated that a primary first molar stainless steel crown provides a desirable retentive contour for placing a stainless steel band. When the inside of the band and the outside band-bearing surfaces of selected crowns were lightly scored with a diamond bur prior to cementation, significantly superior retention was observed.
- **Sasa et al.**[17] reported a median survival time (MST) of 13 months for Band and Loop space maintainer cemented using glass ionomer luting cement.
- **Emine Sen Tunc et al**. reported that Band and Loop space maintainer had a relatively low rate of failure compared to other studies, with only one failure occurring after 9 months.
- **Wright** and **Kennedy**:[18,19] Band and Loop type of space maintainers are one of the most frequently used appliances.
- **Baroni et al.,**[20] **Rajab** (2002), and **Fathian et al.:**[21] Band and loops are been used since long as a space maintainer with good high success rates.

- **Kirzioglu et al.** (2004)**:** In spite of good patient compliance, disintegration of cement, solder failure, caries formation along the margins of the band, and long construction time are some of the disadvantages associated with them.
- **Croll**[22] in 1983: The use of either zinc phosphate or polycarboxylate cement to attach Band and Loop space maintainer was recommended.
- **Garg et al.**[14] and ***Subramanium* et al.** (2008) showed failure of FRCR due to the debonding of enamel composite because of its placement on primary teeth; primary teeth show presence of prismless enamel areas which had negative influence on the resin retention.
- **Setia et al.**[23] comparing band and loop, Ribbond and Super splint, found super splint to be least successful space maintainer in terms of long-term retention and gingival health.
- **Simon et al.**[24] (2012) made a modification as the band and half loop (occasionally referred to as a "one-armed bandit") is a premade appliance with a 0.036 wire that has already been soldered to the lingual surface of the band. Once the correct band size has been selected, the wire is bent to contact the adjacent abutment tooth and cemented. It allows chairside fabrication and delivery.

LINGUAL ARCH SPACE MAINTAINER

It is a bilateral, nonfunctional, passive/active, mandibular fixed appliance. It is the most effective appliance of space maintenance and minor tooth movement in lower arch **(Fig. 35.19).**

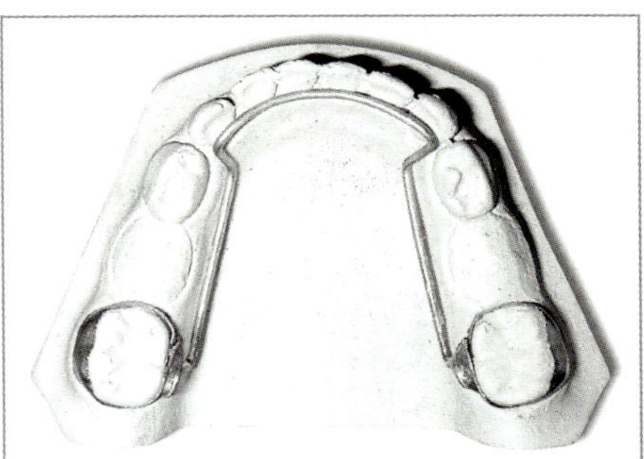

Fig. 35.19: Lingual arch.

Indication

- The appliance is usually indicated to preserve the space created by multiple loss of primary molars when there is no loss of space in the arch. The use of the lingual arch is a good preventive measure, since it helps in maintaining the arch perimeter by preventing both mesial drifting and lingual movement of the molar teeth and also lingual collapse of the anterior teeth.
- Bilateral loss of primary molars after eruption of lower lateral incisors.
- Unilateral loss of primary molars after eruption of lower lateral incisors.
- Minor space regaining.

Contraindication

It is not used before eruption of permanent incisors because the permanent incisor tooth buds develop and erupt somewhat lingual to their primary precursors and the design of conventional mandibular lingual arch might interfere with their eruption.

Design of the Wire Loop

Arch design should be directed toward minimizing the maintenance problems. The arch wire should contact the erupted permanent incisors at the cingulum. Arch wire should be located 2 mm below the gingival margin or edentulous ridge in the posterior regions to prevent distortion under process of mastication and should be located 1–2 mm lingual to the posterior teeth to permit satisfactory eruption of the bicuspids in a buccolingual plane. The arch wire should meet the band at the mesiobuccal cusp, and at the same time, place the soldered joint in the middle third of the band to avoid occlusal interference **(Figs. 35.20A to D).**

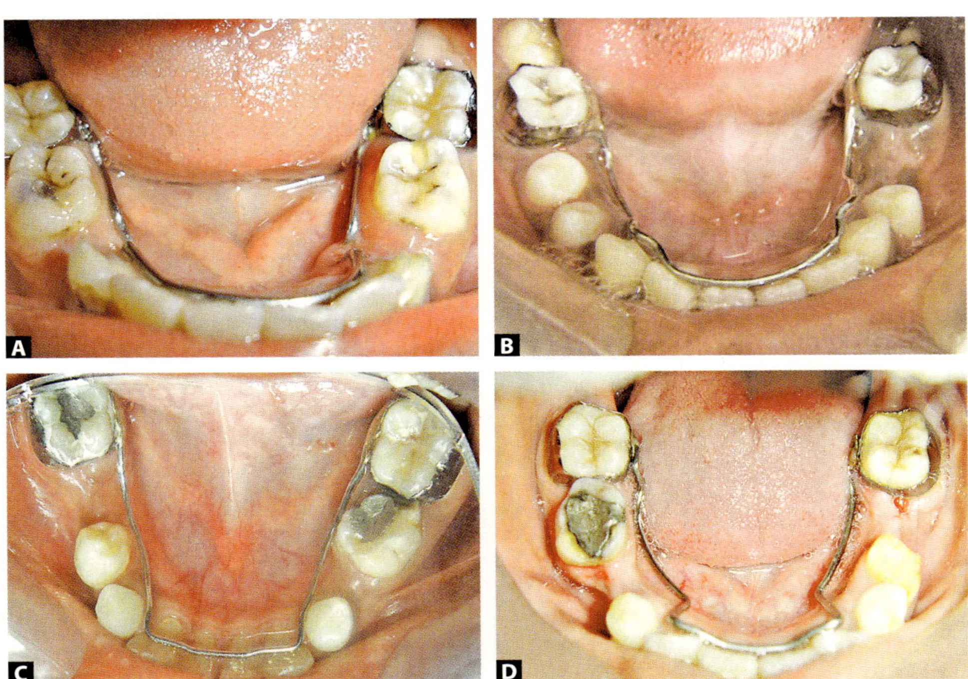

Figs. 35.20A to D: Design of the wire loop.

Advantages

- Many modifications are possible.
- Can also be used to regain space.
- Arch holding space maintainer.
- Passive lingual arch can preserve the E space which can be utilised for minor lower anterior crowding.
- The LLA restricts vertical eruption of the mandibular molars, If employed early in a patient exhibiting excessive vertical growth tendencies, it may have this additional beneficial effect.
- Less likely to interfere with the typical increase in intercanine distance that takes place as a child transitions from mixed to permanent dentition.
- It also has the capacity to relieve potential crowding by allowing incisors to drift distally into the Leeway space as it resists mesial movement of the permanent first molars.

Disadvantages

- Construction is difficult.
- More chances of distortion of appliance by tongue pressure.
- May cause unwanted movements.
- Increased incidence of caries development.
- Habitual fiddling with tongue: wires should be in close adaptation with tooth and soft tissue.
- Increased chance of impaction of teeth distal to 6.

Modifications in Design of Lingual Arch

- **Hotz lingual arch**—with U-loop used for space regaining.
- **Removable lingual arch:** The removable lingual arch wire has precision fitting shafts that fit into corresponding sheaths on the molar bands. It is used as an active appliance or as a device to maintain the arch perimeter.
- **Omega bends**—in canine region to prevent interference.
- **Weldable lingual arch space maintainer: Chawla et al.** in 1984 advocated soldering of wire on the lingual side of the band and also use canine spurs.

Guidelines for successful case selection and treatment with lingual arch

- *The patient should be a Class I dentally and skeletally.*
- *In Class II and III cases, the use of the LLA should form part of a comprehensive orthodontic treatment plan.*
- *The patient's oral hygiene should be impeccable.*
- *Late mixed dentition treatment is appropriate. The mandibular arch must be intact i.e no tooth loss or improperly contoured interproximal restorations. In the case of spontaneous loss of the primary canines, the LLA should be placed within one month of the primary tooth exfoliating.*
- *The amount of anterior crowding must be less than five mm.*
- *The patient should have a pantomograph taken in order that the developing dentition may be assessed.*
- *Prior to proceeding with the treatment, the second molars should be carefully assessed for impaction potential. An intermolar angle of 200 or more should be regarded as a warning sign and other forms of treatment should be investigated and / or considered.*
- *The cooperation of the patient after the appliance has been fitted is very important.*
- *The risks associated with 'fiddling' should be made clear to both the patient and parents.*
- *The importance of regular follow up appointments, at least once every three months needs to be stressed, in order to check the appliance for signs of distortion as well as for regular six-monthly removal and recementation of the LLA.*
- *The appliance is removed once the premolars and canines have fully erupted.*

NANCE PALATAL ARCH SPACE MAINTAINER

Bilateral, nonfunctional, passive, maxillary fixed appliance that does not contact the anterior teeth but approximates the anterior palate via an acrylic button that contacts the palatal tissue, which provides resistance to the anterior movement of posterior teeth in a horizontal direction. This appliance was developed by **Nance** in 1947, and he initially named it "Preventive lingual wire" **(Figs. 35.21A to C)**.

Indications

Nance palatal arch may be used in maintaining the maxillary first permanent molar positioning when there is bilateral premature loss of primary teeth with no loss of space in arch and a favorable mixed dentition analysis.

Design of the Wire Loop

The arch wire extends anteriorly without touching against the surface of the primary molars; as the successor bicuspids usually are broader buccolingually, and the wire could deflect them from their natural position. At the rugae area, a small U-shaped bend should be incorporated in the wire, which is approximately 1–2 mm away from the soft tissue. The bend will enhance the retention of acrylic to the wire. The acrylic button, 0.5 in in diameter, is placed usually on the descending portion of the palatal vault 1–2 mm below the incisive papilla.

Advantages

Can be used with multiple modifications like modified Nance appliance for unilateral molar distalization; Esthetic Nance

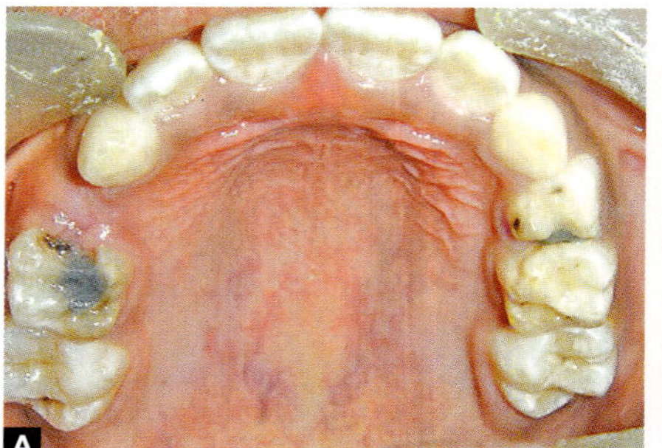

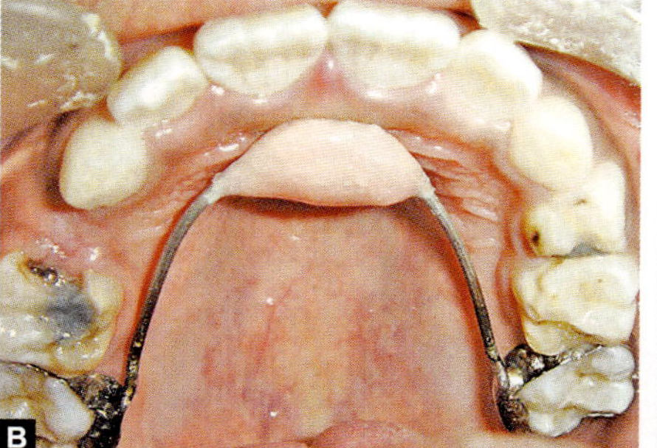

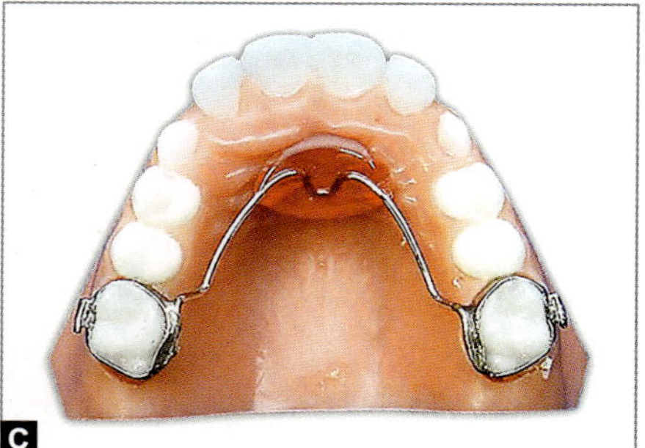

Figs. 35.21A to C: Nance palatal arch space maintainer.

palatal arch with with the attachment of teeth in anterior region to serve as space maintainer and also for anterior esthetics or even Nance to correct crossbite.

Disadvantages

- May cause tissue hyperplasia.
- Irritation to palatal tissues.
- Pressure effects.
- Cannot be used in patients allergic to acrylic.
- Impingement of the button against the palatal tissue can cause irritation, degeneration from the pressure, and lack of hygiene in the area of the rugae.

Controversy

The Nance anterior acrylic component may not contribute to the anchorage of the appliance as once thought. If it is constructed a minimal distance away from the palate to allow proper hygiene and yet it is crucial for space maintenance, then it would be expected to allow space loss to occur according to the gap between the button and the tissue no matter how small this may be.

TRANSPALATAL ARCH

Unilateral, nonfunctional, passive, maxillary fixed appliance that has been recommended for stabilizing the maxillary first permanent molars when primary molars require extraction. This was first reported by **Goshgarian** in 1972 and the construction was described by **Hill et al.** (1975) and **Tsamtsouries** and **White** (1977).

Indications

- The best indication for transpalatal arch is when one side of arch is intact and several primary teeth on the other side are missing.
- To establish and maintain arch widths.
- Derotate unilaterally or bilaterally rotated molars.
- Control upper molar eruption.
- Correct unilateral crossbites for maxillary expansion and buccal root torque of upper molars.
- Correct mesiodistal asymmetries.

Design of the Wire Loop

- The original design included a straight bar extending across the palate **(Fig. 35.22A)**. It should be referred to as the transpalatal bar. A variation of the bar and the type most frequently used is called the Goshgarian appliance or, more commonly, the transpalatal arch.
- The transpalatal arch runs directly across the palatal vault avoiding contact with the soft tissues. U-shaped bend must be given to the wire in middle of palate [can be given mesially **(Fig. 35.22B)** or distally **(Fig. 35.22C)**] if any manipulation is required. As it approaches the mesial part of the palatal surface of the band, the wire should be bent to the distal part of the band to assure a better joint.
- The TPA offers the option of expansion, rotation, contraction, and torque of the molars due to an omega loop in the center of the vault. It is constructed from a 0.036-inch (0.9 mm) stainless steel wire. The central loop is oriented either mesially or distally.

Rationale

When permanent maxillary molars move anteriorly, they rotate mesiolingually around the large lingual root. The space between the buccal and lingual cortical plates becomes narrow anterior to the first molar roots, preventing the molar from advancing directly and limiting its movement to a rotation. The large lingual root contacts the lingual plate and acts as a pivot, allowing the 2 buccal roots to rotate mesiolingually. The TPA reduces anterior molar movement by coupling the right and left permanent molars together and, thus, preventing any possibility of rotations.

Advantages

- Used in multiple unilateral loss.
- Can be used for expansion.

Disadvantage

Both molars may tip together.

DISTAL SHOE SPACE MAINTAINER

Distal shoe appliance is otherwise known as the intra-alveolar appliance **(Fig. 35.23)**. One of the early designs of distal shoe space maintainers was **Willet's** distal shoe. This appliance is rarely used these days because of the increased cost of the materials, difficulties in tooth preparation, and more complicated fabrication procedure. The appliance, which is in practice, is **Roche's** distal shoe or modifications of it using crown and band appliances with a distal intragingival extension.

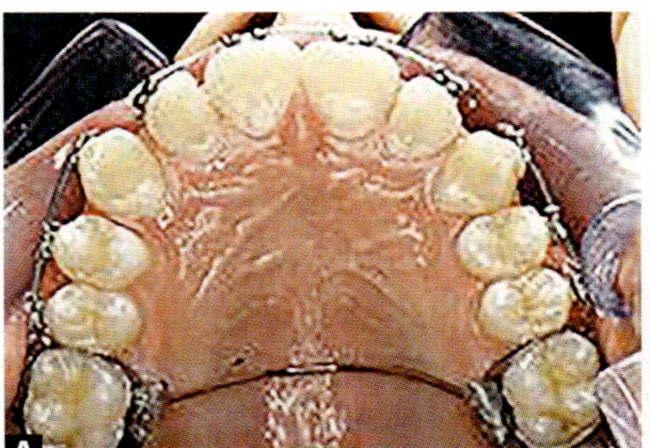

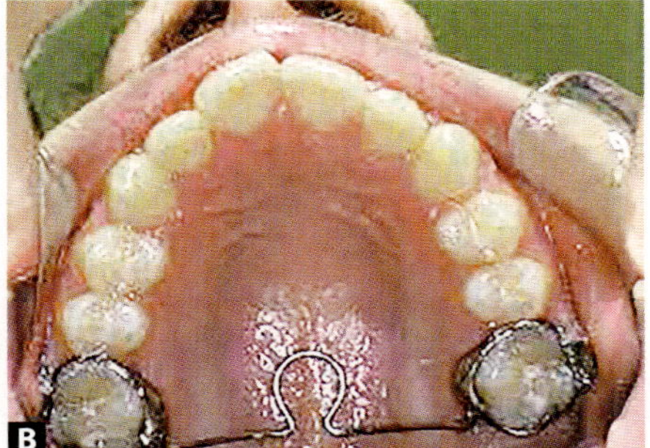

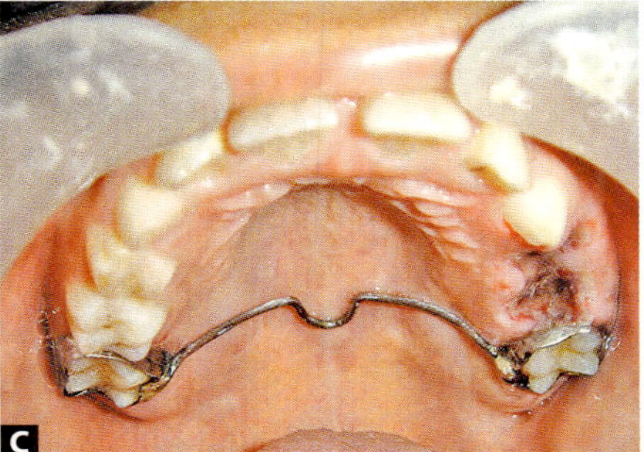

Figs. 35.22 A to C: (A) Transpalatal bar; (B) Mesial transpalatal arch; (C) Distal transpalatal arch.

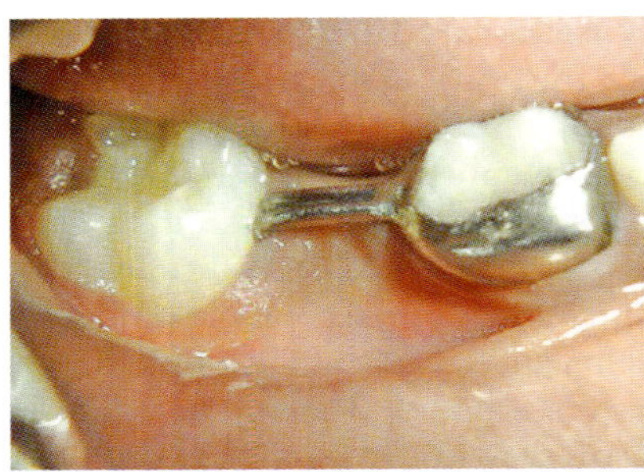

Fig. 35.23: Distal shoe space maintainer.

Roche's appliance offers a V-shaped end, which offers a broader surface and helps prevent rotations. The broader surface also holds a greater chance of success if the unerupted tooth is positioned buccally or lingually in the dental arch. Distal surface of the second primary molar provides a guide for unerupted first permanent molar. When the second primary molar is removed prior to the eruption of first permanent molar, the intra-alveolar appliance provides greater control of the path of eruption of the unerupted tooth and prevents undesirable mesial migration.

Indications

- Premature loss or extraction of the second primary molar prior to the eruption of the first permanent molar.
- Advanced root resorption and periapical bone destruction of the second primary molar prior to eruption of the first permanent molar.
- A primary second molar with advanced caries that is not restorable.
- Ectopic eruption of the permanent first molar.
- Ankylosis of the primary second molar.

Contraindications

- Inadequate abutments due to multiple losses of teeth.
- Poor oral hygiene.
- Lack of parent and patient cooperation.
- Medically compromized patients like patients with congenital heart disease, kidney problems, juvenile diabetes, history of rheumatic fever, generalized debilitation, and hemophiliacs.
- Congenitally missing first permanent molar.

Design of the Wire Loop

Using first primary molar as abutment, the stainless steel band is adapted. If the morphology of tooth does not permit easy placement and adaptation of band, then the tooth is prepared for stainless steel crown and on that band is fitted. An alginate impression is made, the band is removed and placed in the impression, and a stone model is prepared. The tissue bearing loop is then contoured with a 0.0040" wire extending distally into the prepared opening on the model, and the free ends of the loop are soldered to the band **(Figs. 35.24A to C)**.

The primary function of the distal shoe appliance is to provide a guide plane for the eruption path of the first permanent molar. To fulfill this purpose successfully, we should have an understanding of the normal paths of eruption of maxillary and mandibular first permanent molar. Because of this, the distal extension of the appliance will differ for upper and lower arches. In the lower arch, the contact area of distal extension of the appliance should have a slight lingual position over the crest of the alveolar ridge in order to engage the mesial contact area of the first permanent molar as it begins its mesial and lingual movements. By contrast, the contact area of distal extension of the maxillary appliance should be slightly facial to the crest of the alveolar ridge. These considerations are important in preventing the erupting permanent molar from slipping contact with the appliance.

The width should closely approximate the normal contact area of the distal surface of the second primary molar being replaced.

Length of the distal extension (horizontal bar) is another decision confronting in determining of the appliance. Problem is simplified somewhat when the second primary molar is still present to serve as a guide on the working model. In this case, the second primary molar should be maintained if possible until the appliance is ready to be sealed. If the second primary molar is already missing, it is recommended the distal surface of the first primary molar and mesial surface of the unerupted first permanent molar be used as guide.

Depth of the gingival extension (vertical bar) is also an important factor. If the extension is left too long, possible harm to the developing second molar may result. If the extension is too short, the first permanent molar could erupt underneath the appliance. A good preoperative radiograph that is slightly under exposed to show the thickness of overlying soft tissue. This will aid in determining the depth of the groove to be cut in working model for constructing the gingival extension. Gingival extension should extend about 1 mm below the mesial marginal of the first permanent molar or just sufficient to capture its mesial surface.

Before final placement of the space maintainer in the mouth, a radiograph is taken to determine whether the

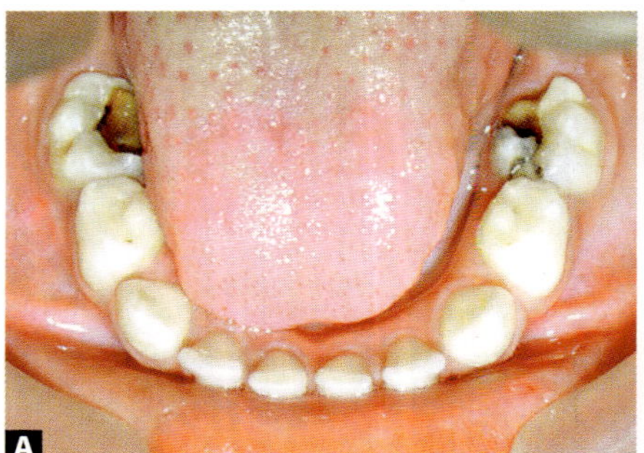

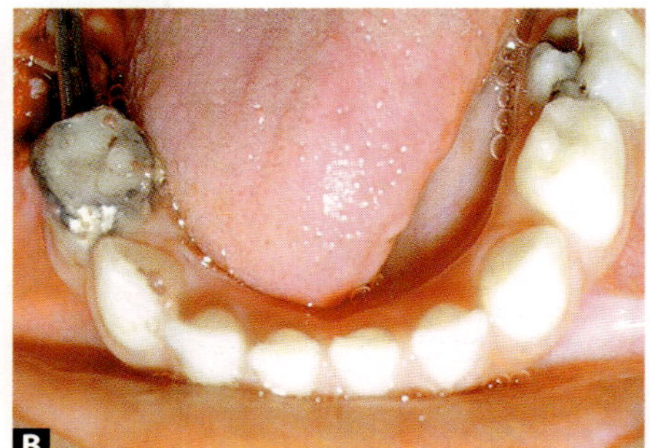

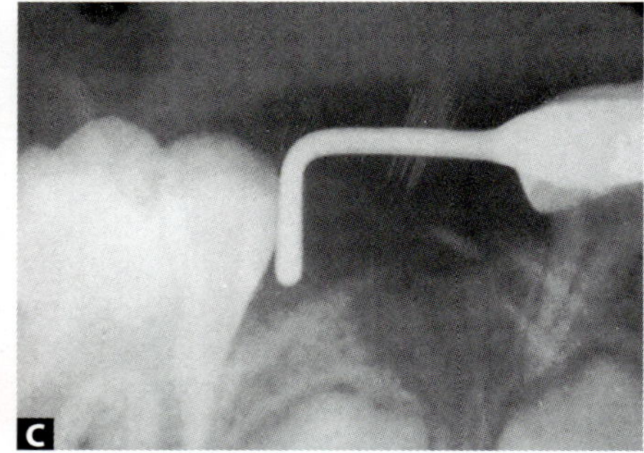

Figs. 35.24A to C: (A) Preoperative presentation; (B) Distal shoe postinsertion after extraction; (C) Radiographic presentation.

tissue extension of the appliance is in proper relationship with the unerupted first permanent molar. Final adjustments in length and contour of the distal shoe can be made at this time. It is best to cement this appliance immediately after the extraction.

Advantages

Only space maintainer, which can be used if there is premature loss of primary second molar before eruption of permanent molars.

Disadvantages

- Can cause deviation of permanent tooth bud.
- May permit tipping if not placed properly.
- Interfere with epithelialization of socket.
- Can cause infection.
- Can only be used in specific patients.
- Retention is not good.
- Construction is difficult.

Modifications in Design of Distal Shoe

- **Gingival saddle appliance (Fig. 35.25):** This is a combination of reverse band and loop and distal shoe where the loop is placed on gingiva and the molar on eruption contact this loop.
- **Levit** (1971) showsan alternative method for construction of distal shoe space maintainer whereby the second primary molar is extracted and the mesial root is ground off. Then the tooth is placed on a previously taken impression. After the stone has set, the primary molar with distal root is removed, and the distal shoe is directly bent down to the distal surface of the artificial distal socket. This eliminates the need for some adjustments in mouth and some X-ray exposure.
- A combination of lingual arch and distal shoe appliance was suggested for use in patients in whom both primary molars are lost and the patient's strong gag reflex prevented the use of a removable appliance.

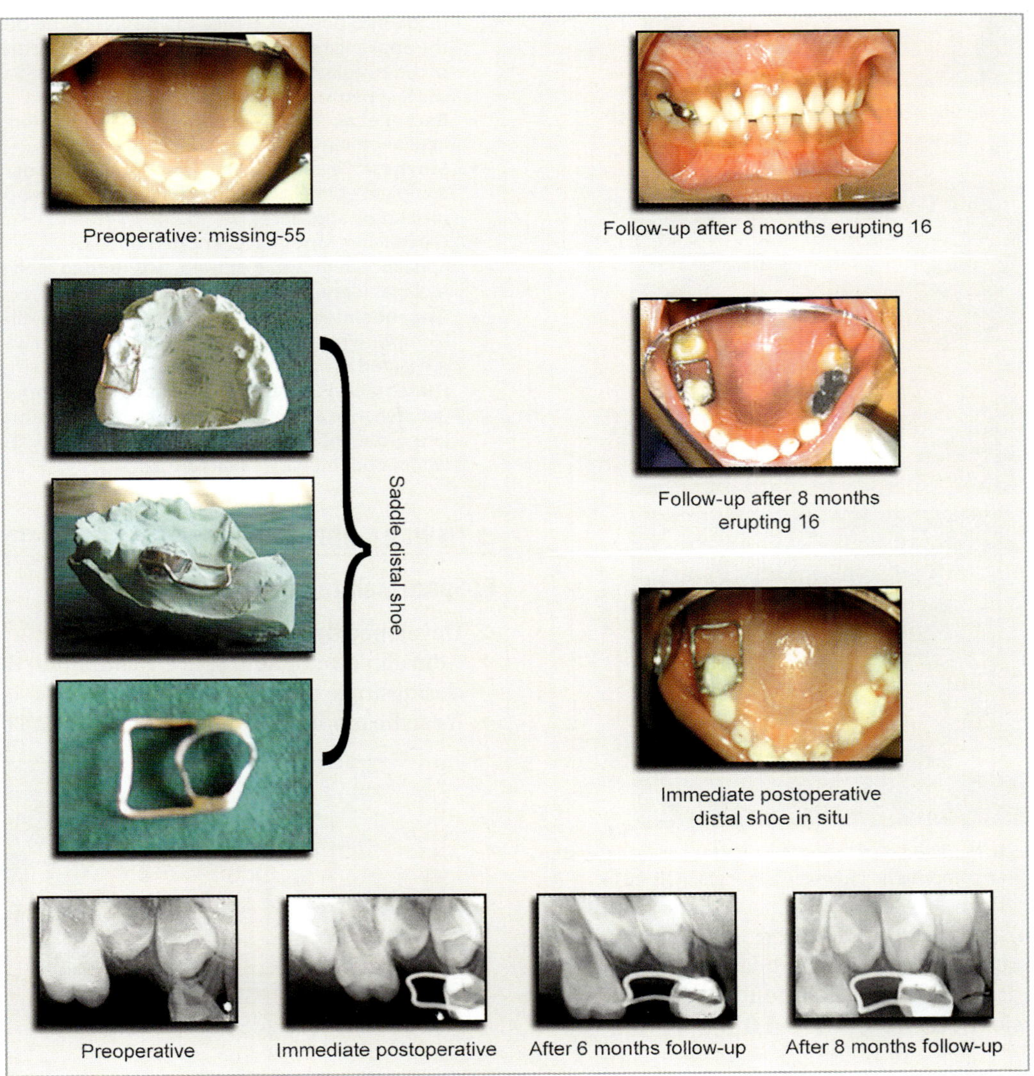

Fig. 35.25: Gingival saddle appliance.

- Placing loops in the horizontal arm of the space maintainer. These loops will permit the precise adjustments needed for accurate placement of molar.
- Space maintainer is placed after signs of eruption of first molar are seen. Vertical extension is short and is not placed intra-alveolarly; it just touches the mesial surface of erupting permanent molar.
- **Bhat et al.**[25] 2014 modified the design of distal shoe space maintainer and fused it with lingual arch in case of early loss of both primary first and second molars unilaterally **(Fig. 35.26).**
- **Chanchala et al.**[26] (2014) modified the design of distal shoe space maintainer in bilateral loss of molars to add circular distal extension with bands on canine and an added functional component **(Figs. 35.27A and B)**.

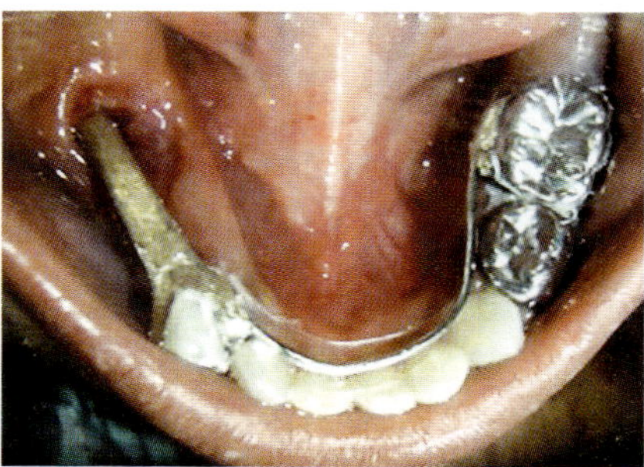

Fig. 35.26: Modified distal shoe with fused lingual arch. (*Source:* Bhat, JCDR, 2014).

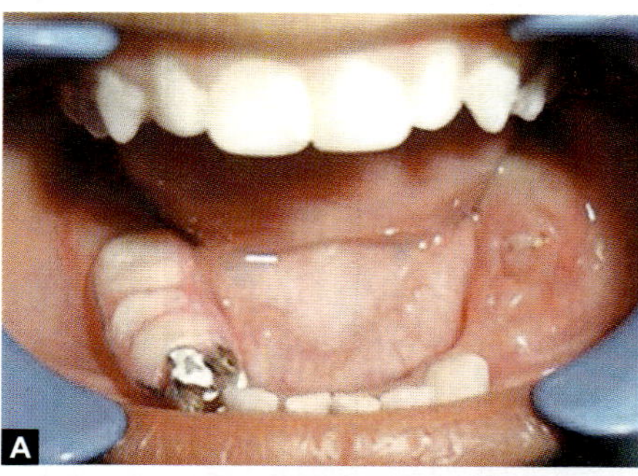

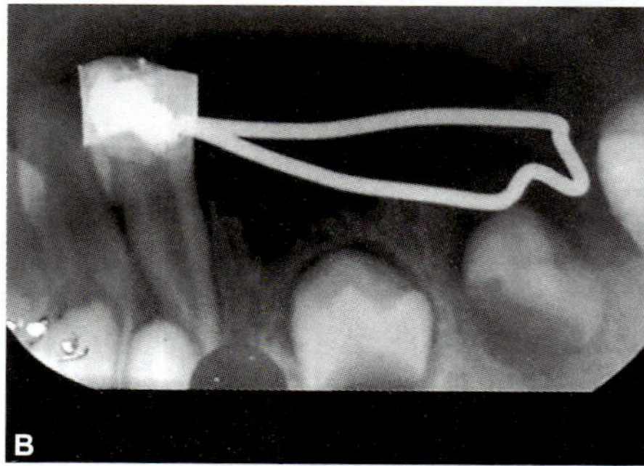

Figs. 35.27A and B: Modified distal shoe with circular distal extension and functional component. (*Source:* Chanchala, JOR, 2014).

- **Somwanshi et al.**[27] 2016 modified the design of distal shoe appliance in case of multiple bilateral loss of teeth by banding and adding lingual component with rectangular distal extensions **(Figs. 35.28A and B)**.

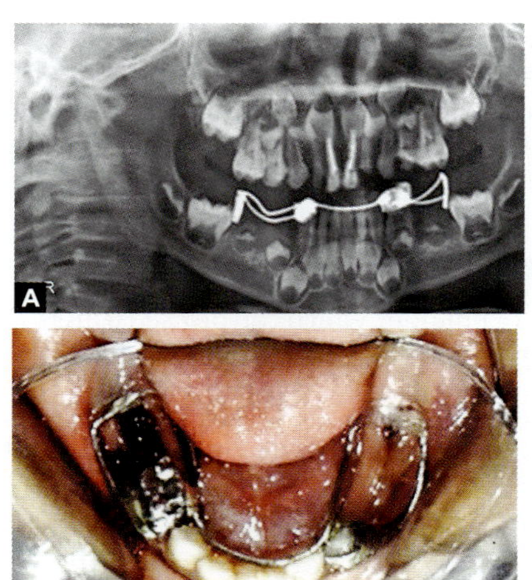

Figs. 35.28A and B: Modified distal shoe with rectangular distal extension and lingual component. (*Source:* Somwanshi, JCDR, 2016).

Research studies regarding distal shoe space maintainers

- **Patil et al**. (2013) explained that in the mandibular arch, the first permanent molar erupts in a lingual and mesial direction using the distal surface of the primary second molar as the buttress to guide into position. Hence the design of the distal extension of the appliance should have a slight lingual position over the crest of the alveolar ridge in order to engage the mesial contact area of the first permanent molar.
- **Barber et al**. (1982) said that there is no need for an intra- alveolar appliance in maxillary arch.
- **Mayhew**[28] evaluated that histologic examination shows that complete epithelialization does not occur after placement of the distal shoe appliance.
- **Carroll** and **Jones** have reported three cases in which a pressure appliance, removable or fixed, was used to guide the permanent molar as it erupted.
- **Gegenheimer** and **Donly** gave a special modification where in along with the gingival extension a distal loop was fabricated and cemented in patient's mouth.
- **Psaltis** and **Fischer** (1982) suggested "an appliance for space maintenance and molar guidance." A combination of lingual arch and distal shoe appliance was suggested for use in patients in whom both primary molars are lost.

NEWER MODIFICATIONS IN SPACE MAINTAINERS

EZ Space Maintainer (Fig. 35.29)

- Developed by **Dr Enis Guray** in 2008.
- Adjustable bondable space maintainer, directly bonded duringsingle office visit.
- It can be modified by including a NiTi coil to regain space.

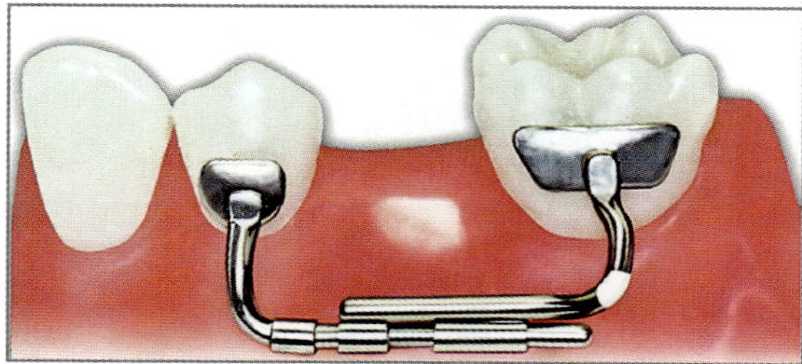

Fig. 35.29: EZ space maintainer.

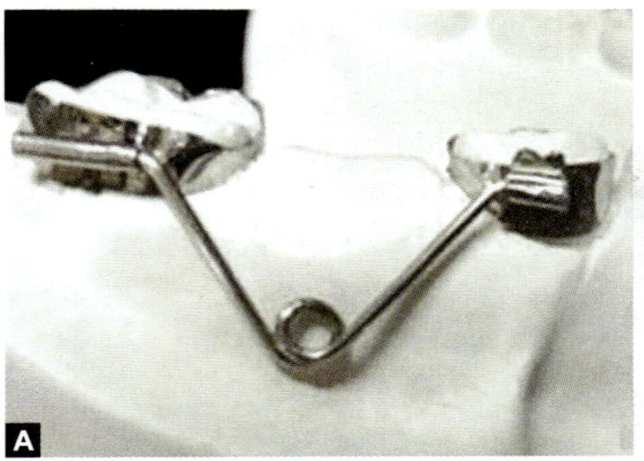
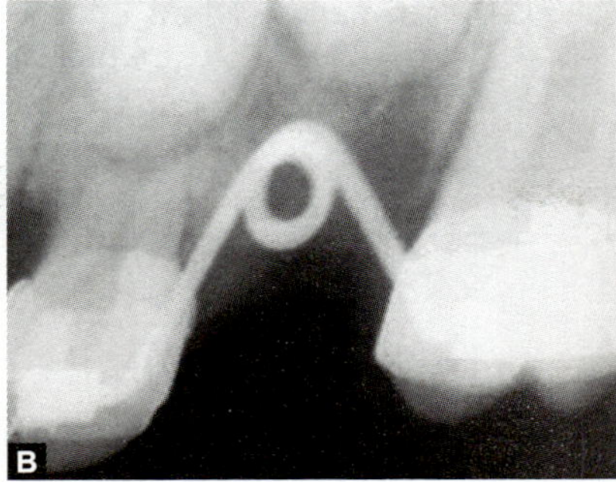
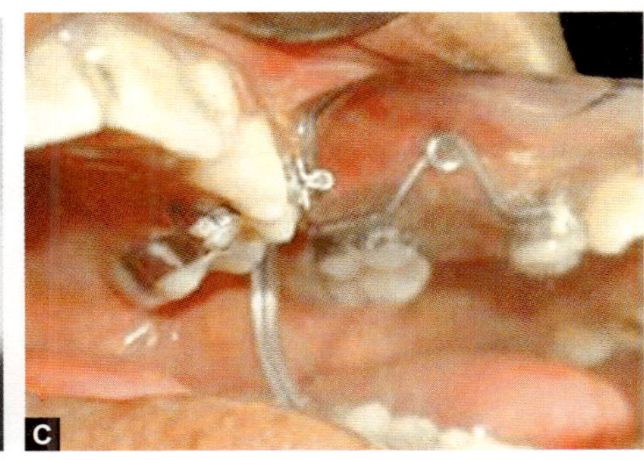

Figs. 35.30A to C: Tube and loop space maintainer.

Tube and Loop Space Maintainer (Figs. 35.30A to C)

- Designed by **Srivastava et al.**[29] in 2017 and termed as "Nikhil appliance".
- Can be given in a single sitting without any laboratory work
- Consists of wire component with helix which is fitted on to the buccal tubes in molars.
- It is an innovative modification of band and loop space maintainer which can be used in single, unilateral tooth loss.

Smart Appliance (Figs. 35.31A to C)

- It is a fixed unilateral space maintainer given by **Mohammed et al.,**[30] in 2020.
- It is indicated in early loss of primary molars and when first permanent molar needs eruption guidance.

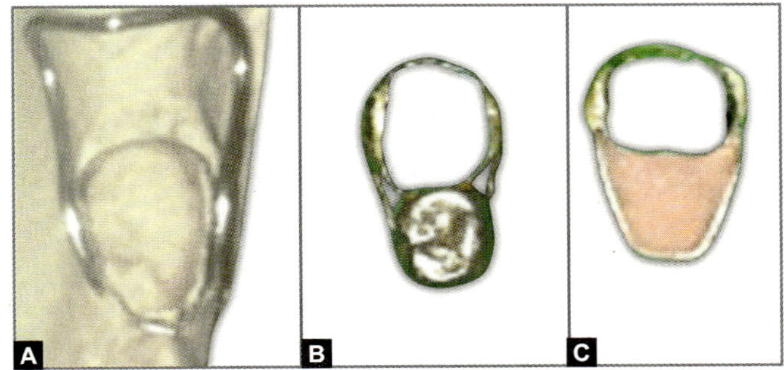

Figs. 35.31A to C: Smart appliance.

- So, it is modification of band and loop space maintainer and distal shoe. Loop is modified by giving disto-labial sloping so as to allow physiologic disto-labial movement of canine. The available space between band and loop is accommodated with stainless steel crown, which restores chewing function along with restricting supraeruption of opposing teeth. The crown is soldered to the band and acrylic is filled on undersurface of crown and loop. When guiding eruption of permanent molar, the same design of loop is placed below the eruption bulge on soft tissue.
- It is given only in cases where permanent first molar has erupted extraosseous by confirming radiographically.
- This supra gingival placement of loop overcomes the drawback of distal shoe and can be indicated in medically compromised patients.
- The appliance requires frequent and long-term follow ups.

Starkey's Appliance (Figs. 35.32A and B)

- It is newer modification of distal shoe space maintainer given by **Tyagi M et al.**[31] in 2021.

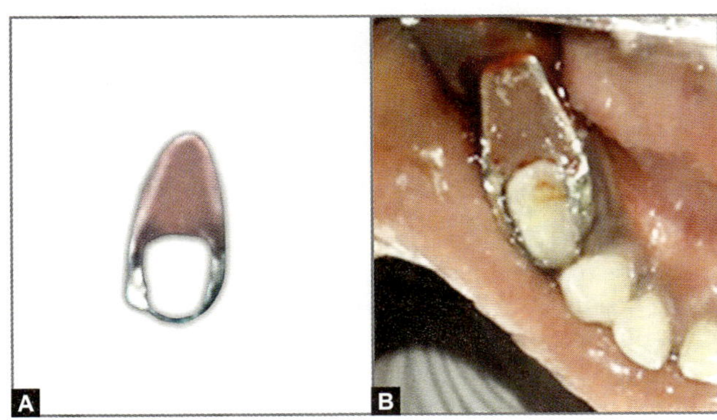

Figs. 35.32A and B: Starkey's appliance.

- Indicated in early loss of primary second molar to guide the eruption of permanent first molar.
- Permanent first molar should pierce the bone and is placed in gingiva. It is also known as eruption guidance appliance.
- The band is soldered on abutment teeth and loop is fabricated from distal surface of abutment teeth till mesial surface of unerupted permanent first molar. The length of loop was evaluated by calculating it on radiograph. Acrylic is pored above the loop till distal extension allowing 1-1.5 mm of acrylic to flow below the mesial marginal ridge of permanent fist molar. The gingival extension is parallel to band and perpendicular to loop.
- The appliance is seated immediately after extraction of primary second molar by placement of acrylic extension in socket.

Fixed Chairside Space Maintainer (Fig. 35.33)

- A novel , acrylic based chairside fixed space maintainer was given by **Yasser R. Souror** [32] in 2019.
- Indicated in early loss of primary second molar.
- The space maintainer is constructed using LACR (Light Cure Acrylic Resin). A pink sheet is used by measuring the distance between the buccal grooves of the lower first permanent molar and distobuccal line angle of the first primary molar using a vernier caliper. The ends upto 3mm on both the sides are weted with bonding agent and light cured for 20 s. Tooth surface is prepared by ,etching,

bonding followed by thin layer of flowable composite on which ends of sheet is adapted and light cured.

- It avoids the need to remove the appliance on following visits for inspection.
- Also it is easy and same day delivery method.

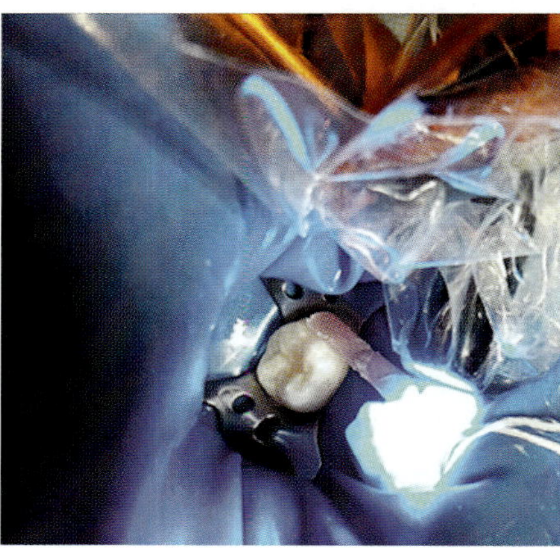

Fig. 35.33: Fixed chairside space maintainer.

Three-dimensional Printed Band and Loop Space Maintainer (Fig. 35.34)

- The use of digital technology in making space maintainer was first used by **Bhagyashri et al.,**[33] in 2022.
- A 3-dimensional model is prepared and then printed using additive process. The whole process of taking impression of the patient, pouring cast, digitalizing it, designing the SM, and printing it by the help of 3D printer increases the precision of the appliance to the next level, minimizing human error.

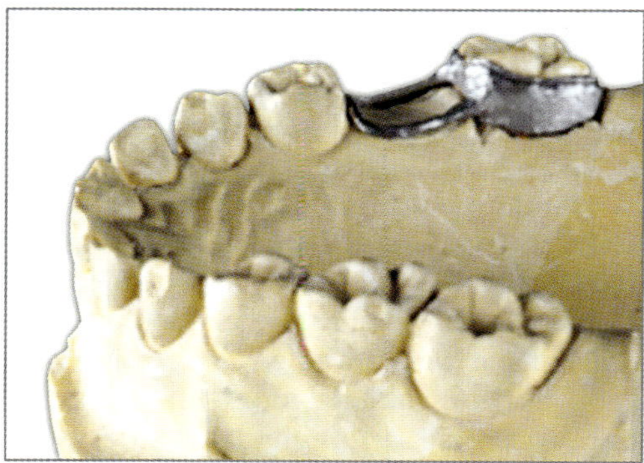

Fig. 35.34: Three dimensional printed band and loop space maintainer.

H-appliance (Fig. 35.35)

- **Pheiroijam et al.**[34] in 2019 introduced a simple "bracket and hook" space maintainer.
- Hook is prepared using 23 gauge stainless steel wire forming two clasp one on both abutment teeth. The mesial end of hook is adapted first and is placed in cervical constriction of molar teeth or by making 0.5mm indentation on distoproximal surface in anterior teeth. The distal end of the loop is inserted in Beggs bracket which is directly bonded on mesio- palatal surface of tooth and at the end of distal hook a pin head clap is formed adapting it to distal interproximal area.
- Disadvantages such as incomplete solder joint, overheating of wire during soldering, breakage of wire at joint during polishing, ill-fitting in patient's mouth, and failure of cementation is overcome by this new design.

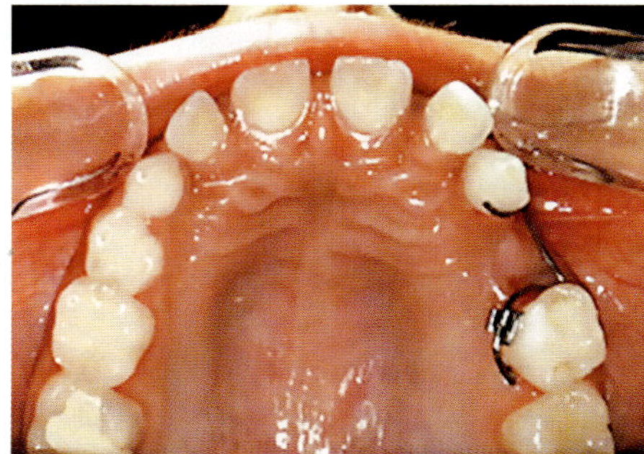

Fig. 35.35: H-appliance.

Bibin Appliance (Fig. 35.36)

- **Bibin et al.,**[35] in 2021 invented a novel patented B-appliance.
- It is pre-fabricated appliance with adjustable arms, capable of fixing it immediately after extraction.
- It overcomes the disadvantages of conventional band and loop along with prevention of supraeruption.
- It has two parts—active and passive arm. Passive arm—made up of stainless steel or any ridged material like composite or plastic. The passive arm has two components: (1) Base and (2) cylindrical tube. Size of the base can be increased or decreased based on the size of the tooth. The Active arm is fabricated using a 21-gauge wire; the one end of the wire is inserted in the buccal or cylindrical tube of the passive arm and cemented with glass ionomer cement (GIC) for a ridged fixation.

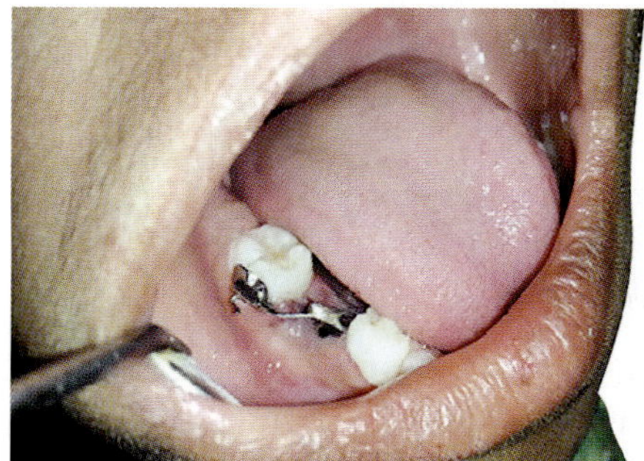

Fig. 35.36: Bibin appliance.

e-Space Maintainer (Kids-e-Dental) (Fig. 35.37)

- To maintain the harmony in the growth and development of jaws we are blessed by nature to have two sets of dentitions. Primary teeth have two indispensable functions of maintaining physiologic space and guiding the eruption of succedaneous teeth in the arches. A sound primary dentition helps in the smooth transition from primary to permanent dentition by preserving the space required for successive permanent dentition. It also helps in mastication, speech, and aesthetics and to maintain arch integrity. Space loss related to arch length and arch perimeter in the maxilla and mandible is a common problem encountered after premature loss of a primary tooth.

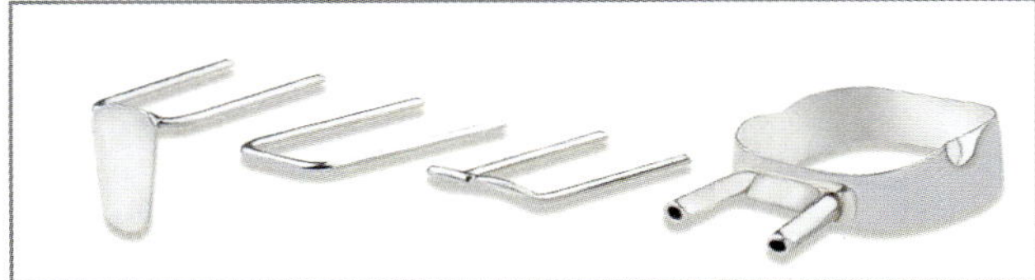

Fig. 35.37: Kids-e preformed space maintainer.

- Maximum space loss usually occurs when permanent molars migrate mesially; resulting in decrease in arch circumference. According to Morrees average arch length of an individual is less at the age of 18 years than at 3 years. Barber believes that our goal should be to prevent arch circumference loss at any cost no matter how miniscule it is. This is where space maintainers have a pivotal role in dentitions that require premature extractions or experience premature exfoliation of primary teeth.
- The safest approach to maintain the arch circumference and prevent future malocclusion is to put an effective, affordable and perdurable space maintainer.

The preformed space maintainer requires following armamentarium.

- Tube crimping plier
- Wire cutter
- Band pusher
- Band adapter
- Preformed bands with attached tube
- Plain loop
- Curved loop
- Distal shoe loop.

Steps in Doing Preformed Space Maintainer

Step 1: Banding—the proper band is selected by trial fitting, and a band is chosen that fits tightly around the tooth and that is well-adapted to the shape of the molar. A band pusher and band adapter is used to fit and adapt the band on tooth.

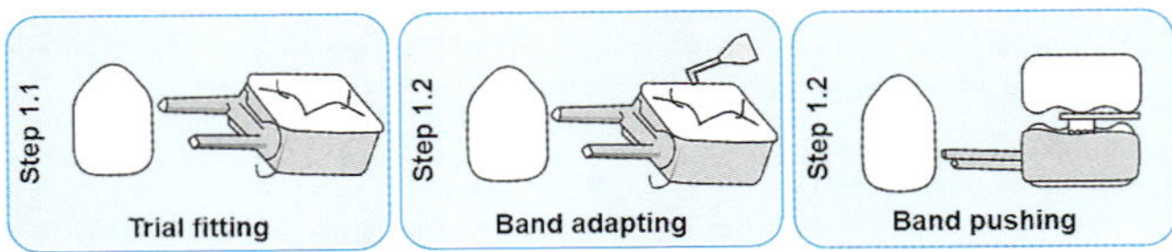

Step 2: Selection of space component—the kit contains three types of space components: Straight loop wire, curved loop wire and distal shoe. Next, a wire loop is selected to act as the spacer. The straight and curved loop is selected for band and loop space maintainer cases and the distal shoe is selected in cases of distal shoe space maintainer.

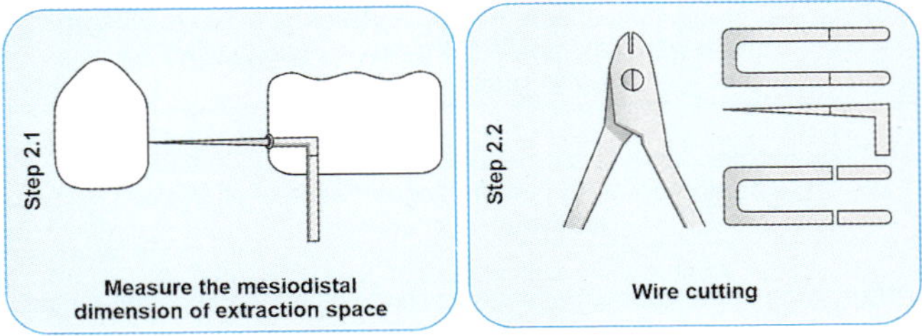

Step 3: Adjusting the space component—according to the extraction space mesiodistal dimension the length of the space component is adjusted. Measure the mesiodistal width intraorally using a straight probe with a rubber stopper. Mark it on the space component and cut it using the cutter provided in the kit. Remove the band from the mouth and slide the wire in the tube of the band. Place the band again on the tooth and check if the space maintainer is fitting properly with space component resting above the contact area of supporting tooth in a passive manner such that it does not slip down.

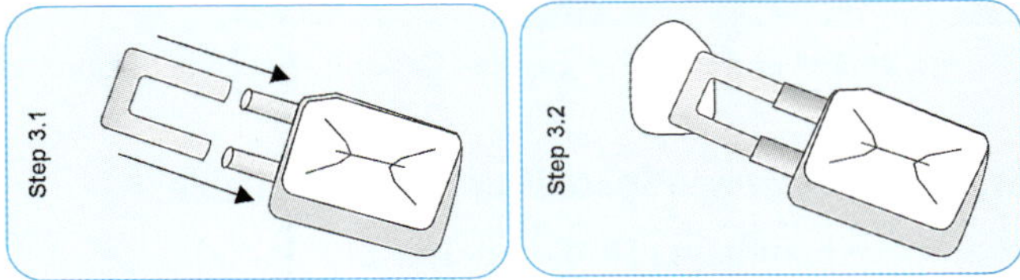

Step 4: Crimping the band tube and space component—using the intraoral crimper crimp the tube in the centre. This will lock the component into the tube.

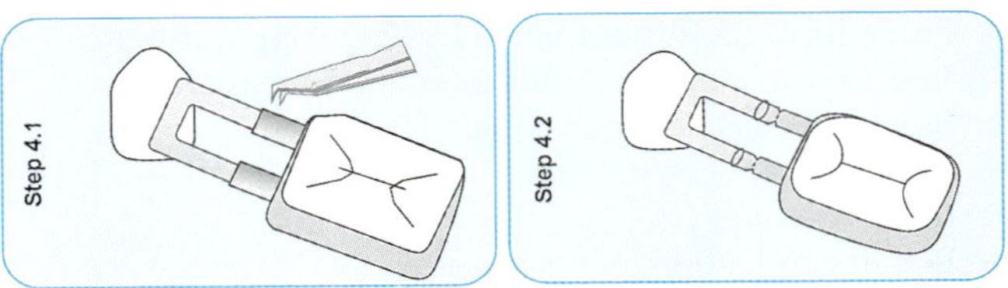

Step 5: Cementation—remove the band and space component and clean with ethanol. Crimp the components again to completely join the tube and space component. Isolate and dry the tooth. Mix luting cement and apply on the inner surface of the band. Seat the band on the tooth using band pusher or band adapter. Remove excess cement after the cement sets.

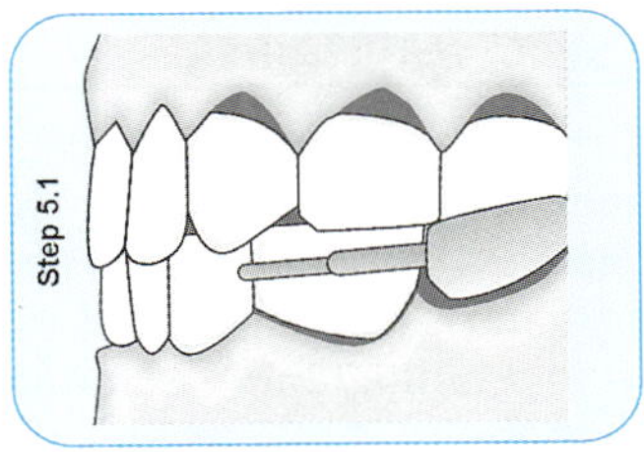

Step 6: Final clinical and radiographic presentation of Kids-e-space maintainers **(Figs. 35.38 to 35.40).**

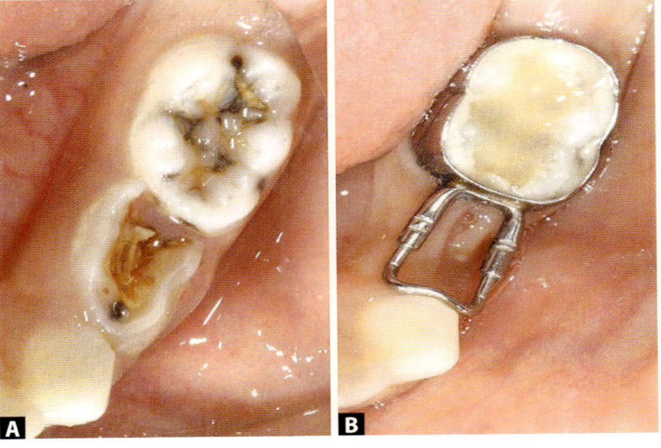

Figs. 35.38A and B: (A) Preoperative; (B) After cementation.

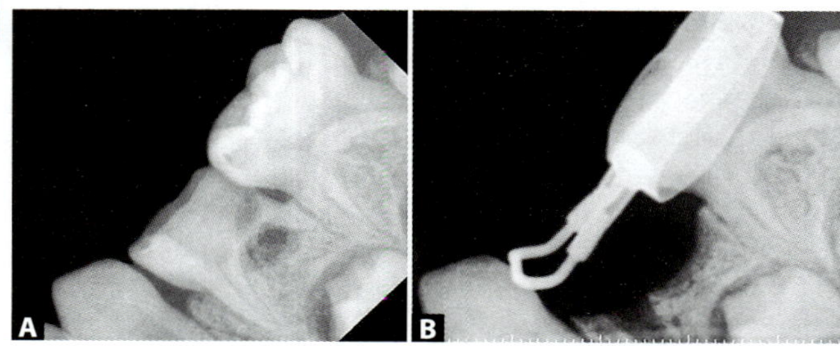

Figs. 35.39A and B: (A) Preoperative IOPA; (B) After cementation.

Brands of Preformed Space Maintainers Available

- e-space maintainer (Kids-e-dental LLP, India)
- Denovo chair side space maintainers (Denovo dental, USA)

Advantages

- It is easy to fabricate
- Procedure can be completed in single appointment
- Reduced cost of the appointment to the patient
- Requires less chair side-time.
- Better patient compliance.
- Inexpensive.
- Repairs and adjustments are easy
- Procedure is under control of the operating dentist
- Can be used easily in sedation cases

Disadvantages

- The loop space is less then 8 mm which can interfere with eruption of premolar
- Initial kit cost is on the higher end

FUNCTIONAL SPACE MAINTAINER

Loss of arch length has been related mainly with tooth migration, following premature loss of primary teeth. This condition has been observed since the 18th century, when **Fauchard** reported it. When a primary tooth is prematurely lost, especially a molar, a careful clinical and radiographic examination should be done, in order to determine the correct treatment to maintain the arch length. When the space for a permanent tooth should be maintained for 2 years or longer, a unilateral fixed space maintainer should always be placed after the premature loss of the second primary molar. There are two methods for constructing a fixed functional space maintainer: Indirect technique and direct technique (double abutment and cantilever).

Indirect Technique

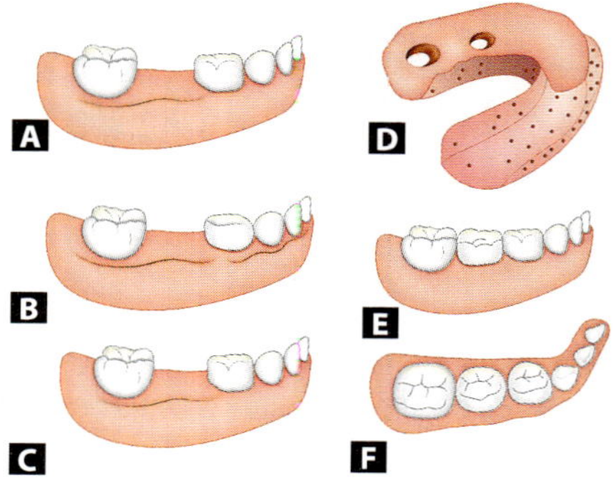

(A) Examine the patient and check occlusion
↓
(B) Prepare the abutment teeth for steel crowns
↓
(C) Adapt steel crowns to the abutment teeth
↓
(D) Compound impression of the quadrant with the crowns in mouth
↓
Place the crowns in the compound and secure when necessary before pouring the model
↓
(E) Solder pontic to abutment teeth and polish space maintainer
↓
(F) Crimp pontic where necessary fill with self-curing acrylic and cement into place

Direct Technique: Double Abutment

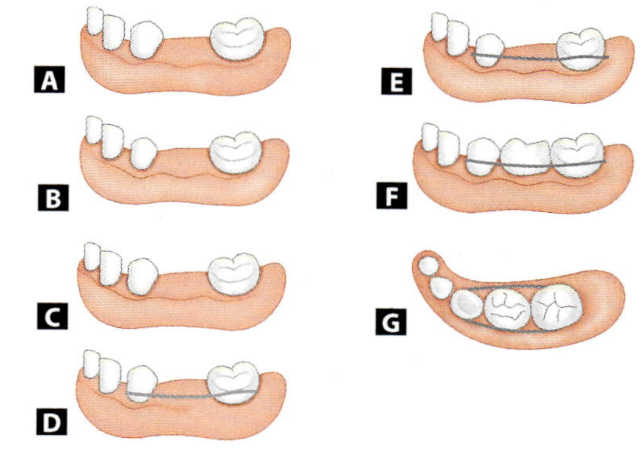

Double abutment
↓
(A) Examine the patient and check occlusion
↓
(B) Prepare the abutment teeth for a steel crowns
↓
(C) Adapt steel crowns to the abutment teeth
↓
(D) Spot weld a two centimeter piece of 0.030 blue elgiloy wire to the buccal occlusal, gingival middle third of the distal stainless steel crown molar
↓
(E) Bend wire to conform to the curve of the arch and cross the buccal middle third of canine
↓
Mark where the wire crosses the canine with a wax pencil
Use pencil marks to relate wire to canine on the welder and spot weld the wire to the canine crown
↓
Try in the stainless crowns with wire to check fit
↓
(F) Select pontic to fit space, trim as necessary, relate to wire and mark with wax pencil. Spot weld pontic to wire.
Try in space maintainer
↓
Take another place of two centimeter piece of 0.030 blue elgiloy wire and pot weld it to the lingual faces of all three stainless steel crowns
↓
After trying in the space maintainer and checking the fit solder all the welded areas and polish
↓
(G) Crimp pontic where necessary fill with self-curing acrylic cement into place

Direct Technique: Cantilever

(A) Cantilever

↓

Examine the patient and check occlusion

↓

No preparation is required because a first permanent molar is used. Adapt stainless steel crown and crimp as necessary

↓

Select a stainless steel crown as a pontic and spot weld one-half centimeter piece of 0.030 blue elgiloy wire to the mesial suface, then bend at a right angle to make occlusal rest on 1st primary molar

↓

(B) Cut off excess wire

↓

(C) Relate pontic to stainless steel crown abutment and mark with pencil

↓

Orient stainless steel crown abutment and pontic on spot welder with pencil marks, weld and try in space maintainer

↓

Solder wire occlusal rest to pontic and to abutment crown and polish

↓

(D) Crimp pontic where necessary fill with self-curing acrylic and cement into place

SPACE MAINTENANCE IN PRIMARY ANTERIOR REGION

The space maintainer consists of artificial teeth (polycarbonate or acrylic) processed onto a lingual arch which in turn is attached to bands for the molars. Stainless steel bands or crowns are fitted to the primary second molars. An arch is constructed and fitted to rest at the base of the cingulum. An attachment post is prepared form 0.028″ wire and soldered to the lingual arch in the site of the missing tooth. The post wire should be placed so that it will lie in the middle of the replacement tooth when the replacement tooth is set in the arch on the model. The post wire should be looped around the lingual arch tightened and held in place, while it is being soldered. Adjoining teeth should be covered with clay and double thickness of aluminum foil to prevent damage during soldering. After soldering the post is bent incisally to conform to the curvature of the arch. The appliance is removed from model, polished, and the tooth is contoured to the gingival contour and positioned in the arch. Crown cutting is then done on this tooth and finally the tooth is built up using composite resin. This is also called **Groper's appliance (Fig. 35.40).**

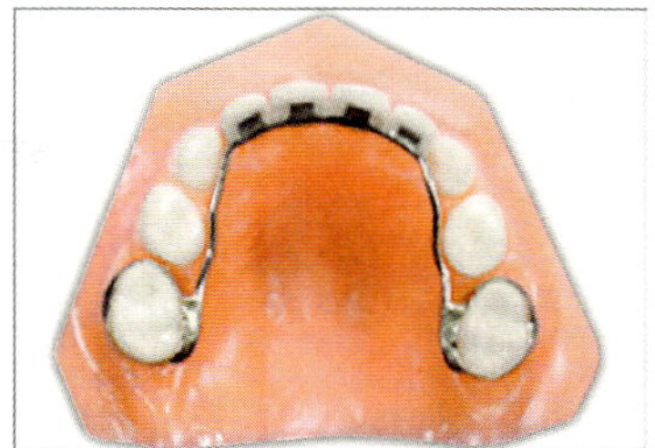

Fig. 35.40: Groper's appliance.

ANTERIOR ESTHETIC FUNCTIONAL SPACE MAINTAINER

Premature loss of primary tooth is one of the most common etiologies for malocclusion. When a primary tooth is lost prematurely, the teeth, present both mesial and distal to the created space, tend to drift in to the space. In the situation where an anterior primary tooth is lost before the schedule, the drifting of adjacent teeth in to the space created rarely occurs but these results into an unesthetic smile and difficulty in biting, that is, loss of function thus making the situation which cannot be left unattended. An esthetic functional space maintainer is thus fabricated to take care of the esthetics and maintain function as well. An alginate impression was made for both maxillary and mandibular arch and was poured in gypsum stone. The shade of the natural teeth was recorded using a proper shade guide. The distance from the distal surface of the maxillary right primary lateral incisor to the distal surface of the maxillary left primary central incisor was measured on the cast and a strip of fiber reinforced composite (FRC) resin was cut of the same length. The FRC strip was adapted over the palatal surface extending from the distal surface of the maxillary right primary left incisor through the distal surface of the maxillary left primary central incisor. Now an acrylic tooth (maxillary right central incisor) of the appropriate shade was selected and was trimmed properly to replace the missing tooth in an esthetic manner. Grooves were made on the palatal surface of the acrylic tooth so as to enhance bonding between the acrylic resin and the composite resin. Now flowable composite was applied throughout the length of the FRC and over the palatal surface of the acrylic tooth **(Figs. 35.41A to C).**

The FRC strip and the acrylic tooth were placed in position over the cast. Care was taken to establish a good contact between the FRC and the acrylic tooth. The FRC and the

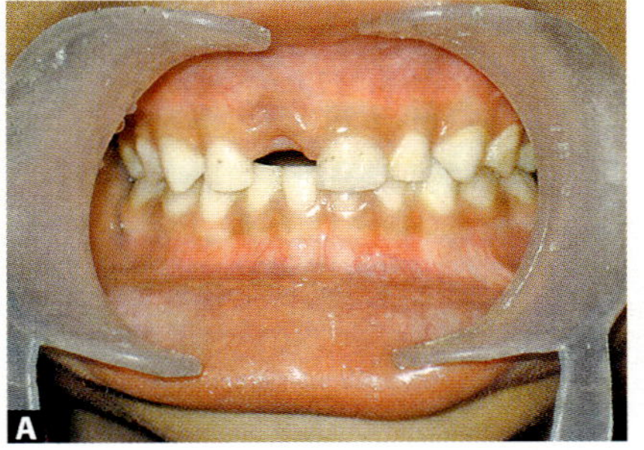

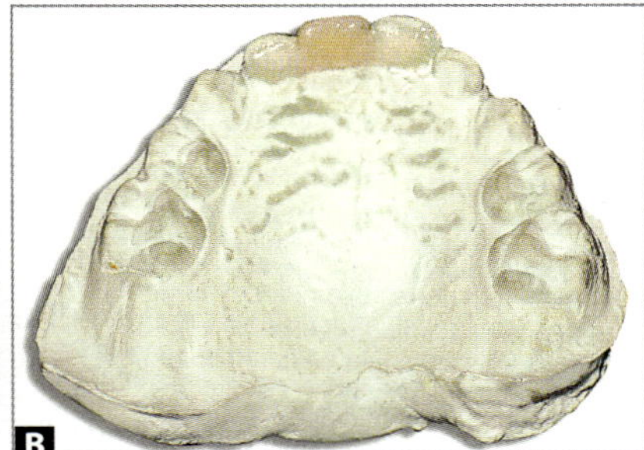

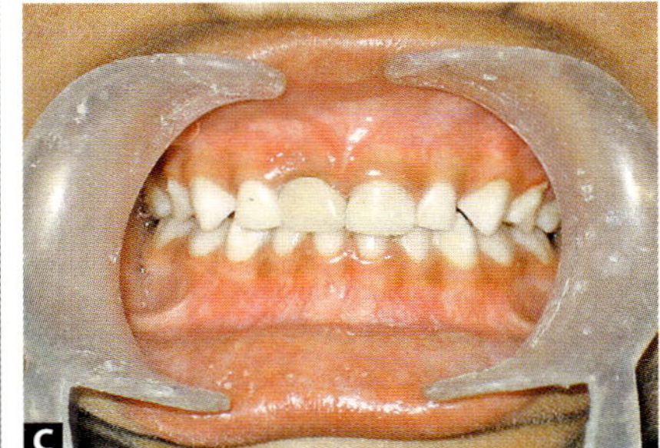

Figs. 35.41A to C: Anterior esthetic functional space maintainer.

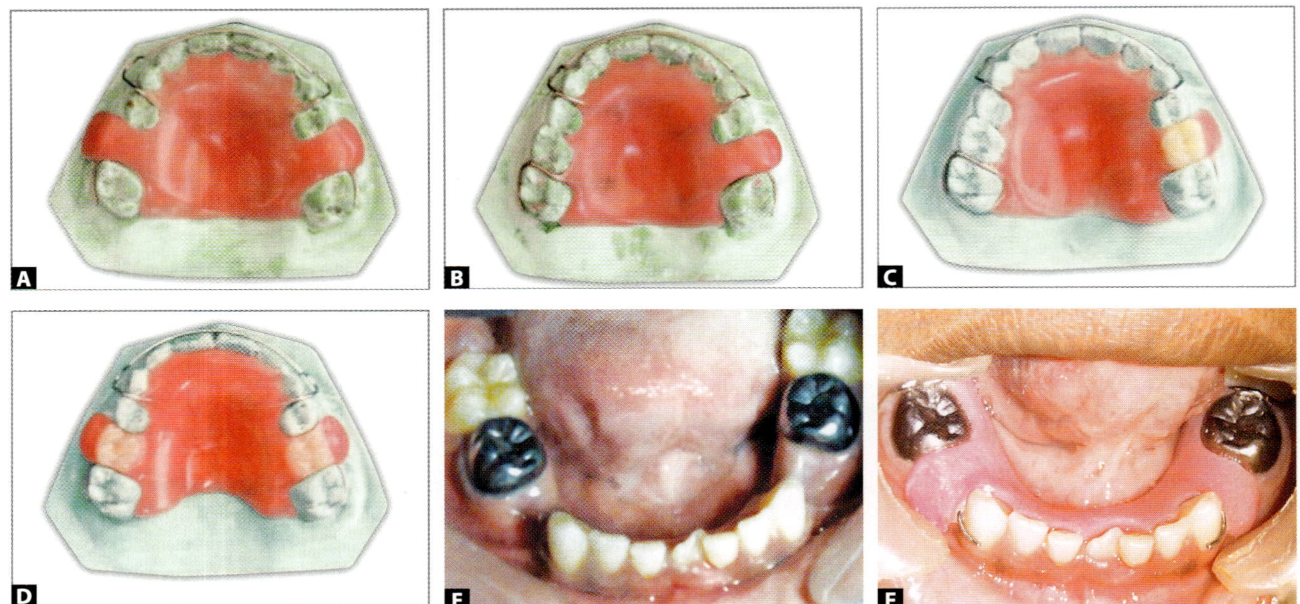

Figs. 35.42A to F: Removable space maintainers: (A) Bilateral nonfunctional space maintainer; (B) Unilateral nonfunctional space maintainer; (C) Unilateral functional removal maintainer; (D) Bilateral functional removal space maintainer; (E and F) Removable space maintainer in a patient.

flowable composite were light cured together from the palatal aspect of the cast. The occlusion was checked over the cast to remove any premature contacts. The appliance was removed from the cast and selective grinding was done wherever necessary. On the next appointment, the appliance was tried in the oral cavity and occlusion was checked for any premature contact. Now the appliance was removed and the palatal surfaces of the tooth on either side of the edentulous space were acid etched. Bonding agent was applied and was cured as per manufacturer's instructions. A thin layer of flowable composite was also applied over the etched surfaces of the abutment teeth. The appliance was placed in position and then the flowable composite was cured using a light curing unit.

REMOVABLE SPACE MAINTAINERS

They are space maintainers that can be removed and reinserted into the oral cavity by the patients **(Figs. 35.42A to F)**.

Indications

- Esthetics is of importance.
- The abutment teeth cannot support a fixed appliance.
- A cleft palate patient.
- Child has reached a mental age of 2.5 years.
- Permanent teeth are not fully erupted for adaptation of bands.
- Multiple loss of primary tooth.

Contraindications

- Lack of patient parent cooperation.
- It the child has not attained a mental age of 2.5 years.
- It the patients are allergic to acrylic materials.
- Epileptic patients.
- Children with possible caries activity.

Advantages of Removable Space Maintainers

- Easy to clean and permit maintenance of proper oral hygiene.
- Restore vertical dimension.
- Help in mastication.
- Post insertion checkup is easy Stimulate eruption of underlying tooth.
- Band construction and elaborate skills and instrumentation are not required.
- Alterations can be made without changing the appliance.

Disadvantages of Removable Space Maintainers

- May be lost or broken by the patient.
- Cannot be used in uncooperative patients.
- Patient may not wear them.
- Lateral jaw growth may be hampered.
- May cause irritation and allergy to underlying tissues.

Research regarding space maintainer

- **Sasa et al.**[17] investigated the success and median survival rate of Band and Loop space maintainers using glass ionomer luting cement for attachment in 40 children (22 females and 18 males) between the ages of 3.4 and 7.3 years. 40% of the Band and Loop space maintainers were successful and 57.5% failed during the study period (40 months). The most common cause of failure was decementation (82% of all failed cases). The overall MST was 19.9 months. Appliances fitted in the maxillary and mandibular left side of the mouth showed a statistically higher survival rate than those fitted in the right side.

- **Quidemat** and **Fayle**[36] in their retrospective study investigated the longevity of 301 space maintainers fitted in 141 patients aged 3.4–22.1 years. Failure occurred in 190 space maintainers (63%), of which 36% were due to cement loss, 24% breakage, 10% design problems, and 9% were lost. Using the life table method, the MST for space maintainers was found to be 7 months. Band and Loop appliances had the highest MST of 13 months, while the lower lingual holding arch (LLHA) had the lowest of 4 months. Unilateral space maintainers survived longer than bilateral space maintainers (MST of 13 vs 5 months).
- **Kundu et al.**[37] conducted a study aimed to evaluate the growth of *Streptococcus mutans*, *Lactobacillus* sp., and *Candida albicans* in saliva during the first 6 months of orthodontic therapy. They concluded that at different time intervals, the total numbers of bacterial count of *Streptococcus mutans* were comparatively higher, followed by *Lactobacillus* sp. and *Candida albicans*.
- **Arikan et al**. (2014): In this study, use of both fixed and removable space maintainers led to an increase in the number of microorganisms in the oral cavity as well as to increases in the periodontal index scores.
- **Uddanwadiker et al.**[38] (2016) did finite element analysis and was applied for evaluation of the deformations on the jaw bone due to a band and loop, Nance appliance, and transpalatal arch space maintainers. The Nance appliance showed the lesser deformation on jawbone than band and loop and transpalatal arch.
- **Dincer et al.**[39] conducted the study to evaluate the effect of removable space maintainers on intercanine arch width increase. Their results indicated that the removable SMs may cease increase in intercanine arch width.
- **Bhaskar** and **Subba Reddy** (2010): They observed that release of nickel and chromium was minimum on 28th day of insertion. The amount released increased proportionally with the number of space maintainers inserted.
- **Mohammad et al.** (2013) evaluated that amount of salivary Ni-Cr released after space maintainer insertion more than stainless steel crowns.
- **Ashish Anand et al.** (2015) explained that release was very much below when compared with the average dietary intake of nickel (300– 500 ppm/day) and for chromium which ranges from 50 to 200 ppm/day which were not capable of causing any toxic effects.
- **Tulunoglu et al.**[40] evaluated the MST of fixed and removable space maintainers. MST of space maintainers was 7.17 months for maxilla and 6.69 months in the mandible. MST was 5.25 months for space maintainers fabricated in both arches.
- **Fathian et al.**[21] did a study over 7 years to assess the survival rates of space maintainers. A total of 63% of all space maintainers lasted their anticipated lifetimes or were still in use. Mean pooled survival times were between 26 and 27 months.
- **Martu et al.**[41] stated that the most common reported reason for failure of fixed space maintainers, such as orthodontic rings, is loosening of the rings and bands.

SPACE REGAINERS

Space maintenance is necessary in early loss of posterior primary teeth because early loss contributes to the development of occlusal disharmonies. However, when space is progressively lost, the therapy should be considered to regain it so that additional disharmonies do not develop. For regaining space or any movement of teeth, the most important procedure is the diagnosis. The attention is not limited to the segment in which tooth is missing.

Considerations for treatment should include the alignment and space needs of other teeth in the arch, the relationships of teeth to denture base, the transverse and sagittal dental relationships, the vertical denture relationships, the skeletal relationships of the denture bases to the cranium, and profile of the soft tissue. The diagnostic aids necessary to develop a database for above consideration include study models, radiographs of all the periapical structures, clinical assessment of facial symmetry, and proportions and possibly cephalometric analysis. It is important to recognize whether teeth have moved bodily into the space or have tipped axially, because forces applied to tip teeth back into a proper alignment are easier to manage than forces required to bodily return teeth to their proper position in the arch. Several problems are associated with the regaining procedures. Usually minimal space loss can be regained better. The space regaining procedure that involves tipping of first permanent molar can be accomplished more easily in the maxillary arch than in the mandibular arch.

Fixed space regainers

- Jaffe's appliance
- Open coil space regainer
- Gerbers space regainer
- Nickel Titanium wire bonded space regainer
- Lingual arch cross bow
- Double banded space regainer
- Sliding loop regainer
- Gurin lock space regainer
- Pendulum appliance
- Hotz lingual arch
- Lip bumper
- Lingual arch with coil spring
- King's appliance

Removable space regainers

- Hawley's appliance with Jack screw
- Split saddle/dumbell spring
- Sling shot space regainer
- Hawley's appliance with finger spring

Jaffe's Appliance

- An appliance for certain minor tooth movement was described by **Paul E Jaffe** in 1963.
- It is useful in the presence of ankylosed tooth, early loss of a primary molar, or an extraction result in filling of adjacent segments into proximal dental area.
- Movement is obtained by the use of light spring pressure against a sliding section or arch.

Open Coil Space Regainer

- It is also called as Herbst space regainer.
- Reciprocal active fixed regainer.
- Used when the first premolar has erupted into the oral cavity.
- A molar band is fitted to the first permanent molar and molar tubes are soldered. Stainless steel wire slightly smaller than tube size is selected and bent into a "U" shape aiming toward the first premolar at a point just below the greatest distal convexity of the first premolar. Spaced coil spring is

A Open coil space regainer in situ

B 35 erupting after regaining space

C Pretreatment

After space regaining

35 erupting after space regaining

D 35 in occlusion

E 9 Oct '04

F 26 April '05

G 26 May '05

H 20 July '05

Figs. 35.43A to H: Space regainer.

cut about 2–3 mm longer than the distance from the anterior stop to the molar tube is used and band is cemented with the coil springs compressed **(Figs. 35.43A to H).**

Gerber's Appliance

- This type of appliance may be fabricated directly in the mouth during or relatively short appointment and requires no lab work.
- A "U" assembly is fitted in tube. Length of the push coil springs is established placing the band-tube-wire assembly in mouth and springs are compressed enough to allow assembly to fit the edentulous area **(Fig. 35.44)**.

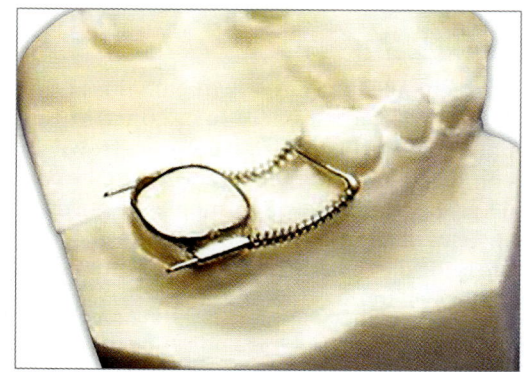

Fig. 35.44: Gerber's appliance.

A seamless orthodontic band or crown is selected for the abutment tooth and fitted

↓

Mesial surface is marked for placement of "U" assembly which may be welded or soldered in place

↓

The "U" section is fitted in the tube, the appliance placed and wire section extended to contact the tooth mesial to edentulous area

↓

Assembly is removed and welded or soldered at this point

↓

If the appliance to be used is a spring loaded space regainer, tube and wire "U" assembly are not welded. An eyelet may be welded to the flattened of the tube next to the band and weldable tube stops are soldered on wire portion and open coil spring sections are cut to fit over wire between "stops" and end of "U" tube

↓

The length of push coil springs is established by placing the band-tube-wire assembly in the mouth, extending the wire to the desired in contact with the mesial tooth and measuring the distance between the tube stops on the wire and the end of "U" tube. To this distance add the amount of space needed to regain, plus 1 to 2 mm. To ensure spring activation, cut springs to this length and compress springs enough to allow the assembly to fit the edentulous area

Hotz Lingual Arch

- It is another method for distalization of molars by **Hitchcock** (1974).
- This is appropriate in a situation where the lower first permanent molar has drifted mesially, but the premolar or cuspid has not drifted distally.
- A "U" loop is incorporated in the arch wire to make it active, which aids in distalization of molar and proclination of the collapsed incisors. The lingual arch provides compound anchorage from all the other teeth which the lingual arch touches. A horizontal spur can be soldered perpendicular to the arch wire contacting the distal surface of the premolar or canine. This compounds the anchorage additionally. The loop on the active side is adjusted periodically once a month **(Fig. 35.45).**

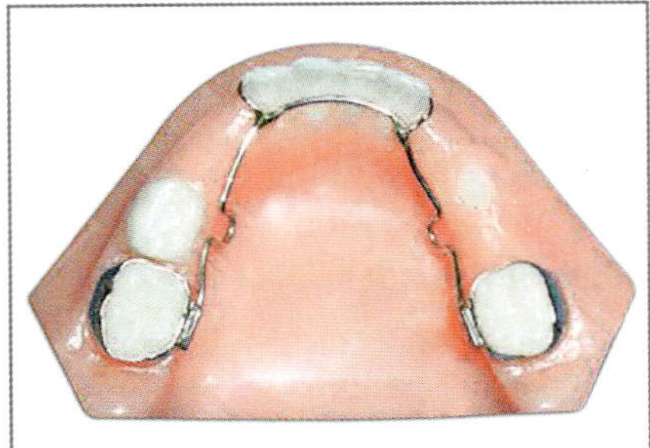

Fig. 35.45: Hotz lingual arch.

Lip Bumper

- The lip bumper is a semifixed type of myofunctional appliance, which can be used in both the arches.
- It harnesses the forces from the lip musculature and transmits them to the molars **(Figs. 35.46A and B).**
- It is used for the space regaining procedures in which bilateral movement is desired.

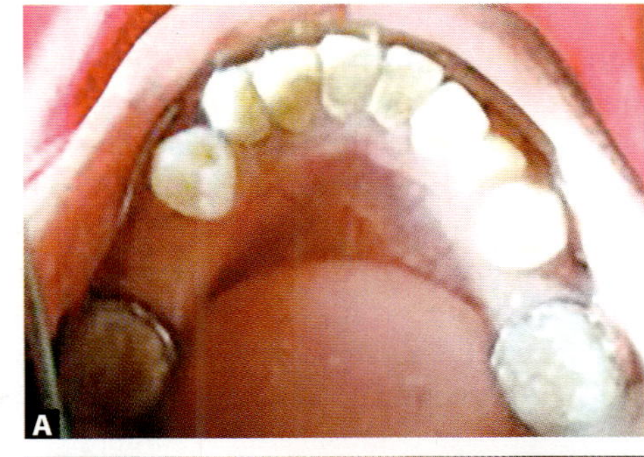

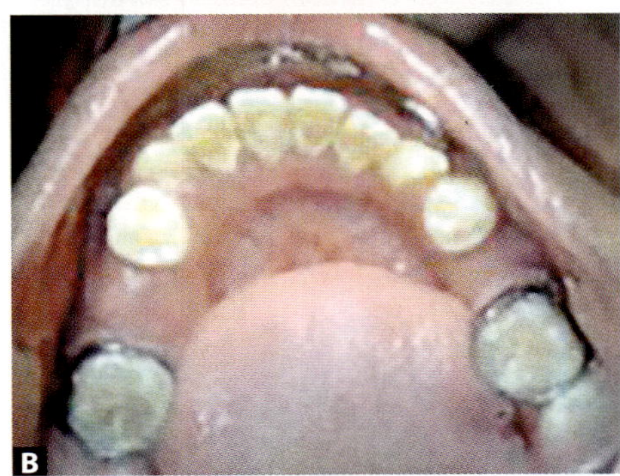

Figs. 35.46A and B: Lip bumper used to regain space.

King's Appliance

- **King** in 1977 described an appliance for regaining of space in both maxillary and mandibular arch.
- The anchorage unit for the mandibular arch is basically a fixed lingual arch with bands fitted on the first primary molar of the treatment side and the first permanent molar on the opposite side. Then an edgewise bracket is spot-welded to the buccal surface of the primary molar band, and the completed anchorage unit is cemented in place. A band with an angulated buccal tube is cemented on the malpositioned molar, and a straight section of wire with an open coil spring is introduced into the buccal tube and ligated into the bracket. The anchorage unit must be modified for the treatment in the maxillary arch **(Fig. 35.47).**

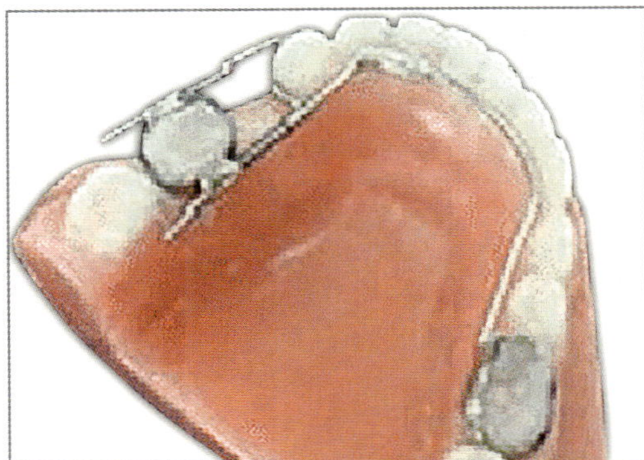

Fig. 35.47: King's appliance.

Sliding Loop Regainer

- It is recommended in cases where space loss occurs due to premature loss of mandibular second primary molar, when both the first molar and first premolar have tipped into the available space.

- The setup applies a constant force to move the first premolar mesially and, with some reciprocal distal movement, move the permanent molar distally.
- It is designed with one band on the permanent molar and two 0.036 inch buccal tubes are welded to the molar band. A loop, similar to the band and loop is fabricated using a 0.036 inch stainless steel wire. An open coil spring of approximately 2 mm in excess of the space to be regained is cut and inserted into the prepared loop. The loop and coil spring component is placed and the loop is slided into the buccal tubes. An occlusal stop is soldered to the loop component of the appliance, and placed in contact with the occlusal surface of the premolar to prevent rotation of the tooth **(Fig. 35.48)**.[42]

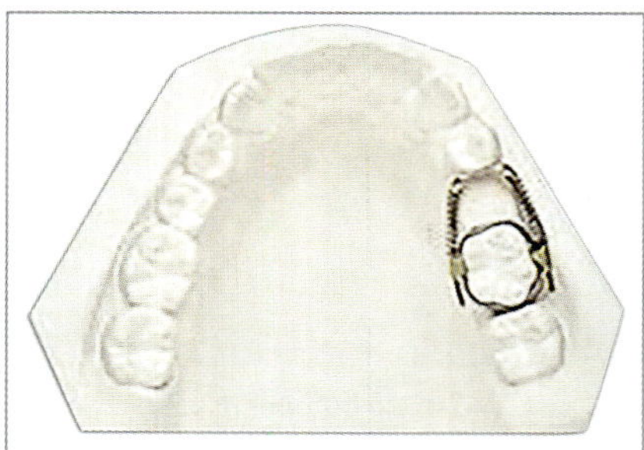

Fig. 35.48: Sliding loop regainer.

Gurin Lock Space Regainer

- It is a unilateral fixed space regainer.
- It is indicated when mesial movement of bicuspid is required without distal movement of the other teeth.
- It consists of bands on the first premolar and molar and a sliding bar soldered to the premolar band. The bar slides into a buccal tube on the molar. This appliance uses a nickel titanium coil spring which is activated by an adjustable Gurin Lock to regain space without tipping or rotating the teeth **(Fig. 35.49)**.[42]

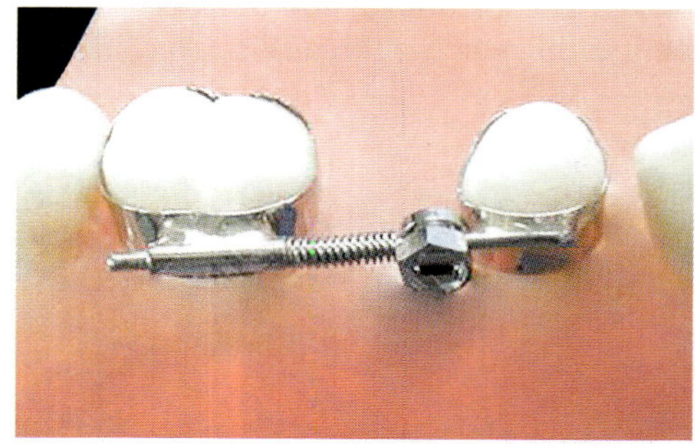

Fig. 35.49: Gurin lock space regainer.

Pendulum Appliance

- The pendulum appliance may be used for unilateral or bilateral distalization of maxillary first molar teeth when mesial drift of upper first molars is present due to early loss of primary molars.
- It can also be used in non-extraction treatment of mild to moderate crowding.
- The pendulum appliance contains an acrylic plate that is retained in place either by clasps to the first premolars or the acrylic is integrated with a metal frame that is soldered to bands on the first premolars. Distalization arms or springs are constructed from 0.6 mm stainless steel round-wire that consists of a closed helix and a U-loop. The purpose of the closed helix is to allow for activation of the distalization arms. The U-loops are incorporated mesial to the molars to allow for adjustment of the axial inclination during distalization. This wire is soldered to molar bands. Typically, an initial activation of 60° to 70° (around the width of one molar) will generate 250 g of force per side. The appliance is activated extraorally and is cemented in place **(Fig. 35.50)**.[43]

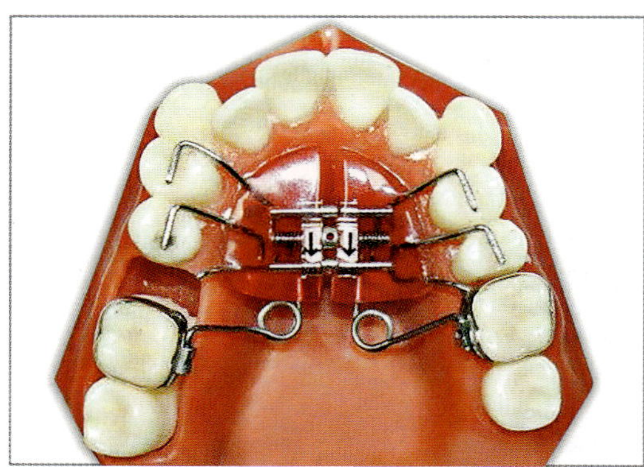

Fig. 35.50: Pendulum appliance.

- **Hilger** (1992) proposed variation in design of pendulum appliance including a lingual sheath on the molar bands allowing intraoral adjustment of the springs, a Nance holding arch or utility arch wires inserted for stabilization while allowing the premolars to drift distally and an expansion screw incorporating in the Nance button allowing space gaining and arch coordination.[44]
- **Nappee MM et al.**[45] (2014) presented a new Pendulum variant using a mini-screw, the "Pendulis". It follows the original concept (titanium-molybdenum alloy distalization springs and polymethyl-methacrylate pellet) but dental support is replaced by a single palatal mini-screw (median in adults, paramedian in children) to which the device is fixed by means of a metal welded cap which can be easily positioned and removed by the practitioner. This appliance allows for better control of the oral hygiene and completely controlled extraoral activation.

Nickel Titanium Wire Bonded Space Regainer

- Modified space regainer is a simple appliance that can be placed chairside in single visit.[46]
- A composite dimple is bonded on the buccal side of permanent first molar and with the help of an explorer, a tunnel is burrowed into the mesial of the dimple. A piece of 0.016" NiTi wire then bonded on the buccal side of primary molar and extended beyond the dimple. After the composite has set on both teeth, direct the free end of wire into the tunnel made in the dimple of first molar. This will give a form of activated loop NiTi wire **(Fig. 35.51)**.
- Over the time the loop returns to its original shape due to the memory properties of NiTi wire, at the same time distalizing and uprighting the first molar.

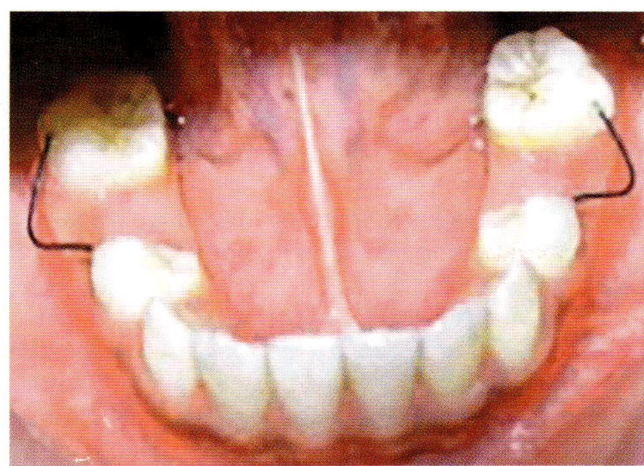

Fig. 35.51: Nickel titanium wire bonded space regainer.

Lingual Arch Cross Bow

- Developed by **Chalakkal et al.**[47]
- It can be used on the lower arch if the first premolar erupts prior to the canine and needs to be distallized to prevent it from encroaching into the canine space **(Figs. 35.52A and B)**.

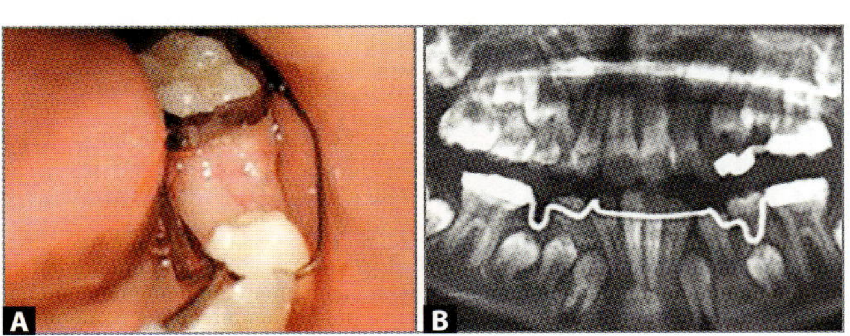

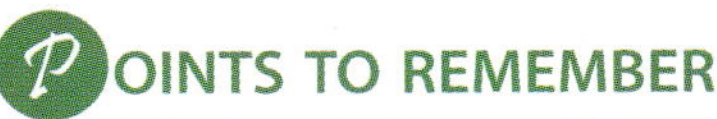

Figs. 35.52A to C: Lingual arch cross bow.

Double Banded Space Regainer

- Developed by **Chalakkal et al.**[47]
- It is used in convention space regaining cases
- Space regained via action of coil springs
- Both the teeth are banded **(Fig. 35.53)**.

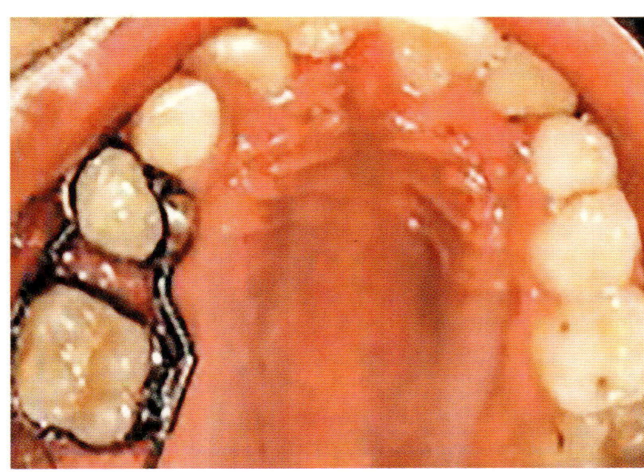

Fig. 35.53: Double banded space regainer.

Anterior Space Regainer

Bayardo in 1986 described an anterior space regainer utilizing direct bond technique. The enamel of the labial surface of left central and right lateral incisors was etched with 35% phosphoric acid and labial tube was individually bonded to each abutment tooth thus causing space regaining.

POINTS TO REMEMBER

- Space maintenance was coined by Brauer in 1941.
- According to Boucher, space maintainer is a fixed or removable appliance designed to preserve the space created by the premature lossof a primary tooth or a group of teeth.
- In the premature loss of first primary molar may be maxillary, mandibular, or both; unilateral or bilateral space maintainers should alwaysbe placed.
- Maximum space is lost during the first 6 months of extraction and most immediate loss is within 76 h. Maxillary spaces close faster as compared to mandibular spaces.
- 1 mm of bone resorbs in 4–5 months and so if the bone is present over the succedaneous tooth it is an indication for space maintainer.
- Space regained by space regainers should be maintained until adjacent permanent teeth have erupted completely and/or until a subsequent comprehensive orthodontic treatment plan is initiated.
- Fixed space maintainers are the appliances, which are fixed onto the teeth and utilize bands or crown for their construction. Reverse bandand loop is given when there is premature loss of primary second molar and the permanent molar have not erupted fully.
- Lingual arch space maintainer is the most effective appliance of space maintenance and minor tooth movement in lower arch.
- Distal shoe space maintainer otherwise known as intra-alveolar appliance, currently in practice is Roche's distal shoe or modifications of it.
- Space maintainer in the primary anterior region consists of artificial teeth (polycarbonate or acrylic) processed onto a lingual arch which inturn in attached to the bands to the molars.

Questionnaire

1. Define space maintenance and explain the factors influencing the placement of space maintainer.
2. Classify space maintainers and give its indications and contraindications.
3. Write a note on arch holding space maintainers.
4. What are the modifications of band and loop space maintainers?
5. Describe in detail the distal shoe space maintainer.
6. Write a note on space regaining.

REFERENCES

1. Cavalcanti AL, Barros de Alencar CR, Medeiros Bezerra PK, Granville-Garcia AF. Prevalence of early loss of primary molars in school children in Campina Grande, Brazil. Pak Oral Dent J. 28:113-6.
2. McDonald RE, Avery DR. Management of space maintenance problems. In: McDonald RE, Avery DR, (Eds). Dentistry for the child and adolescent. St. Louis: The CV Mosby Company; 1994. pp. 707-43.
3. Richardson M. The relationship between the relative amount of space present in the deciduous dental arch and the rate of degree of

space closure subsequent to the extraction of the deciduous molar. Dent Pract Dent Rec. 1965;16:111.

4. Stewart R, Barber T. Pediatric dentistry, scientific foundation and clinical practice. C.V. Mosby; 1982.
5. Tunison W, Flores-Mir C, ElBadrawy H, Nassar U, El-Bialy T. Dental arch space changes following premature loss of primary first molars: a systematic review. Pediatr Dent. 2008;30:297-302.
6. Padma Kumari B, Retnakumari N. Loss of space and changes in the dental arch after premature loss of the lower primary molar: a longitudinal study. J Indian Soc Pedod Prev Dent. 2006:24 (2); 90-6.
7. Laing E, Ashley P, Naini FB. Space maintenance. Int J Paediatr Dent. 2009;19(3): 155-62.
8. Breakspear EK. Further observations on early loss or deciduous molars. Dent Pract Dent Record. 1961;11:233.
9. Breakspear EK. Sequelae of early loss of deciduous molars. Dental Record. 1951;71:127-34.
10. Clinch L. A longitudinal study of the results of premature extraction of deciduous teeth between 3–4 and 13–14 years of age. Pract Dent Record. 1959;9:109.
11. Moyers RE. Handbook of orthodontics, 4th edition; 1988.
12. Rapp R, Demiroz I. A new design for space maintainers replacing prematurely lost first primary molars. Pediatr Dent. 1983;5:131-4.
13. Savitri R, Latha A, Punitha K, Ramya M. Mayne's appliance- guidance of eruption: a case report. Int J Med Dent Case Rep. pp. 1-3.
14. Garg A, Samadi F, Jaiswal JN, Saha S. 'Metal to resin': a comparative evaluation of conventional band and loop space maintainer with the fiber reinforced composite resin space maintainer in children. J Indian Soc Pedod Prev Dent. 2014;32:111-6.
15. Prajapati D, Nayak R, Kashyap N, Kappadi D. Band and loop redefined—the NIMS modification. Unique J Med Dent Sci. 2013;1:46-7.
16. Pushpalatha C, Mala Devi M, Punitha K, Shwetha G. Custom modified band and loop space maintainer—a case report. J Dent Orofacial Res. 2016;12.
17. Sasa IS, Hasan AA, Quidemat MA. Longevity of band and loop space maintainers using glass ionomer cement: a prospective study. Eur Arch Paediatr Dent. 2009;10:6-10.
18. Wright GZ, Kennedy DB. Space control in primary and mixed dentitions. Dent Clin North Am. 1978;22:579-602.
19. Wright GZ, Kennedy DB. Space control in the primary and mixed dentitions. Oral Health. 1981;71:65-75.
20. Baroni D, Ranchini A, Rimondini L. Survival of different type of space maintainers. 1994;16:360-1.
21. Fathian M, et al. Laboratory-made space maintainers: a 7-year retrospective study from private pediatric dental practice. Pediatr Dent. 2007;29.
22. Croll TP, Sexton TC. Distal extension space maintainer: a new technique. Quint Int. 1981;12:1075-80.
23. Setia V, Pandit IK, Shrivastav N. Banded vs bonded space maintainer. Int J Clin Pediatr Dent. 2014;7:97-104.
24. SimonT, Nwabueze I, Oueis H, StengerJ. Space maintenance in the primary and mixed dentitions. J Mich Dent Assoc. 2012;94:38-40.
25. Bhat PK, Navin HK, Idris M, Christopher P, Rai N. Modified distal shoe appliance for premature loss of multiple deciduous molars: a case report. J Clin Diagn Res. 2014;8:ZD43–ZD45.
26. Chanchala HP, Nagaratna PJ, Rashmi S, Godhi BS. Fixed functional distal shoe appliance for bilateral loss of deciduous molars. J Orofac Res. 2014;4:130-2.
27. Somwanshi YI, Katre AN, Jawdekar AM. Modified distal shoe appliance for multiple loss of first and second primary molars. J Clin Diagn Res. 2016;10:ZJ03–ZJ04.
28. Mayhew MJ. Tissue response to appliance in monkeys. Pediatr Dent. 1984;6:148-52.
29. Srivastava N, Grover J, Panthri P. Space maintenance with an innovative "tube and loop" space maintainer (Nikhil appliance). Int J Clin Pediatr Dent. 2016;9:86-9.
30. Zameer M, Dawood T, Basheer SN, Peeran SW, Peeran SA, Birajdar SB, et al. Clinical technique: Space maintenance Following the Premature Loss of Primary Molars using Innovative Fixed Unilateral Space Maintainers (Smart Appliances). Int J Dentistry Oral Sci. 2020;7(12):968-71.
31. Tyagi M, Srivastava N, Kaushik N, Rana V. Effectiveness of Starkey's appliance as space maintainer; a 21 months clinical follow up. Int J Med Dent Case Rep. 2021;8:1-3.
32. Souror YR, Khawandanah MS, Allam SE, Alaishan RA. Case report: A novel, fixed chairside space maintainer. Int J PedodRehabil. 2019;4:80-3.
33. Pawar BA. Maintenance of space by innovative three-dimensional-printed band and loop space maintainer. J Indian Soc PedodPrev Dent. 2019;37:205-8.
34. Singh PH. Simplify your space maintenance with the new H-appliance: A case report. Int J Med Dent Case Rep. 2019;6:1-3.
35. Emmanuel BJ, Raja J, Senthil M, Manzoor R. A novel patented readymade space maintainer – Bibin appliance: A case report. Int J Med Dent Case Rep. 2021;8:1-3.
36. Quidemat MA, Fayle SA. The longevity of space maintainers: a retrospective study. Pediatr Dent. 1998;20:267-72.
37. Kundu R, Tripathi AM, Jaiswal JN, et al. Effect of fixed space maintainers and removable appliances on oral microflora in children: an in vivo study. J Indian Soc Pedod Prev Dent. 2016;34:3-9.
38. Uddanwadiker R, Patil PG. Dentistry. 2013;3:3.
39. Dincer M, et al. J Clin Pediatr Dent. 1996;21:47-50.
40. Tulunoglu O, Ulusu T, Genç Y. An evaluation of survival of space maintainers: a six-year follow-up study. J Contemp Dent Pract. 2005;6:74-84.
41. Martu L, Luchian L, Danila C, Martu C, Barca E, Beldiman MA. The influence of manufacturing and material quality on space maintainers longevity. 2015: 1294-8.
42. Bahreman A. Early-Age Orthodontic Treatment. First edition, chapter, 4, 73-104. Quintessence books.
43. Cetlin NM, Ten Hoeve A. Nonextraction treatment. J Clin Orthod. 1983; 17:396-413.
44. Hilgers JJ. The pendulum appliance for Class II noncompliance therapy. J Clin Orthod. 1992; 26:706-14.
45. Nappee MM, Nappee FJ, Kerbrat JB, Goudot P. The Pendulis appliance: a palatal miniscrew supported molar distalization device. Orthod Fr. 2014; 85(3):265-73.
46. Negi KS. NiTi bonded space regainer/maintainer. J Indian Soc Pedod Prev Dent. 2010;28.
47. Chalakkal P, Thomas AM, Akkara F, Pavaskar R. New design space regainers: 'lingual arch crossbow' and 'double banded space regainer'. J Indian Soc Pedod Prev Dent. 2012;30:161-5..

FURTHER READING

1. Arikan V, Kizilci E, Ozalp N, Ozcelik B. Effects of fixed and removable space maintainers on plaque accumulation, periodontal health, candidal and Enterococcus faecalis carriage. Med Princ Pract. 2015;24:311-7.
2. Baume LJ. Physiologic tooth migration and its significance for development of occlusion. J Dent Res. 1950;29:123.
3. Beena, JP. Distal shoe, an effective space maintainer for premature loss of primary mandibular second molar - A case report. Int J Clin Prev Dent. 2011;7:209-212.
4. Brill WA. The distal shoe space maintainer: chairside fabrication and clinical performance. Pediatr Dent. 2002;24:561-5.
5. Dimond Jr H. A nickel titanium space regainer retainer. J Clin Orthod. 2001;35:767-8.
6. Following the premature loss of primary molars using innovative fixed unilateral space maintainers (smart appliances). Int J Dentistry Oral Sci. 2020;7(12):968-71.
7. Gerber WE. Facile space maintainer. J Am Dent Assoc. 1964;69: 691-4.
8. Graber TM. Orthodontics Principles and Practice, 3rd edition. WB Saunders; 1998.
9. Guideline on management of the developing dentition and occlusion in pediatric dentistry. Am Acad Pediatr Dent. 2014.
10. Hicks EP. Treatment planning for the distal shoe space maintainer. Dent Clin North Am. 1973;17:135-50.
11. Irwin RD, Meerold JS, Richardson A. Mixed dentition analysis: a review of methods and their accuracy. Int J Pediatr Dent. 1995;5:137-42.

12. Jitesh S, Mathew MG. Space maintainer: A review. Drug invention today. 2019; 11 (Spl issue): 21-5.
13. Kargul B, Caglar E, Kabalay U. Glass fiber-reinforced composite resin as fixed space maintainers in children: 12-month clinical follow-up. J Dent Child. 2005;72:109-12.
14. Martinez NP, Elsbach HG. Functional maintenance of arch length. J Dent Child. 1984;pp.190-3.
15. Miyamoto W, Chung CS, Yee PK. Effect of premature loss of primary canines and molars on malocclusion of the permanent dentition. J Dent Res. 1976;55:584-90.
16. Nayak UA, Louis J, Sajeev R, Peter J. Band and loop space maintainer—made easy. J Indian Soc Ped Prev Dent. 2004;22:134-6.
17. Patil VH, Trasad V, Hugar SM. Distal shoe: a review of literature. Int J Sci Res. 2015;4.
18. Proffit WR. Treatment of nonskeletal problems in preadolescent children. In: Proffit WR, editor. Contemporary orthodontics. St. Louis: The CV Mosby Company; 1986. pp. 312-53.
19. Tondon S. Textbook of paedodontics. 2nd edn. Paras Publication; 2009.
20. Ulusoy AT, Cehreli ZC. Provisional use of a natural tooth crown following failure of replantation: a case report. Dent Traumatol. 2008;24:96-9.
21. Uppal A, Singh R. Space regainers: A review. International Journal of Applied Dental Sciences. 2020; 6(2): 654-60.
22. Waggoner WF, Kupietzky A. Anterior aesthetic fixed appliances for the preschooler: considerations and a technique for placement. Pediatr Dent. 2000;23:147-50.
23. Warren JJ, Bishara SE. Comparison of dental arch measurements in the primary dentition between contemporary and historic samples. Am J Orthod Dentofacial Orthop. 2001;119:211-5.
24. Willett RC. Premature loss of primary teeth. Angle Orthod. 1933;3:106.
25. Willett RC. Preventive orthodontics. J Am Dent Assoc. 1936;23:2257.
26. Yeluri R, Munshi AK. Fibre reinforced composite loop space maintainer: an alternative to the conventional band and loop. Contemp Clin Dent. 2012;3:S26-8.
27. Zameer M, Dawood T, Basheer SN, Peeran SW, Peeran SA, Birajdar SB, et al. Clinical Technique: Space Maintenance. Int J Dentistry Oral Sci. 2020;7(12):968-71.

Serial Extractions

Nikhil Marwah, Siddharth Mehta

Chapter Outline

Serial extraction procedures have been of interest to dentists for many years. The term serial extraction describes an orthodontic treatment procedure that involves the orderly removal of selected deciduous and permanent teeth in a predetermined sequence (**Dewel**, 1969). Serial extraction is an interceptive orthodontic procedure usually initiated in the early mixed dentition when one can recognize and anticipate potential irregularities in the dentofacial complex and is corrected by a procedure that includes the planned extraction of certain deciduous teeth and later specific permanent teeth in an orderly sequence and predetermined pattern to guide the erupting permanent teeth into a more favorable position. Every serial extraction diagnosis is based on the promise that future growth will be inadequate to accommodate all of the teeth in a normal alignment. Serial extraction should be diagnosed in the early mixed dentition period and is most effective when undertaken in Class I malocclusions.

Serial extraction *can be defined as the correctly timed removal of certain deciduous and permanent teeth in mixed dentition cases with dentoalveolar disproportion in order to alleviate crowding of incisor teeth; allow unerupted teeth to guide themselves into improved positions; lessen (or eliminate) the period of active appliance therapy.*

PRINCIPLES OF SERIAL EXTRACTION

The treatment objective for a serial extraction is to intercept an arch length deficiency problem to reduce or eliminate the need for extensive appliance therapy.

History of serial extraction

Year	*Name*	*Findings*
1600s	**Paisson**	The first person who pointed the extraction procedure in order to improve the irregular alignment and crowding of teeth
1743	**Bunon**	In his "Essay on the diseases of the teeth," he proposed the removal of deciduous teeth to achieve a better alignment of permanent teeth
1929	**Kjellgren**	Coined the term "serial extraction" to describe a procedure where some deciduous teeth followed by permanent teeth were extracted to guide the rest of the teeth into normal occlusion
1940	**Nance**	Presented clinics on his technique of "Planned and progressive extraction" and has been called as the father of serial extraction philosophy in the United States
1941	**Hotz**	Named the procedure "Guidance of eruption." According to him, the term guidance of eruption is comprehensive and encompasses all measures available for influencing tooth eruption. Active supervision of teeth by extraction.

Arch Length: Tooth Material Discrepancy

- Whenever there is an excess of tooth material as compared to the arch length, it is advisable to reduce the tooth material in order to achieve stable results.
- This principle is utilized in serial extraction procedures where tooth material is reduced by selective extraction of

teeth so that the rest of the teeth can be guided to normal occlusion.

Physiologic Tooth Movement

Human dentition shows a physiologic tendency to move towards an extraction space. Thus by selective removal of some teeth, the rest of the teeth which are in the process of eruption are guided by the natural forces into the extraction space.

INDICATIONS

Serial extraction procedure is generally indicated when there is severe discrepancy between total tooth material and basal bones in patients having Class I malocclusion and having good facial profile. The severity of the crowding should be such that mixed dentition analysis should indicate a discrepancy of at least 8–10 mm excess tooth material in an unmutilated mandibular arch. The indication for doing a serial extraction must correspond to the patient's needs and biologic characteristics and must fulfill the desired objectives. Indications of this procedure are as follows:

- Premature loss of deciduous teeth.
- Arch length deficiency and tooth size discrepancy.
- Absence of physiologic spacing.
- Lingual eruption of lateral incisors.
- Unilateral deciduous canine loss and midline shifting.
- Canines erupting mesial to the lateral incisors.
- Mesial drift of buccal segment.
- Abnormal eruption direction and eruption sequence.
- Gingival recession on labially displaced incisors.
- Flaring, ectopic eruption, ankylosis, etc.
- Abnormal or asymmetric primary canine root resorption.
- Crowded maxillary and mandibular incisors with extreme labial proclination.
- Deleterious oral habits.
- Class I malocclusion showing harmony between skeletal and muscular system.

CONTRAINDICATIONS

- Congenitally absent/missing lower second premolars.
- Extensive caries of permanent first molars.
- Severe class II and III malocclusions of dental as well as skeletal origin.
- Unilateral congenital absence of teeth.
- Abnormal tooth size, shape, color, etc.
- Cleft lip and cleft palate cases.
- Reverse overjet, deep bite, open bite, rotation, gross malposition, crossbite, etc.
- Spaced dentition.
- Class I malocclusions with minimal space deficiency.
- Mild disproportion between arch length and tooth material that can be treated by proximal stripping.

ADVANTAGES

- Treatment is more physiologic as it involves guidance of teeth into normal positions making use of the physiologic forces.
- The removal of deciduous canine allows spontaneous alignment of crowded incisors which simplify later appliance treatment.
- The extraction of first premolar before crowding allows permanent canines to drift into natural alignment without any appliance.
- It lessens the period of future appliance therapy and cost of treatment.
- Psychological trauma associated with malocclusion can be avoided by treatment of the malocclusion at an early age.
- Better oral hygiene is possible thereby reducing the risk of caries.
- Health of investing tissues is preserved.
- Lesser retention period is indicated at the completion of treatment.

DISADVANTAGES

- This procedure cannot be applied in class II and III malocclusion cases. It is avoided in class II division 2. Serial extraction may cause an increase in overbite.
- Psychological trauma: It is unpleasant for a child to have four teeth extracted each time or at three or four occasions.
- If extractions are carried out too early, this result in space loss or delayed eruption of permanent successors.
- Lower permanent canines may erupt ahead of first premolar into extraction space of the first deciduous molar, impacting premolar and making its removal difficult.
- Quite frequently patients require appliance treatment.
- There is no single approach that can be universally applied to all patients.
- Each patient has to be assessed and a suitable extraction timetable has to be planned.
- Treatment time is prolonged as the treatment is carried out in stages spread over 2–3 years. It requires the patient to visit the dentist often.
- Thus, patient cooperation is needed.
- As extraction spaces are created that close gradually, the patient has a tendency of developing tongue thrust.
- Ditching or space can exist between the canine and second premolar.

TECHNIQUE AND STAGES IN SERIAL EXTRACTION THERAPY

Diagnosis and Treatment Plan

- Deciding on the timing and the sequencing for extracting primary and permanent teeth is the key to success. The technique of serial extraction usually involves a period of incisor adjustment followed by a period of canine adjustment.
- Diagnostic records are obtained by study model, periapical radiographs, panoramic and cephalometric radiographs.
- The diagnostic exercise prior to treatment should involve comprehensive assessment of the dental, skeletal, and soft tissues. A tooth material arch length discrepancy must ideally exist. According to most authors, an arch length deficiency of not less than 5–7 mm should exist to undertake this procedure.

- Study model analysis should be carried out to determine the arch length discrepancy.
- Carey's analysis in the lower arch and arch perimeter analysis in the upper arch should be carried out. Mixed dentition analysis helps in determining the space required for the erupting buccal teeth.
- The eruption status of the dentition is evaluated from an OPG.
- The skeletal tissue assessment should involve comprehensive cephalometric examination to study the underlying skeletal relation.
- The soft tissue assessment by clinical examination and cephalograms help in the diagnosis.

Removal of Deciduous Canine

- The purpose is to permit the eruption and optimal alignment of lateral incisors. It prevents the mesial migration of canines into severe malpositions.
- The four deciduous canines are removed as upper permanent lateral incisors are erupting (at about 8.5 years of age).
- The alignment of incisors should improve at the expense of space for permanent canine.

Removal of First Deciduous Molars

- The first deciduous molars are removed in order to encourage the early eruption of first premolar.
- This will be most successful if premolar roots have half formed (at about 9.5 years of age). It is desirable that the first premolar should erupt in advance of canines, although this is often not in the case of lower arch. It is sometimes done earlier in the mandible than maxilla to enhance early eruption of lower first premolar. If the mandibular canine is erupting ahead of the mandibular first premolar, either of two procedures should be carried out.
  - In a combined procedure, extract deciduous mandibular first molars and surgically remove the unerupted permanent first premolar, or
  - To avoid the surgical procedure, extract the deciduous mandibular first molars and, approximately 6 months later, remove the deciduous mandibular second molars. This allows the unerupted first premolars to move distally in the alveolar bone as the canine erupts.

Removal of Erupting First Premolars

- When the upper permanent canine has just emerged through oral mucosa, the first premolar should be extracted.
- This is the most important stage of serial extraction procedure, and it is essential to recheck that the case is suitable for treatment by extraction of first premolars.
- All teeth must be present and sound, and the permanent canines must be mesially inclined. There must be crowding sufficient to justify the extraction of first premolars.

Desired outcome for selection of teeth for extraction

- Extraction of all primary canines will produce maximum amounts of self-improvement in crowding with greatest interception of lingual crossbite in anterior region.
- Extracting all primary first molars produces earliest eruption of first premolars but reduces speed and amount of improvement in anterior crowding and position due to retention of canine that it has limited application.
- Extracting canines and primary first molars is a compromise between rapid improvement in and desired early eruption of anteriors due to simultaneous first premolar eruption. Due to this extraction sequence, reduced distal translation occurs.
- Enucleation of buds of permanent canines permits maximum distal translation of first premolars, which is undesirable in certain cases because it reduces resistance value of anterior teeth for final space closure.

TWEED'S TECHNIQUE FOR SERIAL EXTRACTION

Tweed in 1966 proposed this extraction sequence **(Fig. 36.1)**. At approximately 8 years of age, all first deciduous molars are extracted. Unless, there is unhealthy soft tissue involvement around the lower incisors, or blocked out maxillary incisors, it is preferable to maintain the deciduous canine to retard the eruption of permanent canines.

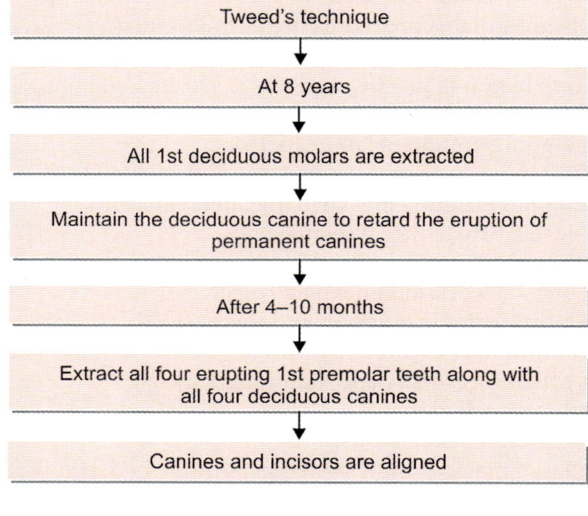

Tweed's technique
At 8 years
All 1st deciduous molars are extracted
Maintain the deciduous canine to retard the eruption of permanent canines
After 4–10 months
Extract all four erupting 1st premolar teeth along with all four deciduous canines
Canines and incisors are aligned

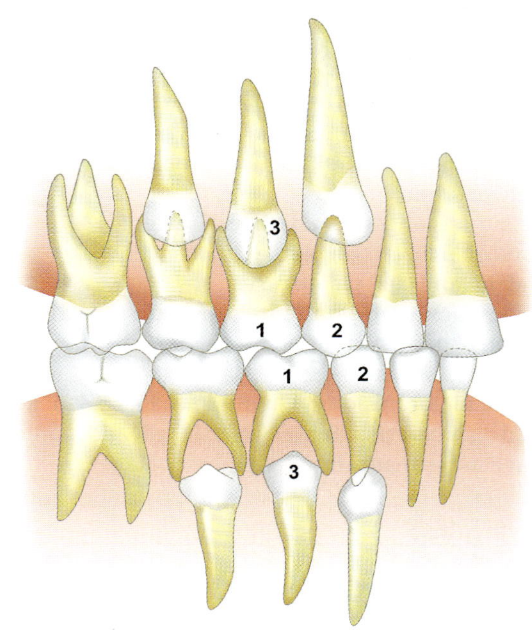

Fig. 36.1: Tweed's method of serial extraction D-C-4.

After 4–10 months of extraction, the first premolar tooth has erupted up to gum level. Do not remove them until their crowns are through alveolar bone. At this time, all four erupting first premolar teeth are removed along with all four deciduous canines. If this is done at least 4–6 months prior to eruption of permanent cuspids, they erupt and migrate posteriorly into good position. The irregularities of mandibular incisors correct themselves.

DEWEL'S METHOD

Dewel has proposed a three-step serial extraction procedure. In the first step, the deciduous canines are extracted to create space for the alignment of the incisors **(Fig. 36.2)**. This step is carried out at 8–9 years of age. A year later, the deciduous first molars are extracted so that the eruption of first premolars is accelerated.

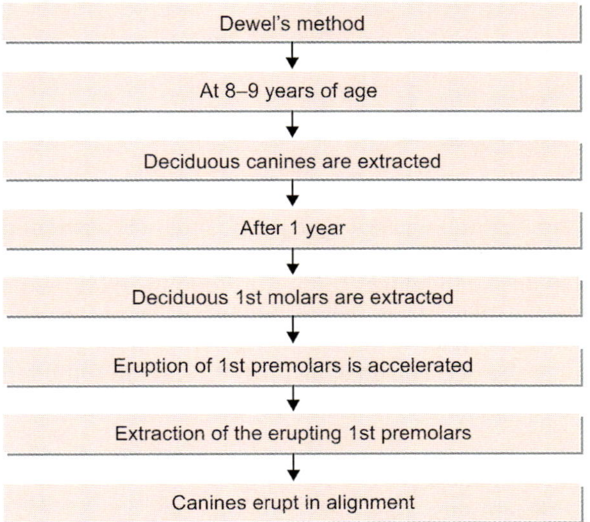

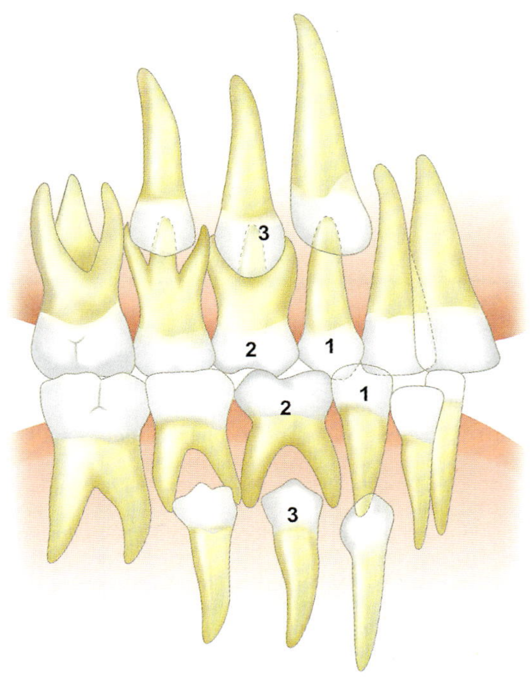

Fig. 36.2: Dewel's method of serial extraction C-D-4.

This is followed by the extraction of the erupting first premolars to permit the permanent canines to erupt in their place. In some cases, a modified Dewel's technique is followed wherein the first premolars are enucleated at the time of extraction of the first deciduous molars. This is frequently necessary in the mandibular arch where the canines often erupt before the first premolars.

NANCE'S METHOD OF SERIAL EXTRACTION

This is similar to the Tweed's technique and involves the extraction of the deciduous first molars followed by the extraction of the first premolars and the deciduous canines **(Fig. 36.3)**.

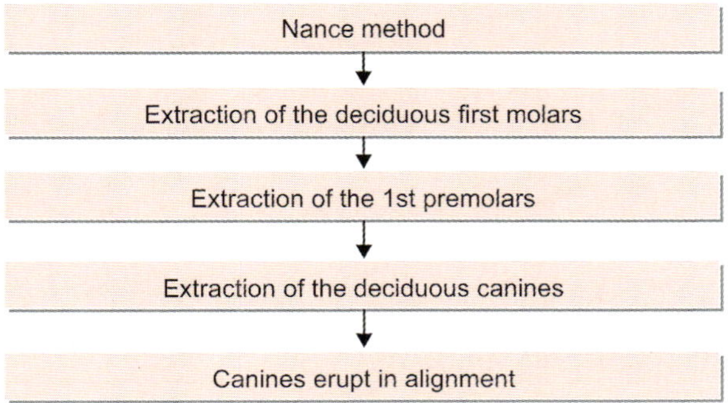

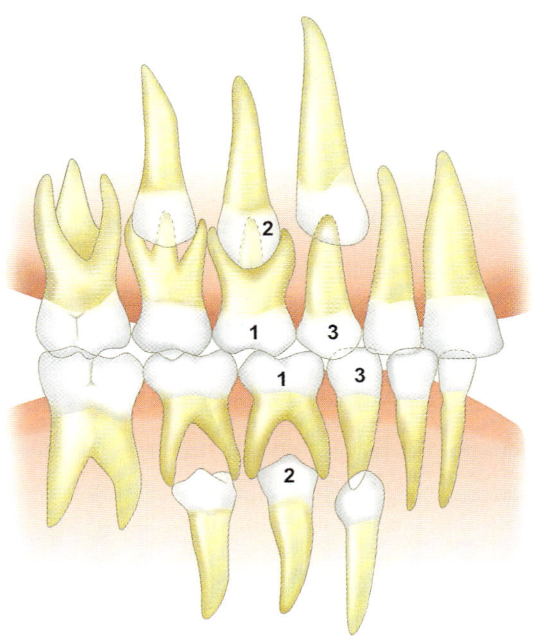

Fig. 36.3: Nance's method of serial extraction D-4-C.

MOYER'S METHOD

Indicated when crowding is seen in central incisor region. First is to extract all deciduous lateral incisors to help in alignment of central incisors. This is followed by extraction of all deciduous canines after 7–8 months to provide space for lateral incisors. After this, extraction of all deciduous first molars is done to stimulate eruption of first premolars. The last sequence is to extract first premolars after 7–8 months, which will not only provide space for canines but also stimulate its eruption **(Fig. 36.4)**.

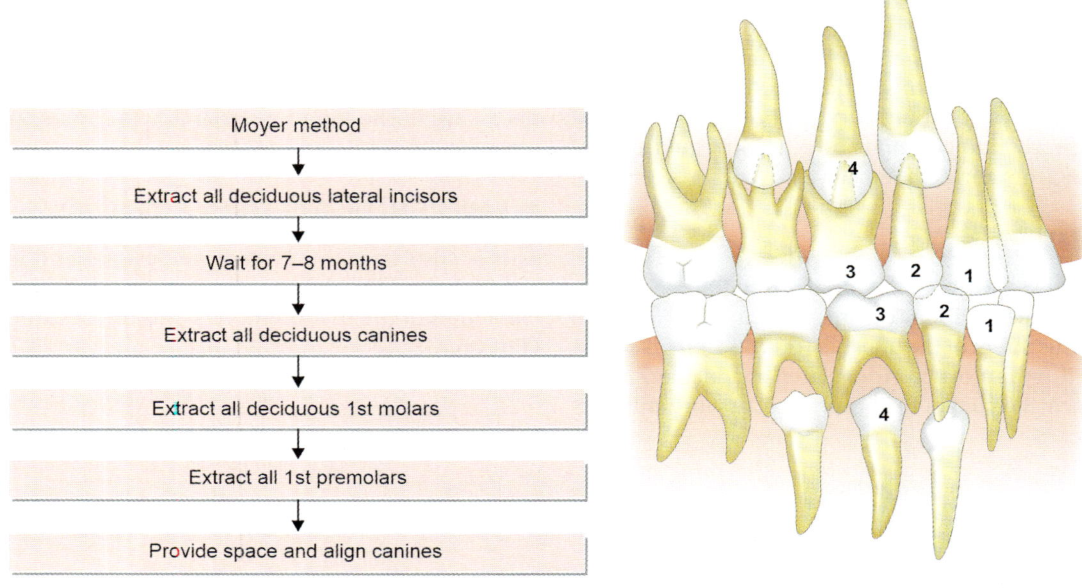

Fig. 36.4: Moyer's method of serial extraction B-C-D-4.

ROLE OF THE PEDODONTIST

Pedodontist and orthodontist are mutually dependent on each other's skills for treatment planning of serial extraction. The ideal plan for the pedodontist is to observe the problem, make a decision that a serial extraction might be appropriate, explain the plan to the patient or parents, and refer the patient to the orthodontist. After having seen the patient and arrived at a decision as to the sequence of extractions and after communicating with the pedodontist, orthodontist should explain the serial extraction plan to the parents as well as advise them that further orthodontic treatment may be needed. At this time, the pedodontist will proceed with the planned sequence of extractions. The pedodontist will thus share in the decision-making process, and the orthodontist does not have a reason to question the decision.

POINTS TO REMEMBER

- Serial extraction can be defined as the correctly timed removal of certain deciduous and permanent teeth in mixed dentition cases with dentoalveolar disproportion in order to alleviate crowding of incisor teeth; allow unerupted teeth to guide themselves into improved positions; lessen (or eliminate) the period of active appliance therapy.
- Kjellgren (1929) proposed the term serial extraction.
- Nance is known as the father of serial extraction.
- Serial extraction procedure is generally indicated when there is severe discrepancy between total tooth material and basal bones in patients having class I malocclusion and having good facial profile. The severity of the crowding should be such that mixed dentition analysis should indicate a discrepancy of at least 8–10 mm excess tooth material.
- Tweed's method of serial extraction D-C-4
- Dewel's method of serial extraction C-D-4
- Nance's method of serial extraction D-4-C
- Moyer's method of serial extraction B-C-D-4

Questionnaire

1. Define serial extraction and give its brief history.
2. Explain Nance's method of serial extraction.
3. Describe Dewel's method of serial extraction.
4. What is Tweed's method of serial extraction?
5. Write a note on Moyer's method of serial extraction.

FURTHER READING

1. Graber TM. Orthodontics: Principles and Practice, 3rd edition. Philadelphia: WB Saunders Co.; 1972. pp. 709-45.
2. Graber TM. Serial extraction: a continuous diagnostic and decisional process. Am J Orthod. 1971;60:541-75.
3. Housten WJB. Walther's Orthodontics Notes, 4th edition. Britol: Wright PSG; 1983. pp. 126-7.
4. Jack G. Dale "Serial extraction part III". J Clin Orthod. 1976. pp. 196-216.
5. Jack G. Dale "Serial extraction part II". J Clin Orthod; 1976. pp. 116-36.
6. Jack G. Dale "Serial extraction part I". J Clin Orthod; 1976. pp. 44-60.
7. Jacobs SG. Reassessment of serial extraction. Aust Orthod J. 1987;10:90-7.
8. Naragond A, Kenganal S. Serial extractions—a review. J Dent Med Sci. 2012;3:40-7.
9. Proffit WR. Contemporary Orthodontics, 2nd edition. Boston: Mosby; 1986.
10. Rani MS. Synopsis of Orthodontics. All India Publications; 1993.
11. Stewart RE. Paediatric dentistry—Scientific Foundation and Clinical Practice, 1st edition. St Louis: CV Mosby Co; 1982.
12. Tweed CH. Clinical Orthodontics, vol. 1. St Louis: CV Mosby Co.; 1966. pp. 261-4.
13. White TC, Gardiner JH. Orthodontics for Dental Students, 3rd edition. London: McMillan Press Ltd.; 1983. pp. 135-8.

CHAPTER

Interceptive Orthodontics

Nikhil Marwah, Shantanu Jain, Deepesh Prajapati, Priya Nagar

Chapter Outline

- Serial Extraction
- Correction of Developing Anterior Crossbite
- Correction of Posterior Crossbite
- Control of Abnormal Habits
- Space Regaining
- Muscle Exercises
- Interception of Skeletal Malrelations
- Removal of Soft Tissue and Bony Barriers

American Association of Orthodontists defined interceptive orthodontics as "*That phase of the science and art of orthodontics employed to recognize and eliminate potential irregularities and malpositions in the developing dentofacial complex.*"

According to **Graber**, interceptive orthodontics refers to the "*Measures undertaken to intercept a malocclusion that has already developed or is developing, and the goal is to restore a normal function.*"

According to **Ackerman** and **Proffit** (1980), interceptive orthodontics can be defined as "*Elimination of existing interferences with the key factors involved in the development of the dentition.*"

Procedures undertaken in interceptive orthodontics
- Serial extraction
- Correction of developing crossbite
- Control of abnormal habits
- Space regaining
- Muscle exercises
- Interception of skeletal malrelation
- Removal of soft tissue or bony barrier to enable eruption of teeth

SERIAL EXTRACTION

- It is an interceptive orthodontic procedure usually initiated in the early mixed dentition.
- Serial extraction is a process of extracting certain deciduous teeth and later specific permanent teeth in an orderly sequence and predetermined pattern to guide the erupting permanent teeth into a more favorable position (Detailed in Chapter 36).
- It is done in cases which show signs of persistent irregularities of teeth due to insufficient space in the arch to accommodate the present amount of tooth substance.

History
- **Kjellgren** (1929), Sweden—coined the term serial extraction
- **Nance** (1940)—termed serial extraction as "Planned progressive extraction" and has been called the "Father of serial extraction"
- **Rudolf Hotz** (1970), Switzerland—termed serial extraction as "Active supervision of teeth by extraction".

Indications

- Class I malocclusion showing harmony between skeletal and muscular system.
- Arch length deficiency as compared to the tooth material.
- Where growth is not enough to overcome tooth material and arch length discrepancy.
- Patients with straight profile and pleasing appearance.

Procedure

The three most popular techniques are:

1. **Dewel's method (CD4):** Removal of deciduous canine → removal of deciduous first molars → removal of erupting first premolars.
2. **Tweed's method (D4C):** Removal of deciduous first molars → removal of erupting first premolars → removal of deciduous canine.
3. **Nance method (D4C):** Removal of deciduous first molars → removal of erupting first premolars → removal of deciduous canine.

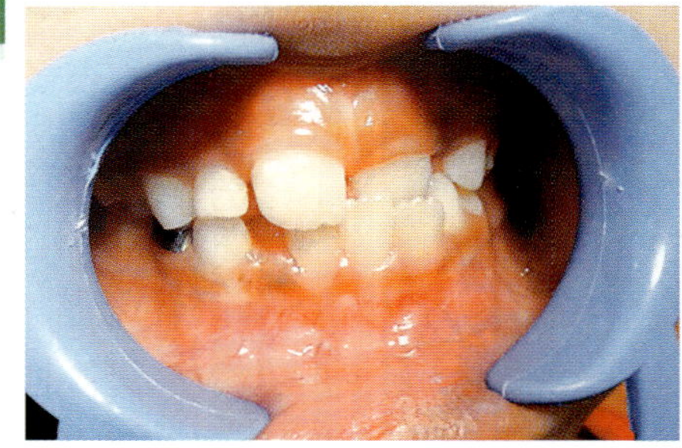

Fig. 37.1: Dentoalveolar crossbite.

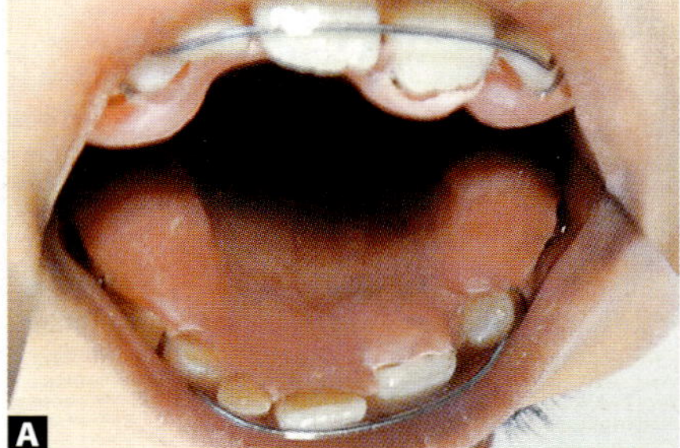

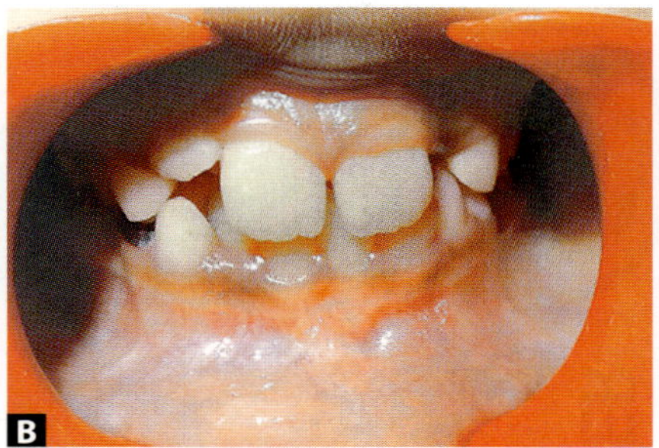

Figs. 37.2A and B: (A) Posterior bite plane with Z spring; (B) Crossbite correction.

CORRECTION OF DEVELOPING ANTERIOR CROSSBITE

- Anterior crossbite is a condition in which one or more maxillary anterior teeth are in lingual relation to the mandibular teeth.
- Anterior crossbites should be intercepted and treated at an early stage because it is a self-perpetuating condition which if not treated early has the potential of growing into skeletal malocclusion and might at a later stage require major orthodontic treatment combined with surgical procedures. It is of three types, viz., dentoalveolar, functional and skeletal anterior crossbite.

Dentoalveolar Anterior Crossbite

- This type is often manifested as one or more inciors in crossbite **(Fig. 37.1)** and usually occurs due to over retained deciduous teeth.
- The most common appliance used for its correction is posterior bite plane with Z spring **(Figs. 37.2A and B).**
- Z spring is fabricated along with Adam's clasp on primary or permanent molars and embedded in acrylic. A labial bow is also incorporated in the appliance to align the upper incisors into their final position after crossbite correction. For first week the appliance is kept passive so that child becomes comfortable in wearing it. The spring is activated every 2 weeks until the crossbite is corrected.

Tongue Blade Therapy

The blade is placed in such a manner that it rests on the mandibular incisors opposing the tooth in crossbite, and the patient is asked to bite with a constant pressure on the tongue blade. If there is adequate space for the tooth in crossbite to be moved into its correct position, the tooth can be guided with the help of the tongue blade **(Figs. 37.3A and B)**.

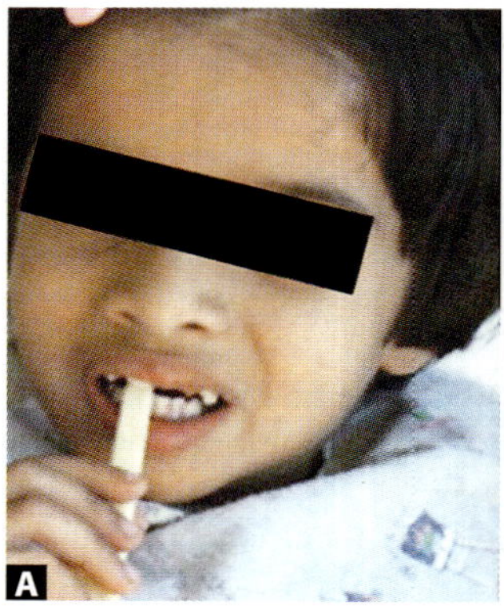

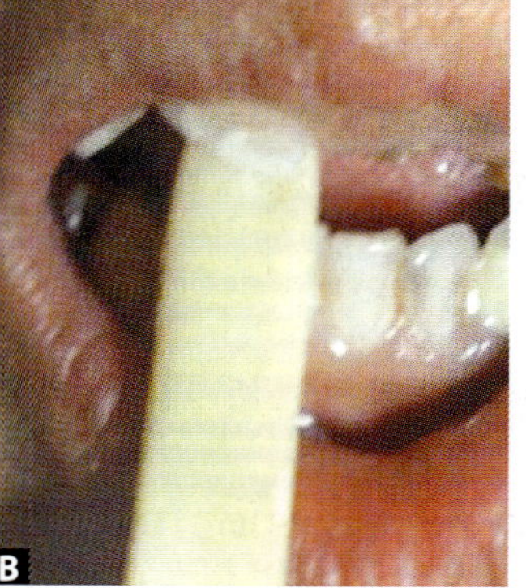

Figs. 37.3A and B: Tongue blade therapy.

The proper use of the tongue blade for an hour or two a day for 10–14 days is sufficient to deflect the lingually erupting tooth into a proper relationship.

Catalan's Appliance (Figs. 37.4A and B)

It is used to correct the crossbite of young patients whose permanent molars have not erupted and deciduous molars are lost. It is used on lower anteriors where the appliance makes use of muscle forces and guides erupting tooth in normal position. When appliance is worn, the teeth can come in contact only in the anterior region during masticatory functions and hence correct the crossbite. It is constructed at 45° angulation on the lower incisors by acrylic or cast metal. A removable appliance of this type requires nearly fulltime wear to be effective and efficient and crossbite can be corrected in total 3 weeks.

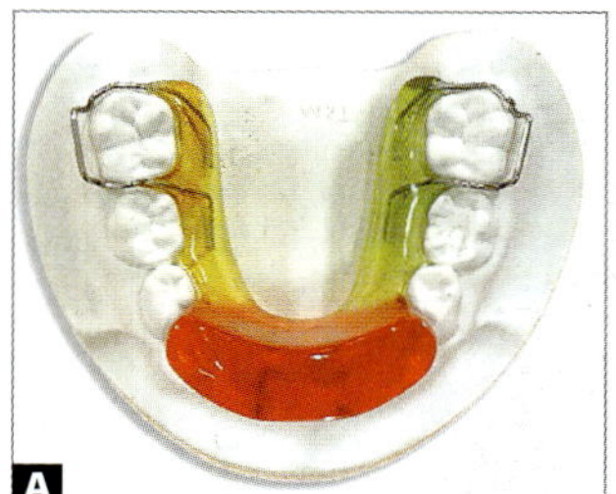

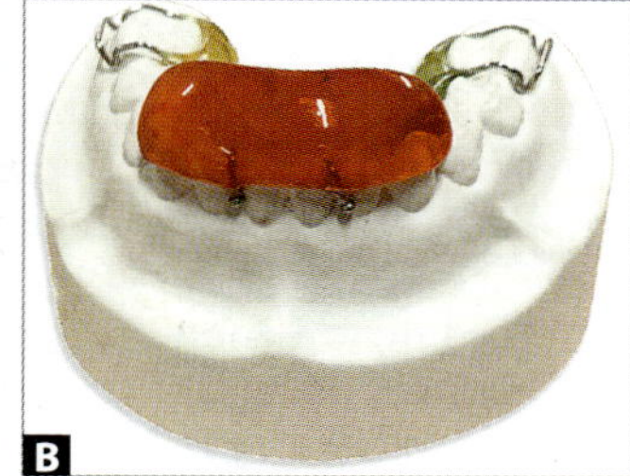

Figs. 37.4A and B: Catalan's appliance.

Reverse Stainless Steel Crown

An anterior stainless steel crown is adapted on the incisor in crossbite and cemented in reverse manner, i.e., the palatal surface of crown faces labial surface of tooth, thus completing the procedure in one appointment. When patient bites on this metal guide plane, the lower incisor moves lingually and upper incisor labially. The patient is recalled after 2 weeks to assess the progress and crown fit. If the crown is found to be loose, it is re-cemented if needed. The crown is removed after the crossbite is corrected.

Fixed Mechanotherapy

- It is also possible to tip the maxillary incisors forward with a 2 × 4 appliance (2 molar bands, 4 bonded incisor brackets) and fixed mechanotherapy with buccal tubes **(Figs. 37.5A to C)**. This may be the best choice for a somewhat older mixed dentition patient with crowding, rotations and more permanent teeth in crossbite.
- After completion of the treatment, fixed lingual arch is placed for 4–6 months or till permanent canines erupt for retention of incisors to their new position.

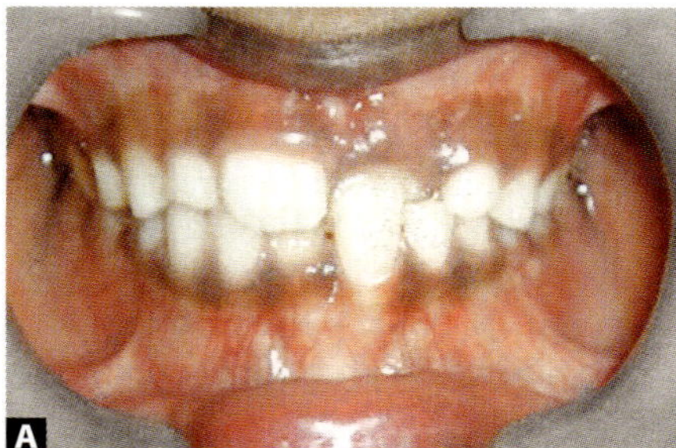
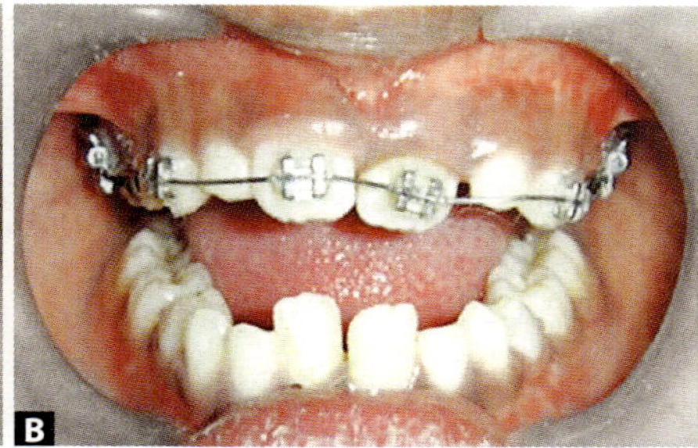
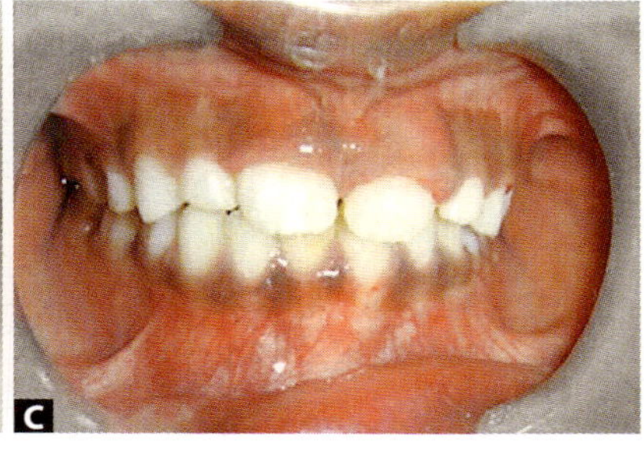

Figs. 37.5A to C: Crossbite correction using fixed mechanotherapy: (A) Preoperative presentation with tooth in crossbite; (B) Placement of fixed appliance; (C) Postoperative photo showing corrected relation.

Functional Anterior Crossbite

- The presence of occlusal prematurities deflects the mandible into a more forward path of closure. So this type of crossbite results from the functional shift of the mandible.
- These are commonly seen in pseudo class III type of malocclusion and are treated by eliminating the occlusal prematurities.

Skeletal Anterior Crossbite

- This occurs due to skeletal discrepancies in growth of maxilla or mandible.
- This type of crossbite usually involves the whole segment instead of one or two teeth **(Fig. 37.6).**

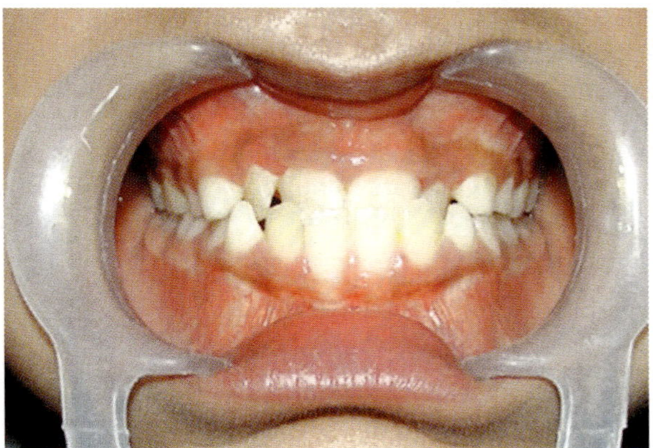

Fig. 37.6: Skeletal crossbite.

- It can be because of maxillary retrognathism or mandibular prognathism or both.
- This type of crossbite is best intercepted by growth modification using myofunctional or orthopedic appliances.

Alternative modalities for anterior crossbite correction

- Essix appliance described by **Sheridan** in 1993 is an esthetic removable device thermoformed from plastic polyester material and is practically invisible, inexpensive and quickly fabricated. It has minimum bulk, superior strength, is retained without clasps, and does not interfere with speech or function.
- **Biradar et al.** In 2011 designed a new method for the correction of anterior crossbite using a modified Essix appliance
- **Liepa et al.** In 2008 described a simple functional appliance for the correction of anterior crossbite involving several teeth called Bruckl appliance. It was constructed using a mandibular Hawley type retainer, inclined plane added to Hawley type retainer and labial bow for retraction of lower incisors. The inclined plane stimulates the forward movement of maxillary incisors which are in crossbite. When activated labial bow acrylic is cut away on the lingual surface of mandibular incisors, the labial bow exerts a retrusive force to upright lower incisors, close spaces, and correct anterior crossbite
- A suitable technique using **Planas direct tracks (PDTs)** has been reported to treat anterior and posterior crossbites in the primary dentition. PDTs are built up with composite on the primary molars, guiding the mandible to slide backward and permitting the tongue to deliver an appropriate force on the maxillary incisors. This brings the maxillary incisors into a normal position and positions the mandible backward in a better sagittal relation with the maxilla in a short period of time
- **Ramirez-Yañez** Evaluated that anterior crossbite was easily treated by restoring the primary maxillary incisors with esthetic pediatric crowns like strip crowns, which were placed in such a manner as to create interference when the teeth were occluded, moving the mandible backward
- **Cheng et al.** In 2017 constructed lingual arch with finger springs which was found effective in anterior crossbite correction regardless of the number of crossbite teeth.

CORRECTION OF POSTERIOR CROSSBITE

There are three types of posterior crossbite generally seen in pediatric patients **(Figs. 37.7A to G).**

1. Lingual crossbite wherein buccal cusps of upper teeth occlude into central groove of lower teeth.
2. Complete lingual crossbite where the buccal surface of maxillary teeth coincides with lingual surface of opposing mandibular teeth.
3. Buccal crossbite where lingual surface of upper teeth occludes against buccal surface of mandibular teeth.

Intermolar Distance

The comparison of intermolar distance between upper and lower molars is important in deciding the amount of maxillary expansion needed to correct crossbite and selection of appliance. The upper intermolar distance is calculated by adding 2 mm to intermolar distance of lower molars. If the amount of maxillary expansion needed is approximately 4–6 mm, it can be achieved by slow expansion for over 3–6 months. For expansion more than 6 mm, rapid expansion is advised by split-acrylic appliance with a jackscrew.

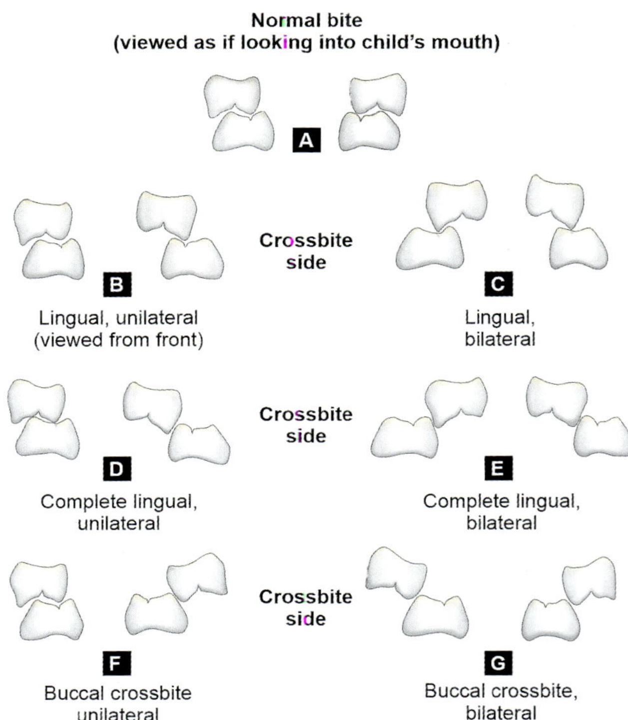

Figs. 37.7A to G: Types of posterior crossbite.

Management

Crossbite Elastics

Single tooth crossbite in molar region can be treated by elastics. A hook or button can be bonded on buccal surface of lower molar and palatal surface of upper molar. An elastic is stretched between the molars in crossbite and worn throughout the day except during meals and brushing. The treatment should not be continued for more than 6 weeks as it can cause extrusion of teeth **(Fig. 37.8)**.

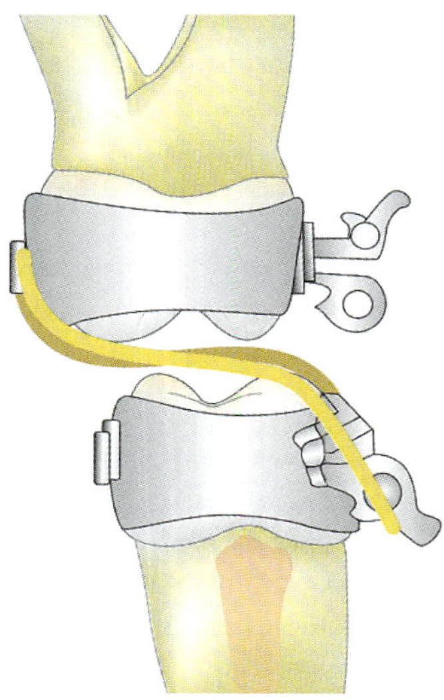

Fig. 37.8: Crossbite elastics.

Quad Helix

This appliance has four helices which increases the length and flexibility of the wire. The wire between two anterior helices is called anterior bridge. The palatal bridge is referred to the wire between anterior and posterior helices. The free wire ends adjacent to posterior helices is called outer arm which is adapted along the palatal surface of upper teeth and soldered to molar bands. The expansion is achieved by opening the helices at regular intervals **(Fig. 37.9)**.

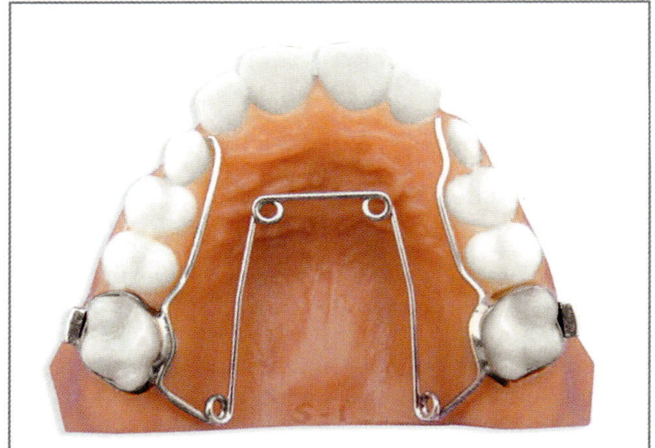

Fig. 37.9: Quad helix.

Porter Appliance

The upper molars are banded and a thick W-shaped wire is adapted on palatal surface. The center of W lies along the palate and free ends are contoured on the palatal surface of molars. For a fixed appliance, the free ends are soldered to molar bands. However, the free ends can be inserted into lingual molar tubes soldered on banded molars to make it a fixed-removable appliance which can be removed by dentist at the time of activation and reinserted. The appliance is mostly recommended in primary dentition and activation is done once a month **(Fig. 37.10)**.

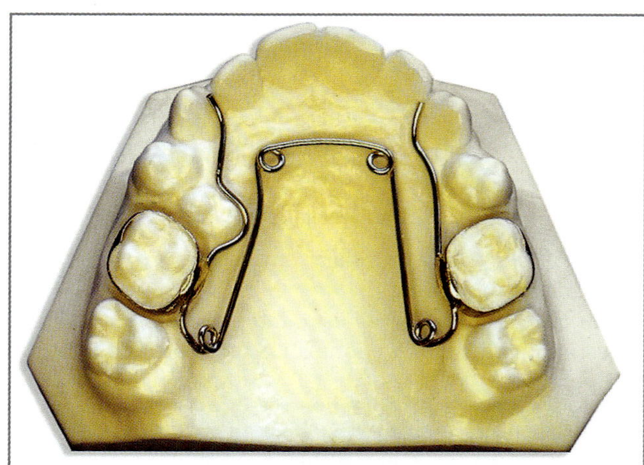

Fig. 37.10: Porter appliance.

Removable Split-Acrylic Expansion Appliance

The appliance consists of Adam's clasps on molars with labial bow and a split acrylic plate with a jack screw or

U-wire embedded along the midline. The jackscrew is placed between upper primary molars and it is easier to activate at home by child's parents. The U-wire is placed with two free ends embedded in acrylic with U-loop of wire free in the midline. It is adjusted by the dentist during treatment. The U-wire appliance is less bulky in palatal area making it more comfortable to wear during speech and swallow. The slow expansion is more comfortable to child and provides better control over treatment outcomes **(Fig. 37.11).**

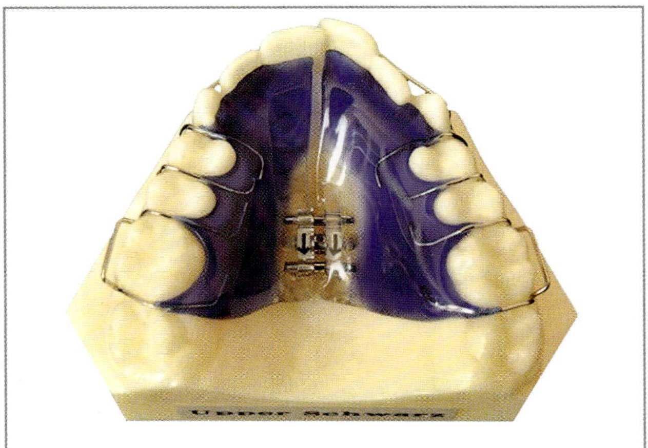

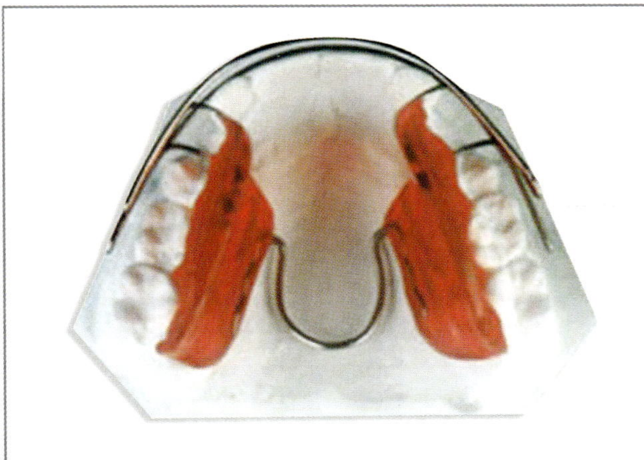

Fig. 37.11: Removable split-acrylic expansion appliance.

Fixed Split-Acrylic Expansion Appliance

Here the upper deciduous second molars are banded and a small loop of wire is soldered on lingual surface of these bands which is later embedded in split-acrylic plate containing jackscrew.

The jackscrew is activated by a pin which is inserted into a hole in jackscrew. The pin is moved anteriorly which rotates the shaft and expands the two halves of acrylic plate. One turn of jack screw pin opens the midline crack by 0.25 mm. The parent is instructed to activate the appliance by 1 turn each week. After 2–3 weeks when the child has adapted the appliance, it can be activated twice weekly.

The upper intermolar distance is recorded at each appointment which helps to monitor the progress of treatment. The same appliance can be used as retainer as itself or with acrylic filled in the midline split for 3 months after completion of treatment **(Fig. 37.12).**

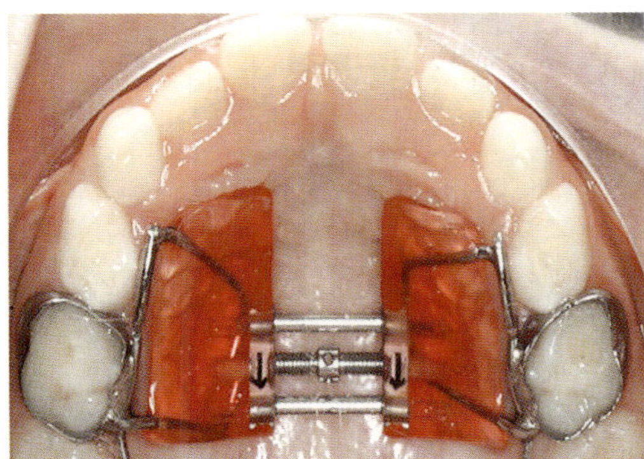

Fig. 37.12: Fixed split-acrylic expansion appliance.

CONTROL OF ABNORMAL HABITS

Habits are referred to certain actions involving the teeth and other oral or perioral structures which are repeated often enough to have a profound and deleterious effect on the dentofacial structures. These deleterious oral habits include thumb sucking, tongue thrusting and mouth breathing **(Fig. 37.13)** (Detailed in Chapter 30).

SPACE REGAINING

- If a primary molar is lost early and space maintainers are not used, a reduction in arch length by mesial migration of the first molar is expected. In such cases the space lost by mesial movement of the first molar can be regained by distalizing it (Detailed in Chapter 35).
- The space regaining procedures are preferably undertaken at an early age prior to the eruption of second molar.

ORAL HABITS

Thumb sucking

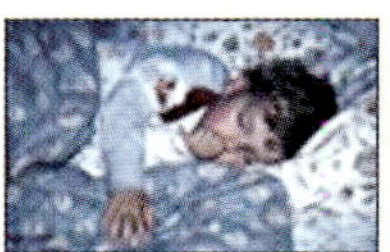

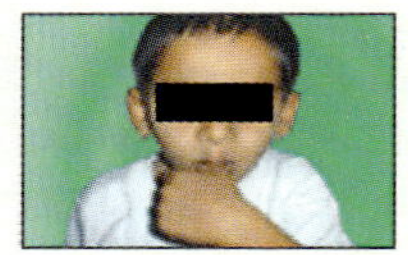

Clinical features:
Posterior crossbite
Dishpan thumb
Hypotonic upperlip
High palatal vault

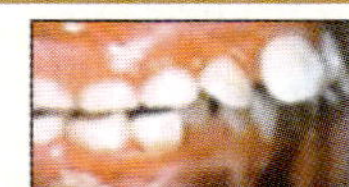

Protruded maxillary incisors

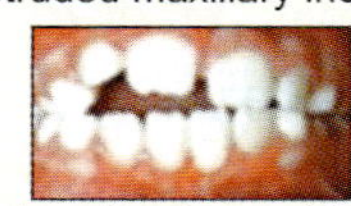

Localized open bite

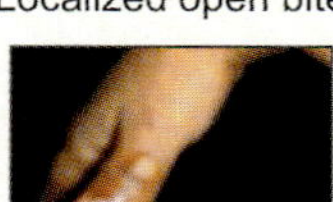

Keratotic lesions on thumb

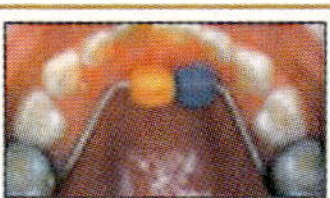

Modified bluegrass appliance

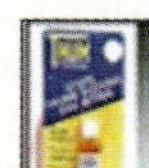

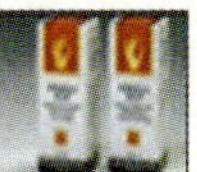

Bitter solutions to prevent sucking

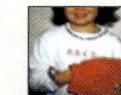

Thumb home concept

Tongue thrusting

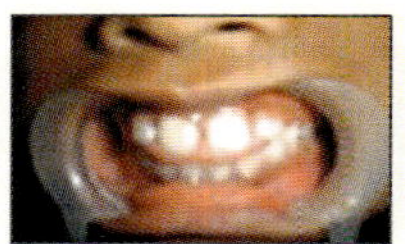

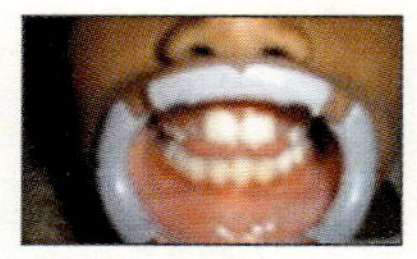

Clinical features:
Proclination of anterior teeth
Midline diastema

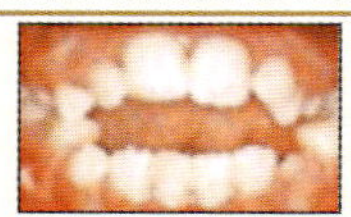

Open bite due to anterior tongue thrust

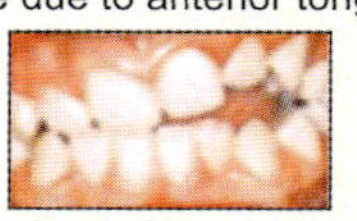

Open bite due to lateral tongue thrust

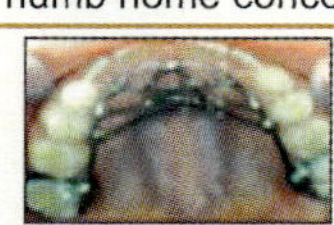

Palatal crib

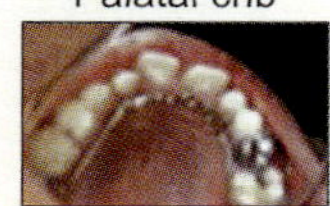

Palatal crib with spikes

Mouth breathing

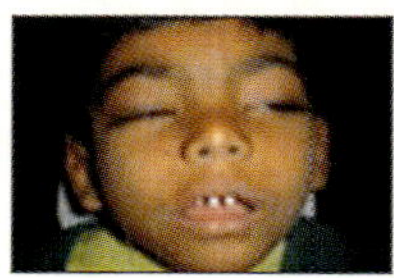

Clinical features:
Long narrow face
Narrow maxillary arch

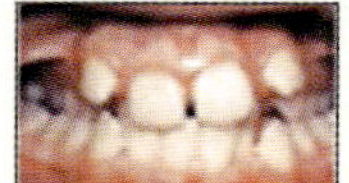

Mouth breathing gingivitis

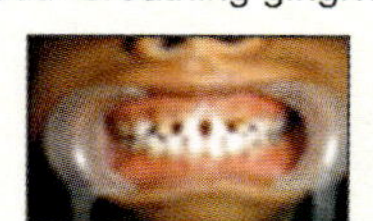

Increased caries incidence

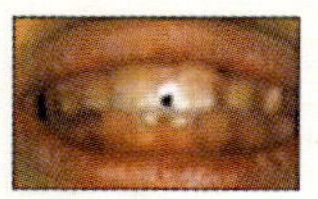

Oral screen

Other management strategies:
Lip exercises
Monobloc activator

Bruxism

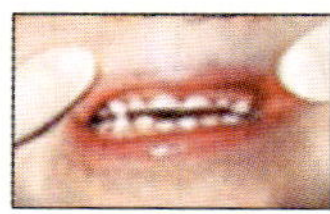

Clinical features:
Worn out occlusal surfaces
Muscle soreness
TMJ pain
Periodontal trauma

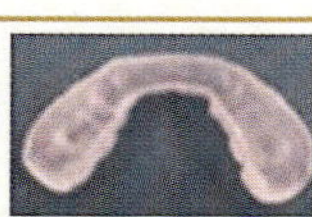

Bite guard

Lip biting

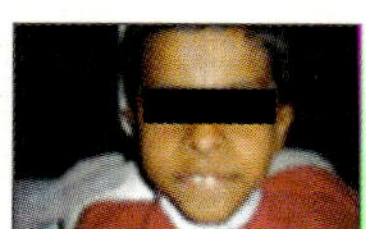

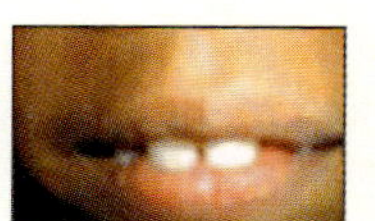

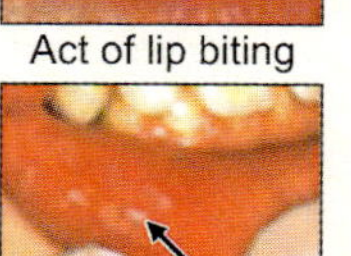

Act of lip biting

Red ulcer formation

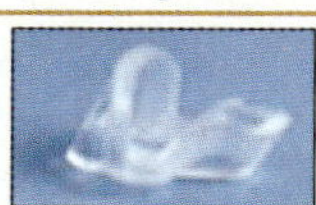

Appliance for localized lip biting

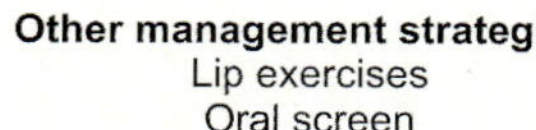

Other management strategies:
Lip exercises
Oral screen

Masochistic habits

(Self-destructive habits)

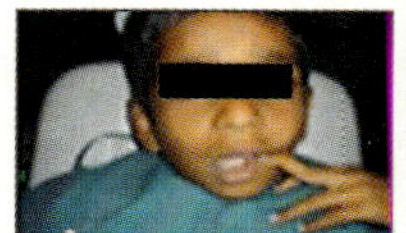

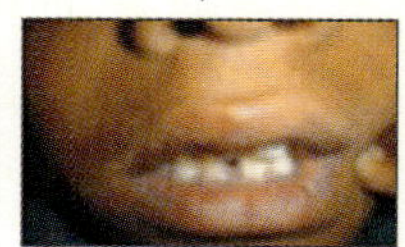

Chewing of inner aspect of cheek

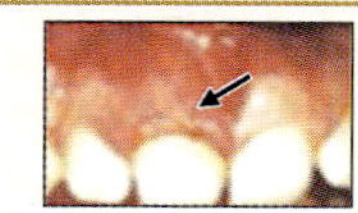

Picking of gingiva with fingernail

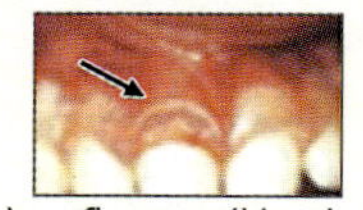

Broken fingernail in gingiva

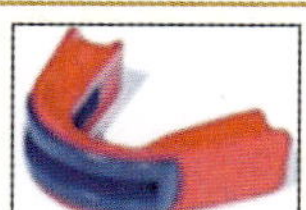

Full mouth guard

Other management strategies:
Psychiatric approach
Oral screen

Fig. 37.13: Common oral habits and rare clinical feature with treatment.

MUSCLE EXERCISES

Exercise for the masseter muscle	Patient is asked to clench the teeth while counting to 10. Now the patient is asked to relax for 10s, and it has to be repeated over a period of time until the masseter muscle feels fatigued
Exercise for the lips (circumoral muscles)	• If the upper lip is hypotonic and flaccid, the child is instructed to extend the upper lip as far as possible curving the vermilion border under and behind the maxillary incisors. This exercise should be done 15–20 min a day for a period of 4–5 months • *Stretching of the upper lip to maintain lip seal:* The patient is asked to hold a thin piece of paper between the lips • If the maxillary incisors are protruded, the lower lip can be used to augment the upper lip exercise. The upper lip is first extended under and behind the maxillary incisors. The vermilion border of the lower lip is then placed against the outside of the extended upper lip and pressed as hard as possible against the upper lip. This type of exercise exerts a strong retracting influence on the maxillary incisors while increasing the tonicity of both upper and lower lips. This exercise is particularly valuable for mouth breathers and should be done for ≥30 min a day • Massaging of the lips • *Button pull exercise:* A button of 1.5 inch diameter is taken and a thread is passed through the button holes. Then, the patient is asked to place the button behind the lips and pull the thread, while restricting it from being pulled out by lip pressure • *Tug-of-war exercise:* This involves use of two buttons, with one placed behind the lips while the other button is held by another person to pull the thread • *Holding and pumping of water back and forth behind the lips:* Patient is asked to hold and pump water back and forth behind the lips until they get tired • For a developing class II division 1 malocclusion, the playing of a wind instrument may be an interceptive procedure
Exercises for the tongue	• *One elastic swallow:* This exercise is used for correction of improper positioning of the tongue. 5/16 inch intraoral elastic is positioned on the tip of the tongue and the patient is asked to raise the tongue and hold the elastic against rugae area and swallow • *Tongue hold exercise:* 5/16 inch intraoral elastic is positioned in a designated spot of the tongue over a prescribed period of time with the lips closed. The patient is then asked to swallow with elastic in place and lips apart • *Two elastic swallow:* Two 5/16 inch elastics are placed on the tongue, one in the midline and the other at the tip and the patient is asked to swallow with the elastics in position • *The hold pull exercise:* The tip of the tongue and the midpoint are made to contact the palate and the mandible is gradually opened. This helps in stretching the lingual frenum

INTERCEPTION OF SKELETAL MALRELATIONS

Skeletal malocclusion if diagnosed at an early age can be intercepted so as to reduce the severity of the malocclusion that may occur. Class II and class III malocclusions are largely maxillomandibular basal malrelationships (Detailed in Chapter 33).

- **Interception of class II malocclusion:** This occurs as a result of either excessive maxillary growth, deficiency in mandibular growth, or a combination of both. Maxillary growth can be restricted by use of face bow with head gear. Mandibular deficiency is usually treated by myofunctional appliances, e.g., FR-II.
- **Interception of class III malocclusions:** This develops as a result of mandibular prognathism, maxillary retrognathism or combination of both. Chin cup with head gear are used to restrict mandibular growth and maxillary deficiency can be intercepted by orthopedic appliance, such as face mask or by means of myofunctional appliances like FR-III.

REMOVAL OF SOFT TISSUE AND BONY BARRIERS

- Over-retained primary teeth, fibrous or bony obstructions, ankylosed primary teeth and supernumerary teeth are causes of noneruption of succedaneous teeth.
- If the permanent tooth fails to erupt because of fibrous or bony obstructions, its eruption may be stimulated by surgically exposing the crown.
- The surgical procedure involves excision of the soft tissue and removal of any bone overlying the crown of the unerupted tooth. The extent of tissue removal should be such that the greatest diameter of the crown of the tooth is exposed.

POINTS TO REMEMBER

- Interceptive orthodontics is defined as "That phase of the science and art of orthodontics employed to recognize and eliminate potential irregularities and malpositions in the developing dentofacial complex".
- Procedures undertaken in interceptive orthodontics are serial extraction, correction of developing crossbite, control of abnormal habits, space regaining, muscle exercises, interception of skeletal malrelation, and removal of soft tissue or bony barrier to enable eruption of teeth.
- Kjellgren (1929), Sweden—coined the term serial extraction.
- Nance (1940) is called the "Father of serial extraction".
- Anterior crossbite is a condition in which one or more maxillary anterior teeth are in lingual relation to the mandibular teeth. It is of three types, viz., dentoalveolar, functional, skeletal anterior crossbite.
- Commonly used space regainers are Gerber space regainer, space regainers using jack screws, space regaining using cantilever spring.

Questionnaire

1. Define interceptive orthodontics and explain its components.
2. What are the treatment options for anterior tooth crossbite?
3. Define serial extraction and its methods.
4. Explain common exercises for orofacial musculature.

FURTHER READING

1. Biradar A, Prakash GS, Manohar MR. Early correction of developing anterior crossbite with modified Essix appliance. J Ind Orthod Soc. 2012;46:159-61.
2. Cheng HC, Shih MJ. Dentofacial changes after anterior crossbite correction using a lingual arch with finger springs. J Dent Sci. 2017(12):70-7.
3. Garvey MT, Barry HJ, Blake M. Supernumerary teeth--an overview of classification, diagnosis and management. J Can Dent Assoc. 1999;65(11):612-6.
4. Gianelly AA. Leeway space and the resolution of crowding in the mixed dentition. Semin Orthod 1995;1:188-194.
5. Gowri Shankar S. Textbook of Orthodontics, 1st edition; 2011.
6. Graber TM. Orthodontics: principles and practice. 3rd ed. Philadelphia, PA; 1972.
7. Guideline on Management of the Developing Dentition and Occlusion in Pediatric Dentistry. American Academy of Pediatric Dentistry: reference manual. 2021;32:6.
8. Kharbanda OP. Diagnosis and management of malocclusion. 2nd edition; 2013.
9. RamirezYañez G. Treatment of anterior crossbite in the primary dentition with esthetic crowns: report of 3 cases. Pediatr Dent. 2011;33:339-42.
10. RamirezYañez GO. Planas' direct tracks as a useful method to correct crossbite in an early age: description of the technique and a case report. J Clin Orthod. 2003;37:294-8.
11. Tondon S. Textbook of pedodontics, 2nd edition. Paras Medical Publisher; 2009.

CHAPTER

Dental Caries

Nikhil Marwah, Puneet Goenka, Deeksha Khurana, Kayalvizhi G

Chapter Outline

Throughout the history of man, diseases have come and diseases have disappeared. For most of the major diseases, it has been possible to clearly identify the means how the disease was brought under control. Such means may include nationwide or even global vaccination programs, change in living conditions with improved nutrition, and noncontaminated drinking water. For other diseases, it may be more difficult to explain the reasons for a change. This is particularly true for diseases with a multifactorial background like dental caries. During the decades of caries decline, a number of actions have been taken to control the disease, and the literature describes numerous studies where one or several factors have been evaluated for their impact. Still, it is difficult to get a full picture of what has happened, as the background is so complex besides so many factors may have been involved both directly and indirectly. The word caries is derived from the Latin word meaning "rot" or "decay." It is akin to the Greek word "Ker" meaning death.

- ***Dental caries*** *is defined as microbial disease of the calcified tissues of teeth that leads to demineralization of the inorganic components and the subsequent breakdown of the organic moieties of enamel and dentin.*
- **Newbrun** (1989): *"Dental caries is defined as a pathological process of localized destruction of tooth tissues by microorganisms".*
- **Shafer** (1993): *"Dental caries is an irreversible microbial disease of the calcified tissues of the teeth, characterized by demineralization of the inorganic portion and destruction of the organic substance of the tooth, which often leads to cavitation".*
- ***Consensus report of a workshop organized by ORCA and cariology research group of IADR (2020):*** *Dental caries is a biofilm mediated, diet modulated, multifactorial, non-communicable dynamic disease resulting in net mineral loss of dental hard tissues. It is determined by biological, behavioral, psychosocial and environmental factors, leading to caries lesion formation.*

CLASSIFICATION OF CARIES

- **According to occurrence:**
  - Primary caries: Original carious lesion **(Fig. 38.1).**
  - Secondary or recurrent caries: Occurring adjacent to an existing restoration or crown **(Fig. 38.2).**
  - Residual caries: Caries left by accident or by operator's intention **(Fig. 38.3)**.
- **According to rate (speed):**
  - Acute or rampant caries: Multiple and extensive carious lesions seen in the same individual, e.g., nursing or baby bottle caries, radiation therapy caries.
  - Chronic or arrested caries: Slow spreading lesions are fairly hard and show brown to black discoloration.
- **According to location:**
  - Pit and fissure **(Fig. 38.4).**
  - Smooth surface **(Fig. 38.5).**
  - Root surface **(Fig. 38.6)**.

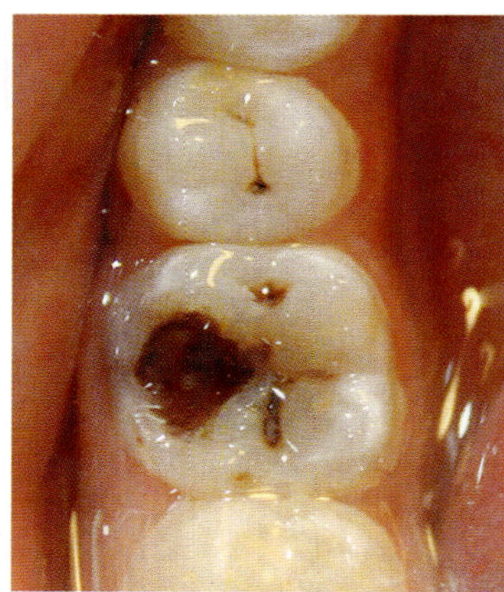

Fig. 38.1: Primary caries.

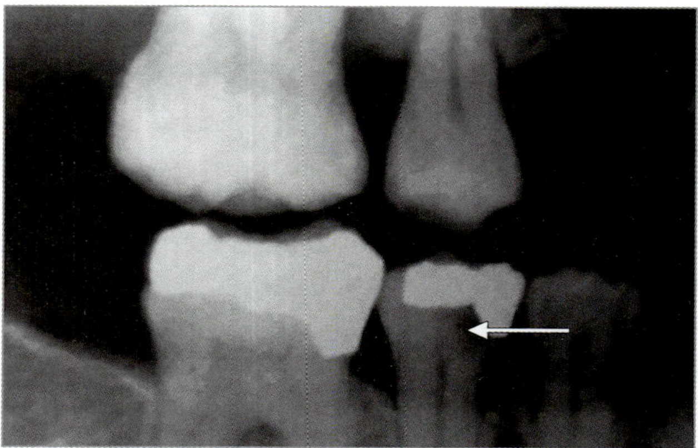

Fig. 38.2: Secondary caries.

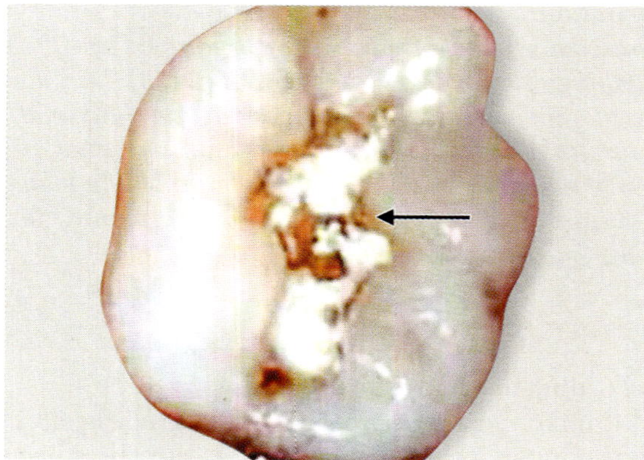

Fig. 38.3: Residual caries.

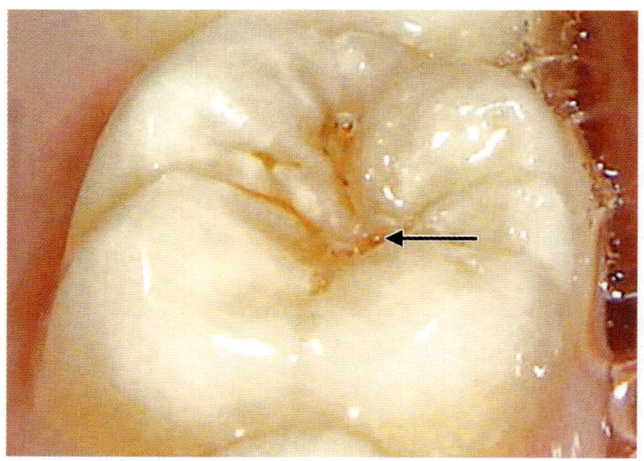

Fig. 38.4: Pit and fissure caries.

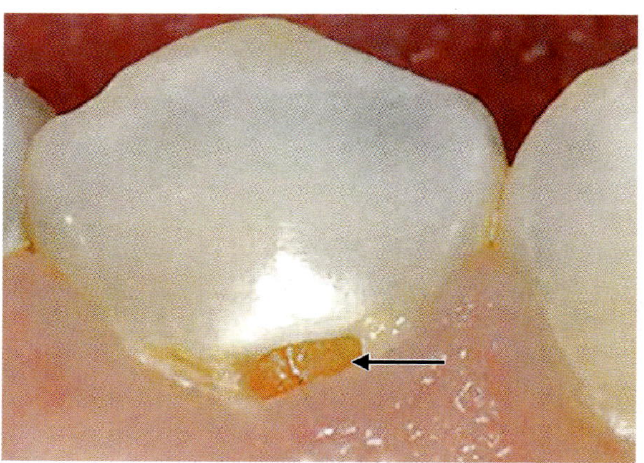

Fig. 38.5: Smooth surface caries.

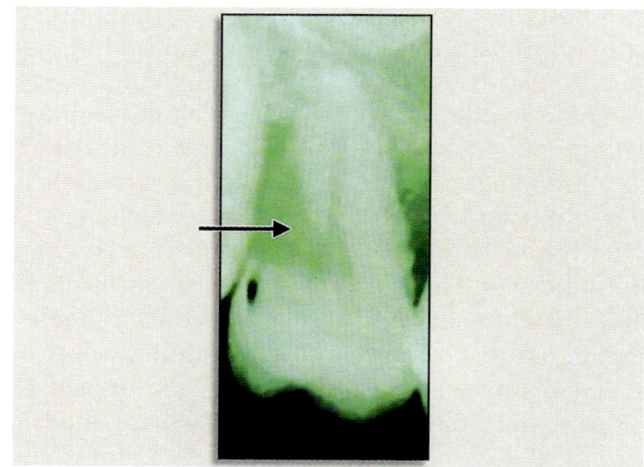

Fig. 38.6: Root surface caries.

- **According to extent:**
  - Incipient caries: It is often reversible and also referred to as non-cavitated carious lesion or white spot lesion—can be remineralized using remineralizing agents without restorative intervention **(Fig. 38.7)**.
  - Cavitated caries: They are non-reversible and usually requires restorative intervention.
- **According to direction:**
  - Forward caries—when caries in enamel is in a V-shape, that is, base pointed toward DEJ.
  - Backward caries—when the more extensive destruction is toward DEJ with small apex.
- **According to age:**
  - Early childhood caries **(Fig. 38.8)**.
  - Adolescent caries.
  - Senile caries.
- **According to surface (Fig. 38.9):**
  - Simple—one surface.
  - Compound—two surfaces.
  - Complex—more than two surfaces.
- **According to type of surface:**
  - Occlusal **(Fig. 38.10)**.
  - Proximal **(Fig. 38.11)**.

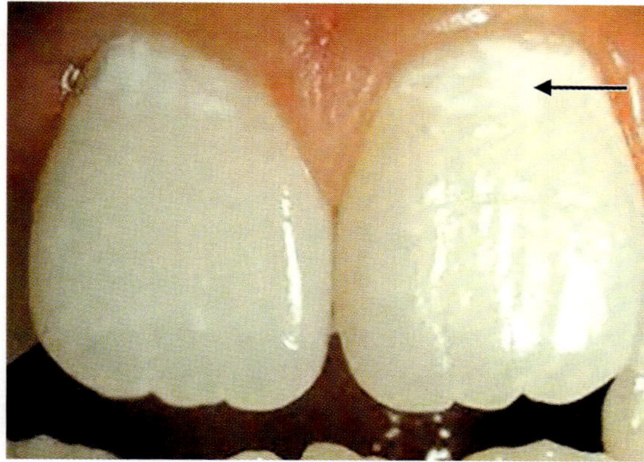

Fig. 38.7: Incipient caries.

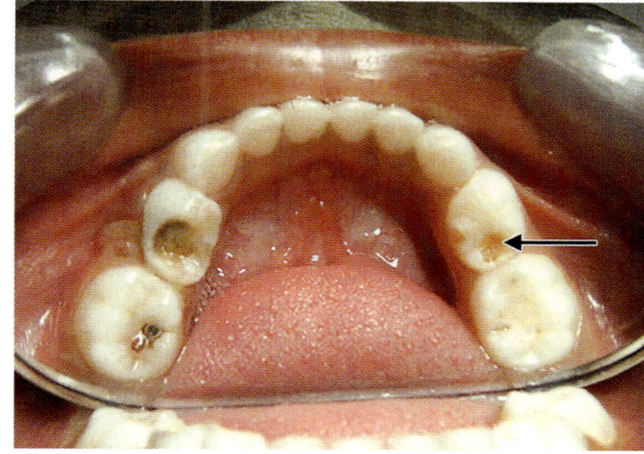

Fig. 38.10: Occlusal caries.

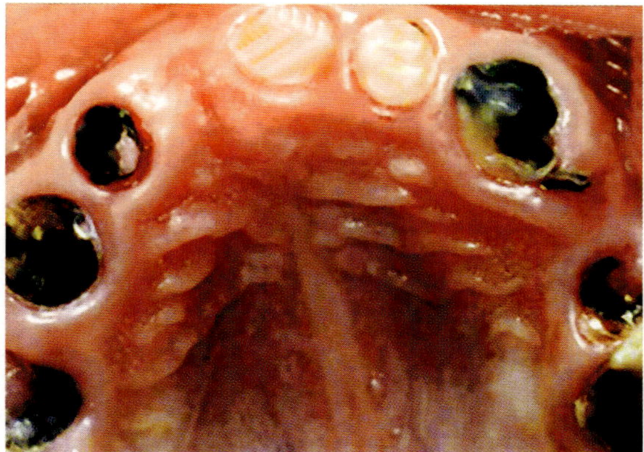

Fig. 38.8: Early childhood caries.

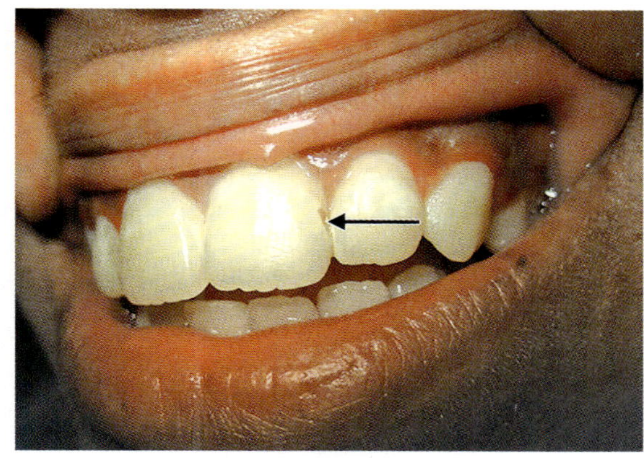

Fig. 38.11: Proximal caries.

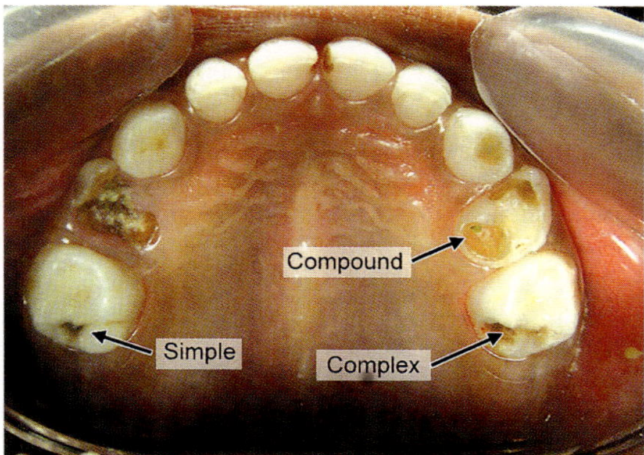

Fig. 38.9: Caries complexity according to surface.

Linear enamel caries (odontoclasia)

An atypical form of dental caries, called linear enamel caries, has been observed in the primary dentition of children, in Latin America and Asian countries.

- **ICDAS (International Caries Detection and Assessment System) (Fig. 38.12):** ICDAS is a simple, evidence-based system for detection and classification of caries in clinical practice, dental research, and dental public health. It provides three levels of caries diagnosis to allow flexibility in implementation.

ICDAS II codes and criteria

Full ICDAS	0	No evidence of caries
	1	Initial caries
	2	Distinct visual change in enamel
	3	Localized enamel breakdown due to caries with no visible dentin
	4	Underlying dark shadow from dentin
	5	Distinct cavity with visible dentin
	6	Extensive distinct cavity with visible dentin
Modified ICDAS	0	No evidence of caries
	A	Initial caries (1+2)
	3	Localized enamel breakdown due to caries with no visible dentin
	4	Underlying dark shadow from dentin
	5	Distinct cavity with visible dentin
	6	Extensive distinct cavity with visible dentin
Merged ICDAS	0	No evidence of caries
	A	Initial caries (1+2)
	B	Moderate caries (3+4)
	C	Extensive caries (5+6)

ICDAS II

Score 0	Score 1	Score 2	Score 3	Score 4	Score 5	Score 6
No visual signs of carious lesions or any enamel defect	First visible changes in the enamel. Visible only after drying with air. Changes in coloration confined to areas of pits	Change in visible enamel even in the presence of moisture. More extensive and not restricted to pits	Destruction located in enamel without visible dentin, discountinuities of enamel surface	Dark shadow on the underlying dentin, with or without localized destruction of enamel	Clear cavity with visible dentin; cavity that involves less than half the tooth surface	Extensive cavity evident in dentin; cavity deep and wide, involves more than half of the tooth

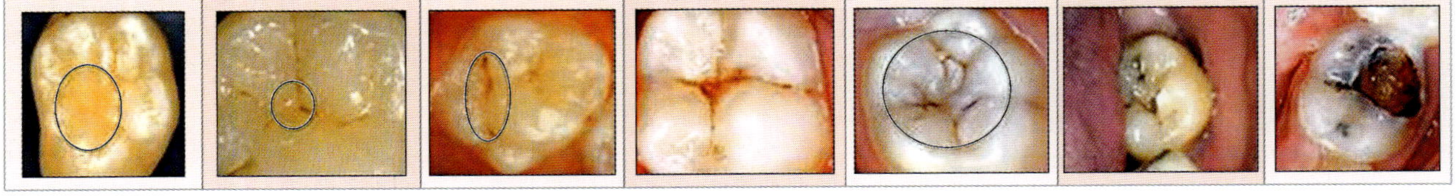

Fig. 38.12: Images of different classification scale established by ICDAS.

Table 38.1: International Caries Detection and Assessment System (ICDAS) codes and American Dental Association (ADA) conversions.

ICDAS Codes						
ICDAS 0	ICDAS 1	ICDAS 2	ICDAS 3	ICDAS 4	ICDAS 5	ICDAS 6
No evidence of caries	Initial caries	Distinct visual change in enamel	Localized enamel breakdown; no visible dentin	Underlying dark shadow from dentin	Distinct cavity with visible dentin	Extensive distinct cavity with visible dentin
ADA caries classification system						
Sound		Initial		Moderate (ICDAS 2-4)		Advanced

- **American Dental Association caries classification system:**
  - **Pit and fissure:** The anatomic pits or fissures of teeth such as occlusal, facial, or lingual surfaces of posterior teeth, or lingual surfaces of maxillary incisors or canines.
  - **Approximal:** The immediate proximity to the contact area of an adjacent tooth surface; may exist on any surface of the tooth.
  - **Cervical and smooth surface:** The cervical area or any other smooth enamel surface of the anatomic crown adjacent to an edentulous space; may exist anywhere around the full circumference of the tooth.
  - **Root:** The root surface apical to the anatomic crown.
- **WHO classification:**

Score	*Criteria*
D0	No lesion or subclinical initial lesions in a dynamic state of progression or regression
D1	Clinically detectable enamel lesions with intact surfaces
D2	Clinically detectable cavities limited to enamel
D3	Clinically detectable lesions penetrating into dentin; surface open or closed
D4	Lesions penetrated into pulp

EPIDEMIOLOGY OF CARIES

- There was no evidence of dental caries in the relatively few teeth found in skull fragments of our earliest known direct ancestors, the Pithecanthropus.
- But there was evidence of fairly extensive decay in Rhodesian man from the Neanderthal age and in prehistoric European of net race, the prevalence being least in prehistoric Asiatic man (2.0 DMF) and most in the Europeans (7.2 DMF). There is also a direct evidence of linking progress of civilization to the number of carious lesions.
- The prevalence and pattern of dental caries did not change significantly during the 2,000 years or more from the beginning of the Iron age to the Medieval period (1066–1500 AD). During this period, the overall caries level was very low, and the most frequent site of caries was the occlusal surface, unlike the pattern in modern man where the carious lesions are at or just below the interproximal contact areas.
- The caries experience varies greatly among countries and even within countries.
- Caries prevalence is generally lowest (0.5–1.7 DMF) for Asian and African countries and highest (12–18 DMF) for the Americans and other Western countries.
- Meta-analysis study of prevalence of dental caries in Indian population showed the overall prevalence of dental caries as 54.16%, whereas age-specific prevalence as 62% in patients above 18 years and 52% among 3–18 years of age.
- According to **Urebia et al.,** the global pooled prevalence of ECC is 48%. The prevalence by continent is Africa: 30%; Americas: 48%; Asia: 52%; Europe: 43%; and Oceania: 82%.

Prevalence rates of caries in Indian children at various ages 5–15 years.

Investigators	*Year*	*Age*	*Place*	*Prevalence (%)*
Shourie	1941	5–6 and 12 years	Delhi	5–6 years: 50.8 12 years: 54.8
Gill	1968	12 years	Lucknow	43.8
Damle et al.	1982	12 years	Haryana	89.5
Tiwari et al.	1985	12 years	Orissa (Odisha)	63.8
Sahoo et al.	1986	12 years	Orissa (Odisha)	67.9
Chawla et al.	1993	12 years	Chandigarh	31.4
Damle and Patel	1994	12 years	Bombay (Mumbai)	80.1
Norboo et al.	1998	5–6/12 years	Leh	5–6 years: 74.6 12 years: 47.7
Venugopal et al.	1998	1–5 years	Mumbai	19.2
Rodriguez and Damle	1998	12 years	Bombay (Mumbai)	63.4
Ali et al.	1998	5–6 years	Akola city	61.4
Menon and Indushekhar	1999	5–6/12 years	Karnataka	2.56 31.0
Gopinath et al.	1999	<5 years	Tamil Nadu	36
Singh et al.	1999	12 years	Haryana	33.1
Kuriakose et al.	1999	<5 years	Kerala	57
Rao et al.	1999	5 years	Moodbidri	76.9
Goel et al.	2000	5–6 years 12–14 years	Puttur, Karnataka	5–6 years: 81.25 12–14 years: 59.6
Chawla et al.	2000	5–6 years	Chandigarh	60.3
Mandal KP et al.	2001	5–6 years	West Bengal	Urban: 52.4 Rural: 48.3
			Odisha	Urban: 56 Rural: 48.7
			Sikkim	Urban: 61.8 Rural: 22
Tiwari et al.	2001	3–7 years	Haryana	34.20
Kulkarni SS et al.	2002	11–15 years	Belagavi	45.12
Dash et al.	2002	5, 8, 11, 15 years	Cuttack (Odisha)	57.9
Saravanan et al.	2003	5/12 years	Pondicherry	5–6 years: 44.4 12 years: 22.3
Jose and king et al.	2003	18–40 months	Kerala	12
Saravanan et al.	2005	5 years	Puducherry	44.4
Kumar et al.	2005	5 years	Chennai	83
Mahejabeen et al.	2006	3–5 years	Hubli, Dharwad city	54.10
Meghashyam et al.	2007	Up to 5 years	Karnataka	75
Tyagi et al.	2008	2–6 years	Davangere	19.2
Saravanan et al.	2008	5–10 years	Chidambaram	Permanent: 71.7 Primary: 26.5
Simratvir et al.	2009	3–6 years	Ludhiana city	52.1
Suma et al.	2010	1–3 years	Bengaluru	15
Singh et al.	2011	5 years	Southwest India	76.3
Acharya and Hiremath et al.	2011	2–3/4–6	Karnataka	45.2
Jaidka et al.	2011	5 years	Meerut	88.5
Mehta et al.	2011	3–5 years	Punjab	43.5
Yashoda et al.	2011	3–5 years	Davangere	45.06
Priyadarshini et al.	2011	24–59 months	Bengaluru	37.30
Bhat PK et al.	2011	10–12	South Bengaluru	5.1
Moses et al.	2011	5–15 years	Chidambaram	63.83
Amith	2011	12–15 years	Maharashtra	64.98
Padma et al.	2011	30–70 months	Andhra Pradesh	63
Phipps et al.	2011	12–71 months	India	62.3

Contd...

Contd...

Investigators	***Year***	***Age***	***Place***	***Prevalence (%)***
Bharadwaj et al.	2012	5 years	Shimla	44.3
Shankar et al.	2012	3–6 years	Bengaluru	58
Retnakumari et al.	2012	12–36 months	Thiruvananthapurum	50.6
Prakash et al.	2012	<5 years	Bengaluru	27.5
Deshpande et al.	2012	36 and 72 months	Rural North Karnataka	40.72
Singh et al.	2012	3 years	Bengaluru	40
Sankeshwari et al.	2012	3–5 years	Belagavi	63.1
Shailee et al.	2012	12/15 years	India	12 years: 32.6 15 years: 42.2
Shingare P et al.	2012	3–14	Raigad Maharashtra	3–6 years: 78.5 7–10 years: 88.61 11–14 years: 73
Peedikayil FC	2013	5–14	Kerala	5–7 years: 40.06 8–10 years: 54.29 11–14 years: 49.11
Gaindhane et al.	2013	43–60 months	Wardha distict	33.48
Shruthi eta l	2013	3–5 years	Kanpur	48
Narang et al.	2013	2–6 years	Lucknow	33
Suprabha et al.	2013	11–13 years	India	59.4
Sarumathi et al.	2013	3–6 years	Chennai	63.4
Joshi et al.	2013	6–12 years	India	69.1
Mittal et al.	2014	5/12 years	Gurugram	5 years: 68.5 12 years: 37.5
Murthy et al.	2014	12–15 years	India	57.9
Mehta and Bhalla et al.	2014	5–6 years	Urban India	38.60
Prabhu et al.	2014	<5 years	KGF	44.34
Anandkrishna	2014	46–71 months	Bengaluru	34
Karunakaran et al.	2014	4–6 years	Namakkal district	65.88
Arora et al.	2014	12	India	57
Sukhabogi et al.	2014	12/15 years	India	12 years: 39.9 15 years: 46.7
Ingle et al.	2014	12–15 years	India	53
Garkoti PD et al.	2015	6–11 years	Haldwani	58.18
Arora B et al.	2015	12 years	Ferozpur city	47.8
Kuriakose et al.	2015	<60 months	Thiruvananthapurum	54.1
Sijlana and pannu et al.	2015	5 years	Haryana	59
Gupta et al.	2015	3–5 years	Uttar Pradesh	45
Sachdeva et al.	2015	<5 years	Haryana	33.85
Sharma KR et al.	2015	5 years	Himachal Pradesh	44.30
Stephen et al.	2015	18–72 months	Salem	15.9
Goel et al.	2015	12/15 years	India	12 years: 34.3 15 years: 46.5
Rajesh SS et al.	2016	3–15 years	South India (Maralur, Tumakuru)	3 years: 32.9 3–5 years: 13.6 6–10 years: 49.7 11–15 years: 25.6
Dash et al.	2016	<5, 5–10, 11–15 years	Chandigarh	5 years: 40.7 5–10 years: 56.2 11–15 years: 34.5
Bhagade et al.	2016	2–4 years	Nagpur	63.8
Shilpashree et al.	2016	3–6 years	Bengaluru	31.40
Hiremath et al.	2016	6–11 years	India	78.9
Koya et al.	2016	24–71 months	India	42
Henry et al.	2016	<3 years	India	40.6
Gopal et al.	2016	3–6	India	27.3
Kottayi et al.	2016	12–15 years	India	3.9

Contd...

Contd...

Investigators	Year	Age	Place	Prevalence (%)
Ponnudurai et al.	2016	6–14 years	India	68.8
Parasuraman G	2017	6–10 years	Tamil Nadu	63.9
Mangla et al.	2017	1–3	India	21
Pal et al.	2017	5–6 years	India	46.6
Shah et al.	2017	5–7 years	India	33.2
Maran et al.	2017	6–12 years	India	73.2
Plaka et al.	2017	12–15 years	India	36.3
Janakiram	2018	5 years, 12 years	India	49
Goenka et al.	2018	5–7 years	India	65.1
Chugh et al.	2018	24–61 months	India	47.3
Vandana et al.	2018	2–6 years	India	38.2
Konde et al.	2018	12 years	India	13.6
Tonpe et al.	2019	3–5 years	India	61.17
Kaur et al.	2020	5–6 years	Patiala, Punjab	52
Kaur et al.	2020	5–6 years	Patiala, Punjab	20
Mulchandani et al.	2021	0–5 years	Bhavnagar, Gujarat	26.31

THEORIES OF DENTAL CARIES

It is clear that fossil teeth provide an accurate record of the state of dentitions of man through the ages. Evidence for caries has been found in *Homosapiens* since Paleolithic times. Numerous references to dental caries, including early theories attempting to explain its etiology, have been found in recorded history of ancient people. A brief review of the history and early theories of the etiology of caries provide an interesting background for the understanding of the current concepts of dental caries.

Legend of the Worm

Probably the earliest reference to tooth decay and toothache came from the ancient Sumerian text known as the "legend of the worm." This text was discovered from an ancient city within the Euphrates Valley of the lower Mesopotamian era, which dates from about 5000 BC. A remedy for toothache, recorded during this period, reads as follows: "Mix beer, the plant sakilbir and oil together, repeat thereon the incantation thrice and put it on the tooth." Chinese and Egyptians used fumigation, which consisted of burning leeks, onions, and *Hyoscyamus*.

Humoral Theory

The legend of the worm faded over the early centuries as the Greek physicians advanced to the humoral theory of caries. The four elemental humors of the body were blood, phlegm, black bile, and yellow bile. An imbalance in these humors resulted in disease. According to **Galen**, the ancient Greek physician and philosopher, "dental caries was produced by internal action of acid and corroding humors." The cure must consist of local or general medicaments according to circumstances and also provide strengthening of the teeth by the use of astringents and tonic remedies.

Vital Theory

It was almost certainly apparent to the early Greek physicians **Hippocrates, Celsius, Galen**, and to more enlightened physicians of the middle ages; the teeth are an integral part of the body and that they were vitally affected by and in turn affected the body. A vital theory of tooth decay was advanced, toward the end of the 18th century, which postulated that tooth decay originated, like bone gangrene, from within the tooth itself.

Chemical Theory

Robertson in 1835 proposed that dental decay was caused by acid formed by fermentation of food particles around teeth. Since fermentation was at this time considered to be a strictly nonvital process, the possibility that microorganisms were involved was not, as yet, recognized.

Parasitic Theory

Long before the demonstration of the germ theory of disease, the possibility that microorganisms can have toxic and destructive effects on tissue was postulated. These postulations spelled the end of the vital theory and gave rise to the idea that chemicals can destroy teeth. In 1843, **Erdl** described filamentous parasites in the membrane removed from teeth. Early microscopic observations of scrapings from teeth and of the carious lesions, by **Antonie van Leeuwenhoek**, indicated that microorganisms were associated with the carious process. A text of what he saw is "I am in the habit of rubbing my teeth with salt in the morning and then rinsing my mouth with water and often after eating, to clean my back teeth with a toothpick, as well as rubbing them hard with a cloth, therefore my teeth back and front remain as clean and white that only a few people of my age can compare with me. Also when I rub my gums with hard salt, they will not bleed. Yet all this does not make my teeth so clean I can see, looking at them with a hollow mirror, that something will stick and grow between the molars, a little white matter, as batter. Observing it I judged that although I could not see anything moving in it there were yet living animalcules in it. I then mixed it several times with pure rain-water, in which there were no animalcules, I then again and again saw that there were many small living animalcules in the said matter, which moved very prettily".

Miller Chemoparasitic Theory

A synthesis of the ideas that acid and microorganisms were involved in the etiology of dental caries occurred in 1889 when **Miller**, an American working at the University of Berlin, published a text entitled "Die Mikroorganismen der Mundhohle." At this time, **Pasteur** had discovered that microorganisms mediate the process of conversion of sucrose to lactic acid. This enabled **Miller** to assign to oral microorganism the role of acid formation and thus assigned a chemical role to flora, which is the basis of his chemoparasitic theory of dental caries.

- The microorganisms of the mouth, by secretion of enzymes or by their own metabolism, degrade the fermentable carbohydrate food material so as to form acids.
- Carbohydrate food material lodged between and on surfaces of teeth is the source of the acid, which demineralizes the lime salts of the tooth.
- The enamel is destroyed by the fermentation of acid and the disintegrated enamel is subsequently mechanically removed by forces of mastication.
- After penetration of the enamel, the dissolution of dentin is brought about in the same manner with the organisms penetrating along the dentinal tubules.
- The final breakdown of dentin results from the secretion of proteolytic enzymes that digest the organic part of dentin and form a cavity.

Miller concluded that caries was caused not by a single species of microorganisms but was related to multiple microbial activities involving acid production and protein degradation. **Miller** summarized his theory as follows: "Dental decay is a chemoparasitic process consisting of two stages: decalcification or softening of the tissues and dissolution of softened residue".

Critique of theory:

- Unable to explain the predilection of specific sites on the tooth to dental caries.
- The initiation of caries on smooth surfaces was not accounted for by this theory.
- Does not explain why some populations are caries free.
- Phenomenon of arrested caries is not explained.
- The concept of tooth resistance while logical did not have any experimental support.

Proteolytic Theory

The surface coverings found on the tooth, in grooves and pits, are organic in nature; also enamel contains small but significant amount of organic material. These observations and the fact that carious lesions are characterized histologically by pigmentation, a phenomenon that was interpreted, without evidence, as being indicative of proteolysis, led to the development of the proteolytic theory espoused primarily by **Gottlieb** (1947), **Frisbie** and **Nuckolls** (1947), and **Pincus** (1950). They described caries like lesions that were initiated by proteolytic activity at a slightly alkaline pH and considered that the process involved depolymerization and liquefaction of the organic matrix of enamel. Gottlieb proposed that microorganisms invade the organic pathways of enamel and initiate caries by proteolytic action. Subsequently, the inorganic salts are dissolved by acidogenic bacteria.

Proteolysis: Chelation Theory

This theory proposed by **Schatz et al.,** in 1955 implies a simultaneous microbial degradation of the organic components (hence, proteolysis) and dissolution of the minerals of the tooth by the process of chelation. According to the proteolytic chelation theory, dental caries results from an initial bacterial and enzymatic, proteolytic action on the organic matter of enamel without preliminary demineralization. Such action, the theory suggests, produces an initial caries lesion and the release of a variety of complexing agents, such as amino acids, polyphosphates, and organic acids. The complexing agents then dissolve the crystalline apatite.

Critique of theory:

- The infecting *Streptococcus* could not hydrolyze gelatin, casein, collagen, or chondroitin. Although proteolysis of the organic matrix of dentin may indeed occur after demineralization, there is no satisfactory evidence to support the claim that the initial attack on enamel is proteolytic.
- Gnotobiotic studies showed that caries can occur in the absence of proteolytic organisms.
- Chemical analysis of early carious enamel lesions show a rise in nitrogen content and a fall in specific gravity that indicate a persistence or increase in organic matter.

Sulfatase Theory

Pincus (1950) advanced the sulfatase theory, whereby bacterial sulfatase hydrolyzes the "mucoitin sulfatase or sulfate" of enamel and the chondroitin sulfate of dentin producing sulfuric acid that, in turn, causes decalcification of the dental tissues.

Complexing and Phosphorylation Theory

It can be readily demonstrated that an uptake of phosphate by plaque bacteria occurs during aerobic and anaerobic glycolysis and the synthesis of polyphosphates. According to this theory, the high bacterial utilization of phosphate in plaque causes a local disturbance in the phosphate equilibrium in the plaque and the tooth enamel resulting in loss of inorganic phosphate from enamel. Soluble calcium complexing compounds produced by bacteria cause further tooth disintegration.

Sucrose-Chelation Theory

Egglers-Lura (1967) proposed that sucrose itself, and not the acid derived from it, can cause dissolution of enamel by forming an ionized Ca saccharate. This theory explains that Ca saccharate and Ca complexing intermediaries require inorganic phosphate which subsequently removed the enamel by phosphorylating enzymes.

Autoimmunity Theory

Burch and Jackson analyzed caries epidemiologic data and suggested that genes, partly inherited and partly mutational, determine whether a site on a tooth is at risk. In dental caries, odontoblasts may be the target cells, which would change the resistance of the enamel to acid attack.

ETIOLOGY OF DENTAL CARIES

Earlier Concept of Dental Caries

In the epidemiological model, a disease state is due to interplay of three primary factors: the host, the agent or recruiting factor, and environmental influences. Applying this to dental caries, **Keyes** and **Jordan** in 1960 gave a model **(Fig. 38.13)** stating that for the initiation and progression of caries interaction between three primary factors is essential: a susceptible host tissue, the tooth; microflora with a cariogenic potential; and a suitable local substrate to meet the requirements of the pathogenic flora.

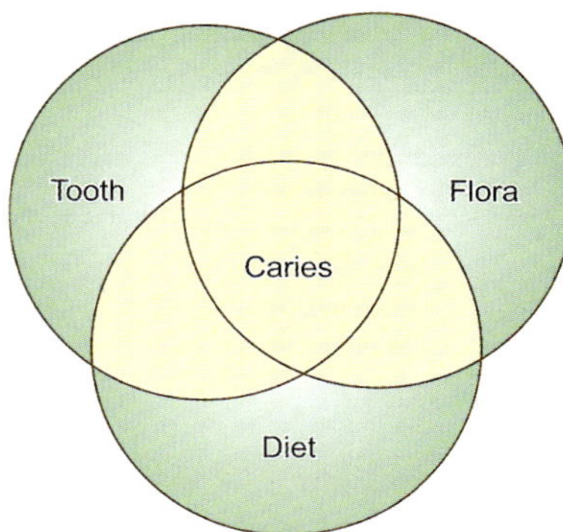

Fig. 38.13: Keyes triad model.

Newbrun modified the Keyes model in 1978 and gave a Newbruns tetrad model **(Fig. 38.14)** where time was added as the fourth factor and proposed that dental caries results from the interaction of oral flora with dietary carbohydrates on the tooth surface over a period of time.

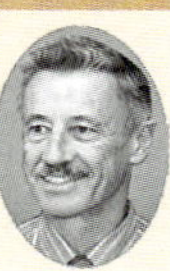

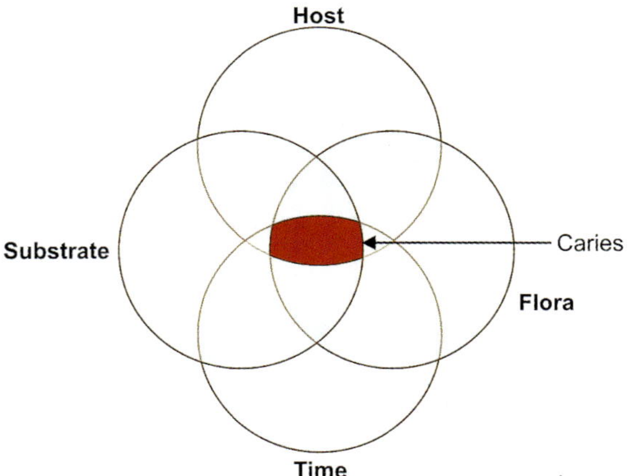

Fig. 38.14: Newbruns tetrad model.

- The tooth is the target tissue destroyed in the dental caries process. The cariogenic oral flora, which is localized to specific sites on teeth, is the agent that produces and secretes the chemical substances that cause the destruction of the inorganic components and the subsequent breakdown of the organic moieties of enamel and dentin. The local substrate provides the nutritional and energy requirement for the oral microflora, thereby permitting them to colonize, grow, and metabolize on selective surfaces of teeth. The third factor, the resistance of the tooth, is obviously important since this determines the overall effects of the attack.

CURRENT CONCEPT OF DENTAL CARIES

As all the individuals with teeth, microbial flora and who are consuming carbohydrates does not develop caries over time. Thus more recently it was postulated that there are several modifying risk and protective factors that influences the onset and progression of the dental caries **(Fig. 38.15)**. This was further modified by **TenCate** in 2009 **(Fig. 38.16)**.

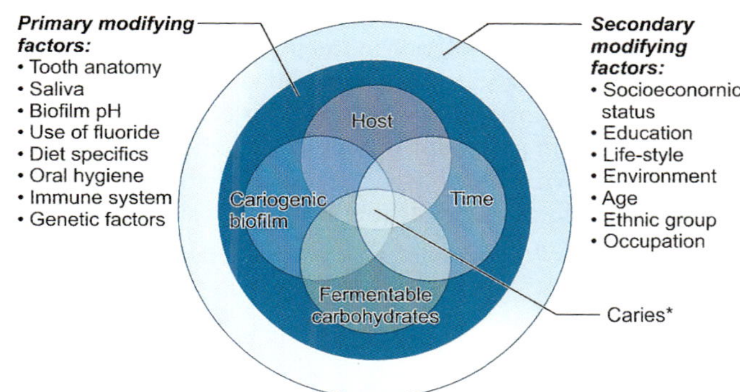

Fig. 38.15: Newer model of caries with primary and secondary factors.

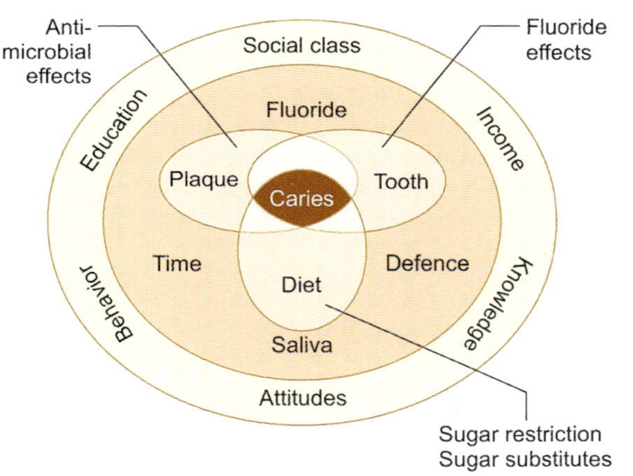

Fig. 38.16: TenCate modifications of Keys model.

ORAL MICROFLORA AND DENTAL CARIES

Carious lesions occur only when a mass of bacteria produces a sufficiently acidic environment that can dissolute the crystalline structure of the tooth. However, the course or progression of the individual carious lesions is not always predictable. Oral bacteria, instead of occurring as individual colonies, are found as members of complex community of multiple species as an aggregate of tightly packed cells held with a sticky matrix. This gelatinous mass of bacteria adhering to the tooth surface is referred to as *Dental Plaque.* Hypothesis concerning the pathogenicity of the plaque is that metabolic activity of the plaque bacteria determines the onset and progression of the carious lesions in the oral cavity.

- **Nonspecific plaque hypothesis:** The traditional hypothesis, which assumes that all plaque is pathogenic. The therapeutic approach with the nonspecific plaque hypothesis will require a complete elimination of plaque which is unrealistic and unachievable even in the most dedicated patients.
- **Specific plaque hypothesis:** Given by **Walter Loesche** in 1976. It suggests that plaque is pathogenic only when signs of associated clinical disease are present. The specific plaque hypothesis advocates elimination of the specific pathogenic organisms, rather than total plaque elimination, thus providing more scientific basis for the treatment of caries.
- **Ecologic plaque hypothesis:** Given by **Marsh** in 1994 and is the most accepted hypothesis. It states that disease is the result of an imbalance in the microflora by ecological stress resulting in an enrichment of certain disease-related microorganisms. Changes in ecological factors like change in pH, redox potential, presence of nutrients, etc., causes virulence of specific microorganism in plaque. This hypothesis suggests that the composition of dental plaque depends on the environment and it is still generally accepted.

The hypothesis that bacteria are a prerequisite for the initiation and progression of dental caries was clinched by **Orland** (1954) at the University of Chicago.

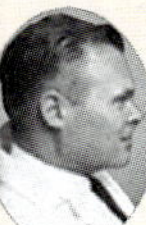

- **Fitzgerald** in 1968 concluded that:
  - Microorganisms are a prerequisite for caries initiation.
  - A single type of organism is capable of inducing caries.
  - The ability of producing acid is prerequisite for caries induction but not all acid-producing organisms are cariogenic.
  - Organisms vary greatly in their capacity (virulence) to induce caries.

Biofilm

The term *plaque biofilm* or *biofilm* is more recently used in place of dental plaque to describe the complex community of microorganisms found in the oral cavity. Biofilm is a highly organized structure composed mainly of bacteria, their by products, extracellular matrix and water. There are around 200 to 300 species of bacteria, protozoa and yeast that are native to human oral cavity. However, group of bacteria which has been largely associated with the dental caries is *Streptococcus* mainly *Streptococcus mutans, Streptococcus salivarius and Streptococcus sanguis.* These bacteria are generally associated with the onset of the carious process and are called as the beginners. Another bacteria *Lactobacilli* has been associated in active progression of cavitated lesions owing to their property of producing high amounts of organic acids in the presence of sucrose. The oral cavity is described as a well-defined ecosystem where different areas of oral cavity owing to their different environment provides habitat to different groups and species of microorganisms.

The tooth surface is covered with the pellicle [acquired enamel pellicle (AEP)] comprising of precipitated salivary glycoproteins, enzymes, and immunoglobulins providing an ideal surface for attachment of many oral microorganisms

↓

First the microorganisms, primarily streptococci, which have receptors for adhesion, adhere to the tooth surface and produce a sticky mass to cohere with each other and form colonies

↓

They then proliferate and spread laterally and away from tooth surface

↓

These colonizers facilitate attachment of spirochetes and filamentous bacteria which otherwise, due to lack of receptors, cannot adhere to the tooth structure

↓

Over the time biofilm community grows many fold thousand cells thick forming structure like corn cobs

↓

Each community of microorganisms create local environment conducive to the successors

↓

As the plaque biofilm matures there is shift to the anaerobic conditions and rapid metabolism of dietary sucrose occurs which causes pH depression at the tooth surface causing dental caries

Tabel 38.2: Oral habitats.

Habitat	***Predominant species***	***Environmental conditions within plaque***
Mucosa	*S. mitis* *S. sanguis* *S. salivarius*	Aerobic pH approximately 7 Oxidation-reduction potential positive
Tongue	*S. salivarius* *S. mutans* *S. sanguis*	Aerobic pH approximately 7 Oxidation-reduction potential positive
Teeth (noncarious)	*S. sanguis*	Aerobic pH 5.5 Oxidation-reduction negative
Gingival crevice	*Fusobacterium* *Spirochaeta* *Actinomyces* *Veillonella*	Anaerobic pH variable Oxidation-reduction very negative
Enamel caries	*S. mutans*	Anaerobic pH <5.5 Oxidation-reduction negative
Dentin caries	*S. mutans* *Lactobacillus*	Anaerobic pH <5.5 Oxidation-reduction negative
Root caries	*Actinomyces*	Anaerobic pH <5.5 Oxidation-reduction negative

DEMINERALIZATION–REMINERALIZATION CONCEPT

- Carious lesions occur when plaque bacteria metabolize refined carbohydrates particularly sucrose and produce organic acids (primarily lactic acid) as a by-product thereby creating a sufficiently acidic environment which can demineralize tooth structure.
- The organic acids dissociate causing the local pH to decline and when the pH decreases to less than 5.5, it overcomes

the buffering capacity of salivary bicarbonate available at the tooth plaque interface thus leading to dissolution of tooth mineral. Thus this pH of 5.5 is considered as the critical pH for enamel.

- However, single event of decreased pH is insufficient to cause apparent changes in the mineral content of the tooth. Frequent episodes of lowered pH, occurring over long periods, results in the characteristic carious lesions. Frequent sucrose exposure causes constant pH depression at the tooth surface resulting in demineralization.
- When there is little availability of carbohydrates, plaque metabolism diminishes causing the pH to increase at the tooth surface. As the local pH increases to greater than 5.5. Remineralization of the tooth structure occurs. Saliva acts as a reservoir of calcium and phosphate ions for the remineralization process.
- As per the availability of dietary sucrose, plaque metabolism changes causing changes in the pH at the tooth surface, thus episodes of exacerbations and remissions of caries activity are seen.
- Dental caries is not a result of a single acid attack caused by the acid formed as a result of fermentation of dietary substrates by the oral microflora. Rather, it is an outcome of the imbalance occurring in the demineralization–remineralization cycle that is continuously operating in the oral cavity.
- This balance is governed by a number of factors which is either caries promoting (promotes demineralization) or caries inhibiting (promotes remineralization) **(Fig. 38.17).**
- An important point to be mentioned is all these factors are present in every individual's oral cavity but in different proportions determining the direction of the demineralization–remineralization cycle.

Pathological factors	Protective factors
• Acid-producing bacteria • Sub-normal saliva flow and/or function • Frequent eating/drinking of fermentable carbohydrates • Poor oral hygiene	• Saliva flow and components • Remineralization (fluoride, calcium, phosphate) • Antibacterials (fluoride, chlorhexidine, xylitol) • Good oral hygiene
Demineralization (caries)	Remineralization (no caries)

Fig. 38.17: Demineralization–remineralization cycle (caries balance).

Stephan's Curve

- In 1940s, **Dr Robert Stephan**, an officer in the US Public Health Service, suggested that there was a continuous change in salivary pH following consumption of foods and beverages, especially with fermentable carbohydrates.
- Stephan curve is a graph **(Fig. 38.18)** published by **Stephan** and **Miller** in 1944 which reflected the fall in salivary pH following a glucose rinse.
- Stephan selected patients who were either caries free or caries inactive or who exhibited various degrees of caries activity. Subjects were asked not to brush their teeth for 3–4 days prior to the measurement of the plaque biofilm pH on the labial surfaces of the anterior teeth. Prior to rinsing

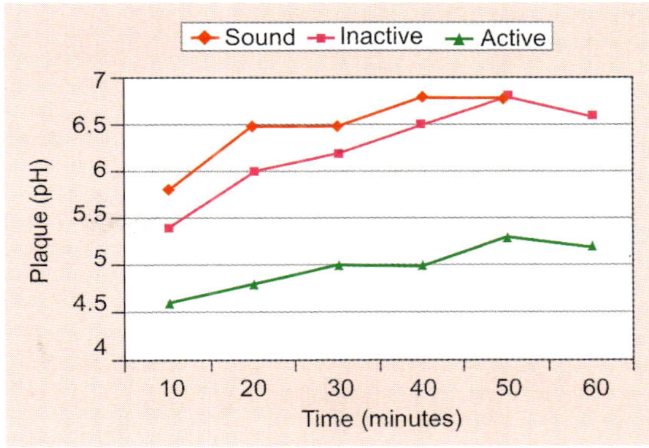

Fig. 38.18: Stephan's curve.

with 10 mL of a 10% glucose solution for 10 seconds, pH readings were obtained. After rinsing with the glucose solution, pH readings were obtained at various time intervals until the pH returned to its original value. The graph has four landmarks, namely, resting pH, the rapid fall in pH, the critical pH, and the recovery phase.

- **Resting plaque pH:** This describes plaque that has not been exposed to fermentable carbohydrates for approximately 2 hours and generally has a pH of between 6 and 7. The resting plaque pH value for an individual tends to be stable and may remain so for long periods. One example of an exception is if antibiotics have been taken, which may alter the oral flora.
- **Decrease in plaque pH:** After exposure of dental plaque to fermentable carbohydrates, the pH decreases rapidly. The rate at which the pH decreases is due in part to the microbial composition of dental plaque. In general, if more acidogenic, aciduric bacteria is present in plaque, the pH would lower more rapidly. The rate of pH decrease is also dependent on the speed with which plaque bacteria are able to metabolize the dietary carbohydrate. While sucrose would be metabolized quickly, prompting a more rapid decrease, larger molecules, like starch, would diffuse into plaque more slowly because it would need to be broken down before it can be assimilated by plaque microbes. Another factor that affects the rate of pH decrease is the buffering capacity of unstimulated saliva. The rate at which plaque pH decreases is also influenced by the density of plaque. Less dense plaque can be penetrated more easily by buffering saliva and oxygen causing slower pH decreases than very dense plaque, which cannot be accessed by saliva and oxygen.
- **Critical pH:** The critical pH is the pH at which saliva no longer remains saturated with calcium and phosphate, thereby permitting the hydroxyapatite in dental enamel to dissolve. It is the highest pH at which there is a net loss of enamel from the teeth, which is generally accepted to be about 5.5 for enamel.
- **Increase in plaque pH:** The low pH remained for some time, taking 30–60 min to return to its normal pH (in the region of 6.3–7.0). Differences were seen between the caries-free group and the caries-active group, with the latter group having significantly lower plaque pH. The gradual recovery of the plaque pH is influenced by various factors. These include the buffering capacity of saliva,

whether fermentable carbohydrate remains in the mouth and the diffusion of acids from plaque into saliva or teeth.

Application of Stephan's curve in day-to-day life:

- **Figure 38.19** shows the plotting of the variation of salivary pH after various meals and snacks.

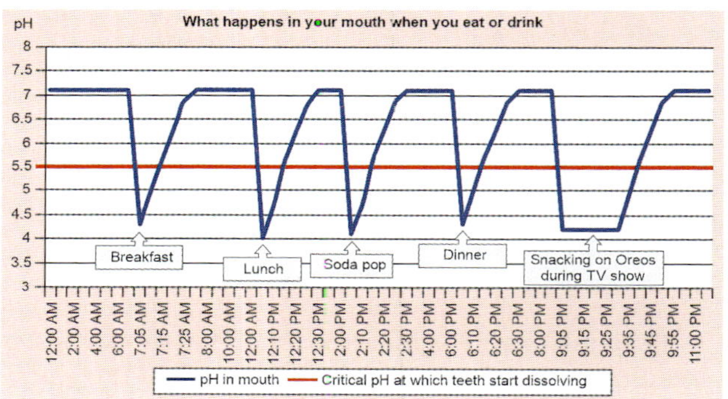

Fig. 38.19: Applicability of Stephan curve in daily routine.

- The initial flat part of the graph represents the resting pH of saliva which is mostly constant for an individual.
- The first dip in the graph represents the fall in salivary pH soon after the breakfast. The degree of fall depends upon the constituents of the breakfast. A breakfast more rich in fermentable carbohydrates will lead to a steeper fall of pH and to a lower level of pH.
- Once the pH goes below the critical pH, the saliva no longer remains saturated with calcium and phosphate ions.
- This results in the shifting of the demineralization–remineralization equilibrium toward demineralization. By the action of buffering agents of saliva and other protective actions like the washing and flushing action of saliva, the pH starts rising. During this event if the pH rises above the critical pH, remineralization of the tooth will start.
- In a situation where an individual consumes snacks before the pH rises above the critical pH (as showed between the lunch and dinner), the salivary pH again falls and does not allow the repair process of remineralization. This outlines the deleterious effect of frequent snacking on the caries process in oral cavity.
- In contrast to this if an individual rinses his oral cavity or brushes his teeth after meals (as showed after dinner), this leads to the flushing out of the acid produced by the microorganisms. In addition, this also lowers the microbial load of the oral cavity and removes the trapped food particles which acts as a reservoir for the substrate required for acid production. All these events result into a steeper rise in the pH, thus exposing the tooth to the acid attack for a lesser time period.
- To conclude all those factors which try to maintain the pH of the oral cavity above the critical pH are caries protective in nature and those which lowers the pH below this level may be considered caries promoting.

HISTOPATHOLOGY OF DENTAL CARIES

Knowledge of the histopathologic features of dental caries is important in detecting and diagnosing the lesion. Familiarity with the shape of lesion is of fundamental importance in understanding the design of cavity preparations.

Enamel Caries

- The first evidence of caries on the smooth enamel surface appears as chalky white opaque areas when air dried and disappear when the tooth surface is rehydrated. The enamel loses its translucency because of the extensive subsurface porosity caused by demineralization. However, the enamel surface is still intact, fairly hard and smooth to touch.
- They are referred to as white spot lesions or incipient carious lesion or noncavitated caries lesion and are usually seen on the facial and lingual surfaces of the teeth and sometimes in proximal surfaces also but difficult to detect.
- These lesions can be distinguished from developmental white spot hypocalcifications of enamel by air drying the surface as hypocalcified enamel is not much affected by the drying and wetting of the surface while these incipient carious lesions disappear totally or partially on hydrated enamel surface.
- These noncavitated lesions of enamel can be remineralized if oral environment is altered. The supersaturation of the saliva with calcium and phosphate ions serves as the driving force for the remineralization process. The corrective measures including plaque removal, local fluoride application or use of other remineralizing agents in form of toothpastes or mousse should be employed.

Zones of enamel caries: Light microscopy studies of carious lesions of enamel without cavitation have revealed four distinct zones, which represent varying degrees of hard tissue transformation. Starting from the advancing front of the lesion, these zones are classified as **(Fig. 38.20)**:

1. *Translucent zone:* The advancing front of a carious lesion is represented by the translucent zone which appears structureless when perfused with quinolone and observed under polarized light. The first discernible signs of enamel breakdown are seen in this area. This zone is not a consistent feature of enamel caries and is only seen when longitudinal ground section of carious teeth is examined. Enamel alteration in this zone results in spaces or pores at junction sites such as the prism boundaries. Microdensitometric and chemical studies

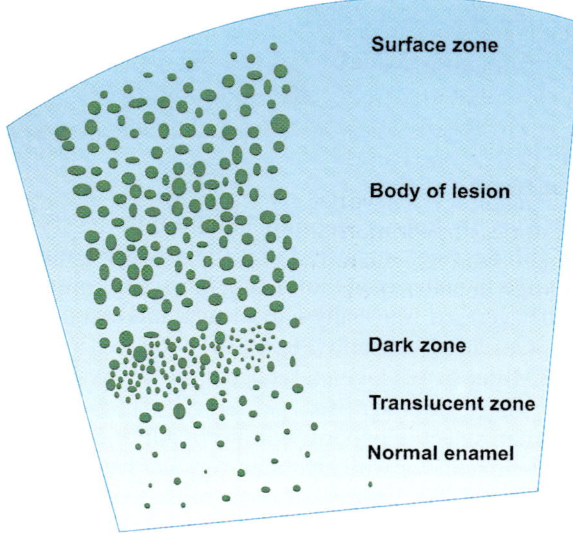

Fig. 38.20: Histopathology of enamel caries.

of this zone indicate some loss of mineral and a resultant pore volume of about 1% as compared to 0.1% in normal enamel. The preferential removal of acid-labile moieties, such as carbonate and magnesium together with calcium and phosphate, is responsible for the increase in porosity but there is no evidence that organic material is removed or significantly altered in the translucent zone.

2. *Dark zone:* The dark zone lies deep to the body of the lesion and just superficial to the translucent zone. This zone is positively birefringent and has a pore volume of 2–4%. This molecular sieving effect permits the micropores to remain filled with air. Light passing through this zone causes the brown discoloration of the dark zone. This is also the reason why the dark zone shows a reversal in its birefringence from negative to positive. Because of this phenomenon, the dark zone is often referred to as the positive zone.
3. *Body of lesion:* Deep to the relatively unaffected enamel surface layer is the body of the carious lesion. Ground sections, when viewed in transmitted light, reveal enhanced striae of Retzius and cross-striations in the enamel prisms. This zone, unlike normal, enamel, is positively birefringent denoting a significant degree of mineral loss. The body of the lesion has a minimum pore volume of 5% at its periphery, and even in a small subclinical lesion, there is a 25% pore volume.
4. *Surface zone:* An important feature of the initial carious lesion is the presence of an apparently intact enamel surface overlying an area of subsurface demineralization. Quantitative studies of the surface layer, 20–100 mm thick, indicate that partial demineralization equivalent to about 1–10% loss of mineral salts has taken place. The surface zone has been defined as the zone of negative birefringence superficial to the positively birefringent body of lesion.

Dentinal Caries

Caries progression in dentin is more rapid than in enamel because of the lower mineral content and tubular structure of the dentin which provides pathway for the ingress of bacteria and its products. So when caries reaches the DEJ lateral spreading of the caries occur, which is seen as V-shaped in cross section with a wide base at the DEJ and the apex directed pulpally.

Zones of Dentinal Caries

Five different zones have been described in carious dentin and these zones appear more distinguished in slowly advancing lesions as compared to rapidly progressing lesions where the difference between the zones becomes less evident. The five zones proceeding from the lesion inward to normal dentin are **(Fig. 38.21)**:

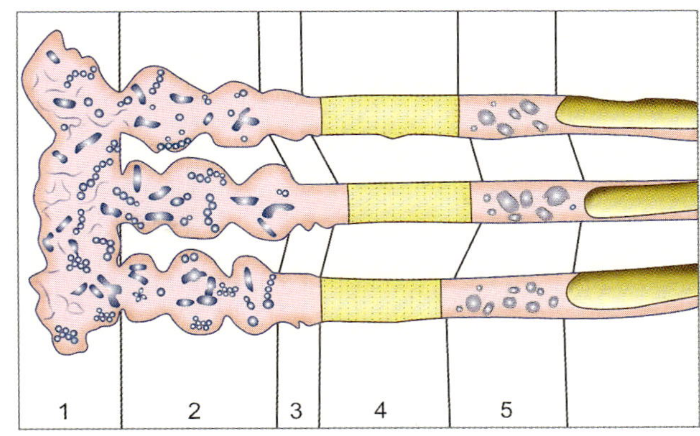

Fig. 38.21: Histopathology of dentinal caries: (1) Zone of decomposed dentin; (2) Zone of bacterial invasion; (3) Zone of transparent dentin; (4) Zone of subtransaprent dentin; (5) Zone of normal dentin.

1. **Zone of decomposed dentin/infected dentin/soft dentin:** It is the outermost zone loaded with bacteria and lacks any recognizable structure, mineral and collagen seem to be absent. Must be removed to ensure sound, successful restoration and to prevent spread of infection.
2. **Zone of bacterial invasion/turbid dentin:** Distorted and widened dentinal tubules filled with bacteria are seen. Mineral content is low and collagen is irreversibly denatured. This zone cannot be remineralized and must be removed before restoration.
3. **Zone of transparent dentin:** Softer than normal dentin due to loss of mineral from the intertubular dentin. Many large crystals are seen in the lumen of the dentinal tubules and the collagen is intact which can serve as a template for remineralization. Bacteria are absent. Stimulation of this region produces pain.
4. **Zone of subtransaprent dentin:** Fine crystals seen in the lumen of dentinal tubules. No bacteria found in this zone. Stimulation of dentin produces pain, and this dentin can remineralize.
5. **Zone of normal dentin:** Deepest area with no crystals in the lumen and tubules show smooth odontoblastic processes. Intact crosslinked collagen and normal dense apatite crystals. No bacteria. Stimulation of the dentin produces sharp pain.

Zone	*Birefringence*	*X-ray*	*Mineral loss (%)*
Translucent	–	Opaque	1.2
Dark	+	Opaque	6
Body of lesion	+	Lucent	24
Surface layer	–	Opaque	10

Clearance from the oral cavity	One of the most important functions of saliva with respect to its role in caries is the removal of bacteria and food debris from the mouth. When saliva is swallowed, any bacteria contained therein are removed from the oral cavity and pass into the stomach. The average unstimulated salivary flow rate is about 0.3 mL/min. Thus, the half-life in the oral cavity for any inert material suspended in saliva is only a few minutes and is certainly very much less than the mean generation time of oral microorganisms
Inorganic constituents of saliva	Na^+, Cl^-, HCO_3, K^+, F^-, Ca, Mg, phosphorus, glucose, ammonia, iodine, etc.
Fluoride concentration of saliva	The level of fluoride ions in ductal saliva is in the range of 0.01–0.03 ppm. Fluoride levels in saliva are largely independent of salivary flow rate and are determined by the amount ingested. Administration of 3.0–10.0 mg of fluoride daily results in a significant increase in fluoride concentration in secretions from the major salivary glands
Calcium and phosphate concentration in saliva	These ions help in remineralization
Salivary proteins with digestive functions	These include α-amylase and other hydrolytic enzymes. The main functions of α-amylase in the oral cavity may be to increase the rate of dissolution and removal of starch-containing food debris retained around the teeth and on the oral mucosa. In addition to α-amylase, small amounts of other enzymes with digestive functions have been detected. These include acid phosphatase, ribonuclease, esterase, aminopeptidase, and glucoronidase
Salivary proteins with protective functions	*Glycoproteins:* They are covalent complexes of protein and carbohydrate. They are usually classified according to the nature of the linkage of the carbohydrate side chain bound to the protein molecule. The most important glycoproteins in saliva that have protective function are the mucinous type
	Salivary agglutinins: Recent evidence indicates that some of the salivary glycoproteins can interact specifically with microorganisms. It has been demonstrated by **Gibbons** and **Spinell** (1970) that salivary glycoproteins can cause an aggregation of various strains of oral microorganisms. Agglutination of microorganisms could either result in their rapid removal from the oral cavity when the saliva is swallowed or, if the agglutinated microorganisms are more adherent, could promote their colonization on epithelial and dental surfaces
Salivary proteins, which inhibit formation of hydroxyapatite	Several salivary proteins bind calcium and inhibit formation of hydroxyapatite. These proteins are statherin and a group of proline-rich proteins *Statherin:* It is a polypeptide of molecular weight 5,380, consisting of 43 amino acids. Statherin, in addition to inhibiting formation of hydroxyapatite, also prevents precipitation of calcium phosphate salts. The physiological advantages of the presence of salivary statherin are that saliva can be supersaturated with respect to hydroxyapatite, thus facilitating remineralization of early carious lesions, without the spontaneous precipitation of calcium phosphate, which would otherwise occur *Proline-rich proteins:* A number of proteins have been isolated from saliva, which is characterized by a high content of proline varying from about 25–40% of the total number of amino acid residues. They inhibit hydroxyapatite formation and constitute a substantial amount of the protein
Buffering capacity	Saliva has three buffering systems, but bicarbonate system is the most powerful of all. The buffering capacity of saliva is a very important property that affects the caries process. The bicarbonate in saliva is able to diffuse into dental plaque of saliva to neutralize the acid formed by microorganisms

DIET AND DENTAL CARIES

Our diet habits have undergone considerable changes, both in quantity and quality, since our evolution. Food can have a two-fold effect because the effects of nutrition are mediated systemically and the effects of diet are manifested locally. The interaction between diet and tooth is of great importance in relation to caries.

Although, it is true that microorganisms are chiefly responsible for caries, the importance of substrate cannot be undermined because microorganisms cannot cause caries without a suitable substrate. The occurrence of caries is dependent on two factors— pre-eruptive (blood, saliva) and posteruptive factors (maturation, mineralization, chelation, plaque, bacteria).

Dietary constituents and dental caries	
Polysaccharides and sugars	The four carbohydrates—starch, sucrose, fructose and glucose—comprise the greatest proportion of foods consumed by man. The main polysaccharide (starch) is not highly cariogenic in man at least in some circumstances. Controlled studies in experimental animals and in humans have confirmed that excessive and frequent use of highly fermentable mono- and disaccharides is correlated with high caries rates. While glucose, fructose, lactose, and mannose have been shown to be cariogenic in animal experiments, they are usually minor constituents of human foods as they are present only in dried fruits, honey, and milk. Sucrose is by far the most common dietary sugar and most cariogenic.
Physical properties of foods and cariogenicity	We know little about the significance of physical properties of foods and their effects on cariogenicity, since few studies involving human subjects have been conducted to explore this relationship. Some important physical properties that determine food texture are: • Mechanical properties: Hardness, cohesiveness, viscosity • Geometric properties: Particle size and shape • Others: Moisture and fat content From a dental standpoint, the physical properties of food may have significance by affecting food retention, food clearance, solubility, and oral hygiene. Obviously, if a type of food is more sticky, there are more chances of getting caries as compared to a food that is readily cleared from oral cavity.
The physical texture and chemical composition of food	It is known to affect salivary flow rates. Saliva that is rapidly flowing is more alkaline than resting saliva and more supersaturated with calcium and phosphate and thus may be more caries inhibitory
Physical properties of food	Those foods that improve the cleansing action and reduce the retention of food within the oral cavity and increase saliva flow are to be encouraged in everyday diets. However, clinical evidence that consumption of these food items will significantly reduce caries per se is lacking
Acidity of foods	Some dietary items are highly acidic and therefore affect, usually in a transient manner, the pH in plaque and saliva. Natural foods, such as lemons, apples, fruit juices, and carbonated beverages, are sufficiently acidic so as to cause demineralization of enamel that is in prolonged contact with them these items, under normal dietary use, are of no consequence in the dental caries process. However, excessive (habitual) use of these foods and beverages may cause etching of enamel with cavitation
Vitamins	Vitamin D and vitamin A are most important with respect to development of teeth. Decrease of vitamin D will lead to calcium and phosphate derangement and, in turn, cause hypoplasia of teeth. Deficiency of vitamin A can lead to changes in ameloblasts, thereby causing alteration in tooth morphology and can also have deleterious effects on salivary glands
Lipids	Fat consumed has been somewhat responsible for anticariogenic effect. This mechanism can be due to protection from demineralization by formation of fatty film in proximal areas

Evidence of Relation between Diet and Caries

The single most important determinant of cariogenicity in the oral cavity is the availability of a suitable local substrate for the oral flora. Some studies have been conducted in human that effectively summarize the diet-caries relation.

Hopewood House Study

- In 1942 an eccentric, wealthy Australian businessman transformed what was formerly a spacious country mansion, Hopewood House, into a "motherhouse" for young children at NSW, Australia. Since the businessman had attributed his own dramatic recovery in health to a drastic change in dietary habits, he stipulated that the children of Hopewood House should be raised on a natural diet that excluded refined carbohydrates.
- The basically vegetarian diet of these children was adequate but spartan porridge, biscuits, wheat gram, fresh and dried fruit, vegetables (cooked and raw), along with butter cheese, eggs, milk, and fruit juices. Vitamin concentrates and an occasional serving of nuts and a sweetening agent such as honey supplemented the meals. The food was uncooked as far as possible in order to retain its natural state.
- The most striking feature of this diet was the notable absence of sugar.
- The fluoride content of the water and food was insignificant, and no tea was consumed. All meals and between meal eating were controlled with great regularity.
- At the end of a 10-year period, the 13-year-old children of Hopewood House had a mean DMF per child of 1.6; the corresponding figure for the general child population of the State of NSW was 10.7. Only 0.4% of the 13-year-old state school children were free from dental caries, whereas 53% of the Hopewood children experienced no caries. The children's oral hygiene was poor, dental calculus was uncommon, but gingivitis was prevalent in about 75% of the children.
- This work shows that in institutionalized children, at least, dental caries can be reduced to insignificant levels by a spartan diet, and without the beneficial influence of fluoride and in the presence of unfavorable oral hygiene.

Vipeholm Study

- In 1939, the Swedish Government requested the Royal Medical Board to investigate the measures that should be taken to reduce the frequency of the most common dental disease in Sweden. This request led to a study at the Vipeholm Hospital, Lund, an institution for mentally disabled individuals, of the relationship between diet and dental caries. The purpose of the study was to find answers to the questions like:

- Does an increase in carbohydrate (mostly sugar) intake cause an increase in dental caries?
- Does a decrease in carbohydrate (sugar) intake produce a decrease in dental caries?

❖ The 436 patients involved in this study were divided into control and six experimental groups. All patients received a diet relatively low in sugar for 1 year, with no sugar in between meals. The groups were divided as:

- *Control groups:* Received a low carbohydrate (mostly starch), high fat diet practically free from refined sugar. Caries activity was almost completely suppressed. After 2 years, this diet was replaced by an ordinary diet to which was added 100 g of sugar a day at meal times, which was accompanied by a small but statistically significant rise in caries activity.
- *Sucrose group:* Received 300 g of sucrose in solution at meal times.
- *Bread group:* 345 g of sweet bread containing 50 g of sugar.
- Chocolate group received the 300 g sugar with meals, which was reduced to 100 g supplemented by 65 g of milk chocolate between meals during the second 2 years.
- *Caramel group:* Received 22 caramels daily in two portions between meals.
- *8-toffee groups:* Received eight toffees in two portions.
- 24-toffee group received 24 toffees between meals.

❖ The main conclusion of the Vipeholm study summarized as:

- The risk of sugar increasing caries activity is great if the sugar is consumed in a form with a strong tendency to be retained on the surfaces of the teeth.
- The risk of sugar increasing caries activity is greatest if the sugar is consumed between meals.
- Increase in caries activity due to the intake of sugar rich foodstuff consumed in a manner favoring caries, the lesion disappear on withdrawal of such foodstuffs from the diet.
- Carious lesions may continue to appear despite the avoidance of refined sugar, maximum restriction of natural sugars, and total dietary carbohydrates.
- The risk of an increase in caries activity is intensified with an increase in the duration of sugar clearance from saliva.

Turku Study

❖ Another large scale and important experiment on caries in human subject was carried out in Turku, Finland and was reported in detail by **Scheinin** and **Makinen** in 1975.

❖ The aim of this study was to compare the cariogenicity of sucrose, fructose, and xylitol.

❖ A total of 125 subjects were divided into three groups on a basis of their own preference. The three groups were as follows: first was sucrose group who received their ordinary sucrose containing diet the second group received xylitol, and the third group, fructose.

❖ The results after 1 year showed that sucrose and fructose had equal cariogenicity, whereas xylitol produced almost no caries. But the second year, caries had continued to increase in the sucrose group but remained unchanged in the fructose group implying that sucrose was more cariogenic than fructose. But the important finding was that in the xylitol group, some early white spot lesions had been remineralized to a point where they could not be scored. These results provided sufficient evidence to link cariogenicity of carbohydrates, especially sucrose.

Experimental Production of Caries in Man

❖ Two such experiments have been tried one in Denmark by **Vonder Fehr** in 1970 and second in Britain by **Edgar** in 1978.

❖ The procedures followed in these studies were nine daily rinses with 10 mL of 50% sucrose and discontinuance of active oral hygiene procedures. White-spot lesions on smooth surfaces were produced in 3 weeks in the experimental group.

❖ At the end of the experiment, meticulous oral hygiene measures were reinstituted along with a daily mouth rinse of 0.2% NaF, which resulted in remineralization of the white spots and a reversal of the caries index scores to the same values as in the control group.

❖ This investigation again produced the required evidence of diet-caries correlation.

Hereditary Fructose Intolerance (HFI)

❖ In 1959, **Froesch** described an inborn error of fructose metabolism transmitted by an autosomal recessive gene. The metabolic error in this condition is due to deficiency of hepatic fructose-1-phosphate aldolase. This causes a cellular accumulation of fructose-1-phosphate, which, in turn, inhibits fructose phosphorylation. This condition results in episodes of pallor, nausea, vomiting, coma, and convulsion following ingestion of fruit containing fructose or cane sugar.

❖ Persons with HFI show a strikingly reduced dental caries experience when compared to a control population of the same age.

FOOD SUGAR SUBSTITUTES

The importance of diet in the development of caries was suspected in antiquity and established in modern times. The process has been shown to be multifactorial in nature, but it has been generally accepted that sugars in the diet are a major contributor to the disease. Sucrose is the most common sugar added to beverages and food products with the consumption in developed countries reported to be 40–60 kg/person/year. In recognition of the caries potential of sucrose, investigators have searched for alternative sweetness. The ideal agent would provide sweetness, but with no unpleasant after-taste, have little or no calories, not be carcinogenic or mutagenic, be economical to produce, and would not be degraded by heat when cooked. Identification of such a product has been challenging. Although several non-nutritive sweetening agents have been marketed, none have processed all of the preferred properties. Some of the agents approved by FDA are:

Aspartame	It is a dipeptide methyl ester, sold under the brand names of NutraSweet and equal. It was discovered in 1965 and is approximately 200 times sweeter than sucrose. Aspartame was approved in 1981 for limited use as a sweetener and extended to a larger market in 1983. Aspartame is the most widely used noncariogenic artificial sweetener. Its primary use is in diet soft drinks, yogurt, puddings, gelatin, and snack foods Aspartame has been shown to have a protective effect against some mycotoxins and is claimed to be safe for use by type II diabetics. But some of the disadvantages of this are reduced number of sickle cells in the blood of patients with homogeneous sickle cells anemia, relative toxic effects on growth, glucose homeostasis, and liver functions with long-term usage
Acesulfame potassium	A non-nutritive produce, approved by the FDA in 1988 for use as a sweetener in dry food products. In 1994 yogurt, refrigerated deserts, syrups, and baked foods were added to the approved list. The use of acesulfame potassium is approved for use in foods, beverages, cosmetics, and pharmaceutical products in >30 countries. Although considered safe for consumption by humans, there have been some health issues raised relative to dose-dependent cytogenetic toxicity
Saccharin	It is 200–500 times sweeter than sucrose and is the oldest of the artificial sweeteners used. It is noncariogenic and noncaloric and is available in liquid and tablet form as a table sweetener but has a slightly bitter aftertaste. But in 1970, saccharin was identified as a potential bladder carcinogen, and its use has hence been limited
Sucralose	It is a non-nutritive, noncaloric, trichlorinated derivative of sucrose. Sucralose is widely used throughout the world in many food products such as tea and coffee sweetener, carbonated and noncarbonated beverages, baked goods, chewing gum and frozen desserts. No health concerns have been reported with it.
Sorbitol	It is a sugar alcohol that occurs naturally in many fruits and berries. It is produced commercially from glucose but is expensive to manufacture. Sorbitol is often used as a "bulk" sweetener in a variety of food substances such as chewing gum, chocolates, and confectionaries. It is half as sweet as sucrose and is considered noncariogenic, but it may be absorbed from the gastrointestinal tract and can cause diarrhea if ingested in large quantities.
Xylitol	It was discovered in wood chips in 1890 and in wheat in 1891. It is a nonfermentable, pleasant tasting, noncariogenic polyol derived from pentose sugar xylose and is relatively expensive to manufacture. Xylitol is as sweet as sucrose and was approved as safe for use in humans in 1986. It is used primarily in chewing gum and possesses approximately the same sweetness potency as sucrose. Recently, xylitol has been credited in reducing the transmission of cariogenic bacteria from mother to infant and has been shown to have bactericidal qualities. The FDA has not yet approved the additional uses of xylitol as a sweetener. However, numerous studies have established the safety for human consumption.
Stevia	It is natural occurring, heat stable sweetener, which is extracted from *Stevia rebaudiana* Bertoni a member of the Chrysanthemum family. The active ingredient, stevioside, is a white crystalline material that contains three glucose molecules and steviol, a diterpenoid carboxylic alcohol. Its sweetness potency is 100–300 times greater than sucrose. Stevia is calorie-free, noncariogenic, and has been used by the indigenous peoples of Paraguay for centuries as a sweetner. It is widely used commercially in Brazil and Japan, and to a lesser extent in China and Germany. In 1995, the FDA approved the importation and use of Stevia as dietary supplement, but not as a sweetener.
Neotame	It is a new product similar in chemical structure to aspartame being developed commercially by the NutraSweet Company. Neotame is a high intensity sweetener reported to have a clean taste with no unpleasant characteristics. It has sweetness potency 6,000–9,000 greater than sucrose and is reported to be heat stable in baking applications. Similar to other sweeteners, the potency of neotame may vary depending upon the food or how it is used. Neotame is reported to be functional and stable in carbonated soft drinks, powdered soft drinks, yellow cake, and yogurt. Neotame has been submitted to the FDA or consideration as a new sweetener in several food categories. However, it has not yet been approved.

GLOBAL DECLINE IN DENTAL CARIES

Has there been a real decline in the prevalence of dental caries? Several excellent reviews have been published during recent years, and there is a general agreement that a marked reduction in caries prevalence has occurred among children in most of the industrialized countries. This is true for countries using water fluoridation as a preventive measure, as well as for countries without such programs.

Global decline in dental caries

- The widespread use of fluoride toothpastes
- Fluoride tablets, fluoride gels
- Fluoride rinsing programs
- Dietary fluoride supplements
- Increased dental awareness
- Availability of dental resources
- Decrease in sugar consumption
- Dental health education programs
- Oral prophylaxis
- Fissure sealants
- Preventive approach in practice
- The widespread use of antibiotics
- Changes in diagnostic criteria
- Herd immunity
- As yet-unknown factors

POINTS TO REMEMBER

- Caries is defined as microbial disease of the calcified tissues of teeth that leads to demineralization of the inorganic components and the subsequent breakdown of the organic moieties of enamel and dentin.
- Classification of caries can be: According to occurrence (primary, secondary or recurrent, residual); according to speed (acute or Rampant, chronic or arrested); according to location (pit and fissure, smooth surface, root surface); according to direction (forward, backward caries); according to age (ECC, adolescent, senile); according to surface (simple, compound, complex). ICDAS, ADA, WHO classification
- Theories of caries: The legend of the worm, humoral theory, vital theory, chemical theory, parasitic theory, Miller's chemoparasitic theory, proteolytic theory, proteolysis-chelation theory, sulfatase theory, complexing and phosphorylation theory.
- Concept of caries was given by Keyes as an epidemiological model which state that a disease state is due to interplay of four primary factors—host, agent, substrate and time. Later Newbrun modified it and added a fourth factor of time to it which is known as Newbrun's Tetrad. Newbrun in 1982 also postulated that many secondary factors also influence the rate of progression of caries **(Fig. 38.14)**.
- Demineralization–remineralization concept is that caries is not a result of a single acid attack caused by the acid formed as a result of fermentation of dietary substrates by the oral microflora. Rather it is an outcome of the imbalance occurring in the demineralization–remineralization cycle that is continuously operating in the oral cavity.
- Stephan curve is a graph published by Stephan and Miller in 1944 which reflected the fall in salivary pH following a glucose rinse.
- Histologically, enamel caries has four zones, viz., translucent zone which is the advancing front of the lesion, dark zone separating the translucent zone from the body of the lesion, body of the carious lesion, which is markedly radiolucent and relatively intact enamel surface layer.
- Histologically, dentinal caries has five zones, viz., zone of decomposed dentin (Infected dentin), bacterial invasion (turbid dentin), transparent dentin, subtransparent dentin and normal dentin.
- Evidence of relation between diet and caries is proved by three landmark studies, namely, Hope Wood House study, Vipeholm study, and Turku study.
- Food sugar substitutes are aspartame, acesulfame potassium, saccharin, sucralose, sorbitol, xylitol, stevia, neotame.
- The research on caries vaccine was pioneered by Martin Taubman and Daniel Smith. The effective molecular targets are adhesions, GtF, and glucan binding proteins, and the most used routes for vaccination are oral, intranasal, tonsillar, and rectal.
- Global decline in dental caries is due to widespread use of fluorides, increased dental awareness, availability of dental resources, decrease in sugar consumption, preventive approach in practice, changes in diagnostic criteria, and herd immunity.

Questionnaire

1. Define and classify dental caries.
2. Epidemiology of caries in India. Describe the theories of dental caries.
3. Explain the current concept of dental caries.
4. What is demineralization and remineralization cycle?
5. Explain Stephan curve with its applicability in daily routine.
6. Histopathology of enamel and dentinal caries.
7. Role of saliva in dental caries.
8. Explain the relation of diet and dental caries.
9. Write a note on food sugar substitutes.
10. Enumerate the reasons for decline in dental caries.
11. Write a note on caries vaccine.

FURTHER READING

1. Akarslan ZZ, et al. Reproducibility and Agreement of Clinical Diagnosis of Occlusal Caries Using Unaided Visual Examination and Operating Microscope. Journal of Canadian Dental Association. 2009;75(6):455.
2. Anderson MH. Changing paradigms in caries management. Curr Opin Dent. 1992:2157-62.
3. Anderson MH. Current concepts of dental caries and its prevention. Oper Dent Suppl. 2001;6:11-8.
4. Clarkson BH. Introduction to cariology. Dent Clin North Am. 1999;43:569-78.
5. Dowd FJ. Saliva and dental caries. Dent Clin North Am. 1999;43:579-97.
6. Ettinger RL. Epidemiology of dental caries: a broad review. Dent Clin North Am. 1999;43:679-94.
7. Featherstone JOB. The science and practice of caries prevention. J Am Dent Assoc. 2000;131:887-99.
8. Fejerskov O. Concepts of dental caries and their consequences for understanding the disease. Community Dent Oral Epidemiol. 1997;25:5-12.
9. Ganesh A, et al. Prevalence of ECC in India: A systematic review. Indian J Pediatrics. 2018.
10. Gugnani N, Pandit IK, Srivastava N, Gupta M, Sharma M. International Caries Detection and Assessment System (ICDAS): A New Concept. International Journal of Clinical Pediatric Dentistry. 2011;4(2):93-100.
11. Jensen ME. Diet and dental caries. Dent Clin North Am. 1999;43:615-33.
12. Kidd EAM. Caries management. Dent Clin North Am. 1999;43:743-64.
13. Machiulskiene V, Campus G, Carvalho JC, et al. Terminology of dental caries and dental caries management. Consensus report of a workshop organised by ORCA and cariology research group of IADR. Caries Res. 2020;54:7-14.
14. Mandel ID. Impact of saliva on dental caries. Compend Suppl. 1989;54:76-81.
15. Mulchandani V, Asna Isani SK, Shah S, Trivedi MV, Joshi A. Prevalence of Early Childhood Caries in 3 to 5 years old Children of Bhavnagar city: A cross-sectional study. Journal of Advanced Health Sciences and Research. 2021;2(1):36.
16. Pandey P, Nandkeoliar T, Tikku A P, Singh D, Singh MK. Prevalence of dental caries in the Indian population: A systematic review and meta-analysis. J Int Soc Prevent Communit Dent. 2021;11:256-65.
17. Pontes, et al. Clinical performance of fluorescence based methods for detection of occlusal caries lesions in primary teeth Braz. Oral Res. 2017;31:e91.
18. Roberts MW, Wright JT. Food sugar substitutes: a brief review for dental clinicians. J Clin Pediatr Dent. 2002;27:1-4.
19. Rugg-Gunn AJ. Diet and dental caries. In: Murray JJ (Ed). The Prevention of Dental Diseases, 2nd edition. Oxford: Oxford University Press; 1989. pp. 4-114.
20. Uribe SE, Innes N, Maldupa I. The global prevalence of early childhood caries: A systematic review with meta-analysis using the WHO diagnostic criteria. International Journal of Paediatric Dentistry; 2021.
21. Vuyyuru CR, Rangari RN, Singaraju GS, Pottem N. Dental Diseases and Factors Defining Utilization of Dental Care Services among Rural Children Aged 12 Years in Nellore District, Andhra Pradesh: A Community-Based Study. J Pharm Bioallied Sci. 2021;13 (Suppl 2):S1422-7.
22. WHO. The etiology and prevention of dental caries. Techn Rep Ser No. 494. Geneva, Switzerland: WHO; 1972. p. 12.

Caries Risk and Activity Assessment

Ashwin Jawdekar, Gargi S Murthy, Nikhil Marwah

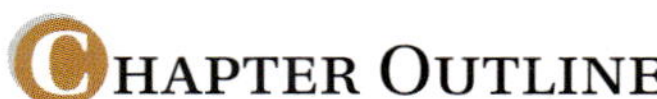

Chapter Outline

The concept of caries risk assessment is, from one point of view, simple and straightforward. The idea is to (1) identify those persons who will most likely develop caries and (2) provide these individuals proper preventive and treatment measures to stop the disease. (3) To determine appropriate recalls (4) for appropriate health economics. Beck's risk model is used when it is important to identify one or more risk factors for the disease so that, likely points for intervention can be planned. A risk model, therefore, should exclude risk predictors such as past disease and number of teeth, as such factors do not cause further disease. A prediction model, on the contrary, is used when one is mainly interested in identifying who is at high risk. The main goal is to maximize sensitivity and specificity of the prediction, so that any good predictor may be included in the model. Caries risk assessment (CRA) is thus "prediction of future caries based on the diagnosis of current disease by evaluation of risk and protective factors for making evidence-based clinical decisions." CRA should be included in a treatment plan in order to facilitate the decision-making process concerning preventive care (both home and office) treatment, recall appointments, etc.

CRA is necessary to identify individuals at risk of developing new lesions as well as for identifying the risk of progression of already present carious lesions in individuals. CRA takes into consideration the risk and protective factors that affect the dynamics of the caries process. CRA is important for making evidence-based clinical decisions.

Broadly speaking, three main approaches for risk assessment are based on—(1) biological factors, (2) socioeconomic factors and (3) past caries experience.

- **Risk:** In epidemiology, is the probability of an event occurring following an exposure.
- **Risk factor**: Factors that increase significantly the risk of onset of a specific disease as proved in well controlled prospective studies.
- **Prognostic risk factor**: Factors that increase significantly the risk of progression of a specific disease as proved in well controlled prospective studies.
- **Risk indicator:** Factors significantly associated with increased prevalence of a specific disease as proved in cross-sectional disease.
- **Caries risk assessment:** Is the consideration of a set of dynamic risk indicators and/factors to guage the likelihood of disease development within some future time frame.
- **Caries activity test** *are defined as tests that estimate the actual state of disease activity (progression/regression).*

RISK ASSESSMENT

Rationale of caries risk assessment

- Caries management limited to restoration of carious teeth without eliminating the caries risk factors will result in failure of treatment as new lesions will appear.
- Caries risk assessment is essential for preventive/nonsurgical approach rather than a restorative/surgical approach.
- Risk assessment enables even high risk children to reach adulthood caries-free.

Uses of caries risk assessment
- Determine the degree of patient's risk for developing dental caries
- Determine the etiological agents responsible for caries in an individual
- Determine if additional diagnostic procedures are required, e.g., diet analysis, salivary analysis
- Helps make preventive and therapeutic recommendations according to the patient's caries risk status.
- Determine need and extent of personalized preventive measures
- Motivation of patient
- Monitor the effectiveness of programs/treatment rendered for an individual
- Criteria for the success of therapeutic measures
- To identify high-risk groups
- Determine need for caries control measures
- Aid in recall appointments
- Aid in selection of patient for caries study
- Helps in efficient allocation of time and resources for oral health programs.

There are at least two different, but related, situations where so-called caries tests are important. The first one concerns the individual treatment of a patient. The tests can provide information about the caries etiological factors that are present. This information can be used to institute the correct and most efficient treatment. Repeated use of the tests can check if the treatment has had the expected effect. The second situation concerns prediction of caries. In most populations, a certain portion develops much more caries than others. If this group can be identified at an early stage, causal treatment measures can be introduced before any irreversible lesions have become established. Both for explaining an ongoing disease, and for the prediction of future disease, a single, simple caries test has often been requested by the profession **(Fig. 39.1)**. Unfortunately, such a test is not available, for the simple reason that dental caries is a complex disease. However, it does not mean that it is impossible to identify and evaluate important risk factors, in order to institute causal treatment directed against the main problems. Thus, the treatment of the caries disease can be based on biological principles and not on chance or beliefs. Such procedures are therefore recommended for anyone who wants to treat the caries as a disease, not only to fill the cavity.

CARIES ACTIVITY TESTS: REQUIREMENTS

These were summarized by Snyder as:
- Should have sound theoretical basis
- Simple
- Easy to perform
- Inexpensive
- Time for test and result should be small
- Should be adaptable for chair-side
- Results should be accurate and reproducible
- Test should have maximal correlation with clinical status
- Should have good validity, reliability, and feasibility.

MICROBIAL TESTS FOR MUTANS STREPTOCOCCI DETECTION

Several methods are available to measure the levels of mutans streptococci in saliva and plaque and on individual tooth surfaces, when such information is needed.

Laboratory Method

- Saliva (or dental plaque) is collected from the individual to be sampled.
- Mixed with a proper transport medium, the sample is sent to a microbiological laboratory.

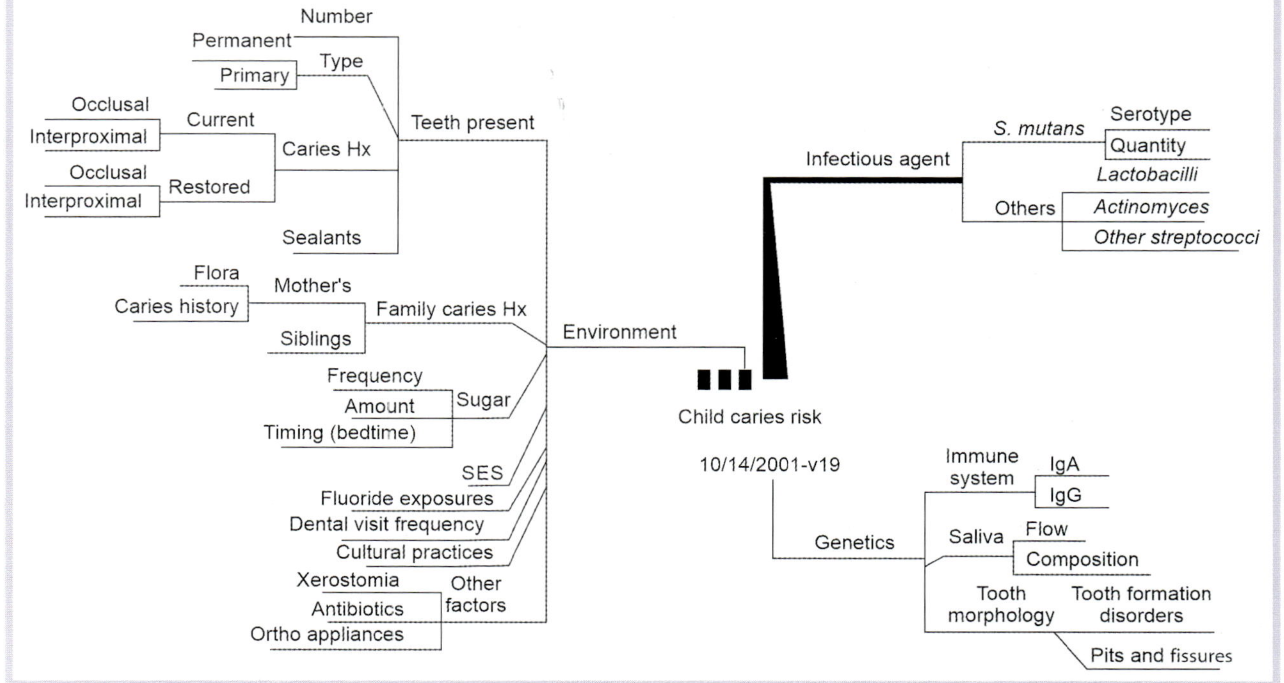

Fig. 39.1: Diagrammatic view of caries risk factors in children using the "nonexclusive" contributory disease model classifications.

- After incubation using a selective medium, mutans colonies on the plates are counted and the results are expressed as number of colony-forming units (CFUs) per mL saliva. A common type of selective agar plate for mutans streptococci is the mitis-salivarius-bacitracin (MSB) agar.
- For screening surveys using agar plates, a simplified method has been described in which wooden spatulas are contaminated by saliva and then directly pressed against selective agar plates. After incubation, the number of colonies on a predetermined area of the agar plate is calculated. Thus, no steps involving transportation, dilution, and plating of saliva are necessary.

Chair-side Method

- The so-called Strip Mutans® test is based on the ability of mutans streptococci to grow on hard surfaces and the use of a selective broth (high sucrose concentration in combination with bacitracin).
- The Dentocult SM-Strip Mutans kit for estimation of mutans streptococci in saliva contains test strips, bacitracin disks, test tubes with broth, paraffin for chewing, and a standard chart to evaluate the level of mutans after incubation.
- The level of mutans streptococci is given as "class" after comparison with a chart, indicating low ("0") to high ("3", equivalent to 10^6 mutans CFU per mL saliva) numbers in saliva. The mutans streptococci colonies will appear on the strip as small blue dots but the color can vary from dark blue to pale blue.

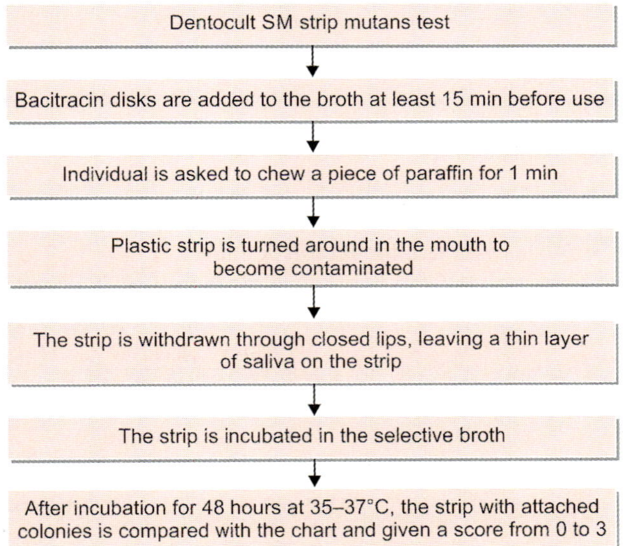

Survey Method

- For field studies, the plates can be placed into plastic bags containing expired air, which are then sealed (Seal- a-Meal) and incubated at 37°C.
- Counts of more than 100 CFU by this method are proportional to greater than 108 CFU of *Streptococcus mutans* per mL of saliva by conventional methods.
- This is a simplified and practical method for field studies.

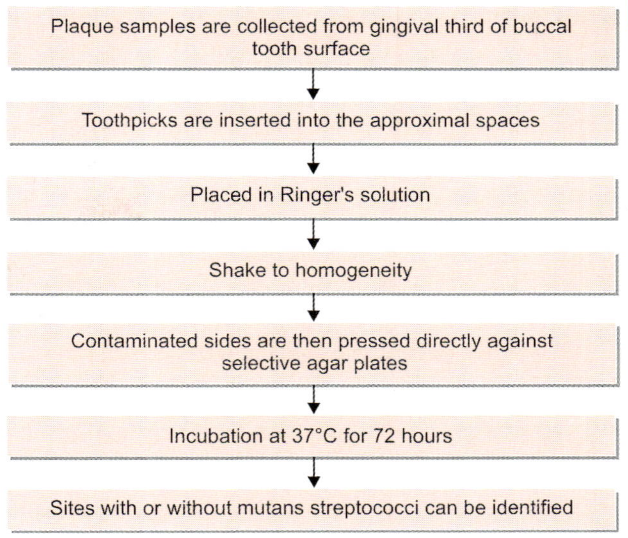

Selective Method

- For the demonstration of mutans streptococci at specific sites, a simple technique has been described by **Kristoffersson** and **Bratthall**.
- This test involves simple screening of diluted plaque sample streaked on a selective culture media.
- Equipment involves sterile toothpicks, sterile Ringer solution, platinum loop, mitis-salivarius agar plates containing sulfadimidine and incubator.

Adherence Method

- Categorizes salivary samples based on ability of *S. mutans* to adhere to glass surfaces when grown in sucrose-containing broth.
- Equipment includes tube to collect saliva, rack to hold culture tubes, disposable pipettes, incubator, and MSB broth (Showa Yakuhin Kako Co. Ltd., Tokyo, Japan). The broth is marketed in a sealed vial, to which is added a strip of paper bearing bacitracin, tellurite, and crystal violet to elute within 10 minutes, after which the broth is ready for use.

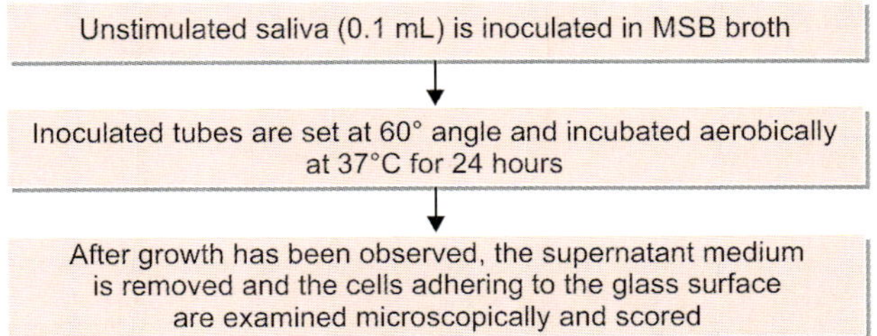

Result of adherence method

+++	*S. mutans* is present at a level higher than 10^5 CFU/mL of whole saliva
–	*S. mutans* is present at less than 10^4 CFU/mL of saliva
Value	***Inference***
–	No growth expressed
+	A few deposits ranging from 1 to 10
++	Scattered deposits of smaller size
+++	Numerous minute deposits with more than 20 large size deposits

MICROBIAL TESTS FOR LACTOBACILLI DETECTION

- This lactobacilli count test was introduced by **Hadley** in 1933.
- The number of lactobacilli in saliva seems to be significantly higher in the early morning, before breakfast, and tooth brushing.

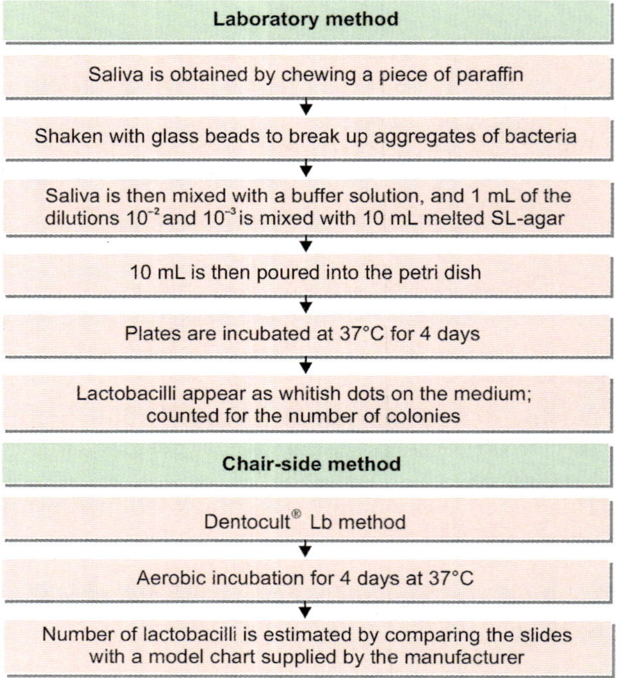

Laboratory method
Saliva is obtained by chewing a piece of paraffin
Shaken with glass beads to break up aggregates of bacteria
Saliva is then mixed with a buffer solution, and 1 mL of the dilutions 10^{-2} and 10^{-3} is mixed with 10 mL melted SL-agar
10 mL is then poured into the petri dish
Plates are incubated at 37°C for 4 days
Lactobacilli appear as whitish dots on the medium; counted for the number of colonies
Chair-side method
Dentocult® Lb method
Aerobic incubation for 4 days at 37°C
Number of lactobacilli is estimated by comparing the slides with a model chart supplied by the manufacturer

- This test estimates the number of acidogenic and aciduric bacteria in the patient's saliva by counting the number of colonies appearing on LBS agar (Rogosa). The total number of colonies on this medium reflects the proportion of the aciduric flora in the saliva.
- The necessary equipment includes saliva-collecting bottles, paraffin, two 9-mL tubes of saline, two agar plates, two bent glass rods, facilities for incubating, and a Quebec counter and pipettes.

Results of lactobacillus count

No. lactobacilli per mL saliva	Caries activity
0–1,000	Little or none
1,000–5,000	Slight
5,000–10,000	Moderate
10,000	Marked

CARIES ACTIVITY TESTS

Snyder Test

- It measures the ability of salivary microorganisms to form organic acids from carbohydrate medium.
- The Snyder test measures the rapidity of acid formation when a sample of stimulated saliva is inoculated into glucose agar adjusted to pH 4.7–5 and with bromocresol green as color indicator.
- The equipment includes saliva-collecting bottles, paraffin, a tube of Snyder glucose agar containing bromocresol green and adjusted to pH 4.7–5, pipettes, and incubating facilities.
- Advantages:
  - Simplicity of equipment testing
  - Less training is needed
  - Cost-effective
  - High correlation between the Snyder acid production test and the lactobacillus plate count

Saliva is collected before breakfast by chewing paraffin
↓
A tube of Snyder glucose agar is melted and then cooled to 50°C
↓
Saliva specimen is shaken vigorously for three minutes
↓
0.2 mL of saliva is pipetted into the tube of agar and immediately mixed by rotating the tube
↓
Agar is allowed to solidify in the tube and is incubated at 37°C
↓
Color change of the indicator is observed after 24, 48 and 72 hours of incubation by comparison with an uninoculated tube against a white background

Results of Snyder test

	24 h	48 h	72 h
Color	If yellow	If yellow	If yellow
Caries activity	Marked	Definite	Limited
Color	If green	If green	If green
Caries activity	Continue to incubate	Continue to incubate	Caries inactive

Alban Test

- It is a simplified substitute for the Snyder test.
- Advantages:
  - Simple
  - Cost-effective
  - Act as a motivational tool for patient
- Color change from blue to yellow is indicative of caries activity.

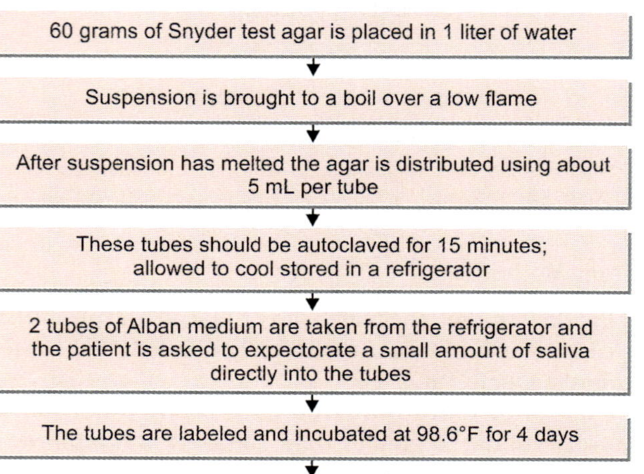

60 grams of Snyder test agar is placed in 1 liter of water
Suspension is brought to a boil over a low flame
After suspension has melted the agar is distributed using about 5 mL per tube
These tubes should be autoclaved for 15 minutes; allowed to cool stored in a refrigerator
2 tubes of Alban medium are taken from the refrigerator and the patient is asked to expectorate a small amount of saliva directly into the tubes
The tubes are labeled and incubated at 98.6°F for 4 days
The tubes are observed daily for color change from blue to green to difinite yellow with decrease in pH

Scoring is based on the depth in medium to which color has changed	
Results of Alban test	
Color change	***Score***
No color change	3/4
Beginning color change	+
One-half color change	++
Three-fourth color change	+++
Total color change to yellow	++++

Swab Test

- This test was developed by **Grainger et al.** in 1965
- This can be used in young and uncooperative patients as there is no need for salivary collection.
- The oral flora is sampled by swabbing the buccal surfaces of the teeth with a cotton applicator which is subsequently incubated for 48 hours.

Result of swab test	
pH	***Caries activity***
4.1	Marked caries activity
4.2–4.4	Active
4.5–4.6	Slightly active
Over 4.6	Caries inactive

Reductase Test

- This test measures the ability of reductase enzyme present in salivary bacteria.
- The test measures the rate at which an indicator molecule, diazoresorcinol, changes from blue to red to colorless on reduction by the mixed salivary flora.
- The reductase test comes in a kit (Treatex, CW Erwin and Co.) which includes calibrated saliva collection tubes with the reagent on the inside of the tube's cap, plus flavored paraffin.

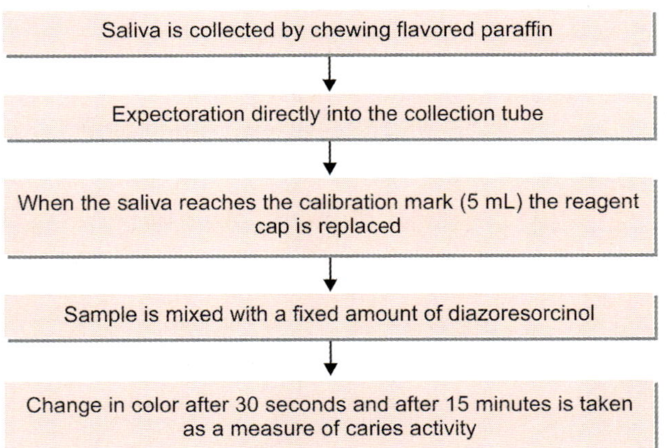

Results of reductase test			
Color	***Time***	***Score***	***Caries activity***
Blue	15 min	1	Non-conducive
Orchid	15 min	2	Slightly conducive
Red	15 min	3	Moderate conducive
Red	Immediate	4	Highly conducive
White	Immediate	5	Extremely conducive

SALIVARY BUFFER CAPACITY TEST

Salivary buffer capacity is important in maintaining a pH level in saliva and plaque which counteracts dissolution of mineral but buffer capacity of whole stimulated saliva is weakly correlated to caries increment; however, below a threshold value, the caries process is facilitated.

- There is a trend of an inverse relationship between buffering capacity of saliva and caries activity.
- The saliva of individuals whose mouths contain a considerable number of carious lesions frequently has a lower acid-buffering capacity than the saliva of those who are relatively caries-free.
- This test, however, does not correlate adequately with caries activity.

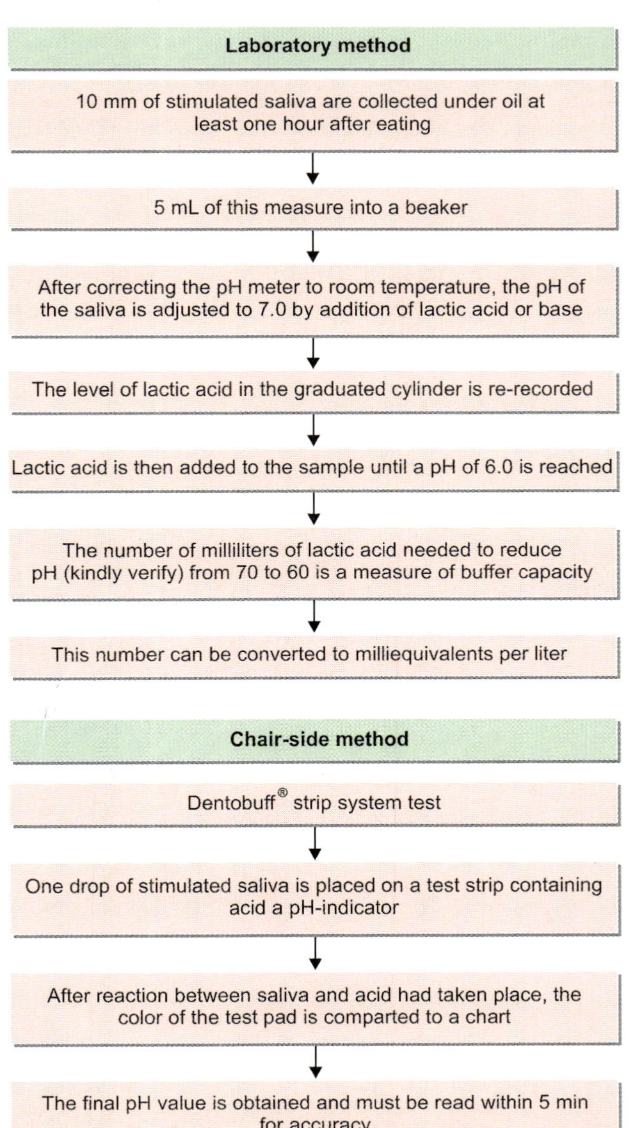

- Buffer capacity can be evaluated by pH or color indicators. The test measures the number of milliliters of acid required to lower the pH of saliva through an arbitrary pH interval, such as from pH 7.0 to 6.0, or the amount of acid or base necessary to bring color indicators to their end point.

- Equipment needed includes a pH meter and titration equipment, 0.05 N lactic acid, 0.05 N base, paraffin, and sterile glass jars containing a small amount of oil.

Result of buffer capacity test	
Buffer capacity	***Color change***
Low buffer capacity	Yellow color
Intermediate buffer capacity	Green color
Normal buffer capacity	Blue color

CARIES-RISK ASSESSMENT TOOLS

The American Academy of Pediatric Dentistry (AAPD) recognizes that caries risk assessment is an essential element of contemporary clinical care for infants, children, and adolescents. Over the past 15 years, strategies for managing dental caries increasingly have emphasized the concept of risk assessment. However, a practical tool for assessing caries risk in infants, children, and adolescents has been lacking. While assessment of caries risk undoubtedly will benefit from emerging science and technologies, the AAPD believes that sufficient evidence exists to support the creation of a framework for classifying caries risk in infants, children and adolescents based on a set of physical, environmental, and general health factors. The **Table 39.1** represents a first step toward incorporating available evidence into a concise, practical tool to assist both dental and nondental health care providers in assessing levels of risk for caries development in infants, children, and adolescents.

Users of the AAPD Caries-risk Assessment Tool (CAT) Must Understand the Following Caveats

- Caries-risk assessment tool (CAT) provides means of classifying dental caries risk at a point in time and therefore should be applied periodically to assess changes in an individual's risk status **(Figs. 39.2 and 39.3)**.
- CAT is intended to be used when clinical guidelines call for caries risk assessment.

Table 39.1: AAPD caries risk assessment- categories.

	Low risk	***Moderate risk***	***High risk***
Clinical conditions	• No decayed teeth in past 24 months • No enamel demineralization (enamel caries "white-spot lesions") • No visible plaque; no gingivitis	• Decayed teeth in the past 24 months • One area of enamel demineralization (enamel caries "white-spot lesions") • Gingivitis	• Decayed teeth in the past 12 months • More than one area of enamel demineralization (enamel caries "white-spot lesions") • Radiographic enamel caries • Visible plaque on anterior (front) teeth • High titers of mutans-streptococci • Wearing dental or orthodontic appliances
Environmental characteristics	• Optimal systemic and topical fluoride exposure • Consumption of simple sugars or foods strongly associated with caries initiation primarily at meal times • Regular use of dental care in an established dental home	• Suboptimal systemic fluoride exposure with optimal topical exposure • Occasional (e.g., 1–2) between meal exposures to simple sugars or foods strongly associated with caries • Mid-level caregiver socioeconomics (e.g., eligible for school lunch program or SCHIP) • Irregular use of dental services	• Enamel hypoplasia • Suboptimal topical fluoride exposure • Frequent (e.g., 3 or more) between meal exposures to simple sugars or foods strongly associated with caries • Low-level caregiver socioeconomic status (e.g., eligible for Medicaid) • No usual source of dental care • Active decay present in the mother of a preschool child
General health conditions			• Children with special healthcare needs • Conditions impacting saliva composition/flow

(SCHIP: State Children's Health Insurance Program)

Name:

Ident.No

Date:

Examiner:

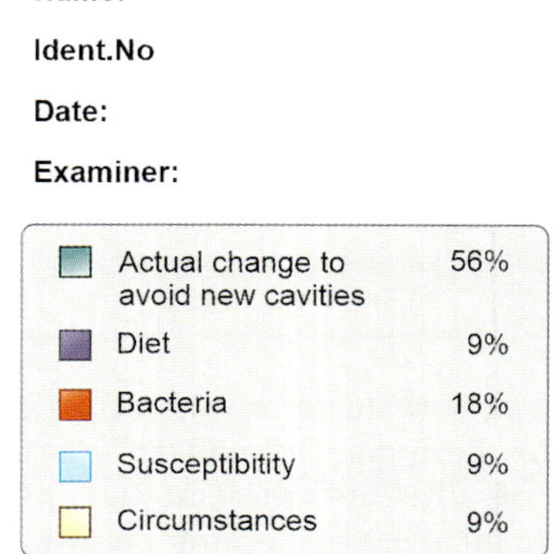

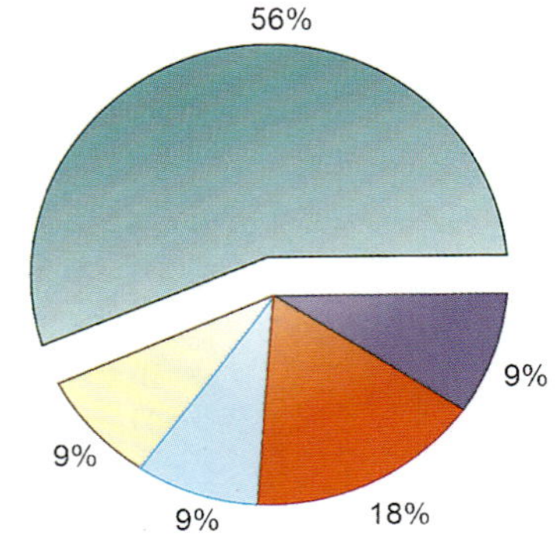

Country/area: Standard set

Group: Standard set

Caries experience	3
Related diseases	0
Diet, contents	1
Diet, frequency	1
Plaque amount	2
Mutans streptococci	2
Fluoride program	2
Saliva secretion	0
Buffer capacity	0
Clinical judgment	1

Fig. 39.2: Cariogram.

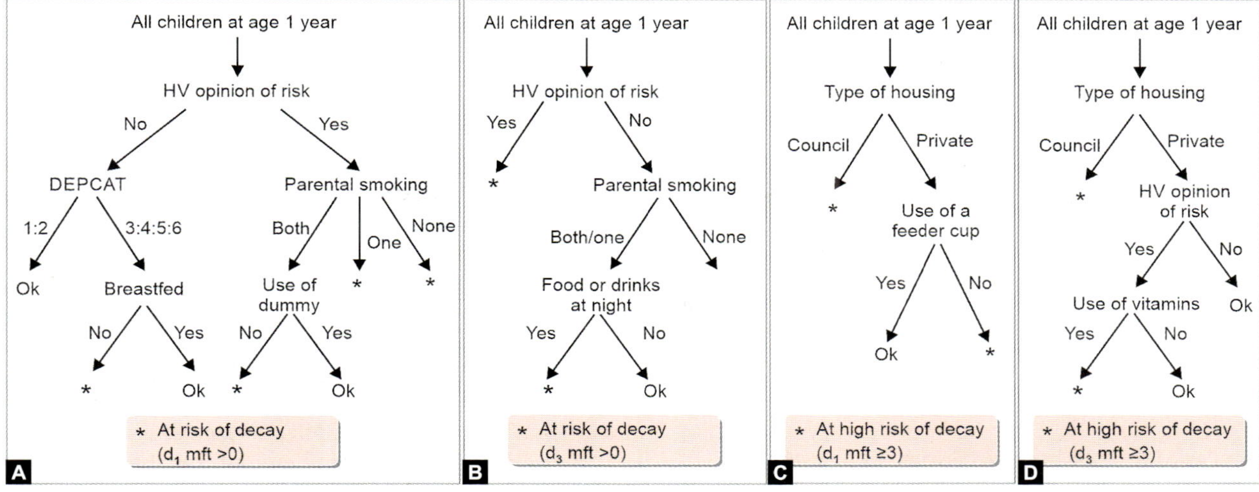

Figs. 39.3A to D: Dundee caries-risk assessment model.

Caries-risk assessment form for 0–5 year olds (for dental providers).

Factors	*High risk*	*Moderate risk*	*Protective*
Biological			
• Mother/primary caregiver has active caries	Yes		
• Parent/caregiver has low socioeconomic status	Yes		
• Child has >3 between meal sugar-containing snacks or beverages per day	Yes		
• Child is put to bed with a bottle containing natural or added sugar	Yes		
• Child has special healthcare needs		Yes	
• Child is a recent immigrant		Yes	
Protective			
• Child receives optimally-fluoridated drinking water or fluoride supplements			Yes
• Child has teeth brushed daily with fluoridated toothpaste			Yes
• Child receives topical fluoride from health professional			Yes
• Child has dental home/regular dental care			Yes
Clinical findings			
• Child has >1 decayed/missing/filled surfaces (dmfs)	Yes		
• Child has active white spot lesions or enamel defects	Yes		
• Child has elevated mutans streptococci levels	Yes		
• Child has plaque on teeth		Yes	

Circling those conditions that apply to a specific patient helps the practitioner and parent understand the factors that contribute to or protect from caries. Risk assessment categorization of low, moderate, or high is based on preponderance of factors for the individual. However, clinical judgment may justify the use of one factor (e.g., frequent exposure to sugar-containing snacks or beverages, more than one dmfs) in determining overall risk.

Overall assessment of the child's dental caries risk: High ☐ Moderate ☐ Low ☐

Caries-risk assessment form for >6 year olds (for dental providers).

Factors	*High risk*	*Moderate risk*	*Protective*
Biological			
• Patient is of low socioeconomic status	Yes		
• Patient has >3 between meal sugar containing snacks or beverages per day	Yes		
• Patient has special healthcare needs		Yes	
• Patient is a recent immigrant		Yes	
Protective	-		
• Patient receives optimally-fluoridated drinking water			Yes
• Patient brushes teeth daily with fluoridated toothpaste			Yes
• Patient receives topical fluoride from health professional			Yes
• Additional home measures (e.g., xylitol, MI paste, antimicrobial)			Yes
• Patient has dental home/regular dental care			Yes
Clinical findings			
• Patient has ≥1 interproximal lesions	Yes		
• Patient has active white spot lesions or enamel defects	Yes		
• Patient has low salivary flow	Yes		
• Patient has defective restorations		Yes	
• Patient wearing an intraoral appliance		Yes	

Circling those conditions that apply to a specific patient helps the practitioner and patient/parent understand the factors that contribute to or protect from caries.Risk assessment categorization of low, moderate, or high is based on preponderance of factors for the individual. However, clinical judgment may justify the use of one factor (e.g., >1 interproximal lesions, low salivary flow) in determining overall risk.

Overall assessment of the dental caries risk: High ☐ Moderate ☐ Low ☐

American Academy of Pediatric Dentistry. Caries-risk assessment and management for infants, children, and adolescents. The Reference Manual of Pediatric Dentistry. Chicago, iii: American Academy of Pediatric Dentistry; 2019:220-4.

- CAT can be used in any clinical setting that allows the assessor to obtain reliable clinical, environmental, and general health information.
- CAT can be used by both dental and nondental personnel. It does not render a diagnosis. However, clinicians using CAT must be familiar with the clinical presentation of dental caries and factors related to caries initiation and progression.
- Because clinicians with various levels of skill working in a variety of settings will use this instrument, advanced technologies such as radiographic assessment and microbiologic testing (shaded areas) have been included but are not essential for using this tool.

AAPD's Caries Risk Assessment Forms (CRA Forms)

- AAPD modified its original CAT into a more sensitive, practical tool to assist dental practitioners and nondental healthcare providers in assessing caries risk in infants, children and adolescents.
- CRA forms for ages 0–5 years and 6 years of age or older are available. Each of the forms contains clinical observations, preventive factors and risk factors arranged into three columns, namely high risk, moderate risk and low risk.
- Patients are classified as low, moderate or high risk depending on where the checked boxes on the form fall and guidelines in the text.
- Clinical judgement may justify use of only one factor in determining overall risk. *Example:* Frequent cariogenic snacks, presence of interproximal caries and decreased salivary flow.

CAMBRA (CARIES MANAGEMENT BY RISK ASSESSMENT)

- This was developed in 2002 and advocated by the California Dental Association **(Table 39.2)**.
- It consists of separate caries-risk assessment forms for dental and medical professionals.
- It is designed to identify risk and protective factors by conducting patient interviews and conducting clinical examinations and bacterial culturing is recommended for children with certain levels or a combination of risk factors.
- The data obtained helps in developing individualized treatment and preventive care recommendations.

CARIOGRAM

- A challenge for the biological factor approach is to correctly summarize the complex picture of the various interrelated caries risk factors, so that it can be easily used by the dental professional routinely in the clinic.
- The pioneering work of **Bo Krasse** and his team at the Dental School in Göteborg laid the foundation for the development of a comprehensive model of the caries risk profile. Building on this work, **Douglas Bratthall** (1997) and workers at the Dental School in Malmö have attempted to make the practical application of risk assessment more accessible by developing a computer-based caries risk assessment model called Cariogram.
- It is a computer program showing a graphical picture that illustrates a possible overall caries risk scenario. The program contains an algorithm that presents a "weighted" analysis of the input data, mainly biological factors. It expresses the extent to which different etiological factors affect caries risk.
- The cariogram identifies the caries risk factors for the individual and provides examples of preventive and treatment strategies to the clinician. The computer version of the cariogram presents a graphical picture that illustrates a possible overall caries risk scenario.

How is a Cariogram Created?

- The patient is examined and data collected for some factors of direct relevance for caries including bacteria, diet, and susceptibility related factors.
- The various factors/variables are given a score according to a predetermined scale and entered in the computer program. According to its built-in formula, the program presents a pie diagram where "bacteria" appears as a red sector, "diet" as a dark blue sector, and "susceptibility"-related factors as a light blue sector. In addition, some "circumstances" are presented as a yellow sector. The four sectors take their shares, and what multifactorial risk assessment is left appears as a green sector and represents the chance of avoiding caries.
- The bigger the green sector, the better from a dental health point of view; small green sector means low chance of

Table 39.2: CAMBRA treatment recommendations based on risk assessment level.

Low risk	*Moderate risk*	*High risk*	*Extreme risk*
OTC toothpaste with fluoride (1,000 to 1,100 ppm fluoride), 2 × daily	• OTC toothpaste with fluoride (1,000 to 1,100 ppm fluoride), 2 × daily • OTC fluoride rinse (0.05% NaF), daily • Xylitol candies or gums, 4 × daily • Alternative regimen: Xylitol candies or gums, 4 × daily Plus: Prescription 5,000 ppm fluoride toothpaste, 2 × daily	• Xylitol candies or gums, 4 × daily • Prescription 5,000 ppm fluoride toothpaste, 2 × daily • Chlorhexidine gluconate (0.12%) rinse 1 × daily for 1 week, every month until the next POE, then reassess • Fluoride varnish applied at first visit and at each POE/CAMBRA recall	• Xylitol candies or gums, 4 × daily • Prescription 5,000 ppm fluoride toothpaste, 2 × daily • Chlorhexidine gluconate (0.12%) rinse 1 × daily for 1 week, every month until the next POE, then reassess • Fluoride varnish applied at first visit and at each POE/CAMBRA recall • Baking soda rinse, 2 tsp. in 8 oz of water, 4–6 × daily

(CAMBRA: caries management by risk assessment; NaF: sodium fluoride; OTC: over-the-counter; POE: periodic oral examination)

Caries-related factors according to the program

Factors	*Comment*	*Information/data needed*
Caries experience	Past caries experience, including cavities, fillings, and missing teeth due to caries. Several new cavities definitely appearing during preceding year should score "3" even if number of filling is low	Decayed missing filled teeth (DMFT), decayed missing filled surfaces (DMFS), new caries experience in the past 1 year
Related general diseases	General disease or conditions associated with dental caries	Medical history, medications
Diet, contents	Estimation of the cariogenicity of the food, in particular fermentable carbohydrate content	Diet history (lactobacillus test count)
Diet, frequency	Estimation of number of meals and snacks per day, mean for a normal day	Questionnaire results (24 h recall or 3 days dietary recall)
Plaque amount	Estimation of hygiene, e.g., according to Silness-Löe plaque index (PI) Crowded teeth leading to difficulties in removing plaque interproximally should be taken into account	PI
Mutans streptococci	Estimation of levels of mutans streptococci (*Streptococcus mutans, Streptococcus sobrinus*) in saliva, e.g., using *Strip mutans* test	Strip mutans test or other similar test
Fluoride program	Estimation of as to what extent fluoride is available in the oral cavity over the coming period of time	Fluoride exposure, interview the patient
Saliva secretion	Estimation of amount of saliva, e.g., using paraffin-stimulated secretion and expressing results as mL saliva per minute	Stimulated saliva test—secretion rate
Saliva buffer capacity	Estimation of capacity of saliva to buffer acids, e.g., using the Dentobuff test	Dentobuff test or other similar test
Clinical judgment	Opinion of dental examiner, "clinical feeling". Examiners own clinical and personal score for the individual patient	Opinion of dental examiner, "clinical feeling". A preset score of 1 comes automatically

avoiding caries = high caries risk. For the other sectors, the smaller the sector, the better from a dental health point of view.

- Cariogram shows if the patient is at a high, intermediate, or at low risk for caries. It also shows the etiological factors responsible for the caries risk of every individual examined. The results also indicate the targeted actions required to improve the situation.
- The cariogram expresses caries risk only.

Evaluation of cariogram

- The dark blue sector "diet" is based on a combination of diet contents and diet frequency
- The red sector "bacteria" is based on a combination of amount of plaque and mutans streptococci
- The light blue sector "susceptibility" is based on a combination of fluoride program, saliva secretion, and saliva buffer capacity
- The yellow sector "circumstances" is based on a combination of caries experience and related diseases
- The green sector shows an estimation of the "chance of avoiding caries".

Advantages

- The model is affordable
- User-friendly
- Easy to understand
- Tool for motivating the patient
- Model can also serve as a support for clinical decision-making when selecting preventive strategies for the patient.

DUNDEE CARIES-RISK ASSESSMENT MODEL

- This is a caries risk assessment model developed in Dundee, Scotland for predicting caries at age 4 years from data collected at age 1 year.
- This model includes risk indicators like previous caries experience, low socioeconomic status, healthcare workers opinion and oral Mutans streptococci counts (if feasible).
- In this model, each recommendation is accompanied by a "strength of evidence" rating.

TRAFFIC LIGHT MATRIX

- This is a commonly used caries risk assessment tool with an objective to alert the clinician regarding the current caries risk status.
- It is based on 19 criteria in five different categories including saliva (6 criteria), plaque (3 criteria), diet (2 criteria), flouride exposure (3 criteria) and modifying factors (5 criteria).
- The risk levels are conveyed by traffic light colors.
  - Red—high
  - Yellow—moderate
  - Green—low
- Advantages:
  - Visual interpretation is simple as it is a color coded model
  - Easy to explain to the patient about the caries risk

Risk Assessment and Referral Tool: CRA-RT

- This tool was introduced in 2020 by researchers from Kerala, India.
- This is a one-dimensional, 11 item tool which assesses the presence/absence of behavioral risk/protective factors by interviewing the mother.
- The cut-off score guides the dental referral of a preschool child by care providers in a community setting.
- Advantages:
  - Can be used in a non-dental, non-medical setting
  - Quick
  - Simple and easy
  - Valid and reliable

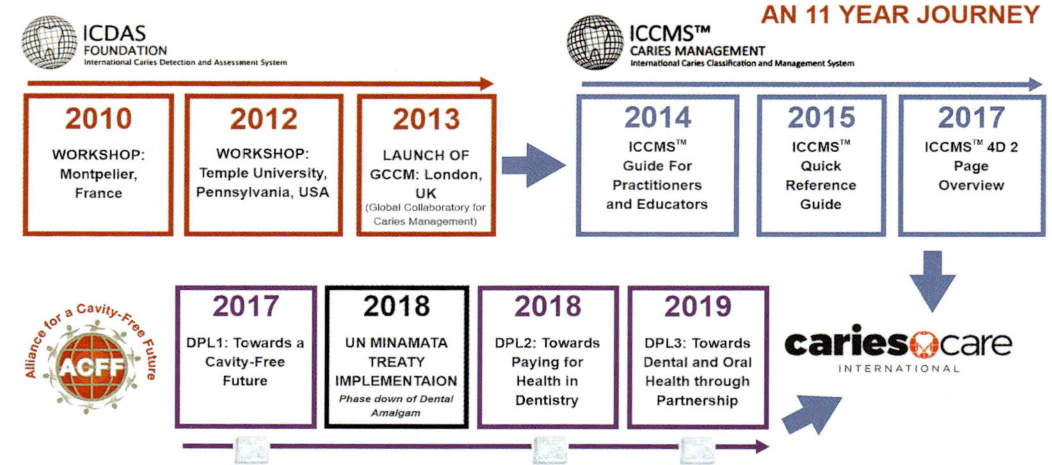

Fig. 39.4: Caries assessment and risk evaluation (CARE).

Caries Assessment and Risk Evaluation (CARE) (Fig. 39.4)

- Evaluating a child's genetic susceptibility to dental caries is valuable in developed societies that have a good dental coverage, adequate fluoride exposure, and where gross malnutrition and negligent oral hygiene are rare. To this effect, researchers at the Division of Diagnostic Sciences of the University of Southern California School of Dentistry developed a novel salivary test for genetic caries risk assessment (CRA) called the CARE test based on the high correlations they found between caries history and quantities of specific oligosaccharides in whole saliva.
- This is probably the only CRA method that can potentially promote caries prevention at the primary level itself (before any carious lesions have appeared), by identifying high caries risk children early and instituting a preemptive aggressive preventive regimen in them.

CRAFT Approach to Caries Management in Children

CRAFT (Caries Risk Assessment for Treatment) is a simple, noninvasive, four-point scale proposed for the prevention and management of caries based on risk assessment in Indian context. For ascertaining the caries-risk in children, parents can be interviewed using the CRAFT questionnaire (presented later). CRAFT can be used as either a physical (print) or a digital tool (android application).

CRAFT Developments

Following are a few significant developments related to the CRAFT over last 6 years.

- CRAFT was conceptualized in 2016 by Dr Ashwin Jawdekar; the first presentation of it was made at the 13th National Post Graduate Convention of the Indian Society of Pediatric and Preventive Dentistry (ISPPD), where the presenter Dr Rinky Thakkar won first prize for the same.
- Dental Council of India adopted CRAFT for consideration during a meeting (DCI WORKSHOP: FIRST DECADE NO DECAY) in February 2018 in Mumbai.
- At the International Academy of Pediatric Dentistry Global Summit on Early Childhood Caries at Bangkok (2018), Dr Ashwin Jawdekar won an award in a presentation on his work on CRAFT.
- A study on the association of CRAFT and Alban test was reported by Thakur, et al (2020) showing positive association.
- Another study showed a significant association between caries risk assessed using CRAFT categorization and OHRQoL of 3–6 year-old children, reported by Iyer and Jawdekar (2021).
- Several studies based on CRAFT are presented at the national conferences of Indian Society of Pedodontics and Preventive Dentistry over the past 6 years.

CRAFT in its first version, was a part of an Android app: **APP4Caries** which also included a Sugar Meter. However, currently the same is unavailable.

HOW to use CRAFT

The CRAFT tool uses a questionnaire that includes different parameters under four domains: Diet, decay status, fluoride exposure and other factors. Based on the available information, caries-risk can be determined which ranges from Very low/No, Low, Moderate, High. A green star is used to indicate 'safety' while a red star for 'risk.'

Dentists can use CRAFT to:
- Understand the caries risk of a child
- Make preventive recommendations to parents
- Devise a treatment plan which includes minimally invasive, restorative and surgical options.

The Android app autoselects the recommendations (for parents as well as dentists) corresponding to each domain based on the risk assessed. A treatment plan with the use of minimum interventional, restorative and surgical approaches can thus be available for each CRAFT risk category.

CRAFT approach allows a dentist to customize a plan with a framework for enhanced patient-participation and behavior-change. On a periodic basis, the CRAFT further allows a dentist to monitor changes in the caries risk and effectiveness of recommended home and office measures, and treatments.

CRAFT Questionnaire

Ask following questions for assessing the risk. Tick appropriately Yes/No

Diet (any Yes indicates risk)

- ≥2 between meal exposures per day of items with
  - Sugar, jaggery or honey (chocolates/soft drink, sweets, cakes, etc.)
  - Starch (chips, wafers)
- Milk bottle
- Syrupy medicines or sweet pills (more than a month)

Fluoride (any two numbers indicate risk)

- Brushing with fluoride-containing toothpaste
- Receiving 6 monthly fluoride application from a dentist
- Using fluoride mouthrinse
- Living in an area with high fluoride water

Decay (any Yes indicates risk)

- Does your child have untreated cavities?
- Did he/she have cavities treated in the past?
- Do you (mother/father) have untreated cavities?

Other (any Yes indicates risk)

- Does your child frequently catch infections or has condition/s suggestive of low immunity? (cold, cough, stomach upset, asthma, etc.)
- Does your child have chalky white or brown patches on the teeth?
- Does your child frequently get a dry mouth?
- Does your child have crowded teeth?

The **Table 39.3** below presents the CRAFT assessment.

Table 39.3: Caries risk assessment for treatment (CRAFT).

Diet	Decay status
• ≥2 exposures per day of sugar or starch containing food items between meals (Yes/No) • Bottle feeding (Yes/No) • Long-term exposure to syrupy medicines or sugar pills (Yes/No)	• Present untreated caries (Yes/No) • Past treated caries (Yes/No) • Parent's caries status (Yes/No)
Fluoride exposure	**Other factors**
• Use of fluoridated toothpaste (Yes/No) • Use of fluoride mouthrinse (Yes/No) • Professional six monthly fluoride application (Yes/No) • Living in area with high/optimally fluoridated water (Yes/No)	• Conditions related to suppressed immunity (asthma, allergies, recurrent respiratory or gastrointestinal infections, etc.) (Yes/No) • Hypomineralization (Yes/No) • Malocclusion/crowding (Yes/No) • Hyposalivation (Yes/No)

Based on the CRAFT assessment, risk of having decayed teeth is shown below:

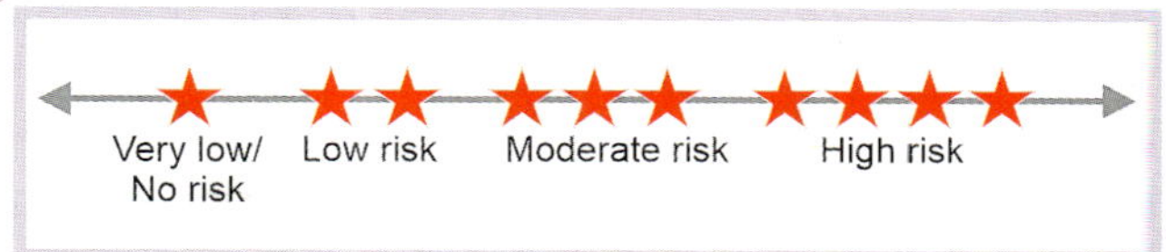

Based on the risk ascertained from the CRAFT, age-appropriate recommendations can be made to parents from the ones listed below:

Diet (Recommendations for Yes ticks):

- Reduce sugar exposure to less than two exposures per day and preferably at meals.
- Stop bottle-feeding of milk or any sweet beverages. Avoid giving milk during or just before sleep. Avoid adding sugar or any sweet additives to milk.
- Consider replacing non-syrupy medicines or sweet pills (Ask the doctor for a suitable alternative, if available).

Fluoride (Recommendations for No ticks):

- Use appropriate fluoride toothpaste for brushing twice daily: non-fluoride for less than 2 year-old, junior fluoride for 2–6 year olds, and regular fluoride for all above 6 years.
- Use fluoride mouthrinse once daily (for all above 6 years).

Decay (Recommendations for Yes ticks):

- Start the treatments for the decayed teeth of the child.
- Follow-up with your dentist at regular intervals (at least once in 6 months).
- Take necessary precautions not to transmit decay-bacteria from parent-to-child (by avoiding sharing spoons or kissing particularly if parents have decayed teeth). Start treatments for decayed teeth of the parent/s.

Other (Recommendations for Yes ticks):

- Consult your family doctor/pediatrician regarding recurrent illnesses, allergies, etc.
- Strengthen the teeth enamel with the use of remineralizing agents (consult your dentist for the same).
- Use hydrating agents, saliva modifier or sugar-free gums (consult your dentist for the same).
- Consider surface modifications or correction of alignment (consult your dentist for the same).

Dentists can also use CRAFT to get comprehensive recommendations for treatments corresponding to risk category from the chart below:

CRAFT Recommendations for dentists

Risk category	*Preventive*	*Restorative/Surgical Measures*	*Follow-up*
Very low/no risk ★	**Home measures—patient counseling related to:** • Dietary advice for sugar reduction and bottle feeding cessation • Age-appropriate tooth-brushing (with fluoride toothpaste) • Fluoride mouthrinse and other remineralizing agents as per the need	None	Six monthly

Contd...

Contd...

Risk category	*Preventive*	*Restorative/Surgical Measures*	*Follow-up*
Low risk ★ ★	**Home measures—patient counseling related to:** • Dietary advice for sugar reduction and bottle feeding cessation • Age-appropriate tooth-brushing (with fluoride toothpaste) • Fluoride mouthrinse and other remineralizing agents as per the need **Office measures—consider minimally invasive approaches:** • Watchful observation for arrested lesions • Fluoride varnish application • Fissure sealants • Silver diamine fluoride	**Consider minimally invasive approaches:** • Surface modification • Selective caries removal and restoration with RMGIC • Fissure sealant • Preventive resin restorations • Smart restorations • Other intracoronal and extracoronal restorations or other treatments only if required	Six monthly
Moderate risk ★ ★ ★	**Home measures—patient counseling related to:** • Dietary advice for sugar reduction and bottle feeding cessation • Age-appropriate tooth-brushing (with fluoride toothpaste) • Fluoride mouthrinse and other remineralizing agents as per the need **Office measures—consider minimally invasive approaches:** • Watchful observation for arrested lesions • Fluoride varnish application • Fissure sealant • Silver diamine fluoride	**Consider minimally invasive as well as restorative/ surgical measures:** • Surface modification • Selective caries removal and restoration with RMGIC • Fissure sealant • Preventive resin restorations • Smart restorations • Other intracoronal and extracoronal restorations • Pulp therapy • Extractions	Three-six monthly
High Risk ★ ★ ★ ★	**Home measures—patient counseling related to:** • Dietary advice for sugar reduction and bottle feeding cessation • Age-appropriate tooth-brushing (with fluoride toothpaste) • Fluoride mouthrinse and other remineralizing agents as per the need **Office measures—consider minimally invasive approaches:** • Watchful observation for arrested lesions • Fluoride varnish application • Fissure sealants • Silver diamine fluoride	**Consider minimally invasive as well as restorative/surgical measures:** • Surface modification • Selective caries removal and restoration with RMGIC • Fissure sealant • Preventive resin restorations • Smart restorations • Other intracoronal and extracoronal restorations • Pulp therapy • Extractions	Three monthly or more frequently

Figures 39.5 to 39.10 shows the workflow of the CRAFT android app.

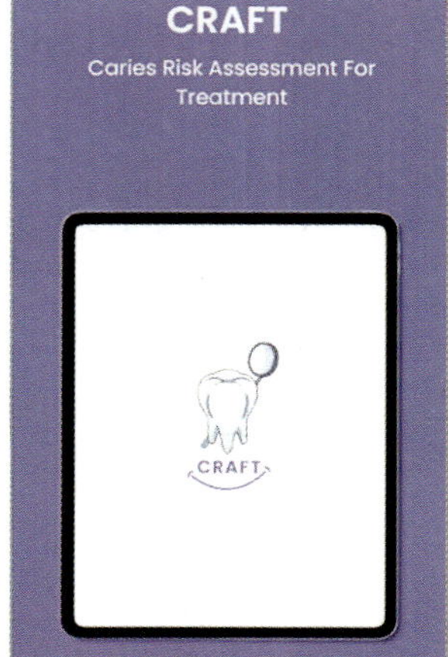

Fig. 39.5: CRAFT app display.

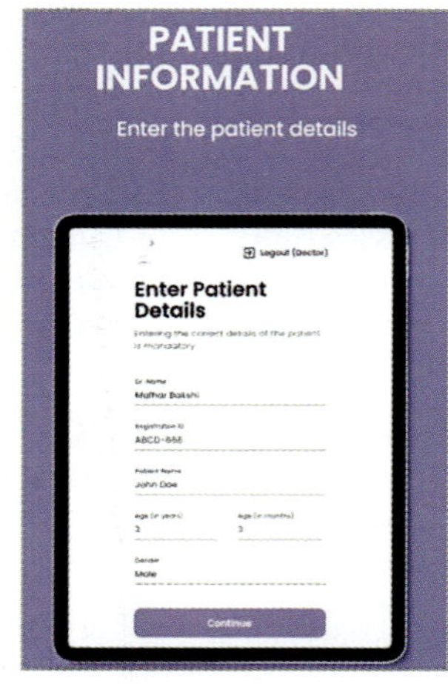

Fig. 39.6: Patient registration.

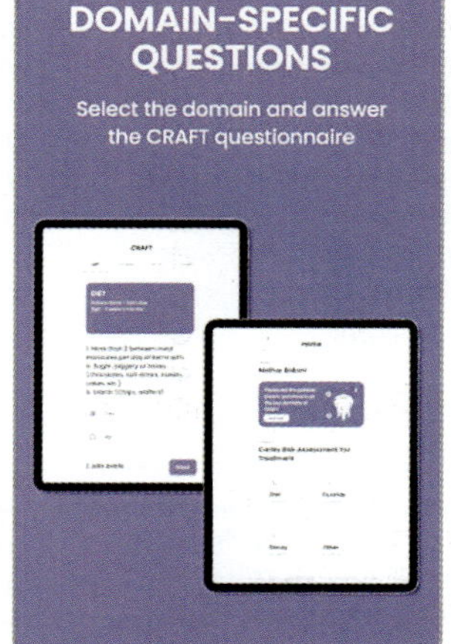

Fig. 39.7: CRAFT questionnaire.

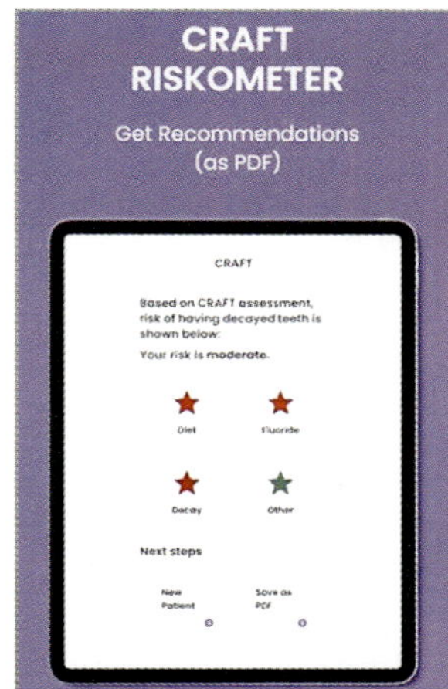

Fig. 39.8: CRAFT risk categorization.

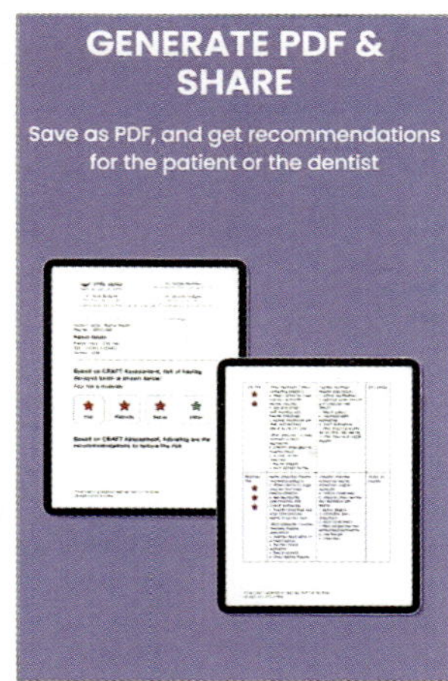

Fig. 39.9: CRAFT PDF for share.

Fig. 39.10: CRAFT scan code for Android app download.

CRAFT Validation/Evaluation Studies

Four preliminary studies have been carried out to evaluate CRAFT in 3-6 year-old otherwise healthy children with caries. In the first, CRAFT scores of children were correlated with their Alban test scores. In the second, CRAFT scores were correlated with the MS colony counts of their mothers. In the third, CRAFT scores were correlated with ECOHIS. In the fourth study, association between caries status and caries risk using CRAFT and reduced cariogram was assessed.

In summary, a CRA tool needs to be simple, practical, evidence-based, inexpensive, and easy for the use of a general dental practitioner. It should be feasible for use at the child's first dental visit and on recall visits. Moreover, it need not include an expensive or elaborate laboratory testing as it may lead to dental care being expensive, and the patient as well as the practitioner may lose interest. A CRA tool must be objective so that precise and customized recommendations can be made as per individual need by the practitioner. Also, the tool should be useful in categorizing the risk, and guide the clinician for interventions and enhance patient participation in the care.

CRAFT evaluation/ validation studies

Objective	***Methodology***	***Key results***	***Conclusion***
To validate CRAFT against Modified Snyder's test (Alban's test) in evaluating caries risk in 3–6 year old children. **Thakur et al.** 2019	A pilot study included 42, healthy 3–6 year old children. Unstimulated midmorning salivary sample was collected just enough to cover the superior surface of the prepared Snyder's medium in test tubes. The length of color change was noted at 24, 48, 72 and 96 hours and compared with the craft score	The mean age of participants was 4.91 ± 0.91 years. Correlation statistic revealed a very high correlation between the Alban score and the craft score (Spearman rho = 0.82.; $p < .05$).	There was a strong correlation between Alban score and CRAFT score.
To determine the association between MS count of mothers and caries risk, using CRAFT, in 3–6 year old children.	32 healthy mother- child pairs were recruited. dmft scores, MS-CFU/mL counts for the mothers and CRAFT and dmft scores for the children were recorded.	There was a low correlation between CRAFT score and mother's colony count (rho = 0.380, $p < .05$) and very low correlation between CRAFT score and mother's DMFT (rho = 0.220; $p < .05$).	There was a positive, but weak association between MS counts of mother and caries risk in children.
To assess the association between dental caries status, risk assessment and OHRQoL in 3–6 year-old children. **Iyer and Jawdekar** (2021)	A cross sectional study was conducted to examine children aged 3–6 years 35 child-parent pair were administered the ECOHIS questionnaire to assess the OHRQoL. The caries status and risk of the child was assessed using dmft, pufa and CRAFT, respectively.	There was a moderate correlation between dmft - ECOHIS score ($r = 0.496$, $p < .01$) Statistically significant difference seen for the frequencies of categories of ECOHIS score with various grades of CRAFT ($p < .05$).	A significant association was seen between caries risk assessed using CRAFT and its impact on OHRQoL.
To assess and compare the association between caries status and caries risk using CRAFT and reduced cariogram.	211 aged 3–6 years were selected. Caries status was assessed as 'dmft'. Caries risk was assessed using CRAFT and reduced cariogram (Internet version 2.01).	The agreement between CRAFT and reduced cariogram, assessed using Cronbach's α was found to be moderate ($\alpha = 0.575$, $p < .05$) when the risk was moderate/intermediate. A significant association was seen with caries status and caries risk as assessed by CRAFT and reduced cariogram.	The two CRA tools, CRAFT and reduced cariogram, showed moderate agreement in caries risk in 3–6 year old children in the category of moderate risk.

POINTS TO REMEMBER

- Caries risk assessment can be defined as a procedure to predict future caries development before the clinical onset of the disease.
- Caries activity test are defined as tests that estimate the actual state of disease activity (progression/regression).
- Caries risk assessment is used to determine need and extent of personalized preventive measures, motivation of patient, monitor the effectiveness of programs, to identify high-risk groups.
- Dentocult SM-Strip mutans is used to measure *Streptococcus mutans* count at chair-side.
- The best evaluated caries activity tests are Snyder, Albans, reductase, and swab test.
- Salivary buffer capacity and pH level in saliva are correlated to caries increment.
- The pioneer of cariogram is Bo Krasse and its development and functionality as a comprehensive model of the caries risk profile was done by Douglas Bratthall (1997).
- Cariogram is a computer program showing a graphical picture that illustrates a possible overall caries risk scenario. It expresses as to what extent different etiological factors of caries affect caries risk and provides examples of preventive and treatment strategies to the clinician.

Questionnaire

1. Define and explain caries risk assessment.
2. What are the microbial tests for mutans streptococci detection?
3. Write a note on Snyder test.
4. What are the color changes in reductase test?
5. Explain salivary buffer capacity test.
6. Describe the cariogram.
7. Explain the various caries risk assessment methods.

FURTHER READING

1. American Academy of Pediatric Dentistry. Caries-risk assessment and management for infants, children, and adolescents. The Reference Manual of Pediatric Dentistry. Chicago, Ill.: American Academy of Pediatric Dentistry; 2021:252-7.
2. Abernathy JR, Graves RC, Bohannan HM, et al. Development and application of a prediction model for dental caries. Community Dent Oral Epidemiol. 1987;15:24-8.
3. Agus H, Schamschula R. Lithium content, buffering capacity and flow rate of saliva and caries experience of Australian children. Caries Res. 1983;17:139-44.
4. Alaluusua S, Kleemola-Kujala E, Gramos L, et al. Salivary caries related tests as predictors of future caries increment in teenagers. A three-year longitudinal study. Oral Microbiol Immunol. 1990;5:77-81.
5. Axelsson P. An introduction to risk prediction and preventive dentistry. Chicago, IL: Quintessence Publishing Co; 2000.
6. Beighton D, Manji F, Baelum V, et al. Associations between salivary levels of Streptococcus mutans, Streptococcus sobrinus, Lactobacilli, and caries experience in Kenyan adolescents. J Dent Res. 1989;68:1242-6.
7. Bratthall D, Hänsel Petersson G, Stjernswärd JR. Assessment of caries risk in the clinic—a modern approach. In: Wilson NHF, Roulet JF, Fuzzi M, editors. Advances in operative dentistry, vol 2. Quintessence Publishing Co, Inc.; 2001. pp. 61-72.
8. Bratthall D, Hänsel Petersson G, Stjernswärd JR. Cariogram. Burt BA. Concepts of risk in dental public health. Community Dent Oral Epidemiol 2005;33(4):240–247. DOI: 10.1111/j.1600-0528.2005.00231.x. www.db.od.mah.se/car/cariogram/cariograminfo. 2004.
9. Douglass CW. Risk assessment in dentistry. J Dent Educ. 1998;62:756-61.
10. Dutchin S, van Houte J. Colonization of teeth in humans by *Streptococcus mutans* as related to its concentration in saliva and host age. Infect Immun. 1978;20:120-5.
11. Eisenberg AD, Mundorff SA, Featherstone JDB, et al. Associations of microbiological factors and plaque index with caries prevalence and water fluoridation status. Oral Microbiol Immunol. 1991;6:139-45.
12. El-Nadeef MA, Bratthall D. Intraindividual variations in counts of mutans streptococci measured by 'Strip mutans' method. Scand J Dent Res. 1990;99:8-12.
13. Ericsson D, Bratthall D. Simplified method to estimate buffer capacity. Scand J Dent Res. 1989;97:405-7.
14. Ericsson Y. Clinical investigation on the salivary buffering action. Acta Odontol Scand. 1959;17:131-65.
15. Ericsson Y, Hardwick L. Individual diagnosis, prognosis and counselling for caries prevention. Caries Res. 1978;12:94-112.
16. Grainger R, Jarrett T, Honey F. Swab test for dental caries activity: an epidemiological survey. J Can Dent Assoc. 1965;31:515-26.
17. Hänsel Petersson G, Bratthall D. Caries risk assessment: a comparison between the computer program "Cariogram", dental hygienists and dentists. Swed Dent J. 2000;24:129-37.
18. Hänsel Petersson G, Twetman S, Bratthall D. Evaluation of a computer program for caries risk assessment in school children. Caries Res. 2002;36:327-40.
19. Iyer CR, Jawdekar AM. "ECC Status, CRAFT Categorization and OHRQL Assessment in 3-6-year-old Children: A Cross-sectional Study". International Journal of Clinical Pediatric Dentistry (Accepted for publication, 2022).
20. Kidd EA. Assessment of caries risk (review). Dent Update. 1998;25:385-90.
21. Larmas MA. A new dip-slide method for the counting of salivary lactobacilli. Proc Finn Dent Soc. 1975;71:31-5.
22. MacRitchie HM, Development of the Dundee Caries Risk Assessment Model (DCRAM)--risk model development using a novel application of CHAID analysis. Community Dent Oral Epidemiol. 2012;40(1):37-45.
23. Newbrun E, Matsukubo T, Hoover CI, et al. Comparison of two screening tests for *Streptococcus mutans* and evaluation of their suitability for mass screenings and private practice. Community Dent Oral Epidemiol. 1984;12:325-31.
24. Pitts NB. Risk assessment and caries prediction. J Dent Educ. 1998;62:762-70.
25. Powell LV. Caries prediction: a review of the literature (review). Community Dent Oral Epidemiol. 1998;26:361-71.
26. Snyder M. Laboratory methods in the clinical evaluation of caries activity. J Am Dent Assoc. 1951;42:400-13.
27. Suneja ES, Suneja B, Tandon B, Philip NI. An overview of caries risk assessment: Rationale, risk indicators, risk assessment methods, and risk-based caries management protocols. Indian J Dent Sci. 2017;9:210-4.
28. Thakkar R, Jawdekar AM. CRAFT- A Proposed Framework for Caries Risk Assessment in Indian Children. EC Paediatrics. 2022;11(3):33-45.
29. Thakur JH, Subhadra HN, Jawdekar A. Evaluation of CRAFT as a Tool for Caries Risk Assessment in 3- to 6-year- old Children and its Validation against Alban's Test: A Pilot Study. Int J ClinPediatr Dent. 2019;12(6):538-42.
30. Twetman. "Caries risk assessment in children: how accurate are we?" European Archives of Paediatric Dentistry. 2015;17(1):27-32.
31. Young DA, Featherstone JD. Implementing caries risk assessment and clinical interventions. Dent Clin North Am. 2010;54(3):495-505. DOI: 10.1016/j.cden.2010.04.002.

CHAPTER

Diagnostic Aids in Dental Caries

Nikhil Marwah

CHAPTER OUTLINE

Childhood is the period of life's greatest physical, psychological, and emotional growth; the child we see today is no longer the same tomorrow. The child patient presents a challenge to the dentist, who must solve the problems of today with an eye to the future and the dental health of an adult. The proper management of dental caries in clinical practice requires an accurate clinical diagnosis. Accurate diagnosis can only be achieved by systematic and methodical collection of data. At the clinical dental practice level, caries diagnosis also has a significant impact since it rules treatment decisions. The diagnosis of early caries lesions has been considered the cornerstone of cost-effective healthcare delivery and quality of dental care. Early diagnosis of the caries lesion is important because the carious process can be modified by preventive treatment so that the lesion does not progress. If the caries disease can be diagnosed at initial stage (e.g., white spot lesion), the balance can be tipped in favor of arrestment of the process by modifying diet, improving plaque control, and appropriate use of fluoride. Using noninvasive quantitative diagnostic methods, it should be possible to detect lesions at an initial stage and subsequently monitor lesion changes overtime during which preventive measures could be introduced.

VISUAL INSPECTION

- Visual inspection, the most ubiquitous caries detection system, is subjective.
- Assessment of features such as color and texture are qualitative in nature. These assessments provide some information on the severity of the disease but fall short of true quantification.
- They are also limited in their detection threshold and their ability to detect early, noncavitated lesions restricted to enamel is poor.
- The clinical accuracy of visual examination with regards to caries detection is only 25–50%.
- **Lussi, Whitehead, Wilson** and **Ricketts** in their respective studies came to the conclusion that visual examination is not an ideal means of diagnosing dental caries as most of the lesions go undetected.

ADA has categorized dental caries as initial, moderate, severe, as follows (**Fisher et al.,** 2012):
- No caries—sound tooth surface with no lesion
- Initial enamel caries—visible noncavitated or cavitated lesion limited to enamel
- Moderate dentin caries—enamel breakdown or loss of root cementum with noncavitated dentin
- Severe dentin caries—extensive cavitation of enamel and dentin

International Caries Detection and Assessment System (ICDAS)
In 2002, ICDAS proposed a classification system for dental caries which continues to remain the leading international system for caries diagnosis even today (ICDAS, 2013):
0—Sound tooth surface
1—First visual change in enamel
2—Distinct visual change in enamel
3—Localized enamel breakdown due to caries with no visible dentin
4—Underlying dark shadow from dentin (with or without enamel breakdown)
5—Distinct cavity with visible dentin—extensive distinct cavity with visible dentin

Visual clinical examination according to Ekstrand et al (1997).

Score	Criteria
0	No or slight change in enamel translucency after prolonged air-drying (5 seconds)
1	Opacity or discoloration hardly visible without drying, but visible after air-drying
2	Opacity or discoloration visible even without air-drying
3	Localized enamel breakdown in opaque or discolored enamel and/or grayish discoloration from the underlying dentin
4	Cavitation in opaque or discolored enamel exposing the dentin

TACTILE EXAMINATION WITH A PROBE

- **GV Black** in1924 suggested the use of a sharp explorer, based on tug back action for diagnosis of dental caries.
- However, tactile examination of dental caries has been criticized because of the possibility of transferring cariogenic microorganisms from one site to another, leading to the fear of further spread of the disease in the same oral cavity.
- Moreover, use of an explorer can cause irreversible damages to the iatrogenic and demineralized tooth structure (**Ekstrand et al.**, 1987; **Stookey**, 2005; **Loesche et al.**, 1979).
- Because of this, a mirror and a blunt probe examination is now advocated **(Fig. 40.1).**

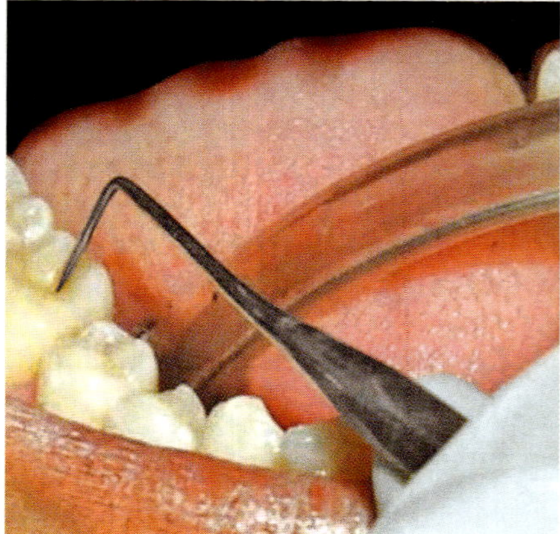

Fig. 40.1: Blunt probe examination.

Diagnostic aids for caries used in Pediatric Dentistry.

Conventional methods	
Visual	• Eyes • Magnifying lens
Tactile sensation	• Probe • Dental floss • Mechanical separation
Illumination	• UV illumination
Dyes	• Basic fuchsin • Procion dyes
Radiography	• Intraoral periapical • Bitewing • Xeroradiography
Recent advances	
Illumination	• FOTI • WFOTI • DIFOTI • Fluorescence camera
Endoscopy	• Endoscopically viewed filtered fluorescence • White light fluorescence • Videoscope
Ultrasonic	• Ultrasonic system scanning acoustic microscope • Ultrasound caries detector
Electrical conductance measurement	• Vanguard electronic caries detector • Caries meter • CarieScan pro
Radiography	• Digital radiography • Digital subtraction radiography • Magnetic resonance microimaging • Photostimulable phosphor radiography • Tuned aperture computed tomography
Lasers	• DIAGNOdent • Dye enhanced laser fluorescence
Miscellaneous	• Species specific monoclonal antibodies • Intraoral television camera • Infrared thermography
Newer alternatives	• Canary system • Midwest caries ID • D-Carie mini • Logicon caries detector • Deep learning-based convolutional • Neural network algorithm • Electronic measurement of caries • Soprolife Spectra caries detection aid • Dexis CariVu • Frequency domain laser-induced • Infrared photothermal radiometry and modulated luminescence • DIAGNOdent pen

(FOTI: fiberoptic transillumination; WFOTI: wavelength-dependent fiberoptic transillumination; DIFOTI: digital imaging fiberoptic transillumination)

DENTAL FLOSS

When a string of unwaxed floss is moved on the carious proximal tooth surfaces, there is resistance on withdrawal and the fibers appear torn.

TOOTH SEPARATION

- Separating the tooth for visualizing the posterior approximal surfaces is now regained popularity.
- This method uses orthodontic modules or bands and achieves slow separation **(Fig. 40.2)**. Taking impressions of the approximal surfaces thus separated have been used to assist in the detection of cavitations.
- Studies have shown that tooth separation has detected more noncavitated enamel lesions than visual-tactile examination without separation or bitewing examination (**Hintze et al.,** 1998; **Pitts** and **Rimmer**, 1992).

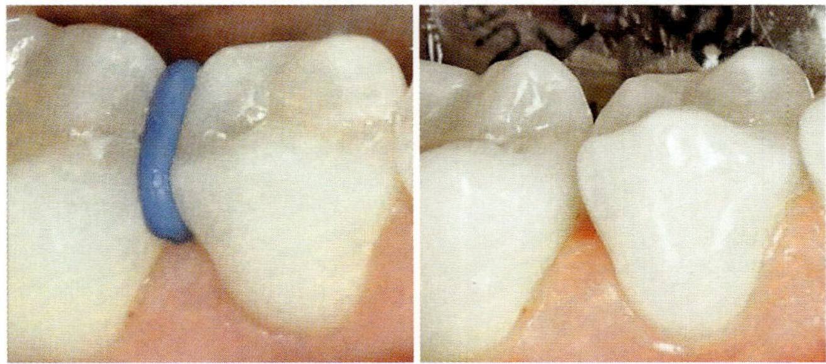

Fig. 40.2: Examination of proximal region after placing separators.

ULTRAVIOLET ILLUMINATION

- Ultraviolet (UV) light has been used to increase the optical contrast between carious lesion and the surrounding soft tissue.
- In area of less mineral content like the carious lesion, the natural fluorescence of tooth enamel as seen under UV illumination is decreased. Under UV illumination, carious lesion appears as a dark spot against fluorescent background **(Fig. 40.3).**

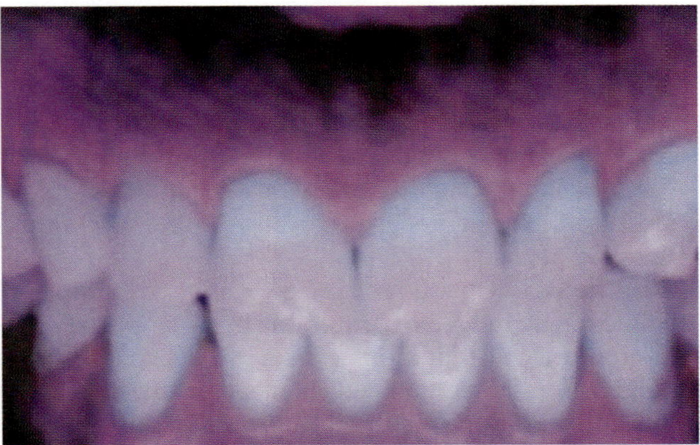

Fig. 40.3: UV Illumination of teeth.

CARIES DETECTOR DYES

- The property of dyes to enhance contrast by their color can be used in clinical dentistry.
- They are applied for about 10s and rinsed off. Any deeply stained tooth structure should be removed, usually with slow speed burs or spoon excavators. They should be applied after you remove all the stained dentin to confirm no residual caries remains in the tooth **(Fig. 40.4)**.

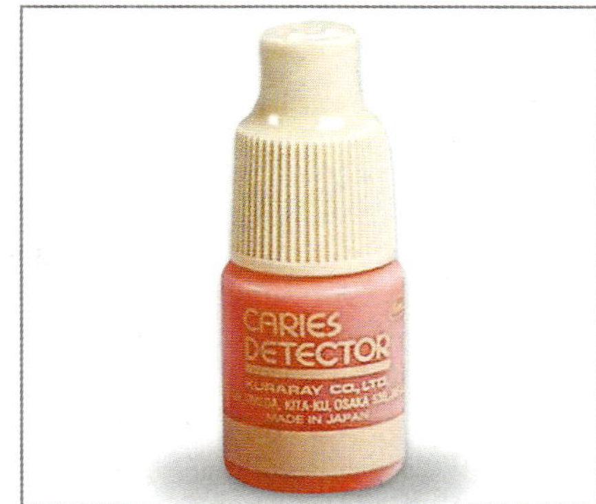

Fig. 40.4: Caries detector dyes.

- Following dyes are used to detect carious enamel specifically:
  - 0.5% basic fuchsin.
  - Procion dyes.
  - 1% acid red in propylene.
  - Methylene blue.
  - Procion dyes react with OH^- and NH^{2+}.

CONVENTIONAL RADIOGRAPHS

- Dental radiographs are indispensable part of the contemporary dentist armamentarium for diagnosis of caries.
- The accuracy of radiographs to diagnose dental caries is between 40% and 65%.
- Rickets, Wenzell found out that radiographs increase the diagnostic ability but only when combined with good visual examination.
- Though conventional radiographs like bitewing and intraoral periapical radiograph are most frequently used for the detection of caries, they may cause overlapping of teeth due to faulty angulations and may also miss the initial lesion. During the primary dentition, the occlusal surface is most susceptible to caries attack, but with the eruption of first permanent molars, the incidence of proximal lesions greatly increases. In such situation, bitewing radiographs are absolutely required to detect proximal lesions in primary molars **(Fig. 40.5)**.
- The limitations of radiographs are that it is not able to differentiate between an active and an arrested caries lesion and also to distinguish a cavitated and a noncavitated lesion.

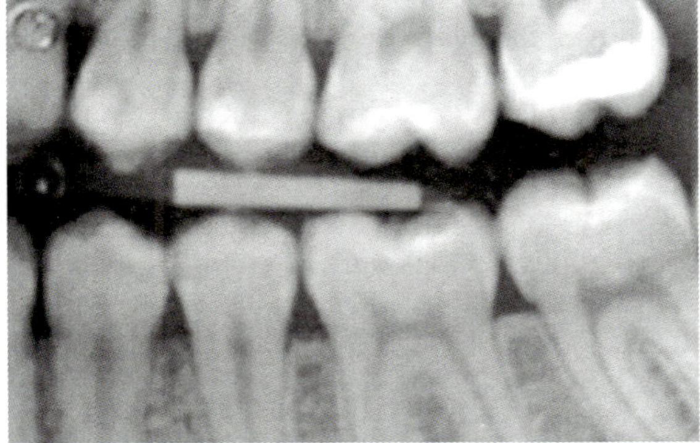

Fig. 40.5: Bitewing radiograph.

ADVANCED DIAGNOSTIC METHODS

Novel diagnostic systems are based upon the measurement of a physical signal—these are surrogate measures of the caries process. Examples of the physical signals that can be used in this way include X-rays, visible light, laser light, electronic current, ultrasound, and possibly surface roughness. For a caries detection device to function, it must be capable of initiating and receiving the signal as well as being able to interpret the strength of the signal in a meaningful way. A range of new caries detection systems have been developed, and these are therefore aimed at augmenting the diagnostic process by facilitating either earlier detection of the disease or enabling it to be quantified in an objective manner.

DIGITAL RADIOGRAPHY

- Digital radiography is a filmless technique for intraoral radiography, utilizes very little of the radiation to which the patient has been exposed, and avoid the need for developing films. This technique has offered the potential to increase the diagnostic yield of dental radiographs.
- **Advantages:**
  - The image is displayed immediately and no need of processing.
  - Reduction in radiation dose.
  - Digital manipulation of the image is possible to enhance the viewing.
  - It can be used as a visual aid to be shown to the patient on the computer screen.
  - It increases the confidence and credibility in the treatment decision-making process.
- **Disadvantages:**
  - The rigidity and thickness of sensor can cause discomfort to the patient.
  - The life span of sensor is unknown.
  - High initial system cost (**van der Stelt**, 2008; **Wenzel**, 1998) (**Bin-Shuwaish et al.,** 2008; **van der Stelt,** 2008; **Wenzel,** 1998).

DIGITAL SUBTRACTION RADIOGRAPHY

- Digital subtraction radiography (DSR) is a more advanced image analysis tools which allows professionals to distinguish small differences between subsequent radiographs that otherwise would have remained unobserved because of over projection of anatomical structures or differences in density that are too small to be recognized by the human eye.
- The procedure is based on the principle that two digital radiographic images obtained under different time intervals, with the same projection geometry, are spatially and densitometrically aligned using specific software.
- If the two digital images are identical, this method will produce an image without details (the result is zero). However, if caries has regressed or progressed in the meantime, the result will be different from zero. When there is caries progression, the outcome will be a value above zero (increase in pixel values). In case of caries regression, the result is opposite, and the outcome will be a value below zero (decrease in pixel values) (**Hekmatian et al.,** 2005).
- The major disadvantage of this technique is very sensitive to any physical noise occurring between the radiographs and even minor changes leads to large errors in the results.

FIBEROPTIC TRANSILLUMINATION

- Fiberoptic transillumination, it is a practical method of imaging teeth in the presence of multiple scattering (**Marcus** and **Friedman**, 1970).
- The illumination is delivered via light source to tooth surface. The light propagates from the fiber illumination a cross tooth tissue on illuminated surfaces. The resulting images of light distribution are then used for diagnosis **(Fig. 40.6)**.

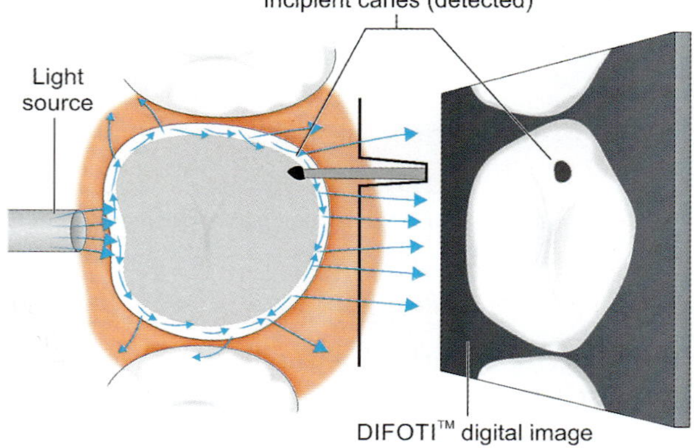

Fig. 40.6: Mechanism of transillumination.

- Carious area appears as darkened shadow that follows the decay (**Oogard** and **Ten Bosch**).
- The equipment includes a 150-W halogen lamp and a rheostat to provide light of maximum intensity. A mouth mirror mounted on steel cuff and fiberoptic probe are placed in embrasure region below contact point to produce a narrow beam for transillumination.
- **Peers et al.,** evaluated FOTI and concluded that it was as accurate as bitewing radiography and superior to visual examination in diagnosis of interproximal caries.
- It is used for diagnosis of caries and identification of necrotic canals.
- Advantages are that it is simple noninvasive examination technique, no radiation hazards, can be used on all surfaces.
- Disadvantage is that the system is subjective rather than objective, as there is no continuous data out putted, and it is not possible to record what is seen in the form of an image.
- Another modification is wavelength-dependent fiberoptic transillumination (WFOTI) which is used for detection of early incipient and approximal carious lesion.

QUANTITATIVE LIGHT-INDUCED FLUORESCENCE

- Fluorescence is a phenomenon by which an object is excited by a particular wavelength of light, and the reflected light is of a larger wavelength. When the excitation light is in the visible spectrum, the fluorescence will be of a different color.

- In the case of the quantitative light-induced fluorescence (QLF), the visible light has a wavelength of 370 nm, which is in the blue region of the spectrum. The resultant autofluorescence of human enamel is then detected by filtering out the excitation light using a band pass filter at >540 nm by a small intraoral camera. This produces an image that is comprised of only green and red channels (the blue having been filtered out) and the predominant color of the enamel is green.
- Demineralization of enamel results in reduction of this auto fluorescence. This loss can be quantified using proprietary software and has been shown to correlate well with actual mineral loss; $r = 0.73–0.86$.
- The QLF equipment is comprised of a light box containing a xenon bulb and a handpiece, similar in appearance to an intraoral camera. Light is passed to the handpiece via a liquid light guide, and the handpiece contains the band pass filter. Live images are displayed via a computer, and accompanying software enables patient's details to be entered and individual images of the teeth of interest to be captured and stored.
- Once an image of a tooth has been captured, the next stage is to analyze any lesions and produce a quantitative assessment of the demineralization status of the tooth. This is undertaken using proprietary software and involves using a patch to define areas of sound enamel around the lesion of interest. Following this the software uses the pixel values of the sound enamel to reconstruct the surface of the tooth and then subtracts those pixels which are considered to be lesion.
- Advantages are high reproducibility, detection of small incipient lesions in enamel and dentin, image storage and transmission, and can act as motivational tool for patient.
- Disadvantage is that it is an isolation sensitive procedure.

FLUORESCENCE CAMERA (VISTA PROOF)

- This device is an intraoral camera which consists of six blue light emitting diodes (LEDs) emitting a 405-nm light, charge-couple device (CCD) sensor, and DBSWIN software for analysis **(Fig. 40.7)**.

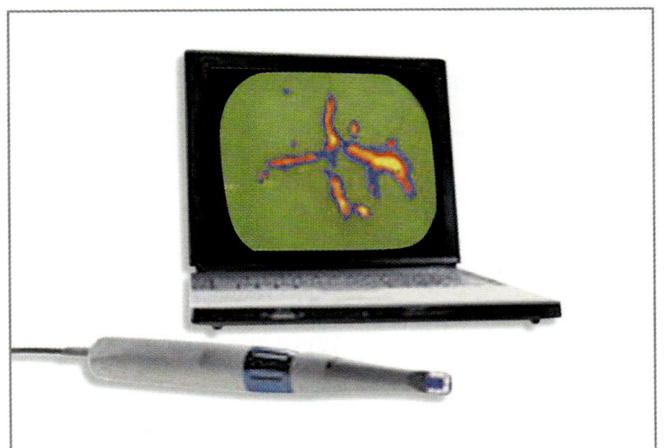

Fig. 40.7: Fluorescence camera.

With this camera, it is possible to digitize the video signal from the dental surface during fluorescence emission using a CCD sensor. On these images, it is possible to see different areas of the dental surface that fluoresce in green (sound dental tissue) and in red (carious dental tissue) (**Thomas**, 2006).

- Advantages include motivation for patient and storage of data.

DIGITAL IMAGING FIBEROPTIC TRANSILLUMINATION

- This was suggested as a tool for caries assessment by **Scheneiderman A.** This was suggested as a tool for caries assessment by **Scheneiderman A et al.,** in 1997.
- This is a new method for detection of dental caries in which the images of teeth are obtained through visible light fibreoptic transillumination and digital CCD camera.
- These images are then sent to a computer for analysis with specific algorithms. These algorithms are developed to facilitate the location and diagnosis of the carious lesion and provide quantitative characterization for monitoring the lesions.
- Advantage is that it can indicate the presence of incipient and recurrent caries even when radiological images fail to show their presence.

LASER FLUORESCENCE (DIAGNODENT)

- The DIAGNOdent (DD) instrument (KaVo, Germany) is another device employing fluorescence to detect the presence of caries **(Fig. 40.8)**.

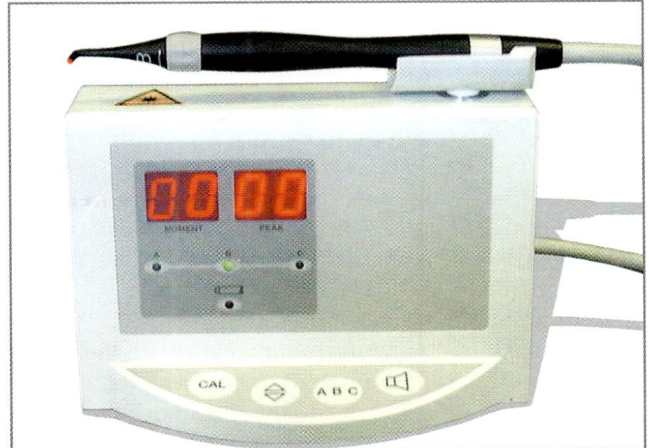

Fig. 40.8: DIAGNOdent.

- Using a small laser, the system produces an excitation wavelength of 655 nm which produces a red-light. This is carried to one of two intraoral tips: one designed for pits and fissures, and the other for smooth surfaces. The tip both emits the excitation light and collects the resultant fluorescence. This is then displayed as a numerical value on two LED displays. The signal comes out as a number on instrument on a scale of 0–99. Higher the number, more is caries **(Fig. 40.9)**.

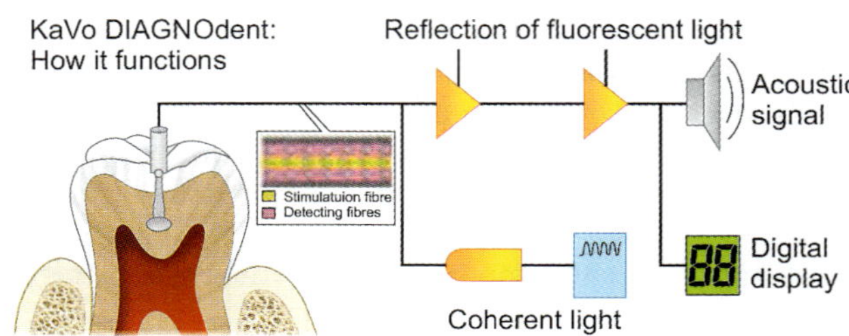

Fig. 40.9: DIAGNOdent working mechanism.

- Principle of DIAGNOdent is based on the fact that the caries induced changes in teeth lead to increased fluorescence at specific excitation wavelength.
- Advantages are early detection of lesion, quantification of caries, and improved diagnostic accuracy.
- Disadvantages are that it cannot detect secondary caries and proximal caries accurately.

Diagnostic interpretations of DIAGNOdent

Signal reading	*Inference*
0–4	No caries, or histological caries limited to outer half of enamel
4.01–10	Histological caries extending beyond the outer half but confined to enamel
10.01–18	Histological dentinal caries limited to outer half of dentin
>18.01	Histological dentinal caries extending into inner half of dentin

ELECTRICAL CONDUCTANCE MEASUREMENT

- The idea of electrical method for caries detection was proposed by **Magitot.**
- It is based on the principle that sound tooth surfaces possess limited conductivity, whereas demineralized or carious enamel act as conductive pathway. Based on the differences in the electrical conductance of carious and sound enamel, two instruments were developed and tested in 1980, i.e., vanguard electronic caries detector and caries meter.
  - **Vanguard electronic caries detector:**
    - Resistance measurements are made between a hand-held connector and probe tip placed in fissure of teeth and superficial saliva is removed to prevent surface conduction.
    - Machine gives a reading on scale of 0-9 which is directly proportional to degree of demineralization.
  - **Caries meter:**
    - Teeth are dried and isolated before starting the treatment. Tooth fissure is moistened with a drop of saliva to ensure good electrical conductance. The resistance measurement is made between probe tip and clip attached to oral electrode and colored lights reflect the status of tooth.
    - Advantage is that it is small, handy, and provides accurate diagnosis.
    - Disadvantages are that area of diagnosis is confined to dimension of probe, it is technique sensitive, and the status of lesion is not known like arrested or active.

Light	*Electric impedance value (K)*	*Status of tooth*	*Recommended treatment*
Green	Above 600K	No caries	No treatment
Yellow	250–600 K	Enamel caries	Observe
Orange	15–250 K	Dentinal caries	Need for restoration
Red	Below 15 K	Pulpal involvement	Pulpal treatment

ULTRASOUND CARIES DETECTOR

- This is a new ultrasonic proximal caries detector that works by transmitting surface ultrasonic waves.
- The ultrasound caries detector (UCD) device is based on pulse-echo method and has software, hardware, and transducer as components. A medical grade silicon wedge is positioned in front of probe to yield surface waves on the tooth surface when the transducer comes in contact with the tooth **(Fig. 40.10)**. This detector records specific profiles of ultrasonic echoes obtained from the enamel surface, dentinoenamel junction, and pulpodentinal junction. Changes in this profile have been described in demineralized lesions, suggesting a substantial difference in the sonic conductivity between sound and demineralized enamel.
- **Matalon et al.,** (2003) compared and found UCD to be superior in sensitivity and specificity as compared to bite wing radiography in detection of approximal caries.

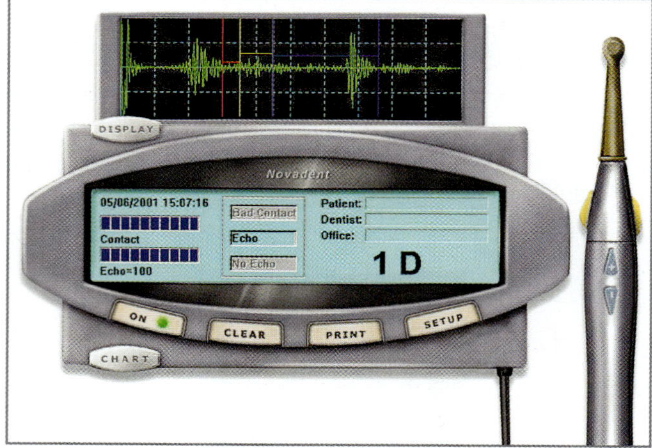

Fig. 40.10: Ultrasound caries detector.

MIDWEST CARIES ID (LED TECHNOLOGY)

- This technology utilizes a handheld device which emits a soft LED between 635 and 880 nm and analyzes the reflectance and refraction of the emitted light from the tooth surface, which is captured by fibreoptics and is converted to electrical signals for analysis **(Fig. 40.11)**.

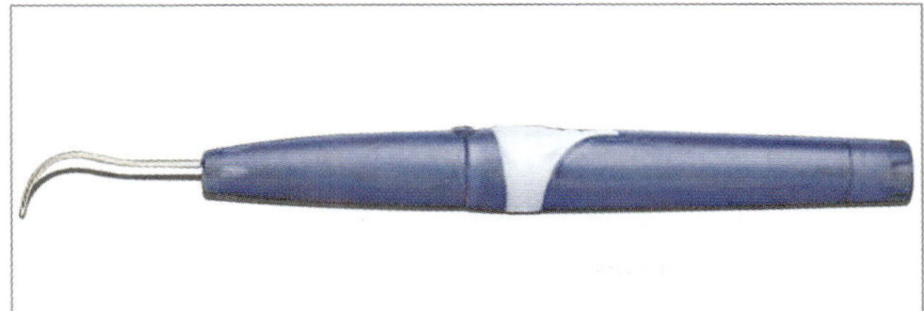

Fig. 40.11: Midwest caries ID.

- The demineralization leads to a change in the LED from green to red with a simultaneous audible signal, which is directly related to the severity of caries lesions.
- Advantage is that sensitivity and specificity is higher than that of DIAGNOdent (**HCiaburro, Krause et al.**).
- Disadvantage is that Midwest Caries ID is notable to differentiate enamel lesions from sound surfaces (**Rodrigues et al.,** 2011).

CARIESCAN PRO

- It involves the passing of an insensitive level of electrical current through the tooth to identify the presence and location of the decay.
- The device is indicated for the detection, diagnosis, and monitoring of primary coronal dental caries (occlusal and accessible smooth surfaces), which are not clearly visible to the human eye.
- This device uses disposable tufted sensors for single use and a test sensor (non-disposable), which is used to check if the device is operating correctly. For assessment of caries, while tufted sensor brush contacts the tooth surface being examined, a soft tissue contact, which is a disposable metal clip that is placed over the lip in the corner of the patient's mouth, connects to the CarieScan via a soft tissue cable to complete the circuit **(Fig. 40.12)**.

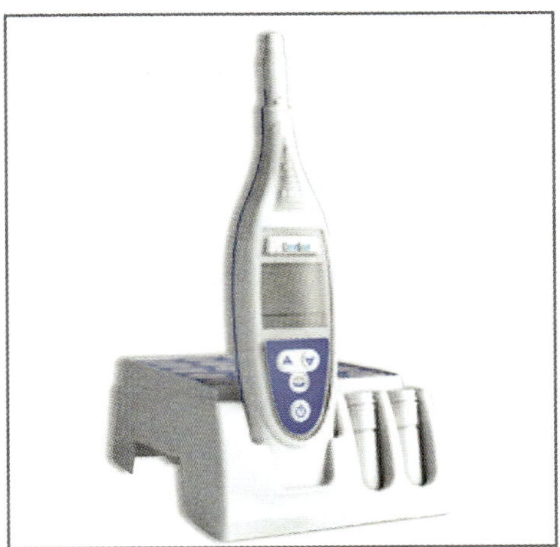

Fig. 40.12: CarieScan Pro.

- During measurement, a green color display indicates sound tooth tissue, while a red color indicates deep caries requiring operative, and a yellow color associated with a range of numerical figures from 1 to 99 depicts varying severity caries, which require only preventive care.
- A systematic review comparing CarieScan with clinical visual examination, bitewing radiograph, and DIAGNOdent reported CarieScan to have a superior sensitivity and specificity (92.5%) over other methods (**JD Bader, DA Shugars, AJ Bonito**).
- Disadvantage is that it cannot be used to assess secondary caries, the integrity of a restoration, dental root caries, and the depth of an excavation within a cavity preparation.

INTRAORAL TELEVISION CAMERA

- Through intraoral television camera (IOTV), the dentist can educate the patient and at the same time can also improve their own diagnostic expertise as they see magnified oral conditions, which are significantly better than direct vision.
- **Forgie et al** (2003) concluded that IOVC can achieve very high level of sensitivity, but this is accompanied with drop in specificity.
- Advantages are increased vision and magnification.
- Disadvantage is loss of specificity.

D-CARIE MINI

- This is a new device introduced by Neks technology in October 2006 at ADA annual session in Las Vegas.
- This was initially developed in Canada.
- This is pen-sized, lightweight, cordless, and fully sterilizable unit that uses laser fluorescence to detect occlusal lesions **(Fig. 40.13).**
- The D-Carie mini has been shown to detect >92% of occlusal caries and over 80% of interproximal caries.
- Approved by FDA in 2007.

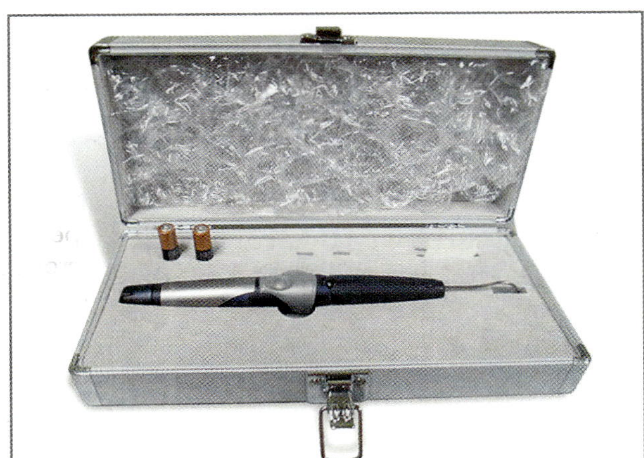

Fig. 40.13: D-Carie mini.

ADVANCED RADIOGRAPHIC TECHNIQUES

- **Magnetic resonance microimaging (MRMI):**
  - The basis of MRMI is that different species of atomic nucleus have different intrinsic nuclear spins. When a magnetic field is applied, the nuclear spins align in a finite number of allowed orientations. If these orientations are perturbed by a pulse of radiofrequency energy, the energy gets absorbed and then retransmitted. The chemical environment of tooth determines the frequency of their transmitted energy peak.
  - Carious regions give an intense image that is readily distinguishable from other soft tissues.

- Advantage is that this technique is noninvasive and allows a specimen to be reimaged after further exposure to clinically relevant environment.
- Major drawbacks include cost and clinical testing.

❖ **Photostimulable phosphor radiography:**
- A latent image is produced by exposing the storage phosphor screen with X-rays.
- Advantages are that it can be used with existing X-ray sources, wider exposure range and transfer of images is possible.
- Disadvantages are high cost and chances of cross infection.

❖ **Tuned aperture computed tomography (TACT):**
- TACT is a new imaging device which enhances the image by decreasing the superimposition of anatomical structures.
- It uses digital radiographic images, and its software correlates these images into layers so that sliced sections can be viewed.
- A series of 8 radiographs can be assimilated one TACT image.
- It is effective in evaluating primary stimulated recurrent caries and simulated osseous defects and can localize a lesion accurately with minimal radiation.

ADVANCED DYE DETECTION TECHNIQUES

❖ **Confocal laser scanning microscopy (CLSM):** This is operated simultaneously with AR and Kr ion lasers, and an appropriate set of filters, the reflection image of the dentin structure, and the fluorescent images of the labelled Carisolv can be recorded simultaneously.

❖ **Dye-enhanced laser fluorescence (DELF):**
- This technique is based on a hypothesis that if a fluorescent dye penetrates a carious lesion, the accuracy of current laser fluorescence for caries detection is enhanced.
- Useful in diagnosis of subsurface lesion.

SPECIES SPECIFIC MONOCLONAL ANTIBODIES

❖ This was given by **Shi et al.,** in 1998, who identified specific monoclonal antibodies that recognize the surface of cariogenic bacteria.

❖ The probes are tagged with fluorescent molecules that measure quantitatively with spectrometer.

❖ They can be used at chairside by dentist and provide instant results.

INFRARED THERMOGRAPHY

❖ Thermal radiation energy travels in the form of waves. It is possible to measure changes in thermal energy when fluid is lost from a lesion by evaporation. The thermal energy emitted by sound tooth structure is compared with that emitted by carious tooth structure.

❖ The technique has been described by **Kaneko et al.,** (1999) and has been proposed as a method of determining lesion activity rather than a method of determining the presence or absence of a lesion.

❖ The clinical data regarding this technique is, however, still insufficient.

MICROTOMOGRAPHY

❖ X-ray microtomography is a miniature version of computerized axial tomography with a resolution in order of micrometers.

❖ It has the ability to accurately measure the linear attenuation coefficient.

❖ From this, the mineral concentration can be computed.

❖ Using microtomography we can form three dimensional images of hard tissues.

OPTICAL COHERENCE TOMOGRAPHY

❖ Optical coherence tomography (OCT) can produce an image of tissue microstructure of the caries lesion to show the changes within and therefore can be compared both qualitatively and quantitatively with histological methods such as microcomputed tomography and transverse microradiography, the current gold standard for measuring demineralization.

❖ OCT creates a two-dimensional map of the tissue microstructure by illuminating the tissue with low power near infrared (NIR) light, collecting the back scattered light, and analyzing the intensity. OCT is based on low coherence interferometry.

❖ Based on the principle, the highest quality image information is in the portion of the detected light that is relatively unscattered and therefore travels the most direct path through the tissue.

CANARY SYSTEM (PTR-LUM)

❖ The Canary System developed by Quantum Dental Technologies takes a different approach to light interacting with teeth. The Canary, using the same type of near infrared laser as DIAGNOdent or Caries ID, rapidly pulses the laser and looks at the interaction of the laser light when the laser is turned off. When pulses of laser light are focused on a tooth, the tooth glows and releases heat. The analysis of the reemitted radiation (luminescence) and the thermal behavior of the emitted infrared photons provides very accurate information about the condition of the tooth. As a lesion grows, there is a corresponding change in the signal. As remineralization progresses, a signal reversal indicates an improvement in the condition of the tooth **(Fig. 40.14)**.

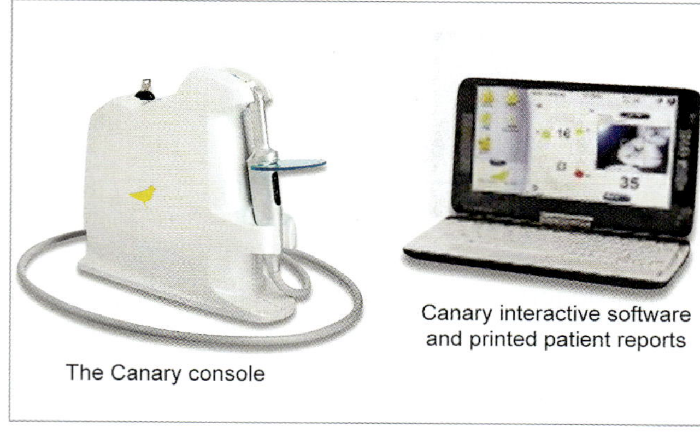

Fig. 40.14: Canary system.

- The temperature rise in the tooth is no >1–2°C which patients cannot detect. There is no alteration of any of the tissues and no safety issues such as those associated with dental X-rays.
- The Canary system is able to see down about 4–5 mm (the average depth of tooth enamel), by changing the cycle or frequency of the laser pulse. Low frequencies about 5 Hz are deep probes because the heat that is generated pulses up and down very slowly, and so it penetrates very deeply into the tooth. High frequencies, around 1,000 Hz are shallow probes.
- The Canary system can detect occlusal pit and fissure caries, smooth surface caries, acid erosion lesion, root caries, interproximal carious lesions, and demineralization and remineralization of early carious lesions.
- This is one of the most challenging clinical situations for all these new technologies is the detection of lesion around restorative materials as the ability of laser light or other forms of energy to penetrate the material is limited. Radiographs can show us defects along the gingival seats of class II restorations, but they can neither examine the walls of the restorations nor the occlusal surfaces. The Canary system using PTR-LUM has shown in preliminary studies the ability to detect lesions around the visible margins of composites.

DEXIS CARIVU

- It uses transillumination technology that makes the enamel appear transparent, while porous lesions trap and absorb light and allow the clinician to see through the tooth, exposing its structure and the development of any carious lesions **(Fig. 40.15)**.
- It uses nonionizing radiation which is ideal for children, pregnant women, and patients who are X-ray averse.
- CariVu is the only detector on the market that detects it all: occlusal, interproximal, and recurrent caries and cracks. It does so using images rather than colors, codes, or sounds. There is no need to clean the tooth surface or calibrate the unit before using.
- CariVu provides easy-to-read images that read like familiar X-ray images-lesions will appear as dark areas.

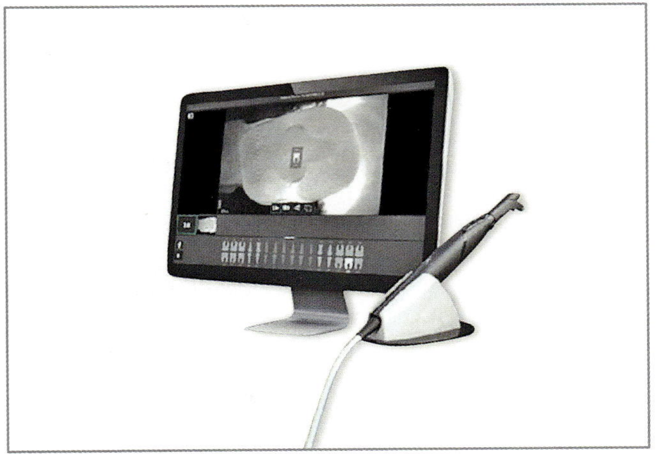

Fig. 40.15: CariVu.

SPECTRA CARIES DETECTION AID

- The Spectra Caries Detection System using fluorescence technology light-emitting diodes (LED) projects high-energy light onto the tooth surface causing cariogenic bacteria to fluoresce red and healthy enamel green **(Fig. 40.16)**.
- The device emits a light with a 400-nm wavelength and filters the fluorescence emitted by the tissue. Specific software then quantifies the fluorescence on a numerical scale from 0 to 5.
- CamX Spectra uses fluorescence to detect caries in fissures and smooth surfaces that may go unnoticed in X-ray images. Detects decay hidden between the margins of existing composite and amalgam restorations.

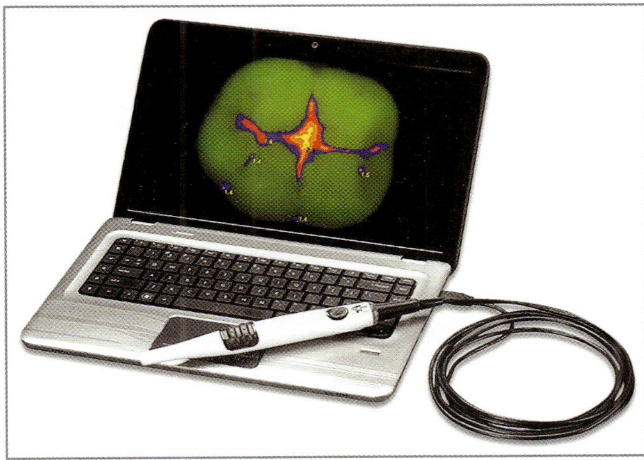

Fig. 40.16: The spectra caries detection system.

FREQUENCY DOMAIN LASER-INDUCED INFRARED PHOTOTHERMAL RADIOMETRY AND MODULATED LUMINESCENCE

- This technology relies on absorption of IR laser light by the tooth with measurement of subsequent temperature change, which is in the 1°C or less range.
- The advantage compared with other methods of detection is that it can perform depth profilometry and very early caries detection and monitoring on tooth surfaces.
- When pulses of laser light hit the tooth surface, the tooth glows (luminescence) and releases heat (photothermal radiometry). It can provide depth profile by varying frequency of laser beam. Detected signal reflects the tooth condition. It detects 50 μ lesion up to 5 mm below the surface.

SOPROLIFE CAMERA

- The SoproLife® camera selectively amplifies fluorescence signals to detect any carious lesion or diseased tissue based on the variation of its autofluorescence compared with the healthy area of the same tooth **(Fig. 40.17)**.
- It (light-emitting diode fluorescence tool) is two devices in one operating as a caries detection device and a high magnification intraoral camera.

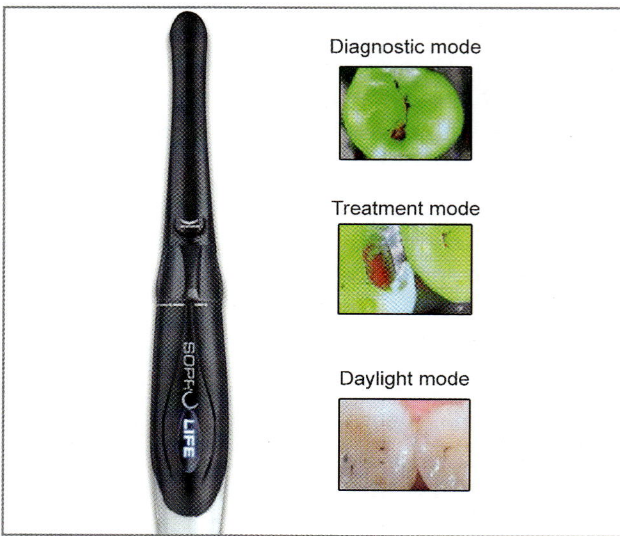

Fig. 40.17: SoproLife® camera.

- It is not software dependent, so it will work with most imaging and practice management software.
- During excavation, the margins of infected and affected dentin are clearly distinguishable, allowing the infected dentin (which shows up bright red) to be removed and the affected dentin (which shows up orange) to be retained to allow the remainder of the tooth to heal.

ELECTRONIC MEASUREMENT OF CARIES

Tooth demineralization due to the caries process causes increased porosity of tooth structure. This porosity contains fluid with ions in it. This increases the electrical conductivity but reduces the electrical impedance (resistance). Electronic countermeasure device uses 23 Hz of fixed frequency of (alternating current) which measures the resistance of tooth, for example, caries meter, vanguard caries detector **(Fig. 40.18)**.

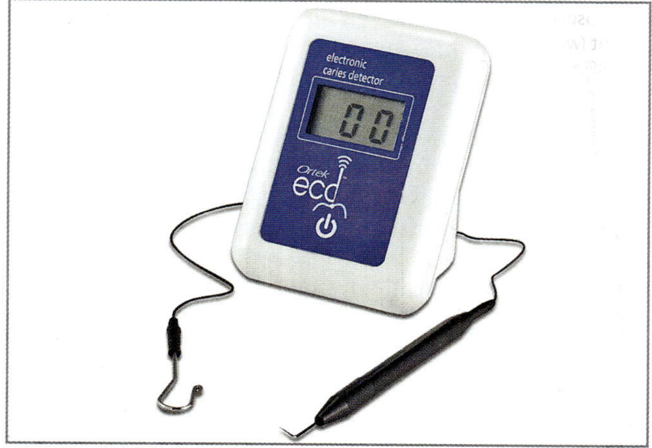

Fig. 40.18: Electronic caries meter.

DEEP LEARNING-BASED CONVOLUTIONAL NEURAL NETWORK ALGORITHM

- Deep convolutional neural networks (CNNs) are a rapidly emerging new area of medical research and have yielded impressive results in diagnosis and prediction in the fields of radiology and pathology.
- These algorithms perform edge detection very efficiently through multiple convolutional and hidden layers with hierarchical feature representations, and deep CNN-based dental caries detector can learn the location and morphological changes of dental carious lesions efficiently and detect them conveniently and reliably.
- Deep learning algorithms, such as ResNet and CapsNet.

LOGICON CARIES DETECTOR

- Logicon Caries Detector™ Software (LCDS, Carestream Dental, GA, USA), the only commercially available computer-aided design, was developed to detect and diagnose dental caries based on traditional algorithms consisting of three-layer forward networks.
- Latest software improvements further enhance the detection process. It applies the algorithm on all eligible interproximal surfaces within a radiograph to generate a view of existing caries, helping the dentist verify manual findings by focusing on surfaces that require further investigation **(Fig. 40.19)**.
- Locate and classify potential proximal caries with a few clicks.
- Save and display selected results for multiple high-risk surfaces on a single radiograph.
- Present more accurate information by indicating penetration depth of caries.

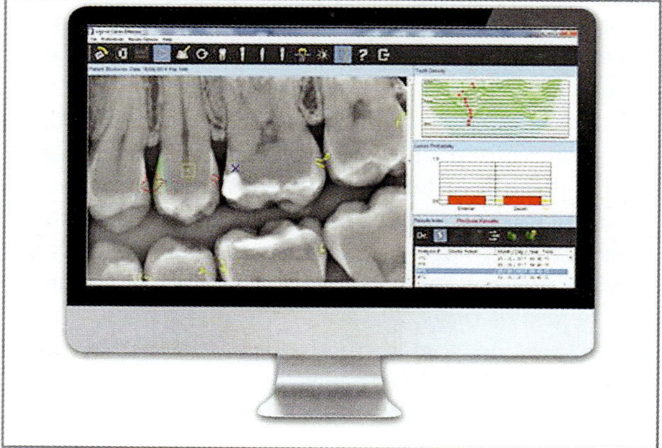

Fig. 40.19: Logicon Caries Detector™ software.

DIAGNODENT PEN

- The second-generation DIAGNOdent laser fluorescence device, better known as the DIAGNOdent Pen (DD Pen). **(Fig. 40.20)**.
- Early, initial caries and hidden caries can be safely detected using the LASER fluorescence technology.
- Children and adolescents in particular have fissure caries in nearly 80% of all cases which can be detected more easily
- Easy detection of the "iceberg" syndrome: 90 % of caries is within the proximal area—they will be detected.
- The DIAGNOdent pen offers the advantage of measuring fluorescence deep within the fissure pattern, since LASER light easily penetrates the enamel and is reflected by even the smallest lesion **(Fig. 40.21)**.

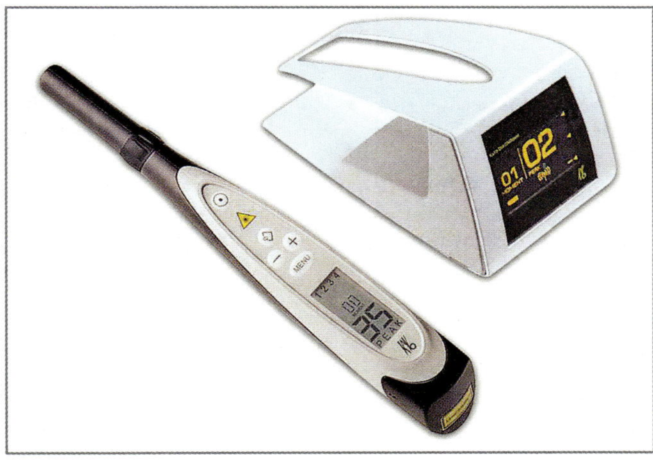

Fig. 40.20: DIAGNOdent pen.

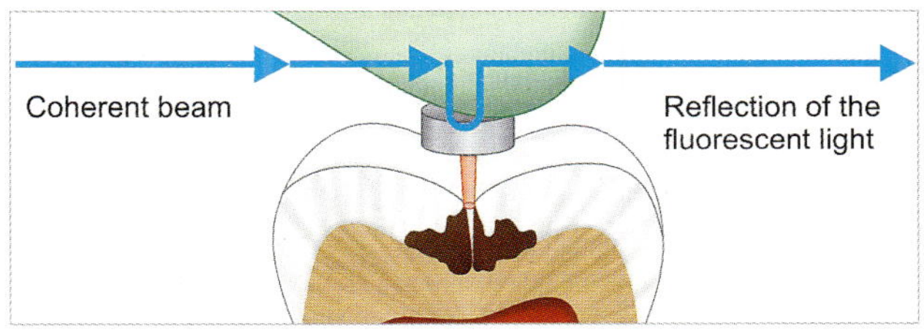

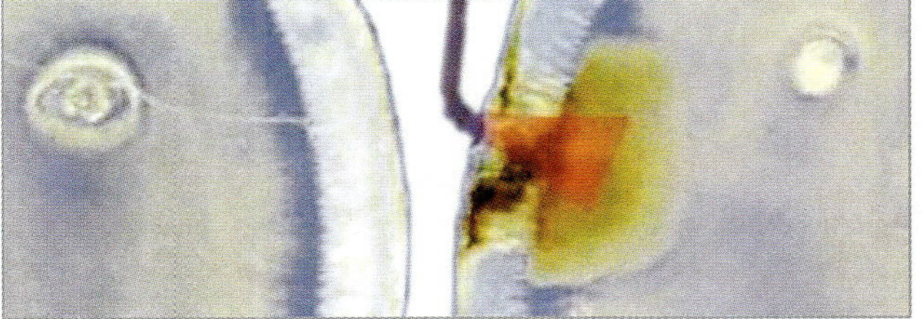

Fig. 40.21: DIAGNOdent pen working mechanism.

SUMMARY OF THE FIVE CURRENTLY AVAILABLE NCDTS ON THE MARKET

Parameter	***Photothermal radiometry and modulated luminescence (PTR/LUM)***	***Fiberoptic and digital fiberoptic transillumination (FOTI and DIFOTI)***	***Quantitative light-induced fluorescence (QLF)***	***Laser fluorescence (LF)***	***Near infrared light transillumination (NIT) and near-infrared reflectance (NIR)***
Commercial product examples	Canary system (Quantum Dental Technologies, Toronto, Canada)	Phatelus optic transillumination light (NSK, Tochigi, Japan) Microlux (AdDent Inc., CT, USA) DiaLUX probe (KaVo Dental GmBH, Biberach, Germany)	The Inspektor™ Pro QLF The Inspektor™ QLF-D Biluminator™ 2+ Qscan™ (Inspektor Research Systems BV, Bussum, The Netherlands)	DIAGNOdent pen (KaVo Dental GmBH, Biberach, Germany)	DIAGNOcam (KaVo Dental GmBH, Biberach, Germany) CariVu (DEXIS, LLC, Hatfield, PA, USA)
Year of introduction	2010	From 1990s	2004	Early 2000s	2012 (Europe) 2013 (USA)
Concept	Conversion of optical energy produced from a laser source into irradiation leading to temperature changes detected by an infrared detector	White light scattering (wavelength = 450–700 nm)	Green and red fluorescence of EDJ after exposure to visible blue light (wavelength ~400–488 nm)	Fluorescence due to bacterial protoporphyrin after the application of red light (wavelength = 655 nm)	Transillumination of near-infrared light (wavelength ~780 nm) using two light emission windows (NIR wavelength = 1310 nm)
Main indication	Proximal caries lesions and cracks	Detection of proximal caries lesions	Smooth (facial) surface lesions	Occlusal caries lesions	Detection of proximal caries lesions in posterior teeth
Caries lesion quantification	Yes	No	Yes	Partial	Partial (Gray scale)
Caries lesion activity determination	No	No	Yes	No	No
Main shortcoming	It is often not possible to correlate the Canary number to results of visual examination or bitewing (BW) radiographs	No lesion quantification, subjective. Potential higher false positive due to difficulty to differentiate between caries lesions and developmental defects and stains, false negative due to large restoration	Not indicated for proximal lesions. Sensitive to the ambient light, difficult accurate repositioning of intraoral camera type devices to take the next image	High values for false positive, no detection of cavitation, no imaging and requires clean teeth and calibration on a sound surface before use	Not indicated for smooth surface on the facial surfaces. No imaging of the caries extension relative to the pulp

Contd...

Contd...

Parameter	Photothermal radiometry and modulated luminescence (PTR/LUM)	Fiberoptic and digital fiberoptic transillumination (FOTI and DIFOTI)	Quantitative light-induced fluorescence (QLF)	Laser fluorescence (LF)	Near infrared light transillumination (NIT) and near-infrared reflectance (NIR)
Main advantage	Does not require a dry field, detection of secondary caries around composite and below resin infiltrants, high repeatability. Connects with practice management software	Affordability, short learning curve, ease of use, applicability in other dental situations	Nondestructive quantification of the physical characteristics of caries lesions, QLF-D advanced device was able to analyze the entire oral cavity extraorally	Caries monitoring possible	NIR with longer wavelengths have no interference from occlusal surface stains, possible to detect caries lesions close to restoration margins, relative ease of use, crack detection, repeatability
Radiation/ hazards	Needs eye protection	None	Needs eye protection	Needs eye protection	None
Occlusal caries	Yes	No	Yes	Yes	Yes
Proximal caries	Yes	Yes	No	Yes	Yes
Facial surface caries	Yes	No	Yes	No	No

It is clear that the differences in caries presentations and behavior in different anatomical sites make it unlikely that any one diagnostic modality will have adequate sensitivity and specificity of detection of carious lesions for all sites. Hence a combination of both conventional and novel diagnostic tools is mandatory to diagnose lesions earlier so that the clinician can restrict to a preventive treatment mode. However, the clinician should be aware of the correct use of the novel diagnostic aids, their advantages and disadvantages, and also should strictly follow the manufacturer instructions. Visual examination remains the method of choice irrespective of surface or dentition and can be adequately supplemented with DIAGNOdent pen especially for primary dentition.

POINTS TO REMEMBER

- Conventional methods of caries diagnosis are visual and tactile examination, radiographs, UV light examination, and use caries detect or dyes.
- DSR is a more advanced image analysis tool which allows professionals to distinguish small differences between subsequent radiographs that otherwise would have remained unobserved because of over projection of anatomical structures or differences in density that are too small to be recognized by the human eye.
- The DIAGNOdent employs fluorescence to detect the presence of caries as it induces changes in teeth lead to increased fluorescence at specific excitation wavelength.
- Caries meter diagnoses caries on the basis of electric impedance.
- UCD is a new ultrasonic proximal caries detect or that works by transmitting surface ultrasonic waves.
- Midwest caries ID is a recent diagnostic aid that analyzes the reflectance and refraction of the emitted light from the tooth surface, which is captured by fiberoptics and is converted to electrical signals for analysis.
- Carie Scan Pro is the most advanced and most accurate development in caries diagnosis which involves the passing of an insensitive level of electrical current through the tooth to identify the presence and location of the decay.
- D-Carie Mini was introduced by Neks technology in 2006 is pen-sized, lightweight, cordless, fully sterilizable unit that uses laser fluorescence to detect occlusal lesions.
- TACT is a new imaging device which enhances the image by decreasing the superimposition of anatomical structures with series of eight radiograph scan be assimilated one TACT image.

Questionnaire

1. Classify the diagnostic aids in dental caries.
2. Write a note on cries detect or dyes.
3. What are the advanced methods of radiographic diagnosis?
4. What is QLF?
5. Explain the principle and working of DIAGNOdent.
6. Describe D-Cariemini and CarieScan pro.
7. Describe canary system of Dexis CariVu.
8. Difference between microtomography and optical coherence tomography.
9. What do you understand by spectra caries detection Aid?
10. Explain in detail about advanced radiographic techniques.
11. Write a note on sporolife camera.

FURTHER READING

1. Abrams SH, Sivagurunathan KS, Silvertown JD, Wong B, Hellen A, Mandelis A, et al. Correlation with caries lesion depth of the canary system, DIAGNOdent and ICDAS II. Open Dent J. 2017;11:679-89.
2. Amaechi BT. Emerging technologies for diagnosis of dental caries: the road so far. J Appl Phys. 2009;105:1020-47.
3. American Dental Association, Council on Access, Prevention, and Interprofessional Relations. Caries diagnosis and risk assessment: a review of preventive strategies and management. J Am Dent Assoc. 1995;126(suppl):1s-24s.
4. Angmar-Månsson B, Al-Khateeb S, Tranaeus S. Quantitative light fluorescence: current research. In: Stookey GK (Ed). Proceedings of 4th annual Indiana conference, early detection of dental caries II. Bloomington: Indiana University School of Dentistry; 2000. pp. 203-18.

5. Angmar-Månsson BE, Al- Khateeb S, Tranaeus S. Caries diagnosis. J Dent Educ. 1998;62:771-80.
6. Bader JD, Shugars DA, Bonito AJ. Systematic reviews of selected dental caries diagnostic and management methods. J Dent Educ. 2001;65:960-8.
7. Fisher J, Glick M. A new model for caries classification and management, FDI World Dental Federation Caries Matrix. J Am Dent Assoc. 2012;143:546-51.
8. Foros P, Oikonomou E, Despina Koletsi D, Rahiotis C. Detection Methods for Early Caries Diagnosis: A Systematic Review and Meta-Analysis. Caries Res. 2021;55:247-59.
9. Foros P, Oikonomou E, Koletsi D, Rahiotis C. Detection methods for early caries diagnosis: A systematic review and meta-analysis. Caries Res. 2021;55:247-59.
10. Gutta A, Merdad HE. In vitro study of the diagnostic performance of the Spectra Caries Detection Aid. J Clin Dent. 2015;26:17-22.
11. He K, Zhang X, Ren S, Sun J. Deep residual learning for image recognition. arXiv; 2015.
12. Hekmatian E, Sharif S, Khodaian N. Literature review: digital subtraction radiography in dentistry. Dent Res J. 2005;2:1-8.
13. Hellen A, Jeon R, Abrams SH, Mandelis A, Amaechi BT. Photothermal and modulated luminescence detection of demineralized tooth restoration interfaces. Abstract # 529, IADR, 2008.
14. Horn AL. Comparison of Dexis CariVu to Traditional Bitewing Radiography for Diagnosis of Interproximal Caries (Doctoral Dissertation, University of Illinois at Chicago).
15. Kockanat A, Unal M. In vivo and in vitro comparison of ICDAS II, DIAGNOdent pen, CarieScan PRO and SoproLife camera for occlusal caries detection in primary molar teeth. Eur J Paediatr Dent. 2017;18:99-104.
16. Lussi A, Imwinkelried S, Pitts N, Longbotton C, Reich E. Performance and reproducibility of a laser fluorescence system for detection of occlusal caries in vitro. Caries Res. 1999;33:261-6.
17. Lussi A. Comparison of different methods for the diagnosis of fissure caries without cavitation. Caries Res. 1993;27:409-16.
18. Nassar HM, Yeslam HE. Current Novel Caries Diagnostic Technologies: Restorative Dentists' Attitude and Use Preferences Healthcare (Basel). 2021;9(10):1387.
19. Patel SA, Shepard WD, Barros JA, Streckfus CF, Quock RL. In vitro evaluation of Midwest Caries ID: A novel light-emitting diode for caries detection. Oper Dent. 2014;39:644-51.
20. Pretty IA. Caries detection and diagnosis: novel technologies. J Dent. 2006;34:727-39.
21. Sasidharan S, Meeral P R. Recent advances in dental caries diagnosis. Int J Community Dent. 2021;9:62-5.
22. Schneiderman A, Elbaum M, Shultz T, et al. Assessment of dental caries with digital imaging fiberoptic transillumination (DIFOTI): in vitro study. Caries Res. 1997;31:103-10.
23. Shi XQ, Welander U, Angmar-Månsson B. Occlusal caries detection with KaVo DIAGNOdent and radiography: an in vitro comparison. Caries Res. 2000;34:151-8.
24. Slimani A, Terrer E, Manton DJ, Tassery H. Carious lesion detection technologies: Factual clinical approaches. Br Dent J. 2020;229: 432-42.
25. Sonick M, Abrahams J, Faiella R. A comparison of the accuracy of periapical, panoramic, and computerized tomographic radiographs in locating the mandibular canal Int J Oral Maxillofac Implants. 1994;9:455.
26. Srilatha A, Doshi D, Kulkarni S, Reddy MP, Bharathi V. Advanced diagnostic aids in dental caries—A Review. J Global Oral Health. 2019;2(2):118-27.
27. Stookey G. Should a dental explorer be used to probe suspected carious lesions? No—use of an explorer can lead to misdiagnosis and disrupt remineralization. J Am Dent Assoc. 2005;136:1527, 1529, 1531.
28. White SC, Yoon DC. Comparative performance of digital and conventional images for detecting proximal surface caries. Dentomaxillofac Radiol. 1997;26:32-8.

CHAPTER

Early Childhood Caries and Rampant Caries

Nikhil Marwah, Gargi S Murthy, Mili Meghpara

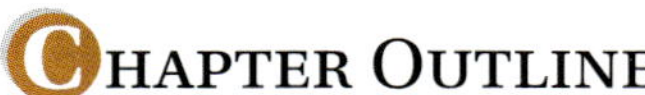

Chapter Outline

- Definitions
- Overview
- Developmental Stages
- Primary Etiological Risk Factors
- Secondary Etiological Risk Factors
- Prevention
- Barriers
- Rampant Caries

Caries in infants and young children was described as early as the middle of the last century. It is also been recognized as a clinical syndrome for decades. **Beltrami** characterized this pattern of early caries in young children in the 1930s as *les dents noire de tout-petits* or literally translated, "black teeth of the very young." In 1962, **Dr Elias Fass** published the first comprehensive description of caries in infants, which he termed as nursing bottle mouth. The first sentence of his paper begins, "Nothing is so shocking to dentist as the examination of child patient suffering from rampant caries," and this is particularly the thought we get on observing a child with nursing caries. Since that first description in 1962, the term nursing bottle mouth has been succeeded by many names, but only recently, have the original concepts been rethought. In 1994, conference at the centers for disease control and prevention recommended the use of a less specific term such as early childhood caries (ECC), because it was the consensus of the attendees that the link between bottle habits and caries was not absolute. However, this term did not negate the basic reasons for tooth demineralization in very young children—extensive exposure to a cariogenic diet and early infection with cariogenic bacteria.

Terminologies for ECC
- Nursing caries: Winter (1966)
- Tooth clearing neglect: Moss (1996)
- Infant and early childhood dental decay: Horowitz (1998)
- ECC: Davies (1998)
- MDSMD: Maternally derived *Streptococcus mutans* disease
- Baby bottle syndrome

DEFINITIONS

Davies (1998):[1] *Complex disease involving maxillary primary incisors within a month after eruption and spreading rapidly to other primary teeth is called childhood caries.*

Abid Ismail (1998):[2] *ECC is defined as occurrence of any sign of dental caries on the tooth surface during first 3 years of life.*

AAPD:[3] *The disease of* ECC *is the presence of* one *or more decayed (noncavitated or cavitated lesions), missing (due to caries), or filled tooth surfaces in any primary tooth in a child 71 months of age or younger. In children younger than 3 years of age, any sign of smooth-surface caries is indicative of severe early childhood caries (S-ECC). From ages 3–5,* one *or more cavitated, missing (due to caries), or filled smooth surfaces in primary maxillary anterior teeth or a decayed, missing, or filled score of ≥4 (age 3), ≥5 (age 4), or ≥6 (age 5) surfaces constitutes S-ECC.*

OVERVIEW

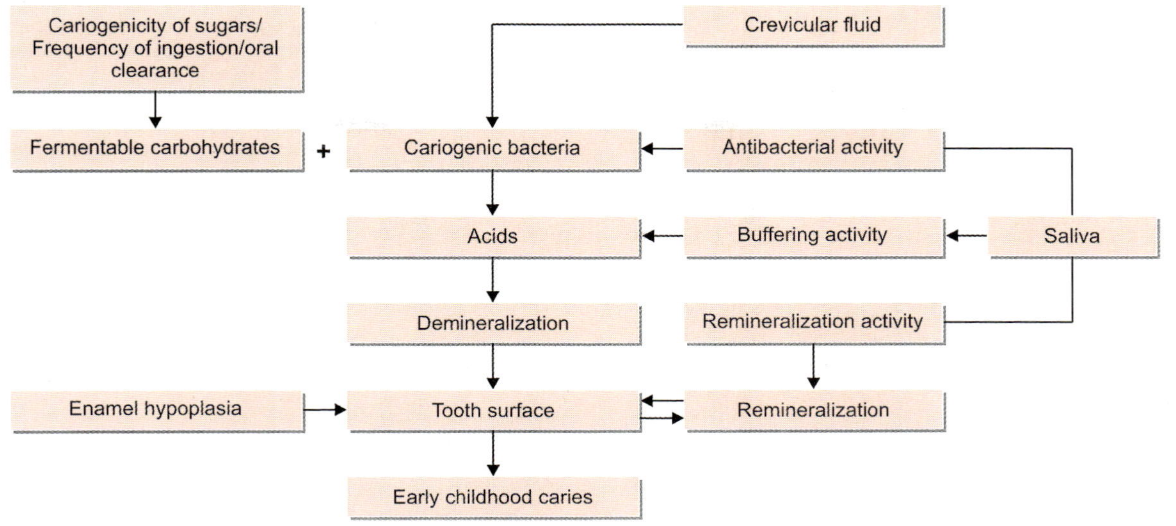

Classification of ECC by Wyne[4]

Type	*Clinical features*
Type I	• Mild-to-moderate • Existence of isolated carious lesion involving molars and incisors • Number of carious teeth increase as cariogenic challenge persists • Cause is usually a combination of cariogenic semisolid food and lack of oral hygiene • Seen in 2–5 years old
Type II	• Moderate-to-severe • Labiolingual carious lesion affecting maxillary incisors • Mandibular incisors are not affected • Use of feeding bottle or at will breastfeeding, or a combination of both with or without poor oral hygiene • Seen soon after eruption of teeth
Type III	• Severe • Carious lesions affecting all the teeth including lower incisors • Cause is cariogenic food and poor oral hygiene • Condition is rampant

AAPD in 2014 modified the definition of ECC

- *ECC is defined as the presence of one or more decayed (noncavitated or cavitated lesions), missing (due to caries), or filled tooth surfaces in any primary tooth in a child under the age of six.*
- *The definition of S-ECC is any sign of smooth-surface caries in a child younger than 3 years of age, and from ages 3–5, one or more cavitated, missing (due to caries), or filled smooth surfaces in primary maxillary anterior teeth, or a decayed, missing, or filled score of ≥4 (age 3), ≥5 (age 4), or ≥6 (age 5).*

DEVELOPMENTAL STAGES

Stage	*Clinical stage*	*Age*	*Features*
Stage I	Initial reversible stage **(Fig. 41.1)** Fig. 41.1: Initial reversible stage.	10–18 months	• Cervically and occasionally interproximal areas of chalky white demineralization • No pain
Stage II	Damaged carious stage **(Fig. 41.2)** Fig. 41.2: Damaged carious stage.	18–24 months	• Lesion in maxillary anterior teeth may spread to dentin and show yellowish brown discoloration • Pains on having cold food items

(Contd...)

(Contd...)

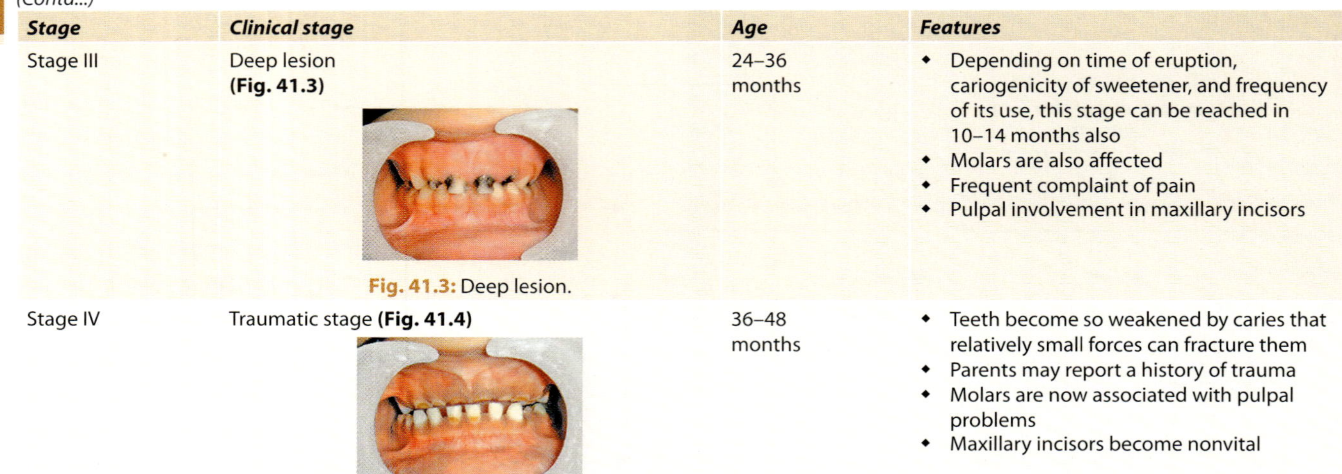

Stage	Clinical stage	Age	Features
Stage III	Deep lesion **(Fig. 41.3)** Fig. 41.3: Deep lesion.	24–36 months	• Depending on time of eruption, cariogenicity of sweetener, and frequency of its use, this stage can be reached in 10–14 months also • Molars are also affected • Frequent complaint of pain • Pulpal involvement in maxillary incisors
Stage IV	Traumatic stage **(Fig. 41.4)** Fig. 41.4: Traumatic stage.	36–48 months	• Teeth become so weakened by caries that relatively small forces can fracture them • Parents may report a history of trauma • Molars are now associated with pulpal problems • Maxillary incisors become nonvital

PRIMARY ETIOLOGICAL RISK FACTORS

Dental decay in infants and babies is now collectively known as ECC. Although the etiology of ECC is similar to that of other types of coronal smooth surface caries, the biology may differ in some respects. The bacterial flora and host defense systems in the young infant are in the process of being established; in addition, the tooth surfaces are newly erupted and immature and may show hypoplastic defects. Thus, in ECC, there may be an unique risk factor in infants and young children.

Dental Plaque

- Dental plaque is a structurally- and functionally-organized biofilm. It has a diverse microbial composition in health which remains relatively stable but changes in carious state.
- Although there are few studies on the formation and development of plaque in young children, relevant information may be extrapolated from *in vivo* studies in young adults.
- Besides modulation of the oral flora, the acquired pellicle has functions such as lubrication, protection from acid attack, prevention of crystal growth on enamel surfaces, and a role in enamel remineralization.
- In the absence of fermentable carbohydrates, organic acids such as acetate, propionate, and butyrate are produced. In contrast, when fermentable carbohydrates are present, lactate is mainly produced, which coincides with a pH drop in plaque.
- Bacteria and their alkaline products provide major contributions to the pH rise in plaque, and the base-generating metabolism of plaque bacteria is considered by many to be a significant determinant for cariogenicity of plaque.
- The presence of visible plaque and its early accumulation have been related to caries occurrence among children.[5] **Alaluusua** and **Malmivirta**[6] found that 91% of the children studied were correctly classified into caries risk groups, based solely on the presence or absence of visible plaque.

Mutans Streptococci

- As in other types of coronal dental decay, the main bacteria implicated in ECC are of the group now termed "mutans streptococci" of which the species *S. mutans* and *S. sobrinus* are most commonly isolated in human dental caries.
- **Virulence of mutans streptococci:** Mutans streptococci possess a wide range of cariogenic traits, which are significant determinants of the cariogenicity of plaque. These characteristics confer them with an ecological advantage over other oral bacteria.
  - Mutans streptococci synthesize α-1,3-rich water insoluble glucans from sucrose (**Tanzer et al.**[7] 1984). In addition to the mediation of irreversible adhesion and colonization of mutans streptococci to the teeth, these glucans increase the thickness of plaque, and result in enhanced rates of sugar diffusion and acid production at the deeper plaque layers (**Van Houte J et al.**,[8] 1985).
  - Synthesize intracellular polysaccharides (IPS), which support continual acid production during periods of low concentration of exogenous substrate. This activity maintains acidogenicity and fosters tooth demineralization during periods of low salivary secretion such as during sleep (**Spatafora G et al.**[9] 1995).
  - Mutans streptococci produce large amounts of acid, particularly lactic acid, which are potent in driving tooth demineralization (**Johnson ED et al.**, 1980).
  - The aciduricity or acid tolerance of the bacteria is extremely high, thus allowing colonization and persistence under cariogenic conditions.
  - Last, it has been suggested that the production of dextranase allows the invasion of mutans streptococci to replace earlier colonizing dextran-producing bacteria such as *S. sanguis* (**Tanzer JM,**[10] 1989).
- **Colonization of mutans streptococci in dental plaque:**
  - Initial attachment of the mutans streptococci is now thought to be independent of sucrose, and mediated by adhesions on the bacterial surface interacting directly with the salivary proteins.

- In the absence of sucrose, other bacteria such as *S. sanguis* have a higher affinity for pellicle-coated teeth than mutans streptococci. But in the presence of fermentable carbohydrates, especially sucrose, mutans streptococci irreversibly adhere to the pellicle through the synthesis of glucans mediated by glucosyltransferases produced by the bacteria (**Bowen WH et al.**, 1991; **Loesche WJ,**[11] 1986).
- *Candida albicans* which is frequently detected in oral cavity of children with ECC, develop a synergistic relationship with S. mutans when a sucrose rich diet is available, boosting formation of plaque biofilms, leading to aggressive onset of ECC. It is also said to be a relevant pathogen in caries progression.

❖ **Establishment of mutans streptococci in infants:**
- Most studies including predentate children show that mutans streptococci are usually not cultured from the oral cavity prior to the eruption of teeth. The reason for the low prevalence in predentate children may be related to the fact that mutans streptococci generally require non-shedding surface to colonize. Thus, the organisms are usually first detected when the first primary teeth emerge into the oral cavity, or when obturators for palatal clefts are inserted.
- The infection rate of mutans streptococci increases with age, as well as the number of teeth present in the infant's mouth. This probably reflects the increasing number of retentive sites for bacterial colonization.
- Infants acquire MS through vertical transmission from the oral cavity of the primary caregiver and horizontal transmission from other individuals in their immediate environment (**Caufield et al.** 2000).
- The age at which mutans streptococci are first acquired in infants is thought to influence their susceptibility to caries, i.e. the earlier colonization, the higher is caries risk (**Berkowitz RJ et al.,**[12] 1980; **Caufield PW,** 1993[13]).
- **Kohler**[14] conducted a study in 4-year-old children and found out that 89% of children colonized with mutans streptococci at the age of 2 years had a higher DMFT as compared to children who were noncolonized.

❖ **Transmission of mutans streptococci:**
- As mutans streptococci are predominantly found in the mouth, transmission is likely to be mediated via the saliva.
- Strong correlation between salivary mutans streptococci counts in mothers and their children have been reported. Salivary concentrations of 10^5 CFU (colony forming units) mutans streptococci/ mm of maternal saliva were associated with a 52% infection rate in their children, compared to only 6% infection rate when the maternal saliva concentration was 10^3 CFU or below (**Berkowitz RJ, et al.**[15] 1981).

Infant Feeding Patterns

- ❖ Reports suggest that putting a child to bed with a baby bottle is a widespread behavior, seen in 18–85% parents. A limited number of studies have examined reported bedtime bottle use in children with and without maxillary anterior decay, but many of these studies have been carried out in the dental office, potentially leading to bias.
- ❖ Although the use of bottle is predominant in children with ECC, but it is not the sole factor. Length of contact with the bottle at night time is also important. Greater length of bottle contact appears to be positively associated with caries.
- ❖ Although commonly believed to be the cause of maxillary anterior caries, use of a bedtime bottle appears to be highly prevalent in children with and without anterior caries, and there is evidence to support the conclusion that use of the bottle beyond the age of 1 is a major caries risk factor. It is seen that children with caries eliminate bottle use 4–7 months later than those without caries (**Marino RV et al.**[16] 1989).
- ❖ Contents of the bottle like sweetened milk, sugared beverages and juices are said to lead to ECC. Also, soda and sports drinks are implicated in ECC.
- ❖ Furthermore, children who are exclusively breastfed also appear to be susceptible to caries. These findings suggest that the role of the bottle in caries development is not as clear as previously thought, and further clarification of the association of infant feeding patterns and caries is required.

Tooth Brushing

- ❖ As ECC starts on surface that can be easily accessed by routine tooth brushing, oral hygiene levels may be associated with caries risk.
- ❖ Increased frequency and better oral hygiene levels are associated with lower caries levels in preschool children.
- ❖ A major problem confronting the investigation of the relationship between tooth brushing and ECC is the methodological issue of assessing the frequency of brushing, quality of plaque removal, and actual levels of oral hygiene.

Salivary Factors

- ❖ Saliva provides the main host defense systems against dental caries. It has major roles in the clearance of foods and the buffering of acid generated by dental plaque.
- ❖ Saliva also mediates selective adhesion and colonization of bacteria on tooth surface and contains several antimicrobial systems, which may aid in the elimination of bacteria.
- ❖ Saliva contains several antimicrobial proteins, including lysozyme, lactoferrin, agglutinins that are likely to be of significance in dental caries.
- ❖ Saliva also contains several organic compounds, which agglutinate oral bacteria and enhance their removal. These agglutinins include mucins, agglutinating glycoproteins, fibronectin, lysozyme, and secretory immunoglobulins.
- ❖ Flow rates of saliva are important as oral clearance, buffering capacity, and antimicrobial activities are largely dependent on this.

Sugars

❖ **General cariogenicity of sugars:**
- Sucrose, glucose, and fructose found in fruit juices and vitamin C drinks as well as in solids are probably the main sugars associated with infant caries.
- Sucrose, the most widely used sugar, is considered the most important in dental caries, as it is the only substrate used for bacterial generation of plaque dextrans (**Newbrun**[17] 1982). This is essential for bacterial adherence and thus facilitates the implantation of cariogenic bacteria in the oral cavity.

- **Frequency of consumption of sugars:**
  - There are now many studies which suggest that children with ECC have a high frequency of sugar consumption, not only of fluids given in the nursing bottle, but also of sweetened solid foods.
  - It is noted that increased frequency of eating sucrose increases the acidity of plaque and enhances the establishment and dominance of the aciduric mutans streptococci. The increased total time sugar is in the mouth increases the potential for enamel demineralization, and there is inadequate time for remineralization by saliva. As a result of this, demineralization becomes the predominant mechanism.

Oral Clearance of Carbohydrates

- In infants with ECC, the sleep time consumption of sugar is another common characteristic. The low salivary flow during sleep decreases oral clearance of the sugars and increases the length of contact time between plaque and substrates, thus increasing the cariogenicity of the substrate significantly.
- In this regard, **Hanaki M,et al.**[18] (1993) reported that clearance of glucose is slowest on the labial surfaces of the maxillary incisors and buccal surface of mandibular molars. These site differences in oral clearance may explain, in part, the distribution of the carious lesions in ECC, which are characteristically localized to the maxillary primary incisors and first molars.

Bovine Milk

- The cariogenicity of milk is often questioned because plain bovine milk is the common fluid placed in the feeding bottle in many cases of ECC and also because prolonged breastfeeding has been putatively associated with ECC.
- But most of the studies prove that milk is not cariogenic, and in fact, it may exhibit some cariostatic effect.
- *In vitro* studies showed that milk decreases the solubility of enamel, and these results have been extended by intraoral cariogenicity tests (ICT), which demonstrated that cheese extracts prevented enamel softening caused by sucrose.
- The mechanisms of protection by milk appear to work are decreasing demineralization and increasing remineralization of enamel, increasing the calcium and phosphate concentrations in plaque and increasing the acid buffering capacity of plaque.
- The main components of milk involved in reducing demineralization and increasing remineralization have been reported to be various forms of casein, namely, μ-casein and sodium caseinate.
- The mechanism involved is that α-casein may concentrate in the acquired pellicle and act as inhibitors of mutans streptococci adherence to saliva-coated hydroxyapatite and also reduce the adherence of *S. mutans* glucosyl transferases to saliva-coated hydroxyapatite (**Reynolds E,**[19] **et al.** 1995).

Human Milk

- There has been a paucity of studies reporting on the cariogenicity of human breast milk.
- Compared to bovine milk, human breast milk has a lower mineral content, higher concentration of lactose (7 vs 3%), and less protein (1.2 vs 3.3 g per 100 mL), but these differences are probably insignificant in terms of cariogenicity (**Drake SJ,** 1976).
- However, the relationship between breastfeeding and dental caries is likely to be complex, and confounded by many biological variables such as mutans streptococci infection, enamel hypoplasia, intake of sugars, as well as social variables such as education and socioeconomic status, which may affect behavior related to oral health.

Fluorides

- Although the benefits of water fluoridation and postnatal fluoride supplementation in the primary dentition are well known, there is minimal information on the cariostatic effects of topical fluoride in the early primary dentition, particularly in the prevention of ECC.
- The topical effects of fluoride are complex, and include changes on the mineral phases, as well the modulation of metabolic effects on mutans streptococci and other bacteria in dental plaque.
- Even at very low concentration, fluoride can affect the demineralizing process in a carious lesion by decreasing the rate of subsurface dissolution and enhancing the deposition of fluoridated apatite in the surface zone.
- In dental plaque, fluoride can act as a direct inhibitor of enzymes, which affects the metabolic activity of mutans streptococci. This reduces the acid tolerance of mutans streptococci by affecting the functioning of proton extruding ATPases, which results in cytoplasmic acidification and inhibition of glycolytic enzymes.

SECONDARY ETIOLOGICAL RISK FACTORS

Immunological Factors

- As the hard dental tissues are immunologically inactive, the host defense mechanism involved in dental caries is centered on the prevention of colonization and pathogenic activity of cariogenic bacteria.
- Host immune mechanisms include specific immune factors derived from saliva (secretory immunoglobulin A, sIgA), or serum and gingival crevicular fluid (immunoglobulin G, IgG) and nonspecific antimicrobial systems derived mainly from saliva.
- sIgA may inhibit bacterial adherence or agglutination, as well as neutralization of bacterial enzymes. Although the protective effects of sIgA in other mucosal areas are well known, there is little evidence that naturally occurring sIgA antibodies protect against dental caries (**Brandtzaeg P,**[20] 1979).

Tooth Maturation and Defects

- An important area in caries etiology, which is currently not well emphasized, is the area of tooth defects. Prevalence of enamel tooth defects in primary teeth range from 6-80%. Enamel tooth defect is said to be the single best predictor of ECC at 3 years (**Oliveira**[21] 2006). Enamel tooth defects are also associated with premature birth and low birth weight which in turn is associated with ECC. (**Lai et al** [22]1997).

- Tooth is most susceptible to caries in the period immediately after eruption and prior to final maturation. Thus, in many infants, a combination of recently erupted immature enamel in an environment of cariogenic flora with frequent ingestion of fermentable carbohydrates would render the tooth particularly susceptible to caries.
- In addition to lack of maturation, the presence of developmental structural defects in enamel may increase the caries risk.

Race and Ethnicity

- Children living in ethnic areas demonstrate an extremely high rate of ECC, ranging from 70% to 80%, despite efforts to educate parents to reduce baby bottle use.
- Single parent and complex family composition increases risk of caries (**Matilda**[23] 2000, **Schrodth and Cheba** 2007).
- South Asian children (6-18mn) where the care givers have prechewing food practices, caries rate is increased. (**Harrison**[24] 2007).
- **Milnes** notes that ECC is so pervasive among these children that parents consider it a normal childhood disease that affects all children. Some of the factors that have been postulated for this increased incidence of ECC are:
  - Increased risk that could be associated with cultural norms including concern for oral health.
  - Prenatal diet that could contribute to enamel hypoplasia.
  - Care of/for primary teeth.
  - Child rearing practices.
  - Access to dental and medical care.
  - Minorities may experience significant barriers to dental care, including cost of care and availability of accessible services.

Acidic Fruit Drink

It is now well known that acid in fruit juices and soft drinks may decrease the oral pH. In the presence of sugars in the drinks, this fall in pH is likely to enhance fermentation of carbohydrates and thus cause more profound enamel demineralization.

Socioeconomic Status

- Social class may influence caries risk in several ways
- Individuals from lower socioeconomic status experience financial, social, and material disadvantages that compromise their ability to care for themselves, obtain professional health care services, and live in a healthy environment, all of which lead to reduced resistance to oral and other diseases.

Dental Knowledge

- Dental knowledge is regarded as an important variable in the etiology of ECC because understanding the relationship between the microbiology of caries, the role of cariogenic foods, and use of baby bottle is necessary for prevention of ECC.
- But contrary to this thinking, there was a very interesting finding in this group, and it was that higher the knowledge of the caregiver more was the incidence of caries.
- Caregiver's who place high value on their own oral health will take children to the dentist (**Sohn** 2007).

Genetic Factors

There is a growing body of evidence suggesting the profound influence of genetic factors in dental caries susceptibility. Several genes and single nucleotide polymorphisms (SNPs) have been associated with early childhood caries. Eg- MMP20 rs1784418 SN single nucleotide polymorphisms (SNPs)'s association with protection against ECC in Saudi preschool children (**Al Marshad LK et al.**[25] 2021), frequency of rs10735810 CC genotype is higher in the high caries risk group Chinese children between 3-5 yrs.(**Qin X et al** [26] 2019).

Association between background factors (socioeconomical status, dietary habits, oral hygiene) and ECC

Authors	*Background factors associated*
Thitasomakul et al. (2009)	• Children aged 12–18 months • Low income • Mothers did not have a daily intake of milk • No calcium during pregnancy • Children who were breastfed • Mother's poor oral health status • Mothers had only primary school education • Mothers with 10 or more decayed teeth
	• Children who were not fed cooked rice or commercial cereal by the age of 3 months • Children who had soft drinks at 9 months • Children who had local traditional desserts at 9 months
	• Children who had started eating vegetables later than 6 months • Sweetened food • Sugary food by the age of 5 months • Soft drinks • Sugary snacks • Children who did not have their teeth brushed at 9 months
Nunn et al. (2009)	• Race • History of a child's visit to the dentist • Parent's education • Annual household income
Barnabé et al. (2010)	• Gini coefficient
Niji et al. (2010)	• Mother's age at childbirth (<22 years) • Frequency of between meal snacks >4 times a day • Child's caries activity tests score at the age of 1.5 years equal to or greater + 1.5
Tyagi (2008)	• Children who were bottle fed • Use of dummy/pacifier
Tiberia et al. (2007)	• Leaving the bottle with the child • Having problems brushing • Holding liquids in the mouth for prolonged time • Being Caucasian
Tellez et al. (2006)	• More grocery stores in the neighborhood—increase in dental caries • More churches in the neighborhood—decrease in dental caries
Feldens et al. (2010)	• Breastfeeding duration • Frequency of breastfeeding • Night-time bottle use for liquids other than milk • High density of sugar • High density of lipids • Maternal schooling • Per capita income • Teeth at 12 months

Stress

- One of the underlying mechanisms that could account for the effects of social class on oral health status is the increased stress experienced in families with financial and social instability related to lower socioeconomic status.
- **Brown** studied the relationship between caries and stress and demonstrated a positive relationship between parent's anxiety about dental treatment and children's caries levels. But the role of stress in ECC bears further investigation, particularly whether stress affects immunology, coping skills or preventive oral health behaviors.

Management

According to the AAPD guidelines, treatment approaches include:

- Chronic disease management aims to sustain oral health in the long term. This includes parent engagement to facilitate and promote preventive measures while encouraging the identification and reduction of individual risk factors.
- Active surveillance emphasizes careful monitoring of caries progression and prevention programs (e.g., frequent fluoride varnish applications) in children with incipient lesions.
- Minimal intervention approaches includes caries arrest with silver diamine fluoride, interim therapeutic restorations (ITR) that temporarily restore teeth in young children until a time when traditional cavity preparation and restoration is possible, and the use of Hall-style crowns.

PREVENTION

Early screening for signs of caries development, starting from the first year of life, could identify infants and babies showing the risk of developing ECC and could also assist in providing information of parents about how to promote oral health and prevent the development of tooth decay. High-risk children should be targeted with a professional preventive program that includes fluoride varnish application, fluoridated dentifrices, fluoride supplements, sealants, diet counseling, and chlorhexidine.

Prevention of ECC also requires addressing the social and economic factors that face many families where ECC is endemic. The education of mothers or caregivers to promote healthy dietary habits in infants has been the main strategy used for the prevention of ECC. There are three general approaches that have been used to prevent ECC; first is the community-based strategy that relies on educating mothers in the hope of influencing their dietary habits as well as those of their infants, second approach is based on the provision of examination and preventive care in dental clinics, the third involves the development of appropriate dietary and self-care habits at home.

According to American Academy of Pediatric Dentistry, the establishment of a dental home when the first tooth erupts is imperative to be able to implement preventive and early intervention treatments before advanced disease becomes established.

Recommendations for preventive maneuvers for early childhood caries

Interventions	*Target*
Chlorhexidine varnish	High-ECC risk groups
Dietary counseling	High-ECC risk groups
Early detection	All infants before the age of 1 year
Education	All infants and babies
Education	High-ECC risk communities
Fluoride supplements	High-ECC risk groups
Fluoride dentifrices	All infants and babies
Fluoride varnish	High-ECC risk groups
Prenatal fluoride supplements	All infants and babies
Sealants	High-ECC risk groups
Water fluoridation	Community
Xylitol substitutes	High-ECC risk groups
Control of mother-infant infection with cariogenic bacteria	High-ECC risk groups

RAPIDD Scale

- The readiness assessment of parents concerning infant dental decay (RAPIDD) Scale was developed to/assess a parent's stage of change precontemplative, contemplative, or action with regard to his/her child's dental health.
- This instrument based on the work by **Prochaska** and **DiClemente** measures pro and con parental beliefs about caring for their child's teeth. Parents in precontemplative stage show low openness and low health score, whereas those in action stage show high scores.
- RAPIDD scale consisted of 38 items with responses on 5-point scale ranging from strongly agree to strongly disagree. The patient or primary caretaker was instructed to select a box under one of the five categories after the interviewer read them the question in their native language. Each of the 38 items was placed into one of four constructs:
  1. Openness to health information.
  2. Valuing dental health.
  3. Convenience and change difficulty.
  4. Child permissiveness. In order to categorize respondents as precontemplators, contemplators, or action individuals, the responses to the questions within each construct were summed, these slimmed values were ranked, and percentiles were calculated for each individual within each construct.
- The RAPIDD instrument is a tool that is used to determine parent's stage of change for their child's oral health. Once a particular stage of change has been established the counselor then determines the best approach to move into next stage.

Community-based Education

- The goal of education is to increase the knowledge of mothers about ECC and to improve the dietary and nutritional habits of infants and mothers. It is assumed that an increase in the knowledge of mothers or caregivers will influence their self-care habits and dietary practices and, in turn, improves the dietary and oral hygiene habits of infants leading to the prevention of ECC.

- Positive changes in infant feeding practices have been found to be modest, even when a community educational program was designed and implemented in collaboration with members of a high ECC risk community.
- One such study was carried out a decade ago in American Indian and Alaskan native communities. The goal of the study was to reduce the number of children with ECC by 50% in a 5-year period. The study sites were divided into three intervention approaches— high, medium and low intensity. In the high-intensity sites, community coordinators of the project and parent volunteers were trained to administer the educational program on site directly by the project development team. In the medium-intensity sites, the coordinators only attended a training session organized by the development team of the project. In low-intensity sites, only the project educational material and guidelines were mailed and no training was provided. The educational program was designed to address the feeding problems identified in the communities—unwillingness of parents to wean children from the bottle, weaning a child to the bottle instead of a cup, and the lack of knowledge about ECC. The program included one-to-one counseling, where volunteers, health professionals, and employees from the community discussed ECC and its prevention with mothers or caregivers. The logo used in the project was appropriately labeled "Stop BBTD" (baby bottle tooth decay). After 3 years, there was 33% reduction in ECC prevalence in high-intensity sites, 18% in medium-intensity sites, and 27% in low-intensity sites.

Prevention of Transmission of Cariogenic Bacteria

- There is evidence that cariogenic bacteria are transmitted from mothers to their infants. Genotypes of mutans streptococci in infants appeared identical to those of the mothers in 71% of mother-infant pairs.
- A nonrandomized study divided mothers who had at least 10^6 mutans streptococci per mm of saliva into test and control groups. The test program included provision of dental education, oral hygiene instruction, dental treatment, tooth cleaning, application of 2% sodium fluoride, fluoride varnish. This program was started when the child was 3–8 months in age and continued until they reached the age of 3 years. On re-examination, it was found that children whose mothers were in the experimental group had a DMFT of 5.2, which was much lower as compared to the DMFT of control group, which was 8.6.[14]

Professional and Home-based Preventive Approaches

- Some of the professionally applied and home-based approaches that could be employed in the prevention of ECC are listed based on risk status **(Table 41.1).**

Table 41.1: Risk-based treatment methodology.

No signs of ECC or low-ECC risk status	***Signs of ECC or high-ECC risk status***
Fluoridated dentifrices	Fluoride varnish
Review of dietary and oral hygiene	Sealants
	Chlorhexidine varnish
	Xylitol pacifiers
	Fluoridated supplements and dentifrices
	Dietary counseling

- Professional treatment for ECC ranges from diet counseling to the prosthodontic rehabilitation of patient. Restorations are accomplished by GIC and composites, endodontic therapy is done as indicated followed by placement of crowns, and grossly decayed teeth are extracted followed by placement of space maintainers **(Figs. 41.5A to F).**

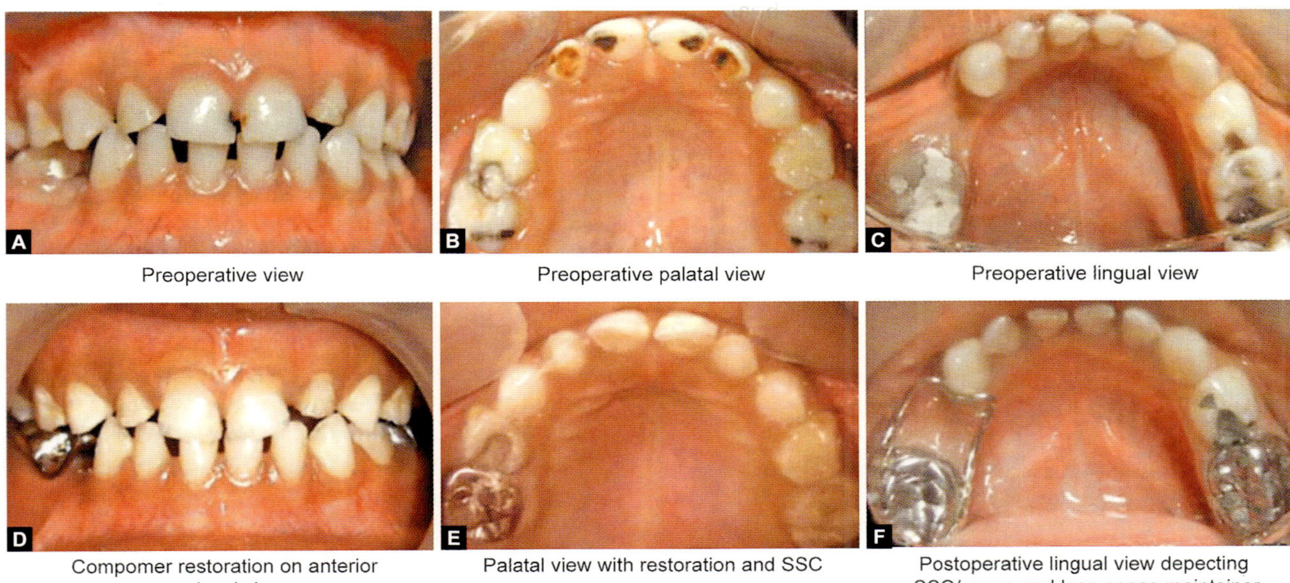

A
Preoperative view
B
Preoperative palatal view
C
Preoperative lingual view
D
Compomer restoration on anterior occlusal view
E
Palatal view with restoration and SSC
F
Postoperative lingual view depecting SSC/crown and loop space maintainer

Figs. 41.5A to F: Full mouth rehabilitation case: (A and B) Compomer restoration of central incisors; (C and D) Pulpectomy done IRT 54, 55 followed by stainless steel crown IRT 55; (E and F) Pulpectomy done IRT 75 and 85 followed by stainless steel crown and band and loop space maintainer IRT 75.

- The use of fluoride is done according to the level of fluoride in water **(Table 41.2)**.

Table 41.2: Recommended fluoride supplemental dosage schedule (mg F/day).

	Fluoride level in water		
Age	<0.3	0.3–0.7	>0.7
0–2	0.25	0.00	0.00
2–3	0.50	0.25	0.00
3–16	1.00	0.50	0.00

BARRIERS

Any proposal to improve social, mental, and physical health of children cannot be successful without adequate funding, political leadership, and support. Some of the potential barriers in providing optimum care for children are:

- Lack of involvement and commitment from dental and other health organizations.
- The dental community lacks a shared vision of the definition of the problem, how to prevent it, and who is responsible for planning and implementation.
- There is no integrated plan to fight the social, economic, and nutritional issues facing people in low socioeconomic group. There is weak direct support for research on epidemiology, etiology, and prevention of ECC.
- Dental health is not a priority of most programs and insurance packages.

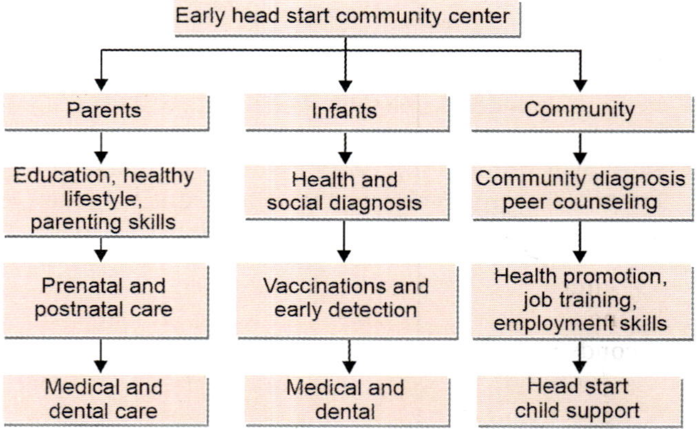

Model for prevention of early childhood caries

The literature on ECC is growing, but before real gains can be accomplished in preventing the onset and progression of ECC, investigators need to come to some consensus on the following issues:

- A definition of ECC specifying what constitutes ECC and its applicable age
- Need for larger, more representative epidemiological studies of ECC using heterogeneous populations.
- Longitudinal studies are needed to assess the natural history for the ECC
- Additional attention is needed to investigate baby bottle usage and its roles in the etiology of ECC
- ECC screening efforts should be integrated with pediatricians
- Additional attention needs to be paid to the role of professional dental care and access to dental care in the incidence, prevalence, and severity of ECC

RAMPANT CARIES

Caries in early stages of life is an unsolved enigma for most of us around the world. Rampant caries is the appearance of more than five new lesions in an individual of any age group in a year whereas nursing caries is any caries which occurs in children or may be attributed to bottle-feeding habit. The essence here is that nursing caries is a type of rampant caries. Nursing bottle caries is characterized by a rampant caries pattern initially involving maxillary deciduous anterior teeth; followed by posterior teeth and mandibular anterior teeth are usually spared. This condition is attributable to frequent prolonged contact with bottle containing sweet beverages or milk.

Massler (1945) *defined rampant caries as suddenly appearing, widespread, rapidly spreading, burrowing type of caries, resulting in early involvement of pulp and affecting those teeth, which are usually regarded as immune to decay.*

Winter et al. (1996) *defined rampant caries as caries of acute onset involving many or all the teeth in areas that are usually not susceptible. They further defined the condition to be associated with rapid destruction of crowns with frequent involvement of dental pulp.*

Terminologies for nursing caries:

- Nursing caries—**Winter** (1966)
- Nursing bottle mouth—**Kroll** (1967)
- Nursing bottle syndrome—**Shelton** (1977)
- Night bottle syndrome—**Dilley** (1980)
- Nursing bottle caries—**Tsintaosaurus** (1986)
- Baby bottle tooth decay—**Min Kelly** (1987)
- Milk bottle syndrome—**Ripa** (1988)

Rampant caries is of the following three types:

1. Nursing bottle rampant caries
2. Adolescent rampant caries and
3. Xerostomia-induced rampant caries

Clinical Appearance

- The pattern of rampant caries in the primary dentition is usually related to the order of tooth eruption with the exception of the mandibular primary incisor. The mandibular incisors are probably more resistant to caries because of their close proximity to the secretions of the submandibular salivary glands as well as the cleansing action of the tongue during the process of suckling the bottle.
- The initial lesion usually appears on the labial surface of the maxillary incisors, close to the gingival margins, as a whitish area of decalcification or pitting of the enamel surface shortly after eruption.
- These lesions soon become pigmented to a light yellow and, at the same time, extend laterally to the proximal surfaces and downward to the incisal edge **(Fig. 41.6)**.
- Less commonly, the decalcification may present initially on the palatal surfaces or even at the incisal edge in some extreme cases.
- At a more advanced stage, the carious process will often extend around the circumference of the tooth, leading to pathologic fracture of the crown on minimal trauma **(Fig. 41.7)**.

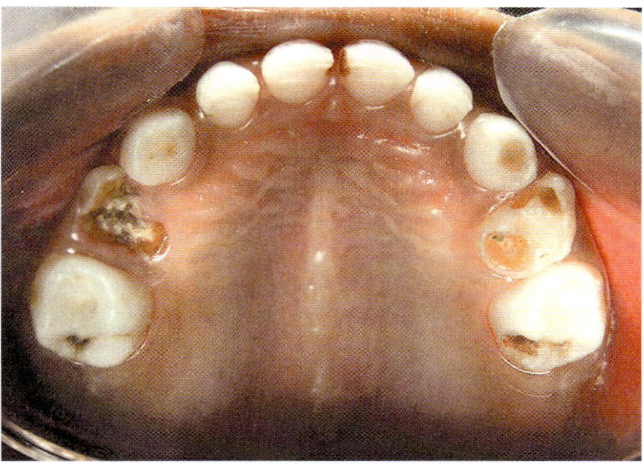

Fig. 41.6: Initial clinical appearance of rampant caries.

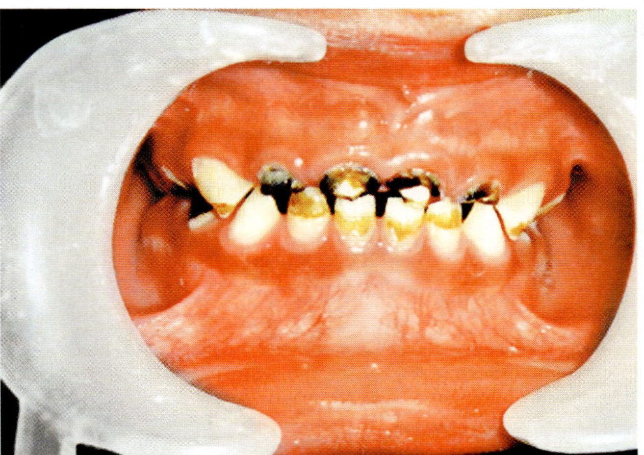

Fig. 41.7: Advanced clinical appearance of rampant caries..

- Other teeth, namely, the first primary molars, the second primary molars, and eventually the canines, will become involved.
- Nursing bottle caries is a form of rampant dental caries in the primary dentition of infants and children. In most cases, the problem is found in an infant who frequently falls asleep with a baby bottle filled with milk or sugar-containing substances like vitamin C syrup, sweetened fruit juice, or even carbonated drinks.
- The condition can also be associated with breastfed infants who have prolonged feeding habits or with children.
- Whose pacifiers are frequently dipped in honey, sugar, or syrup.
- The decrease in salivary flow rate during sleep, as well as the pooling of sweet fluids around the teeth, results in a highly cariogenic environment.
- Rampant caries may also occur in the permanent dentition of teenagers, because of their frequent intake of cariogenic snacks and sweet drinks between meals. Typical rampant caries in adolescents is characterized by buccal and lingual caries of premolars and molars and proximal and labial caries in the mandibular incisors.
- A specific form of rampant caries may occur in children and adolescents who have a greatly reduced salivary flow as a result of radiotherapy for the treatment of cancer of the head and neck region or as a result of the surgical removal of neoplasm in the oral cavity; this is called radiation caries.

Prevention and Treatment

- The type of treatment instituted for patients with rampant caries depends on the patients and parents motivation toward dental treatment, the extent of the decay, and the age and cooperation of the child. These factors should be assessed during the child's first few visits to the dentist.
- Initial treatment, including provisional restorations, diet assessment, oral hygiene instruction, and home and professional fluoride treatments, should be performed before any comprehensive restorative treatment commences.
- Caries stabilization and provisional restorations should be placed in symptom-free teeth with established dentinal caries to minimize the risk of pulpal exposure in the future and to improve function. However, in patients presenting with acute and severe signs and symptoms of gross caries, pain, abscess, sinus or facial swelling, immediate treatment is indicated.
- Because diet is one of the major factors in the initiation and development of caries, a dietary assessment should form a fundamental part of the examination. Parents should be educated to reduce the frequency of sucrose consumption by their child, especially between meals. Consumption of sugar-containing foods and beverages should be restricted to meal times. Parents can be instructed to record the amount and quantities of food and beverages consumed during and between meals for three consecutive days. Dietary vitamin supplements as well as oral medications must also be included.
- If bottle-feeding is still being practiced, particularly at night, it should be stopped by gradually diluting the bottle contents with water as well as decreasing the amount of added sugar over a 2 or 3-week period and finally substituting the bottle with a feeding cup.
- Young adults usually brush their teeth for less than 40 seconds and spend only 30% of the time on the caries-susceptible surfaces. Therefore, it is important to teach children the proper techniques of toothbrushing at different age groups. Generally speaking, children under the age of 8 years can best manage the circular scrub technique under parental supervision, whereas after the age of 11–12 years, the Bass technique can be taught.
- Both systemic and topical fluoride treatments are useful for preventing dental caries; the choice depends on the level of fluoride in the drinking water and the stage of development of the dentition **(Table 41.3)**. Children with a primary dentition will benefit from both fluoride tablets and the use of a small amount of fluoride toothpaste. The child should be encouraged to chew or suck the tablet, preferably at bedtime. This provides a topical effect on dental enamel of the erupted teeth followed by a systemic effect on developing enamel after swallowing.
- Once rampant caries is under control, comprehensive restorative treatment can be carried out **(Fig. 41.8)**. If the patient is seen at an early stage, when caries is still in the incipient or white spot stage, and there is minimal

Table 41.3: Fluoride treatment for children with rampant caries (0.3–0.7 ppm water fluoride level).

Type	*0–2 years*	*2–3 years*	*3–13 years*	*>13 years*
Dietary fluoride supplement	Not indicated	0.25 mg F daily	0.5 mg F daily	Not indicated
Operator-applied topical fluoride	APF topical solution or gel, 1.23% F, applied four times a year	APF topical solution or gel, 1.23% F, applied four times a year	APF topical solution or gel 1.23% F, applied four times a year	APF topical solution or gel, 1.23% F, applied four times a year
Self-applied topical fluoride	Not indicated	Not indicated	Self-application of gel-tray daily for approximately 4 weeks, thereafter continue with a daily fluoride rinse (0.05% NaF)	Self-application of gel-tray daily for approximately 4 weeks, thereafter continue with a daily fluoride rinse (0.05% NaF)
Fluoride dentifrice	Brush with F-containing dentifrice	Brush with F-containing dentifrice	Brush with F-containing dentifrice	Brush with F-containing dentifrice

(APF: acidulated phosphate fluoride; NaF: sodium fluoride)

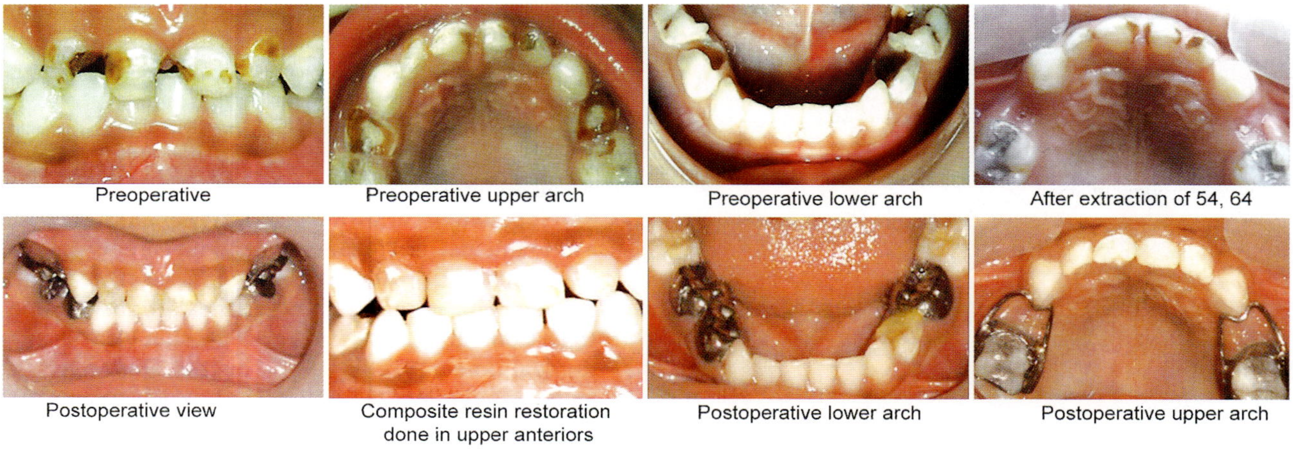

Preoperative

Preoperative upper arch

Preoperative lower arch

After extraction of 54, 64

Postoperative view

Composite resin restoration done in upper anteriors

Postoperative lower arch

Postoperative upper arch

Fig. 41.8: Full mouth rehabilitation of rampant caries patient.

or no loss of enamel surface integrity, an improvement in oral hygiene technique, a change in dietary habits, and weekly home or professionally applied topical fluoride therapy will help arrest the lesions, and the need for restorations may be obviated. Unfortunately, dental treatment is only sought for most children with rampant caries when extensive cavitation has occurred and restorative treatment is required. Acid-etched composite resin restorations can be used to restore anterior maxillary teeth whereas pedo-form strip crowns, which are more esthetic, functional, and durable, are indicated in anterior teeth with gross caries and extensive coronal destruction. Alternatively, glass-ionomer cement, which adheres to enamel and dentin as well as releases fluoride, can also be used as the restorative material; however, the results are esthetically less pleasing than those achieved with composite resin restorations. Acid-etched composite resin restorations, glass-ionomer-silver cermet cements, and stainless steel crowns can be used to store the posterior teeth. Depending on the extent of the lesions, pulpotomies, pulpectomies, or extraction may be indicated. Where extractions of teeth have been carried out, a prosthesis should be provided for maintenance, function, and esthetics. Rampant caries is a distressing clinical condition confronting the child, parents and dentist. With the advances in knowledge about the etiology and pathogenesis of dental caries, rampant caries can now be prevented.

Age-specific Prevention of Rampant Caries

Dentition: 0–5 years	
Advice therapy	Diet counseling with parents on good nursing techniques • Toothpaste • Fluoride tablets, if in area without water fluoridation • Professional topical fluoride application every 6 months
Control	• Oral hygiene instructions to parents • Toothbrushing with parental supervision • 6-month recall

(Contd...)

(Contd...)

Dentition: 5–12 years	
Advice therapy	Diet counseling with parents and patients ◆ Toothpaste ◆ Fluoride tablets up to 8 years if in area without water fluoridation ◆ Mouth rinse ◆ Professional topical fluoride application every 6 months
Control	◆ Oral hygiene instructions to patient ◆ Toothbrushing without parental supervision ◆ Sealants ◆ 6-month recall
Permanent dentition: 12 years onward	
Advice therapy	Diet counseling with parents and patients ◆ Toothpaste ◆ Mouth rinse ◆ Professional topical fluoride application every 6 months ◆ Oral hygiene instructions to patient
Control	◆ Toothbrushing ◆ Interdental cleaning with floss ◆ Sealants

The Rampant Caries Control Program (RCCP)[27] was established in January 2003 at the University of Iowa College of Dentistry to manage patients with high caries activity, with the goal of helping them control the disease throughout life.

It has three phases:

I. Phase I disease control has three important components: (1) acute/emergency treatment, (2) operative treatment, and (3) chemotherapeutic agents and preventive treatment. The first component, acute/emergency treatment, such as root canal therapy, is provided only if necessary to address emergency needs. Extractions are also completed for any tooth that cannot be restored.

II. Operative treatment, the second component, is based on caries management by individual risk assessment. This phase consists of caries risk assessment, caries removal and placement of transitional restorations, and sealants.

III. In the third component—chemotherapeutic agents and preventive treatment—individualized prevention is provided at both the dental visit and through home care.

Successful management of rampant caries depends on a coordinated team approach among the pediatrician, pediatric dentist, parents, and child. The pediatrician should educate the parents about good nursing and dietary habits and the importance of good oral hygiene to their child's teeth and should encourage parents to bring their child to the dental office before he or she is 12 months of age for a screening examination and counseling, because pediatricians are often the first medical personnel to see the newborn baby. Pediatric dentists, who are more experienced in the implementation of preventive and restorative dentistry to infants and young children, should play a vital role in the management of rampant caries in children. However, interest and cooperation from the parents and children are equally important. Consequently, educational efforts should be emphasized and reinforced, especially in areas where the prevalence of rampant caries is high.

POINTS TO REMEMBER

- First terminology used for ECC was nursing caries by Winter (1966).
- The term ECC was given by Davies (1998).
- The newest term according to its causative agent is called MDSMD—maternally derived S. mutans disease.
- The disease of ECC is defined as presence of one or more decayed, missing or filled tooth surfaces in any primary tooth in a child 71 months of age or younger.
- The various stages in development of ECC lesion are initial reversible stage, damaged carious stage, deep lesion, traumatic stage.
- Risk factors for ECC include dental plaque, mutans streptococci, stress, dental knowledge, socioeconomic status, race and ethnicity, tooth maturation and defects, immunological factors, bovine milk, oral clearance of carbohydrates, cariogenicity of sugars, tooth brushing, and infant feeding patterns.
- Mutans streptococci is most prevalent in dental caries because it synthesize α-1,3-rich water insoluble glucans from sucrose which increase the thickness of plaque, and result in enhanced rates of sugar diffusion and acid production at the deeper plaque layers; IPS, which support continual acid production; produce large amounts of lactic acid, which are potent in driving tooth demineralization; production of dextranase allows the invasion of mutans streptococci to replace earlier colonizing dextran-producing bacteria such as Streptococcus sanguinis; mutans streptococci irreversibly adhere to the pellicle through the synthesis of glucans mediated by glucosyltransferases produced by the bacteria.
- Use of baby bottle is not the sole factor for ECC. Length of contact with the bottle at night-time is also important. Greater length of bottle contact appears to be positively associated with caries. Use of the bottle beyond the age of 1 is a major caries risk factor.
- Milk is not cariogenic, and in fact, it may exhibit some cariostatic effect.
- Nursing bottle caries is a type of rampant caries.
- Massler (1945) defined rampant caries as suddenly appearing, widespread, rapidly spreading, burrowing type of caries, resulting in early involvement of pulp and affecting those teeth, which are usually regarded as immune to decay.
- Initial lesion appears on the labial surface of the maxillary incisor as a whitish area of decalcification. In advanced stage, the carious process will often extend around the circumference of the tooth, leading to pathologic fracture in anterior teeth and deep caries in posterior teeth.
- A specific form of rampant caries may occur in children who have a greatly reduced salivary flow as a result of radiotherapy; this is called radiation caries.
- The treatment for rampant caries extends from dietary counseling to endodontic therapy followed by crowns.

Questionnaire

1. Define and classify early childhood caries.
2. What are the developmental stages of ECC?
3. Explain the primary and secondary etiological factors of ECC.
4. Describe the role of mutans streptococci in ECC.
5. Describe the management of a child with ECC.
6. What are the barriers in treatment of caries?
7. Explain the fluoride protocol for ECC patients.
8. Define rampant caries.
9. Give the clinical features and treatment options for rampant caries.
10. What is the fluoride regimen for children with rampant caries?

REFERENCES

1. Davies GN. Early childhood caries: a synopsis. Community Dent Oral Epidemiol. 1998;26(Suppl 1):106-16.
2. Selwitz RH, Ismail AI, Pitts AI. Dental caries. Lancet. 2007;369:51-9.
3. American Academy of Pediatric Dentistry. Symposium on the prevention of oral disease in children and adolescents. Chicago, IL, November 11-12, 2005: conference papers. Pediatr Dent. 2006;28:96-198.
4. Wyne AH. Early childhood caries: nomenclature and case definition. Community Dent Oral Epidemiol. 1999;27:313-5.
5. Tinanoff N, Kanellis MJ, Vargas CM. Current understanding of the epidemiology mechanisms, and prevention of dental caries in preschool children. Pediatr Dent. 2002;24:543-51.
6. Alaluusua S, Malmivirta R. Early plaque accumulation, a sign for caries risk in young children. Community Dent Oral Epidemiol. 1994;22:273-6.
7. Tanzer JM, Freedman ML, Fitzgerald RJ. Virulence of mutants defective in glycosyltransferase, dextran-mediated aggregation, or dextran activity. In: Mergenhagen S, Rosan B, editors. Molecular basis of oral microbial adhesion. Washington, DC: American Society for Microbiology; 1984. pp. 204-11.
8. Van Houte J, Russo J, Prostak KS. Increased pH-lowering ability of *Streptococcus mutans* cell masses associated with extracellular glucan-rich matrix and the mechanisms involved. J Dent Res. 1989;68:4511-9.
9. Spatafora G, Rohrer K, Barnard D, Michalek S. A *Streptococcus mutans* mutant that synthesizes elevated levels of intracellular polysaccharide in hypercariogenic *in vivo*. Infect Immun. 1995;63:2556-63.
10. Tanzer JM. On changing the cariogenic chemistry of coronal plaque. J Dent Res. 1989;68(Spec Iss):1576-87.
11. Loesche WJ. Role of *Streptococcus mutans* in human dental decay. Microbiol Rev. 1986;50:353-80.
12. Berkowitz RJ, Jordan HV, White G. The early establishment of *Streptococcus mutans* in the mouth of infants. Arch Oral Biol. 1975;20:171-4.
13. Caufield PW, Cutter GR, Dasanayake AP. Initial acquisition of mutans streptococci by infants: evidence for a discrete window of infectivity. J Dent Res. 1993;72:37-45.
14. Kohler B, Andreen I, Johnson B. Earlier is the colonization of mutans streptococci higher is the incidence of caries in a 4-year-old children. Oral Microbiol Immunol. 1988;3:14-7.
15. Berkovitz RJ, Turner G, Green P. Maternal salivary levels of mutans and primary oral infections in infants. Arch Oral Biol. 1981; 26:17-9.
16. Marino RV, Bomze K, Scholl TO, Anhalt H. Nursing bottle caries: characteristics of children at risk. Clin Pediatr. 1989;28:129-31.
17. Newbrun E. Sugar and dental caries: a review of human studies. Science. 1982;217:418-23.
18. Hanaki M, Nakagaki H, Nakamura H, et al. Glucose clearance from different surfaces of human central incisors and the first molars. Arch Oral Biol. 1993;38:479-82.
19. Reynolds EC, Cain CJ, Webber FL, et al. Anticariogenicity of calcium phosphate complexes of tryptic casein phosphopeptides in the rat. J Dent Res. 1995;74:1272-9.
20. Brandtzaeg P. The oral secretory immune system with special emphasis on its relation to dental caries. Proc Finn Dent Soc. 1979. pp.71-84 .
21. Oliveira AFB, Chaves AMB, Rosenblatt A. The Influence of Enamel Defects on the Development of Early Childhood Caries in a Population with Low Socioeconomic Status: A Longitudinal Study. Caries Res 2006;40:296-302.
22. Lai PY, Seow WK, Tudehope DI, Rogers Y. Enamel hypoplasia and dental caries in very-low birthweight children: a case-controlled, longitudinal study. Pediatr Dent. 1997;19(1):42-9.
23. Mattilda M, Rautava P, Sillanpaa M, Paunio P. 2000. Caries in 5 year old children and associations with family related factors. J Dent Res. 79(3):875-81.
24. Harrison R, Benton T, Everson-Stewart S, Weinstein P. Effect of motivational interviewing on rates of early childhood caries: a randomized trial. Pediatr Dent. 2007;29(1):16-22.
25. AlMarshad LK, AlJobair AM, Al-Anazi MR, et al. Association of polymorphisms in genes involved in enamel formation, taste preference and immune response with early childhood caries in Saudi pre-school children. Saudi Journal of Biological Sciences. 2021;28(4):2388-2395.
26. Qin X, Shao L, Zhang L, Ma L, Xiong S. Investigation of interaction between vitamin D receptor gene polymorphisms and environmental factors in early childhood caries in Chinese children. Biomed Res Int. 2019;2019:431.
27. Guzmán-Armstrong S, Warren JJ. Management of high caries risk and high caries activity patients: rampant caries control program (RCCP). J Dent Educ. 2007;71:767-75.

FURTHER READING

1. American Academy of Pediatric Dentistry. Infant oral health care. Pediatr Dent. 1994;16:29.
2. American Academy of Pediatric Dentistry. Policy on early childhood caries (ECC): Unique challenges and treatment options. The Reference Manual of Pediatric Dentistry. Chicago, Ill.: American Academy of Pediatric Dentistry; 2021:85-6.
3. Berkowitz RJ, Jordan HV, White G. The early establishment of Streptococcus mutans in the mouth of infants. Arch Oral Biol. 1975;20:171-4.
4. Berkowitz RJ, Turner J, Green P. Maternal salivary levels of Streptococcus mutans and primary oral infection of infants. Arch Oral Biol. 1981;26:147-9.
5. Boue D, Armau E, Tiraby G. A bacteriological study of rampant caries in children. J Dent Res. 1987;66:23-8.
6. Darke SJ. Human milk versus cow's milk. J Hum Nutr. 1976;30:233-8.
7. Derkson GD, Ponti P. Nursing bottle syndrome: prevalence and etiology in a non-fluoridated city. J Can Dent Assoc. 1982;48:389-93.
8. Fass EN. Is bottle feeding of milk a factor in dental caries? Dent Child. 1962;29:245-51.
9. Firestone AR. Effects of increasing contact time of sucrose solution of powdered sucrose on plague pH *in vivo*. J Dent Res. 1982;61:124-34.
10. Hackett AF, Rugg-Gunn AJ, Murray JJ, et al. Can breastfeeding cause dental caries? Hum Nutr Appl Nutr. 1984;38:23-8.
11. Hamada S, Slade HD. Biology, immunology and cariogenicity of Streptococcus mutans. Microbiol Rev. 1980;44:331-84.
12. Ismail AI. Fluoride supplements: current effectiveness, side effects and recommendations. Community Dent Oral Epidemiol. 1994;22:164-72.
13. Johnsen DC, Gerstenmaier JH, DiSantis TA, et al. Susceptibility of nursing-caries children to future approximal molar decay. Pediatr Dent. 1986;8:168-70.
14. Keyes PH, Jordan HV. Factors influencing the initial transmission and inhibition of dental caries. In: Harris RS(Ed). Mechanisms of Hard Tissue Destruction. New York, NY: NY Acad. Pr.; 1963.pp. 261-83.
15. Kohler B, Andreen I, Jonsson B, et al. Effect or caries preventive measure on Streptococcus mutans and Lactobacilli in selected mothers. Scand J Dent Res. 1982;90:102-8.
16. Kohler B, Birkhed D, Olsson S. Acid production of human strains of *Streptococcus mutans* and *Streptococcus sobrinus*. Caries Res. 1995;29:402-6.

17. Kotlow LA. Breastfeeding: a cause of dental caries in children. J Dent Child. 1977;44:192-3.
18. Mandal ID. Functions of saliva. Dent Res. 1987;66:623-7.
19. Marino RV, Bomze K, Scholl TO, et al. Nursing bottle caries, characteristics of children at risk. Clin Pediatr. 1989;28: 129-31.
20. Milnes AR, Bowden GHW. The microflora associated with developing lesions of nursing caries. Caries Res. 1985;19:289-97.
21. National Foundation of Dentistry for the Handicapped. A guide to the use of fluoride for the prevention of dental caries with alternative recommendations for patients with handicaps. J Am Dent Assoc. 1986;113:515,522,531,535.
22. Richardson BD, Cleaton-Jones PE, McInnes PM, et al. Infant feeding practices and nursing bottle caries. J Dent Child. 1981;48:423-9.
23. Ripa JW. Nursing caries: a comprehensive review. Pediatr Dent. 1988;10:268-82.
24. Rugg-Gunn AJ. Fluorides in the prevention of caries in the preschool children. J Dent. 1990;18:304-7.
25. Seow WK. Bottle caries: a challenge for preventive dentistry. Dent Today. 1987;3:1-9.
26. Van Houte J, Gibbs G, Butera C. Oral flora of children with "nursing bottle caries". J Dent Res. 1982;61:382-5.
27. Van Houte J. Bacterial specificity in the etiology of dental caries. Int Dent J. 1980;30:305-26.
28. Winter GB, Hamilton MC, James PMC. The role of the comforter as an aetiological factor in rampant caries of the deciduous teeth. Arch Dis Child. 1966;41:202-12.
29. Winter GB, Hamilton MC, James PMC. Role of the comforter as an etiological factor in rampant caries of the deciduous dentition. Arch Dis Child 1966;417:207-21.

CHAPTER 42

Molar Incisor Hypomineralization

Ramesh K, Seema Bargale, Maya Ramesh, Nidhi Gupta

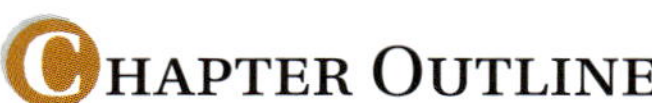

CHAPTER OUTLINE

- Evolution of Terminology
- Histopathology
- Etiological Factors
- Prevalence and Global Impact
- Clinical Presentation
- Differential Diagnosis
- Clinical Management

A developmental dental defect of enamel is one of the clinical challenges, which can affect the quality of life, as well as pose treatment challenges. Molar incisor hypomineralization (MIH) is one such defect, which is showing an increasing trend in the last two decades. Disturbances arising during any of the stages of enamel formation are exhibited as hypomineralized and hypoplastic defects. In 1982 FDI coined two distinct terminologies for the defects in enamel as: (1) Qualitative defect of enamel with clinically abnormal translucency of enamel as in case of MIH; (2) Quantitative defect of enamel as in enamel hypoplasia **(Fig. 42.1).**

Molar incisor hypomineralization (MIH) is a human dentition developmental abnormality that damages the enamel of the first permanent molars and can also affect the incisors. The second permanent molars and premolars are usually unaffected. Hypomineralized second primary molars (HSPMs) have been linked to MIH, and HSPMs can be used as a predictor of MIH.

Molar incisor hypomineralization *is a systemic disorder defined as a qualitative enamel deficiency of systemic origin that affects at least one first permanent molar and can also be associated with permanent incisors.*

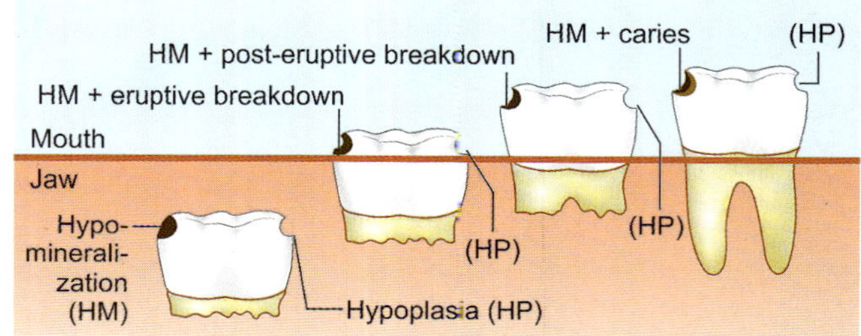

Fig. 42.1: Difference between hypoplasia and hypomineralization.

Weerheijm KL et al., *defined it as hypomineralization of systemic origin, presenting as demarcated, qualitative defects of enamel of one to four first permanent molars frequently associated with affected incisors.*

EVOLUTION OF TERMINOLOGY

Since roughly 1970, this illness has been recognized and characterized using a number of terminologies like non-fluoride enamel opacities, internal enamel hypoplasia, non-endemic mottling of enamel, idiopathic enamel opacities and cheese molars. In 2001 **Weerheijm KL et al.,**[1] came out with a distinct terminology MIH and it is still the most used term.

HISTOPATHOLOGY

The enamel matrix serves as a molecular framework and an essential step for the arrangement of the crystals in the enamel. This crystal skeleton, arranges the phosphate and calcium ions as hydroxyapatite. Approximately, the time taken for enamel formation is close to one thousand days, of which two-third is dedicated for the maturation process. The very important stage in child's life is the duration up to the age of one year, during which the maturation process takes place for the permanent first molars, incisors and primary second molars. Time taken for maturation is also slightly more for the molars compared to the incisors, so the chances of involvement of only permanent molars are very high when compared to the permanent incisors.

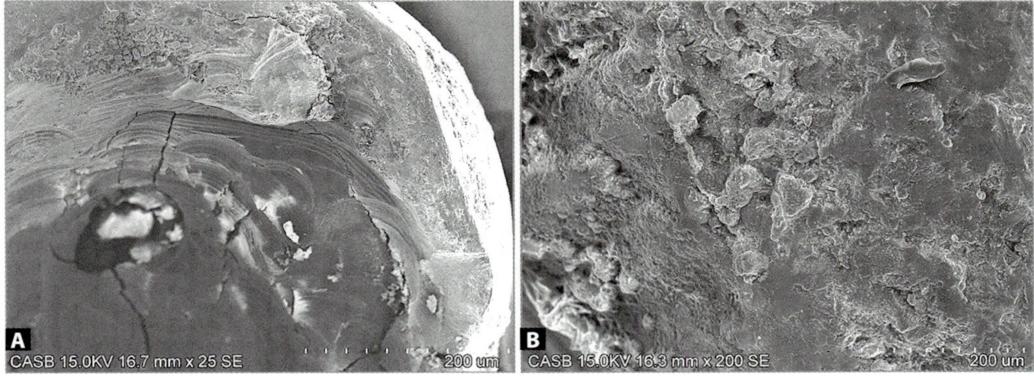

Figs. 42.2A and B: SEM of surface of MIH showing loose and less dense prism.

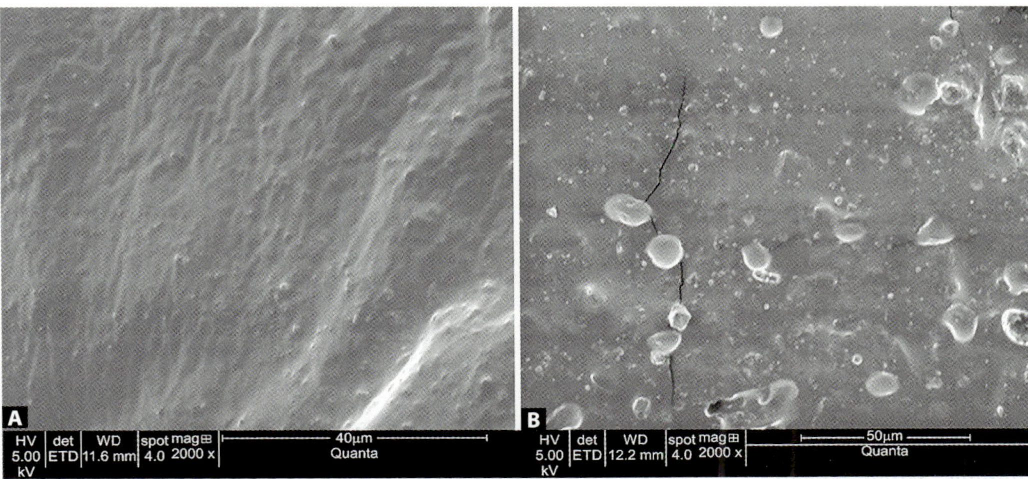

Figs. 42.3A and B: SEM enamel permeability of normal enamel and of MIH.

- A significant loss of mineral content in MIH affected area compared to the adjacent normal enamel.
- The Ca:P ratio was not found to be altered much compared to the normal enamel.
- The enamel permeability on MIH affected teeth was assessed with SEM, there was presence of high amount of droplets on the surface of MIH affected teeth when compared to the adjacent normal enamel.
- An increase in enamel permeability, which can contribute as one of the risk factor for dental caries.[2]
- Presence of more protein content in severe MIH.[3]
- When the amount of carbon content was evaluated, it was found to have more carbon and carbonate concentration in MIH affected area compared to the normal enamel.[3]
- **MIH and enamel:** Several researchers have explored the surface of enamel in MIH, which has shown high percentage of porosity ranging from 5% to 25 % compared to the adjacent normal enamel **(Figs. 42.2A and B)**. Scanning electron microscopic images under magnification showed less dense prism structures, which are loosely packed with partial loss of prismatic patterns, less distinct prism borders, more marked interprismatic space, and wider sheath regions. It has also shown high enamel permeability compared to the adjacent normal enamel in SEM studies **(Figs. 42.3A and B)**. The mechanical properties of enamel are depleted compared to the healthy enamel, leading to failure of retention of restorations. There is also lack of hardness and modulus of elasticity of enamel, the property that is caused due to the alteration in the mineral density.
- **MIH and pulp dentin complex:** Dentine sensitivity is one of the chief complaints in children with MIH. As enamel is more porous in nature it exposes the dentin to various thermal, mechanical and osmochemical stimuli. This can also favor ingress of bacterial contaminants leading to a state of hyperemic pulp, thereby resulting in chronic inflammation of the pulp. This can further cause morphological and cytochemical neuronal changes, with an overexpressed dentin sensitivity. This is exhibited in children as difficulty in brushing of teeth affected with MIH leading to early involvement of dental caries.

ETIOLOGICAL FACTORS (GEMS)

- Unlike other dental diseases, etiology of MIH is also considered to be of multifactorial with genetic, environmental, medical and systemic factors **(Table 42.1)**. It can be caused due to a single or multiple factors occurring at a specific time of tooth formation.
- In a quest to identify the main etiology for MIH, it has been observed in recent research that there exists no single

Table 42.1: Various etiological factors of MIH.

Genetic	Environmental	Medical	Systemic
D1X gene	Nutritional deficiency	Preterm baby	Severe malnutrition
RUNX2 gene	Low socioeconomic status	Prolonged delivery cyanosis	Maternal diabetes
Kallikrein 4	Vaccines	Neonatal hypocalcemia, vitamin D deficiency	Thyroid and parathyroid problems
MMP-20 (enamelysin protein)	Dioxins in breast milk	Febrile illness	Chronic systemic diseases
	Antibiotics	Respiratory and infectious diseases, chickenpox	Bilirubinemia

causative factor and mostly its complex in nature with a significant contribution from genetic factors.[4]

- A recent gene study evaluating various genes *AMELX, ENAM, AMBN* and *MMP20* involved in amelogenesis have shown a strong genetic association.[5]
- Combination of genetic predisposition, environmental and systemic causes would be expected to affect teeth in a stable, temporal pattern. The number of teeth, degree of involvement of MIH and variable lesion presentation and characteristics between teeth and within single teeth remain uncertain.[6]
- Evidences were inconclusive when it is related to prenatal factors except in case of some unspecified maternal illness. The perinatal conditions includes hypoxia, cesarean section and premature birth and postnatal factors like chronic medical conditions like measles, urinary tract infection, bronchitis, otitis media, gastric disorders and respiratory diseases like asthma and pneumonia.
- Childhood fever and use of antibiotics also contribute to the etiology.
- Maternal factors like prolonged breastfeeding, low birth weight, smoking, alcohol consumption were not associated with MIH.
- Thus it can be concluded that systemic and epigenetic/genetic factors acting synergistically or additively is the likely cause of MIH.[7]

PREVALENCE AND GLOBAL IMPACT OF MIH

- MIH affects 3–40% of the population; with the global prevalence reported around 12.9% (11.7–14.3%).
- The prevalence reports from India ranges from 2% to 27%.
- The most involved tooth is 95%.
- First permanent molars followed by the permanent incisors.
- Female and male predilection ranged from 0.81% to 1.04%.
- Treatment needs was seen in 23.5–31.7%.
- Prevalence of MIH is assessed with different scoring criteria but the most reliable and appropriate method of evaluation is by using the European Academy of Pediatric Dentistry (EAPD) by **Ghanim et al**,.[8] 2011 and the scoring criteria was further modified to quantify the severity, the number of involved teeth, type and extent of the MIH in 2015 **(Table 42.2)**.

Table 42.2: EAPD Criteria for data recording of MIH (Ghanim et al. 2015[8]).

MIH/HSPM clinical data recording sheet— First permanent molars, permanent incisors, and second primary molars (short form)
0 = No visible enamel defect
1 = Enamel defect, not MIH/HSPM
2 = White/creamy or yellow/brown demarcated opacities
3 = PEB
4 = Atypical restoration
5 = Atypical caries
6 = Missing sue to MIH/HSPM
7 = Cannot be scored*
MIH/HSPM clinical data recording sheet—permanent and primary dentitions (long form)
0 = No visible enamel defect
1 = Enamel defect, not MIH/ HSPM
11 = Diffuse Opacities
12 = Hypoplasia
13 = Amelogenesis imperfecta
14 = Hypomineralization defect (not MIH/HSPM)
2 = Demarcated opacities
21 = White/creamy demarcated opacities
22 = Yellow/brown demarcated opacities
3 = PEB
4 = Atypical restoration
5 = Atypical caries
6 = Missing sue to MIH/HSPM
7 = Cannot be scored*
Lesion Extension Criteria (Index teeth only, scores 2 to 6)
I = Less than 1/3rd of tooth affected
II = Atleast 1/3rd but less than 2/3rd of the tooth affected
III = Atleast 2/3rd of the tooth affected

CLINICAL PRESENTATION OF MIH

- MIH presents clinically as white opaque to yellowish brown areas with a characteristic feature of well-demarcated and distinct borders from the adjacent normal enamel **(Fig. 42.4)**. Discoloration of the affected areas is caused by a change in the optical character of the hypomineralized enamel due to a decrease in mineral content and an increase in protein and water content. The color of the enamel might alter from white opaque lesions to a creamy yellow or brown color.
- One of the characteristic feature noticed in porous enamel, especially in the molars, is the post-enamel

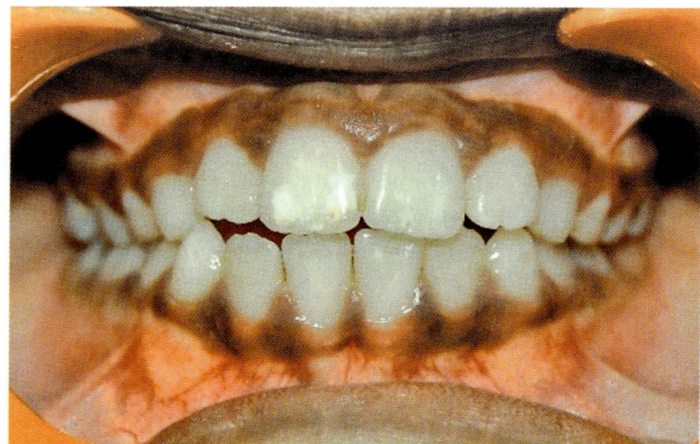

Fig. 42.4: Mild MIH in anteriors.

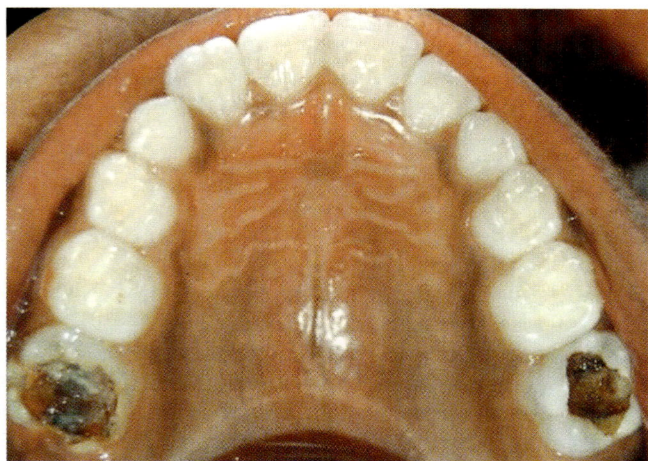
Fig. 42.5: MIH with PEB in permanent molars.

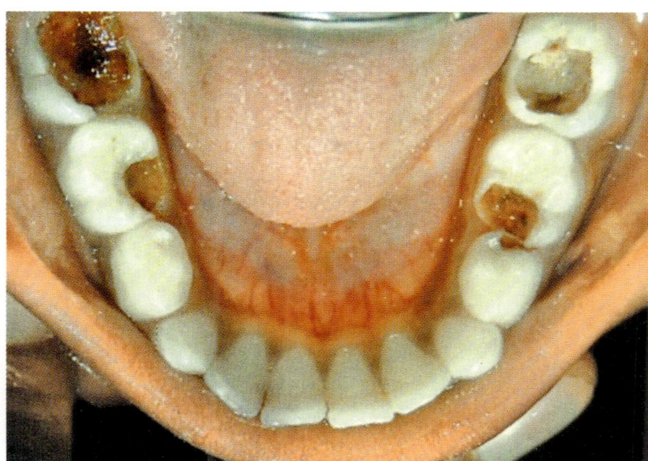
Fig. 42.6: HSPM in primary second molars with PEB.

breakdown (PEB) caused due to masticatory stress **(Fig. 42.5)**. It is usually associated with severe sensitivity and if left unattended over long time, usually presents clinically as dental caries overriding the MIH defect, with gross destruction of the tooth structure and pulpal involvement.

- In the anteriors it is usually presented as labial lesions, giving rise to cosmetic concerns with minimal or nil breakdown.
- Demarcated white/yellow/brown opacities usually limited to incisal or cuspal one third, rarely involving cervical one-third.
- Rapid caries progression—because of the porous and friable enamel structure.
- Adhesion of restoration material is poor.
- A combination of hypersensitivity and rapidly progressing caries causes chronic inflammation of the pulp, preventing effective local anesthesia.

Hypomineralized second primary molar (HSPM)/deciduous molar hypomineralization (DMH)

- A condition involving the primary second molar is also seen with similar clinical characteristics of MIH **(Fig. 42.6)**.
- Clinical appearance of HSPM can be white, creamy, yellow or brown in color similar to MIH.
- The brown darker opacities are more prone for post-eruption breakdown compared to white opacities.
- The surface is often smooth and shiny with well-defined borders with normal enamel.
- The recent studies reported an overall prevalence of HSPM between 1.6% and 20.4%.
- The mineral content of teeth with HSPM when evaluated showed around 20% lower mineral content compared to the adjacent normal enamel.[9] There was strong reduction of around 20–22% mineral content in the yellow or brown discolored enamel, while the white opacities did not differ in the mineral content.[10] (**Singh R et al.,** IJCPD13(5)2021).
- The relationship between HSPM and MIH was evaluated and there has been a strong association between them, a child with HSPM has around five times more chances to get MIH, thus HSPM can be considered as a valuable predictor of MIH. More involvement of molars with HSPM has a higher odd ratio for MIH.[11] (**Singh R et al.,** JASi 69(3)2020)

Lygidakis et al.[12] (2010) classification of MIH	
Mild	Demarcated enamel opacities without enamel breakdown. Occasional sensitivity to external stimuli (e.g., air) but not brushing mild esthetic concerns on discoloration of incisors
Severe	Demarcated enamel opacities with breakdown caries persistent/spontaneous hypersensitivity affecting function (e.g., brushing) strong aesthetic concerns that may have socio-psychological impact

Mathu-Muju and Wright[13] (2006) classification of MIH	
Mild	No caries associated with the affected enamel, no hypersensitivity, the demarcated opacities located at non-stress bearing areas, and incisor involvement is usually mild
Moderate	The post-eruptive enamel breakdown limited to one or two surfaces without cuspal involvement, atypical restorations can be needed, and normal dental sensitivity. The demarcated opacities present on molars and incisors
Severe	Post-eruptive enamel breakdown, crown destruction, caries associated with affected enamel, history of dental sensitivity, and esthetic concerns.

Teixeira et al.[14] (2018) classification of MIH

	Mild	***Moderate***	***Severe***
Crown appearance	Demarcated opacities not involving the load-bearing area of the molars	Intact atypical restoration	Post-eruptive enamel breakdown
Enamel loss	Isolated opacities	Involvement of occlusal or incisal one-third of teeth, but without initial post-eruptive enamel breakdown	Post-eruptive enamel breakdown, usually severe
Caries	No associated caries	Caries limited to one or two surfaces and without cuspal involvement, and possible post-eruptive enamel breakdown	Substantial progression of caries
Sensitivity	Normal dental sensitivity	Child usually exhibits normal dental sensitivity	A history of dental sensitivity
Esthetics	No parental concerns	Parental concerns	Parental concerns

Weerheijm et al.[1] (2001) judgement criteria for diagnosing MIH	
Key clinical feature	***Description of MIH***
Demarcated opacities	• Clearly demarcated opacities • Variability in color and size • Defects less than 1 mm not to be reported
Posteruptive enamel breakdown (PEB)	• Defect of the surface after eruption of the tooth • Loss of enamel from an initially formed surface after tooth eruption • Frequently associated with a pre-existing demarcated opacity
Atypical restorations	• Size and shape of restorations not conforming to the caries picture • Frequently extends to the buccal and palatal/lingual surfaces • Frequently associated with an opacity at the margin of the restoration • For incisors, a buccal restoration can be noticed not related to trauma
Extraction of molars due to MIH	• Absence of a first permanent molar should be related to the other teeth of the dentition • Opacities or atypical restorations in the other first permanent molars combined with absence of a first permanent molar • Absence of first permanent molars in an otherwise sound dentition in combination with demarcated opacities on the incisors
Failure of eruption of a molar or an incisor	• First permanent molar or the incisor to be examined are not yet erupted

DIFFERENTIAL DIAGNOSIS

Diagnosing MIH can be difficult, and clinicians may confuse MIH with other developmental defects of enamel such as fluorosis or amelogenesis imperfecta. The diagnosis of MIH can be further complicated if the tooth begins to decay as the tooth is erupting, thereby destroying the affected crown structure. It is, however, important to accurately diagnosis MIH so that the different approaches for managing the condition can be implemented to achieve optimal treatment outcomes. Clinical evaluation for the presence of MIH ideally involves examining the four first permanent molars and eight permanent incisors. The examination should be performed when the teeth are clean and moist. They are examined for the presence of demarcated changes in enamel color and translucency (opacities) and areas of enamel loss that most often occur in the affected molars. The clinical differentiation of MIH from other developmental defects of enamel (DDE) is described in **Table 42.3**.

MANAGEMENT OF MIH

The age of the child's teeth determines the treatment possibilities. Because damaged teeth are significantly more likely to develop carious lesions and post-eruptive breakdown due to increased porosity, caries prevention is always critical in the early post-eruptive period. In later stages of growth, the enamel matures, and if prevention is successful and the enamel surface is preserved, the relative value of prevention decreases in comparison to the requirement for restorative treatment. MIH teeth are more susceptible to disintegration and carious lesion development, intensive prevention should begin as soon as they emerge.

Pain: One of the major problems associated with MIH is chronic hypersensitivity, restricting routine oral hygiene measures, problems associated with the intake of cold and warm food. This is exhibited as severe chronic pain associated with sudden anxiety episodes, causing behavioral problems and obtaining cooperation for dental treatment. Most of the dentists treating MIH experience difficulties in providing painless treatment due to lack of achieving effective local anesthesia. This is mainly due to the chronic inflammation of pulp a state of hyperemic pulp caused due to the thermal, physical and chemical stimuli to the exposed dentin.

- Stick to basic protocols for behavioral management used in pediatric dentistry.
- Confidence building measures with minimal invasive screening without using air blowing.
- Use of alternate delivery system like STA (single tooth anesthesia) or Quick sleeper system.

Preventive measures should be based on individual patient factors like caries risk, PEB, any symptoms and their severity, and the extent/severity of the demarcated lesions.

- The effectiveness of topical fluoride in the form of concentrated varnishes and gels has shown that the

Table 42.3: Differential diagnosis for MIH.

Molar and incisor hypomineralization	• White, creamy, or yellow-brown opacities • Affects one or more than one first permanent molars and often associated with permanent incisors, while other teeth are not affected • Lesion >1 mm • Asymmetrical pattern • Caries often present • Post-eruptive enamel breakdown
Amelogenesis imperfecta	• Often with a family history • Affects primary and permanent dentitions • Possibility of enamel resorption and ankylosis • Possibility of anterior open bite • Possibility for agenesis of second molars
Fluorosis	• With a history of fluoride intake during tooth development • Primary dentition is usually not affected, but all permanent tooth usually tend to be involved • Symmetrical and bilateral pattern • Caries resistant
White spot lesions	• Occur in the cervical areas of teeth because of plaque accumulation in this area
Traumatic hypomineralization	• History of injury to the affected deciduous tooth • Often limited to one tooth • Asymmetrical pattern

fluoride ions act as a reservoir, which can be positioned as fluorapatite during remineralization. This gives beneficial effects like reduces teeth sensitivity and increases resistance to demineralization.[15]

- Early introduction of CPP-ACP has been found to very effective in terms of remineralization at early stage lesions, especially in a newly erupted immature teeth.[16] This action is achieved by nanocomplex CPP-ACP by increasing the bioavailability of Ca and P in the saliva for remineralizing MIH affected surface.[12]
- For reducing caries risk dietary counseling and fluoride toothpastes with at least 1450 ppm F are recommended.

Clinical Considerations for Treatment

- **Bonding:** Use of 5% NaOCl for 60 seconds after etching enhances the bonding in enamel of MIH, by removal of excess protein content.[17] It is strongly recommended to use self-etch adhesive, attributing to the fact that without rinsing the residual water interference is eliminated.[18] Acetone-containing adhesive solutions have also shown good results.
- **Analgesia:** Premedication prior to use of local anesthesia, alternatives like articaine in dilution 1:400,000.
- **Pit and fissure sealants:** Use GIC based sealants for patients with porous enamel surfaces and resin-based fissure sealants with adhesive treatment for intact hypomineralized molars.
- **Anterior esthetic treatment:** For creamy-whitish flaws, micro-abrasion with 18% hydrochloric or 37.5% phosphoric acid and pumice may yield acceptable results. Combining micro-abrasion with bleaching may be used to treat more severe enamel abnormalities. For brownish-yellow flaws, 'in-office' bleaching with 10% carbamide peroxide may be considered. Use of resin infiltration as a treatment mode have given physical benefits in addition to esthetics. There is a notable increase in the resistance to demineralization and microhardness.[19]
- **Treatment for posterior teeth:** All porous enamel should be removed from the cavity until resistance to the bur or probe is felt. Restorations made of GIC or resin-modified GIC should only be used as a temporary solution. For up to three surface build-ups, resin composite restorations are indicated. In severely damaged MIH molars, preformed metal crowns can be used successfully with good long-term survival rates and in older children, non-precious metal, gold, or tooth-colored indirect onlays can be used.
- **Anterior teeth:** Treatment decisions are based on the severity of the condition:
  - Resin perfusion
  - Microabrasion
  - Bleaching
  - Resin infiltration
  - Resin composition restorations
  - Composite veneers
- **Posterior teeth:** Treatment decisions are based on the severity of the condition:
  - Desensitizing toothpaste
  - Fluoride varnish
  - Sealants
  - GIC or RMGIC as temporary restorations (1–2 weeks) to reduce tooth sensitivity
  - Resin composite restorations
  - Full-coverage restorations (e.g., stainless steel crowns)
  - Extraction

New MIH treatment needs index (Table 42.4): Based on the treatment needs for MIH a newly developed index was formulated by **Steffen et al.**, a part of the concept developed by **Wuerzburg**. This index describes the data's like treatment needs with the severity of MIH. This is based on two key symptoms experienced like hypersensitivity and PEB.[20]

Table 42.4: Molar and incisor hypomineralization treatment need index.[20]

Score	Definition
0	No MIH
1	MIH without hypersensitivity and without defect
2	MIH without hypersensitivity, but with defect
2a	<1/3 defect extension
2b	>1/3, but <2/3 defect extension
2c	>2/3 defect extension and/or defect close to the pulp requiring extraction or atypical restoration
3	MIH with hypersensitivity, but without defect
4	MIH with hypersensitivity and with defect
4a	<1/3 defect extension
4b	>1/3, but <2/3 defect extension
4c	>2/3 defect extension and/or defect close to the pulp requiring extraction or atypical restoration

Psychosocial Aspects of MIH on Children

- Young children (8–10 years of age) with moderate/severe MIH may experience significantly poorer quality of life than their peers, which is attributed to the functional limitations.
- Negative impacts relating to the social and emotional effects of having visible incisor opacities have also been highlighted, as children may be embarrassed to show their teeth in normal social encounters.[21]
- **Hasmun et al.,** carried out a prospective study in which aesthetic treatment was provided to children with MIH who were reportedly upset by the appearance of their anterior opacities. One month following minimally invasive intervention, children reported significantly improved self-esteem.

Questionnaire

1. What is MIH?
2. What is HSPM?
3. What's the difference between hypoplasia and hypomineralization?
4. How do you differentiate all developmental defects of enamel clinically?
5. What is the cause of pain in MIH?
6. What is PEB?
7. What are the clinical types of MIH?
8. During which stage of amelogenesis does MIH arise?
9. What are the treatment modalities available for MIH?
10. What is the reason for pulpal pain in MIH?

11. How do you manage pain and hypersensitivity in MIH?
12. What is atypical restoration?
13. What is ideal the timing for extraction of MIH molars with poor prognosis?
14. Discuss in detail about the molar incisor hypomineralization.
15. Explain the etiological factors for the MIH.
16. What are the clinical factors to be considered while examination for MIH?
17. Classification for diagnosis of molar incisor hypomineralization.
18. What are the differential diagnosis of MIH?
19. Discuss about the treatment modalities for MIH cases.

REFERENCES

1. Weerheijm KL, Jalevik B, Alaluusua S. Molar-incisor hypomineralization. Caries Res. 2001;35:390-1.
2. Krishnan R, Wadei MM, Qahthani MT, Albeshri E, Ramesh M, Assiri YH, et al. Assessment of Enamel Permeability Using Scanning Electron Microscopy in Permanent Teeth with and without Molar Incisor Hypomineralization—An In Vivo Study. J Clin of Diagn Res. 2020;14(2):ZC18-ZC22.
3. Crombie FA, Manton DJ, Palamara JE, Zalizniak I, Cochrane NJ, Reynolds EC. Characterisation of developmentally hypomineralised human enamel. J Dent. 2013;41:611-8.
4. Vieira AR, Kup E. On the etiology of molar-incisor hypomineralization. Caries Res. 2016;50(2):166-9.
5. Jeremias F, Pierri RAG, Souza JF, Fragelli CMB, Restrepo M, Finoti LS, et al. Family-based genetic association for molar-incisor hypomineralization. Caries Res. 2016;50(3):310-8.
6. Vieira AR, Manton DJ. On the variable clinical presentation of molar-incisor hypomineralization. Caries Res. 2019;53(4):482-8.
7. Bussaneli DG, Vieira AR, Santos-Pinto L, Restrepo M. Molar-incisor hypomineralization: an updated view for aetiology 20 years later. Eur Arch Paediatr Dent. 2022;23(1):193-8.
8. Ghanim A, Morgan M, Mariño R, Bailey D, Manton D. Molar-incisor hypomineralization: Prevalence and defect characteristics in Iraqi children. Int J Paediatr Dent. 2011;21:413-21.
9. Kar S, Sakar S, Mukherjee A. Prevalence and distribution of developmental defects of enamel in the primary dentition of IVF children of West Bengal. J Clin Diagn Res. 2014;8:ZC73-6.
10. Wagner Y. Developmental defects of enamel in primary teeth-findings of a regional German birth cohort study. BMC Oral Health. 2017;17:10.
11. Elfrink MEC, ten Cate JM, Jaddoe VWV, Hofman A, Moll HA, Veerkamp JSJ. Deciduous molar hypomineralization and molar incisor hypomineralization. J Dent Res. 2012;91(6):551-5.
12. Lygidakis NA. Treatment modalities in children with teeth affected by molar-incisor enamel hypomineralization (MIH): a systematic review. Eur Arch Paediatr Dent. 2010;11:65-74.
13. Mathu-Muju K, Wright J T. Diagnosis and treatment of molar incisor hypomineralization. Compend Contin Educ Dent. 2006;27(11): 604-10.
14. Teixeira RJPB, Andrade NS, Queiroz LCC, Mendes FM, Moura MS, Moura LFAD, et al. Exploring the association between genetic and environmental factors and molar incisor hypomineralization: evidence from a twin study. Int J Paediatr Dent. 2018;28(2): 198-206.
15. William V, Messer LB, Burrow MF. Molar incisor hypomineralization: review and recommendations for clinical management. Pediatr Dent. 2006;28:224-32.
16. Baroni C, Marchionni S. MIH supplementation strategies: prospective clinical and laboratory trial. J Dent Res. 2011;90:371-6.
17. Chay PL, Manton DJ, Palamara JE. The effect of resin infiltration and oxidative pre-treatment on microshear bond strength of resin composite to hypomineralised enamel. Int J Paediatr Dent. 2014;24:252-67.
18. William V, Burrow MF, Palamara JE, Messer LB. Microshear bond strength of resin composite to teeth affected by molar hypomineralization using 2 adhesive systems. Pediatr Dent. 2006;28:233-41.
19. Paris S, Schwendicke F, Seddig S, Mueller WD, Dorfer C, Meyer-Lueckel H. Micro-hardness and mineral loss of enamel lesions after infiltration with various resins: influence of infiltrant composition and application frequency in vitro. J Dent. 2013;41(6):543-8.
20. Steffen R, Kramer N, Bekes K. The Wurzburg MIH concept: the MIH treatment need index (MIH TNI): A new index to assess and plan treatment in patients with molar incisior hypomineralization (MIH). Eur Arch Paediatr Dent. 2017;18(5):355-61.
21. Rodd HD, Graham A, Tajmehr N, Timms L, Hasmun N. Molar Incisor Hypomineralisation: Current Knowledge and Practice. International Dental Journal. 2021;71:285-91.

FURTHER READING

1. Almuallem Z, Busuttil-Naudi A. Molar incisor hypomineralisation (MIH)—an overview. Br Dent J. 2018;225:601-9.
2. Almulhim B. Molar and Incisor Hypomineralization. JNMA. 2021;59 (235):295-302.
3. Bozal CB, Kaplan A, Ortolani A, Cortese SG, Biondi AM. Ultrastructure of the surface of dental enamel with molar incisor hypomineralization (MIH) with and without acid etching. Acta Odontol Latinoam. 2015;28:192-8.
4. Bussaneli DG, Vieira AR, Santos-Pinto L, Restrepo M. Molar-incisor hypomineralisation: an updated view for aetiology 20 years later. Eur Arch Paediatr Dent. 2022;23(1):193-8.
5. Costa-Silva CM, de Paula JS, Ambrosano GMB, Mialhe FL. Influence of deciduous molar hypomineralization on the development of molar-incisor hypomineralization. Braz J Oral Sci. 2013;12(4):335-8.
6. Crombie F, Manton D, Kilpatrick N. Aetiology of molar-incisor hypomineralization: a critical review. Int J Paediatr Dent. 2009;19(2):73-83.
7. Garot E, Denis A, Delbos Y, Manton D, Silva M, Rouas P. Are hypomineralised lesions on second primary molars (HSPM) a predictive sign of molar incisor hypomineralisation (MIH)? A systematic review and a meta-analysis. J Dent. 2018;72:8-13.
8. Garot E, Rouas P, Somani C, Taylor GD, Wong F, Lygidakis NA. An update of the aetiological factors involved in molar incisor hypomineralisation (MIH): a systematic review and meta-analysis. Eur Arch Paediatr Dent. 2022;23(1):23-38.
9. Ghanim A, Elfrink M, Weerheijm K, Marinõ1 R, Manton D. A practical method for use in epidemiological studies on enamel hypomineralisation. Eur Arch Paediatr Dent. 2015; 16:235-46.
10. Krishnan R, Ramesh M, Chalakkal P. Prevalence and characteristics of MIH in school children residing in an endemic fluorosis area of India: an epidemiological study. Eur Arch Paediatr Dent. 2015;16:455-60.
11. Krishnan R, Ramesh M. Molar incisor hypomineralisation: A review of its current concepts and management. SRM J Res Dent Sci. 2014;5:248-52.
12. Lopes LB, Machado V, Mascarenhas P, Mendes JJ, Botelho J. The prevalence of molar-incisor hypomineralization: a systematic review and meta-analysis. Sci Rep. 2021;11(1):22405.
13. Lygidakis NA, Garot E, Somani C, Taylor GD, Rouas P, Wong FSL. Best clinical practice guidance for clinicians dealing with children presenting with molar-incisor-hypomineralisation (MIH): an updated European Academy of Paediatric Dentistry policy document. Eur Arch Paediatr Dent. 2022;23(1):3-21.
14. Mahoney EK, Rohanizadeh R, Ismail FS, Kilpatrick NM, Swain MV. Mechanical properties and microstructure of hypomineralised enamel of permanent teeth. Biomaterials. 2004;25:5091-100.
15. Marcenes W, Kassebaum NJ, Bernabé E, Flaxman A, Naghavi M, Lopez A, et al. Global burden of oral conditions in 1990-2010: a systematic analysis. J Dent Res. 2013;92(7):592-7.
16. Mittal N, Sharma BB. Hypomineralised second primary molars: prevalence, defect characteristics, and possible association with molar incisor Hypomineralisation in Indian children. Eur Arch Paediatr Dent. 2015;16(6):441-7.
17. Ogden AR, Pinhasi R, White WJ. Nothing new under the heavens: MIH in the past? Eur Arch Paediatr Dent. 2008;9(4):166-71.
18. Schwendicke F, Elhennawy K, Reda S, Bekes K, Manton DJ, Krois J. Corrigendum to "Global burden of molar incisor hypomineralization." J Dent. 2019;80:89-92.

CHAPTER

Chemomechanical Caries Removal

Nikhil Marwah, Nikita Gupta

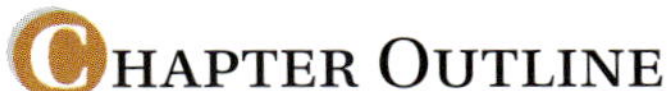

Chapter Outline

- Caridex®
- Carisolv®
- Papaćarie Gel®
- Carie Care Gel™
- BRIX 3000 Gel™

Caries continues to affect a significant portion of the world population and treatment of the decay is associated with pain in many patients. Conventional caries removal and cavity preparation entail the use of burs. Disadvantages of this system include: (1) the perception by patients that drilling is unpleasant, (2) local anesthesia is frequently required (3)drilling can cause deleterious thermal effects, (4) drilling can also cause pressure effects on the pulp, and (5) the use of a handpiece may result in removal of softened, but uninfected dentin, resulting in an excessive loss of sound tooth tissue. As a result, there is a growing demand for procedures or materials that facilitate caries management.

The chemomechanical method for caries removal was developed to overcome these shortcomings. It is not only more comfortable for the patient but also able to better preserve the healthy tissue. According to **Banerjee et al.**, the chemomechanical method is an effective alternative for caries removal, because it brings together atraumatic characteristics and bactericide/bacteriostatic action. The method was created so as that an active ingredient would soften the predegraded collagen of the lesion without pain or undesirable effects to adjacent healthy tissues.

In 1975, **Habib et al.,** introduced a method using 5% sodium hypochlorite to remove carious tissues and since then, many studies have attempted to improve this early technique. The sole use of 5% sodium hypochlorite was known to be toxic and aggressive to adjacent healthy tissues. Therefore, a new solution was developed adding sodium hydroxide, sodium chloride, and glycine to the 5% sodium hypochlorite. This modified formula was known as GK-101, and it was comprised of N-monochloroglycine. It was more effective than the hypochlorite alone but was very slow in carious tissue removal. Also, at the time of the introduction of GK-101, the use of adhesive dental materials was not common, and dentists still prepared teeth according to Black's cavity design. The approach of Extension for Prevention by **Sir GV Black** was necessary at that time since there was no other valid alternative. Therefore, the use of a method that only removed carious dentin could not significantly reduce the need of drilling to create mechanical retention. But it's time to move from "Extension for Prevention" to "Prevention for Extension".

Advantages of chemomechanical caries removal

- Its proven effectiveness
- Method's safety
- Elimination of local anesthesia and bur
- Lower anxiety built in patients
- Conservation of the sound tissue
- Only demineralized dentin containing denatured collagen is affected
- Gel consistency implies control of the application and reduces the risk of spillage

CARIDEX®

- Caridex™ (National Patent Medical Products Inc) was later developed by **CM Habib** by replacing glycine with aminobutyric acid and upgraded GK-101 to GK-101E and the product then being *N*-monochloroaminobutyric acid.
- **Krogman, Goldman** published first report on this material in 1975 and it gained Food and Drug Administration (FDA) approval in 1984. It was initially introduced in the US market in 1985.
- The system involved the intermittent application of pre-heated *N*-monochloro-dl-2-aminobutyric acid (GK-101E) to the carious lesion. The solution was claimed to cause disruption of collagen in the carious dentin, thus

facilitating its removal. The mechanism of softening involved chlorination of remaining partially degraded dentinal collagen and the conversion of hydroxyproline to pyrrole-2-carboxylic acid, which initiated disruption of the altered collagen fibers in the caries.

- Caridex was not widely adopted, possibly due to the expense, additional clinical time and the bulky Caridex delivery system, which consisted of a reservoir, a heater, a pump, and a handpiece with an applicator tip. It also transpired that conventional tooth preparation was significantly faster in removing caries than the Caridex system. However, Caridex did demonstrate the possible potential for chemomechanical caries removal and laid foundation for further research.

CARISOLV®

- During the 1980s studies at the universities by Malmö,Huddinge at Chalmers Technical University in Göteborg was directed toward a more efficient and effective chemomechanical caries removal system than Caridex®.
- **Chriser Hedwards** with **LarsStrid** of Medi Team (Dentalutveckling Göteberg AB) collaborated with **Dan Ericson** and **Rolf Bornstein** in Sweden in January 1998 led to the development of a new patented system for chemomechanical caries removal called Carisolv® **(Fig. 43.1)**.

Indications for use

- Where the preservation of tooth structure is important
- The removal of root/cervical caries
- The management of coronal caries with cavitation
- The removal of caries at the margins of crowns and bridge abutments
- The completion of tunnel preparations
- Where local anesthesia is contraindicated
- The care of caries in dentally anxious patients, notably needle phobics
- Management of primary carious lesions in deciduous teeth
- Atraumatic restorative technique procedures
- Caries management in patients with special needs

- It was initially approved for clinical use in dental practice by the Swedish counterpart to the FDA and was then, introduced to the European market as a successor to the Caridex™ system. Carisolv™ key difference to other products already in the market was the use of three amino viz lysine, leucine, and glutamic acid instead of the amino butyric acid. These amino acids counter-acted the sodium hypochlorite aggressive behavior at the oral tissues.
- Despite its effectiveness, Carisolv™ was not a blockbuster mainly because it required extensive training and registration of professionals and customized instruments which increased the cost of the solution. As a result, few people had access to the Carisolv™ solution.

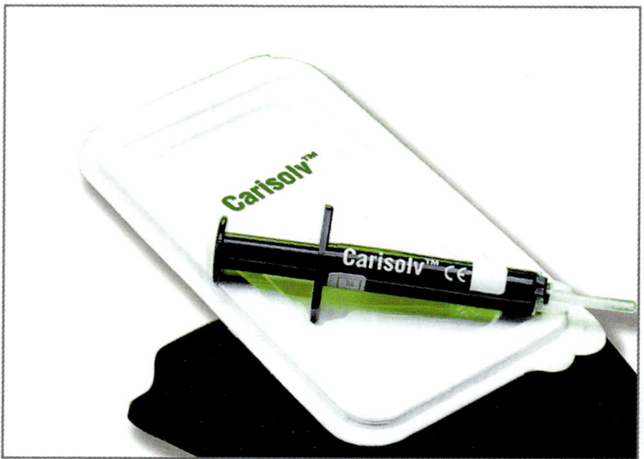

Fig. 43.1: Carisolv.

Constituents of Carisolv®

The formulation of Carisolv® is isotonic in nature and consists of the following:

- Available as single mix or multimix syringes **(Figs. 43.2 and 43.3):**
  - *Syringe one:* Sodium hypochlorite (0.5%).
  - *Syringe two:* Three amino acids (glutamic acid, leucine, lysine).

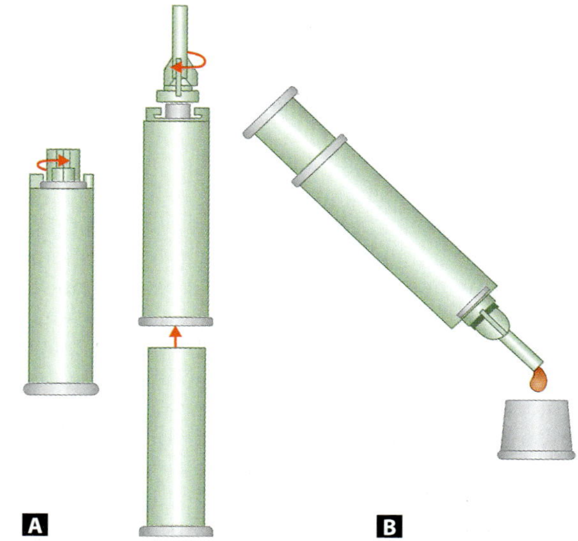

Figs. 43.2A and B: Single mix syringes: (A) Join and mix the syringe; (B) Mix both components and pour.

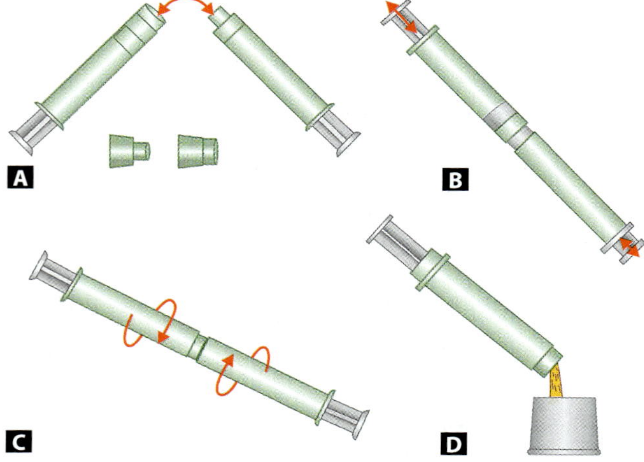

Figs. 43.3A to D: Multi-mix syringes: (A) Join the two syringes; (B) Thoroughly mix of the two syringes; (C) Separate the syringes; (D) Pour the Carisolv mix.

- *Gel substance:* Carboxymethyl cellulose.
- *Adjunct:* Sodium chloride/sodium hydroxide.

- *Vehicle:* Saline solution.
- *Coloring indicator:* Red.

Advantages

- Three amino acids are incorporated instead of one, and the different changes have improved the interaction with the degraded collagen within the lesion, thus increasing the efficacy.
- Carisolv® has a higher viscosity, which allows for the application of higher concentrations of amino acids and sodium hypochlorite without increasing the total amount of fluid used, therefore reducing the total volume required.
- The solution does not need to be heated, or applied through a pump mechanism.
- The increased viscosity of Carisolv® enhances precision placement.
- The overall stability is increased, giving an improved shelf-life.

Mode of Action (Figs. 43.4A to D)

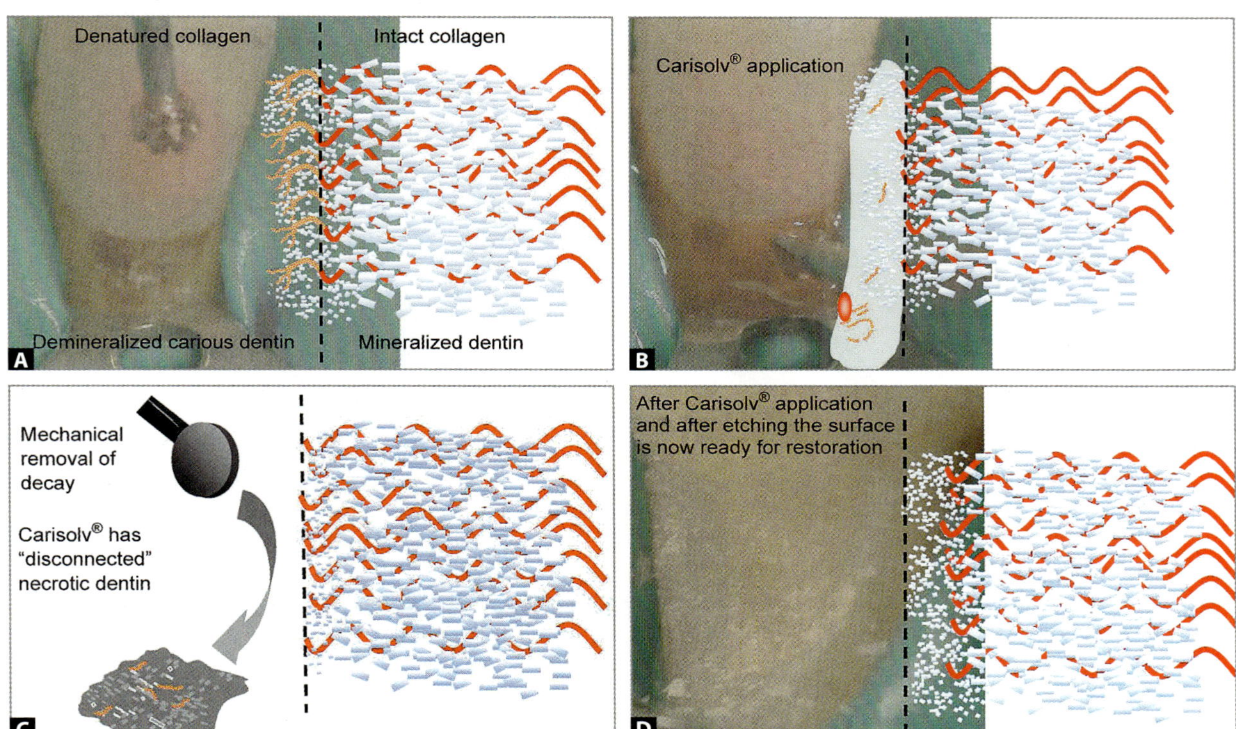

Figs. 43.4A to D: Mode of action of Carisolv®.

When the Carisolv® gel is mixed, the amino acids bind chlorine and form chloramines at high pH

↓

The softening effect on the carious tissue is the result of several reactions that act in concert to disrupt the fiber structure of collagen

↓

The three amino acids are differently charged, which allow for an electrostatic attraction to different areas of the proteins in the carious dentin

↓

The peptide chains of all proteins, including collagen, are made up of hydrophic and hydrophobic patches. So, each of the three chloroamino acids in Carisolv® electrostatically attracts one these patches, effectively bringing reactive power to the full length of the target, the collagen fiber, while minimizing unwanted side-reactions from hypochlorite

↓

The formation of chloramines reduces the reactivity of the chlorine without altering its chemical function. Moreover, chlorinated amino acids are probably able to disrupt the several types of electrostatic bond that hold the fibrous structure together

↓

The chemical result of these processes is a breakdown of degraded collagen characteristically found in the demineralized portion of a carious lesion

↓

The gel softens only the carious dentin, while healthy tissue is unaffected. The degraded collagen has an open structure and is therefore more susceptible to further breakdown by chloramines

↓

The porous nature of demineralized dentin allows Carisolv® to penetrate. The unaffected collagen is more resistant to degradation, but the framework of degraded collagen in the porous mineral is broken down and can easily be scraped off–sound and carious dentin become easily separable clinically—the carious dentin is easier to dislodge than the sound dentin

Hand Instruments

To ensure the most effective removal when the Carisolv® gel has softened the carious dentin, specially designed instruments and tips have been developed. They are atraumatic, help to preserve tissue,and speed up the treatment. The tips have different shapes and sizes to suit cavities of all kinds. Hand instruments can be classified as:

- **Depending upon type of tips (Fig. 43.5):**
  - *Instruments with permanent tips:* The instrument tips are paired together in double ended Carisolv® instruments.
  - *Instruments with interchangeable tips:* A single handle can be used with a range of different interchangeable Carisolv® instruments.

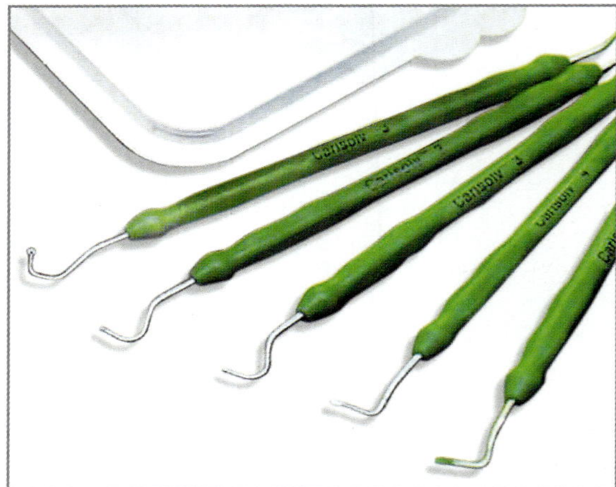

Fig. 43.5: Hand instruments.

- **Standard instrument classification (Fig. 43.6):**
  - *Carisolv® hand instrument1(extra bend; star 3, flat 0):* Primarily used for crown margins and are as that are difficult to access.
  - *Carisolv® hand instrument 2 (multistar, star 3):* The basic instrument to apply gel and start removing caries. The multistar tip promotes penetration of the gel. When getting closer to healthy dentin, use the star-shaped tip, scraping in all directions with its four-pronged design.

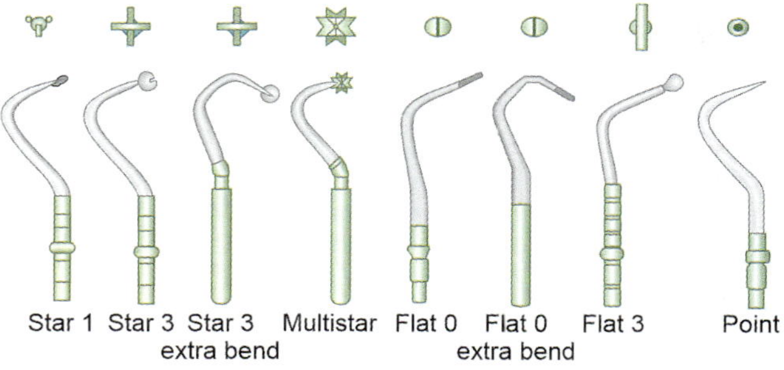

Fig. 43.6: Tips of hand instruments.

  - *Carisolv® hand instrument 3 (star 2, star 1):* To remove caries in smaller cavities; for example, root caries or deciduous teeth.
  - *Carisolv® hand instrument 4 (flat 3, flat 2):* To be used, for example, close to the pulp and to remove the softened carious dentin from the cavity.
  - *Carisolv® hand instrument 5 (flat 1, flat 0):* Flat 0 and flat 1 are used to remove caries at the dentinoenamel junction.

PowerDrive™

- It is a combined electronic instrument for power-operated, minimally invasive caries removal with Carisolv® and for endodontic treatment **(Fig. 43.7).**
- Selective and precise—removes only carious dentin.
- Fast, simple, and efficient removal of caries.
- Power Drive™ operates with high tissue control and at a low sound level.
- Patients can operate the control unit themselves.
- Useful for patients with dental phobia.

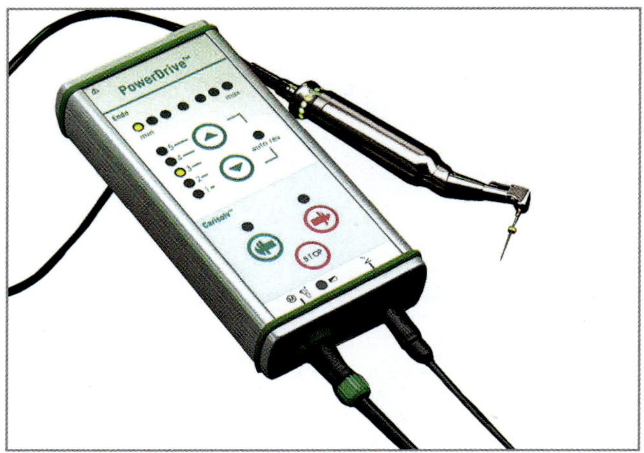

Fig. 43.7: PowerDrive™.

Clinical Procedure of Caries Removal with Carisolv (Fig. 43.8)

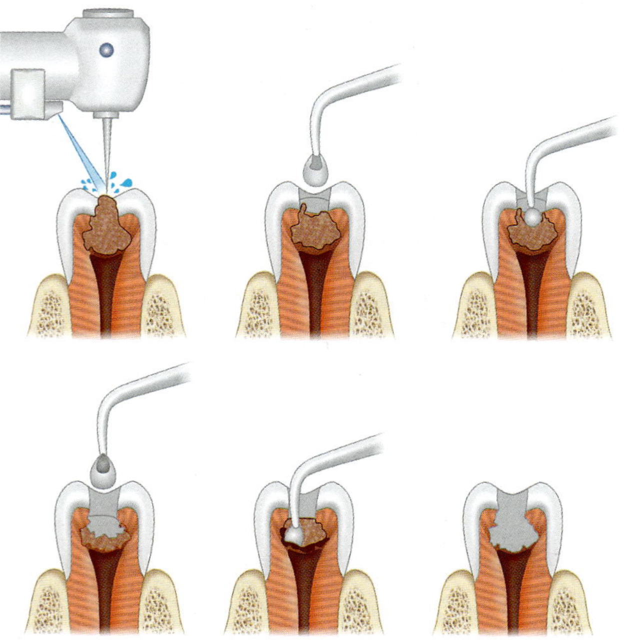

Fig. 43.8: Cavity preparation using Carisolv®.

Treatment of Children using Carisolv®

The clinical procedure undertaken is the same, but there are a few behavioral modifications that have to be made:
- Do not to rush.
- Be sure to give the gel 30 seconds to react.
- Keep the patient well-informed during the treatment.
- If the patient experiences any pain, check that the cavity is completely covered with gel and consider the potential benefit of local anesthesia.
- It is very important not to work with too much force—use speed and not pressure in your movement of the Carisolv® instruments.
- Rub/massage the gel into the carious lesion.

Mix the two components of Carisolv® (NaOCl and amino acid solution) thoroughly according to the instructions is included with the package. Put the required amount of gel into a suitable container

↓

Use a Carisolv® instrument to pick up the gel and apply it to the carious dentin

↓

Soak the caries generously

↓

Wait for at least 30 seconds, for the chemical process to soften the caries

↓

Select a power drive TM tip a Carisolv® hand instrument to match the size, position and accessiblility of the cavity

↓

Scrape off the superficial softened carious dentin. The hand instrument with the multistar tip may facilitate the early penetration of the gel. Work carefully using scraping or rotating movements

↓

Remove the softened carious dentin with the instrument. Avoid flushing or drying the cavity

↓

Keep the lesion soaked with and continue scraping. 30 seconds of waiting time is needed

↓

Repeat until the gel no longer turns cloudy and the surface feels hard using the instrument

↓

Check extra carefully for caries at the dentinoenamel junction. If you are using a drill to adjust the periphery before filling. This can be done while the gel is still in the cavity

↓

When the cavity feels free from caries, remove the gel and wipe the cavity with a moistened cotton pellet or rinse it with lukewarm water, inspect and check it with a sharp probe

↓

If the cavity is not free from caries, apply new gel and continue scraping

↓

If necessary the periphery of the cavity should be adjusted using hand instruments or the drill

↓

Restore the tooth with a suitable filling material according to the manufacturer's instructions for use

Research studies regarding use of Carisolv®

- **KumarJ et al.**[1] in 2012 compared the clinical efficiency of chemomechanical caries removal using Carisolv® and Papacarie® a papain gel and concluded that the time for caries removal with Carisolv® and Papacarie® were, respectively,11.67 ± 3.25 min and 10.48 ± 2.96 min. The mean volume of carious tissue removed

Contd...

Contd...

with Papacarie® was higher than that with Carisolv®; however,the difference was not significant.
- **El-Tekeya et al.**[2] in 2012 compared the effectiveness of two chemomechanical caries removal methods on residual bacteria in dentin of primary teeth and concluded that Papacarie is significantly more efficient in reducing the residual cariogenic bacteria in the dentin of primary teeth versus both Carisolv and the hand excavation method.
- **Pires Corrêa FN et al.**[3] in 2007 compared chemical and conventional caries removal technique in primary teeth and found that the microhardness of the dentin remaining after removal with arotary cutting instrument and chemomechanical removal (Carisolv® and Papacarie®) was similar.
- **Bohari MR et al.**[4] in 2012 clinically evaluated the three methods of caries removal, conventional, chemomechanical, and LASER technique, and found that Airotor and laser irradiation were more efficient and less time-consuming methods of caries excavation in primary teeth, whereas, chemomechanical and laser irradiation were less painful techniques, as experienced by young children.
- **Pandit IK et al.**[5] in 2007 conducted an in vivo study comparing the different methods of caries removal was done in children of age group 6–9 years. Caries removal was done by hand instruments, Airotor and Carisolv. The efficacy, time taken, and pain experienced by the patient during caries removal was evaluated. The results showed that Airotor was the most efficient method (mean value 0.38), while Carisolv was the least painful (mean value 0.080) and the most time-consuming method (534.8 seconds).

Comparison of Caridex® and Carisolv®

Characteristic	*Caridex®*	*Carisolv®*
Solution 1	1% NaOCl	0.5% NaOCl
Solution 2	0.1 M aminobutyric acid Glycine NaCl 0.1 M NaOH	0.1 M glutamic acid Leucine/lysine NaCl NaOH
Dye	–	Erythrocin (pink)
pH	11	11
Physical properties	Liquid	Gel
Volume needed	100–500 mL	0.2–1.0 mL
Time required	30–45 min	5–15 min
Equipment	Applicator unit	Basic hand instruments
Active time after mixing	1 hour	20 min

PAPAĆARIE GEL

- In 2003, a research project in Brazil led to the development of a new formula to universalize the use of chemomechanical method for caries removal and promote its use in public health. The new formula was commercially known as Papacarie® **(Fig. 43.9).**
- It is basically comprised of papain, chloramines, toluidine blue, salts, thickening vehicle, which together are responsible for the Papacarie's bactericide, bacteriostatic, and anti-inflammatory characteristics.

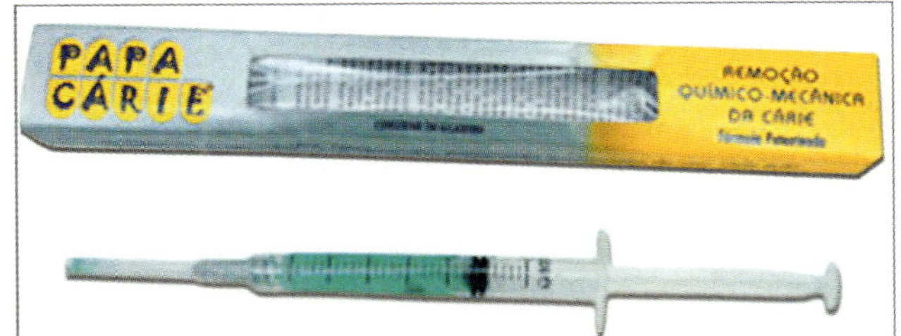

Fig. 43.9: Papacarie gel.

- Papain comes from the latex of the leaves and fruits of the green adult papaya. *Carica papaya*, for instance, is cultivated in tropical regions,such as Brazil, India, South Africa, and Hawaii, and is largely used in the food, beverage, and drug industries.
- Papain accelerates the cicatricial process and according to Mandelbaum, papain is indicated in all phases of the cicatricial process, and it promotes chemical debridement, granulation and epithelialization, stimulation of the tensile strength of the scars.
- Papain interacts with the exposed collagen causing the dissolution of minerals from the dentin and bacteria, thus making the infected dentin more softened, which facilitates its removal with the use of non-cutting instruments and without anesthesia and rotary instruments. It acts by breaking the partially degraded collagen molecules. The action of Papaćarie causes cleavage of the polypeptide chains and hydrolysis the crosslinks of collagen. Right after degradation, oxygen is freed, this explains the appearance of bubbles on the surface during a clinical procedure.
- According to **Flindt**, papain acts only on damaged tissue due to the absence of an antiplasmatic protease, the alpha-1-antitrypsine that hinders its proteolytic action in tissues considered normal.
- **Dawkins** showed that *Carica papaya* has bactericide and bacteriostatic properties which inhibit growth of Gram-positive and Gram-negative organisms. **Pereira et al.** used samples of infected dentin cultivated in brain-heart infusion (BHI) broth in Petri dish to assess the Papacarie antimicrobial activity. The results showed the largest Papacarie activity was in case of *Streptococcus* and *Lactobacillus.*

Clinical Procedure

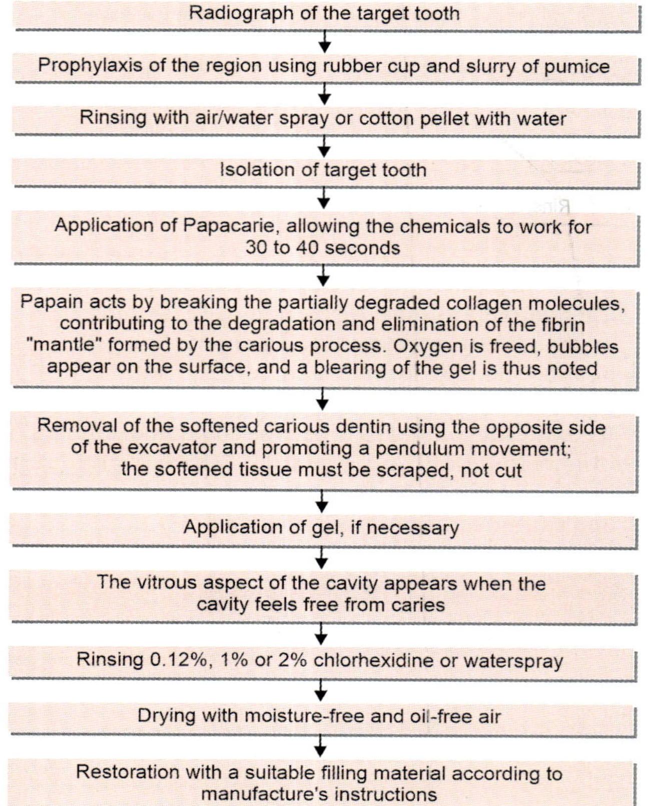

Radiograph of the target tooth
Prophylaxis of the region using rubber cup and slurry of pumice
Rinsing with air/water spray or cotton pellet with water
Isolation of target tooth
Application of Papacarie, allowing the chemicals to work for 30 to 40 seconds
Papain acts by breaking the partially degraded collagen molecules, contributing to the degradation and elimination of the fibrin "mantle" formed by the carious process. Oxygen is freed, bubbles appear on the surface, and a blearing of the gel is thus noted
Removal of the softened carious dentin using the opposite side of the excavator and promoting a pendulum movement; the softened tissue must be scraped, not cut
Application of gel, if necessary
The vitrous aspect of the cavity appears when the cavity feels free from caries
Rinsing 0.12%, 1% or 2% chlorhexidine or waterspray
Drying with moisture-free and oil-free air
Restoration with a suitable filling material according to manufacture's instructions

Research studies regarding use of Papacarie®

- **JawaD et al.**[6] in 2010 compared *in vitro* the efficacy of chemomechanical caries removal agent (Papacarie) and conventional method of caries removal and found that complete removal of caries was achieved significantly in both the methods, there was less marked destruction of dentinal tubules in chemomechanical caries removal method by Papacarie. Thus, Papacarie is recommended as an efficient, easy to perform, comfortable and less destructive solution for the patient seeking an alternative to the conventional method.
- **Bussadori**[7] observed through an electronic scanning microscope that in conventional techniques for decayed tissue removal in permanent teeth with caries (using diamond points and /or burs), dentin surfaces showed a residual smear layer, whereas while using Papacarie, there was more preservation of dentin structure and bacterial removal.
- An *in vitro* evaluation done by **Bussadori** and **Martins**[8] of Papacarie cytotoxicity using fibroblast culture in different concentrations (2%, 4%, 6%, 8%, and 10%) of papain led to the finding that the same was not cytotoxic. Hence, Papacarie was proved to be safe to be used in pediatric patients.
- According to **Flindt**,[9] papain acts only on damaged tissue due to the absence of an anti-plasmatic protease, α-l-antitrypsin,that hinders its proteolytic action in tissues considered normal.
- **Pereira**[10] emphasize that the dentin remaining pattern after removing caries with Papaćarie is completely different from that found after caries removal with a high rotation diamond point drill.

CARIE CARE GEL

- In 2010, with the intention of presenting a new agent that cost less than Papacarie and is easily available, a new chemomechanical caries removal system, Carie Care™, **(Fig. 43.10)** was launched in India.
- Carie Care, a product that has been locally introduced has as its main active ingredient from papaya extract, an endoprotien, chloramines and dye.
- Papain in papaya extract acts as a debris removing agent, with no harmful effect on sound dental tissues because of the enzyme specificity. In addition to papain, the chloramines present in the product have the potential of dissolving carious dentin by means of chlorination of the partially degraded collagen. This mechanism affects the collagen structure, dissolving hydrogen bonds, soften the carious dentin and thus facilitating tissue removal.
- In addition, the preparation contains specific percentages of essential clove oil from plant sources, which has anti-inflammatory, analgesic, and mild anesthetic effect which

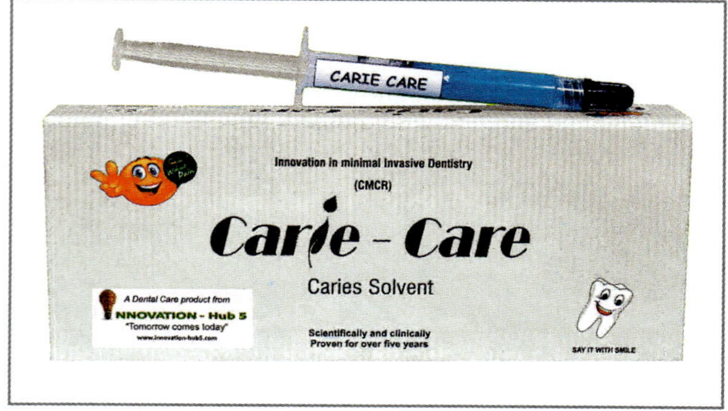

Fig. 43.10: Carie Care gel.

will reduce the pain perception during the operative procedure.

- ❖ The preparation also contains explicit gelling agent in accurate percentage to offer exact consistency to the gel in order that when applied there is no spill over.
- ❖ **Venkataraghavan K et al.** noticed that the color and taste of the gel was well appreciated by the patients. In addition to these, it is more cost-effective, as compared to other agents, and does not require ant specialized equipment or special training during application.

Clinical Procedure

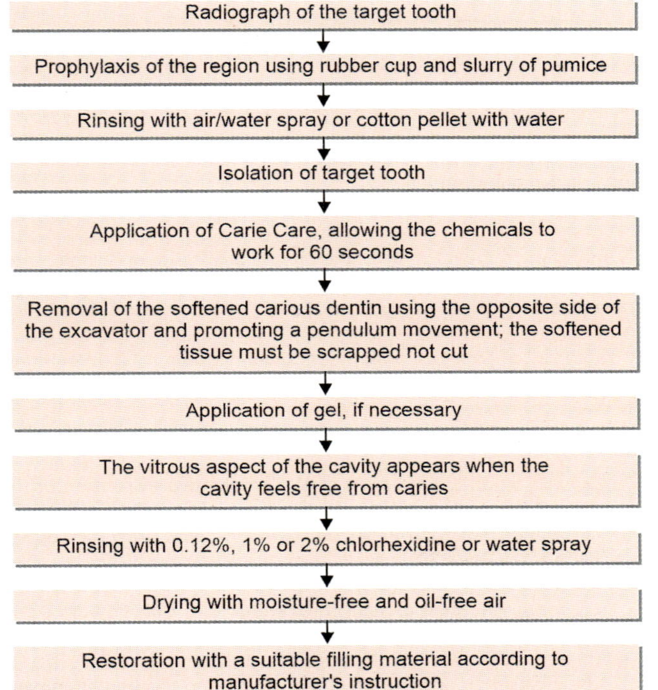
Radiograph of the target tooth
Prophylaxis of the region using rubber cup and slurry of pumice
Rinsing with air/water spray or cotton pellet with water
Isolation of target tooth
Application of Carie Care, allowing the chemicals to work for 60 seconds
Removal of the softened carious dentin using the opposite side of the excavator and promoting a pendulum movement; the softened tissue must be scrapped not cut
Application of gel, if necessary
The vitrous aspect of the cavity appears when the cavity feels free from caries
Rinsing with 0.12%, 1% or 2% chlorhexidine or water spray
Drying with moisture-free and oil-free air
Restoration with a suitable filling material according to manufacturer's instruction

Research studies regarding use of Carie Care™

- **Venkataraghavan K et al.**[11] observed that as it does not contain sodium hypochlorite, so there is no chance of irritation even if the gel comes in contact with the adjacent soft tissues. Hence, this agent can be used for caries removal in proximal lesions also.
- **Hosoyo Y et al.**[12] in his in-vitro study showed that chemomechanically treated dentin have more surface energy, greater affinity for adhesive material, and better bonding than conventionally treated dentin.
- **Kush et al.**[13] when assessed the antimicrobial action, the Carie Care demonstrated significant antimicrobial action on the growth of *Aggregatibacter actinomycetemcomitans* when compared with Papacarie Duo.
- **Shivasharan et al.**[14] clinically evaluated the efficiency of caries removal using Carie Care compared to the SmartPrep burs for complete caries excavation. The differences between complete caries excavation, pain reaction and need for local anesthesia using both the techniques were statistically insignificant. Whereas the time taken for caries removal using Carie-Care was significantly less than Smart burs. Hence it was concluded that both the techniques can be used effectively for caries excavation in primary teeth.

BRIX 3000 GEL

- ❖ In 2016, a new material had been found in Argentina, named Brix 3000 (**Fig. 43.11**), also papain based, obtained from leaves latex and fruits of green papaya that acts as a chemical debriding agent.

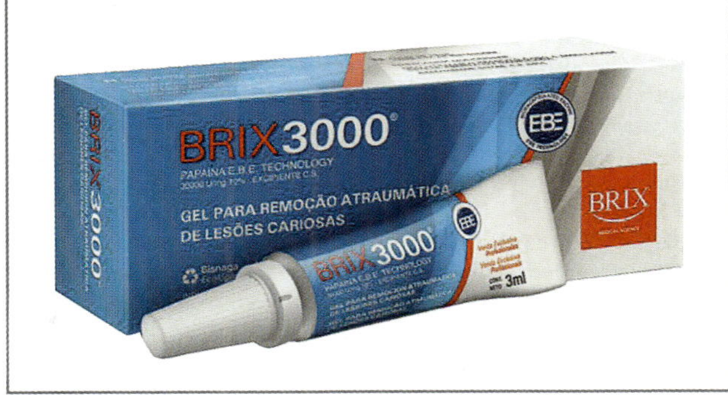
BRIX3000
PAPAINA E.B.E. TECHNOLOGY
GEL PARA REMOÇÃO ATRAUMÁTICA DE LESÕES CARIOSAS
EBE
BRIX
3ml

Fig. 43.11: BRIX 3000 gel.

- ❖ The differential of this product from other is the amount papain used (3000 U/mg in a concentration of 10%) and the bioencapsulation by EBE technology (encapsulated buffer emulsion), which gives the gel the ideal pH to immobolize the enzymes and liberate them at the moment of exerting its proteolysis on the collagen, and the enzymatic activity supplied the Brix agent by many effective properties included the higher proteolysis effectiveness and greater antibacterial and antifungal potency with an increase in the antiseptic effect on tissue.
- ❖ **Felizardo et al.** verified the efficacy of Brix 3000 and concluded that the use of enzymatic papain gel was an efficient alternative for caries removal, easy to use, and preserve to the maximum healthy dental structure, showing promise to be used as atraumatic caries removal technique.

Clinical Procedure

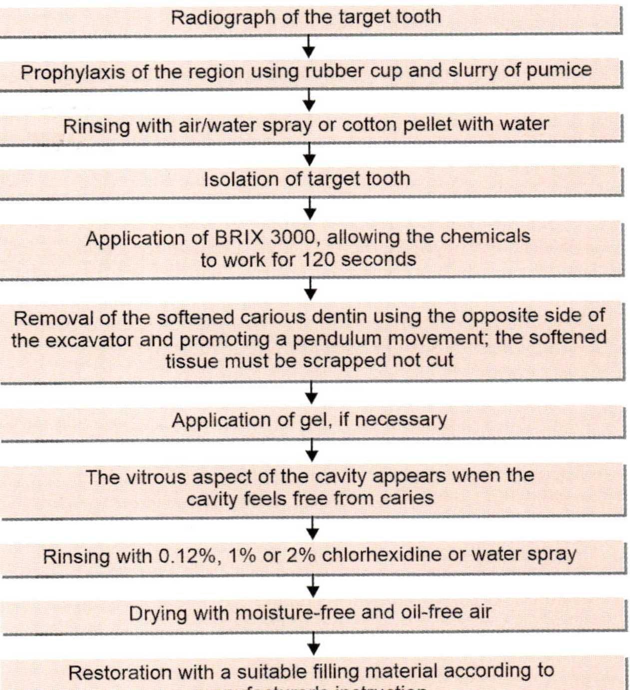
Radiograph of the target tooth
Prophylaxis of the region using rubber cup and slurry of pumice
Rinsing with air/water spray or cotton pellet with water
Isolation of target tooth
Application of BRIX 3000, allowing the chemicals to work for 120 seconds
Removal of the softened carious dentin using the opposite side of the excavator and promoting a pendulum movement; the softened tissue must be scrapped not cut
Application of gel, if necessary
The vitrous aspect of the cavity appears when the cavity feels free from caries
Rinsing with 0.12%, 1% or 2% chlorhexidine or water spray
Drying with moisture-free and oil-free air
Restoration with a suitable filling material according to manufacturer's instruction

Research studies regarding use of BRIX 3000™

- **Ismail MMM et al.**[15] compared the conventional drilling method and BRIX 3000 on pain reaction during caries removal and stated that the anxiety rating scale during the period of treatment showed the percentage of the negative behavior in the chemomechanical caries removal method was less than the percentage of the ceramic bur; and BRIX 3000 was more comfortable than the conventional rotary instrument (ceramic bur), that reduced the need for local anesthesia and the use of the drill.
- **Torresi and Bseremi**[16] verified the efficacy of BRIX 3000 for the removal of carious tissue comparing 75 patients treated with the mechanical chemical agent and 75 by the traditional rotary method. It was found that the gel was effective for 62 patients (82.7%) with a single application of the product.
- **Alkouhli MM et al.**[17] compared and evaluated the effectiveness of BRIX 3000™ and 2.25% sodium hypochlorite gel with conventional rotary instrumentation method in caries excavation of primary molars and found that CMCR agents are effective in removing the carious dentine of primary teeth without negatively affecting the cooperation of children.

POINTS TO REMEMBER

- GK-101 was the first chemomechanical agent for caries removal.
- Advantages of chemomechanical caries removal are safety, elimination of local anesthesia and bur, lower anxiety, conservation of the sound tissue.
- Caridex™ was developed by CM Habib from a formula made of N-monochloroglycine and aminobutyric acid and was called as GK-101E. Disadvantages of this were expense, additional time consumption, and bulky armamentarium.
- Chriser Hedwards with Lars Strid of MediTeam collaborated with Dan Ericson and Rolf Bornstein in Sweden in January 1998 to develop Cariosolv®.
- Indications for Cariosolv® are where the preservation of tooth structure is important, removal of root caries, removal of caries at the margins of crowns and bridge abutments, tunnel preparations, when local anesthesia is contraindicated, needle phobics, management of primary carious lesions in deciduous teeth. Cariosolv® can be used with either hand instruments or Power DriveTM which is a combined electronic instrument for power-operated, minimally invasive caries removal.
- A new type of chemomechanical agent was developed in Brazil in 2003 comprised of papain, chloramines, toluidine blue, salts, thickening vehicle, and called as papain gel.

Questionnaire

1. What are the indications and advantages of chemomechanical caries removal?
2. Write a note on Caridex®.
3. Describe the composition, instrumentation, mode of action and clinical procedure for application of Cariosolv®.
4. Compare all the chemomechanical caries removal agents and write in detail about your choice of agent.
5. Write a short note on Brix 2000.
6. Describe in detail about papacarie gel and its advantage over other.

REFERENCES

1. Kumar J, Nayak M, Prasad KL, Gupta N. A comparative study of the clinical efficiency of chemomechanical caries removal using Carisolv® and Papacarie®—a papain gel. Indian J DentRes. 2012;23(5):697.
2. El-Tekeya M, El-Habashy L, Mokhles N, El-Kimary E. Effectiveness of 2 chemomechanical caries removal methods on residual bacteria in dentin of primary teeth. Pediatr Dent. 2012;34:325-30.
3. Pires Corrêa FN, Oliveira Rocha RD, Rodrigues Filho LE, Muench A, Delgado Rodrigues CR. Chemical versus conventional caries removal techniques in primary teeth: a microhardness study. J Clin Pediatr Dent. 2007;31:187-92.
4. Bohari MR, Chunawalla YK, Ahmed BM. Clinical evaluation of caries removal in primary teeth using conventional, chemomechanical and laser technique: an in vivo study. J Contemp Dent Pract. 2012;13(1):40-7.
5. Pandit IK, Srivastava N, Gugnani N, Gupta M, Verma L. Various methods of caries removal in children: a comparative clinical study. J Indian Soc Pedod Prev Dent. 2007;25:93.
6. Jawa D, Singh S, Somani R, et al. Comparative evaluation of the efficacy of chemomechanical caries removal agent (Papacarie) and conventional method of caries removal: an invitro study. J Indian Soc Pedod Prev Dent. 2010;28:73.
7. Bussadori SK, Castro LC, Galvyo AC. Papain gel: a new chemomechanical caries removal agent. J Clin Pediatr Dent. 2005;30:115-9.
8. Bussadori SK, Silva LR, Guedes CC. Utilization of Papacarie for chemical and mechanical removal of decayed tooth in atraumatic restorative technique (ART): minimum invention technique for treatment of deep dental decay. 2005. pp.391-400.
9. Flindt M. Health and safety aspects of working with enzymes. Process Biochem. 1979;13:3-7.
10. Pereira SA, Silva LR, Motta LJ, Bussadori SK. Chemomechanical caries removal with Papaćarie gel. RGO, 2004;52(5): 385-88.
11. Venkataraghavan K, Kush A, Lakshminarayana C, Diwakar L, Ravikumar P, Patil S, et al. Chemomechanical caries removal: A review & study of an indigenously developed agent (Carie CareTM Gel) in children. J Int Oral Health. 2013;5:84-90.
12. Hosoya Y, Shinkawa H, Marshal GW. Influence of Carisolv on resin adhesion for two different adhesive systems to sound human primary dentin and young permanent dentin. J Dent. 2005;33:283-91.
13. Kush A, Thakur R, Patil SS, Paul ST, Kakanur M. Evaluation of antimicrobial action of Carie Care™ and Papacarie Duo™ on *Aggregatibacter actinomycetemcomitans* a major periodontal pathogen using polymerase chain reaction. Contemp Clin Dent. 2015;6:534-8.
14. Shivasharan PR, Farhin AK, Wakpanjar MM, Shetty A. Clinical Evaluation of Caries Removal in Primary Teeth Using Carie-care and Smart Prep Burs: An In vivo Study. Indian J Oral Health Res. 2016;2:27-31.
15. Ismail MMM, Al Haider AH. Evaluation of the efficacy of caries removal using papain gel (Brix 3000) and smart preparation bur (in vivo comparative study). J Pharm Sci & Res. 2019;11(2):444-49.

16. Torresi FN, Besereni L. Effectiveness method of chemomechanical removal of dental caries as papain in adults, J. Rev Assoc Paul cir Dent. 2017;71(3):266-9.
17. Alkhouli MM, Al Nesser SF, Bshara NG, Almidani AN, Comisi JC. Comparing the efficacies of two chemo-mechanical caries removal agents (2.25% sodium hypochlorite gel and brix 3000), in caries removal and patient cooperation: A randomized controlled clinical trial. J Dent. 2020; Article ID: 103280.

FURTHER READING

1. Chemomechanical caries removal: a comprehensive review of the literature. Int Dent J. 2001;51:291-9.
2. Ericson D, Zimmerman M, Raber H, et al. Clinical evaluation of efficacy and safety of a new method for chemomechanical removal of caries. Caries Res. 1999;33:171-7.
3. Hannig M. Effect of Carisolv™ solution on sound, demineralized and denatured dentin—an ultrastructural investigation. Clin Oral Invest. 1999;3:155-9.
4. Kimmel JR, Smith EL. Crystalline papain: preparation, specificity and activation. J Bio Chem. 1954;207:514-73.
5. OsatoJA, Santiago LA, Remo GM, Cuadra MS, Mori A. Antimicrobial and antioxidant activities of unripe papaya. LifeSci.1999;53: 1383-9.
6. Wennerburg A, Sawasa T, Kultje C. The influence of Carisolv on enamel and dentin surface topography. Eur J Oral Sci.1999; 106:1-10.
7. Yip HK, Samaranayake LP. Caries removal techniques and instrumentation: are view. Clin Oral Invest.1998;2:148-54.
8. Zu-Qian G, Qian-Min C, Wei S. The clinical application of the chemomechanical caries removal system (Caridex): a comparative study. Compend Contin Educ Dent.1987;8:638-40.

CHAPTER

Pediatric Operative Dentistry

Nikhil Marwah, Raghunath Reddy MH

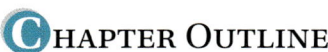

Chapter Outline

- Classification of Cavity Preparation
- Principles of Cavity Preparation
- Modifications of Cavity Preparation in Primary Teeth
- Matrix
- Wedges
- Rubber Dam
- Air Abrasion (Microabrasion and Kinetic Cavity Preparation)

Operative dentistry *is the art and science of the diagnosis, treatment, and prognosis of defects of teeth that do not require full coverage restorations for correction. Such treatment should result in the restoration of proper tooth form, function, and esthetics while maintaining the physiologic integrity of the teeth in harmonious relationship with the adjacent hard and soft tissues, all of which should enhance the general health and welfare of the patient.*

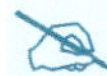

Pediatric operative dentistry is a dynamic combination of ever improving materials and new techniques. In 1924, **GV Black** *outlined several steps for the preparation of carious permanent teeth to receive an amalgam restoration. Same steps have been adopted, though slightly modified for the restoration of primary teeth.*

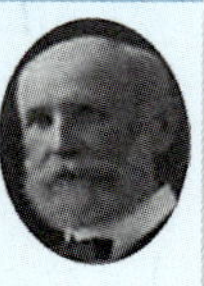

No longer is it excusable to provide substandard care for primary teeth on the basis that they will exfoliate, ignoring the duration required for the restoration and value of teeth in maintaining arch integrity. Moreover, ignoring and neglecting dental caries in primary dentition sends a wrong message that teeth are not important. Before going in the details of pediatric operative dentistry, one must first realize that the primary teeth vary considerably from their permanent counterparts, not only in morphology but also in composition. These differences are tabulated in **Table 44.1**.

CLASSIFICATION OF CAVITY PREPARATION

Black's Classification

- **Class I:** All pit and fissure lesions on occlusal surface of premolars and molars, lesions on occlusal two-third of the facial and lingual surfaces of molars, and lesions on lingual surface of maxillary incisors.

Importance of primary teeth
- Help in mastication
- Speech-premature loss of maxillary primary anteriors before the age of 3 years results in impairment of speech that may last later in life
- Maintenance and improvement of appearance (esthetics)
- Maintenance of arch length
- Prevent development of abnormal oral habits like tongue thrusting
- Prevent psychological effects associated with premature tooth loss

- **Class II:** Lesions on the proximal surfaces of posterior teeth.
- **Class III:** Lesions on the proximal surfaces of anterior teeth that do not involve the incisal angle.
- **Class IV:** Lesions on the proximal surfaces of anterior teeth that involve the incisal edge.
- **Class V:** Lesions on the gingival third of the facial or lingual surfaces of all teeth.
- **Class VI:** Lesions on the incisal edge of anterior teeth or the occlusal cusp tips of posterior teeth **(Simon's** modification).

Table 44.1: Differences between deciduous and permanent teeth.

Deciduous dentition	*Permanent dentition*
General differences	
1. 20 in number	1. 32 in number
2. Do not have premolars	2. Have 8 premolars
3. Only two molars are present	3. Third molar is also present (can we put it as dental formula)
4. White in color	4. Less white as compared to primary teeth
Morphological differences (crown)	
5. Crowns are more bulbous	5. Less bulbous
6. Broad contact area between the teeth	6. Contact point is present
7. Enamel–dentin junction is more sinuous and the enamel end abruptly	7. Enamel ends in a gradual manner
8. Buccal and lingual surfaces of primary molars are flat	8. Buccal and lingual surfaces are rounded
9. Buccal and lingual surfaces of first molar converge toward the occlusal surface, so the buccolingual diameter is much less than cervical diameter	9. There is no such convergence of the buccal and lingual surfaces, so the buccolingual diameter is more than cervical diameter
10. Primary teeth have marked constriction at the neck	10. Less constriction
11. Mamelons are absent	11. Mamelons are present in anterior teeth
12. Enamel cap end in a marked ridge	12. Enamel cap end in a feather-edge
13. Enamel is thin but shows consistent depth (1 mm)	13. Thicker enamel of varying depth
14. Show more attrition	14. Less attrition
15. Less tooth structure covering the pulp	15. There is more covering of enamel and dentin
16. Enamel rods at cervix slope occlusally	16. Enamel rods at cervix slope gingivally
17. The mineral content of enamel is more organic	17. Less organic content than primary tooth
18. All primary teeth show neonatal line	18. Only first molars exhibit neonatal line
19. Dentinoenamel junction is flat	19. Dentinoenamel junction is scalloped
20. Crowns are wider in mesiodistal diameter as compared to cervico-occlusal height	20. Crowns are larger cervico-occlusally than mesiodistally
21. Occlusal table is narrow	21. Occlusal table is wider
Morphological differences (root)	
22. Roots of primary teeth are long and slender	22. Roots are short and robust
23. Roots have a short trunk	23. Larger undivided portion of root is present
24. Roots are more divergent and flaring, as they have to accommodate the permanent tooth bud	24. Roots are less divergent and do not flare to a great degree
25. Undergo physiologic resorption	25. Do not undergo physiologic resorption, only pathologic changes can take place
Histological differences	
26. Presence of a cap-like zone of reticular and collagenous fibers	26. No such zone present
Pulpal differences	
27. Greater thickness of dentin over the pulpal wall at occlusal fossa	27. Less covering of dentin
28. Pulp chambers are large	28. Small sized pulp chambers
29. Pulp horns are higher, especially the mesial pulp horn in case of primary first molar	29. Pulp horns are low
30. Accessory canals in the primary teeth are located in the furcation area	30. Accessory canals in the primary teeth are located in the root apices
31. No regressive changes can be seen	31. Regressive changes in the form of calcifications and pulp stones are seen
32. Root canals are ribbon like	32. Root canals are more tortuous and curved
33. Enlarged apical foramen	33. Constricted apical foramen
34. Abundant blood supply	34. Less blood supply as compared to primary teeth
35. Response to external stimuli is typical inflammatory reaction	35. Response is by calcification or calcific scarring
36. Nerve fibers terminate in odontoblastic region as free nerve endings	36. Nerve fibers end among odontoblasts and beyond predentin
37. Density of innervation is less, so the teeth are less sensitive to operative procedures	37. Density of innervation is greater, thereby leading to more sensitivity
38. Reparative dentin formation below arrested caries is more extensive	38. Less reparative dentin formation as compared to primary teeth
39. Poor localization of infection and inflammation	39. Better localization of infection and inflammation

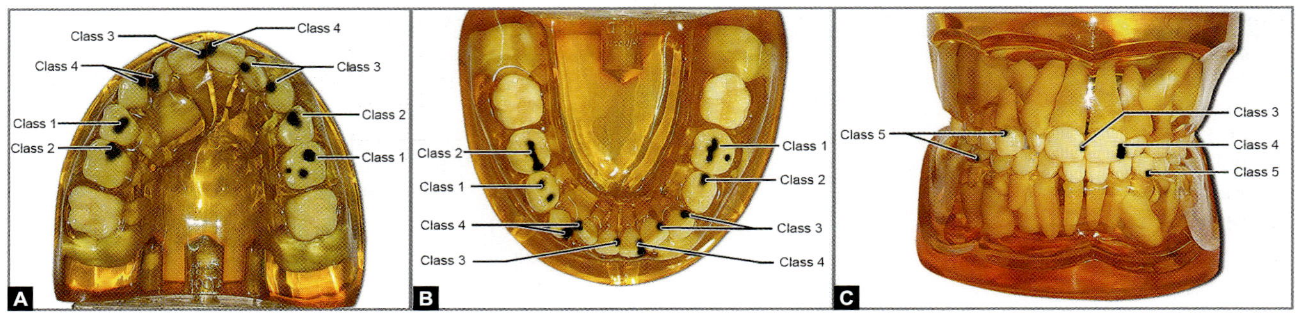

Figs. 44.1A to c: Finn's modification of GV Black's classification of dental caries for primary teeth.

Finn's Modification for Primary Teeth (Figs. 44.1A to c)

- **Class I:** Pit and fissure cavities on occlusal surface of molars and the buccal and lingual pits of all teeth.
- **Class II:** Cavities on the proximal surfaces of posterior teeth with access established from occlusal surface.
- **Class III:** Cavities on the proximal surfaces of anterior teeth that may or may not involve the labial or lingual extension.
- **Class IV:** Restorations on the proximal surfaces of anterior teeth that involve the incisal edge.
- **Class V:** Cavities on the cervical third of all teeth, including proximal surfaces where the marginal ridge is not included in cavity preparation.

Mount and Hume's Classification

This is a new system that identifies the site as well as the complexity of the lesion.

- **Site I:** Pits and fissure on occlusal surfaces
- **Site II:** Proximal areas just below the contact point
- **Site III:** Cervical one-third of crown
- **Size I:** Minimal involvement of dentin
- **Size II:** Moderate involvement of dentin but remaining tooth structure strong enough to support restoration
- **Size III:** Large cavity with weakened tooth structure
- **Size IV:** Extensive caries with loss of bulk of tooth structure.

PRINCIPLES OF CAVITY PREPARATION

Although the Black's principles of cavity preparation are now not being used, a brief mention of these principles is a must before we explain newer principles of "constriction for conviction," "minimal intervention," and "ART."

Initial Tooth Preparation

Initial tooth preparation is at a specific limited depth so as to provide access to the caries or defect, reach sound tooth structures (except for later removal of infected dentin on the pulpal or cranial walls), resist fracture of the tooth or restorative material from masticatory forces principally directed along the long axis of the tooth, and retain the restorative material in the tooth.

- **Step 1 (Outline form and initial depth):** Defined as the location that the peripheries of the completed tooth preparation will occupy on tooth surfaces.
- **Step 2 (Primary resistance form):** That shape and placement of the preparation walls that best enable both the restoration and the tooth to withstand, without fracture, masticatory forces delivered principally in the long axis of the tooth.
- **Step 3 (Primary retention form):** It is that shape or form of the conventional preparation that resist displacement or removal of the restoration from tipping or lifting forces.
- **Step 4 (Convenience form):** That shape or form of the preparation that provides for adequate observation, accessibility, and ease of operation in preparing and restoring the tooth.

Final Tooth Preparation

- **Step 5:** Removal of any remaining infected dentin and old restorative material, if indicated.
- **Step 6:** Pulp protection if indicated.
- **Step 7 (Secondary resistance and retention forms):** Many preparations require additional retentive features. When tooth preparation includes both occlusal and proximal surfaces, each of those areas should have independent retention and resistances features. For example, locks for amalgam, grooves for cast metal, and skirts for cast restorations.
- **Step 8 (Procedures for finishing external walls):** It is the further development, when indicated of a specific cavosurface design and degree of smoothness or roughness that produces the maximum effectiveness of the restorative material being used. The objectives are to create best marginal seal possible between the restorative material and tooth structure, afford a smooth marginal junction and provide maximum strength of both the restorative material and tooth.
- **Step 9 (Final procedures):** Cleansing, inspecting, and sealing. Includes removing all chips and loose debris that have accumulated, drying the preparation and making a final complete inspection of the preparation for any remaining infected dentin, unsound enamel margins or any condition that renders the preparation unacceptable to receive the restorative material.

Kidd and **Smith** (1994) recommended that during cavity preparation, the following sequence should be followed:

- Gain access to the caries
- Excavate all caries

- Consider design of the cavity in relation to:
  - Final choice of the material
  - Retention of the restoration
  - Protection of the remaining tooth structure
  - Optimal strength of the restoration
  - Shape and protection of cavity margins
  - Refine and debride the cavity
  - Placement of restoration.

MODIFICATIONS OF CAVITY PREPARATION IN PRIMARY TEETH

Owing to multiple anatomical, morphological, and histological differences between the primary and permanent teeth, the cavity preparation among the two also varies greatly. Some of the common modifications in case of primary teeth are:

Class I: Cavity Preparation (Figs. 44.2 and 44.3)

- Due to narrow occlusal table, the buccolingual dimensions of occlusal part of cavity are reduced.
- The chance of inadvertent pulp exposure is minimized by limiting the cavity to 0.5 mm pulpal to enamelo-dentinal junction.
- Maximum intercuspal cavity width should be limited.
- Walls of preparation should be parallel or slightly convergent occlusally.
- The central pit of lower first primary molar usually becomes carious before mesial pit, which decays less frequently. The outline form should be limited to central pit; it is adjacent buccal and lingual grooves and distal triangular fossa. It is advisable not to cross ridge to join mesiobuccal and mesiolingual cusp because of its proximity to pulp horns. Pulpal roof in primary teeth is concave as compared to permanent teeth where it is nearly flat so cavity floor should be kept little concave.
- Depth should be just 0.5 mm into the dentin, so the total depth from the cavosurface should not be more than 1.5–2.0 mm.
- Include all pits and fissures and lateral extension should be such so as to just accommodate the amalgam condenser.
- Flat or slightly concave pulpal floor with rounded line and point angles.
- While extending laterally on the buccal side, bur should be kept parallel to the buccal surface, and while extending lingually, bur should be parallel to lingual surface. This makes the occlusal convergence without much cutting.

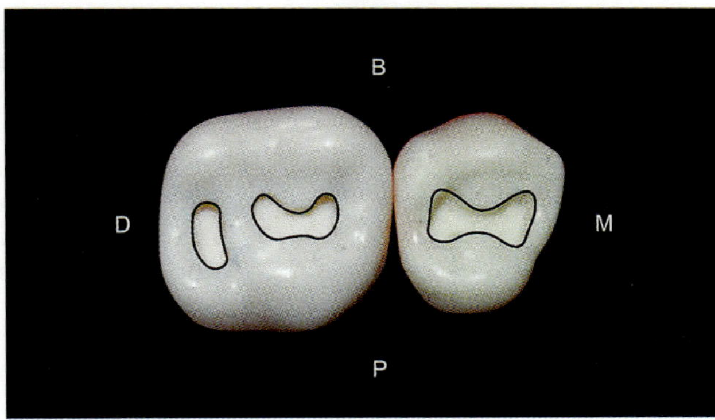

Fig. 44.2: Occlusal view of primary maxillary first and second molar showing class 1 cavity preparation.

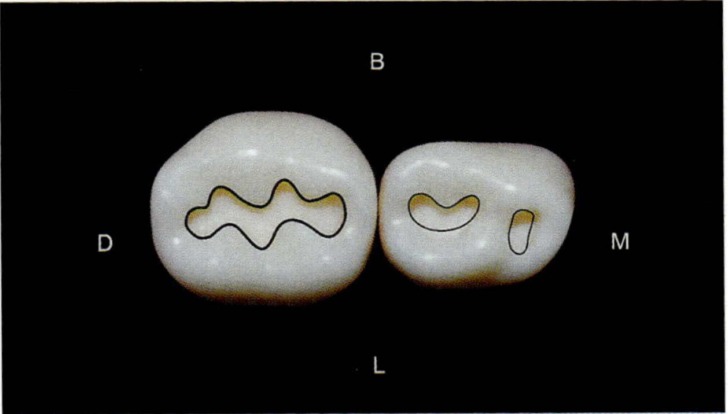

Fig. 44.3: Occlusal view of primary mandibular first and second molar showing class 1 cavity preparation.

Class II: Cavity Preparation

- **Occlusal box:** Same principles applied as for class I, but extension of outline is different for different teeth:
  - **For all first primary molars:** Extend the occlusal box half the way mesiodistally in a dovetail-like fashion.
  - **For mandibular second primary molars:** All pits and fissure should be included in preparation.
  - **For maxillary second primary molars:** Nearest occlusal pit should be involved. Oblique ridge should not be involved until undermined by the caries.
- Sharp cavosurface angle.
- Rounded/bevelled/grooved axiopulpal line angle in order to reduce stresses on this point and to allow greater bulk of material. Isthmus width should be half the intercuspal width.
- **Proximal box:** Greater width of the proximal box in order to keep the cavity margins in the self-cleansing areas. More buccolingual extension of the gingival floor or seat.
- Occlusal convergence.
- Axial wall should follow the contour of the external surface.
- The direction of enamel roads at the cervical line is either horizontal or occlusal, and therefore gingival bevel is not given while preparing class II cavity.
- Retention grooves should not be given.
- **Kennedy** (1997) contraindicated the idea of dovetail lock. He said that when occlusal fissure are prepared, this does not result in straight-line cavity that would require dovetail lock, instead it produces a curved shape that itself provides retention. Hence, if the dovetail was given, it would lead to unnecessary cutting of sound tooth structure.
- The distance between mesial surface of lower first mandibular molar and pulp horn is only 1.6 mm. Although 1.5 mm depth has been suggested for class I cavity, establishing this depth may lead to pulp exposure, and hence Rodda recommended 1 mm of depth.

The cavity designs for the proximal box are explained in the **Figures 44.4 to 44.11.**

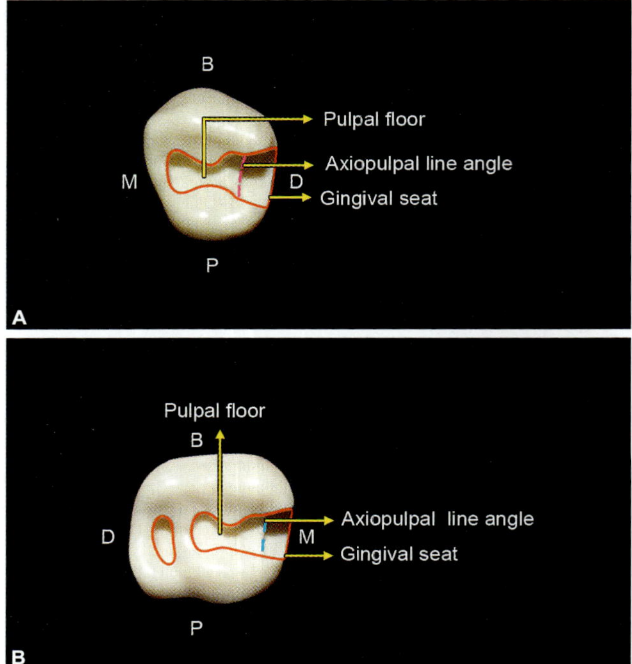

Figs. 44.4A and B: (A) Occlusal view of primary maxillary first molar showing class 2 cavity preparation; (B) Occlusal view of primary maxillary second molar showing class 2 cavity preparation.

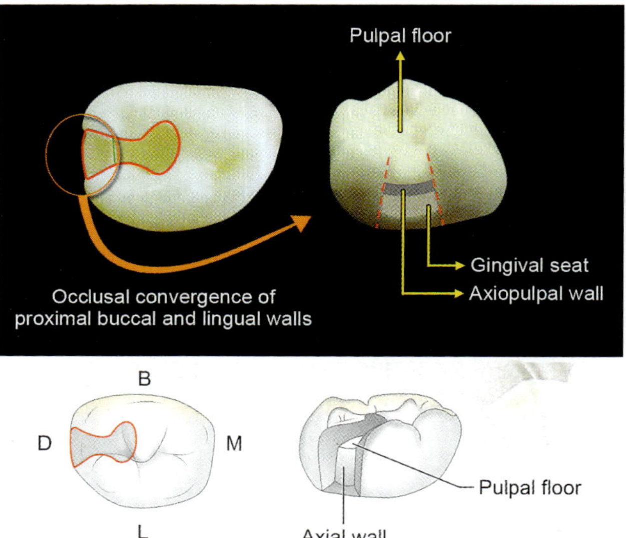

Fig. 44.5: Occlusal and proximal view of primary mandibular first molar showing class 2 cavity preparation.

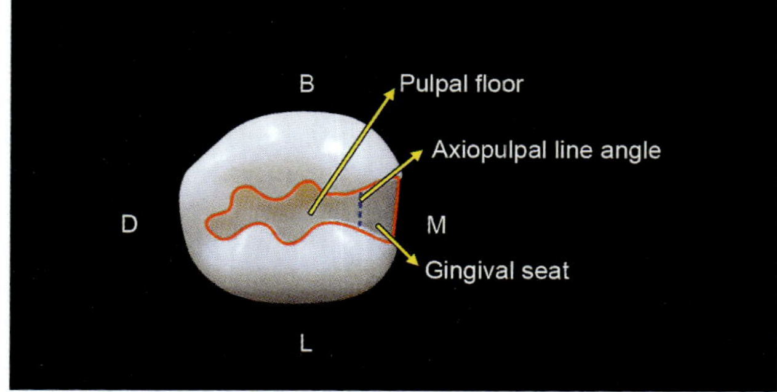

Fig. 44.6: Occlusal view of primary mandibular second molar showing class 2 cavity preparation.

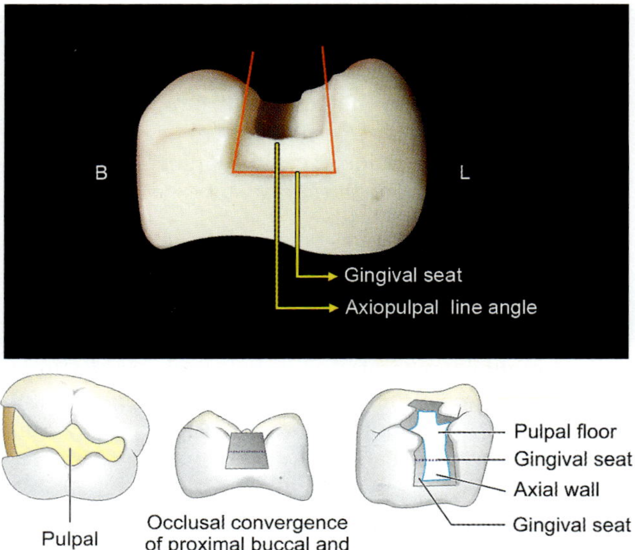

Fig. 44.7: Proximal view of primary mandibular second molar showing class 2 cavity preparation.

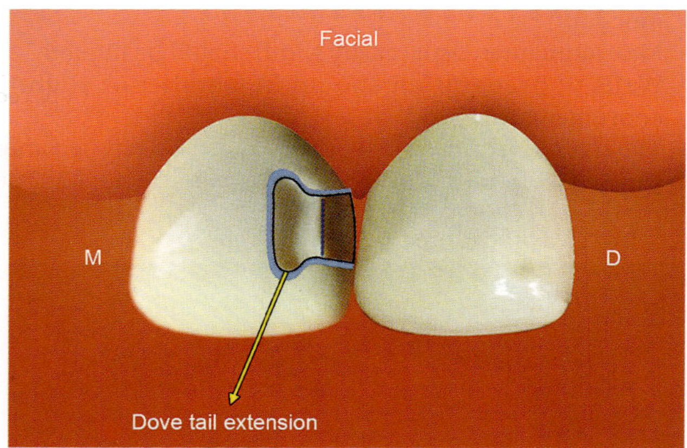

Fig. 44.8: Labial view of primary maxillary central incisor showing class 3 cavity preparation with labial dove tail extension. Dove tail extension provides additional retention.

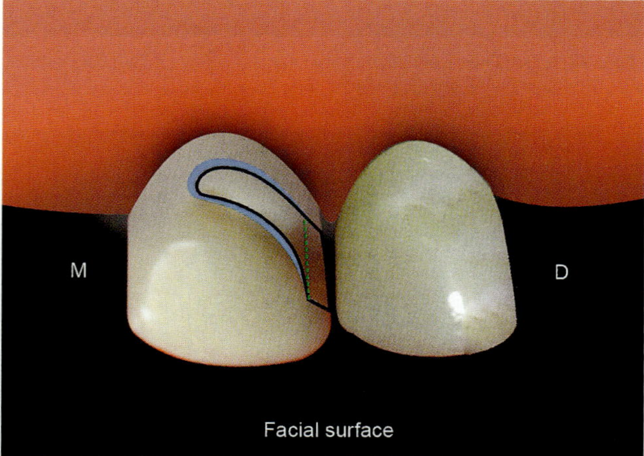

Fig. 44.9: Labial view of primary maxillary central incisor showing modified class 3 cavity preparation for decalcification of gingival one third of the tooth along with proximal caries. A short bevel is placed along the cavosurface margin.

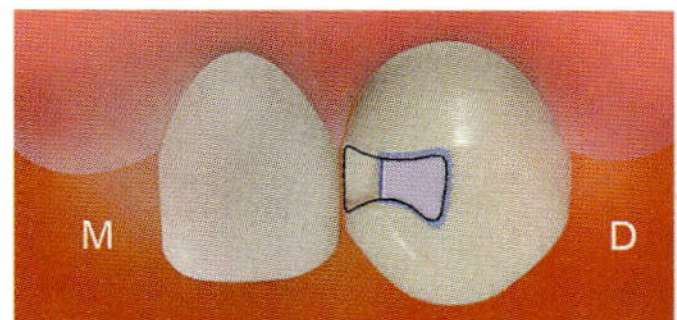

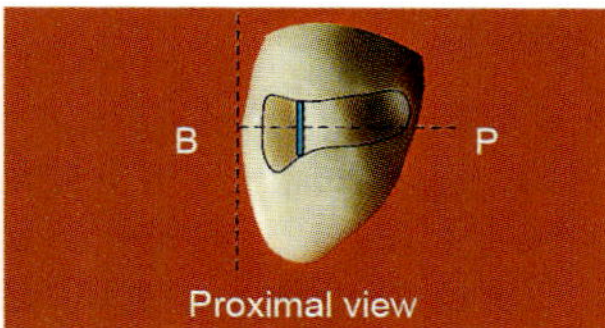

Fig. 44.10: Labial and proximal view of primary maxillary canine showing class 3 cavity preparation with labial dove tail extension. Proximal box is placed perpendicular to tangent line drawn on labial side. A short bevel is placed along the cavosurface margin.

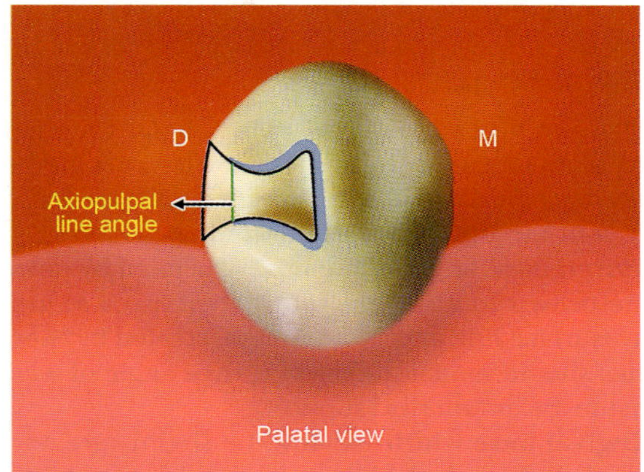

Fig. 44.11: Palatal view of primary mandibular canine showing class 3 cavity preparation with palatal dove tail extension.A short bevel is placed along the cavosurface margin.

MATRIX

Matricing is a procedure whereby a temporary wall is created opposite the axial wall surrounding the areas of tooth structure lost during preparation. The appliance used for building these walls is called matrix **(Fig. 44.12)**.

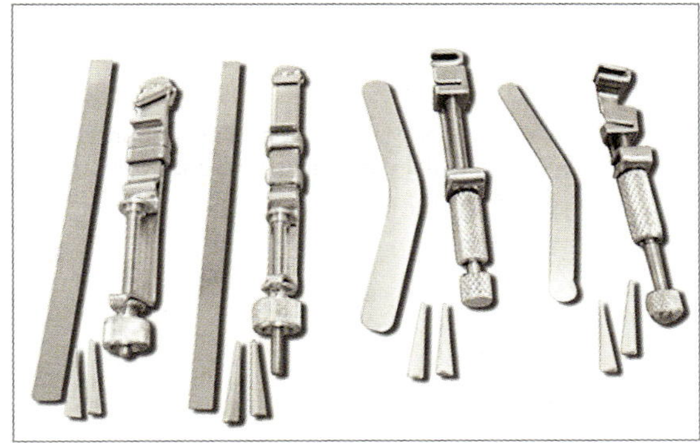

Fig. 44.12: Matrix band and retainers.

Rationale for Using Matrix

- Accurate reproduction of contour of teeth
- To prevent interproximal excess
- To establish tight contact areas
- To maintain integrity of normal gingival papillae
- To maintain arch dimensions in primary dentition.

Functions of Matrix

- To replace the missing wall
- Close adaptation of restorative material
- Retain restorative material during placement
- Allows restoration of contact point and external crown contour
- Isolation of cavity.

Ideal Requirements of Matrix

- Rigid to allow condensation
- Promote desired contour
- Should form positive contact with tooth
- Should be of minimal thickness
- Compatible with restorative material
- Easy of application
- Economical.

Classification of Matrix

According to place of application	• Posterior—t-band, tofflemire • Anterior—celluloid matrix
According to constituents	• Metallic—ivory No. 1, ivory No. 8, tofflemire • Nonmetallic—Mylar strips
According to presence or absence of retainer	• With retainer—ivory No. 1, ivory No. 8 • Without retainer—S-band
According to form	• Anatomical—celluloid crown form • Nonanatomical—ivory No. 1
According to patent	• Patent—ivory No. 1 • Nonpatent—celluloid crown form
According to use	• Universal—ivory No. 8, tofflemire • Unilateral—ivory No. 1

Recent Modifications in Matrix

- **Sectional matrix:** This system is easy to place, gives a large preparation area, thus reducing the working time. An added advantage of this system is that both mesial and distal proximal restorations can be accomplished by one matrix placement **(Fig. 44.13)**.

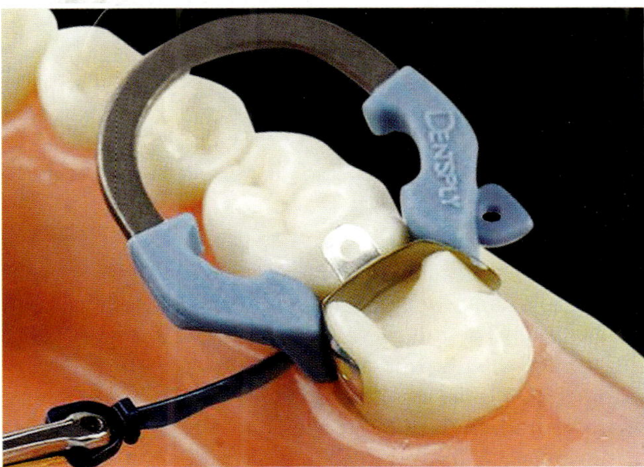

Fig. 44.13: Sectional matrix.

- **SmartView matrix system:** The SmartView matrix system also comes with SmartBands sectional matrices and titanium instruments. The SmartBands have a nonstick surface, are anatomically contoured, and integrate a reinforced placement tab while the instruments are made of high-grade, blue titanium. The specially designed titanium instruments are strong, durable, and lightweight. These are mostly used for composite restorations **(Fig. 44.14)**.

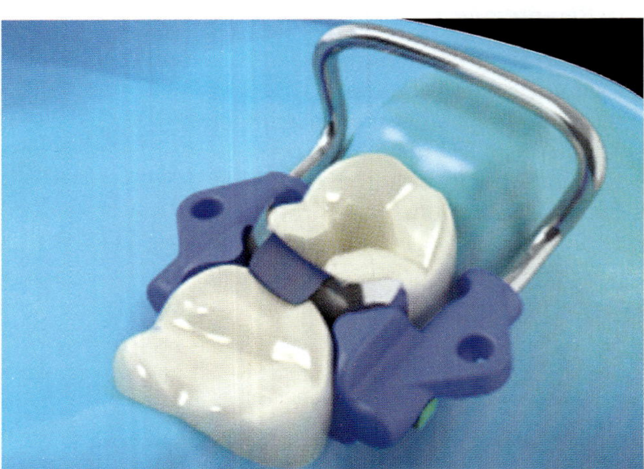

Fig. 44.14: SmartView matrix.

WEDGES

- It is used along with the matrix to prevent gingival overhangs of restorations. It is defined as a piece of wood, metal, etc., one end of which is an acute angled edge formed by two converging planes used to tighten or exert force in various ways **(Fig. 44.15)**.

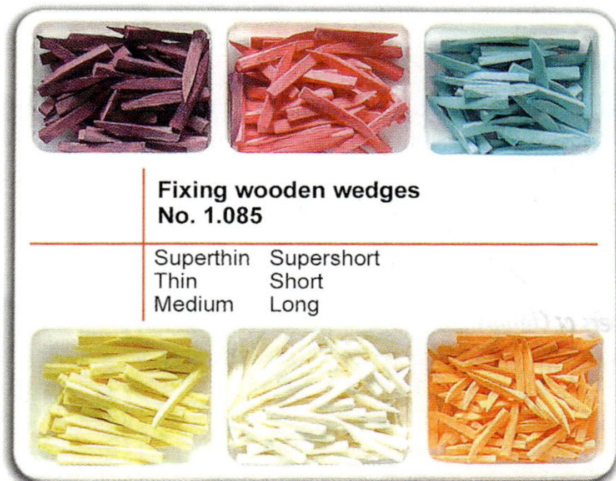

Fixing wooden wedges
No. 1.085
Superthin Supershort
Thin Short
Medium Long

Fig. 44.15: Wedges.

- The earliest description of wedges is during 1883 when wedges of boxwood, orangewood, and balsam wood are described. The metal wedges came into existence a little later, and the first one was Ottolenghi steel wedge.
- In 1960, **Messing** elaborated the disadvantages of preformed chair side wedges and **Produits Dentaires** introduced anatomical PD silver wedges that even had a hole for the floss.
- Currently all types of wedges like plastic, metal, wood, and celluloid are available depending upon side and type of tooth. The newest type of wedge is the light reflecting one introduced by Luci-Wedge, Hawe-Neos dental, Switzerland.

Types

- **According to anatomy:**
  - Anatomical—in shape of embrasure
  - Nonanatomical—round.
- **According to material used:**
  - Wooden—can be made of either hard or soft wood
  - Plastic—available in various shapes.
- **According to color:**
  - Colored—all types
  - Light reflecting—to be used with composites.

Selection of Wedges

A wedge should compress the matrix band to remaining healthy tooth structure through its entire buccolingual length apically to gingival cavosurface line angle. To select a correct wedge, four variables are to be selected:

1. **Convergence angle of the base**—dictated by tangential line drawn to adjacent tooth structures at gingival cavosurface line angles. The angle created by these two lines should match the convergence angle of wedge to ensure maximum rigid support.
2. **Gingival base width**—should be slightly greater than interdental space width in order to achieve stability.
3. **Wedge height**—is critical to establish contact point.
4. Concavity of side walls—dictates proximal contour of the restored tooth surface.

Ideal requirements of wedges

- Easy to apply and withdraw
- Should be of the shape of embrasure
- Should not cause deformation of matrix
- Be disposable
- Be radiopaque
- Be rigid
- Nontoxic and nonirritant
- Stable in oral fluids.

Functions

- Assures close adaptation of matrix band to tooth
- Prevents gingival overhang
- Assures proper health of interdental col
- Tooth separation
- Stabilization of band
- Absorbs fluid

Different placements of wedging (single, double, wedge wedging, and piggyback wedging).

RUBBER DAM

The need to work under dry conditions, free of saliva, has been recognized for centuries, and the idea of using a sheet of rubber to isolate the tooth dates almost 150 years. The introduction of this notion is attributed to a young American dentist from New York, ***Sanford Christie Barnum****, who in 1864 demonstrated for the first time the advantages of isolating the tooth with a rubber sheet. At that time, keeping the rubber in place around the tooth was problematic, but things soon improved a few years later, when in 1882,* ***SS White*** *introduced a rubber dam punch similar to that used still now. In the same year,* ***Dr Delous Palmer*** *introduced a set of metal clamps which could be used for different teeth.*

Advantages (Ballal et al., 2013)

- Dry clean operating field
- Access with visibility
- Moisture control
- Retraction of soft tissue
- Aseptic environment
- Improved properties of dental materials
- Protection of patient and operator
- Prevents aspiration or swallowing of small instruments and restorative materials
- Prevents tissue irritation by etchant
- Prevents tissue damage by rotary burs and sharp objects
- Effective infection control—aerosol prevention
- Reduce patient conversation
- Retainer provides some amount of mouth opening
- Quadrant restorative procedures are facilitated
- Minimization of mouth breathing.

Disadvantages

- Patient acceptance
- Poorly retentive clamps
- Trauma to tissues
- Frame can cause pressure marks on face
- Latex allergy
- Buildup of saliva
- Partially erupted tooth cannot receive a retainer
- Psychological intolerance.

Contraindications

- Absolute contraindication is known allergy to latex
- Patients with respiratory problems
- Patient at risk with transient bacteremia
- Severe gingival disease.

Euphemisms used for preparation of child for rubber dam placement		
Raincoat	–	Rubber dam sheet
Hanger	–	Frame
Clip	–	Clamp

Armamentarium

The entire armamentarium for the rubber dam placement is supplied as a package either for permanent or deciduous dentition. This contains rubber dam sheets, clamps for all teeth, template, retainer, rubber dam punch, retraction cord, and frame **(Figs. 44.16A to E)**.

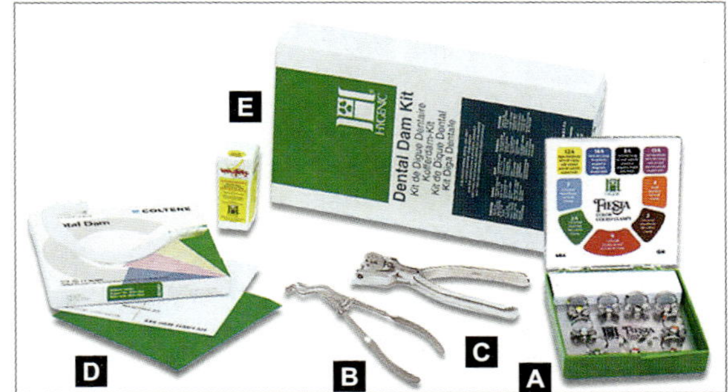

Figs. 44.16A to E: Rubber dam armamentarium. (A) Rubber dam clamps; (B) Rubber dam retainer forcep; (C) Rubber dam punch; (D) Rubber dam sheets; (E) Retraction cord.

Rubber Dam Sheets (Fig. 44.17)

- Available sizes are: 5″ × 5″ or 6″ × 6″
- Available thickness are:
  - Thin—0.15 mm
  - Medium—0.2 mm
  - Heavy—0.25 mm
  - Extra heavy—0.30 mm
  - Special heavy—0.35 mm
- Available colors are green, blue, black, pink, and dark blue.
- Also available in different flavors like mint, banana, and strawberry.
- The rubber dam sheet has a dark side and a shiny side. The shiny side is always toward the tissues so that the dam can pass easily over them with minimal irritation, whereas the dull side should be toward the occlusal aspect so that no light reflects from it to obstruct vision.
- The raw material—as with latex gloves—is the sap of the native rubber tree. Chemically, the substance is a cis-1,4 polyisoprene
- Other materials used for rubber dam are artificial latex (Isodam nonlatex) or latex-free rubber dam material (Flexidam nonlatex).

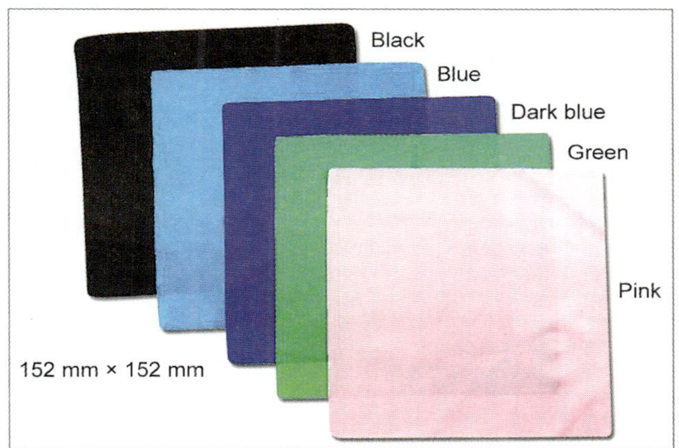

Fig. 44.17: Rubber dam sheet.

Retainers or Clamps

- It has four prongs and two jaws that are connected by a bow as shown **(Fig. 44.18)**.
- Various types and sizes are present for each tooth.
- Its use is to anchor the most posterior tooth to be isolated and also to retract gingival tissue
- Can be classified as wingless or winged

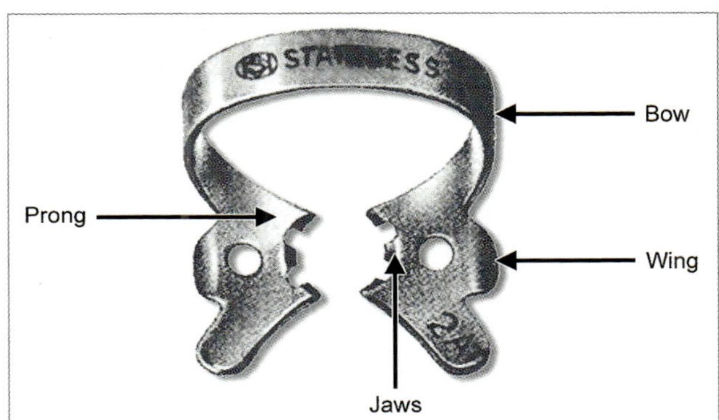

Fig. 44.18: Parts of clamp.

Modifications of clamps

- **Clamp with long guard extension**
  - Clamp with long guard extension has a larger wing which is used for retraction of the tongue.
  - These clamps retract and protect the cheek and tongue along with isolation.
  - They can be used with gauze or cotton rolls just for the retraction of tongue and cheek (**Sauveur**, 1997).

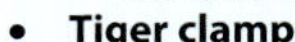

- **Tiger clamp**
  - Tiger clamps are clamps with serrated jaws.
  - These serrations increase the stabilization of the clamp on the partially erupted or broken down teeth.

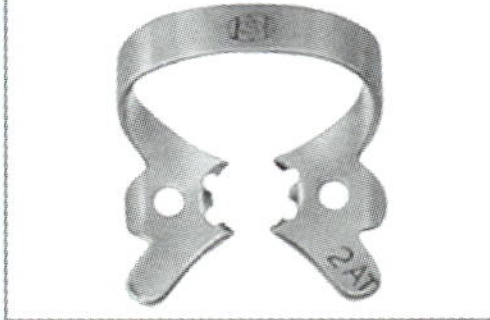

- **S-G (Silker-Glickman) clamp**
  - S-G clamp is a clamp with anterior extension which allows for retraction of the dam around a severely broken down tooth, and the clamp itself is placed on a tooth proximal to the one being treated.
  - It is made from durable cast stainless steel, which is autoclavable, corrosion-resistant, flexible and long lasting.
  - It is ideal clamp for molar isolation.

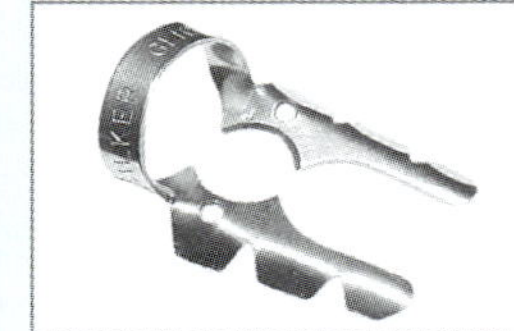

- **Super clamp (Dent Corp Research and Development, NY, USA)**
  - Super clamp comes with a pre-cut rubber dam material designed to fit the clamp.
  - It is very simple to use, quick and easy to place.
  - It allows for easy evacuation of oral fluids with a saliva ejector or a high-volume evacuator, and also can be used without the rubber dam to protect only the tongue and soft tissues.
  - The clamp is made out of a thin, flexible stainless steel.
  - Disadvantage is that, it cannot be used for anterior teeth.
  - It comes in three sizes: L—large clamp for molars, M—medium clamp which can also be used for molars and S—small clamp which can be used for premolars (**Scardina**, 2009).

Rubber Dam Retaining Forceps

- Used for placement and removal of clamps **(Figs. 44.19A to C)**.
- This instrument is necessary to open the clamp and position it around the tooth.
- The ivory forceps are preferable, because they allow the dentist to apply direct pressure toward the gum, which is frequently necessary to position the clamp securely below the bulge of the tooth crown.

Rubber Dam Punch

- It is a precision instrument having a rotating metal table with six holes of varying sizes and a tapered, sharp, pointed plunger **(Figs. 44.20A and B)**.
- It is used to make round holes of different diameters (0.7–2 mm).
- The largest hole being for molars and the smallest for mandibular incisors.

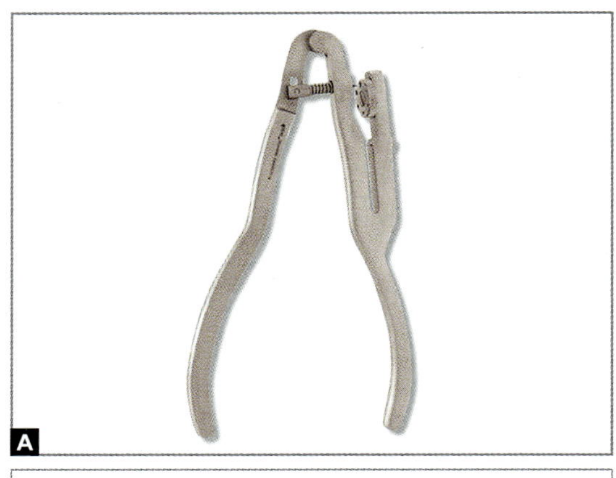

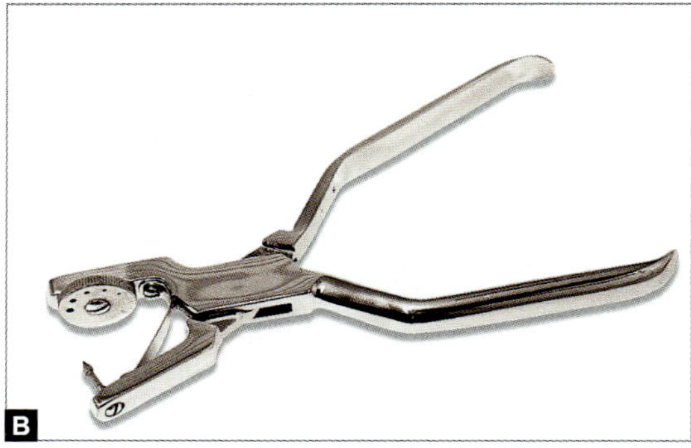

Figs. 44.20A and B: (A) IRDP rubber dam punch; (B) Ainsworth rubber dam punch.

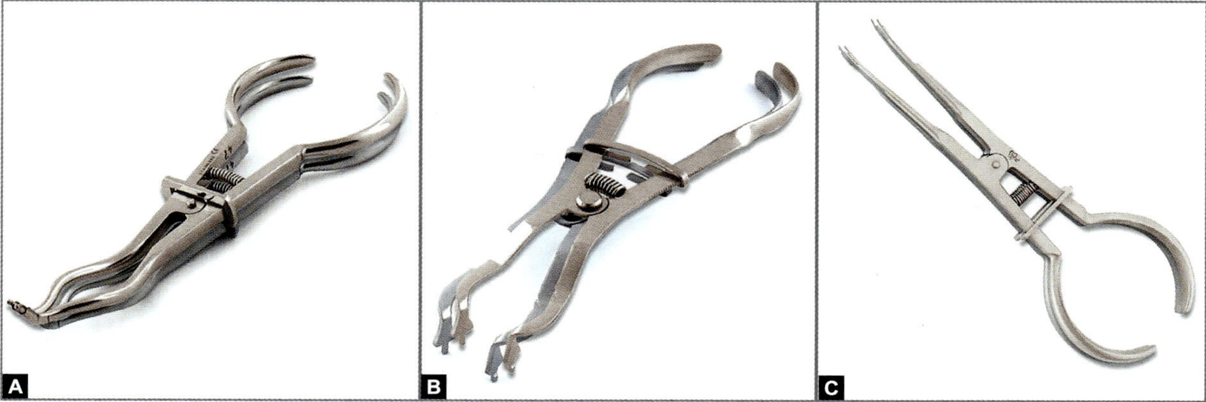

Figs. 44.19A to C: Rubber dam retainer forceps: (A) Brewer rubber dam forcep; (B) IV type rubber dam forcep; (C) University of Washington rubber dam forcep.

Rubber Dam Frame

- This is necessary to maintain tension in the dam so that the lips and cheeks may be retracted
- It holds and positions the border of rubber dam
- It is of two types:
  1. Metallic—**Young's** frame **(Fig. 44.21)**
  2. Plastic—**Nygaard-Ostby frame (Fig. 44.22)**, **Starlite Visi frame (Fig. 44.23)**, **LeCadre Articule frame (Fig. 44.24)**.

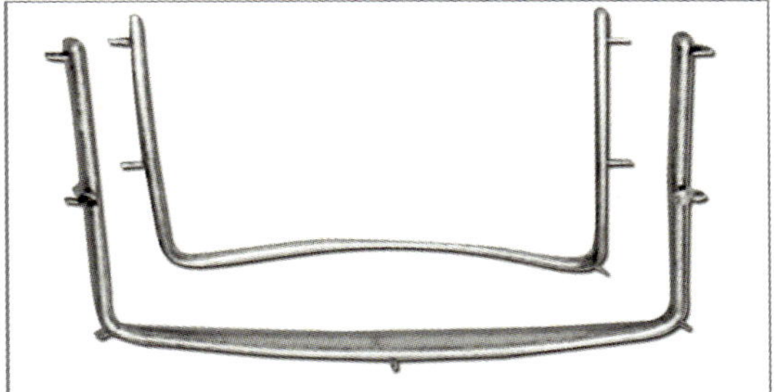

Fig. 44.21: Young's frame.

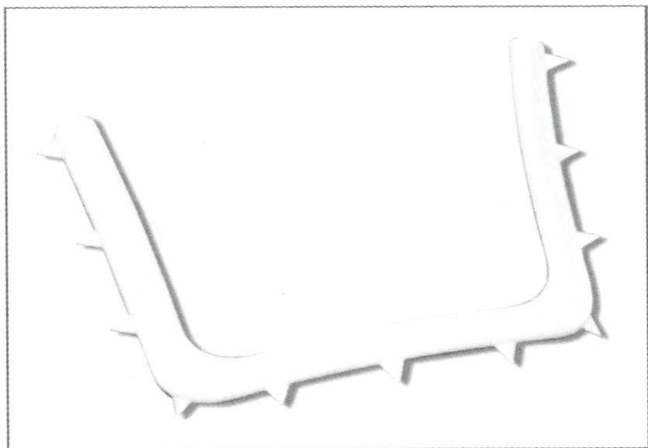

Fig. 44.22: Nygaard-Ostby frame.

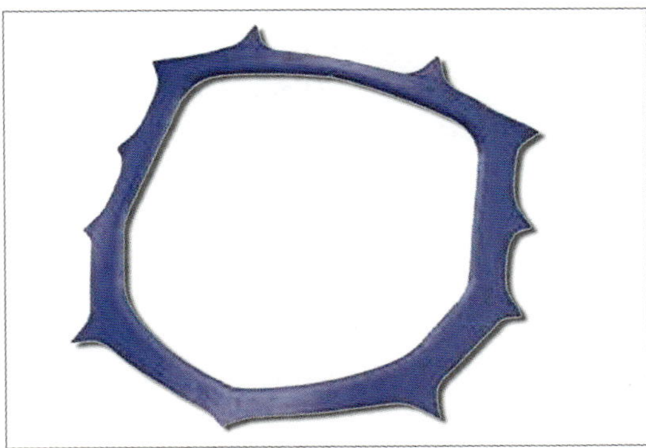

Fig. 44.23: Starlite Visi frame.

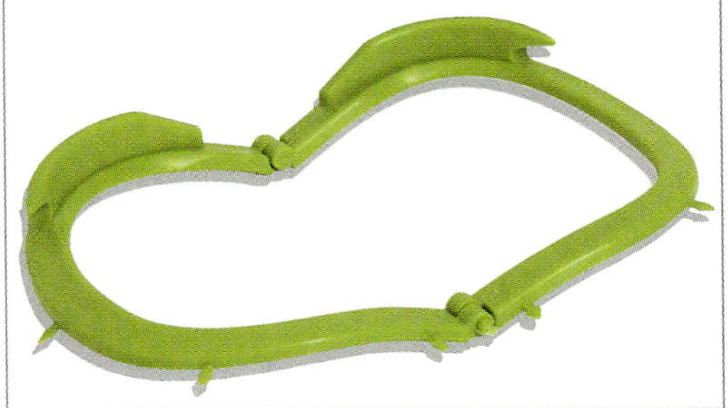

Fig. 44.24: LeCadre Articule frame.

YUNAD: Young's Universally Adjustable Rubber Dam Frame

- This frame has been named as YUNAD frame. It is named as YUNAD because it is a modification to Young frame (Y) and it is universally (UN) adjustable (AD) in nature (patent pending).
- It is designed by **Dr T Pavani.**
- **Ahlers MO** proposed safe T frame to overcome this tautness however the frame was not adjustable.
- Advantage of right sized frame for an individual is that it reduces the tautness in dam sheet and stabilizes dislodgment of clamp.

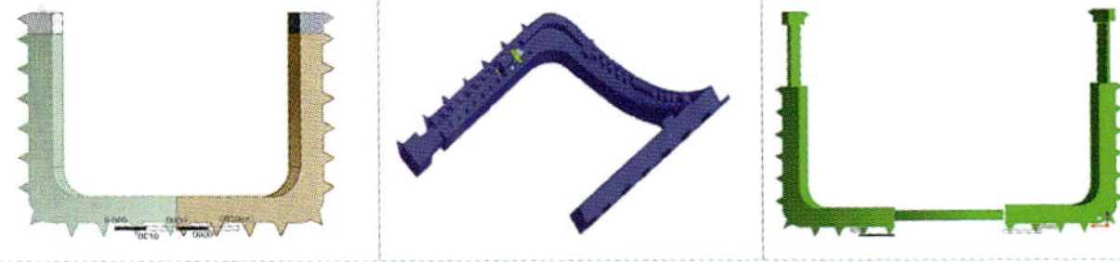

- Frame parameters:
  - The YUNAD frame is comprised of two L shaped components, each having a vertical and horizontal arm. Both the vertical and horizontal arms are adjustable by a slide with lock mechanism. The YUNAD frame had been designed in such a way that on compression the vertical length of the frame is 7 cm and horizontal length is 7.5 cm. On extending the adjustable arm that is within the vertical arm of the L shaped component, it measures a maximum length of 13 cm and the lower part of the entire unit is curved so as to accommodate the chin.
  - This frame has been designed in such a way that it has smaller vertical and horizontal dimensions when it is in its compressed position than the conventional pedo-frames available and has a greater vertical and horizontal dimensions when it is expanded to its maximum than the existing adult frames.
- Advantages:
  - Reduces tautness in the dam sheet, thereby increases stability
  - Right size of frame avoids injury to eyes
  - The sharp edges are broad and not pointed but still will stabilize sheet on edges.
  - One frame for all
  - Autoclavable
- Disadvantages:
  - The wear and tear of slide and lock mechanism
  - Expensive

The Safe-T-frame (Sigma Dental Systems)

- Composed of two hinged frame members whose snapshot-locking mechanism securely clamps the rubber dam sheet inplace.
- This concept also makes it possible to retain the traditional U-formed frame geometry and dimensions and offers a secure fit without-stretching the rubber dam sheet. It also has a further advantage of, raised edges of the frame which provide a barrier around the sheet preventing fluids from escaping on to the patient.

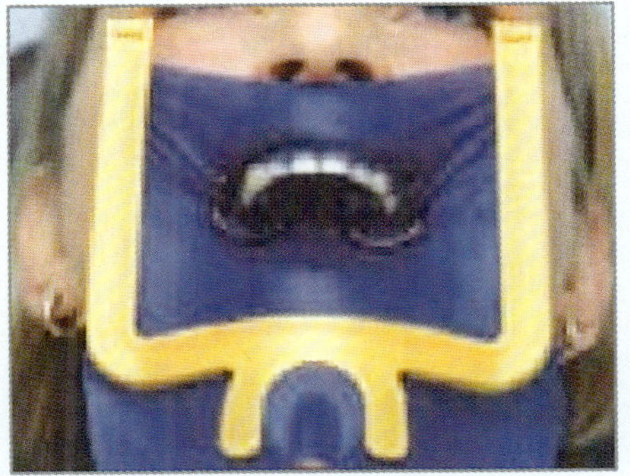

Rubber Dam Napkin

It is placed between rubber dam and patient's skin. It has the following uses:
- Prevents allergy
- Acts as a cushion
- Prevents pressure marks on patient's cheeks
- Convenient method for wiping the patient's lips on removal of dam.

Adjuncts

- **Lubricant:** To facilitate passing of dam through posterior contacts and also help the dam to pass over clamps. It is also applied over patient's tissues to prevent injury and dryness. Commonly used lubricants are soap solution, petroleum jelly, and cocoa butter.
  - **Dental floss:** To secure the rubber dam
  - **Rubber dam template:** To check for exact placement of rubber dam **(Fig. 44.25)**.

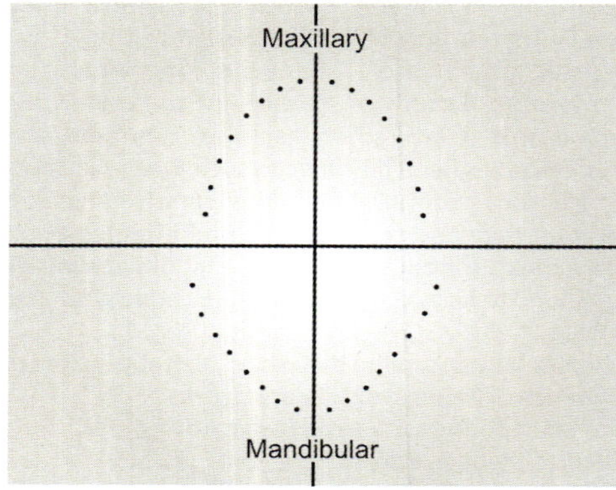

Fig. 44.25: Rubber dam template.

  - **Cushees:** These are soft thermoplastic cashew-shaped nodules which are grooved on their inner surface and act as rubber dam clamp cushions **(Fig. 44.26)**. It is slipped over the tooth attachment blade of clamp prior to clamp application. It increases patient comfort through elimination of contact of steel clamp with gingiva or tooth enamel, and thus helps to protect the natural tooth structure and costly restorations. It also enhances rubber dam seal to limit leaking from above or below the dam and reduces clamp slippage. They are sterilizable and reusable and are available in two sizes: yellow for anterior and bicuspid clamps and blue for molar clamps.

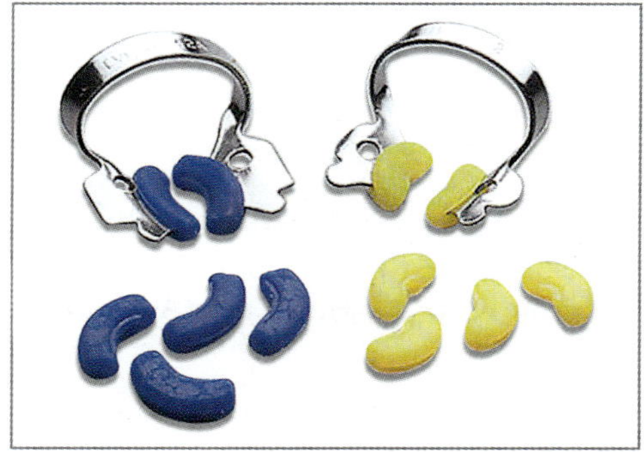

Fig. 44.26: Rubber dam cushees.

- **Wedjets (hygenic):** These are stretchable elastic stabilizing cords made from natural latex rubber and used as a rubber dam retainer **(Fig. 44.27)**. These are a faster and easier method of retaining the rubber dam than using conventional clamps. It is placed like dental floss over the rubber dam in the interproximal areas of the teeth, holding the rubber dam in position. It is available in extra small, small and large sizes. It reduces patient trauma and discomfort caused by metal clamps and are especially used in the isolation of anterior teeth.

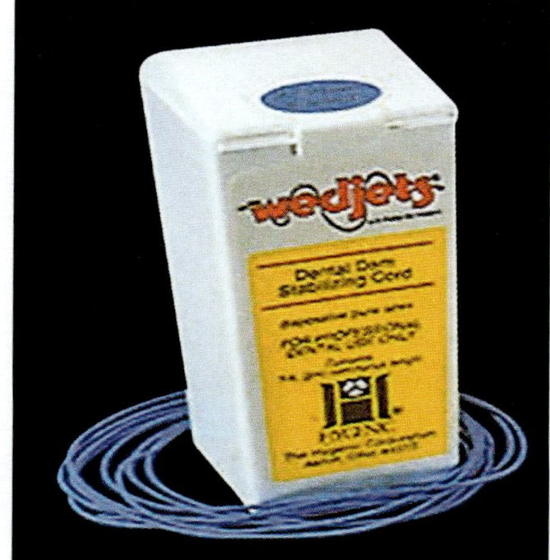

Fig. 44.27: Rubber dam wedjets.

Misadventures and Complications

- Trauma to lips and gingiva
- Poor clamp selection leading to laceration of gingiva
- Loss of springiness of clamp may lead to loss of retention
- Pressure marks on face
- High dam can block nasal passage
- Worn out clamps can fracture during treatment.

Procedures for Placement of Rubber Dam (Figs. 44.28A to C)

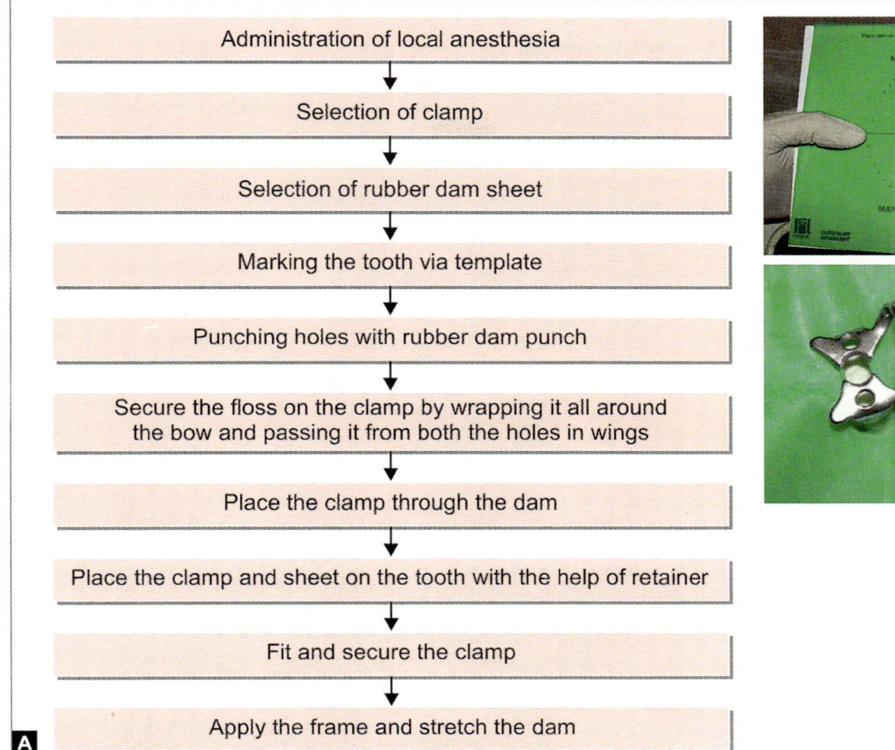
Administration of local anesthesia
Selection of clamp
Selection of rubber dam sheet
Marking the tooth via template
Punching holes with rubber dam punch
Secure the floss on the clamp by wrapping it all around the bow and passing it from both the holes in wings
Place the clamp through the dam
Place the clamp and sheet on the tooth with the help of retainer
Fit and secure the clamp
Apply the frame and stretch the dam
A

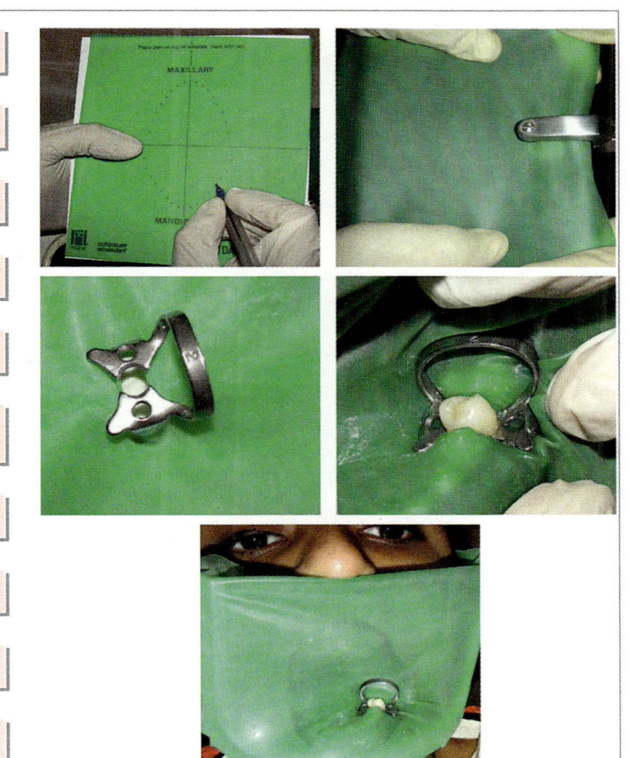
MAXILLARY

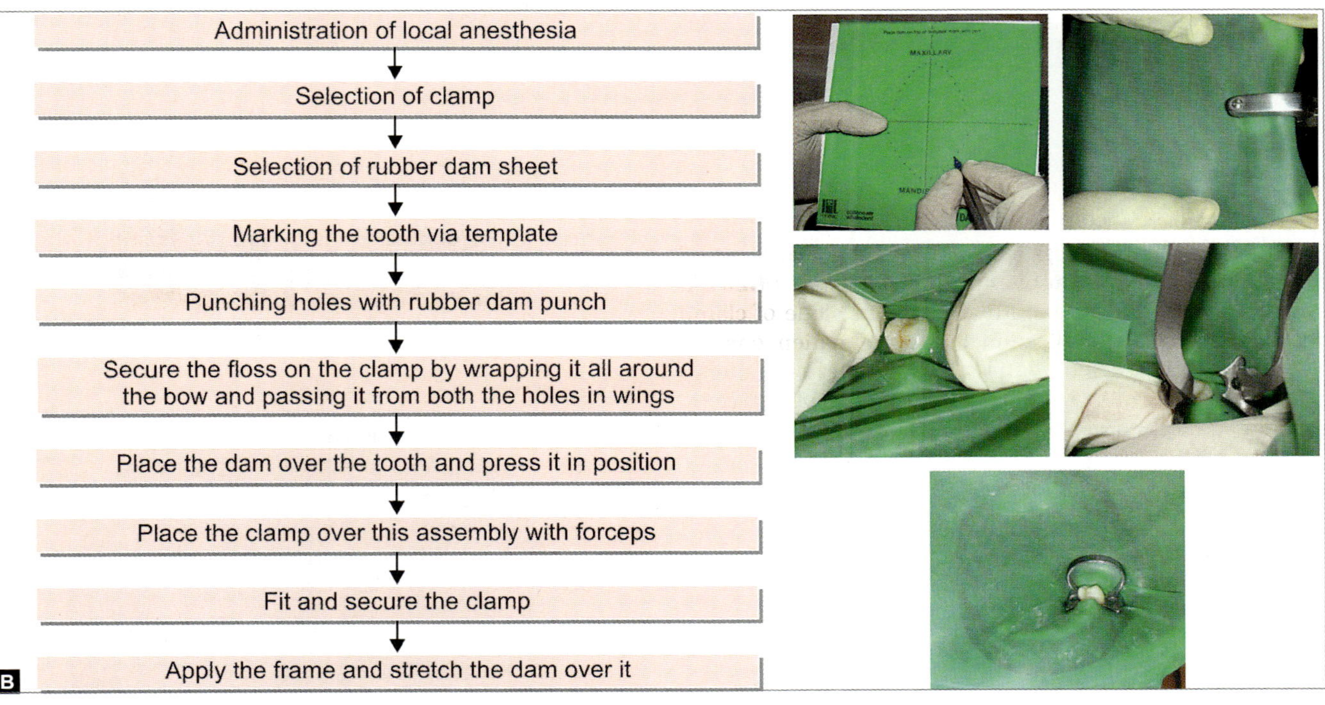
Administration of local anesthesia
Selection of clamp
Selection of rubber dam sheet
Marking the tooth via template
Punching holes with rubber dam punch
Secure the floss on the clamp by wrapping it all around the bow and passing it from both the holes in wings
Place the dam over the tooth and press it in position
Place the clamp over this assembly with forceps
Fit and secure the clamp
Apply the frame and stretch the dam over it
B
MAXILLARY

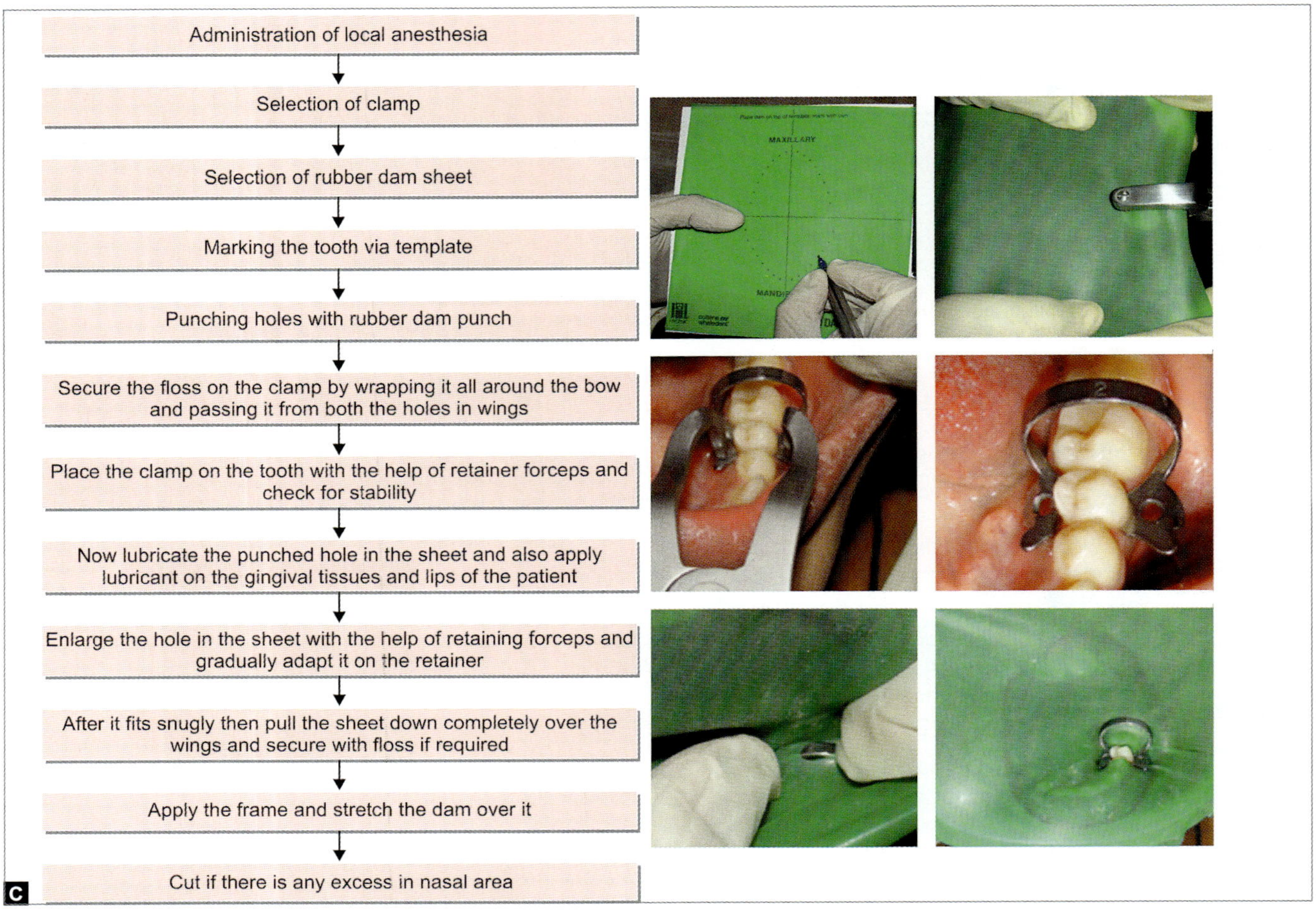

Administration of local anesthesia

↓

Selection of clamp

↓

Selection of rubber dam sheet

↓

Marking the tooth via template

↓

Punching holes with rubber dam punch

↓

Secure the floss on the clamp by wrapping it all around the bow and passing it from both the holes in wings

↓

Place the clamp on the tooth with the help of retainer forceps and check for stability

↓

Now lubricate the punched hole in the sheet and also apply lubricant on the gingival tissues and lips of the patient

↓

Enlarge the hole in the sheet with the help of retaining forceps and gradually adapt it on the retainer

↓

After it fits snugly then pull the sheet down completely over the wings and secure with floss if required

↓

Apply the frame and stretch the dam over it

↓

Cut if there is any excess in nasal area

C

Figs. 44.28A to C: Rubber dam placement procedures.

Recent Modifications

Quick Dam or InstaDam

- These are new types of rubber dams that have preattached frame
- Ease of application
- Minimal time consumption in placement
- Use of X-ray is more simplified with this type of dam
- They can either have a rectangle or circle pattern **(Fig. 44.29)**
- Disposable

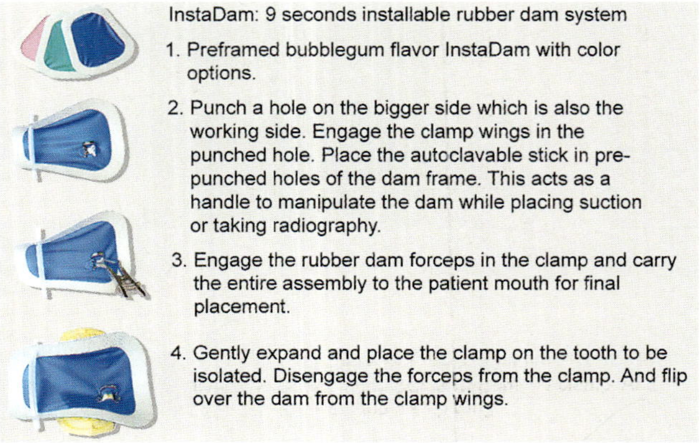

InstaDam: 9 seconds installable rubber dam system

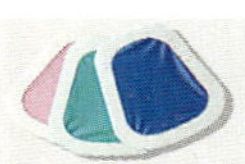

1. Preframed bubblegum flavor InstaDam with color options.
2. Punch a hole on the bigger side which is also the working side. Engage the clamp wings in the punched hole. Place the autoclavable stick in pre-punched holes of the dam frame. This acts as a handle to manipulate the dam while placing suction or taking radiography.
3. Engage the rubber dam forceps in the clamp and carry the entire assembly to the patient mouth for final placement.

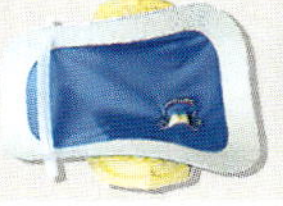

4. Gently expand and place the clamp on the tooth to be isolated. Disengage the forceps from the clamp. And flip over the dam from the clamp wings.

Fig. 44.29: InstaDam. (*Source:* Navadha ENT, Mumbai, Maharashtra).

OptraDam

- This is a type of quick dam for anterior segment where it can be fixed directly without use of any retainer clamps **(Fig. 44.30)**.
- Its method of application is quiet simple **(Fig. 44.31)**.

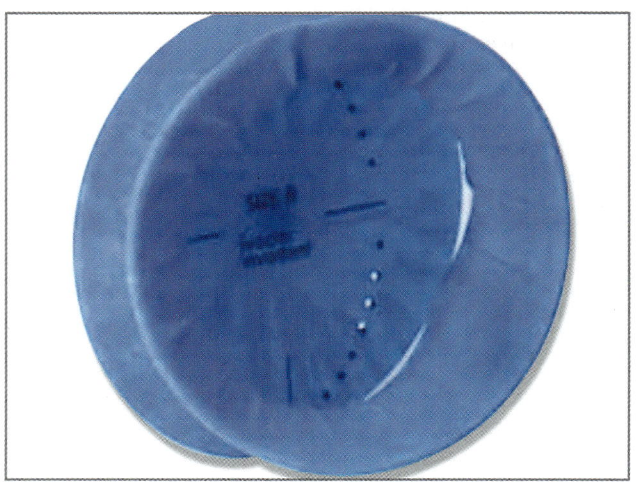

Fig. 44.30: OptraDam.

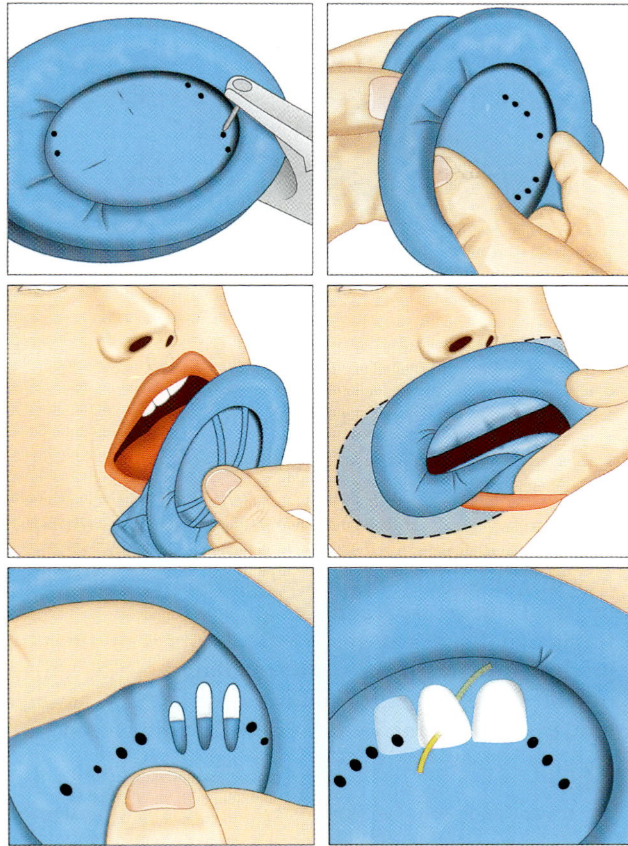

Fig. 44.31: Placement of OptraDam.

Split Dam Technique

- Isolation of badly broken down tooth is challenging as there might not be sufficient tooth structure to permit four-point stable contact around tooth and retain the clamp. In such cases, split dam technique is advised.
- In this technique, the rubber dam clamp is placed on the neighboring tooth. Two holes are punched approximately 5 mm apart and linked up by removing the rubber between them with scissors or by punching the third hole to connect the first two holes.
- The rubber dam is stretched over the rubber dam clamps or the teeth, and then the frame is placed to secure the sheet. The exposed area between the teeth is then sealed with a caulking agent like OraSeal. This ensures that there is no leakage.

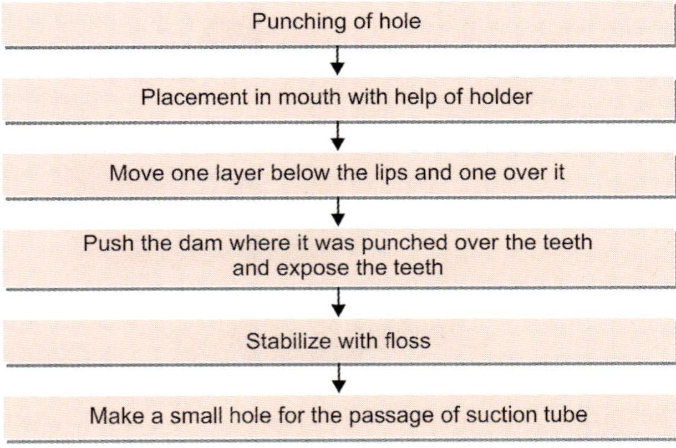

Derma Dam (UltraDent Products. Inc, USA)

Derma Dam is also a nonlatex dam which removes the possibility of latex reactions. It has allow content of surface proteins and has an advantage of having low dermatitis potential, reduced allergic reactions and greater tear resistance **(Fig. 44.32)**.

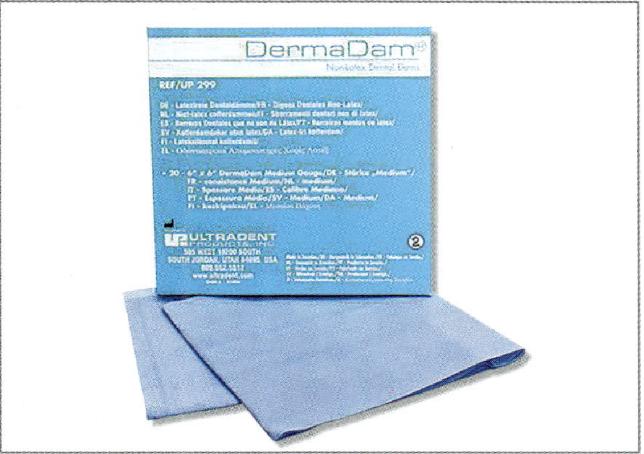

Fig. 44.32: Derma Dam.

Flexi Dam (Coltène/Whaledent)

- Flexi Dam is an elastic non latex dental dam made from an elastic plastomer **(Fig. 44.33)**.
- It can be elongated more than 1000% before tearing.
- It is more tenacious than latex dam and is simple to place.

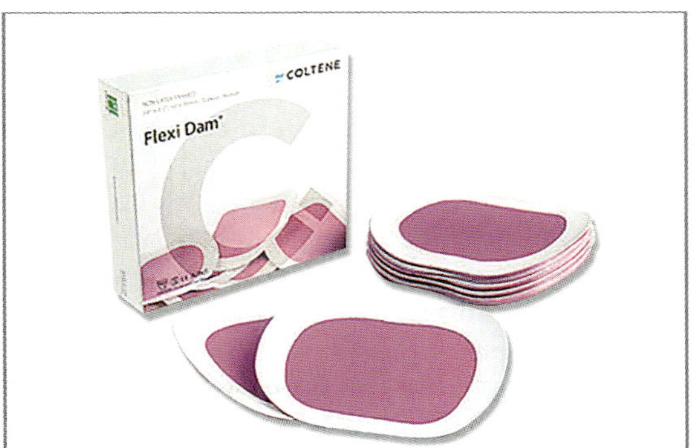

Fig. 44.33: Flexi Dam.

HandiDam (Aseptico)

- HandiDam is a preframed rubber dam which eliminates the need for traditional frames **(Fig. 44.34)**.
- It is quick and easy to place and allows easy access to oral cavity during the root canal procedure.

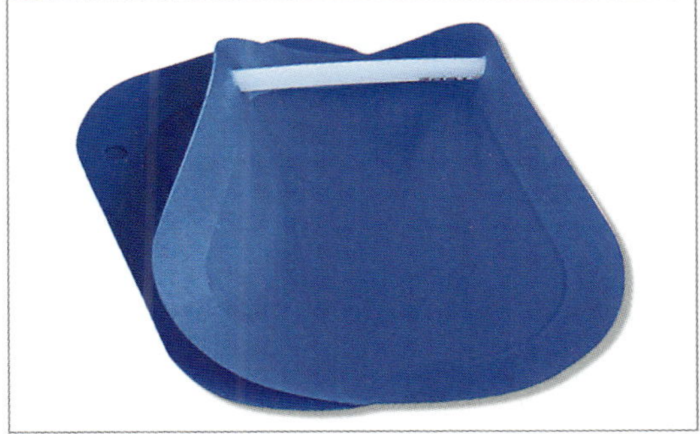

Fig. 44.34: HandiDam.

Dry Dam

- Dry dam is an alternative type of rubber dam which does not require a frame.
- It consists of a small rubber sheet set in the center of an absorbent paper with light elastics on either side to pass over the ears **(Fig. 44.35)**. It fits like a face mask with an absorbent lining to give patient comfort and reduced risk of allergic reaction.

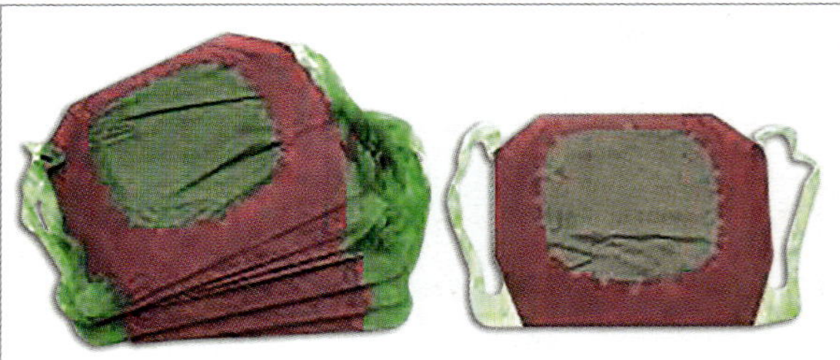

Fig. 44.35: Dry Dam.

- It is available in medium and thin varieties.
- It is useful for quickly isolating anterior teeth but it is not useful for isolation of posterior teeth.

OptiDam (Kerr)

- OptiDam is the first rubber dam with 3-dimensional shape and nipple design. The 3-dimensional shape of OptiDam and the anatomical frame shape match the contours of the mouth **(Fig. 44.36)**.
- This allows greater access and improved visibility to the working area. It also reduces tension resulting in easier rubber dam application and low risk of clamp displacement. OptiDam involves much less preparatory work than for conventional rubber dams, i.e., no marking of the tooth position because of outward oriented nipples and no hole-punching procedures as the nipples are easily cut. It offers maximum patient comfort and allows them to breath with no pressure around the nasal area.
- OptiDam is available in two versions—anterior and posterior.

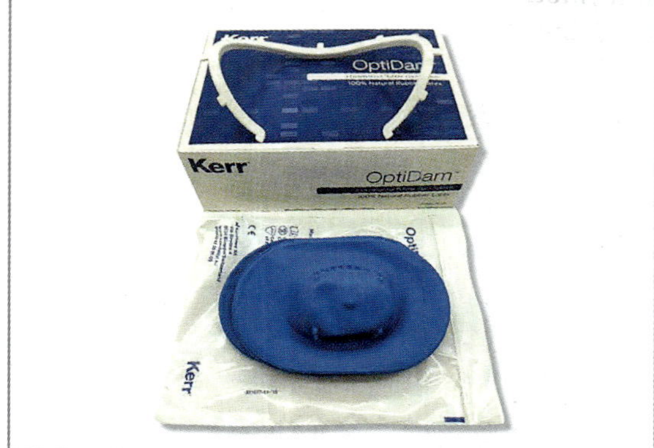

Fig. 44.36: OptiDam.

Kool Dam (Pulpdent Corporation)

- It is a light cured material applied on the gingiva or tooth surfaces prior to power bleaching, sand blasting or other procedures requiring intraoral protection or isolation.
- It is also called as liquid rubber dam **(Fig. 44.37)**.

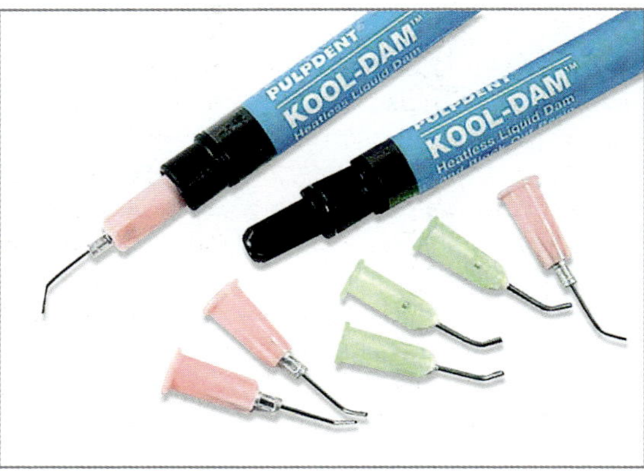

Fig. 44.37: Kool dam.

- *Because of its low exothermic reaction, it eliminates burning and pain, thus assuring patient comfort. It remains flexible after curing and has good tear resistance. It is moisture friendly and works well in the oral environment*
- A similar resin product called as OpalDam is manufactured by UltraDent Incorporation.
- It has two disadvantages. Firstly, being resin based, it produces heat when cured, and can thus cause discomfort or pain to the patient. Secondly, some of these products tend to displace and not stay where they are placed.

> **OraSeal®**
> OraSeal® caulking and OraSeal® Putty are especially designed, cellulose-based caulking and block-out materials that are syringe delivered to seal rubber dams to optimize tissue isolation, to block out undercuts associated with large gingival embrasures, and to prevent displacement during intraoral pick-up of anchoring attachments.

Fast Dam

- Anatomically shaped fast dam is designed to provide a superior means of maintaining a dry quadrant field **(Fig. 44.38)**.
- It can be used in place of cotton rolls to retract the cheek and tongue while maintaining a dry field.
- Continuous aspiration is achieved by means of 17 suction holes along the perimeter, eliminating the need to change saturated cotton rolls while retracting the cheek and tongue.
- Fast dam fits into the valve of all standard saliva ejectors.

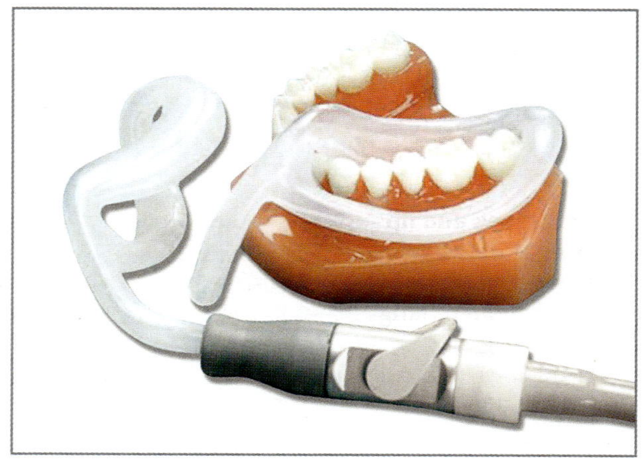

Fig. 44.38: Fast dam.

Isolite System

- The Isolite is a new dental device that simultaneously delivers continuous throat protection, illumination, retraction and isolation **(Fig. 44.39)**.
- It has a unique soft, flexible mouthpiece which isolates maxillary and mandibular quadrants simultaneously, retracts and protects the soft tissues from accidental damage from high-speed turbines, delivers shadow less illumination and continuously aspirates fluids and prevents the aspiration of foreign objects.
- It can be particularly useful in young people with incompletely erupted teeth.

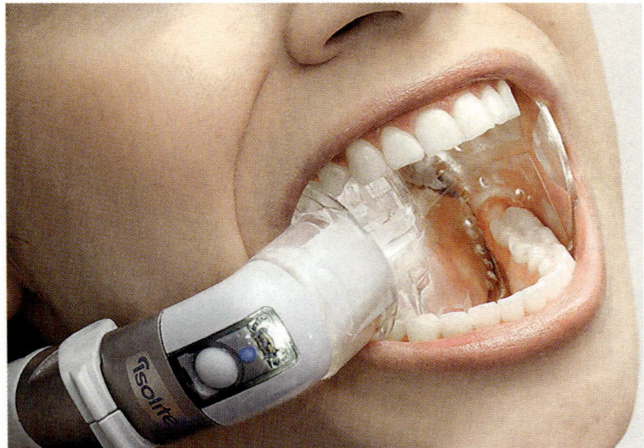

Fig. 44.39: Isolite system.

Isodry System

- A similar device, to Isolite system which performs the same function, but requires external lighting **(Fig. 44.40)**.
- It disadvantages are significantly more expensive than the rubber dam, does not provide the color contrast with the teeth, may cause damage to the gingiva, since it does not seal the gingiva.

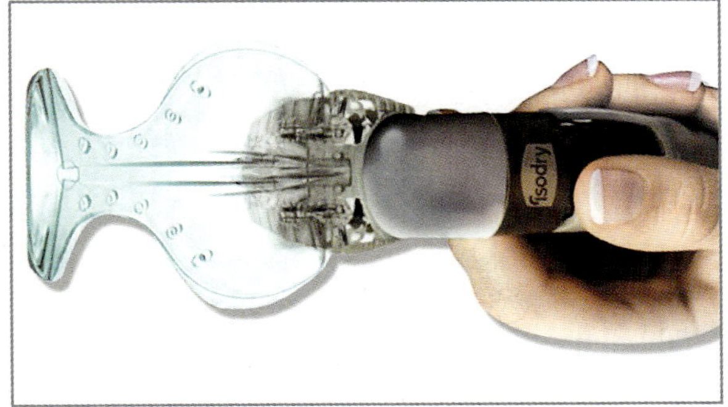

Fig. 44.40: Isodry system.

Intraoral cheek and lip retractor mouth opener tool:

- This is an intraoral tool that gives an unobstructed view of the operative field **(Fig. 44.41)**.
- It avoids patient fatigue and allows a relaxing treatment session.
- It also allows retraction of the tongue to avoid any injury intraoperatively.
- It is autoclavable.
- It is a cost-effective option for isolation and retraction.

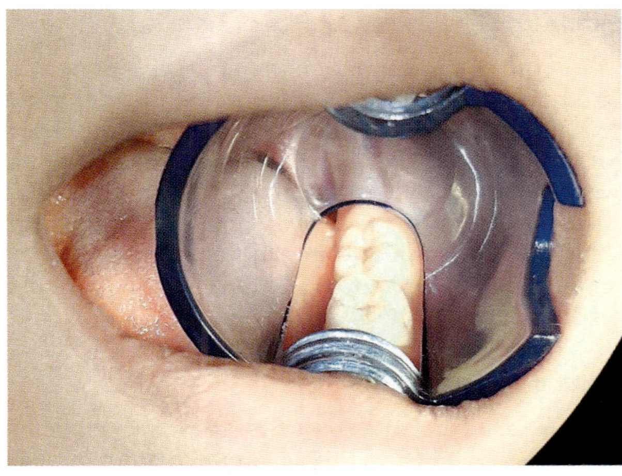

Fig. 44.41: Intraoral cheek and lip retractor mouth opener tool. *(Pic courtesy:* Keyur Chauhan, Ahmedabad).

AIR ABRASION (MICROABRASION AND KINETIC CAVITY PREPARATION)

The study of the use of air abrasion technology for dental applications initiated by **Dr Robert Black** of Corpus Christi Texas in the 1940s was successfully introduced in 1951 with the Airdent air abrasion unit (SS White). In spite of showing promising results, the concept did not gain popularity due to three major factors. First, air abrasion was not able to prepare cavities with well-defined walls and margins, and the materials during that time (mostly amalgam and direct or indirect gold) demanded such preparations since the concept of bonding had not been introduced. Second, the introduction of the air turbine handpiece in the late 1950s made conventional cavity preparations less time consuming. Third, as high-velocity suction had not been developed, evacuation of the powder was difficult.

Though the basic concept of the air abrasion device has remained the same, it has experienced a rebirth not due to changes in the device per se but due to improvements in bonding, restorative materials, isolation, and high volume suction. Air abrasion can be best described as a pseudomechanical, nonrotary method of cutting and removing dental hard tissue. The terms "micro air-abrasion" and "kinetic cavity preparation" have been used synonymously to describe air abrasion.

Advantages

There are many advantages to the patient when the dentist uses air abrasion:

- It is painless
- Local anesthesia is rarely needed
- It works quickly and the tooth with a small lesion is ready to restore in seconds
- It work quietly without the whine of the all too familiar dental headpiece
- There is no vibration or pressure to cause micro-fractures that weaken tooth
- There is no production of heat to damage the dental pulp
- Lesser sound tooth structure is removed.

Principle

- Air abrasion for restoration preparation removes tooth structure using a stream of aluminum oxide particles generated from compressed air or bottled carbon dioxide or nitrogen gas. The abrasive particles strike the tooth with high velocity and remove small amounts of tooth structure.
- Efficiency of removal is relative to the hardness of the tissue or material being removed and the operating parameters of the air abrasion device.

Operating Parameters

- A number of air abrasion systems are available today such as the PrepMaster (Groman Inc.), Airbrator (North Bay/Bioscience, LLC), PrepStart, and PrepAir (Danville Engineering) all of which work on the same principle. Some like the RONDOflex plus (KaVo) work on the principle of air abrasion technology with water spray.
- Generally, air pressures range from 40 psi to 160 psi. The recommended levels are at 100 psi for cutting and 80 psi for surface etching.
- The most common particle sizes are either 27 or 50 μm in diameter. The larger particles allow the clinician to work faster but will result in comparatively larger sized cavity preparations than those with the 27 μm particles. Higher particle flow rate will allow more particles to abrade the working surface faster.
- The speed of the abrasive particles when they hit the tooth depends upon the gas pressure, nozzle diameter, particle size, and distance from the surface.
- Typical operating distances from the tooth range from 0.5 mm to 2 mm. Further distances produce a more diffuse stream that results in a diminished cutting ability.

Precautions

- Need to protect patient with glasses, rubber dam if possible
- Dental team needs masks and glasses
- Stop frequently to check the progress
- Start with low pressure and low power then increase as needed
- Hold tip 1–2 mm away from tooth at a 45° angle then activate
- Always keep tip moving
- Requires external suction and air evacuation for the room
- Use disposable mirrors
- Like any air stream air abrasion can cause subcutaneous emphysema.

Clinical Uses

- Classes I, II, III, IV, and V cavity preparations
- Sealants and preventive restorations
- Repair of composite and porcelain especially margin of veneers
- Removal of composite and amalgam.

Procedure

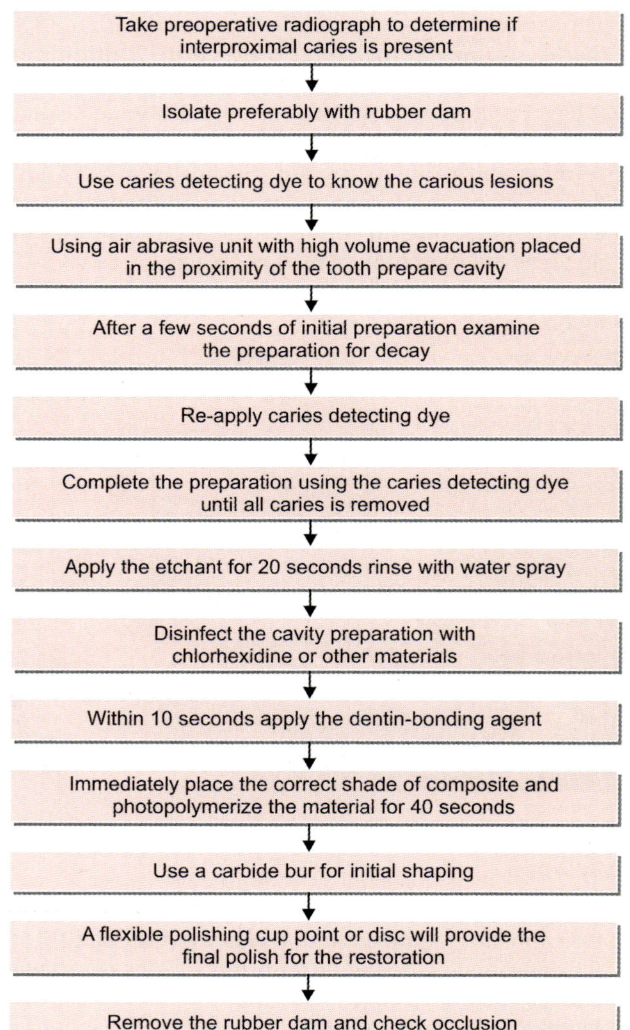
Take preoperative radiograph to determine if interproximal caries is present
Isolate preferably with rubber dam
Use caries detecting dye to know the carious lesions
Using air abrasive unit with high volume evacuation placed in the proximity of the tooth prepare cavity
After a few seconds of initial preparation examine the preparation for decay
Re-apply caries detecting dye
Complete the preparation using the caries detecting dye until all caries is removed
Apply the etchant for 20 seconds rinse with water spray
Disinfect the cavity preparation with chlorhexidine or other materials
Within 10 seconds apply the dentin-bonding agent
Immediately place the correct shade of composite and photopolymerize the material for 40 seconds
Use a carbide bur for initial shaping
A flexible polishing cup point or disc will provide the final polish for the restoration
Remove the rubber dam and check occlusion

Accessories for Air Abrasion System

- Grades of the powder particles
- Various tip diameter sizes and tip angulations
- Air abrasion resistant intraoral mirror
- Sand trap traps the abrasive particles from where they can be evacuated through the suction
- Power plus booster recompresses the compressed air up to 135 psi to increase the air pressure
- Disposable air abrasion handpiece—Airbrator® (North Bay/Bioscience, LLC)
- Super high volume evacuation systems—RapidVac™ (Union Medical Evacuation System)
- MicroVibe tip generates mechanical vibrations that help resin penetrate narrow gaps.
- The first air abrasion system was introduced in 1951 as Airdent air abrasion unit (SS White)
- RONDOflex plus (KaVo) uses air abrasion technology with water spray.

POINTS TO REMEMBER

- Operative dentistry is the art and science of the diagnosis, treatment, and prognosis of defects of teeth that do not require full coverage restorations for correction. Such treatment should result in the restoration of proper tooth form, function, and esthetics while maintaining the physiologic integrity of the teeth in harmonious relationship with the adjacent hard and soft tissues, all of which should enhance the general health and welfare of the patient.
- GV Black in 1924 outlined the classification of cavity preparation into five types, and later on the sixth modification was added by Simon.
- Finn classification is used for pediatric dentistry.
- Mount and Hume classification exemplifies the complexity of lesion.
- In the principles of tooth preparation, initial tooth preparation includes outline form, resistance form, retention form, convenience form, whereas final tooth preparation includes removal of any remaining infected dentin and old restorative material, pulp protection, secondary resistance, and retention forms, procedures for finishing external walls and cleansing, inspecting, sealing.
- Modifications in class i cavity preparation for primary teeth includes narrow occlusal table, limiting the cavity to 0.5 mm pulpal to enamelodentinal junction, walls of preparation should be parallel or slightly convergent occlusally, flat or slightly concave pulpal floor with rounded line and point angles.
- Modifications in class ii cavity preparation for primary teeth includes rounded axiopulpal line angle, isthmus width should be half the intercuspal width, greater width of the proximal box, occlusal convergence, gingival bevel is not given, dovetail lock should be present.
- Matricing is a procedure whereby a temporary wall is created opposite the axial wall surrounding the areas of tooth structure lost during preparation. Conventional matrix retainers are ivory No. 1 and 8, tofflemire matrix retainer. The newer modifications are sectional matrix, Palodent plus that can be used on both side in a single placement and SmartView which can be used for composites.
- SC Barnum in 1864 discovered the rubber dam and Delous Palmer discovered the rubber dam retainers. The main advantages of rubber dam are dry clean operating field, access with visibility, moisture control, retraction of soft tissue, aseptic environment, and prevent aspiration or swallowing of small instruments and restorative materials.
- The armamentarium for the rubber dam placement contains rubber dam sheets, clamps for all teeth, template, retainer, rubber dam punch, retraction cord, and frame.
- Rubber dam frames include metallic (Young frame) and plastic (Nygaard Ostby, Starlite Visi, Lecadre Articule). Dr Robert Black in the 1940s introduced air abrasion.

Questionnaire

1. Define operative dentistry and give the importance of primary teeth.
2. Differentiate between primary and permanent teeth.
3. Classify cavity preparation and the principles of cavity preparation.
4. What is matricing? Enumerate the new systems.
5. Describe rubber dam components and its placement techniques.
6. What is air abrasion technology?

FURTHER READING

1. Ballal, Vasudev. Safety tools in endodontics. Saudi Endodontic Journal. 2013;3:95.
2. Ballal NV, Khandeelwal D, Saraswathi MV. Rubber dam in endodontics: An overview of recent advances. Int J Clin Dent. 2013;1(4):39.
3. Banerjee A, Watson TF. Air abrasion: its uses and abuses. Dent Update. 2002;29:340-6.
4. Baum L, Phillips RW, Lund MR. Textbook of Operative Dentistry. Philadelphia: WB Saunders; 1981. pp. 295-8.
5. Bennett N. The science and practice of dental surgery, volume 11. Oxford: Oxford Medical Publications; 1931. pp. 795-9.
6. Black CV. Operative dentistry, volume II, 5th edition. Chicago: Medico-Dental Publishing Co.; 1922. pp. 262-3.
7. Christensen G. Cavity preparation: cutting or abrasion? J Am Dent Assoc. 1996;127:1651-4.
8. Clark TD, Mjorl A. Current teaching of cariology in North American dental schools. Oper Dent. 2001;26: 412-8.
9. Curzon MEJ, Roberts JF, Kennedy DB. Kennedy's paediatric operative dentistry, 4th edition. California: Wright; 1996.
10. Elderton RJ. The prevalence of failure of restorations: a literature review. J Dent. 1976;4:207-10.
11. Gilmore HW, Lund MR, Bales OJ, et al. Operative dentistry, volume 51, 4th edition. Louis: CV Mosby Co.; 1982. pp. 139-40.
12. Gordan VV. Clinical evaluation of replacement of Class V resin based composite restorations. J Dent. 2001;29:485-8.
13. Harris CA. The Principles and Practice of Dentistry, 11th edition. Philadelphia: Blakistan Sons and Co; 188S.
14. Heasman P. Master dentistry, restorative dentistry. Paediatr Dent Orthod. 2004;2:172-3.
15. Jørgensen KD, Wakumoto S. Occlusal amalgam fillings: marginal defects and secondary caries. Odontol Tidskr. 1968;73:43-54.
16. Kamann WK. The rubber dam: the change in indications and techniques. Schweiz Monatsschr Zahnmed. 1998;108:771-81.
17. Klausner LH, Green TG, Charbeneau GT. Placement and replacement of amalgam restorations: a challenge for the profession. Oper Dent. 1987;12:105-12.
18. McComb D. Systematic review of conservative operative caries management strategies. J Dent Educ. 2001;65:1154-61.
19. Messing J. A new style of interdental wedge. Br Dent J. 1960;108:18-9.
20. Mjorl A. Placement and replacement of restorations. Oper Dent. 1981;6:49-54.
21. Murdoch-Kinch CA, McLean ME. Minimally invasive dentistry. J Am Dent Assoc. 2003;134:87-95.
22. Ottolengui R. Methods of filling teeth. Philadelphia: 55 White; 1891.
23. Preto R. Biological restorations as a treatment option for primary molars with extensive coronal destruction. Braz Dent J; 2007. p. 18.
24. Qualtrough AJE, Wilson NHF. History, development of interproximal wedges in clinical practice. Dent Update. 1991.pp.66-70.
25. Rainey J. Air abrasion: an emerging standard of care in conservative operative dentistry. Dent Clin North Am. 2002;46:185-209.
26. Ryge G. Biological evaluation of dental materials. In: Proceedings of the 50th anniversary symposium on dental materials research national bureau of standards special publication 352 dental materials research; June 1972.
27. Sengupta A, Pandit V, Gandhe P, Gujrathi N, Chaubey S. Rubber Dam International Journal of Current Research. 2019;11(10):7708-14.
28. Taft J. A Practical Treatise on Operative Dentistry, 4th edition. London: T Ruber; 1883.
29. van Pelt AW. Kinetic cavity preparation. Ned Tijdschr Tandheelkd. 2000;107:67.
30. White JM, Eakle SW. Rationale and treatment approach in minimally invasive dentistry. J Am Dent Assoc. 2000;131:18S.

CHAPTER

Commonly Used Restorative Materials in Pediatric Dentistry

Deepak Raisinghani, Nikhil Marwah, Sonu Acharya

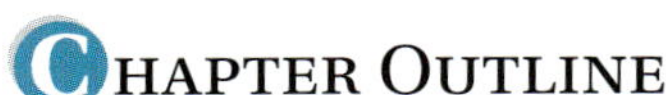

CHAPTER OUTLINE

- Silver Amalgam
- Bonded Amalgam Restoration
- Composite
- Calcium Hydroxide
- Glass Ionomer Cements
- Zirconomer

SILVER AMALGAM

Dentists have used it for restoring teeth for more than 150 years. The popularity of dental amalgam likely will continue to decline as the longevity of these other materials and their suitability as general amalgam replacements in the dentition is demonstrated. Dental amalgam is produced by mixing liquid mercury with solid particles of an alloy of silver, tin, copper, and sometimes zinc, palladium, indium, and selenium. This combination of solid metals is known as the amalgam alloy.

Classification

- **Based on copper content:**
  - *High copper content:* Copper content more than 12%
  - *Low copper content:* Copper content less than 6%.
- **Based on zinc content:**
  - Zinc-containing alloy with more than 0.01% zinc
  - Zinc-free alloys with less than 0.01% zinc.
- **Based on particle shape and type:**
  - *Lathe-cut:* Irregularly-shaped filings produced by cutting an ingot of alloy on a lathe.
  - *Spherical particle:* Produced by atomizing the alloy, whilst still liquid into a stream of inert gas.
  - *Admixed:* It contains both lathe-cut and spherical particles.

Physical Properties

- **Compressive strength (after 24 hours):**
  - Resistance to compression forces is the most favorable strength characteristic of amalgam.
  - The high-copper unicompositional materials have the highest early-compressive strengths of more than 250 MPa at 1 hour.
  - The compressive strength at 1 hour was lowest for lathe-cut alloy (45 Mpa).
  - High values for early-compressive strength are an advantage for an amalgam, because they reduce the possibility of fracture by prematurely high contact stresses from the patient before the final strength is reached.
- **Tensile strength:** Tensile strengths are only a fraction of their compressive strengths; therefore, cavity designs should be constructed to reduce tensile stresses resulting from biting forces.
- **Transverse strength:**
  - These values are sometimes referred to as the modulus of rupture.
  - Because amalgams are brittle materials, they can withstand little deformation during transverse strength testing. The main factors related to the high values of deformation are: (1) the slow rates of load application, (2) high creep of the specific amalgam, and (3) higher temperature of testing.
- **Elastic modulus:**
  - When the elastic modulus is determined at low rates of loading, such as 0.025–0.125 mm/min, values in the range of 11–20 GPa are obtained.
  - High-copper alloys tend to be stiffer than low-copper alloys.
- **Creep:**
  - The higher the creep magnitude, the greater the degree of marginal deterioration.
  - The highest value of 6.3% was found for the low-copper cut alloy, and the lowest values (0.05–0.09%) were determined for the high-copper unicompositional spherical alloys.

- **Corrosion:**
  - Corrosion is the progressive destruction of a metal by chemical or electrochemical reaction with its environment. Excessive corrosion can lead to increased porosity, reduced marginal integrity, loss of strength, and the release of metallic products into the oral environment.
  - The presence of a relatively high percentage of tin in low copper alloys reduces the corrosion resistance. The average depth of corrosion for most amalgam alloys is 100–500 pm.

Clinical Considerations

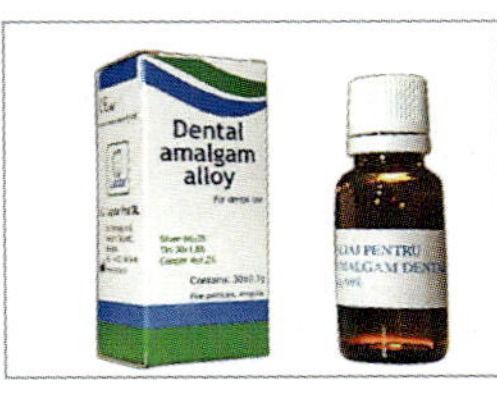

- Recommended mercury alloy ratios for most modern lathe-cut alloys is approximately 1:1, or 50% mercury and in case of spherical alloys, the recommended amount of mercury is closer to 42%, because spherical particles have lower surface/volume to completely wet the particles.
- Alloy and mercury were mixed by hand with a mortar and pestle or in an amalgamator. This process is called trituration. As alloy particles are coated with a film of oxide, which is difficult for the mercury to penetrate, this film must be rubbed off so that a clean surface of alloy can come in contact with mercury. The removal of oxide layer by abrasion is done by trituration.
- Amalgamation occurs when mercury contacts the surface of silver tin alloy particles. When powder is triturated, the silver and tin in the outer portion of the particles dissolve into mercury. Mercury has limited solubility for silver 0.035 wt% and tin. When the solubility in mercury is exceeded, crystals of two binary compounds precipitate into the mercury forming γ_1 (Ag_2Hg_3) and γ_2 (Sn7 Hg). Because the solubility of silver in mercury is much lower than that of tin, 0.6 γ_1 phase precipitate first and γ_2 phase precipitate later.
- Immediately after trituration, the alloy powder coexists with the liquid mercury, giving the mix a plastic consistency. γ_1 and γ_2 crystals grow as the remaining mercury dissolves the alloy particles.
- The next step in amalgamation is mulling, which is rubbing of the mixture to remove excess mercury and give a cohesive form. This is done by squeezing the mixture with a muslin cloth to drain out the extra mercury.
- As the mercury disappears, the amalgam hardens and is ready for condensation in the cavity. Ag-Sn-Cu alloy particles + Hg $\rightarrow \gamma_1$ + h + unconsumed alloy particles.

Indication of Amalgam

- Moderate-to-large restorations
- Restorations that are not in highly esthetic areas of the mouth
- Restorations that have heavy occlusal contacts
- Restorations that cannot be well-isolated
- Restorations that extend onto the root surface
- Foundations
- Abutment teeth for a removable partial denture
- Temporary or caries control restorations.

Contraindication of Amalgam

- Esthetically prominent areas of posterior teeth
- Small-to-moderate Classes I and II restorations that can be well-isolated
- Small Class VI restorations.

Mercury Toxicity

- The initiation of toxic effects of mercury was first evaluated in fishermen when they contacted Minamata disease due to excess mercury in water.
- Mercury penetrates from the restoration into tooth structure. An analysis of dentin underlying amalgam restorations reveals the presence of mercury, which in part may account for a subsequent discoloration of the tooth. Use of radioactive mercury in silver amalgam has also revealed that some mercury might even reach the pulp.
- The maximum level of occupational exposure considered safe is 50 µg of mercury per cubic meter of air per day.
- Amalgam tattoo is a common pitfall of the amalgam restoration.

Advantages of amalgam	*Disadvantages of amalgam*
• Ease of use	• Noninsulating
• High tensile strength	• Nonesthetic
• Excellent wear resistance	• Less conservative
• Favorable long-term clinical research results	• Weakens tooth structure
• Lower cost than for composite restorations	• More technique sensitive
	• More difficult tooth preparation
	• Initial marginal leakage

Operatory Prevention

- The operatory should be well-ventilated.
- All excess mercury, including waste, disposable capsules, and amalgam removed during condensation should be collected and stored in well-sealed containers containing water.
- Proper disposal through reputable dental vendors is mandatory to prevent environmental pollution.
- Amalgam scrap and materials contaminated with mercury or amalgam should not be incinerated or subjected to heat sterilization.
- If mercury comes in contact with the skin, the skin should be washed with soap and water.
- Use of carpeting is limited as it may incorporate mercury vapors and waste.

BONDED AMALGAM RESTORATION

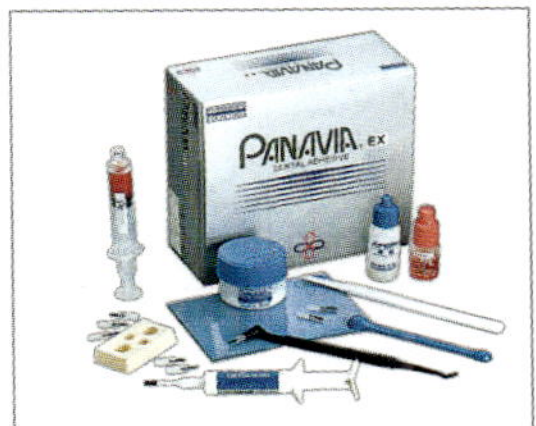

Recent concepts have suggested that posterior composite resin restorations may replace amalgam as a restorative material. Concern regarding mercury toxicity and greater interest in improved esthetics has encouraged a move away from amalgam as the material of choice for posterior restorations. However, some of the physical properties of composite resins used in the restoration of posterior teeth, combined with problems associated with technique sensitivity during placement, have led some to question their widespread use. The bonded amalgam restoration resulted from technology developed for use with resin-retained prostheses. Panavia EX (Kuraray), a chemically active resin that bonds to both enamel and metal, is one such material. Amalgam bond (Parkell) is an alternative material that has been developed specifically for bonding amalgam to etched enamel and dentin.

Properties

- Bonded amalgam restorations have significant advantages over both conventional amalgam restorations and posterior composite resin restorations.
- **Cavity design:** Conventional amalgam restorations are retained by mechanical retention like undercut cavity design but bonded amalgam incorporation technique reduces the need for removal of sound tooth tissue to create mechanical retention.
- **Handing properties:** Good esthetics and the ability to bond to enamel and dentin by the acid-etch technique, with and without bonding resins.
- **Polymerization contraction:** No polymerization contraction.
- **Marginal leaking:** Marginal leakage and loss of marginal integrity around conventional amalgam restorations have been recognized as serious disadvantages. Bonded amalgam restorations, however, show significantly less marginal leakage than conventional amalgam restorations.
- **Cuspal flexure:** The use of bonded restorations in posterior teeth has been shown to reduce cuspal flexure and increase the structural integrity of the tooth when compared to conventional restorations.

Clinical Technique

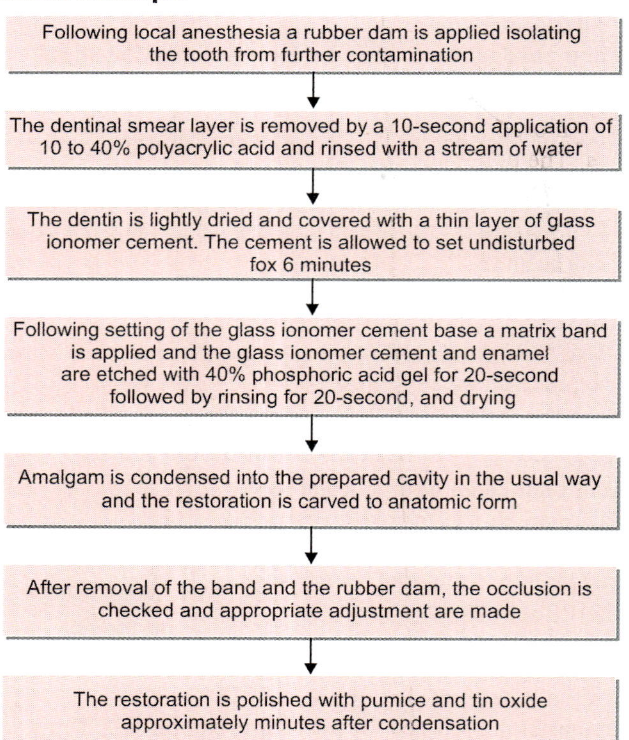

Following local anesthesia a rubber dam is applied isolating the tooth from further contamination
The dentinal smear layer is removed by a 10-second application of 10 to 40% polyacrylic acid and rinsed with a stream of water
The dentin is lightly dried and covered with a thin layer of glass ionomer cement. The cement is allowed to set undisturbed fox 6 minutes
Following setting of the glass ionomer cement base a matrix band is applied and the glass ionomer cement and enamel are etched with 40% phosphoric acid gel for 20-second followed by rinsing for 20-second, and drying
Amalgam is condensed into the prepared cavity in the usual way and the restoration is carved to anatomic form
After removal of the band and the rubber dam, the occlusion is checked and appropriate adjustment are made
The restoration is polished with pumice and tin oxide approximately minutes after condensation

COMPOSITE

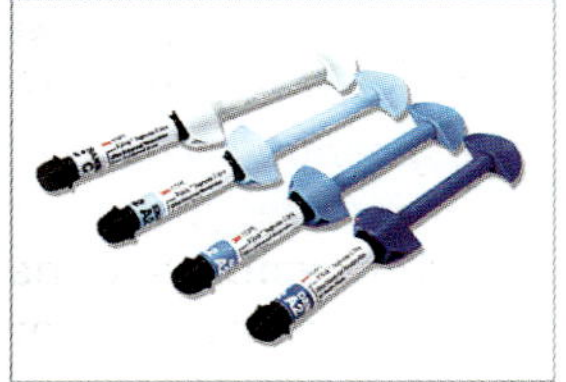

In material science, a composite is a mixture produced from at least two of the different classes of materials, i.e., metals, ceramics, and polymers. **Dental composites** are *complex, tooth-colored filling materials composed of synthetic polymers, particulate ceramic reinforcing fillers, molecules which promote or modify the polymerization reaction that produces the cross-linked polymer matrix from the dimethacrylate resin monomers, and silane-coupling agents which bond the reinforcing fillers to the polymer matrix.*

Composite (componere = to combine) is the universally used tooth-colored direct restorative material developed in 1962 by combining dimethacrylates (epoxy resin and methacrylic acid) with silinized quartz powder by **Bowen (1963).**

Classification of composites according to filler particles (Lutz and Philips, 1983)

Filler	*Macro-filler (>10 µm)*	*Macro-filler (0.01–0.1 µm)*	*Micro-filter complexes*	
Composite type	Macro-filler composite	Hybrid composite	Homogenic micro-filler composite	Inhomogenic micro-filler composite
Properties	+ Physical properties	+ Radiopacity	+ Polishability	+ Polishability
	+ Radiopacity	+ Polishability	– Wear resistance	+ Esthetics
	– Polishability	+ Physical properties	– Water absorption	– Physical properties
	– Wear resistance	– Polymerization shrinkage	– Radiopacity – Polymerization shrinkage	
Purpose	Core build-up material under indirect restoration? No longer indicated	All classes of restoration	Small anterior restorations Class V	Small anterior restorations Class V
Example	Prisma-Fil®	Tetric Ceram®	Palfique®	Filtek Al 10®

+: Positive property, performance acceptable
–: Negative property, performance unacceptable

Properties of Composites

- **Linear coefficient of thermal expansion (LCTE):** It is the rate of dimensional change of a material per unit change in temperature. The closer the LCTE of the material is to the LCTE of enamel, the less chance there is for creating voids or openings at the junction of the material and the tooth when temperature changes occur. The LCTE of improved composites is approximately three times that of tooth structure.
- **Water absorption:** When a restorative material absorbs water, its properties change, and therefore, its effectiveness as a restorative material is usually diminished. Materials with higher filler contents exhibit lower water absorption values.

- **Wear resistance:** It refers to a material's ability to resist surface loss as a result of abrasive contact with opposing tooth structure, restorative material, food boli, and such items as toothbrush bristles and toothpicks. Wear resistance of composite materials is generally good.
- **Surface texture:** It is the smoothness of the surface of the restorative material. Microfill composites offer the smoothest restorative surface; hybrid composites also provide surface textures that are both esthetic and compatible with soft tissues.
- **Radiopacity:** Esthetic restorative materials must be sufficiently radiopaque, so that the radiolucent image of recurrent caries around or under a restoration can be more easily seen in a radiograph. Most composites contain radiopaque fillers, such as barium glass, to make the material radiopaque.
- **Modulus of elasticity:** It is the stiffness of a material. A material having a higher modulus is more rigid; conversely, a material with a lower modulus is more flexible. A microfill composite material with greater flexibility may perform better in certain Class V restorations than a more rigid hybrid composite.
- **Solubility:** It is the loss in weight per unit surface area or volume due to dissolution or disintegration of a material in oral fluids, over time, at a given temperature. Composite materials do not demonstrate any clinically relevant solubility.
- **Polymerization:** Full polymerization of the material is determined by the degree of conversion of monomers into polymers, indicating the number of methacrylate groups that have reacted with each other during the conversion process. The factors that influence the degree of conversion of the composite are given in **Table 45.1**.

Table 45.1: Factors that influence the composite resin polymerization process.

Factor	*Clinical repercussions*
Curing time	It depends on—resin shade, light intensity, box deep, resin thickness, curing through tooth structure. Composite filling
Shade of resin	Darker composite shades cure more slowly and less deeply than lighter shades (60 seconds at a maximum depth of 0.5 mm)
Temperature	Composite at room temperature cure more completely and rapidly
Thickness of resin	Optimum thickness is 1–2 mm
Type of filler	Microfine composites are more difficult to cure than heavily loaded composites
Distance between light and resin	Optimum distance <1 mm, with the light positioned 90° degrees from the composite surface
Light source quality	Wavelength between 400 nm and 500 nm. A power density about 600 mW/cm^2 is required to ensure that 400 mW/cm^2 reaches the first increment of composite in a posterior box
Polymerization shrinkage	Depends on the amount of organic phase

Classification of composites according to matrix components

Matrix	*Chemical system*	*Group*	*Example of material*
Conventional matrix	Pure methacrylate	Hybrid composite	Tetric EvoCerarm®
		Nano composite	Filtek supreme XT®
Inorganic matrix	Inorganic polycondensate	Ormocers	Admira® Definite®
Acid modified methacrylate	Polar groups	Compomers	Dyract eXtra®
Ring opening epoxide	Cationic polymerization	Silorans	Filtek Silorane®

Types of Composite

- **Hybrid composite resins:**
  - These composites are so called, because they are made up of polymer groups (organic phase) reinforced by an inorganic phase, comprising 60% or more of the total content. It is composed of glasses of different compositions and sizes, with particle sizes ranging from 0.6 to 1 μm and containing 0.04 μm sized colloidal silica.
  - The character is tic properties of these materials are availability of a wide range of colors and ability to mimic the dental structure, less curing shrinkage, low water absorption, excellent polishing and texturing properties, abrasion and wear very similar to that of tooth structures, similar thermal expansion coefficient to that of teeth, universal formulas for both the anterior and posterior sector, different degrees of opaqueness and translucency in different tones and fluorescence.

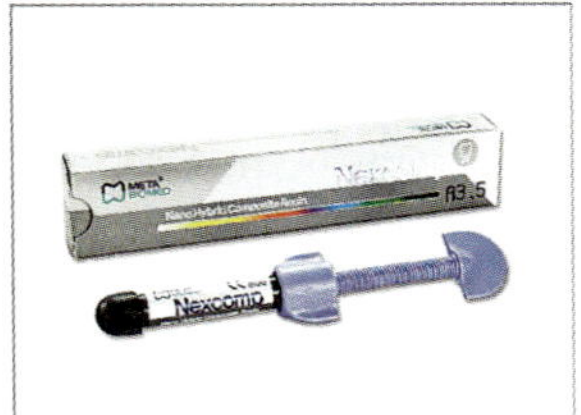

- **Flowable composites:**
  - These are low-viscosity composite resins, making them more fluid than conventional composite resins.
  - The percentage of inorganic filler is lower and some substances or rheological modifiers which are mainly intended to improve handling properties have been removed from their composition.
  - Their main advantages are—high wettability of the tooth surface, ensuring penetration into every irregularity; ability to form layers of minimum thickness, so improving or eliminating air inclusion or entrapment; radiopaqueness and availability in different colors.
  - The drawbacks are—high curing shrinkage, due to lower filler load, and weaker mechanical properties.
  - These are indicated in Class V restorations, cervical wear processes and minimal occlusal restorations or as liner materials in Class I or II cavities or areas of cavitated enamel.

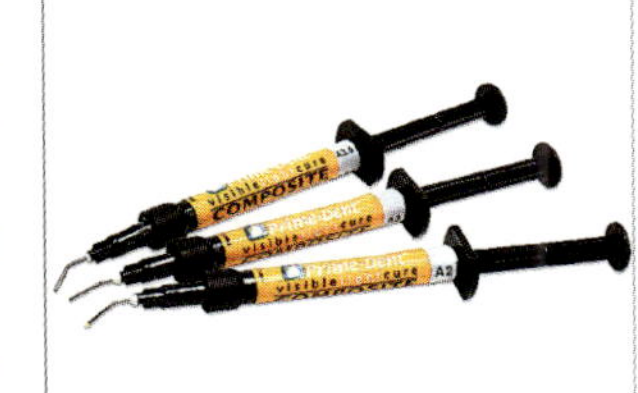

- **Condensable composites:**
  - Condensable composites are composite resins with a high percentage of filler.

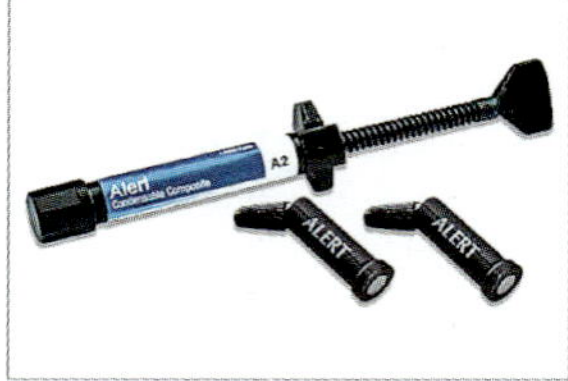

  - The advantages are—condensability (like silver amalgam), greater ease in achieving a good contact point, and better reproduction of occlusal anatomy.
  - Their main disadvantages are—difficulties in adaptation between one composite layer and another, difficult handling and poor esthetics in anterior teeth.
  - Indication is Class II cavity restoration in order to achieve a better contact point.
- **Ormocers:**
  - Ormocers, a word originally derived from organically modified ceramic, were originally developed for science and technology (e.g., for special surfaces like protective coatings, nonstick surfaces, antistatic coatings, and nonreflective coatings).

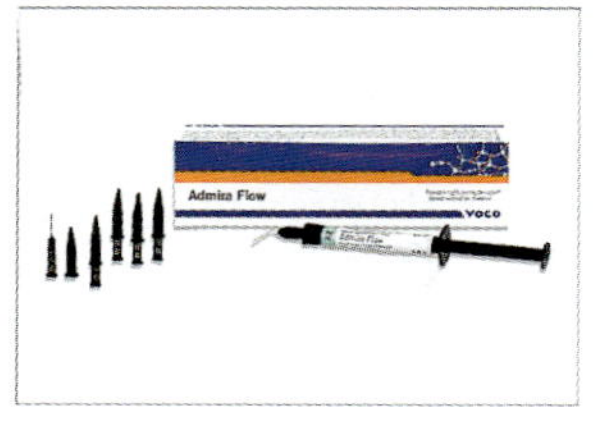

  - The organic polymers influence the polarity, the ability to cross link, hardness, and optical behavior.
  - The glass and ceramic components (inorganic constituents) are responsible for thermal expansion and chemical stability.
  - The polysiloxanes influence the elasticity, interface properties, and processing.
  - **Bottenberg et al. (2009)** compared Admira®
  - (ormocer) and Tetric Ceram® (hybrid composite) and found no difference.
  - Ormocers have a reduced polymerization shrinkage compared to hybrid composites **(Yap and Soh, 2004).**
- **Compomer:**
  - The word "Compomer" comes from composite and glass ionomer
  - The material itself is a poly-acrylic or polycarboxylic acid-modified composite. Compomer are composed of composite and glass ionomer components in an attempt to take advantage of the desirable qualities of both materials—the fluoride release and ease of use of the glass ionomers and the superior material qualities and esthetics of the composites.

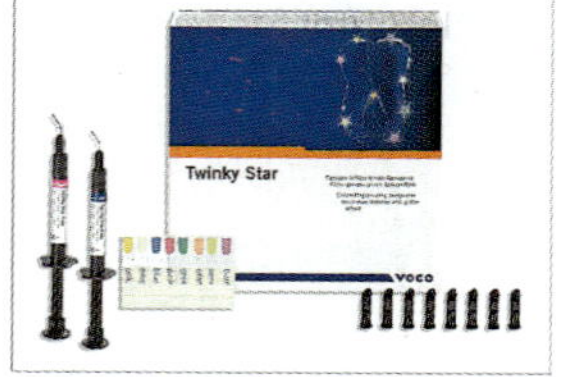

  - Compomer restorations have been shown to have insufficient retention without pretreatment of the dental hard tissue with an adhesive system **(Folwaczny et al.,** 2001; **Moodley and Grobler,** 2003**).**
  - Compomer is most suitable for restorations in the deciduous dentition due to their low abrasion resistance **(Zantner et al.,** 2004; **Krämer et al.,** 2006**).**
  - In cervical restorations, compomer restorations performed better than resin-modified glass ionomers but not as well as hybrid composites **(Folwaczny et al.,** 2000**).**
  - The fluoride release of compomer increased quickly initially (24 hours), but decreased equally quickly. The ability of compomer (Dyract eXtraR)® to be recharged with fluoride from its environment resulting in longer lasting caries prevention has been discussed by **Vieira et al.,** 1999.
- **Silorane:**
  - The name of this material class refers to its chemical composition from silox- anes and oxirans.

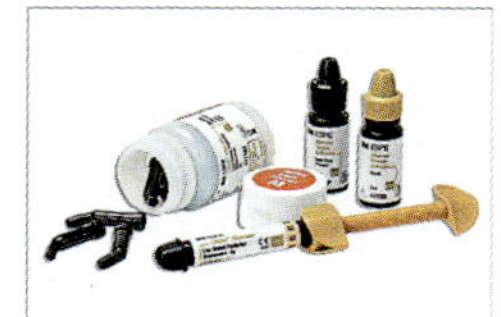

  - This product class aims to have lower shrinkage, longer resistance to fading, and less marginal discoloration.
  - The fillers in Filtek Silorane®, the only silorane material in the market at the moment, consist of 0.1–2.0 µm quartz particles and radiopaque yttrium fluoride.
  - The adhesion of streptococci observed on the surface of silorane restorations was low, may be because of its hydrophobic properties (**Bürgers et al.,** 2009).
- **Nanocomposite:**
  - Nanotechnology may provide composite resins with a dramatically smaller filler particle size that can be dissolved in higher concentrations and polymerized into the resin system.

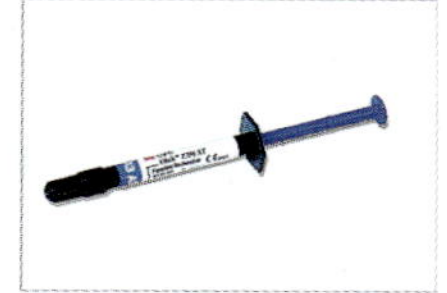

  - The molecules in these materials can be designed to be compatible when coupled with a polymer and provide unique characteristics (i.e. physical, mechanical, optical).
  - Nanotechnology can, however, improve this continuity between the tooth structure and the nano-sized filler particle and provide a more stable and natural interface between the mineralized hard tissues of the tooth and these advanced restorative biomaterials.
- **Antimicrobial composite:**
  - Silver and titanium particles were introduced into dental composites, respectively, to introduce antimicrobial properties and enhance the biocompatibility of the composites. Several reports have described the incorporation of a methacryloyloxy-dodecyl-pyridinium-bromide monomer in composite resins that showed no release of the incorporated monomer but still exhibited antibacterial properties.

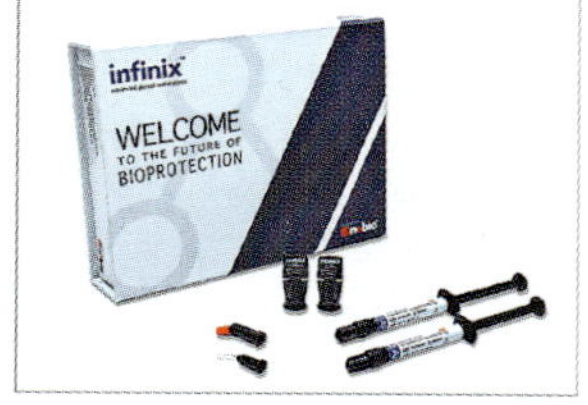

- **Stimuli responsive composite:**
  - Stimuli-responsive materials possess properties that may be considerably changed in a controlled fashion by external stimuli such as changes of temperature, mechanical stress, pH, moisture or electric or magnetic fields.
  - Stimuli-responsive dental composites may be quite useful, for example, for "release-on-command" of

antimicrobial compounds or fluoride to fight microbes or secondary caries, respectively.

- **Fiber reinforced composite:**
  - It consists of fiber material held together by resin matrix. They are structural materials that have at least 2 district constituents—the reinforcing component which provides strength and stiffness and the surrounding matrix supports the reinforcements and provides work ability.

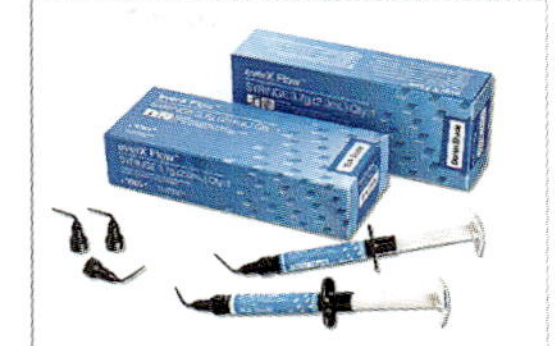

  - In dental applications, polymeric or resin matrices reinforced with glass, polyethylene or carbon fibres are most common.
  - *Characteristics of FRCs:* Good overall mechanical properties, superior strength, non corrosive properties, radiolucency, good bonding properties, good flexural strength.
  - Application of FRCs in dentistry:
    - Crown framework
    - Anterior or posterior fixed prosthesis
    - Chairside tooth replacements
    - Appliances like periodontal splints
    - Endodontic posts fabrication
- **Self healing composite:**
  - Epoxy resin composite was one of the first self-repairing or self-healing synthetic materials which shows some similarities to resin-based dental material.
  - If a crack occurs in the epoxy composite material, some of the microcapsules are destroyed near the crack and release the resin. The cracks were filed by resin and reacts with a Grubbs catalyst dispersed in the epoxy composite, which results in polymerization of the resin and repair of the crack.

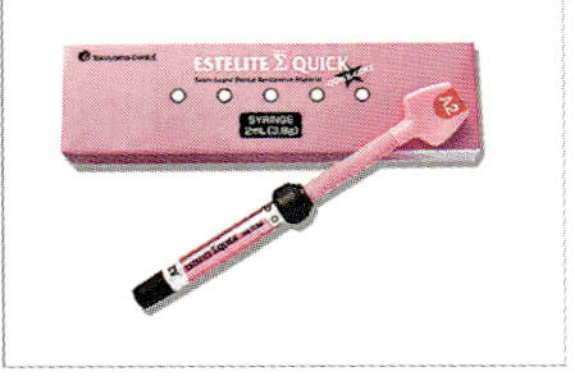

Indications	*Contraindications*

• Classes I, II, III, IV, V, and VI restorations
• Foundations or core build-ups
• Sealants
• Preventive resin restorations
• Esthetic enhancement procedures
  » Partial veneers
  » Full veneers
  » Tooth contour modifications
  » Diastema closures
• Cements (for indirect restorations)
• Temporary restorations
• Periodontal splinting
	• If the operating site cannot be isolated from contamination by oral fluids
	• If all of the occlusal load will be on the restorative material
	• Economics
	• Restorations that extend onto the root surface may result in less than ideal marginal integrity

Advantages	*Disadvantages*
• Esthetic • Conservative of tooth structure removal • Tooth preparation is simple • Have low thermal conductivity • Used almost universally • Bonded to tooth structure • Repairable	• May have a gap formation • Time-consuming • Costly • Establishing proximal contacts, axial contours, embrasures may be more difficult • Technique sensitive • Exhibit greater occlusal wear in areas of high occlusal stress • Marginal leakage can occur

CALCIUM HYDROXIDE

Limestone is a natural rock mainly composed of calcium carbonate ($CaCO_3$) which forms when the $CaCO_3$ solution existing in mountain and sea water becomes crystallized **(Alliet** and **VandeVoorde,** 1988**)**. The calcium oxide (CaO) formed is called "quicklime" and has a strong corrosive ability. Calcium hydroxide is a white odorless powder with the formula $Ca(OH)_2$ and a molecular weight of 74.08. It has low solubility in water which decreases as the temperature rises; it has a high pH (about 12.5±12.8) and is insoluble in alcohol. This low solubility is, in turn, a good clinical characteristic, because a long period is necessary before it becomes soluble in tissue fluids when in direct contact with vital tissues.

The earliest reference to calcium hydroxide has been attributed to **Nygren** (1838) for the treatment of the "fistula dentalis" but its introduction to dentistry of is credited to **Hermann** (1936). Calcium hydroxide was introduced in United States by **Teuscher** and **Zander** in 1938 and is since then being used as a pulpal medicament. Although the overall mechanisms of action of calcium hydroxide are not fully understood, many articles have been published describing its biological properties, role of the high pH and the ionic activity in the healing process, diffusion through dentinal tubules, and influence on apical microleakage.

Properties
- Arrangement is amorphous matrix, crystalline fillers
- Bonding = covalent; ionic
- Setting reaction = acid–base reaction
- Insulator for thermal and electrical conductivity
- Solubility: 0.3–0.5
- Elastic modulus is 588
- Compressive strength more than 24 hours is 138.

Mechanism of Action of Calcium Hydroxide

- **Mechanism of action (MOA) of hydroxyl ions on bacteria:** Calcium hydroxide is an antibacterial agent due to its elevated pH which influences the specific activity of the proteins of the membrane with a combination with specific chemical groups and can lead to alterations in the ionization state of organic components, depending on pH, there will be an intense transfer of available nutrients through membrane, inducing inhibition and toxic effect on cell. Thus, the influence of elevated pH (12.6) of OH- ions, transfer capacity, and permeability of cytoplasmic membrane explains the action of calcium hydroxide on bacteria, this is known as lipidic peroxidation.

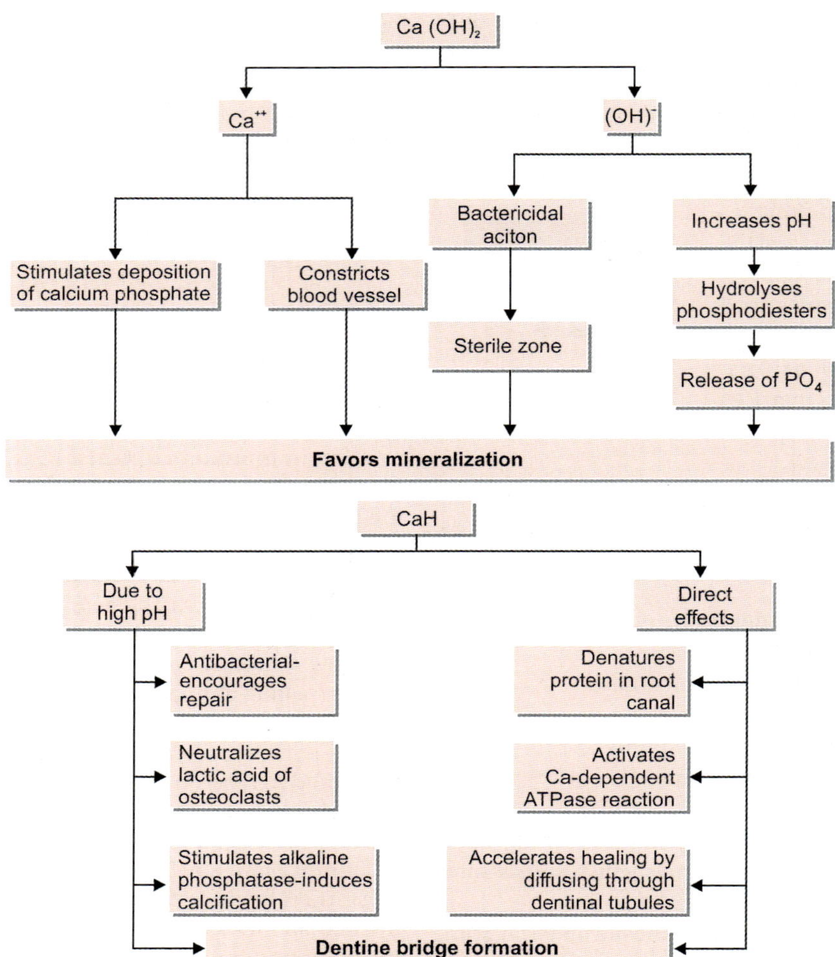

- **Mechanism of action on tissues:** Elevated pH of calcium hydroxide activates alkaline phosphatase from the tissue. This is hydrolytic enzyme that liberates phosphate from esters of phosphates. This phosphate ion, once free, reacts with calcium ion from the blood stream to form a precipitate, calcium phosphate, in the organic matrix. This precipitate is the molecular unit of hydroxyapatite. Calcium hydroxide when in direct contact with adjacent tissue gives origin to a zone of necrosis through rupture of glycoproteins resulting in protein degeneration within 7–10 days.

Uses of Calcium Hydroxide

- **Calcium hydroxide as a cavity liner:**
  - Calcium hydroxide cements are used for lining specific areas of deep cavities.
  - Calcium hydroxide cavity liners are provided as pastes that set to a hard mass when mixed. The base paste of a typical product contains calcium tungstate, tribasic calcium phosphate, and zinc oxide in glycol salicylate. The catalyst paste contains calcium hydroxide, zinc oxide, and zinc stearate in ethylene toluene sulfonamide. The ingredients responsible for setting are calcium hydroxide and a salicylate, which react to form an amorphous calcium disalicylate. Fillers such as calcium tungstate or barium sulfate provide radiopacity.

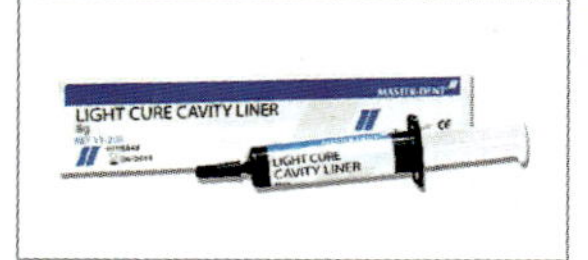

  - A light-cured calcium hydroxide liner consists of calcium hydroxide and barium sulfate dispersed in an urethane dimethacrylate resin.
  - Calcium hydroxide (self-cured) liners have low values of tensile strength and compressive strength, or elastic modulus, compared with high-strength bases.

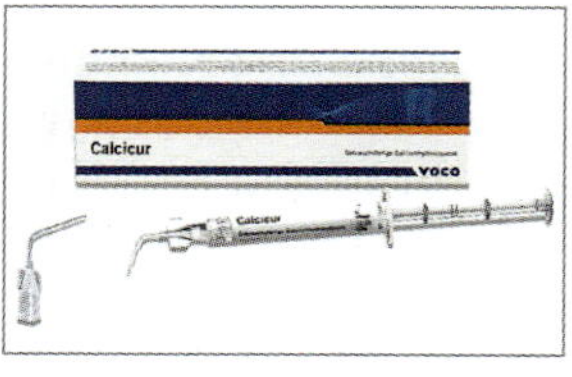

- **Calcium hydroxide as an intracanal medicament:**
  - It is the most commonly used dressing for treatment of the vital pulp.
  - It also plays a major role as an intervisit dressing in the disinfection of the root canal system.
  - Calcium hydroxide cannot be categorized as a conventional antiseptic, but it kills bacteria in root canal space.
  - Calcium hydroxide is normally used as slurry of calcium hydroxide in a water base paste.

- Calcium hydroxide is a slowly working antiseptic and direct contact experiments *in vitro* require 24 hours contact period for complete kill of enterococci and reduce the effect of the remaining cell wall material.

❖ **Calcium hydroxide as an endodontic sealer:**

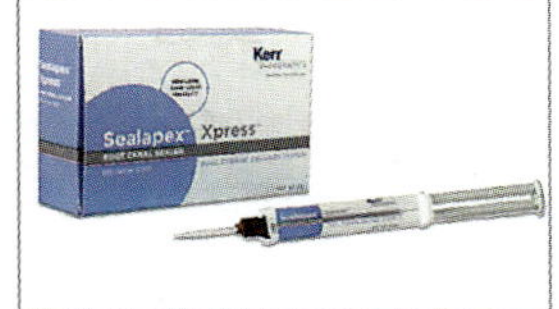

- In the root canal obturation, sealer plays an important role, as it fills the gap between the walls of the prepared dentine and the gutta-percha.
- Recently introduced several calcium hydroxide sealers are Sealapex (Kerr), Apexkit (Vivadent).

❖ **Calcium hydroxide as a pulp capping agent:**

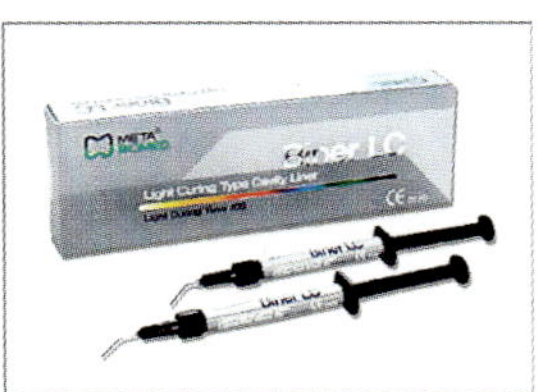

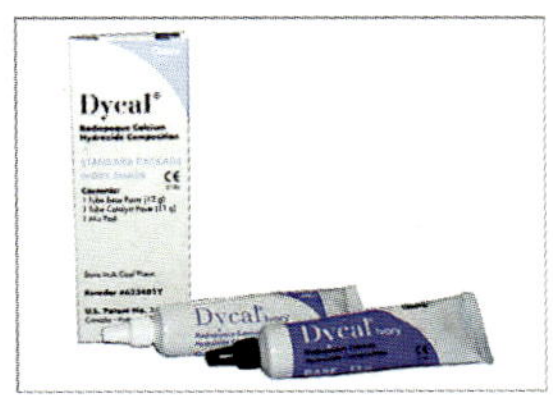

- Calcium hydroxide is generally accepted as the material of choice for pulp capping.
- Histologically, there is a complete dentinal bridging with healthy radicular pulp under calcium hydroxide dressings.
- When calcium hydroxide is applied directly to pulp tissue, there is necrosis of adjacent pulp tissue and an inflammation of contiguous tissue. Dentinal bridge formation occurs at the junction of necrotic tissue and vital inflamed tissue. Beneath the region of necrosis, cells of underlying pulp tissue differentiate into odontoblasts and elaborate dentin matrix.
- Three main calcium hydroxide products for pulp capping are Pulpadent, Dycal, and Hydrex (MPC).

❖ **Calcium hydroxide in apexification:**

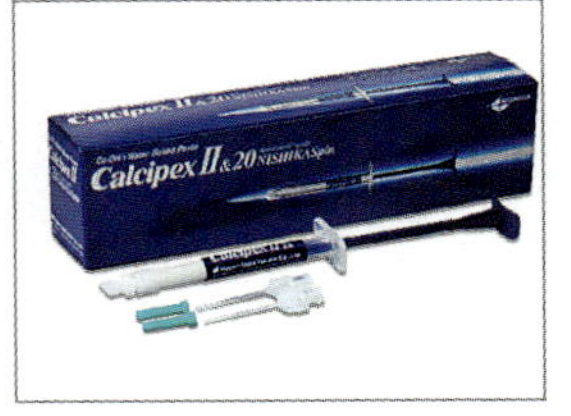

- In apexification technique, canal is cleaned and disinfected; when tooth is free of signs and symptoms of infection, the canal is dried and filled with stiff mix of calcium hydroxide and camphorated p-monochlorophenol (CMCP).
- Commercial paste of calcium hydroxide like Calasept, Pulpdent, and Metapex may be used to fill the canals.
- Histologically, the formation of osteodentin after placement of calcium hydroxide paste immediately on conclusion of a vital pulpectomy has been reported. There appears to be a differentiation of adjacent connective tissue cells; there is also deposition of calcified tissue adjacent to the filling material. The calcified material is continuous with lateral root surfaces; the closure of apex may be partial or complete but consistently has minute communications with the periapical tissue.

❖ **Calcium hydroxide in pulpotomy:**

- It is the most recommended pulpotomy medicament for pulpally involved vital young permanent tooth with incomplete apices.
- It is acceptable because it promoted reparative dentin bridge formation and thus pulp vitality is maintained.

❖ Three histologic zones under calcium hydroxide in 4–9 days:

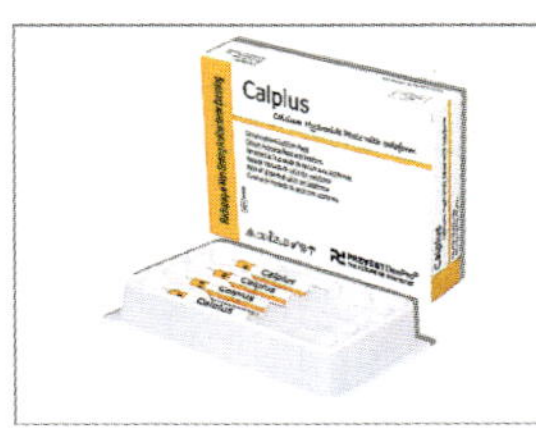

1. Coagulation necrosis
2. Deep-staining areas with varied osteodentin
3. Relatively normal pulp tissue, slightly hyperemic and underlying an odontoblastic layer.

❖ **Calcium hydroxide in weeping canals:**

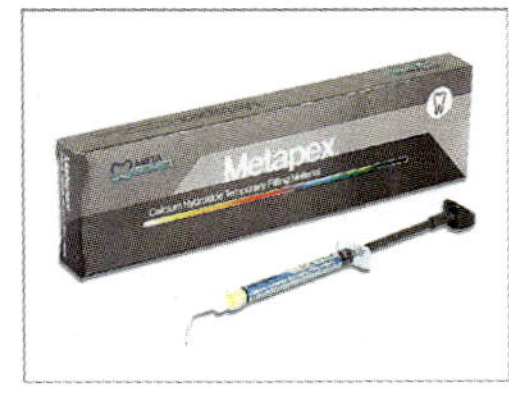

- Sometimes a tooth undergoing root canal treatment shows constant clear or reddish exudate associated with periapical radiolucency. Tooth can be asymptomatic or tender on percussion, but when opened in next appointment, exudates stop, but again reappear in next appointment, this is known as "weeping canal".
- In these cases, tooth with exudates is not ready for obturation, since culture reports normally show negative bacterial growth so, antibiotics are of no help. For such teeth, dry the canals with sterile absorbent paper points and place calcium hydroxide in canal which helps in controlling the exudates because pH of periapical tissues is acidic in weeping stage which gets converted into basic pH by calcium hydroxide.

Advantages of calcium hydroxide	***Disadvantages of calcium hydroxide***
• Initially bactericidal then bacteriostatic	• Associated with primary tooth resorption
• Promotes healing and repair	• Dissolve after 1 year with cavosurface dissolution
• High pH stimulates fibroblasts	• May degrade during acid etching
• Neutralizes low pH of acids	• Degrades upon tooth flexure
• Stops internal resorption	• Marginal failure with amalgam condensation
• Inexpensive and easy to use	• Does not adhere to dentin or resin restoration

GLASS IONOMER CEMENTS

Glass ionomer cements (GICs) were developed in an attempt to capitalize on the favorable properties of both silicate and polycarboxylate cements. Unfortunately, the first generation materials had severe limitations. Excessive opacity, limited shade selection, mixing and handling problems, and a troublesome clinical technique quickly doused the enthusiasm surrounding this new product. As a result, glass ionomer has struggled to gain popularity even though continued research and development has produced a clinically useful restorative material.

Development

- **1969:** First developed by **AD Wilson** and **BE Kent**
- **1973:** First material marketed (ASPA IV) (USA 1977)
- **1975:** First luting material
- **1978:** Cermet ionomer cements
- **1982:** Water-activated cements
- **1986:** Resin-modified cements
- **1988–89:** First commercial product from 3M (Vitrebond™)
- **1990–93:** Several"Resin-Ionomer Hybrid" liners and restoratives introduced
- **1994:** Resin-glass ionomer hybrids officially names"Resin Modified Glass Ionomer Cements" at the International Symposium on Glass Ionomer Cements
- **1995–Present:** Introduction of compomers and packable glass ionomers.

Properties of Glass Ionomer Cement

- Low solubility
- Coefficient of thermal expansion similar to dentin
- Fluoride release and fluoride recharge
- High compressive strengths
- Bonds to tooth structure by primarily chemical (calcium-carboxyl groups), micromechanical
- Low flexural strength
- Low shear strength
- Dimensional change (slight expansion) (shrinks on setting, expands with water sorption)
- Brittle
- Lacks translucency
- Rough surface texture
- Biocompatible to tissues.

Composition of Glass Ionomer Cement

Liquid

- Polyacid (acrylic, maleic, itaconic)
- Water
- Comonomer: D-Tartaric: accelerates set, increases working time, translucency, and strength
- Recently added: Polyvinyl phosphoric acid.

Composition property of GIC hybrid composite

Property	*GIC*	*Hybrid composite*
Compressive strength (MPa)	Up to 200	350–500
Tensile strength (MPa)	15	34–62
Modulus of elasticity (MPa)	20,000	13,500–18,000
Coefficient of thermal expansion ($\times 10^{-5}$/°C)	10.2–11.4	25–38
Thermal diffusivity (mm^2/sec)	0.198	0.675

(GIC: glass ionomer cement)

Powder

- Alumina (Al_2O_3)
  - 16.6%
  - Forms the skeletal structure
  - Increase opacity
- Silica (SiO_2)
  - 29%
  - Increase translucency
- Calcium fluoride (CaF_2)
  - 34.2%

Classification of glass ionomer cement

According to Philips	*According to Sturdvent*	*According to Wilson and McLean*

Type I—Luting
Type II—Restorative
Type III—Liner and base
	• Traditional or conventional
	• Metal -modified GIC
	  » Cermets
	  » Miracle mix
	• Light- cured GIC
	• Hybrid (resin modifiesd GIC)
	• Polyacid -modified resin composites
		• Type I— Luting
		• Type II
		  » Esthetic filling material
		  » Bis-reinforced filling material
		• Type III—Lining base and fissure sealant

According to Davidson and Major	***According to GJ Mount***	***According to intended applications (Figs. 45.1A to I)***

• Conventional/traditional
  » Glass ionomer for direct restorations
  » Metal reinforced GIC
  » High viscosity GIC
  » Low viscosity GIC
  » Base/Lliner
  » Luting
• Resin modified GIC
  » Restorative
  » Base/Liner
  » Pit and fissure sealant
  » Luting
  » Orthodonic cementation material
• Polyoid modified resin composites/ compomers
	• Glass ionomer cements
	  » Glass polyalkenoates
	  » Glass polyphosphonates
	  » Rein modified GIC
	  » Polyacid modified composite resin
	• Auto cure
	• Dual cure
	• Tri cure
	• Type I–Luting
	• Type II–Restorative
	  1. Restorative esthetic
	  2. Restorative reinforced
	• Type III–Lining or base
		• Type I—Luting
		• Type II—Restorative
		• Type III—Fast setting lining
		• Type IV—Fissure sealants
		• Type V—Orthodontic cements
		• Type VI—Core build up material
		• Type VII—Command set
		• Type VIII—GIC for ART
		• Type IX—Geriatric and pediatric

According to McLean, Nicholson and Wilson		***Based on chemical constituents of cement***

• Glass ionomer cement
  » Glass polyalkenoates
  » Glass polyphosphonates
• Resin modified GIC
• Polyacid modified GIC
		• Conventional
		• Metal reinforced
		  » Miracle mix
		  » Cermets
		• Resin modified

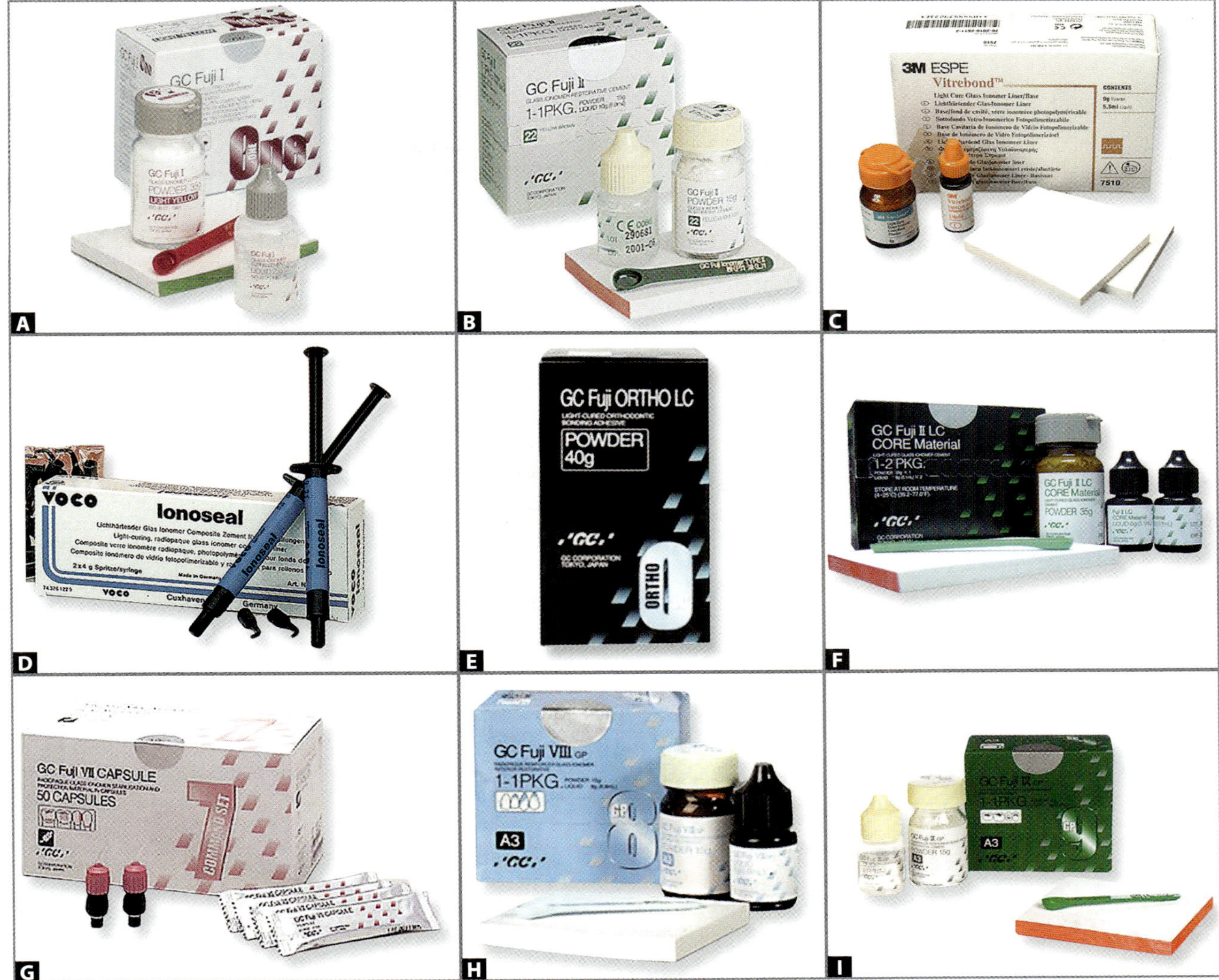

Figs. 45.1A to I: (A) Type I, luting; (B) Type II, restorative; (C) Type III, fast setting lining; (D) Type IV, fissure sealants; (E) Type V, orthodontic cements; (F) Type VI, core build-up material; (G) Type VII, command set; (H) Type VIII, GIC for ART; (I) Type IX, geriatric and pediatric. (ART: atraumatic restorative treatment; GIC: glass ionomer cement)

- Increases opacity
- Acts as flux
- Aluminum phosphates ($AlPO_4$)
  - 9.9%
  - Decrease melting temperature
  - Increase translucency
- Cryolite (Na_3AlF_6)
  - 5%
  - Increases opacity
  - Acts as flux.
- Other ions: NA^+, K^+, Ca^+, Sr^{+3}
- Fluoride
  - Decrease fusion
  - Anticariogenecity
  - Increase translucency.

Powder is basically an acid soluble calcium aluminosilicate glass containing fluoride. It is formed by fusing silica and alumina and calcium fluorite, metal oxides, and metal phosphates at 11,000–15,000°C and then pouring the melt onto a metal plate/into water. The glass formed is crushed, milled, and ground to a form powder of 20–50-u size depending on what it's going to be used for.

Dispensing of Glass Ionomer Cement

- Conventional GICs are supplied as powder and a liquid system
- The dispensing and mixing of the powder and liquid are critical and may introduce a considerable variability in the mechanical and physicochemical properties of the set cement **(Figs. 45.2A to C)**.
- The variation in different types of GIC (lining/ restorative/ luting) is based on the particle size of power only. All the other constituents as well as liquid are the same for all.
- Powder liquid ratio for luting 1.5:1 and for restoration is 3:1.

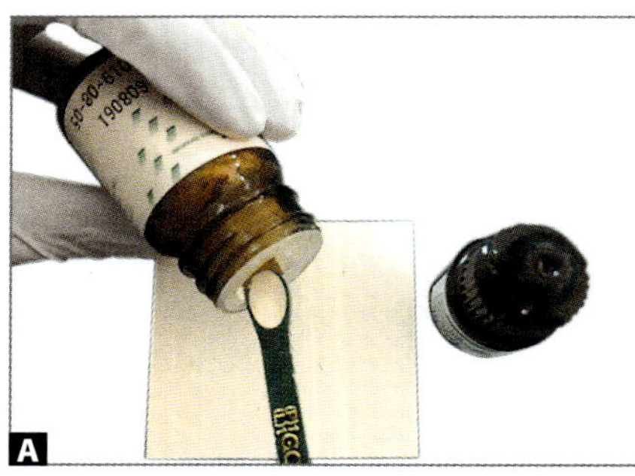

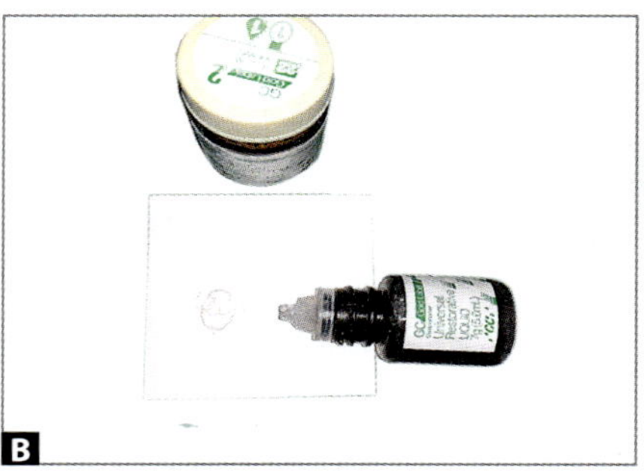

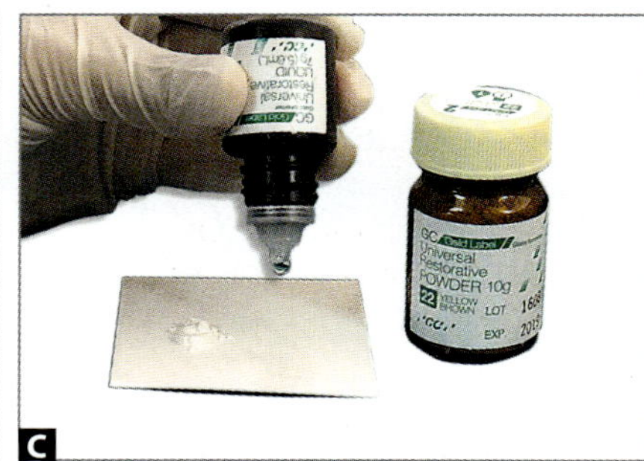

Figs. 45.2A to C: (A) Fill the spoon with powder to exact measure without excess; (B) Tilt the bottle so as to avoid any air bubbles; (C) Pour from the bottle holding it vertically.

Setting Reaction of Glass Ionomer Cement (Fig. 45.3)

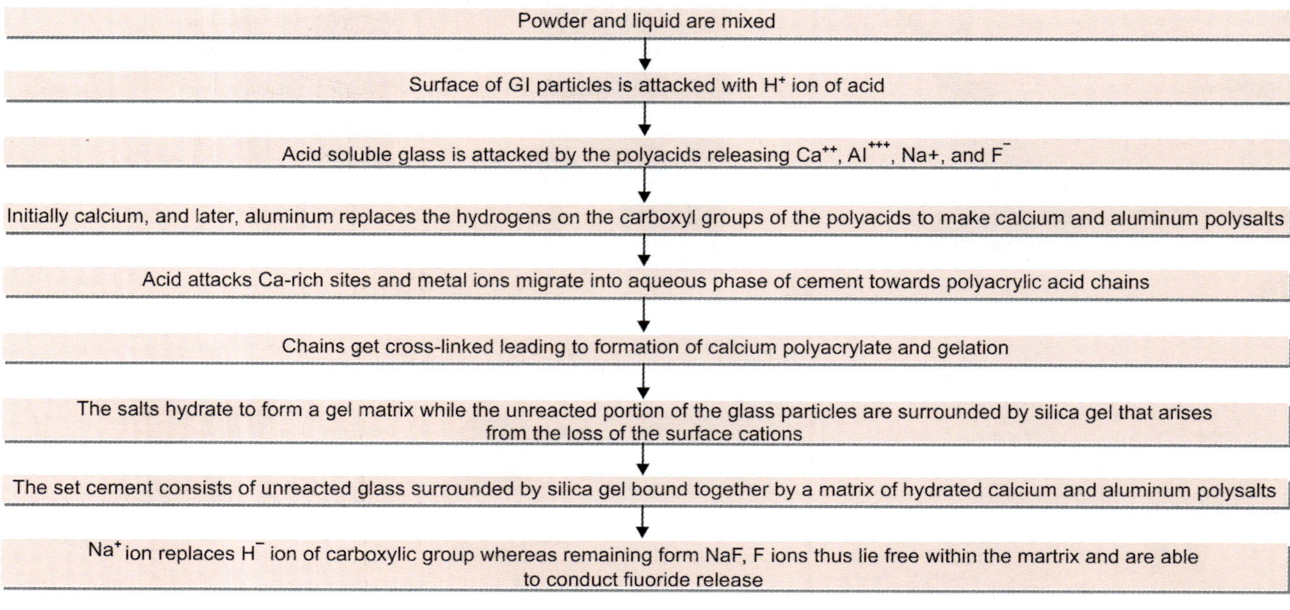

Powder and liquid are mixed
Surface of GI particles is attacked with H^+ ion of acid
Acid soluble glass is attacked by the polyacids releasing Ca^{++}, Al^{+++}, Na+, and F^-
Initially calcium, and later, aluminum replaces the hydrogens on the carboxyl groups of the polyacids to make calcium and aluminum polysalts
Acid attacks Ca-rich sites and metal ions migrate into aqueous phase of cement towards polyacrylic acid chains
Chains get cross-linked leading to formation of calcium polyacrylate and gelation
The salts hydrate to form a gel matrix while the unreacted portion of the glass particles are surrounded by silica gel that arises from the loss of the surface cations
The set cement consists of unreacted glass surrounded by silica gel bound together by a matrix of hydrated calcium and aluminum polysalts
Na^+ ion replaces H^- ion of carboxylic group whereas remaining form NaF, F ions thus lie free within the martrix and are able to conduct fiuoride release

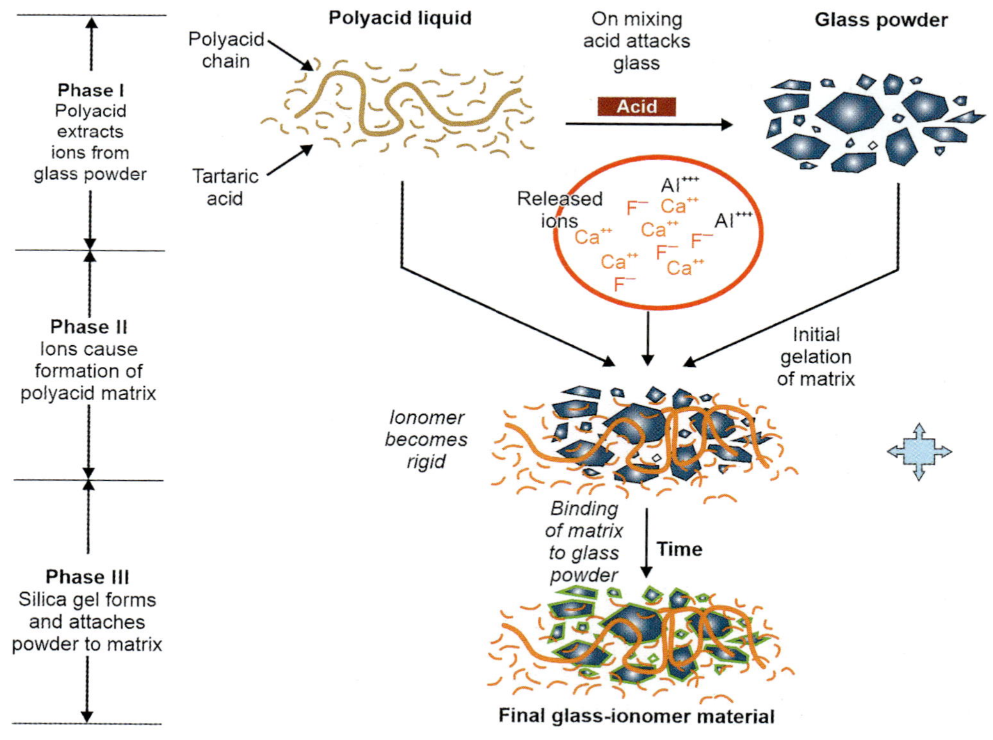

Fig. 45.3: Setting reaction of GIC. (GIC: glass ionomer cement).

Indications

- Nonstress bearing areas
- Classes III and V restorations in adults
- Classes I and II restorations in primary dentition
- Temporary or "caries control" restorations
- Crown margin repairs
- Cement base under amalgam, resin, ceramics, direct, and indirect gold
- Core build-ups when at least three walls of tooth are remaining (after crown preparation).

Contraindications

- High-stress applications
- Classes IV and II restorations
- Cusp replacement
- Core build-ups with less than three sound walls remaining.

Advantages

- Bonds to enamel and dentin
- Significant fluoride release can be recharged
- Coefficient of thermal expansion similar to tooth structure
- Tooth colored
- Low thermal conductivity.

Disadvantages

- Opacity higher than resin
- Less polishability than resin
- Poor wear resistance
- Brittle, poor tensile strength
- Poor longevity in xerostomic patients.

Recent Developments of Glass Ionomer Cement

- **Modified powder—liquid system:**
  - The rational of this development was to enhance the manual mixing procedure with a product with improved handling features and high reproducibility of dosing.
  - To be able to accomplish, this task specialized processing procedure for powder was followed (specialized granulates).
  - This system has improved wetting of the powder by the liquid rendering the mixing process much easier and faster.
- **Capsules:**
  - The GIC in the form of capsule system is a modern application method, which simplifies and allows procedures to be performed with greater ease and efficiency.

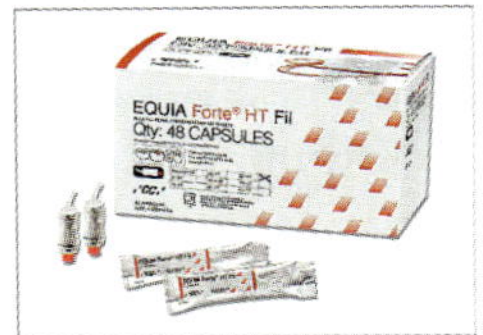

  - These capsules contain premeasured glass ionomer powder and liquid, which ensures correct ratio, consistency of mix and a predictable result.
  - These capsules have angled nozzles that act as a syringe for accurate placement of the material into a cavity or a crown for cementation.
- **Paste–paste dispensing system:**

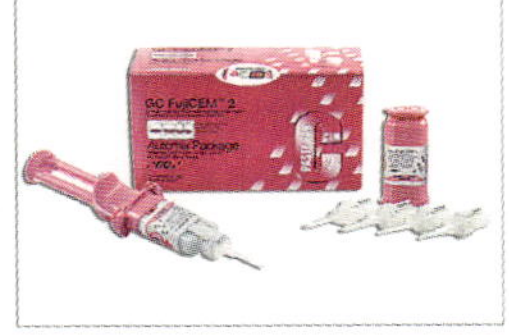

  - This is the latest development in the GIC technology. This dispensing system was designed with the objectives of providing optimum ratio, easy mixing, easy placement, total reliability, using a specially designed cartridge and an easy-to- use material dispenser.
  - In order to provide the material in a paste–paste consistency, an ultrafine glass powder was designed specifically. The low particle size provides the mixed cement with a thixotropic creamy consistency.

Modifications of Glass Ionomer Cement

- **Metal-modified glass ionomer:**
  - *Silver alloy admix (silver amalgam alloy particles mixed with glass particles)*
    - The addition of metal powders or fibers to GICs can improve strength; **Sced** and **Wilson** found that metal fibers were best for increasing flexural strength.

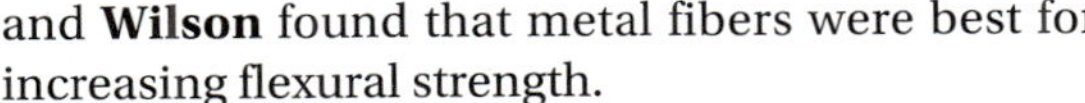

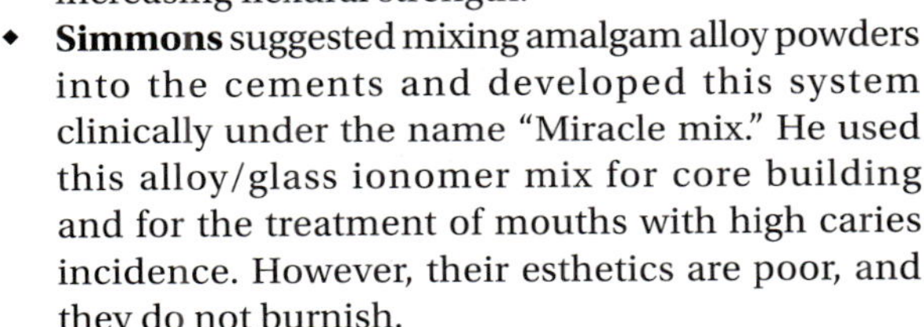

    - **Simmons** suggested mixing amalgam alloy powders into the cements and developed this system clinically under the name "Miracle mix." He used this alloy/glass ionomer mix for core building and for the treatment of mouths with high caries incidence. However, their esthetics are poor, and they do not burnish.

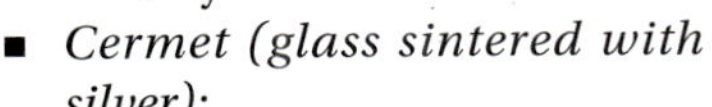

  - *Cermet (glass sintered with silver):*

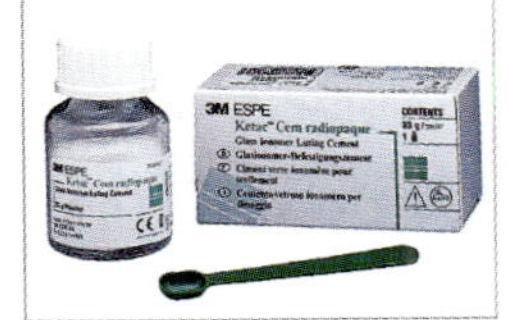

    - The solution to the problem of improving resistance to abrasion was the development of Cermet ionomer cements by **McLean** and **Gasser**. By sintering the metal and glass powders together, strong bonding of the metal to the glass was achieved.
    - Cermet ionomer cements have greatly improved resistance to abrasion when compared with GICs and their flexural strength is also higher.
    - However, their strength is still insufficient to replace amalgam alloys and their use should be confined to low-stress-bearing cavity preparations.
- **Resin-modified glass ionomer:**
  - Visible light cure glass ionomers, hybrid glass ionomers
    - Despite all the improvements, the two problems of conventional GICs still remained—moisture sensitivity and lack of command cure. To overcome these problems, attempts have been made to combine glass ionomer chemistry with the well-known chemistry of composite resins.
    - So, resin modification of GIC was designed to produce favorable physical properties similar to those of resin composites while maintaining the basic features of the conventional GIC.

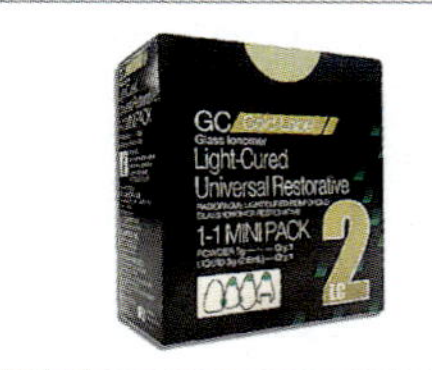

- In these newer materials, the fundamental acid/base curing reaction is supplemented by a second curing process, which is initiated by light or chemical.
- These products are considered to be dual-cure cements if only one polymerization mechanism is used; if both mechanisms are used, they are considered to be tri-cure cements.
- In their simplest form, these are GICs with the addition of a small quantity of a resin such as hydroxyethyl methacrylate (HEMA) or Bis-GMA in the liquid. More complex materials have been developed by modifications of the polyacid with side chains that can be polymerized by a light- curing mechanism.
- The first commercial RMGICs were liners, Vitrebond (3M).

❖ **"High strength," "packable," or "high viscosity" glass ionomers:**

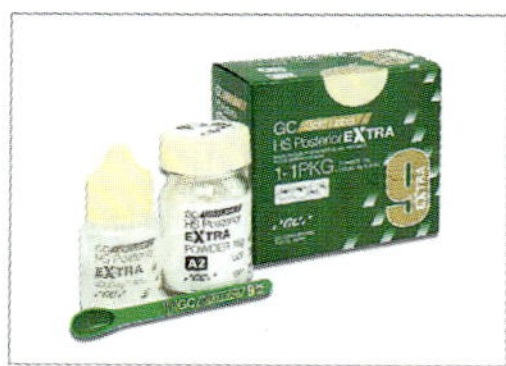

- These glass ionomers are particularly useful for atraumatic restorative treatment technique (ART).
- They were designed as an alternative to amalgam for posterior preventive restorations.
- Examples of highly viscous GICs are Fuji IX and Ketac Molar.
- These cements set only by a conventional neutralization reaction but have properties that exceed those of the resin-modified systems. Setting is rapid, early moisture sensitivity is considerably reduced, and solubility in oral fluids is very low.

❖ **Giomer:**

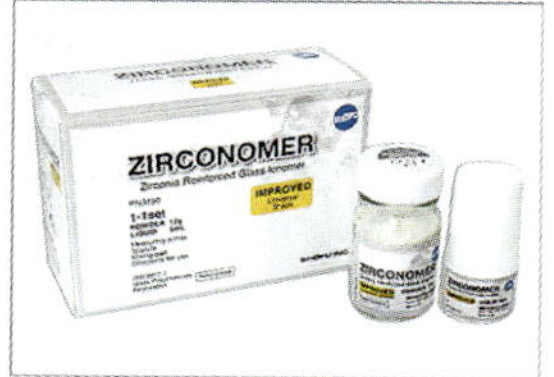

- It is a recently introduced hybrid esthetic restorative material based on prereact-ed glass ionomer technology (PRG).
- Chemically, it is fluoro-aluminosilicate glass reacted with polyalkenoic acid in water prior to inclusion into silica filled urethane resin.
- These are mainly indicated for restoration of root caries, cervical caries, class V cavities, and also in restoration of primary teeth.
- Its advantages include—continuous fluoride release, clinical stability, high biocompatibility, highly esthetic, and ease of bonding.

❖ **Nanoionomer GIC:**

- The incorporation of nanoparticles (the average particle size of glass ionomer particles were around 10–20 μm) into glass powder of glass ionomers led to wider particle size distribution, which resulted in higher mechanical values. Consequently, they can occupy the empty spaces between the glass ionomer particles and act as reinforcing material in the composition of the GICs.

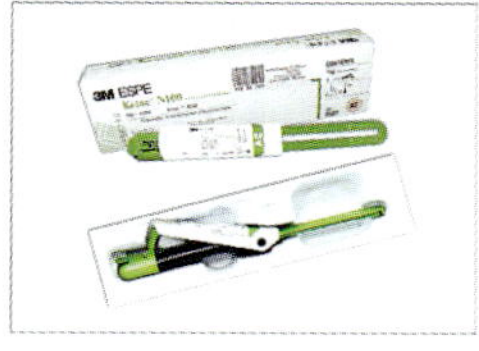

- The nanofiller components of nanoionomers also enhance some physical properties of the hardened restorative. Its bonding mechanism should be attributed to micromechanical interlocking provided by the surface roughness, most likely combined with chemical interaction through its acrylic or itaconic acid copolymers.
- Their most important advantages are superb polish, excellent esthetics, and improved wear resistance.
- The clinical indications are primary teeth restorations; transitional restorations; small Class I restorations; sandwich restorations; Classes III and V restorations; core build-ups.

❖ **The low viscosity/flowable GIC**

- To overcome the shortcomings faced by fluoride releasing material, a new material has been developed for fluoride release. Greater the fluoride release in a material, more open is the structure resulting in low strength. In order to improve the strength of these fluoride containing materials, if they are made more dense and strong, then the efficacy of F release is decreased. Soon after placement, there is sudden burst of fluoride release followed by a rapid decline in ion release rate.

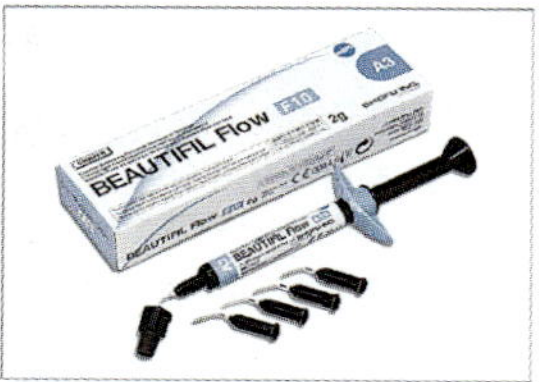

- This modified GIC has 2 part: Restorative part and Charge part. The restorative part is used the usual way when the 1st burst of fluoride is expelled, the therapeutic potential of the restoration spent. The material is given a second fluoride charge by using a gel material that replenishes the fluoride site in the restoration by ion exchange and recovers the fluoride release and therapeutic potential of the restoration.
- Uses are as pit and fissure sealant, lining, endodontic sealers, sealing of hypersensitive cervical areas.
- Eg: Fuji lining LC, Fuji III and IV, Ketac-Endo.

ZIRCONOMER

❖ *Zirconomer* defines a new class of restorative glass ionomer that promises the strength and durability of amalgam with the protective benefits of glass ionomer while completely eliminating the hazard of mercury. The inclusion of zirconia fillers in the glass component of *zirconomer* reinforces the structural integrity of the restoration and imparts superior mechanical properties for the restoration of posterior load bearing areas where the conventional restorative of choice is amalgam.

❖ Zirconomer is developed to exhibit strength that is consistent with amalgam, through a rigorous manufacturing technique. The glass component of this high-strength glass ionomer undergoes finely controlled micronization to achieve optimum particle size and characteristics. The homogeneous incorporation of zirconia particles in the glass component further reinforces the material for lasting durability and high tolerance to occlusal load. The polyalkenoic acid and the glass components have been specially processed to impart superior mechanical and handling qualities to this high-strength glass ionomer.

- It is also called—*the white amalgam*.

Indications

- Classes I and II cavities
- Structural base in sandwich restorations
- All classes of cavities where radiopacity is a prime requirement
- Core build-up under indirect restorations
- Root surfaces where overdentures rest
- Pediatric and geriatric restorations
- Long-term temporary replacement for fractured cusps
- Fractured amalgam restoration
- Suitable for ART techniques.

Advantages

- Reinforced with special zirconia fillers to match the strength and durability of amalgam
- Sustained high fluoride release
- Packable and condensable like amalgam without the hazard of mercury
- High flexural modulus and compressive strength ensures longevity in stress bearing areas
- Chemically bonds to enamel/dentin and has tooth-like coefficient of thermal expansion
- Adequate working time with snap-set reaction
- Easy mixing and handling characteristics minimize chair time and enables ease of bulk placement
- Excellent resistance to abrasion and erosion.

Bioactive Restorative Materials in Pediatric Dentistry

- They can be defined as "a material that forms a surface layer of a material similar to apatite in the presence of an inorganic phosphate solution" or as materials those can elicit a response in host.
- In 1950s the term biomimmetic was used by biomedical engineer Otto Schmitt who emphasised on the biological mechanisms of products that immitate nature.
- Larry Hench introdyced bioglass in 1969 which had silicate glass causing bioactivity.
- Properties: The calcium silicate and calcium aluminate cements combine several properties unlike most other dental materials.
  - The cements set with water, are dimensionally stable, and form alkaline hydroxide within the hydrated cement matrix.
  - Being stable in moisture is a tremendous benefit for dental applications.
  - Lack of expansion or contraction helps seal the area of the tooth anatomy that is being replaced with cement, whereas the common, polymer-based, dental restoratives shrink.
  - The high pH provides antimicrobial action on planktonic bacteria and yeast, although insufficient to destroy tenacious biofilms.
  - Most importantly, the calcium cements release calcium and hydroxide ions from their surface on contact with moist tissues. The calcium and hydroxide ions from the cement react with the phosphate ions in tissue fluids and precipitate a thin layer of a calcium phosphate compound, a process known as biomineralization. This surficial precipitate is akin to HA, the ceramic constituent of bones and teeth.
- Some newer bioactive restorative materials are Biodentine, Bioaggregate, BioRoot RCS, calcium-enriched mixture cement, Endo-CPM, Endocem, EndoSequence, EndoBinder, EndoSeal MTA, iRoot, MicroMega MTA, MTA Bio, MTA Fillapex, MTA Plus, NeoMTA Plus, OrthoMTA, Quick-Set, RetroMTA, Tech Biosealer and Theracal LC.
- Bioaggregate (Innovative Bioceramic Inc. Vancouver, British Columbia, Canada) contains di/tricalcium silicate and tantalum oxide for radiopacity. This kit contain water to be mixed with powder.
- Biodentine (Septodont, France) is stated to be the first di/tricalcium silicate cement with zirconia as radiopacifier. The powder in Biodentine also contains calcium chloride so as to accelerate the setting time.
- Theracal LC (Bisco, USA) material mostly contains resins with 45% "hydraulic cement", which may contain barium zirconate. Setting time is fast (0.3 minutes) as its light cured.
- Endocem (Maruchi, South Korea) is described as an MTA derived cement.It contains fine silica partices as di/tricalcium silicate.
- Retro MTA (BioMTA, South Korea) is a fast setting cement conatining calcium carbonate, silicon dioxide, aluminium oxide and calcium zirconia complex.

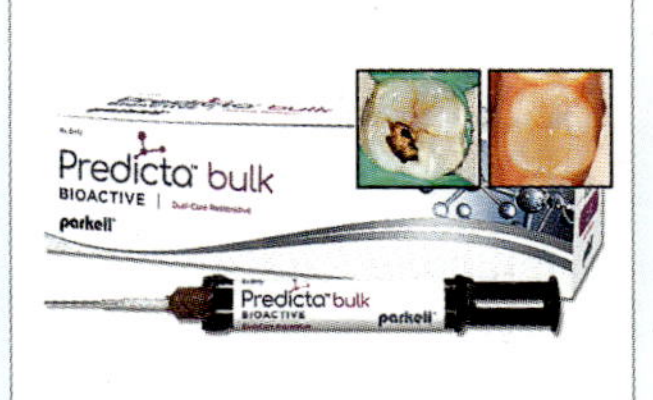

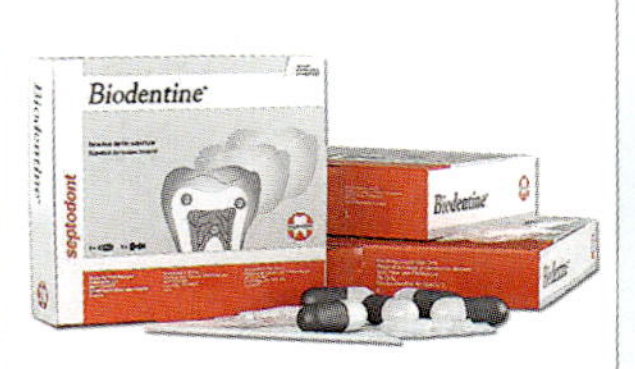

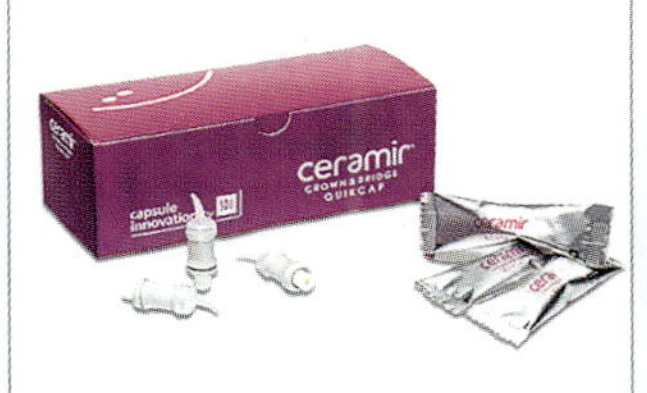

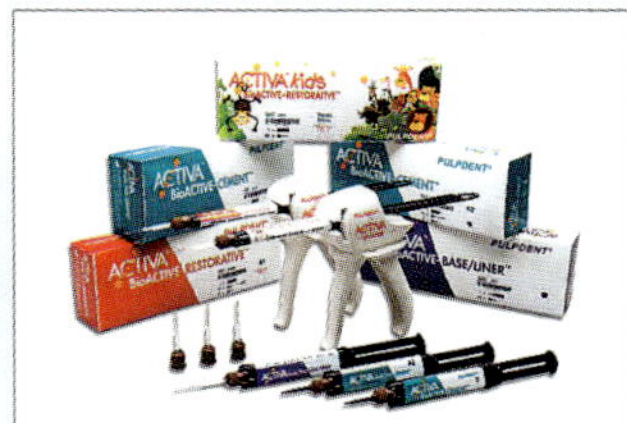

POINTS TO REMEMBER

- Dentists have used silver amalgam as a restorative material for more than 150 years.
- Corrosion is the progressive destruction of a metal by chemical or electrochemical reaction with its environment. Recommended mercury–alloy ratios for most modern lathe-cut alloys is 1:1, or 50% mercury.
- The initiation of toxic effects of mercury was first evaluated in fishermen due to excess mercury in water. The maximum safe level of occupational exposure to mercury is 50 µg.
- Composite is the universally used tooth-colored direct restorative material developed in 1962 by combining dimethacrylates with silanized quartz powder by Bowen (1963).
- Ormocers, a word originally derived from organically modified ceramics, were originally developed for science and technology.
- Ormocers have a reduced polymerization shrinkage compared to hybrid composites. The word "Compomer" comes from composite and glass ionomer.
- Calcium hydroxide was introduced to dentistry by Hermann in 1936.
- Bioactive dental materials are the future of dentistry. These materials show biomineralization (precipitation of hydroxyapatite [HA]) phenomena and produce ions that stimulate cytokines for healing of pulp tissue.

Questionnaire

1. Classify amalgam and write a note on its clinical application.
2. Write about mercury toxicity.
3. Describe waste management of amalgam and other restorative materials.
4. Classify composites and explain its various types.
5. What are the uses, advantages, and disadvantage of calcium hydroxide?
6. Describe the role of calcium hydroxide in endodontics.
7. Classify GIC and give its composition.
8. What are the modifications of GIC?
9. Define bioactive dental materials.
10. Describe the various bioactive dental materials.
11. Explain the various uses of bioactive dental materials.
12. Advantages and disadvantages of bioactive dental materials.
13. Future research on dental materials, in relation to pediatric dentistry.

FURTHER READING

1. American Dental Association/National Institute of Dental Research. 1991 Symposium on esthetic restorative materials. Chicago: American Dental Association; 1993. p. 167.
2. Benly P. Recent advances in composite –A review. J Pharm Sci Res. 2016;8(8): 881-83.
3. Camilleri J. Staining potential of neo MTA Plus, MTA Plus, and biodentine used for pulpotomy procedures. J Endod. 2015;41(7):1139-45.
4. Care L, Davidson J. Advances in glass ionomer cement. J Minim Interv Dent. 2009;2(1).
5. Craig RG (Ed). Restorative Dental Materials, 10th edition. St. Louis: Mosby; 1997.
6. Dhoot R, Bhondwe S, Mahajan V, LonareS, Rana K. Advances in glass ionomer cement(GIC): A review. IOSR – J Dent Med Sci2016;15(11): 124-26.
7. Farhad A, Mohammadi Z. Calcium hydroxide: a review. Int Dent J. 2005;55:293-301.
8. Heinemann S, Rossler S, Lemm M, Ruhnow M, Nies B. Properties of injectable ready-to-use calcium phosphate cement based on water-immiscible liquid. Acta Biomater. 2013;9(4):6199-207.
9. Hench LL. Chronology of bioactive glass development and clinical applications. New J Glass Ceram. 2013;3(2):67-73.
10. Hickel, et al. New direct restorative materials. Int Dent J. 1998;8:3-16.
11. Jo SB, Kim HK, Lee HN, Kim Y-J, Dev Patel K, Campbell Knowles J, et al. Physical properties and biofunctionalities of bioactive root canal sealers in vitro. Nanomaterials (Basel). 2020;10(9):1750.
12. Kumar A, Tekriwal S, Rajkumar B, GuptaV, Rastogi R. A review on fibre reinforced composite resins. Annals Prosthot Rest Dent. 2016;2(1): 11-16.
13. Lahari K, Jaidka S, Somani R, RevelliA, Kumar D, Jaidka R. Recent advances in composite restorations. Int J Adv Res. 2019;7(10): 761-79.
14. Lyapina MG, Tzekova M, Dencheva M, et al. Nano-glass ionomer cements in restorative dentistry. J IMAB. 2016;22:1160-5.
15. Mohammed M, Saujanya KP, Jain D, et al. Role of calcium hydroxide in endodontics: a review. Glob J Med Public Health. 2012;1:66-72.
16. Morfis AS, Sykaras S. Clinical use of calcium hydroxide in dentistry—review. Hell Stomatol Chron. 1987;31:169-75.
17. Mount GJ. Glass-ionomer cements past present and future. Oper Dent. 1994;19:82-90.
18. Rozaidah T. Dental composites: a review. J Nihon Univ Sch Dent. 1993;35:161-70.
19. Siboni F, Taddei P, Zamparini F, Prati C, Gandolfi MG. Properties of BioRoot RCS, a tricalcium silicate endodontic sealer modified with povidone and polycarboxylate. Int Endod J. 2017;50(Suppl 2): e120-36.
20. Sidhu SK, Nicholson JW. A review of glass ionomer cements for clinical dentistry. J Funct Biomater. 2016;7: E16.
21. Singh P, Kumar N, Singh R, et al. Overview and recent advances in composite resin: a review. Int J Sci Stud. 2015;3: 169-72.
22. Tay KCY, Loushine BA, Oxford C, Kapur R, Primus CM, Gutmann JL, et al. In vitro evaluation of a Ceramicrete-based root-end filling material. J Endod. 2007;33(12):1438-43.
23. Tiskaya M, Al-Eesa NA, Wong FSL, Hill RG. Characterization of the bioactivity of two commercial composites. Dent Mater. 2019;35(12):1757-68.
24. Torabinejad M, Watson TF, Pitt Ford TR. Sealing ability of a mineral trioxide aggregate when used as a root end filling material. J Endod. 1993;19(12):591-5.
25. Tyas MJ. Reaction and discussion. Clinical performance of glass ionomer cements. Symposiurn on esthetic restorative materials. Chicago IL: American Dental Association; 1991.
26. White SR, Sottos NR, Geubelle PH,Moore JS, Kessler MR, Sriram SR et al. Autonomic healing of polymer composites. Nature. 2001;409: 794-97.
27. Willems G, Lambrechts P, Braem M, Vanherle G. Composite resins in the 21st century. Quintessence Int. 1993;24: 641-58.
28. Wilson AD, Kent BE. The glass-ionomer cement: a new translucent dental filling material. J Chem Technol Biotechnol. 1971;21:313.

Concepts of Minimal Intervention: Cavity Design Modifications, Minimally Invasive Preparation Techniques, ART and SDF

Sivakumar Nuvvula, Mridula Goswami, Dhanraj Kalaivanan, Debarchhana Jena, Deval Kumar Arora, Lalitha Jairam

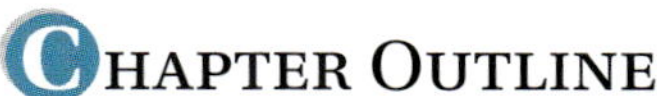

Chapter Outline

The term minimal intervention is relatively new in dentistry and has been introduced to suggest to the profession that it is time for change in the principles of operative dentistry. Preservation and maintenance of good oral health is the prime objective of every pediatric dentist. Dental caries is the most common childhood disease and multiple etiological factors, including biological, genetic, nutritional, socioeconomic, cultural, and environmental, etc., contribute for it. Treatment of dental caries is dependent on the stage of caries progression. Minimally invasive dentistry (MID), has been introduced as a new approach for addressing caries and carious lesions through minimally invasive techniques for the preservation of tooth. The original approach to the treatment of caries was purely surgical. It was thought that the only effective method of eliminating the disease was to completely remove all of the demineralized areas of tooth structure and rebuild it with an inert restoration that would simply obturate the cavity. The margin of the cavity had to be placed on a so-called caries-free surface to avoid the risk of further plaque accumulation that could lead to recurrence of the disease. This led to the development of a standardized system of intervention regardless of the size and extent of the original lesion. Even the smallest area of demineralization required the removal of a standard amount of sound tooth structure to prevent progression. Cavity designs were classified and standardized, and sound natural tooth structure was sacrificed in the name of geometric perfection to accommodate the shortcomings of the restorative material. A number of problems arise from this approach. First, it fails to recognize that cavitation is essentially a symptom of a bacterial disease. Second, it denies the ability of the tooth structure to remineralize and heal. Once tooth structure is removed, for whatever reason, it cannot be remineralized, and the original form, anatomy, esthetics and strength are lost forever.

The concept of preventive dentistry was developed on the basis of demineralization, but, with the poor understanding of remineralization at that time. However, the full cycle was not appreciated. The philosophy of minimal intervention dentistry has now risen in an attempt to combine all the existing knowledge of prevention, remineralization, ion exchange, healing, and adhesion with the objective of reducing carious damage in the simplest and least invasive manner possible thereby reducing procedural time, pain, stress and anxiety of the pediatric patients.

PRINCIPLES OF MINIMAL INTERVENTION

The surgical approach has been proven to be inefficient and destructive and is obviously maximally interventionist. A recent policy document produced by the World Dental Federation suggested that there are four basic principles that must be applied to fulfill the description of minimal intervention dentistry.

1. **Control the disease through reduction of cariogenic flora**: Only in the absence of disease will restorative dentistry succeed. This is why control of the disease is the primary focus, and only when such control has been achieved, will it be possible to offer long-term repair of the damage. Correct diagnostic procedures must be carried out for every patient at-risk to determine the potential for carious activity. Modification of the oral microflora is essential in the initial stage, and a number of oral lavages are available to modify the balance of the oral flora although chlorhexidine is probably the most effective of these.
   - *Diagnosis of initial carious lesion:* The purpose is to detect visual changes in color, translucency and structure of the enamel, level of demineralization,

brown or white stains, plaque biofilm and the gingival pathology at suspected sites. A blunt/rounded probe or a periodontal probe can be used, for the examination.

- *Clinical parameters that indicate and determine the status of single carious lesion are:*
  - The appearance of the lesion determines the severity.
  - The position of the lesion determines the possibility of plaque build-up.
  - Tactile perceptions on probing determines the presence of surface deposits and roughness of the enamel indirectly showing the level of demineralization and damage.
  - Presence or absence of gingival bleeding on probing determines the status of the gingival health.
- *Extensive clinical observation of initial carious lesion:* International Caries Detection and Assessment System (ICDAS). The classification defines six codes. Initial carious lesions are mainly explained by Code 1 and 2. Recent addition in the caries diagnostic aids has made the diagnosis of early carious lesion easy and more accurate.
- *Assessment of individual caries risk:* Caries risk is the probability of future caries development. American Academy of Pediatric Dentistry recognizes that caries-risk assessment and management protocols can assist clinicians with decisions regarding treatment option and are important elements of holistic care for infants, children, and adolescents. It includes both primary and secondary disease.
- *Direct risk factors for caries development and progression:* Amount of plaque deposition, type of bacteria, dietary pattern, frequency of carbohydrate intake on daily basis, saliva amount, saliva buffer capacity, exposure to fluorides.
- *Indirect risk factors for caries*: Socioeconomic background and general health of the child.

2. **Remineralize early lesions:** Remineralization should be recognized and utilized as far as possible for any tooth that has been subject to attack by caries, because there is no real substitute for natural tooth structure. It has been known for many years that "white-spot" lesions on the visible surfaces of teeth can be remineralized and repaired. Successful remineralization requires intensive patient education and cooperation; the patient must have a full understanding of the implication of food types, the need for plaque removal, and the possible need for additional oral lavages for control of bacterial populations (Dealt in detail in Chapter 47).
   - *Requirements of an ideal remineralization material:*
     - It should deliver calcium and phosphate by diffusing into the subsurface
     - It should not deliver excess of calcium ions
     - It should not favor any calculus formation
     - It should work at an acidic pH
     - It should boost the remineralizing properties of saliva
     - It should benefit over conventional fluoride therapy for novel materials.
3. **Perform minimal intervention surgical procedures, as required:** If the disease has progressed to cavitation on the tooth surface, it is no longer possible to completely control plaque accumulation without some degree of surgical intervention. In view of the potential for remineralization and healing, a minimal intervention approach is encouraged. The principle of preservation of natural tooth structure should dominate decisions about both new and old lesions.
   - *Radiographic evaluation of proximal caries* also adds to better diagnosis and appropriate treatment plan. Early proximal lesions are the lesions with radiolucency in the inner half of enamel, at dentoenamel junction or even slightly into the dentin, but with little or no evidence of cavitation. The radiographic changes in proximal lesions can be assessed following the classification given by **Ben and Dankel et al.**

     E1 = Radiolucency detected in outer 1/2 of enamel
     E2 = Radiolucency detected in inner 1/2 of enamel
     D1 = Radiolucency detected in outer 1/3 of dentin
     D2 = Radiolucency detected in middle 1/3 of dentin
     D3 = Radiolucency detected in inner 1/3 of dentin
4. **Repair, rather than replace, defective restorations:** The replacement of any failed restoration will also lead to further loss of tooth structure and subsequent weakening of the remaining crown. This steady progression should be limited as far as possible; with the advent of adhesion, biomimetic materials, and minimal intervention cavity designs, it is often possible to repair, rather than replace, a restoration that has suffered a limited failure.

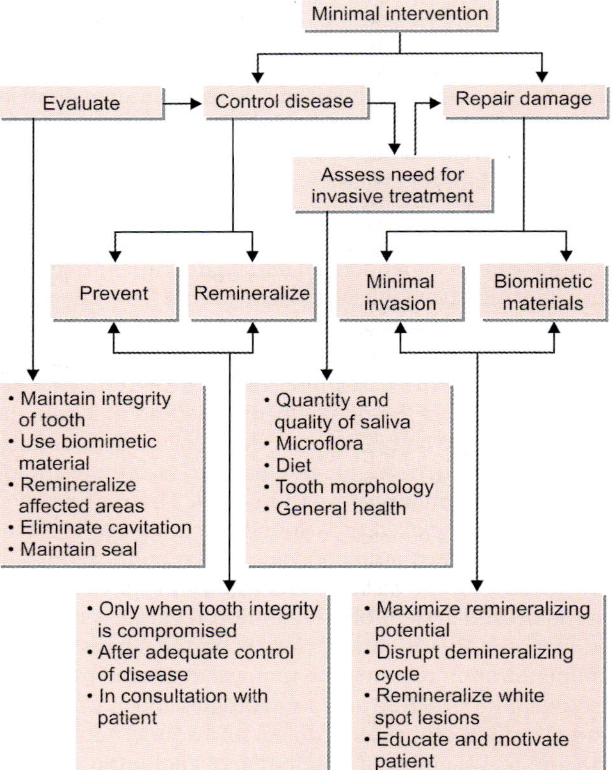

CAVITY DESIGN MODIFICATIONS

It is apparent that it should now be possible to review the **GV Black** approach to cavity design and be far more conservative in removing natural tooth structure. Minimal intervention cavity designs have been discussed for more than 20 years (**Knight** 1984; **Hunt** 1984) and a new classification that encourages the profession to see operative dentistry in a new light has been proposed (**Mount** and **Hume**, 1997). The **GV Black** classification does not address this new philosophy; thus, it is in the interest of both the patient and operator to adopt a new method. The proposed classification takes into account the fact that there are only three surfaces of the crown of a tooth that can be subject to caries attacks. These surfaces are:

- **Site 1:** Pits and fissures on the occlusal surface of posterior teeth and other defects on otherwise smooth enamel surfaces.
- **Site 2:** Contact areas between any pair of teeth, anteriors or posteriors.
- **Site 3:** Cervical areas related to gingival tissues, including exposed root surfaces.

A neglected lesion will continue to extend in an area of demineralization in relation to one of the sites noted above. As it extends, so will the complexities of the restoration increase. The sizes that can be readily identified include:

- **Size 0:** Initial lesion at any site can be identified but has not yet resulted in surface cavitation. It can possibly be healed.
- **Size 1:** Smallest minimal lesion requiring operative intervention. The cavity is into dentin just beyond healing through remineralization.
- **Size 2:** Moderate-size cavity. There is still sufficient sound tooth structure to maintain the integrity of the remaining crown.
- **Size 3:** The cavity needs to be modified and enlarged to provide some protection for the remaining crown from the occlusal load. There is already a split at the base of a cusp or, if not protected, a split will likely develop.
- **Size 4:** The cavity is now extensive, following the loss of a cusp from a posterior tooth or an incisal edge from an anterior.

Site 1, Size 0	The concept of the fissure seal, as discussed by **Simonsen** (1989) and others, is particularly sound in a newly erupted tooth. Sealing a deep fissure before it becomes partially occluded by plaque and pellicle, and in advance of demineralization into dentin, has an acceptable clinical history (**Feigal**, 1998; **Ekstrand**, 1998). The earliest fissure sealants were unfilled or lightly filled resins, but recent research has shown that there are some doubts about the integrity of the acid etch union between resin and enamel in these regions. It has been shown that a glass ionomer will successfully occlude such a fissure (**Wilson** and **McLean**, 1988). This is now being termed "fissure protection" to differentiate it from a "resin seal".
Site 1, Size 1	As the fissure walls become demineralized, the dentin will become involved as well. This may pose a rather dangerous situation because there is often some difficulty in diagnosing the presence of a dentin lesion. Radiographs will not show this early lesion very clearly and laser detector and electrical impedance machines have limitations. In the presence of strong, fluoridated enamel, the occlusal surface entry to the lesion will remain limited, and bacteria-laden plaque can be forced down into a defective fissure. Under these circumstances, dentin involvement can become advanced before symptoms are noted. The fissure system is a complex series of pits and fissures; therefore, a carious defect will often be limited to a very restricted area, leaving the remaining fissure system sound and uninvolved. This means that only the carious defect needs to be instrumented. However, prudence suggests that minor apparent defects should be explored in a very conservative manner before sealing the fissure system.
Site 1, Size 2	In this classification, the lesion will either have progressed to some degree or it may represent replacement of a failed Class I restoration. The same conservative principles should apply, as discussed above, in as much as it is only necessary to deal with the carious lesion, and there is no need to open up the remaining fissures any further. If there is any part of the fissure system that is in doubt, it can be explored very conservatively, but there is no doubt that it is sufficient to seal the fissures, and any carious process below will be arrested. However, the occlusal involvement will be more extensive and, if there is any doubt about the ability of the glass ionomer to withstand the occlusal load, it can be cut back conservatively and laminated with resin composite.
Site 1, Sizes 3, 4	When a restoration requires replacement, the existing cavity will be relatively large. The previous surgical approach to cavity design required the removal of all infected tooth structure and softened affected dentin on floor of the cavity and also required removal of all unsupported enamel on the occlusal surface. Consequently, there was a potential for loss of occlusal contact with the opposing tooth. To avoid such procedures a temporary restoration is placed over the carious structure, and this helps in remineralizing the lesion and decreasing pulpal inflammation. Glass ionomer should be used for the transitional restoration following removal of infected layer of dentin from the surface of a large cavity. It will adhere to both enamel and dentin through an ion- exchange mechanism, thus eliminating microleakage. It will also adhere to the collagen of demineralized dentin on the cavity floor through either hydrogen bonding or metallic-ion bridging. In the absence of bacterial activity, the pulpal inflammation will subside. In the presence of water from the positive dentinal fluid flow that follows, there will be calcium, phosphate, and fluoride ions exchanged between the glass ionomer and the demineralized dentin. Further ions will be available from the pulpal fluid, and the dentin will remineralize.
Site 2, Size 0	It should be noted that radiographic evidence of demineralization at the contact area does not necessarily mean that there is cavitation on the proximal surface and, in the absence of cavitation, it is often possible to heal the lesion. In fact, proximal lesions progress very slowly because that surface is not under masticatory load and is, to a degree, protected from traumatic damage (**Pitts**, 1983; **Shwartz**, 1984). In contrast to the occlusal fissure lesion, it may take up to 4 years to penetrate the full thickness of the enamel and an additional 4 years to progress through the dentin to the pulp.
Site 2, Size 3, 4	The principles for the restoration of an extensive proximal lesion are essentially the same as those for an occlusal lesion. In gaining access to the affected demineralized dentin, there is no need to remove enamel just because it appears to be unsupported according to the old surgical principles. However, the walls of the cavity should be cleaned of all infected dentin to allow development of the full ion-exchange adhesion with the glass ionomer. Demineralized dentin can remain on both the axial and pulpal walls on the assumption that it will remineralize under the influence of the glass ionomer. First increment should be placed and tamped over the entire floor of the cavity using a small, dry plastic sponge. A further increment must be applied, and if the size of the cavity requires it, this one should be tamped in as well to adapt it properly to the walls. The cavity must be overfilled, the glass ionomer allowed to set, and lastly, the occlusion adjusted. With active caries, this restoration may be regarded as a long-term transitional restoration, destined to be replaced after 3 months or more, by which time the caries should be controlled. On the other hand, if the glass ionomer is intended to complete the restoration at the same appointment, it should be allowed to set before trimming it back and repreparing the cavity for resin composite to be laminated over it.

Enamel Cavity

Enamel rods located at occlusal fissures accumulate at their top centripetally and are supported at the bottom by dentin. Therefore, if restoration is placed in a cavity limited to the enamel layer, it will be supported indirectly by the surrounding bottom layer of dentin irrespective of brittleness of enamel. The key advantages of enamel cavity preparation in children are painless preparation method, which reduces anxiety and fear of the child. Also allows minimum tooth structure loss. Thereby original strength of the tooth is maintained to maximum.

Tunnel Cavity Preparation

- This is indicated if the cavity is small and if placed 2–2.5 mm below the marginal ridge.
- The aim is to develop an access via the occlusal aspect so as to preserve the strength of marginal ridge and also to prevent formation of proximal cavity **(Fig. 46.1).**
- The early proximal lesion on a posterior tooth will commence in enamel immediately below the contact area because this is where plaque will accumulate and mature. As the lesion develops, some degree of breakdown and cavitation of the enamel will eventually occur, but this will remain confined to the area below the contact until it is quite advanced. There will generally be a zone of demineralized enamel surrounding the cavitation, but as long as the surface is smooth, this remains capable of remineralization in the presence of fluoride. The contact area may remain sound and the marginal ridge may be quite strong, provided the lesion is more than 2.5 mm below the crest of the marginal ridge (**Wilson** and **McLean**, 1988).
- Access to the lesion through the occlusal surface should be limited to the extent required to achieve visibility and should be undertaken from an area that is not under direct occlusal load.
- Fossa immediately next to medial marginal ridge is the most suitable position for entry.
- Glass ionomer is best suited for such cavities as it readily flows into a small cavity and has the ability to remineralize the enamel margins and any dentin on axial wall.

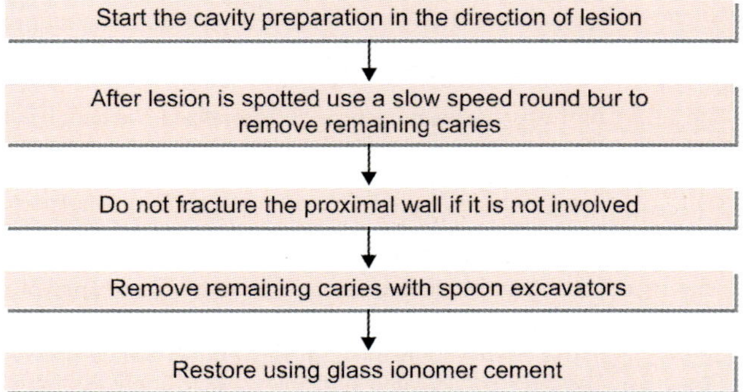

Start the cavity preparation in the direction of lesion
After lesion is spotted use a slow speed round bur to remove remaining caries
Do not fracture the proximal wall if it is not involved
Remove remaining caries with spoon excavators
Restore using glass ionomer cement

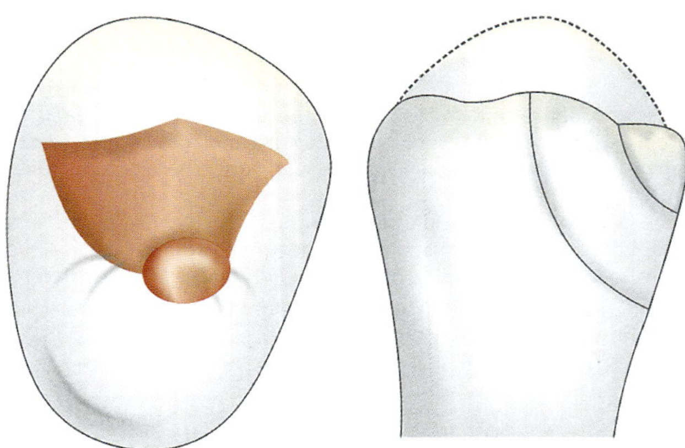

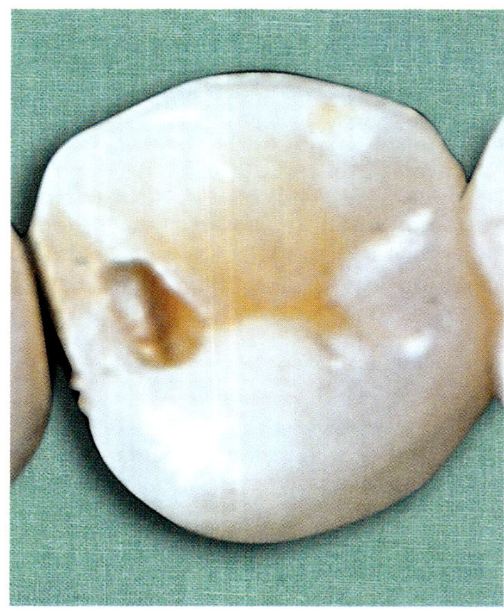

Fig. 46.1: Tunnel cavity preparation.

Slot Cavity Preparation

- As the name denotes, it is creation of a small slot on the proximal aspect of posterior teeth
- Indicated if there is a small lesion involving the area of or below the marginal ridge only in deciduous teeth
- The outline form will be dictated entirely by the extent of the breakdown of the enamel, removing only that which is friable and easily eliminated without applying undue pressure. Retention will be through adhesion, so it is only necessary to clean the walls around the full circumference of the lesion, leaving the axial wall because it will be affected by dentin only
- Cavity preparation is done only on the proximal aspect after establishing entry over marginal ridge, and the extent of cavity is defined by the extent of the lesion with the intention to preserve as much tooth as possible **(Fig. 46.2)**
- The material of choice is glass ionomer, but resin composite may be a useful material because on many occasions, there will be an enamel margin around the full circumference.

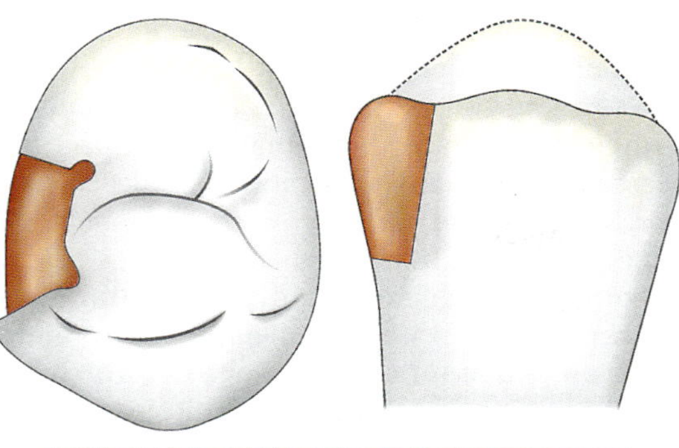

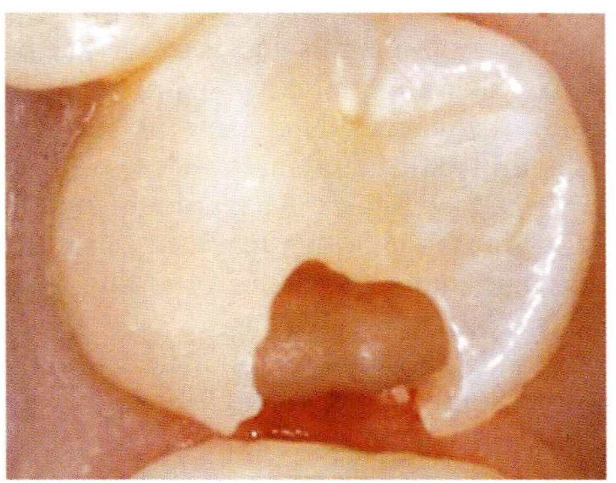

Fig. 46.2: Slot cavity preparation.

PROXIMAL APPROACH

- This is a very conservative approach used when the proximal surface of a tooth becomes accessible at the time of cavity preparation in an adjacent tooth. The lesion may have been revealed through radiographs, or it may be noted only during cavity preparation.
- The larger cavity in the adjacent tooth will normally need to be of reasonably generous proportions to allow room to maneuver, but when such an approach is possible, it leads to considerable conservation of natural tooth structure. It is only necessary to remove enamel that is broken down beyond remineralization. There will often be a residual area of demineralized enamel around the circumference of the lesion, and this should be retained because it is quite capable of being remineralized **(Fig. 46.3)**. As this entire restoration will be hidden by adjacent tooth, it is essential to use a radiopaque material. Glass ionomer is preferred because the limited access will make it difficult to assure full polymerization of the resin through light activation.
- It is apparent that it is time for a change in operative dentistry. It is not possible to really imitate natural tooth structure on a long-term basis, so it is best that it be retained as far as possible. Therapeutic methods for the control of the disease are available, and these should be the first line of defense. In the presence of early carious lesions, there is no justification for removal of tooth structure simply to provide a theoretic resistance to further carious attack or to develop mechanical retention for restorative materials. It is important that the profession embraces modern science and move into the new century.

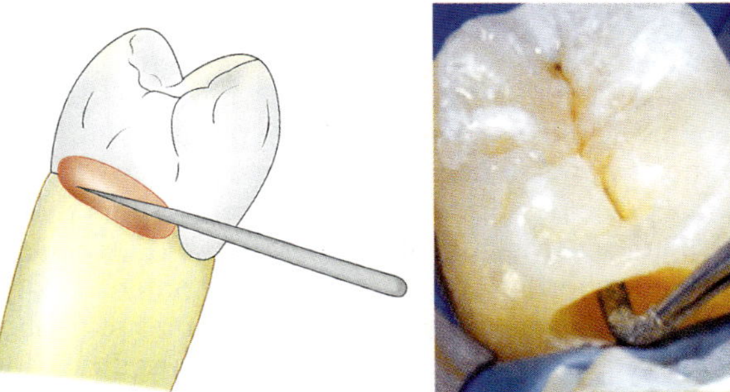

Fig. 46.3: Proximal approach.

MINIMALLY INVASIVE PREPARATION TECHNIQUES

- **Mechanical systems**
  - *Atraumatic restorative treatment:* The atraumatic restorative treatment (ART) is a technique that involves removal of carious tissues using hand instruments alone and restoring the cavity with an adhesive substance. Glass ionomer cement is currently the most popular restorative material.
  - *Smart burs:* The development of a technology for removing caries-infected dentin while conserving caries-affected dentin is one of the major goals of modern dentistry. It is for this reason that the use of a polymer bur has brought to reality an innovative, recently proposed self-limiting notion in mechanical caries eradication. The paddle-shaped bur is made of medical-grade polyether-ketone-ketone (PEKK) with a unique flute design and a hardness and wear resistance that allows it to remove only the soft caries-infected dentin while keeping the caries-affected dentin intact. The bur, which is only used at low speeds (500–800 rpm), quickly dulls and vibrates as it comes into contact with the more calcified caries-affected dentin.
- **Sonic oscillating systems**
  - A good alternative to traditional cavity preparation would usher in the use of ultrasonic devices since they do not create the high-pitched sound that irritates patients and are less expensive than lasers.
  - The study of this approach has been limited to work done in the 1950s by **Nielsen et al.**, who suggested that an ultrasonic tool may be used to cut tooth tissue. He created a magnetostrictive instrument that oscillates at a frequency of 25 kHz. The cutting action was achieved by the high-speed oscillations of the cutting tip, when this was combined with thick aluminium oxide and water slurry the kinetic energy of water molecules was transferred to the tooth surface via the abrasive used.
  - Sonic cavity preparation techniques available are SONIC flex system and CVDentus® system
- **Chemomechanical systems**
  - There is an increasing desire for processes or materials that make caries control easier in today's world. Chemomechanical caries removal is one such alternative treatment. It is a method for less invasive, soft dentin caries removal based on biological principles (**Zinc et al.**, 1988).
  - Chemomechanical caries removal is a noninvasive treatment that uses a chemical substance to remove infected dentin. This procedure not only removes infected tissues, but also protects the healthy tooth

structure, preventing pulp irritation and patient discomfort. This is can also be observed as a dissolution-based approach to caries eradication.

- Instead of drilling, this procedure removes soft carious structure with the help of a chemical agent and an atraumatic mechanical force. Materials that adhere to the dentin surface, like as composite resins or glass ionomer, are required to restore cavities produced with this approach. Caridex, Carisolv, Papacarie and Brix 3000 are among the commercially marketed products.

❖ **Kinetic system**

- Dr Robert Black introduced air abrasion, also known as advanced particle beam technology or microabrasive technology, in 1943. Cutting dental hard tissues with air-abrasion is a pseudo-mechanical, non-rotary approach. It removes tooth structure by utilizing the kinetic energy of alumina particles entrained in a high-velocity stream of air. Air abrasive procedures are well suited for restorations using modern day bonded resin materials, and they improve restorative lifespan.
- When highly energetic abrasive particles are directed towards healthy enamel or dentine, the substrate absorbs the kinetic energy and quickly cuts or abrades. As a result, the technique is also known as kinetic cavity preparation.
- The quantity of tooth removal and depth of penetration are affected by a number of factors such as air pressure, particle size, quantity of particles going through the nozzle, handpiece nozzle diameter, nozzle angulation, distance from object, and time of exposure to the object.
- Air pressures typically range from 40 to 160 psi. For cutting, 100 psi is recommended, while for surface etching, 80 psi is advised. Particles with diameters of 27 µm or 50 µm are the most prevalent. The larger particles allow the clinician to operate more quickly, but they also result in larger cavity preparations. More particles will abrade the working surface faster with a higher particle flow rate. Though exposure to aluminium oxide particles is a risk, adequate evacuation with high-volume suction eliminates it; however, patients with known respiratory disorders, such as asthma, should exercise caution.

❖ **Hydrokinetic systems**

- Light Amplification by Stimulated Emission of Radiation is an acronym for LASER. A laser device consists of a lasing material confined within an optical cavity and an external energy source to maintain a population inversion, allowing for stimulated emission of a given wavelength, resulting in a monochromatic, collimated, and coherent beam of light.
- To ensure that the laser energy reaches the target site, two delivery mechanisms were used. One, is a flexible hollow wave guide or tube with a mirror finish on the inside. The laser energy is reflected along this tube before exiting through a handpiece at the surgical end, where the beam strikes the tissue without making contact.
- A glass fiber optic cable is the second delivery system. This cable has the potential to be more flexible than the waveguide. With the naked end protruding, the fiber fits snuggly into a handpiece. It can be used in a contact or noncontact mode; however, it is most commonly utilized in a contact mode, touching the surgical site directly. As a function of time, the dental laser can emit light energy in two modes: constant on or pulsed on and off.

❖ **Ozone**

- Ozone is a thermodynamically unstable oxygen compound that decomposes to create molecular oxygen and atomic oxygen, both of which are very reactive. It oxidizes all non-noble metals instantly and attacks many organic compounds as a radical. Apart from fluorine, this makes ozone one of the most powerful oxidants. Because ozone is such a potent oxidant, it successfully eliminates bacteria, fungus, viruses, and parasites at far lower concentrations than chlorine, and without the hazardous side effects.
- The use of ozone gas in dentistry has been recommended for the sterilization of cavities, root canals, periodontal pockets, and herpetic lesions.
- Additionally, in dentistry, ozonated water is used to promote homeostasis, increase local oxygen supply, and reduce bacterial development. Theoretically, ozone can lower the bacterial count in active carious lesions, halting the advancement of caries and potentially preventing or delaying the need for dental restorations. As a result, it offers a wide range of possible applications in dental sciences. Ozone therapy can be used to treat cavities, chronic periodontitis, endodontic treatment and root canal disinfection, infections following tooth extractions, persistent wound healing deficiencies following radiotherapy, aphthae, and mycoses, among other things.

❖ **Vector system**

- The vector system is a novel approach that combines ultrasonic effects of quartz crystal suspension and the microabrasive action of the same. This approach helps in microinvasive preparation, contouring, and finishing of the tooth material and nonmetal restorations using specially designed metal tools and abrasive slurry of silicon carbide.
- The device generates ultrasonic vibrations, which are transformed by a resonating ring into a vertically deflected horizontal oscillation. As a result, the instrument tip moves parallel to the root surface, making it ideal for use with hydroxyl-apatite or silicon-carbide-based irrigation fluids. Therapy with the vector system has been demonstrated to be less painful than treatment with traditional systems since vibrations are not applied horizontally to the root surface.

❖ **Plasma**

- Following solids, liquids, and gases, plasma is the fourth state of matter. When gases are stimulated to the point where electrons fly off from part or all of their atoms, this substance is created. In 1929, an American chemist named Irving Langmuir registered the name.
- Plasma has added benefits when it comes to treating cavities rather than drilling into them. When the plasma jet shoots, it charges oxygen gas in the surrounding air, resulting in highly reactive molecules capable of

breaking down bacteria's defenses. These reactive oxygen species can penetrate and destroy bacterial cell walls.

- **Caries infiltration system**
  - Recently, caries infiltration, a minimally invasive method for smooth surface white spot lesions, has been developed. By filling and reinforcing the pore system of a non-cavitated white spot, or incipient proximal lesions, with a light curable resin, this approach and product, created to bridge the gap between prevention and restoration. The chameleon effect is created by the infiltrating resin, which has a high refractive index and does not require shade matching.

ATRAUMATIC RESTORATIVE TREATMENT

The atraumatic restorative treatment (ART) is a procedure based on removing carious tooth tissues using hand instruments alone and restoring the cavity with an adhesive restorative material. Another terminology used for ART is alternate restorative treatment. Usually, carious lesions are left untreated in children of underprivileged communities of developing and underdeveloped countries mainly because of financial problems and lack of awareness. Over the last two to three decades, although dental caries has decreased substantially in the few industrialized countries but from a global perspective, it still remains a widespread problem. The treatment requires qualified personnel and expensive equipment. The absence of clean and pressurized water and irregular supply of electricity makes it impossible for the oral healthcare personnel to work efficiently. A group in Zimbabwe and another in Thailand began experimentation to check longevity and efficiency of ART, and their results were so encouraging that the system has been adopted by the World Health Organization (WHO) and is being promoted worldwide as a useful technique for communities that lack regular dental facilities. A new method was presented for treating dental caries, which involved neither drill or water nor electricity at the headquarters of the WHO, Geneva, on World Health Day (April 8, 1994).

The Operator's Work Posture and Positions

- The work posture and position of the operator should provide the best view of the inside of the patient's mouth. At the same time, both patient and operator should be comfortable.
- The operator sits firmly on the stool, with straight back, thighs parallel to the floor and both feet flat on the floor. The head and neck should be still, the line between the eyes horizontal and the head bent slightly forward to look at the patient's mouth.
- The height of the stool must then be adjusted so that the operator can see the patient's teeth clearly.
- The distance from the operator's eye to patient's tooth is usually between 30 cm and 35 cm. The operator should be positioned behind the head of the patient. The exact position will depend on the area of the patient's mouth to be treated **(Fig. 46.4)**.

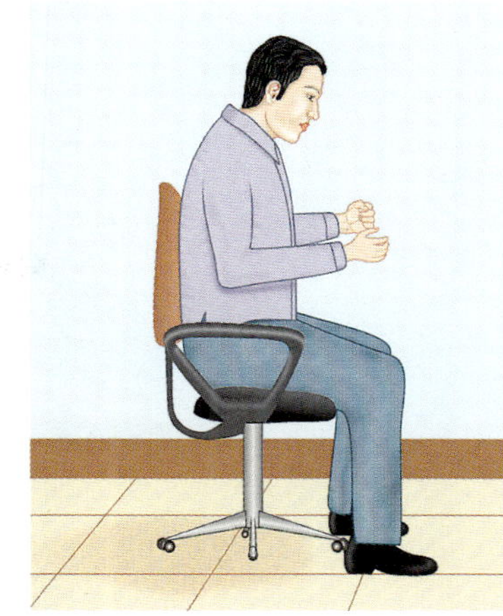

Fig. 46.4: The operator's work posture and position.

Assistance

- Oral care is best provided by a team consisting of an operator and an assistant.
- When treating patients, particularly children, using ART, it is a great advantage if another person can mix the glass-ionomer cement. This allows the operator to concentrate on the cavity and maintain effective saliva control. The assistant works at the left side of a right-handed operator and does not change position **(Fig. 46.5)**. The assistant should sit as close to the patient as possible, facing the patient's mouth.
- The assistant's head should be 10–15 cm higher than the operator, so that the assistant can also see the operating field and can pass the correct instruments when needed.

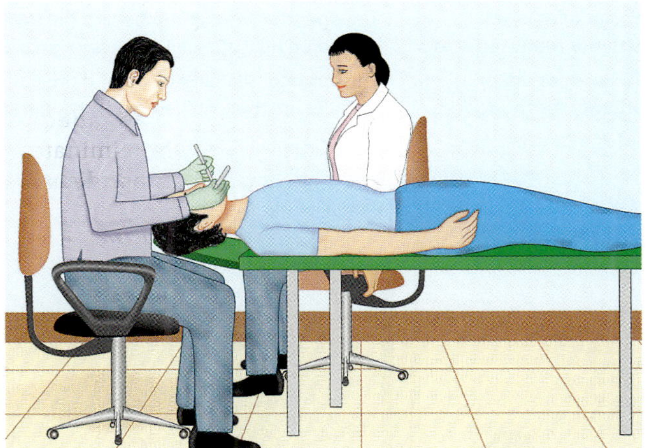

Fig. 46.5: With assistance.

Patient Position

As with any other oral treatment, ART requires correct patient and operator positions. A patient lying on the back on a flat surface will provide safe and secure body support and comfortable and stable position for lengthy periods of time **(Fig. 46.6)**.

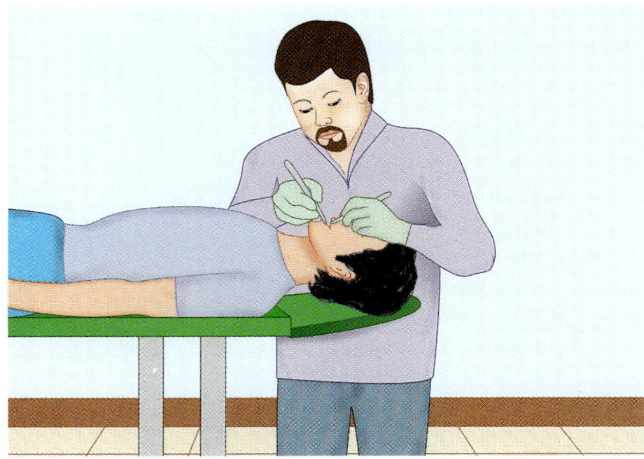

Fig. 46.6: Patient position.

Operating Positions (According to Right-handed Dentist) (Figs. 46.7A and B)

Position for upper right posterior tooth surfaces	The operator sits directly behind the patient's head. Mirror vision is used and the patient's head is tilted backward with the mouth fully open. Turning the patient's head will depend on the surfaces to be treated, i.e., for a palatal surface of an upper right molar-patient's head is turned slightly to the right, for a buccal surface of an upper right molar- patient's head is turned slightly to the left
Position for upper left posterior tooth surfaces	For occlusal and buccal surfaces, the operator sits directly behind the patient's head. Tilt the patient's head backward and turn it slightly to the right with the mouth fully open for occlusal and partly closed for buccal surfaces. For working on the palatal surface, the operator sits slightly to the right of the patient's head. Tilt the patient's head backward and turn it slightly to the left with the mouth fully open for direct vision
Position for lower left posterior tooth surface	The operator sits to the right rear of the patient's head. The patient's head is placed in the central position and tilted slightly forward. For occlusal and buccal surfaces, turn the head slightly to the right. The mouth should be fully open for occlusal views and partly closed for buccal surfaces to allow access for the mouth mirror. Direct vision may be used for most of the teeth
Position for lower right posterior tooth surfaces	The operator sits to the right rear of the patient's head, which should be tilted forward. For occlusal and lingual working surfaces, turn the head slightly to the right with the mouth fully open for direct vision. To view the buccal surfaces, turn the head slightly to the left with the mouth partly closed to allow access for the mouth mirror and hand instruments
Position for lower anterior tooth surfaces	The operator sits directly behind the patient's head. Tilt the patient's head forward in the central position. The mouth should be fully open and direct vision is used
Position for upper anterior tooth surfaces	The operator sits directly behind the patient. Tilt the patient's head backward with the mouth open. The buccal surfaces are then viewed directly and the lingual surfaces are viewed through the mouth mirror

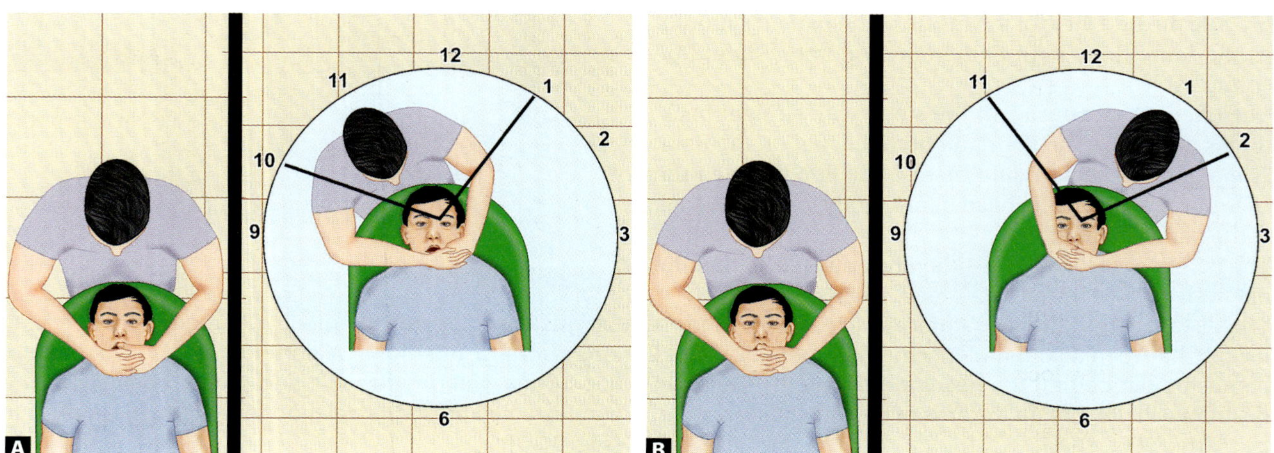

Figs. 46.7A and B: (A) Operating positions for right-handed dentist; (B) Operating positions for left-handed dentist.

Operating Light

- Good vision is essential for working in the oral cavity.
- The light source can be the sun (natural) or artificial. Artificial light is more reliable and constant than natural light and can also be focused on a particular spot. Therefore, in a field setting, a portable light source is recommended, e.g., a headlamp, glasses with a light source attached, or a light attached to the mouth mirror.

Essential Instruments and Materials

The success of any treatment depends on the operator knowing the functions of the various instruments and using them correctly. Following instruments and materials are used for ART:

Mouth mirror	This instrument is used to reflect light onto the field of operation, to view the cavity indirectly, and to retract the cheek or tongue
Explorer	This instrument is used to identify the presence of soft carious dentin
Tweezers	This instrument is used for carrying cotton wool rolls, cotton wool pellets, wedges, and articulation paper from the tray to the mouth and back
Spoon excavator	This instrument is used for removing soft carious dentin
Dental hatchet	This instrument is used for widening the entrance to the cavity, for slicing away thin unsupported and carious enamel left after carious dentin has been removed
Carver	This double-ended instrument has two functions. The blunt end is used for inserting the mixed glass-ionomer into the cleaned cavity and into pits and fissures. The sharp end is designed to remove excess restorative material and to shape the glass-ionomer
Mixing pad and spatula	These are necessary for mixing glass ionomer cement
Cotton wool rolls	These are used to absorb saliva, so that the tooth to be treated can be kept dry
Cotton wool pellets	These are used for cleaning cavities. They are available in various sizes
Petroleum jelly	This material is used to keep moisture away from the glass-ionomer restoration and to prevent the examination glove from sticking to the glass-ionomer as it sets hard
Plastic mylar strip wedges	This material is used for contouring the proximal surface of multiple surface restorations. These are used to hold the plastic strip close to the shape of the proximal surface of a tooth so that restorative material is not forced between the gums and teeth.

Arrangements in the Mouth

- A very important aspect for the success of ART is control of saliva around the tooth being treated.
- Cotton wool rolls quite effective at absorbing saliva and can provide short-term protection from moisture or saliva. Rolls can be either bought or prepared form bulk cotton dressing pack. The location in the mouth and method of placement of cotton wool rolls is described below:
  - *Upper teeth*: Retract the lip and cheek with the mouth mirror to make space between the cheek and teeth for the cotton wool roll. Place the cotton roll in position with a slight rotating action from the tooth toward the gingiva. This will help prevent the cotton wool roll from coming out easily.
  - *Lower teeth*: Ask the patient to stick the tongue out. Push the tongue aside with the mouth mirror. Place a cotton wool roll on each side of the floor of the mouth. Then ask the patient to retract the tongue back to its normal position.

Procedure for Atraumatic Restorative Treatment (Figs. 46.8A to H)

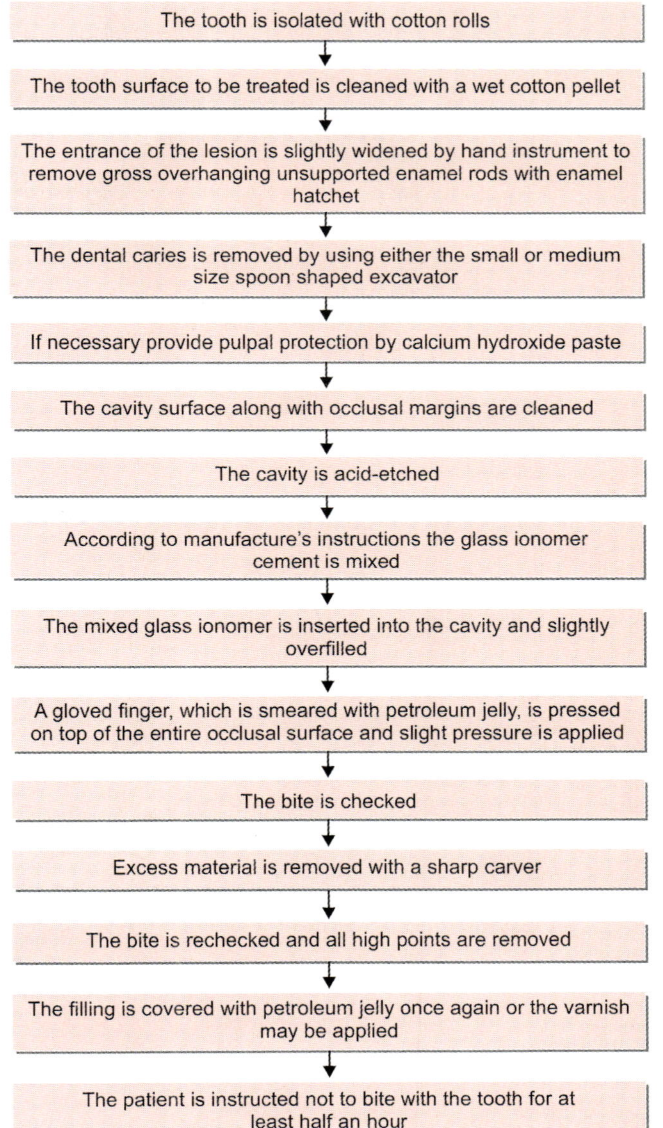

The tooth is isolated with cotton rolls
The tooth surface to be treated is cleaned with a wet cotton pellet
The entrance of the lesion is slightly widened by hand instrument to remove gross overhanging unsupported enamel rods with enamel hatchet
The dental caries is removed by using either the small or medium size spoon shaped excavator
If necessary provide pulpal protection by calcium hydroxide paste
The cavity surface along with occlusal margins are cleaned
The cavity is acid-etched
According to manufacture's instructions the glass ionomer cement is mixed
The mixed glass ionomer is inserted into the cavity and slightly overfilled
A gloved finger, which is smeared with petroleum jelly, is pressed on top of the entire occlusal surface and slight pressure is applied
The bite is checked
Excess material is removed with a sharp carver
The bite is rechecked and all high points are removed
The filling is covered with petroleum jelly once again or the varnish may be applied
The patient is instructed not to bite with the tooth for at least half an hour

Advantages of ART

- Easily available inexpensive hand instruments are used rather than the expensive electrically driven dental equipment. As it is almost a painless procedure, the need for local anesthesia is eliminated or minimized.
- ART involves the removal of only decalcified tooth tissues, which results in relatively small cavities and conserves sound tooth tissue as much as possible.

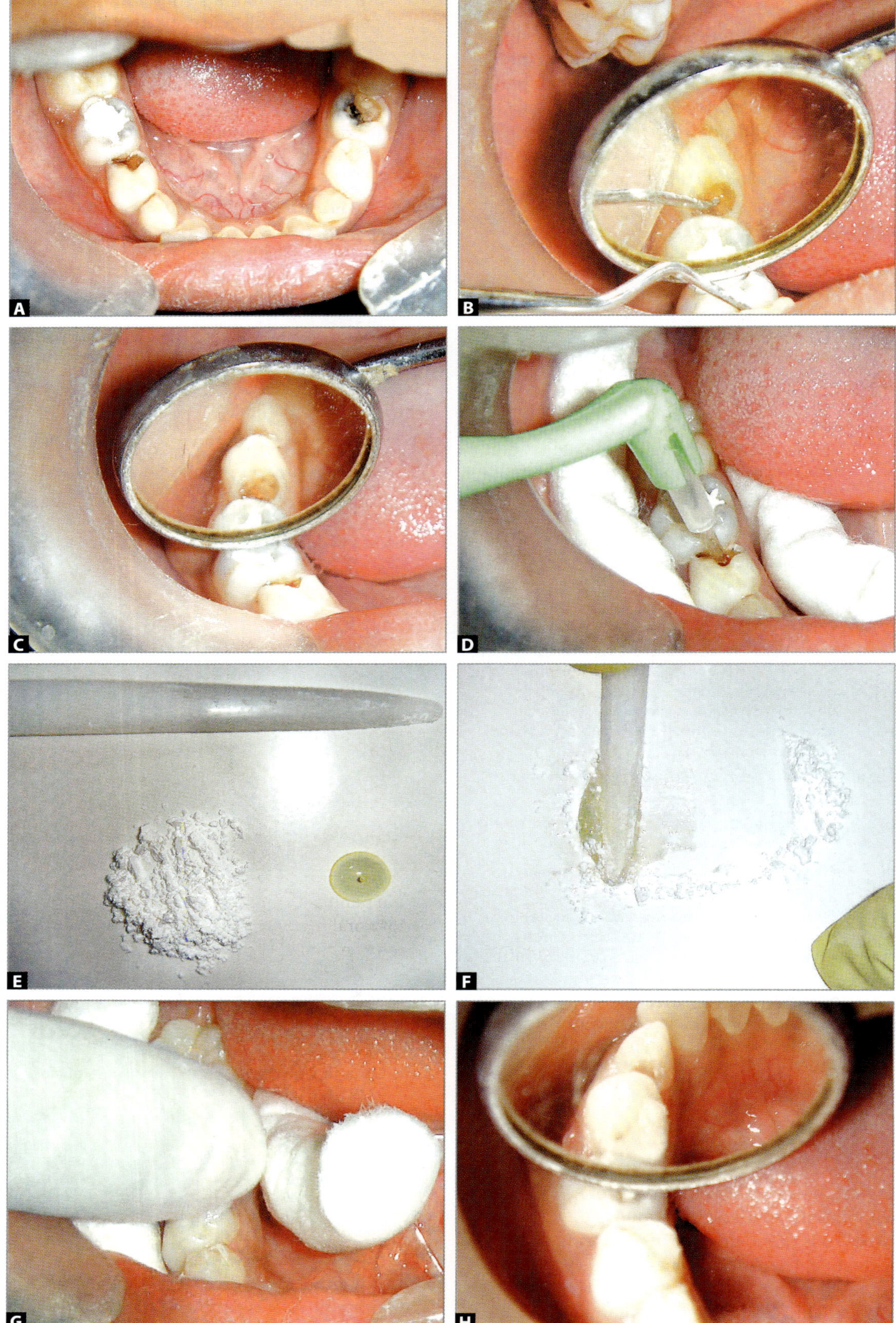

Figs. 46.8A to H: (A) Preoperative; (B) Excavation of caries; (C) Cavity after caries removal; (D) Cavity conditioning; (E) Dispensing of glass ionomer cement; (F) Mixing of glass ionomer cement; (G) Insertion of glass ionomer cement; (H) Restored cavity.

- Sound tooth tissue need not be cut for retention of filling material. The retention is obtained by the microtags produced due to etching and also because of the chemical adhesion of glass ionomer restorative material with cavity walls.
- A practice of straightforward and simple infection control is used without the need to use autoclaved hand pieces.
- The leaching of fluoride from glass ionomer probably remineralizes sterile demineralized dentin and prevents development of secondary caries.
- The combined preventive and curative treatment can be done in one appointment. Repairing of defects in the restoration can be easily done.
- It is less expensive and less time consuming as in one sitting several fillings can be done.
- One of the greatest advantages of ART is that it enables the oral health workers to reach people who otherwise never would have received any oral health service.

Disadvantages of ART

- ART restorations are not long lasting. The average life is 2 years depending upon the rate of caries activity of the individual oral cavity.
- As fundamental principles of cavity preparation are not followed, all oral health workers may not accept it.
- Because of the low wear resistance and low strength of the existing glass ionomer materials their use is limited to small and medium sized one surface cavity only.
- The continuous use of hand instruments over long period of time may result in hand fatigue.
- A relatively unstandardized mix of glass ionomer may be produced due to hand mixing.

Material Usage for Atraumatic Restorative Treatment

The reasons for using hand instruments rather electrically driven handpiece

- It makes restorative care accessible to all population groups.
- The use of a biological approach, which requires minimal cavity preparation that conserves sound tooth. The low cost of hand instruments compared to electrically driven dental equipment.
- The limitation of pain that reduces the need for local anesthesia to a minimum and reduce psychological trauma to patients. Simplified infection control; hand instruments can be easily cleaned and sterilized after every patient.

The Reasons for Using Glass Ionomer

- As the glass ionomer chemically bonds to both enamel and dentin, the need to cut sound tooth tissue to prepare the cavity is reduced.
- Fluoride is released from the restoration to prevent secondary caries.
- Glass ionomer is biocompatible, does not cause any irritation to pulp and gingival, and has a coefficient of thermal expansion similar to tooth structure.

ART sealants

Sealing of pit and fissures which are susceptible to caries is an effective preventive measure. The conventional pit and fissure technique involves the use of resins requiring utmost moisture control and curing. To overcome these disadvantages, ART sealants have emerged as a successful alternative. Application of a high viscosity GIC is done by a press finger method. This ensures that the material flows into the fissures efficiently. The success rates of ART sealants have shown to be comparable to resin-based sealants thereby making it an alternative choice especially in cases where isolation will be a challenge in un-cooperative children or special healthcare need individuals.

Applications of ART in a Dental Clinic

- In a dental set up, the importance of ART will be in handling an anxious or un un-cooperative child wherein there is almost no possibility in maintaining moisture control. In such situations, ART will be a simple and effective option which will alleviate fears due to airotor and sound of suction in an anxious child.
- The SMART technique will be particularly useful in cases of high caries risk individuals, medically compromised children, patients who cannot tolerate invasive procedures such as use of airotor and anxious children.
- ART sealants have shown excellent results in terms of longevity and caries prevention as compared to conventional resin-based sealants. The ease of application, less technique sensitiveness, fewer steps in placing GIC, lesser treatment time and good clinical outcomes makes GIC based ART sealant a valuable choice while treating a patient in a dental clinic setup.

As ART is based on modern concepts of cavity preparation where minimal intervention and invasion is emphasized; this approach is applicable also in the industrialized countries for special groups such as the physically and mentally handicapped and the elderly. In 2000, the division of public oral health implemented a training, research, and service program in the ART approach. The aim was the promotion of ART in public health services, private oral healthcare services, tertiary oral health training institutions, and health services for refugee communities.

A revolution in dentistry!! It may be too early to say, but *Grossman* sums it up: "There are always detractors who pooh-pooh at new techniques, but the ART approach at present serves a purpose. It is minimally invasive by saving tooth and maximally preventive by preventing further decay. It is a wonderful way of introducing a nervous patient to dental care, thereby laying the foundation for a lifetime of good oral health care".

SILVER DIAMINE FLUORIDE

Our knowledge of caries has shifted significantly, from a bacterial-driven disease process to a biofilm-mediated disease process. The traditional, surgical approach to carious lesion excision has now been replaced by the rise of minimal invasive dentistry (MID), which aims to preserve good tooth structure utilizing noninvasive procedures. Silver Diamine Fluoride (SDF) had attracted increased contemporary attention due to its efficacy in arresting the progression of dental caries. In 2014, Food and Drug Administration (FDA) approved a commercially available SDF product as a Class II medical device to treat dentin hypersensitivity and later in 2016, the US FDA declared SDF as 'Breakthrough therapy' to arrest dental caries. Caries arresting treatment using SDF can be provided at professional and community levels on regular intervals.

Various organizations recommend the use of Silver Diamine Fluoride (SDF), through their guidelines. AAPD Guidelines (2017), ADA Guidelines (2016), IAPD Guidelines (2020).

History:

- 1891—Stebbins—silver nitrate—arresting caries lesions over 3 year period.
- Percy Howe—Boston, Forsyth University—added ammonia—to stabilize the Silver nitrate -Howe's solution
- 1969—first research on SDF—Osaka University Japan
- 1970—Western Australia School Dental Service—Silver fluoride application followed by Stannous Fluoride application
- 20th century—Japanese—Ohagura dye used in rituals—reduced caries incidence
- 2014—August—US FDA cleared SDF as Class II medical product to treat dentin hypersensitivity
- 2016—October—US FDA - 'Breakthrough Therapy'– to arrest dental caries

First research on SDF was conducted in 1969 at Osaka University in Japan. The powerful antimicrobial properties of silver with the benefits of a high dose of fluoride were combined and this formulation also resulted in a precipitate that occluded dentinal tubules and reduced the hypersensitivity. In due course "diammine silver fluoride" was granted approval as a cariostatic agent from the Central Pharmaceutical Council of the Ministry of Health and Welfare of Japan and marketed as Saforide (Toyo Seiyaku Kasei Co. Ltd., Osaka, Japan).

This compound, AgF (NH_3), is commonly misspelled or misinterpreted as silver diamine fluoride, however, the correct terminology is silver diammine fluoride as it contains two ammine groups (NH_3), not two amine groups (NH_2). The use of the term "diamine" became wide in use, and has become the accepted form both in the scientific and marketing literature.

Based on many studies all over the world, a concentration of 38% SDF was found to be superior at arresting caries compared to lower concentrations of 10% or 12%. SDF was superior at arresting dental caries and preventing new caries compared to fluoride varnish alone, interim therapeutic restorations (ITR) with fluoride-releasing glass ionomer cement (GIC) or other economical interventions such as chlorhexidine and oral hygiene instruction. However, when SDF was used as a fissure sealant for noncavitated molars, it did not perform better or equal to glass ionomers or resin sealants. Multiple applications of SDF were found to be better at arresting dental caries than one-time placement. There was no data on the optimal frequency and time interval between these applications, however, an application every 6–12 months is recommended.

Silver diamine fluoride gained clearance from the US FDA as a Class II medical device in August 2014. Similar to 5% sodium fluoride varnish, its approval for use to treat dentin hypersensitivity in adults aged 21 and older. Its capacity to block dentin tubules endorsed it to be classified as a medical device, rather than a drug. The FDA awarded SDF the designation of in October 2016, based on its arrest of dental decay in children and adults, a first for an oral health therapy.

Thus, SDF is identified as a drug "to treat a serious or life-threatening disease or condition" and affirms that the drug may demonstrate substantial improvement over existing therapies based on preliminary clinical evidence. The oral disease is also categorized as a serious medical condition for the first time and raised its importance as a substantial public health issue.

Composition of SDF

Silver Diamine Fluoride (SDF) is commonly used in the concentration of 38%. The most accepted composition is described here, but components may vary as per the brand and commercial product.

Silver	24–28%
Ammonia	7.5–11.0%
Fluoride	5–6 % (approx. 44,800 ppm)
Deionized water	<62.5%
Colouring	<1%

Mechanism of Action of SDF

Silver diamine fluoride is an exceptional caries-arresting agent due to the antibacterial properties of silver, the resulting precipitated barrier, and the high dose of fluoride delivered. The two main components, fluoride and silver, are made soluble in water by the addition of ammonia. While metallic silver is inert, silver ions are broad-spectrum antimicrobial with high biocompatibility and low toxicity in humans.

These ions act as tiny "silver bullets" that damage and degrade bacterial cell walls, disrupt bacterial DNA synthesis and replication, and disrupt intracellular metabolic activity, eventually leading to cell death. The slain bacteria further act as a carrier for silver ions and can kill living bacteria nearby in a process known as the "zombie effect."

The fluoride penetrates deeper into the tooth with SDF as compared with other fluoride solutions, creating a fluoride reservoir in the tooth structure. The fluoride component of SDF contributes to remineralization and fluorapatite formation, producing harder, more caries-resistant tooth structures. To date, this medicament has the highest concentration of fluoride ions available in the market. The 5% SDF solution contains 44,800 fluoride parts per million (ppm), almost twice that of 5% sodium fluoride varnish which contains 22,600 ppm. The 5% SDF reacts with calcium and phosphate ions to produce fluorohydroxyapatite crystals, which are less susceptible to solubility and essential to tooth remineralization. Despite the high concentration, the small amount required to be effective suggests that SDF is well within the margin of safety for use.

Once applied, a physical barrier precipitates out of the clear solution onto the carious lesion. Two resultant products, silver phosphate (Ag_3PO_4), which acts a reservoir of phosphate ions, and calcium fluoride (CaF_2), which acts as a pH-regulated fluoride supply during cariogenic challenge. It is hypothesized that silver fills the microtubules, further sealing the tooth from disease. Free silver ions in the lesion, demineralized crevices or craze lines are reduced by the environmental oxygen and turn the lesion black, which is the major side effect of this medicament. A study reported that parent acceptability of the black staining was low for anterior teeth (29.7%) but acceptance increased if the choice was between SDF application and treatment under general anesthesia (60.3%).

Indications

Case selection criteria: SDF has shown success in anti-caries therapy benefiting children of all age groups and adolescents.

- To arrest caries of the primary teeth in precooperative children who are unable to sit in the dental chair for longer treatment periods.
- As an interim treatment in cavitated lesion in children with special needs.
- Multiple cavitated lesions that are difficult to treat in one visit.
- To arrest caries in people who are unable to access dental treatment or tolerate conventional dental care such as people with intellectual/developmental disabilities
- Immunocompromised patients as these patients have a much higher risk of systemic infection arising from untreated dental caries.

Tooth selection criteria:

- No spontaneous pain
- No clinical signs of pulpal inflammation
- Cavitated lesions that do not invade the pulp. Radiographs may be taken to assess depth if necessary.
- Cavitated caries lesions on any surface that can be reached with a brush for the application of SDF as part of non-restorative caries control.

Contraindications

- Silver Diamine Fluoride (SDF) cannot be used in teeth with pulpitis or pulpal necrosis. It is not indicated in teeth with deep lesions where the carious dentin has been excavated, due to the ammonia content and high pH of SDF, which may create a pulpal reaction.
- The contraindications of SDF include individuals with a silver allergy, those with open oral lesions and teeth with irreversible pulpitis.
- SDF can irritate already sensitive oral lesions (e.g., herpetic gingivostomatitis, ulcerative gingivitis) and should be used with caution until the symptoms subside. Symptomatic treatment of the mucosa is advised.

Technique of Silver Diamine Fluoride Application (Figs. 46.9A to C)

- Protect the skin and lips with a protective covering (cocoa butter or vaseline) to prevent black discoloration of the lips and soft tissues.
- Use cotton rolls to isolate the regions to be treated.
- Apply a protective coating, such as cocoa butter, to the gingival tissues, being careful not to cover the surfaces of carious tooth lesions.
- Remove gross debris from the cavitated lesion to improve SDF contact with denatured dentin; carious dentin excavation is not required.
- One drop may be enough for 5 to 8 teeth. Microbrush application is advised.
- Dry lesion with gently compressed air flow
- Before applying, dip the brush, bend it, and dab it on the side of a plastic dappen dish to remove excess liquid, then apply for at least one minute.

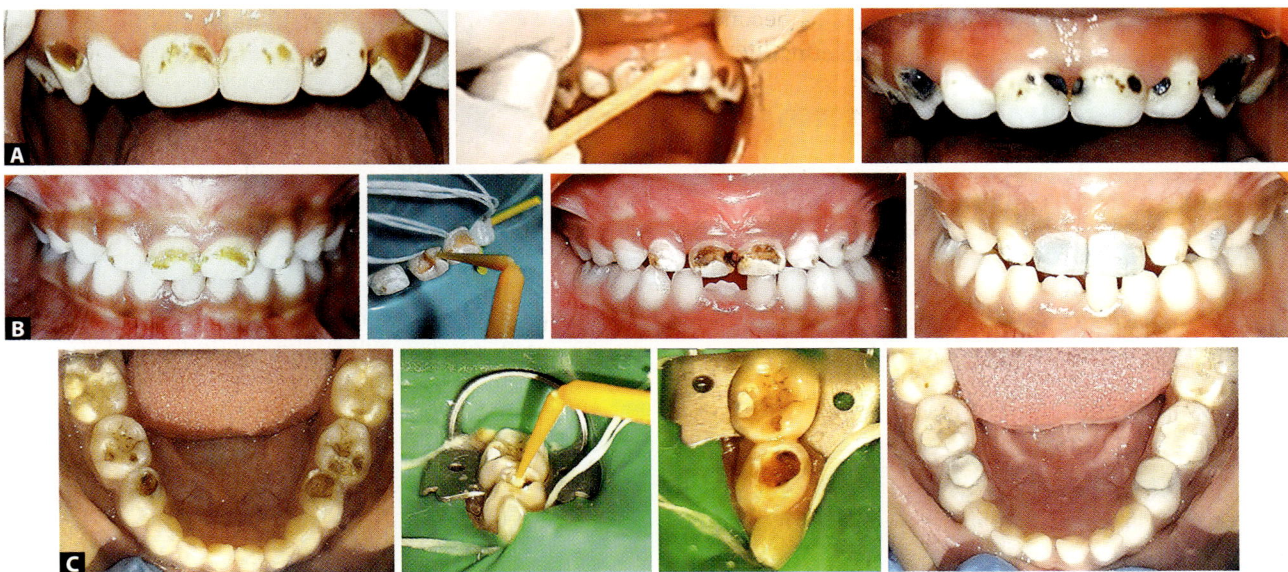

Figs. 46.9A to O: (A) SDF anterior case with carious teeth and SDF application; (B) SDF posterior case with SDF application and silver modified atraumatic restorative technique (SMART); (C) SDF anterior case with SMART.

- Use mild air to dry the medication. Isolate for at least 3 minutes.
- The entire dentition may be treated with 5% NAF varnish to help prevent caries on teeth and sites not treated with SDF.

Follow up period after SDF application:

- Follow up after two to four weeks recommended after every application
- Check for consistency of the applied lesions. Reapplication may be recommended in cases at recall visits based on activity and hardness of the caries lesion.
- Biannual application is recommended rather than a single application in non-restorative caries control therapy.
- For teeth with large carious lesions approximating the pulp, adjunctive restorative procedures (GIC or composite resins) to SDF should be considered to maximize its effectiveness, as it does not restore form and function. However, the silver particles that may extend into the dentin tubules could create some bonding problems for subsequent composite resin restorations placed over SDF-treated tooth structures. Placement of GIC over the SDF-treated lesion is termed as silver modified atraumatic restorative technique (SMART).

Superfloss technique of SDF for proximal lesions:

Interproximal lesions are challenging to control and arrest due to difficulty in access, limited salivary access and poor flossing compliance in children. SDF could be applied in such delveloping proximal lesions involving dentin or enamel using a superfloss and microbrush. To avoid the death spiral of restorations, incipient proximal lesions confined to enamel can also be benefitted by SDF.

Advantages of SDF

- SDF is a safe material.
- It has a simple chairside technique with less sensitive application procedure. A simple paint on technique for children is very useful.
- SDF is an efficient and effective material to arrest dental caries.
- The application of SDF is painless.
- SDF is noninvasive in nature.
- SDF is not expensive.
- It has minimal requirement for personnel time and training.
- It aids in preventing newer carious lesions.
- It provides a great alternative to procedures when time and cooperation in a child are a issue in the dental set up.
- It does not require local anesthesia administration.
- It has no risk of infection.
- It has a good safety margin as no case of toxicity reported. Silver allergy is very rare.

Disadvantages of SDF

- Black staining
  - The disadvantage of using SDF to stop caries is that the lesions will be stained black; as a result, some children and their parents may be dissatisfied with the aesthetics of this treatment outcome.
  - It has been proposed that when carious dentin is exposed to SDF, silver phosphate is produced, which is insoluble. Silver phosphate is yellow when originally created, but quickly turns black when exposed to light or reducing chemicals.
- Its application may sometimes give a metallic taste.
- It does not restore the form and/or function of decayed teeth.
- Gingival and mucosal inflammation
  - In most situations, the damage is temporary, and the afflicted tissue turns white, but it heals within 1–2 days.
- SDF can discolor the skin and clothes
  - The stain left by SDF on the skin, while not painful, cannot be wiped away and takes a long time to remove. If skin or clothes have been soiled, the following method to remove the stain: (a) If discoloration occurs quickly, rinse with running water, soap, or ammonia water. (b) If the discoloration persists, use a solution of sodium hypochlorite or a bleaching powder (with caution in dyed cloth).

Commercially Available Products of SDF and their Fluoride Concentrations (Figs. 46.9A to G)

- e-SDF 38%/44,800- 51,370 ppm F/Kids-e-dental Llp, Mumbai, India
- Cariclear 38%/44,800 ppm/Ammdent, Chandigarh, India
- Kedo SDF 38%/44,800 ppm Chennai, Tamil Nadu, India
- Saforide 38%/45,283 ppm F/Toyo Seiyaku Kasei, Osaka, Japan
- Advantage arrest/38.3–43.2% w/v,/ (expected 45,283 to 51,013 ppm F)/Elevate Oral Care, WestPalm Beach, FL, USA/Riva star 30–35%/(44,800 ppm)/SDI Dental Ltd, Australia
- Topamine 38%/(54,400 ppm F)/Dentalife Australia Pty. Ltd/ Ancárie12%/14,170 ppm/Maquira, Maringá,PR, Brazil
- Ancárie 30%/35,426 ppm F/Maquira, Maringá,PR,Brazil
- Cariestop 12%14,170 ppm F/Biodinâmica, Ibiporã, PR, Brazil
- Cariestop 30%/35,426 ppm F/Biodinâmica, Ibiporã, PR,Brazil/ Cariostatic 10%/Inondonlaboratorio, Brazil
- Fagamin 38%/44,800 ppm F/Tedequim SRL,Argentina
- Fluoroplat 38%/NaF laboratorio, Argentina

Advancements in SDF

- SDF with Potassium Iodide: After applying SDF to the tooth structure, the remaining free silver ions in solution would react with potassium iodide to precipitate creamy white silver iodide crystals. As a result, free silver ions are no longer available in the mouth to react with sulfur and other chemicals to produce black precipitates within the teeth.
- SDF is now being tested in gel form in advanced research.
- A new technique involving SDF application followed by light curing is being tested.

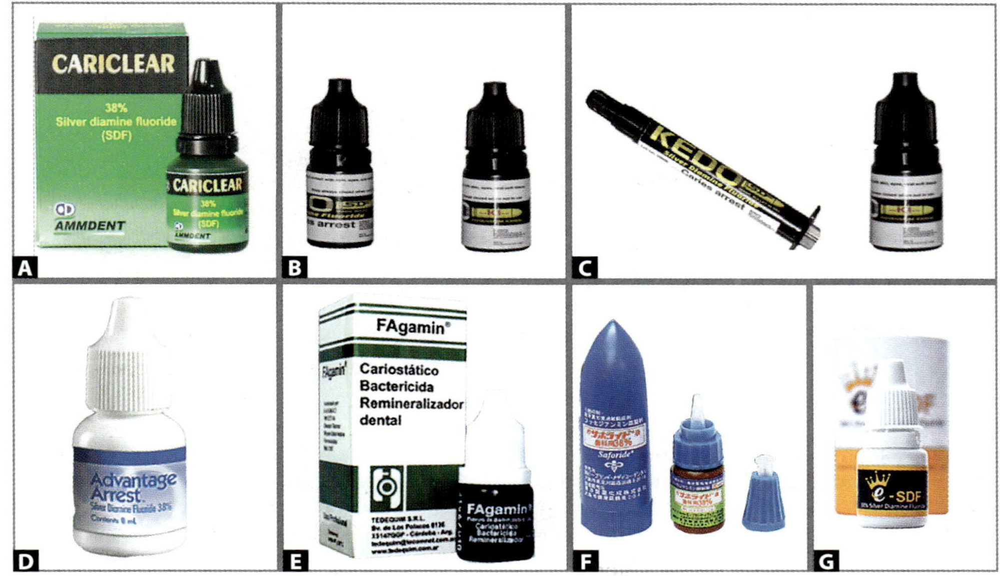

Figs. 46.9A to G: Commercially available SDF: (A) Carieclear SDF; (B) Kedo SDF (Liquid Form); (C) Kedo SDF (Gel Form); (D) Advantage Arrest; (E) FAgmin; (F) Saforide; (G) Kids-e- SDF.

POINTS TO REMEMBER

- Preservation of tooth structure and maintenance of occlusal relationships are essential in the design and construction of all restorations.
- Extension for prevention is no longer a valid concept, and focus is shifted to preservation with use of adhesive materials. Concept of minimal intervention was initiated by Knight and Hunt (1984), and the classification was proposed by Mount and Hume.
- Principles of minimal intervention include—control the disease through reduction of cryogenic flora; remineralize early lesions; perform minimal intervention surgical procedures, as required; repair, rather than replace, defective restorations. Tunnel cavity design is indicated if the cavity is small and if placed 2–2.5 mm below the marginal ridge. The aim is to develop an access via the occlusal aspect so as to preserve the strength of marginal ridge and also to prevent formation of proximal cavity.
- Slot cavity design is creation of a small slot on the proximal aspect of posterior teeth and is indicated if there is a small lesion involving the area of or below the marginal ridge only in deciduous teeth.
- Proximal cavity design approach is a conservative approach used when the proximal surface of a tooth becomes accessible at the time of cavity preparation in an adjacent tooth.
- The atraumatic restorative treatment (ART) is a procedure based on removing carious tooth tissues using hand instruments alone and restoring the cavity with an adhesive restorative material. Another terminology used for ART is alternate restorative treatment.
- Adapted by WHO on World Health Day, April 8, 1994.
- The distance from the operator's eye to patient's tooth is usually between 30 and 35 cm. The operator should be positioned behind the head of the patient.
- A patient lying on the back on a flat surface will provide safe and secure body support and comfortable and stable position for lengthy periods of time.
- The assistant works at the left side of a right-handed operator.
- Advantages of ART are inexpensive hand instruments, painless procedure, involves the removal of only decalcified tooth tissues, fluoride effect, less expensive, and less time-consuming.
- SMART has emerged as a paradigm shift in managing carious lesions especially when the generation of aerosols is undesirable.
- ART sealants in a valuable option in preventive care for un-cooperative children and individuals with special healthcare needs.
- First documented usage of silver compounds in dentistry was reported by Stebbins.
- In the mid-20th century, Yamaga and co-workers reported that low caries progression in "*Ohaguro*" communities was due to an active ingredient, SDF.
- First research on SDF was conducted in 1969 at Osaka University in Japan.
- Silver diammine fluoride as it contains two ammine groups (NH_3), not two amine groups (NH_2).
- Placement of GIC over the SDF-treated lesion is termed as silver modified atraumatic restorative technique (SMART).
- The US FDA declares SDF as 'Breakthrough Therapy' to arrest Dental Caries, in 2016.
- Silver diamine fluoride can be used in management of interproximal lesions—Superfloss technique
- Light curing—no influence on antimicrobial activity of SDF.

Questionnaire

1. Define, classify, and explain the concept of minimal intervention.
2. What is Mount and Hume's classification?
3. Explain the design of tunnel cavity preparation.
4. Write a note on slot cavity design.
5. What is proximal approach of cavity preparation?
6. Define ART and explain the working positions of operator.
7. What are the instruments and materials of ART?
8. Describe the procedure of ART.
9. Newer concepts in ART.
10. Discuss the use of SDF in Pediatric Dentistry.

FURTHER READING

1. American Academy of Pediatric Dentistry. Guideline on caries-risk assessment and management for infants, children, and adolescents. Pediatr Dent. 2013;35:E157-64.
2. Axelsson P. An introduction to risk prediction and preventive dentistry. Illinois: Quintessence Publishing Co Ltd; 1999. p. 7.
3. Banerjee A, Watson TF, Kidd EAM. Dentine caries excavation: review of current clinical techniques. British Dental Journal. 2000;188(9): 476-82.
4. Bansal M, Gupta C. Air Abrasion --An approach to minimal invasive dentistry. Guident. 2012;5(3):79-80.
5. Baum L, Phillips RW, Lund MR. Textbook of operative dentistry. Philadelphia: WB Saunders; 1981. pp. 295-8.
6. Bhatiya P, Thosa N. Minimal invasive dentistry --An emerging trend in pediatric dentistry: A review. Int J Contemp Dent Med Rev. 2015, Article ID: 320115, 2015. doi: 10.15713/ins.ijcdmr. 51.
7. Black CV. Operative Dentistry, volume 2, 5th edition. Chicago: Medico-Dental Publishing Co.; 1922. pp. 262-3.
8. Black GV. A work on operative dentistry: the technical procedures in filling teeth. Chicago, IL: Medico-Dental Publishing Company; 1917.
9. Burgess JO, Vaghela PM. Silver diamine fluoride: a successful anticarious solution with limits. Adv Dent Res. 2018;29:131-4.
10. Coluzzi DJ. Fundamentals of dental lasers: science and instruments. Dental Clinics of North America. 2004;48(4):751-70.
11. Crystal YO, Marghalani AA, Ureles SD, et al. Use of silver diamine fluoride for dental caries management in children and adolescents, including those with special health care needs. Pediatr Dent. 2017;39(5):E135-45.
12. Curzon MEJ, Roberts JF, Kennedy DB. Kennedy's Paediatric Operative Dentistry, 4th edition; Wright, Oxford, 1996. pp. 32-3.
13. Frencken JE, Peters MC, Manton DJ, Leal SC, Gordan VV, Eden E. Minimal intervention dentistry for managing dental caries --A review: Report of a FDI task group. Int Dent J. 2012;62:223-43.
14. Frencken JE. The state-of-the-art of ART sealants. Dental update. 2014;41(2):119-24.
15. Ganesh M, Parikh D. Chemomechanical caries removal (CMCR) agents: Review and clinical application in primary teeth. Journal of Dentistry and Oral Hygiene. 2011;3(3):34-45.
16. Gao SS, Zhao IS, Duffin S, et al. Revitalising silver nitrate for caries management. Int J Environ Res Public Health. 2018;15(1):E80.
17. Gupta M, Abhishek. Ozone: An Emerging Prospect in Dentistry. Indian Journal of Dental Sciences. 2012;1(4):47-50.
18. Haiat A, Ngo HC, Samaranayake LP, Fakhruddin KS. The effect of the combined use of silver diamine fluoride and potassium iodide in disrupting the plaque biofilm microbiome and alleviating tooth discoloration: A systematic review. PLoS ONE. 2021;16(6):e0252734.
19. Hasselrot L. Tunnel restorations in permanent teeth. A 7-year follow-up. Swed Dent J. 1998;22:1-7.
20. Hegde VS, Khatavkar RA. A new dimension to conservative dentistry: Air abrasion. Journal of Conservative Dentistry. 2010;13(1):4-8.
21. Horst JA, Ellenikiotis H, Milgrom PL. UCSF protocol for caries arrest using silver diamine fluoride: rationale, indications and consent. J Calif Dent Assoc. 2016;44(1):16-28.
22. http:// SMART BURS/procedure-without-la-cutting-that-is.html
23. http://www.dentaid.org/data/dentaid/downloads/ART_Manual_English.
24. http://www.dentistrytoday.com/restorative/minimally-invasive-dentistry/1492
25. Hunt PR. A modified Class II cavity preparation for glassionomer restorative materials. Quintessence Int. 1984;15:1011-8.
26. Innes NP, Evans DJ, Stirrups DR. The hall technique; a randomized controlled clinical trial of a novel method of managing carious primary molars in general dental practice: Acceptability of the technique and outcomes at 23 months. BMC Oral Health. 2007;7:18.
27. Jayesh R, Ramakrishan D. Minimal-Invasive Methods of Cavity Preparation. European J of Molecular and Clinical Medicine. 2020;7(3):2068-78.
28. Josgrilberg EB, Guimarães MS, Pansani CA, Cordeiro RCL. Influence of the power level of an ultra-sonic system on dental cavity preparation. Brazilian Oral Research 2007;21(4):362-7.
29. Knight GM. The use of adhesive materials in the conservative restoration of selected posterior teeth. Aust Dent J. 1984;29:324-31.
30. Kotlow LA. Lasers in pediatric dentistry. Dental Clinics of North America. 2004;48(4):889-922.
31. Makkar S, Makkar M. Ozone --Treating Dental Infections. Indian Journal of Somatology. 2011;2(4):256-59.
32. Modasia R, Modasia D. Application of silver diamine fluoride as part of the Atraumatic Restorative Technique. BDJ Student. 2021;28(2): 42-3.
33. Mount GJ, Hume WR. A revised classification of carious lesions by site and size. Quintessence Int. 1997;28:301-3.
34. Mount GJ, Hume WR. Preservation and restoration of tooth structure, Chapter 11. London: Mosby International; 1998. p. 129.
35. Mount GJ, Ngo H. Minimal intervention: a new concept for operative dentistry. Quintessence Int. 2000;31:527-33.
36. Mount GJ. Longevity in glass-ionomer restorations: review of a successful technique. Quintessence Int. 1997;28:643-50.
37. Nairn HF Wilson. Minimally Invasive Dentistry --The Management of Caries. 1st edition. Quintessence Pub Co; 2007.
38. Schwarz I. The Vector System: an Ultrasonic Device for Periodontal Treatment. Periodontology. 2004;1(2):181-5.
39. Seifo N, Cassie H, RadfordJR, Innes NPT. Silver diamine fluoride for managing carious lesions: an umbrella review. BMC Oral Health. 2019;19(1):145.
40. Silva NFRA, Carvalho RM, Pegoraro LF, Tay FR, Thompson VP. Evaluation of Self-limiting Concept in Dentinal Caries Removal. Journal of Dental Research 2006;85(3):282-6.
41. Smales RJ, Yip HK. The atraumatic restorative treatment (ART) approach for primary teeth: review of literature. Pediatr Dent. 2000;22(4):294-8.
42. Smales RJ, Yip HK. The atraumatic restorative treatment (ART) approach for the management dental caries. Quintessence Int. 2002;33(6):407-32.
43. Smitha T, Chaitanya Babu N. Plasma in dentistry: an update. Indian Journal of Dental Advancement. 2010;2(2):132-5.
44. Taft J. A Practical Treatise on Operative Dentistry, 4th edition. London: T Ruber; 1883. pp. 118-23.
45. Tascón J. Atraumatic restorative treatment to control dental caries: history, characteristics, and contributions of the technique. Rev Panam Salud Publica. 2005;17(2):110-5.
46. Trask PA. Silver diamine fluoride: it's about time! J Calif Dent Assoc. 2016;44(3):151.
47. Vanderlei AD, Borges AL, Cavalcant BN, Rode SM. Ultrasonic versus high-speed cavity preparation: Analysis of increases in pulpal temperature and time to complete preparation. Journal of Prosthetic Dentistry. 2008;100(2):107-10.
48. Yildirim M, Seymen F, Keklikoglu N. The Evaluation of the Vector System in Removal of Carious Tissue. International Journal of Dentistry. 2010:1-6.
49. Zaeneldin A, Yu OY, Chu CH. Effect of silver diamine fluoride on vital dental pulp: A systematic review. J Dent. 2022;119:104066.

CHAPTER

Remineralization in Pediatric Dentistry

Shradha Jain, Yash Shah, Megha Gupta

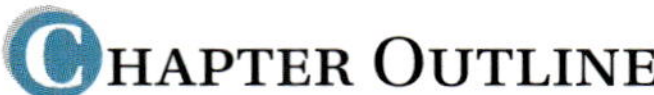

CHAPTER OUTLINE

- Concept of Remineralization and Demineralization
- Fluoride Remineralizing Agents
- Alpha Tricalcium Phosphate
- Amorphous Calcium Phosphate
- Casein Phosphopeptide–Amorphous Calcium Phosphate
- Dicalcium Phosphate Dihydrate
- Bioactive Glass
- Nanoparticles for Remineralization
- Other Remineralizing Agents
- Resin Infiltration
- Microabrasion Remineralization Technique

The goal of modern dentistry is to manage non-cavitated caries lesions non-invasively through remineralization in an attempt to prevent disease progression and improve aesthetics, strength, and function. It is a natural repair mechanism to restore the minerals again, in ionic forms, to the hydroxyapatite (HAP) crystal lattice.

Numerous types of remineralizing agents and remineralizing techniques have been researched and are being used clinically, with significantly predictable positive results. The recent researches on remineralization are based on biomimetic remineralization materials, having the capability to create apatite crystals within the completely demineralized collagen fibers. A range of novel calcium-phosphate-based remineralization delivery systems have also been developed for clinical application. These delivery systems include crystalline, unstabilized amorphous, or stabilized amorphous formulations of calcium phosphate. Biomimetic approaches to stabilization of bioavailable calcium, phosphate, and fluoride ions and the localization of these ions to non-cavitated caries lesions for controlled remineralization show promise for the non-invasive management of dental caries.

Remineralization *is defined as the process whereby calcium and phosphate ions are supplied from a source external to the tooth to promote ion deposition into crystal voids in demineralized enamel, to produce net mineral gain.*

Demineralization *is the loss of calcified material from the structure of tooth. Demineralization process involves loss of minerals at the advancing front of the lesion, at a depth below the enamel surface, with the transport of acid ions from the plaque to the advancing front and mineral ions from advancing front towards plaque.*

CONCEPT OF REMINERALIZATION AND DEMINERALIZATION

Sound enamel is acellular tissue containing 80-90% by volume of carbonated calcium hydroxyapatite an inorganic material and remaining 10-20% of fluid and proteinaceous organic material . The parallel arrangement of enamel prisms forms an intercrystalline space which provides diffusion path for enamel caries. Acids produced by fermentation of carbohydrate enters enamel and reacts with the hydroxyapatite mineral, this reaction releases mineral ions in the solution resulting in demineralization and formation of subsurface lesion **(Fig. 47.1)**.

$$Ca_{10}(PO_4)\ 6\ (OH)_2 + 14\ H^+ \rightarrow 10\ Ca^+ + 6\ H_2\ PO_4^- + H_2\ O$$

Dissolution of mineral in the acidic solution is due to:

- The hydrogen ions remove hydroxyl ions to form water, as follows: $H^+ + OH^- = H_2O$. Therefore, as the [H+] increases in an acid solution, the [OH–] must decrease in a reciprocal manner.
- Lower the pH, the lower the concentration of PO_4^{3-}, the only species that contributes to the IAP of HA.
- Thus, as any solution is acidified, the calcium concentration is unaffected but the concentrations of both OH– and PO_4^{3-}

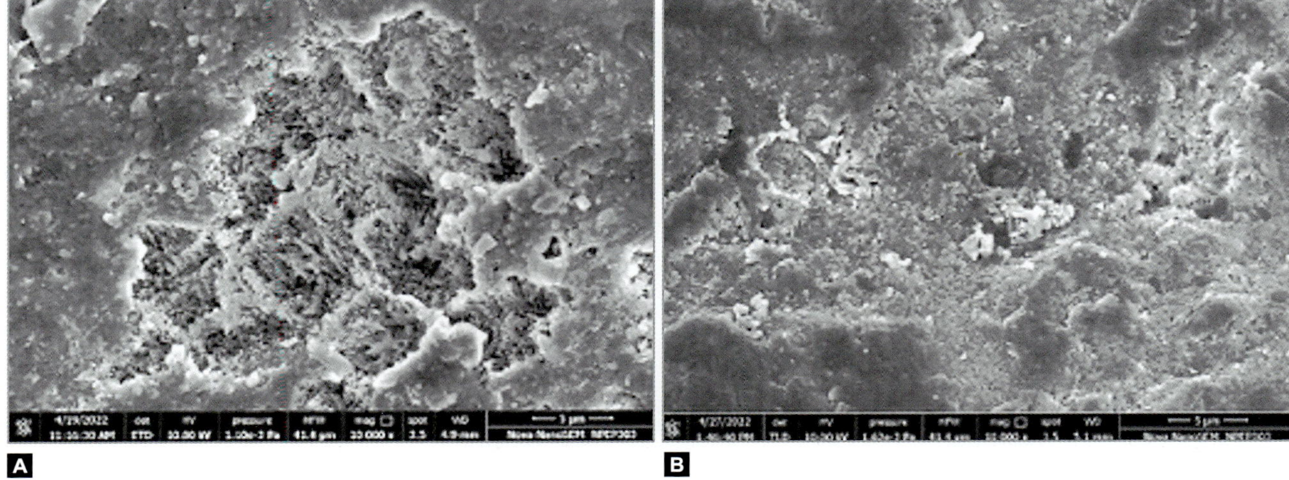

Figs. 47.1A and B: Concept of remineralization and demineralization: (A) Remineralization; (B) Demineralization.

are reduced and so, therefore, is the IAP, often to a value less than the Ksp.

$$IAP = (Ca^{2+})_{10}(PO_4^{3-})_6(OH^-)_2$$

$$(Ca^{2+})_{10}(PO_4^{3-})_6(OH^-)_2 < Ksp \text{ (tooth mineral)} = \text{Demineralization}$$

$$(Ca^{2+})_{10}(PO_4^{3-})_6(OH^-)_2 > Ksp \text{ (tooth mineral)} = \text{Remineralization}$$

- Increase in calcium and phosphate in oral fluid drives remineralization of subsurface lesion.

Degree of saturation

Ratio of ionic product of a substance in the solution (IAP) to its ionic product at saturation (Ksp)

DS = [IAP (ionic activity product in solution)\Ksp (ionic activity product at saturation)]1/9

Ksp = Concentration of ions to the power in saturated solution

It is a constant value Ksp (carbonated -HAP) = 4.57×10^{-49}

IAP = ion concentration in solution

DS = 1 saturation condition (IAP = Ksp)

DS<1 solution undersaturated with respect to mineral (IAP < Ksp) → Demineralization

DS>1 solution supersaturated with respect to mineral (IAP > Ksp) → Remineralization

Critical pH[1]

- It is the pH at which a solution is just saturated with respect to a particular mineral.

If solution pH > critical pH= supersaturation = mineral precipitate

If solution pH < critical pH = undersaturated = mineral dissolve

$$\text{Precipitation} \rightleftarrows \text{Dissolution}$$

$$Ca_{10}(PO_4)_6(OH)_2 \rightleftarrows 10Ca^{2+} + 6PO_4^{3-} + 2OH^-$$

$$\text{Solid} \rightleftarrows \text{Solution}$$

Pathophysiology of Remineralization[2]

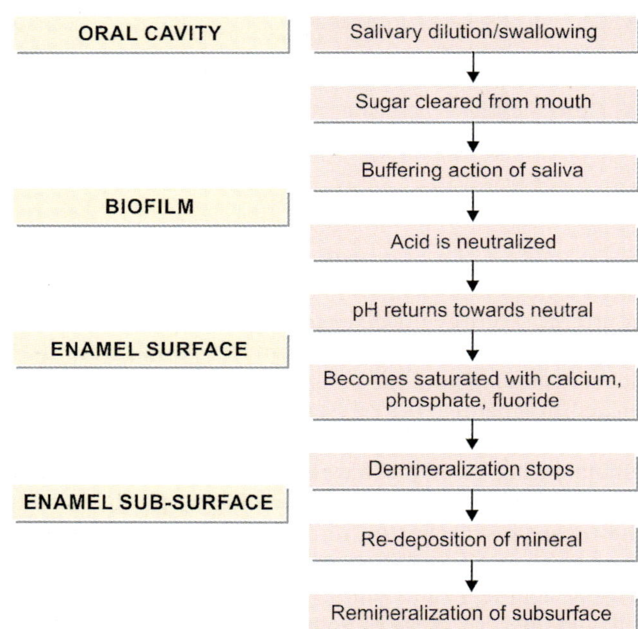

Susceptibility of primary Enamel to demineralization and remineralization: Some factors makes primary teeth more susceptible to caries when they erupt as mentioned below:[3]

- Enamel of primary teeth is thinner (1.1–2.6 mm), more permeable, softer and easily worn compared to permanent teeth.
- Density of enamel decreases towards dentino-enamel junction resulting in increase in porosity, fluid and organic material away from surface.
- Enamel crystals are larger with smaller or no prisms in enamel, which are non-homogenously arranged.
- Carbonate content is higher in primary teeth, so the solubility of enamel is greater.
- Primary enamel is deficient in phosphate.

- Fluoride concentration in outer layer is lower than permanent teeth.

Remineralizing Agents

Previously most recommended treatment approach was periodic application of fluoride and varnish but current approach to halt the progress of demineralization is by application of remineralizing agents. It is most preferred non-invasive method over operative procedures. Arrest of incipient lesion at early stage, results in reprecipitation of mineral back to demineralized subsurface to remineralize. Clinically remineralization of enamel can be evaluated by enamel hardness and shine. In terms of evaluation shallow enamel lesions represent full enamel recovery and arrested lesion represent negligible remineralization. Treatment of proximal incipient caries is fluoride therapy, but if caries advances further restorative treatment has to be done. So, management of proximal incipient lesion lies between preventive and invasive treatment options.[4]

Ideal requirements of a remineralizing agent

1. Should deliver calcium and phosphate into the subsurface
2. Should not deliver any excess of calcium
3. Should not favor calculus formation
4. Should work at an acidic pH so as to stop demineralization during a carious attack
5. Works in xerostomia patients
6. Boosts remineralizing properties of saliva
7. For novel materials, shows a benefit over fluoride.

Indications of remineralization[5]

1. An adjunct preventive therapy to reduce caries in high-risk patients
2. Reduce dental erosion in patients with gastric reflux or other disorders
3. To reduce decalcification in orthodontic patients
4. To repair enamel in cases involving white-spot lesions
5. Orthodontic decalcification or fluorosis or before and after teeth whitening and to desensitize sensitive teeth.

Classification of remineralizing agents[6]

1. Fluorides
2. Non-fluoride remineralizing agents
   - Calcium phosphate based agents
     - Alpha tricalcium phosphate (TCP) and beta TCP (β-TCP)
     - Amorphous calcium phosphate
     - CPP–ACP
     - Dicalcium phosphate dihydrate (DCPD)
   - Bioactive glass (sodium calcium phosphosilicate)
   - Nanoparticles for remineralization
     - Calcium fluoride nanoparticles
     - Calcium phosphate-based nanomaterials
     - Nano HAP particles
     - ACP nanoparticles
     - Nano-bioactive glass materials
   - Miscellaneous
     - Grape seed extract
     - Xylitol
     - Arginine
     - Theobromine
     - Polydopamine
     - PA
     - Self-assembling peptides
     - Electric field-induced remineralization

FLUORIDE BASED REMINERALIZING AGENTS

Topical and systemic fluoride administration post eruption has ability to reduce incidence of caries. Professionally applied agents such as varnish, gels, fluoride releasing restorative materials and personally applied agents like dentifrices and mouth rinse help in this type of remineralization.

Sodium fluoride	*Directly provides free fluoride*
Sodium monofluorophosphate	Fluoride of choice when calcium containing abrasives are used. The fluoride released is absorbed to the mineral surface, as a CaF_2 or a CaF_2-like deposit, in free or bound form.
Stannous fluoride	Provides fluoride and stannous ions where the latter act as an antimicrobial agent

Mechanism of remineralization:

- Highly electronegative fluoride ion retains on dental hard tissue, the oral mucosa and in the dental plaque to decrease demineralization and enhance remineralization.
- Adsorbed fluoride ion on dental mineral attracts calcium ion, which then attract phosphate ions, this results in formation of fluorapatite crystal, which is less soluble than carbonated hydroxyapatite mineral. Fluorapatite prevents diffusion of acid and prevents enamel dissolution.[7]
- Fluoride speeds up remineralization by growth of new fluorapatite **(Figs. 47.2A and B)**.
- It inhibits activity of acid producing carious bacteria, by interfering in glycolytic pathway.

Studies regarding remineralization with fluoride[8]

- **Fowler et al.** found that toothpaste formulations containing 1426 ppm F as sodium fluoride or 1400 ppm F as amine fluoride gave a significant protection of enamel from erosive acid challenges in vitro compared to 0 ppm F placebo toothpaste.
- According to **Pradubboon et al.**, 0.05 NaF mouth rinse combined with twice-daily regular use of fluoride toothpaste, when used twice daily, effectively enhances the remineralization of incipient caries.
- An in vivo study by **Mehta et al.** using a single application of a light curable fluoride varnish (Clinpro T) has proven its effectiveness in preventing demineralization.
- Uptake of calcium can be enhanced with the use of titanium fluoride (TiF).
- Fluoride varnish is superior to chlorhexidine.

Non-fluoridated Remineralizing Agents

Ability of fluoride to speed up remineralization is dependent on availability of calcium and phosphate ions thus limiting remineralization to their availability. Fluoride is least effective in pit fissure caries than smooth surface caries and excess of fluoride leads to dental as well as skeletal fluorosis. These limitations have prompted to search for safer alternative for remineralization, shifting towards non-fluoridated agents.

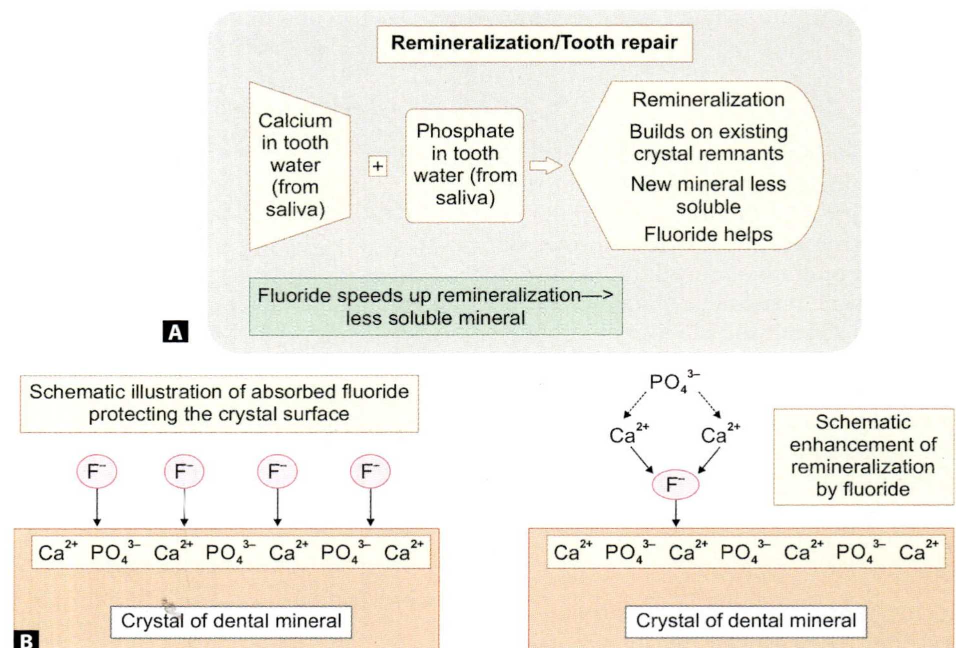

Figs. 47.2A and B: (A) Schematic illustration of fluoride ions protecting surface; (B) Schematic illustration of remineralization by fluoride ions.

Calcium Phosphate Compounds

- Calcium phosphate is the principal form of calcium found in bovine milk and blood. It is a major component of hydroxyapatite (HA) crystals. Concentrations of calcium and phosphate in saliva and plaque play a key role in tooth demineralization and remineralization processes.
- The plaque fluid contains Ca/P ratio approximately 0.3 and enamel remineralization can be obtained with a calcium/phosphate ratio of 1.6, so additional calcium supply will enhance enamel remineralization.

Tricalcium Phosphate (TCP)

- It has the chemical formula $Ca_3(PO_4)_2$, and exists in two forms, alpha and beta.
- Alpha TCP is formed when human enamel is heated to high temperatures. It is a relatively insoluble material in aqueous environments.
- Crystalline beta TCP can be formed by combining calcium carbonate and calcium hydrogen phosphate, and heating the mixture to over 100°C for 1 day, to give a flaky, stiff powder.
- Beta TCP is less soluble than alpha TCP, and thus in an unmodified form is less likely to provide bioavailable calcium. It is used in products such Cerasorb®, Bio-Resorb® and Biovision®.
- Higher amount of calcium and fluoride forms calcium fluoride during storage, which renders the fluoride less effective in preventing tooth decay. TCP can protect unwanted interactions with fluoride. This protected calcium additive works with fluoride to initiate high-quality mineral growth thus acting as a catalyst to enhance remineralization and build a high-quality, acid-resistant mineral.
- *Mechanism of remineralization:* The structure of TCP is similar to hydroxyapatite, once the functionalized calcium ions are released, they readily interact with the tooth surface and subsurface. It possesses unique calcium environments capable of reacting with fluoride and enamel. While the phosphate floats free, these exposed calcium environments are protected, preventing the calcium from prematurely interacting with fluoride's finally comes into contact with the tooth surface and gets moistened by saliva, the protective barrier breaks down, making the calcium, phosphate and fluoride ions available to the teeth. The fluoride and calcium then react with weakened enamel to provide a seed for enhanced mineral growth relative to fluoride alone **(Fig. 47.3)**.
- *Clinical applications*: TCP provides catalytic amounts of calcium to boost fluoride efficacy and may be well designed to coexist with fluoride in a mouth rinse or dentifrice because it will not react before reaching the tooth surface.
  - 3M™ ESPE™ Clinpro™ 5000 (1.1% Sodium Fluoride) Anti-Cavity Toothpaste with TCP provided superior protection against lesion initiation and progression[9] **(Fig. 47.4A)**.
  - 5% Sodium White Varnish, can help decrease hypersensitivity by depositing high-quality, acid-resistant mineral that occludes exposed dentinal tubules **(Fig. 47.4B)**.
  - 3M™ ESPE™ Clinpro™ 5000 toothpaste reduced the average lesion depth by more than 10%, demonstrating remineralization was occurring deep in the lesion with the most severe damage and thus provides superior remineralization at both the enamel surface and deep within the lesion.

Functionalized tricalcium phosphate

"Smart" calcium phosphate system is a new hybrid material created with a milling technique that fuses beta tricalcium phosphate (ß-TCP) and sodium lauryl sulfate or fumaric acid. This blending results in "functionalized" calcium and a "free" phosphate, designed to increase the efficacy of fluoride remineralization.

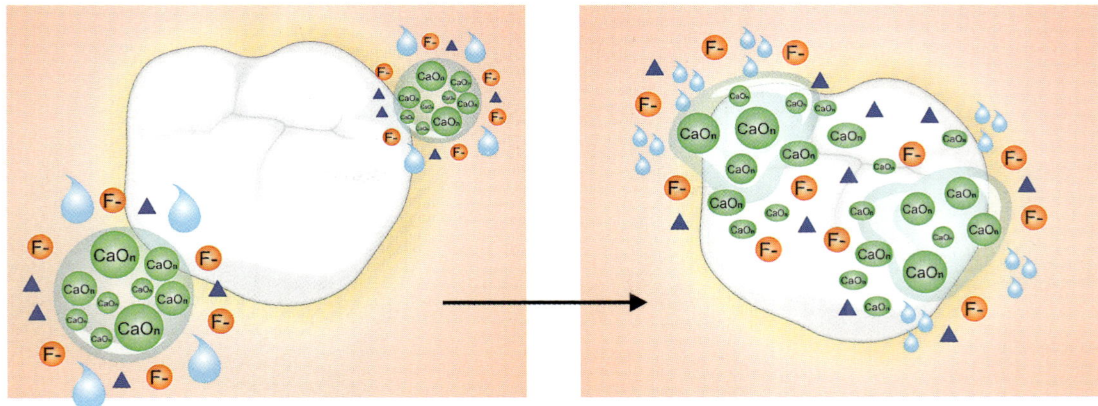

Fig. 47.3: Mechanism of remineralization by TCP.

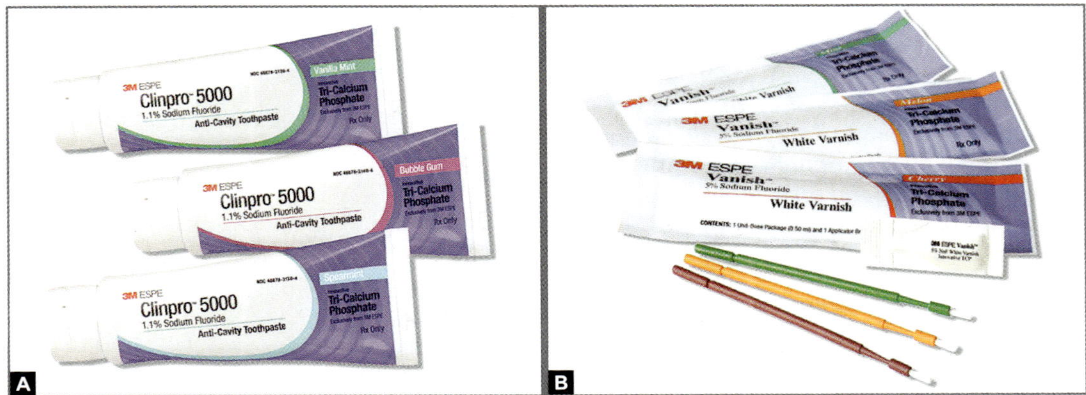

Figs. 47.4A and B: TCP containing formulations: (A) Clinpro™ 5000. 1.1% sodium fluoride anti-cavity toothpaste; (B) Vanish™. 5% sodium fluoride white varnish with TCP.

Amorphous Calcium Phosphate (ACP)

- ACP was first described by **Aaron S Posner** in the mid 1960s and its technology was developed by **Dr Ming S Tung.**[10]
- In 1999, ACP was incorporated into toothpaste called Enamelon and later reintroduced in 2004 as Enamel Care toothpaste.
- *Properties of ACP*:
  - Non-crystalline ACP highly reacts with body fluid, resulting fast apatite reprecipitation.
  - Better osteoconductivity than hydroxyapatite (HAP).
  - Better biodegradability than tricalcium phosphate.
  - Good bioactivity but no cytotoxicity.
  - High solubility under oral conditions.
  - Ability to rapidly hydrolyze to form apatite
- *Mechanism of remineralization*: The ACP technology requires a two-phase delivery system to keep the calcium and phosphorous components from reacting with each other before use. The current sources of calcium and phosphorous are two salts, calcium sulfate and dipotassium phosphate. When the two salts are mixed, they rapidly form ACP or, in the presence of fluoride ions, amorphous calcium fluoride phosphate (ACFP) that can precipitate on to the tooth surface. This precipitated ACP can then readily dissolve into the saliva and can be available for tooth remineralization. These phases (ACP and ACFP) are potentially very unstable and may rapidly transform into a more thermodynamically stable, crystalline phase such as hydroxyapatite and fluorhydroxyapatite; thus, it has lower substantivity.[11]
- *Clinical applications:* Enamelon consists of unstabilized calcium and phosphate salts with sodium fluoride. The calcium salts are separated from the phosphate salts and sodium fluoride by a plastic divider in the centre of the toothpaste tube **(Fig. 47.5A)**. Enamelon™ is that calcium and phosphate are not stabilized, allowing the two ions to combine into insoluble precipitates before they come into contact with saliva or enamel.[12]
- ACP-containing material, NiteWhite™ claims to "rebuild tooth enamel **(Fig. 47.5 B)**. However there is no published evidence in the current dental literature to support claims of subsurface remineralization or reversal of white spot lesions.

Dicalcium Phosphate Dihydrate (DCPD)

- Dicalcium phosphate dihydrate is a calcium phosphate with high solubility that can deliver bioavailable calcium and phosphate.
- *Mechanism of remineralization:* DCPD dissolves in saliva and releases calcium ions, increase in calcium ion

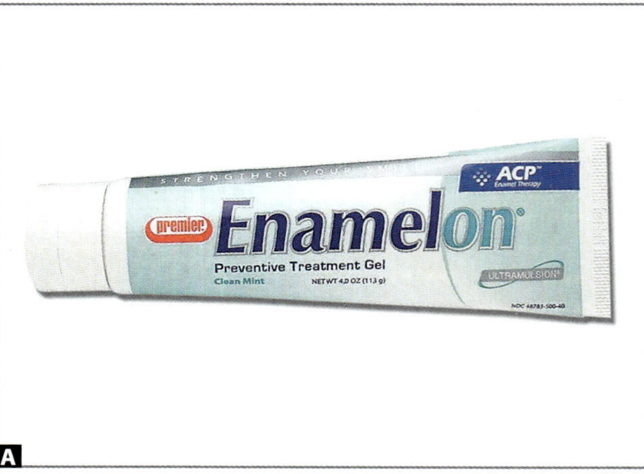

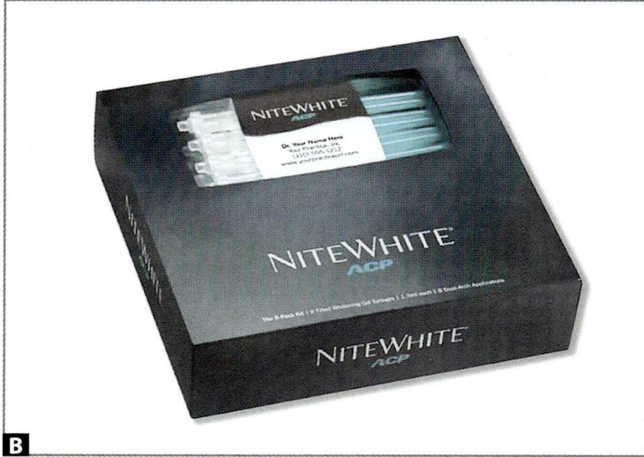

Figs. 47.5A and B: ACP containing formulations.

concentration promotes remineralization. These calcium ion acts as carrier of fluoride toward tooth surface and forms Fluoroapatite, replenishing lost mineral.

- Inclusion of DCPD in a dentifrice increases the levels of free calcium ions in plaque fluid, and these remain elevated for up to 12h after brushing, when compared to conventional silica dentifrices. Also, there is enhanced calcium incorporation into enamel from DCPD and increased levels are detected in plaque up to 18 h.[13,14]

Casein Phosphopeptide–Amorphous Calcium Phosphate (CPP-ACP)

- **Eric Reynolds** and coworkers at the University of Melbourne Australia developed this technology.
- The casein phosphopeptides (CPP) are produced from a tryptic digest of the milk protein casein, then aggregated with calcium phosphate and purified by ultrafiltration.
- CPP consisting of multiple phosphoseryl residues, which provide stability to, calcium and phosphate ions and forms CPP stabilized CPP-ACP complex in both acidic and basic pH and in presence of fluoride forming CCP-ACPF complex **(Fig. 47.6)**[15] (**Adamson and Reynolds**, 1996).
- *Properties of CPP*[15]
  - CPP is a peptide, which contains elements that can bind calcium.
  - Casein phosphopeptide can stabilize calcium phosphate present in the solution as amorphous calcium phosphate and help the ACP to bind with the dental enamel.
  - The ability of casein phosphopeptide to integrate in the pellicle decrease the count of *S. mutans*.
  - CPP–ACP has role in reversal of the early white spot lesion.
- *Mechanism of remineralization*: Calcium phosphate is normally insoluble and forms a crystalline structure at neutral pH. However, the CPP keeps the calcium and phosphate in an amorphous, non-crystalline state. In this amorphous state, calcium and phosphate ions can enter the tooth enamel. CPP-ACP and CPP-ACFP complexes provide bioavailable calcium and phosphate ions at the tooth surface, thus inhibiting demineralization and favoring remineralization **(Fig. 47.7)**.[16]

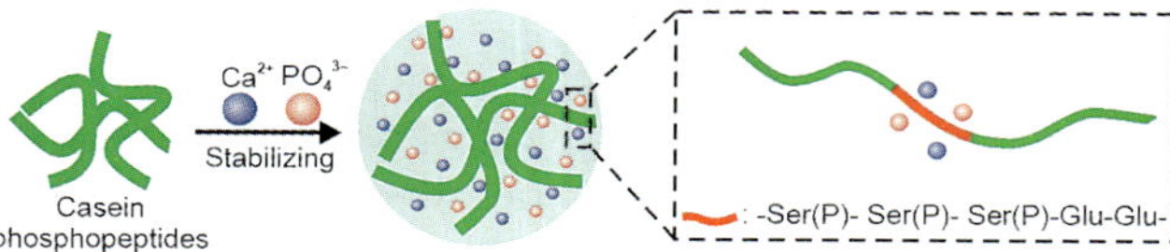

Fig. 47.6: CPP-ACP complex.

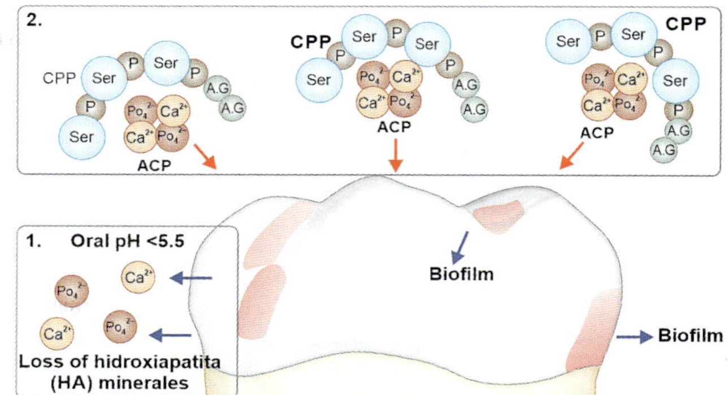

Fig. 47.7: CPP-ACP remineralization: 1. Oral pH <5.5 induces loss of hydroxyapatite (HA) minerals. 2. Saturation of the oral environment and biofilm with Ca^{2+} and PO_4^{3-} ions, promoting the dental remineralization process.

- *Indications of CPP-ACP*[17]
  - Tooth Mousse is a safe product to use especially in young children under 2 years of age with early childhood caries.
  - Used for patients with special needs.
  - Used for high caries-risk patients in an attempt to remineralize early enamel lesions.
  - Used in cases of molar incisor hypomineralization (MIH) for remineralizing hypoplastic molars and white spot lesions.
  - Used in cases of erosion whereby it neutralizes acid challenges from internal and external acid sources.
  - Used in patients with orthodontic appliances for the purpose of caries prevention and prevention/remineralization of white spot lesions.
  - Used to reduce dentinal sensitivity
  - Used as a substitute for toothpaste in those allergic to commercial toothpastes.

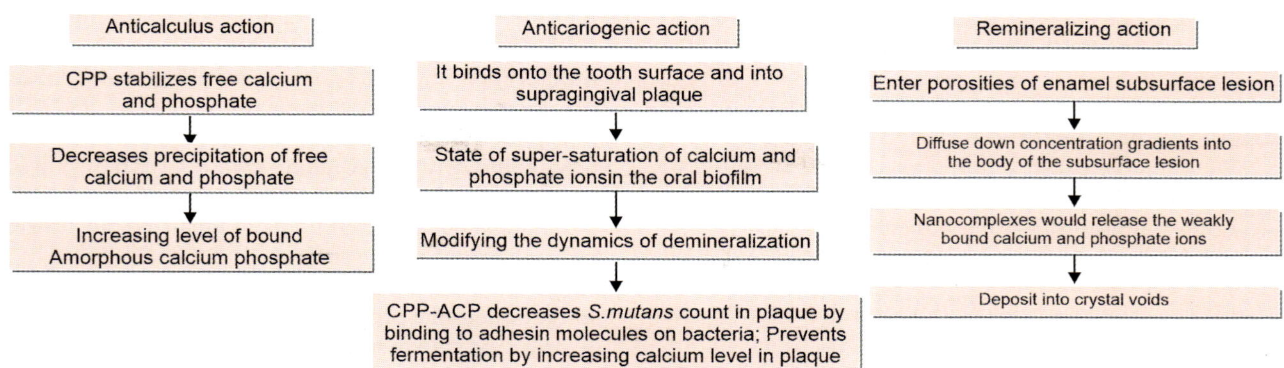
CPP-ACP
Anticalculus action
CPP stabilizes free calcium and phosphate
Decreases precipitation of free calcium and phosphate
Increasing level of bound Amorphous calcium phosphate
Anticariogenic action
It binds onto the tooth surface and into supragingival plaque
State of super-saturation of calcium and phosphate ionsin the oral biofilm
Modifying the dynamics of demineralization
CPP-ACP decreases S.mutans count in plaque by binding to adhesin molecules on bacteria; Prevents fermentation by increasing calcium level in plaque
Remineralizing action
Enter porosities of enamel subsurface lesion
Diffuse down concentration gradients into the body of the subsurface lesion
Nanocomplexes would release the weakly bound calcium and phosphate ions
Deposit into crystal voids

Table 47.1: Dental products containing CPP-ACP, ACP, CPP-ACPF.

Active ingredients	*Trademark (manufacturer)*	*Commercial presentation*
CPP-ACP	MI Paste™ (GC)/Tooth Mousse™ (GC)	Topical paste
CPP-ACP	Trident Xtra Care® (Adams)	Chewing gum
CPP-ACP	Trident Total® (Adams)	Chewing gum
CPP-ACP	FUJIVII™ EP (GC)	Glass ionomer cement
CPP-ACPF	MI Paste plus™ (GC)/Tooth Mousse plus™ (GC)	Topical paste
CPP-ACPF	MI Varnish™ (GC)	Varnish
ACP	NiteWhite™ (Phillips)	Tooth bleaching gel
ACP	DayWhite™ (Phillips)	Tooth bleaching gel
ACP	Aegis® Ortho (Bosworth Co)	Dental adhesive
ACP	Aegis® Pit and Fissure Sealant (Bosworth Co)	Pit and fissure sealant
ACP	Relief® ACP (Phillips)	Tooth desensitizing gel
ACP	Enamelon® (Premier)	Toothpaste

- *Contraindication*: CPP–ACP is a milk product, hence it cannot be given to patients having intolerance to milk.
- *Mode of delivery of CPP-ACP* **(Table 47.1)**
  - *Chewing gums:* Chewing of CPP-ACP sugar-free gum promotes prebiosis and oral homeostasis. CPP-ACP chewing gum produced increase in salivary buffer capacity when compared to xylitol-containing chewing gum.[18] The CPP–ACP chewing gum is marketed as GC Recaldent™ or Trident White™.

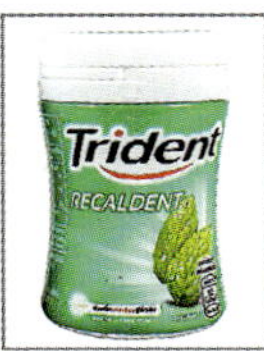
Trident
RECALDENT

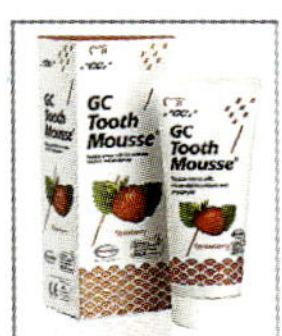
GC Tooth Mousse
GC Tooth Mousse

  - *Tooth crèmes:* Tooth mousse contains 10% w/v CPP-ACP. The release of ions at oral pH was approximately 95 % after 15 minutes (**Paterson et al.**, 2008). This rapid release means that when the crème is applied to tooth surfaces there will be a rapid increase in calcium ion concentration in the plaque fluid and saliva. Tooth Mousse protects enamel surface by providing resistance from acid, and recovery of surface microhardness after acid exposure (**Kargul et al.**[19] 2012). Tooth mousse plus with additional fluoride ion into CPP-ACP produce a novel amorphous calcium fluoride (CPP-ACPF). This phase is responsible for additive anticariogenic effect due to formation of fluoroapatite. CPP is able to stabilize amorphous calcium fluoride phosphate (CPP-ACFP), which allows additive effects on remineralization compared with the fluoride or CPP-ACP alone (**Cochrane et al.**[20] 2006). Tooth Mousse elevated plaque pH levels for the first 48 hours, but Tooth Mousse Plus elevated plaque pH until 96 hours (**Heshmat et al.**[21] 2013).

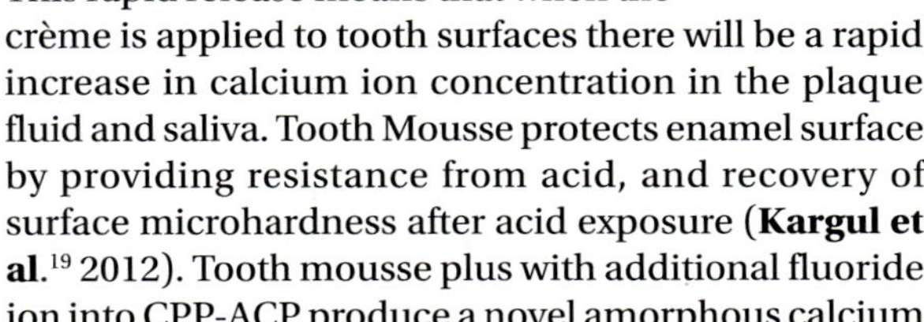

    - *Home application of Tooth crèmes:* It can be applied directly with clean finger onto the teeth, smeared over all surfaces, and left in place to slowly dissolve overnight. Any material that is swallowed is completely safe and will contribute toward dietary calcium.
    - *Professional application of Tooth crèmes:* Arrested white spot lesions should have a surface etching treatment before remineralization with Recaldent products. Such a treatment, either alone or combined with gentle pumicing, will remove approximately 30 microns of surface enamel, but will not cause further mineral loss from the subsurface zone of the white spot lesion.
  - *Mouth rinses:* The contents of calcium and inorganic phosphate in supragingival plaque increased after use

of the CPP-ACP mouthwash for a three-day clinical trial.

- *Lozenges:* Lozenges are also a suitable vehicle for to promote enamel remineralization through delivery of CPP-ACP.
- *Dentifrices:* The addition of 2% CPP–ACP to the 1100 ppm fluoride dentifrice showed superior enamel subsurface remineralization. According to **Kumar et al** application of CPP–ACP after the use of fluoride toothpaste is the most effective method for remineralization. So it is recommended that CPP-ACP should be used as a self-applied topical coating after the teeth have been brushed with a fluoridated toothpaste by children who have a high caries risk.[22]
- *Varnish:* MI varnish™ with RECALDENT consists of CPP-ACP and 5% NaF (22,600-ppm fluoride). The application leaves a film of varnish on tooth surfaces and remains on teeth for approximately four hours. It is indicated for hypersensitive teeth and on white-spot lesions in orthodontic patients. According to **Prabhakar et al.,**[23] (2019) the inclusion of CPPACP in MI varnish® (GC America Inc., Alsip, IL, USA) has been proven to inhibit enamel demineralization to a much greater extent than fluoride varnishes without CPPACP. High water solubility and relatively neutral conditions of the CPP–ACP complexes contribute to fast release of the ions from MI varnish.[24]

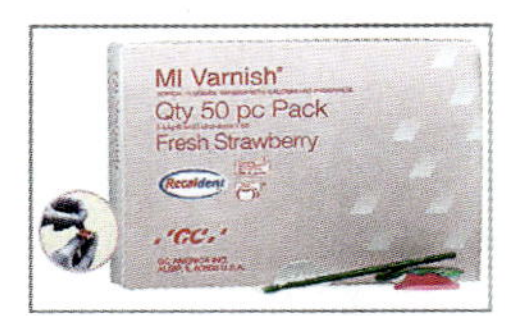

Research on CPP-ACP

- **Choi et al.**[25] concluded that the depth of penetration of the remineralizing ions (Ca & P) in CPP-ACP paste is related to the depth of demineralized enamel (approximately 1050~1350 μ). The Ca and P levels of remineralized enamels in higher than those of the sound enamels in 1, 2 weeks.
- **Reynolds et al.**[26] evaluated that CPP-ACP was superior to that achieved with other forms of calcium in remineralizing enamel subsurface lesions.
- **Rose et al.**[27] studied that CPP-ACP binds with about twice the affinity of the bacterial cells for calcium. Application of CPP-ACP to plaque may cause a transient rise in plaque fluid free calcium, which may assist remineralization.
- **Palaniswamy et al.**[24] conducted a study to evaluate remineralizing potential of bioactive glasses (BAGS) and amorphous calcium phosphate-casein phosphopeptide (ACP-CPP) on early enamel lesion and found that increase in the micro hardness was in 10 days with BAGS compared to 15 days in ACP-CPP group.
- **Munjal et al.** concluded that CPP-ACP therapy to be used minimum for 12 weeks is highly recommended as post-orthodontic treatment need in management of smooth surface white spot lesions on teeth undergoing fixed orthodontic therapy.

Bioactive Materials

- *A **bioactive material** is defined as a material that stimulates a beneficial response from the body, particularly bonding to host bone tissue and to the formation of a calcium phosphate layer on a material surface."*
- *Mechanism of action*: BG-45S5 is inorganic amorphous, calcium, sodium phospho-silicate material, which contains five-fold ratio of Ca/P. These ions interact in presence of saliva and precipitates calcium phosphate. In the presence of saliva releases sodium, in the oral fluids replacing hydrogen ion resulting in increase in pH. Increased alkalinity leads to the release of calcium, phosphate, and silica ions forming a robust HA-like layer (crystalline hydroxycarbonate apatite). Exchange of ions leads to formation of silica rich layer formed on the surface of bioactive glass which helps to localized calcium and phosphate ions on the surface.
- *Properties*:
  - Antimicrobial property
  - High net gain in mineral content
  - Improved lesion depth reduction
  - Reduction in organic content of enamel
  - Increased rate of mineralization
- NovaMin® is composed primarily of calcium, sodium, phosphorus, and silica. According to in vivo study by **Burwell AK et al.** NovaMin has ability to prevent demineralization and promote remineralization. **Wang et al.** compared remineralization potential of Calcium sodium phosphosilicate group (CSP, NovaMin®), Colgate Sensitive Pro-Relief and GC Tooth Mousse and concluded that higher potential of remineralization in NovaMin®.
- BioMinF is a bioglass-containing dentifrice with a composition of calcium, phosphate, and fluoride. According to **Joiner et al.** Fluorapatite formed from BioMinF is more resistant to the action of extrinsic and intrinsic acids. **Abdul Majeed et al.** compared BioMinF® toothpaste with NovaMin® and concluded that former contains high fluoride contents and greater potential to promote the remineralization of demineralized human enamel.

Nanomaterials

- **Richard Feynman** gave the concept of nanotechnology, in which material in range of 1–100 nm are incorporated in adhesives or resins. Adhesive nanomaterials will prevent breakdown of collagen improving durability of bonding and resin nanomaterials will release Ca^{2+} and PO_4^{3-} in low pH enhancing remineralization.[28]
- **Nano particulate hydroxyapatite (NHAP):** Remineralization occurs because of stable release of Ca^{2+} and PO_4^{3-} from NHAP. **Leitune VC et al.** concluded that Total etch adhesive containing NHAP increases bond strength of teeth. **Bossu, M et al.** evaluated both in vivo and in vitro results on primary teeth and proved the ability of NHAP in caries prevention.
- **Nanosized calcium fluoride ($NCaF_2$):** Prolonged release of fluoride from $NCaF_2$ materials provides better level of F to promote remineralization. **Yi J et al.** studied white spot lesion using $NCaF_2$-containing cement found increase in enamel hardness (56%) and decreased in lesion depth (43%).
- **Nanosized amorphous calcium phosphate particle (NACP):** Provide resistance to dental caries in acidic environment by releasing higher levels of Ca^{2+} and PO_4^{3-} transforming acidic environment towards alkalinity.

- **Bioactive glass nanoparticle (NBG):** Mineralized layer with a porous network is formed with release of Ca^{2+} and PO_4^{3-} which prevent breakdown of collogen, creates high alkaline pH, that promote antibacterial action by release of Ag^{+}.
- **Calcium phosphate-based nanomaterials:** It includes nanoparticles of HAP, TCP, and ACP as sources to release calcium/phosphate ions and increase the supersaturation of HAP in carious lesions.

Miscellaneous Agents

- **Grape seed extract**
  - Grape seed extract (GSE) has a high proanthocyanidin (PA) content.
  - PA-treated collagen matrices are non-toxic and inhibit the enzymatic activity of glucosyl transferase, F-ATPase and amylase.
  - **Epasinghe et al**. proved synergistic effect of PA when combined with CPP amorphous calcium fluoride phosphate (CPP-ACFP) on remineralization of artificial root.
- **Arginine**
  - Arginine is a semi-essential amino acid available in micromolar concentrations in saliva.
  - It effectively maintains healthy oral biofilms by improving pH homeostasis through modulation of the oral microbial community.
  - It is selectively metabolized by arginine deaminase system to ammonia that elevates biofilm pH to counter acidic microenvironments by cariogenic pathogen Streptococcus mutans.
  - In-vitro studies have shown that when used in combination with fluoride, arginine significantly increased fluoride uptake compared with fluoride alone, and lesions treated with arginine containing toothpaste also showed superior fluoride uptake.
- **Xylitol**
  - Xylitol is tooth friendly carbohydrate, which is resistant to fermentation by *Streptococcus*.
  - Available in mints or gum so that it will promote remineralization by activating buffering action due to increase in salivary flow.
  - Its mechanism is as follows:[29]

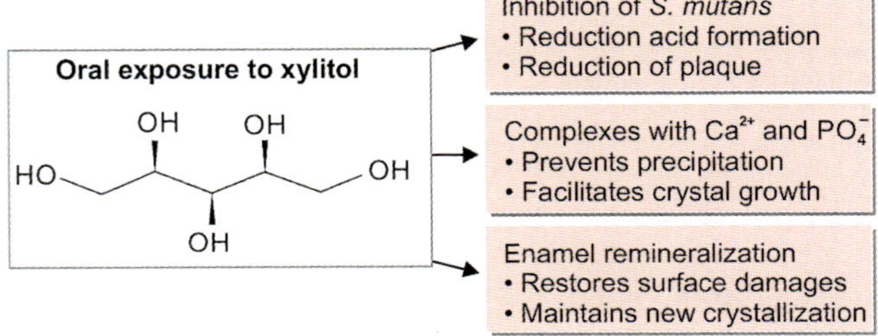

  - **Milburn et al**. compared fluoride release from Enamel Pro®, Duraphat® with varnish containing xylitol-coated calcium and phosphate and found greatest initial fluoride release in the first four hours in xylitol varnish.
- **Theobromine: A Tooth friendly chocolate**[30]
  - This commercially available toothpaste (Théodent) contains Theobromine, a bitter alkaloid of cacao plant with chemical formula $C_7H_8N_4O_2$. It is present in chocolate, as well as in tea leaves and kola nut.
  - Cocoa powder can vary in amount of theobromine from 1.2 to 2.4%.
  - Cocoa bean husk has shown anti-glucosyltransferase activity and antibacterial activity.
  - Theobromine stimulated the growth of new enamel. It allows for calcium and phosphate from saliva to come together in large unit crystal that is four times the size of hydroxyapatite. It has shown to improve microhardness of tooth enamel, which can enhance resistance to tooth decay.
  - Surface microhardness values showed that 200 mg/L theobromine protected enamel more than 100 mg/L.
  - The application of theobromine on enamel surface results in a very smooth surface by process of remineralization.
  - It is without any ill effects and will cause no harm if swallowed.
  - According to **Sadeghpour et al.**[31] Theobromine protected teeth from caries better than fluoride. The amount of Theobromine in a one-ounce dark chocolate bar has a better effect on tooth hardness than a 1.1% prescription sodium fluoride treatment.
  - **Tamara Yuanita, et al** (2020) in his comparative study found that Theobromine gel has higher enamel hardness than CPP-ACP.
- **Polydopamines**
  - PDA has a lattice structure similar to that of hydroxyapatite and participates in strong binding with calcium ions and phosphate ions, which can promote the formation of biomimetic hydroxyapatite in artificial saliva.
  - The oxidative polymerization of dopamine in aqueous solutions spontaneously forms polydopamine, mimicking DOPA, which exhibits a strong adhesive property to various substrates under wet conditions.
  - In demineralized dentin, the collagen fibers when coated with polydopamine, remineralization was promoted, which shows that polydopamine binding to collagen fiber act as a new nucleation site that will be favorable for HA crystal growth.
- **Electric field-induced remineralization**
  - **Wu et al.**[32] have introduced this technique to remineralize the completely demineralized dentin collagen matrix and also to shorten the mineralization time, which it achieved in the absence of both calcium phosphates and their analogs with the help of electrophoresis. Electrophoresis can transport ions more rapidly through a gel or solution than diffusion alone and can be used to accelerate HA formation in agarose hydrogels for the synthesis of HA–agarose hybrid materials.
  - Enables ion migration in a specific one-dimensional direction and promote crystal growth.

- Promote the diffusion of calcium and phosphate ions into the interior of the demineralized collagen matrix to induce collagen fibril remineralization.
- Accelerate the speed of mineralization

❖ **Polyamide poly (amidoamine) (PAMAM)**

- Dendrimers are nano-polymer with good biocompatibility, low toxicity and non-immunogenicity. It has both antibacterial and remineralization potential by modifying the terminal group.
- PAMAM–OH macromolecules bound to collagen fibrils within the tubules through size-exclusion features of collagen fibrils and electrostatic interactions. Then the templates served as a nucleation site to attract calcium ions through calcium complexation by both amide groups and hydroxy groups. Then the calcium ions attracted phosphate ions to form HA. The stable intratubular minerals could resist the acid attack, which ensured that the dentinal tubule occlusion was effective under acidic oral environment (**Liang et al.**).[33]
- PAMAM+NACP together showed synergistic effects and produced triple benefits: Excellent nucleation templates, superior acid neutralization, and ions release leading to much greater remineralization capacity.

RESIN INFILTRATION

❖ Resin infiltration is a technique that creates a diffusion barrier within the lesion without establishing any material on the enamel surface. It is an attempt to reduce lesion progression by sealing diffusion pores within the body of enamel caries by infiltration with a low viscosity resin.[34]

❖ This concept has been modified and commercially developed in Germany for the management of smooth surface and proximal non-cavitated caries lesions.

❖ Icon® is marketed in two different forms: proximal surface and vestibular surface kits. The usage for both is similar except for the need for separation in the case of proximal lesion treatment (**Fig. 47.8**).

❖ Icon® infiltrates the lesion, makes the bacteria inactive and prevents caries progression.

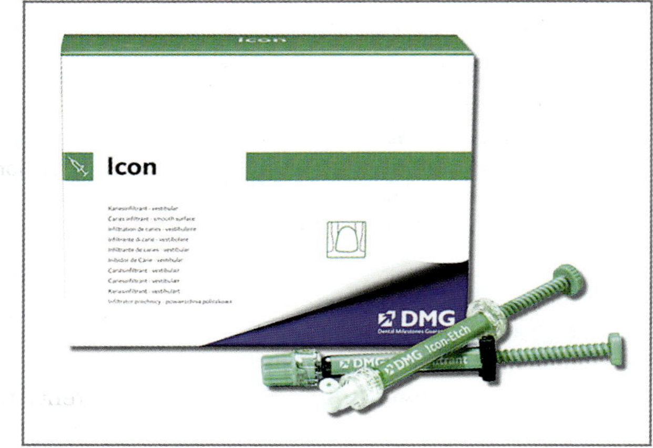

Fig. 47.8: Icon®.

Technique (Figs. 47.9A to F)

Surface of the teeth is cleaned and prepared with 15% hydrochloric acid for 2 minutes. If the lesion is very deep, then it is advisable to sandblast the white area prior to applying the hydrochloric acid to the tooth. The sandblasting helps to open up the enamel tubules so that better penetration can be achieved

↓

Ethanol wet bonding technique is used to desiccate the surface by applying 99% ethanol (Icon Dry) for 30 seconds followed by air-drying. This will coax hydrophobic monomers to infiltrate into demineralized wet enamel or dentine, and improve the efficacy of penetration of the hydrophobic infiltrate (TEGDMA) to get a well-defined, resin-infiltrated layer.

↓

This technique involves slowly replacing water within the demineralized collagen matrix with ascending concentrations of ethanol, allowing the latter to penetrate the collagen matrix without causing additional shrinkage of the interfibrillar spaces, thus preventing the phase separation of hydrophobic resin monomers

↓

Icon resin, composed of tetraethylene glycol dimethacrylate, is applied on the lesion surface using a microbrush and allowed to penetrate for three minutes.

↓

The excess is removed using a cotton roll and light cured

↓

Repeated application for another one minute is performed and then the resin is light cured again. The resin is applied twice because of the shrinkage of the material after the first application, resulting in the generation of space that can be then occluded by a second application.

↓

The excess resin is then removed and the surface is polished

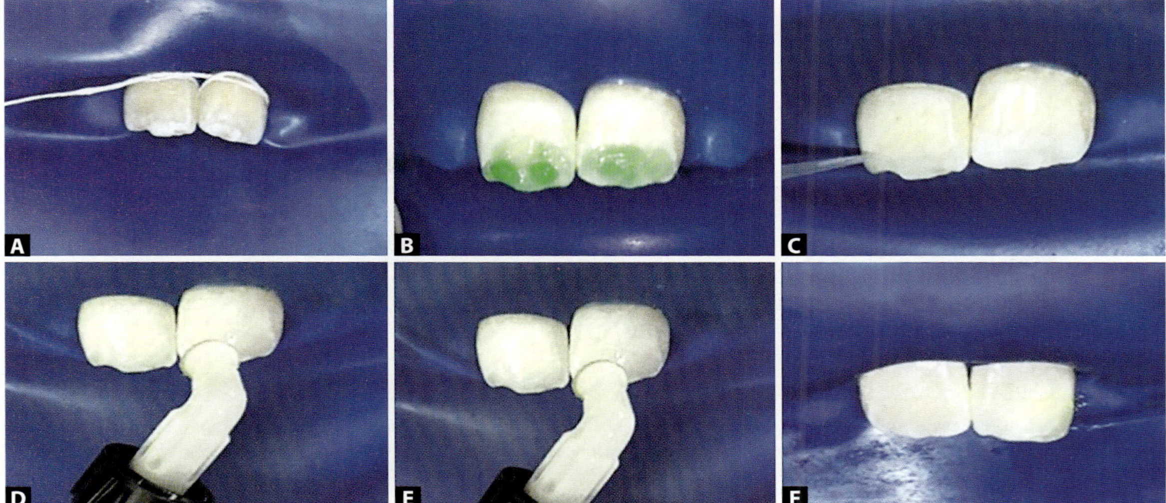

Figs. 47.9A to F: Steps of resin infiltration (Icon) procedure: (A) Isolation using rubber dam; (B) Application of Icon-etch for 2 min; (C) Apply Icon dry for 30s; (D) Apply icon-infiltrant for 3 min; (E) Replace applicator tip, apply icon infiltrant for 1 min, remove access and floss, light cure for 40 second and polish; (F) Postoperative image after polishing.

Advantages

- The enamel lesions lose their whitish appearance when their microporosities are filled with the resin and look similar to sound enamel. This occurs as the difference in the refractive indices between porosities and enamel is negligible.
- Noninvasive treatment, achieved in a single visit.
- Minimized risk of secondary caries; and no risk of postoperative sensitivity and pulpal inflammation.
- Improved esthetic outcome with high acceptance when used as a "masking" resin on demineralized labial surfaces
- Permanent occlusion of superficial micropores and cavities and obturation of porous, deeply demineralized areas.

Limitations

- Strict dry field is required.
- Not effective in deep lesions, as the greater the depth of the carious lesion, the lower will be the probability of achieving a complete infiltration.
- Extensive lesions are also associated with higher polymerization shrinkage and the consequent appearance of porosities and cracks.

Resin Infiltration in Primary Teeth

- The management of non-cavitated caries lesions using the resin infiltration technique in primary teeth differs from that in permanent teeth as primary enamel is less mineralized, more porous and aprismatic when compared to permanent enamel. As a result, the diffusion coefficient seems to be greater in primary enamel.
- The proximal surface layer is less mineralized and thinner in primary molars compared to the permanent ones and thus, the rate of progression of proximal caries in primary molars is significantly higher than that in the permanent ones.
- **Paris S et al.**[35] found that primary teeth exhibited better infiltrate penetration than permanent teeth, after 1 minute application of resin. About 3–5 minutes are required to almost completely infiltrate a natural lesion in permanent teeth with a lesion extended to the inner half of enamel, whereas, 1 min application resulted in only superficial infiltration.
- **Ekstrand et al.**[36] Proximal caries in primary molars treated by resin infiltration and fluoride varnish progressed significantly lesser (23%) than those treated with fluoride varnish only (61%) after one year.

MICROABRASION REMINERALIZATION TECHNIQUE (Mab-Re)

- Term Mab-Re is given by **Deshpande AN et al.**[37] in 2017.
- Microabrasion is accompanied by the application of remineralizing agents on the tooth surface. This remineralizing agent releases ions that fill the Microabrasion-generated micro tags.
- The most widely used enamel process for the microabrasion-remineralization (Mab-Re) technique is micro-abrasion along with application of CPP-ACP cream.
- Advantages
  - It is a promising way of restoring the intrinsic enamel stains and fixing the irregularities without removing or compromising the sound tooth structure.
  - Sensitivity due to acid etching, which was also taken care of with the use of CPP-ACP cream.
  - More secure oral atmosphere and patient compliance.
- The procedure of micro abrasion remineralization (Mab-Re) may be a very promising way to cope with certain stains, abnormalities, developmental defects, and lesions following orthodontic operation **(Figs. 47.10A to D)**.

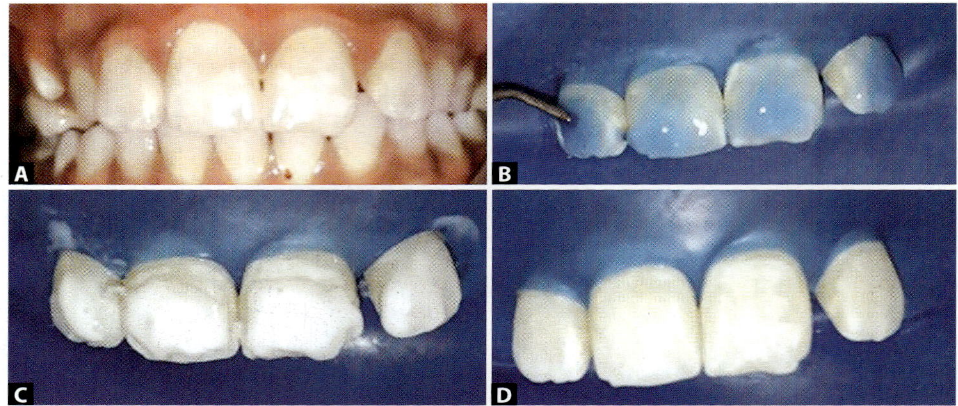

Figs. 47.10 A to D: Steps of micro abrasion remineralization using Tooth Mousse: (A) Hypoplastic lesion seen on 11, 21; (B) Rubber dam isolation and application of Etchant (37% phosphoric acid) for 30 seconds; (C) Application of tooth mousse remineralizing agent for 4 min; (D) Postoperative photograph.

REFERENCES

1. Garg P, Tyagi S, Sinha D, Singh U. An update on remineralizing agents. Journal of Interdisciplinary Dentistry. 2013, 3; 151-8.
2. Pitts, N. B. et al. Dental caries. Nat. Rev. Dis. Primers. 2017, 3; 17030.
3. Robinson C, Shore RC, Brookes SJ, Strafford S, Wood SR, Kirkham J. The chemistry of enamel caries. Crit Rev Oral Biol Med. 2000;11(4): 481-95.
4. Belli R, Rahiotis C, Schubert EW, Baratieri LN, Petschelt A, Lohbauer U. Wear and morphology of infiltrated white spot lesions. J Dent. 2011;39(5):376-85.
5. Pande P, Rana V, Srivastava N, Kaushik N. A compendium on remineralizing agents in dentistry. Int J Appl Dent Sci. 2020; 6 (1):247-250.
6. Arifa MK, Ephraim R, Rajamani T. Recent advances in dental hard tissue remineralization: A review of literature. Int J Clin Pediatr Dent. 2019;12 (2):139-144.
7. Featherstone JD. Dental caries: a dynamic disease process. Aust Dent J. 2008; 53 (3): 286-91.
8. Pannu, R, Berwal V. Remineralization - An evolving concept: A review. Journal of Advanced Medical and Dental Sciences Research. 2017: 5 (11), 60-63.
9. Featherstone JDB, Rapozo-Hilo M, Le C. Inhibition of demineralization and promotion of remineralization by 5000 ppm F dentifrices. 2012;46(2):118-29.
10. Tung MS, Eichmiller FC. Dental applications of amorphous calcium phosphates. J Clin Dent. 2003; 10:1-6.
11. Zhao, et al. Amorphous calcium phosphate and its application in dentistry. Chemistry Central Journal. 2011;5:40.
12. Thompson A, Grant LP, Tanzer JM. Model for assessment of carious lesion remineralization, and remineralization by a novel toothpaste. J Clin Dent. 1999;10 (1SpecNo):34-9.
13. Arifa MK, Ephraim R, Rajamani T. Recent advances in dental hard tissue remineralization: A review of literature. Int J Clin Pediatr Dent. 2019;12(2):139-44.
14. Goswami M, Saha S, Telgi C. Latest developments in non-fluoridated remineralizing technologies. Journal of the Indian Society of Pedodontics and Preventive Dentistry. 2012;30.
15. Yan J, Yang H, Luo T, Hua F, He H. Application of amorphous calcium phosphate agents in the prevention and treatment of enamel demineralization. Front Bioeng Biotechnol. 2022, 10:853436.
16. Madrid-Troconis Cristhian Camilo, Perez-Puello Sthefanie del Carmen. Casein phosphopeptide-amorphous calcium phosphate nanocomplex (CPP-ACP) in dentistry: state of the art. Rev Fac Odontol Univ Antioq. 2019; 30(2): 248-62.
17. Al-Batayneh, Ola. The clinical applications of tooth mousse TM and CPP-ACP products in caries prevention: evidence- based recommendations. Smile Dental Journal. 2009;4: 8-12.
18. Hegde RJ, Thakkar JB. Comparative evaluation of the effects of casein phosphopeptide-amorphous calcium phosphate (CPP-ACP) and xylitol-containing chewing gum on salivary flow rate, pH and buffering capacity in children: An in vivo study. J Indian Soc Pedod Prev Dent. 2017; 35:332-7.
19. Kargul B. Remineralization potential of theobromine, APF gel and CPP-ACP: pilot study. J Dent Res. 2012, 91 (Spec Issue C): 623.
20. N.J. Cochrane. QLF and TMR analysis of CPP-ACFP remineralized enamel in vitro. J Dent Res. 2006, 85 (Spec Issue B): 0192.
21. Heshmat H. Effect of GC tooth mousse and MI paste plus on dental plaque acidity. J Dent Res. 2013, 92 (Spec Issue B): 82902.
22. Reynolds EC, Cai F, Cochrane NJ, Shen P, Walker GD, Morgan MV, et al. Fluoride and casein phosphopeptideamorphous calcium phosphate. J Dent Res. 2008;87(4):3448.
23. Attiguppe P, Malik N, Ballal S, Naik SV. CPPACP and fluoride: A synergism to combat caries. Int J Clin Pediatr Dent. 2019; 12:1205.
24. Nadar BG, Yavagal PC, Velangi CS, Yavagal CM, Basavaraj SP. Efficacy of casein phosphopeptideamorphous calcium phosphate varnish in remineralizing white spot lesions: A systematic review and metaanalysis. Dent Res J. 2022; 19:48.
25. Han Ju Choi, Yeong Chul Choi, Kwang-Chul Kim, Sung-Chul Choi. Remineralization depth of CPP-ACP on demineralization human enamel in vitro. J Korean Acad Pediatr Dent. 2008;35(2).
26. Reynolds EC. Improved plaque uptake and enamel remineralization by fluoride with CPP-ACP. Dent Res. 2006;85 (Spec Issue B):2538.
27. Rose RK. Binding characteristics of streptococcus mutans for calcium and casein phosphopeptide. Caries Res. 2000; 34 (5): 427-31.
28. Chen H, Gu L, Liao B, Zhou X, Cheng L, Ren B. Advances of anti-caries nanomaterials. Molecules. 2020; 25 (21): 5047.
29. Auerkari EI, Soufyan A, Alkatiri F, Verisqa F, Megantoro A, Sumawinata N, Mangundjaja S. Effect of xylitol on remineralization of demineralized dental enamel. International Journal of Clinical Preventive Dentistry. 2010;6(2).
30. Sudharsana A. Tooth friendly chocolate. Journal of Pharmaceutical Science and Research. 2014; 7(1):49.
31. Arman S. A neural network analysis of theobromine vs. fluoride on theenamel surface of human teeth. Diss Abstr Int. 2007;68(Suppl B):150.
32. Wu XT, Cao Y, Mei ML, Chen JL, Li QL, Chu CH. An electrophoresis-aided biomineralization system for regenerating dentin- and enamel-like microstructures for the self-healing of tooth defects. Cryst Growth Des. 2014; 14:5537-48.
33. Liang K, et al. Effective dentinal tubule occlusion induced by polyhydroxy-terminated PAMAM dendrimer in vitro. RSC Adv. 2014; 4:43496-503.
34. Manoharan V, Arun Kumar S, Arumugam SB, Anand V, Krishnamoorthy S, Methippara JJ. Is resin infiltration a microinvasive approach to white lesions of calcified tooth structures?: a systemic review. Int J Clin Pediatr Dent. 2019; 12(1): 53-8.
35. Paris S, Meyer-Lueckel H, et al. Resin infiltration of artificial enamel caries lesions with experimental light curing resins. Dent Mater J. 2007;26(4):582-8.
36. Ekstrand K, Martignon S, et al. The non-operative resin treatment of proximal caries lesions. Dent Update. 2012;39(9):614-6.
37. Deshpande AN, Joshi NH, Pradhan NR, Raol RY. Microabrasion-remineralization (MAb-Re): An innovative approach for dental fluorosis. J Indian Soc Pedod Prev Dent. 2017;35(4):38.

CHAPTER

Stainless Steel Crowns in Pediatric Dentistry; Conventional and Hall Technique

Nikhil Marwah, Anshula Deshpande, Sonali Saha, Nirmala SVSG, Ravi GR, Ravichandra KS

CHAPTER OUTLINE

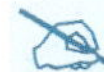

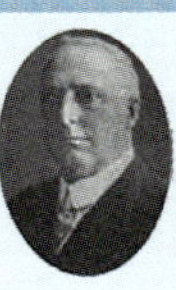

Rehabilitation of grossly lost tooth structure in primary or young permanent teeth by means of stainless steel crowns (SSCs) has become a viable assistance to Pediatric Dentist ever since Rocky Mountain Company introduced them in 1947 but familiarized by **Humphrey** and **Engel** in 1950s.[1-3]

Stainless steel crowns *can be defined as prefabricated crown forms that are adapted to individual teeth and cemented with a biocompatible luting agent.*[4] The distinctive anatomical characteristics of primary teeth, petite lifespan of primary teeth in the oral cavity, short attention span of the child, prolonged duration, and intricate treatment planning involved in preparation of Willets inlay or cast crown restorations favors SSCs as an alternative in Pediatric Dentistry. This chapter will attempt to make a comprehensive review of the SSC.

History of stainless steel crowns

- 1947: Rocky Mountain Company introduced crowns
- 1950: **Humphrey** and **Engel** popularized SSC
- 1971: **Mink and Hill** advised SSC modification for over and undersized crowns.
- 1977: **McEvory** advised modification of SSC technique for SSC with arch length or space loss
- 1980 to 1990: Various pre-veneered stainless steel crowns (PVSSC) were introduced
- 1981: **Nash** advocated modification of SSC for adjacent crowns placement
- 1983: **Hartman** advised veneered SSC technique for esthetic anterior crown restoration
- 2006: Hall technique was introduced by **Dr Norna Hall** for SSC adaptation on carious tooth without tooth preparation

INDICATIONS OF STAINLESS STEEL CROWNS

- *Extensive caries:* If the caries is involving three or more surfaces, this leads to insufficient tooth structure to hold a restoration, and in such cases crown proves to be more cost-effective and prevents further damage.
- *Extensive decalcification*: On any one surface like proximal; is also an indication as it might lead to space loss at a later stage.
- *Rampant caries*: In such cases, there is need for multiple restorations on a single tooth, so it is much cost-effective and much less traumatic to place an SSC on the tooth.
- *Recurrent caries*: Placement of crown will also help in removing the possibility of recurrent caries around existing restoration.
- *After pulp therapy*: Following pulp therapy, the tooth structure is weakened due to removal of dentin. Such teeth are prone to fractures and hence crown coverage is mandatory to avoid it (**Duggal and Curzon**, 1989).
- *Inherited or acquired enamel defects*, for example, hypoplasia, amelogenesis imperfecta (permanent and primary teeth): Such patients have a tendency to fracture teeth while normal eating practices alongwith the common associated pain. It is imperative to provide crown for these patients to avoid pain and fracture and also restore the vertical dimension.
- *Intermediate restoration*: In children with class II division 1 malocclusion with hypoplastic or carious molar, this can be planned till eruption of premolar and second molars.

- *Fractures of permanent and primary incisors*: If an incisor is fractured, crowns in anterior teeth can be given as a temporary dressing to cover the exposed dentin.
- *Severe bruxism*: When teeth show extreme wear and tear owing to bruxism, crown is a good restorative choice. This is because SSC can neither wear down nor fracture and at the same time restore lost vertical dimension.
- *Correction of crossbite*: Can be used for single tooth crossbite correction (**Croll and Lieberman**, 1999).
- *Abutment teeth to prosthesis*: These are useful extracoronal restorations in abutment teeth to removable prosthesis.
- *As part of a space maintainer*: Crowns can be a part of crown and loop or crown band and loop space maintainer.

Indications for permanent molar teeth
- Interim restoration of a broken-down or traumatized tooth
- When financial considerations are a concern
- Teeth with developmental defects (dentin dysplasia, sensitivity)
- Restoration of a permanent molar which requires full coverage but is only partially erupted
- Young permanent molars following endodontic treatment

Indications for anterior primary teeth
- Interim restoration traumatized tooth
- When financial considerations are a concern
- Morphological and occlusal considerations

CONTRAINDICATIONS FOR STAINLESS STEEL CROWNS

- Primary molars close to exfoliation
- Primary molars near exfoliation
- Teeth that exhibit mobility
- Teeth which are not restorable
- Patients with known nickel allergy (**Hensten and Petersen** 1992).

CLASSIFICATION OF STAINLESS STEEL CROWNS

According to trimming **(Figs. 48.1A to C)**	• *Untrimmed crowns*: These crowns are neither trimmed nor contoured and require lot of adaptation, thus are time consuming, e.g., the Rocky Mountain crowns • *Pretrimmed crowns*: These crowns have straight, non-contoured sides but are festooned to follow at line parallel to the gingival crest. They still require contouring and some trimming, e.g., Unitek, 3M, Denovo crowns. • *Precontoured crowns*: These crowns are festooned and are also pre-contoured though a minimal amount of festooning and trimming may be necessary, e.g., 3M, Prime Pedo, Rainbow Crowns, Hu Friedy crowns
According to composition **(Figs. 48.2A to D)**	• Stainless steel crowns—18-8 Austenitic stainless steel (67% iron, 18% chromium, 8% nickel), e.g., Unitek stainless steel crowns, 3M crowns, Rainbow crowns • Nickel-chromium crowns—nickel chrome alloy (70% nickel, 15% chromium, 10% iron), e.g., Ni-chro-ion crowns, Inconel • Tin-base crowns (tin—96%, silver alloy—4%), e.g., Henry Schein crowns, 3M Isoform crowns • Aluminum-base crowns manganese—1.2%, magnesium—10%, iron—0.7%, silicon—0.3%, copper—0.25%), e.g., Parkell crowns
According to position **(Fig. 48.3)**	• Crowns for posterior teeth, e.g., Unitek stainless steel crowns, 3M Co, Prime Pedo, Rainbow crowns, Hu Friedy crowns • Crowns for anterior teeth, e.g., Unitek crowns, Nu smile SSC
According to company	• The Rocky Mountains, Prime Pedo, 3M, Prime Pedo, Rainbow crowns, Hu Friedy crowns
According to occlusal anatomy	Ion—compact occlusal anatomy Unitek—best occlusal anatomy Rocky mountains—occlusally small Ormco—smallest and least occlusally carved Rainbow/Prime Pedo/3M/Hu Friedy—most acceptable occlusal anatomy

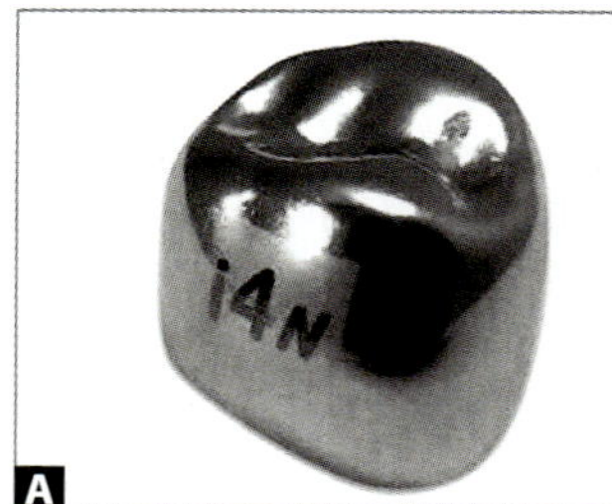

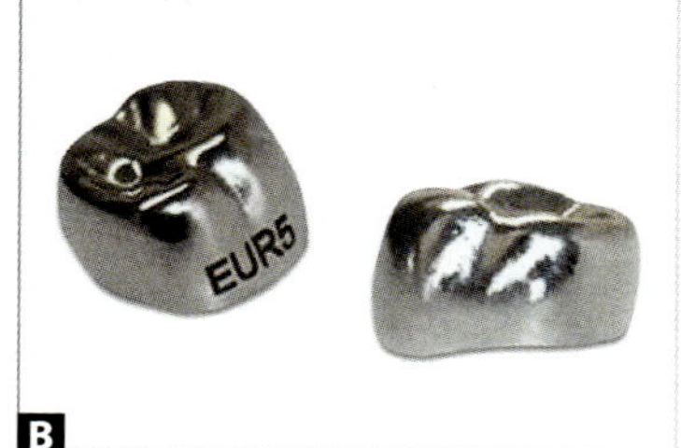

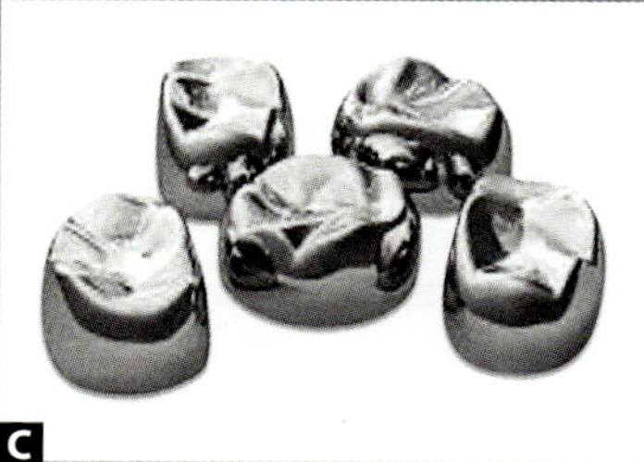

Figs. 48.1A to C: Crowns according to the trim: (A) Untrimmed; (B) Pretrimmed; (C) Precontoured.

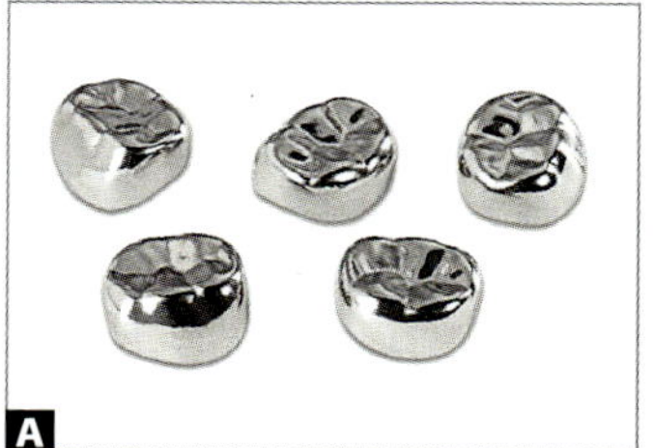

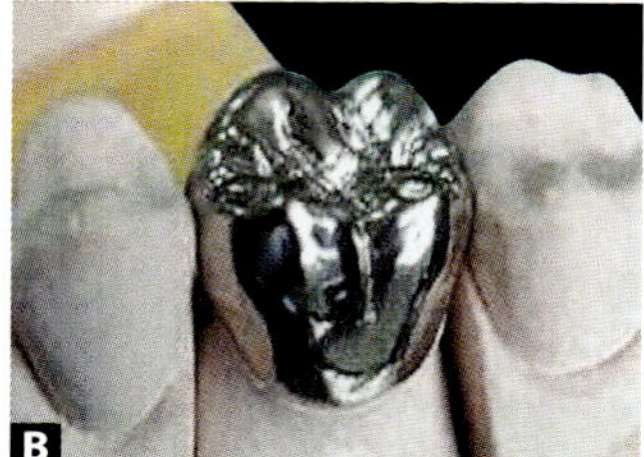

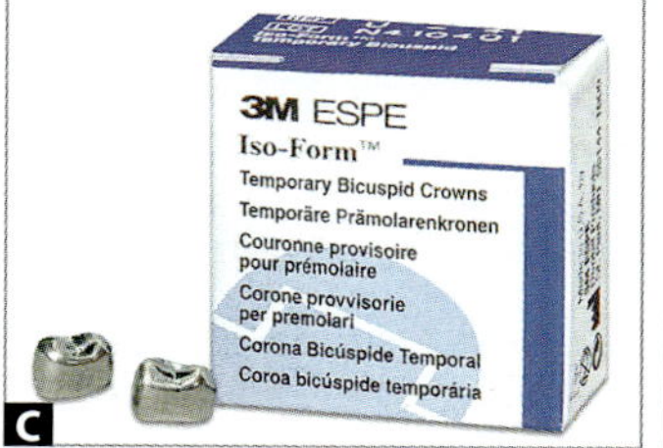

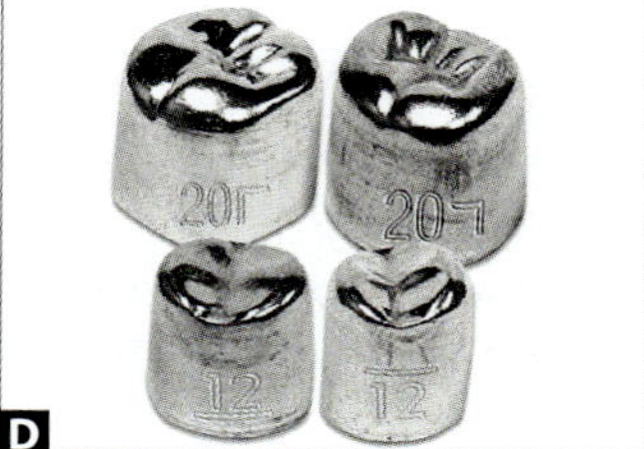

Figs. 48.2A to D: Crowns according to the composition: (A) Stainless steel crowns; (B) Nickel–chromium crowns; (C) Tin-based crowns; (D) Aluminium-based crowns.

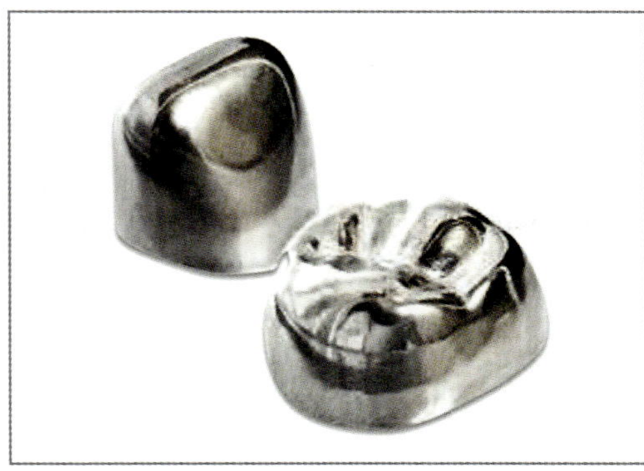

Fig. 48.3: Crowns according to the location.

COMPOSITION OF STAINLESS STEEL CROWNS

Stainless Steel Crowns (18–8 Crowns)

- Stainless steel is low-carbon alloy steel that contain more than or equal to 11.5% chromium.
- The term "stainless steel" is used when the chromium content exceeds 11% and is generally in the range of 12–30%.
- SSC contain about 18% chromium and 8% nickel as well as small amounts of other elements and are considered as 18-8 stainless steel.
- There are three general classes of stainless steel: The heat hardenable 400 series martensitic types, the non-heat hardenable 400 series ferrite types, the austenitic types of chromium nickel-manganese 200 series and chromium nickel 300 series.
- The austenitic types have high ductility, low yield strength, and high ultimate strength, which make them outstanding for deep drawing and forming procedures. They are readily welded and can be work hardened to high levels. The austenitic types provide the best corrosion resistance of all of the stainless steels, particularly when they have been annealed to dissolve chromium carbides and then rapidly quenched to retain the carbon in solution. This property is used during contouring when the crown is work hardened and re-adapted during fit.
- Chromium contributes to the formation of a very thin surface film, probably oxide that protects against corrosive attack.

Iron	67%
Chromium	17–19%
Nickel	10–13%
Minor elements	4%

Nickel-Base Crowns

- These are ion crowns constructed of Inconel 600, a relatively new addition to the category of preformed crowns, and are primarily nickel-chromium.
- The metallurgic characteristics of the nickel-chromium alloy permit these crowns to be strain hardened during manufacture. Higher hardness renders the ion crown more difficult to contour and adapt to the prepared tooth.

Nickel	76%
Chromium	15%
Iron	8%
Carbon	0.08%
Manganese	0.35%
Silicon	0.2%

CONVENTIONAL APPROACH FOR PLACEMENT OF STAINLESS STEEL CROWNS

The initial crown preparation was suggested by **Mink** and **Bennett**.[5] Other techniques frequently quoted in the literature include the simplified ones presented by **Rapp** and **Castaldi**[6] but none have been as comprehensive and successful as Mink technique. The current approach of **Keneddy** is based on the original Mink and Bennett concepts and requires both tooth and crown reduction.

Armamentarium

- **Burs and stones (Fig. 48.4):**
  - No. 169L or No. 69L FG
  - No. 6 or No. 8 RA
  - No. 330 FG
  - Tapered diamond FG
  - Round bur
  - Flame-shaped diamond bur
  - Long thin tapered
  - Green stone or heatless stone/rubber wheel
  - Rough polishing wheel
  - Wire wheel-for finishing crown

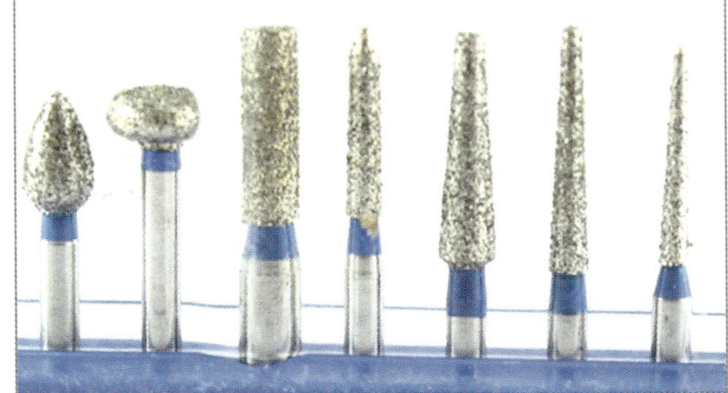

Fig. 48.4: Burs used for tooth preparation in SSC.

- **Pliers**—Hoe pliers, No. 114 Johnson contouring pliers, No. 417 Crimping pliers, No. 112 Ball and socket pliers **(Figs. 48.5A to E) (Table 48.1).**
- Scaler or any sharp instrument.
- Crown and bridge scissors.
- Crown seater and remover.
- For cementation: Luting cement, mixing pad, spatula.
- Miscellaneous: Articulating paper, bitewax, glass marking pencil, glass slab.

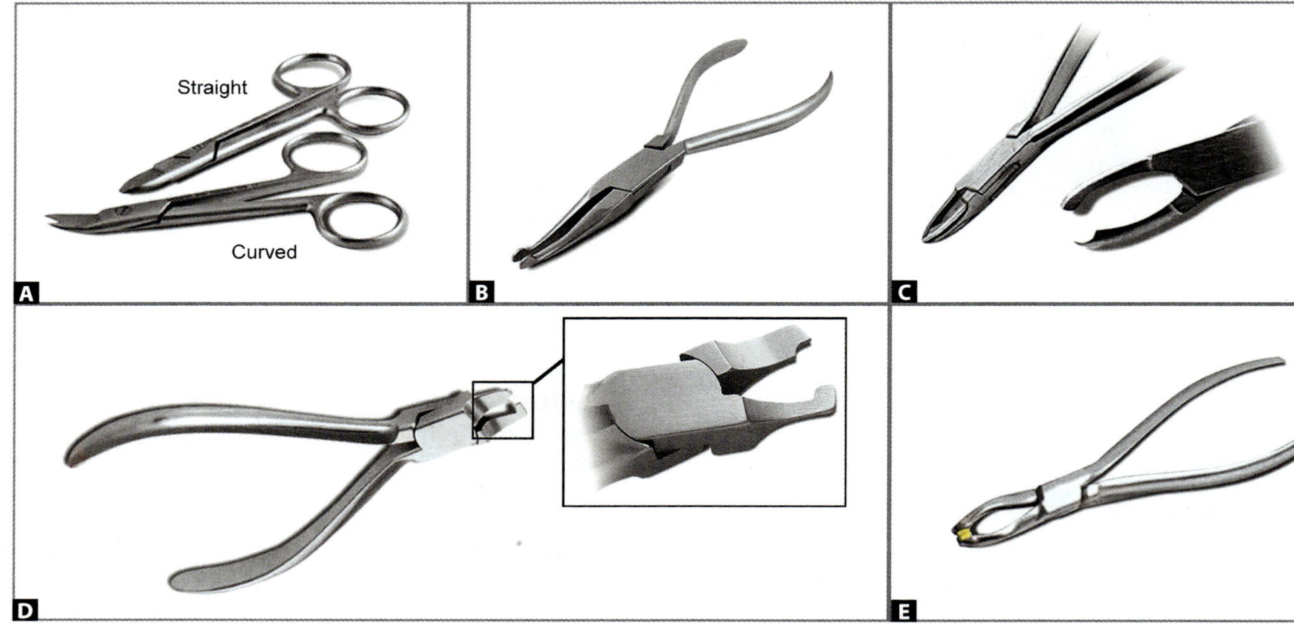

Figs. 48.5A to E: Armamentarium for stainless steel crowns: (A) Crown cutting scissors; (B) Straight hoe pliers; (C) Contouring pliers; (D) Crimping pliers; (E) Crown remover.

Table 48.1: Pliers and scissors markings as per company.

Hu-Friedy	*GDC*
Slim Crown and Band Contouring Pliers 678-221MC	Johnson Contouring 3000/59
Band Crimping Pliers 678-225	Crown Crimping Plier 3000/225
Curved Crown and Gold Scissors SCGC	Crown and Band TC Curved 12.0 CM S5039

Evaluation of Preoperative Occlusion

- The objective is to replicate the existing occlusion after the SSC placement.
- Dental midline, cusp-fossa relationships bilaterally must be assessed.
- Before starting the tooth preparation, we should evaluate the occlusion by visual examination and transfer this relation onto the bite wax by asking the patient to bite on it.

Crown Selection

- The main considerations in selecting the proper SSC are—adequate mesiodistal (MD) diameter, light resistance to seating and proper occlusal height.
- A crown should be somewhat larger than the tooth to which it is being adapted, especially when the gingival part of the crown is trimmed and crimped. The goal is to select the smallest crown that completely covers the preparation and establish proper proximal contacts.
- Any of the following three different methods can be used for crown selection with predictable success:
  1. Trial and error method by arbitrarily selecting different sizes.
  2. Measuring the internal MD measurement by using a boley gauge or vernier calipers **(Fig. 48.6)**.
  3. By using charts **(Table 48.2)**.
- Pick the crown with the help of sterile tweezers or thumb forceps **(Fig. 48.7)**.

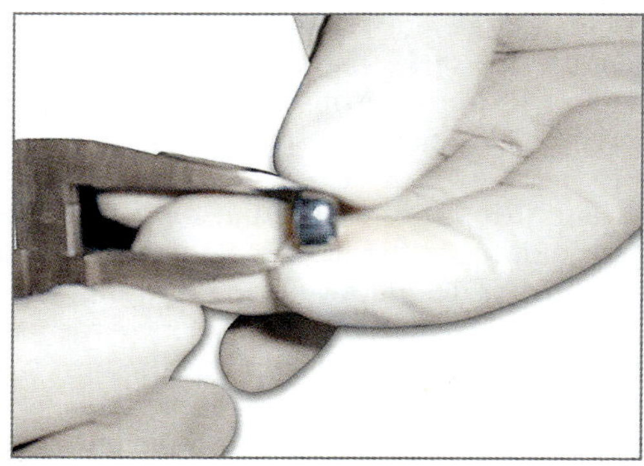

Fig. 48.6: Measuring of crown diameter with the help of caliper.

Table 48.2: Average sizes for SSC.

Tooth	*Sizes available*	*Width range (mm)*
Upper 1st primary molar	2–7	7.2–9.2
Upper 2nd primary molar	2–7	9.2–11.2
Lower 1st primary molar	2–7	7.4–9.4
Lower 2nd primary molar	2–7	9.4–11.4
Upper 1st permanent molar	2–7	10.7–12.8
Lower 1st permanent molar	2–7	10.8–12.8

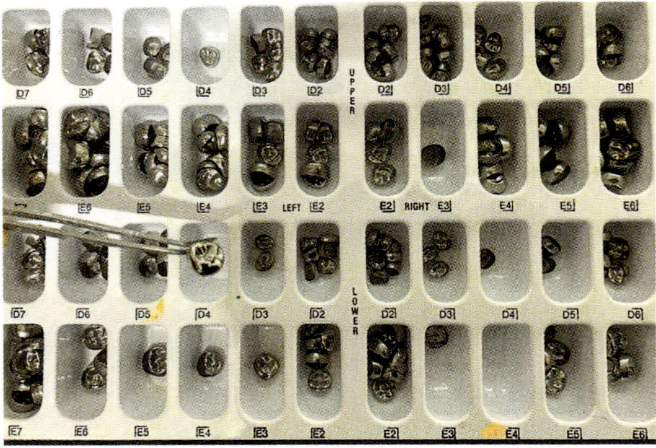

Fig. 48.7: Picking of selected crown from the box.

Occlusal Reduction

- Start the occlusal reduction with pear-shaped (American football shaped) bur. Reduce the occlusion by about 1.0–1.5 mm uniformly along the cuspal structure so as to create a reduced tooth but the same occlusal anatomy **(Figs. 48.8A to D).**
- The reduction is determined by comparing the marginal ridges of adjacent teeth.
- Occlusal reduction to be done prior to proximal to avoid invisibility of preparation areas due to blood contamination. **Full et al**. (1974) considered that occlusal preparation should be done first to allow better access to the proximal areas of the tooth, while other authors suggest the proximal reduction before the occlusal surface.
- **Mathewson, Pinkham and Mink and Bennet** proposed proximal reduction first followed by occlusal, whereas **Stewart, Welbury, Forrester and Brocre** proposed occlusal reduction first followed by proximal.
- **Humphrey** (1950) advocated that cusps should be reduced only if necessary.
- **Rapp** (1966) had concluded that preparation height should be 4 mm from gingival margin.
- **Mink** and **Bennett** (1968) advocated 1–1.5 mm uniform occlusal reduction.
- **Matthewson et al** (1974) proposed 1–1.5 mm occlusal reduction.
- **Troutman** and **Kennedy** (1976) advised 1.5–2 mm occlusal reduction.

Proximal Reduction

- The proximal reduction is done with the help of tapering fissure and needle burs with the main objective of breaking the contact.
- Slice the mesial and distal surfaces with needle-shaped bur and then break the contact between the teeth with tapering fissure (No.169L) bur.
- Hold the bur slightly at an angle to the long axis of the tooth and extend the slice to the buccal and lingual line angles giving 2–5° taper **(Figs. 48.9A to D).**
- The objective is to produce near vertical reduction with the gingival margin of the preparation to be a feather (knife) edge without any shoulder or ledge. Excessive taper may reduce retention, while a shoulder or ledge may pose difficulty in seating the crown (**Myers,** 1976).[7]
- Avoid bur damage or marks on adjacent teeth. Some other methods of prevention of damage to adjacent teeth include cutting with safe-sided disks, use of separators or wedges, and by placement of band material between the cutting surfaces.

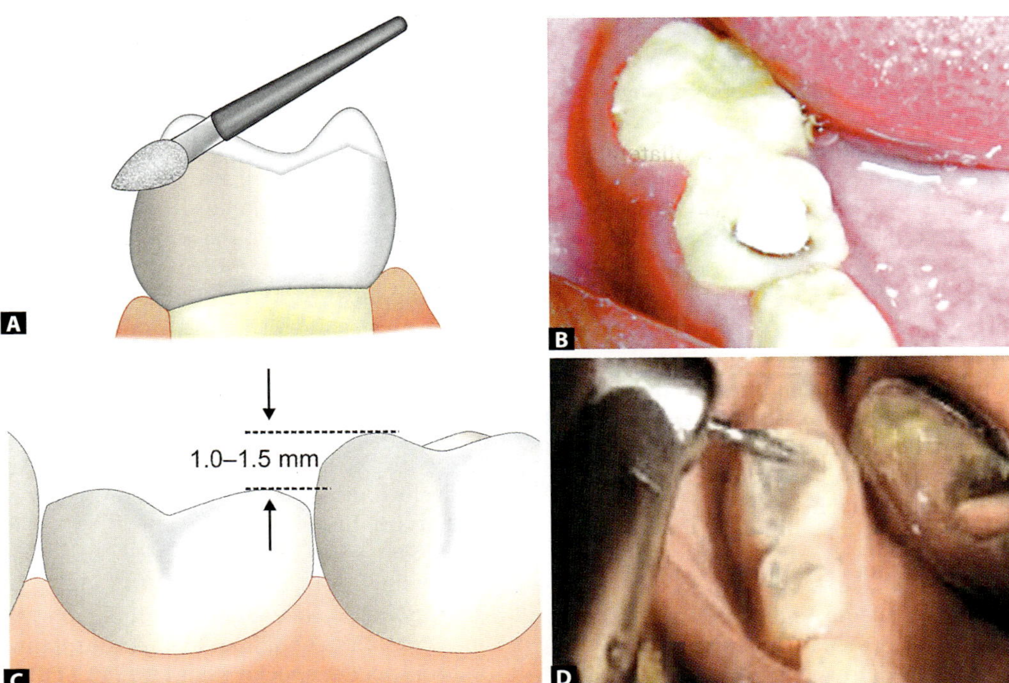

Figs. 48.8A to D: (A) Diagrammatic representation of occlusal reduction; (B) Post-occlusal reduction view; (C) Diagrammatic representation of cutting dimensions; (D) Occlusal reduction in primary mandibular second molar.

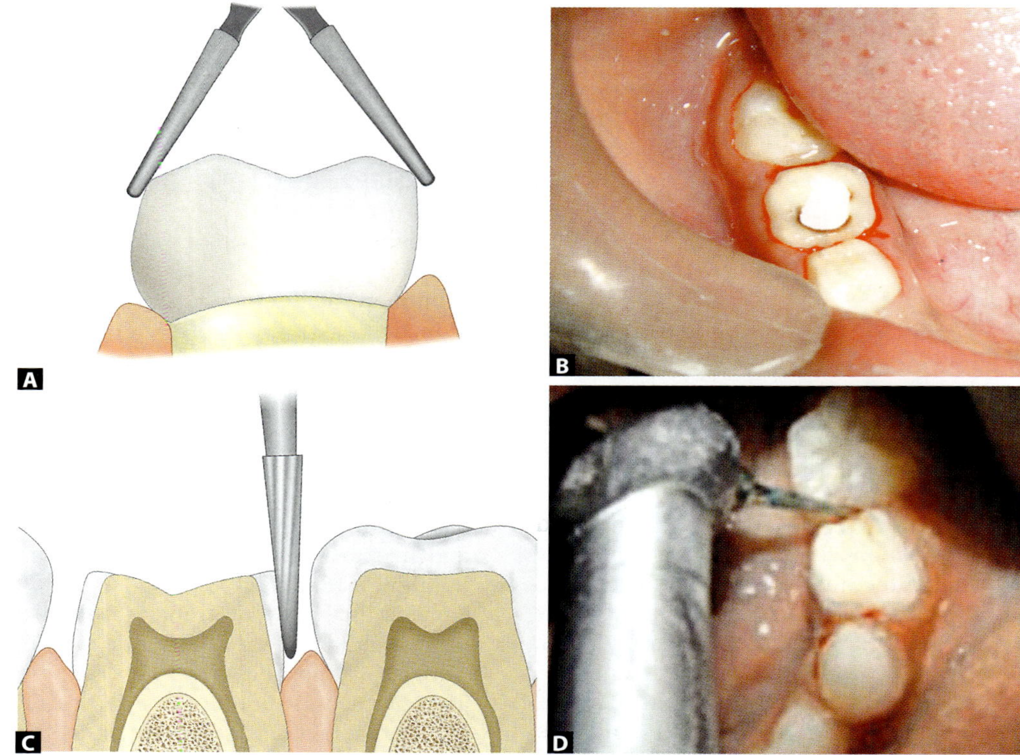

Figs. 48.9A to D: (A) Diagrammatic representation of proximal reduction; (B) Post-proximal reduction view; (C) Diagrammatic representation of cutting dimensions; (D) Proximal reduction in primary mandibular second molar.

Buccal/Lingual Reduction

- Buccal and lingual reduction is optional. Although SSCs require no reduction on the buccal or lingual aspect, some authors feel that it is needed due to the space usage.
- Tongue is very critical to anything extra near it, even as mall piece of food on the lingual aspect will trouble tongue, and it will keep on touching it till it gets dislodged. So even if we place a well-finished 0.05 mm worth of crown structure in the lingual aspect without cutting, it will be perceived by the tongue as extra, and it will hence act to dislodge it. It is therefore necessary according to these authors to reduce at least 0.5 mm buccal and lingual surface also.
- The preparation is confined to occlusal one-third only using the taper fissure bur at a 30–45° angle to the occlusal surface. Natural undercuts on the buccal and lingual surfaces are retained in this way which aid in the retention of the crown.
- **Duggal** and **Curzon** suggested trying selected crown for size before carrying out lingual or buccal reduction.
- **Mathewson et al** (1974), **Andlaw** and **Rock** (1984) suggested that buccolingual reduction is not done for retention, and is undertaken only if the buccal or lingual bulges obstruct crown placement.

Finishing of Tooth Reduction

- Reduce and round off all line angles and sharp corners of the preparation with the help of finishing burs.
- The occlusal as well as the proximal aspect must be rounded off but with utmost care so as to avoid any further reduction.

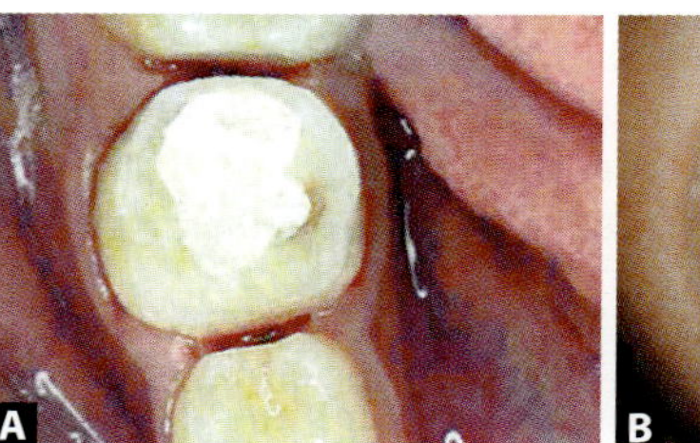

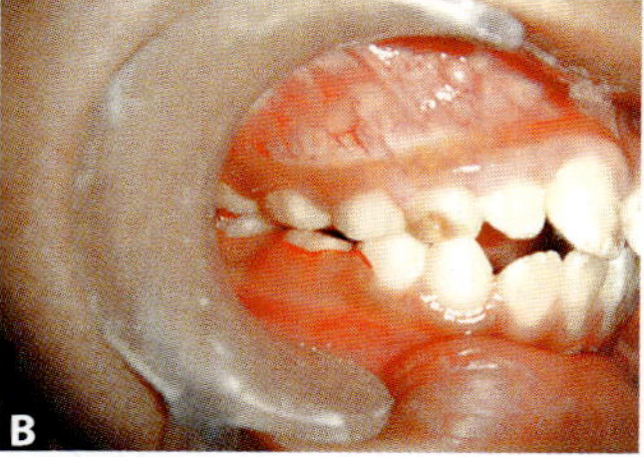

Figs. 48.10A and B: (A) Top view of finished tooth preparation; (B) Side view of the finished tooth preparation.

- Verify the occlusion and proximal contacts **(Figs. 48.10A and B).** There should be a gap of 1–1.5 mm between the prepared tooth and the opposing tooth during occlusion. This is verified by marginal ridge of the adjacent tooth. Verify the proximal cutting by passing a thin probe onto the mesial and distal sides and feel for ledges.

Crown Attachment

- This is the most critical step in usage of SSC by Pediatric Dentist so as to prevent any type of injury to child like accidental ingestion or inhalation of crown due to slippage.
- This can be achieved by:
  - Soldering a hook on the lingual aspect of crown to which floss is tied **(Fig. 48.11A).**
  - Soldering a lingual attachment to which floss is tied.
  - Attachment of floss to crown structures on the buccal aspect by special glues **(Fig. 48.11B).**
  - Prefabricated crowns with rings (Kids crown) **(Fig. 48.11C).**

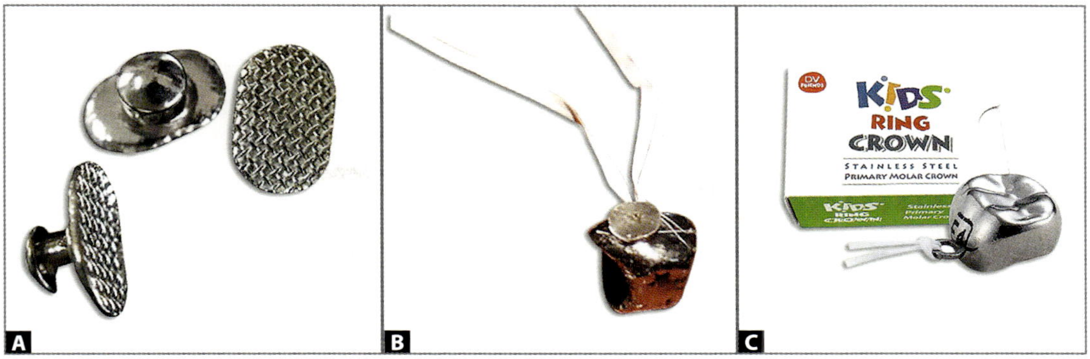

Figs. 48.11A to C: (A) Lingual attachments of SSC; (B) Attaching of floss to SSC; (C) Pre-fabricated attachments of SSC.

Crown Adaptation—Festooning and Initial Fit

- If rubber dam is being used, it is necessary to remove it at this stage.
- Festooning of the proximal surface should be performed before trying the crown as it will facilitate in ease of placement and will limit false blanching signs.
- The buccal and lingual gingiva around second primary molars and the lingual marginal gingiva of first primary molars resemble smile (∪), while the buccal marginal gingiva mimic 'S' shape that looks stretched (~). The proximal contours of all the primary molars look like frown (∩). The gingival margins of the trimmed crowns must correspond to their respective gingival margins of the tooth.
- Place the crown on the lingual side and rotate it toward the buccal side **(Fig. 48.12A)**.
- The crown should fit loosely, with 2–3 mm excess gingivally. With a scaler, scratch around the gingival margin on the crown or mark with a glass marking pencil. This scratch line indicates the gingival line and the gingival contour, as well as the portion of the crown to be removed.
- Remove the crown from the prepared tooth, exposing the scratch line and with the help of crown and bridge scissors, cut the crown 1 mm below the scratch line **(Fig. 48.12B)**.
- Now smoothen the edges with finishing burs **(Fig. 48.12C)**.

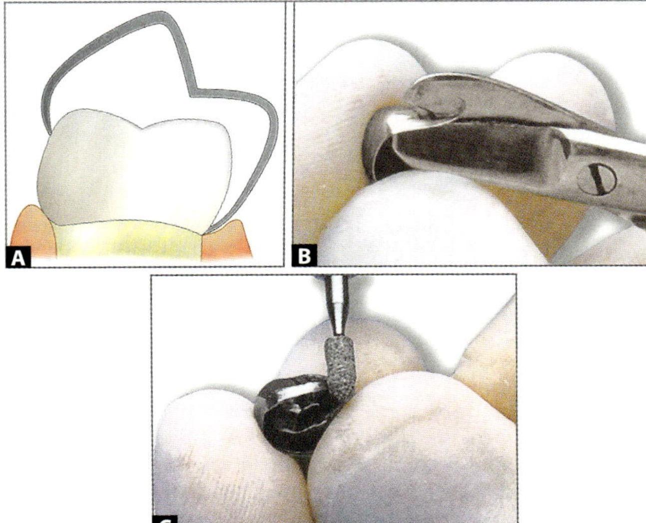

Figs. 48.12A to C: Crown adaptation: (A) Check fit of crown; (B) Trimming of excess crown; (C) Finishing of crown.

- Retry the crown on the tooth. If there is blanching of the gingiva, it may be necessary to rescribe the crown and retrim it in areas where blanching is visible.
- Check the gingival extent of crown with the help of probe; it should not be more than 1 mm on buccal aspect and 0.5 mm on the lingual side.
- **Spedding**[8] described two principles pertaining to length and gingival margins of the crowns for better adaptation of the crowns to the teeth. The goal is to extend the crown 1 mm beneath the free margin of the gingival sulcus and to approximate the gingival margins of the crown to the gingival crest around the tooth. The subgingival placement of crown margin is justified since for primary teeth the buccal, lingual, and proximal contours are just above the gingival crest, and the objective is to engage the crown in natural undercuts.

Contouring

- The next step in adaptation is to contour the crown with pliers so as to reciprocate the original contour of the tooth.
- Most of the crowns provided today are pre-contoured but minimal contouring aids in better anatomy, hence better retention and its obvious advantages.
- Contouring is done with the help of No. 114 Johnson contouring pliers. A ball and socket pliers is used to contour the buccal and lingual surfaces by holding the crown firmly with the pliers, and force is exerted from the opposite side of the crown to bend the gingival one third of the crown inward **(Fig. 48.13)**.

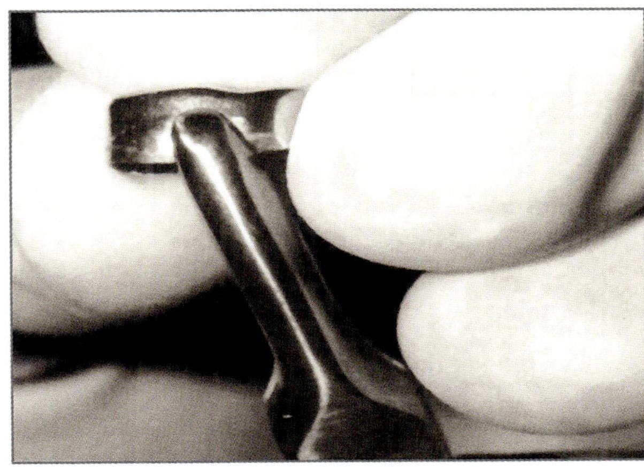

Fig. 48.13: Contouring the crown.

- The advantage of contouring is that the crown gets work hardened by manipulation and becomes more retentive.

Crimping of the Crown

- This is very important to the gingival health of the supporting tissue as a poorly adapted crown will serve as a collection point for bacteria, contributing to recurrent caries or incipient periodontal disease.
- Using the No. 417 crimping pliers, the crown is crimped in the gingival third.
- The procedure of crimping is that the pliers must be "walked" through the entire crown continuously without lifting. After completion of crimping, there will be a gradual bend in the gingival third of crown **(Fig. 48.14)**. This can be more appreciated on a glass slab.
- The uses of crimping are protection of soft tissues, prevention of leakage of cements, prevention of contamination and adequate retention.

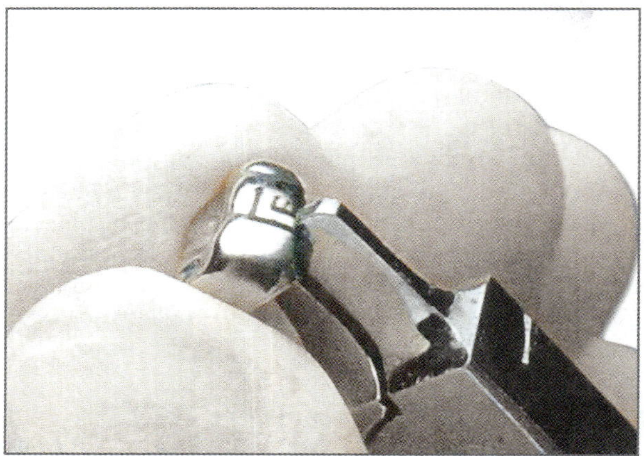

Fig. 48.14: Crimping the crown.

CHECKING THE FINAL FIT

- After the contouring and crimping is complete, retry the crown and with an explorer, check all the margins for adaptation **(Figs. 48.15A and B).**
- Seat the crown in a lingual to buccal direction, and it should snap into position under firm finger pressure. The quality of retention of crown is directly dependent on its snugly fit into the tooth.
- This is the best time to evaluate occlusal harmony and compare it with preoperative occlusion.
- After final adaptation, check for any destabilization or rocking of crown by pressing an explorer on the occlusal aspect to apply load.
- Critical evaluation of blanching all around the tooth structure must be done, and a pre-cementation radiograph must be taken at this stage.

Crown Finishing

- The finishing of the margins of the crown form is done using a green stone held at angle to the margin.
- A slow speed handpiece will give better and produce a sharp feather edge margin that can be closely adapted to the prepared tooth at the gingival margin.

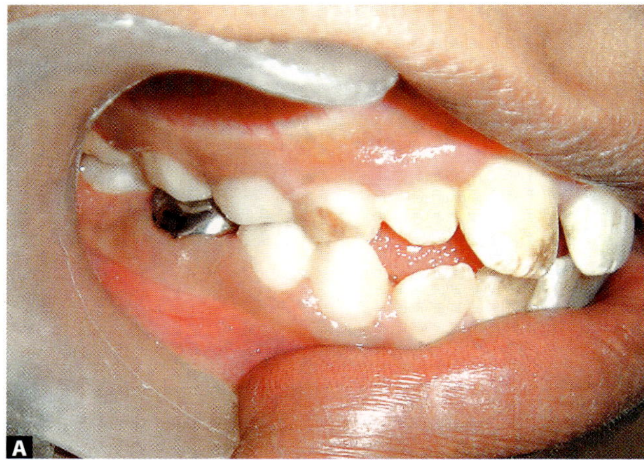

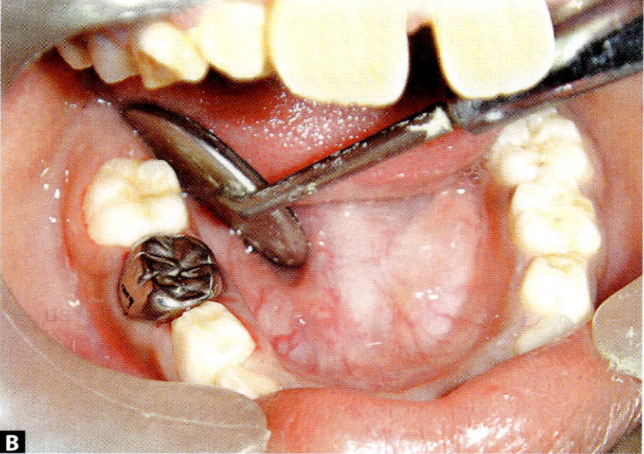

Figs. 48.15A and B: Final fit of stainless steel crowns: (A) Final occlusion; (B) Intraoral view of SSC.

- Crown is then smoothened with finishing burs and polished with rubber wheel or rouge.

Crown Cementation

- Remove, clean, and dry the crown as well as the tooth surface. Isolate with cotton and instruct the patient not to close the mouth.
- **Myers** (1983) has advocated the application of varnish before cementing crown especially in case of a vital tooth to prevent any postoperative sensitivity due to exposed tubules.
- Mix the luting cement and load onto the crown with the help of non-sticky instruments. At least two-third of the crown must be filled with the luting consistency of cement **(Fig. 48.16A)**.
- The commonly used cements are zinc phosphate, zinc oxide eugenol, reinforced zinc oxide eugenol, poly carboxylate cement and GICs.
- Seat the crown, usually first on the lingual side and then the buccal side at the same time supporting the child's mandible with one hand as you seat the crown. Ask the patient to bite slowly so as to seat the crown completely in accurate position.
- Remove excess cement with a scaler or explorer after it has set and gently but firmly check all the areas of the gingival sulcus for retained cement **(Fig. 48.16B)**.

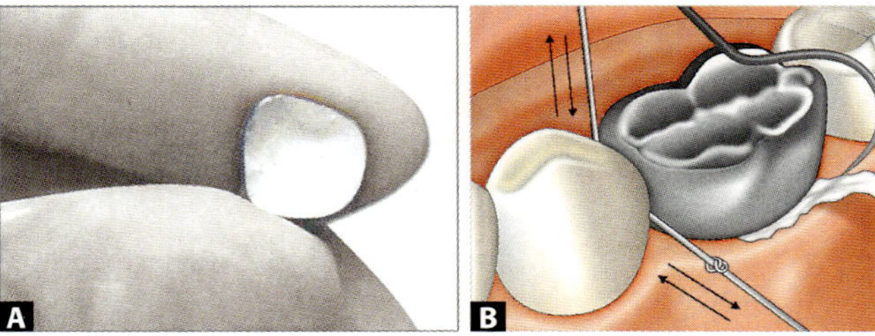

Figs. 48.16A and B: Cementation of crown: (A) Loading of crown for cementation; (B) Removal of excess cement.

Polishing of SSC and Discharge of Patient

- Polish the crown with acidulated phosphate fluoride prophylaxis paste prior to discharging the patient. It is best to evaluate the occlusion and fit again at this stage.
- After the cement sets, it is advisable to move a waxed floss in the interproximal aspect to check for any excess cement as it may cause irritation and inflammation of tissues.
- A completely cleaned, shining crown is shown to the child for appreciation and positive reinforcement.

CLINICAL MODIFICATIONS OF STAINLESS STEEL CROWNS

Pre-Veneered Stainless Steel Crowns

- **Lopez-Loverich et al** (2015) evaluated the retention of SSC versus preveneered crowns on primary anterior teeth and concluded that there was "good crown retention rates for both crown types with no statistically significant difference between them."
- *O'Connell et al (2014) evaluated the clinical performance of two brands of stainless steel veneered molar crowns after three years (NuSmile crowns and Kinder Krowns). The study found that the primary problem with resin-veneered crowns used in posterior primary molars was facing fracture. In addition, when the adjacent tooth was missing, fracture was more likely to occur, possibly due to the increased force of occlusion on the veneered crown.*

Adjacent Stainless Steel Crowns

- **Nash** described additional reduction of adjacent proximal surfaces of teeth when adjacent teeth are to be restored with SSC simultaneously.
- When more than one SSC needs to be done in a quadrant, one crown is finished and cemented before proceeding to next one because if both are prepared at one time, it might lead to encroachment of space for either one of them **(Fig. 48.17)**.

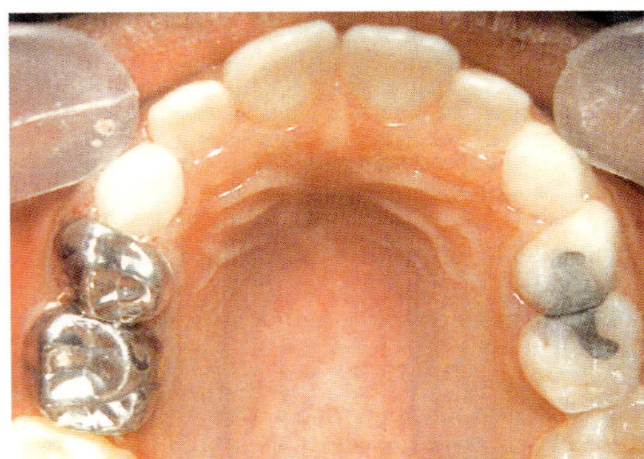

Fig. 48.17: Two adjacent crowns.

- When an SSC and a class II amalgam restoration are to be done at one appointment, the crown is finished first and then the restoration is done. After the crown is cemented, clean the excess cement from and around the crown. Adapt and wedge a matrix band and now insert an amalgam restoration. The SSC is used as guide in reproducing the anatomy and morphology of the silver amalgam restoration **(Fig. 48.18)**.

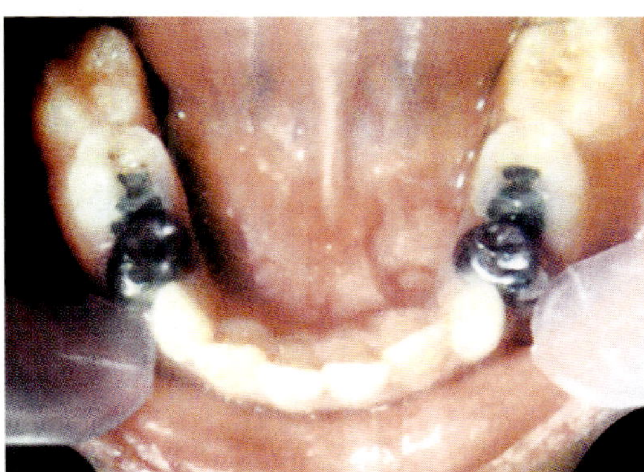

Fig. 48.18: Crown with amalgam restoration.

Adjacent Stainless Steel Crowns with Arch Length Loss

- Extensive and long-standing carious lesions can cause a shift of primary teeth into the interproximal contact areas. With this MD dimension loss, it is very difficult to restore the lost arch length.
- Usually, crowns will adjust to the tooth preparation individually but cannot be placed at the same time because of the mesial drift of the adjacent teeth. The crown preparations must be reduced further. Now flatten the contacts of the crowns by using the Hoe pliers **(Fig. 48.19)**.

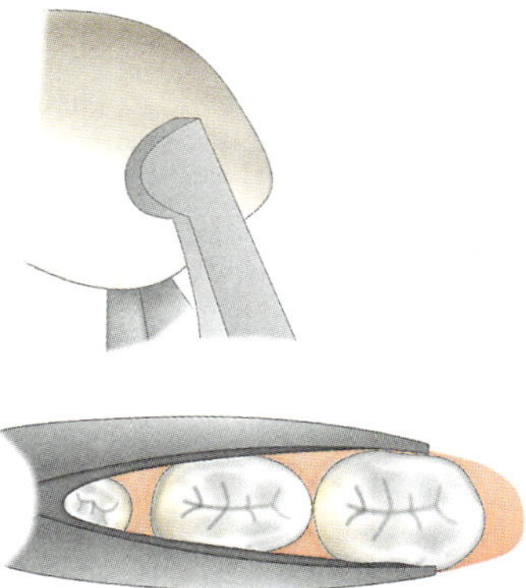

Fig. 48.19: Manipulation of crowns in arch length loss.

- **Myers** suggested modifications of SSC in the case of arch length loss where he told that more than usual reduction in the tooth to be crowned can be done so as to enable the crown to fit into the available MD space.

Oversized/Undersized Crown

Mink and **Hill**[9] described modification of crowns for smaller or larger teeth. A larger crown can be altered by cutting the edges, overlapping, and welding them to reduce the crown circumference so as to fit a smaller tooth **(Fig. 48.20)**.

Similarly, the circumference of a smaller crown can be increased to fit a larger tooth by cutting the edges and welding an additional piece of orthodontic band material **(Fig. 48.21)**.

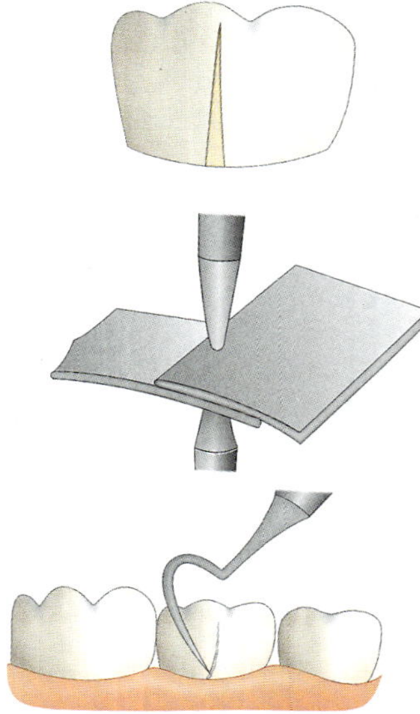

Fig. 48.20: Oversized crown.

Oversized Crown

Try the crown on the tooth
↓
Use a pair of scissors to cut the crown from the gingival to the occlusal surface, either buccally or lingually
↓
Pinch the crown together, in effect reducing the crown size
↓
Again, try the crown on the tooth. The gingival margins of the crown should approximate the gingival margins of the tooth
↓
The cut edges can then be repositioned and spot-welded
↓
Polish the soldered areas
↓
Check the crown for marginal adaptation, contour, crimp, and cement the crown

Undersized Crown

Check the crown on the tooth
↓
Cut a V-shaped groove in the crown on the buccal or lingual side
↓
Try the crown on the tooth for fit
↓
Spot-weld a strip of orthodontic band material over the V-shaped groove in the crown
↓
Retry the crown on the tooth
↓
Solder, adapt, contour, and crimp the crown
↓
Polish the soldered area and cement the crown

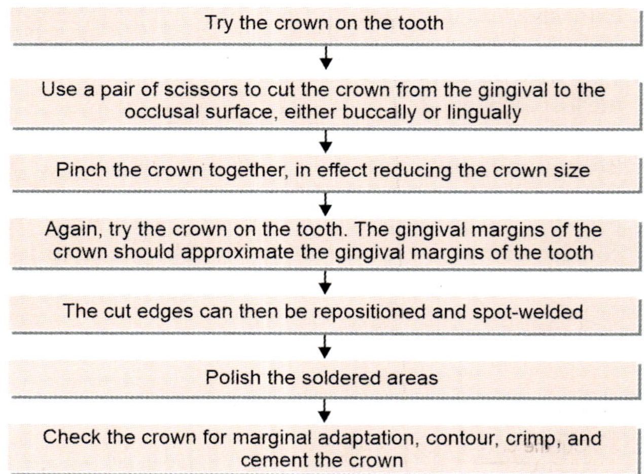

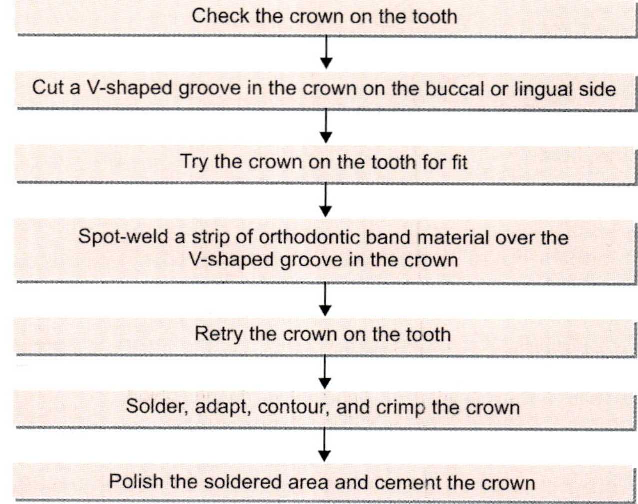

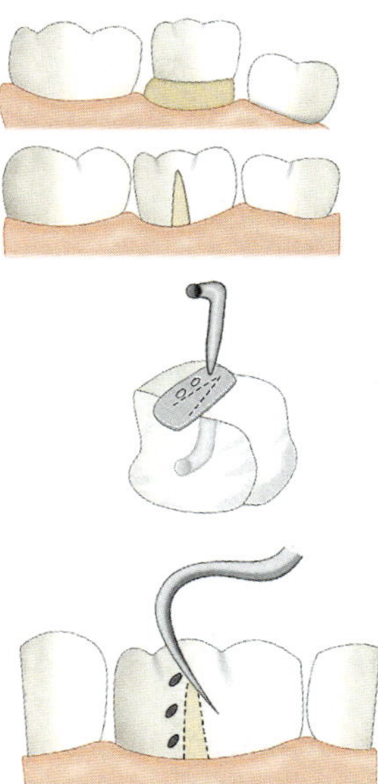

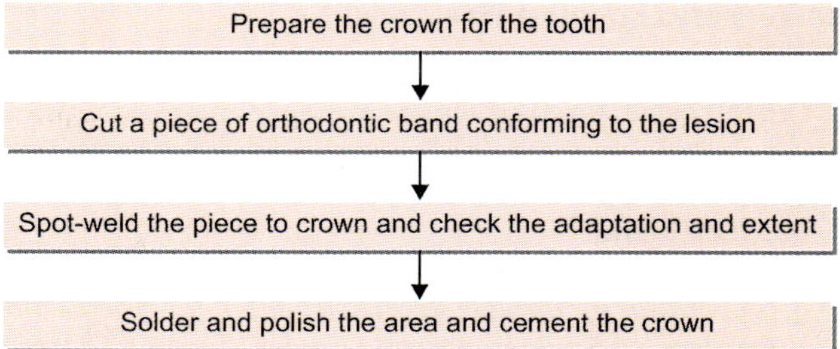

Fig. 48.21: Undersized crown.

Crown Extension for Deep Proximal Lesions

Prepare the crown for the tooth
↓
Cut a piece of orthodontic band conforming to the lesion
↓
Spot-weld the piece to crown and check the adaptation and extent
↓
Solder and polish the area and cement the crown

Other Suggested Modifications

- **Hartmann**[10] advocated esthetic modification of SSC by cutting away the labial metal, leaving a labial window that is restored with composite resin (CR). This restoration is called open-face SSC.
- **McEvoy**[11] recommended that primary maxillary first molar crown can be used to restore the morphologically altered primary mandibular first molar of the opposite side.
- **Croll**[12] described a technique of increasing the occlusal thickness of crown to compensate for the wear in children with grinding habits.
- In the cases of lower molar with lesser MD dimension, upper molar crown can be used as modification.
- **MS Duggal** concluded that the crown can be rotated mesiobuccally.

Consideration for successful use of SSC
- Removal of caries, and where needed, appropriate pulpal therapy.
- Optimum reduction of tooth structure for adequate crown retention.
- Lack of damage to adjacent teeth after opening interproximal contacts.
- Selection of appropriately sized crown to maintain arch length.
- Accurate marginal adaptation and gingival health.
- Good functional occlusion.
- Optimum cementation procedure.

Advantages of stainless steel crown

- Can be completed in a single appointment.
- Less time consuming than cast restorations.
- No need for laboratory procedures.
- Less sensitive to moisture.
- Less prone to fractures.
- Longevity.
- Durable as compared to multisurface restorations.
- Cost effective.
- Premature contacts are well tolerated by the child.
- Comfortable to the patient.

Disadvantages of stainless steel crown

- Significant amount of tooth structure is removed.
- Unesthetic.
- Poor marginal adaptation may cause gingivitis.
- Gingival inflammation due to excess unremoved cement.
- Over hanging distal margins may cause impaction of permanent first molars.

COMPLICATIONS ASSOCIATED WITH SSC

- **Interproximal ledge:** A ledge will be produced instead of a shoulder free interproximal slice if the angulation of the tapered fissure bur is incorrect.
  - Reason: Occurs if the angle of the tapered fissure bur is incorrect.
  - Result: Failure to remove the ledge causes difficulty in seating the crown.
  - Rectify: Extend the slice subgingivally by holding the thin tapered bur parallel to the long axis of the tooth.
  - Precaution: Interproximal slice is difficult when the adjacent tooth is partly erupted and in poorly established contact areas, in such a case, delay the crowning.
- **Crown tilt:** This is seen if complete lingual or buccal wall is destructed by caries or improper use of cutting instrument. The disadvantage of this is that supraeruption of the opposing tooth may occur.
  - Reason: Destruction of buccal or lingual wall by caries or over instrumentation.
  - Result: Tilting occurs towards the deficient side.
  - Rectify: Placement of amalgam alloy or GIC prior to crowning.
  - Clinical significance: Supraeruption of the opposing tooth may occur.
- **Poor margins:** When the crown is poorly adapted, its marginal integrity is reduced. This can lead to recurrent caries, plaque accumulation and subsequent gingivitis.
- **Inhalation or ingestion of crown:** This may happen because of slippage from hand or by jerky reaction of patient. If this occurs, attempt can be made to remove the crown by holding the child upside down as soon as possible. If this is unsuccessful, medical referral should be done for an immediate chest X-ray to verify if the crown is in lungs or in alimentary tract.
- **Overextension of crown:**
  - Reason: Insufficient trimming of crown.
  - Result: Identified with gingival blanching leading to loss of periodontal attachment and periodontal problems due to food lodgment.
  - Rectify: By identifying adequate 1 mm gingival extension of the crown margin, scratching the line, trimming the excess and crimping followed by polishing.

LONGEVITY OF STAINLESS STEEL CROWNS

Study	*Multisurface amalgam teeth number*	*Multisurface amalgam teeth failure*	*PMC teeth number*	*PMC teeth failure*	*Duration (years)*
Braff (1975)	150	131 (87%)	76	19 (25%)	2.5
Dawson (1981)	102	72 (71%)	64	8 (13%)	2
Messer et al (1988)	1177	255 (22%)	331	40 (12%)	5
Roberts (1990)	706	82 (12%)	673	13 (2%)	10
Einwag (1996)	66	38 (58%)	66	4 (6%)	8
Total	2201	578 (26%)	1210	84 (7%)	5

Summary of Crown Placement Procedure (Fig. 48.22)

Select a crown according to mesiodistal diameter
↓
Pick the crown with the help of sterile tweezers or thumb forceps
↓
Evaluate the occlusion
↓
Administration of local anesthesia
↓
Occlusal reduction of 1.0 to 1.5 mm with pear-shaped bur
↓
Proximal reduction with needle-shaped bur break contact and establish 2 to 5 taper
↓
Reduce and round off all line angles with finishing burs
↓
Verify the occlusion and proximal contacts
↓
Attachment of floss to crown by glue
↓
Try the crown on the tooth
↓
Festooning on the proximal surface should be performed
↓
Place the crown
↓
Scratch around the gingival margin on the crown or mark with a glass marking pencil
↓
Cut the crown 1 mm below the scratch line with scissors
↓
Smoothen the edges with finishing burs
↓
Contour the crown
↓
Crimping of the crown in the gingival third
↓
Finish the margins of the crown using a green stone to produce a sharp feather-edge margin
↓
Crown is smoothened with finishing burs
↓
Polished with rubber wheel or rouge
↓
Precementation radiograph
↓
Mix and load luting cement onto the crown
↓
Seat the crown and ask the patient to bite slowly
↓
Remove excess cement
↓
Polish the crown with acidulated phosphate fluoride prophylaxis paste

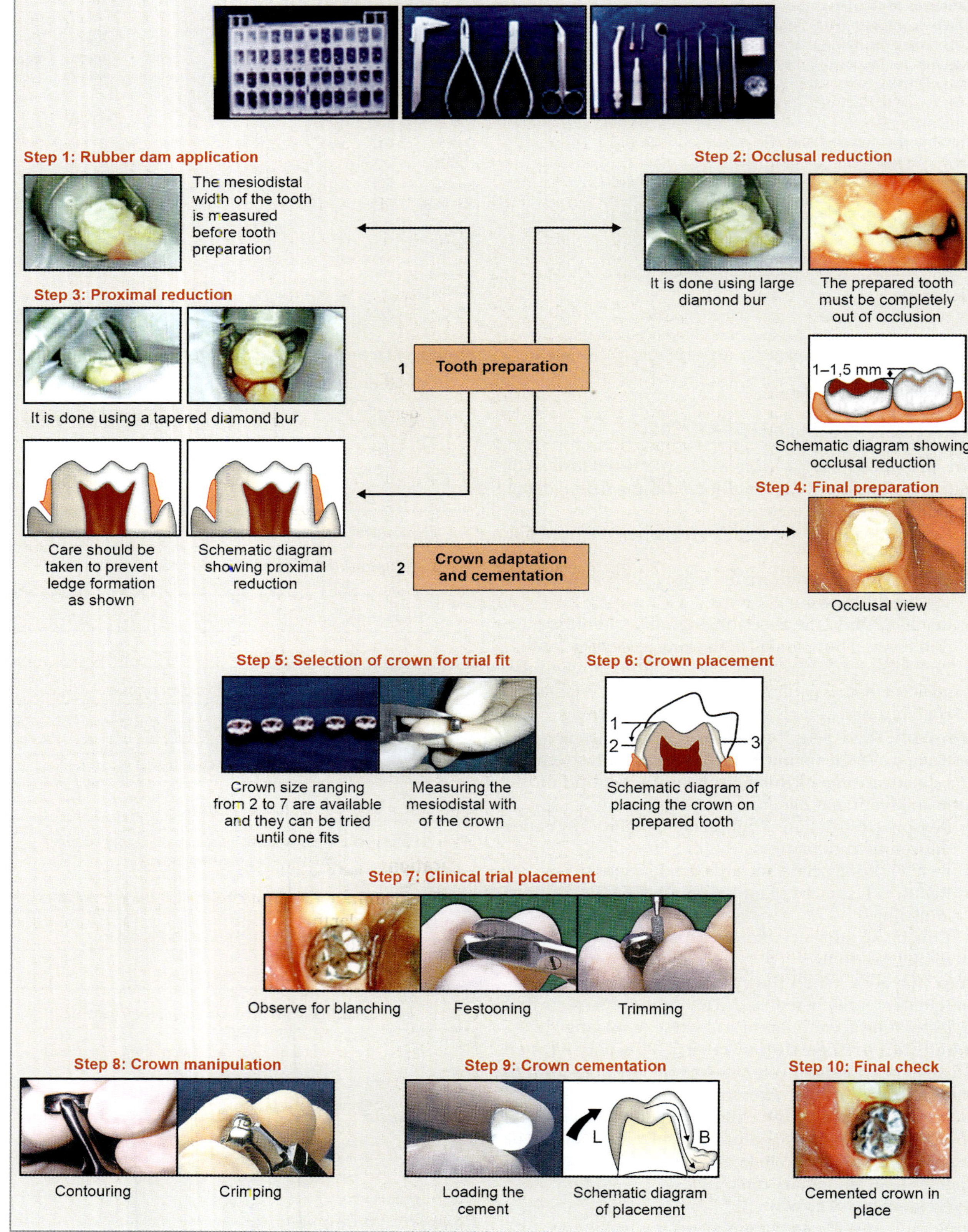
Step 1: Rubber dam application
The mesiodistal width of the tooth is measured before tooth preparation
Step 2: Occlusal reduction
It is done using large diamond bur
The prepared tooth must be completely out of occlusion
Step 3: Proximal reduction
It is done using a tapered diamond bur
1
Tooth preparation
1–1,5 mm
Schematic diagram showing occlusal reduction
Step 4: Final preparation
Care should be taken to prevent ledge formation as shown
Schematic diagram showing proximal reduction
2
Crown adaptation and cementation
Occlusal view
Step 5: Selection of crown for trial fit
Step 6: Crown placement
1
2
3
Crown size ranging from 2 to 7 are available and they can be tried until one fits
Measuring the mesiodistal with of the crown
Schematic diagram of placing the crown on prepared tooth
Step 7: Clinical trial placement
Observe for blanching
Festooning
Trimming
Step 8: Crown manipulation
Step 9: Crown cementation
Step 10: Final check
L
B
Contouring
Crimping
Loading the cement
Schematic diagram of placement
Cemented crown in place

Fig. 48.22: Step-wise stainless steel crown preparation.

Research pertaining to use of SSC

- A comparative review by **Randall**[13] encompassing five clinical studies on the performance of SSCs with that of multisurface amalgam restorations concluded that the crowns were superior to multisurface amalgam restorations.
- **Seale**[14] compiled scientific evidence favoring the SSC as restoration of choice in children with high-risk for caries.
- **Rector**[15] and **Noffsinger**[16] confirmed that the cement retention of the crown is critical than mechanical retention. However, clinical studies are not available to determine the differences, if any, between various types of cement as well as types of preparation.
- **Ludwig et al**[17] (2014) compared the clinical and radiographic success of SSC used to restore primary molars with caries lesions, placed by means of both the traditional technique (involving complete caries removal and tooth reduction before placement of the SSC) and the Hall technique (involving no caries removal, no crown preparation, and no use of local anesthetic before placement of the SSC) and showed similar success rate for SSC placed with the traditional technique or the Hall technique.
- **Memarpour et al**[18] (2015) studied that when SSC margins overlaid the restoration materials, cavity restoration with amalgam or GIC before SSC placement led to less microleakage and material loss.
- **Afshar et al**[19] (2015) did a study to compare the buccolingual (BL) and MD dimensions of primary molars with those of SSC in an Iranian population and observed that best adaptation was seen in second lower molars, and the least adaptations were seen in first and second upper molars.
- **Prabhakar et al**[20] (2017) compared the effectiveness of preformed zirconia crowns with the gold standard SSC for the restoration of primary teeth through a finite element analysis and concluded that even at maximal physiologic masticatory force levels, a grossly destructed tooth restored with preformed zirconia crown can with stand stress better than a tooth restored with SSC.
- **Ushton et al**[21] (2011) explored the use of the SSC in dentistry today. They reviewed the indications, techniques for placement, advantages, and drawbacks when compared to alternative restorative materials and concluded that regardless of personal opinion, the SSC should continue to be recognized for its efficiency, cost-effectiveness, and successful treatment modality.
- **Mata et al**[22] (2006) evaluated amalgam restorations versus SSCs in the primary dentition. The scientific literature provides evidence that SSCs demonstrate greater longevity and reduced need for retreatment, compared to multisurface amalgam restorations. There is high-level evidence for the use of SSCs because of their cost-effectiveness, ease of placement, and longevity.
- **Pathak et al**[23] (2016) compared the retentive strength of two dual-polymerized self-adhesive resin cements (RelyX U200, 3M ESPE and Smart Cem2, Dentsply Caulk) and a resin-modified glass ionomer cement (RMGIC; RelyX Luting2, 3M ESPE) on SSC. They concluded that retentive strength of dual-polymerized self-adhesive resin cements was better than RMGIC, and Rely XU200 significantly improved crown retention when compared with Smart Cem2 and RelyX Luting2.
- **Subramaniam et al**[24] (2010) evaluated and compared the retentive strength of three luting cements and concluded that retentive strength of adhesive resin cement and RMGIC was significantly higher than that of the conventional GIC.
- **Veerabadhran et al**[25] (2012) conducted a study to find out the effect of retentive groove, sandblasting, and cement type on the retentive strength of SSCs in primary second molars. It was found that the crowns luted with RMGIC offered better retentive strength of crowns than GICs and SSCs which were cemented without sandblasting showed higher mean retentive strength than with sandblasting of crowns. The presence of groove did not influence the retentive strength of SSCs.
- **Yilmaz et al**[26] (2011) did a study to determine the wear of SSCs in children and compare the extent of microleakage in SSCs that had been repaired using either a cermet GIC or a packable CR and concluded that the occlusal surfaces of SSCs for first and second primary molars display wear. Although perforated SSCs can be repaired using either a cermet GIC or a packable CR, less microleakage occurs in SSCs that were repaired with a cermet GIC than those with a packable CR.
- **Einwag et al**[27] (1996) evaluated that two alternative methods of restoring primary teeth that had multisurface lesions were examined in a clinical longitudinal study. In a paired comparison, SSCs proved far superior to multisurface amalgam restorations with respect to both lifespan and replacement rate. SSCs are not only more acceptable to the patient and more cost-effective but also more acceptable to the dentist because of the comparatively simple procedures involved in restoring even severely affected primary molars.

HALL TECHNIQUE FOR PLACEMENT OF STAINLESS STEEL CROWNS

- The Hall technique is a conservative alternative treatment for carious primary molars named after **Dr Norna Hall**, a general dental practitioner from Scotland, who developed and used the technique for over 15 years until she retired in 2006.[28]
- The Hall technique involves the use of SSC to seal over caries lesions on primary molars by using glass ionomer cement; it involves no caries removal, no crown preparation and no administration of local anesthetic.
- Restoring the carious primary molar in children using the "Hall technique (HT)" is an internationally controversial but evidence-based new treatment modality. It started in the United Kingdom (UK) in 2007 where it is now considered the "Gold Standard" for managing the multi-surface asymptomatic carious primary molars.
- Hall technique was introduced to the undergraduate Pediatric Dentistry curriculum in 2010 in UK and New Zealand dental schools, and in some dental schools across Europe.

Indications

- The main indication for the Hall technique is caries in a primary molar that does not extend further than the middle third of dentin and that has no signs or symptoms of pulpal involvement.
- A recent radiograph of the tooth must show a clear band of dentin between the advancing decay and the pulp and there must be no evidence of inter-radicular radiolucency.
- Class I lesion, non-cavitated, if patient unable to accept fissure sealant.
- Conventional restoration Class I lesion, cavitated, if patient unable to accept partial caries removal technique.
- Conventional restoration Class II lesions, cavitated or non-cavitated.

Contraindications

- The Hall technique is contraindicated where a tooth is so broken down as to be unrestorable with a PMC; if there is no obvious clear band of dentin evident on the radiograph; or if there is any evidence, radiographically or clinically, of irreversible pulpitis.

- Teeth with signs or symptoms of irreversible pulpitis, or dental sepsis (pulpal pathosis).
- Teeth with clinical or radiographic signs of pulpal exposure, or periradicular pathology.
- Patients at risk of infective endocarditis.

Clinical Procedure

- **Armamentarium**
  - Mirror.
  - Straight probe to remove separators, if used.
  - Excavator to remove crown if necessary, and useful for cement removal.
  - Flat plastic carrier to load crown with cement.
  - Cotton rolls for child to bite down on and push crown over tooth, and to wipe away cement.
  - Band forming pliers can be useful for adjusting crowns, particularly where the primary molar has lost length mesiodistally due to caries.
  - Gauze to protect the airway and wipe off excess cement.
  - Elastoplast to secure the crown for airway protection.
- **Clinical steps**
  - **Assessing the tooth shape, contact points/areas and the occlusion**
    - *Tight contact points, and their management with separators*
      - Hall crowns can often be fitted successfully to primary molars which are in contact with adjacent teeth, as there is some elasticity in the periodontal ligament which can absorb the displacement necessary to fit the crown. However, much depends on the willingness of the child to bite the crown into place, and on the shape of the contact point.
      - Some teeth have very broad contact points, which can make fitting crowns difficult. In such cases, placing orthodontic separators through the mesial and distal contacts can be useful when fitting crowns with the Hall technique, although it does mean the patient will have to make a second visit.
      - Two lengths of dental floss should be threaded through the separator. The separator should then be stretched taut, and "flossed" through the contact point briskly and firmly until the leading edge only is felt "popping through" the contact point. The floss should then be removed, and the patient seen 3 to 5 days later for removal of the separator **(Figs. 48.23A to C)**.

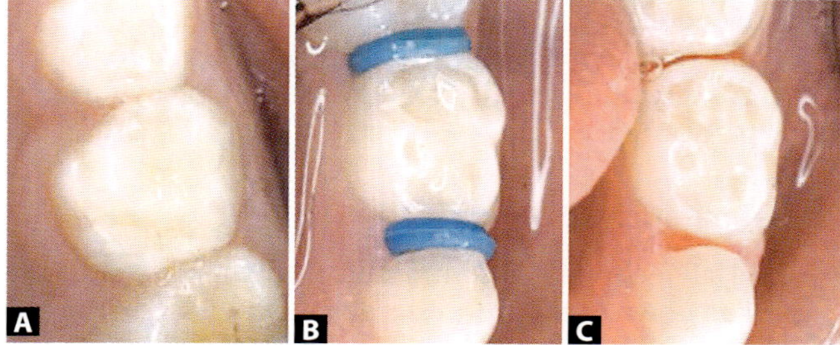

Figs. 48.23A to C: Use of separators to create space for SSC in tight contacts: (A) Tight contacts; (B) Placement of separators; (C) Spacing in the proximal aspect post-separator removal.

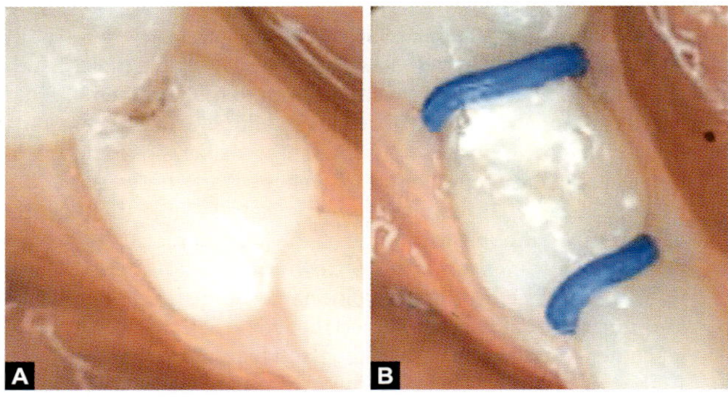

Figs. 48.24A and B: Excavation of a distal cavity on a mandibular first primary molar is followed by placement of a celluloid matrix strip and a temporary dressing, allowing separators to be placed 10 minutes later.

    - *Crown morphology and marginal ridge breakdown*
      - Often where there is marginal ridge breakdown in one molar, there can be migration of the adjacent molar into the cavitated area. The picture below shows an example of this. If the missing tooth walls are imagined, they will be seen to overlap. This can make placing a Hall crown difficult without making some adjustments to the tooth itself or the crown.
      - One way to solve this issue is placement of a temporary restoration to rebuild the marginal ridge and allow a separator to be placed to make space for the crown to be fitted **(Figs. 48.24A and B)**.
      - Second method is by adjusting the crown with band forming pliers being used to adjust the crown margins and the effect of rotating them 180 degrees to "pinch in" a concavity to accommodate the intruding marginal ridge of an adjacent tooth.
      - Trying a different crown.
      - Carrying out some tooth preparation; however, this will usually require the use of local anesthesia
    - *Assessing the occlusion*
      - Before fitting a Hall crown, firstly we must measure the anterior overbite in order to assess the degree of propping of the bite following fitting of the crown and secondly to check the buccal relationship of the tooth to be crowned with its opposing number to ensure there is no laterally displacing contact following fitting of the crown.
- **Protecting the airway**
  - It is also important, before the crown is placed, to ensure there will be no danger of the child inhaling or swallowing a loose crown (the same precautions as should be taken when fitting a conventional crown).
  - This is most easily done by sitting the child upright.
  - However, for maxillary teeth, working with the child seated upright means that the optimum operator working position has to be compromised. For mandibular teeth, the operator can simply move to the front or side of the child.
  - A gauze swab square can be placed between the tongue and the tooth where the crown is to be fitted. It should extend to the palate and round the back of the mouth in front of the fauces **(Fig. 48.25A)**.

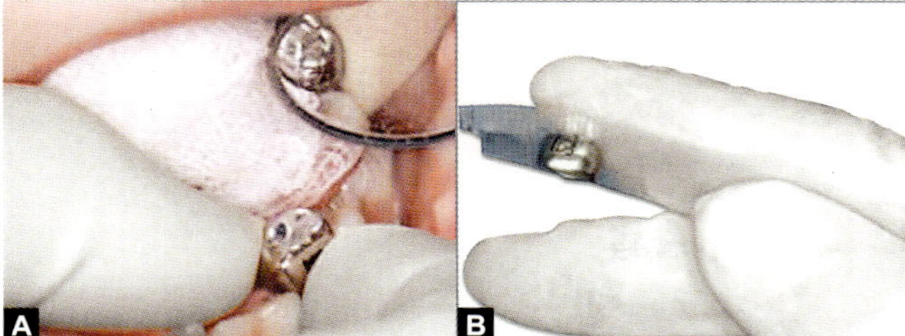

Figs. 48.25A and B: Airway protection: (A) Use of gauze; (B) Use of micropore tape.

- A piece of micropore tape, doubled back on itself for part of its length, can be used to secure the crown **(Fig. 48.25B)**.

❖ **Sizing a crown**
- Select different sizes o f crowns until you find one which covers all the cusps, and approaches the contact points, with a slight feeling of "spring back" **(Fig. 48.26).**
- You should aim to fit the smallest size of crown which will seat.
- Do not be tempted to fully seat the crown through the contact points before cementation; they can be very difficult to remove.

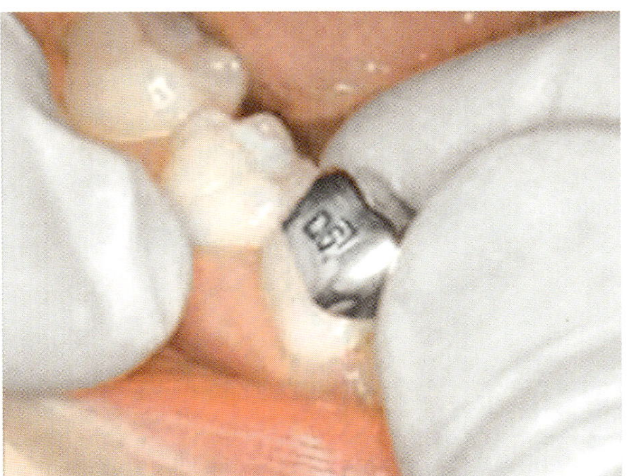

Fig. 48.26: Sizing the crown.

❖ **Loading the crown with cement**
- Following try in, dry the inside of the crown, using the end of a cotton roll.
- Load the crown generously (it should be at least two thirds full) with a glass ionomer luting cement. Take care fill the crown from the base upwards and ensure that there is cement around all the walls. Be careful to avoid air blows and voids **(Fig. 48.27).**

❖ **Fitting the crown, and first stage seating**
- Place the crown over the tooth.
- Some clinicians will seat the crown with firm finger pressure alone. For mandibular teeth, a useful method is to place your thumb on the occlusal surface of the crown, with the four fingers of your hand placed under the border of the mandible to spread the force as you apply firm pressure with your thumb. For maxillary teeth, the child's head may be supported by the back of the dental chair, or sometimes by placing your other forearm gently on the top of their head to balance the force applied when fitting the crown **(Fig. 48.28)**.

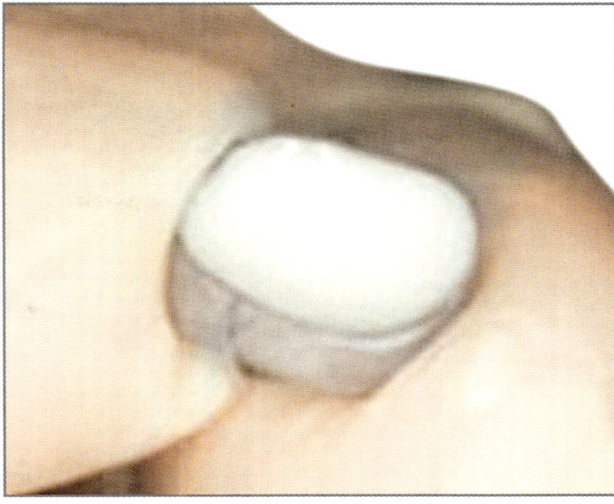

Fig. 48.27: Loading the crown.

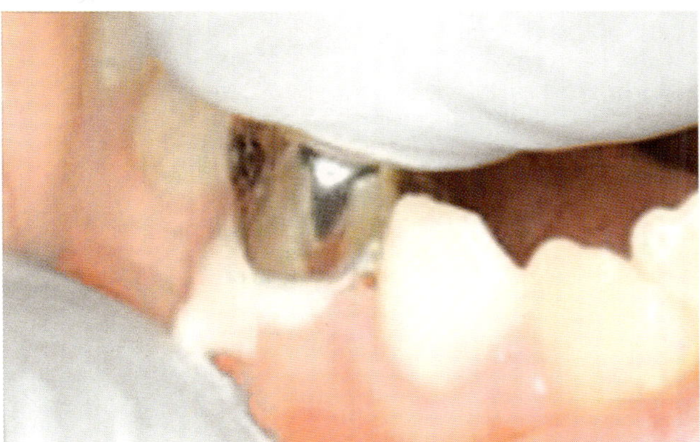

Fig. 48.28: Fitting of crown.

- Some clinicians partially seat the crown until it engages with the contact points, allowing the finger to be removed without risk of the crown falling off, and the child then being encouraged to bite the crown into place.

❖ **Wipe the excess cement away, check fit and second stage seating**
- As soon as the crown is fitted, the child should be asked to open to allow the crown position to be checked and excess glass ionomer can be wiped away.
- If the crown is fitting satisfactorily, the child should be asked to bite firmly on the crown for 2–3 minutes, or the crown should be held down with firm finger pressure as an alternative. Often the crown will seat a little further, expressing more cement. This is possibly due to accommodation to the displacing pressure by the adjacent teeth **(Fig. 48.29).**

❖ **Final clearance of cement, check occlusion**
- Remove excess cement, flossing between the contacts **(Fig. 48.30A)**.
- Blanching usually disappears within minutes **(Fig. 48.30B)**.
- The occlusal discrepancy should resolve in a few weeks.

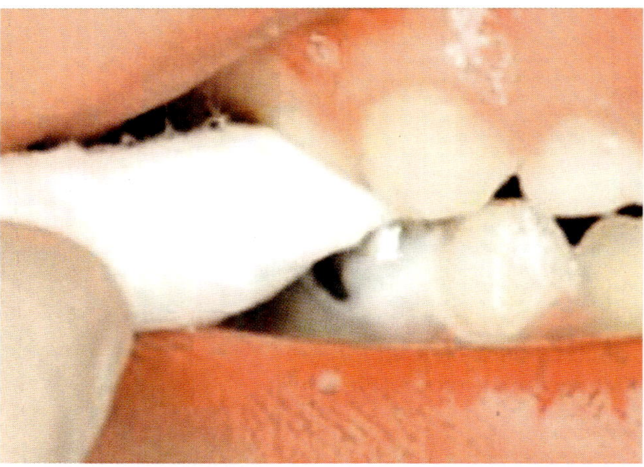

Fig. 48.29: Second stage seating.

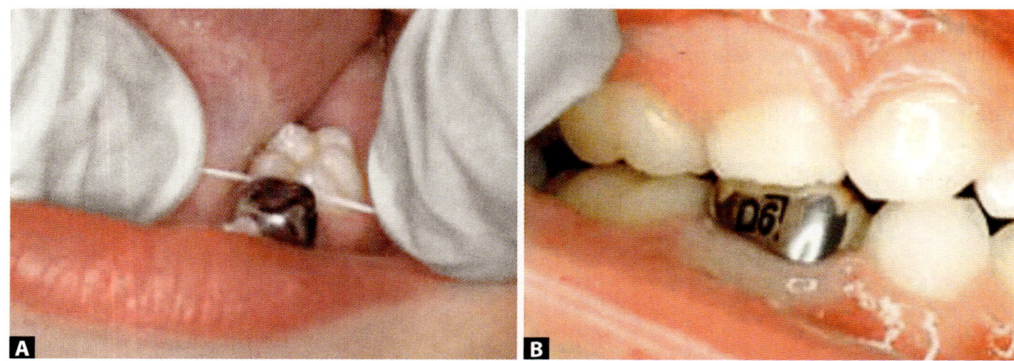

Figs. 48.30A and B: (A) Removal of excess cement with floss; (B) Final occlusion and check.

Advantages

- ❖ Improve compliance in young children and reduce anxiety associated with dental treatment.
- ❖ Increase the use of SSC by clinicians.
- ❖ Avoid negative child health impacts and costs of repeat treatment.
- ❖ Reduce tooth extractions and extensive treatment.
- ❖ In conjunction with a preventive program.

Special considerations for Hall technique

- Hall crowns should not be fitted to opposing (occluding) teeth at the same appointment. The occlusion should have re-established, with bilateral contacts, before opposing crowns are fitted.
- However, if a primary molar on either side of the same arch or diagonally opposite teeth in different arches, i.e., a maxillary left primary molar and a mandibular right primary molar, then these can be fitted at the same appointment
- It is usually not possible to fit a crown using the Hall technique to both primary molars in the same quadrant at the same appointment; adjacent primary molars requiring Hall crowns should have them fitted at separate appointments.
- If the crown does not seat sufficiently, then remove it using the excavator before the cement sets.
- The Hall technique is not a "fit and forget" technique. Patients should be reviewed on a normal recall schedule, with radiographic examination in line with current recommendations, and the Hall technique should be used in conjunction with a full preventive program.

Research studies regarding Hall technique

- **Clark et al** (2017) study provides evidence of high clinical and radiographic success rates for SSCs placed on primary molars with the Hall technique.
- **Boyd et al** (2018) concluded that there was a much higher success rate in the children treated with Hall technique than plastic restorative material
- **Ludwig et al** (2014) evaluated that similar success rate for SSCs placed with the traditional technique or the Hall technique.
- **Roberts A et al** (2018) concluded that Hall technique was widely used among specialist pediatric dentists in the UK.

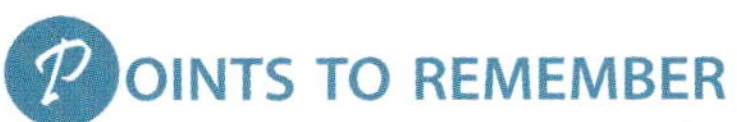

POINTS TO REMEMBER

- Stainless steel crowns can be defined as prefabricated crown forms that are adapted to individual teeth and cemented with a biocompatible luting agent.
- Humphrey was the one who popularized SSC.
- Mink and Bennett gave the method of tooth and crown preparation for SSC.
- Indications of SSC include extensive caries, rampant caries, after pulp therapy, acquired enamel defects, intermediate restoration, fractures of permanent and primary incisors, severe bruxism, abutment teeth to prosthesis, and as part of a space maintainer.
- Stainless steel crowns can be divided according to trimming, composition, company, position, and occlusal anatomy. Untrimmed crowns are neither trimmed nor contoured, e.g., the Rocky Mountains; pretrimmed crowns are non-contoured but are festooned, e.g., 3 M; pre-contoured crowns are festooned and precontoured, e.g., Ni-Chro Ion crowns.
- Hall method of SSCs placement is based on no cutting approach and was named after Dr Norna Hall. It is mainly indicated in class I noncavitated lesion where in the child is unable to accept fissure sealant. It involves selection of smallest crown that covers all the surfaces, and its directly fitting it onto the tooth without any tooth or crown preparation. Convention procedure for placement of SSC involves occlusal reduction, proximal reduction, finishing, and rounding of all sharp margins, trimming of crown, festooning, contouring, crimping, and cementation.
- Occlusal reduction is done with pear-shaped bur, and about 1.0–1.5 mm reduction is done uniformly along the cuspal structure.
- Proximal reduction is done to create a 2–5° taper and break contact. Contouring is done with the help of No. 114 Johnson contouring pliers.
- Crimping is done using the No. 417 crimping pliers where in the crown is crimped in the gingival third. The uses of crimping are protection of soft tissues, prevention of leakage of cements, prevention of contamination, and adequate retention.
- Complications of SSCs are interproximal ledge formation, crown tilt, poor margins, inhalation, or ingestion of crown.

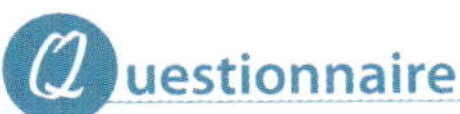

Questionnaire

1. Give the indication and classification of stainless steel crown.
2. What is Hall's approach for placement of stainless steel crown?
3. Describe in detail the procedure of stainless steel crown placement.
4. How is crimping accomplished and what are its uses?
5. Explain the modifications of stainless steel crown.
6. What are the complications associated with stainless steel crown?

REFERENCES

1. Pokorney RL. Stainless steel preformed crowns. Rev Dent Lib. 1965;15:20-6.
2. Humphrey WP. Use of chromic steel in children's dentistry. Dent Surv. 1950;26:945-7.
3. Engel RJ. Chrome steel as used in children's dentistry. Chron Omaha Dist Dent Soc. 1950;13:255-8.
4. Academy of Pediatric Dentistry. Specialissue. Reference Manual. 2020;21:105.
5. Mink JR, Bennett IC. The stainless steel crown. J Dent Child. 1968;35:186.
6. Rapp R. A simplified yet precise technique for the placement of stainless steel crowns on primary teeth. J Dent Child. 1966;33:101.
7. Myers DR. The restoration of primary molars with stainless steel crown. J Dent Child. 1976;43:406-9.
8. Spedding RH. Two principles for improving the adaptation of stainless steel crowns to primary molars. Dent Clin North Am. 1984;28(1):157-75.
9. Mink JR, Hill CJ. Modifications of stainless steel crown forprimary teeth. J Dent Child. 1971;38:197-205.
10. Hartmann CR. The open-face stainless steel crown: anesthetic technique. J Dent Child. 1983;50:31-3.
11. McEvoy SA. Approximating stainless steel crowns in space-lossquadrants. J Dent Child. 1977;44:105-7.
12. Croll TP. Increasing occlusal surface thickness of stainless steel crowns: a clinical technique. Pediatr Dent. 1982;2(4):297-9.
13. Randall RC. Preformed metal crowns for primary and permanent molar teeth: review of the literature. Pediatr Dent. 2002;24:489-500.
14. Seale NS. The use of stainless steel crowns. Pediatr Dent. 2002;24: 501-5.
15. Rector. JA, Mitchell RJ, Spedding RH. The influence of tooth preparation and crown manipulation on the mechanical retention of SS crowns. J Dent Child. 1985;52:422-7.
16. Noffsinger DP, Jedrychowski JR, Caputo AA. Effect of polycarboxylate and glass ionomer cements on stainless steel crown retention. J Pediatr Dent. 1983;5:68-71.
17. Ludwig KH, Fontana M, Vinson LA, et al. The success of stainless steel crowns placed with the Hall technique. A retrospective study. JADA. 2014;145:1248-53.
18. Memarpour M, Derafshi R, Razavi M. Comparison of microleakage from stainless steel crowns margins used with different restorative materials: an in vitro study. Dent Res J. 2016;13:7-12.
19. Afshar H, Sabeti AK, Shahrabi M. Comparison of primary molar crown dimensions with stainless steel crowns in a sample of Iranian children. J Dent Res Dent Clin Dent Prospect. 2015;9:86-91.
20. Prabhakar AR, Chakraborty A, Nadig B, et al. Finite element stress analysis of restored primary teeth: a comparative evaluation between stainless steel crowns and preformed zirconia crowns. Int J Oral Health Sci. 2017;7:10-5.
21. Ushton KA, Estrella MR. The stainless steel crown debate: friend or foe? J Mich Dent Assoc. 2011;93:42-6.
22. Mata AF, Bebermeyer RD. Stainless steel crowns versus amalgams in the primary dentition and decision-making inclinical practice. Gen Dent. 2006;54:347-50.
23. Pathak S, Shashibhushan KK, Poornima P, et al. In vitro evaluation of stainless steel crowns cemented with resin-modified glass ionomer and two new self-adhesive resin cements. Int J Clin Pediatr Dent. 2016;9:197-200.
24. Subramaniam P, Kondae S, Gupta KK. Retentive strength ofluting cements for stainless steel crowns: an in vitro study. J Clin Pediatr Dent. 2010;34:309-12.
25. Veerabadhran MM, Reddy V, Nayak UA, et al. The effect of retentive groove, sand blasting and cement type on the retentive strength of stainless steel crowns in primary second molars --an in vitro comparative study. J Indian Soc Pedod Prev Dent. 2012; 30:19-26.
26. Yilmaz Y, Kara NB, Yilmaz A, et al. Wear and repair of stainless steel crowns. Eur J Paediatr Dent. 2011;12:25-30.
27. Einwag J, Dünninger P. Stainless steel crown versus multisurface amalgam restorations: an 8-year longitudinal clinical study. Quintessence Int. 1996;27:321-3.
28. The hall technique manual Scottish dental. www.scottishdental.org/index.

FURTHER READING

1. Boyd DH, Page LF, Thomson WM. The Hall technique and conventional restorative treatment in New Zealand children's primary oral health care--clinical outcomes at two years. International Journal of Paediatric Dentistry. 2018;28(2):180-8.
2. Calache H, Martin R. The Hall Technique--A Minimally Invasive, Anxiety Reducing Method of Managing Dental Caries in Primary Molars.
3. Clark W, Geneser M, Owais A, Kanellis M, Qian F. Success rates of Hall technique crowns in primary molars: a retrospective pilot study. Gen Dent. 2017;65(5):32-5
4. Clemens A, Walkar D, Pinkham JR. Stainless steel crown for deciduous molars. JADA. 1974;89:360-4.
5. Fuks AB, Ram D, Eidelman E. Clinical performance of esthetic posterior crowns in primary molars: a pilot study. Pediatr Dent.1999;2:445-8.
6. Goldberg NL. The stainless steel crowns in pediatric dentistry. Dent Dig. 1969;75:351-5.
7. Helm HW. Simplified procedure for stainless steel crowns in pedodontics. J Can Dent Assoc. 1963;29:369.
8. Henderson HZ. Evaluation of the preformed stainless steel crown. J Dent Child. 1973;40:353-8.
9. Innes NPT, Stirrups DR, Evans DJP, et al. A novel technique using preformed metal crowns for man aging carious primary molars in general practice --a retrospective analysis. Br Dent J.2006;200:451-4.
10. Kennedy DB. The stainless steel crown. In: Kennedy DB (Ed). Pediatric operative dentistry. Bristol: J Wright and Sons Ltd.;1976.
11. Kumar A, Gupta H, Yadav CS, Rastogi S. The hall technique in paediatric dentistry: a review of the literature and an "all hall" case report with a-24 month follow up. Sultan Qaboos University Medical Journal. 2013;13(3):368-70.
12. Ludwig KH, Fontana M, Vinson LA, Platt JA, Dean JA. The success of stainless steel crowns placed with the Hall technique: a retrospective study. The Journal of the American Dental Association. 2014;145(12):1248-53.
13. Roberts A, McKay A, Albadri S. The use of Hall technique preformed metal crowns by specialist paediatric dentists in the UK. British Dental Journal. 2018;224(1):48.
14. Troutman KC, Reisbick MH. Steel crowns. In: Stewart RE, Barber TK, Troutman KC, Wei SHY (Eds). Pediatric dentistry: scientific foundations and clinical practice. St. Louis: CV Mosby Co.; 1982.
15. Wei SHY. Stainless steel crowns. Pediatric dentistry: total patient care. Philadelphia: Leas and Febiger; 1988.

CHAPTER

Esthetic Crowns in Pediatric Dentistry

Ravi GR, Nikhil Marwah, Suzan Sahana, Mukul Jain, Amol Patil

Chapter Outline

- Facial Cutout Stainless Steel Crowns
- Pre-veneered Stainless Steel Crowns
- Cheng Crowns
- Dura Crowns
- Kinder Krowns
- Pedo Pearls
- Polycarbonate Crowns
- Strip Crowns
- Shell Crowns
- Pedo Jacket Crowns
- Art Glass Crowns
- Figaro Crowns
- Edelweiss Pediatric Crowns
- Zirconia Crowns
- Bioflex Crowns

The healthy oral cavity is a primary requisite for beautiful looks. Despite the fact that it is largely preventable, dental caries is the most common chronic disease of childhood. Clinical examination of early childhood caries (ECC) discloses a distinctive pattern, and the teeth most often involved are the maxillary central incisors, lateral incisors, and the maxillary and mandibular first primary molars. The maxillary primary incisors are the most severely affected with deep carious lesions usually involving the pulp. In extreme cases, ECC can even lead to total loss of the crown structure. The early loss of primary anterior teeth may result in reduced masticatory efficiency, loss of vertical dimension, development of parafunctional habits (tongue thrusting, speech problems), esthetic-functional problems such as malocclusion and space loss, and psychologic problems that can interfere in the personality and behavioral development of the child. In addition, trauma to primary anterior teeth can result in displacement injuries such as luxation, uncomplicated or complicated crown fractures, or discoloration of teeth. In any of these clinical situations, parents often seek for esthetic rehabilitation of the primary teeth of their children.

Esthetic requirement of severely mutilated primary anterior teeth in the case of early childhood caries has been a challenge to pediatric dentist. In the last half century, the emphasis on treatment of extensively decayed primary teeth shifted from extraction to restoration. Early restorations consisted of placement of stainless steel bands or crowns on severely decayed teeth. While functional, they were unesthetic and their use was limited to posterior teeth. Over the last two decades, there has been an explosive interest by adults in esthetic restoration of their compromised dentition. Similarly, a higher esthetic standard is expected by parents for restoration of their children's carious teeth. With the growing awareness of the esthetic options available, there is a greater demand for solutions to unsightly problems such as early childhood caries, malformed and discolored teeth, hypoplastic defects, tooth fractures and bruxism in children. This chapter highlights the different materials available and the various means of approach in restoring primary anterior teeth.

Among restorative treatment options, biological and resin composite restoration either by means of direct or indirect technique and prefabricated crown are mentioned in the literature. Severely decayed primary teeth in anterior region may not be able to withstand occlusal forces if restored with conventional cements. Therefore, the use of full coverage anterior crowns in such cases is more cost-effective and a viable option. Treatment for restoring primary anterior teeth is shown in **Flowchart 49.1**.

Flowchart 49.1: Treatment for restoring primary anterior teeth.

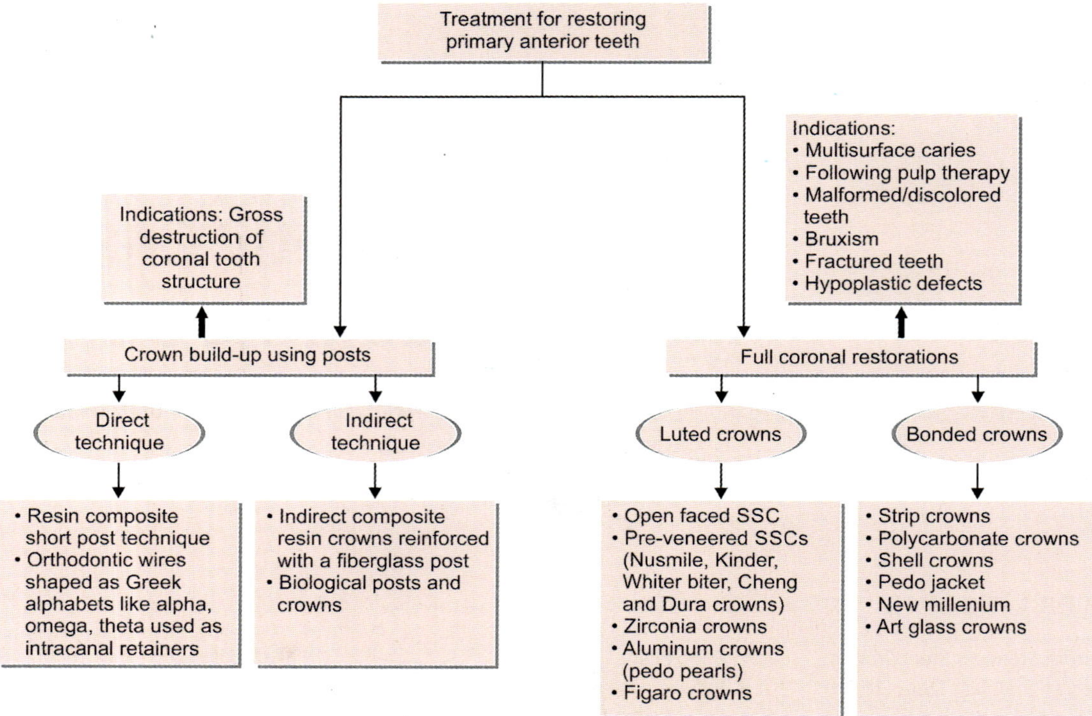

FACIAL CUTOUT STAINLESS STEEL CROWNS

- These are indicated in maxillary canines where strength is a major requirement as compared to esthetics.
- The labial portion of anterior SSC is removed, and composite is placed in the labial fenestration of SSC as a facing, thereby providing adequate strength and acceptable esthetics.
- Although there is an improvement in the appearance, the technique is time consuming and metal margins are still visible. The disadvantage of these crowns is that they are not easily removed.

Technique (Figs. 49.1A to I)

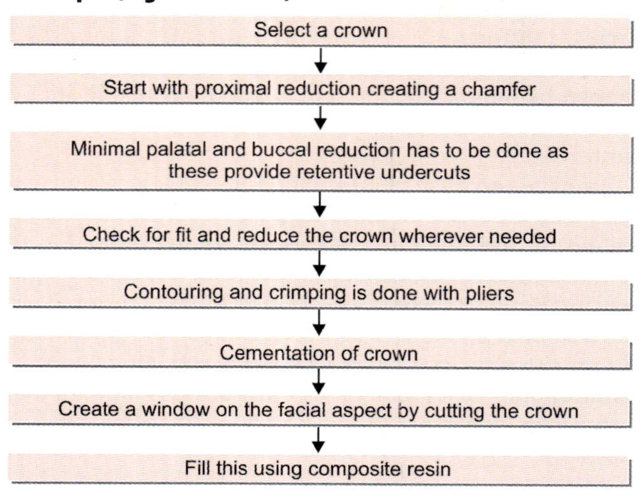

Select a crown
Start with proximal reduction creating a chamfer
Minimal palatal and buccal reduction has to be done as these provide retentive undercuts
Check for fit and reduce the crown wherever needed
Contouring and crimping is done with pliers
Cementation of crown
Create a window on the facial aspect by cutting the crown
Fill this using composite resin

PRE-VENEERED STAINLESS STEEL CROWNS

- In these crowns, the composite resins and thermoplastics are bonded to the metal.
- This type of pre-veneered crown was developed to serve as a convenient, durable, reliable, and esthetic solution to the difficult challenge of restoring severely carious primary incisors **(Figs. 49.2A to G)**.
- Various commercially available veneered SSCs include—Cheng crowns, Kinder krowns, Nu Smile and Whiter biter, Pedo Compu crowns, and Dura crowns.
- The drawbacks of these types of crowns are limited crimp ability as crimping of the metal portion will weaken the esthetic facing and may lead to premature failure, require more aggressive tooth reduction, and the shape of the pre-veneered SSCs (PVSSCs) is not alterable.
- The advantages are esthetics, full coverage, ease to place, and satisfaction for the child and parent.

CHENG CROWNS

- Cheng crowns **(Fig. 49.3)** made their public debut in1987.
- These are stainless steel pediatric anterior crowns faced with a high-quality composite, mesh-based with a light cured composite. It presents a unique solution for natural looking stain resistant crowns.
- It is available for the right and left central and lateral as well as cuspids. It is available in short and regular lengths and sizes suitable for centrals, lateral, and cuspids.
- Most crown procedures can be completed in one patient visit and with less patient discomfort. They can undergo

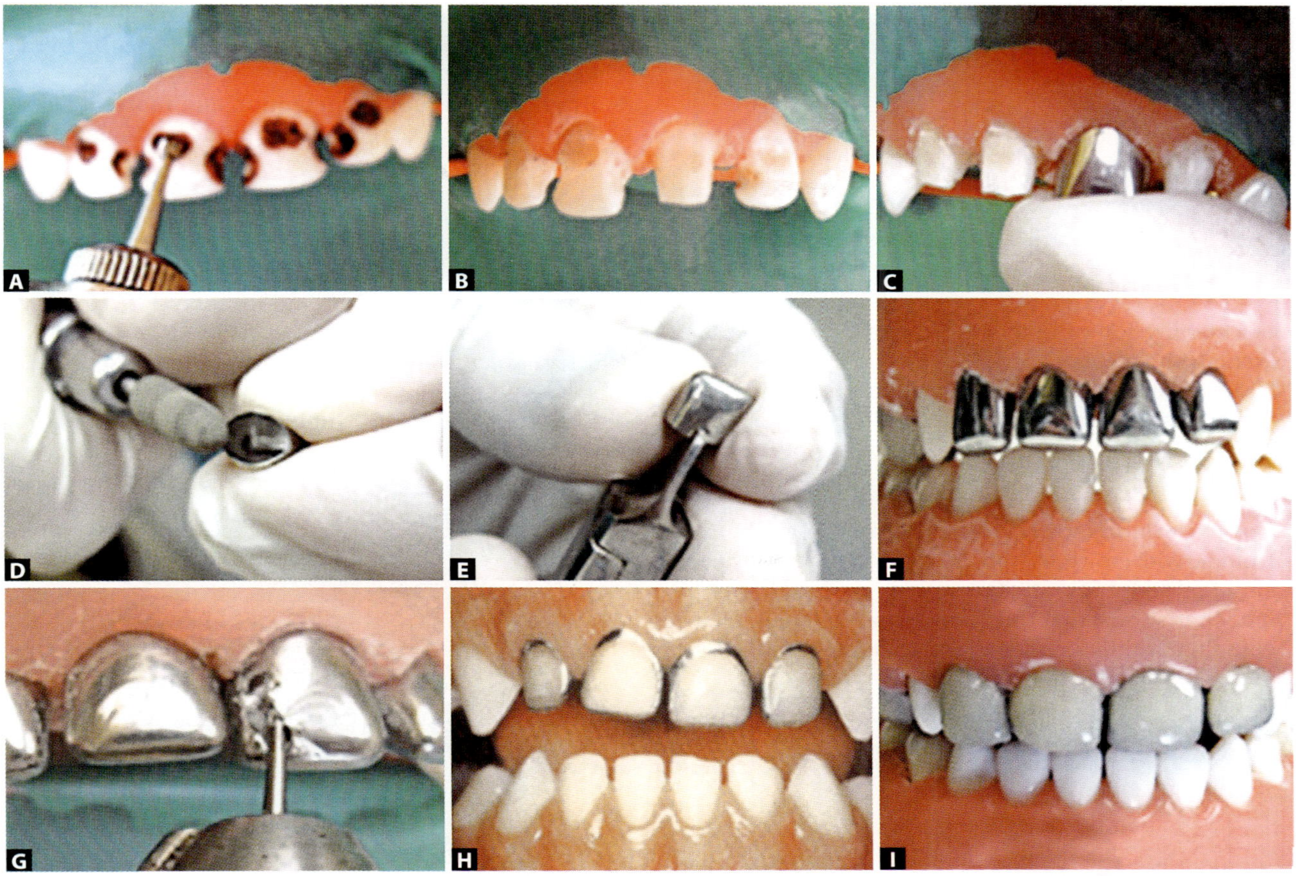

Figs. 49.1A to I: Placement of stainless steel crown with composite facing: (A) Remove decay with slow speed handpiece; (B) After restoration or RCT reduce the facial surface by 1 mm and lingual by 0.5 mm creating a feather edge gingival margin; (C) Try the crown; (D) Trim the crown for fit; (E) Contour and crimp the crown for snug fit; (F) Cement the crowns; (G) Cut a facial window; (H) Trim and smoothen the edges; (I) Restore with composite facing. (*Source:* With permission from Schwartz S. Full coverage esthetic restoration of anterior primary teeth. Crest® Oral-B®at dental care. com. In:Continuing education course. 2012.pp. 1-25).

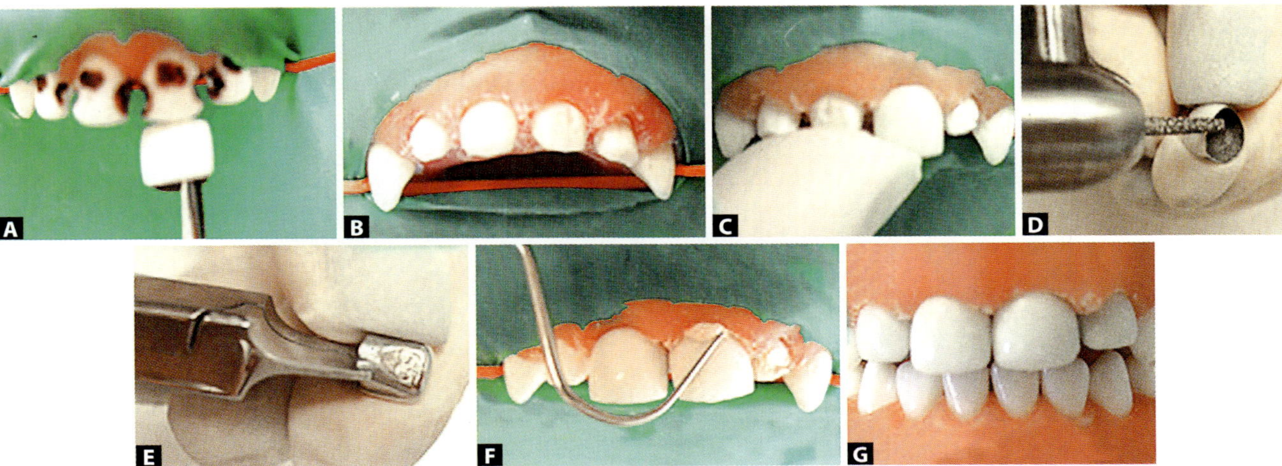

Figs. 49.2A to G: Placement of pre-veneered stainless steel crown: (A) Select the crown; (B) Prepare the tooth; (C) Refine the prep; (D) Trim the crown; (E) Crimp the crown; (F) Cement the crown; (G) Cemented crowns in place. (*Source:* With permission from Schwartz S. Full coverage esthetic restoration of anterior primary teeth. Crest® Oral-B® at dentalcare.com. In: Continuing education course. 2012. pp.1-25).

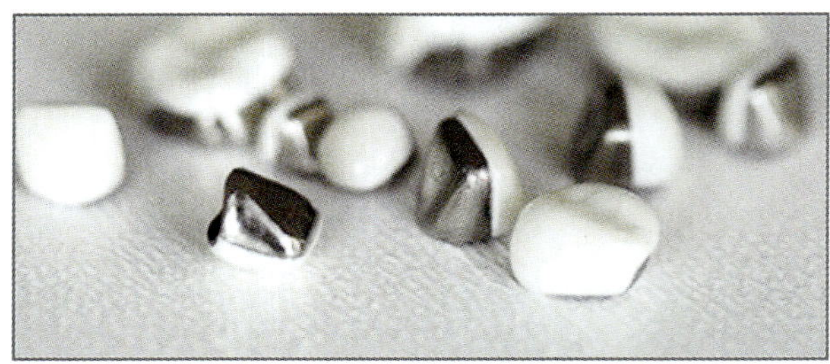
Fig. 49.3: Cheng crowns.

heat sterilization without significant effect on their bond strength and color.

- Disadvantages of all pre-veneered crowns are fracture of veneers during crimping and they are expensive.

DURA CROWNS

- Crowns can be crimped labially and lingually, can be easily trimmed with crown scissors, easily festooned, and has got a full-knife edge **(Fig. 49.4)**.
- Study has shown that these crowns with veneer facings were significantly more retentive than the non-veneered ones when cement and crimping were combined.

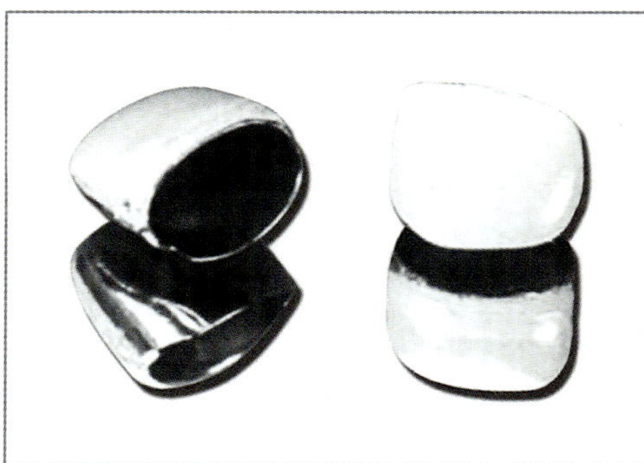
Fig. 49.4: Dura crowns.

KINDER KROWNS™

- Kinder Krowns offer the most natural shades and contour available for the pediatric patient **(Fig. 49.5)**.
- The great depth and vitality from the life-like composite reveal a natural smile without the bulky "Chiclet" look of other restorations.

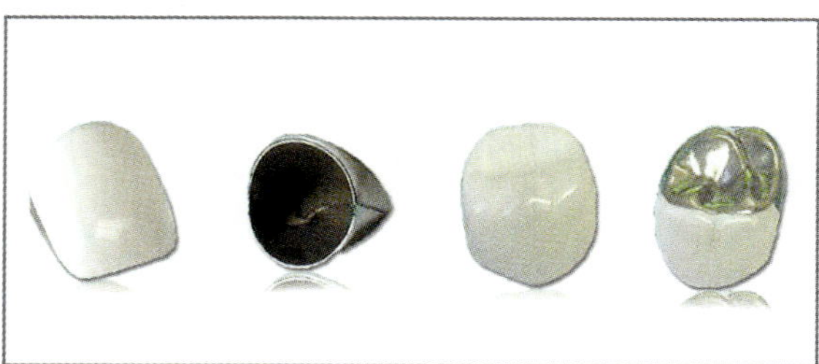
Fig. 49.5: Kinder Krowns™.

- They come in two esthetically pleasing shades, Pedo 1 and Pedo 2. The Pedo 2 shade is the most natural shade while Pedo1shade is for those cases when the bleached white shade is wanted.
- Kinder Krowns™ are designed with Incisa Lock™—the optimal union of state-of-the-art bonding procedures and mechanical retention.
- By adding mechanical retention and more composite, Kinder Krowns™ are strong without sacrificing form or function.

PEDO PEARLS™

- These are beautiful heavy gauge aluminum crowns coated with US Food and Drug Administration (FDA) food grade powder coating and epoxy resin **(Fig. 49.6)**.
- They have universal anatomy and so can be used on either side.
- Easy to cut and crimp, without chipping or peeling.
- Composite can be added if required.
- Disadvantages are less durability and softer crowns.

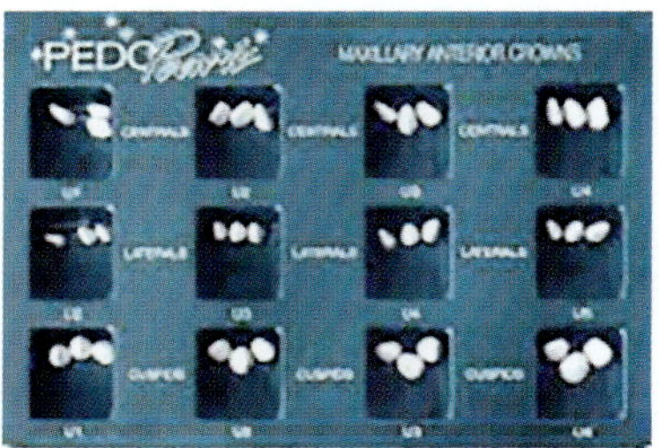

Fig. 49.6: Pedo pearls™.

POLYCARBONATE CROWNS

- Polycarbonates are aromatic linear polyesters of carbonic acid.
- They exhibit high impact strength and rigidity and are termed thermoplastic resins since they are molded as solids by heat and pressure into the desired form.
- It is esthetic than SSC, easy to trim, and can be adjusted with pliers **(Fig. 49.7)**.
- These crowns do not resist strong abrasive forces thus leading to occasional fracture; hence it is contraindicated in cases of severe bruxism and deep bite. Advantages are that they are extremely stable dimensionally and unaffected by acids, ether, and alcohol. Disadvantage is their poor abrasion resistance.

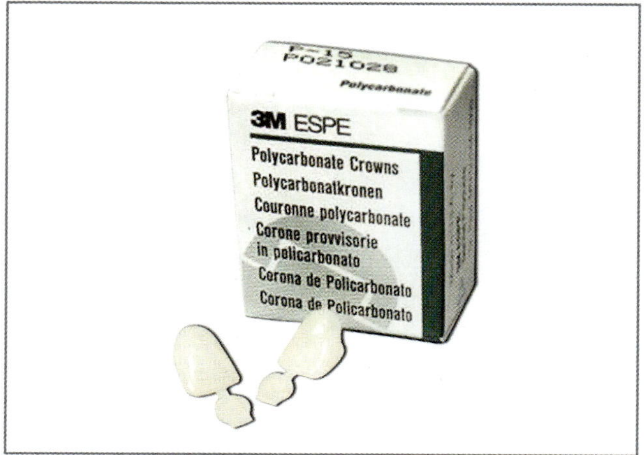

Fig. 49.7: Polycarbonate crowns.

Indications

- ❖ Full coverage restoration of primary maxillary anterior teeth with extensive caries
- ❖ Early childhood caries
- ❖ Deformities in structure of teeth
- ❖ Discolored teeth.

Contraindications

- ❖ Deep bite
- ❖ Bruxism
- ❖ High functionality of teeth.

Technique (Figs. 49.8A to F)

Correct size crown is selected by measuring the mesiodistal width at the level of the contact point of the prepared tooth or by measuring the width of the contralateral tooth in the same arch

↓

Cervical crown margin is trimmed to the required contour with crown scissors or by grinding with a trimming bur or stone

↓

The crown is then lined with acrylic or composite material. If cold cure acrylic is to be used, the material should be poured into the crown after mixing and, once the "dough" stage is reached, seated over the preparation. Prior to seating the crown, the preparation and surrounding gingiva should be lubricated with water or saliva

↓

As the acrylic starts to set, the crown should be removed from the preparation and reseated a number of times. Removal of the crown during polymerization of the acrylic resin helps to dissipate heat build–up from the exothermic reaction and prevent locking into undercuts

↓

Lining a polycarbonate crown will ensure good marginal adaptation to the preparation. Cold cure acrylics chemically bond with polycarbonate crowns. Composite materials need some retention, by mechanically roughening the inside crown surface. A chemical bond to composite can be obtained by priming the fitting surface of the polycarbonate with methyl methacrylate liquid

↓

After the lining material has set, the crown is removed from the tooth and the margins carefully trimmed and finished. It is important that an accurate fit is obtained at the preparation margin to maintain gingival health

↓

After checking the fit and occlusion, the polycarbonate crown should be cemented using proprietary temporary luting cement and the excess removed

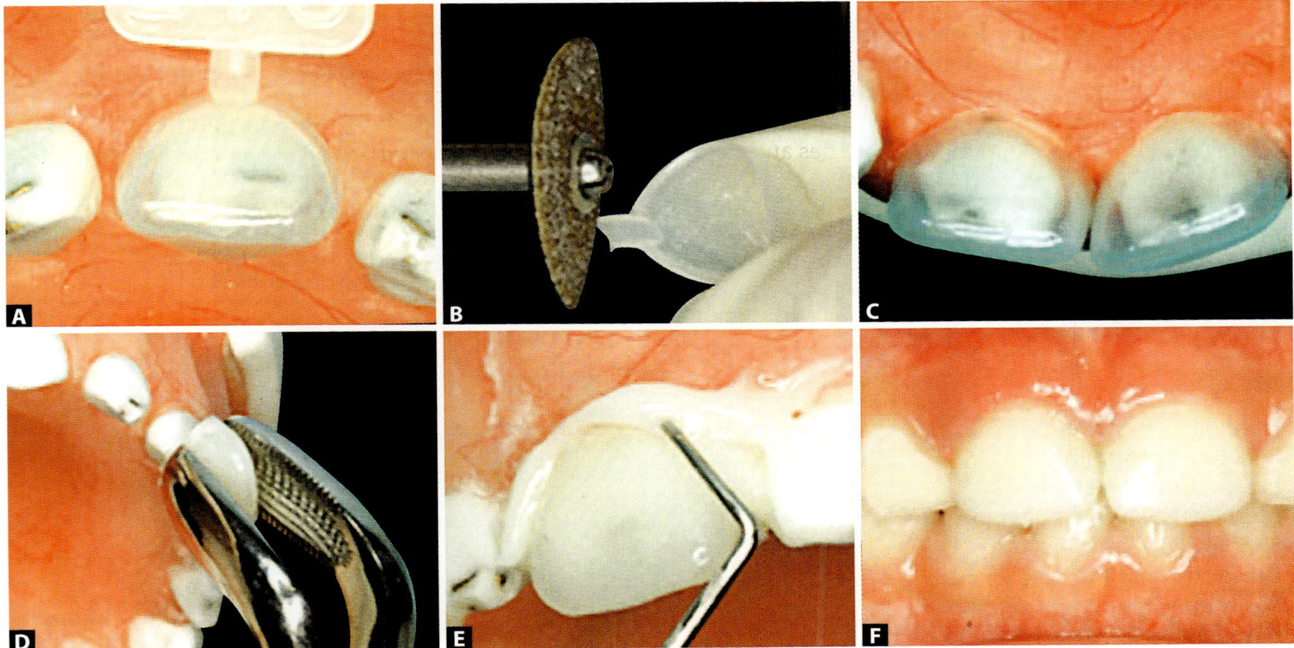

Figs. 49.8A to F: Placement of polycarbonate crowns: (A) Following reduction of 2 mm, try the crown; (B) Trim the crown; (C) Check for subgingival fit of crown; (D) Remove the crown for final inspection; (E) Cement crowns; (F) Final fit of crown. (*Source:* With permission from Schwartz S. Full coverage esthetic restoration of anterior primary teeth. Crest® OralB® at dentalcare.com. In: Continuing education course. 2012.pp.1-25).

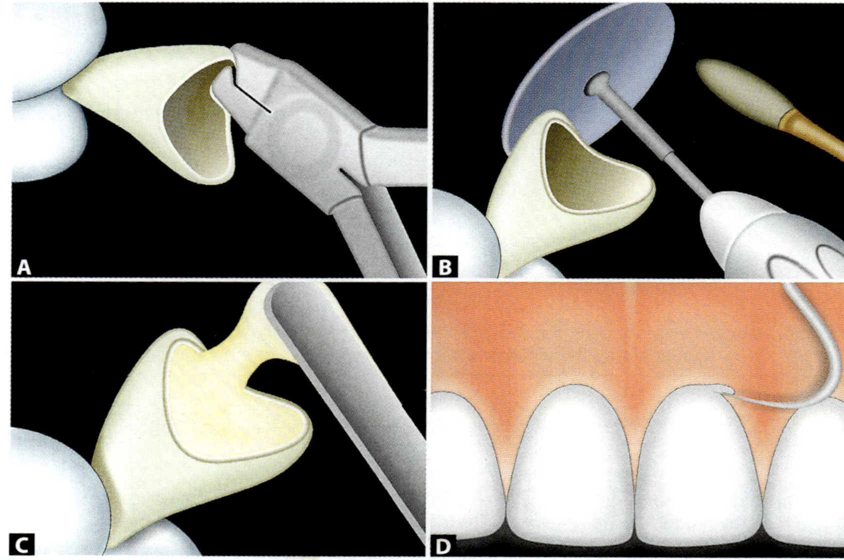

Figs. 49.9A to D: Placement of modified polycarbonate crowns.

Modified Polycarbonate Crowns

- 3M ESPE polycarbonate prefabricated crowns **(Figs.49.9 A to D).**
- The crowns are made of a polycarbonate resin incorporating microglass fibers which not only permit crown adjustment with pliers but also give these crowns good durability and strength.
- They are time saver as they are easy to trim with dental burs or crown scissors and can then be easily adjusted with pliers.
- Crown composition permits crown adjustment.
- Provides good durability and strength.
- Smooth surface finish for patient comfort and to help minimize plaque build-up.
- They have good an atomic form and esthetics.
- They are manufactured in an universal shade which is translucent enough to allow shade adjustment by the type of lining material used.

STRIP CROWNS

These are celluloid crown forms that are the most effective for use in pediatric patients with extensive caries in anterior teeth. These are commonly used crown forms filled with composite and bonded on the tooth.

Advantages

- Easy to place and remove
- Less time consuming
- Parent/patient pleasing
- Ideal for ankylosed tooth build ups
- Simple to fit and trim
- Removal is fast and easy
- Easily matches natural dentition
- Easy shade control with composite
- Superior esthetic quality
- Large selection of size
- Easy to repair.

Technique (Figs. 49.10A to R)

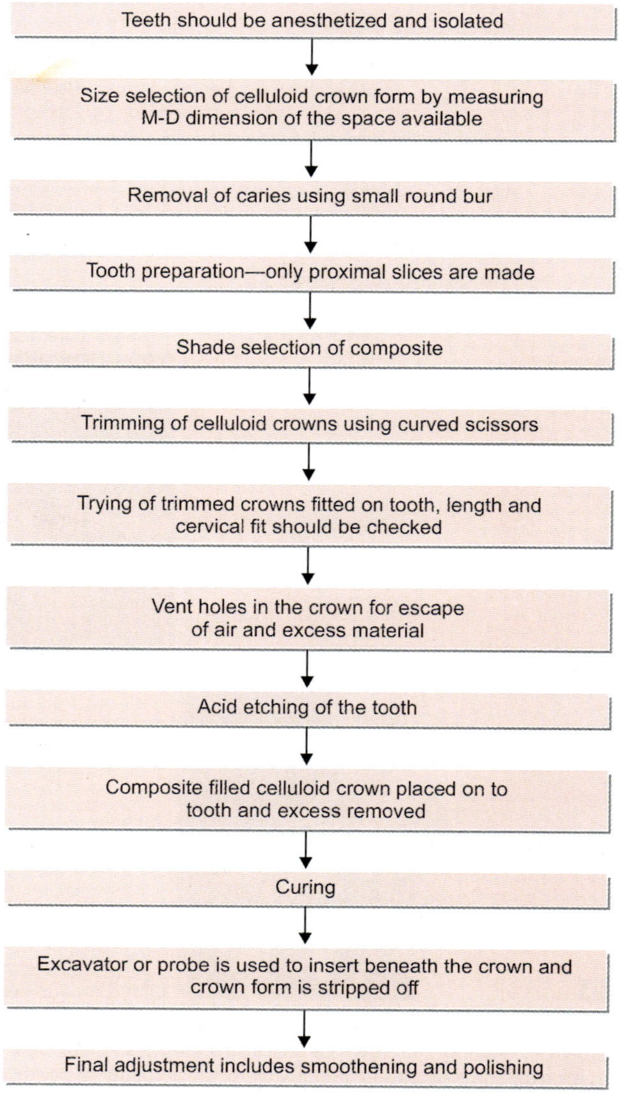

Teeth should be anesthetized and isolated
Size selection of celluloid crown form by measuring M-D dimension of the space available
Removal of caries using small round bur
Tooth preparation—only proximal slices are made
Shade selection of composite
Trimming of celluloid crowns using curved scissors
Trying of trimmed crowns fitted on tooth, length and cervical fit should be checked
Vent holes in the crown for escape of air and excess material
Acid etching of the tooth
Composite filled celluloid crown placed on to tooth and excess removed
Curing
Excavator or probe is used to insert beneath the crown and crown form is stripped off
Final adjustment includes smoothening and polishing

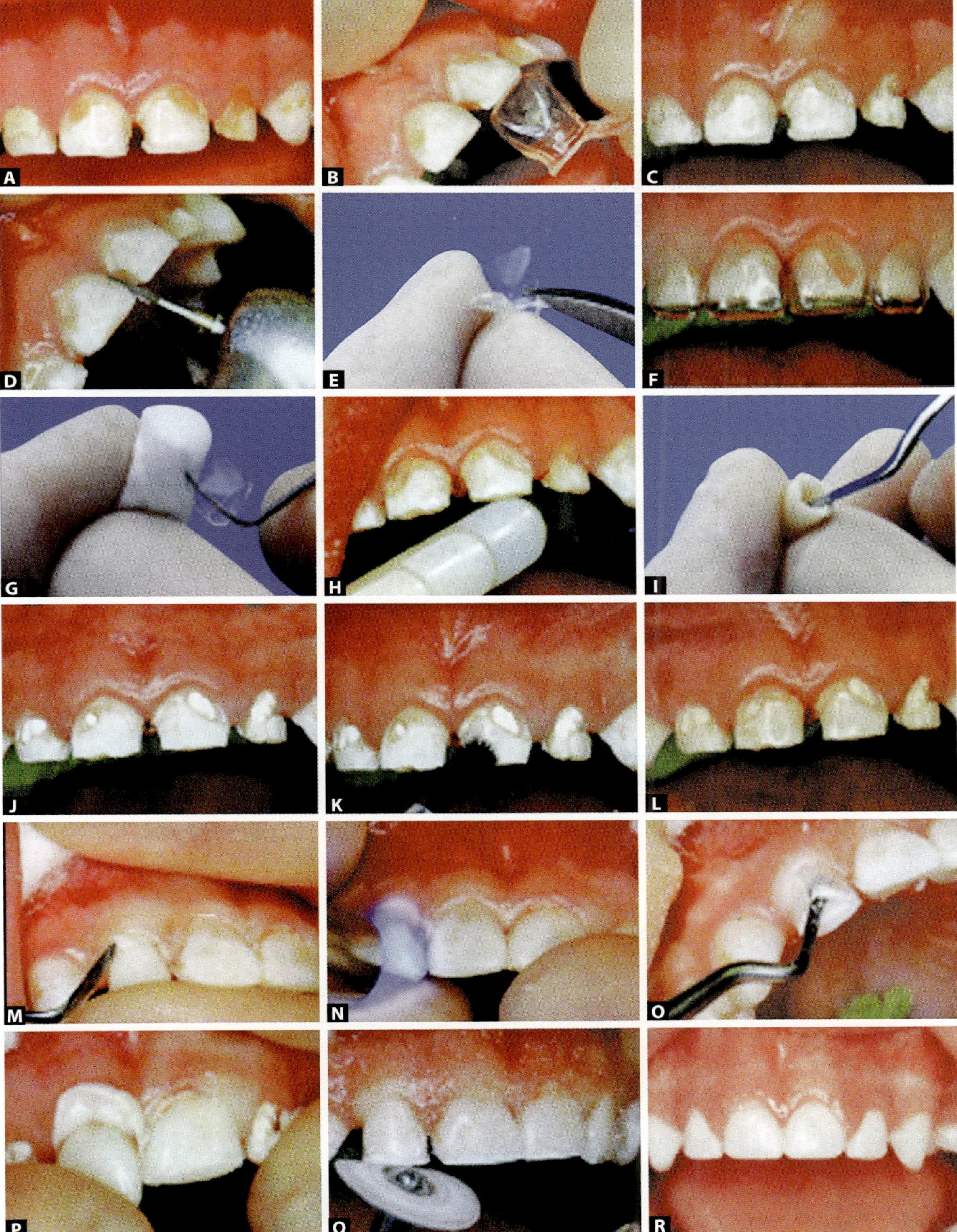

Figs. 49.10A to R: Strip crown placement: (A) Carious anterior teeth should be anesthetized and properly isolated; (B) Size of celluloid crown form is selected by measuring mesiodistal diameter of teeth; (C) Caries is removed using a small round bur in a slow speed handpiece; (D) Teeth are then prepared using tapered diamond or tungsten carbide bur. Incisal, mesial, and distal sides are prepared; (E) Celluloid crowns are trimmed using curved scissors. Care should be taken not to distort the crown form; (F) Trimmed crown forms are fitted onto prepared incisors. Length and cervical fit should be checked; (G) Vent holes are made in the mesial and distal corners of the incisal edge to allow air and excess composite resin to escape; (H) Proper shade of composite resin is chosen; (I) Composite resin is squeezed into the crown form and hollowed in the center to reduce the excess; (J) Teeth are etched for 1 minute with a proprietary etchant, washed, and dried to get frosty appearance; (K) Bonding agent is applied and curved for 15 seconds; (L) A proprietary calcium hydroxide paste or glass ionomer cement is applied to the pulpal wall of exposed dentin; (M) Excess resin is removed from the edges which makes the final finish easier; (N) Composite resin is cured for1minute, labially and palatally; (O) An excavator or probe is inserted beneath the edge of the celluloid and the crown form is stripped off; (P) Crown forms containing composite are firmly seated on the prepared teeth. Excess pressure should not be applied; (Q) Smooth and polish the crowns; (R) Labial view of the finished crown restoration.

SHELL CROWNS

- A novel technique for esthetic rehabilitation of the maxillary anterior teeth with custom made composite shell crowns with an indirect approach.
- Perfection of the restoration using a silicone positioner.
- Indirect approach so most of the work is done on the cast thereby reducing the chair side time.

Technique (Figs. 49.11A to F)

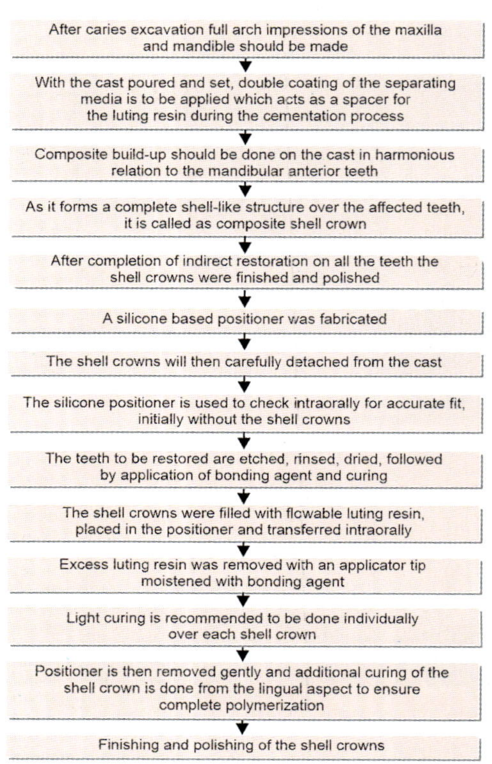

After caries excavation full arch impressions of the maxilla and mandible should be made
With the cast poured and set, double coating of the separating media is to be applied which acts as a spacer for the luting resin during the cementation process
Composite build-up should be done on the cast in harmonious relation to the mandibular anterior teeth
As it forms a complete shell-like structure over the affected teeth, it is called as composite shell crown
After completion of indirect restoration on all the teeth the shell crowns were finished and polished
A silicone based positioner was fabricated
The shell crowns will then carefully detached from the cast
The silicone positioner is used to check intraorally for accurate fit, initially without the shell crowns
The teeth to be restored are etched, rinsed, dried, followed by application of bonding agent and curing
The shell crowns were filled with flowable luting resin, placed in the positioner and transferred intraorally
Excess luting resin was removed with an applicator tip moistened with bonding agent
Light curing is recommended to be done individually over each shell crown
Positioner is then removed gently and additional curing of the shell crown is done from the lingual aspect to ensure complete polymerization
Finishing and polishing of the shell crowns

PEDO JACKET CROWNS

- It is a tooth colored copolyester material which is filled with resin and left on tooth after polymerization instead of being removed **(Fig. 49.12)**.
- It does not split, stain, or crack.
- Crowns can be easily trimmed with scissors.
- Disadvantage is that only one size is available.

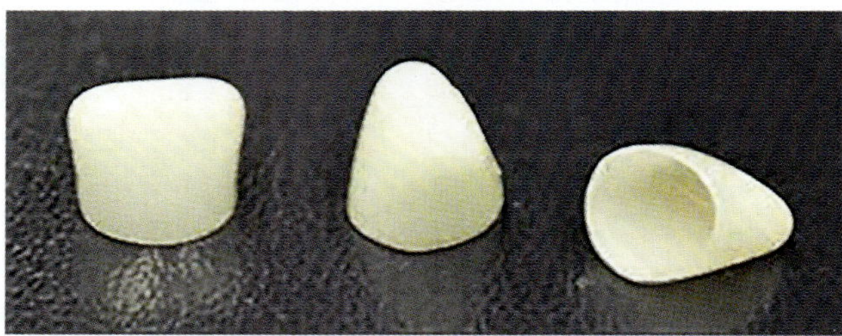

Fig. 49.12: Pedo jacket crowns.

ART GLASS CROWNS

- These are the only patented, preformed crowns for pediatric usage.
- Art glass contains multifunctional methacrylate (methacrylates with multiple reaction sites); which has the ability to form three-dimensional molecular networks with a highly cross-linked structure. The total filler content of Art glass is only 75% (55% microglass and 20% silica filler), but when the matrix is cured, the amorphous, highly cross-linked organic glass forms, which we call polymer glass that is one of the toughest materials available to dentistry.
- Wear of Art glass is similar to enamel and kind to opposing dentition. High inorganic filler makes Art glass color stable and plaque resistant. Matched to the Vita shade system, simplifies shade selection.

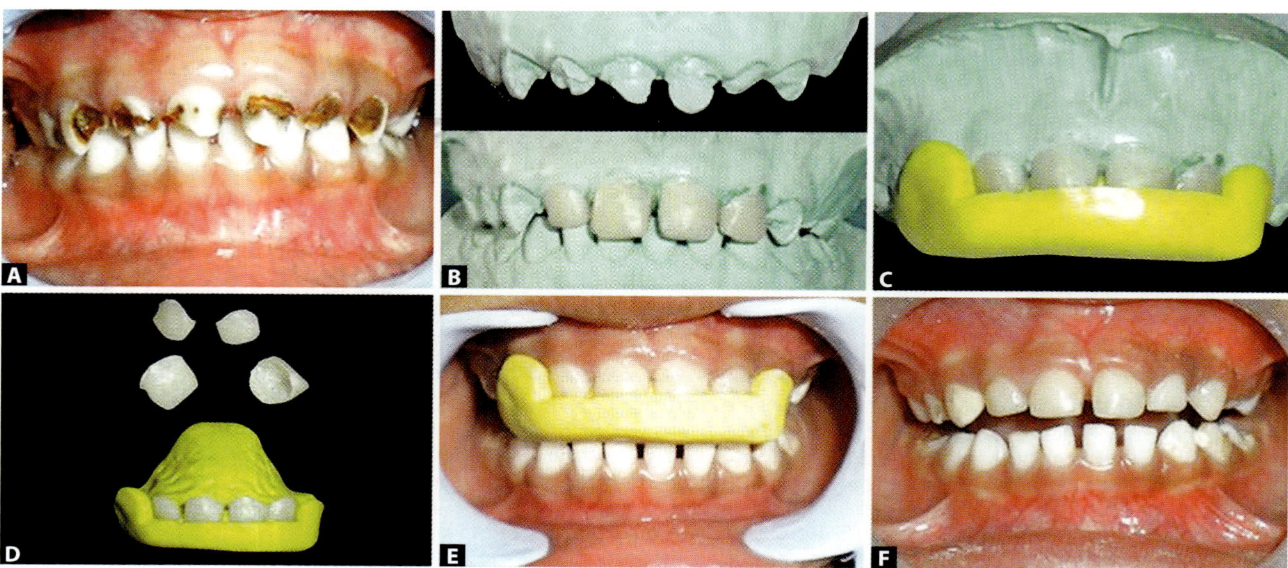

Figs. 49.11A to F: Placement of shell crowns: (A) Clinical presentation of caries; (B) Composite build upon cast after excavation and impression; (C) Fabrication of silicone positioner; (D) Shell crowns seated in position; (E) Cementation of crown using positioner; (F) Completely rehabilitated anterior segment with composite shell crowns. (*Source:* With permission from Murthy PS, Deshmukh S. Indirect composite shell crown: anesthetic restorative option for mutilated primary anterior teeth. J Adv Oral Res. 2013; 4:29-32).

- Flexural strength over 50% higher than porcelain, less chance of fracture. Easily adjusted or repaired intra orally, less chair time for dentists.
- Provides the esthetics and lasting qualities of porcelain. Offers the ease and bond ability of a composite **(Fig. 49.13)**.

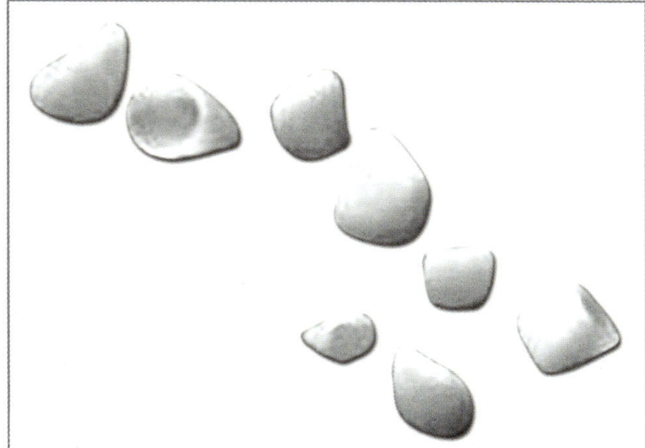

Fig. 49.13: Art glass crowns.

FIGARO CROWNS

- Prefabricated Figaro crowns have been introduced for the treatment of primary teeth in 2018. Figaro Crowns are made in the U.S.A. and possess all ISO and the FDA Certifications **(Fig. 49.14)**.
- They are available in 5 sizes for each tooth and in universal style for lower incisors
- The name was derived by following line—"The Fiber Glass Revolution has begun."

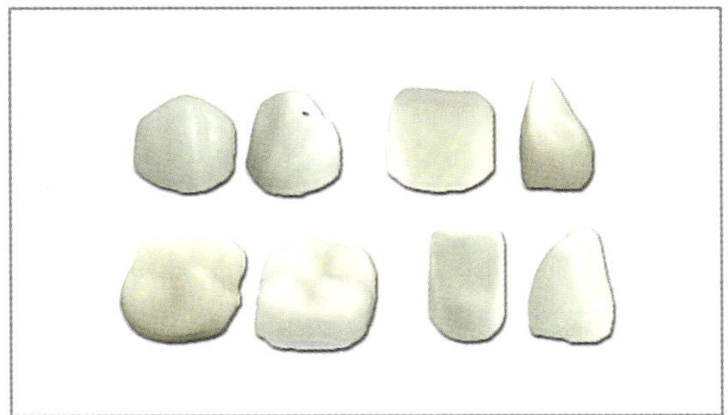

Fig. 49.14: Figaro™ crowns.

Composition

- These crowns utilise either fiberglass or quartz fibers embedded with an outer cosmetic composite resin material. The fibers, one of the components of Figaro crowns are basically fiberglass but the variety of fibers are used including quartz fibers, carbon fibers and aramid fibers such as Dupoint Kevlar brand fibers.
- Fiberglass herein is intended to encompass a wide range of fibers that may be woven into mesh sheets imparting strength.
- Figaro crown utilizes Titanium oxide, $TiO2$ (0.3–1.2 micrometers in size) as its suitable colorant.

Properties and Preparation

- The strength and biocompatibility with a degree of flexibility are much closer to tooth structure.
- Due to flex fit technology, Figaro crowns require less tooth preparation as compared to Zirconia crowns and cementation can be done using Glass ionomer cement.
- Wall thickness of this crown is 0.5–1 mm which is very close to stainless steel.
- Preparation for tooth reduction is still similar to stainless steel with no subgingival preparation so the tooth preparation is less aggressive.
- Figaro crowns are designed to not be crimped due to their pre-beveled margins.
- Its Flex-Fit technology ensures snug friction fit.

Advantages

- One of the remarkable advantages of this crown is the strength and biocompatibility with a degree of flexibility, which is much closer to tooth structure than stainless steel and zirconia crowns.
- Replication of the true anatomy of a natural tooth.
- Not technique sensitive.
- Less aggressive tooth preparation.
- Snug fit.

Disadvantages

- Color change after some months of placement
- Fracture failures
- Microleakage

EDELWEISS PEDIATRIC CROWNS

- Introduced in 2018, Edelweiss pediatric crowns are the recent additions to the array of pediatric esthetic full coverage restorations **(Fig. 49.15)**.
- These are made of densely filled composite with layer-sintered barium glass.
- Edelweiss pediatric crowns are prefabricated crowns that are contoured to mimic the anatomy of the primary tooth

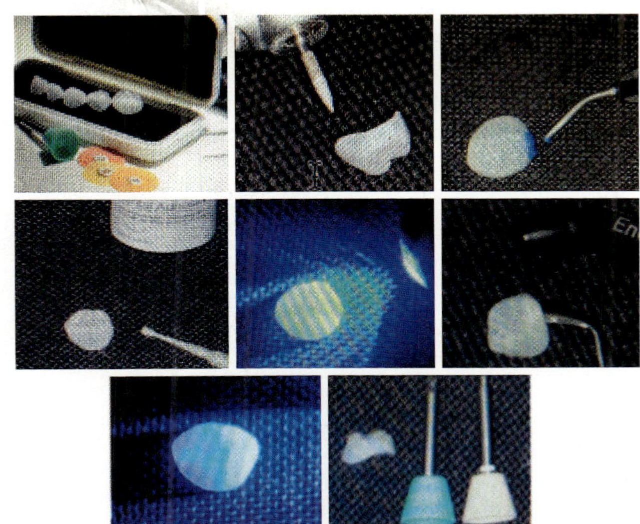

Fig. 49.15: Edelweiss pediatric crowns.

and are supplied in various sizes for both anterior and posterior teeth for different clinical situations. These are available in small, medium and large sizes and offer sizing guides for easy selection of crowns.

- The edelweiss pediatric crowns imitates the form of natural primary teeth well and mimics the anatomy of the primary tooth. The mesial and distal margins follow the natural gingival margin of the primary teeth, minimizing excessive tooth reduction and removing the need to take margins subgingival unless caries dictates extension. Furthermore, because of the minimal preparation needed, there is no risk of iatrogenic damage to pulp tissue of the primary tooth **(Fig. 49.16).**
- The crown needs slight roughening on the inside followed by etch and bond application and then bonded to the tooth with composite.
- Antibacterial, plaque resistant and biocompatible
- Advantage
  - Easy-to-remove, as they can be cut in a way similar to dentine.
  - Very little occlusal adjustment is needed.
  - Preserving the natural tooth structure
  - Natural abrasion and the flexural modulus is similar to that of a natural tooth
  - Highly esthetic
  - Excellent bond to tooth structure
  - Less time needed to place crowns
  - Cost effective
- Mechanical properties
  - Low shrinkage due to nanotechnology and high amount of filler 83%
  - Good abrasion resistance
  - Very good physical and mechanical properties
  - Antibacterial surface due to zinc and fluorine particles in the filler
  - Easy polishing
  - Natural fluorescence and opalescence
- Indications
  - Anterior and posterior restorations
  - Discoloration of primary teeth
  - Congenitally malformed primary incisors
  - Primary teeth affected by localized or generalized developmental defects
  - Poor enamel quality
  - Following pulp therapy procedures
  - Fractured primary teeth following trauma

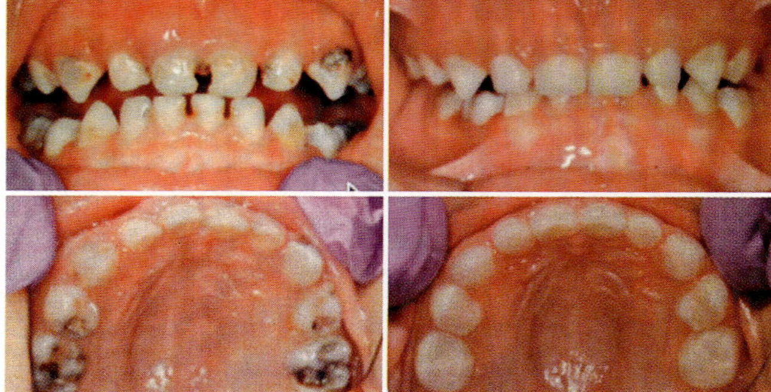

Fig. 49.16: Clinical case of edelweiss pediatric crowns.

  - As an abutment for a space maintainer or denture
  - Severe bruxism
- Contraindications
  - Physiological root-resorption
  - Primary tooth with higher mobility
  - Patient non-cooperation or non-compliance
  - Allergy to any of the ingredients

ZIRCONIA CROWNS

Esthetic treatment of severely decayed primary teeth is one of the greatest challenges to pediatric dentists. In the last half century, the emphasis on treatment of extensively decayed primary teeth shifted from extraction to restoration. Early restorations consisted of placement of stainless steel crowns (SCCs) on severely decayed teeth. While functional, they were unesthetic and their use was limited to posterior teeth. A higher esthetic standard is expected by parents for restoration of their children's carious teeth. Thus, the choice of full coverage restorations for primary teeth must provide an esthetic appearance in addition to restoring function and durability. Endowed with properties of superior biocompatibility, tooth color, adequate mechanical strength, and toughness along with good chemical and dimensional stability, preformed zirconia crowns are being evaluated as an alternative to preformed SCCs, pre-veneered crowns and strip crowns.

- In 2006, **Dr John Hansen** and **Dr Jeffrey Fisher** founded EZPEDO, Inc in USA and developed world's first pediatric zirconia crown. In 2007, they developed the first prototype and in 2008 the first preformed zirconia crown was fitted in child's mouth. In 2010, they offered the crowns for sale. In 2017, the company changed the name to Sprig.
- In 2012, Nu Smile from USA introduced full coverage zirconia crown system with featuring exclusive try-in crowns.
- In2012, Kinder Krowns from USA also introduced preformed zirconia crowns.
- In 2017, Kids-e-Crown: The first indigenously made crown in India were introduced as first smart pediatric zirconia crowns.

Properties

- Prefabricated monolith zirconia crowns are made of yttrium-stabilized zirconium and are either milled or injection molded.
- Zirconia (zirconiumioxide, ZrO_2), also named as "ceramic steel", has optimum properties for dental use—superior toughness, strength, and fatigue resistance, in addition to excellent wear properties and biocompatibility.
- It has excellent resistance to chemicals and corrosion, low thermal conductivity, electrical insulation, coefficient of thermal expansion similar to iron, and modulus of elasticity similar to steel.
- Zirconia offers many benefits, including far greater flexural strength than that of a natural tooth, autoclavability, and a superior esthetics. About 5 and 10 times, the amount of force is required to cause fracture of zirconia crown than

the mean maximum biting force in the molar areas of children aged 10–12 years.

Indications

- Restoring tooth defects requiring esthetics
- Tooth with large carious lesion
- Teeth with hypoplastic defects or with developmental anomalies such as dentinogenesis or amelogenesis imperfecta
- Teeth that have undergone pulp therapy
- Fractured teeth
- Extensive tooth loss due to bruxism, attrition or abrasion
- Patient allergic to nickel and contraindicated for SSC
- Minimum 2 mm of supragingival healthy tooth structure.

Contraindications

- Crowded dentition
- Uncooperative child
- Subgingival soft caries
- If a space maintainer or orthodontic appliance requires soldering to be done on crown.

Different Company Zirconia Crowns with Details of Design

- **NuSmile Zirconia crowns:** They are scientifically developed using CT and digital scans of natural primary teeth. They have 0.2 mm margins and come in two natural pedo shades (light and extra light) for more precise color matching. Company makes narrow first primary molars for easier placement in crowded cases. There are 0–6 sizes for upper anteriors and lower canines whereas lower incisors have 1–4 universal sizes. In posteriors, there are 1–7 sizes. It is also provided with Nu Smile Try-In Crown to check fitting prior to final cementation. This feature not only saves clinicians chairside time but also eliminates extra steps and disinfection of crown and improves bonding of zirconia to luting cement.
- **Kinder Krowns Zirconia crowns:** It has internal retention system (retention bands) which locks the restoration after cementation. Fine-feathered margin of zirconia Kinder Krown makes the emergence profile for the crown as natural as possible. It is available in two sizes—midsize and regular size. Mid-sizes redesigned to alleviate seating issues in situations when you are placing crowns back-to-back or when your patients have experienced major space loss. The mid-sized crowns have same bucco-lingual width as their regular size counterpart, but the mesial-distal has been reduced to allow for easier position placement. They make LP-Less Prep™ design that requires less reduction and time to place. They have both universal and left or right anterior crown option. The central and lateral have 1–6 sizes. Canines have 1–6 regular sizes and0.5–5.5 mid-sizes. Posteriors have2–7 regular sizes and1.5–6.5 mid-sizes.
- **EZ Pedo Crowns:**They are pioneers of preformed zirconia crowns technology. They have flat fit inter proximal contours making side by side placement with zirconia easier. It comes with the patented retention technology, Zir-Lock Ultra, i.e., retentive grooves which extent all the way to the crown margins, preventing cement washout, prevents entry of harmful bacteria, moreover it provides two times more surface area for bonding. Additional retention is provided through blasting with aluminum oxide.
- **Kids-e-crown:** The posterior crowns have inner flat occlusal table with uniform axial walls. There are micro-mechanical boxes for retention. The wall thickness is 0.2 mm and margins are 0.2 mm. Anteriors are universal in design. The sizes for anteriors are 0–5and posteriors there are five regular sizes 2–6 and three narrow sizes 3–5. The narrow sizes are mid-sizes with broader buccolingual dimension for proximal lesions and space loss cases. The labeling of the crowns is permanently embossed inside the crown.
- **Signature crown:** It has a 0.2 mm feather edge margin and 0.5 mm over all thickness. Permanent laser engraved labeling. Posterior crowns have flat distal proximal wall of primary first molar and mesial flat proximal wall of primary second molar with no narrow crowns. In anteriors, both universal contoured and left/right side options are available. There are 1–6 posterior and 1–4 anterior sizes with no space loss crowns. The company does not make canine crowns.

Technique (Figs. 49.17 to 49.20)

- **Step 1(Crown selection):** Select appropriate size of crown measuring mesiodistal width.
- **Step 2 (Incisal and occlusal reduction):** Reduce 1.5–2 mm incisally using donut shape bur following the incisal plane.
- Make flat occlusal preparation of 1.5–2 mm using donut shape bur. Nu Smile advocates making sloped occlusal pattern following cuspal inclines, whereas Kinder Krown, Sprig, and Kids-e advocate flat preparation.
- **Step 3 (Supragingival reduction):** Make a chamfer finish line of 0.5–1 mm on all four sides of crown equi-gingival using chamfer bur. If contact is tight use taper bur to break contact.
- **Step 4(Supragingival reduction):** Using a taper bur, remove the chamfer finish line going 1–2 mm subgingival making a feather edge or no finish line.
- **Step 5 (Check fit and bleeding control):** Check for passive fit of selected crown. Control bleeding using pressure or hemostat.
- **Step 6 (Cementation):** Clean the crown under tap water and with alcohol to remove blood and saliva. Air dry the crown and completely fill it with luting cement and cement the crown under finger pressure until the cement sets. Not to tell the patient to bite till the cement sets as there are chances that the crown can fracture. Remove excess cement using explorer and floss. Take X-ray to check for any residual cement.
- **Modifying Zirconia crowns:** Diamond burs can be used to trim zirconia crowns with soft intermittent motion and water irrigation. They can be reduced cervically. Any trimming done on the crown should be followed by polishings in unpolished zirconia can abrade the opposing tooth. Using burs on sintered zirconia crowns can lead to microcracks development and increased chances of fracture of crowns.

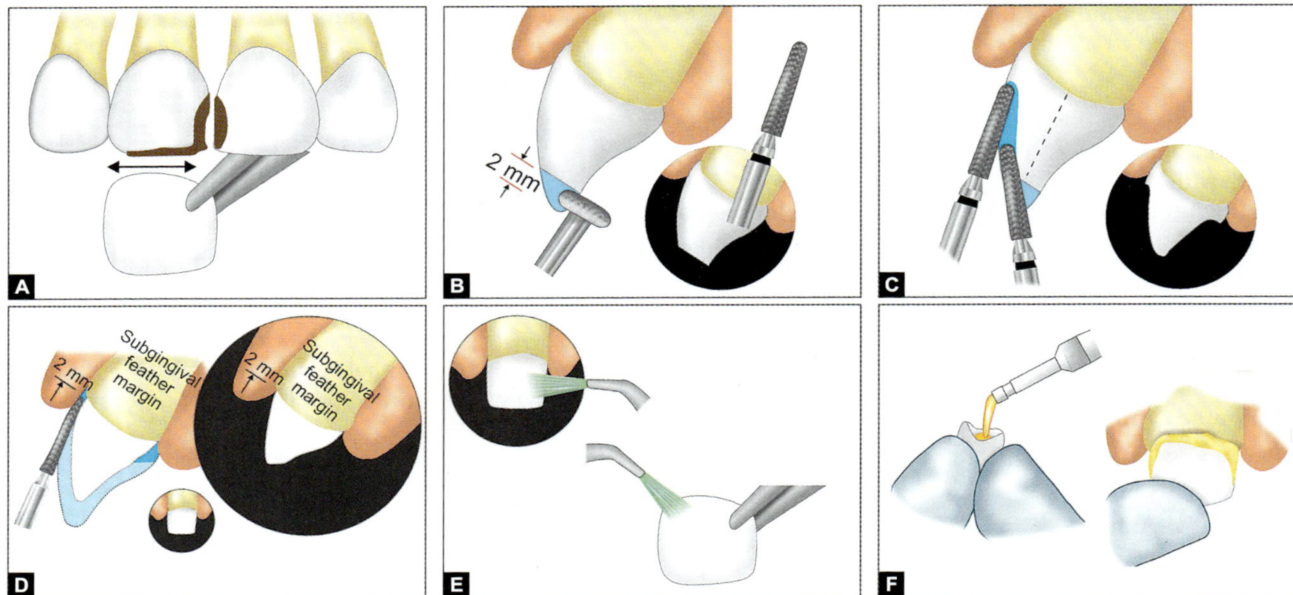

Figs. 49.17A to F: Anterior preparation technique: (A) Crown selection; (B) Incisal preparation; (C) Supragingival preparation; (D) Subgingival preparation; (E) Check fit and preparation; (F) Cementation.

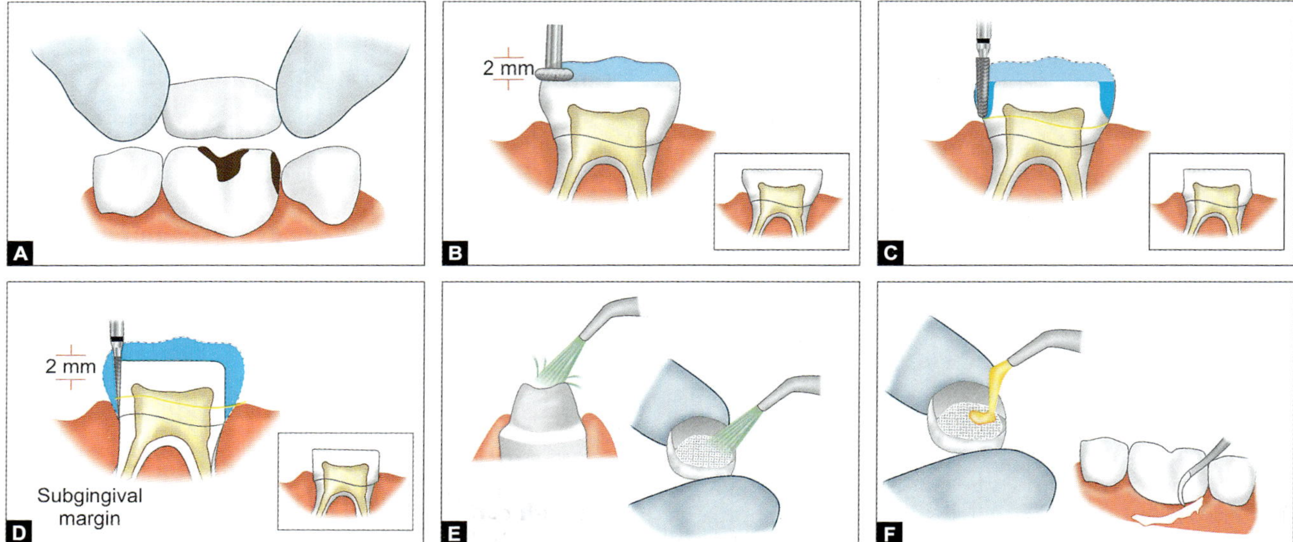

Figs. 49.18A to F: Posterior preparation technique: (A) Crown selection; (B) Occlusal preparation; (C) Supragingival preparation; (D) Subgingival preparation; (E) Check fit and preparation; (F) Cementation.

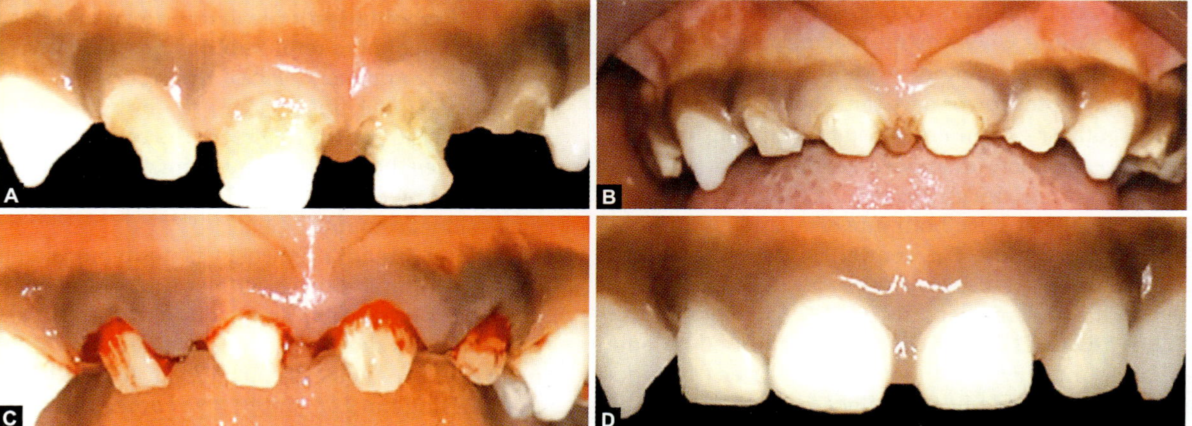

Figs. 49.19A to D: Anterior crown preparation: (A) Preoperative; (B) Supragingival preparation; (C) Subgingival preparation; (D) Postoperative view. *(Pic courtesy:* Dr Mukul Jain, Kids-e-crown).

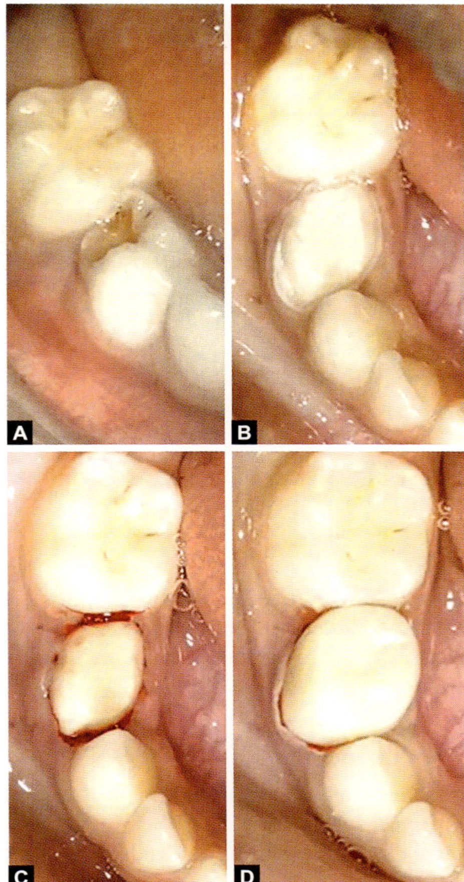

Figs. 49.20A to D: Posterior crown preparation: (A) Preoperative; (B) Supragingival preparation; (C) Subgingival preparation; (D) Postoperative view. (*Pic courtesy:* Dr Mukul Jain, Kids-e-Crown).

Advantages

- They are highly esthetic, with greater durability than composite strip crowns and pre-veneered crowns.
- Highly biocompatible and as strong as steel.
- High acceptance by patients and parents.
- They are not as technique sensitive as composite strip crowns, as the fabricated crown is cemented rather than bonding.
- They take a bit longer to place than SSCs; about the same as pre-veneered crowns and less than open-faced SSCs.
- Zirconia crowns will not chip as the pre-veneered SSCs do on occasion.
- Do not discolor and break down overtime like resin strip crowns.
- Can be autoclaved without any changes in property.

Disadvantages

- They are thicker than other crowns, therefore greater tooth reduction is required.
- Subgingival preparation leads to bleeding, which can hamper bonding strength of luting cement.
- Brittle—can fracture if not handled properly.
- Unlike SSCs, they cannot be crimped and contoured.
- High cost as more number of sizes required.
- Abrasion of opposite natural tooth if not polished properly.
- Shade options are limited.

BIOFLEX CROWNS

The biggest challenge in Pediatric Dentistry is managing child's behavior and fulfilling parent's expectations. To overcome such challenges, we need faster techniques and natural looking restorations. A ideal full coverage restoration in Pediatric Dentistry should be esthetic, durable, economical and not technique sensitive.

Stainless steel crowns are gold standard for full coverage restoration in Pediatric Dentistry with the advantages of ease of doing and durability. To overcome metallic look of stainless steel crowns zirconia crowns were introduce, but they require lot of tooth preparation.

Recently, Bioflex crowns were introduced for primary teeth in 2022 by Kids-e-Dental LLP, India. Bioflex crowns are world's first flexible, durable, self-adaptable and esthetic preformed pediatric crowns which offer properties of both stainless steel crowns and zirconia crowns.

Features

- **Flexi fit:** They are flexible crowns and can be easily contoured and trimmed. The crown fit to tooth preparation is snug fit and not passive like zirconia crowns.
- **Esthetic:** These tooth colored crowns are mono-chromatic and opaque.
- **Self-adapt technology:** The crowns bend at the area of high occlusion and self-adapt to new occlusion after cementation of the crowns. But the crowns should not be kept high clinically and require occlusion preparation.
- **Radio-opaque:** The crown borders are radio-opaque and walls look radio lucent in the radiograph making the evaluation of direct and indirect pulp capping possible.
- **Durable:** There are self-adaptable to the occlusal forces with good abrasion resistance and load bearing capacity.
- Bio-compatible
- **Rough cementing surface:** The inner surface is sand blasted for better retenzion
- **Laser marking:** Clinically, the laser marking is not visible as it is done on cementing surface and looks natural in patience oral cavity.

Composition

Made up of high strength hybrid resin polymer used in the medical field requiring high strength, flexibility and durability. They are metal and Bis-GMA free.

Clinical Procedure Protocol for Bioflex Crowns (Figs. 49.21A to H)

Step 1

Maintain cuspal inclines and reduce the occlusal surface by 1.00–1.5 mm, including the central groove.

Step 2

Buccal/lingual reduction—confined to the occlusal third.

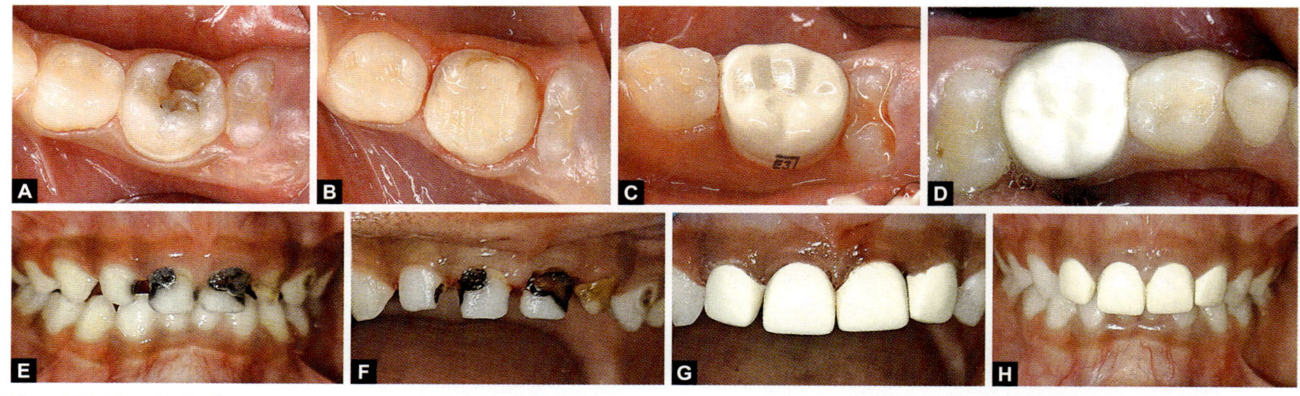

Figs. 49.21A to H: Bioflex crowns: (A) Preoperative; (B) Tooth preparation; (C) Immediate postoperative; (D) 1 month follow-up; (E) Preoperative; (F) Preparation; (G) Immediate postoperative; (H) 6 months follow-up. (*Pic courtesy:* Dr Meenakshi Kher and Dr Milind Shah).

Step 3

Proximal preparation—around 0.5 mm just enough to clear the contact area

Step 4

Rounding off all line angles.

Step 5

Seating the crown from lingual to buccal direction to achieve snug fit. Check occlusion and don't keep the occlusion high.

Crimping is not recommended but slight contouring can be carried out by using Howes plier. If crown is high trimming can be done using curved scissors and then finishing and polishing with either stone or rubber wheel.

Step 6

About 1/2 or 2/3rd of crown is filled with self- setting resin modified glass ionomer cement or glass ionomer type I can be used. Light cured cements are not recommended. Remove excess cement using floss or explorer.

Limitations

- Not as esthetic as zirconia crowns as shade it is mono chromatic.
- Long-term clinical research required.

POINTS TO REMEMBER

- Facial cut out SSCs are indicated in maxillary canines where strength is a major requirement as compared to esthetics. The labial portion of anterior SSC is removed, and composite is placed in the labial fenestration of SSC as a facing, thereby providing adequate strength and acceptable esthetics.
- Pre-veneered SSC are crowns in which the composite resins and thermoplastics are bonded to the metal. This type of crown was developed to serve as a convenient, durable, reliable, and esthetic solution to the difficult challenge of restoring severely carious primary incisors. Various commercially available veneered SSCs include Cheng crowns, Kinder krowns, Nu Smile and Whiter biter, Pedo Compu crowns, and Dura crowns.
- Polycarbonate crowns are esthetic than SSC, easy to trim, and can be adjusted with pliers, but they have poor abrasion resistance.
- Strip crowns are celluloid crown forms that are the most effective for use in pediatric patients with extensive caries in anterior teeth. These are commonly used crown forms filled with composite and bonded on the tooth. Advantages are easy to place and remove, less time consuming, matches natural dentition, superior esthetic quality, and large selection of size.
- Shell crown is a novel technique for esthetic rehabilitation of the maxillary anterior teeth with custom made composite crowns with an indirect approach.
- Some recent modifications of anterior crowns are Pedo Jacket (it is a tooth colored copolyester material which is filled with resin and left on tooth after polymerization instead of being removed); New Millennium (crowns are made up of laboratory enhanced composite resin material) and Art glass crowns.
- Art glass crowns are the only patented, preformed crowns for pediatric usage. They are made up of microglass and silica-filler and have the ability to form three-dimensional molecular networks with a highly crosslinked structure. It provides esthetics of porcelain and bond ability of a composite.
- Preformed zirconia crowns are passive fit.
- Tooth reduction is more while doing a zirconia crown on a primary teeth as compared to stainless steel crown. There are two steps in preparation supragingival and subgingival feather edge or no margin.
- Preformed zirconia crowns have excellent biocompatibility.

Questionnaire

1. What are the options for restoring primary anterior teeth?
2. Describe stainless steel crowns for anterior teeth and their modifications.
3. Write a note on polycarbonate crowns.
4. Describe the indications, advantages, and the technique for placement of strip crowns.
5. What are Art-glass crowns?
6. Explain the procedure of fabrication of shell crowns?
7. Write a short note on pre-formed zirconia crowns in pediatric dentistry?
8. Write in detail preparation technique pre-formed zirconia crowns in pediatric dentistry?
9. What are the indications and contraindications of zirconia crowns in pediatric dentistry?

FURTHER READING

1. AAPD. Reference Manual, Clinical Guidelines. 2011:12;33(6).
2. Arens D. The role of bleaching in esthetics. Dent Clin North Am. 1989;33:319-36.
3. As per the Information provided by- Manufacturer Kids-e-dental LLP, Santacruz, Mumbai, India
4. Austinglas tech.com [Internet]. Austin,TX: GlastechInc.; C2001 [Cited 2010 Feb 11]. Availablefrom:http://www.austinglastech.com/comp.htm.
5. Baker LH, Moon P, Mourino AP. Retention of esthetic veneers on primary stainless steel crowns. ASDC J Dent Child.1996;63:185-9.
6. Breakthrough in Pediatric Dentistry: Direct system Pediatric crowns-edelweiss dentistry. Retreived 6 Ocober 2020. Available from: https://www.edelweissdentistry.com/wpontent/uploads/2020/03/EW_PediatricCrown_Brochure_02_2020_EN_compressed.pd
7. Chakraborty S DA, Agarwala P, Zahir S, Lahiri PK, Kundu GK. Esthetic rehabilitation of decayed primary incisors using figaro crowns and strip crowns. IJDSIR. 2019;2(2):490-4.
8. Cohn C. Pre-veneered stainless steel crowns—an esthetic alternative. ADA CERP. 2012.
9. Croll TP, Helpin ML. Preformed resin-veneered stainless steel crowns for restoration of primary incisors. Quintessence Int.1996;27:309-13.
10. Croll TP. Primary incisor restoration using resin veneered stainless steel crowns. J Dent Child. 1998;65:89-95.
11. Donly KJ, Sasa I, Contreras CI, Mendez MJC. Prospective Randomized Clinical Trial of Primary Molar Crowns: 24-Month Results. Pediatr Dent. 2018;40(4):253-8. PMID: 30345963.
12. El-Habashy LM, El Meligy OA. Fiberglass crowns versus preformed metal crowns in pulpotomized primary molars: a randomized controlled clinical trial. Quintessence Int. 2020;51(10):844-852. doi: 10.3290/j.qi.a45169. PMID: 32901239.
13. Ghosh A, Jalan P, Zahir S, Kundu G. Figaro crowns: A promising alternative for esthetic and functional rehabilitation of decayed primary incisors: A case report. IDA WB. 2019; 35:335.
14. Guelmann M, Gehring DF, Turner C. Retention of veneered stainless steel crowns on replicated typodont primary incisors: an in vitro study. Pediatr Dent. 2003;25:275-8.
15. Kavya KG, Anegundi RT, Tavargeri AK, Trasad V, Patil SB. An update on aesthetic crowns. Austin J Dent. 2020; 7(3): 1143.
16. Kilpatrick NM. Durability of restorations in primary molars. J Dent. 1993;21:67-73.
17. Kupietzky A, et al. The clinical and radiographic success of bonded resin composite strip crowns for primary incisors. Pediatr Dent. 2003;25:577-81.
18. Kupietzky A, Waggoner WF, Galea J. The clinical and radio-graphic success of bonded resin composite strip crowns for primary incisors. Pediatr Dent. 2003; 25:577-81.
19. Lee JK. Restoration of primary anterior teeth: review of the literature. Pediatr Dent. 2002;24:506-10.
20. Luke LS, Reisbick MH. Steel crowns. In: Stewart RE, Barber TK, Troutman KC, Wei SHY (Eds). Pediatric Dentistry: Scientific Foundations and Clinical Practice. St Louis: CV Mosby Co.;1982.
21. MacLean JK, Champagne CE, Waggoner WF, et al. Clinical outcomes for primary anterior teeth treated with pre-veneered stainless-steel crowns. Pediatr Dent. 2007;29:377-81.
22. MacLean JK, et al. Clinical outcomes for primary anterior teeth treated with preveneered stainless steel crowns. Pediatric Dent. 2007;29:377-81.
23. MandrolipS. Biologic restoration of primary anterior teeth: a case report. J Indian Soc Pedod Prev Dent. 2003; 21:95-7.
24. Mathew MG, Roopa KB, Soni AJ, Khan MM, Kauser A. Evaluation of clinical success, parental and child satisfaction of stainless steel crowns and zirconia crowns in primary molars. J Family Med Prim Care. 2020;9:1418-23.
25. MendesFM, DeBenedetto MS,del Conte Zardetto CG, et al. Resin composite restoration in primary anterior teeth using short-post technique and strip crowns: a case report. Quintessence Int. 2004; 35:689-92.
26. MesserLB, Levering NJ. The durability of primary molar restorations: II. Observations and predictions of success of stainless steel crowns. Pediatr Dent. 1988;10:81-5.
27. Moodley D, Gupta K, Stephan L. Edelweiss PEDIATRIC CROWNs: A new and innovative approach to restoring paediatric teeth. 2019.
28. Mortada A, King NM. A simplified technique for the restoration of severely mutilated primary anterior teeth. J Clin Pediatr Dent. 2004;28:187-92.
29. Murthy PS, Deshmukh S. Indirect composite shell crown: anesthetic restorative option for mutilated primary anterior teeth. J Adv Oral Res. 2013;4:29-32.
30. Niharika, Biswas R, Galui S, Saha S, Sarkar S. Aesthetic rehabilitation of decayed maxillary primary incisors using figaro crowns -a case report. IDA, W.B. 2019:35(3): 16-19.
31. Peretz B, Ram D. Restorative material for children's teeth: preferences of parents and children. J Dent Child. 2002;69:243-8.
32. Planells del Pozo P, Fuks AB. Zirconia crowns—An esthetic and resistant restorative alternative for ECC affected primary teeth. J Clin Pediatr Dent. 2014;38:193-5.
33. Ram D, Fuks AB, Eidelman E. Long-term clinical performance of esthetic primary molar crowns. Pediatr Dent. 2003; 25:582-4.
34. Randall RC. Preformed metal crowns for primary and permanent molar teeth: review of the literature. Pediatr Dent. 2002;24:489-500.
35. Randal RC, Vrijhoef MM, Wilson NH. Efficacy of preformed metal crowns vs. amalgam restorations in primary molars: a systematic review. J Am Dent Assoc. 2000;31:337-43.
36. Roberts C, Lee JY, Wright JT. Clinical evaluation of and parental satisfaction with resin-faced stainless steel crowns. Pediatr Dent. 2001; 23:28-31.
37. Roberts JF, Sherriff M. The fate and survival of amalgam and preformed crown molar restorations placed in a specialist paediatric dental practice. Br Dent J. 1990; 169:237-44.
38. Sahana S, Vasa AAK, Sekhar R. Esthetic crowns for primary teeth: a review. Ann Essences Dent. 2010; 2:87-93.
39. Schwartz S. Full coverage esthetic restoration of anterior primary teeth. Dental Continuing Education Course. 2012. pp.1-25.
40. Seale NS. The use of stainless steel crowns. Pediatr Dent. 2002; 24:501-5.
41. Shah PV, Lee JY, Wright JT. Clinical success and parental satisfaction with anterior pre-veneered primary stainless steel crowns. Pediatr Dent. 2004; 26: 391-5.
42. Sharaf AA. The application of fiber core posts in restoring badly destroyed primary incisors. J Clin Pediatr Dent. 2002;26:217-24.
43. Sztyler K, Wiglusz RJ, Dobrzynski M. Review on preformed crowns in pediatric dentistry-the composition and application. Materials (Basel). 2022;15(6):2081. doi: 10.3390/ma15062081. PMID: 35329535; PMCID: PMC8950869
44. Talekar AL, Chaudhari GS, Waggoner WF, Chunawalla YK. An 18-month prospective randomized clinical trial comparing zirconia crowns with glass-reinforced fiber composite crowns in primary molar teeth. Pediatr Dent. 2021;43(5):355-362. PMID: 34654496.
45. Usha M, Deepak V, Venkat S, et al. Treatment of severely mutilated incisors: a challenge to the pedodontist. J Indian Soc Pedod Prev Dent. 2007;25: S34-6.
46. Waggoner WF. Restoring primary anterior teeth: review. Pediatr Dent. 2002; 24:511-6.
47. Wei SHY, King NM. Stainless steel crowns. In: Wei SHY (Ed). Pediatric dentistry: Total Patient Care. Philadelphia: Lea & Febiger. 1988. pp. 224-31.
48. Yilmaz Y, Guler C. Evaluation of different sterilization and disinfection methods on commercially made preformed crowns. J Indian Soc Pedod Prev Dent. 2008; 26:162-7.
49. Yilmaz Y, Gurbuz T, Eyuboglu O, et al. There pair of pre-veneered posterior stainless steel crowns. Pediatr Dent. 2008;30:429-35.
50. Zimmerman JA, Feigal RJ, Till MJ, et al. Parental attitudes on restorative materials as factors influencing current use in pediatric dentistry. Pediatr Dent. 2009; 31:63-70.

CHAPTER 50

Pulp and Periapical Diseases

Nikhil Marwah, Naveen Manuja, Shrishty Chalana

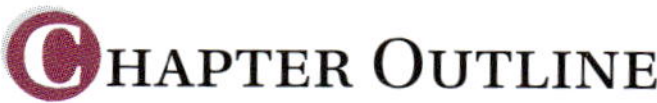

Chapter Outline

- General Features of Pulp
- Primary Root Canal Morphology
- Pulp Diseases
- Periapical Lesions
- Diagnosis of Pulp Pathology

Toothache has been a scourge to mankind from the earliest times. Chinese and Egyptians were the first to describe caries and alveolar abscess, whereas Greeks and Romans were the initiators of pulpal treatment by cauterization using hot needle, boiling oil, and fermentation of opium. Special problems in dealing with primary dentition are due to differences in pulp anatomy, differences in pulp response, and changes caused by normal receptive process. With the advances in material, instruments, and technique, some sort of success has been tried to achieve in pediatric endodontics over the past decades.

GENERAL FEATURES OF PULP

The dental pulp occupies the center of each tooth and consists of soft connective tissue. Primary teeth have 20 pulp organs, their shape confines to the tooth with the mean volume of a single pulp being 0.01 cm^3.

Coronal Pulp

Coronal pulp is located in center of the crown and resembles outer surface of coronal dentin. It has six surfaces, namely, buccal, lingual, occlusal, mesial, distal, and the floor. Due to continuous deposition of dentin, coronal pulp becomes smaller with age.

Radicular Pulp

This extends from cervical region of the pulp to the root apex. It is single in anterior and multiple in posterior teeth. It also decreases with age due to continuous deposition of dentin.

Apical Foramen

Average size of this foramen in maxillary anteriors is 0.4 mm and 0.3 mm in mandibular anteriors. The location and shape of apical foramen depends on the functional influence, for example, if tooth migrates, the apical foramen exerts pressure causing resorption. At the same time cementum is laid on opposite side, this is called apical foramen relocation. The mean maximum and minimum diameter of the minor apical foramina ranged from 0.158 to 0.323 mm. The most common minor apical foramen shape was oval (81%). Frequency of accessory foramina was between 2% and 41% for the various tooth types. The frequency of deviation of the minor apical foramina from the anatomic apex varied from 43% to 83% and the distance of deviation in all the teeth was between 0.052 and 2.921 mm.

Accessory Canals

These are seen laterally in the apical third of root. Exact mechanism is not known, but these are due to premature loss of root sheath cells.

Ahmed and **Abbott** accessory root formation usually occurs through two ways, either by splitting the Hertwig epithelial root sheath (HERS) to form two similar roots or by folding of the HERS to form an independent root which may have various morphological roots.

Primary Pulp Organs

These function for short period of time (average—8.3 years) and are divided into three periods:

Pulp Organ Growth

Takes place during the time the crown and roots are developing (1 year).

Pulp Maturation

Time period after root is completed until root resorption begins (3 years).

Pulp Regression

Beginning of root resorption till exfoliation (3–6 years).

Permanent Pulp Organs

Pulp of permanent teeth requires 12 years to develop and maxillary arch requires longer time to complete each process than the mandibular arch.

PRIMARY ROOT CANAL MORPHOLOGY

Maintenance of pediatric dental integrity is important for ensuring correct tooth spacing, mastication, phonation, esthetics, and prevention of psychological effects due to tooth loss. The roots of the primary teeth are formed completely approximately 16–20 months following eruption, and the form and shape of the root canals roughly correspond to the form and shape of the external anatomy of the teeth. There are different patterns that that be observed in case of root canals. Differentiation of a root into separate canals, as in the mesial root of the mandibular molars, occurs by continued deposition of dentin. This narrows the isthmus between the walls of the canals and continues until the formation of dentin islands in the root canal and eventual division of the root into separate canals. The main goal of root canal therapy for deciduous teeth is to clean the root canals of infected tissues; therefore, knowledge of the size, morphology, and variation of the root canals of a primary tooth is useful in visualizing the pulp cavity during treatment.

Vertucci Classification

Classification of Vertucci (type I–type VIII) and additional classification of Sert et al. (type IX)

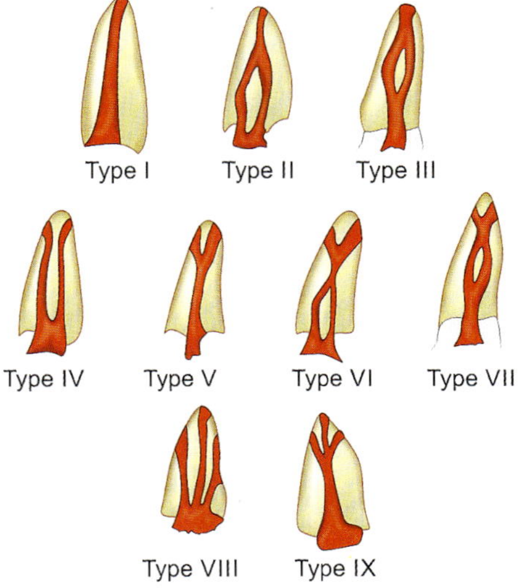

GENERAL FEATURES OF THE PULP CAVITIES OF DECIDUOUS TEETH (FIGS. 50.1 A AND B)

- Smaller depth of dentin between the pulp chamber and the enamel, especially in the mandibular second deciduous molar.
- Very thin, highly projecting pulp horns in the molars, especially mesial.
- The pulp chamber is relatively larger than in the corresponding permanent tooth as a result of the thinner dentin walls which enclose it.
- There are no clearly defined root canal entrances.
- Long root canals in the molars, the root canals are often irregular and ribbon-like.
- The root canals of the deciduous molars diverge greatly.
- Thin enamel.

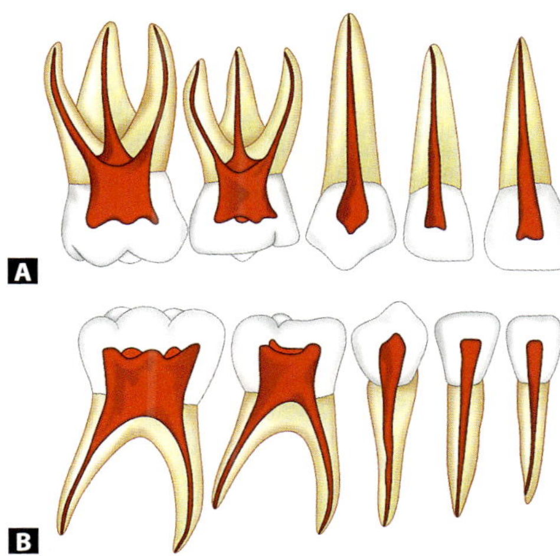

Figs. 50.1A and B: Pulp cavities of the deciduous teeth.

DECIDUOUS INCISORS

The simple pulp chamber of this tooth is fan-shaped when viewed from the labial aspect and corresponds with the shape of the crown. It is relatively wider than that of the permanent incisor and extends further incisally so that the pulp lies closer under the thin enamel covering the crown. Pulp exposures during even the most simple clinical cavity preparations occur quite frequently because of this. The pulp horns are less pointed than in the permanent incisors. The pulp chamber is wedge-shaped labiolingually and becomes narrower at the incisive edge.

The root canal is wide and splays out more than in the permanent incisors resulting in a relatively wider apical cross section, without a clearly defined apical constriction. The root canal is widest labiolingually so that the mesiodistal flattening results occasionally in a partial division of the canal into two canals separated by a mesiodistal dentin dividing wall. In most cases, however, the deciduous incisors have only one root canal with an oval cross-section, ending in a relatively wide apical foramen. The apical third of the root is perforated by many accessory canals.

Maxillary Central Incisor

The pulp chamber and canals resemble the exterior form of the tooth. The pulp chamber has three small projections on its incisal border and tapers evenly toward the cervix, with no distinct constriction at its junction with the pulp canal. The pulp canal varies from a round shape to a slight labiolingual compression but in either case tapers evenly toward the apex **(Fig. 50.2)**.

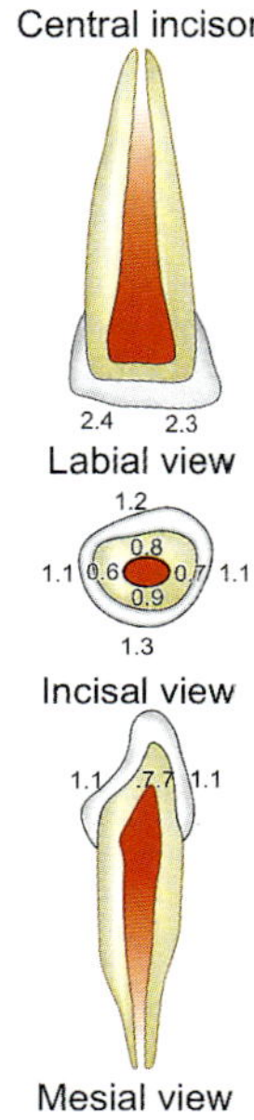

Fig. 50.2: Maxillary central incisor.

Maxillary Lateral Incisor

The pulp morphology is similar to that of the central incisor, but there is generally a demarcation between the pulp chamber and the pulp canal **(Fig. 50.3)**.

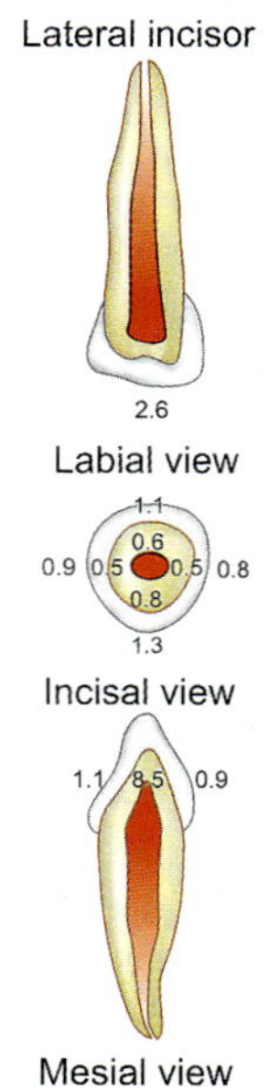

Fig. 50.3: Maxillary lateral incisor.

Mandibular Central Incisor

The pulp chamber conforms to the external anatomy of the crown, and there is usually a definite constriction between the pulp chamber and the pulp canal. The pulp canal tapers evenly toward the apex **(Fig. 50.4)**.

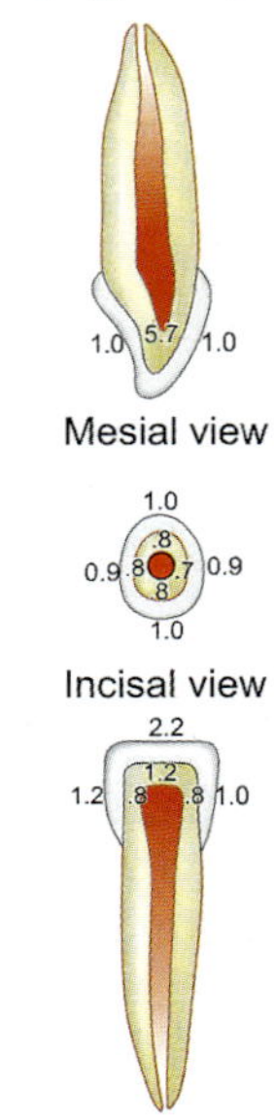

Fig. 50.4: Mandibular central incisor.

Mandibular Lateral Incisor

The pulp chamber and canal generally conform to the external morphology of the tooth. There is no constriction between the pulp chamber and pulp canal such as that found in the mandibular central incisor **(Fig. 50.5)**.

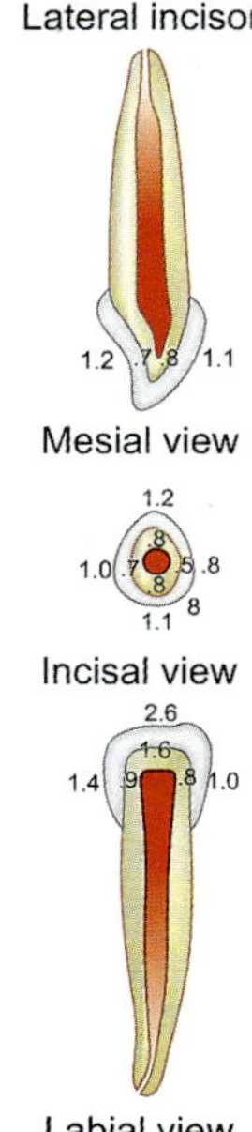

Fig. 50.5: Mandibular lateral incisor.

DECIDUOUS CANINE

The pulp chamber of this tooth is similar in many ways to that of the deciduous incisors, except that it has a single pulp horn, corresponding with the external morphology of the crown. There is no obvious morphological border between the pulp chamber and the root canal, so that the entire pulp cavity tapers evenly from the roof of the pulp chamber to the root apex, without being interrupted by constrictions.

In cross-section, the root canal appears flattened on the mesial and distal sides giving it a slightly oval shape. The root canal of this tooth is longer than that of all the other deciduous teeth and ends in an obvious apical foramen with many small accessory apical canals. The apical third tends to curve distally. The root canal is proportionally longer relative to the crown height, than in the permanent canines. As is the case with all deciduous teeth, the dentin between the pulp chamber and the enamel layer covering the crown is much less than in the permanent canine.

Maxillary Canine

Pulp morphology shows three projections at the incisal aspect of the pulp chamber; the central is the largest and longest, followed by the distal and mesial projections. There is little demarcation between the pulp chamber and the root canal, which tapers evenly as it approaches the apex **(Fig. 50.6)**.

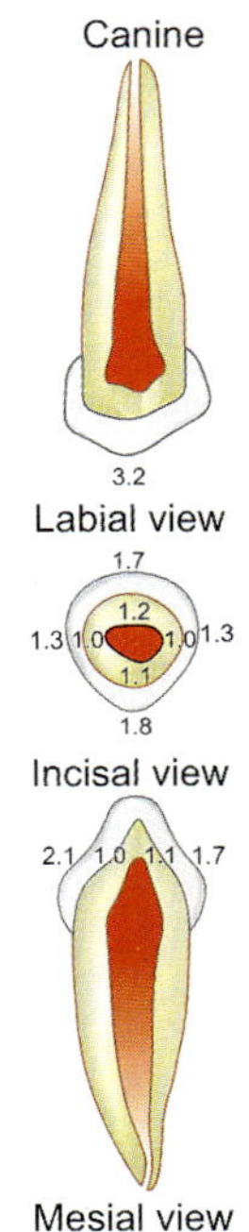

Fig. 50.6: Maxillary canine.

Mandibular Canine

The pulp morphology conforms to the external morphology of the tooth, with no demarcation between the pulp chamber and pulp canal **(Fig. 50.7)**.

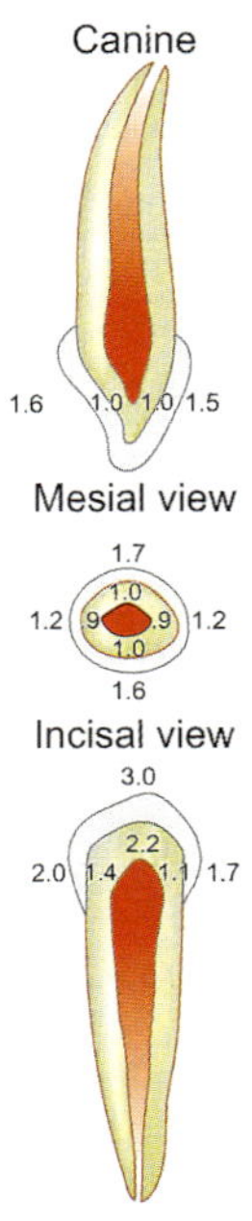

Fig. 50.7: Mandibular canine.

DECIDUOUS MOLARS

The pulp chamber of these teeth is very large relative to the external dimensions of the crown. This is especially true of the mandibular second molar. The dentin and enamel walls of these teeth are fairly thin, and the distance between the pulp horns and the enamel surface is sometimes as little as 2 mm. Special "Eastman" burs are often advised for the preparation of cavities in deciduous molars in the hope of reducing the chances of pulp exposure during treatment.

The pulp chamber has the same number of pulp horns as there are cusps on the crown, and these extend quite far under the cusps. This is especially true of the mesial pulp horns, the most obvious example of which is present in the second molars. The root canals are irregular, often ribbon-like and much more complicated than those in the permanent molars. The root furcation is very close to the level of the cementoenamel junction, so that lateral perforation is a risk at this pain during endodontic treatment.

Maxillary First Molar

The coronal pulp morphology is similar to the external form. There are generally three pulp horns; the mesiobuccal is the largest, followed by mesiolingual and the distobuccal. There are three pulp canals corresponding to the three roots. According to **Hibbard** and **Ireland** and **Barker** variations from this basic pulp canal anatomy are fairly common. The most frequently found are anastomoses and branching in the apical region, often connecting the lingual and distobuccal pulp canals **(Fig. 50.8)**.

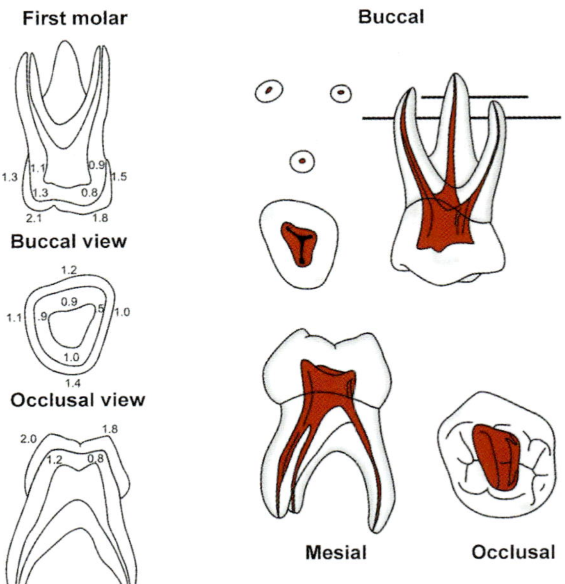

Fig. 50.8: Maxillary first molar.

Maxillary Second Molar

The pulp morphology shows a pulp chamber that conforms to the external contours of the crown. There is one pulp horn corresponding to each cusp; the mesiobuccal is the largest, followed by the mesiolingual, distobuccal, and distolingual. The pulp canals do not show a high incidence of branching and anastomosing such as is seen in the maxillary first primary molar **(Fig. 50.9)**.

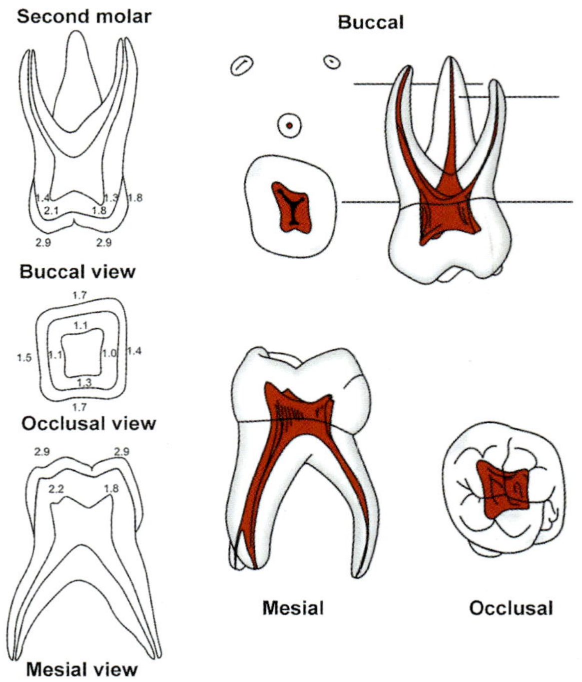

Fig. 50.9: Maxillary second molar.

Mandibular First Molar

The pulp chamber is typical, with four pulp horns, the mesiobuccal the largest and longest. There are generally three pulp canals—distal, mesiobuccal and mesiolingual. The two mesial canals generally extend from the chamber separately or in a ribbon shape but usually become more confluent via branching and anastomosing as they approach the apex **(Fig. 50.10)**.

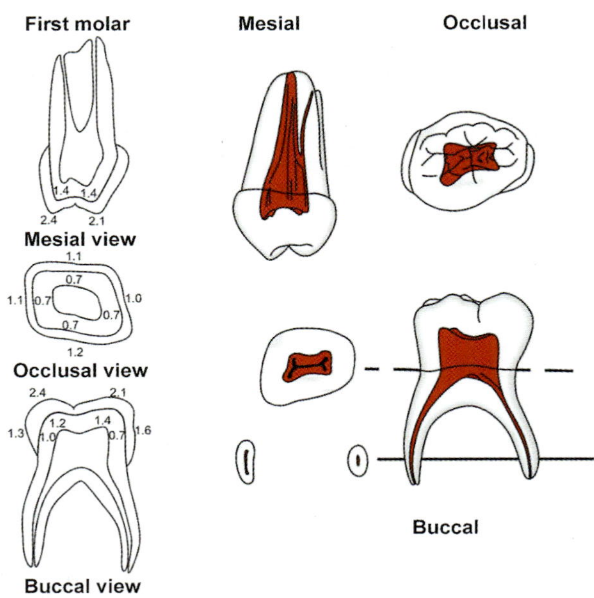

Fig. 50.10: Mandibular first molar.

Mandibular Second Molar

The pulp morphology generally shows a pulp chamber with five pulp horns and three pulp canals. The mesiobuccal and mesiolingual pulp horns are the largest and longest.

The mesiobuccal and mesiolingual pulp canals are usually confluent and ribbon-shaped as they leave the chamber but divide into separate canals with occasional branching as they approach the apex **(Fig. 50.11)**.

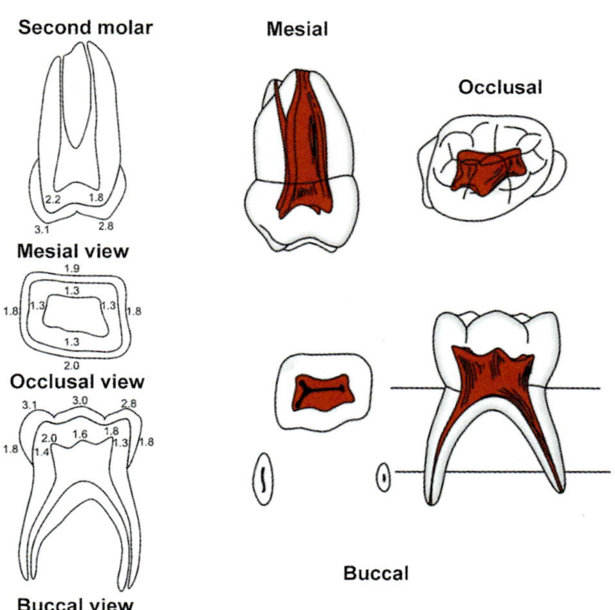

Fig. 50.11: Mandibular second molar.

PULP DISEASES

The dental pulp consists of loose connective tissue interspersed with tiny blood vessels, myelinated and unmyelinated nerves, and lymphatics. The cellular components of pulp consist of odontoblasts, fibroblasts, undifferentiated cells, and certain cells from immune system. The pulp responds to changes in environment in the same way as any other loose connective tissue. However, lack of collateral circulation, presence of dentin forming cells (odontoblasts), and its encasement in unyielding hard tissue (dentin) make its inflammatory response unique from any other organ in the human body.

Etiology of Pulp Diseases

The most common cause of pulp and periapical diseases is the presence of microorganisms within the involved tooth. However, there are several other factors which may affect the health of pulp. These may broadly be classified into:

- **Bacterial:** Via direct invasion or indirectly by its toxins.
- **Mechanical:** Trauma, attrition, abrasion, erosion, cavity preparation, crown preparation, orthodontic movement, osteotomy, barodontalgia and cracked tooth.
- **Thermal:** Friction during tooth cutting, exothermic reaction of dental materials, conduction of heat in deep fillings, and laser burn.
- **Electrical:** Galvanism.
- **Chemical:** Etchants, cements, cavity disinfectants, and desiccants.

<table>
<tr><td>Dentinal hypersensitivity</td><td>
• When pain occurs with thermal, chemical, tactile, or osmotic stimuli associated with exposed dentine, the diagnosis is dentine sensitivity
• The pain is consistent with an exaggerated response of the normal pulpo-dentinal complex, and it is severe and sharp on application of the stimulus to the exposed dentine
• Nonetheless, there is no lingering discomfort once the stimulus is removed
• Not only do the nerves in these exposed tubules respond to hot and cold and sweet and sour but also to scratching with a fingernail or during tooth brushing. For this reason, patients often avoid brushing the area. This only worsens the situation from plaque build-up
Treatment
• An insulating cement base under amalgam fillings will prevent the shock of hot or cold to the pulp. Eventually, irritation dentin will build-up to protect the pulp from thermal shock
• Marginal microleakage around restorations may also lead to hypersensitivity. Replacement of restoration in such cases leads to alleviation of symptoms
• In order to further desensitize the exposed dentin, dentifrices may be prescribed which reduce pain by nerve desensitization or by occluding dentinal tubules.
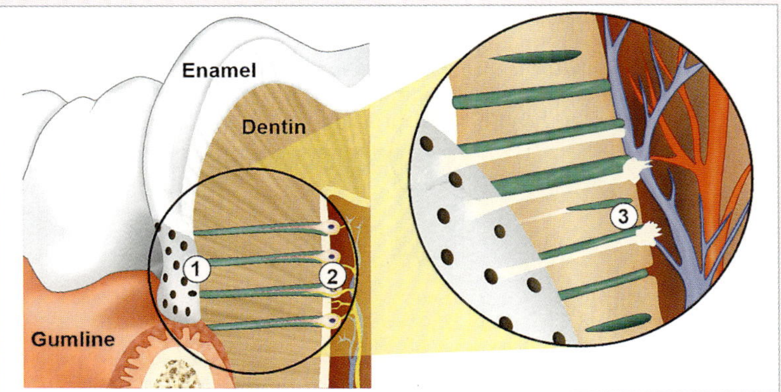

</td></tr>
<tr><td>Reversible pulpitis</td><td>
• It is one of the earliest form of pulpitis is also referred to as "pulp hyperemia".
• Pulp with reversible pulpitis has mild inflammation, and it is capable of healing once the irritating stimulus has been removed
• Pain is only felt when a stimulus (usually cold or sweet foods but sometimes heat) is applied to the tooth, and the pain ceases within a few seconds or immediately upon removal of the stimulus. This is due to the movement of dentinal fluid toward the pulpal tissue
• The pain is short and sharp in nature, but it is never spontaneous
• Occurs due to stimulation of A delta fibers.
• There are no radiographic changes evident in the periapical region
Treatment
• As Grossman has stated, "The best treatment for reversible pulpitis is its prevention." Removal of noxious stimulus generally is sufficient to allow the pulp to return back to its healthy state.
</td></tr>
</table>

Contd...

Irreversible pulpitis	• In case of irreversible pulpitis, the pulp has been damaged beyond repair, and even the removal of the noxious stimulus will not allow its proper healing. The pulp generally degenerates progressively, causing necrosis and reactive destruction • One of the classic symptoms of irreversible pulpitis is lingering pain induced by thermal stimuli • The initial reaction is a very sharp pain to hot or cold stimuli followed by dull ache or a throbbing pain for minutes to hours after the stimulus is removed • Pain increases on bending or lying down • Spontaneous pain is another hallmark feature of irreversible pulpitis • Pain may be intermittent or continuous which occurs due to stimulation of C- fibers. • If the periapical tissues are involved, the tooth is tender to percussion • In most cases, radiographs are not useful in diagnosis, but they can be helpful in identifying the possible cause of the disease, e.g., associated caries, or fracture of tooth, etc. ***Treatment*** The treatment options are: • Pulp or endodontic therapy (tooth restorable) • Extraction otherwise (unrestorable) 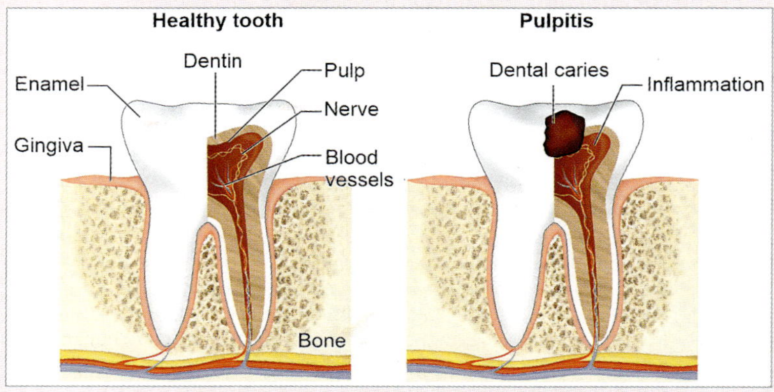
Hyperplastic pulpitis	• Hyperplastic pulpitis (pulp polyp) is a productive inflammatory response of pulp • It usually involves chronically inflamed young pulp, widely exposed by caries on its occlusal aspect • It is characterized by a reddish cauliflower like growth of inflamed connective tissue rising out of the carious crown. The tissue is mostly firm, insensitive to the touch, and occasionally may cause mild discomfort during mastication • Often covered with epithelium, it resembles a pyogenic granuloma of the gingiva from which it may be easily differentiated by lifting it away from the walls with a spoon excavator to view the pedicle of its origin • The tooth will respond to pulp testing which is often delayed. • No significant radiographic changes (except for the cause of the problem—e.g., caries, fractured restoration, etc.) are evident unless there is also periapical involvement ***Treatment*** • Frequently, the teeth involved in hyperplastic pulpitis are so badly decayed that restoration is virtually impossible, and extraction is usually indicated • On the other hand, if the tooth is restorable, pulp or endodontic therapy is recommended 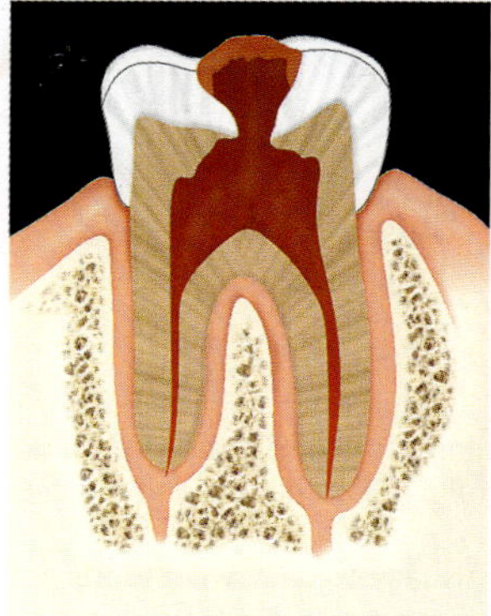 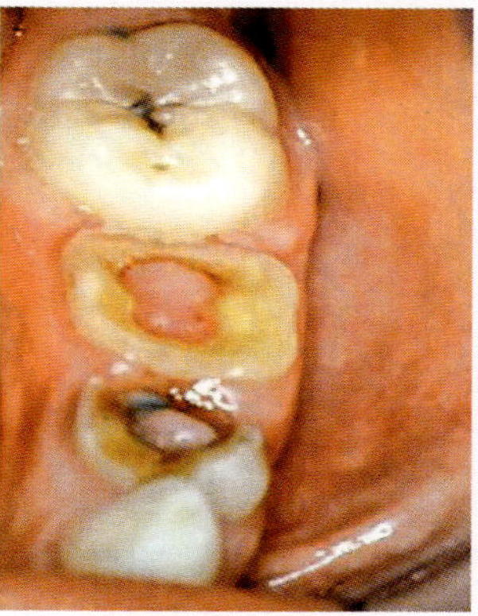

Contd...

Necrobiosis (partial necrosis)	• A tooth with necrobiosis has both inflamed and necrotic (usually infected) pulp tissue. The necrotic tissue may be in the coronal portion of the pulp (e.g., pulp chamber) with the inflamed tissue apically, or the different tissue states may exist in different canals of a multi-canal tooth. The symptoms may be mild with intermittent painful episodes.
Necrosis	• There are no true symptoms of complete pulp necrosis for the simple reason that the pulp, together with its sensory nerves, is totally destroyed • Pain usually does not present unless the periodontal ligament (PDL) is affected. However, if only partial necrosis has occurred, the patient may have some mild pain and discomfort • A routine radiographic survey or coronal discoloration may present the first indication that something is amiss in the case of the tooth with a necrotic pulp • On questioning, the history may reveal past trauma, previous episodes of pain, or history of restorations and caries • The radiograph may be helpful if a periradicular lesion exists because it generally indicates associated pulp death. Per se, no changes in the canal are noted radiographically to indicate necrosis ***Treatment*** • If the tooth is salvageable, endodontic therapy is indicated, else extraction is the only solution 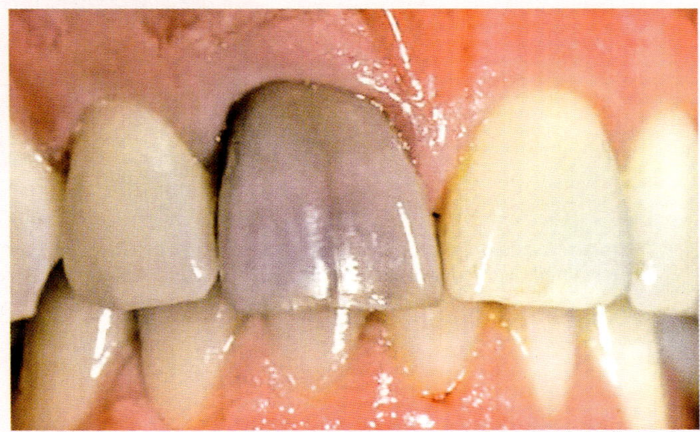
Internal resorption	• The term internal resorption is applied to the destruction of predentin and dentin • Often only recognized during a routine radiographic examination, it is asymptomatic and unidentifiable clinically until the lesion has progressed considerably • It may begin anywhere in the pulp space and if left untreated can perforate either above bone or into the PDL within bone • When confined to the crown, enough tooth structure may be destroyed for the pulp to show through the enamel—hence the synonym for internal resorption, "pink tooth" • The etiology is unclear, but it is probably due to a metaplastic change or activation of dentinoclasts within the inflamed pulp tissue • History of impact trauma has often been found to be associated with internal resorption ***Treatment*** • Since the pulp tissue cells are responsible for the destructive process, its removal by endodontic therapy arrests any further resorption. 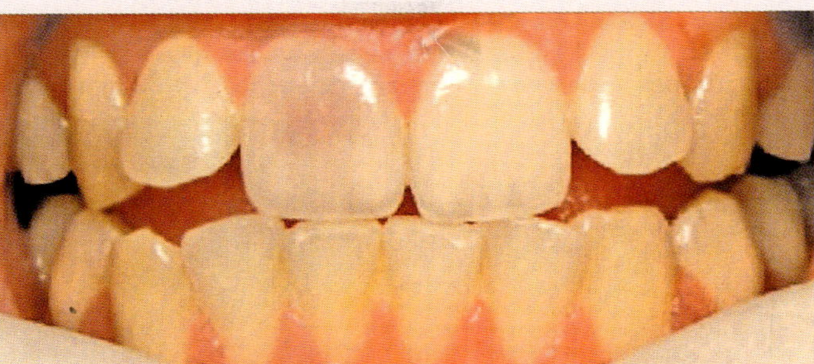

Contd...

Pulp degenerations	• The pulp will usually respond to noxious stimuli by becoming inflamed, but it may also respond by degeneration which includes atrophy and fibrosis and calcification. Although these changes are not evident clinically, it is appropriate to discuss these changes along with other pulp diseases • ***Atrophy*** is a normal physiologic process that occurs with age and is asymptomatic. The cellularity of the pulp tissue is decreased with an increase in intercellular material. Pulp sensitivity tests responses may be normal or delayed. No significant radiographic or clinical signs are present.

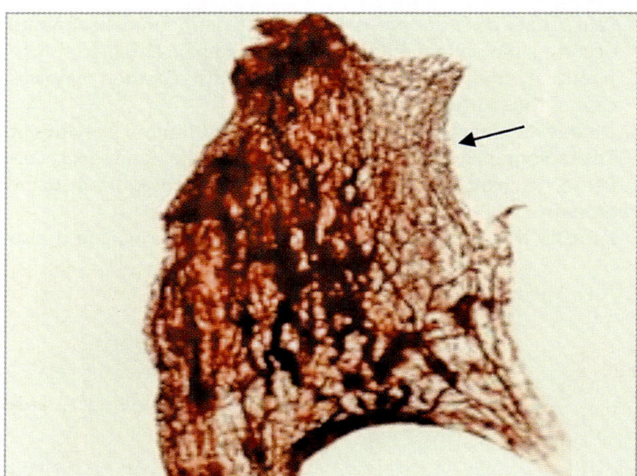

• ***Fibrosis:*** As the pulp atrophies, there may also be fibrosis of the pulp tissue, and the extent of this will be largely determined by the number of irritant episodes suffered by that particular pulp throughout its history.

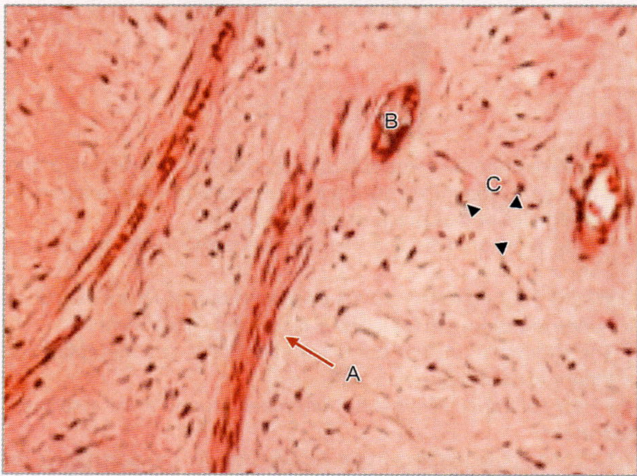

• ***Calcification:*** In calcific degeneration, pulp tissue is replaced with calcific material. It may occur anywhere in the pulp space and may be diffused or localized (pulp stones). Teeth with calcifications are usually asymptomatic. There are usually no or delayed response to electrical test. Radiographically, there is no evidence of the usual pulp chamber outline and the root canal may appear narrow or it may not be evident at all.

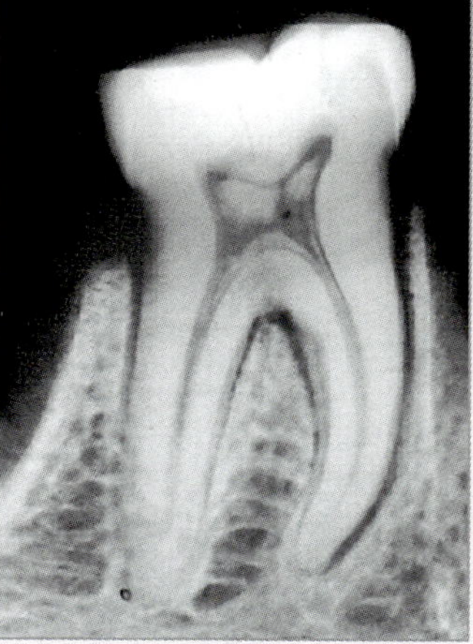

PERIAPICAL LESIONS

Teeth with normal periradicular tissues are nonsensitive to percussion and palpation testing. Radiographically, periradicular tissues are normal with an intact lamina dura and a uniform PDL space. Exposure of the dental pulp to bacteria and their by-products, acting as antigens, may elicit nonspecific inflammatory responses as well as specific immunological reactions in the periradicular tissues and cause the periapical lesion. These periapical lesions resulting from necrotic dental pulp are among the most frequently occurring pathologies found in alveolar bone.

As already mentioned in case of pulpal diseases, the various lesions described below are interrelated, and if allowed to progress undeterred, one may lead to another.

Acute apical periodontitis

- It is painful inflammation of the periodontal tissues. Usually, a result of microbes spreading from root canal to periapical tissues. Other reasons include trauma, irritation to periapical area
- The patient will generally complain of discomfort to biting or chewing
- Sensitivity to percussion is a hallmark diagnostic test result of acute periradicular periodontitis
- Tooth is usually not sensitive to hot or cold
- Depending on the cause of inflammation, it may or may not respond to vitality tests
- Palpation testing may or may not produce a sensitive response
- Radiographically, the PDL space may appear normal, widened, or there may be a distinct radiolucency

Treatment

- Determination of cause and relieving the symptoms. In case it is because of pulpal involvement, endodontic therapy is indicated

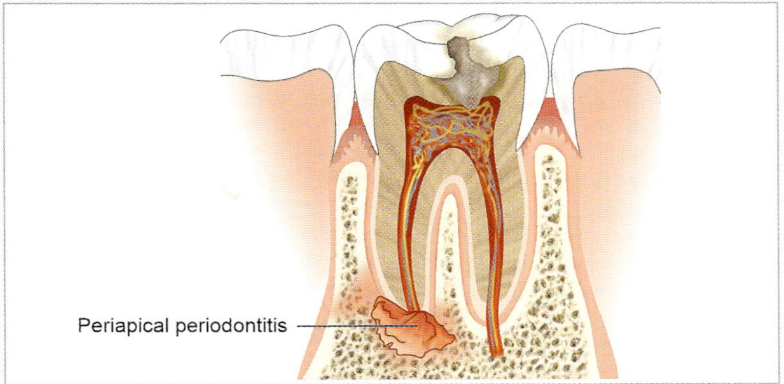

Acute periapical abscess

- It refers to painful localized collection of pus in the periapical connective tissue
- It is characterized by rapid onset, spontaneous pain, pus formation, and often swelling of the associated tissues
- Depending upon the location of the apices of the tooth and muscle attachments, a swelling will usually develop in the buccal vestibule, on the lingual or palatal, or as a facial space infection
- Percussion testing produces a response that is usually exquisitely sensitive. Palpation testing may produce a sensitive response
- The tooth gives negative response to vitality test
- Radiographically, the PDL space may be widened, or demonstrate a distinct radiolucency

Treatment

- Endodontic treatment concomitant with the drainage of abscess. Suitable measures must also be taken to control any systemic manifestations

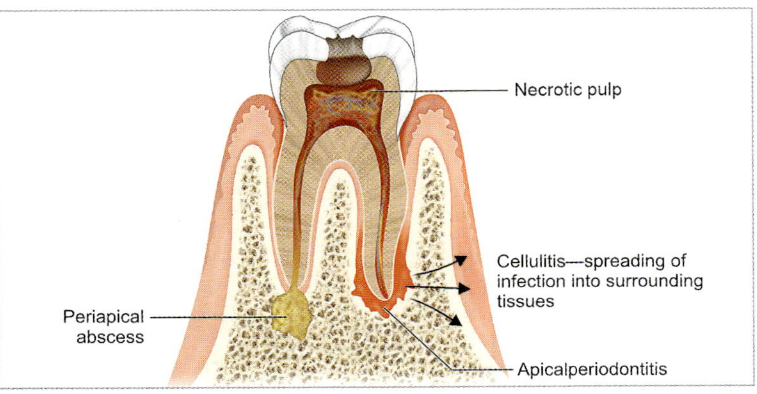

Contd...

Chronic periradicular abscess (suppurative periradicular periodontitis)	• An inflammatory reaction to pulpal infection and necrosis characterized by gradual onset, little or no discomfort, and intermittent discharge of pus through an associated sinus tract • The resultant inflammatory process causes periradicular bone resorption that manifests as periradicular radiolucency on the radiograph • Clinically, the patient is asymptomatic or very rarely has mild pain and the lesion is detected with a routine radiograph • Percussion and palpation testing produce nonsensitive responses • Tooth generally responds negatively to vitality tests • Radiographically there will be a sign of radiolucency indicating osseous destruction ***Treatment*** • Endodontic therapy if the tooth can be restored otherwise extraction • The sinus tract does not generally require any special treatment 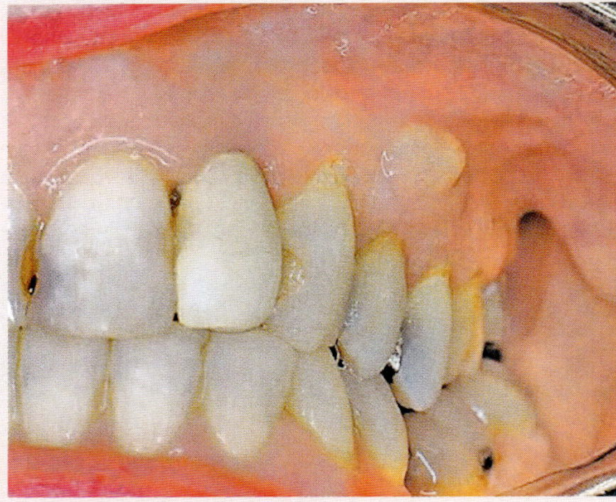
Recrudescent abscess	• It refers to an acute exacerbation arising from a pre-existing chronic lesion • Also known as "Phoenix Abscess". • Immediately following endodontic therapy • Inadequate debridement during the endodontic procedure • Tooth feels elevated in its socket • The tooth is severely tender • Palpation may produce positive response with signs of inflammation evident on overlying mucosa • Negative response to electric pulp testing (EPT) • The radiograph shows a well-defined radiolucency ***Treatment*** • The treatment options are similar to that of acute alveolar abscess
Focal sclerosing osteomyelitis (condensing osteitis)	• The involved tooth will have an etiologic factor for low-grade, chronic inflammation such as a necrotic pulp, extensive restorative history, or a crack • The patient may be asymptomatic or demonstrate a wide range of pulpal symptoms • EPT and thermal tests may or may not be responsive • Percussion and palpation testing may or may not be sensitive • Radiographically, the involved tooth will present with increased radiodensity and opacity around one or more of the roots ***Treatment*** • These periradicular radiodensities resolve gradually after endodontic therapy 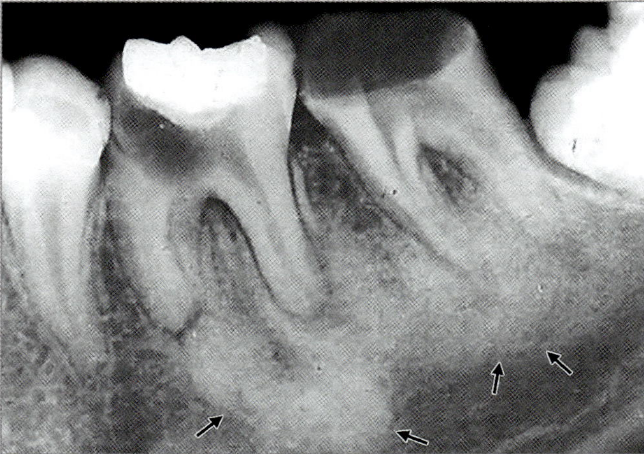

Contd...

Periapical granuloma	• This disease entity is characterized by growth of granulation tissue in relation to the periodontium at the apex in response continued bacterial irritation • Patient usually is asymptomatic • The tooth is generally nonvital and not responsive to percussion • Although there is a growth of granulation tissue in the area, there is rarely any swelling or expansion of cortical plates • Radiograph shows loss of lamina dura and diffused periapical radiolucency ***Treatment*** • Pulp or endodontic therapy of the concerned tooth 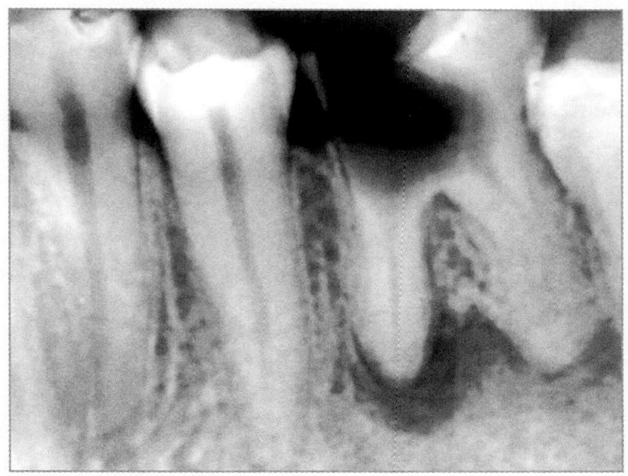
Periapical cyst	• The radicular cyst is a chronic inflammatory lesion with a closed pathologic cavity, lined either partially or completely by epithelium • A cyst may develop in relation to an infected tooth due to continuous irritation and stimulation of epithelial rests of Malassez, which are normally present in the PDL • Majority of cases of periapical cyst are asymptomatic. The tooth is seldom painful or sensitive to percussion • Pressure due to growth of the cyst may make it obvious as a swelling or cause movement of the root • Radiograph shows a distinct rarefaction at the apex with a thin radiopaque border ***Treatment*** Treatment of periapical cyst is conservative initially by root canal treatment. Surgical intervention is advisable only if the conservative means fail. There are two options: 1. Conservative approach by pulp or endodontic therapy and regular follow-ups. During recall visits observe for regression of the cyst. If the cyst does not regress, surgical intervention is advised 2. Pulp or endodontic therapy immediately followed by surgical intervention 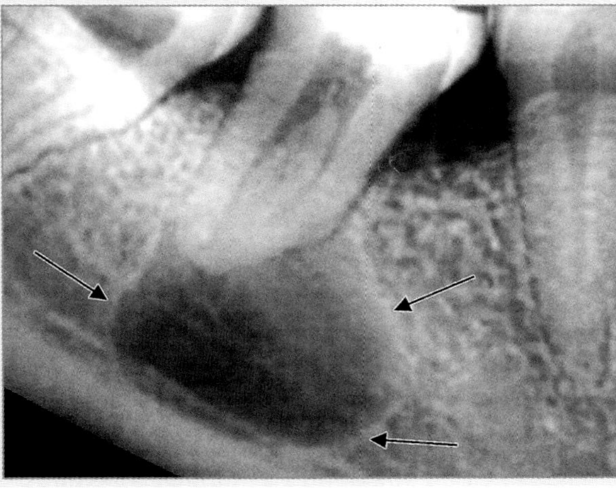

DIAGNOSIS OF PULP PATHOLOGY

Pain

An accurate history must be obtained of the type of pain, duration, frequency, location, spread, aggregating and relieving factors. In young children, the pain history should not be considered as a sole criterion in diagnosing pulpal conditions.

Nerve Fibers in Dental Pulp (Table 50.1)

- The pulp contains two types of sensory nerve fibers—myelinated (A fibers) and unmyelinated (C fibers).
- Approximately, 80% of the nerves of the pulp are C fibers and the rest are Aδ fibers.
- The relatively late appearance of A fibers in the pulp may help to explain why the electric pulp test tends to be unreliable in young teeth, as A fibers are more easily electrically stimulated than C fibers.

Table 50.1: Fibers associated with dental pain.

A delta fibers		*C Fibers*
2-5 µm	Diameter	0.3-2.1 µm
5-30 m/s	Conduction velocity	0.4-2 m/s
Yes, No	Myelinated	No
Subodontoblastic	Location	Near the blood vessels throughout the pulp
Sharp, pricking, unpleasant, bearable	Pain characteristics	Lingering, throbbing unbearable

Mode

Is the onset spontaneous or provoked?

Periodicity

Do symptoms have temporal pattern or are they sporadic or occasional? Early pulpitis—symptoms seen in evening or after meal.

Frequency

Have the symptoms persisted since they began or have they been intermittent?

Duration

How long do symptoms last when they occur?

Quality of Pain

Dull and aching—pain of bony origin. Throbbing, pounding, and pulsing—pain of vascular origin sharp, recurrent. Stabbing—pathosis of nerve root complexes, irreversible pulpitis.

Postural Change

Pain accentuated by bending over, blowing the nose—maxillary sinus involvement.

Time of Day

Pain in the masticatory muscles on working may indicate occlusal disharmony or temporomandibular joint (TMJ) dysfunction or possible acute pulpalgia.

Hormonal

Menstrual toothache occurs due to increase in body fluid retention. Teeth may ache and become tender on percussion. Symptoms disappear when cycle ends.

Types of Pain

- **Momentary pain:** Immediate response to hot or cold that disappears on removal of the stimulus indicates that the pathosis is limited to the coronal pulp.
- **Persistent pain:** Pain from thermal stimuli would indicate widespread inflammation of the pulp, extending into the radicular filaments.
- **Spontaneous pain:** Throbbing, constant pain that may keep the patient awake at night. This type of pain indicates pulpal damage—irreversible pulpitis.
- **Provoked pain:** Stimulated by thermal, chemical, or mechanical irritant and is eliminated when noxious stimulus is removed. Indicates dentine sensitivity due to deep carious lesion or faulty restoration. Pulp is in reversible stage.

Visual and Tactile Examination

This is one of the simplest tests, but most often it is done casually during examination, and as a result, valid information is lost. A thorough visual, tactile examination of hard and soft tissue relies on checking the three Cs, that is—color, contour, and consistency.

Mobility

Mobility in a primary tooth may result from physiological or pathological cause. Tooth mobility is directly proportional to the integrity of the attachment apparatus. Clinician should use two mouth mirror handles to apply alternating lateral forces in a facial lingual direction to observe the degree of mobility of the tooth.

Grading of mobility

	Wyman's index (1975)
0	Horizontal <0.2 mm
1	Horizontal 0.2–1 mm
2	Horizontal 1–2 mm
3	Horizontal >2 mm and vertically

Percussion

Pain from pressure on a tooth indicates that periodontal ligament is inflamed. The normal approach is to use blunt end of the instrument in children. A useful clinical test is to apply finger pressure to the tooth and check the child's response by watching the eyes.

Palpation

Simple test done with fingertips using light pressure to examine tissue consistency and pain response. It determines presence, intensity, and location of pain and presence of bony crepitus.

Radiographs

Recent preoperative radiographs are prerequisites to pulp therapy in primary and young permanent teeth. It demonstrates pathological conditions and position of the succedaneous permanent tooth. These will dictate the decision on performing pulp therapy for primary tooth.

The Exposure Site

The size of the exposure site and the nature of exudate expressed from it are useful diagnostic aids. Light red blood that can be arrested easily is associated with inflammation that is limited to the coronal pulp in primary teeth. Deep red blood histologically indicates that inflammation has extended into the root canals of primary molars.

Pulp Testing

Pulp testing is widely used to assess vitality of mature permanent teeth, but these are not reliable in deciduous teeth as fear of unknown makes child patient apprehensive of the electric vitalometer and may give inaccurate results. Another reason is that newly erupted teeth may have incomplete innervation and therefore may not give correct results. The detailed overview of pulp testing has been explained in Chapter 52.

POINTS TO REMEMBER

- Average size of apical foramen in maxillary anteriors is 0.4 mm, and in mandibular anteriors is 0.3 mm. Accessory canals are seen laterally in the apical third of root due to premature loss of root sheath cells.
- Primary pulp organs function for short period of time of average—8.3 years.
- In the case of incisors, pulp chamber is fan-shaped when viewed from the labial aspect and corresponds with the shape of the crown. It is relatively wider than that of the permanent incisor and extends further incisally so that the pulp lies closer under the thin enamel covering the crown.
- The root canal is wide and splays out more than in the permanent incisors resulting in a relatively wider apical cross-section, without a clearly defined apical constriction.
- The pulp chamber of canines is similar in many ways to that of the deciduous incisors, except that it has a single pulp horn corresponding with the external morphology of the crown.
- The root canal of this tooth is longer than that of all the other deciduous teeth and ends in an obvious apical foramen with many small accessory apical canals. the apical third tends to curve distally.
- The pulp chamber of molars is very large relative to the external dimensions of the crown. this is especially true of the mandibular second molar.
- The pulp chamber has the same number of pulp horns as there are cusps on the crown, and these extend quite far under the cusps.
- The root canals are irregular, often ribbon-like, and much more complicated than those in the permanent molars.
- Diseases of pulp include hypersensitivity, reversible pulpitis, irreversible pulpitis, hyperplastic pulpitis, necrosis, and pulp degeneration.
- Diseases of periapical tissues include—acute apical periodontitis, acute periapical abscess, chronic periradicular abscess (suppurative periradicular periodontitis), recrudescent abscess, focal sclerosing osteomyelitis (condensing osteitis), periapical granuloma, and periapical cyst.
- Reversible pulpitis is characterized when pain is only felt when a stimulus is applied to the tooth, and the pain ceases within a few seconds or immediately upon removal of the stimulus.
- One of the classic symptoms of irreversible pulpitis is lingering pain induced by thermal stimuli. The initial reaction is a very sharp pain to hot or cold stimuli followed by dull ache or a throbbing pain for minutes to hours after the stimulus is removed.
- Hyperplastic pulpitis (pulp polyp) is a productive inflammatory response of pulp. It involves chronically inflamed young pulp, widely exposed by caries on its occlusal aspect.
- The term internal resorption is applied to the destruction of predentin and dentin and is only recognized during a routine radiographic examination.
- Acute apical periodontitis is painful inflammation of the periodontal tissues.
- Acute periapical abscess refers to painful localized collection of pus in the periapical connective tissue.
- Chronic periradicular abscess is an inflammatory reaction to pulpal infection and necrosis characterized by gradual onset, and intermittent discharge of pus through an associated sinus tract.
- Recrudescent abscess refers to an acute exacerbation arising from a preexisting chronic lesion.
- In focal sclerosing osteomyelitis (condensing osteitis), the involved tooth will have an etiologic factor for low-grade, chronic inflammation such as a necrotic pulp, extensive restorative history, or a crack.
- Periapical cyst is a chronic inflammatory lesion with a closed pathologic cavity, lined either partially or completely by epithelium.

Questionnaire

1. Explain the diseases of pulp.
2. Describe the diseases of periapical tissues.
3. What are the methods for diagnosis of pulp and periapical pathologies?
4. What are the features of deciduous pulp cavity?
5. Describe the endodontic morphology of deciduous dentition.

FURTHER READING

1. Ahmed HM, Abbott PV. Accessory roots in maxillary molar teeth: a review and endodontic considerations. Aust Dent J. 2012; 57:123-31.
2. Ali SG, Mulay S. Pulpitis: A review. IOSR J Dent Med Sci. 2015;14(8):92-7.
3. Barker BCW, Parsons KC, Williams GL, et al. Anatomy of root canals. IV deciduous teeth. Aust Dent J. 1975; 20:101-6.
4. Camp J. Pediatric endodontics: endodontic treatment for the primary and young permanent dentition. In: Cohen S, Burns

RC (Eds). Pathways of the Pulp, 8th edition. St. Louis: Mosby YearbookYearbook, Inc; 2002.
5. Chaudhary M, Chaudhary SD. Essentials of Pediatric Oral Pathology, 1st edition. Jaypee Brothers Publication, New Delhi. 2011.
6. Fuks AB. Pulp therapy for the primary dentition. In: Pinkham JR, Casamassimo PS, Fields HW, McTigue DJ, Nowak A (Eds). Pediatric Dentistry: Infancy Through the Adolescence, 3rd edition. Philadelphia, PA: WB Saunders Co; 1999.
7. Graunaite I, Lodiene G, Maciulskiene V. Pathogenesis of apical periodontitis: A literature review. J Oral Maxillofac Res. 2011;2(4) e1:1-15.
8. Gupta D, Grewal N. Root canal configuration of deciduous mandibular first molars: an in vitro study. J Indian Soc Pedod Prev Dent. 2005; 23:134-7.
9. Gutmann JL, Baumgartner JC, Gluskin AH, Hartwell GR, Walton RE. Identify and define all diagnostic terms for periapical/ periradicular health and disease states. J Endod. 2009;35(12):1658-74.
10. Hibbard ED, Ireland RL. Morphology of the root canals of the primary molar teeth. J Dent Child. 1957; 24:250-7.
11. Lyroudia KM, Dourou VI, Pantelidou OC, Labrianidis T, Pitas IK. Internal root resorption studied by radiography, stereo microscope, scanning electron microscope and computerized 3D reconstructive method. Dent Traumatol. 2002; 18:148-52.
12. McDonald RE, Avery DR, Dean JA. Treatment of deep caries, vital pulp exposure, and pulpless teeth: In: McDonald RE, Avery DR, Dean JA (Eds). Dentistry for the Child and Adolescent, 8th edition. St. Louis: Mosby Inc.; 2004.
13. Murray PE, About I, Franquin JC, et al. Restorative pulpal and repair responses. J Am Dent Assoc. 2001;132: 482-91.
14. Patel S, Ricucci D, Durak C, Tay F. Internal root resorption: A review. J Endod. 2010;36(7):1107-21.
15. Singh G, Paul R S, Arora A, Kumar S, Jindal L, Raina S. Disease of Pulp and Periradicular Tissue: An Overview. J Curr Med Res Opin. 2020;11(0):652-64.
16. Woelfel JB. Dental Anatomy: Its Relevance to Dentistry, 4th edition. Philadelphia, PA: Lea & Febiger; 1990. pp. 201-30.
17. Zircher E. The Anatomy of the Root Canals of the Teeth of the Deciduous Dentition, and of the First Permanent Molars. New York: William Wood & Co; 1925.
18. Zoremchhingi, Joseph T, Varma B, et al. A study of root canal morphology of human primary molars using computerized tomography: an in vitro study. J Indian Soc Pedod Prev Dent. 2005; 23:7-12.

CHAPTER

Concepts of Revascularization and Pulp Regeneration

Pradnya Kathe, Prachi Mital, Shivani Mathur, Vinita Goyel

CHAPTER OUTLINE

Regenerative endodontics is a very interesting and emerging field in dentistry which has received a great deal of research in the past two decades. Revascularization of pulp is perhaps one of the most important focuses in regenerative research. Pulp revascularization is definitely a very promising and an innovative treatment concept especially in the immature necrotic tooth. It has the potential to create a paradigm shift in the endodontic management of young permanent teeth in the field of pediatric dentistry.

Terms like regenerative endodontics and Pulp revascularization must be well defined initially, and their close relationship stressed. The term REP has been used in the later sections synonymously with revascularization, which may cause confusion to readers.

Dental regeneration *can be defined as the process by which specialized dental tissues are replaced by the recruitment, proliferation, migration, and differentiation of dental stem cells.*[1]

Pulp revascularization *in the simplest terms may be defined as reintroduction of vascularity in the root canal system.*[2]

Lenzi and **Trope**[3] suggested the term revitalization as being more appropriate because it is descriptive of the nonspecific vital tissue that forms in the root canal.

RATIONALE FOR REVASCULARIZATION

Unlike the mature permanent tooth, in which the pulp is completely necrosed before the infection reaches the periapical tissues, in an immature tooth the open apex facilitates for large communication between pulp and apical tissues and therefore potential vital pulp cells remain in spite of progression of infection to the periapical tissue **(Figs. 51.1A to E)**. It is this entity of cells that are the primary targets of all revascularization procedures. The abundance of vascular supply in such teeth coupled with successful disinfection of the infected pulp would create an environment for the proliferation of the potential vital pulp stem cells to recreate new tissue in the pulp space. Hence achieving asepsis with effective medicaments is critical to pulp revascularization or maturogenesis.[4]

The necrotic uninfected pulp may be used as a scaffold for the ingrowth of the new tissue from the periapical area. Lately autologous platelet-rich plasma (PRP) is gaining grounds for use as scaffold.

History of Revascularization Procedures

Nygaard-ostby and **Hjortdal**[5] pioneered regenerative procedures way back in 1960s. In 1971, **Nygaard-ostby** and **Hjortdal** evaluated the role of the blood clot in healing. **Yanpiset** and **Trope**[6] carried out pulp revascularization in replanted immature dogteeth. **Iwaya** and **colleagues**[7] in 2001 showed the revascularization potential of an immature permanent tooth and this basically renewed the interest in revascularization procedures.

Trope[8] in 2007 showed successful revascularization of the necrotic infected pulp space of an immature permanent maxillary central incisor induced *in vivo* by stimulation of a blood clot from the periapical tissues. Based on their findings, the authors predicted replacement of existing traditional techniques such as apexification by induction of a hard tissue barrier via $Ca(OH)_2$ or mineral trioxide aggregate (MTA) with pulp revascularization procedures if proven successful in controlled research models.

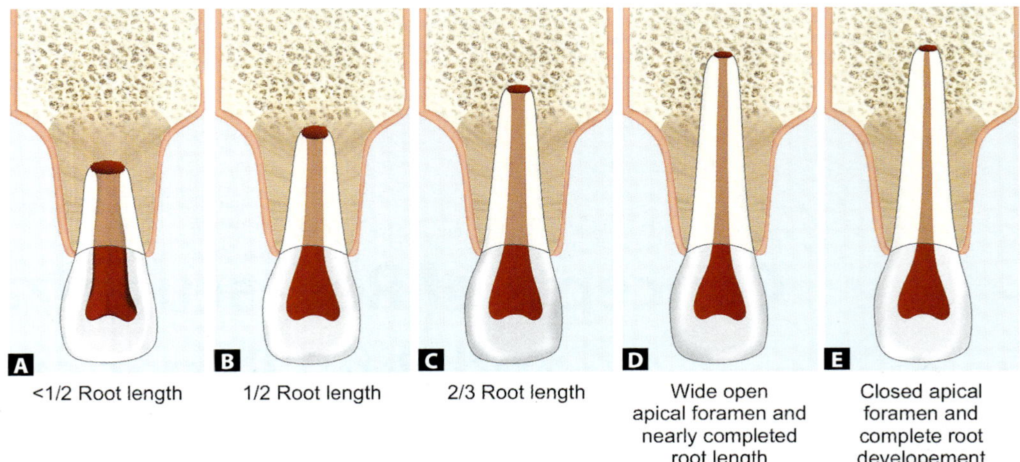

Figs. 51.1A to E: Cvek's classification.

BASIC PRINCIPLES OF REVASCULARIZATION PROCEDURE

Banchs and Trope[9]

They described the following three goals for regenerative endodontic procedures (REPs) as basis of successful revascularization of an immature tooth.

1. The first requirement is elimination of bacteria by effective canal disinfection.
2. The second condition is the creation of a scaffold for the ingrowth of new tissue.
3. The third prerequisite is the prevention of bacterial reinfection with creation of a bacteria-tight seal.

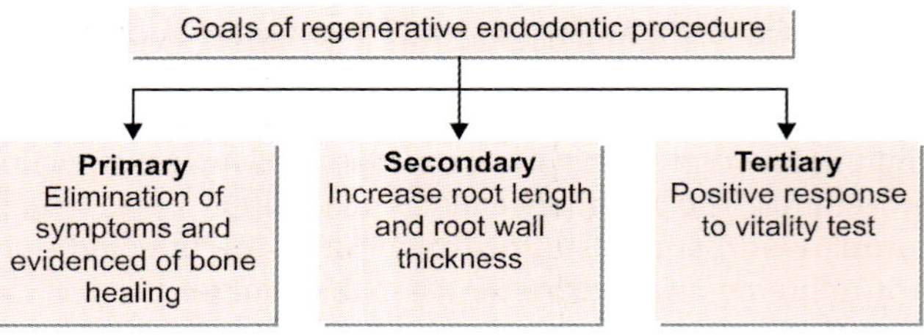

THE BIOLOGICAL CONCEPT OF REGENERATIVE ENDODONTICS

It involves the triad of tissue regeneration:

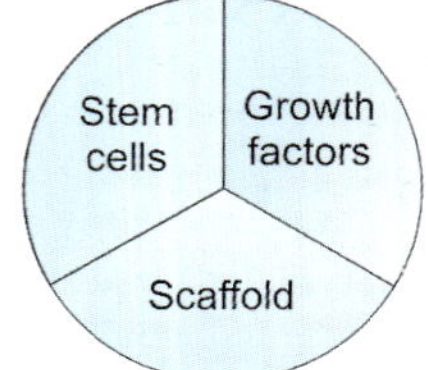

Stem Cells

These are undifferentiated cells with self-renewal and differentiation property. Though the sources of stem cells in the oral cavity are multiple, the stem cells from apical papilla (SCAP) have received special attention in the field of pulpal revascularization. Other types of stem cells include—dental follicle stem cells (DFSCs), dental pulp stem cells (DPSCs), periodontal ligament stem cells (PDLSCs), stem cells from human exfoliated deciduous teeth (SHED), salivary gland stem cells (SGSCs), the induced blood clot via over instrumentation of the canals contains stem cells. Its reported that the blood collected from the canals contain 400–600 times more mesenchymal stem cell markers while compared to the systemic blood **(Fig. 51.2).**

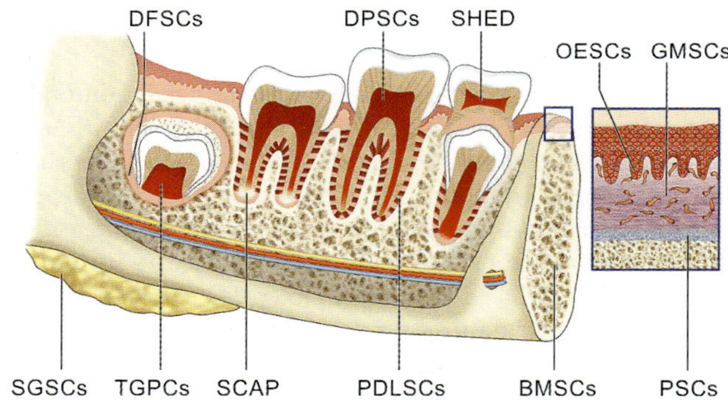

Fig. 51.2: Stem cells in oral cavity.

Scaffolds

The purpose of the scaffolds is to provide three-dimensional structures for stem cells to proliferate and differentiate into the desired cells. They should also promote cell-biomaterial interactions, cell adhesion, and extracellular matrix deposition while permitting the sufficient transport of required gases, nutrients and regulatory factors **(Fig. 51.3).**

The ideal properties of the scaffold include:

- Should have high porosity and an adequate pore size to facilitate cell seeding and diffusion.
- Should allow effective transport of nutrients, oxygen, and waste.
- Should be biodegradable (rate of biodegradation should coincide with the rate of tissue formation) and biocompatible.
- Should have adequate physical and mechanical strength.

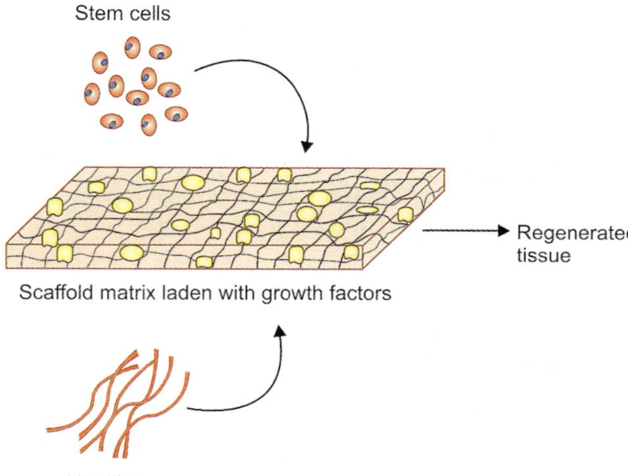

Fig. 51.3: Diagrammatic representation of scaffold.

Various scaffolds which can be used are given below:

Biological/natural	*Synthetic/artificial*
Blood clot	Polymers-Polylactic acid
Platelet-rich plasma (PRP)	Polyglycolic acid
Platelet-rich fibrin (PRF)	Bioceramics-calcium
Collagen	Phosphate, bioactive glass
Chitosan	Glass ceramics
Glycosaminoglycans	
Demineralized dentine matrix	

- **Blood clot:** Most of the REPs use blood clot as the scaffold, however it is considered to promote healing rather than to result in regeneration of the tissues. Blood clot has got cytokines and growth factors in low concentration. Blood clot contains huge number of haemopoetic cells that can undergo cell death with time and release toxins causing stem cell death. Therefore, it is not considered ideal scaffold.
- **PRP:** PRP is a first generation platelet aggregate and is potential addendum/substitute scaffold with a rich source of growth factors. Platelet concentration in PRP exceeds 1 million/mL, which is 5 times more than that of the normal platelet count. The various growth factors present in PRP include PDGF, TGF-b, IGF, VEGF, EGF, which are released via degranulation of alpha granules of platelets. It's easy to prepare, however requires to draw blood in young patients and reagents to prepare PRP. There are less number of cytokines in PRP than in PRF and healing is also slower when compared to PRF. The treatment cost can be more compared to that using blood clot.
- **PRF:** It is also known as Choukroun's PRF and is a second generation platelet aggregate. It is instantaneously obtained by centrifuging the drawn blood from the patient without adding anticoagulant. Thus, soon when the blood comes in contact with the glass surface of the test tube coagulation starts. The PRF has 3D structure and is a rich source of growth factors (PDGF, TGF-β1 and IGF) and cytokines. All the components either together or individually promote healing and angiogenesis. It can be considered as an ideal biomaterial for pulp-dentine regeneration. However, the drawback of using PRP and PRF is the intravenous collection of blood, which is difficult in children, and lack of mechanical strength to support coronal restoration.
- **Collagen:** It constitutes the extracellular matrix of all the tissues and is responsible for the tensile strength of the same. The various advantages of collagen as a scaffold for REPs include—biocompatibility, biodegradability, high alkaline phosphatase activity (thus exhibits good blastic/forming activity), easy placement of cells and growth factors along with the easy replacement with natural tissues after its degradation. Collagen forms the hard and soft tissue which simulates the natural extracellular matrix of dentine when used for REPs. It's available in various forms via gels, sponges and sheets. However rapid degradation and contraction are the undesirable properties of collagen.
- **Chitosan:** Chitin, present in the exoskeleton of crustaceans and cell walls of some fungi undergoes deacetylation to form Chitosan. Ability of chitosan to form porous scaffold makes it is to be used in REPs. Its biocompatible, biodegradable and has high alkaline phosphatase activity (thus exhibits good blastic/forming activity). It shows antibacterial activity too. Chitosan is hydrophilic allowing easy cell attachment and proliferation and it can be molded to the required shape. But chitosan scaffold is weak and may show inconsistent behavior with the inoculated cells. Probable toxicity post chemical modification of chitosan is also a concern.
- **Glycosoaminoglycans:** One of the glycosaminoglycans present in the extracellular matrix is hyaluronic acid (HA). It is bioactive and has properties of osteogenesis and chondrogenesis. When used for REPs, it can even promote odontogenesis by forming pulp-dentine complex. The properties of HA are biocompatibility, biodegradability, bioactive, nonimmunogenecity, wound healing ability, nonthrombogenicity and high water solubility. The high water solubility makes it loose the structural integrity in aqueous environment. This demerit can be overcome by using cross-linked HA. HA is available in either injectable scaffold form or as a sponge.
- **Demineralized dentin matrix:** The demineralized matrix of dentin contains huge collagenous and noncollagenous proteins. It is nonimmunogenic, biocompatible and causes odontogenesis and osteogenesis. But obtaining demineralized dentine matrix is a time consuming procedure.
- **Polymers:** Various polymers used as scaffolds in REPs include polylactic acid (PLA), poly-l-lactic acid (PLLA), polyglycolic acid (PGA) and polyepsiloncaprolactone (PCL). These being the synthetic polymers are biocompatible, biodegradable by simple hydrolysis and allow controlled alteration of degradation rate, porosity, microstructure and stiffness. However, they can evoke acute inflammatory reactions in the host.
- **Bioceramics:** This category includes calcium/phosphate materials (β-TCP or HA), bioactive glasses and glass ceramics. Most common biomaterials in use are calcium phosphate-based (Ca-P) bioceramics. They are thought to provide favorable 3D scaffold for human dental pulp

stem cell (hDPSC) growth and odontogenic differentiation. The demerits of this category of scaffolds include lack of organic phase, slow degradation rate, brittleness and difficult fabrication.

Growth Factors

Regulation of the transplanted cells or endogenous cells in pulp-dentine complex is done by growth factors by influencing cell migration, proliferation and differentiation. They belong to the class of polypeptides or proteins and various examples include platelet-derived growth factor (PDGF), transforming growth factor (TGF), bone morphogenetic protein (BMP), vascular endothelial growth factor (VEGF), fibroblast growth factor (FGF) and insulin-like growth factor (IGF).

	Source	*Activity*	*Use*
BMP	Bone matrix	Differentiation of osteoblast-mineralization of bone	Make stem cells- synthesize mineralized matrix
CSF (colony stimulating factor)	Wide range of cells	Proliferate specific pluripotent bone stem cells	Increases stem cells number
FGF (fibroblast growth factor)	Wide range of cells	Proliferate fibroblast and other cells	Increases stem cells
IL1-13	Leucocytes	Stimulate humoral and cellular immune response	Promotes inflammatory activity
TGF	Dentin matrix and helper cells NK cells	Anti-inflammatory, promotes wound healing, inhibit macrophage and decrease lymphocyte proliferation	Promotes mineralization of pulp tissue

CLINICAL CONSIDERATIONS FOR A REGENERATIVE ENDODONTIC PROCEDURE[10]

These considerations mentioned below, laid down by the American Association of Endodontists (AAE), should be seen as one possible source of information **(Figs. 51.4A to E and 51.5A to I).**

A. Case Selection

- Any tooth with open apex, incompletely formed roots, necrotic pulp is suitable candidate for regeneration.
- Pulp space is not needed for post and core or any final restoration.
- Patient or the parent should be compliant with frequent follow-ups.
- No allergies to any of materials should be present.

B. Informed Consent

It is the clinician's duty to disclose all material information necessary to make an informed decision. It should include following details:

- Number of appointments should be explained to patient, parent or the guardian as it may require two or more appointments with frequent follow-ups.
- Explaining the adverse effects like staining of the tooth, Pain or infection can occur anytime during the treatment, lack of response to treatment.
- Discussing alternative treatment plans with the patient example MTA apexification, no treatment or extraction.

C. First Appointment: Access and Disinfection

- Anesthetize and isolate the tooth with rubber dam.
- Access opening is made.
- Working length determined by using small file.
- Slowly irrigate the root canal system by using a lower concentration of 1.5% Sodium hypochlorite by using sidevent irrigation needle or EndoVac and then irrigated with saline.
- Use of chlorhexidine is avoided as it is cytotoxic to stem cells and also it does not have tissue-dissolving property.
- Dry the canals with paper point.
- Calcium hydroxide or triple antibiotic paste (1:1:1 ciprofloxacin: metronidazole: minocycline) is placed in the canal as a light medicament. Triple antibiotic paste has potential to cause staining of teeth due to presence

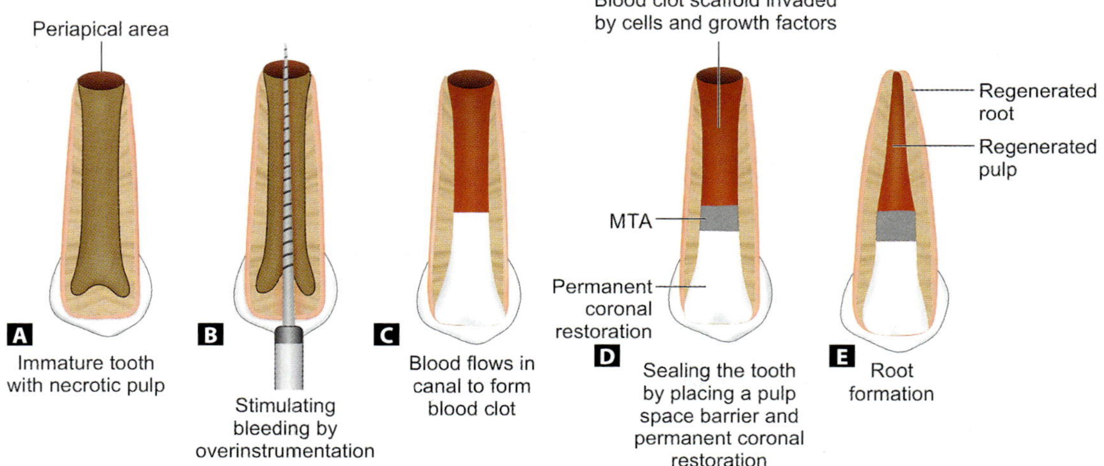

Figs. 51.4A to E: Diagrammatic representation of steps in regeneration procedure.

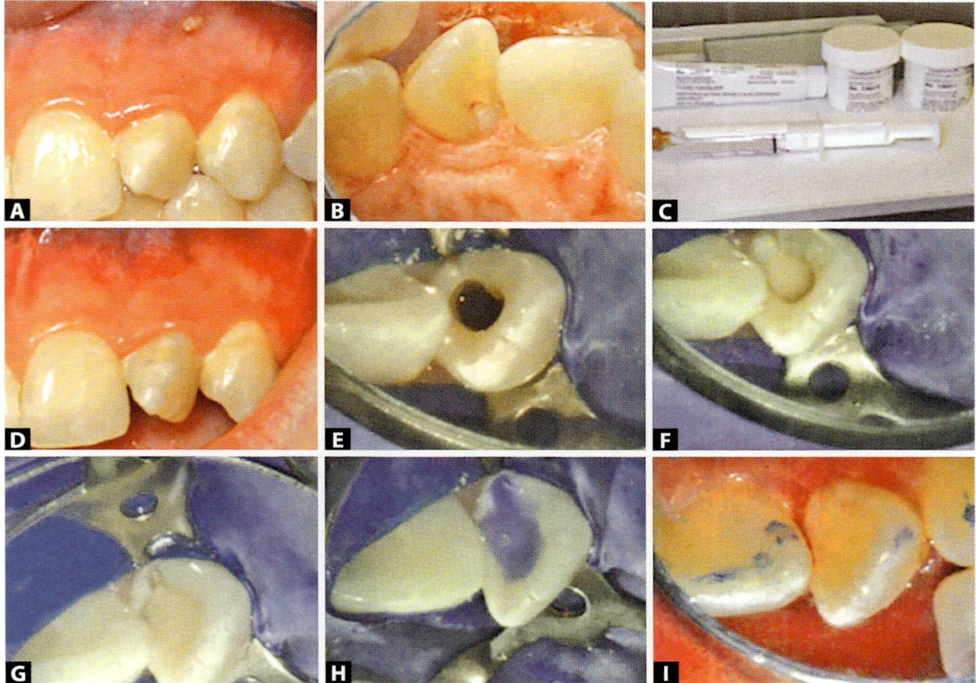

Figs. 51.5A to I: A modified protocol using autologous fibrin matrix (AFM) or platelet-rich plasma (PRP). (A) Case presents with a diagnosis of necrosis with chronic apical abscess on the lateral incisor. Note presence of sinus tract; (B) The dens invaginatus can be appreciated on lingual aspect of tooth; (C) New antibiotic protocol in esthetic area using 2 MIX or double antibiotic paste and the macrogol and propylene glycol carrier (MP); (D) Absence of both sinus tract and coronal staining; (E) AFM or PRP placed in canal; (F) Collatape placed over PRP; (G) Resin modified glass ionomer was placed over Collatape and the enamel was beveled; (H) Etched with composite; (I) Restored with composite.

of minocycline. To avoid this staining, either double antibiotic paste without minocycline paste or substitution of minocycline for other antibiotics (such as amoxicillin, clindamycin; cefaclor) or application of dentin bonding agent to seal the pulp chamber can be done.

- Access cavity is sealed temporarily using either cavit, Glass ionomer or any other temporary material.
- **The Antibiotic Paste:** Hoshino et al.[21] have shown the effectiveness of 3 MIX or triple antibiotic paste both in vitro and in vivo. The triple antibiotic paste mix (1:1:1 by volume of ciprofloxacin/metronidazole/minocycline) is used. The pills are to be crushed with a mortar and pestle and mixed together as slurry with macrogol ointment and propylene glycol. Minocycline has long been known to stain dentin.

D. Second Appointment: Stimulate, Scaffold, and Seal

- Patient is recalled after 2–4 weeks after first appointment.
- Clinical examination is done to evaluate for any signs and symptoms of infection. If present, then again repeat the intracanal medicament.
- Local anesthesia without vasoconstrictor is given so that bleeding can be induced later.
- 3% Mepivacaine should be used as it will facilitate triggering of bleeding in the canal.
- Isolate the tooth with rubber dam.
- Coronal access is reestablished again and tooth is irrigated slowly with either 17% EDTA or saline.
- Use of sodium hypochlorite in second visit is avoided as it may be cytotoxic to stem cells.
- Canals are dried with paper point.
- Bleeding is induced by inserting small file 1–2 mm beyond apical foramen with the aim of filling the entire canal with blood till the level of the cementoenamel junction.
- Once the blood clot is formed, a resorbable matrix such as CollaPlug™, Collacote™, CollaTape™ over the blood clot is placed that serve as internal matrix for palcement of 3 mm of MTA.
- A 3–4 mm layer of glass ionomer followed by composite restoration is applied to seal the coronal portion.
- Follow-up after 3 months and 6 months and yearly till 4 years is advised.

Torabinejad and **Turman**[11] reported a case in which no bleeding was evoked, but instead they hypothesized that the PRP (a form of AFM) injected into the canal-attracted stem cells into the canal system. They concluded that whatever tissue was produced in the canal was result of the presence of AFM.

Chueh and **Huang**[12] gave some general expectations for the progress of REPs. They observed radiographic evidence of bony healing in 3–21 months (mean 8 months), and radiographic evidence of root development in 10–29 months (mean 16 months). These results suggest that radiographic evidence of healing and root development should occur within 2 years. Signs and symptoms such as pain, soft tissue swelling, or increasing radiolucency indicate failure of procedure and will likely obviate alternative treatment such as artificial apical barrier with MTA or extraction.

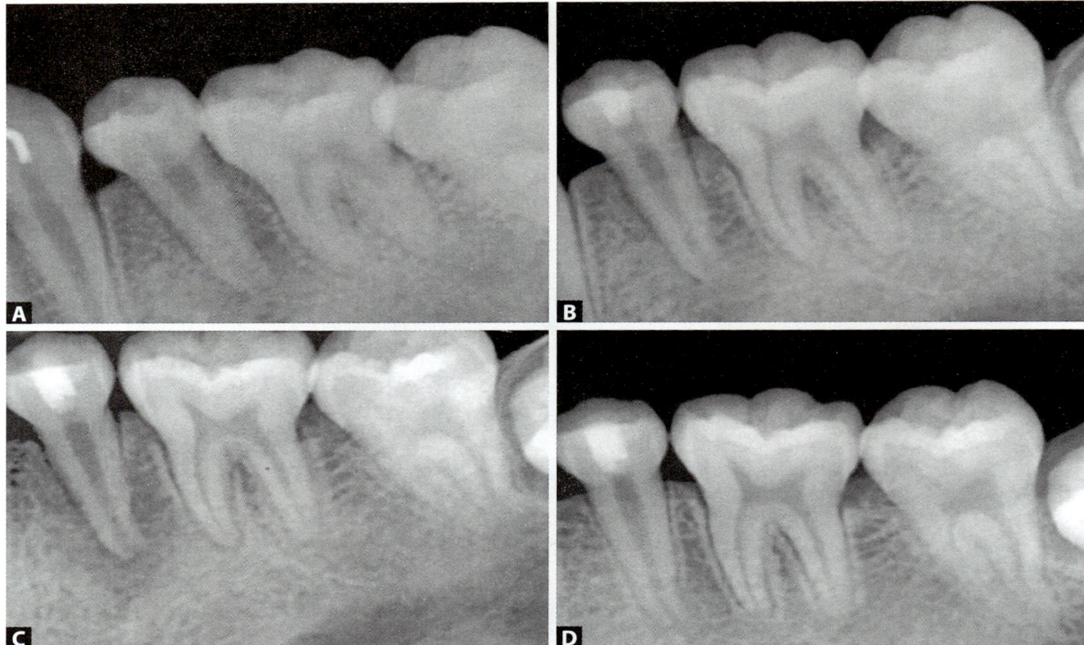

Figs. 51.6A to D: Radiographic presentation of pulp regeneration.

Overview of Clinical Cases

- Following points to be taken into account before considering any case for revascularization as suggested by **Garcia-Goday** and **Murray**[13]**:**
  - Presence of necrosis or infection
  - Periodontal status
  - Presence of periapical lesions
  - Stage of root development
  - Vitality status
  - Patient's age and health status.

In general, most of the in vivo cases (by **Banch** and **Trope; Ikawa et al.**) have shown consistent principles **(Figs. 51.6A to D and 51.7A to E):**

- First, most of the patients have been young (6–18 years old). Age may play a role in stem cell population and regenerative potential. **Kling et al.**[14] suggested that the size of the apical opening has an effect on the successful revascularization of avulsed immature permanent teeth and, by extrapolation, it is thought that an open apex may be part of the age predilection of successful REPs. Not only is it generally accepted that a short and open root is more conducive to ingrowth of tissues, but it is suggested that a short and open apex may indicate the increased presence and numbers of stem cells of the apical papilla (SCAP).
- Another principle, which is often counterintuitive to most clinicians, is the absence of instrumentation of the dentinal walls. In most cases, the disinfection approach was chemical (using either an antibiotic paste or calcium hydroxide) rather than chemomechanical. It is thought that the presence of the non-infected necrotic pulp as well as the induced blood clot scaffold may have been essential in providing a lattice for progenitor cell growth.[15]
- In addition, many of these cases have reported some vital tissue at the apical portion of the canal and most cases reported presence of a blood clot or other protein scaffold. There is some suggestion that outcomes may be significantly different between teeth that have some vital tissue in the apical portion of the canal versus those teeth in which the pulp has been lost.[16]

Notable Considerations in Revascularization Procedures

- It has been noted that REP in replanted avulsed teeth demonstrate a greater likelihood of revascularization.[14] This finding suggests that revascularization of necrotic pulps with fully formed (closed) apices might require instrumentation of the tooth apex to approximately 1–2 mm in apical diameter to allow systemic bleeding into root canal systems.
- The development of regenerative endodontic procedures may require reexamination of many of the closely held precepts of traditional endodontic procedures. The revascularization method assumes that the root canal space has been disinfected and that the formation of a blood clot yields a matrix (e.g., fibrin) that traps cells capable of initiating new tissue formation.
- It is not clear that the regenerated tissue's phenotype resembles dental pulp; however, case reports published to date do demonstrate continued root formation and the restoration of a positive response to thermal pulp testing.
- Another important point is that young adult patients generally have a greater capacity for healing.[17]

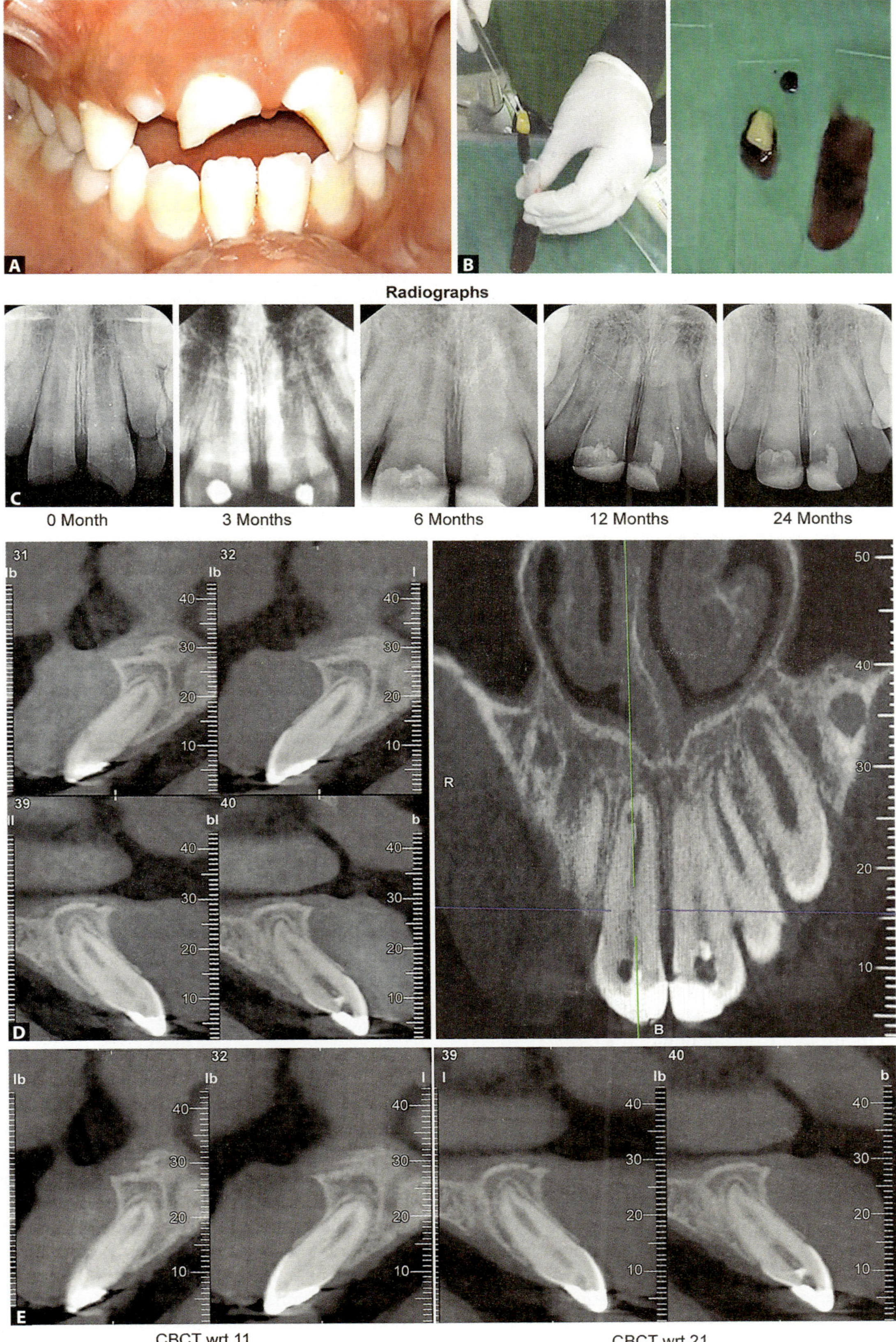

Figs. 51.7 A to E: Case description: 7-year-old male patient with history of trauma 2 months back; 11, 21 Ellis Class 3 fracture; Regeneration using platelet-rich fibrin (PRF): (A) Preoperative picture; (B) Platelet rich-fibrin; (C) Serial radiographs depict completion of root formation; (D and E) CBCT images shows 3D image of root completion wrt 11, 21.

HISTOLOGY OF THE REGENERATED TISSUE

The reported outcome from case reports or series showing continued root development after revitalization or regeneration procedures, although encouraging. But are not sufficient to demonstrate regeneration of pulp tissue. In a recent review by **Andreasen** and **Bakland**[18] based on an analysis of more than 1,200 traumatized teeth and 370 autotransplanted premolars, four types of healing outcomes following regeneration procedures have been discussed:

1. Revascularization of the pulp with accelerated dentin formation leading to pulp canal obliteration (PCO)
2. Ingrowth of cementum and periodontal ligament (PDL)
3. Ingrowth of cementum, PDL, and bone
4. Ingrowth of bone and bone marrow.

There is a lack of histologic data on human teeth following intentional revitalization procedures, making it impossible to determine with any certainty the type of tissue occupying the canal space. Results from animal studies may provide a glimpse into possible outcomes in human teeth following revitalization procedures. A recent study by **Wang** and et al.[19] on immature necrotic teeth of dogs that underwent revitalization procedures demonstrated the presence of intracanal cementum on the dentinal walls and cementum on the apical portion of the root. In addition, some of the teeth had evidence of intracanal bone or bone-like tissue and connective tissue similar to the PDL. The evidence from this study on dogs suggests that the tissue in the canal space may be closer to extracanal tissues than pulp tissue. Another animal study demonstrated that it may be possible to obtain pulp-like tissue after a revitalization procedure. **Huang et al.**[20] subcutaneously implanted 6–7 mm long human tooth fragments containing dental stem cells seeded onto a poly (D, L, -lactide-co-glycolide) (PLG) scaffold into immunodeficient mice. Three to four months after the transplantation, the tooth fragments were harvested. The histology revealed the formation of well-vascularized soft tissue in the root canal space, and a continuous layer of dentin-like tissue lined with odontoblast-like cells. Recently **Torabinejad et al. (2014)** made an interesting finding regarding the histology of the regenerated pulp tissue. They reported a case in which regenerated vital pulp tissue was removed in a young patient who developed mild symptoms of tenderness and insisted on root canal treatment. Examination of the tissue removed from the root canal revealed the presence of a vital pulp-like vital connective tissue. There was no evidence of bone in the specimen. Very few inflammatory cells were noted in the periphery of the specimen. They concluded that pulp-like tissue can be generated in a human tooth with the use of PRP as a scaffold in regenerative endodontic procedures.

PROBLEMS ENCOUNTERED DURING REVASCULARIZATION PROCEDURE

- **Tooth discoloration:** The bluish discoloration or staining was reported to be caused by the presence of minocycline above the CEJ. Even if extreme care was taken not to have any antibiotic paste coronal to the CEJ, discoloration still occurred. **Hoshino et al.**[21] recognized that minocycline caused pigmentation, and they suggested that it could be replaced with amoxicillin, cefaclor, cefroxadine, fosfomycin, or rokitamycin. It was found that the combination of metronidazole and ciprofloxacin with any of these antibiotics was just as effective in sterilizing endodontically treated teeth. Thus, minocycline was replaced by cefaclor, a second generation cephalosporin. This change resolved the staining problem for the cases that followed, and at the same time maintained control of the dental infections. **Reynolds et al.**[22] described a modified technique to avoid undesired crown discoloration that involved sealing the dentinal tubules of the chamber with bonded composite resin, thus avoiding any contact between the triple antibiotic paste and the dentinal walls. **Jong-Hyun et al.** applied dentin bonding adhesive to the root canal walls before introducing the antibiotic paste. A visual assessment of the color change showed that the bonding agent was effective in preventing discoloration. Another approach to prevent discoloration is to place a Root Canal Projector (CJM Engineering Inc, Santa Barbara, CA, USA) into the access, seal the coronal dentin with composite, and then remove the projector and place the triple antibiotic paste in the canal. In cases of crown discoloration, treatment by intracoronal bleaching with sodium perborate should be considered. Minocycline was replaced by cefaclor, a second generation cephalosporin. This change resolved the staining problem for the cases that followed, and at the same time-maintained control of the dental infections.
- **Failure to produce significant bleeding:** It was found that the induction of a significant blood clot was difficult to achieve. The blood clot serves to allow the migration of stem cells along the canal; consequently, it was assumed that the absence of a blood clot would impede such a migration and thus, adversely affects the treatment.
  - It was hypothesized that the absence of significant bleeding was caused by the epinephrine in the local anesthetic solution. Bleeding was consistently induced once local anesthetic without a vasoconstrictor was used.
  - Another technique that proved useful in inducing bleeding involved overinstrumenting beyond the apex with a slightly bent endodontic file that was dipped in a calcium chelator 17% EDTA (Pulpdent Corp, Watertown, Mass, USA).
  - Both techniques were used successfully.
- **Collapse of the MTA material into the canal:** According to the revascularization protocol, MTA material is to be inserted on top of the newly formed blood clot. The MTA has a setting time of over 2.5 hours and attains an ideal seal at 48 hours. Often, the blood clot is not strong enough to hold the MTA, resulting in a collapse of the MTA within the root canal. It was found that placing a collagen matrix, CoUaplug® above the blood clot served as a solid absorbable matrix against which the MTA could be packed.
- **Potential for allergic reactions:** A potentially more serious consequence of using antibiotics in the canal space is an allergic reaction. Allergic reactions have been reported after topical use of the antibiotics in the triple antibiotic paste. There are no reports, however, of allergic reactions after the use of these antibiotics in root canals. Nonetheless, patients and guardians should be informed of the possibility of a reaction and asked about related allergies.
- **Failure of the apical bone to heal and/or tissue to grow into the canal space:** This may be evidenced

radiographically by a persistent or enlarging apical radiolucency, and/or the lack of root development. One should expect to see apical bone healing at approximately 8 months after the completion of treatment, and root development at approximately 16 months. Additionally, a sign of treatment failure would be radiographic evidence of root resorption. Persistent pain, swelling, or sinus tract would also indicate failure of the treatment. If any of these signs or symptoms should occur, alternative treatments should be considered, including apexification, nonsurgical root canal treatment, or extraction.

It is important to emphasize to the parents that success could only be achieved after a longer period, such as 2 years, and to adhere closely to the protocol. The number of follow-up appointments may appear redundant, but it is a new procedure that should benefit from a well-grounded protocol. In the near future, with the accumulation of successful treatments, it is felt that fewer visits may be necessary. The subject of revascularization has been presented mainly by the endodontic community. Often, clinicians, such as pediatric dentists, are the first to receive children with necrotic immature permanent teeth. This approach is new, and, as in any new treatment, obstacles are encountered. Changes were made from the initial protocol and were able to produce more predictable outcomes. In the objective of providing evidence-based guidelines, further research is needed pertaining to the various antibiotic medications, cements and matrices that can be used for dental pulp-tissue engineering.

MERITS OF REVASCULARIZATION

There are several advantages to a revascularization approach:

- The approach is technically simple and can be completed using currently available instruments and medicaments without expensive biotechnology.
- The regeneration of tissue in root canal systems by a patient's own blood cells avoids the possibility of immune rejection and pathogen transmission from replacing the pulp with a tissue-engineered construct. The case reports of a blood clot having the capacity to regenerate pulp tissue are exciting, but caution is required, because the source of the regenerated tissue has not been identified. However, plasma-derived fibrin clots are being used for development as scaffolds in several studies. Enlargement of the apical foramen is also necessary to promote vascularization and to maintain initial cell viability via nutrient diffusion. Cells must have an available supply of oxygen; therefore, it is likely that cells in the coronal portion of the root canal system either would not survive or would survive under hypoxic conditions.[23]
- Lateral walls of the root are reinforced with deposition of dentin and hard tissue which is thick compared to the thin, fragile dentin and fracture prone roots formed by apexification/apexogenesis.

LIMITATIONS OF REVASCULARIZATION PROCEDURES

- Generally, tissue engineering does not rely on blood clot formation, because the concentration and composition of cells trapped in the fibrin clot is unpredictable. This is a critical limitation to a blood clot revascularization approach, because tissue engineering is founded on the delivery of effective concentrations and compositions of cells to restore function. It is very possible that variations in cell concentration and composition, particularly in older patients (where circulating stem cell concentrations may be lower) may lead to variations in treatment outcome.[24]
- In some cases, the whole canal may get calcified.
- Difficult to achieve it in fully formed permanent teeth (in which some clinicians have tried pulp revascularization by enlarging the apical foramen). Enlargement of the apical foramen is necessary to promote vascularization and to maintain initial cell viability via nutrient diffusion. Related to this point, cells must have an available supply of oxygen; therefore, it is likely that cells in the coronal portion of the root canal system either would not survive or would survive under hypoxic conditions before angiogenesis.
- Development of resistant bacterial strains (due to long-term use of antimicrobial agents).
- Allergic reaction to intracanal medicament.
- Potential risk of necrosis, if tissue is reinfected.
- Minimal case reports published to date.

Goals of apexogenesis as given by Webber:
- Sustaining a viable Hertwig's epithelial root sheath (HERS), thus maintaining a favorable crown/root ratio
- Maintenance of pulpal vitality, thus reinforcing thin dentinal root canal walls
- Promoting root end closure
- Creating a dentinal bridge at the site of pulpotomy.

Although the healing potential of pulp has long been recognized, the nature and the intensity of infection are still the determining factors for the outcome of pulp recovery. Due to the improved regimen of canal disinfection, it seems to be the right time to establish a new protocol for treating these infected and avulsed young teeth. At the same time, clinical research is needed to provide information on the success rate and prognosis of this treatment modality. Although many drawbacks have been noted in the revascularization concept, it definitely is a very promising technique. The procedure is very simple in terms of materials and technique making it very feasible in routine clinical practice.

POINTS TO REMEMBER

- Revascularization technique is an innovative, simple procedure for treatment of immature necrotic teeth.
- It may be considered as an alternative to traditional apexification procedures using calcium hydroxide or MTA.
- Not suitable for teeth that require post and core procedures in future.
- Younger the patient better are the results of revascularization.
- Apical foramen that are open more than 1 mm show better results due to better access to pluripotent cells in the apical papilla.
- Minimum canal wall instrumentation key to success of the procedure.
- Antibiotic paste should be freshly prepared for each case.
- Revascularization procedure can be performed successfully in multirooted teeth also.

Questionnaire

1. What is the difference between pulp regeneration and revascularization?
2. What are triads of tissue regeneration?
3. What is the procedure for revascularization and what are its limitations?

REFERENCES

1. Mathieu S, El-Battari A, Dejou J, et al. Role of injured endothelial cells in the recruitment of human pulp cells. Arch Oral Biol. 2005;50:109-13.
2. Hargreaves KM, Law AS. Regenerative endodontics. In: Hargreaves KM, Cohen S (Eds). Cohen's Pathways of the Pulp, 10th edition. St Louis (MO): Mosby Elsevier;2011. pp. 602-19.
3. Lenzi R, Trope M. Revitalization procedures in two traumatized incisors with different biological outcomes. J Endod. 2012;38:411-4.
4. Sakthi S, Bharadwaj SL. Pulp revascularisation in pediatric dentistry. J dent. 2012;1(1).
5. Nygaard-Ostby B, Hjortdal O. Tissue formation in the root canal following pulp removal. Scand J Dent Res. 1971;79:333-49.
6. Yanpiset K, Trope M. Pulp revascularization of replanted immature dog teeth after different treatment methods. Endod Dent Traumatol. 2000;16:211-7.
7. Iwaya SI, Ikawa M, Kubota M. Revascularization of an immature permanent tooth with apical periodontitis and sinus tract. Dent Traumatol. 2001;17:185-7.
8. Thibodeau B, Trope M. Pulp revascularization of a necrotic infected immature permanent tooth: case report and review of the literature. Pediatr Dent. 2007;29:47-50.
9. Banchs F, Trope M. Revascularization of immature permanent teeth with apical periodontitis: new treatment protocol? J Endod. 2004;30(4):196-200.
10. American Association of Endodontists. (2013). Considerations for a Regenerative Endodontics Procedure.
11. Torabinejad M, Turman M. Revitalization of tooth with necrotic pulp and open apex by using platelet-rich plasma: a case report. J Endod. 2011;37:265-8.
12. Chueh LH, Huang GT. Immature teeth with periradicular periodontitis or abscess undergoing apexogenesis: a paradigm shift. J Endod. 2006;32(12):1205-13.
13. Garcia-Godoy F, Murray PE. Recommendations for using regenerative endodontic procedures in permanent immature traumatized teeth. Dent Traumatol. 2012;28(l):33-41.
14. Kling M, Cvek M, Mejare I. Rate and predictability of pulp revascularization in therapeutically reimplanted permanent incisors. Endod Dent Traumatol. 1986;2:83-9.
15. Banchs F, Trope M. Revascularization of immature permanent teeth with apical periodontitis: new treatment protocol? J Endod. 2004;30(4):196-200.
16. Geisler TM. Clinical considerations form regenerative endodontic procedures. Dent Clin N Am. 2012;56:603-26.
17. Amler MH. The age factor in human extraction wound healing. J Oral Surg. 1977;35:193-7.
18. Andreasen JO, Bakland LK. Pulp regeneration after non- infected and infected necrosis, what type of tissue do we want? A review. Dent Traumatol. 2011;28(1):13-8.
19. Wang X, Thibodeau B, Trope M, et al. Histologic characterization of regenerated tissues in canal space after the revitalization/ revascularization procedure of immature dog teeth with apical periodontitis. J Endod. 2010;36(1):56-63.
20. Huang GT, Yamaza T, Shea LD, et al. Stem/progenitor cell- mediated de novo regeneration of dental pulp with newly deposited continuous layer of dentin in an in vivo model. Tissue Eng. 2010;16:605-15.
21. Hoshino E, Kurihara-Ando N, Sato I, et al. In vitro antibacterial susceptibility of bacteria taken from infected root dentine to a mixture of ciprofloxacin, metronidazole and minocycline. Int Endod J. 1996;29:125-30.
22. Reynolds K, Johnson JD, Gohenca N. Pulp revascularization of necrotic bilateral bicuspids using a modified novel technique to eliminate potential coronal discoloration: a case report. Int Endod J. 2009;42:84-92.
23. Dewan RG, Kochhar R, Bhandari PP, et al. Indian Journal of Dental Sciences. 2013;51(2).
24. Murray PE, Garcia-Godoy F, Hargreaves KM. Regenerative endodontics: a review of current status and a call for action. J Endod. 2007;33:377-90.

FURTHER READING

1. Amler MH. The age factor in human extraction wound healing. J Oral Surg. 1977;35:193-7.
2. Andreasen JO, Bakland LK. Pulp regeneration after non- infected and infected necrosis, what type of tissue do we want? A review. Dent Traumatol. 2011;28(1):13-8.
3. Banchs F, Trope M. Revascularization of immature permanent teeth with apical periodontitis: new treatment protocol? J Endod. 2004;30(4):196-200.
4. Dabbagh B, Alvaro E, Vu DD, et al. Clinical complications in the revascularization of immature necrotic permanent teeth. Pediatr Dent. 2012;34;414-7.
5. Gathani KM, Raghavendra SS. Scaffolds in regenerative endodontics: A review. Dent Res J (Isfahan). 2016;13(5): 379-386.
6. Geisler TM. Clinical considerations form regenerative endodontic procedures. Dent Clin N Am. 2012;56:603-26.
7. Hargreaves KM, Diogenes A, Teixeira FB. Treatment options: biological basis of regenerative endodontic procedures. J Endod. 2013;39(3 Suppl): S30-43.
8. Huang GT, Sonoyama W, Liu Y, Liu H, Wang S, Shi S. The hidden treasure in apical papilla: the potential role in pulp/ dentin regeneration and bioroot engineering. J Endod. 2008;34(6):645-51.
9. Huang GT, Yamaza T, Shea LD, et al. Stem/progenitor cell- mediated de novo regeneration of dental pulp with newly deposited continuous layer of dentin in an in vivo model. Tissue Eng. 2010;16:605-15.
10. Kim JH, Kim Y, Shin SJ, et al. Tooth discoloration of immature permanent incisor associated with triple antibiotic therapy: a case report. J Endod. 2010;36:1086-91.
11. Law AS. Outcomes of regenerative endodontic procedures. Dent Clin N Am. 2012;56:627-37.
12. Lovelace TW, Henry MA, Hargreaves KM. Evaluation of clinically delivered SCAP cells in regenerative endodontic procedures. J Endod. 2010;36:554.
13. Nosrat A, Seifi A, Asgary S. Regenerative endodontic treatment (revascularization for necrotic immature permanent molars: a review and report of two cases with a new biomaterial. J Endod. 2011;37:562-7.
14. Petrino JA, Boda KK, Shambarger S, et al. Challenges in regenerative endodontics: a case series. J Endod. 2010;36:536-41.
15. Plascencia H, Díaz M, Gascón G, Garduño S, Guerrero-Bobadilla C, Márquez-De Alba S, González-Barba G. Management of permanent teeth with necrotic pulps and open apices according to the stage of root development. Journal of clinical and experimental dentistry. 2017 Nov;9(11): e1329.
16. Shah N, Logani A, Bhaskar U, et al. Efficacy of revascularization to induce apexification/apexogenesis in infected, nonvital, immature teeth: a pilot clinical study. J Endod. 2008;34:919-25.
17. Smith A. Dentin formation and repair. In: Hargreaves KM, Goodis HE (Eds). Seltzer and Bender's Dental Pulp, 3rd edition. Chicago: Quintessence Publishing;2002. pp. 41-62.
18. Trevino EG, Patwardhan AN, Henry MA, et al. Effect of irrigants on the survival of human stem cells of the apical papilla in a platelet rich plasma scaffold in human root tips. J Endod. 2011;37:1109-15.
19. Wang X, Thibodeau B, Trope M, et al. Histologic characterization of regenerated tissues in canal space after the revitalization/ revascularization procedure of immature dog teeth with apical periodontitis. J Endod. 2010;36(1):56-63.

CHAPTER

Diagnostic Pulp Testing

Nikhil Marwah, Naveen Manuja

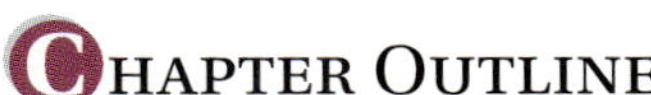

CHAPTER OUTLINE

Dental pulp tests are investigations that provide valuable diagnostic and treatment planning information to the dental clinician. If pathosis is present, pulp testing combined with information taken from the history, examination, and other investigations such as radiographs leads to the diagnosis of the underlying disease which can usually be reached relatively easily.

CLASSIFICATION OF PULP TESTING

Pulp tests are broadly classified according to the component that they test like blood supply, nerve supply, etc.

Pulp Vitality Testing

- Assessment of the pulp's blood supply.
- Pulp tissue may have an adequate vascular supply but is not necessarily innervated. Hence, most of the current pulp testing modalities do not directly assess the pulp vascularity, and this is exemplified by clinical observations that traumatized teeth can have no response to a stimulus (such as cold) for a period of time following injury.
- Done by laser Doppler and pulse oximeter.

Pulp Sensibility Testing

- Assessment of the pulp's sensory response.
- Sensibility is defined as the ability to respond to a stimulus, and hence this is an accurate and appropriate term for the typical and common clinical pulp tests such as thermal and electric tests given that they do not detect or measure blood supply to the dental pulp.

Pulp Sensitivity Testing

- Condition of the pulp being very responsive to a stimulus.
- Thermal and electric pulp tests are not sensitivity tests although they can be used as sensitivity tests when attempting to diagnose a tooth with pulpitis since such teeth are more responsive than normal.
- If the pulp responds to a stimulus (indicating that there is innervation), clinicians generally assume that the pulp has a viable blood supply and it is either healthy or inflamed, depending on the nature of the response (with respect to pain, duration, and so forth), the history, and the other findings. The three types of responses can be summarized:
  - The pulp is deemed normal when there is a response to the stimulus provided by the sensibility test, and this response is not pronounced or exaggerated, and it does not linger.
  - Pulpitis is present when there is an exaggerated response that produces pain. Typically, mild pain of short duration is considered to indicate reversible pulpitis, while severe pain that lingers indicates irreversible pulpitis.
  - The absence of responses to sensibility tests is usually associated with the likelihood of pulp necrosis; the tooth is pulpless or has had previous root canal therapy.

Classification of Pulp Testing Methods

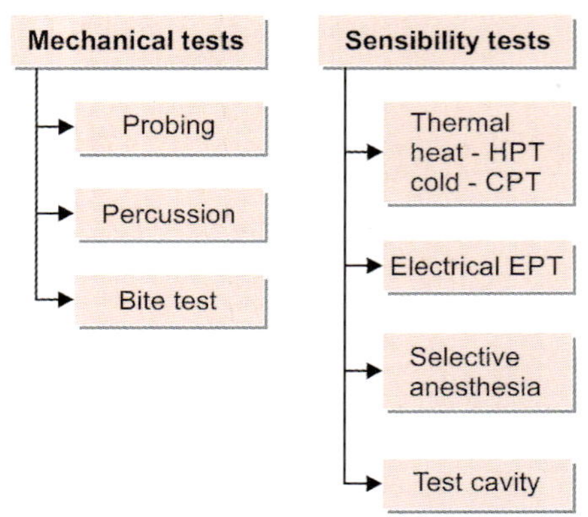

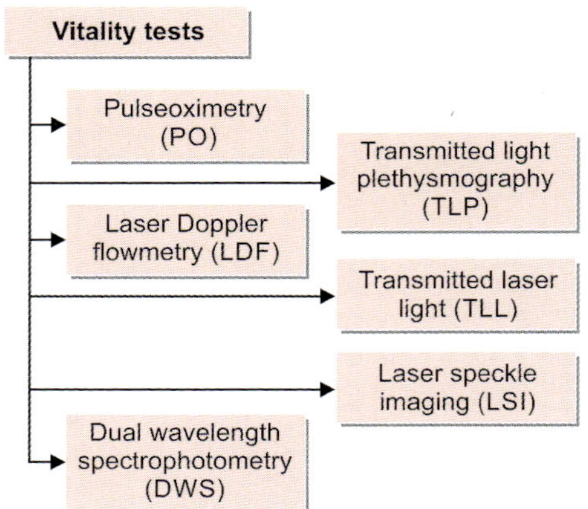

THERMAL TESTS

This was first reported by **Jack** in 1899, and it involved application of agents to the teeth to increase or decrease temperature and to stimulate pulp sensory responses through thermal conduction. Although these techniques may be primate and old, they are still useful in diagnosis of pulp sensibility.

Responses to thermal test:
- No response—nonvital pulp
- Mild—moderate pain subsides in 1–2 seconds—normal
- Strong—momentary pain subsides in 1–2 seconds—reversible pulpitis
- Moderate to strong painful response that lingers for several seconds after the stimulus has been removed—irreversible pulpitis.

Cold Tests

- Cold thermal testing causes contraction of the dentinal fluid within the dentinal tubules, resulting in a rapid outward flow of fluid within the patent tubules. This rapid movement of dentinal fluid results in "hydrodynamic forces" acting on the ä nerve fibers within the pulp-dentine complex, leading to a sharp sensation lasting for the duration of the thermal test.
- A variety of cold tests may be employed; the major difference between them is the degree of cold that is applied to the tooth.
- Ideally, cold testing should be used in conjunction with an electric pulp tester so that the results from one test will verify the findings of the other test.
- If a mature, nontraumatized tooth does not respond either to electric pulp testing (EPT) or cold, the tooth may be considered nonvital. However, caution should be exercised when testing multirooted teeth, as they may respond positively to cold, even though only one root actually contains vital pulp tissue. The cold test alone may be used to differentiate between reversible and irreversible pulpitis. Overall, cold tests appear to be more reliable than heat tests. Furthermore, there is a general consensus that the colder the stimulus, the more effective the assessment of tooth innervation status.
- Ethyl chloride and ice have been popular in the past, but CO_2 snow and other refrigerants such as dichlorodifluoromethane (DDM) have been shown to be effective and superior to ice and ethyl chloride.

Ice

- This is perhaps the simplest cold testing agent requiring practically zero cost to prepare, and it can be made in a standard household freezer. A common way to make ice in useful sizes and dimensions involves freezing water in empty local anesthetic cartridges.
- Direct application of ice can be difficult and problematic, and hence pencil sticks of ice would be useful.
- Application is done for 5 seconds on the facial surface of teeth **(Fig. 52.1)**.

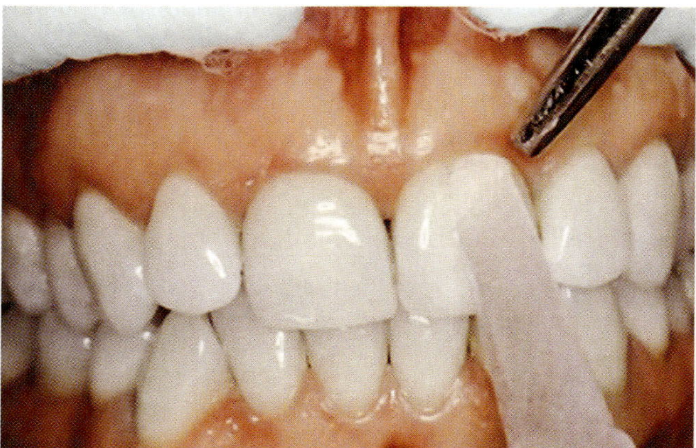

Fig. 52.1: Cold test with ice stick. (*Source:* Iraqi Dental Academy).

Refrigerant Spray

- Due to its ease of storage, relatively cheap cost, and simple application technique, refrigerant spray is widely used in clinical settings.
- More effective agents such as DDM have superseded traditional refrigerants such as ethyl chloride. However, DDM, being a chlorofluorocarbon, has decreased in popularity and market availability due to environmental concerns of atmospheric ozone layer depletion. Consequently, manufacturers have replaced DDM with other gases, including tetrafluoroethane (TFE) or

a propane/butane/isobutane gas mixture stored in a pressurized can (Endo Frost, Germany).

- The application of the refrigerant spray requires a carrier such as a cotton pellet saturated with the substance prior to direct contact with the teeth as described by Jones **(Fig. 52.2)**.
- Refrigerant sprays have also been shown to evoke faster pulp responses by 1–3 seconds.

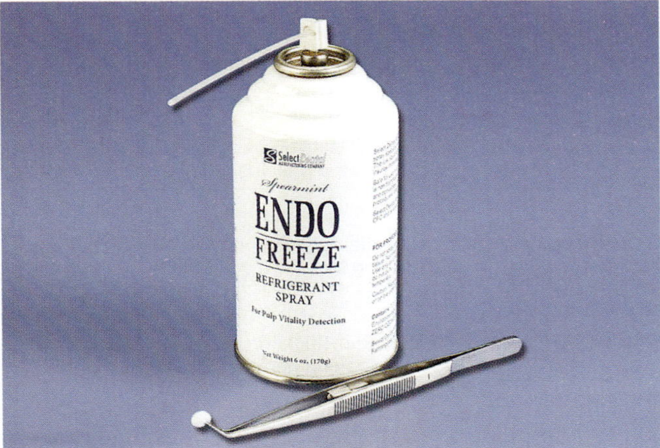

Fig. 52.2: Refrigerant spray.

Carbon Dioxide Snow

- CO_2 snow, or dry ice, is prepared from a pressurized liquid CO_2 cylinder using a commercially available apparatus known as the Odontotest (Fricar AG Zurich, Switzerland). This involves the liquid CO_2 being forced through a small orifice such that when it comes under atmospheric pressure, most of the liquid will be converted into dry ice.
- The dry ice is collected in a "pencil stick" form that can then be applied to one tooth at a time with the aid of the supplied plunger.

Heat Test

- Heat testing can be undertaken using gutta-percha sticks **(Fig. 52.3)** or compound material heated to melting temperature and directly applied to the tooth being tested with lubricant in order to facilitate removal of the material; heated ball-ended metallic instruments placed near the tooth (but without touching the tooth surface); battery-powered controlled heating instruments such as Touch 'n Heat.
- This test may be difficult to use on posterior teeth because of limited access.
- The major disadvantage of this method is that excessive heating may result in pulp damage.
- Prolonged heat application will result in biphasic stimulation of Ad fibers initially, followed by the pulpal C fibers. Activation of C fibers may result in a lingering pain; therefore, heat tests should be applied for no more than 5 seconds.

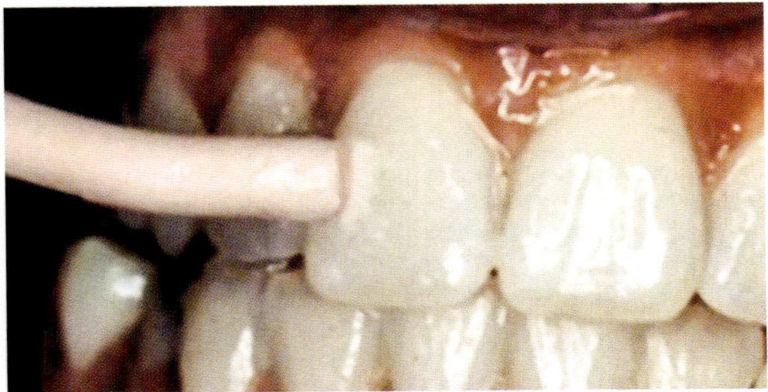

Fig. 52.3: Heat test with gutta-percha stick. (*Pic courtesy:* pocketdentistry.com).

ELECTRIC PULP TESTING

The use of electricity in dentistry is attributed to **Magitot** and described in his book Treatise on Dental Caries published in France in 1867 (cited in Prinz, 1919). Later, **Marshall** (1891) and **Woodward** in 1896 used electricity to demonstrate vital and nonvital pulps. **Roentgen** in 1895 was probably the first to introduce the use of electricity clinically for diagnosing diseases of the pulp (**Grossman,** 1976). In 1901, investigators in Europe attempted to standardize the instrument used for electrical stimulation of the dental pulp, and in the same year, Futy used a device where the primary current of an induction coil fed two electrodes. One was held in the patient's hand, and the other applied to the tooth with a platinum pin covered with water-saturated cotton. Futy observed that normal teeth reacted when moist; devitalized teeth did not react, even to much greater amounts of current; teeth with inflamed pulps had a much lower threshold of irritability, requiring less current for a response; teeth with normal enamel responded best when tested near the neck of the tooth. Over the years, many studies were done to analyze the effect of EPT like **Kaletsky** and **Furedi** (1936), **Stephan** (1937), **Ziskin** and **Zegarelli** (1945). **Seltzer et al.** showed that "*the electric pulp test was of some value in suggesting the possibility of an inflammatory state, but it was far from definitive.*" In the 1970s, EPT regained popularity when new designs of instrument were introduced which were monopolar and battery operated. Currently, testers have many different electric impulses and have digital read out for ease of application (**Dummer et al.,** 1986) **(Fig. 52.4)**.

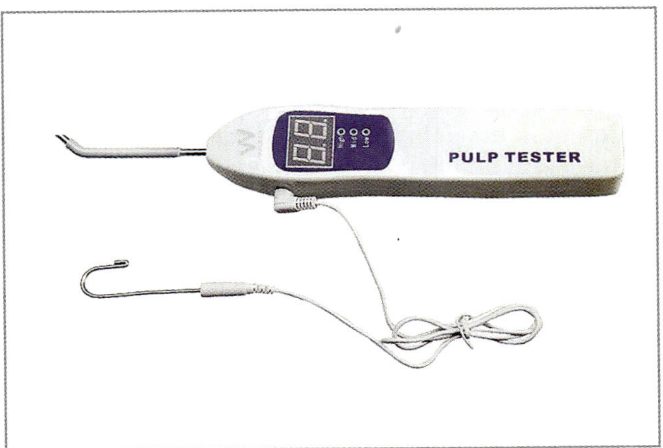

Fig. 52.4: Electric pulp tester

Working Principle

- Electric pulp testing works on the premise that electrical stimuli cause an ionic change across the neural membrane, thereby inducing an action potential with a rapid hopping action at the nodes of Ranvier in myelinated nerves.
- The pathway for the electric current is thought to be from the probe tip of the test device to the tooth, along the lines of the enamel prisms and dentine tubules, and then through the pulp tissue. The "circuit" is completed via the patient wearing a lip clip or by touching the probe handle with his/her hand **(Fig. 52.5)**.

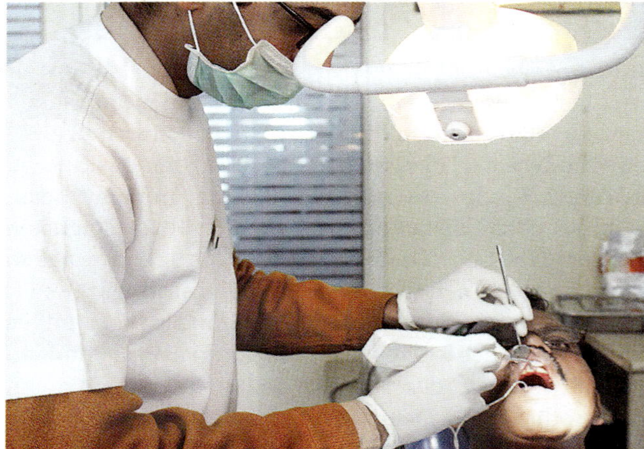

Fig. 52.5: Procedure of performing electric pulp testing.

- A "tingling" sensation will be felt by the patient once the increasing voltage reaches the pain threshold, but this threshold level varies between patients and teeth and is affected by factors such as individual age, pain perception, tooth surface conduction, and resistance.
- In order to ensure that the appropriate current pathway is followed, correct placement of the EPT probe tip flat against the contact area and having a conducting medium such as toothpaste between the probe tip and the tooth surface is essential.
- **Jacobson** found in an in vitro experiment involving incisors and premolars that placing the probe tip labially within the incisal or occlusal, two-thirds of the crown gave more consistent results.

Limitations of EPT

- Electric pulp testing depends on the vital sensory fibers present in the pulp. Its disadvantage is that it does not provide any information about the vascular supply of pulp, which is a true determinant of pulp vitality.
- Electric pulp tests are known to be unreliable in many instances, producing false results in healthy immature teeth with incompletely formed roots which may be erupting since these teeth may take up to 5 years before the maximum number of myelinated fibers reaches the pulp-dentin border at the plexus of Raschkow.
- Recently traumatized teeth undergoing pulp repair may also have false results and thus may not respond to EPT. In humans, many clinical observations from dental trauma studies have indicated that it can take pulps a minimum of 4–6 weeks following trauma for sufficient recovery of sensation to obtain valid pulp testing results. Theories proposed by Öhman for this loss of pulp sensibility include pressure or tension on the nerve fibers, blood vessel rupture, and ischemic injury. It is then assumed that these effects were reversible in the cases where the pulp sensation recovered. **Pileggi et al.** have shown that 10–12 days are required for the sensory component of the pulp to start to respond EPT again as damage from trauma heals.

Describe the test to the patient in a way that will reduce anxiety

↓

Isolate the area of teeth to be tested with cotton rolls and saliva ejectors and air-dry all the teeth

↓

Check the electric pulp tester for function and determine that current is passing through the electrode

↓

Apply an electrolyte on the teeth electrode and place it against the dried enamel

↓

Retract the patient's cheek or lip away from the tooth electrode with the free hand. This will complete the electric circuit

↓

Introduce minimal current onto the tooth and increase the current slowly asking the patient to indicate when any 'tingling or warmth' sensation occurs

↓

Record the results according to the numeric scale

- They are not recommended for use on crowned teeth or in patients wearing orthodontic bands.
- Anxious or young patients may have a premature or false-positive response due to the expectation of feeling an unpleasant sensation.
- **False-positive response:** This means that the pulp is necrotic, yet the patient will signal that there is sensation in the tooth. This may be due to electrode contact with a metal restoration or the gingiva, patient's anxiety, liquefaction necrosis, and failure to isolate tooth before testing.
- **False-negative response:** This means that the pulp is vital, yet the patients will be unresponsive to electric pulp tests. This may be seen in inadequate contact between the electrode and enamel, recently traumatized tooth, calcification of root canal, recently erupted tooth with an immature apex, partial necrosis, and in a patient who has been heavily premedicated with analgesics, narcotics, or alcohol tranquillizers.

Nagarathna et al. (2015)[1] conducted a study to assess the efficiency and reliability of thermal and electrical pulp tests in primary teeth and found that the highest accuracy rate was calculated for EPT (0.814) followed by cold test (0.777) and heat test (0.759).

Shahi et al. (2015)[2] conducted an in vivo study to evaluate and compare pulse oximeter and conventional pulp testing method (EPT) to assess pulp vitality in primary second molar and young permanent first molar and concluded that pulse oximeter was more sensitive and specific than electric pulp test.

SAFETY CONCERNS OF PULP SENSIBILITY TESTS

Safety Concerns of Heat Tests

- The temperature of melting gutta-percha used in pulp testing is approximately 78–150°C.
- **Zach et al.** noted that an increase of 11°C that occurs during restorative procedures without adequate cooling can harm the pulp. Therefore, prolonged contact with heat is a safety concern.
- An in vitro study by **Fuss et al.** showed that heat testing using gutta-percha increased pulp temperature by less than 2°C with less than 5 seconds of application—a temperature change that is unlikely to have caused pulp damage.

Safety Concerns of Cold Tests

- Concerns have been raised in the past about the possible damaging effects of cold testing agents.
- **Lutz et al.** found that cracks may be formed on enamel surfaces from direct CO_2 snow contact.
- However, subsequent studies by **Peters et al.** and **Fuss et al.** concluded that these concerns were insignificant.

Safety Concerns of EPT

In EPT, the current produced by the testing device may cause danger to patients who have cardiac pacemakers, with the risk of precipitating cardiac arrhythmia via pacemaker interference, but more recent studies have shown no interference from EPT or similar electrical dental devices.

PULP VITALITY TESTS

Laser Doppler Flowmetry

- It is a new method of evaluating pulp vitality by measuring the velocity of RBC in capillaries.
- The laser Doppler flowmetry (LDF) technique was first described in dental literature in 1986 by **Gazelius et al.**
- A near infrared with a wavelength of 632.8 nm is produced by 1 mW helium neon laser within the flowmeter, and this is transmitted along a flexible fiber optical conductor inside a specially designed round dental probe with a diameter of 2 mm.
- This electro-optical technique uses a laser source that is aimed at the pulp, and the laser light travels to the pulp using the dentinal tubules as guides. The backscattered reflected light from circulating blood cells is Doppler-shifted and has a different frequency to the static surrounding tissues. The total backscattered light is processed to produce an output signal. The signal is commonly recorded as the concentration and velocity (flux) of cells using an arbitrary term "perfusion units" (PU), where 2.5 V of blood flow is equivalent to 250 PU **(Fig. 52.6)**.
- In order to record the Doppler shift of the blood cells, both the probe and tooth need to be completely still. Hence, a stabilizing splint made of polyvinyl siloxane or acrylic is usually used.
- Two to three millimeter from the gingival margin is the ideal position for the probe tip as this creates a balance between minimizing the noise and having a recognizable signal volume.

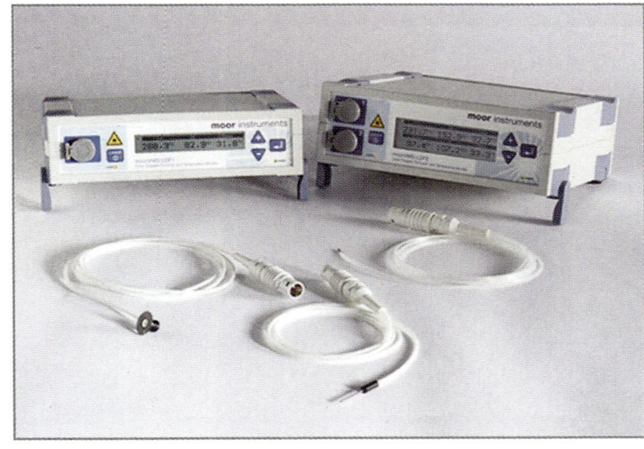

Fig. 52.6: Laser Doppler flowmeter.

- There have been differing views with regards to the accuracy of pulp testing using LDF, given that false results suggesting no blood flow are possible when the laser pathway is interfered with or obstructed. Likewise, the amount of signal contamination from nonpulp sources, primarily the periodontium, can lead to false readings suggesting the presence of pulp blood flow.

Limitations of LDF

- Contamination noise due to backscattered light from periodontal tissues (Akpinar et al., 2004) is impossible to eliminate in LDF even if it is covered with PVS splint.
- The closer the probe is positioned to the gingival margin, the higher the signal output due to greater pulp tissue volume will be but the potential gingival contamination is also higher (Ramsay, Artun and Martinen, 1991).
- Heithersay (Marin, Bartold and Heithersay, 1997) reported a case where traumatized upper central incisor teeth had stained and subsequently returned to normal colour, it was noticed that LDF readings were zero while the tooth was discoloured by blood products.

Pulse Oximetry

- This is an oxygen saturation monitoring device widely used in medical practice for recording blood oxygen saturation levels during the administration of intravenous anesthesia.
- It was invented by **Aoyagi** in the early 1970s.
- Pulse oximetry is an entirely objective test, requiring no subjective response from the patient.
- The pulse oximeter **(Fig. 52.7)** sensor consists of two light-emitting diodes, one to transmit red light (640 nm) and the other to transmit infrared light (940 nm), and a photodetector on the opposite side of the vascular bed. The light emitting diode transmits light through a vascular bed such as the finger or ear. Oxygenated hemoglobin and deoxygenated hemoglobin absorb different amounts of red/infrared light. The pulsatile change in the blood volume causes periodic changes in the amount of red/infrared light absorbed by the vascular bed before reaching the photodetector. The relationship between the pulsatile change in the absorption of red light and the pulsatile change in the absorption of infrared light is analyzed by

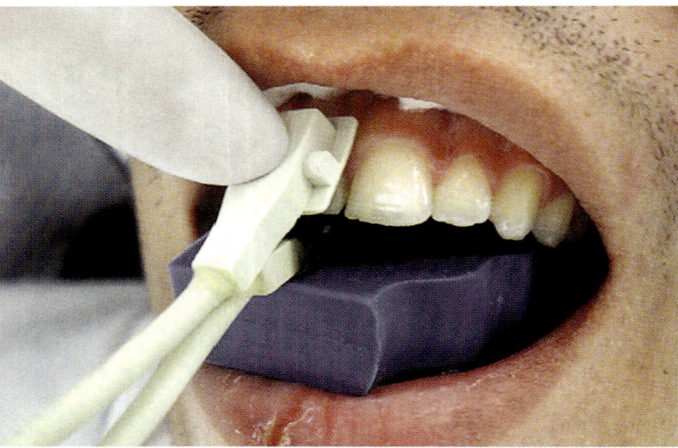

Fig. 52.7: Pulse oximeter.

the pulse oximeter to determine the saturation of arterial blood.

- Compared to laser Doppler flowmeters, pulse oximeters are relatively inexpensive.
- An in vitro study by **Noblett et al.** compared pulse oximetry with blood gas saturation in a simulated pulp blood flow model and showed promising results.

Principle:

- The principle of this is based on Beer's law which relates the absorption of light; by a solute to its concentration and optical properties at a given wavelength. In the red region, oxyhaemoglobin absorbs less light than deoxyhemoglobin and vice versa in case of infrared region. The system has a probe which contains a diode that limits light in two different wavelengths. **(Fig. 52.8)**
  1. Red lights (660 mm)
  2. Infrared light (850 mm)

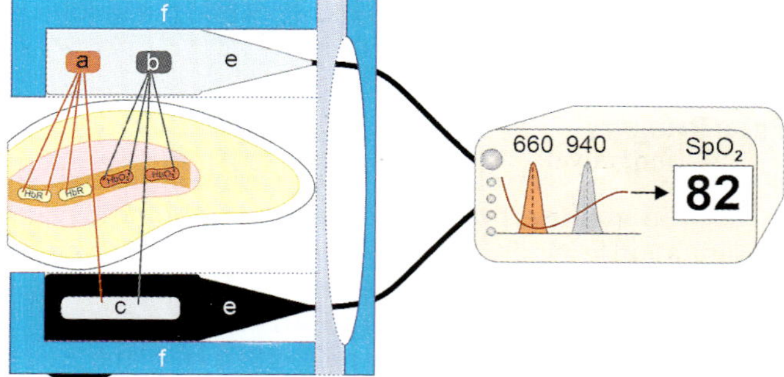

Fig. 52.8: Principle of pulse oximeter.

Limitations

Include the background absorption associated with venous blood and tissue constituents, in addition to this there are chances for refraction and reflection of light that may add on-to its disadvantage.

Laser Speckle Imaging

- Laser speckle imaging enables the differentiation between the absence and presence of perfusion and has the advantage that it is relatively insensitive to the angle of incidence of the laser light, which suggests that the precise positioning

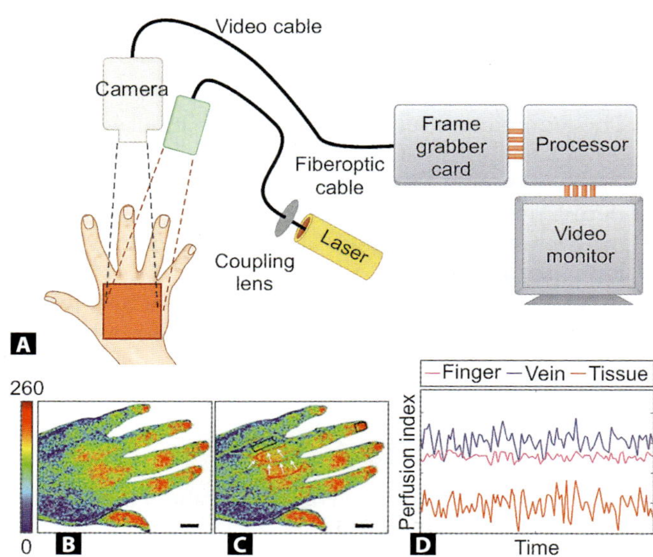

Figs. 52.9A to D: Laser speckle imaging.

of an eventual probe design in the mouth is unnecessary to enable the accurate interrogation of the pulpal chamber for the presence of blood flow **(Figs. 52.9A to D).**

- Recently, an upgraded version of LSI—the polarized laser speckle contrast imaging (LSCI) system—has shown improvement in pulpal blood flow monitorization, being able to detect a wider range of blood flow velocity and smaller changes of blood flow.

EXPERIMENTAL NONINVASIVE VITALITY/SENSIBILITY TESTS

Transmitted Laser Light

- It is an experimental variation to LDF, aimed at eliminating the non-pulp signals.
- Transmitted laser light (TLL) uses similar sending or receiving probes as conventional LDF, but the probes are separate. Thus, the laser beam is passed through from the labial or buccal side of the tooth to the receiver probe which is situated on the palatal or lingual side of the tooth.
- The limitations with TLL are the same as with any laser technology where obstruction and/or interference from within the tooth structure will affect the results.

Transillumination

- This utilizes a strong light source which identifies color changes that may indicate pulp pathosis.
- This technique may not be useful in large posterior teeth and especially in teeth with large restorations. However, it is a helpful adjunct to conventional pulp tests, and it can help to identify cracks in teeth **(Fig. 52.10)**.

Ultraviolet Light Photography

- It examines different fluorescence patterns that may allow additional contrast of otherwise more difficult to observe visible changes.
- It has similar limitations as transillumination, and it is only an adjunct to conventional pulp tests, at best.

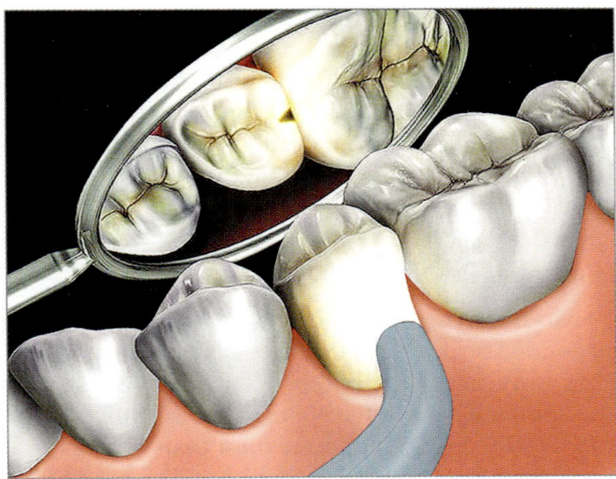
Fig. 52.10: Transillumination.

Surface Temperature Measurement

- It has not found practical clinical use in pulp testing, even though there have been reports that a measurable temperature difference can be found over time in teeth with healthy pulps in contrast to teeth with diseased pulps.
- Potential interfering factors such as breathing by the patient and the lengthy time required for this technique are the major drawbacks.

Physiometric Tests

Taylor in 1960 coined the word "physiometric" to describe such tests that assess the state of the pulpal circulation, rather than the integrity of the nervous tissue thus providing valuable information.

Photoplethysmography

- This was given by **Reich** in 1952.
- This method involves passing light on the tooth and measuring the existing wavelengths using a photocell and galvanometer.
- If a tooth with an intact blood supply is warmed, there should be vascular dilatation, and this would register as a current from the photocell **(Fig. 52.11).**

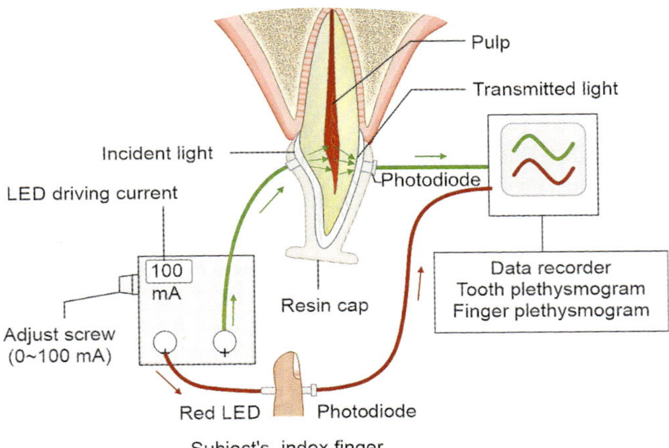

Fig. 52.11: Photoplethysmography.

Thermography

- A hot object emits infrared radiation in proportion to its temperature. Measurement of this radiation may provide information on pulpal circulation.
- Temperature measurement, as a diagnostic procedure for human teeth, has been described with the use of thermistors infrared thermography, and liquid crystals.
- The underlying principle was that teeth with an intact pulp blood supply (vital/healthy pulp tissue) had a warmer tooth surface temperature compared with teeth that had no blood supply.
- The disadvantages of using this technique are that the teeth must be isolated with rubber dam, after which a period of acclimatization is necessary prior to imaging and requires the subjects to be at rest for 1 hour prior to testing.

Light Photoplethysmography

- It is a noninvasive technique used to monitor pulpal blood flow and has been successfully applied in animal and human studies.
- It has been suggested that transmitted light photoplethysmography (TLP) incurs less signal contamination from the periodontal blood flow than is the case for LDF; however, studies have to be evaluated before it can be put to practice.

Dual Wavelength Spectrometry

- Measures blood oxygenation changes within the capillary bed of dental tissue and thus is not dependent on a pulsatile blood flow.
- Helps to differentiate reproductive readings between a pulp chamber of a vital and non-vital tooth.
- In young children, where there are avulsed and replanted teeth with open apices, the blood supply is regained within the first 20 days after replantation but nerve supply lags behind. Repeated readings are taken in such cases up to 40 days to ensure an increase in blood oxygenated level that means the healing process has occurred; the pulp of such teeth has also started to recover (Kayalvizhi and Subramaniyan, 2011) (R. Rajakeerthi and Ms, 2019).

Hughes Probeye Camera

This is used in detecting temperature changes as small as 0.1°C hence can be used to measure pulp vitality experimentally.

The use of 4300 Thermal Hughes Probeye Video System (Hughes Aircraft Co., Carlsbad, CA) was reported in 1989 by **Pogrel et al.** and was found to be sensitive enough to measure temperature differences as low as 0.1°C. Newer, less cumbersome, and easier to use models are now available.

EXPERIMENTAL INVASIVE VITALITY/SENSIBILITY TESTS

Test Cavity

- Given by **Seltzer** and **Bender** in 1975.
- This test is performed when other methods have failed.
- The test cavity is made by drilling the enamel dentin junction of an unanesthetized tooth using a slow speed

handpiece without water coolant. If patient feels sensitivity, it is an indication of pulpvitality.

- This test may serve as a last resort in testing for pulp vitality. It is only considered when the results of all other tests have proved inconclusive. Its value in clinical practice has been largely anecdotal as there is no evidence base to support its effectiveness.

Anesthetic Testing

- Given by **Grossman** in 1978.
- If the patient continues to have vague, diffuse, strong pain, and prior testing has been inconclusive, intraligamentary anesthesia may be used to identify the source of pain.
- When dental symptoms are poorly localized or referred, an accurate diagnosis is extremely difficult. Sometimes, patients may not even able to specify whether the symptoms are from the maxillary or mandibular arch. In such cases, and where pulp testing has proved inconclusive, an anesthetic test may be helpful.
- The technique is as follows: using either infiltration or an intraligamentary injection, the most posterior tooth in the area suspected of causing the pain is anesthetized. If pain persists once the tooth has been fully anesthetized, the tooth immediately mesial to it is then anesthetized, and so on, until the pain disappears. If the source of the pain cannot be even localized to the upper or lower jaw, an inferior alveolar nerve block injection is given; cessation of pain indicates involvement of a mandibular tooth.
- This approach has an advantage over a test cavity, which may incur iatrogenic damage.

Pulp Hemogram

- Suggested by **Guthrie** and **Baume** in 1966.
- It was suggested that taking the first drop of blood from an exposed pulp and subjecting it to a differential white cell count might be useful in diagnosis of pulpal conditions.

Comparison between pulp vitality tests and pulp sensibility tests in references to the studies.

Comparative studies of pulp testing		
Tests	***Sensitivity***	***Specificity***
CPT (Cold pulp test) (Kim el al., 2015)	0.86	0.84
HPT (Heat pulp test) (Kim el al., 2015)	0.77	0.66
EPT (electric pulp test) (Evans el al., 1999)	0.72	0.92
LDF (Laser Doppler flowmetry) (Kim el al., 2015)	0.92	0.95
Heated GP (Evans et al., 1999)	0.86	0.41
Ethyl Chloride (Evans el al., 1999)	0.83	0.93

LIMITATIONS OF PULP TESTING

False-positive Results

- A false-positive response is where a nonvital tooth appears to respond positively to testing.
- This may occur in anxious or young patients who may report a premature response because they are anticipating an unpleasant sensation.
- Necrotic breakdown products in one part of a root canal system can conduct electric currents to viable nerve tissue in adjacent areas, thereby resulting in a false-positive result.
- Contact with metal restorations may also result in conduction of the current to the periodontium, giving a false vital response; the same may occur with inadequately dried teeth.

False-negative Results

- A false-negative result means that a vital tooth has not responded positively to testing.
- This may be seen in teeth with incomplete root development, which have a higher threshold to testing, and require a stronger stimulation than normal to elicit a response.
- Following injury, traumatized teeth may not respond to thermal or EPT due to nerve rupture. The pulps of these teeth, however, may still be vital as their blood vessels remain intact or have revascularized. Therefore, traumatized teeth should always be carefully monitored at periodic intervals as their nerve fibers may subsequently regain function.
- Patients with psychotic disorders may not respond to pulp testing.

Sensitivity and Specificity

- Sensitivity denotes the ability of a test to detect disease in patients who actually have the disease. Thus, the sensitivity of a pulp vitality test indicates the test's ability to identify nonvital teeth. It is defined as the ratio of the number of persons with a positive test result who have the disease divided by the total number of persons with the disease who were tested. A test with a sensitivity of 0.80 therefore has an 80% chance of achieving a positive result when individuals with the disease are tested.
- Specificity, on the other hand, describes the ability of a test to detect the absence of disease. Thus, specificity of a pulpvitality test indicates the test's ability to identify vital teeth. It is defined as the ratio of the number of patients with a negative test result who do not have disease divided by the total number of tested patients without the disease. A test with a specificity of 0.80 has an 80% chance of returning negative results when performed on persons without the disease.

Correlation with Pulp Histopathology

Conservative procedures, aimed at preserving pulp vitality, can only be effective if the status of the pulp is accurately assessed. Responses to vitality testing, however, correlate poorly with histological findings.

Objectivity

- **Ingle** and **Beveridge** have proposed that patient's responses to pulp testing procedures may be considered objective.
- The use of a "control" tooth, on the opposite side of the mouth, has been proposed to remove subjectivity from

an individual's response. This approach, however, is still open to criticism as there is no way of knowing whether the "control" tooth itself is normal.

Reproducibility

- **Reiss** and **Furedi** have reported that patients respond differently to pulp tests on different days, and at different hours of the same day.
- Reproducibility of pulp testing is therefore an area for concern and may relate to the variable state of mind of the patient as well as the lack of intrinsic accuracy of several types of commercial electrical pulp testers.

Unpleasant Sensation

- All methods of pulp testing require the patient to indicate when he or she feels a sensation.
- **Naylor** and **Greenwood** consider that pain is the only sensation elicited by stimulation of pulpal nerves.
- **Mumford** and **Newton** reported that patients use many words other than "pain" to describe the sensation. In most cases, however, the resultant sensation is perceived as "unpleasant".

Effect of Dental Development

- Many authors have observed that erupting teeth show an increased threshold value to EPT or may give no response, even though their vitality is assured.
- Sensitivity to electrical stimulation appears to be related to the stage of root development.
- **Fulling** and **Andreasen** found that thermal testing with carbon dioxide snow gave consistently positive responses irrespective of the stage of dental development.

Effect of Drugs

Several authors have stated that sedative, tranquillizing, or analgesic medications increase the threshold of stimulation of pulpal nerves in some patients.

Effect of Periodontal Disease

There are conflicting reports as to the effect of periodontal disease on pulp testing responses. No increase in pulpal stimulus threshold has been reported in the presence of periodontal disease or bone loss.

Effect of Trauma

- Several authors have highlighted the unpredictable response of a tooth to pulp testing following trauma.
- Immediately following traumatic injury, teeth often fail to respond to conventional pulp testing methods due to temporary loss of response caused by injury, inflammation, pressure, or tension to apical nerve fibers. It may take 8 weeks, or longer, before a normal pulpal response can be elicited.
- **Bhaskar** and **Rappaport** found vital pulp tissue in a series of 25 teeth which has sustained trauma and did respond to conventional vitality tests. They concluded that conventional pulp tests are simply tests of sensitivity and, as such, have questionable value in predicting pulp vitality. For this reason, they recommended that endodontic therapy be delayed in the case of traumatized teeth, and the pulp tissue considered vital in the absence of sinus tract or periapical radiolucency.
- A more accurate assessment of pulp vitality would be made by determining the presence of a functioning blood supply, thus allowing the healing potential to be evaluated at an earlier stage.

Limitations in Children

According to **Mumford**, pulp testing in children below the age of 10 years is unreliable because children may not cooperate for the test. The incomplete innervations of newly erupted teeth may affect the results (as neural sensitivity in primary teeth varies with the stage of root development and resorption). They may elicit false-positive or false-negative results if the dentist asks the child leading questions, and also the unpleasant stimuli produced by the tester may affect behavior management or cooperative problems with pediatric patients. Though the use of traditional tests helps establish an empirical diagnosis, none of these tests are completely reliable. Thus, the validity of children's response in pulp vitality testing has been questioned.

Pulp test selection chart for different clinical situations in primary teeth.

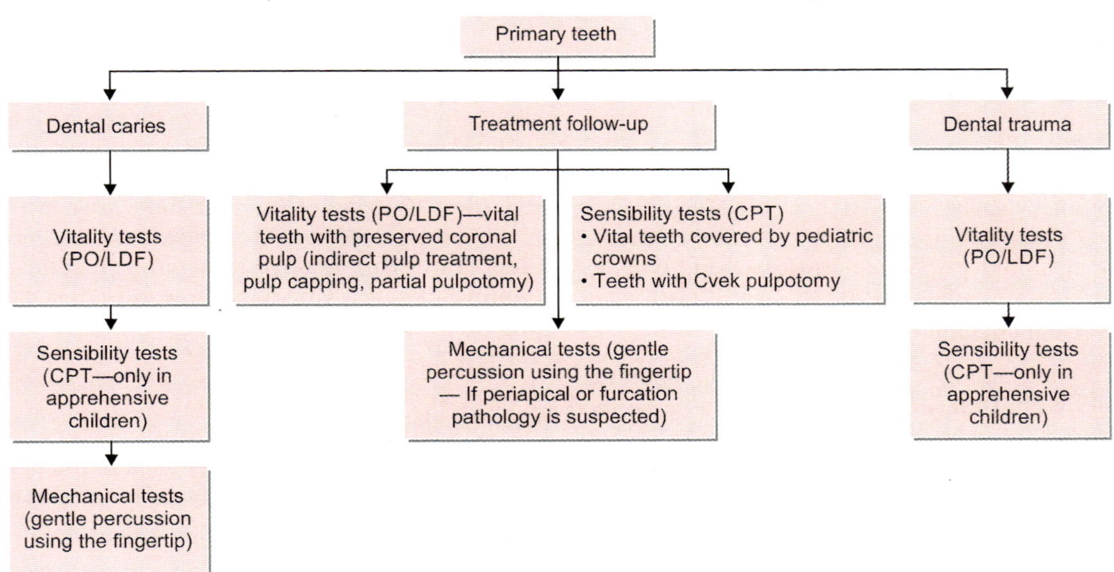

Pulp test selection chart for different clinical situations in immature permanent teeth.

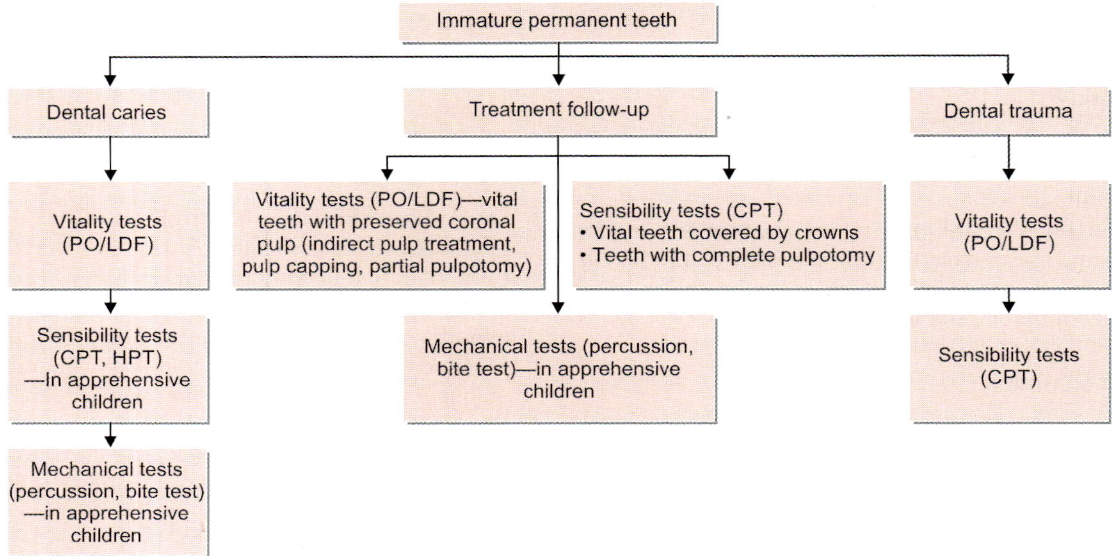

RECENT DEVELOPMENTS IN PULP TESTING

Detection of Interleukins

Interleukins are involved in modulating bone cell activity. Interleukin-1 (IL-1) has been shown to be potent stimuli of bone resorption in organ culture. This hormone-peptide is produced primarily by monocytes and macrophages. Diverse inflammatory cell types are clearly present in periapical lesions. Periapical samples exhibited significant activity of IL-1β (mean 604.4 ± 563.0 pg/mg protein), whereas normal pulp had no activity.[3]

Gas Desaturation

Goho conducted a study on permanent and deciduous teeth and found that SaO_2 on average was in the range of 93–94% in comparison to the SaO_2 taken from index fingers, which is approximately 97%.

Thermographic Imaging

A color image is produced which indicates a relative difference in temperature in both superficial and deep areas. Computer-controlled infrared thermographic imaging (TI) is another noninvasive method of recording the surface temperature of the body. It is highly sensitive and has been used extensively in nonmedical military applications. Computerized infrared TI for human teeth is under investigation to assess pulp vitality.[5]

Optical Reflection Vitalometry

Work started in the late 1990s, and a preliminary report was published in 1997 by **Oikarinen et al.** This method is another non-invasive method to detect pulp vitality. One can "see" the pulse of the pulp or the oral mucosa. This device, too, is yet to be clinically accepted and commercially available.[6]

Cholesteric Liquid Crystals

Cholesteric crystals are a type of "liquid" crystal, that is, ordered fluids, with a helical structure ordered along the long axis known as chiral-nematic liquid crystals. Due to their fluidity, these are easily influenced by temperature or pressure. **Howell et al.** in Lexington 1970 found that nonvital teeth have lower temperature than vital teeth. They used cholesteric compounds that were in a 10% solution in a chlorinated hydrocarbon solvent. When applied to the tooth surface, the crystals went through color changes that were compared with adjacent or contralateral teeth. Their usage in detecting pulp vitality is based on the principle that the teeth in intact pulp blood supply have a higher tooth surface temperature compared with teeth that had no blood supply.[7]

Color Power Doppler

Color power Doppler flowmetry allows the presence and direction of the blood flow within the tissue of interest to be observed. The intensity of the Doppler signal is represented by changes in real time on a graph (Doppler) and is also shown in the form of color spots on the gray-scale image (color). Positive Doppler shifts are caused by the blood moving toward the transducer and are represented in red, whereas negative Doppler shifts are caused by blood moving in the opposite direction and are represented in blue. Power Doppler is associated with color Doppler to improve its sensitivity to low flow rates. It is based on the integrated power spectrum and can disclose the minor vessels.[8]

Radiolabeled Microsphere

Pulpal blood flow has been estimated in intact teeth using radiolabeled microspheres and found to be in the range 20–60 mL/min/100 g tissue. Measurements from exposed pulp indicate that the tissue fluid pressure is high and pulsatile. Furthermore, micropuncture studies have shown that the arteriolar pressure is lower and the venular pressure higher than in other tissues.[9]

Xenon 133 Isotope

The tooth to be tested has to be injected with 0.2-mCi Xenon 133 in saline by a buccal intraligament injection. Radiation counts were detected from teeth using a small cadmium telluride radiation probe. Pulpless teeth had relatively constant counts for the duration of the experiment (200–300). In vital teeth, the initial counts were much higher (718–981) than a gradual decrease that occurs with time. Thus, it is possible to differentiate between vital and pulpless teeth as it checks the status of pulpal blood flow by measuring the washout of Xenon 133.[10]

Recent studies have shown that blood circulation and not innervation is the most accurate determinant in assessing pulp vitality, as it provides an objective differentiation between necrotic and vital pulp tissues. The unpredictability of testing tooth pulp nerve response is well-recognized. When nerve sensations are inhibited or abolished in the tooth, traditional tests are of little value, but method based upon the pulpal vasculature response is a better option. Finally, one should consider recent methods of pulp vitality testing that attempt to measure the pulpal condition objectively.

POINTS TO REMEMBER

- Pulp vitality testing is assessment of the pulp's blood supply and is done by laser Doppler and pulse oximeter.
- Pulp sensibility testing is assessment of the pulp's sensory response and is done by thermal and electric tests.
- Pulp sensitivity testing checks the responsive of pulp to a stimulus.
- Thermal tests were first reported by Jack in 1899.
- Ice, ethyl chloride, CO_2 snow, DDM are used for cold tests.
- Heat test can be done either by heated gutta-percha sticks or by heated ball burnisher. EPT was initiated by Magitot.
- In the case of trauma, we must wait for 4–6 weeks before conducting pulp vitality tests as it is the minimum time required for pulp to heal.
- Laser Doppler flowmetry is a new method of evaluating pulp vitality by measuring the velocity of RBC in capillaries and was described in dental literature in 1986 by Gazelius et al.
- Pulse oximetry measures the blood oxygen saturation levels.
- Some recent advancements in pulp diagnosis are TLL, transillumination, ultraviolet light photography, surface temperature measurement, photoplethysmography, thermography, TLP, dual wavelength spectrometry, Hughes Probeye camera.

Questionnaire

1. Define and classify pulp testing.
2. Write a note on thermal tests of pulp vitality.
3. Explain electric pulp testing with its principle and procedure.
4. Describe pulp vitality tests.
5. What are the recent modifications in the area of pulp testing?
6. Enumerate and explain the limitations of pulp testing.

REFERENCES

1. Nagarathna C, Shakuntala BS, Jaiganesh I. Efficiency and reliability of thermal and electrical tests to evaluate pulp status in primary teeth with assessment of anxiety levels in children. J Clin Pediatr Dent. 2015;39:447-51.
2. Shahi P, Sood PB, Sharma A, et al. Comparative study of pulp vitality in primary and young permanent molars in human children with pulse oximeter and electric pulp tester. Int J Clin Pediatr Dent. 2015;8:94-8.
3. Barkhordar RA, Hussain MZ, Hayashi C. Detection of interleukin-1 beta in human periapical lesions. Oral Surg Oral Med Oral Pathol Oral Radiol. 1992;73:334-6.
4. Goho C. Pulse oximetry evaluation of vitality in primary and immature permanent teeth. Pediatr Dent. 1999;21:125-7.
5. Kells BE, Kennedy JG, Biagioni PA, et al. Computerised infrared thermographic imaging and pulpal blood flow: Part A protocol for thermal imaging of human teeth. Int Endod J. 2000;33:442-7.
6. Oikarinen KS, Kainulainen V, Särkelä V, et al. Information of circulation from soft tissue and dental pulp by means of pulsatile reflected light: further development of optical pulp vitalometry. Oral Surg Oral Med Oral Pathol Oral Radiol Endod. 1997;84:315-20.
7. Howell RM, Duell RC, Mullaney TP. The determination of pulp vitality by thermographic means using cholesteric liquid crystals. A preliminary study. Oral Surg Oral Med Oral Pathol. 1970;29:763-8.
8. Ford TR, Patel S. Technical equipment for assessment of dental pulp status. Endod Topics. 2004;7:2.
9. Matthews B, Andrew D. Microvascular architecture and exchange in teeth. Microcirculation. 1995;2:305-13.
10. Trope M, Jaggi J, Barnett F, et al. Vitality testing of teeth with a radiation probe using 133 xenon radioisotope. Dent Traumatol. 1986;2:215-8.

FURTHER READING

1. Alghaithy RA, Qualtrough AJE. Pulp sensibility and vitality tests for diagnosing pulpal health in permanent teeth: A critical review. Int. Endod J. 2017;50:135–42.
2. Bhaskar SN, Rappaport HM. Dental vitality tests and pulp status. J Am Dent Assoc. 1973;86:409-11.
3. Brännström M. The hydrodynamics of the dental tubule and pulp fluid: its significance in relation to dentinal sensitivity. Annu Meet Am Inst Oral Biol. 1966;23:219.
4. Chambers G. The role and methods of pulp testing in oral diagnosis: a review. Int Endod J. 1982;15:1-15.
5. Chen E, Paul V. Dental pulp testing: a review. Int J Dent. 2009;2009:1-12.
6. Dummer PM, Hicks R, Huws D. Clinical signs and symptoms in pulp disease. Int Endod J. 1980;13:27-35.
7. Ehrmann EH. Pulp testers and pulp testing with particular reference to the use of dry ice. Aust Dent J. 1977;22:272-9.
8. Farias T, Lima R, Luize S, Kelly T, Silva L, Jo et al. Vitality Tests for Pulp Diagnosis of Traumatized Teeth: A Systematic Review. J. Endod. 2021;45:490–499.

9. Fathima T, Ezhilarasan AD. Pulp Testing: A Literature Review. Annals of R.S.C.B. 2021;25(3):704-23.
10. Foreman PC. Ultraviolet light as an aid to endodontic diagnosis. Int Endod J. 1983;16:121-6.
11. Fuhr K, Scherer W. Prüfmethodik und Ergebnisse vergleichender Utersuchungen zur vitalitätsprüfung von Zähnen. Dtsch Zahnarztl Z. 1968;23:1344-9.
12. Fulling HJ, Andreasen JO. Influence of maturation status and tooth type of permanent teeth upon electrometric and thermal pulp testing. Scand J Dent Res. 1976;4:286-90.
13. Gazelius B, Lindh-Strömberg U, Pettersson H, et al. Laser Doppler technique: a future diagnostic tool for tooth pulp vitality. Int Endod J. 1993;26:8-9.
14. Gazelius B, Olgart L, Edwall B, et al. Noninvasive recording of blood flow in human dental pulp. Endod Dent Traumatol. 1986;2:219-21.
15. Ghouth N, Duggal MS, BaniHani A, Nazzal H. The diagnostic accuracy of laser Doppler flowmetry in assessing pulp blood flow in permanent teeth: A systematic review. Dent. Traumatol. 2018;34:311–9.
16. Gopikrishna V, Pradeep G, Venkateshbabu N. Assessment of pulp vitality: a review. Int J Paediatr Dent. 2009;19:3-15.
17. Hill CM. The efficacy of transillumination in vitality tests. Int Endod J. 1986;19:198-201.
18. Igna A, Mircioaga D, Boariu M, Stratul SI. A Diagnostic Insight of Dental Pulp Testing Methods in Pediatric Dentistry. Medicina 2022;58(665):1-13.
19. Kayalvizhi G, Subramaniyan B. Traditional pulp vitality testing methods: an overview of their limitations. J Oral Health Comm Dent. 2011;5:12-4.
20. Lutz F, Mormann W, Lutz T. Enamel cracks caused by vitality tests with carbon dioxide snow. SSO Schweiz Monatsschr Zahnheilkd. 1974;84:709-25.
21. Mumford J. Evaluation of gutta-percha and ethyl chloride in pulp testing. Br Dent J. 1964;116:338-42.
22. Mumford JM. Thermal and electrical stimulation of teeth in the diagnosis of pulpal and periapical disease. Proc R Soc Med. 1967;60:197-200.
23. Penna KJ, Sadoff RS. Simplified approach to use of electrical pulp tester. N Y State Dent J. 1995;61:30-1.
24. Peters DD, Baumgartner JC, Lorton L. Adult pulpal diagnosis. Evaluation of the positive and negative responses to cold and electrical pulp tests. J Endod. 1994;20:506-11.
25. Petersson K, Soderstrom C, Kiani-Anaraki M, et al. Evaluation of the ability of thermal and electrical tests to register pulp vitality. Dent Traumatol. 1999;15:127-31.
26. Radhakrishnan S, Munshi AK, Hegde AM. Pulse oximetry: a diagnostic instrument in pulpal vitality testing. J Clin Pediatr Dent. 2002;26:141-5.
27. Ramsay DS, Artun J, Martinen SS. Reliability of pulpal blood- flow measurements utilizing laser Doppler flowmetry. J Dent Res. 1991;70:1427-30.
28. Rowe H, Pitt Ford TR. The assessment of pulpal vitality. Int Endod J. 1990;23:77-83.
29. Sasano T, Onodera D, Hashimoto K, et al. Possible application of transmitted laser light for the assessment of human pulp vitality—Part 2: Increased laser power for enhanced detection of pulpal blood flow. Dent Traumatol. 2005;21: 37-41.
30. Seltzer S, Bender IB, Ziontz M. The dynamics of pulp inflammation: correlations between diagnostic data and actual histologic findings in the pulp. Oral Surg Oral Med Oral Pathol. 1963;16:969-77.
31. Shoher I, Mahler Y, Samueloff S. Dental pulp photo- plethysmography in human beings. Oral Surg Oral Med Oral Pathol. 1973;36:915-21.
32. Stoops LC, Scott Jr D. Measurement of tooth temperature as a means of determining pulp vitality. J Endod. 1976;2: 141-5.
33. Tomer AK, Raina AA, Ayub FB, Bhatt M. Recent advances in pulp vitality testing: A review. Int J Appl Dent Sci. 2019;5(3):08-12.
34. Xu, F, Xie C, Zhang Y, Shi G, Shi J, Xu X, Zhao Y, Zhu Y, He X. Vertically Polarized Laser Speckle Contrast Imaging to Monitor Blood Flow in Pulp. J Mod Opt. 2021;68:1075–82.
35. Zach L. Pulp lability and repair;effect of restorative procedures. Oral Surg Oral Med Oral Pathol. 1972;33:111-21.
36. Öhman A. Healing and sensitivity to pain in young replanted human teeth. An experimental, clinical, and histological study. Odontol Tidskr. 1965;73:166-227.

CHAPTER

Endodontic Armamentarium

Satish Vishwanathaiah, Nikhil Marwah, Vineeta Nikhil, PR Geetha Priya

CHAPTER OUTLINE

Preparation of the root canal system is recognized as being one of the most important stages in root canal treatment. It includes the removal of vital and necrotic tissues from the root canal system, along with infected root dentin and, in cases of retreatment, the removal of metallic and non-metallic obstacles. Although mechanical preparation and chemical disinfection cannot be considered separately and are commonly referred to as chemomechanical or biomechanical preparation, the following chapter is intended to focus on the endodontic armamentarium only.

Although **Fauchard**, one of the founders of modern dentistry described instruments for trephination of teeth, preparation of root canals and cauterization of pulps in his book *"Le Chirurgien Dentiste"*, no systematic description of preparation of the root canal system could be found in the literature at that time. First endodontic hand instrument has been developed by **Edward Maynard**. Notching a round wire (in the beginning watch springs, later piano wires), he created small needles for extirpation of pulp tissue. In 1852, **Arthur** used small files for root canal enlargement and in 1915 the K file were introduced. The standardization of instruments was first proposed in 1929 by **Trebitsch** and by **Ingle** in 1958, but International Organization for Standardization (ISO) specifications for endodontic instruments were published in 1974.

GOALS OF MECHANICAL ROOT CANAL PREPARATION

As stated earlier, mechanical instrumentation of the root canal system is an important phase of root canal preparation as it creates the space that allows irrigants and antibacterial medicaments to more effectively eradicate bacteria and eliminate bacterial byproducts. However, it remains one of the most difficult tasks in endodontic therapy. The major goals of root canal preparation are:

- Removal of vital and necrotic tissue from the main root canal
- Creation of sufficient space for irrigation and medication
- Preservation of the integrity and location of the apical canal anatomy
- Avoidance of iatrogenic damage to the canal system and root structure
- Facilitation of canal filling
- Avoidance of further irritation and/or infection of the periradicular tissues
- Preservation of sound root dentin to allow long-term function of the tooth.

CLASSIFICATION OF ENDODONTIC INSTRUMENTS

According to Function by Grossman

- Exploring instruments, e.g., smooth broaches, endodontic explorer.
- Debridement instruments, e.g., barbed broaches, rasp for removal of pulp tissue.
- Cleaning and shaping instruments, e.g., files, reamers.
- Obturating instruments, e.g., spreaders, pluggers to fill root canal with obturating material.

Based on use by ISO–FDI (3630-5)

- **ISO Group I:** Hand use only, e.g., K-files, H-files, broach, pluggers, spreader.
- **ISO Group II:** Non rotary endodontic instrument:
  - Engine driven instruments, e.g., Reciprocating file, self-adjusting file.
  - Ultrasonic and sonic instruments, e.g., Rispi sonic, Helio sonic, EndoActivator, Ultra X.
- **ISO Group III:** Rotary endodontic instruments used with a handpiece:
  - Slow speed stainless steel instruments, e.g., GG drills, peeso reamer.
  - NiTi rotary instruments e.g., ProTaper Universal file, Hyflex CM
- **ISO Group IV:** Engine driven adapting itself to the canal anatomy, e.g., Self-adjusting file (SAF) system.
- **ISO Group V:** Engine driven reciprocating instruments, e.g., Wave One.
- **ISO Group VI:** Sonic and ultrasonic instruments.

ISO STANDARDIZATION OF ENDODONTIC INSTRUMENTS (FIGS. 53.1 TO 53.3)

To standardize the length, diameter, taper of instruments, **Ingle and Levine** suggested few guidelines:

- The numbering of instruments shall be from 10 to 100 with an increase of 5 units till number 60 and then 10 units till 100.
  Revision: Smaller instruments number 6 and 8 and larger instrument above 100 till 140 were added.
- The number of instrument designates the tip size of instrument in 100th of millimeter, e.g., 30 number instrument has tip size of 0.3 mm (D1).
- With every mm the diameter of instrument increase by 0.02 mm from tip to end of cutting blade (D2). The diameter at D2 is D1+0.32 mm.
  Revision: The D1 was later revised to D0 and D2 to D16.
- The instruments shall be color coded.

MISCELLANEOUS ENDODONTIC INSTRUMENTS

- **Plastic instruments:** It has two ends; the first is used to carry temporary filling material. The opposite end is used as a plugger to condense cement and base materials in the root canal.

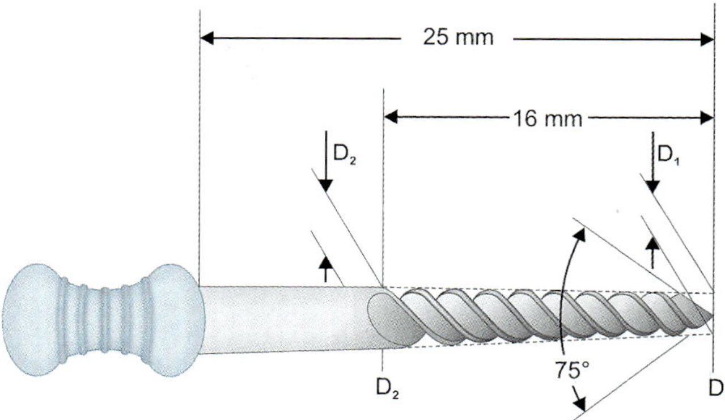

Fig. 53.1: Original ISO standardization given by Ingle and Levine (1958).

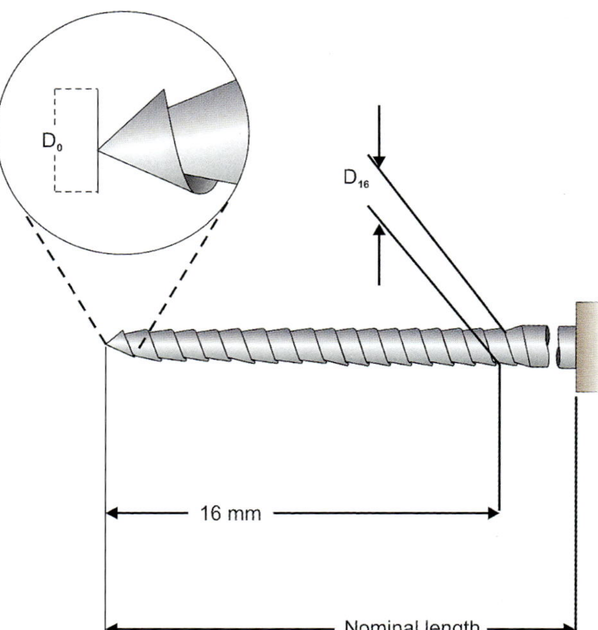

Fig. 53.2: New standardization proposed in 2002 (No. from 6 to 140/ D_1 became D_0/D_2 became D_{16}/Half sizes in 0.02 flare were introduced like 12.5, 17.5/Ni-Ti Profile named 0.29 series).

Color code	ISO size	d.± 0.02 mm	d.± 0.02 mm
	006	0.06	0.38
	008	0.08	0.40
	010	0.10	0.42
	015	0.15	0.47
	020	0.20	0.52
	025	0.25	0.57
	030	0.30	0.62
	035	0.35	0.67
	040	0.40	0.72
	045	0.45	0.77
	050	0.50	0.82
	055	0.55	0.87
	060	0.60	0.92
	070	0.70	1.02
	080	0.80	1.12
	090	0.90	1.22
	100	1.00	1.32
	110	1.10	1.42
	120	1.20	1.52
	130	1.30	1.62
	140	1.40	1.72

Fig. 53.3: Color coding of files according to new standardization.

- **Endodontic locking pliers (tweezer):** It has a lock that allows materials to be held without continuous finger pressure; also it has a groove which facilitates holding guttapercha and absorbing points.

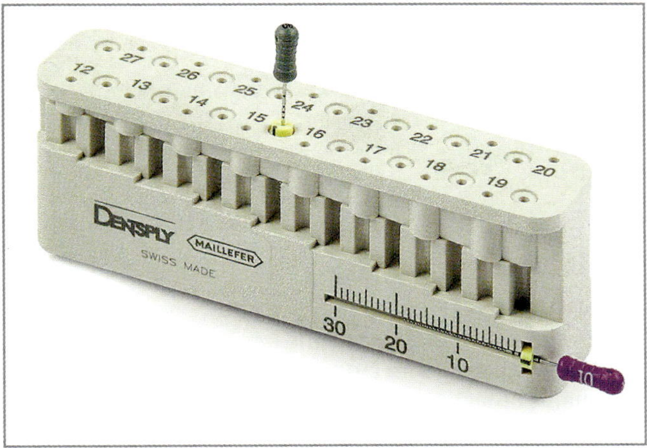

Fig. 53.4: Endodontic block.

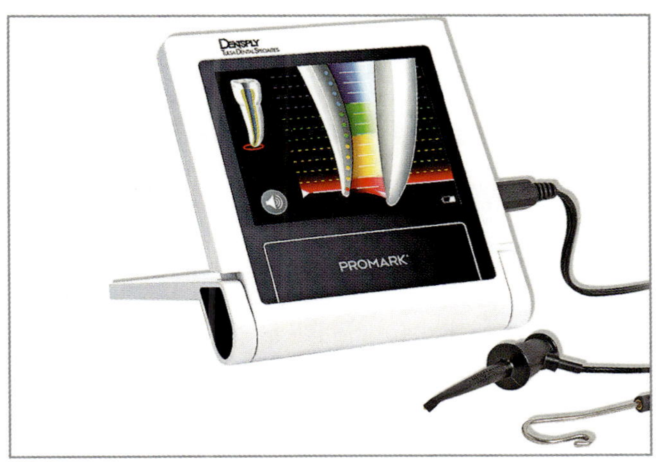

Fig. 53.6: Electronic apex locator.

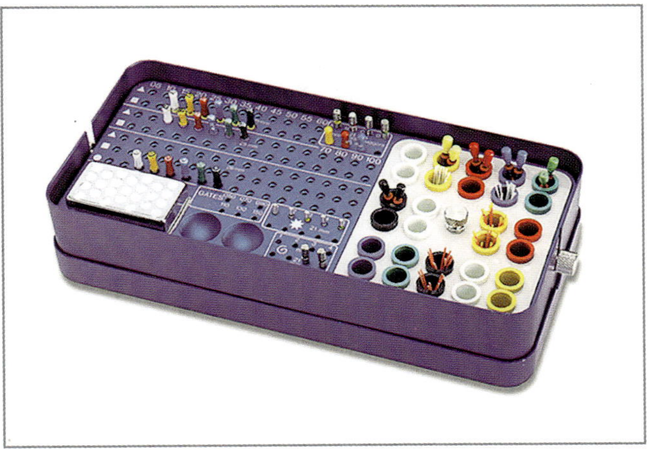

Fig. 53.5: Endodontic instrument box.

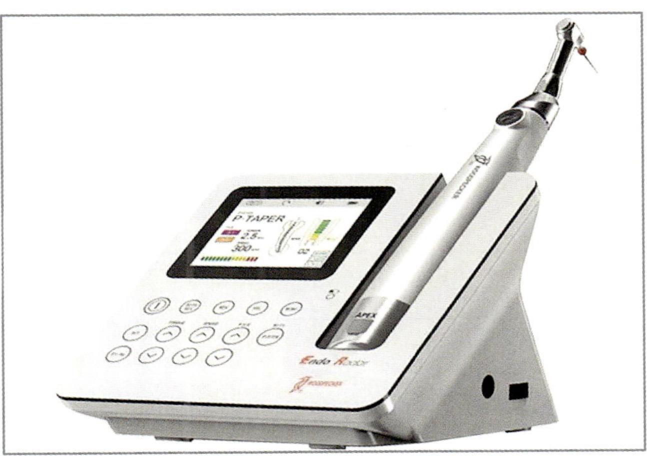

Fig. 53.7: Endo motor.

- **Endodontic block (Fig. 53.4):** It is a convenient plastic device for setting a precise working length for both reamers and file as well as gutta-percha points.
- **Endodontic Instrument organizer (endodontic box) (Fig. 53.5):** It is used for arrangement of reamers and files according to the size and length. The organizer provides holes for the files to be placed vertically.
- **Endodontic syringe:** It is used to carry irrigating solution into the root canal. The tip of the needle varies in design, e.g., notched, beveled, side vented etc. Both close and open-ended needles can be used, but close-ended minimizes the chances of inadvertent extrusion of irrigant in periapical area.
- **Electronic apex locator (Fig. 53.6)**: It is an electronic device used to determine the working length electronically, e.g., Root ZX, Propex, Canal Pro.
- **Endo motor (Fig. 53.7):** It is a motor which supply controlled and precise torque to an endodontic handpiece thus provide cutting speed with prevention of instrument separation, e.g., X-Smart Endo motor, Canal Pro CL2.
- **Transfer sponge:** It is sponge saturated with disinfectant solution. The reamers and files can be placed in it after being used.
- **Rubber/silicon stopper:** It is used to mark the length of the tooth on reamers and files; it should be perpendicular to the long axis of the instrument. It may be of different shape-round, square, triangle or tear with a marking which helps to mark the direction of curvature of canal.

ACCESS PREPARATION INSTRUMENTS

- These are the instruments used for preparation of access cavity:
  - Rotary instruments, e.g., round diamond bur, tapered diamond bur, combination of round and tapered bur **(Fig. 53.8)**, Endo Z bur **(Fig. 53.9)**, Gates Glidden drills **(Fig. 53.10)**
  - Ultrasonic instruments, e.g., Start-X tips **(Fig. 53.11)**.

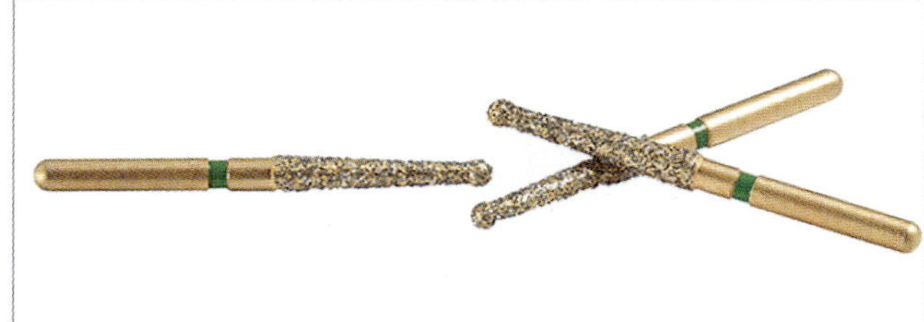

Fig. 53.8: Endo access bur.

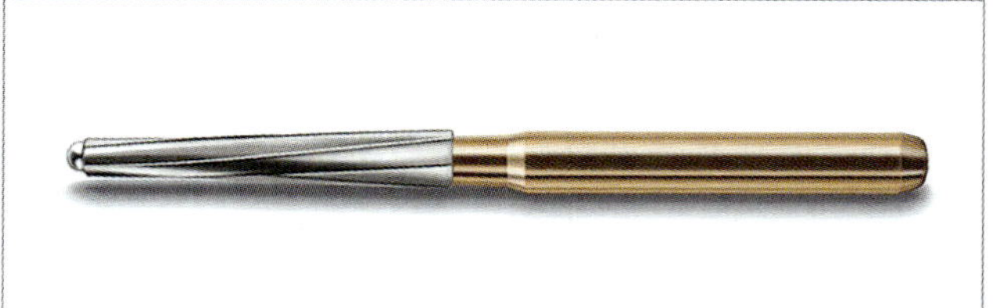

Fig. 53.9: Endo Z bur.

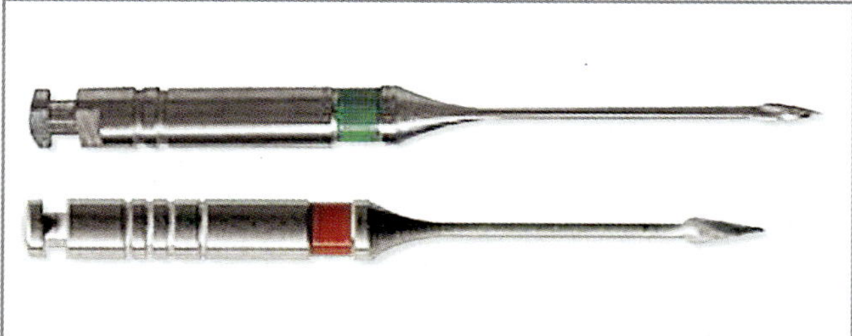

Fig. 53.10: Gates Glidden drill.

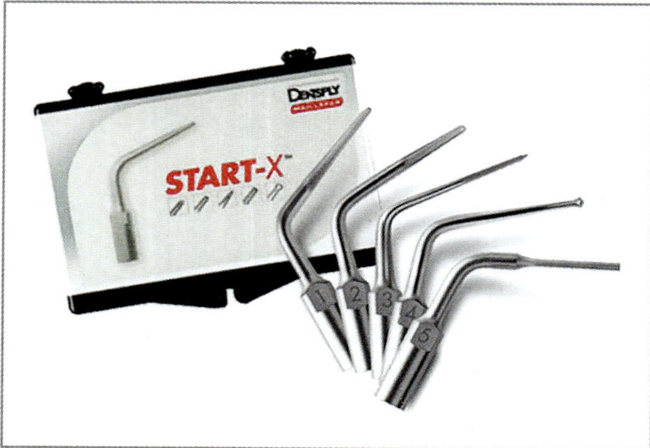

Fig. 53.11: Start X tips.

EXPLORING ENDODONTIC INSTRUMENTS

These are used to locate the root canal orifice and to determine or assist in obtaining patency of root canal, e.g., smooth broach and endodontic explorer.

Endodontic Explorer

It is a double ended instrument which is used to locate and enlarge the root canal orifice. The different angulation of shank at both ends make it suitable for both anterior and posterior application. The tip is strong and sharp (e.g., DG-16) **(Fig. 53.12).**

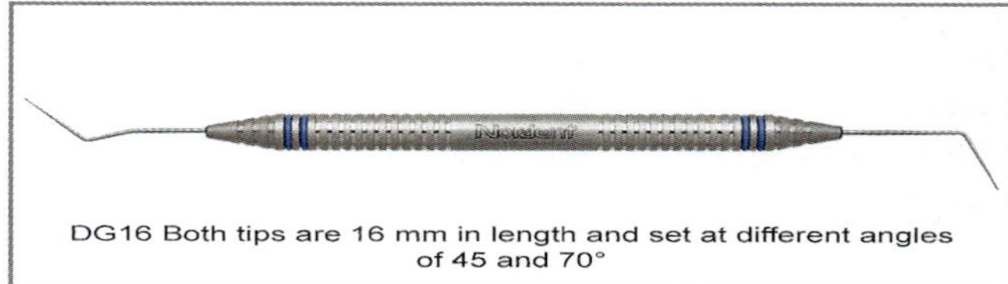

DG16 Both tips are 16 mm in length and set at different angles of 45 and 70°

Fig. 53.12: DG-16 Endodontic explorer.

Smooth Broaches

- Also called as Miller needles.
- These are smooth, pointed and tapered with either round, pentagonal or square cross-section **(Fig. 53.13).**
- Smooth broaches are useful as pathfinder in curved fine canals because of their flexibility and fine diameter.

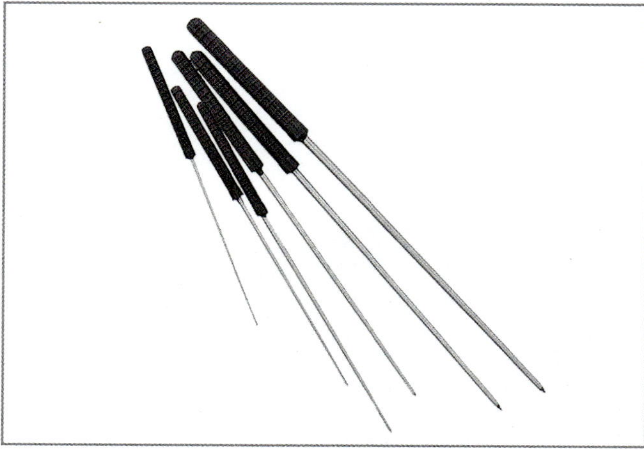

Fig. 53.13: Smooth broach.

DEBRIDEMENT INSTRUMENTS

The instruments which are used to extirpate the pulp from the root canal or from pulp chamber or necrotic tooth debris.

Endodontic Excavator

- It is larger than spoon excavator and is used to allow excavation of the contents of the pulp chamber **(Fig. 53.14).**
- It is also used in curettage of periapical lesions in surgical endodontics.

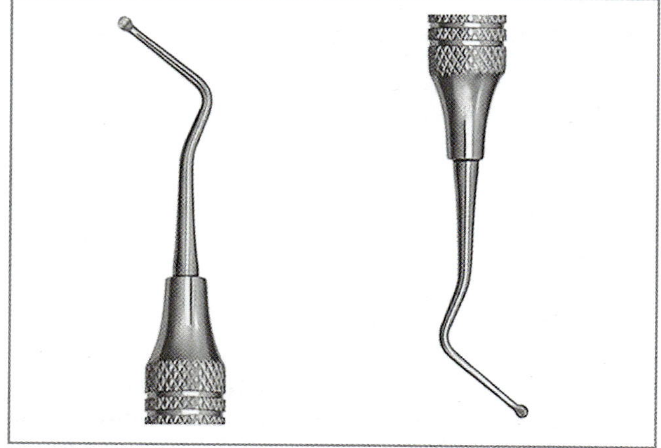

Fig. 53.14: Endodontic excavator.

Barbed Broaches

- It is a short-handled instrument with a shaft having projections directed obliquely towards the handle **(Fig. 53.15).**
- It is used to extirpate pulp in the root canal, remove cotton and paper points from the root canal, and loosen debris in necrotic canals.
- It is manufactured from a tapered round soft steel wire of varying diameter into which, angle cuts are made to produce barbs.
- The disadvantage of this instrument is that it can be used in straight canals and not in the blunt canals.

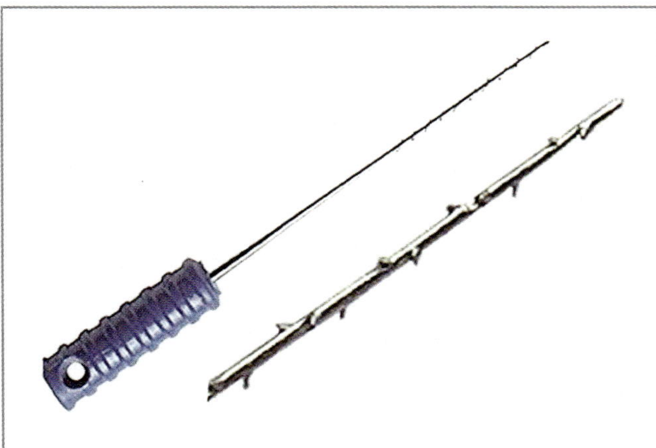

Fig. 53.15: Barbed broach.

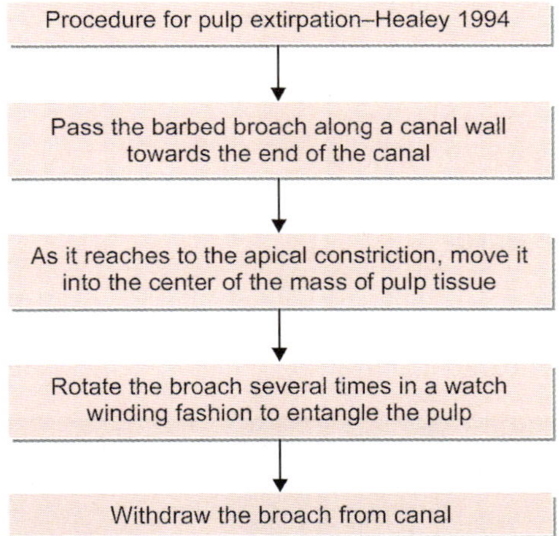

Procedure for pulp extirpation–Healey 1994
Pass the barbed broach along a canal wall towards the end of the canal
As it reaches to the apical constriction, move it into the center of the mass of pulp tissue
Rotate the broach several times in a watch winding fashion to entangle the pulp
Withdraw the broach from canal

CLEANING AND SHAPING INSTRUMENTS

These instruments are used to shape the root canal laterally and apically. These include K-files, H-files, reamers, and Ni-Ti files. Although the basic function of all files is the same they however differ in design, number of flutes, and cross-section which is directly proportional to the action and cutting efficiency of each of these cleaning and shaping instruments **(Fig. 53.16)**.

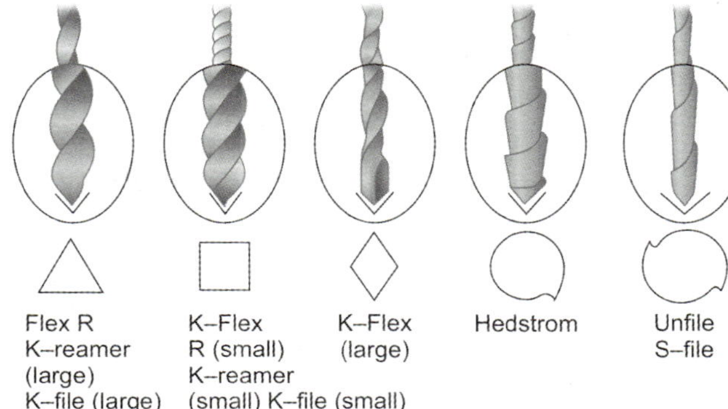

Fig. 53.16: Variable flute designs of files and their cross-section.

K-files

- Designed as early as 1904 by **Kerr**
- Originally made from a square or triangular blank, machine twisted to form a tight spiral with more cutting flutes than a reamer **(Fig. 53.17)**
- 1½–2½ flutes/mm
- Less susceptible to breakage
- Decreased flexibility
- Lesser cutting efficiency
- Rasping or pulling action.

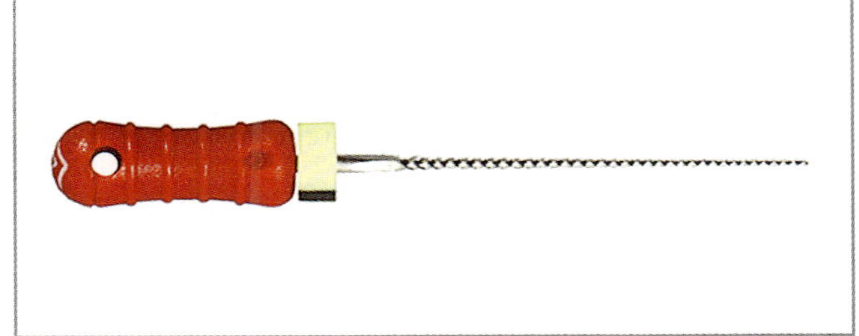

Fig. 53.17: K-file.

Modifications of K-file

- **K-flex file:** It is introduced in 1982. It is made of a diamond or rhomboid Cross-section bar. This instrument is more flexible because of decreased cross-section diameter. The rhomboidal blank produces alternating high and low flutes those are supposed to make the instrument more efficient to remove debris. It is available in stainless steel and Ni-Ti types.
- **Flex-O file:** This employs a more flexible type of file which does not fracture easily. These instruments are developed from triangular cross-section bar. They have 1.81 flutes/mm, hence have more cutting efficiency.
- **Triple-flex:** These have more flutes than reamer but less than K-file. These are made of stainless steel and have trangular cross-section.

Reamer

- They are constructed from a square or triangular blank, twisted into a spiral but with fewer cutting flutes than a file **(Fig. 53.18)**

- It cuts only dentin if it is rotated
- ½–1 flute/mm
- More cutting efficiency
- Pushing, rotating, and retracting action.

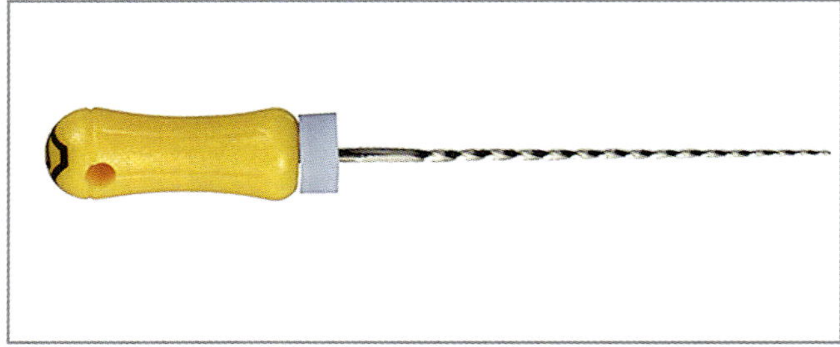

Fig. 53.18: K-reamer.

H-files

- They are called Hedstrom files
- They are made of stainless steel and are machined from a round-tapered blank **(Fig. 53.19)**
- They have good cutting efficiency and are used in pulling action
- They are flexible and are indicated in tortuous canals as in primary teeth
- The procedure for shaping using H-files is that file is inserted into the root canal to the apex, laterally pressed against one side of the canal wall, and withdrawn with a pulling motion to file the dentinal wall
- Kennedy strongly recommended use of H-files in primary teeth, since they remove hard tissue only on withdrawal which prevents pushing the infected material through the apices
- Sizes—0.10–1.40 mm and Tip size—0.15–0.60 mm
- The main disadvantage of H-files is that they tend to fracture.

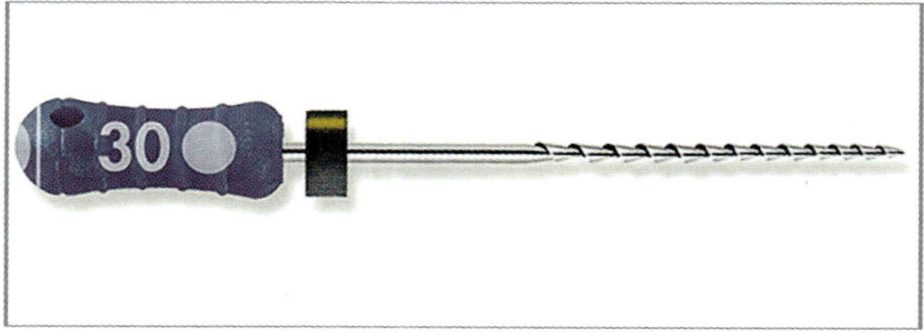

Fig. 53.19: H-file.

Modifications of H-file

- **Safety H-files:** Introduced by **Kerr** manufacturing Co. in 1998. A noncutting side characterizes the spiral of the working end of these files with smoothened edges to prevent ledging in curved canals. A flat side on the handle orients the operation to the smoothened edge of the instrument while using it in the root canal.
- **Sharpie® Hedstrom files:** These are designed for teeth with irregular walls or for removing instruments from a canal.
- **Miltex® Hi-5® files:** These are designed with helically ground flutes and pentagonal cross-section which is good for penetration in small or calcified canals.

Nickel–Titanium Files

- They are introduced by **Elizabeth S Bair** in 1999–2000. They have nickel (55%) and titanium (45%)
- The flexibility and the instrument design allow the files to closely follow the original root canal path **(Fig. 53.20)**
- The tortuous and irregular canal walls of primary molars are effectively cleaned with Ni-Ti files since the clockwise motion of the rotary files pulls pulpal tissue and dentin out of the canal as the files are engaged.

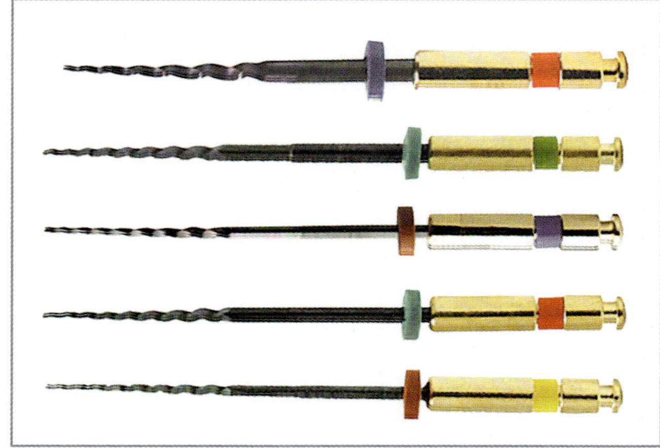

Fig. 53.20: Nickel -titanium files.

Advantages

- Tissue and debris are more easily and quickly removed
- Faster results
- Allows easy access to all canals
- It possess a memory effect.

Disadvantages

- Cost
- Learning the technique.

Retreatment Files

These files are used during nonsurgical endodontic retreatment for removal of obturating material, e.g., Hyflex Remover, ProTaper Universal Retreatment files **(Fig. 53.21).**

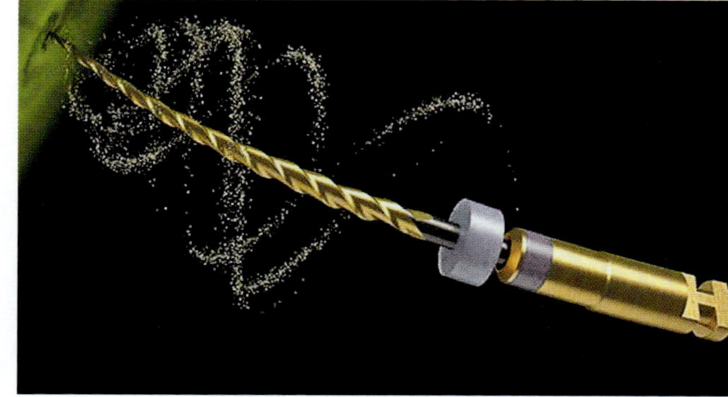

Fig. 53.21: Retreatment file.

IRRIGATION

The success of endodontic treatment depends on the eradication of microbes from the root canal system and prevention of reinfection. The main goal of instrumentation is to facilitate effective irrigation, disinfection, and filling. There is no single irrigating solution that alone sufficiently covers all the functions required from an irrigant. Optimal irrigation is based on the combined use of two or several irrigating solutions, in a specific sequence, to predictably obtain the goals of safe and effective irrigation. Irrigants have traditionally been delivered into the root canal space using syringes and metal needles of different size and tip design.

Desired functions of irrigating solutions:

- Washing action (helps remove debris)
- Reduce instrument friction during preparation (lubricant)
- Facilitate dentin removal (lubricant)
- Dissolve inorganic tissue (dentin)
- Penetrate to canal periphery
- Dissolve organic matter (dentin collagen, pulp tissue, biofilm)
- Kill bacteria and yeasts (also in biofilm)
- Do not irritate or damage vital periapical tissue, no caustic or cytotoxic effects
- Do not weaken tooth structure.

Irrigating solutions:

- **Sodium hypochlorite (NaOCl)** is the most popular irrigating solution. NaOCl ionizes in water into Na_1 and the hypochlorite ion, OCl, establishing an equilibrium with hypochlorous acid (HOCl). Hypochlorous acid is responsible for the antibacterial activity and disrupts several vital functions of the microbial cell, resulting in cell death. Although hypochlorite alone does not remove the smear layer, it affects the organic part of the smear layer, making its complete removal possible by subsequent irrigation with ethylenediaminetetraacetic acid (EDTA) or citric acid (CA). However, continuous irrigation and time are important factors for the effectiveness of hypochlorite. It should be used throughout the instrumentation phase.
- **EDTA and CA:** Complete cleaning of the root canal system.
- requires the use of irrigants that dissolve organic and inorganic material. EDTA and CA effectively dissolve inorganic material, including hydroxyapatite. They have little or no effect on organic tissue and alone they do not have antibacterial activity, despite some conflicting reports on EDTA. EDTA and CA are used for 2–3 minutes at the end of instrumentation and after NaOCl irrigation. Removal of the smear layer by EDTA or CA improves the antibacterial effect of locally used disinfecting agents in deeper layers of dentin.
- **Chlorhexidine digluconate (CHX)** is widely used in disinfection.
- in dentistry because of its good antimicrobial activity. It has gained considerable popularity in endodontics as an irrigating solution and as an intracanal medicament. CHX does not possess some of the undesired characteristics of sodium hypochlorite (i.e. bad smell and strong irritation to periapical tissues). However, CHX has no tissue-dissolving capability and therefore it cannot replace NaOCl. In high concentrations, CHX causes coagulation of intracellular components. One of the reasons for the popularity of CHX is its substantivity (i.e. continued antimicrobial effect), because CHX binds to hard tissue and remains antimicrobial.

Irrigation Devices and Techniques[1]

The effectiveness and safety of irrigation depends on the means of delivery. Traditionally, irrigation has been performed with a plastic syringe and an open-ended needle into the canal space. An increasing number of novel needle-tip designs and equipment are emerging in an effort to better address the challenges of irrigation.

Syringes

Plastic syringes of different sizes (1–20 mL) are most commonly used for irrigation. Although large volume syringes potentially allow some time-savings, they are more difficult to control for pressure and accidents may happen. Therefore, to maximize safety and control, use of 1–5 mL syringes is recommended instead of the larger ones. All syringes for endodontic irrigation must have a Luer-Lok design. Because of the chemical reactions between many irrigants, separate syringes should be used for each solution.

Needles

Although 25-gauge needles were common place for endodontic irrigation a few years ago, they were first replaced by 27-G needles, now 30-G and even 31-G needles are taking over for routine use in irrigation. As 27-G corresponds to ISO size 0.42 and 30 G to size 0.31, smaller needle sizes are preferred. Several studies have shown that the irrigant has only a limited effect beyond the tip of the needle because of the dead-water zone or sometimes air bubbles in the apical root canal, which prevent apical penetration of the solution. However, although the smaller needles allow delivery of the irrigant close to the apex, this is not without safety concerns. Several modifications of the needle-tip design have been introduced in recent years to facilitate effectiveness and minimize safety risks.

EndoActivator (Advanced Endodontics, Santa Barbara, CA, USA)

A new type of irrigation facilitator. It is based on sonic vibration (up to 10,000 cpm) of a plastic tip in the root canal. The system has three different sizes of tips that are easily attached (snap-on) to the handpiece that creates the sonic vibrations. **(Fig. 53.22)** EndoActivator does not deliver new irrigant to the canal but it facilitates the penetration and renewal of the irrigant in the canal. Two recent studies have indicated that the use of EndoActivator facilitates irrigant penetration and mechanical cleansing compared with needle irrigation, with no increase in the risk of irrigant extrusion through the apex.

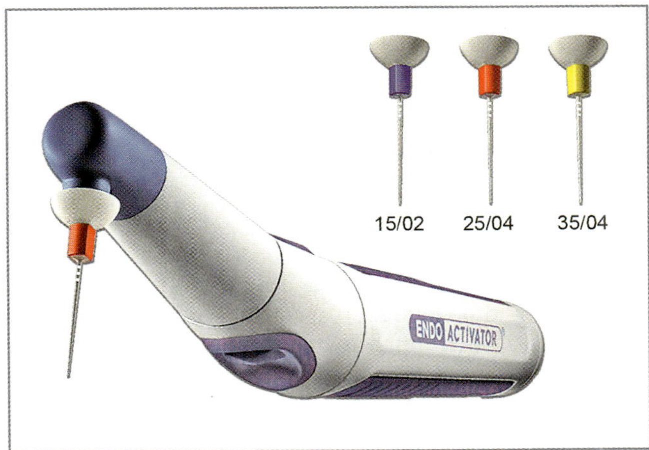

Fig. 53.22: EndoActivator.

Vibringe (Vibringe BV, Amsterdam, The Netherlands)

A new sonic irrigation system that combines battery-driven vibrations (9000 cpm) with manually operated irrigation of the root canal. Vibringe uses the traditional type of syringe or needle delivery but adds sonic vibration **(Fig. 53.23)**.

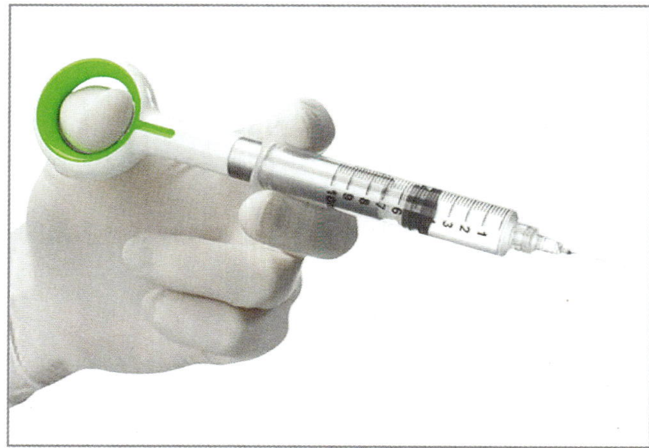

Fig. 53.23: Vibringe.

RinsEndo system (Durr Dental Co)

Based on a pressure-suction mechanism with approximately 100 cycles per minute. A study of the safety of several irrigation systems reported that the risk of overirrigation was comparable with manual and RinsEndo irrigation, but higher than with EndoActivator or the EndoVac system **(Fig. 53.24)**.

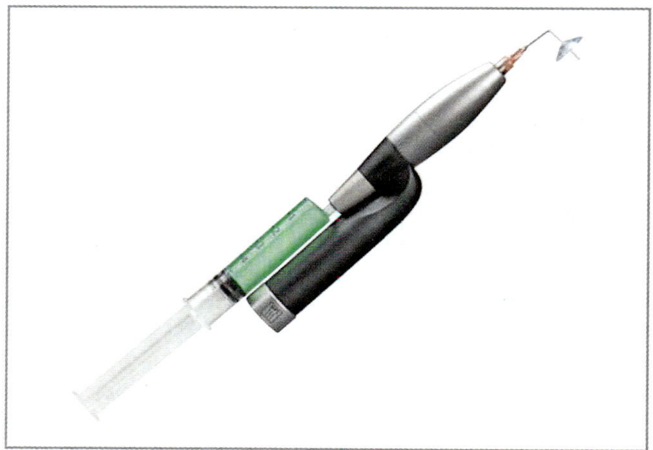

Fig. 53.24: RinsEndo irrigation.

EndoVac (Discus Dental, Culver City, CA, USA)

Represents a novel approach to irrigation as, instead of delivering the irrigant through the needle, the EndoVac system is based on a negative-pressure approach whereby the irrigant placed in the pulp chamber is sucked down the root canal and back up again through a thin needle with a special design **(Fig. 53.25)**. There is evidence that, compared with traditional needle irrigation and some other systems, the EndoVac system lowers the risks associated with irrigation close to the apical foramen considerably.

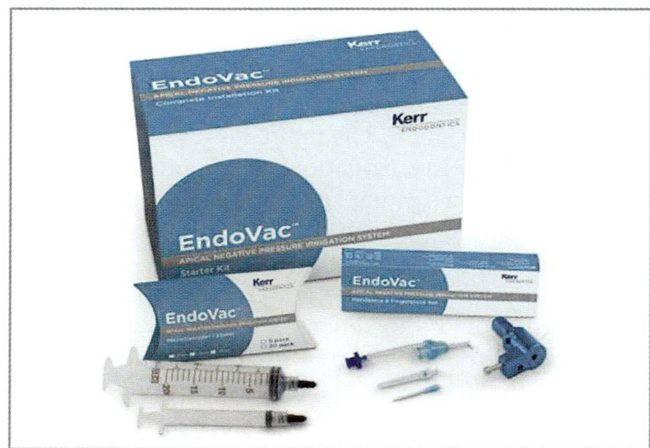

Fig. 53.25: EndoVac system.

Ultrasound

The use of ultrasonic energy for cleaning of the root canal and to facilitate disinfection has a long history in endodontics. The comparative effectiveness of ultrasonics and hand-instrumentation techniques has been evaluated in several earlier studies. Most of these studies concluded that ultrasonics, together with an irrigant, contributed to a better cleaning of the root canal system than irrigation and hand-instrumentation alone. Cavitation and acoustic streaming of the irrigant contribute to the biologic chemical activity for maximum effectiveness. Ultrasonic files (e.g. U File by Mani) must have free movement in the canal without making contact with the canal wall to work effectively.

OBTURATING INSTRUMENTS

The function of these instruments is to pack root canal with obturating material or help in accomplishing the task. These include—spreaders, pluggers and lentulo spirals.

Spreader

- Smooth, long tapered and pointed end instrument.
- These are used to compact gutta-percha to the walls of root canal in lateral compaction technique.
- It can be classified as hand spreader **(Fig. 53.26)** and finger spreader **(Fig. 53.27)**. Finger spreader is like files and is smaller and shorter to be used in posterior teeth.

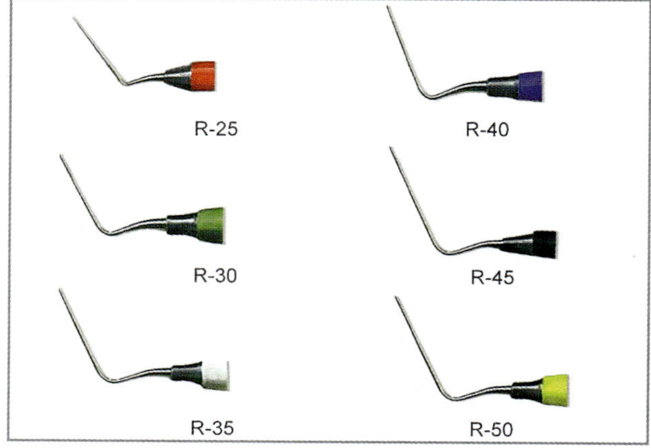

Fig. 53.26: Hand spreader.

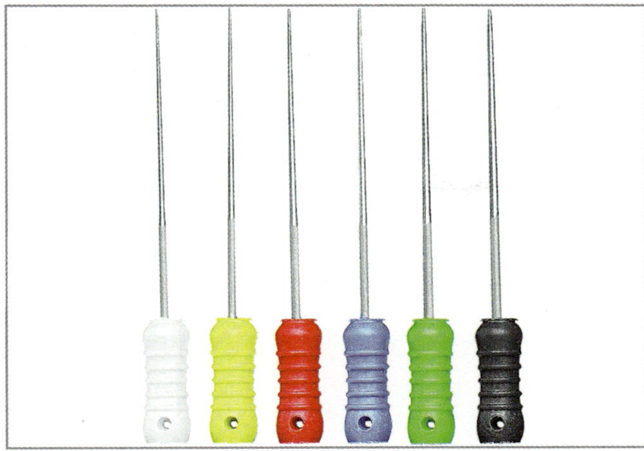

Fig. 53.27: Finger spreader.

Plugger

- Long and blunt flat tip blade instrument used for vertical condensation of the obturating material.
- **It is of two types:** Long-handled **(Fig. 53.28)** and finger-type **(Fig. 53.29)**.

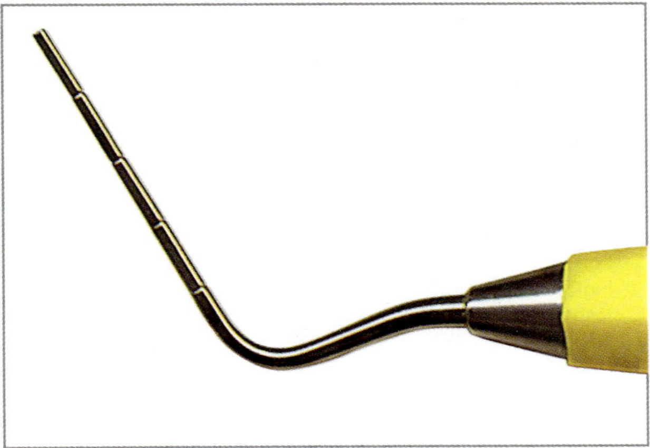

Fig. 53.28: Hand plugger.

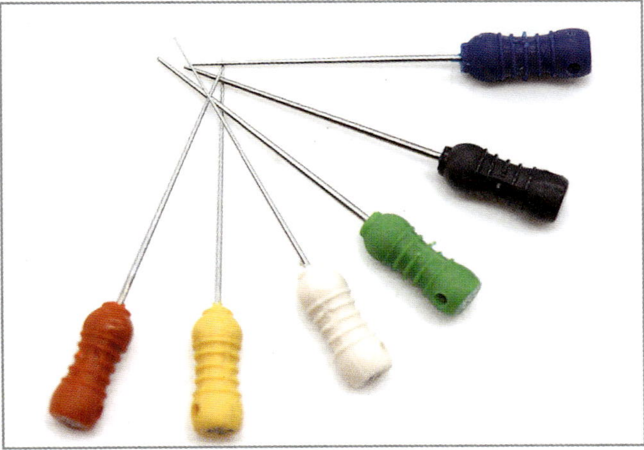

Fig. 53.29: Finger plugger.

Lentulo Spiral

- Function is placement of sealer cement and intracanal medicament in canal **(Fig. 53.30).**
- Also used in obturation of primary teeth with paste system.
- It can be used as handheld or in a slow speed handpiece.
- They have reverse spiral shape which enables easy insertion of material in canal. Advantage is ease of work and minimal time consumption.
- Disadvantage is breakage or frocking of spiral.

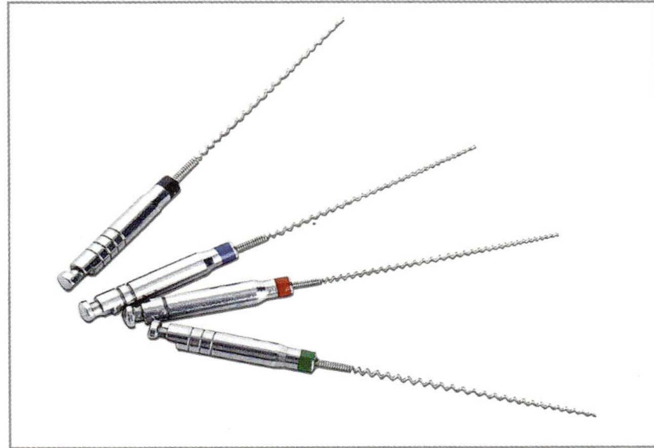

Fig. 53.30: Lentulo spiral.

ENDODONTIC SURGERY INSTRUMENTS

These are instruments that are utilized during endodontic surgery, e.g., Impact Air 45° handpiece, Stropko irrigator, microsuction, root end preparation tips etc.

Impact Air 45° Handpiece

This handpiece has a unique 45° angled head, which allows maximum accessibility and visibility. It's another uniqueness is that the air is exhausted through the back of the handpiece. Both these features make is suitable for use in endodontic surgery.

Stropko Irrigator

The Stropko irrigator provides precise control of air and/or water, which is particularly important for rinsing and drying precisely after staining root-end preparation for unexcelled vision during endodontic surgery especially under microscope.

Root End Preparation Tips

These are ultrasonic tips that are modified to enable them to prepare root-end cavities after root end preparation. These tips can be made up of either stainless steel or diamond coated or zirconium nitride coated.

POINTS TO REMEMBER

- First endodontic hand instrument has been developed by Edward Maynard.
- Arthur, 1852 was the first to use files.
- K-file was introduced in 1915.
- The standardization of instruments was first proposed in 1929 by Trebitsch and by Ingle in 1958.
- A new standardization of instruments was proposed in 2002 which changed the numbers, added new components like half diameters and protaper files.
- The major goals of root canal preparation are removal of vital and necrotic tissue from the main root canal, creation of sufficient space for irrigation and medication, and preservation of the integrity and location of the apical canal anatomy.
- Exploring instruments: smooth broaches; debridement instruments: barbed broaches; Cleaning and shaping instruments: files; Obturating instruments: spreaders, pluggers.
- Endodontic explorer is used to locate the root canal orifices. Smooth broaches are useful as pathfinder in curved fine canals. Barbed broaches are used to extirpate pulp in the root canal.
- K-files were designed as early as 1904 by Kerr and made from a square or triangular blank. They have less cutting efficiency and flexibility but are less susceptible to breakage.
- Newer modification of K-files include K-Flex file and Flex-O file which have better cutting efficiency.
- H-files are machined from a round tapered blank, work on pulling action and have high flexibility and cutting efficiency.
- Kennedy strongly recommends use of H-files in primary teeth, since they remove hard tissue only on withdrawal which prevents pushing the infected material through the apices.
- Nickel–titanium files were introduced by Elizabeth S Bair in 1999–2000. These have shape memory and the instrument design allow the files to closely follow the original root canal path.
- Obturating instruments are used to pack root canal with obturating material or help in accomplishing the task. These include spreader, pluggers and lentulo spirals.

Questionnaire

1. Classify endodontic instruments and outline the goals of biomechanical preparation.
2. Explain the concept of ISO standardization of endodontic instruments.
3. Write a note on broaches.
4. What are the recent modifications of K-files?
5. Explain and differentiate between K-files, H-files, reamers, and Ni-Ti files.
6. What are obturating instruments?

REFERENCE

1. Markus Haspasalo, Ya Shen, Wei Qian, Yuan Gao. Irrigation in Endodontics. Dent Clin N Am. 2010;54:291-312.

FURTHER READING

1. Anthony LP, Grossman LI. A brief history of root canal therapy in the United States. J Am Dent Assoc. 1945;32: 43-50.
2. Briseno BM, Sonnabend E. The influence of different root canal instruments on root canal preparation: an in vitro study. Int Endod J. 1991;24:15-23.
3. Bryant ST, Dummer PMH, Pitoni C, et al. Shaping ability of 0.04 and 0.06 taper profile rotary nickel–titanium instruments in simulated root canals. Int Endod J. 1999;32:155-64.
4. Bryant ST, Thompson SA, Al-Omari MAO, et al. Shaping ability of profile rotary nickel–titanium instruments with ISO sized tips in simulated root canals: Part 1. Int Endod J. 1998a;31:275-81.
5. Curson I. History and endodontics. Dent Pract. 1965;15:435-9.
6. Fauchard P. (1733) Tractat von den Zähnen. Reprint. Hüthig- Verlag; Heidelberg: 1984. p. 111.
7. Grossman LI. Pioneers in endodontics. J Endod. 1987;13:409-15.
8. Haapasalo M, Shen Y, Qian W, et al. Irrigation in Endodontics. Dent Clin N Am. 2010;54:291-312.
9. Ingle JI. A standardized endodontic technique using newly designed instruments and filling materials. Oral Surg Oral Med Oral Pathol. 1961;14:83-91.
10. Lilley JD. Endodontic instrumentation before 1800. J Br Endod Soc. 1976;9:67-70.
11. Ruddle C. Cleaning and shaping the root canal system. In: Cohen S, Burns R (Eds). Pathways of the Pulp, 8th edition. Mosby: St Louis, MO; 2002. pp. 231-92.
12. Schilder H. Cleaning and shaping the root canal. Dent Clin North Am. 1974;18:269-96.
13. Walia H, Brantley WA, Gerstein H. An initial investigation of bending and torsional properties of nitinol root canal files. J Endod. 1988;14:346-51.

CHAPTER

Pulp Therapy for Vital Teeth

Nikhil Marwah, Nikhil Srivastava, Satish Vishwanathaiah, Ravi GR, Srishty Chalana

CHAPTER OUTLINE

Vital pulp therapy (VPT) is defined as a treatment modality aims to preserve and maintain pulp tissue that has been compromised but not destroyed by caries, trauma, or restorative procedures in a healthy state. The indications, and type of pulpal therapy are based on the status of the pulp tissue which is classified as: normal pulp (symptom-free and normally responsive to vitality testing), reversible pulpitis (pulp is capable of healing), symptomatic or asymptomatic irreversible pulpitis (vital inflamed pulp is incapable of healing), or necrotic pulp.

Pulp exposure of the dental pulp exists when the continuity of the dentin surrounding the pulp is broken by physical or bacterial means leading to direct communication between the pulp and external environment. **Pieter Van Forest** was the first to speak about root canal therapy and in 1910 **Glove** designed instruments that could prepare a canal to a certain size and taper. The objectives of pulp therapy are conservation of the tooth in a healthy state of functioning as an integral component of the dentition; preservation of the arch space; enhance esthetics, mastication; help in maintenance of a healthy oral environment; prevention of deleterious effects on the succedaneous tooth, and the periapical tissue.

INDIRECT PULP THERAPY

- **Indirect pulp therapy** *is defined as a procedure wherein small amount of carious dentin is retained in deep areas of cavity to avoid exposure of pulp, followed by placement of a suitable medicament and restorative material that seals off the carious dentin and encourages pulp recovery* **(Ingle).**
- *A procedure in which only the gross caries is removed from the lesion and the cavity is sealed for a time with a biocompatible material is referred to as indirect pulp treatment* **(McDonald).**
- **Besic** *in 1943 studied the fate of bacteria sealed in dental cavities. His method involved what has become known as the indirect pulp capping.*

Objectives of indirect pulp therapy (IPT):
These were given by ***Eidelman*** *in 1965:*
- Arresting the carious process
- Promoting dentin sclerosis
- Stimulating formation of tertiary dentin
- Remineralization of carious dentin.

- **Ricketts et al.** *stated that "in deep lesions, partial caries removal is preferable to complete caries removal to reduce the risk of carious exposure".*
- *In 1961,* **Damle SG** *termed IPT as "Reconstructed Dentin" to prevent pulp exposure.*
- *According to* **AAPD**—*indirect pulp capping—a procedure performed in a tooth without a deep carious lesion approximating the pulp but without signs or symptoms of pulp degeneration. Indirect pulp treatment is indicated in permanent tooth diagnosed with normal pulp with no sign or symptoms of pulpitis or with a diagnosis of reversible pulpitis.*

Rationale

- Its rationale is that carious dentin consists of two distinct layers. An outer layer that is irreversibly denatured, infected, non-remineralizable and should be removed and an inner layer that is reversibly denatured, not infected, remineralizable and should be preserved.

- Removing the outer layers of the carious dentin that contain the majority of the microorganisms thus reducing the continued demineralization of the deeper dentin layers from bacterial toxins and sealing the lesion to allow the pulp to regenerate reparative dentin.

Layers of Carious Dentin

Outer layer	*Middle layer*	*Inner layer*
Necrotic, soft, brown dentin outer layer	A firm (leathery), discolored dentin layer	A hard, discolored dentin deep layer
Teaming with bacteria	Fewer bacteria	Minimal amount of bacterial invasion
Not painful to remove	Painful to remove	Painful to instrumentation

Indications of IPT

History	*Clinical examination*	*Radiographic examination*
• Mild pain associated with eating • Negative history of spontaneous, extreme pain	• Deep carious lesions, which are close to, but not involving the pulp in vital primary or young permanent teeth • No mobility • When pulp inflammation is seen as nominal and there is a definite layer of affected dentin after removal of infected dentin	• Normal lamina dura and periodontal ligament (PDL) space • No radiolucency in the bone around the apices of the roots or in the furcation

Contraindications of IPT

History	*Clinical examination*	*Radiographic examination*
• Sharp, penetrating pulpalgia indicating acute pulpal inflammation • Prolonged spontaneous pain particularly at night	• Mobility of the tooth • Discoloration of the tooth • Negative reaction of electric pulp testing	• Definite pulp exposure • Interrupted or break in lamina dura • Radiolucency about the apices of the roots • Widened periodontal • ligament space

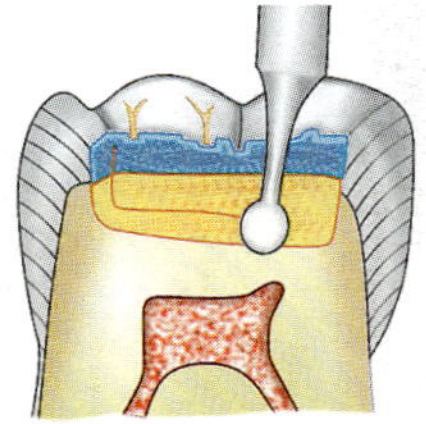

Remove the caries with a slow-speed bur

A

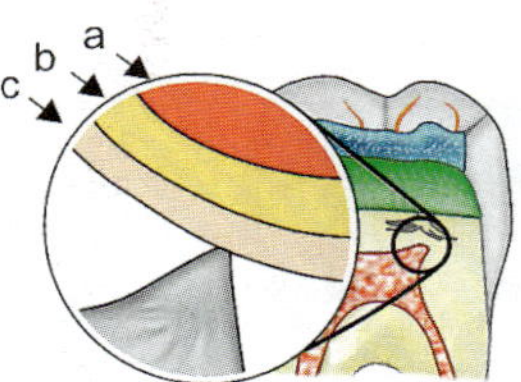

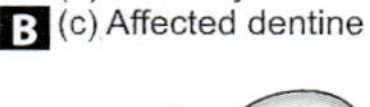

The three layers of carious dentin:
(a) Necrotic tissue/infected dentine
(b) Leathery infected dentine
B (c) Affected dentine

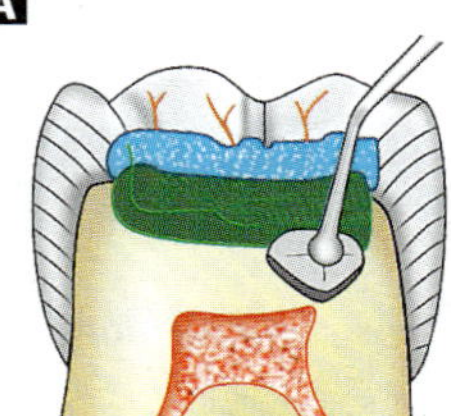

Place calcium hydroxide over the carious dentin

C

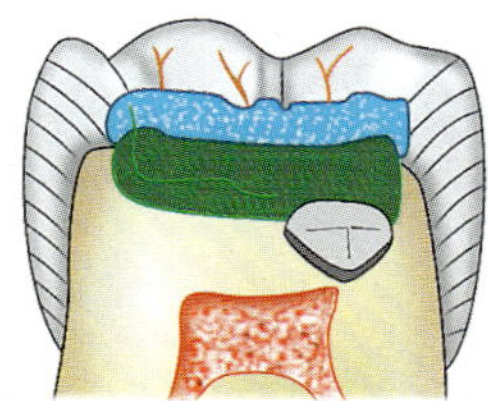

D Final restoration in place

Figs. 54.1A to D: Procedure of indirect pulp therapy.

Treatment Procedure (Figs. 54.1A to D)

The earlier approach was the two-appointment procedure, but now single session is preferred as:

- The re-entry to remove the residual minimal carious dentin may not be necessary if the final restoration maintains a seal and the tooth is asymptomatic.
- After cavity preparation, if all the carious dentin was removed except the portion that would expose the pulp, re-entry might be unnecessary.

If pulp exposure occurs during re-entry, the main objective of IPC is compromised. So, a more invasive vital pulp therapy technique has to be done or would be indicated.

Using polyamide burs or smart burs:

- After gaining access to the carious layer.
- Polyamide burs are used, which remove only the infected dentin
- The burs wear off when reached the affected dentin
- This reduces the risk of pulp exposure
- Once reached affected dentin, place calcium hydroxide
- Base is built up with GIC or reinforced ZoE cement
- Final restoration is placed

Procedure of application of pulp capping agent:

- Most frequently used material for indirect pulp therapy is Dycal (calcium hydroxide). This is supplied as two-paste system, one containing base (brown) (titanium dioxide in glycol salicylate) and the other catalyst (white) (calcium hydroxide and zinc oxide in ethyl toluene sulfonamide)
- One drop of each paste is dispensed in the mixing pad. Now the catalyst paste (white) is lifted with a blunt probe and carried to the cavity where it is spread all over the cavity floor only. In similar fashion the base paste (brown) is taken to the cavity and the two pastes are then mixed in the cavity and spread evenly with the help of ball burnisher. This not only evenly mixes the pastes but also allows a uniform thickness to be attained in cavity. Although Dycal can be mixed on the pad and carried to the cavity also the above-described method is more convenient as Dycal sets very fast after mixing.

Sequelae/Outcome of IPT

Three distinct types of new dentin formation take place:[1]

1. Cellular fibrillar dentin—first 2 months.
2. Globular dentin—3 months.
3. Tubular dentin (uniform mineralized dentin): One-fifth of reparative dentin formation begins in less than 30 days. After 3 months, 0.1 mm is formed.

Stepwise excavation technique: The basic difference between stepwise excavation technique and indirect pulp treatment (IPT) is that in IPT re-entry may or may not be attempted but in stepwise excavation re-entry is attempted at various intervals.

Guidelines for stepwise excavation:[2]

- Deep lesion considered likely to result in pulp exposure if treated by a single and terminal excavation. Evaluated by X-ray, the dentinal lesion involves three-fourths or more of the dentin thickness.
- No history of pretreatment symptoms such as spontaneous pain and provoked pulpal pain. However, mild to moderate pain on thermal stimulation is accepted.
- Positive pulp sensibility tested by an electric pulp tester, thermal stimulation, or test cavity.
- Pretreatment radiograph that rules out apical pathosis.
- Finish the peripheral excavation of the cavity followed by a central excavation removing the outermost necrotic and infected demineralized dentin, in order that a provisional restoration can be properly placed.
- Do not excavate as closely as possible during the first step, thereby reducing the risk of pulp exposure.
- Select a provisional restorative material based on the length of the treatment interval, ranging between 6 months and 8 months.
- The final excavation is often less invasive than expected, as a result of the altered dentinal changes gained during the treatment interval.
  Procedure is very similar to IPT except the less invasive first step.

Research studies regarding IPT:

- **Mathur et al.**[3] in 2017 compared the efficacy of calcium hydroxide (setting type), glass ionomer cement (GIC) (Type VII), and mineral trioxide aggregate as an indirect pulp capping agent and found that all are equally as suitable as IPC agents suggesting mineral gain.
- **Korwar A et al.**[4] in 2015 studied the pulp response of two high fluoride releasing materials silver diamine fluoride (SDF) and Type VII GIC when used as IPT materials and concluded that both are equally effective in tertiary dentin formation.
- According to **Coll JA**[5] (2008) IPT has been shown to have a lower cost, higher success long-term, better exfoliation pattern, and better success treating reversible pulpitis than pulpotomy.
- **Sujlana A et al.**[6] in 2017 conducted as study on direct pulp capping (DPC) in primary teeth and concluded that DPC should not be disregarded as a treatment option in primary teeth. With regard to the pulp capping material of choice, calcium hydroxide still remains the "gold standard" for DPC in primary teeth and is even the active product providing success with mineral trioxide aggregate (MTA).
- **Parisay I et al.**[7] IPC is a favorable technique for treating primary teeth with deep caries without exposure of the reversibly inflamed pulp; it offers the advantages of lower cost, long-term higher success rate, and better exfoliation pattern. In the review several studies showed a success rate of **IDPC** have been reported to be higher than 90% in primary teeth.

DIRECT PULP THERAPY (PULP CAPPING)

It is defined by **Kopel** *(1992) as the placement of a medicament or nonmedicated material on a pulp that has been exposed in course of excavating the last portions of deep dentinal caries or as a result of trauma.*

Objective

To create new dentin in the area of the exposure and subsequent healing of the pulp.

Rationale

To achieve a biologic closure of the exposure site by deposition of hard tissue barrier (dentin bridge) between pulp tissue and capping material thus walling off the exposure site.

Indications

- Small mechanical exposure surrounded by sound dentin in asymptomatic vital primary teeth or young permanent teeth. Exposure should have bright red hemorrhage that is easily controlled by dry cotton pellet with minimal pressure.
- True pinpoint exposure.

Contraindications

- Severe toothache at night
- Spontaneous pain
- Tooth mobility
- Radiographic appearance of pulp, periradicular degeneration
- Excess of hemorrhage at the time of exposure
- Serous exudate from the exposure
- External or internal root resorption
- Swelling or fistula.

Treatment considerations

- **Debridement:** Necrotic and infected dentin chips have to be removed else they will invariably be pushed into the exposed pulp during last stages of caries removal and impede healing and increase pulpal inflammation.
- **Hemorrhage and clotting:** A blood clot should not be allowed to form at the exposure site because it may impede pulpal healing or formation of reparative dentin.
- **Bacterial contamination:** Once all the caries or debris is removed, the cavity should be irrigated with saline, if not the debris may interfere with healing.
- **Exposure enlargement:** The exposure site must be enlarged because:
  - It removes inflammation and infected tissue in the exposed area.
  - It facilitates washing away carious and noncarious debris.
  - It allows a closer contact of more capping medicament material to the actual pulp tissue.

Technique of Direct Pulp Therapy (Figs. 54.2A to C)

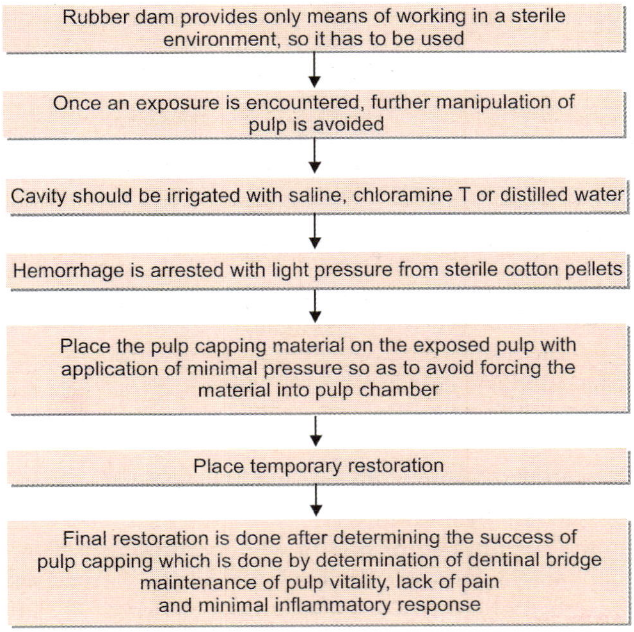

Rubber dam provides only means of working in a sterile environment, so it has to be used

↓

Once an exposure is encountered, further manipulation of pulp is avoided

↓

Cavity should be irrigated with saline, chloramine T or distilled water

↓

Hemorrhage is arrested with light pressure from sterile cotton pellets

↓

Place the pulp capping material on the exposed pulp with application of minimal pressure so as to avoid forcing the material into pulp chamber

↓

Place temporary restoration

↓

Final restoration is done after determining the success of pulp capping which is done by determination of dentinal bridge maintenance of pulp vitality, lack of pain and minimal inflammatory response

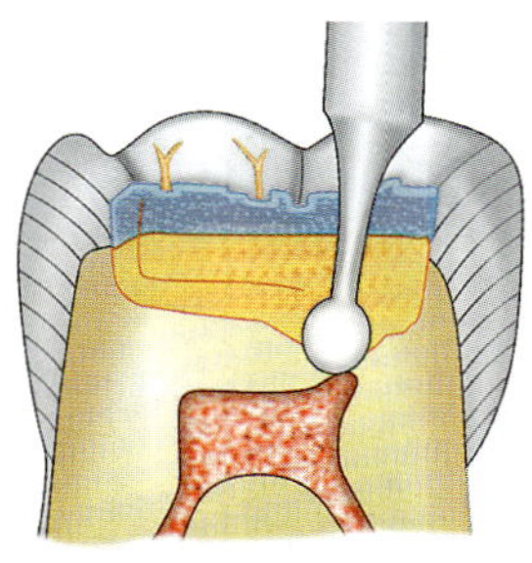

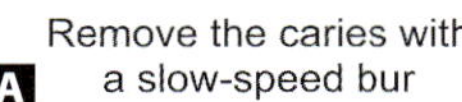

A

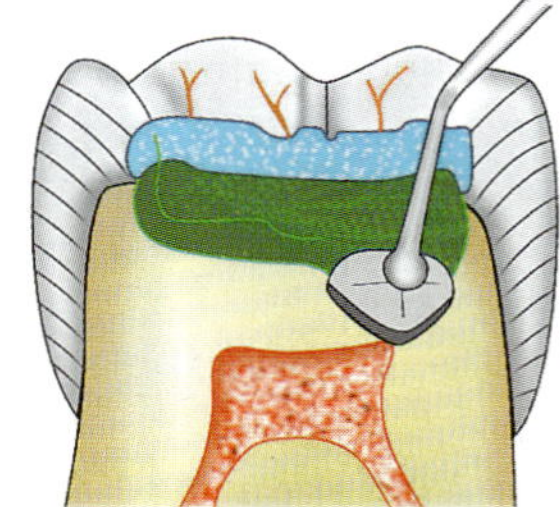

Place pulp capping agent over the exposed pulp

B

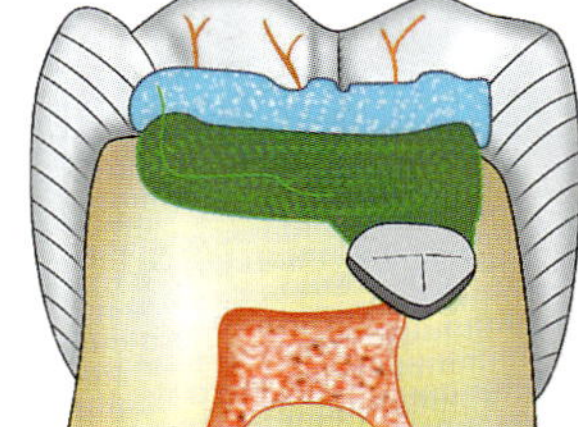

C Direct pulp capping

Figs. 54.2A to C: Direct pulp therapy.

Histological Changes after Pulp Therapy (Fig. 54.3)

These were illustrated by **Glass** and **Zander** in 1949.

- **After 24 hours:** Necrotic zone adjacent to calcium hydroxide paste is separated from healthy pulp tissue by a deep staining basophilic layer.

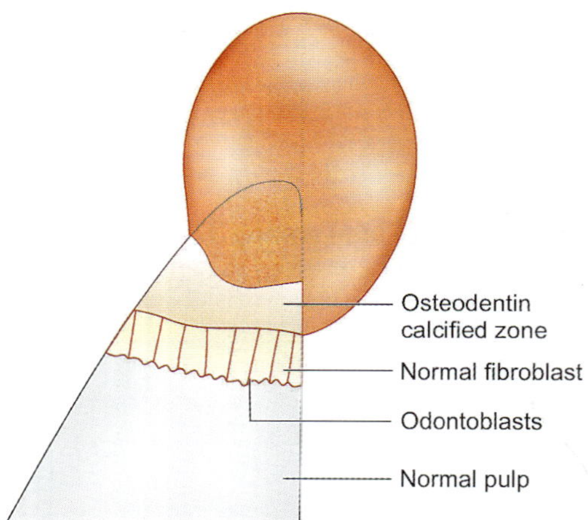

Fig. 54.3: Zone of histological changes.

- **After 7 days:** Increase in cellular and fibroblastic activity
- **After 14 days:** Partly calcified fibrous tissue lined by odontoblastic cells is seen below the calcium potentiate zone; disappearance of necrotic zone.
- **After 28 days:** Zone of new dentin.

Medications and Materials Used for Pulp Capping

1. **Calcium hydroxide:**
   - Calcium hydroxide is a white, crystalline, slightly soluble basic salt that dissociates into calcium ions and hydroxyl ions in solution and exhibits a high alkalinity (pH 11). It is used in both setting and non-setting forms in dentistry. Dentists also use calcium hydroxide because of its antimicrobial properties and its ability to induce hard tissue formation.
   - Calcium hydroxide forms a dentin bridge when placed in contact with pulpal tissues (**Rasmussen P, Mjor IA**, 1971).[8]
   - Initially, a necrotic zone is formed adjacent to the material, and, depending on the pH of the calcium hydroxide material, a dentin bridge is formed directly against the necrotic zone. Under this, the tissue differentiates into odontoblasts, which then elaborate into matrix.
   - The necrotic zone is resorbed and replaced by a dentin bridge; however, this barrier is not always complete (**Holland R et al.** 1979).[9]
   - An enzyme involved in mineralization. (**Foreman PC, Barnes IE**, 1990; **Heithersay GS**, 1978; **Siqueira JF Jr, Lopes HP**, 1999).[10-12] Several theories exist as to how calcium hydroxide induces hard tissue formation. These include the high alkalinity (pH of 11), which produces a favorable environment for the activation of alkaline phosphatase.
   - Some common calcium hydroxide agents used for direct pulp capping are calcium hydroxide powder with distilled water, pulpdent (52.5% calcium hydroxide in an aqueous sol. of methyl cellulose), Dycal, and Hydrex (calcium hydroxide, barium sulfate, titanium dioxide).
2. **Corticosteroids and antibiotics:**
   - **Brosch JW** introduced this combination in 1966.
   - These agents include neomycin and hydrocortisone; ledermix [$Ca(OH)_2$ and prednisolone], penicillin or vancomycin with $Ca(OH)_2$.
3. **Inert materials:**
   - Isobutyl cyanoacrylate and tricalcium phosphate ceramic.
4. **Collagen fibers:**
   - Collagen fibers influence mineralization and are less irritant than $Ca(OH)_2$ with dentin bridge formation in 8 weeks.
5. **4-META adhesive:**
   - The main advantage of 4-META adhesive is that it can soak into the pulp, polymerize there and form a hybrid layer with the pulp thereby providing adequate sealing.
6. **Direct bonding:**
   - Recent advances in total etch direct bonding have evoked an interest in application for pulp therapy. The attractiveness of these systems is that a polygenic film can be layered over an exposure site without displacing pulp tissue and onto surrounding dentin where it penetrates the tubules. The adhesive film is cured by light and acts as a barrier as a composite resin is gently spread over the pulp onto the surrounding dentin.[13]
7. **Isobutyl cyanoacrylate:**
   - **Berkman** in 1971 used it as capping agent and proved it to be an excellent hemostatic agent as well as a reparative dentin bridge stimulator.
   - The disadvantage of this material is that it is cytotoxic when freshly polymerized.

8. **Denatured albumin:**
   - This protein has calcium-binding properties.
   - If a pulp exposure is capped with a protein, the protein may become a matrix for calcification, thereby increasing the chances of biologic obliteration.
9. **Mineral trioxide aggregate:**
   - Mineral trioxide aggregate has demonstrated the ability to induce hard tissue formation in pulpal tissues and it promotes rapid cell growth.
   - Histologic evaluation of pulpal tissue demonstrated that MTA produces a thicker dentinal bridge, less inflammation, less hyperemia and less pulpal necrosis compared with calcium hydroxide. MTA also appears to induce the formation of a dentin bridge at a faster rate than does calcium hydroxide.
   - The process by which MTA acts to induce dentin bridge formation, however, is not known. **Ford et al.**[14] theorized that the tricalcium oxide in MTA reacts with tissue fluids to form calcium hydroxide, resulting in hard tissue formation in a manner similar to that of calcium hydroxide.
   - **Caicedo et al.** (2006) demonstrated good pulp response in primary teeth after direct pulp capping MTA.
   - According to **Farsi et al.**[15] (2006) and **Bogen et al.**[16] (2008) they have shown high success rate in pulp capping nearly about 93–98%.
10. **Laser:**
    - **Andreas Meritz** in 1998 evaluated the effect of laser on direct pulp capping and reported a success rate of 89%.
11. **Bone morphogenic protein:**
    - **Urist** discovered bone morphogenic protein (BMP) in 1965.
    - He observed that demineralized bone matrix could stimulate new bone formation when implanted to ectopic sites such as muscles. He also observed that demineralized dentin also had inductive properties and it forms both bone and dentin.
    - The implications for pulp therapy are immense as it is capable of inducing reparative dentin.
    - They concluded that recombinant human osteogenic protein-1 in a collagen carrier matrix appeared to be suitable as bioactive capping agent for surgically exposed dental pulp.
12. **TheraCal-LC**
    - TheraCal-LC is a new light-cured resin-modified calcium silicate-filled base/liner that is suggested for direct and indirect pulp treatments. TheraCal-LC consists of Portland cement, polyethylene glycol dimethacrylate polymerizable methacrylate monomers, and barium zirconate.
    - It has high ability to release calcium ions that trigger proliferation and differentiation of pulpal tissues and stimulate hard tissue formation.
    - TheraCal-LC has improved physical properties, enhanced durability, increased stability, and reduced solubility and is as effective against *S. mutans* as calcium hydroxide.
    - Compressive strength of TheraCal-LC is considered the greatest among MTA and Biodentine.
    - TheraCal-LC is opaque whitish in color. Therefore, it should be applied in a thin layer to avoid affecting the shade of final restoration.
13. **Chlorhexidine gluconate with resin-modified glass ionomer or with calcium hydroxide**
    - The American Academy of Pediatric Dentistry published an article that studied the success of IPT performed using 2% CHX together with RMGI in primary molars. Their goal of disinfection was to sterilize any residual bacteria after removal of infected dentine. Their results showed that using 2% CHX with RMGI may contribute to the success of IPT.

Limitation of direct pulp therapy in primary teeth:
Direct pulp capping is primarily contraindicated in primary teeth, however, recently lasers are the only option that have demonstrated success of direct pulp capping in primary teeth. Some of the reasons for this contraindication are:
- As the inherent potential of primary tooth cells is to resorb the tooth hence more odontoclasts are present as compared to odontoblasts. So when pulp capping material is placed it stimulates the undifferentiated mesenchymal cells that differentiate into odontoclastic cells. These cells exert their resorptive potential which leads to internal resorption.
- High cellular content, abundant blood supply and consequently faster inflammatory response and poor localization of infection are some of the other reasons that direct pulp capping is contraindicated in primary teeth.

Table 54.1: Bioinductive materials used for pulp capping.[17]

	Material					
	MTA					
Property	***ProRoot MTA***	***MTA angelus***	***RetroMTA***	***Biodentine***	***TheraCal LC***	***Activa bioactive base/liner***
Release date	***1999***	***2001***	***2014***	***2011***	***2011***	***2014***
Composition	Powder: Tricalcium silicate, dicalcium silicate, tricalcium aluminate, bismuth oxide, gypsum Liquid: Water	Powder: tricalcium silicate, dicalcium silicate, tricalcium aluminate, silicon oxide, potassium oxide, aluminum oxide, sodium oxide, iron oxide, calcium oxide, bismuth oxide,	Powder: calcium carbonate, silicon dioxide, aluminum oxide, calcium zirconia complex Liquid: Water	Powder: tricalcium silicate, dicalcium silicate, caldum oxide, caldum carbonate, zirconium oxide, iron oxide Liquid: calcium chloride, water-soluble polymer, water	Light-curing single paste: resin bis-phenyl glycidyl methacrylate (BisGMA) & polyethylene glycol dimethacrylate (PEGD) modified calcium silicate filled with CaO,	Diurethane dimethacrylate. bis (2-(methacryloyloxy) ethyl) phosphate, barium glass, ionomer glass, polyacrylic acid/ maleic acid copolymer, dual-cure chemistry, sodium fluoride, colorants

Contd...

Property	Material					
	MTA					
	ProRoot MTA	***MTA angelus***	***RetroMTA***	***Biodentine***	***TheraCal LC***	***Activa bioactive base/liner***
		magnesium oxide, insoluble residues of crystalline silica Liquid: Water			calcium silicate particles (type III Portland cement), Sr glass, fumed silica, barium sulfate, barium zirconate	
Color	***White***	***White***	***White***	***White***	***White***	***Tooth-shade***
Mixing	0.5 g pouches of powder + pre-measured unit dose of water (mixed manually)	Powder + liquid (mixed manually)	0.3 g pouches of powder + 3 drops of water (mixed manually)	0.7 g capsule of powder + 5 drops of liquid (30 s; 4000-4200 rpm)	Dispensed directly from a flowable syringe (no mixing)	Two-paste system dispensed directly from an automix syringe
Setting reaction		Hydration reaction				3 setting mechanisms: - self-cure - light-cure (20 s) - acid–base reaction
	MTA + water → calcium hydroxide + calcium silicate hydrate			Tricalcium silicate + water → hydrated calcium silicate gel + calcium hydroxide	Light-cure (20 s)	

Table 54.2: Key properties of bio-inductive materials used in vital pulp treatment (VPT)—clinical manipulation and performance.

Property		Material					
		MTA					
		ProRoot MTA	***MTA Angelus***	***RetroMTA***	***Biodentine***	***TheraCal LC***	***Activa bioactive base/liner***
Discoloration of tooth structure		+	+	+	-		
Final setting time (min)		261 ± 21[40] 228.33 ± 2.88[37]	24.0[38] 48.3 ± 4[41,42] 83.66 ± 17.61[39]	12.66 ± 3.05 [39]	45.0[43] 85.66 ± 6.03[37]	Immediate	25-3.0
Single visit treatment		-	-	-	+	+	+
Handling		+	+	+	++	+++	+++
Consistency			Granular, initial looseness		Uniform, putty-like	Flowable	Flowable
Cytotoxicity		NA	NA	NA	NA	Observed	Observed
Radiopacity (mm Al)		6.4–8.5[44]	4.5–5.96[44]	4.07 ± 0.20[45] 3.01 ± 0.09[46]	1.5-4.1[43,44] 2.79 ± 0.22[47]	2.17 ± 0.17[47]	NA
Solubility at 24 h (%)		1.735 ± 0.328[48] 10.89 ± 0.48[26]	29.55 ± 2.35[26]	1.447 ± 0.201[48]	11.83 ± 0.52[26]	2.75 ± 1.04[26]	NA
	After 24 h	0[49]	NA	1.15 ± 0.32[50]	1.01 ± 0.13[50]	0.44 ± 0.20[50] 0.09 ± 0.20[51]	NA
Bond strength to dentine (MPa)	After 7 days	0.85 ± 1.42[49]	NA	NA	9.75 ± 2.19[49]	NA	NA
	After 14 days	4.96 ±4.54[49]	NA	NA	9.34 ± 1.01[49]	NA	23.7 ± 17.8[52] after 28 days after DBA application
SBS to composite after 24 h (MPa)	Methacrylate-based composites	8.9 ± 5.7[53]	11.40 ± 3.19[54] SE DBA (7th generation)	4.71 ± 2.35[55] SE DBA (7th generation)	17.7 ± 62[53]	19.3 ± 8.4[56]	NA
	Silorane-based composites	7.4 ± 3.3[53]	NA	NA	8.0 ± 3.6[53]	3.6 ± 2.5[56]	
Clinical success rate in VPT (%)			80–97[31,57,58] (up to 9-10 years)		73096	NA	NA
Cost of single package		€45 for 0.5 g	€50 for 1 g	€14 for 0.3 g	€10 for a 0.7g capsule	€20 for a 1g syringe	€90 for a 7 mL syringe
Approximate cost per application (€)		22.5	12.5	14	10	5	3.5

NA—not available; SE—self-etch; DBA—dentin bonding agent.

Table 54.3: Interfacial properties of bio-active materials.

Property		Material					
		MTA					
		ProRoot MTA	MTA Angelus	RetroMTA	Biodentine	TheraCal LC	Activa bioactive base/ liner
Marginal seal to dentine		• Chemical and/or micromechanical adhesion • Penetration in dentinal tubules				• Low 5BS due to polymerization shrinkage • Poor chemical or micromechanical adhesion	• Poor chemical or micromechanical adhesion due to lack of self-adhesive properties • Good seal after DBA application
pH Intially/Endpoint		9.93/8.00[45] 12.48/11.56[73] 10.99/7.20[26]	10.48-9.45.[74] 11.71-10.57[73] 11.31-8.94[26]	9.93/7.9[45]	11.98/11.16[75] 11.63/9.21[26]	10.66/9.85[73] 8.54/8.00[26]	8.00
Calcium release (ppm)		15.7-27.4[26]	11.7-55.1[26]	NA	18.0-95.3[26]	12.6-34.2[26]	NA
Pulp/dentine treatment		Rinse with 2.6-5.0% NaOCl	-	-	Hemostasia	Hemostasis	lightly dry, DBA for higher SBS[52] (E&R DBA not required act to manufacturer)
Response of the pulp		• Non-inflammatory reaction, • Increase in TGF-β1, • Non-toxic to pulp cells, • Favorable odontoblastic layer formation			• Non-inflammatory reaction, • Increase in TGF-β1, • Non-toxic to pulp cells, • Well-arranged odontoblasts	• Mild chronic inflammation, • Toxic to pulp fibroblasts, • Less favourable odontoblastic layer formation	• Biointeractive, • Toxic to pulp cells due to resin component?
Hard tissue barrier quality		• Regular • Homogenous • Uniform thickness • Lacks characteristics of natural dentine			• Complete dentin bridge formation • Regular • Uniform thickness	• Low quality calcific barrier • Inferior dented bridge formation • Reduced dentin bridge thickness	NA
Surface treatment composite placement	Recommended by manufacturer	37% H_3PO_4(15s) DBA	-	-	DBA	DBA	ACTIVA BioACTIVE RESTORATIVE or DBA + composite[52]
	Recommended by research	E&R DBA[76-78] 9% HF (90s), Silane[82]	E&R DBA[76-78] (after 72 h) 50-µAl_2O_3 (15 s, 7 mm distance)[54]		2-SE DBA[79,80]	E&R DBA (higher SBS)[81]	NA
Maturation period			≥ days[83,84] 1 year[85]		72 h[86] >2 weeks[87,88]		NA

NA—not available; E&R—etch and rinse; 2-SE—two-step self-etch; DBA—dentine bonding agent; SBS—shear bond strength.

PULPOTOMY

- It is the surgical removal of coronal pulp of a recently exposed tooth with an objective to relieve pain in patients with acute pulpalgia and preserving the vitality of radicular pulp, thereby maintaining the tooth in the dental arch.
- **Finn** (1995) defined it as the complete surgical removal of the coronal portion of the dental pulp, followed by placement of a suitable dressing or medicament tha*t will promote healing and preserve vitality of the tooth.*
- **American Academy of Pediatric Dentistry (1998)** defined pulpotomy as the amputation of affected, infected coronal portion of the dental pulp preserving the vitality and function of the remaining part of radicular pulp.

Rationale (Figs. 54.4A to D)

- Radicular pulp is healthy and capable of healing after surgical amputation of the infected coronal pulp.
- Preserves vitality of the radicular pulp.
- Maintains tooth in a physiologic condition.

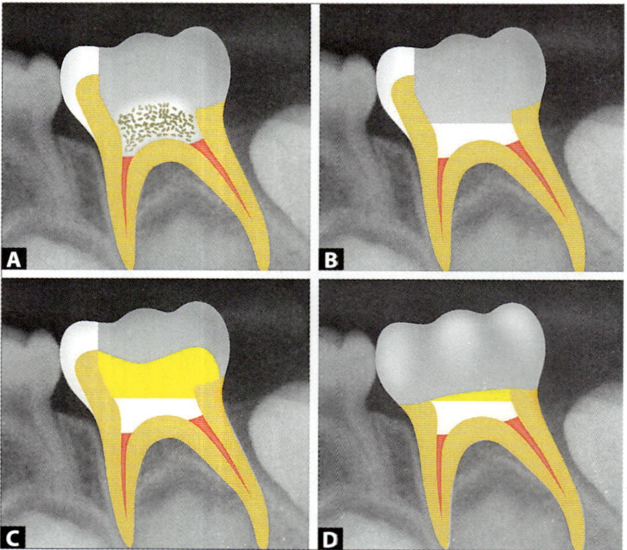

Figs. 54.4A to D: Pulpotomy: (A) Carious tooth; (B) Pulpotomized tooth; (C) Tooth restored; (D) Complete rehabilitation with SSC.

Indications of Pulpotomy

- Vital pulp exposure, mechanical or traumatic in which inflammation is considered to be confined to coronal pulp only.
- Carious exposure (1–2 mm) without any history of spontaneous pain.
- In young permanent tooth with vital exposed pulp and incompletely formed apices.

Contraindications of Pulpotomy

- History of spontaneous toothache.
- Tenderness on percussion.
- Root resorption more than one-third of root length.
- Large carious lesion with nonrestorable crown.
- Highly viscous, sluggish hemorrhage from canal orifice, which is uncontrollable.
- Medical contradictions like heart disease, immunocom promised patient.
- Swelling or fistula.
- External or internal resorption.
- Pathological mobility.
- Calcification of pulp.

Classification of pulpotomy (Ranly)

Types	*Other name*	*Features*	*Examples*
Vital pulpotomy			
Devitalization	Mummification, cauterization	It is intended to destroy or mummify the adjacent vital tissue	*Single sitting:* • Formocresol • Electrosurgery • Laser *Two stages:* • GysiTriopaste • Easlick's formaldehyde • Paraform devitalizing paste.
Preservation	Minimal devitalization, noninductive	This implies maintaining the maximum vital tissue, with no induction of reparative dentin	• ZnO eugenol • Glutaraldehyde • Ferric sulfate
Regeneration	Inductive, reparative	This has formation of dentin bridge	• $Ca(OH)_2$* • Bone morphogenic protein • Mineral trioxide aggregate • Enriched collagen • Freezed dried bone • Osteogenic protein.
Nonvital pulpotomy			
Mortal pulpotomy	—	It is done in compromised cases	• Beechwood cresol • Formocresol

** The AAPD's Use of Vital Pulp Therapies in Primary Teeth with Deep Caries Lesions recommended against the use of calcium hydroxide for pulpotomy.*

Formocresol Pulpotomy/Single-stage Pulpotomy

Formocresol was introduced by **Buckley** in 1904 and since then a lot of modifications have been tried and advocated regarding the techniques of formocresol pulpotomies.

Criteria for case selection (Heilig J et al. 1984 and Waterhouse et al. 2000):
- Teeth with deep carious lesion (radiographically the caries should be approximating to the pulp). Teeth should be restorable after completion of the procedure.
- Absence of symptoms indicative of advanced pulpal inflammation such as spontaneous pain or history of nocturnal pain. Absence of clinical signs or symptoms.
- Absence of clinical or radiographic signs of pulpal necrosis, i.e., furcation involvement, periapical pathology, internal resorption, calcification in canal.

- Hemorrhage should stop within five minutes from the amputated pulp stumps using a sterile pledget of moist cotton. After assessment of clinical and radiographical criteria, single visit pulpotomy procedure was performed on the selected molars.

- **Sweet** (1936): Formulated multi-visit technique.
- **Doyle** (1962): Advocated two-sitting procedure (complete devitalization).
- **Spedding** (1965): Gave 5 minutes protocol (partial devitalization).
- **Venham** (1967): Proposed 15 seconds procedure.
- Direct comparison of two and single visit formocresol pulpotomy in primary molar was made by **Redig** (1968) and concluded that neither was superior.
- Current concept uses 4 minutes of application time.

Composition of Formocresol: Buckley's Formula

- Cresol—35%.
- Glycerol—15%.
- Formaldehyde—19%.
- Water—31%.

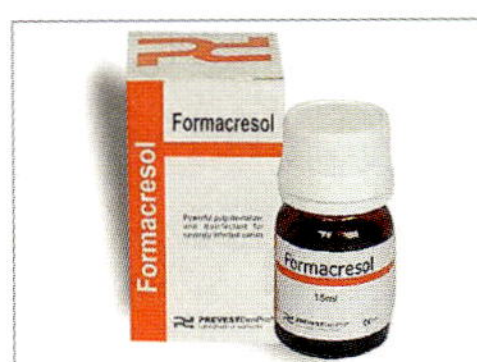

Preparation of Formocresol

Currently we use 1/5th conc. of Buckley's formula, which is prepared by the following method:

Dilute 3 parts (90 mL) glycerine with 1 part (30 mL) diluted sterile water

↓

Add 1 part [30 mL] Formocresol to 4 parts diluent

↓

Add 30 mL of Formocresol to 120 mL of diluent to obtain 150 mL of dilute formocresol, i.e., 1/5th strength.

Mechanism of Action of Formocresol

It prevents tissue autolysis by bonding to the proteins. This bonding is of peptide groups of side chain amino acids and is a reversible process accomplished without changing the basic structure of protein molecules.

Histological Changes

- These were demonstrated by **Mass** and **Zilbermann**[18] in 1933 and also by **Massler** and **Mansokhani** in 1959 **(Fig. 54.5)**. Immediately the pulp becomes fibrous and acidophillic.

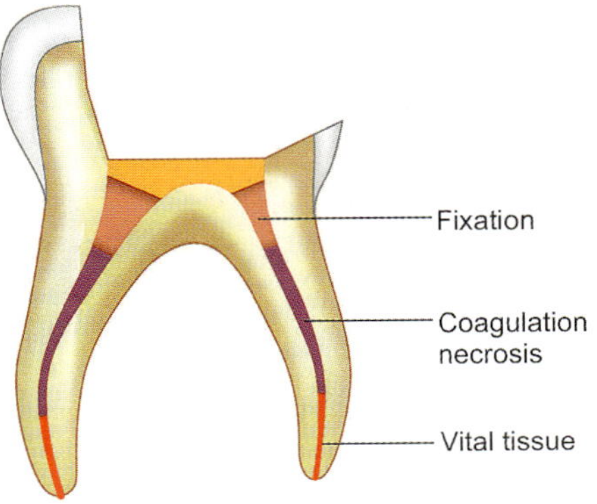

Fig. 54.5: Zones after fixing with formocresol.

- 7–14 days: Three zones appear:
  1. A broad eosinophilic zone of fixation.
  2. A broad pale-staining zone of atrophy with poor cellular definition.
  3. A broad zone of inflammation extending apically into normal pulp tissue.
- One year
  - Progressive apical movement of these zones with only acidophilic zone left at the end of 1 year.

Procedure of Formocresol Pulpotomy (Figs. 54.6A to G)

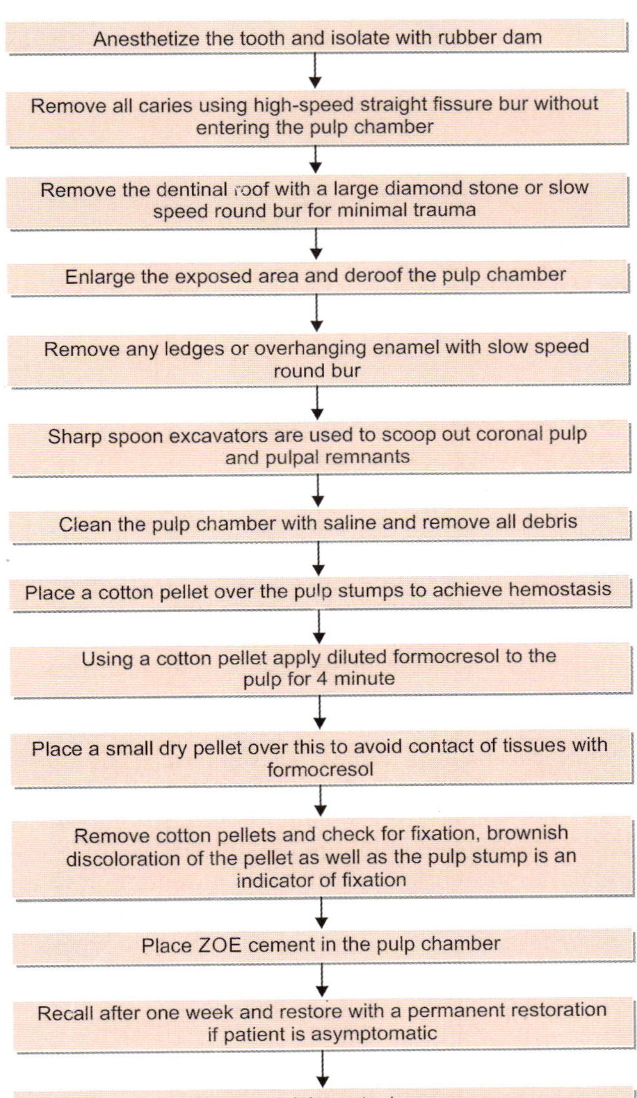

Anesthetize the tooth and isolate with rubber dam
Remove all caries using high-speed straight fissure bur without entering the pulp chamber
Remove the dentinal roof with a large diamond stone or slow speed round bur for minimal trauma
Enlarge the exposed area and deroof the pulp chamber
Remove any ledges or overhanging enamel with slow speed round bur
Sharp spoon excavators are used to scoop out coronal pulp and pulpal remnants
Clean the pulp chamber with saline and remove all debris
Place a cotton pellet over the pulp stumps to achieve hemostasis
Using a cotton pellet apply diluted formocresol to the pulp for 4 minute
Place a small dry pellet over this to avoid contact of tissues with formocresol
Remove cotton pellets and check for fixation, brownish discoloration of the pellet as well as the pulp stump is an indicator of fixation
Place ZOE cement in the pulp chamber
Recall after one week and restore with a permanent restoration if patient is asymptomatic
Place a stainless steel crown

Concerns about Formocresol

- **Toxicity:** Formocresol and formaldehyde have shown to be cytotoxic, mutagenic, and carcinogenic in animal experiments by **Lewis** in 1981. But **Ranly** calculated that over 3,000 pulpotomies must be performed in the same individual for formocresol to reach toxic level.
- **Systemic distribution: Myers** in 1978 demonstrated systemic distribution of radioisotope-labeled formaldehyde. When used in pulpotomies in animals,

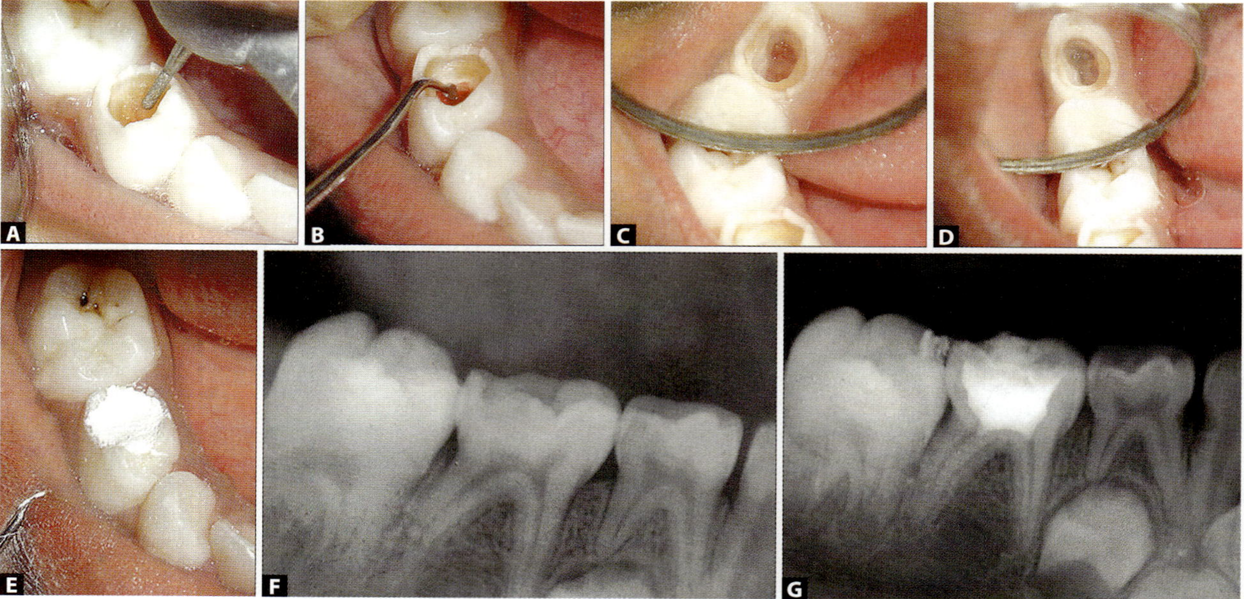

Figs. 54.6E to G: Procedure of pulpotomy: (A) Cavity preparation; (B) Excavating coronal pulp; (C) After complete removal of coronal pulp; (D) Post-formocresol fixation; (E) Temporization of cavity; (F) Preoperative X-ray of mandibular second molar showing carious lesion; (G) Postoperative X-ray after pulpotomy.

labelled formaldehyde has been found in periodontal ligament, bone, dentine, and urine.

- **Antigenicity: Thoden Valzen** in 1977 has shown immunogenic potential of formaldehyde in rabbits, dogs, and guinea pigs.
- **Mutagenicity and cytogenicity: Nongentini** in 1980 postulated that mutational changes were achieved by application of formaldehyde and cytogenicity for 15 minutes, in monkey kidney cells. Formaldehyde denaturates nucleic acids by forming methylol derivatives that renders genetic machinery inoperable. It may also affect biosynthesis and cell reproduction by interacting with DNA and RNA. **Milnes** 2006,[19] published an extensive and detailed review of the more recent research on the metabolism, pharmacokinetics, and carcinogenicity of formaldehyde and concluded that formaldehyde is not a potent human carcinogen under conditions of low exposure. He concluded that extrapolation of these research results to pediatric dentistry suggests an inconsequential risk of carcinogenesis associated with formaldehyde use in pediatric pulp therapy.

Modified Formocresol Pulpotomy

- This technique was used by **Trask** (1972) in young permanent molars that have to be retained for a short period of time only.
- The technique is identical to that described for primary teeth, except that the formocresol pellet is sealed permanently in the tooth.

Two-visit Devitalization Pulpotomy

This is two-stage procedure involving the use of paraformaldehyde to fix the entire coronal and radicular pulp tissue in two visits.

Indications

- There is evidence of sluggish bleeding at the amputation site that is difficult to control.
- Pus in the chamber, but none at the amputation site.
- There is thickening of the PDL.
- History of pain.

Contraindications

- Nonrestorable tooth.
- Tooth with necrotic pulp.

Procedure

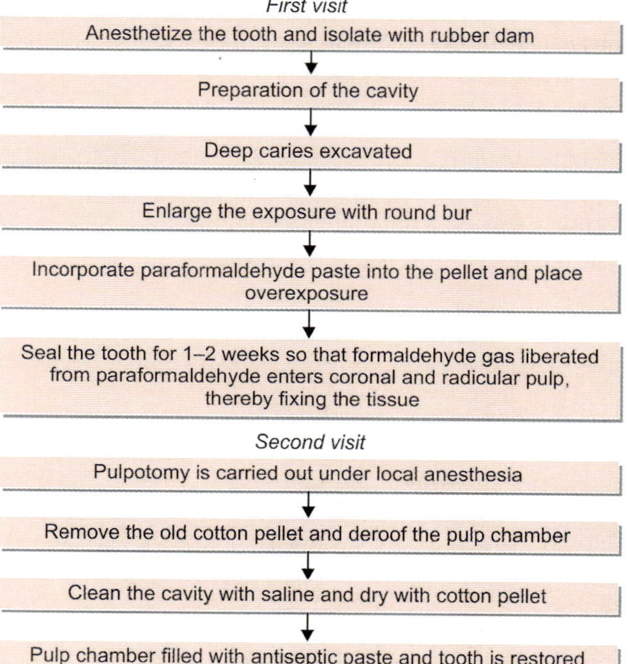

First visit
Anesthetize the tooth and isolate with rubber dam
Preparation of the cavity
Deep caries excavated
Enlarge the exposure with round bur
Incorporate paraformaldehyde paste into the pellet and place overexposure
Seal the tooth for 1–2 weeks so that formaldehyde gas liberated from paraformaldehyde enters coronal and radicular pulp, thereby fixing the tissue
Second visit
Pulpotomy is carried out under local anesthesia
Remove the old cotton pellet and deroof the pulp chamber
Clean the cavity with saline and dry with cotton pellet
Pulp chamber filled with antiseptic paste and tooth is restored

Materials used for two-visit pulpotomy

Gysitriopaste	*Easlick's paraform-aldehyde paste*	*Paraform devitalizing paste*
• Tricresol	• Paraformaldehyde	• Paraformaldehyde
• Cresol	• Procaine base	• Lignocaine
• Glycerin	• Powdered asbestos	• Propylene glycol
• Paraformal-dehyde	• Petroleum jelly	• Carbowax
• Zinc oxide eugenol (ZOE)		• Carmine to color

Research studies regarding formocresol pulpotomy:

- In 1956, **Nacht**[20] undertook study using formaldehyde paste and found that the teeth were maintained in good clinical condition for approximately 2 years and reported evidence of resorption and a lack of clinical symptoms over a 5 years period.
- **Emmerson et al.**[21] reported a histologic study. They reported that immediately, below the amputation area, there was a homogeneous yellow-stained area, and below that area was a normal-appearing fixed zone of pulp tissue. Below the fixed zone, there was evidence of degenerated odontoblasts and linear pulp calcification. The authors also reported that, throughout the pulp, there was an absence of inflammatory cells, with no evidence of resorption or metaplastic changes.
- **Fuks** and **Bimstein**[22] observed clinically and radiographically that children treated with pulpotomies using a 1:5 dilution of formocresol had a clinical success of 94.3% and concluded that in that 1:5 dilution of formocresol was an effective alternate medicament for primary vital pulpotomy procedures in children.
- **Coll J A et al.**[23] , 2017, in their systematic review and meta-analysis reported high rate of success and quality with MTA and Formocresol pulpotomy techniques
- **Rajasekharan et al.**[24] , 2018, in their review reported a short initial setting time, superior flexural strength and better sealing abilities of biodentine when compared to MTA, proves to be a better material by overcoming the drawbacks of MTA.

Success rate of formocresol pulpotomies

Author	*Observation time*	*Clinical success*	*Radiographic success*
Doyl et al. (1962)	5–18 months	100	-
Morawa et al. (1974)	6–60 months	98	98
Mejare (1979)	60 months	55	55
Fuks et al. (1996)	33 months	85	78
Ibricevic and Al-Jame (2003)	48 months	97	91
Subramaniam et al. (2009)	24 months	100	85
Hugar and Deshpande (2010)	36 months	100	96
Yildiz and Tosun (2014)	30 months	100	95

Glutaraldehyde Pulpotomy

- It was first suggested by **S Gravenmade** and was introduced by **Kopel** in 1979.
- He suggested that inflamed tissue that produces toxic by-products should be fixed, rather than being treated with strong disinfectants. He felt that satisfactory fixation with formocresol required an excessive amount of medication, as well as longer period of interaction but glutaraldehyde solution might replace formocresol in endodontics, because it appears to have fixative properties with less destruction of tissue and at the same time appears to be bactericidal.

Mechanism of Action

- 2% glutaraldehyde produces rapid surface fixation of the underlying pulpal tissue.
- A narrow zone of eosinophilic, stained, and compressed fixed tissue is found directly beneath the area of application, which blends into vital normal appearing tissue apically.
- With time, the glutaraldehyde fixed zone is replaced by macrophagic action with dense collagenous tissue, thus the entire root canal tissue is vital.[22]

Advantages of Glutaraldehyde over Formocresol

- It is bifunctional reagent, which allows it to form strong intra- and intermolecular protein bonds leading to superior fixation by cross linkage.
- It is excellent antimicrobial.
- Superior fixative properties, self-limiting penetration.
- Causes less necrosis of the pulpal tissue.
- Causes less dystrophic calcification in pulp canals.
- Less toxicity does not perfuse through the pulp tissue to the apex.
- Demonstrates less systemic distribution.
- It is low tissue binding, readily metabolized, eliminated in urine, and expired in gases—90% of the drug is gone in 3 days.
- Mutagenicity and antigenicity—less as compared to formocresol.

Research studies using glutaraldehyde pulpotomy:

- **Garcia-Godoy**[25] used a 2% buffered glutaraldehyde solution on pulpotomies in children and reported the technique to be clinically and radiographically successful 98% of the time.
- **Fuks et al.**[26] reported that the use of a 2% buffered glutaraldehyde solution in primary molars in children was clinically and radiographically successful 94% of the time after six months; then, the success rate decreased to 90% after 12 months.
- **Davis et al.**[27] reported a histological study that compared 5% buffered glutaraldehyde to 2% diluted formocresol as medicaments on treated teeth. They reported that glutaraldehyde showed less penetration than formocresol; that only mild inflammation was seen in the glutaraldehyde group and was confined to the middle third of the radicular tissue, with only limited necrosis; and that the apical tissue was still vital in 78% of the cases.

Success rate of glutaraldehyde pulpotomies

Author	*Observation time*	*Clinical success*	*Radiographic success*
Kopel et al. (1980)	0–12 months	100	-
Garcia-Godoy (1985)	48 months	98	-
Tsai et al. (1993)	36 months	98	79
Havale et al. (2013)	12 months	100	83

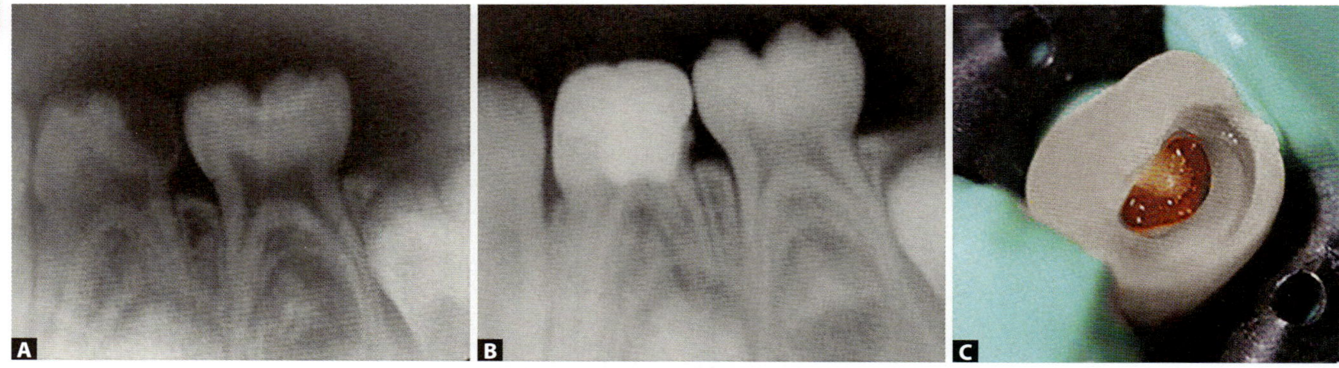

Figs. 54.7A to C: Ferric sulfate pulpotomy: (A) Preoperative radiograph; (B) Postoperative radiograph; (C) Pulpal appearance after application of agent.

Ferric Sulfate Pulpotomy

- Ferric sulfate (FS) a nonaldehyde chemical has received attention recently as a pulpotomy agent.
- The methods of pulpotomy are similar to formocresol pulpotomy with the only difference in the agent used **(Figs. 54.7A to C).**
- Ferric sulfate as a 15.5% solution has been commonly used as a coagulative and hemostatic retraction agent for crown and bridge impressions and is slightly acidic.
- The mechanism of action is still debated but agglutination of blood proteins results from the reaction of blood with both ferric and sulfate ions. The agglutinated proteins form plugs to occlude the capillary orifices.
- Ferric sulfate as a pulpotomy agent on the theory that its mechanism of controlling hemorrhage might minimize the chances for inflammation and internal resorption.

Research studies of ferric sulfate pulpotomy:
- **Ranly** proposed that metal protein clot at the surface of the pulp stump acts as a barrier to irritating components of the subbase.
- **Fuks**[28] (1997) showed 93% of success rate of FS when compared with formocresol pulpotomy which showed 84% of success rate.
- **Smith**[29] (2000) reported a clinical success rate of 99% but radiographic success rate of 74% in FS pulpotomy.
- **Markovic et al.** (2005) showed 91% success rate with formocresol and 89% success rate with FS pulpotomy.

Success rate of FS pulpotomies

Author	*Observation time*	*Clinical success*	*Radiographic success*
Fei et al. (1990)	12 months	100	97
Papagiannoulis et al. (2002)	36 months	90	74
Yadav et al. (2014)	9 months	86	80
Yildiz and Tosun (2014)	30 months	95	85

Laser Pulpotomy

- The use of lasers in pulpotomy was based on their ability of rapid control of bleeding and coagulation.
- In 1985, **Ebimara** reported the effects of Nd: YAG laser on the wound healing of amputed pulps using Nd: YAG laser at 20 Hz and placing intermediate restorative material (IRM) paste.
- Many authors have compared various lasers in the endodontic use and have used CO_2 or Nd: YAG or diode lasers.

Procedure (Figs. 54.8A to C)

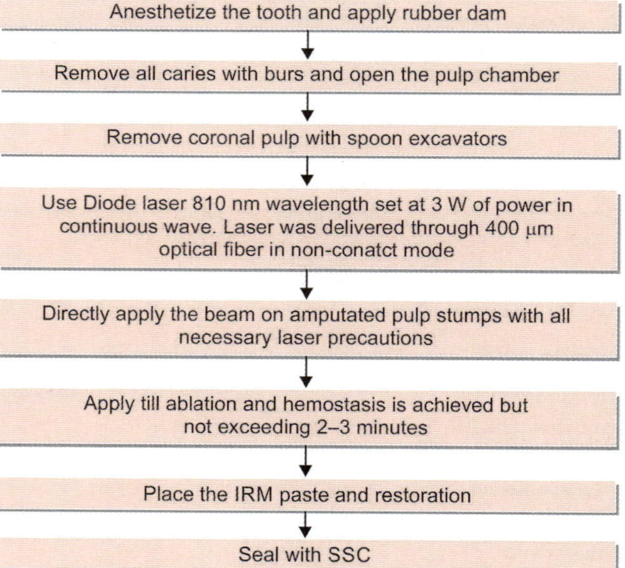

Anesthetize the tooth and apply rubber dam
Remove all caries with burs and open the pulp chamber
Remove coronal pulp with spoon excavators
Use Diode laser 810 nm wavelength set at 3 W of power in continuous wave. Laser was delivered through 400 μm optical fiber in non-conatct mode
Directly apply the beam on amputated pulp stumps with all necessary laser precautions
Apply till ablation and hemostasis is achieved but not exceeding 2–3 minutes
Place the IRM paste and restoration
Seal with SSC

Liu JF[30] (2006) compared the effects of Nd:YAG laser pulpotomy with formocresol on human primary teeth. In the Nd:YAG laser group, clinical success was 97%, and radiographic success was 94%. Whereas in formocresol pulpotomy, the success rates were 85% and 78%, respectively.

Electrosurgical Pulpotomy

Mark was the first US dentist routinely to perform electrosurgical pulpotomies in 1993 with a success rate of 99% for primary molars.

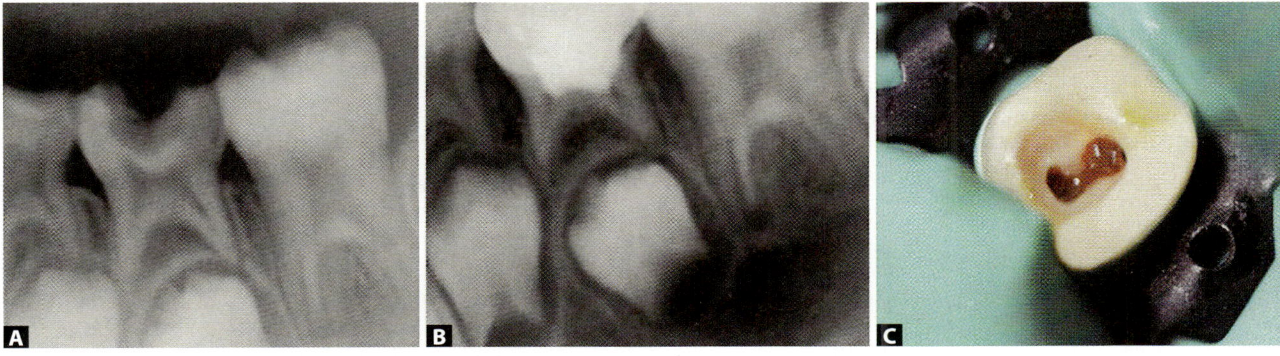

Figs. 54.8A to C: Laser pulpotomy. (A) Preoperative radiograph; (B) Postoperative radiograph; (C) Pulpal appearance after application of laser.

Procedure

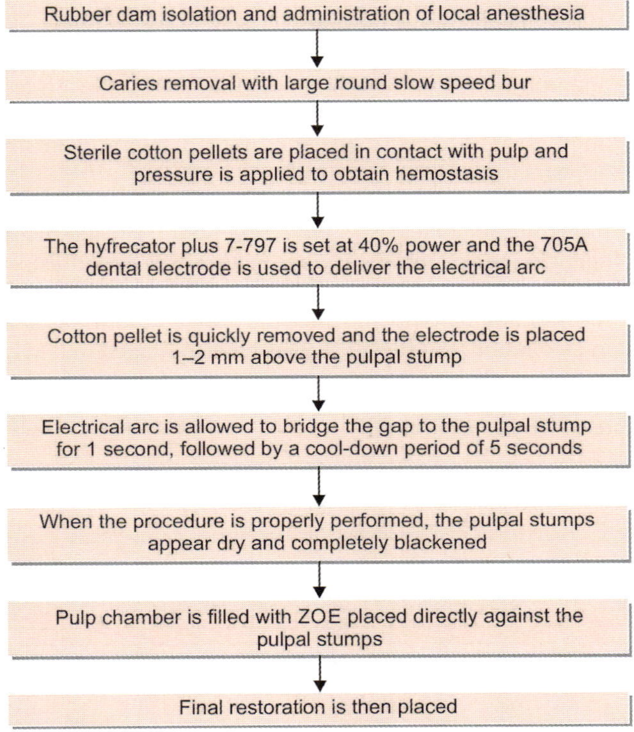

Rubber dam isolation and administration of local anesthesia
Caries removal with large round slow speed bur
Sterile cotton pellets are placed in contact with pulp and pressure is applied to obtain hemostasis
The hyfrecator plus 7-797 is set at 40% power and the 705A dental electrode is used to deliver the electrical arc
Cotton pellet is quickly removed and the electrode is placed 1–2 mm above the pulpal stump
Electrical arc is allowed to bridge the gap to the pulpal stump for 1 second, followed by a cool-down period of 5 seconds
When the procedure is properly performed, the pulpal stumps appear dry and completely blackened
Pulp chamber is filled with ZOE placed directly against the pulpal stumps
Final restoration is then placed

Cvek's Pulpotomy

- This is also called as calcium hydroxide pulpotomy or young permanent partial pulpotomy.
- This was proposed by **Mejare** and **Cvek**[31] in 1978.
- Indicated in young permanent teeth where the pulp is exposed by mechanical or bacterial means and the remaining radicular tissue is judged vital by clinical and radiographic criteria whereas the root closure is not complete.
- **Sari S,** 2002 performed Cvek pulpotomy in immature permanent incisor with 5-year follow-up and noticed tooth remained symptom-free with subsequent apical closure.
- Rationale:
  - To preserve vitality of radicular pulp and allow for normal root closure.

Procedure (Figs. 54.9A to E)

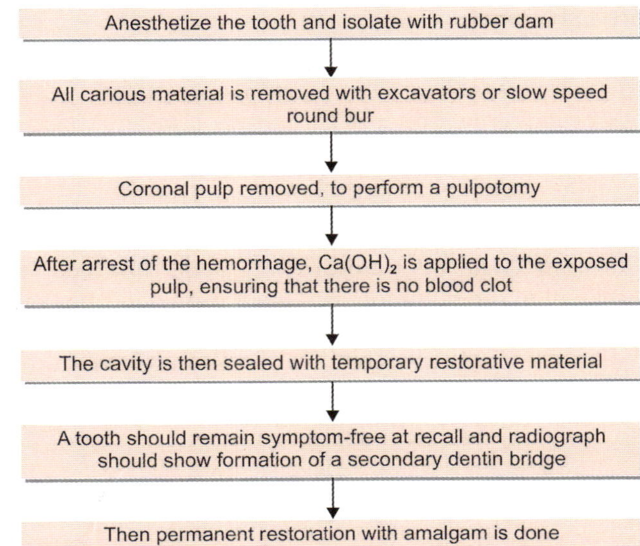

Anesthetize the tooth and isolate with rubber dam
All carious material is removed with excavators or slow speed round bur
Coronal pulp removed, to perform a pulpotomy
After arrest of the hemorrhage, $Ca(OH)_2$ is applied to the exposed pulp, ensuring that there is no blood clot
The cavity is then sealed with temporary restorative material
A tooth should remain symptom-free at recall and radiograph should show formation of a secondary dentin bridge
Then permanent restoration with amalgam is done

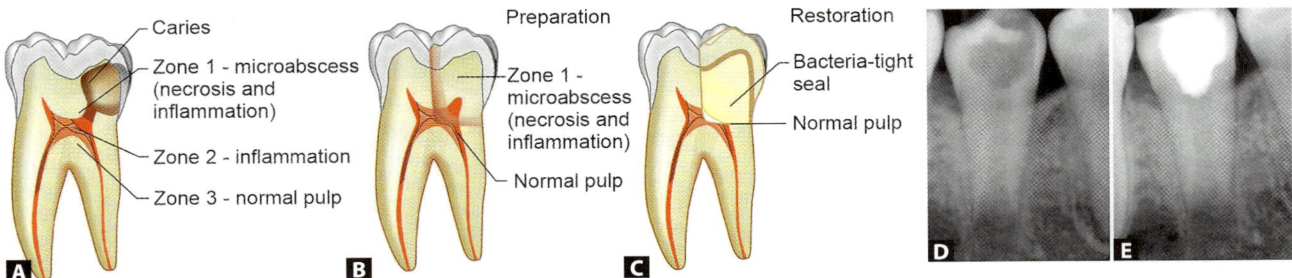

Figs. 54.9A to E: Cvek's pulpotomy: (A) Diagrammatic description of inflammation extending till pulp; (B) Extension of preparation; (C) Placement of calcium hydroxide on the partial amputated pulp; (D) Preoperative X-ray of lesion; (E) Postoperative appearance of Cvek's pulpotomy.

Mortal Pulpotomy

- It is also called nonvital pulpotomy.
- Ideally, nonvital tooth should be treated by pulpectomy, but sometimes it is impracticable due to non-negotiable root canals and limited patient cooperation, mortal pulpotomy is indicated for such patients.

Procedure

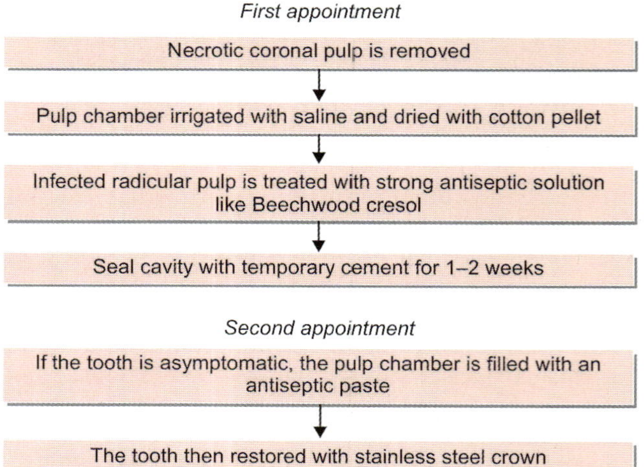

First appointment
Necrotic coronal pulp is removed
Pulp chamber irrigated with saline and dried with cotton pellet
Infected radicular pulp is treated with strong antiseptic solution like Beechwood cresol
Seal cavity with temporary cement for 1–2 weeks
Second appointment
If the tooth is asymptomatic, the pulp chamber is filled with an antiseptic paste
The tooth then restored with stainless steel crown

CURRENT CONCEPTS IN PULPOTOMY

Portland Cement

- Pulpotomies with Portland cement as a medicament in human primary molars were performed by Conti.
- MTA and Portland cement had the same clinical, biological, and mechanical characteristics. The only difference was bismuth oxide was added to MTA for improved radiopacity.
- **Sakai et al.**[32] compared the clinical and radiographic effectiveness of MTA and Portland cement as pulp dressing agents in carious primary teeth. They reported that all of the pulpotomized teeth were clinically and radiographically successful at 2 years. The authors reported that no statistically significant difference regarding dentin bridge formation was found between the groups throughout the follow-up period.

Mineral Trioxide Aggregate (MTA)

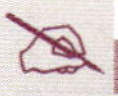

Torabinejad described the physical and chemical properties of MTA in 1995.

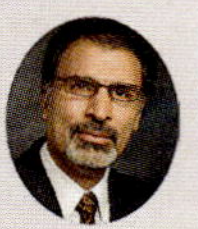

- It is an ash colored powder made primarily of fine hydrophilic particles of tricalcium aluminate, tricalcium silicate, silicate oxide, tricalcium oxide, and bismuth oxide is added for radio-opacity. Hydration of the powder results in a colloidal gel composed of calcium oxide crystals in an amorphous structure. This gel solidifies into a hard structure in less than 3 hours.

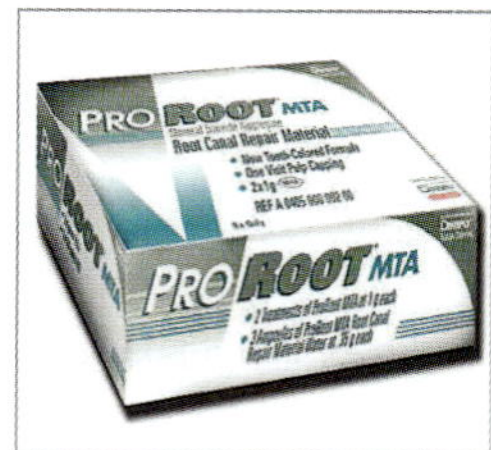

- It has a compressive strength equal to ZOE with polymer reinforcement (IRM).

Properties of Mineral Trioxide Aggregate

- It is biocompatible material, and its sealing ability is better than that of amalgam or ZOE.
- Initial pH is 10.2 and set pH is 12.5.
- The setting time of cement is 4 hours.
- The compressive strength is 70 MPa, which is comparable with that of IRM.
- Low cytotoxicity—it presents with minimal inflammation if extended beyond the apex.
- Mineral trioxide aggregate has demonstrated the ability to induce hardtissue formation in pulpal tissues and it promotes rapid cell growth.
- According to **Torabinejad et al.**[33] MTA has an antibacterial effect on some facultative bacteria but no effect on strict anaerobic bacteria. This limited antibacterial effect is less than that demonstrated by calcium hydroxide pastes. The ability of MTA to resist the penetration of microorganisms appears to be high.
- The use of MTA as an agent for pulp capping or for providing apical seal is well-documented.[34] The use of this agent in pulp capping was doubted as it was hypothesized that the hard tissue barrier formed by MTA could deflect the permanent tooth bud once the primary tooth was near to exfoliation. But recent studies have indicated that MTA can be used successfully as a pulpotomy agent also.

Procedure (Figs. 54.10A and B)

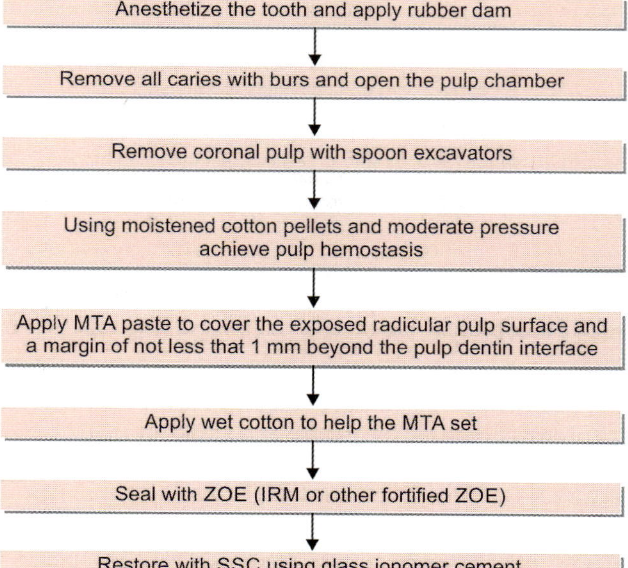

Apply MTA paste to cover the exposed radicular pulp surface and a margin of not less that 1 mm beyond the pulp dentin interface
Apply wet cotton to help the MTA set
Seal with ZOE (IRM or other fortified ZOE)

Research studies regarding MTA pulpotomy:

- **Cuisia**[35] **et al.** (2001) conducted pulpotomy in 60 molars and showed clinical success rate was 93% for formocresol and 97% for MTA, whereas the radiographic success was 77% for formocresol and 93% for MTA.
- **Agamy**[36] **et al.** (2004) conducted a clinical trial and compared gray MTA, white MTA, and formocresol in 72 molars of 24 children. They found 100% clinical and radiographic success rate with MTA and 90% success rate with formocresol.

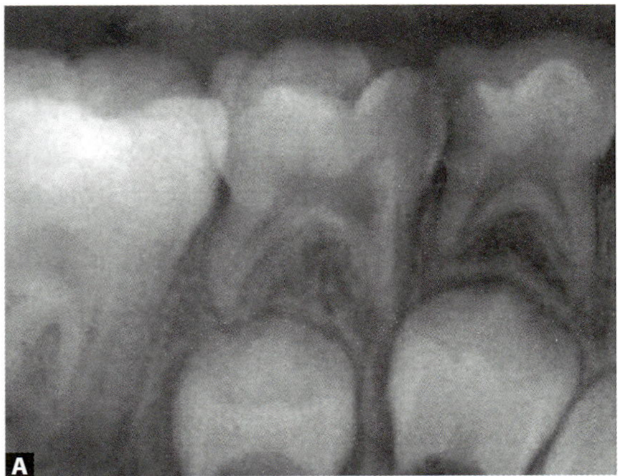

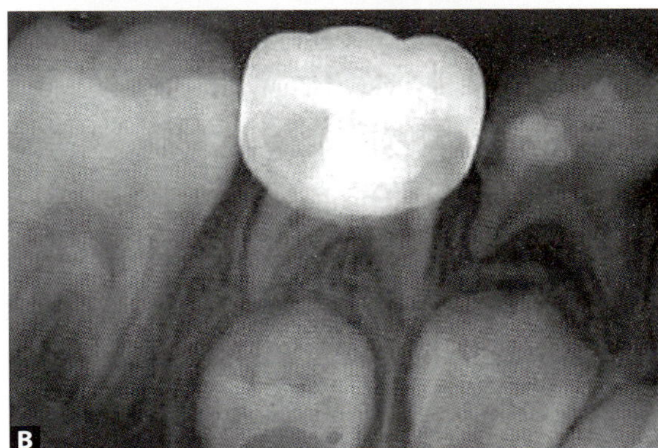

Figs. 54.10A and B: Mineral trioxide aggregate pulpotomy.

- **Naik** and **Hedge**[37] (2005) showed 100% clinical and radiographic success rate both with formocresol and MTA.
- **Godhi B**[38] **et al.** (2011) evaluated the effects of MTA and formocresol on vital pulp after pulpotomy of primary molars and concluded that MTA has more success rate as compared to formocresol.
- **Sonmez et al.**[39] did comparison of four pulpotomy techniques (formocresol, ferric sulfate, calcium hydroxide ($Ca(OH)_2$), and MTA) as pulp dressing agents in pulpotomized primary molars with clinical and radiographic examinations every 6 months over 2 years. The success rates were 76.9% for formocresol, 73.3% for ferric sulfate, 46.1% for $Ca(OH)_2$, and 66.6% for MTA.
- **Shirvani A et al.**[40] compared MTA versus formocresol pulpotomy via meta-analysis of randomized clinical trials and concluded that MTA is more effective.

Success rate of MTA pulpotomies

Author	*Observation time*	*Clinical success*	*Radiographic success*
Agamy et al. (2004)	12 months	100	100
Holan et al. (2005)	74 months	97	97
Subramaniam et al. (2009)	24 months	100	95
Hugar and Deshpande (2010)	36 months	100	100
Olatosi et al. (2015)	12 months	100	96

Nanohydroxyapatite and Bone Morphogenic Protein

- Appeared to be biocompatible and produced no pulpal reaction.
- Studies only done in animals and no human trials yet.

Calcium-enriched Mixture

Malekafzali et al. compared calcium-enriched mixture cement and MTA as pulp dressing biomaterials in vital pulpotomies of carious primary molars and concluded that it can be used and has similar properties to MTA.

Allium Sativum Oil

- **Mohammad et al.**[41] compared the clinical and radiographic effects of *A. sativum* oil and those of formocresol in vital pulpotomies of primary teeth.
- *A. sativum* oil had good healing potential, leaving the remaining pulp tissue functioning and healthy and is a biocompatible material that is compatible with vital human pulp tissue.

Lyophilized Freeze-dried Platelet with Calcium Hydroxide

- These compounds act as signaling proteins that could be directly involved in the regulation of cell proliferation, migration, and extracellular matrix production in the dental pulp.
- A lyophilized freeze-dried platelet-derived preparation is containing transforming growth factor (TGF), platelet derived growth factor (PDGF), bone morphogenetic proteins (BMPs), and insulin growth factor (IGF).
- These proteins have been used extensively in oral and maxillofacial reconstruction, adjunctive procedures related to the placement of osseointegrated implant in humans and periodontal regeneration.

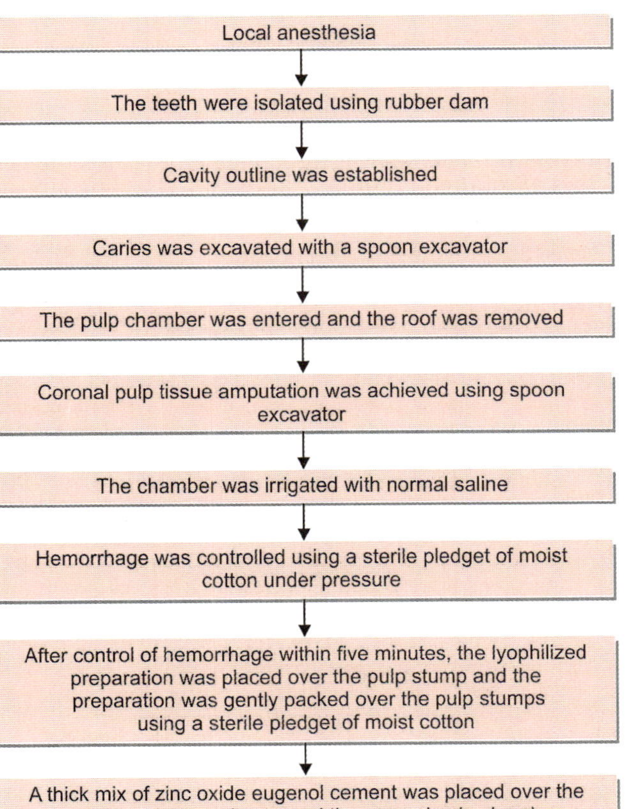

Research regarding lyophilized freeze-dried platelet with pulpotomy agent:

- Animal and human in vivo and in vitro studies have shown that these proteins stimulate differentiated cell of pulp to differentiate into odontoblast to deposit a layer of cementum.
- **Kalaskar R** and **Damle SG** (2004)[42] evaluate the potential of lyophilized freeze-dried platelet with calcium hydroxide as pulpotomy agent and found out that it had 100% success.

Enamel Matrix Derivative

- Enamel matrix derivate (EMD) is obtained from embryonic enamel as amelogenin has been demonstrated in vitro to be capable of stimulating periodontal ligament cell proliferation sooner when compared to gingival fibroblasts and bone cells.
- The ability of EMD to facilitate regenerative processes in mesenchymal tissues is well-established. The EMD-induced processes mimic parts of normal odontogenesis. It is believed that the EMD proteins participate in the reciprocal ectodermal-mesenchymal signaling that control and pattern these processes. Based on these observations, it has been suggested that amelogenin participates in the differentiation of odontoblasts and the subsequent predentin formation.
- Emdogain gel (Straumann, Switzerland) has been successfully employed for pulpotomies in uninfected teeth in animal studies. EMD components act as a signal for induction of mesenchymal cell differentiation, maturation and biomineralization.
- Form a stable extracellular matrix that provides a beneficial and protective pulp environment.
- Emdogain is a bio inductive material that is compatible with vital human tissues.
- It offers a good healing potential and is capable of inducing dentin formation leaving the remaining pulp tissue healthy and functioning.
- Emdogain may act in a multitude of ways on mesenchymal cells that provide pulp protection.

Research regarding EMD as pulpotomy agent:

- According to **Nakamura et al.**[43] when a pulp wound is exposed to EMD, substantial steps occur in a process resembling classic wound healing with subsequent neogenesis of normal pulp tissues and repair of dental pulp which includes rapid fibrodentin matrix formation and subsequent reparative dentinogenesis. The pulp matrix itself showed homogeneous fibrous deposition together with reparative dentin islands. The formation of new dentin started from within the pulp at some distance from the amputated site. There was also a marked tendency for angiogenesis in the deeper parts of the pulps, indicating an increased level of cell growth and/or metabolism. After the initial phase of healing in these teeth, a web of odontoblast-like cells was also observed growing from the central part of the pulp toward the pulp chamber walls, forming a dentin bridge. The EMD-induced hard tissue closely resembled osteodentin early in the process and later became more like secondary dentin.
- **Jumana et al.**[44] reported the clinical success of 93% using Emdogain for pulpotomy.

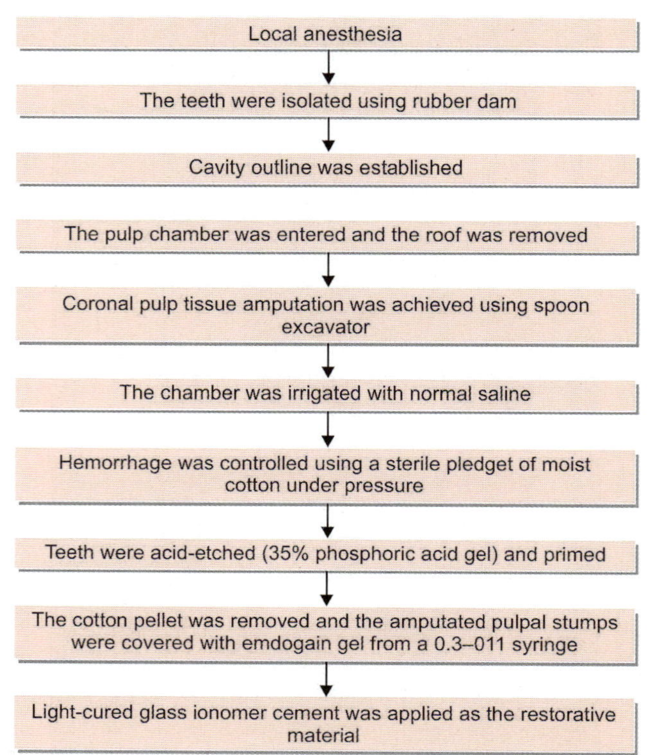

Propolis

- It is a wax-cum-resin substance that is produced by bees
- It is shown to have antibacterial, antiviral, antifungal, immunostimulation hypotensive, and cytostatic activity mainly due to the presence of lavonoids (2-phenyl-1,4-benzopyrone), aromatic acids, and esters. As an anti-inflammatory agent, it inhibits prostaglandin synthesis.

- **Carmen et al.** compared the effectiveness of 10% propolis tincture and formocresol pulpotomy in primary molars and showed that 10% propolis tincture was as effective as FC.
- **Lima et al.** following histological analysis concluded that the inflammatory response was less severe, the area of pulp necrosis was smaller, and more frequent formation of a mineralized tissue barrier was evident.

Ankaferd Blood Stopper (ABS)

- It is an herbal extract obtained from five different plants: *Thymus vulgaris, Glycyrrhiza glabra, Vitis vinifera, Alpinia officinarum*, and *Urtica dioica*.
- The possible mechanism is explained by **Goker et al.**[45] who concluded that following application of ABS, it forms an encapsulated protein network that provides focal points for vital erythrocyte aggregation. ABS-induced protein network formation with blood cells particularly erythrocytes cover the primary and secondary hemostatic system without disturbing individual coagulation factors.

Platelet-rich Plasma

- It was introduced by **Marx** in 1998 for reconstruction of mandibular defects, and it represents a relatively new biotechnology that is part of the growing interest in tissue engineering and cellular therapy

- Platelet-rich plasma (PRP) gel is an autologous modification of fibrin glue obtained from autologous blood used to deliver growth factors in high concentrations.
- It is an autologous concentration of human platelets in a small volume of plasma, mimics the coagulation cascade, leading to formation of fibrin clot, which consolidates and adheres to application site.
- Its biocompatible and biodegradable properties prevent tissue necrosis and extensive fibrosis and promote healing.
- Platelet-rich plasma has been found to work via three mechanisms: Increase in local cell division; Inhibition of excess inflammation by decreasing early macrophage proliferation, and degranulation of the agranules in platelets.

Rani et al.[46] concluded that PRP was found to be an ideal material for pulpotomy with low toxic effect, increased tissue regenerating properties, and good clinical results.

Pulpotec

- It is a newly available radiopaque, non-resorbable paste that is used for pulpotomy treatment. It is available as powder liquid system (Products Dentaires SA, Vevey, Switzerland)
- Powder consists of polyoxymethylene, iodoform and liquid consists of dexamethasone acetate, formaldehyde, phenol, and guaiacol.
- Its mode of action is by cicatrization of the pulpal stump at the chamber-canal interface, while maintaining the structure of underlying pulp.

Calcium Phosphate Cement

- Several formulations of calcium phosphate cement (CPC) have been successfully designed for various orthopedic and dental applications.
- Calcium phosphate cement possesses the combination of biocompatibility, osteoconductivity, and mouldability along with being nontoxic and nonimmunogenic.
- Chitra-CPC is a new CPC formulation with good rheological properties developed in India.

Ratnakumari et al.[47] used chitra-CPC and reported favorable results with mild pulpal inflammation and improved quality of dentin bridge formation.

Biodentine

- Bioceramic materials in pediatric endodontics, now can be safely considered as a munificent entity which has changed the prognosis of many cases which were once considered as unsalvageable.
- Biodentine new bioactive calcium silicate-based cement has been recently launched in the dental market as a 'dentin substitute'.
- This new biologically active material aids its penetration through opened dentinal tubules to crystallize interlocking with dentin and provide mechanical properties. Biodentine has been formulated using MTA-based cement technology and hence, claims improvements of some of the properties such as physical qualities and handling **(Table 54.4)**, including its other wide range of applications like endodontic repair and pulp capping in restorative dentistry.

Table 54.4: Setting time and porosity characteristics of MTA and biodentine.

Material	*Initial setting time (minutes)*	*Final setting time (minutes)*	*Porosity characteristics [density (g/cm²)]*
MTA (ProRoot)	70	175	1.882 (0.002)
Biodentine	6	10.1	2.260 (0.002)

- **Bogen G et al.** in a study have shown that the dynamic interaction of Biodentine with the dentin and pulp tissue interface stimulates pulp cell recruitment and differentiation, upregulates transformation factors (gene expression), and promotes dentinogenesis.[48]
- Biodentine is available in the form of a capsule containing the ideal ratio of its powder and liquid. The composition of powder is tricalcium silicate ($3CaO.SiO_2$) (main core material), dicalcium silicate ($2CaO.SiO_2$) (second core material), calcium carbonate ($CaCO_2$) (filler), zirconium oxide (ZnO_2) (radio-opacifier), iron oxide (coloring agent) **(Table 54.5)** while the liquid contains calcium chloride which acts as an accelerator, hydrosoluble polymer function as water reducing agent and water.

Table 54.5: Composition of biodentine.

Powder	*Percentage*
Tricalcium silicate ($3CaO.SIO_2$) (main core material)	80.1
Dicalcium silicate ($2CaO.SIO_2$) (second core material)	–
Calcium carbonate ($CaCO_2$) (filler)	14.9
Zirconium oxide (ZnO_2) (radioopacifier)	5
Iron oxide (coulouring agent)	–

Procedure

After hemostasis

↓

Biodentine (Septodont, Saint Maur des Fosse's, France) is mixed according to the manufacturer's instructions and applied (First, the Biodentine capsule is struck gently on a solid surface and then mix the powder inside, further mix with 5 droplets of liquid for 30 seconds using a triturator)

↓

The Biodentine mixture is condensed to the pulp stumps using an amalgam carrier and moistened cotton pellet

↓

The cavity is filled with Biodentine after waiting time of 9–12 minutes

↓

Restore by using a stainless steel crown and cemented with glass ionomer cement

Uses

Biodentine has been reported to be successful in certain unconventional circumstances which include pulpotomy after several days of traumatic pulp exposure, single visit apexification, massive resorptive lesion with multiple perforations, combined endodontic periodontic lesion and incomplete vertical root fracture.

Research studies regarding biodentine:
- **Rajasekharan et al.**[24] highlights Biodentine's spectrum of clinical applications in pediatric dentistry per se and overall, in endodontics, restorative dentistry and dental traumatology.
- **Kusum et al.**[49] evaluated 25 primary molars in 3- to 10-year-old children were treated with Biodentine and MTA and showed 92 and 80% radiographic success respectively after 9 months follow-up and 100% clinical success was observed in both the groups.
- In the study by **Niranjani et al.**[50], no statistically significant difference was observed between MTA and Biodentine as a pulpotomy medicament after 6 months follow-up.
- **Togaru et al.**[51], evaluated 90 decayed primary molars that required pulpotomy treatment with either Biodentine or MTA. Both the groups showed a 95.5% success rate at the end of 12 months.
- **Rajasekharan S et al.**[52] did RCT of 25 primary molars treated with Biodentine, reported 95.2% clinical and 94.4% radiographic success after 18 months. In both RCTs, clinical and radiographic findings did not show any significant difference between Biodentine and MTA.

Some Alternative Herbal Therapies

- **Honey:** Natural products have been used for several years in folk medicine. Among the natural products, medicinal importance of honey has been well documented in the literature as it has been known to possess antimicrobial as well as wound healing property. It has an excellent antimicrobial and wound healing property. Honey is used to treat various oral lesions such as lichen planus, candidiasis, and stomatitis. Kumari et al.[53] evaluated the efficacy of honey as a pulpotomy agent and found very promising results both clinically and radiographically.
- **Turmeric:** It is a natural anti-inflammatory and antioxidant which is widely used as an ayurvedic medicine. **Purohit et al.**[54] in their study found a good clinical and radiographic success with turmeric powder in 6-month follow-up.
- **Aloe vera:** It has got various properties such as immunomodulatory, antiviral and anti-inflammatory, antibacterial, antifungal as well as protective nature against a broad range of microorganisms. **Gupta et al.**[55] evaluated the effect of freshly extracted *A. vera* gel from its leaves as a pulpotomy agent in primary molar teeth and found a good clinical and radiographic success.

APEXOGENESIS

It is defined as the treatment of a vital pulp by capping or pulpotomy in order to permit continued growth of the root and closure of the open apex.

Rationale

Maintenance of integrity of the radicular pulp tissue to allow for continued root growth.

Indications

- Indicated for traumatized or pulpally involved vital permanent tooth when root apex is incompletely formed.
- No history of spontaneous pain.
- No sensitivity on percussion.
- No hemorrhage.
- Normal radiographic appearance.

Contraindications

- Evidence that radicular pulp has undergone degenera tive changes.
- Purulent drainage.
- History of prolonged pain.
- Necrotic debris in canal.
- Periapical radiolucency.

Procedure (Figs. 54.11A to C)

Application of rubber dam following local anesthesia

↓

Remove all of carious tooth structure and open up the pulp chamber

↓

Remove coronal pulp tissue with excavators, care is taken to prevent damage to radicular pulp

↓

Rinse all the residual debris and control hemorrhage by placement of a moist cotton pellet over the amputed pulp

↓

$Ca(OH)_2$ mixture is placed over the pulp stumps, followed by temporary restoration

↓

Follow-up radiographs are taken periodically to check the root development

↓

Once root development is complete, the conventional root canal treatment is done

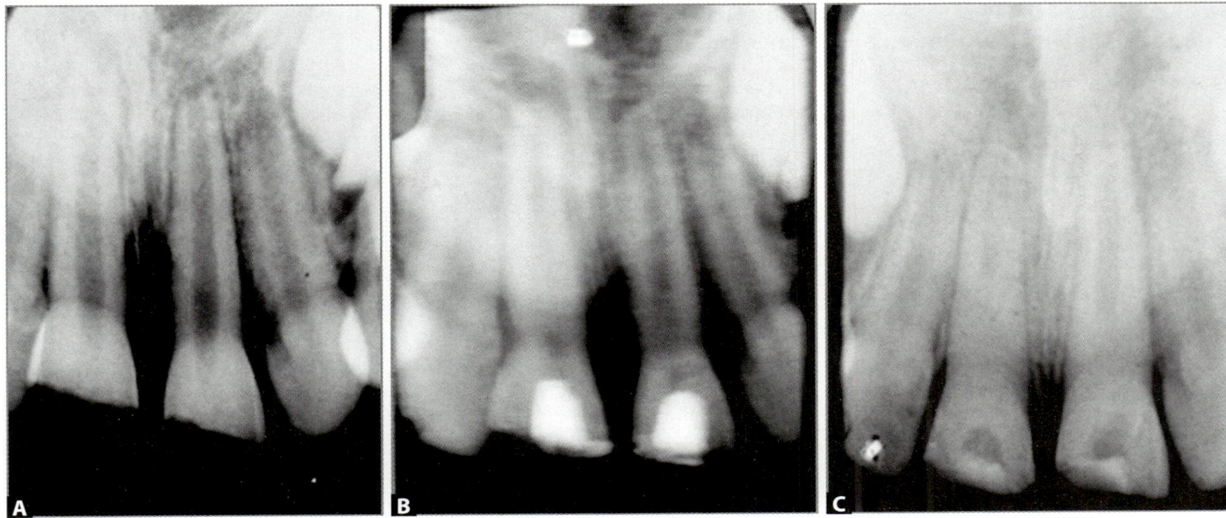

Figs. 54.11A to C: Apexogenesis. (A) Traumatic injury to young permanent teeth; (B) Calcium hydroxide apexogenesis done; (C) Continued root growth with maintenance of vitality.

Recent research regarding pulpotomy in primary teeth:

- **Erdem AP et al.[56] (2011)** evaluated the total success rates of MTA, FS, and FC as pulpotomy agents in primary molars and concluded that both MTA and FS showed comparable results to FC and can be used an alternative pulpotomy agents.
- **Alam F et al.[57] (2013)** carried out a study to compare the effectiveness of dilute FC and FS in the pulpotomies of 60 primary molars clinically and radiographically after 3 and 5 months and concluded that both the agents have similar outcomes but FS being nontoxic, can be used as an alternative to FC for pulpotomy.
- **Yildiz E et al.[58] (2014)** conducted a study to evaluate four different pulpotomy medicaments (FC: formocresol, FS: ferric sulfate, CH: calcium hydroxide, and MTA: mineral trioxide aggregate) in primary molars. At 30 months, clinical success rates were 100%, 95.2%, 96.4%, and 85% in the FC, FS, MTA, and CH groups, respectively. In radiographic analysis, the MTA group had the highest (96.4%), and the CH group had the lowest success rate (85%). So, it was concluded that FS and MTA can be used as an alternative to FC pulpotomy.
- **Gupta G et al.[59] (2015)** also had conducted a study on laser pulpotomy, FS pulpotomy, and electrosurgical pulpotomy in human primary molars for 12 months and stated that laser is an effective alternative to conventional techniques.
- **Niranjani K et al.[60] (2015)** carried out a study to evaluate the success and efficacy of MTA, lasers and biodentine as pulpotomy agents both clinically and radiographically for 6 months in 60 primary molars and it was concluded that pulpotomies performed with either MTA, laser or biodentine are equally efficient with similar clinical or radiographic success and hence can be considered as alternatives to FC.
- **Akhtar M et al.[61] (2016)** conducted a study to compare biodentine as pulpotomy agent to FC clinically and radiographically for 6 months on 122 patients and concluded that Biodentine™ as a pulpotomy agent has a high success rate and should be routinely used in practice for the treatment of carious primary molars.
- **Purohit RN et al.[54] (2017)** conducted a study to evaluate clinical and radiological outcomes of turmeric powder as pulpotomy agent in primary molars. Results showed significant success rate clinically (93.34%) and radiographically (100%) after 6 months follow-up. Thus, it was concluded that turmeric powder can be used as a pulpotomy agent, but further studies are required in this area.
- **Hugar SM et al.[62] (2017)** conducted a study to compare the clinical and radiographic success of FC, propolis extract, turmeric gel, and CH on primary molars and were evaluated for 1, 3, and 6 months. Results showed comparable outcomes to FC. The clinical success rate was found to be 100% except for CH where it was 80% and the radiographic success rate was 93.3%, 86.7%, 73.3% and 100% for propolis extract, turmeric gel, CH, and FC, respectively. Therefore, the study concluded that the materials used in the study have given a comparable result to FC suggesting their use as pulpotomy agent.
- **Kumari KK et al.[53] (2017)** conducted in vivo study to evaluate and compare the clinical and radiographic success of honey and FC as pulpotomy agents in primary molars in children aged 3–8 years. Clinically, both the groups showed 100% success during the follow-up periods, but radiographic success was 86.9% and 77.2% after 12 months, respectively.
- **Li Y et al.[63] (2014)** compared with traditional root canal therapy, stem cell-based therapies initiate a new approach to treating dental pulp diseases. The development of teeth depends on many kinds of stem cells and some of which still exist after the formation of the root, creating a chance for the tooth to regenerate itself when it stops developing due to infection or trauma.
- **Mousivand S et al.[64] (2021)** evaluated the outcome of apexogenesis with mineral trioxide aggregate (MTA) in traumatized anterior and carious posterior teeth over 5 years and found that success rate of apexogenesis using MTA in immature teeth was relatively high.

Review of guidance for the selection of regenerative endodontics, apexogenesis, apexification, pulpotomy, and other endodontic treatments for immature permanent teeth[65]

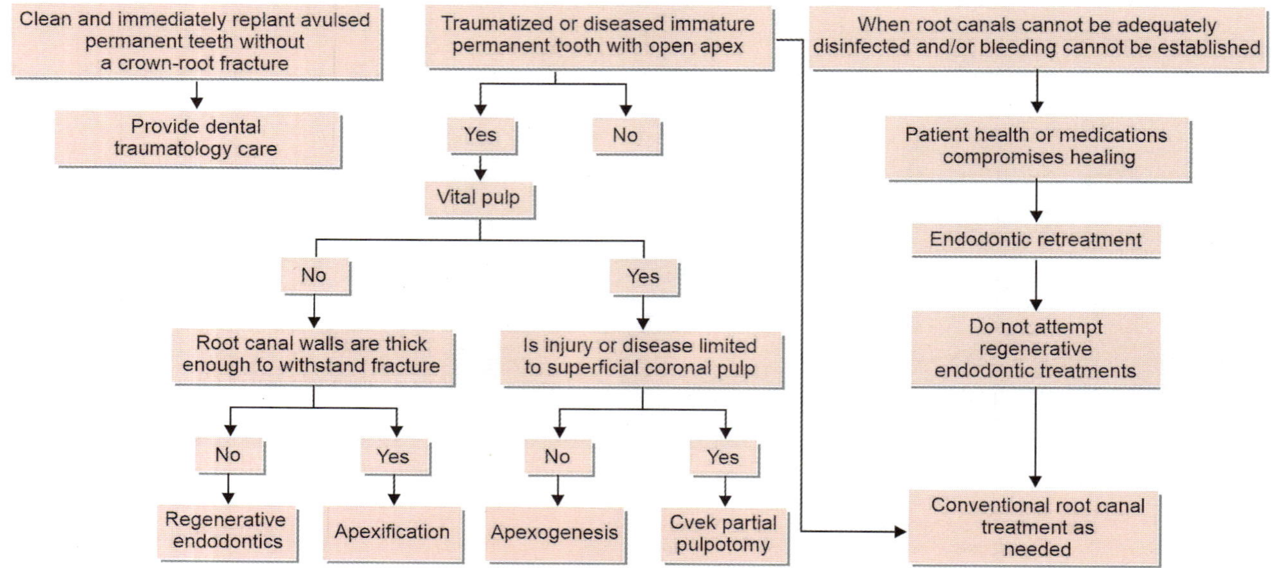

POINTS TO REMEMBER

- Indirect pulp capping is defined as a procedure wherein small amount of carious dentin is retained in deep areas of cavity to avoid exposure of pulp, followed by placement of a suitable medicament and restorative material that seals off the carious dentin and encourages pulp recovery.
- Direct pulp capping is defined by Kopel (1992) as the placement of a medicament or nonmedicated material on a pulp that has been exposed in course of excavating the last portions of deep dentinal caries or as a result of trauma.
- Finn (1995) defined pulpotomy as the complete removal of the coronal portion of the dental pulp, followed by placement of a suitable dressing or medicament that will promote healing and preserve vitality of the tooth.
- Objectives of indirect pulp capping are arresting the carious process, promoting dentin sclerosis, stimulating formation of tertiary dentin and remineralization of carious dentin.
- Indication for direct pulp capping is small mechanical exposure surrounded by sound dentin in asymptomatic vital primary teeth or young permanent teeth.
- Medications used for pulp capping are CH, corticosteroids and antibiotics, collagen fibers, 4-meta adhesive, direct bonding, isobutyl cyanoacrylate, MTA, laser and BMP.
- Direct pulp capping is primarily contraindicated in primary teeth, however, recently lasers are the only option that have demonstrated success of direct pulp capping in primary teeth. As the inherent potential of primary tooth cells is to resorb the tooth hence more odontoclasts are present as compared to odontoblasts. So when pulp capping material is placed it stimulates the undifferentiated mesenchymal cells that differentiate into odontoclastic cells. These cells exert their resorptive potential which leads to internal resorption.
- Types of pulpotomy: Devitalization—formocresol; preservation—glutaraldehyde and ferric sulfate; regeneration—CH, BMP, and MTA; mortal pulpotomy—Beechwood cresol.
- Indication of pulpotomy is mechanical pulp exposure in primary teeth.
- Formocresol was introduced by Buckley in 1904 its composition is cresol—35%, glycerol—15%, formaldehyde—19%, and water—31%.
- Current newer materials for pulpotomy are MTA, lypholized platelet, and enamel matrix derivatives.

Questionnaire

1. Define indirect pulp capping and explain its procedure.
2. What are the materials used for direct pulp capping?
3. Why is direct pulp capping contraindicated in primary teeth?
4. Write a note on Cvek's pulpotomy.
5. Give the definition, indication, contraindications and classification of pulpotomy.
6. Describe the procedure of formocresol pulpotomy.
7. What are the newer materials used for pulpotomy?
8. Write a note on MTA.

REFERENCES

1. Stewart DJ, Kramer IRH. Effects of calcium hydroxide on the unexposed pulp. J Dent Res. 1958;37:758.
2. Bjørndal L. Indirect pulp therapy and stepwise excavation. J Endod. 2008;34(7):S29-33.
3. Mathur VP, Dhillon JK, Logani A, et al. Evaluation of indirect pulp capping using three different materials: A randomized control trial using cone-beam computed tomography. Indian J Dent Res. 2016;27(6):623.
4. Korwar A, Sharma S, Logani A, et al. Pulp response to high fluoride releasing glass ionomer, silver diamine fluoride, and calcium hydroxide used for indirect pulp treatment: an in-vivo comparative study. Contemp Clin Dent. 2015;6(3):288-92.
5. Coll JA. Indirect pulp capping and primary teeth: is the primary tooth pulpotomy out of date? J Endod. 2008;34(7):S34-9.
6. Sujlana A, Pannu PK. Direct pulp capping: A treatment option in primary teeth? Pediatric Dental J. 2017;27(1):1-7.
7. Parisay I, Ghoddusi J, Forghani M. A review on vital pulp therapy in primary teeth. Iran Endod J. 2015;10(1):6-15.
8. Rasmussen P, Mjor IA. Calcium hydroxide as an ectopic bone inductor in rats. Scand J Dent Res. 1971;79(1):24-30.

9. Holland R, de Souza V, de Mello W, et al. Permeability of the hard tissue bridge formed after pulpotomy with calcium hydroxide: a histologic study. JADA. 1979;99:472-5.
10. Foreman PC, Barnes IE. Review of calcium hydroxide. Int Endod J. 1990;23:283-97.
11. Heithersay GS. Calcium hydroxide in the treatment of pulpless teeth with associated pathology. J Br Endod Soc. 1975;8(2):74-93.
12. Siqueira JF Jr, Lopes HP. Mechanisms of antimicrobial activity of calcium hydroxide: a critical review. Int Endod J. 1999;32:361-9.
13. Falster CA, Araujo FB, Straffon LH, et al. Indirect pulp treatment: In vivo outcomes of an adhesive resin system vs calcium hydroxide for protection of the dentin-pulp complex. Pediatr Dent. 2002;24(3):241-8.
14. Ford TR, Torabinejad M, Abedi HR, et al. Using mineral trioxide aggregate as a pulp-capping material. JADA. 1996;127:1491-4.
15. Farsi N, Alamoudi N, Balto K, et al. Clinical assessment of mineral trioxide aggregate (MTA) as direct pulp capping in young permanent teeth. J Clin Pediatr Dent. 2006;31:72-6.
16. Bogen G. Direct pulp capping with mineral trioxide aggregate: an observational study. J Am Dent Assoc. 2008;139:305-15.
17. Kunert M, Lukomska-Szymanska M. Bio-Inductive Materials in Direct and Indirect Pulp Capping—A Review Article. Materials 2020;13(5):1204.
18. Mass E, Zilberman U. Clinical and radiographic evaluation of partial pulpotomy in carious exposures of permanent molars. Pediatr Dent. 1993;15(4):257-9.
19. Milnes AR. Persuasive evidence that formocresol use in pediatric dentistry is safe. J Can Den Assoc. 2006;72:247-8.
20. Nacht MA. Devitalizing technic for pulpotomy in primary molars. ASDC J Dent Child. 1956;23(1st quart):45.
21. Emmerson C, Miyamoto O, Sweet C, et al. Pulpal changes following formocresol applications on rat molars and human primary teeth. JS Calif Dent Assoc. 1959;27:309-23.
22. Fuks AB, Bimstein E. Clinical evaluation of diluted formocresol pulpotomies in primary teeth of school children. Pediatr Dent. 1981;3(4):321-4.
23. Coll JA, Seale NS, Vargas K, Marghalani AA, Al Shamali S, Graham L. Primary Tooth Vital Pulp Therapy: A Systematic Review and Meta-analysis. Pediatr Dent. 2017;39(1):16-123.
24. Rajasekharan S, Martens LC, Cauwels RG, Anthonappa RP. Biodentine™ Material Characteristics and Clinical Applications: A 3-year Literature Review and Update. Eur Arch. Paediatr Dent. 2018;19:1-22.
25. Garcia-Godoy F. A 42-month clinical evaluation of glutaraldehyde pulpotomies in primary teeth. J Pedod. 1985;10(2):148-55.
26. Fuks A, Bimstein E, Klein H. Assessment of a 2% buffered glutaraldehyde solution in pulpotomized primary teeth of school children: a preliminary report. J Pedod. 1985;10(4):323-30.
27. Davis M, Myers R, Switkes M. Glutaraldehyde: an alternative to formocresol for vital pulp therapy. ASDC J Dent Child. 1981;49(3):176-80.
28. Fuks AB. Pulp therapy for the primary dentition. In: Pinkham JR, Casamassimo PS, Fields HW, McTigue DJ, Nowak A (Eds). Pediatric Dentistry: Infancy Through Adolescence, 3rd edition. Philadelphia, Pa: WB Saunders Co; 1999.
29. Smith DR. Ferric sulfate pulpotomies in primary molars, a retrospective study. AAPD. 2000;22:3.
30. Liu JF. Effects of Nd: YAG laser pulpotomy on human primary molars. J Endod. 2006;32:404-7.
31. Cvek M. A clinical report on partial pulpotomy and capping with calcium hydroxide in permanent incisors with complicated crown fractures. J Endod. 1978;4(8):232-7.
32. Sakai VT, Moretti AB, Oliveira TM, et al. Pulpotomy of human primary molars with MTA and Portland cement: a randomised controlled trial. Br Dent J. 2009;207(3):128-9.
33. Torabinejad M, Hong CU, Pitt Ford TR, et al. Antibacterial effects of some root end filling materials. J Endod.1995;21:403-6.
34. Torabinejad M, Chivian N. Clinical applications of mineral trioxide aggregate. J Endod. 1999;25(3):197-205.
35. Cuisia ZE, Musselman R, Schneider P, et al. A study of mineral trioxide aggregate pulpotomies in primary molars. Pediatr Dent. 2001;23:168.
36. Agamy HA, Bakry NS, Mounir MM, et al. Comparison of mineral trioxide aggregate and formocresol as pulp- capping agents in pulpotomized primary teeth. Pediatr Dent. 2004;26:302-9.
37. Naik S, Hegde AM. Mineral trioxide aggregate as a pulpotomy agent in primary molars: an in vivo study. J Indian Soc Pedod Prev Dent. 2005;23:13-6.
38. Godhi B, Sood PB, Sharma A. Effects of mineral trioxide aggregate and formocresol on vital pulp after pulpotomy of primary molars: An in vivo study. Contemp Clin Dent. 2011;2:296-301.
39. Sonmez D, Sari S, Cetinbas T. A Comparison of four pulpotomy techniques in primary molars: a long-term follow-up. J Endod. 2008;34(8):950-5.
40. Shirvani A, Asgary S. Mineral trioxide aggregate versus formocresol pulpotomy: A systematic review and meta-analysis of randomized clinical trials. Clin Oral Investig. 2014;18:1023-30.
41. Mohammad SG, Raheel SA, Baroudi K. Clinical and radiographic evaluation of Allium sativum oil as a new medicament for vital pulp treatment of primary teeth. J Int Oral Health. 2014;6(6):32-6.
42. Kalaskar RR, Damle SG. Comparative evaluation of lyophilized freeze dried platelet derived preparation with calcium hydroxide as pulpotomy agents in primary molars. J Indian Soc Pedod Prev Dent. 2004;22(1):24-9.
43. Nakamura Y, Hammarstrom L, Matsumoto K, et al. The induction of reparative dentine by enamel proteins. Int J Endod. 2002;35:407-17.
44. Jumana S, Ahmed M, Nadia W, et al. Comparison of enamel matrix derivative versus formocresol as pulpotomy agents in the primary dentition. J Endod. 2008;34:284-7.
45. Goker H, Haznedaroglu IC, Ercetin S, et al. Haemostatic actions of the folkloric medicinal plant extracts Ankaferd Blood Stopper. J Int Med Res. 2008;36:163-70.
46. Rani S, Iram Z, Shipra J. Platelet rich plasma-a healing aid and perfect enhancement factor: review and case report. Int J Clin Pediatr Dent. 2011;4:69-75.
47. Ratnakumari N, Bijimol T. A histological comparison of pulpal response to Chitra-CPC and formocresol used as pulpotomy agents. Int J Clin Pediatr Dent. 2012;5:6-13.
48. Bogen G, Chandler N. Pulp preservation in immature permanent teeth. Endod Topics. 2010;23(1):131-52. https:// doi.org/10.1111/j.1601-1546.2012.00286.x
49. Kusum B, Rakesh K, Richa K. Clinical and radiographical evaluation of mineral trioxide aggregate, Biodentine and propolis as pulpotomy medicaments in primary teeth. Restor Dent Endod. 2015;40:276–85.
50. Niranjani K, Prasad MG, Vasa AA, et al. Clinical evaluation of success of primary teeth pulpotomy using mineral trioxide aggregate((R)), laser and Biodentine(TM)—an in vivo study. J Clin Diagn Res. 2015;9:35–7.
51. Togaru H, Muppa R, Srinivas N, et al. Clinical and radiographic evaluation of success of two commercially available pulpotomy agents in primary teeth: an in vivo study. J Contemp Dent Pract. 2016;17:557–63.
52. Rajasekharan S, Martens L, Vandenbulcke J, et al. Efficacy of three different pulpotomy agents in primary molars—a randomised control trial. Int Endod J. 2016;50:215–28.
53. Kumari K, Sridevi E, Sai Sankar A, Gopal A, Pranitha K, Manoj Kumar M. Evaluation of honey as a new medicament for vital pulp therapy in primary teeth. SRM Journal of Research in Dental Sciences. 2017;8(2):58-63.
54. Purohit R, Bhatt M,Purohit K, Acharya J, Kumar R, Garg R. Clinical and radiological evaluation of turmeric powder as a pulpotomy medicament in primary teeth: An in vivo Study. International Journal of Clinical Pediatric Dentistry. 2017;10:37-40.
55. Gupta N, Bhat M, Devi P, Girish. Aloe-Vera: A Nature's Gift to Children. International Journal of Clinical Pediatric Dentistry. 2010 May-Aug;3(2):87-92.
56. Erdem AP, Guven Y, Balli B, et al. Success rates of mineral trioxide aggregate, ferric sulfate, and formocresol pulpotomies: a 24-month study. Pediatr Dent. 2011;33(2):165-70.

57. Alam F, Khattak YK, Rehman SU. Ferric sulphate versus formocresol in pulpotomies of primary molars. JKCD. 2013;4(1):2-6.
58. Yildiz E, Tosun G. Evaluation of formocresol, calcium hydroxide, ferric sulfate, and MTA primary molar pulpotomies. Eur J Dent. 2014;8(2):234-40.
59. Gupta G, Rana V, Shrivastava N, et al. Laser pulpotomy- an effective alternative to conventional techniques: a 12 months clinicoradiographic study. Int J Pediatr Dent. 2015;8(1):18-21.
60. Niranjani K, GhanshyamPrasad M, Vasa AAK, et al. Clinical evaluation of success of primary teeth pulpotomy using mineral trioxide aggregate, laser and Biodentine™- an in vivo study. J Clin Diagn Res. 2015;9(4):35-7.
61. Akhtar M, Rana SAA, Rana MJA, et al. Clinical and radiological success rates of biodentine for pulpotomy in children. Int J Contemp Med Res. 2016;3(8):2334-6.
62. Hugar SM, Kukreja P, Hugar SS, et al. Comparative evaluation of clinical and radiographic success of formocresol, propolis, turmeric gel and calcium hydroxide on pulpotomized primary molars: a preliminary study. Int J Clin Pediatr Dent. 2017;10(1):18-23.
63. Li Y, Shu LH, Yan M, et al. Adult stem cell-based apexogenesis. World J Methodol. 2014;4(2):99-108.
64. Shima M, Mahshid S, Saeed M, Niloufar K. Evaluation of the outcome of apexogenesis in traumatised anterior and carious posterior teeth using mineral trioxide aggregate: a 5-year retrospective study. Australian Endodontic Journal, October 2021.
65. American Academy of Pediatric Dentistry. Pulp therapy for primary and immature permanent teeth. The Reference Manual of Pediatric Dentistry. Chicago, Ill. American Academy of Pediatric Dentistry; 2021:399-407.

CHAPTER

Pulp Therapy for Nonvital Teeth

Nikhil Marwah, Satish Vishwanathaiah, Nikhil Srivastava, Prachi Mital, Srishty Chalana

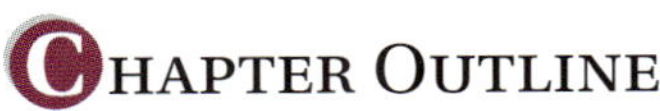

CHAPTER OUTLINE

- Single Visit Pulpectomy
- Multiple Visit Pulpectomy
- Obturation
- Apexification
- Frank's Criteria for Apexification

The concept of pediatric endodontics being divided into vital and nonvital pulp therapy has been outlined by most of the guidelines of pulp therapy [American Academy of Pediatric Dentistry (AAPD), UK, etc.]. Their basic recommendation is that if the infection has spread to radicular pulp and the tooth is showing signs of irreversible pulpitis, then such teeth be termed as nonvital. The recommended treatment for such cases is pulpectomy for primary teeth, apexification for young permanent teeth, and root canal treatment (RCT) for permanent teeth.

The historical view has never been in favor of pulpectomy in primary teeth. **Cohen** stated that primary teeth were not suitable for proper biomechanical endodontic procedures. **Massler** felt that only the most dedicated of pediatric dentists should attempt endodontic procedures on primary teeth. **Brauer** claimed that endodontic procedures were impractical in children. However, as time passed by, the views changed and pulpectomy became an essential part of treatment. **Rabinowitch** published an extensively documented study of 1,363 root canals on nonvital primary molars and reported that an average of 5.5 visits was required for nonperiapically involved teeth, and 7.7 visits were required for teeth with periapical involvement.

Although pulpectomy is the total removal of the pulp tissue from the root canals, this cannot be achieved in primary dentition, because of the complexity and irregularity of the canals, accessory canals, ever present resorption, and inability to determine an anatomical apex, therefore, the term pulpectomy should not be used, but rather the term pulp canal therapy should be used.

- **Mathewson** (1995) *defined it as the complete removal of the necrotic pulp from the root canals of primary teeth and filling them with an inert resorbable material so as to maintain the tooth in the dental arch.*
- **Finn** *defines pulpectomy as removal of all pulpal tissue from the coronal and radicular portions of the tooth.*

Objectives of pulpectomy:
- Maintain the tooth free of infection
- Biomechanically cleanse and obturate the root canals
- Promote physiologic root resorption
- Hold the space for the erupting permanent tooth.

Indications of pulpectomy

General indications
- Patient should be in good general health with no serious disease
- Maximum cooperation of patient and parents.

Clinical indications
- All teeth with pulpal involvement in which inflammation/infection has spread beyond the coronal pulp are the candidates of pulpectomy whether vital or non-vital.
- A restorable tooth with necrosed or irreversibly inflamed pulp.
- A tooth previously planned for a pulpotomy that shows uncontrolled pulpal hemorrhage
- Pulpless primary anterior teeth when speech, esthetics are a factor.

Radiographic Indications
- Adequate periodontal and bony support.

Contraindications of pulpectomy

General contraindications
- Young patient with systemic illness such as congenital ischemic heart disease, leukemia
- Children on long-term corticosteroids therapy.

Clinical contraindications
- Loss of bone support (excessive tooth mobility)
- Communication between the roof of the pulp chamber and the region of furcation
- A non-restorable tooth: Insufficient tooth structure to allow isolation by rubber dam and extracoronal restoration.

Radiographic contraindications
- External root resorption
- Internal root resorption in the apical third of the root
- Radicular cyst, dentigerous/follicular cyst in association with the primary tooth
- Interradicular radiolucency that communicates with the gingival sulcus.

SINGLE VISIT PULPECTOMY

This is carried out as an extension of pulpotomy procedure, probably on the spot decision when hemorrhage from amputated pulp stumps is uncontrollable, but the tooth does not show any periapical changes.

Indications

- Large carious exposure with frank involvement of radicular pulp but without any periapical changes
- Primary teeth with inflammation extending beyond coronal pulp, indicated by hemorrhage from the amputated radicular stumps that is dark red, slowly oozing and uncontrollable.

Single Sitting Pulpectomy

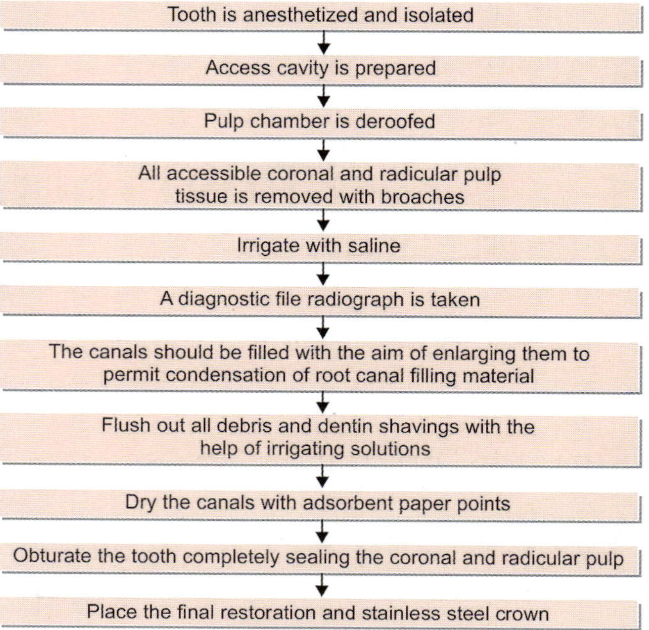

Tooth is anesthetized and isolated
Access cavity is prepared
Pulp chamber is deroofed
All accessible coronal and radicular pulp tissue is removed with broaches
Irrigate with saline
A diagnostic file radiograph is taken
The canals should be filled with the aim of enlarging them to permit condensation of root canal filling material
Flush out all debris and dentin shavings with the help of irrigating solutions
Dry the canals with adsorbent paper points
Obturate the tooth completely sealing the coronal and radicular pulp
Place the final restoration and stainless steel crown

Procedure (Figs. 55.1A to J)

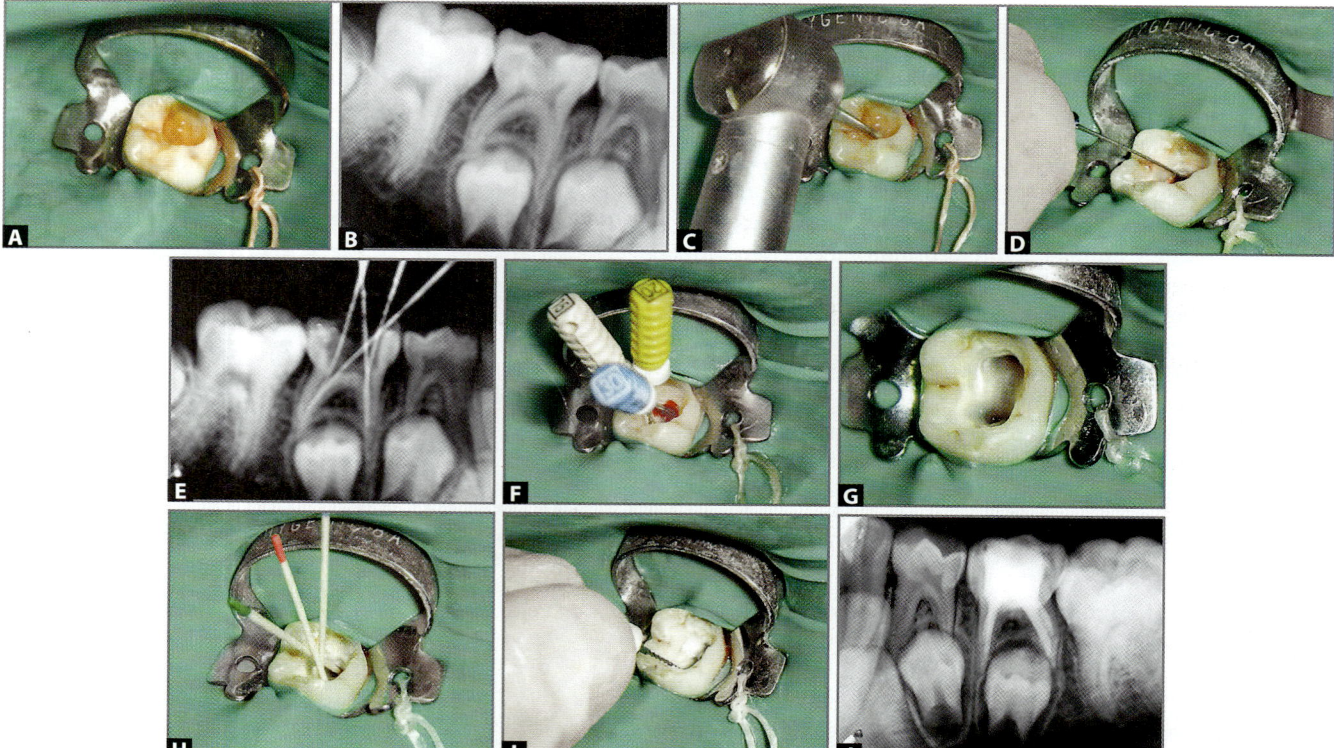

Figs. 55.1A to J: (A) Preoperative carious tooth; (B) Preoperative radiograph; (C) Access opening; (D) Pulp extirpation with broach; (E) Working length radiograph; (F) Biomechanical preparation; Pulpectomy in primary teeth: (G) Clean and enlarged canals; (H) Drying of canals with paper point; (I) Obturating the canals; and (J) Postoperative X-ray.

MULTIPLE VISIT PULPECTOMY

Indications

- Given by **Paterson** and **Curzon** in 1992
- Indicated where infection, an abscess or chronic sinus exists
- Nonvital primary teeth
- Teeth with necrotic pulp and periapical involvement.

Procedure

First Appointment (Access Opening)

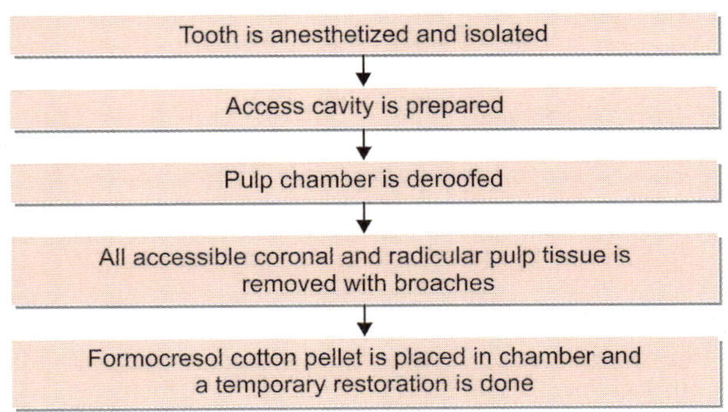

Second Appointment (Cleaning and Shaping)

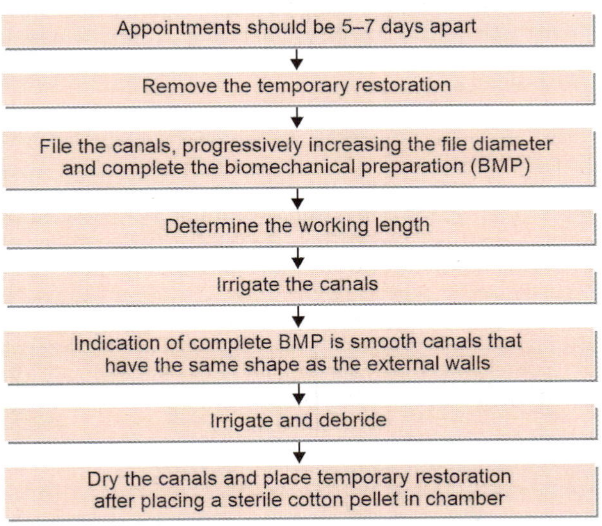

Appointments should be 5–7 days apart
Remove the temporary restoration
File the canals, progressively increasing the file diameter and complete the biomechanical preparation (BMP)
Determine the working length
Irrigate the canals
Indication of complete BMP is smooth canals that have the same shape as the external walls
Irrigate and debride
Dry the canals and place temporary restoration after placing a sterile cotton pellet in chamber

Third Appointment (Obturation)

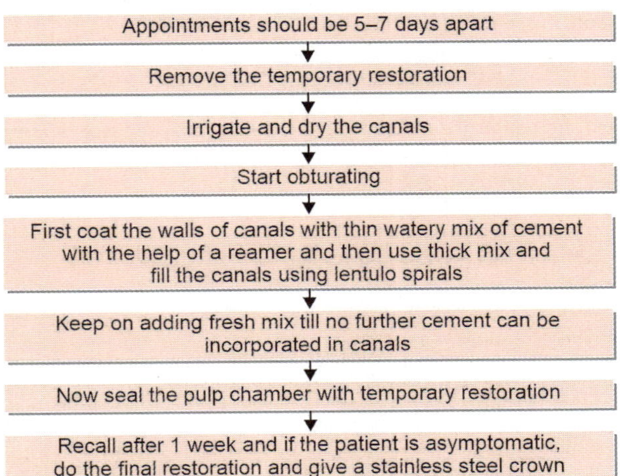

Appointments should be 5–7 days apart
Remove the temporary restoration
Irrigate and dry the canals
Start obturating
First coat the walls of canals with thin watery mix of cement with the help of a reamer and then use thick mix and fill the canals using lentulo spirals
Keep on adding fresh mix till no further cement can be incorporated in canals
Now seal the pulp chamber with temporary restoration
Recall after 1 week and if the patient is asymptomatic, do the final restoration and give a stainless steel crown

OBTURATION

The aim of obturating the root canal system is to provide an airtight seal to prevent recontamination of the canal from either apical or coronal leakage, and to isolate and neutralize any remaining pulpal tissue or bacteria.

Techniques of Obturation

Several techniques have been used for the filling of material into primary teeth root canals, but an ideal technique is one that offers consistency, is easy to use, and can be mastered by the user. Some of the techniques for primary tooth obturation are (**Mahajan et al.**)[1] as follows:

Endodontic Pressure Syringe

It was developed by **Greenberg** and the technique was described by **Spedding** and **Krakow** in 1965. This apparatus consists of a syringe barrel, threaded plunger, wrench, and threaded needle. Needle is placed 1 mm short of apex and with a slow withdrawing type of motion, the needle is withdrawn 3 mm with each quarter turn of the screw until the canal is visibly filled at the orifice. Disadvantages include overfill, more time consumption, and more voids.

Mechanical Syringe

This method was proposed by **Greenberg** in 1971. Cement is loaded into the syringe with 30 G needle as per the manufactures recommendation and expressed into the canal. Press using continuous pressure while withdrawing the needle.

Jiffy Tubes

This technique was popularized by **Riffcin** in 1980. The standardized mixture of zinc oxide eugenol (ZOE) is loaded into the tube and is placed into the canal orifice and the material expressed into the canal with a downward squeezing motion until the orifice appears visibly filled.

Tuberculin Syringe

Syringe utilized by **Aylard** and **Johnson**[2] in 1987 was a standard 26 G, 3/8th inch needle. Material was expressed into the canal by slow finger pressure on the plunger until the canal was visibly filled at the orifice. The disadvantage of the tuberculin syringe technique is the difficulty of separating the tip during injection, which may compromise optimal filling and increase the presence of voids.

Incremental Filling Technique

This was first used by **Gould**[3] in 1972. Endodontic plugger, corresponding to the size of the canal with rubber stop, is used to place a thick mixture of cement into the canal. Thick mixture was prepared into a flame shape corresponding to size and shape of the canal and then tapped gently into the apical area with the help of plugger. Its disadvantages are poor consistency of material and voids due to incomplete condensation.

Reamer Technique

A reamer coated with ZOE paste was inserted into the canal with clockwise rotation, accompanied by a vibratory motion to allow the material to reach the apex, and then withdrawn from the canal, while simultaneously continuing the clockwise rotary motion.

Insulin Syringe Technique

As described by **Nagar et al.**[4] a homogeneous mixture of ZOE, according to manufacturer's instructions is loaded into the insulin syringe and a stopper is used after assessing the working length of the canal. The needle is inserted into the canal and kept about 2 mm short of apex. The material is then pressed into the canal and while doing so the needle is retrieved from the canal outward while continuing to press the material inside.

Disposable Injection Technique

24 gauge needle is used to carry zinc oxide eugenol material in canal with adjusted stopper to working length and the material is gently pushed into the canal till the material is seen flowing out of the canal orifice, after this, needle is gradually withdrawn while pushing the material till the needle reaches the pulp chamber.

NaviTip

Recently, a thin and flexible metal tip was introduced, viz. NaviTip (Ultradent), in the market to deliver root canal sealer. This NaviTip comes in different lengths and a rubber stop may be adjusted to it. Endoseal, a syringe delivered ZOE-based canal sealer, can be expressed by the NaviTip system.

Bidirectional Spiral

Dr Barry Musikant (1998) developed a new obturation technique with bidirectional spiral. This technique ensures that a minimal amount of obturating material will past the apex. This controlled coverage is achieved because the spirals at the coronal end of the instrument spin the material down the shaft toward the apex, while the spirals at the apical end spin the material upward toward the coronal end.

Pastinject (Micromega)

It is a specially designed paste carrier with flattened blades, which improves material placement into the root canal. In a study conducted by **Grover et al.**[5] it was concluded that among lentulo spirals, bidirectional spiral, pastinject, and pressure syringe, the pastinject technique has proved to be the most effective, yielding a higher number of optimally filled canals and minimal voids, combined with easier placement of the material into the canals.

Lentulo Spiral Technique

This was advocated by **Kopel** in 1970. Lentulo spiral was dipped into the mixture and then introduced into the canal to its predetermined length and rotated in the canal. Additional amount of paste is added into the canal, till it is filled. The first step is to take the lentulo spiral of one size smaller than your last fill. This is followed by coating the canals with very thin mixture of obturating material. This then is followed up by final insertion of obturating material in thick consistency in specified motion in slow speed. The two precautions to be taken are: (1) first to always work short of working length and (2) second the motion should only be initiated when we enter canal orifice. This technique has been documented to be one of the best methods of primary tooth obturation with respect to consistency, voids and filling optimization. The disadvantages are overfill and breakage of instrument, both of which can be avoided if used with proper indication and precaution.

Research regarding techniques of pulpectomy:

- **Aylard and Johnson**[2] and **Dandashi et al.**[6] evaluated root canal obturation methods in primary teeth in vitro and concluded that the lentulo spiral mounted in a slow-speed handpiece was superior in filling straight and curved root canals of primary teeth.
- **Torres et al.**[7] also concluded that calcium hydroxide [$Ca(OH)_2$] radiodensity in a curved canal was significantly greater using a lentulo spiral-only technique.
- **Sigurdsson et al.**[8] reported that application with a lentulo spiral was more homogeneous than injection of $Ca(OH)_2$ paste.
- **Deonízio et al.**[9] reported that the 15,000 rpm speed was more effective in filling the apical third and 5,000 rpm speed was more effective in filling the cervical and middle thirds in their study utilizing lentulo spirals at different speeds for filling the root canal with $Ca(OH)_2$ paste.
- **Memarpur M. et al.**[10] concluded that an optimal filling result was obtained more frequently with the Lentulo instrument than with the packing technique.
- **Other techniques**: Amalgam plugger by **Nosonwitz** (1960) and **King** (1984), paper points by **Spedding** (1973), and plugging action with wet cotton pellet by **Donnenberg** (1974), incremental filling with reamer.
- **Aminabadi et al.**[11] in their systematic review and meta-analysis concluded that lowest overfilling rate was related to plugger and handheld Lentulo spiral techniques for ZOE and calcium hydroxide pastes respectively
- **Nagaveni et al.**[12] studied Volumetric evaluation of ZOE using 5 different obturation methods using CBCT scan and concluded that lentulo spiral mounted to handpiece showed the best technique.
- **Singh et al.**[13] studied volumetric evaluation of four obturating techniques in primary teeth using cone beam computed tomography and showed navitip system and endodontic pressure syringe showed the best root canal obturation, with the nearest to complete filling of the volumes of prepared root canals, while the insulin syringe was least effective.

Ideal requirements of root canal filling material

Given by **Castagnola:**

- The material should resorb with the same rate as the primary tooth root resorbs
- It should neither irritate the periapical tissues nor coagulate any organic remnants in the canal
- It should have a stable disinfecting power
- Any surplus material passed beyond the apex should be resorbed easily
- It should be inserted easily into the root canal and also removed easily if necessary
- It should not be soluble in water
- It should not discolor the tooth
- It should be radiopaque
- It should be harmless to the adjacent tooth germ.

According to **Rabinowitch:**

- It should not irritate the periapical tissues nor coagulate any organic remnants in the canal.
- It should have a stable disinfecting power.
- Excess pressed beyond the apex should be resorbed easily.
- It should be inserted easily into the root canal and removed easily if necessary.
- It should adhere to the walls of the canal and should not shrink.

- It should not be soluble in water.
- It should not discolour the tooth.
- It should be radiopaque.
- It should induce vital periapical tissue to seal the canal with calcified or connective tissue.
- It should be harmless to the adjacent tooth germ.
- It should not set to a hard mass, which could deflect an erupting permanent tooth.

According to **Rifkin**:

- Should be Resorbable
- Should have an Antiseptic property
- Noninflammatory and nonirritating to the underlying permanent tooth germ,
- Good Radiopacity for visualization on radiographs,
- Ease of insertion and ease of removal.
- Should not cause any tooth discoloration.

Materials used for Obturation

A wide variety of materials have been used for obturation of primary teeth with varying success **(Table 55.1)**.[14]

Materials	*Composition*
Zinc oxide eugenol	Zinc oxide powder + eugenol oil
Calcium hydroxide	–
Iodoform	Derivative of iodine
Vitapex	Calcium hydroxide + iodoform + oil additives
Walkhoff paste	Parachlorophenol + camphor + menthol
KRI paste	Iodoform + camphor + parachlorophenol + menthol
Maisto paste	Zinc oxide + iodoform + thymol + chlorophenol camphor + lanolin
Mineral trioxide aggregate	Tricalcium aluminate + tricalcium silicate + silicate oxide + tricalcium oxide + bismuth oxide
Endoflas	Barium sulfate + calcium hydroxide + iodoform + zinc oxide eugenol
Guedes pinto paste	Rifocort + idoform + camphorated parachlorophenol
CTZ Paste:	chloramphenicol 500 mg+tetracycline 500 mg + zinc oxide 1000 mg + eugenol 1 drop
Chitra HAP-Fil	Hydroxyapatite - Iodoform paste
Calen paste	2.5 g calcium hydroxide, 0.5 g zinc oxide, 0.05 g colophony, and 1.75 mL polyethylene glycol

Zinc Oxide Eugenol

- Most commonly used.
- **Bonastre** (1837) discovered ZOE and it was subsequently used in dentistry by **Chisholm** (1876).
- Zinc oxide eugenol pastes the first root canal filling material to be recommended for primary teeth, as described by **Sweet** in 1930.
- Zinc oxide eugenol is said to have anti-inflammatory and analgesic properties.
- Its limitations are slow resorption, irritation to the periapical tissues, necrosis of bone and cementum, and alter the path of erupting teeth.
- When ZOE mixture is used, thin mixture is used to coat the walls of the canal, followed by a thick mixture that can be manually condensed into the lumen of the canal.
- **Barr et al.**[15] showed 82.3% clinical success rate, **Gould**[3] showed 86.1%, and **Coll et al.**[16] showed 86.1% clinical success rate.
- **Barcelos et al.**[17] showed 85% of clinical success with ZOE but the overfilling was evident even after evaluation period.

Research regarding use of ZOE as pulpectomy obturation material:

- **Praveen et al.**[18] concluded that excess material forced through the apex during filling procedures can remain in the apical tissue during the process of physiological root resorption and it takes few months or even years to resorb.
- **Hashieh et al.**[19] studied the beneficial effects of eugenol. The amount of eugenol released in the periapical zone immediately after placement was 10–4 and falls to 10–6 after 24 h, reaching zero after 1 month. Within these concentrations, eugenol is said to have anti-inflammatory and analgesic properties that are very useful after a pulpectomy procedure.
- **Al-Ostwani et al.**[20] used a combination of zinc oxide + propolis (ZOP) and concluded that there was acceptable clinical and radiographic success rate with faster resorption seen in some cases.
- **Chandra et al.**[21] used a combination of zinc oxide + ozonated oil and evaluated that this combination has biological properties such as bactericidal action, debriding effect, angiogenesis stimulation capacity, and high oxidizing power, and after 12-month follow-up, there was progressive bone regeneration at the periapical region with good clinical and radiographic success rate.

Table 55.1: Summary of the success rates of pulpectomy procedures in primary molars using different filling materials.

Investigator	*Year*	*Follow-up (months)*	*Number of teeth examined*	*Filling material*	*Success rate (%)*
Rabinowitch	1953	N/A	1,363	Black ZOE	99.5% (calculated)
Gould	1972	7–26	29	ZOE	82.9% (calculated)
Fuchino et al.	1978	1–19	130	Vitapex®	86.2–97.7%
Rifkin	1980	12	26	KRI	89.0%
Hideki et al.	1981	24–54	183	Vitapex®	93.5%
Coll et al.	1985	6–36	33	ZOE	80.5%
Coll et al.	1985	60–82	29	ZOE	86.1%
Garcia-Godoy	1987	6–24	55	KRI	95.6%
Reyes	1989	6–24	53	KRI + FC + $Ca(OH)_2$	100.0%
Barr et al.	1991	12–74	62	ZOE + FC	82.3%
Holan et al.	1993	6–48	34	ZOE	65%
Holan et al.	1993	6–48	44	KRI	84%
Coll et al.	1999	3–22	33	Vitapex®	100%
Fuks et al.	2002	6–52	55	Endoflas	70%

($Ca(OH)_2$: calcium hydroxide; ZOE: zinc oxide eugenol)

- **Chawla et al.**[22] used a mixture of ZOE + $Ca(OH)_2$ + sodium fluoride $Ca(OH)_2$ and concluded that addition of fluoride was seen to give this material a resorption rate that matched the resorption rate of primary teeth.
- **Jeeva PP et al.**[23] used hydroxy apatite based pulpectomy medicament "Chitra HAP - Fil" is compared with Zinc oxide eugenol, Metapex to evaluate cytotoxicity and antimicrobial activity by in-vitro methods. Results showed that Metapex is significantly least toxic than Chitra HAP-Fil which was less cytotoxic than ZOE.
- **Khairwa et al.**[24] used zinc oxide and aloe vera as obturating material and concluded that endodontic treatment using a mixture of zinc oxide powder and aloe vera gel in primary teeth has shown good clinical and radiographic success. A detailed observational study with longer follow-up will highlight the benefits of aloe vera in primary teeth as an obturating medium.
- **Rewal et al.**[25] they compared the success rate of zinc oxide eugenol and endoflas, former showing success rate of 83% and latter 100% and concluded by sayinf endoflas has better results than ZOE, so former should be used as obturating material in deciduous teeth.
- **Pinto et al.**[26] compared success rate of ZOE and calen paste thickened with zinc oxide. High success rate with calen/zo was seen as this material prevented pathologic root resorption and induced new bone.
- **Cerqueira et al.**[27] confirms that Guedes pinto paste had a favorable antimicrobial activity along with an exceptional diffusion capability against all the microorganisms. Antimicrobial action of GP occurred in decreasing order against: *Bacillus subtilis, Streptococcus oralis, Streptococcus mutans, Staphylococcus epidermis, Escherichia coli, Staphylococcus aureus* and *Enterococcus faecalis.*

Iodoform Paste

- Iodoform has been added to various obturating material to improve the properties as these pastes are bactericidal.
- Castagnola showed that iodoform pastes are bactericidal to microorganisms in the root canal.
- Its disadvantages include yellowish discoloration of the tooth and irritation to periapical tissues.
- It is commercially available as Walkhoff paste, Maisto paste and Guedes-Pinto paste **(Table 55.2)**.

Table 55.2: Components of Guedes-Pinto paste proposad in 1981.

GPP Components	*Composition (per grarn)*	*Physical aspect*	*Property*
Rifocort® Merrel Leppetit	• Prednisolone acetate (corticosteroid) (5 mg)—anti-inflammatory • Rifamycin sodium salt-antibiotic • Propilenglicol–vehicle • Macrogol (polyethylene-glycol)–vehicle	Ointment	Anti-inflammatory Antibiotic
Camphorated parachloropheool (Biodinâmica)	(proportion 3:7) '30% parachlorophenol 70% camphor	Liquid	Antimicrobial Analgesic
Iodoform (K-Dent)	Iodine	Powder	Antimicrobial

Shows authors and their observations for zinc oxide eugenol.

Authors	*Observations*
Allen[8]	Speculated that the resorption rate of zinc oxide eugenol (ZOE) and the root differed, resulting in small areas of ZOE paste possibly being retained.
Barker and Lockett[6]	Material when extruded from the apex cause a mild foreign body reaction.
Barker and Lockett[6] **Speddlng**[11] **Mortazavi and Mesbahi**[2]	Stated that extruded ZOE resisted resorption and took months or even years to resorb.
Coll and Sadrian[17]	Pulpectomized teeth rarely exfoliate later than normal and timing of exfoliation was not related to retention of ZOE paste. Anterior cross-bite, palatal eruption, and ectopic eruption of the succedaneous tooth following ZOE pulpectomy.
Colletai.[15]	Reported that when ZOE extrudes, it develops a fibrous capsule that prevents resorption of the material. Thus, it has a slow rate of resorption and has a tendency to be retained even after tooth exfoliation. Areas of cementum resorption were evident, periodontal ligament exhibited intense and moderate thickening. Dentin resorption was not observed, whereas bone resorption was found.
Cox et al.[7]	Zinc oxide powder had no inhibitory effect and the addition of eugenol to zinc oxide retarded the growth of only the gram-positive organisms. The inclusion of zinc acetate as a setting accelerator inhibited both gram-positive and gram-negative bacteria.
Erasquin et al.[5]	Reported that the canals overfilled with (ZOE) are not recommended because it irritates the periapical tissues and causes necrosis of bone and cementum.
Haitz et al.[16] **Coll and Sadrían**[17]	Observed deflection of permanent tooth eruption in 20% of pulpectomized tooth that were extracted.
Garcla-Godoy,[12] **Ranly and Garcla-Godoy,**[13] **Praveen et al.**[14]	Reported deflection of developing permanent tooth bud because of Its hardness.
Hashieh et al.[20]	Studied the beneficial effects of eugenol. The amount of eugenol released in the periapical zone immediately after placement was 10-4 and falls to 10-6 after 24 hours, reaching zero after one month. Within these concentrations eugenol is said to have anti inflammatory and analgesic properties that are very useful after a pulpectomy procedure.
Holan and Fuks[4]**; Moskovitz and Samara**[10]	Malformation of successor is attributed to the cytotoxic and neurotoxic nature of eugenol.
Jerrell and Ronk[9]	Reported a case of developmental arrest of a premolar following overfilling of the root canal of the second primary molar using zinc oxide-eugenol/formocresol paste.
Loevy[18]	Premolars erupt early after primary teeth pulpotomies. Possibly a mild chronic inflammation exists in periapical area of some pulpectomies judged successful that is not clinically evident. This could cause premature eruption of succedaneous tooth and uneven resorption of pulpectomy treated tooth.
Praveen et al.[14]**; Sunitha et al.**[21]	Excess material forced through the apex during filling procedures can remain in the apical tissue during the process of physiological root resorption and it takes few months or even years to resorb.

Shows zinc oxide combinations with other materials.

Combination	Author	Observation
Zinc oxide + Propolis (ZOP)	**Al-Ostwani et al.[26]**	ZOP paste was synthesized by mixing 50% zinc oxide powder with 50% hydrolytic propolis. Triera was acceptable clinical and radiographic success rate with faster resorption seen in some cases.
Zinc oxide + Ozonated oil	**Chandra et al.[25]**	It has biological properties such as, bactericidal action, debriding effect, angiogenesis stimulation capacity and high oxidizing power (**Guinesi et al.,** 2011). After 12 months follow-up there was progressive bone regeneration at the periapical region with good clinical and radiographic success rate.
Zinc oxide eugenol (ZOE) + Calcium hydroxide [(CA(OH)$_2$] + Sodium fluoride	**Chawla et al.[23]**	Ca(OH)$_2$– demerit of resorbing at a faster rate than the physiologic root resorption. To overcome this filling material incorporated with fluoride was utilized. The addition of fluoride was seen to give this material a resorption rate that matched the resorption rate of primary teeth.
Iodoformized ZOE	**Garcia-Godoy[12]**	It was found to be effective for both aerobic and anaerobic bacteria with a maximum sustaining period of 10 days.
Zinc oxide + Calen paste	**Pinto et al.[24]**	Clinical and radiographic outcomes for calen/zo were equal to ZOE after 18 months, suggesting that both the materials can be indicated for obturation of primary teeth
Zinc oxide + Calcium hydroxide	**Praveen et al.[14]**	Obturated material remained up to the apex of root canals till the beginning of physiologic root resorption and was found to resorb at the same rate as that of primary teeth
Zinc oxide eugenol + Aldehydes	**Praveen et al.[14]; Chawla et al.[22]**	The addition of these compounds neither increased the success rate nor made the material more resorbable as compared to zinc oxide eugenol alone

Calcium Hydroxide

- Since its introduction by **Herman** Ca(OH)$_2$ has been used in various forms in dentistry. In present generation, Ca(OH)$_2$ has been used as a prime root filling material for primary teeth. It is commercially available as Vitapex® and Metapex®.
- Antibacterial effect is primarily due to the liberation of hydroxyl ions and inactivation of enzymes in the bacterial cytoplasmic membrane.
- The rate of resorption of the material from within the canals is faster than the rate of physiologic root resorption. When used in primary teeth with hyperemic pulp, Ca(OH)$_2$ comes in contact with some vital pulp tissue remnants and can trigger the cascade of inflammatory root resorption.
- Studies have reported a success rate of 80–90%.

Hollow Tube Effect

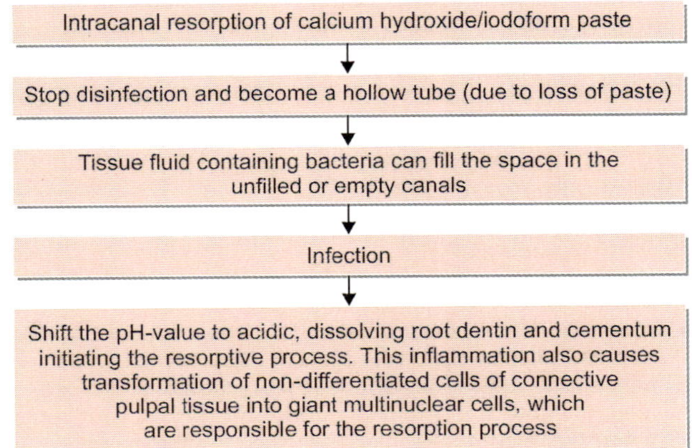
Intracanal resorption of calcium hydroxide/iodoform paste
Stop disinfection and become a hollow tube (due to loss of paste)
Tissue fluid containing bacteria can fill the space in the unfilled or empty canals
Infection
Shift the pH-value to acidic, dissolving root dentin and cementum initiating the resorptive process. This inflammation also causes transformation of non-differentiated cells of connective pulpal tissue into giant multinuclear cells, which are responsible for the resorption process

Calcium Hydroxide Combinations

- Metapex (Meta Biomed) and Vitapex (Neo Dental Chemical Products Co., Ltd, Tokyo, Japan).
- When extruded into furcal or apical areas, it can either be diffused away or resorbed in part by macrophages, in a short time as 1 or 2 weeks and causes no foreign body reaction.
- **Nurko et al.**[28] and **Kawakami et al.**[29] have reported favorable results with Vitapex® for root canal filling of primary teeth with a success rate ranging from 96 to 100%.
- **Barcelos et al.**[17] not only showed 89% of clinical success with vitapex but also showed evident resorption of material which was overfilled.

Showing antibacterial properties of Metapex reported by various authors.

Authors	Observations
Kriplani et al.[46]; Harini priya et al. [52]	Metapex has lowest antibacterial activity when compared to ZOE, Vitapex and Calcium hydroxide. However, it showed moderate activity against *Streptococcus pyogenes, Staphylococcus aureus, Enterococcus feacalis, Escherichia coli* and *Pseudomonas aeruginosa* but failed to inhibit *Candida albicans*. So, it was concluded from their study that ZOE>vitapex>Ca(OH)$_2$>metapex.
Seow et al.[56]	The weak antimicrobial activity of metapex may be partially explained by the facts that calcium hydroxide, an ingredient of metapex has been demonstrated to interfere with the antiseptic capacity of dyadic combinations of endodontic medicaments
Tchaou et al.[50]	Calcium hydroxide with iodoform had exhibited no antimicrobial activity

Showing antibacterial properties of Vitapex reported by various authors.	
Authors	***Observations***
Kripani et al.[46]; Harini prlya et al.[52]	Metapex has lowest antibacterial activity when compared to ZOE, Vitapex and Calcium hydroxide. However, it showed moderate activity against *Streptococcus pyogenes, Staphylococcus aureus, Enterococcus feacalis, Escherichia coli* and *Pseudomonas aeruginosa* but failed to inhibit *Candida albicans*. So, it was concluded from their study that ZOE>vitapex>$Ca(OH)_2$>metapex.
Seow et al.[56]	The weak antimicrobial activity of metapex may be partially explained by the facts that calcium hydroxide, an ingredient of metapex has been demonstrated to interfere with the antiseptic capacity of dyadic combinations of endodontic medicaments
Tchaou et al.[50]	Calcium hydroxide with iodoform had exhibited no antimicrobial activity

Endoflas

- Endoflas is a resorbable paste produced in South America which contains components similar to that of Vitapex, zinc oxide, and eugenol.
- This paste is obtained by mixing a powder containing tri-iodomethane and iodine dibutilorthocresol (40.6%), zinc oxide (56.5%), $Ca(OH)_2$ (1.07%), and barium sulfate (1.63%) with a liquid consisting of eugenol and paramonochlorophenol.
- The advantages are that they are hydrophilic, so used in humid canals, provide a good seal, has the ability to disinfect dentinal tubules due to its broad spectrum of antibacterial activity, and is biocompatible.
- **Ramar et al.**[30] showed 100% clinical success and 81.1% radiographic success

Authors	***Observations***
Hegde et al.[59]	Endoflas™ moderately inhibited the gram-negative and gram-positive organisms and showed strong inhibition of *Candida albicans*
Pelczar et al.[58]	The high antimicrobial activity of Endoflas™ was probably due to the presence of iodoform and eugenol, both of which have antibacterial action. Eugenol acts by protein denaturation, while iodoform is an oxidizing agent. Even after the material sets, surface hydrolysis of the chelate (zinc eugenolate) results in release of eugenol, thus

Endoflas-Chlorophenol-Free (CF)

Endoflas-chlorophenol-free (CF) was developed which is free of chlorophenol so that fixation effect which may affect the osteoblast cells is removed so as to avoid the radiolucent lesions following endodontic treatment of primary teeth.

Calen Paste with Zinc Oxide

- Calen paste is radiopaque $Ca(OH)_2$.
- Studies reveal that this combination prevented pathologic root resorption and induced new bone formation and addition of zinc oxide provides better consistency to the paste.

Pulpotec

- Pulpotec has antiseptic, antibacterial and anti-inflammatory properties with iodoform as main component.
- Pulpotec can be used in the teeth showing bone lesion and help in reduction of clinical signs of infection and can be used for treatment for necrotic primary teeth in pediatric dentistry.

Aloe vera

- Aloe vera is an herbal and naturally found material and it enhances various phases of wound healing process, such as macrophage recruitment, collagen synthesis and wound contraction.
- **Khairwa et al.**[24] evaluated clinical and radiographic success of zinc oxide combined with aloe vera and showed good success rate. They reported that this material can be used as an alternative for ZOE.

Zinc-Oxide Ozonated Oil

- Ozone is gaseous, energized form of oxygen which is a strong oxidizing agent responsible for remarkable bactericidal and fungicidal effects.
- In the study conducted by **Chandra et al.**[21] there was good clinical success rate at 12-month follow-up, which was attributed to the antibacterial and excellent healing properties of ozone peroxides. Accordingly, the authors have concluded that it can be considered as a good combination with ZOE.

Lesion Sterilization and Tissue Repair (LSTR)

- This concept was developed by Niigata University School of Dentistry.
- The theory behind lesion sterilization and tissue repair (LSTR) is that the repair of damaged tissue might occur if lesions are disinfected.
- This has also been referred to noninstrumentation endodontic treatment (NIET) which uses triple antibiotic paste mixture of metronidazole, ciprofloxacin, and minocycline.
- The walls of access cavity are chemically cleaned with ethylenediaminetetraacetic acid (EDTA) after mechanical debridement and pulpal floor is covered with three mixture antibiotic paste.
- The material can produce vascular changes in pulp, involving inflammation and formation of granulation tissue with accompanying metaplasia of the connective tissue and macrophages to form osteoclast like multinucleated giant odontoclasts. The remaining vital pulp cells proliferate and develop new pulp tissue into the coronal pulp chamber, so called pulp revascularization.

Research regarding LSTR:

- **Hoshino et al.**[31] reported that, rifampicin the component of four mixture causes discoloration of tooth.
- **Pinky et al.**[32] concluded that the antibiotics were mixed in the ratio of 1:3:3. One part ciprofloxacin, three parts metronidazole and minocycline. They also concluded that ornidazole could replace metronidazole as it had longer duration of action, with better efficacy and slower metabolism compared to metronidazole.

- **Trairatvorakul and Detsomboonrat**[33] concluded that three mixture cannot replace conventional root canal treatment.
- **Grewal et al**, [34] evaluated and compared root resorption rate of mandibular primary molars treated with alternative lesion sterilization and tissue repair and conventional endodontic treatment.
- **Agarwal etal,** [35] performed systematic review comparing LSTR and Vitapex and found that there is no difference in the success rate. At 12 months, clinically, there was no difference in the outcomes of both groups but radiographically, statistically significant difference in root resorption between treated teeth and their controls in both the groups was observed. At 36 months, interradicular bone resorption around the crown of succedaneous teeth and their delayed eruption was noted in LSTR group. LSTR therapy could be a viable treatment modality for infected/nonvital primary molars with poor prognosis and intended to be maintained for shorter duration in the oral cavity as natural space maintainers.
- **Shankar et al,**[36] compared clinical and radiographic efficacy of 1 mg/mL and 1 g/mL concentrations of modified triple antibiotic pastes containing ciprofloxacin, metronidazole, and clindamycin. Both the groups showed similar clinical success rate with no statistically significant difference.
- **Shindova**[37] in their review suggested that Knowledge of the composition and characteristics of the available obturating materials is a useful advantage to dentists to address the functional problems associated with endodontic infections in very young patients. Future studies should also seek and compare the long-term effects of the use of traditional and alternative intracanal materials.

Recent research studies regarding pulpectomy:

- **Navit et al.**[38] in 2016 did a study with an aim to assess the antimicrobial efficacy of different obturating materials used in pediatric dentistry. The results concluded that endoflas > ZOE > $Ca(OH)_2$ + chlorhexidine > $Ca(OH)_2$ + iodoform + distilled water ~ Metapex > saline.
- **Walia et al.**[39] in 2016 did a study on the state of pulp before the treatment and concluded that type of obturating paste can be a factor in the accelerated root resorption in primary teeth undergoing pulpectomy.
- **Pandranki et al.**[40] conducted study using three different methods of obturation of primary molars with endoflas was used, viz. (1) endodontic pluggers, (2) lentulo spirals and (3) NaviTips. The study concluded that motor driven lentulo spiral and pluggers were almost equally efficient to fill endoflas to an optimal level, devoid of voids, and both were considered better compared to NaviTip system.
- **Rawi**[41] conducted a study with an aim to apply blood clot technique for nonvital deciduous molars using MTA and concluded that "induction of periapical bleeding into the canal space is a necessary step in regenerative endodontic procedures of nonvital teeth and the blood clots in the canal spaces could serve as a matrix or scaffold to promote pulp tissue wound healing and brought mesenchymal stem cells from periapical area into the canal space".

APEXIFICATION

- A method of inducing apical closure by the formation of osteocementum or similar hard tissues or continued apical development of the root of an incompletely formed tooth with non-vital pulp **(Fig. 55.3)**.
- **Cohen** *It is defined as a method to induce development of the root apex of an immature pulpless tooth by formation of osteocementum/bone-like tissue.*
- **Morse et al.** (1990) *Apexification is a method of inducing apical closure through the formation of mineralized tissue in the apical pulp region of a nonvital tooth with an incompletely formed root and an open apex.*

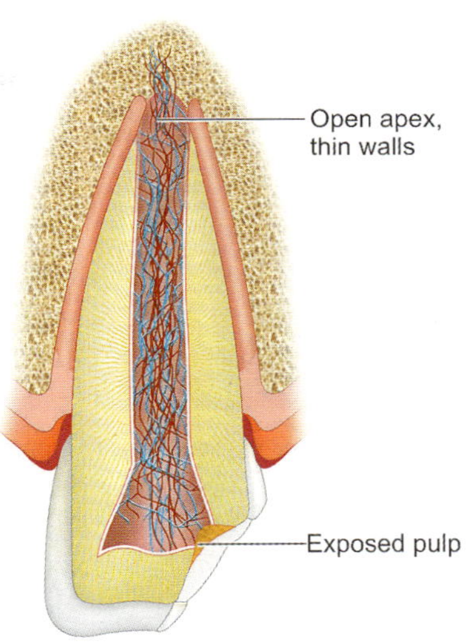

Fig. 55.3: Diagrammatic representation of open apex.

Objective

To induce either closure of open apical third of root canal or the formation of an apical calcific barrier against which obturation can be achieved.

Indication

- For nonvital permanent teeth with open apex.

Rationale

- When the pulp of an immature tooth becomes dead either due to trauma or caries, its Hertwig's epithelial sheath stops its function of root end formation. These teeth present with blunderbuss canals in which obturation by orthograde methods is nearly impossible. By the introduction of suitable medicament, apical barrier is produced at the same time length of the root is increased and canal is then obturated using thermoplasticized tech.

Types of Apex in Immature Teeth

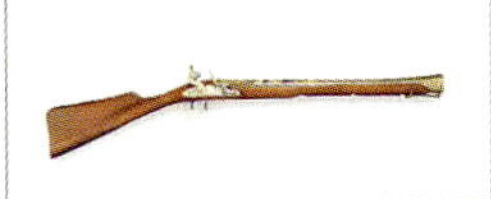

- Divergent walls with wide funnel shaped apical foramen also termed as blunderbuss apex
- Parallel or convergent walls also known as non bunderbuss apex.
- The term blunderbuss implies to an 18th century weapon with a short and wide barrel. It originates from the Dutch word 'DONDERBUS' which means 'thunder gun.'

Causes of Open Apex (Fig. 55.4)

- Caries
- Trauma
- Dentin dysplasia
- Root resoption
- Overinstrumentation
- Root end resection.

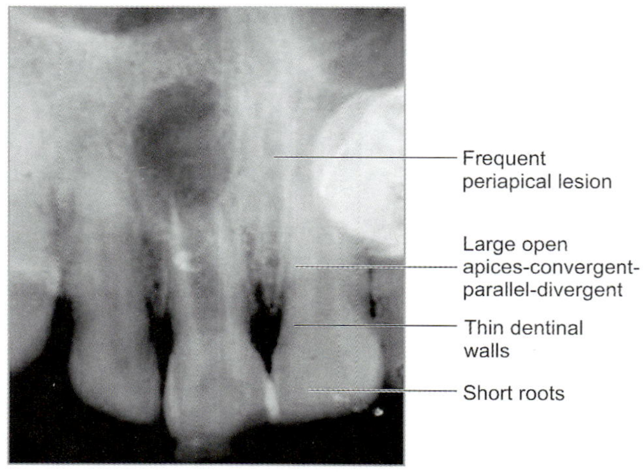

Fig. 55.4: Problems associated with Open Apex.

Difficulties Encountered While Treating Open Apex

- Disinfection of canals: There is high chance for extrusion of irrigants especially sodium hypochlorite (NaOCl). Therefore, copious irrigation with low concentration of sodium hypochlorite is done in such cases (0.5%).
- Thin roots-increased risk for fracture of teeth. Therefore, aggressive use of endodontic files should be avoided.
- Optimal sealing of rootcanal becomes difficult as no apical stop exist.

Materials Used

- Calcium hydroxide
- Mineral trioxide aggregate.
- Biodentine
- Bioceramic materials.

Calcium Hydroxide Apexification

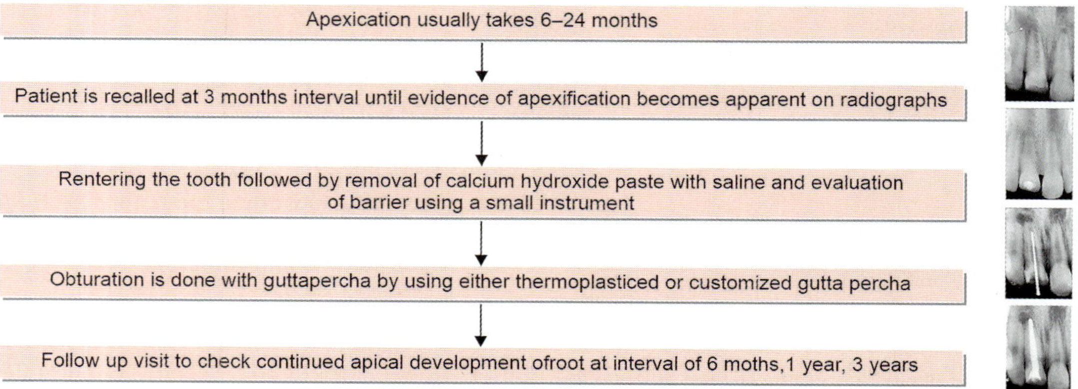

Apexication usually takes 6–24 months
Patient is recalled at 3 months interval until evidence of apexification becomes apparent on radiographs
Rentering the tooth followed by removal of calcium hydroxide paste with saline and evaluation of barrier using a small instrument
Obturation is done with guttapercha by using either thermoplasticed or customized gutta percha
Follow up visit to check continued apical development ofroot at interval of 6 moths,1 year, 3 years

Note

- If any signs of pain, swelling, infection is seen during this phase then canal is again thoroughly cleaned and disinfected and filled with calcium hydroxide paste.
- If apical barrier is not formed or inadequate then calcium hydroxide is repeated and patient is recalled until the barrier formation is achieved.

MTA Apexification

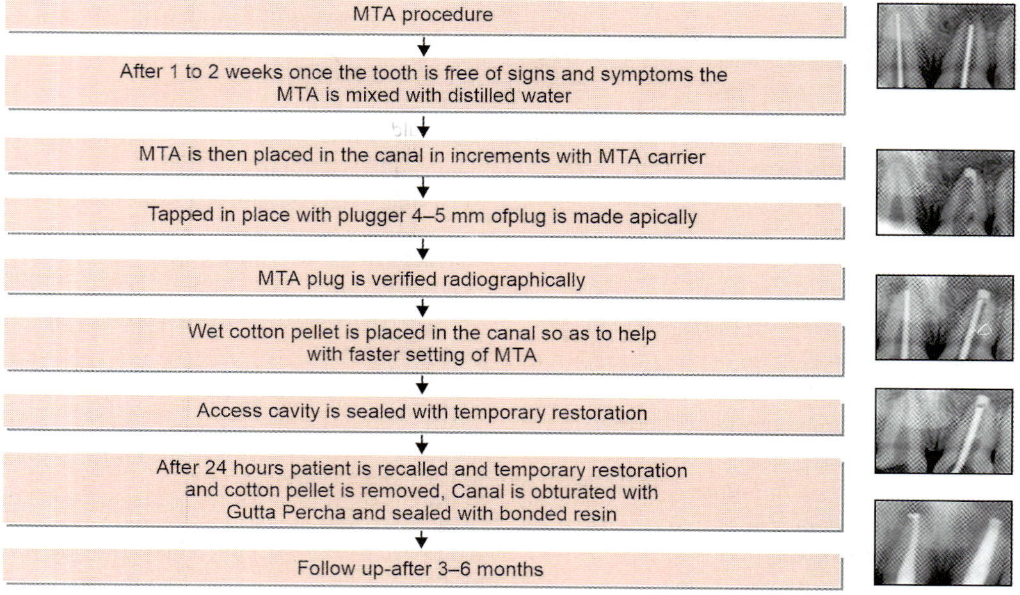

MTA procedure
After 1 to 2 weeks once the tooth is free of signs and symptoms the MTA is mixed with distilled water
MTA is then placed in the canal in increments with MTA carrier
Tapped in place with plugger 4–5 mm ofplug is made apically
MTA plug is verified radiographically
Wet cotton pellet is placed in the canal so as to help with faster setting of MTA
Access cavity is sealed with temporary restoration
After 24 hours patient is recalled and temporary restoration and cotton pellet is removed, Canal is obturated with Gutta Percha and sealed with bonded resin
Follow up-after 3–6 months

FRANK'S CRITERIA FOR APEXIFICATION (FIG. 55.5)

- Apex is closed, through minimum recession of the canal
  - Continued closure of canal and apex at a normal appearance
- Apex is closed with no change in root space
  - A dome shaped apical closure with the canal retaining a blunderbuss appearance

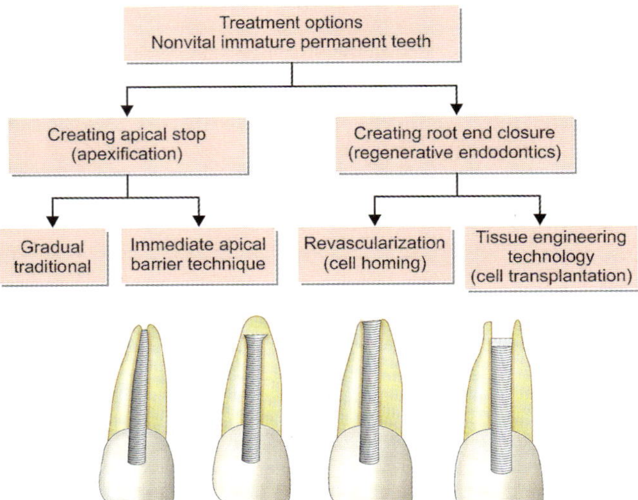

Fig. 55.5: Frank's criteria.

- Radiographically apparent calcific bridge at the apex
  - No apparent radiographic changes but a positive stop in the apical area
- There is no radiographic evidence of apical closure, but upon clinical instrumentation, there is definite stop at the apex, indicating calcific repair.
  - A positive stop and radiographic evidence of a barrier coronal to the anatomic apex of tooth
- **Shaik et al.**[42] 2021, compared success rates of MTA , Endosequence bioceramic root repair and Calcium hydroxide materials for apexification and revealed that all three of these biomaterials had similar success rates above 90%
- **Guerrero et al.**[43], 2018 opined that multiple appointments to replace calcium hydroxide was a draw back when compared to MTA which needed only to be applied once.

POINTS TO REMEMBER

- Mathewson (1995) defined pulpectomy as the complete removal of the necrotic pulp from the root canals of primary teeth and filling them with an inert resorbable material so as to maintain the tooth in the dental arch.
- Clinical indications for single-sitting pulpectomy is large carious exposure with Frank involvement of radicular pulp but without any periapical changes and for multiple-sitting pulpectomy are primary teeth with pulpal necrosis or periapical changes.
- Obturation of root canal system is done to prevent recontamination of the canal from either apical or coronal leakage and to isolate and neutralize any remaining pulpal tissue or bacteria. Various obturation methods are endodontic pressure syringe by Spedding and Krakow (1965), mechanical syringe by Greenberg (1971), tuberculin syringe by Aylard and Johnson,[2] jiffy tubes by Riffcin (1980), incremental filling with plugger, lentulo spiral technique by Kopel (1970), amalgam plugger by Nosonwitz (1960) and King (1984), paper points by Spedding (1973), plugging action with wet cotton pellet by Donnenberg (1974), and incremental filling with reamer.
- Materials used for obturation are ZOE, $Ca(OH)_2$, Vitapex®, Walkhoff paste, KRI paste, Maisto paste, mineral trioxide aggregate, and Endoflas.
- Apexification is a method of inducing apical closure by formation of a mineralized tissue in the apical region of a nonvital permanent tooth with an incompletely formed root apex. Indicated for nonvital permanent teeth with open apex (blunderbuss canals).
- Frank's criteria for apexification is apex is closed, through minimum recession of the canal; apex is closed with no change in root space; radiographically apparent calcific bridge at the apex; there is no radiographic evidence of apical closure, but upon clinical instrumentation, there is definite stop at the apex, indicating calcific repair.

Questionnaire

1. Define pulpectomy and give its indications and contraindications.
2. Explain the procedure of pulpectomy.
3. Enumerate materials used for obturation of primary teeth and explain its ideal properties.
4. What are the techniques used for obturation of primary teeth?
5. Differentiate between apexogenesis and apexification.
6. What is the procedure of apexification?
7. Write a note on Frank's criteria of apexification.

REFERENCES

1. Mahajan N, Bansal A. Various obturation methods used in deciduous teeth. Int J Med Dent Sci. 2015;4:708-13.
2. Aylard SR, Johnson R. Assessment of filling techniques for primary teeth. Pediatr Dent. 1987;9:195-8.
3. Gould JM. Root canal therapy for infected primary molar teeth: preliminary report. J Dent Child. 1972;39:269-73.
4. Nagar P, Araali V, Ninawe N. An alternative obturating technique using insulin syringe delivery system to traditional reamer: an in-vivo study. J Dent Oral Biosci. 2011;2: 7-19.
5. Grover R, Mehra M, Pandit IK, et al. Clinical efficacy of various root canal obturating methods in primary teeth: a comparative study. Eur J Paediatr Dent. 2013;14:104-8.
6. Dandashi MB, Nazif MM, Zullo T, et al. An in vitro comparison of three endodontic techniques for primary incisors. Pediatr Dent. 1993;15:254-6.
7. Torres CP, Apicella MJ, Yancich PP, et al. Intracanal placement of calcium hydroxide: a comparison of techniques, revisited. J Endod. 2004;30:225-7.
8. Sigurdsson A, Stancill R, Madison S. Intracanal placement of Ca(OH)2: a comparison of techniques. J Endod. 1992;18:367-70.
9. Deonízio MD, Sydney GB, Batista A, et al. Root canal filling with calcium hydroxide paste using Lentulo spiral at different speeds. Dent Press Endod. 2011;1:58-63.

10. Memarpour M, Shahidi S, Meshki R. Comparison of different obturation techniques for primary molars by digital radiography. Pediatr Dent. 2013;35:236-40.
11. Aminabadi NA, Asl Aminabadi N, Jamali Z, Shirazi S. Primary tooth pulpectomy overfilling by different placement techniques: A systematic review and meta-analysis. J Dent Res Dent Clin Dent Prospects. 2020 Fall;14(4):250-61.
12. Nagaveni NB, Yadav S, Poornima P, Bharath KP, Mathew MG, Naveen Kumar PG. Volumetric evaluation of various obturation techniques in primary teeth using cone beam computed tomography - An in vitro study. J Indian Soc Pedod Prev Dent. 2017;35(3):244-48.
13. Singh A, Gupta N, Agarwal N, Kumar D, Anand A. A Comparative Volumetric Evaluation of Four Obturating Techniques in Primary Teeth Using Cone Beam Computed Tomography. Pediatr Dent. 2017 Mar 15;39(2):11-16.
14. Rajsheker S, Mallineni SK, Nuvvula S. Obturating materials used for pulpectomy in primary teeth—a mini review. J Dent Craniofac Res. 2018;3:3.
15. Barr ES, Flaitz CM, Hicks JM. A retrospective radiographic evaluation of primary molar pulpectomies. Pediatr Dent. 1991;13:4-9.
16. Coll JA, Josell S, Casper JS. Evaluation of a one-appointment formocresol pulpectomy technique for primary molars. Pediatr Dent. 1985;7:123-9.
17. Barcelos R, Santos MP, Primo LG, et al. ZOE paste pulpectomies outcome in primary teeth: a systematic review. J Clin Pediatr Dent. 2011;35:241-8.
18. Praveen P, Anantharaj A, Karthik V, et al. A review of the obturating material for primary teeth. SRM Univ J Dent Sci. 2011;1:1-3.
19. Hashieh IA, Ponnmel L, Camps J. Concentration of eugenol apically released from ZnO E based sealers. J Endod. 1999;22:713-5.
20. Al-Ostwani AO, Al-Monaqel BM, Al-Tinawi MK. A clinical and radiographic study of four different root canal fillings in primary molars. J Indian Soc Pedod Prev Dent. 2016;34:55-9.
21. Chandra SP, Chandrasekhar R, Uloopi KS, et al. Success of root fillings with zinc oxide–ozonated oil in primary molars: preliminary results. Eur Arch Paediatr Dent. 2014;15:191-5.
22. Chawla HS, Setia S, Gupta N, et al. Evaluation of a mixture of zinc oxide, calcium hydroxide, and sodium fluoride as a new root canal filling material for primary teeth. J Indian Soc Pedod Prev Dent. 2008;26:53-8.
23. Jeeva PP, Retnakumari N. In-vitro comparision of cytotoxicity and anti-microbial activity of three pulpectomy medicaments- Zinc oxide euginol,Metapex and Chitra HAP – Fill. IOSR Journal of Dental and Medical Sciences. 2014; 13(2):40-7.
24. Khairwa A, Bhat M, Sharma R, et al. Clinical and radiographic evaluation of zinc oxide with aloe vera as an obturating material in pulpectomy: an in vivo study. J Indian Soc Pedod Prev Dent. 2014;32:33-8.
25. Rewal N, Thakur AS, Sachdev V, Mahajan N. Comparison of Endoflass and Zoe as root canal fillng material in primary dentition. JISPPD. 2014;32: 317-21.
26. Pinto DN, Sousa DL, Araujo RB, Moreira JJ. 18 month clinical and radiographic evaluation of two root canal filling materials in primary teeth with pulp necrosis secondary to trauma. Dent Traumat. 2011;3: 221-24.
27. Cerqueira DF, Moura AC, Santos EM, Guedes Pinto. Cytotoxicity, histopathological and clinical aspect of endodontic iodoform paste used in Pediatrc Dentistry. J Clin Ped Dent 2007;32:105-10.
28. Nurko C, Garcia-Godoy F. Evaluation of a calcium hydroxide/ iodoform paste (Vitapex) in root canal therapy for primary teeth. J Clin Pediatr Dent. 1999;23:289-94.
29. Kawakami T, Nakamura C, Eda S. Effects of the penetration of a root canal filling material into the mandibular canal. Tissue reaction to the material. Endod Dent Traumatol. 1991;7:36-41.
30. Ramar K, Mungara J. Clinical and radiographical evaluation of pulpectomies using three root canal filling materials: an in vivo study. J Indian Soc Pedod Prev Dent. 2010;28:25-9.
31. Hoshino E, Kurihara-Ando N, Sato I. In-vitro antibacterial susceptibility of bacteria taken from infected root dentine to a mixture of ciprofloxacin, metronidazole and minocycline. Int Endod J. 1996;29:125-30.
32. Pinky C, Shashibhushan KK, Subbareddy VV. Endodontic treatment of necrosed primary teeth using two different combinations of antibacterial drugs: an in vivo study. J Indian Soc Pedod Prev Dent. 2011;29:121-7.
33. Trairatvorakul C, Detsomboonrat P. Success rates of a mixture of ciprofloxacin, metronidazole, and minocycline antibiotics used in the non-instrumentation endodontic treatment of mandibular primary molars with carious pulpal involvement. Int J Paediatr Dent. 2012;22:217-27.
34. Grewal N, Sharma N, Chawla S. Comparison of resorption rate of primary teeth treated with alternative lesion sterilization and tissue repair and conventional endodontic treatment: An in vivo randomized clinical trial. J Indian Soc Pedod Prev Dent. 2018;36(3):262-7.
35. Agarwal SR, Bendgude VD, Kakodkar P. Evaluation of Success Rate of Lesion Sterilization and Tissue Repair Compared to Vitapex in Pulpally Involved Primary Teeth: A Systematic Review. J Conserv Dent. 2019;22(6):510-15.
36. Shankar K, Ramkumar H, Dhakshinamoorthy S, Paulindraraj S, Jayakaran TG, Bommareddy CS. Comparison of Modified Triple Antibiotic Paste in Two Concentrations for Lesion Sterilization and Tissue Repair in Primary Molars: An In Vivo Interventional Randomized Clinical Trial. Int J Clin Pediatr Dent. 2021;14(3):388-392.
37. Shindova M. Root canal filling materials in primary teeth - review. Folia Med (Plovdiv). 2021;63(5):657-662.
38. Navit S, Jaiswal N, Khan SA, et al. Antimicrobial efficacy of contemporary obturating materials used in primary teeth—an in-vitro study. J Clin Diagn Res. 2016;10: ZC09-12.
39. Walia T. Pulpectomy in hyperemic pulp and accelerated root resorption in primary teeth: a review with associated case report. J Indian Soc Pedod Prev Dent. 2014;32:255-61.
40. Pandranki J, Chitturi RR, Vanga NV, et al. A comparative assessment of different techniques for obturation with endoflas in primary molars: an in vivo study. Indian J Dent Res. 2017;28:44-8.
41. Rawi B. A new era in treatment of non-vital primary molars: one year follow-up study. Dentistry. 2018;8:468.
42. Shaik I, Dasari B, Kolichala R, Doos M, Qadri F, Arokiyasamy JL. et al. Comparison of the success rate of mineral trioxide aggregate, endosequence bioceramic root repair material, and calcium hydroxide for apexification of immature permanent teeth: systematic review and meta-analysis. Journal of Pharmacy & Bioallied Sciences, 2021;13(Suppl 1):S43-S47.
43. Guerrero F, Mandoza A, Rivas D, Asipiazu K. Apexification: A sysytemic review. J Cons Dent 2018;21: 462-5

FURTHER READING

1. AAPD guidelines
2. Camp J. Pediatric endodontics: endodontic treatment for the primary and young permanent dentition. In: Cohen S, Burns RC (Eds). Pathways of the Pulp, 8th edition. St. Louis: Mosby;2002.
3. McDonald RE, Avery DR, Dean JA. Treatment of deep caries, vital pulp exposure, and pulpless teeth: In: McDonald RE, Avery DR, Dean JA (Eds). Dentistry for the Child and Adolescent, 8th edition. St. Louis: Mosby;2004.

CHAPTER

Rotary Endodontics in Primary Molars

Thejokrishna Pammi, Satish Vishwanathaiah, Manu Bansal, Abhishek Khairwa, Rajesh Kumar, Nilesh Rathi, Ganesh J

CHAPTER OUTLINE

Over the decades premature exfoliation of primary teeth due to necrosis of pulp of deciduous tooth is considered one of the main concern in Pediatric Dentistry. Recently pulpectomy gained the popularity as the choice of treatment over the extraction for such tooth to maintain them in the arch. In pediatric endodontics time efficacy is very important due to unpredictability of the patient and difficulty of root canal morphology. Endodontics in primary teeth can be challenging and time consuming, especially during canal preparation which is considered as one of the most important steps in root canal therapy. Although root canal instrumentation is performed widely with hand instruments, the time efficacy and patient cooperation is still the challenge. To overcome such challenges rotary endodontic systems are introduced in Pediatric Dentistry.

Barr (2000) introduced the rotary endodontics in pediatric dentistry. Endodontic treatment in primary molars has experienced continuous evolutions with advent to science and technology. We have observed, from extraction as solution to pulp involved primary tooth to use of hand files in similar to permanent teeth endodontics, gradually evolved to rotary files.

We have applied the science evolved from permanent tooth endodontics to primary molars since the beginning. We employed all instruments used in permanent tooth to primary tooth. Be it hand files, instruments or rotary files. Considering that rotary files are more convenient to use and can facilitate root canal treatment, their application may be more appropriate in children with behavior management problems.

But the dynamics that operate in primary tooth endodontics are different form that in permanent tooth. Permanent tooth endodontics is primary concerned with biomechanical preparation creating pathway to reach the complex apical delta, followed by disinfection and preparation of apex so as to provide way to root canal sealer and gutta-percha leading to hermetic seal.

CLASSIFICATION AND DEVELOPMENT OF ROTARY SYSTEMS

The first description of the use of rotary devices was given by **Oltramare**. He reported the use of fine needles with a rectangular cross-section, which could be mounted into a dental handpiece. In 1889, **William H Rollins** developed the first endodontic handpiece for automated root canal preparation. In 1928, the 'cursor filing contra-angle' was developed by the Austrian company W&H (Bürmoos, Austria). This handpiece created a combined rotational and vertical motion of the file. Finally, endodontic handpieces became popular in Europe with the marketing of the Racer-handpiece (W&H) in 1958 and the Giromatic (Micro-Méga, Besançon, France) in 1964. A period of modified endodontic handpieces began with the introduction of the Canal Finder System (SET, Gröbenzell, Germany) by Levy. Some of the rotary systems are developed over period of time.

Rotary FRF system.		
Handpiece	***Manufacturer***	***Mode of action***
	Conventional systems	
Racer	Cardex, via W&H, Bürmoos, Austria	Vertical movement
Giromatic	Micro-Méga, Besançon, France	Reciprocal rotation (90°)
Endo-Gripper	Moyco Union Broach, Montgomeryville, PA, USA	Reciprocal rotation (90°)
Endolift	Sybron Endo, Orange, CA, USA	Vertical movement + reciprocal rotation (90°)
	Flexible systems	
Excalibur	W&H	Lateral oscillations (2000 Hz, 1.4–2 mm amplitude)
Endoplaner	Microna, Spreitenbach, Switzerland	Vertical motion + free rotation
Canal-Finder-system	SET, Gröbenzell, Munich	Vertical movement (0.3–1 mm) + free rotation under friction
	Sonic systems	
Sonic Air 3000	Micro-Méga	
Endostar 5	Medidenta Int, Woodside, NY, USA	6,000 Hz
	Ultrasonic systems	
Cavi-Endo	Dentsply DeTrey	Magnetostrictive 25,000 Hz
	Ni-Ti systems	
Lightspeed	Lightspeed, San Antonio TX, USA	Rotation (360°)
ProTaper	Dentsply Maillefer, Ballaigues, Switzerland	Rotation (360°)
K3	Sybron Endo	Rotation (360°)
Profile 0.04 and 0.06	Dentsply Maillefer	Rotation (360°), taper 0.4–0.8
HERO 642	Micro-Mega	Rotation (360°), taper 0.02–0.06

Light-speed instrument	***ProFile instrument***	***GT rotary instrument***	***K3 instrument***	***HERO instrument***	***Race instrument***	***ProTaper instrument***
• Appeared like Gates-Glidden drill • Used in beginning of 1990 • Low torque handpiece at 1500 rpm • Disadvantage is too many instruments in sequence	• First rotary Ni-Ti • Developed in 1994 • Blunt noncutting tip • Used at high torque of 150–300 rpm • Disadvantage of high fracture incidence	Noncutting end with variable tapers	• Designed by McSpadden • 0.02–0.06 tapers • Better cutting efficiency • 350–500 rpm	• Second generation that put positive rake angle in its design Looks like H-file • High torque low speed at 300–600 rpm • Available in sizes of 25–40 with variable tapers • New version is HERO Shaper	• Appears like reamer with alternate cutting edges • Triangular and square taper • Advantage is more flexibility • Noncutting tip • Operates with low torque handpiece at 600–700 rpm	• Design has variable taper along the length • Triangular cross-section • Appears like modified K-file • Comprises of 3 files each of shaping and finishing type • High torque 150–300 rpm

Generations of Rotary Systems

1st generation files	***2nd generation files***	***3rd generation files***	***4th generation files***	***5th generation files***
Passive cutting radial lands	Active cutting edges	Reduces cyclic fatigue	Single-file technique	Safest, most efficient, and simplest file systems
Fixed tapers of 4% and 6%	Mitigate taper lock	Reduced broken files	Due to its compressible open tube design, it exert uniform pressure on the dentinal walls, regardless of the cross-sectional configuration of the canal	Offset design in the file minimize the engagement between the file and dentin, enhances auguring debris out of a canal and improves flexibility along the active portion of a ProTaperNext file
Numerous files to achieve the preparation objectives	Fixed tapered design	Heat treatment technology, twisted file	Have a reciprocating movement that is equal clockwise and counterclockwise rotation and requires more inward pressure to progress	Offset design and produce a mechanical wave of motion that travels along the active length of the file

ROTARY INSTRUMENT DESIGN

Tip Design

Tip of a instrument: Guide the file through the canal and enlarges the canal.

Two Types

1. **Active/cutting tip:**
   - It has cutting edges on its surface helps to shape the narrow, calcified canals.
   - Disadvantage of accidental apical perforation or transportation.
   - E.g., Quantec file.
2. **Passive/non-cutting tip:** No cutting edges present create a concentric circle at the end of the root.
   E.g., Profile, GT, lightspeed.

Instrument Taper

Taper denotes the per millimeter increase in file diameter from the tip towards the file handle.

Types

1. **Constant taper:** E.g., Profile system.
2. **Varying or graduating taper:** E.g., Quantec system.
3. **Progressive taper:** E.g., ProTaper system.

As the taper increases diameter of instrument increase and it leads to increase in the rigidity of instrument.

Feature is incorporated to:
- Reduce canal transportation
- Screwing in forces
- Supports the cutting edge
- Limits the depth of cut.

Flute

It is the groove in the working surface used to collect soft tissue and dentin chips removed from the wall of the canal.

The effectiveness of the flute depends on its depth, width, configuration, and surface finish.

Radial Land

The surface that projects axially from the central axis as far as the cutting edge between the flutes.

Functions

- Prevents "screwing in" of the file
- Supports the cutting edge
- Limits the depth of cut
- Reduces the propagation of microcracks on its circumference.
- Maintains the file in the center of root canal

Helix/Helical Angle

The angle the cutting-edge forms with the long axis of the file.

Constant Helical Angle

- Cutting efficiency is less
- More debris accumulation especially on coronal portion of instrument
- More susceptible to "Screwing In" effect

Variable Helical Angle

- Better cutting efficiency
- Better debris removal
- Less chances of "Screwing In" effect

Rake Angle

Rake angle is the angle formed by the leading edge and the long axis of the file.

Positive/Cutting Rake Angle

Angle formed by the leading edge and the surface to be cut (its tangent) is obtuse.

Negative/Scrapping Rake Angle

If the angle formed by the leading edge and the surface to be cut is acute.

Composition and Properties of Some Ni-Ti Files Used in Rotary Endodontics

NiTi system	*Alloy*	*Composition*	*Properties*	*Recommended use*
Hyflex CM	CM wire	Martensite with different amounts of austenite and R-phase	• No superelasticity • High resistance to cyclic fatigue • Increased flexibility	• Severely curved canals • Bypassing ledges
Hyflex EDM	CM wire; EDM technology	No austenite phase	• Increased cutting efficiency • Increased cyclic fatigue resistance	• Straighter canals • Used in combination with Hyflex CM in severely curved canals
BT-RaCe	Conventional Ni-Ti	Austenite-electropolished	• Triangular cross-section • Booster tip	• Conservative instrumentation of all types of canals • Original canal shape maintained
Vortex Blue and ProTaper Gold	M-wire	Martensite TiO_2 layer on surface	• Shape memory • Superelasticity • Increased cyclic fatigue resistance	• Severely curved canals • Bypassing ledges
XP-endo Shaper XP-endo Finisher	Max-wire		• High resistance to cyclic fatigue • Superelasticity • Shape memory	• Complex root canal morphology
2Shape	T-wire		• Asymmetric cross-section • Additional cutting edges	• Complex root canal morphology
One Curve	C wire		• Increased flexibility • Better cyclic fatigue resistance	• Complex root canal morphology

Pitch

The pitch of the file is the distance between a point on the leading edge and the corresponding point on the adjacent leading edge.

The smaller the pitch or the shorter the distance between corresponding points, the more spirals the file will have and the greater the helix angle will be.

Most files have a variable pitch, that changes along the working surface.

ROTARY ENDODONTICS IN PRIMARY TOOTH

The objective of use of rotary files in primary molars is different from permanent molars. Root canal debridement is primary objective of root canal instrumentation in primary molars, whereas in permanent teeth it is biomechanical preparation leading to ideal shaping of canals to receive gutta-percha.

Ideal Requisites of Pediatric Rotary Files

- It should have optimum length for preparation of canal with no excess length.
- It should be flexible to maintain the canal centricity.
- Effective debridement of the root canal without weakening the tooth structure or endangering the underlining permanent teeth (**Lin** et al. 2006).

Rationale of Rotary Endodontics[1,2]

- Instrumentation time is reduced.
- Improved cleaning efficiency.
- Comfortable for the patient.
- It changes the morphology of primary root canals from ribbon shaped irregular root canal to conical shape, which favors higher density and quality of root canal filling.
- The extrusion of debris apically is less in rotary as compared to hand K-files.

Types of Rotary Endodontics System for Primary Tooth

The generations of files that are frequently used for permanent teeth have limitations while using them in primary teeth as they have thinner curved roots with ribbon-shaped morphology increasing the chance of lateral perforation. Apart from this, the longer file length makes it difficult to work in pediatric patient and this created the requirement of pediatric endodontic rotary files. Some systems that were used for pediatric endodontics are ProFile 0.4 (Dentsply), ProTaper (Dentsply) **(Figs. 56.1A to C)**, HERO 642 (Micro-Méga) **(Figs. 56.2A to C)**. The disadvantage initially permanent tooth rotary instruments/files with taper varying from 11 to 19% were employed **(Figs. 56.3A and B)**, primarily due to nonavailability of lower taper files.

With increased evidence of their safety in primary molars, rotary files specifically for primary molars began to develop. Currently most rotary instruments are less taper (4–12%) M type of Ni-Ti alloy, augmenting endurance to cyclic fatigue and fracture, adding more safety features to the files. Rotary files for primary tooth are available in India, with lengths varying from 12 to 18 mm and taper 2 to 12%.

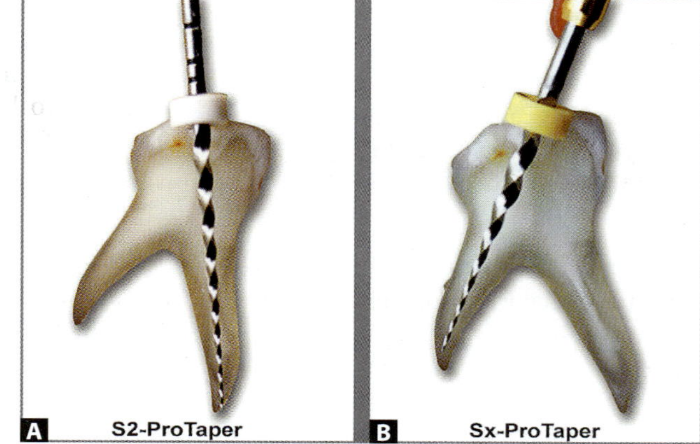

Figs. 56.3A and B: ProTaper S files.

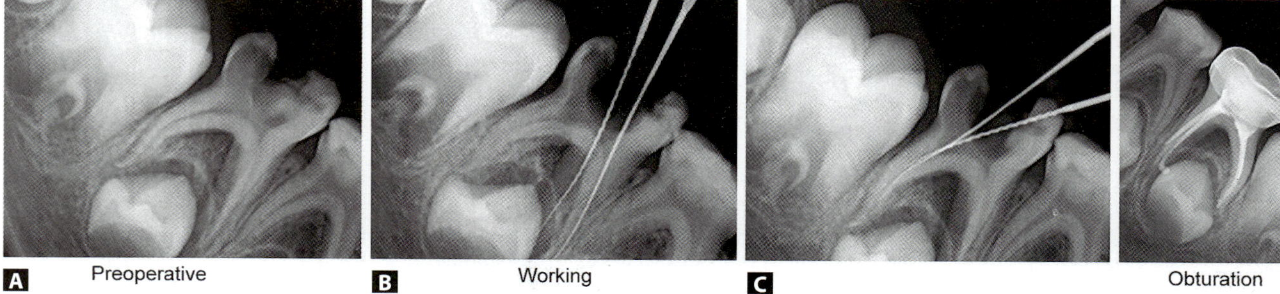

Figs. 56.1A to C: Case with protaper. (*Picture courtesy:* Dr Parth Shah).

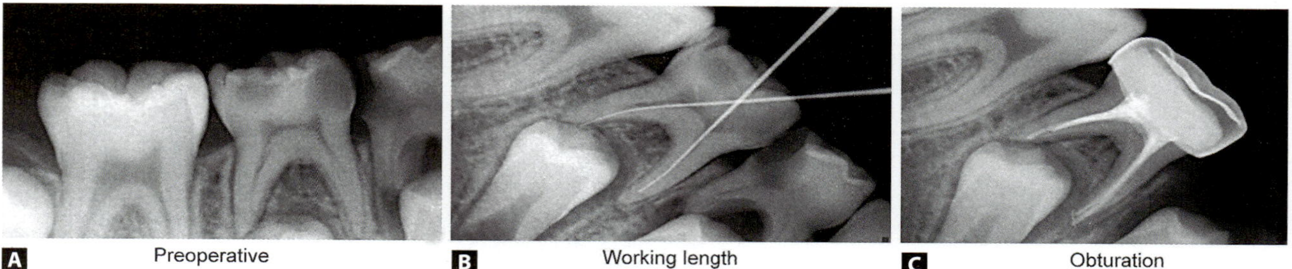

Figs. 56.2A to C: Case with HERO shaper. (*Pic courtesy:* Dr Parth Shah).

The systems which are currently used for primary tooth:

- Kedo S—Primary rotary files:
  - Kedo S rotary files—1st generation Kedo S file system
  - Kedo SG rotary files—2st generation Kedo S file system
  - Kedo SG blue file—3st generation Kedo S file system
  - Kedo S square—4st generation Kedo S file system
- Prime pedo
- Pro-AF-Baby-Gold rotary files
- Pro-AF Baby blue file system
- DXL Pro™ files

Working Length Establishment in Primary Tooth[3]

In primary tooth, we have a dynamically shifting apex related to time. This is the zone consisting of odontoclastic cells along with granulation tissue. It is noninflammatory and histological part of healthy apex in primary tooth. That is responsible for physiologic resorption. Similar situation in permanent tooth apex is seen only in pathologic conditions.

Therefore, biomechanical shaping of canals as in permanent tooth endodontics cannot be applied here. Instrumenting the dynamically shifting apex is not prudent. Over instrumentation can trigger foreign body reaction leading to accelerated root resorption, chronic periapical irritation/infection and sometimes accompanied injury to successor. Hence, limiting the working length by 1–2 mm of radiographic apex assures safety in primary tooth endodontics. So, a trial length is obtained by measuring the tooth on the preoperative radiograph and subtracting 1–2 mm. A small diameter file is placed into the canal to the trial length and another exposure taken from which the working length is determined. Whenever possible, all radiographs should be taken utilizing the paralleling technique in order to minimize distortions. The working length should be 1–2 mm short of the radiographic apex ideally. If obvious signs of root resorption are present, it may be necessary to further shorten the working length by an additional 1–2 mm in order to avoid overextension of the instruments into the periapical tissues.

For ensuring safety all endodontic treatment to be done under rubber dam. In cases where rubber dam application is not feasible, then use #25, 2% gutta-percha cones to verify tentative working length. Always tag hand files with at least 15–20 cm length dental floss or nylon thread, to retrieve incase of accidental ingestion or aspiration of files.

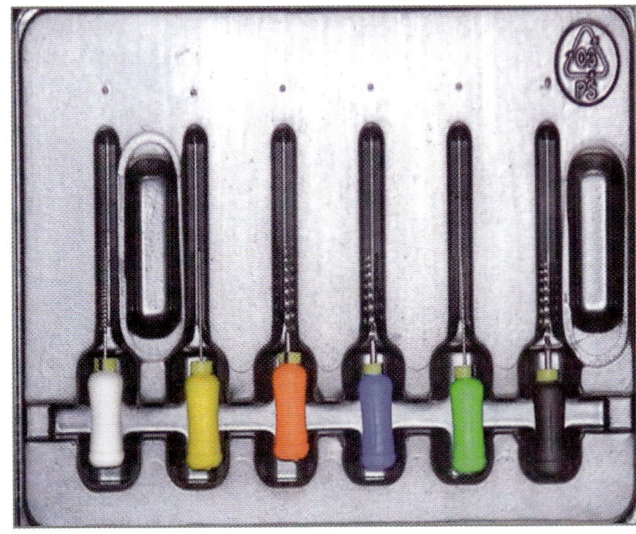

Fig. 56.4: Kedo-SH.

KEDO FILES

Kedo files was introduced by Ganesh Jeevanandan in the year 2016. Kedo file system consists of hand files and rotary files which are exclusive designed for primary teeth. Kedo rotary file system consist of Kedo-S, Kedo-SG and Kedo-SG blue. These Ni-Ti rotary files with variably variable taper designs providing the flexibility and efficiency to achieve consistently successful cleaning and shaping.

Kedo hand system	*Kedo rotary system*
• Kedo-SH	• Kedo-S
	• Kedo-SG
	• Kedo-SG blue

Kedo-SH Files

Kedo-SH **(Fig. 56.4)** is a hand file system which consist of series of files. The file system consists of P1, P2, P3 stainless steel files and D1, E1 and U1 nickel-titanium files. The total length of the file is 16 mm with a flute length of 12 mm. **Table 56.2** shows features of Kedo-SH files.

Table 56.2: Features of Kedo-SH files.

File series	*File design*	*Color*	*Tip diameter*	*Taper*	*Material used*	*Use*
P1	K- file	White	0.15	2%	Stainless-steel	Initial patency of molar canals
P2	H-file	Yellow	0.20	2%	Stainless-steel	Pulp extirpation in molar canals
P3	H-file	Green	0.35	2%	Stainless-steel	Patency/pulp extirpation in anterior canals
D1	Triangular	Red	0.25	4–8% VV taper	Nickel-titanium	Shaping of narrower molar canals
E1	Triangular	Blue	0.30	4–8% VV taper	Nickel-titanium	Shaping of wider molar canals
U1	Triangular	Black	0.40	4–8% VV taper	Nickel-titanium	Shaping of anterior teeth

Technique Using Kedo-SH Files (Figs. 56.5A and B)

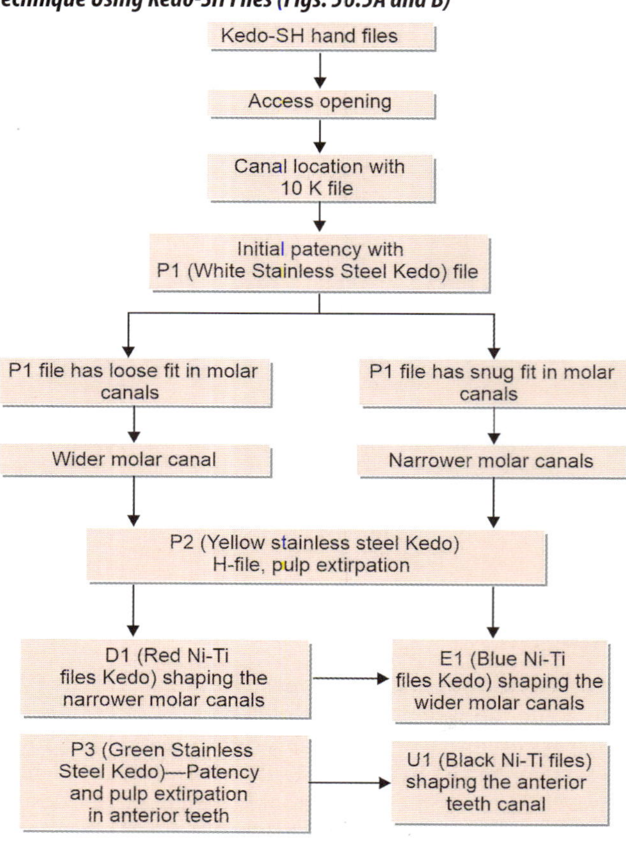

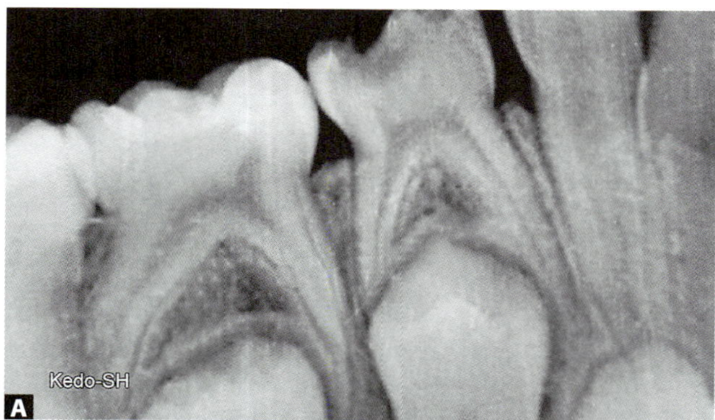

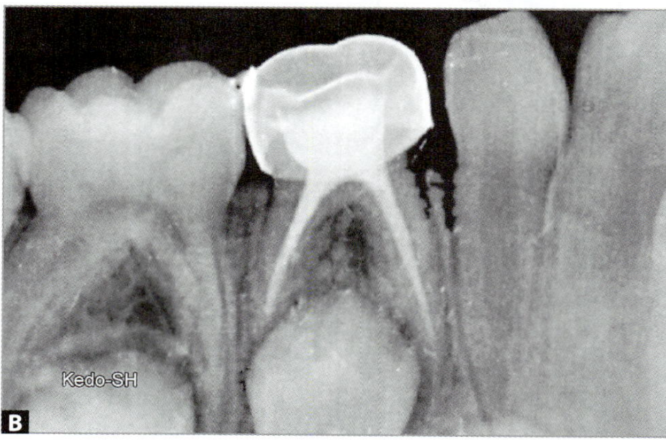

Figs. 56.5A and B: Case for Kedo-SH files. (*Pic courtesy*: Dr Ganesh Jeevanandan).

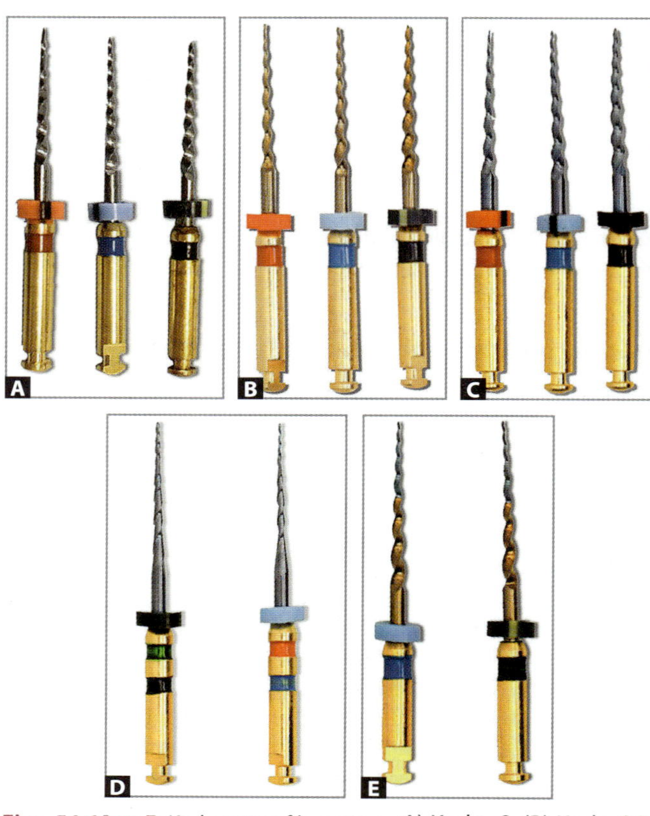

Figs. 56.6A to E: Kedo rotary file system: (A) Kedo- S; (B) Kedo-SG; (C) Kedo-SG blue; (D) Kedo-S square (E) Kedo-S plus.

Kedo Rotary

Kedo rotary file system **(Figs. 56.6A to E)** consist of Kedo-S, Kedo-SG, Kedo-SG blue, Kedo-S square, Kedo-S plus. These Ni-Ti rotary files with variably variable taper designs providing the flexibility and efficiency to achieve consistently successful cleaning and shaping. **Table 56.3** shows comparison of different Kedo rotary files.

Technique for Using Kedo Rotary Files (Figs. 56.7A and B)

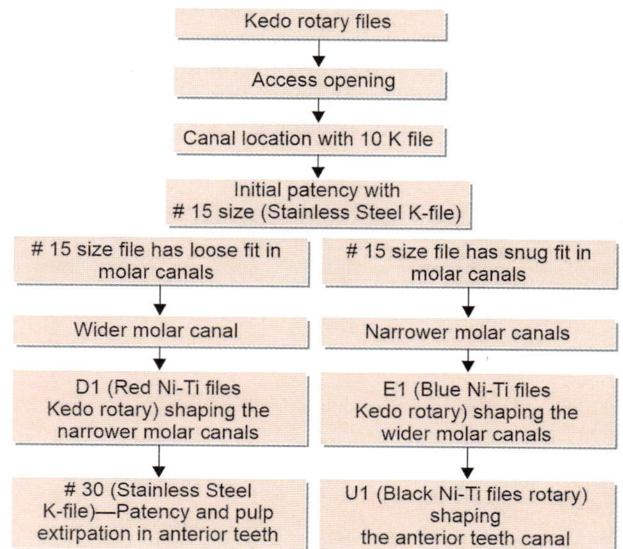

Table 56.3: Comparison of Kedo rotary files.

Features	*Kedo-S*	*Kedo-SG*	*Kedo-SG blue*	*Kedo-S square*	*Kedo-S plus*
Length	16 mm length,12 mm flutes	16 mm length,12 mm flutes	16 mm length,12 mm flutes	16 mm length,12 mm flutes	16 mm length,12 mm flutes
Taper	4–8% variably variable taper	4–8% variably variable taper	4–8% variably variable taper	4–8% variably variable taper	4–8% variably variable taper
Metallurgy	Nickel-Titanium rigid	Nickel-Titanium heat treated: Controlled memory	Nickel-Titanium heat treated with blue titanium oxide layer: Controlled memory	Nickel-Titanium heat treated with blue titanium oxide layer: Controlled memory	Nickel-Titanium heat treated with blue titanium oxide layer: Controlled memory
File series	D1, E1 and U1	D1, E1 and U1	D1, E1 and U1	P1 and A1	D1, E1 and U1
Color coded	D1-Red, E1-Blue and U1-Black	D1-Red, E1-Blue and U1-Black	D1-Red, E1-Blue and U1-Black	P1-Red and Blue A1-Green and Black	P1+-Blue A1+-Black
Tip diameter	D1-0.25, E1-0.30 and U1-0.40	D1-0.25, E1-0.30 and U1-0.40	D1-0.25, E1-0.30 and U1-0.40	P1-0.28 and A1-0.38	P1+-0.28 and A1+-0.38
Clinical use	D1–Narrower molar canals E1–Wider molar canals U1–Anterior canals	D1–Narrower molar canals E1–Wider molar canals U1–Anterior canals	D1–Narrower molar canals E1–Wider molar canals U1–Anterior canals	P1– Molar canals and A1–Anterior canals	P1+-Molar canals and A1+-Anterior canals

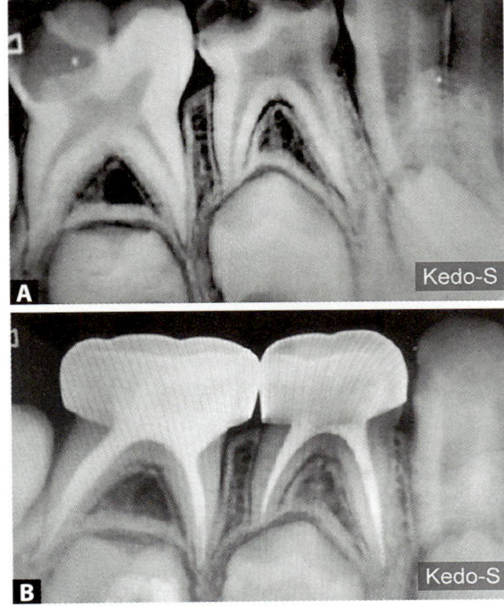

Figs. 56.7A and B: Case for kedo rotary files. (*Pic courtesy:* Dr Ganesh Jeevanandan).

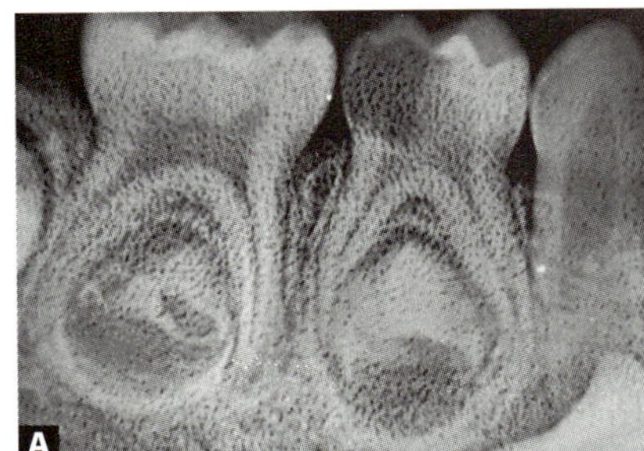

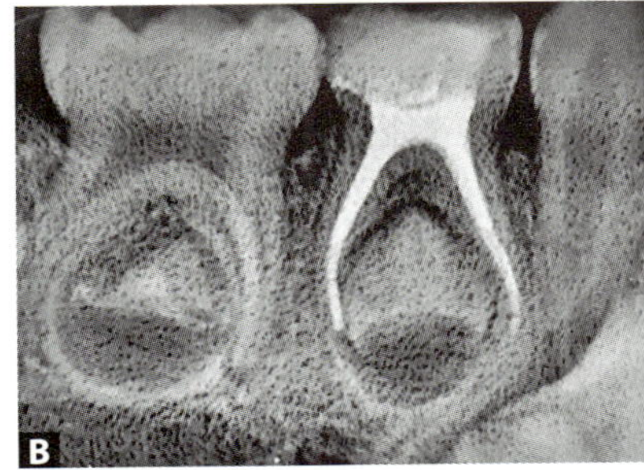

Figs. 56.8A and B: Case for Kedo-S square and Kedo-S plus rotary files. (*Pic courtesy:* Dr Ganesh Jeevanandan).

Technique for Using Kedo- S Square and Kedo-S Plus Rotary Files (Figs. 56.8A and B)

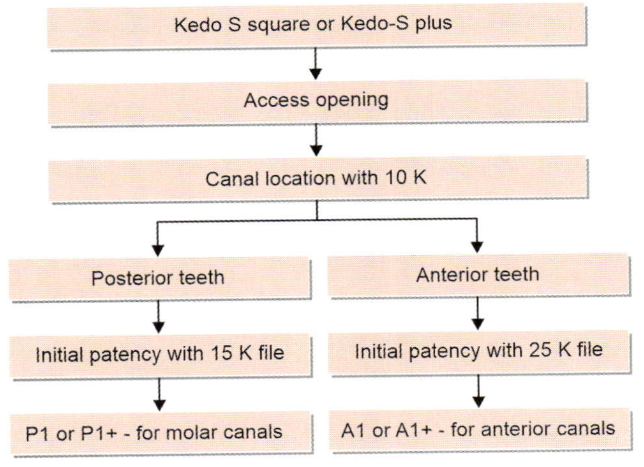

PRIME PEDO FILES

Prime Pedo rotary files **(Figs. 56.9A and B)** were developed by **Thejokrishna Pammi** and produced in 2016 and available in India since 2017. It is three files system, Starter (12%/16 mm/#17), P1: 6%/18 mm/#15, P2: 6%/18 mm/#25. About 6% taper offers optimum flare in canal preparation in primary molars to facilitate irrigation and debridement as well prevents weakening and inadvertent perforation of canal walls that happens commonly with higher taper instruments.

Procedures (Fig. 56.10)

Following stringent case selection and standard access cavity and pulp extirpation, establish working length 1.0–2 mm short of radiographic apex.

- Set the speed 200–400 rpm and torque 2–4 N/cm. Using starter file enlarge the orifice and gain entry into canal,

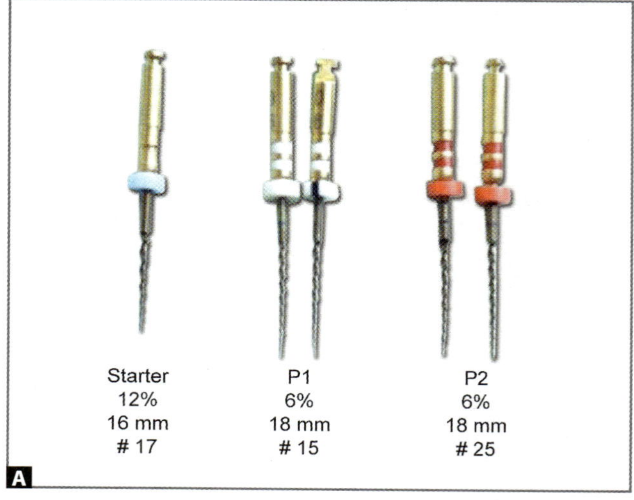

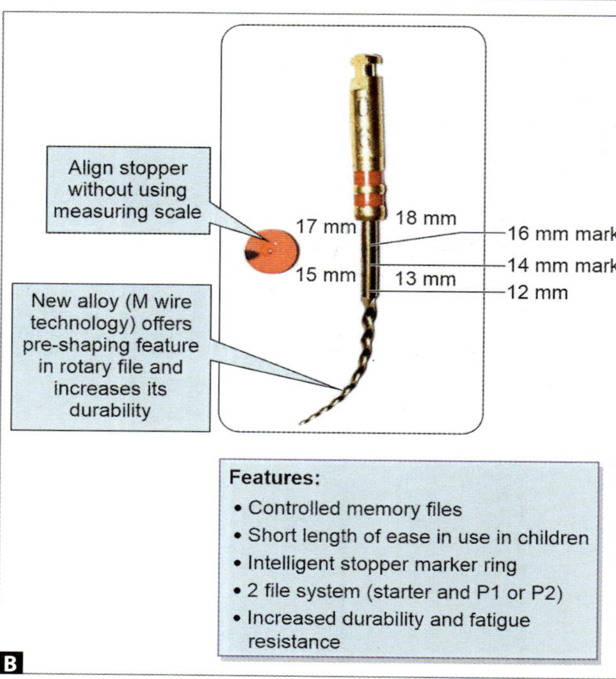

Figs. 56.9A and B: (A) Prime pedo rotary files; (B) Features of controlled memory rotary files (Prime pedo).

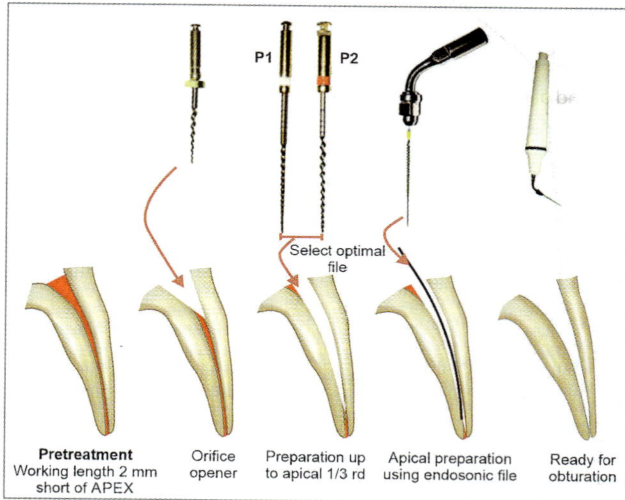

Fig. 56.10: Diagrammatic representation of procedures.

- Select P1 for thin canals like MB2 (mesio-buccal) of maxillary primary second molar or ML (mesio-lingual) canal of mandibular primary first molar, followed by P2 up to established working length.
- Precurve the instrument as suitable, enter the orifice of canal and activate engine.
- The taper of instrument creates a pathway to carry intracanal irrigant to apical 1/3rd, leading to efficient chemomechanical debridement of apical 1/3rd.
- Sodium hypochlorite as intracanal lubricant is advisable, never use rotary file in dry canal. Never inject sodium hypochlorite to the root canal; it may diffuse to periapical region leading post-treatment complication and morbidity.
- Activation of sodium hypochlorite through endosonic files or hand instrument agitation is must to achieve optimal root canal debridement. Endosonic files give continuous jet of water during use, saving time. The complex root canal architecture of primary molars can be debrided by chemomechanical means only, never solely by rotary or hand instruments.
- Hand instrument like H-files will required debride few inaccessible areas like isthmus region in C-shaped canal.
- At least 15 mL of normal saline or metronidazole infusion as final irrigant per canal is advised in last stage of root canal debridement.
- Dry the canal using paper points and use injectable calcium hydroxide paste or suitable intracanal medicaments or alternatives followed by stainless steel crown.
  - Parent has to be informed about need to monitor endodontic treatment in primary molars is more than permanent teeth due to continuous physiologic root resorption and shifting apex. Especially following human Intervention in such regions, it mandatory to monitor.
  - It is prudent of have radiographic follow-up; immediate post-treatment 1-3-6 monthly and later annually.

Technique for Using Prime pedo Files (Figs. 56.11A to D)

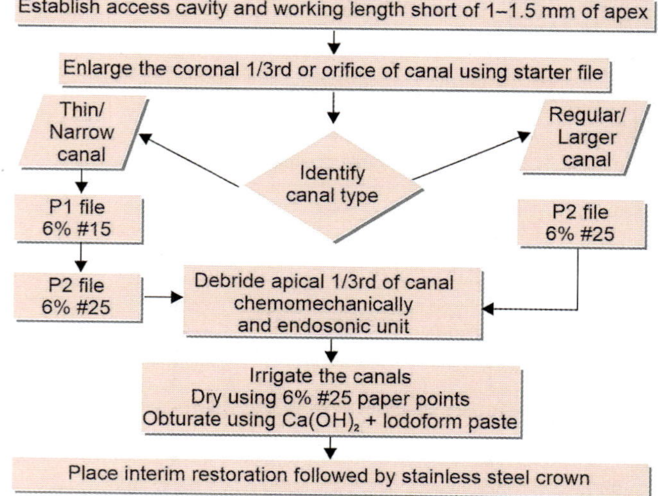

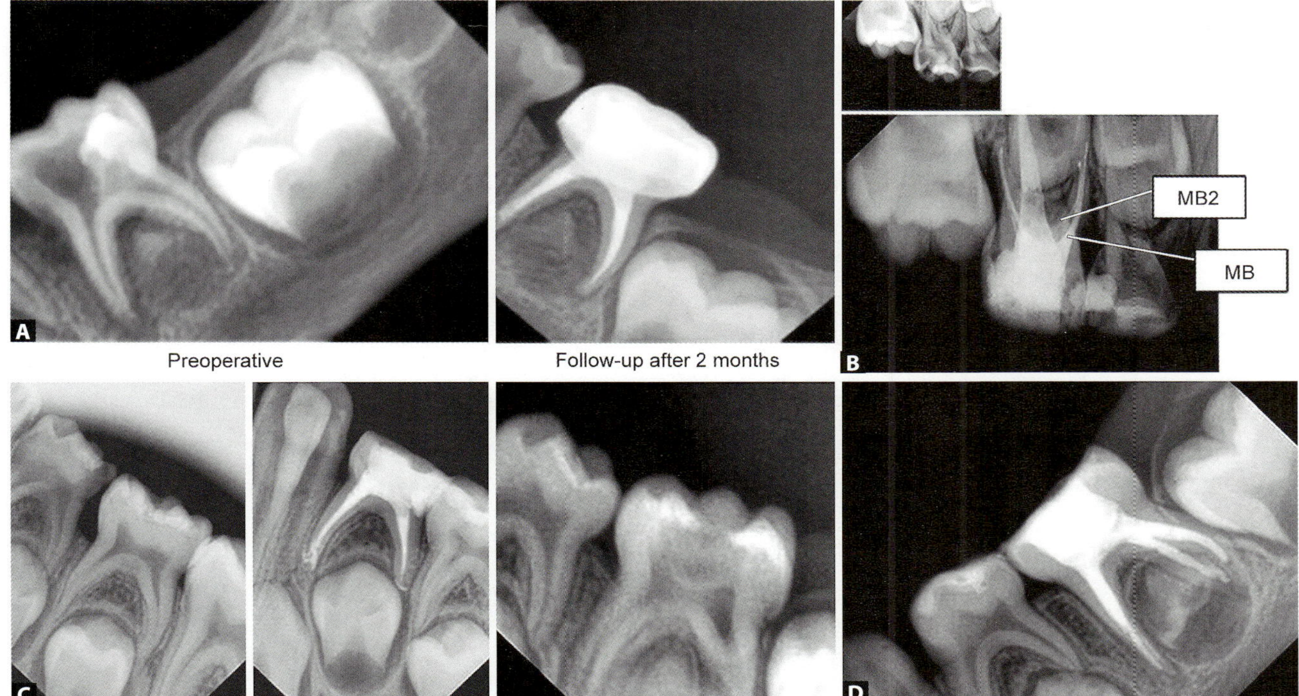

Figs. 56.11A to D: Cases with Prime pedo file: (A) Mandibular second molar; (B) Maxillary second primary molar; (c) Mandibular first primary molar; (D) Mandibular second primary molar. (*Pic courtesy:* Dr Thejokrishna Pammi).

Note

- The Ni-Ti files with a conic predefined form should be used witha low-speed handpiece (1;64 or 1:32 reduction gear or with endomotor system) with continuous torque 2–4 N/cm and 200–400 rpm, obtaining a conical and smooth root canal that facilitates sealing of the root canal system.
- It is not necessary to use a "crown-down" instrumentation technique in primary teeth since the dentin cuts more easily than in permanent teeth.
- Care must be taken not to enter the primary root canal more than twice with each rotary file, for over preparation can leadto unexpected lateral perforation, especially in severely curved canals.
- Do not be tempted to drive in more that estimated working length. The design of files is triangular (Prime pedo files) in cross-section which will get pulled in or screwed in during use. Slowerspeed setting are recommended for better control.
- It is prudent to under prepare or under obturate with the developing successor present apically.

PRO-AF-BABY-GOLD FILES

Pro-AF-Baby-files **(Fig. 56.12)** is marketed by Dantalyze and consists of 5 files. B2, B3, B4 and B5 **(Table 56.4)**. It is a versatile pediatric rotary file system marketed by DentAlyze. It is gold heat-treated, controlled memory Ni-Ti file with a triangular cross-section. It is highly flexible and resistant to fracture. It is duly designed to confirm multiple variations in the width of the apex as in resorbing root and in narrow canals. It is available in a set of five files namely 20/0.04, 25/0.04, 25/0.06, 30/0.04, for posterior teeth, and 40/0.04 for anterior teeth. The selection of the file confirming the canal morphology ensures adequate shaping without compromising on the dentin of the canal. 4% #30 rotary or hand files do not cause any canal perforation.

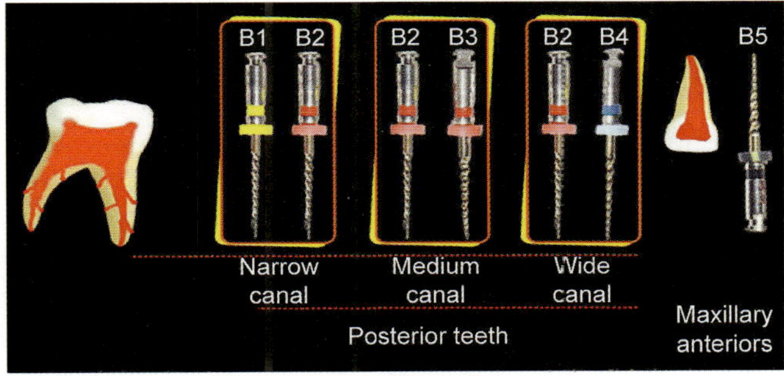

Figs. 56.12: Pro-AF-Baby-files.

Table 56.4: Describing features of Pro-AF-Baby-files.

Type of canal	*Type of files for instrumentation*	*Instrument code*
MB, ML, DB narrow canals	# 20/04, # 25/04	B1, B2
MB, ML, DB medium canals	# 25/04, # 25/06	B2, B3
Distal and palatal wide canals	# 25/04, # 30/04	B3, B4
Maxillary anteriors	# 30/04/ # 40/04	B4, B

Advantages

- The wider canals are cleaned with 6% taper files and canals with wider apex are prepared by #30/0.04 or #40/0.04.
- It has excellent canal centricity with the least extrusion of debris as compared to other files (**Jain S** et al., 2020).
- It has achieved better quality of obturation (**Shah HS**, 2021).
- Improved canal centricity (**Rathi N** et al., 2021).
- Sequential enlargement of the canal reduces the chance of file separation, and ledge formation.

Technique to Use Pro-AF-Baby-Files (Figs. 56.13A and B)

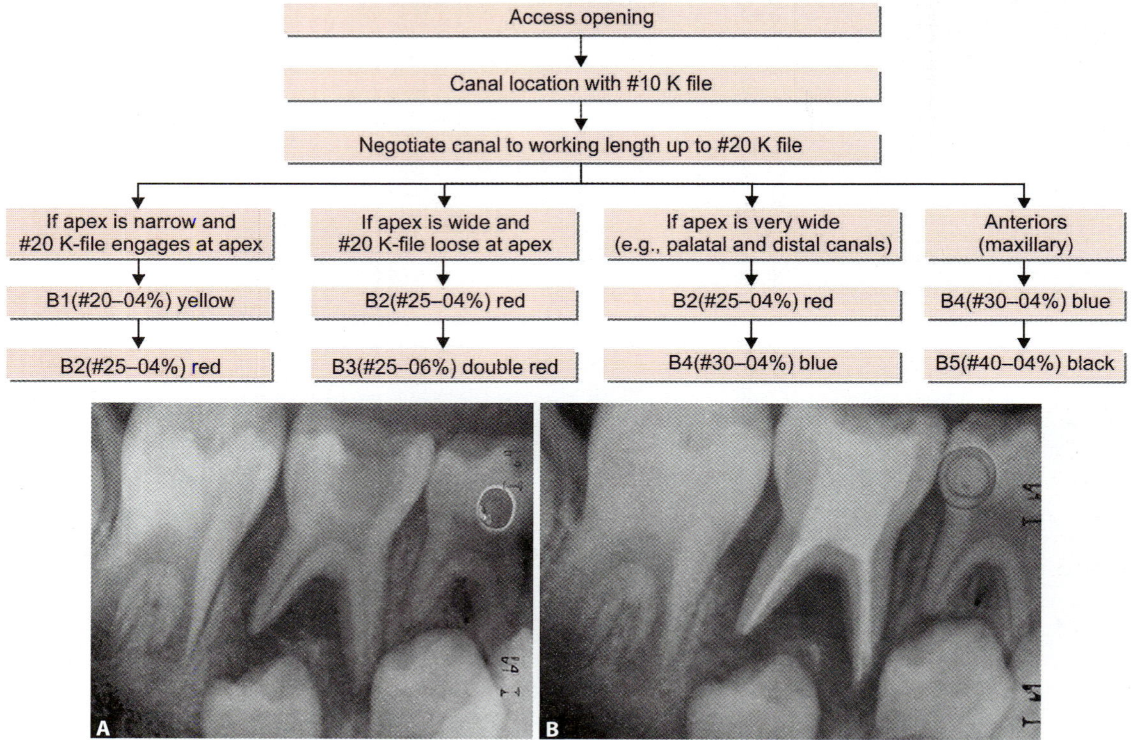

Figs. 56.13A and B: Case for Pro-AF-Baby-files. (*Pic courtesy:* Dr Nilesh Rathi).

Baby Blue Files

It is a newly patented pediatric endodontic file system marketed by DentAlyze, comprising of a set of three files having two different cross-sections. It has a blue heat treatment for improving flexural strength. The first file, "Foster file" is a variable taper file designed to cater to two purposes in a single go. In the apical 4 mm length, it creates a glide path with the tip size of 0.17 mm and the coronal 9 mm is serving to enlarge the orifice. The second and third files are 28/0.05 and 38/0.05 having constant taper with modified tip and double S cross-section **(Fig. 56.14)**.

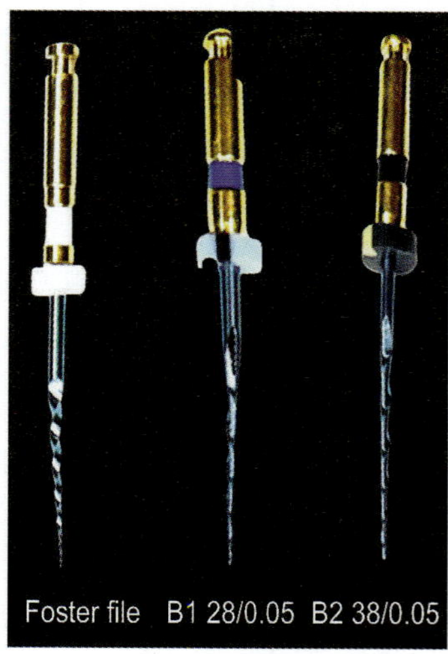

Fig. 56.14: Pro-AF-Baby Blue files.

Advantages of the System

Characteristic features	*Properties*	*Clinical implication*
Foster file	• Glide path in apical • Orifice opener in coronal	• Avoid ledge preparation even in a narrow canal • Adequate extirpation of the pulp
Metallurgy	Blue heat treatment	High fracture resistance
Double S cross-section	• Increased flexibility • Large relief area • Wider core • Two-point contact	• Minimal chance of fracture • Conservative preparation of the canal with optimum shaping and complete removal of the pulp • Acts like a rotating H file
Modified tip	Conical noncutting tip	Least extrusion of the debris
Length	17 mm	Optimum length for comfort and precision

Protocol for Use (Figs. 56.15A and B)

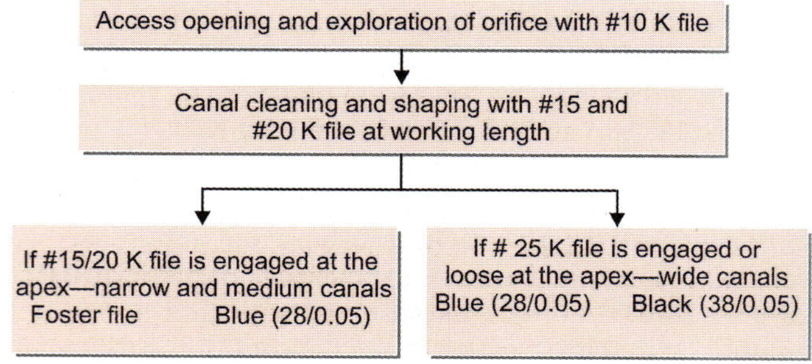

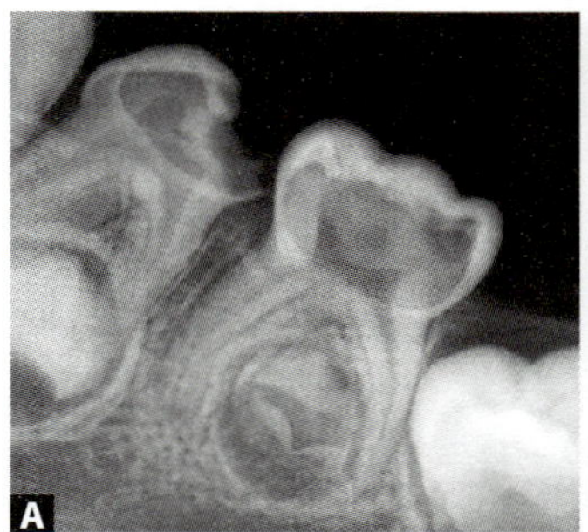

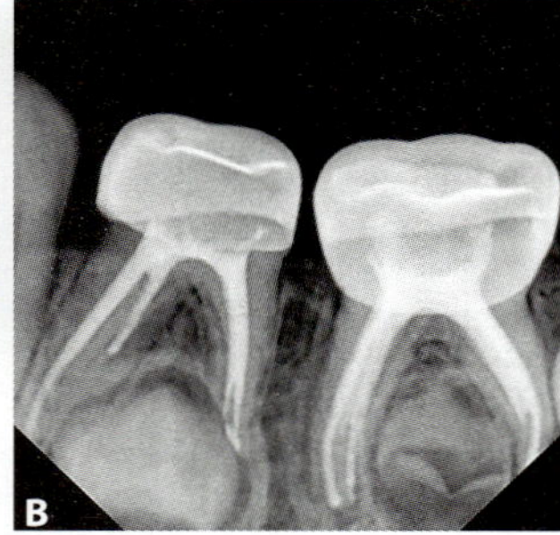

Figs. 56.15A and B: Case for Pro-Af-Baby Blue files. (*Pic courtesy:* Dr Nilesh Rathi).

PRECAUTIONS FOR ROTARY SYSTEM

- Irrigation and keeping a moist canal is the most important in rotary endodontics as instrumenting dry canals can result in broken file tips, especially in the smaller size files.
- Frequently inspect each file for flute unwinding or distortion and discard immediately. If no flute distortion is detected discard the files after use in five primary teeth.
- Always use a straight-line access.
- Use minimal or no pressure on the handpiece while filing.
- No skipping of files should be done and they should be used in correct sequence.
- The file should be inserted and ejected from the canals while in rotation as stopping or starting of files in canals can cause file fracture.

Basic Rule for Rotary Instrumentation

	Do's	*Dont's*
Case selection	Gradual curves, glide path confirmed with straight sixe no, 20 K file	Acute coronal curves and other anatomical variations
Glide path	Confirm a patent canal to the level the rotary should follow	Unknown canal conditions ahead of the rotary instrument
Speed	Low (250 rpm)	High (>350 rpm)
Torque	Dependent on file, low for smaller diameter taper governed by motor or tactile feedback	Uniformely low or always high; reliance on torque controlled motor
Hand movement	Pecking for radial landed files, brushing for nonlanded files	Forcing the file apically

CLEANING OF ROTARY Ni-Ti ENDODONTIC INSTRUMENT

The protocol comprises of:

- Vigorous strokes in a scouring sponge soaked in 0.2% chlorhexidine solution. Around 30 minutes pre-soak in an enzymatic cleaning solution.
- 15 minutes of ultrasonication in the same solution. Around 20 seconds rinse in running tap water.

Advantages of Rotary

- Tissue and debris are more easily and quickly removed
- The nickel-titanium files are flexible, allowing easy access to all canals
- Nickel-titanium files do not need to be precurved
- Nickel-titanium rotary files follow original root canal anatomy
- Prepared canals are funnel shaped, resulting in a more predictable uniform paste fill;
- Ni-Tis are available in various length
- Shorter instrumentation time than manual techniques, which is a relevant factor in pediatric dentistry because it allows faster procedures while maintaining quality and safety thereby reducing the patient's as well as operator's fatigue.

Disadvantages of Rotary

- Cost of the endomotor and handpiece;
- Increased cost of Ni-Ti endodontic files;
- Cyclic fatigue of endodontic instruments;
- Endodontic instruments are prone to fracture;
- Learning the technique.

Root canals of deciduous teeth can instrument by manual or rotary or combination (hybrid) techniques. Rotary technique generates more uniform—well controlled forces that results in optimal dentin removal, resulting in uniform root canal preparation and presents shortest instrumentation time. It shall not be surprising that rotary endodontics will soon make manual technique adjuvant or obsolete. With almost a decade experience of use of rotary instruments in children and observation during follow-up examinations, we conclude that following stringent case selection, adhere to standard operation protocol of instrument selection and sequence of it use and follow-up with radiographic examination will deliver predictable success in pulpectomy in primary molars.

POINTS TO REMEMBER

- The first description of the use of rotary devices was given by Oltramare.
- William H Rollins developed the first endodontic handpiece for automated root canal preparation. Cursor filing contraangle was first handpiece.
- Ni-Ti rotary systems included light-speed instrument, Pro file instrument, GT rotary instrument, K3 instrument, HERO instrument, Race instrument and ProTaper instrument.
- HERO shaper is 2nd generation instrument that puts positive rake angle in its design.
- ProTaper is the recent-most rotary system. It has variable taper along the length and appears like modified K-file.
- The technique recommended for deciduous teeth uses 4% taper instruments in narrow canals and 6% taper can be used in larger canals.
- The S2 file has a tip size of 20 and an apical taper of 4%, which approximates the root canal size of primary molars.
- It is necessary to use an additional H-file (No. 20 or No. 30) combined with copious sodium hypochlorite irrigation to remove any loose pulp tissue with a brushing motion.

Questionnaire

1. Classify rotary endodontic systems.
2. Describe the technique of biomechanical preparation using ProTaper rotary system in children.
3. What are the different rotary systems used in primary tooth?
4. What are the precautions to be exercised while using rotary system in children?
5. What are the recent modifications in rotary endodontics?

REFERENCES

1. Crespo S, Cortes O, Garcia C, Perez L. Comparison between rotary and manual instrumentation in primary teeth. J Clin Pediatr Dent. 2008;32:295-8.
2. Topçuogìu G, Topcçuogìlu, HS, Akpek F. Evaluation of apically extruded debris during root canal preparation in primary molar teeth using three different rotary systems and hand files. Int J Paediatr Dent. 2016;26:357-3.
3. Goerig AC, Camp JH. Root canal treatment in primary teeth: a review. Pediatr Dent. 1983;5(1):33-7.

FURTHER READING

1. Barr B, Barr N. Posterior pulpectomies: using rotary files. Children's Dentistry a partnership newsletter. 1999;6:1-3.
2. Barr ES, Kleier DJ, Barr NV. Use of Nickel-Titanium rotary files for root canal preparation in primary teeth. Pediatr Dent. 1999;21:453-4.
3. Barr ES, Kleier DJ, Barr NV. Use of Nickel-Titanium rotary files for root canal preparation in primary teeth. Pediatr Dent. 2000;22:77-8.
4. Coleman CL, Svec T, Wang M, Suchina J, Glickmaan GN. Stainless steel versus nickel-titanium K-files: analysis of instrumentation in curved canal. J Endod. 1995;2:237.
5. Glossen CR, Haller RH, Dove SB, Del Rio CE. A comparison of root canal preparations using Ni-Ti hand, Ni-Ti engine drive, and K flex endodontic instruments. J Endod. 1995;21: 146-51.
6. Guelzow A, Stamn O, Martus, Kielbassa AM. Comparative study of six rotary Nickel-Titanium systems and hand instrumentation for root canal preparation. Int Endod J. 2005;38(10):743-52.
7. Hulsman M, Herbst U, Schafers F. Comparative study of root-canal preparation using Light and Quantec SC rotary Ni-Ti instruments. Int Endod J. 2003;36(11):748-56.
8. Kuo CI, Wang YL, et al. Application of Ni-Ti rotary files for pulpectomy in primary molars. J Dent Sci. 2006;1:10-15.
9. Leonardo MR, Leanardo RT. Sistemas rotatorios em endondontia-instrumentos de Niquel-Titanio. Artes Medicas. Sao Paula: 2002.
10. Linsuwanont P, Parashos P, Messer HH. Cleaning of rotary nickel-titanium endodontic instruments. Aus Dent J. 2004;49:1.
11. McDonald RE, Avery DR. Dentistry for the child and adolescent 7th Ed. Mosby. St Louis: 2004.
12. Pettiette MT, Metzger Z, Phillips C, Trope M. Endodontic complications of root canal therapy performed by dental students with stainless steel K files and Nickel-Titanium hand files. J Endod. 1999;25:230-4.
13. Short JA, Morgan LA, Baumgartner JC. A comparison of canal centering ability of four instrumentation techniques. J Endod. 1997;23: 503-7.
14. Silva LAB, Leonardo MR, Filho PN, Tanomaru JMG. Comparison of rotary and manual instrumentation techniques on cleaning capacity and instrumentation time in deciduous molars. J Dent Child. 2004;71:45-7.
15. Walia HM, Brantley WA, Gerstein H. An Initial investigation of the bending and torsional properties of Nitinol root canal files. J Endod. 1988;14:346-51.
16. Zmener O, Balbacham L. Effectiveness of Nickel- Titanium files for preparing curved root canals. Endod Dent Tramatol. 1995;11:121-3.

CHAPTER 57

Normal Features of Gingiva

Ravi GR, Mayur Kaushik, Noopur Kaushik, Karthik Krishna M

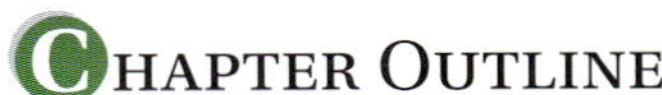

CHAPTER OUTLINE

- Macroscopic Appearance of the Periodontium

The periodontium is the foundation for the dentition. The components of periodontium—the alveolar mucosa, gingiva, cementum, periodontal ligament, and alveolar bone, serve as the supporting apparatus for the teeth in function and in occlusal relationships. By learning the fine knitting details of its embryonic origin, composition, histological and clinical appearance with normal physiologic variations, it enables us to develop an understanding of their relationships in health and to understand the processes that occur in pathology. This will include macroscopic, microscopic, and radiographic details of the components of the periodontium. The knowledge of the details of the tissue compartments, the cells which are involved, and how the cellular products and the cells interact will provide a greater understanding of the functions of the periodontium. Thus, it is important to know about the anatomy and physiology of the healthy periodontium and its relationship to the natural dentition, jaws, and the oral environment.

MACROSCOPIC APPEARANCE OF THE PERIODONTIUM

The periodontium is composed of the gingiva, alveolar mucosa, cementum, periodontal ligament, and alveolar bone **(Figs. 57.1A and B)**. The gingiva is firmly bound to the underlying bone and is continuous with the alveolar mucosa that is situated apically and is unbound. The border of these two tissue types is clearly demarcated and is called the mucogingival junction. There is no mucogingival junction on the palatal aspect of the maxilla as the gingiva is continuous with the palatal mucosa.

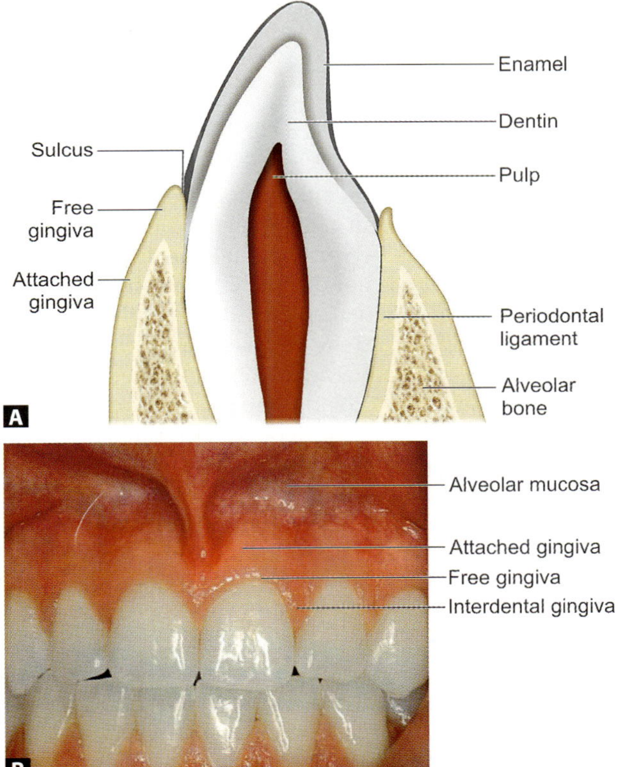

Figs. 57.1A and B: Components of the periodontium. (*Source:* Garant, 2003).

The gingiva consists of a free gingival margin and attached gingiva **(Figs. 57.2A and B)**. The free gingival margin is situated about 2 mm coronal to the cementoenamel junction (CEJ) of the tooth and the attached gingiva extends from the base of the free gingiva to the mucogingival junction. The gingiva is typically pink in color but may vary due to

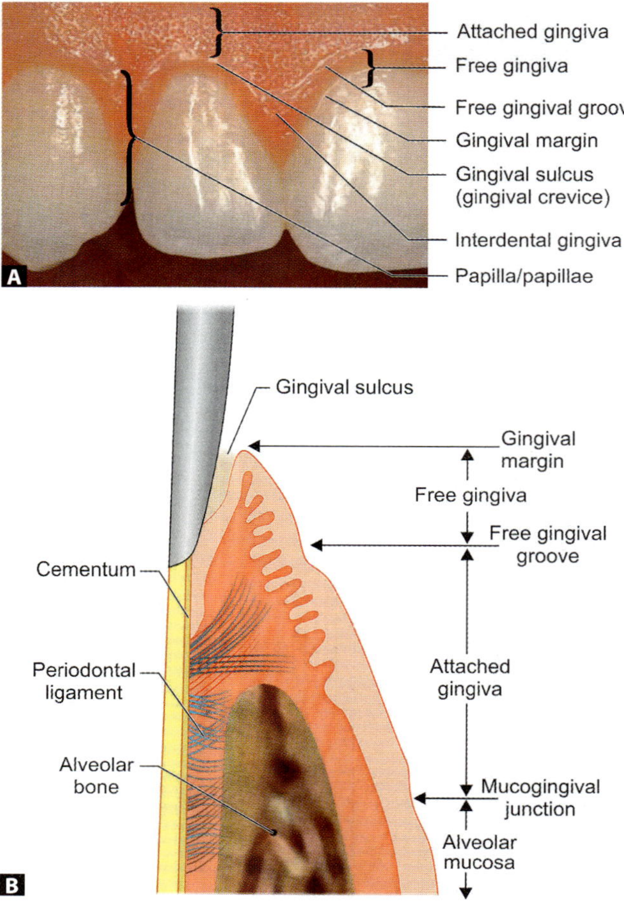

Figs. 57.2A and B: Parts of gingiva.

physiologic pigmentation among some races. Unattached portion of the gingiva that surrounds the tooth in the region of the CEJ is called as free or marginal gingiva. It fits closely around the tooth but is not directly attached to it and forms soft tissue wall of gingival sulcus. It meets the tooth in a thin rounded edge called the gingival margin which follows the contours of the teeth. The free and attached portions of gingiva are generally not clearly demarcated from each other, although sometimes a linear depression termed as the 'free gingival groove' separates them.

The gingival sulcus is a narrow space bound by the tooth surface and inner lining of free gingiva. Its clinical depth can be measured with a periodontal probe and serves as a standard diagnostic tool in the detection of periodontal disease.

Attached gingiva is tightly connected to the cementum on the cervical third of the root and to the periosteum (connective tissue cover) of the alveolar bone. The width of the attached gingiva varies with the location in the oral cavity as well as with physiologic age. The facial gingiva is typically widest in the incisor region and narrowest in the premolar region for the maxillary arch and ranges from 1 to 9 mm. In the mandible also, the attached facial gingiva is narrowest at the premolar and canine region. When the lingual attached gingiva was examined, it was found that the widest areas were on the mandibular molars and the narrowest were on the incisor and canine regions, about 1.8 mm. There is a general increase of width of the attached gingiva from the primary to permanent dentition as well as with increasing age. This occurs due to the compensatory eruption of teeth in response to occlusal tooth wear. The attached gingiva allows the gingival tissue to withstand mechanical forces of mastication, tooth brushing, and prevents free gingiva from being pulled away from the tooth when tension is applied to the alveolar mucosa.

The tissue that resides in the interproximal embrasure is called the interproximal papilla. The shape of this tissue is influenced by the shape of the interproximal contact, the width of the interproximal area, and the position of the CEJ of the involved teeth. The shape of this papilla varies from triangular and knife-edge in the anterior regions with point sized contacts of the teeth to broader and more square shaped tissue in the posterior sextants due to the teeth having broad contact areas. Also present in the wider papillary areas is the col, a valley-like structure situated apical to the contact area **(Fig. 57.3)**. The epithelium of the col lacks keratinization, making this region more susceptible to bacterial penetration and onset of periodontal inflammation. This phenomenon is attributed to the clinical occurrence of swollen and inflamed interdental papillae in early gingivitis.

The texture of the gingiva varies with age and is typically smooth in infancy, stippled from 3 years onwards, and again becomes smoother with advanced age. Stippled tissue has a texture similar to the kind of an orange peel and its presence does not necessarily mean healthy gingiva **(Fig. 57.4)**.

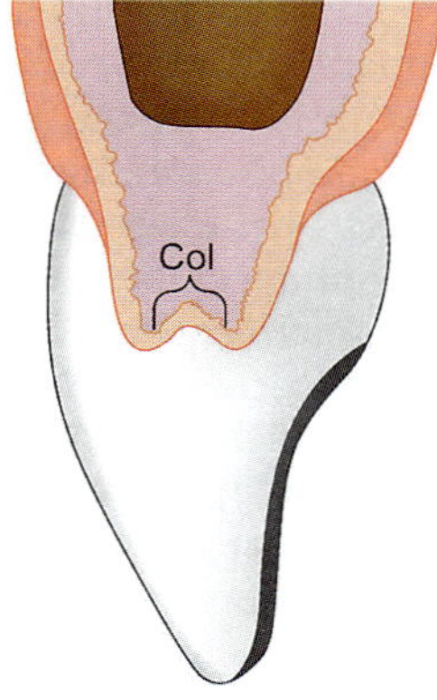

Fig. 57.3: Interdental col. (*Source:* Garant, 2003).

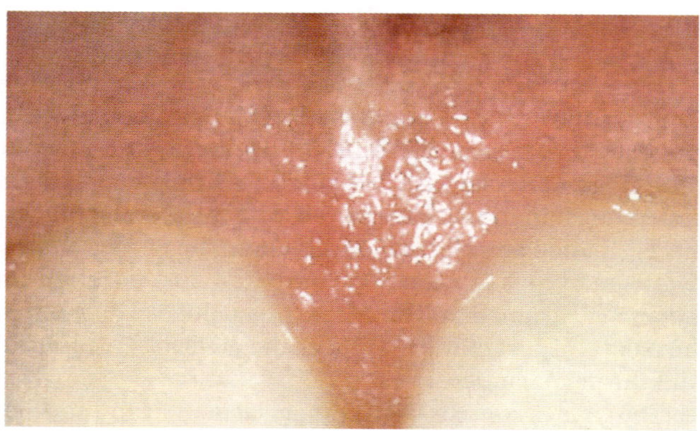

Fig. 57.4: Stippling of gingival tissue.

Studies on Normal Features of the Gingiva in Children

- **Ihn- Ah Yoo** *conducted a study on children in Korea and concluded that—the mean width of attached gingiva of the children aged 6–12 years proved to be wider in the maxilla than in the mandible when the same teeth on both jaws were compared. In case of the primary teeth, the widest width was found in the areas of maxillary primary lateral incisors and maxillary primary canines (3.50 mm) and the narrowest zone was noted in the area of mandibular first primary molars (1.34 mm). In the permanent dentition, the greatest width was found in the areas of maxillary permanent lateral incisors (3.00 mm) and the narrowest zone in mandibular first premolars (0.55 mm). At the age of tooth change, the attached gingivae of primary teeth were wider than those of successive permanent teeth except for maxillary central incisors of boys. The maximum in the frequency of mucogingival problems was found in the areas of upper and lower first primary molars of primary dentition, and in the upper and lower first premolars of permanent dentition regardless of sex.*
- **Takashi Hanioka et al.,** *2005 conducted a case-control study to investigate the relationship between gingival pigmentation in children and passive smoking. The findings suggested that excessive pigmentation in the gingiva of children is associated with passive smoking. The visible pigmentation effect in gingiva of children could be useful in terms of parental education.*
- **Bimstein E, Peretz B, and Holan G,** *2003 conducted study to describe the prevalence of gingival stippling in children of various ages. The authors concluded that Stippling was evident from 3 years of age and thereafter and no particular changes were observed with the increasing age or gender. Stippling was more evident in maxillary arch than the mandibular arch, which was not statistically significant.*

Differentiating Features of Gingiva in Children and Adults
Clinical Features **(Figs. 57.5A and B)**

Characteristic	***Children***	***Adult***
Color	Pale pink	Coral pink
Surface	Smooth	Stippled
Gingiva margin	Thick and round	Knife-edged
Free gingiva	Para-keratinized or nonkeratinized saddle area	Nonkeratinized saddle area
Interdental gingiva	Interdental clefts present	Clefts not present
Attached gingiva	Retrocuspid papilla present	Retrocuspid papilla absent
Sulcus depth	2.1–2.3 mm	2–6 mm
Alveolar mucosa	Red, thin, and vascular	Pink
Periodontal ligament	Wide	Narrow
Collagen bundles	More hydrated and less differentiated	More differentiated
Polypeptide chains	Normal cross-linking	Tight cross-linking
Ground substance	Low ratio of collagen to ground substance	Ground substance to collagen ratio normal
Fibers	Gingival fibers are immature	Mature and organized

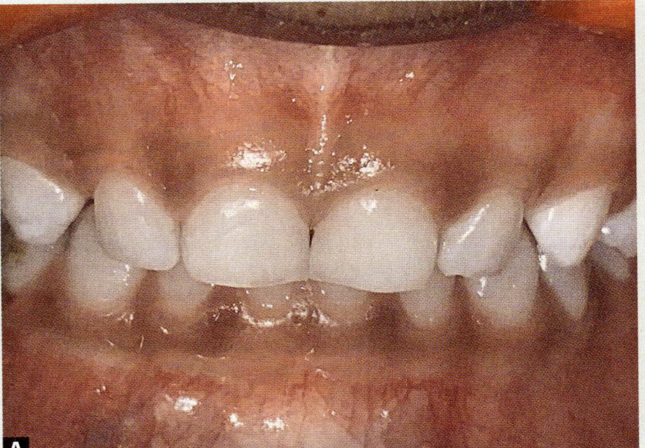

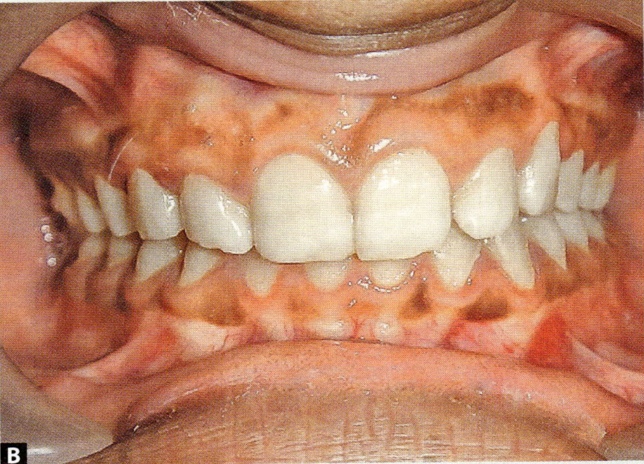

Figs. 57.5A and B: Gingiva of children and adults.

Radiological features (Figs. 57.6 A and B)		
Trabeculae	Thick trabeculae with large marrow spaces	More trabeculae with less marrow spaces
Lamina dura	Prominent	Thin
Interdental septa	Flat	Pointed

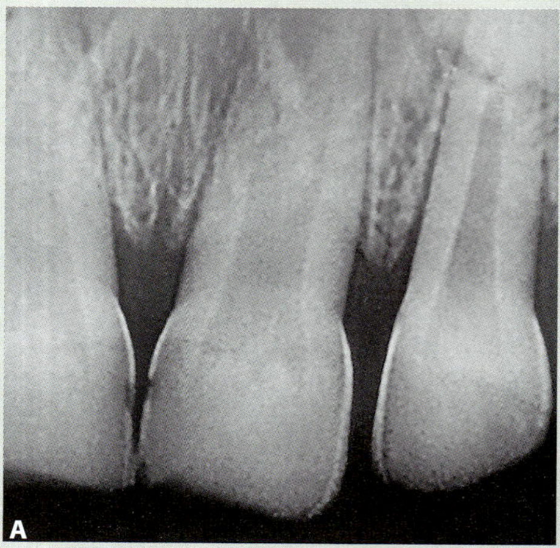

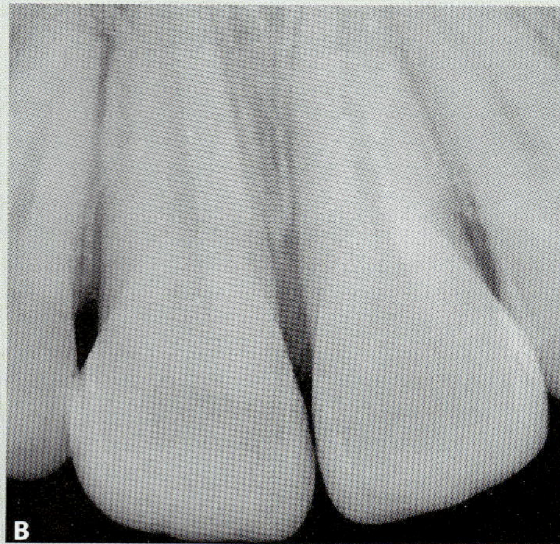

Figs. 57.6A and B: Radiograph of primary and permanent teeth.

Clinical Significance

- In children there is normal spacing present in the dentition which makes the appearance of the interdental papillae to be relatively flatter than the adult gingivae.
- The responsibility of plaque control can be shared by both patient/Professional by use of mechanical and pharmaceutical methods, especially under 7 years of age as child does not have enough manual dexterity to effectively brush his /her teeth.
- Absence of stippling is indicative of gingivitis (after 5 years of age).
- During adaptation of stainless-steel band care must be taken to follow the gingival contour especially on proximal surface in order to prevent injury to underlying Interproximal gingiva (= Col).
- Use of interdental aids such as floss should be reserved for adolescent with manual dexterity (in order to prevent injury to gingiva).
- Depth of gingival sulcus has to be considered during placement of subgingival restoration/crown margins. Extending such margins beyond the sulcus depth will lead to impingement of the tissue, resulting in gingival inflammation/recession.
- Proper contact area with adjacent teeth needs to be pre-planned during placement of crowns or restorations as it will affect the characteristics of the underlying col region.

POINTS TO REMEMBER

- The components of periodontium—the alveolar mucosa, gingiva, cementum, periodontal ligament, and alveolar bone.
- The width of the attached gingiva varies with the location in the oral cavity as well as with physiologic age.
- There is a general increase of width of the attached gingiva from the primary to permanent dentition as well as with increasing age.
- Average sulcus depths in primary dentition range from 1–2 mm, with a tendency to increase during transition to permanent dentition.
- The tissue that resides in the interproximal embrasure is called the interproximal papilla.

Questionnaire

1. Describe the features of children's gingiva.
2. Write the differentiating features of children and adult gingiva.

FURTHER READING

1. Ainamo J, Löe H. Anatomical characteristics of gingiva: A clinical and microscopic study of the free and attached gingiva. J Periodontol. 1966;37(1):5-13.
2. Bimstein E, Eidelman E. Morphological changes in the attached and keratinized gingiva and gingival sulcus in the mixed dentition period: A 5-year longitudinal study. J Clin Periodontol. 1988;15:175-9.
3. Bimstein E, Peretz B, Holan G. Prevalence of gingival stippling in children. J Clin Pediatr Dent. 2003;27:163-5.
4. Hanioka T, Tanaka K, Ojima M, Yuuki K. Association of melanin pigmentation in the gingiva of children with parents who smoke. Pediatrics. 2005;116(2): e186-90.
5. Orban B. Clinical and histologic study of the surface characteristics of the gingiva. Oral Surg Oral Med Oral Pathol. 1948;1(9):827-41.
6. Saario M, Ainamo A, Mattila K, et al. The width of radiologically-defined attached gingiva over permanent teeth in children. J Clin Periodontol. 1994;21:666-9.

CHAPTER

Gingivitis in Children

Ravi GR, Mandeep S Virdi, Mayur Kaushik, Noopur Kaushik, Karthik Krishna M

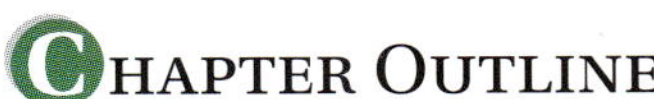

CHAPTER OUTLINE

- Stages of Gingivitis
- Types of Gingivitis in Children

Gingivitis or inflammation of the gingiva is the most common oral disease in children and adolescents. It is characterized by the presence of gingival inflammation without detectable bone loss or clinical attachment loss. The causes and risks are as varied in children as in adults and range from local to systemic causes. The most important local predisposing factor in children however is poor oral hygiene. This chapter aims to discuss the various forms of gingivitis encountered in children and adolescents.

STAGES OF GINGIVITIS

Page and **Schroeder** (1976) reported the sequence of changes during the development of gingivitis and periodontitis under four stages, according to prominent histopathological signs **(Table 58.1)**.

1. **Stage 1:** Initial lesion, which occurs within 2–4 days after allowing plaque to accumulate, an increased volume of junctional epithelium (JE) is occupied by polymorphonuclear leukocytes (PMNL). Blood vessels subjacent to the JE become dilated and exhibit increased permeability. A small cellular infiltrate of PMNL and mononuclear cells forms and collagen content in the infiltrated areas markedly decreases.
2. **Stage 2:** Early stage gingivitis, which is about 4–7 days after plaque accumulation. Evolves in humans at this stage, the differentiating sign being accumulation of large numbers of lymphocytes as an enlarged infiltrate in the connective tissue.
3. **Stage 3:** In Established stage, which is about 2–3 weeks of plaque accumulation, there is preponderance of plasma cells in an expanded inflammatory lesion with continuance of earlier changes. The established lesion may persist for a long time before becoming "aggressive" and progressing to the advanced lesion.
4. **Stage 4:** Advanced lesion, the infiltrate is dominated by plasma cells. Collagen destruction continues with loss of alveolar bone and apical migration of JE, with "pocket" formation now being apparent. Throughout the sequence, viable bacteria remain outside the gingiva, on the surface of the tooth and in the periodontal pocket against, but not invading the soft tissue.

TYPES OF GINGIVITIS IN CHILDREN

Plaque-induced Gingivitis

- This type of gingivitis is associated primarily with dental plaque accumulation due to poor oral hygiene **(Fig. 58.1)**.
- It is regarded as the most common periodontal disease in children.

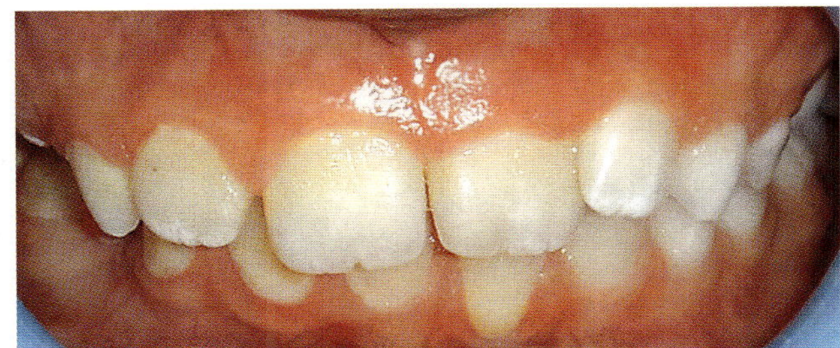

Fig. 58.1: Plaque-induced gingivitis.

Table 58.1: Stages of gingivitis.

Stages	Days	Vascular changes	Predominant immune cells	Clinical findings	
Stage I	2–4	↑ Permeability of vascular bed	Polymorphonuclear leukocytes (PMNL)	↑ Gingival fluid flow	
Stage II	4–7	Vascular proliferation	Lymphocytes	Erythema and bleeding on probing	
Stage III	14–21	Stage II + blood stasis	Plasma cells and B lymphocyte	Change in color, size, texture, etc.	
Stage IV	>month	Degeneration	Plasma cell	Loss of connective tissue attachment and alveolar bone	

- Plaque-induced gingivitis has a tendency to occur more frequently with increasing age with, highest prevalence seen during puberty. This condition is usually less severe in intensity as compared to that in adults.
- Calculus deposits are rarely seen in younger children but may increase with age.
- Increased subgingival levels of *Actinomyces* sp., *Capnocytophaga* sp., *Leptotrichia* sp., and *Selenomonas* sp. are associated with plaque-induced gingivitis.
- The extent of inflammation maybe modified by conditions associated with hormonal changes, e.g., Puberty (refer below), diabetes mellitus, etc.
- Plaque-induced gingivitis usually can be treated with professional cleaning of the teeth and improvement of oral hygiene of the child.

Incipient Gingivitis

- Considered as precursor of full-fledged gingivitis, it is characterized by limited areas of mild inflammation, clinically evident as mild redness and/or delayed bleeding.
- It may rapidly progress to localized gingivitis if untreated.

Gingivitis due to Habit

Gingivitis is a very common finding in the maxillary anterior region in individuals with mouth breathing habit. This habit is common among young children and it predisposes to dryness of the gingival when the lubricating effect of saliva is absent **(Fig. 58.2)**.

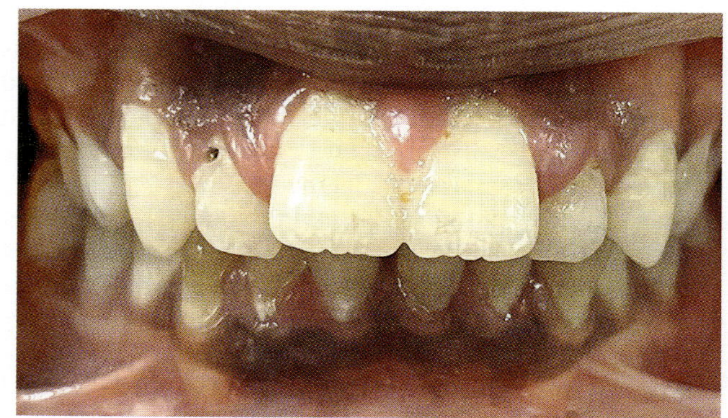

Fig. 58.2: Mouth breather gingiva.

Eruption Gingivitis

- The erupting primary or permanent tooth pushes onto the overlying soft tissue resulting a bulge that is quite firm. Sometimes this bulge maybe filled with blood and appear as a purplish tumor, known as ***eruption cyst***.
- It most commonly occurs in primary and permanent first molar regions.
- The gingival margin of an erupting tooth may appear reddish and edematous. This occurs due to poor oral hygiene because of discomfort during tooth cleaning and results in plaque accumulation and inflammation.
- This aspect in combination with prominence of the underlying tooth structure may give an appearance of severe enlargement.

Orthodontic Appliance Induced Enlargement

- Fixed orthodontic appliances can cause difficulty in plaque removal resulting in gingival enlargement. Changes usually occur by 2 months of appliance placement.
- However, this situation is temporary and limited only to gingival tissues. Sometimes, bulky tissue may interfere with oral functions or impede further orthodontic treatment. Such cases may be resolved with gingivoplasty.

Infective Gingivitis

These are of viral or bacterial origin and caused by viruses or bacteria, which are normal commensals of the oral cavity becoming virulent when present in high proportions.

Herpetic Gingivostomatitis

- It affects both the gingiva and other parts of the oral mucous membrane. It is commonly seen in children less than 3 years of age.
- It is caused by the herpes simplex virus type 1.
- Infection usually follows bouts of childhood fevers such as malaria, measles, and chickenpox. The onset is preceded by a prodromal period with symptoms such as irritability, malaise, vomiting, and fever and the appearance of small vesicles which rupture to reveal small yellowish painful ulcers with erythematous margins **(Fig. 58.3)**.

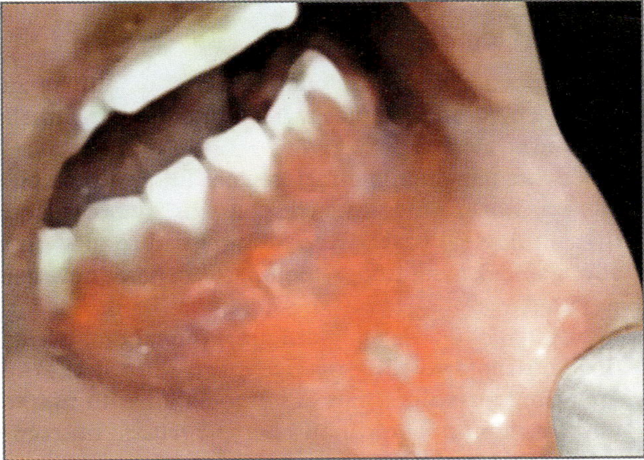

Fig. 58.3: Herpetic gingivostomatitis.

- The condition is associated with drooling of saliva, inability to chew and swallow, and the child may become increasingly uncooperative during tooth brushing.
- The condition is self-limiting and the management is to encourage bed rest, plenty of fluid, and maintenance of good oral hygiene through gentle debridement. Analgesics are prescribed to relieve the pain and application of a mild topical anesthetic gel has been found useful in young children.

Human Immunodeficiency Virus-associated Gingivitis

- Oral manifestations of human immunodeficiency virus (HIV) disease are an important part of the natural history of HIV disease.
- Many studies have reported that hairy leukoplakia, pseudomembranous candidiasis, Kaposi sarcoma, non-Hodgkin's lymphoma, linear gingival erythema, necrotizing ulcerative gingivitis, and periodontitis were common lesions seen in patients with HIV infection and acquired immune deficiency syndrome (AIDS).

Acute Necrotizing Ulcerative Gingivitis

- Acute necrotizing ulcerative gingivitis is (ANUG) used to be known as "trench mouth" because it was seen frequently in soldiers occupying trenches during the World War I and was also called "Vincent's angina", after the French physician **Henri Vincent** (1862–1950).
- This is an acute multiple bacterial infection of the gingivae.
- The lesion starts at the interdental papillae, spreading along the gingival margins and if untreated, starts to destroy the underlying connective tissue and bone. There is a characteristic necrotic odor associated with this condition and the mouth becomes progressively painful with sloughing off, of the necrotic ulcers on the gingivae. The ulcers become erythematous and bleed following minimal trauma, especially tooth brushing **(Fig. 58.4)**.

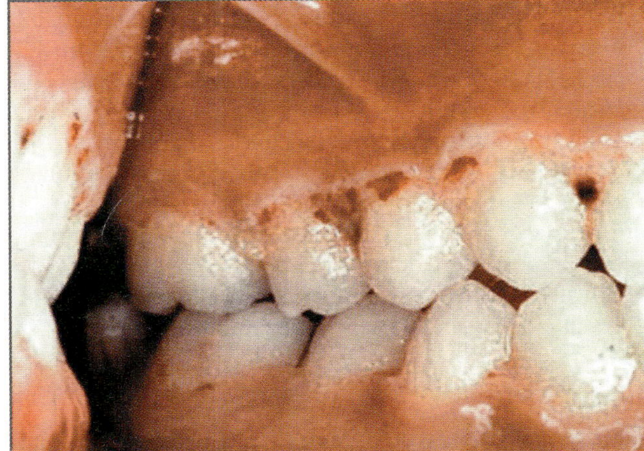

Fig. 58.4: Acute necrotizing ulcerative gingivitis.

- Regional lymph nodes are enlarged and tender.
- If untreated, destruction of the soft tissues of the mouth and cheek and facial bones result, a condition referred to as Cancrum Oris or Noma.

- It occurs with low frequency (<1%) in children in developed countries, but still seen in higher proportions (2–5%) in children and adolescents in developing countries in Africa, Asia, and South America.
- Predisposing factors include poor oral hygiene, malnutrition, depressed immunity, and long-term hospitalization.
- The bacteria implicated earlier were *Fusobacteria fusiformis* and *Borrelia vincentii*. However, modern electron microscope studies have shown the lesion to be colonized by various species of gram-negative anaerobes and spirochaetes such as *Treponema* species, *Bacteroides, Veillonella, Fusobacteria* and *Actinomyces.*
- The treatment of choice is regular gentle debridement of the gingiva and irrigation with an oxidizing antiseptic such as hydrogen peroxide, until the infection clears. Diet and oral hygiene counseling is also useful and should be followed up to ensure speedy healing.

Malnutrition-induced Gingivitis

- Adolescence is a time of rapid growth, independent food choices, and food fads. It is also a period of heightened caries activity as a result of increased intake of cariogenic substances and inattentiveness to oral hygiene procedures.
- There is evidence that different foods, such as dietary proteins and carbohydrates can affect the buffering capacity of saliva and protein deficiency influences markedly the composition of whole saliva in man.

Pubertal Gingivitis

- A higher amount of plaque has also been found in the primary dentition compared with the mixed and permanent dentitions, but the prevalence and severity of inflammation of the oral tissues (gingivitis and periodontitis) is low in healthy young children and gradually increases with increasing age.
- Pubertal gingivitis has been seen with increasing frequency in young teenagers and has been ascribed to the "rush" of sex hormones, which also affects the reaction of tissues to corticosteroids.
- The condition ranges from localized inflammation of one or two papillary gingivae, also called "gingival epulis", to generalize marginal gingivitis.
- It primarily manifests as an interproximal inflammation with increased bleeding tendency.
- However, removal of dental deposits and improvement in oral hygiene usually resolve the condition.

Drug-induced Gingivitis

- Abnormal gingival enlargement may occur due to intake of certain drugs. Three classes of drugs have been proven till date to cause enlargement:
  - Anticonvulsants, e.g., phenytoin
  - Calcium channel blockers, e.g., nifedipine
  - Immunosuppresants, e.g., cyclosporine
- Gingival enlargement is the most significant oral finding and can occur in up to 50% of patients
- Early research showed an increase in the number of fibroblasts in the patients receiving dialntin and thus, it is often known as Phenytoin induced gingival overgrowth (PIGO).
- It develops as early as 2–3 weeks after the initiation of therapy and peaks at 18–24 months. The initial clinical appearance is painless enlargement of interproximal gingiva and in severe cases complete enlargement of buccal and lingual, both anterior an posterior segment occurs which is fibrotic in nature.
- In cases where the oral hygiene is good and food debris and plaque are not allowed to accumulate, this side effect of anticonvulsive therapy is not so significant.
- Difficulty in brushing in this condition could result in increased plaque accumulation and inflammation.
- Prolonged medication with these drugs may result in severe enlargement that sometimes entirely covers the teeth **(Fig. 58.5)**.
- Treatment includes alternation of drug followed by meticulous oral prophylaxis and in severe cases where the enlarged tissue interferes with function and esthetics, surgical resection is advised.

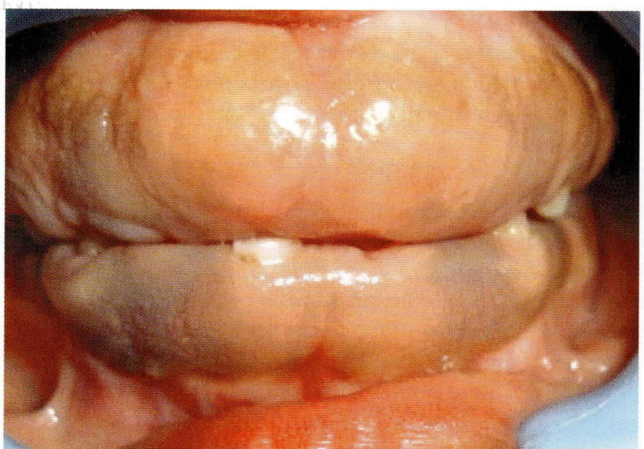

Fig. 58.5: Drug-induced gingivitis.

Plasma Cell Gingivitis

- Plasma cell gingivitis is characterized by diffuse and massive infiltration of plasma cells into the subepithelial gingival tissue.
- It is a rare benign inflammatory condition with no clear etiology, but an exaggerated response to bacterial plaque, immunological reaction to allergens in food such as strong spices, medications, toothpaste, or herbs have been reported.
- In affected children, standard professional oral hygiene procedures and nonsurgical periodontal therapy including antimicrobials are associated with marked improvement of clinical and patient related outcomes **(Figs. 58.6A and B)**.

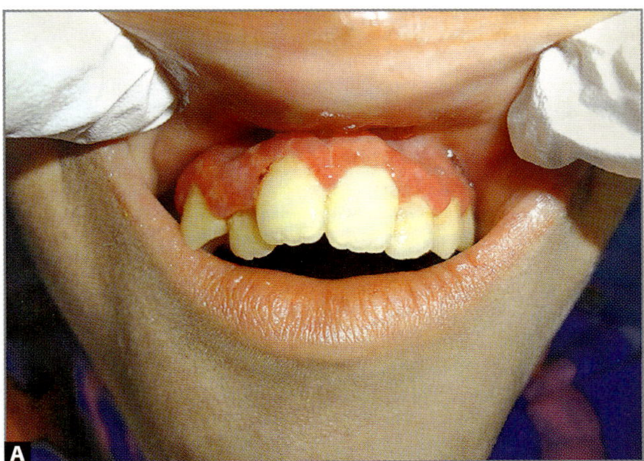

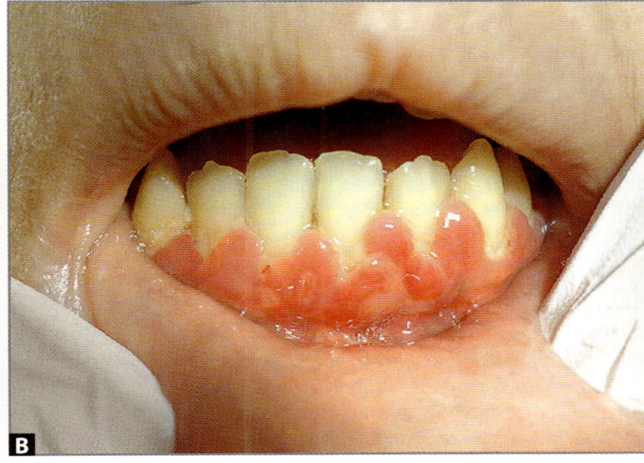

Figs. 58.6A and B: Plasma cell gingivitis–clinical presentation. (*Pic courtesy:* Shivalingu MM, Rathnakara SH, Khanum N, Basappa S. Plasma cell gingivitis: A rare and perplexing entity. J Indian Acad Oral Med Radiol [serial online] 2016 [cited 2022 Sep 23];28:94-7).

Allergy and Gingival Inflammation

- This type of gingivitis is seen in children, in which allergies are recorded due to pollens. The increase in gingival inflammation is attributed to both plaque accumulation and allergic reactions.
- **Matsson and Moller** studied the degree of gingival inflammation in children with allergies to pollen. The results indicated an enhanced gingival inflammatory reaction in the allergic children during the pollen seasons.

Localized Juvenile Spongiotic Gingival Hyperplasia

- This is a recently discovered condition with unknown pathology.
- Lesions present as localized areas appearing as reddish, elevated patches on the attached gingiva that bleed on slight provocation.
- Most cases have been observed in 8–14 year age range with a site predilection for anterior labial gingiva.

Several factors such as genetics, systemic conditions, medications, diet, and individual host response to infection have been identified in the etiology of gingivitis in children. However, the most significant facilitating factor is dental plaque which could be controlled by mechanical means and use of topical chemical agents.

Clinical Significance

- Plaque-induced gingivitis/gingivitis associated with poor oral hygiene is prevalent in children and adolescents and is quickly reversible and can be treated with a good oral prophylactic treatment i.e., good toothbrushing and flossing techniques, to keep the teeth free of bacterial plaque.
- Mild eruption gingivitis requires no treatment other than improved oral hygiene. The greatest increase in the incidence of gingivitis in children is often seen in the 6–7 year age group when the permanent begin to erupt. This increase in gingivitis apparently occurs because the gingival margin receives no protection from the coronal contour of the tooth during the early stage of active eruption, and the continual impingement of food on the gingivae causes the inflammatory process.
- ANUG is rare in preschool children and the use of mild oxidising mouth rinses after each meal and twice chlorhexidine aids in overcoming the infection.
- In cases of puberty induced gingivitis, the treatment should be directed towards improved oral hygiene, removal of all irritants, and dietary changes to ensure adequate nutritional status.
- Substitution of drug and oral hygiene prophylaxis should be the first line of treatment in cases of drug induced gingival enlargement.
- Gingivectomy/gingivoplasty is advocated in cases of moderate—severe gingival inflammation after proper oral prophylaxis along with 2 weeks of chemical therapy. If done immediately it may lead to over resection of enlarged fibrous gingiva, further leading to recession.
- Gingival zenith is important, especially in cases of anterior gingivectomy and is slightly lower in children as compared to adult.

POINTS TO REMEMBER

- Gingivitis or inflammation of the gingiva is characterized by the presence of gingival inflammation without detectable bone loss or clinical attachment loss.
- Stages of gingivitis were given by Page and Schroeder (1976) as initial lesion, early stage, established stage, advanced lesion.
- Different types of gingivitis in children are plaque-induced gingivitis, eruption gingivitis, infective gingivitis, herpetic gingivostomatitis, HIV-associated gingivitis, ANUG, malnutrition-induced gingivitis, pubertal gingivitis, drug-induced gingivitis, and plasma cell gingivitis.
- Plaque-induced gingivitis is seen most commonly in children.
- Eruption gingivitis is gingival inflammation occurring around an erupting permanent tooth.

- Herpetic gingivostomatitis is commonly seen in children less than 3 years of age and occurs due to herpes simplex virus type 1. Its ulcers are small yellowish painful ulcers with erythematous margins.
- Acute necrotizing ulcerative gingivitis is an acute multiple bacterial infection of the gingiva whose predisposing factors include poor oral hygiene, malnutrition, depressed immunity and long-term hospitalization and causative bacteria include *Fusobacteria fusiformis*, *Borrelia vincentii*, and *Treponema* species.
- Pubertal gingivitis is the reaction of tissues to corticosteroids.
- Drug-induced gingivitis is the outcome of antiepileptic therapy with phenytoin or immunosuppressive therapy with systemic cyclosporine.

Questionnaire

1. Define gingivitis and explain its stages.
2. What are the different types of gingivitis seen in children?
3. Write a note on herpetic gingivostomatitis.
4. Explain the etiology, clinical features and treatment of ANUG.
5. Management of drug-induced gingival enlargement.

FURTHER READING

1. Agarwal PK, Agarwal KN, Agarwal DK. Biochemical changes in saliva of malnourished children. Am J Clin Nutr. 1984;39:181-4.
2. Agnihotri R, Bhat KM, Bhat GS, et al. Periodontal management of a patient with severe aplastic anemia: a case report. Spec Care Dentist. 2009;29:141-4.
3. Balasubramaniam R, Sollecito TP, Stoopler ET. Oral health considerations in muscular dystrophies. Spec Care Dentist. 2008;28:243-53.
4. Brennan MT, Sankar V, Baccaglini L. Oral manifestations in patients with aplastic anemia. Oral Surg Oral Med Oral Pathol Oral Radiol Endod. 2001;92:503-8.
5. Crielaard W, Zaura E, Schuller AA, et al. Exploring the oral microbiota of children at various developmental stages of their dentition in relation to their oral health. BMC Med Genomics. 2011;4:22.
6. Gafan GP, Lucas VF, Roberts GJ, et al. Prevalence of periodontal pathogens in dental plaque of children. J Clin Microbiol. 2004;42: 4141-6.
7. Hart TC. Genetic aspects of periodontal diseases. In: Bimstein E, Needleman HL, Karinbux N, Van Dyke TE (Eds). Periodontal and Gingival Health and Diseases. London, England: Children, Adolescents and Young Adults. Martin Dunitz Ltd; 2001. pp. 189-204.
8. Lovegrove JM. Dental plaque revisited: bacteria associated with periodontal disease. JNZ Soc Periodontol. 2004;87:7-21.
9. Matsson L, Möller C. Gingival inflammatory reactions in children with rhinoconjunctivitis due to birch pollinosis. Scand J Dent Res. 1990;98(6):504-9.
10. Matsson L. Factors influencing the susceptibility to gingivitis during childhood–a review. Int J Paediatr Dent. 1993;3:119-27.
11. Oh TJ, Eber R, Wang HL. Periodontal disease in the child and adolescent. J Clin Periodontol. 2002;29:400-10.
12. Okada M, Kobayashi M, Hino T, et al. Clinical periodontal findings and microflora profiles in children with chronic neutropenia under supervised oral hygiene. J Periodontol. 2001;72:945-52.
13. Oredugba F, Ayanbadejo P. (2012). Gingivitis in Children and Adolescents. [online] Available from: https://www.intechopen.com/books/oral-health-care-pediatric-research- epidemiology-and-clinical-practices/gingivitis-in-children-and-adolescents [Accessed April 2018].
14. Oredugba FA, Akindayomi Y. Oral health status and treatment needs of children and young adults attending a day centre for individuals with special needs. Bio Med Central Oral Health. 2008;8:30.
15. Oredugba FA. Comparative oral health of children and adolescents with cerebral palsy and controls. J Disabil Oral Health. 2011;12:81-7.
16. Oredugba FA. Use of oral health care services and oral findings in children with special needs in Lagos, Nigeria. Spec Care Dent. 2006;26:59-65.
17. Page RC, Shroeder HE. Pathogenesis of inflammatory periodontal disease. Lab Invest. 1976;33:235-49.
18. Papaioannou W, Gizani S, Haffajee AD, et al. The microbiota on different oral surfaces in healthy children. Oral Microbiol Immunol. 2009;24:183-9.
19. Perdikogianni H, Papaioannou W, Nakou M, et al. Periodontal and microbiological parameters in children and adolescents with cleft lip and/palate. Int J Paediatr Dent. 2009;19:455-67.
20. Research, Science and Therapy Committee Guidelines of the American Academy of Periodontology. Periodontal diseases of children and adolescents. J Periodontol 2003;74:1696-1704.

Periodontal Diseases in Children

Ravi GR, Karthik Krishna M, Mayur Kaushik, Noopur Kaushik

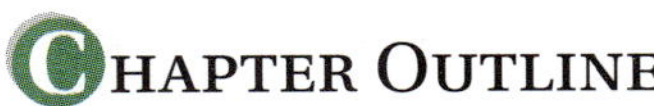

CHAPTER OUTLINE

- Classification of Periodontal Diseases
- Types of Periodontitis in Children and Adolescents
- Microbiology of Periodontitis
- Etiopathogenesis
- Influences of Systemic Diseases on Periodontitis in Children and Adolescents

The term "periodontal disease" may encompass all pathological conditions of the periodontal tissues. Inflammatory lesion recognized by research as color change and/or by bleeding on gentle probing within the gingival sulcus or pocket orifice along with loss of support of the affected tooth, i.e., destruction of the tooth-attached fibers and the bone into which they are inserted, is also present, the condition is characterized as periodontitis. Apart from examination of gingiva, the examination of periodontium is also very crucial in children and adolescents as these entities exhibit plethora of variations physiologically and as well as pathologically. A thorough knowledge about these will enable the novice in diagnosing and executing appropriate intervention. This chapter highlights the normal and as well as various pathological conditions that are encountered by the clinician in a day-to-day practice.

CLASSIFICATION OF PERIODONTAL DISEASES

According to American Academy of Periodontology

The classification of the periodontal diseases has under-gone considerable iterations over the years. Based on the World Workshop in Clinical Periodontics in 1989, the American Academy of Periodontology proposed the classification of periodontitis **(Table 59.1)**.

Table 59.1: Classification of periodontitis by American Academy of Periodontology.

1977	*1986*	*1989*
• Juvenile periodontitis • Chronic marginal periodontitis	• Juvenile periodontitis » Prepubertal » Localized juvenile periodontitis » Generalized juvenile periodontitis • Adult periodontitis • Necrotizing ulcerative gingivo-periodontitis • Refractory periodontitis	• Early-onset periodontitis » Prepubertal periodontitis ◊ Localized ◊ Generalized » Juvenile periodontitis ◊ Localized ◊ Generalized » Rapidly progressive periodontitis • Adult periodontitis • Necrotizing ulcerative periodontitis • Refractory periodontitis • Periodontitis associated with systemic disease

According to European Society of Periodontology

The consensus by the first European Workshop on Periodontology in 1993 reached a conclusion that the existing disease classifications were unsatisfactory due to: (1) extensive overlap; (2) the necessity to assume what the previous disease progression had been (progressive periodontitis); (3) the lack of detailed information on the quality of treatment previously provided and the patient's compliance and tissue response (refractory) and (4) the lack of a consistent basis for classification. The recommendation was that classification should be based on causative factors and host-response factors.

- Early-onset periodontitis
- Adult periodontitis
- Necrotizing periodontitis.

According to International Workshop for a Classification of Periodontal Diseases and Conditions (1999)

- Gingival diseases
  - Dental plaque-induced gingival diseases
  - Nonplaque-induced gingival lesions
- Chronic periodontitis [slight: >1–2 mm clinical attachment loss (CAL); moderate: 3–4 mm CAL; and severe: >5 mm CAL]
  - Localized
  - Generalized (>30% of sites are involved)
- Aggressive periodontitis (slight: 1–2 mm CAL; moderate: 3–4 mm CAL; and severe: >5 mm CAL)
  - Localized
  - Generalized (>30% of sites are involved)
- Periodontitis as a manifestation of systemic diseases
  - Associated with hematological disorders
  - Associated with genetic disorders
  - Not otherwise specified
- Necrotizing periodontal diseases
  - Necrotizing ulcerative gingivitis
  - Necrotizing ulcerative periodontitis
- Abscesses of the periodontium
  - Gingival abscess
  - Periodontal abscess
  - Pericoronal abscess
- Periodontitis associated with endodontic lesions
  - Combined periodontic-endodontic lesions
- Developmental or acquired deformities and conditions
  - Localized tooth-related factors that modify or predispose to plaque-induced gingival diseases/periodontitis
  - Mucogingival deformities and conditions around teeth
  - Mucogingival deformities and conditions on edentulous ridges
  - Occlusal trauma

- In 2017 the American Academy of Periodontology (AAP) and European Federation of Periodontology (EFP) co-presented the new classification for periodontal and peri-implant diseases and conditions at the World Workshop
- The new classification replaced the terms 'chronic' and 'aggressive' used in the Armitage model as periodontitis is a broad spectrum of a single disease, and not two distinct ones.
- There was also the addition of staging and grading the disease

TYPES OF PERIODONTITIS IN CHILDREN AND ADOLESCENTS

Early-onset Periodontitis

- The term early-onset periodontitis is usually diagnosed in patients under the age of 35 years.
- The destruction of the periodontium is advanced for the age of onset of the condition.
- Early-onset periodontitis has a tendency to aggregate in families **(Table 59.2)**.

Prepubertal Periodontitis

- Extremely rare category of periodontitis, usually having an onset during or soon after the eruption of the deciduous teeth.
- Both familial clustering of prepubertal periodontitis and a higher incidence in females have been documented.
- The associated plaque deposits are moderate and there is little inflammation of the gingivae, but bleeding upon probing is present at affected sites.
- There are no associated systemic conditions, and patients do not suffer from frequent upper respiratory tract infections. The destruction is not as rapid as in the generalized form, and the condition usually responds to treatment.

Localized Early-onset Periodontitis

- This form of early-onset periodontitis is also referred to as localized juvenile periodontitis.
- According to **Hart et al.,** diagnosis of localized early-onset periodontitis is based on attachment loss of more than 4 mm on at least two permanent 1st molars and incisors (one of which must be a 1st permanent molar).
- Not more than two other permanent teeth, which are not 1st permanent molars or incisors, should be affected. Most striking feature is the presence of deep pockets.
- Another striking feature is the arc-shaped defect seen in OPG of the patient extending from distal of 2nd premolar to mesial aspect of second molar on both the sides.
- Premature and excessive mobility of maxillary and mandibular primary incisors and 1st primary molars are seen.
- As the disease progresses, other symptoms may arise, deep, dull, and radiating pain during mastication may be observed.

Table 59.2: Comparison of key types of periodontitis that can affect adolescents.

		Early-onset periodontitis	
	Incipient adult periodontitis	***Localized***	***Generalized***
Age of onset	May begin in early teens	Puberty or later. Bone loss may be detectable in deciduous dentition	Puberty or later but usually before age 35 years
Clinical presentation	Loss of attachment of 1 mm or 2 mm. first molars, incisors commonly affected on mesial and distal sites, but other teeth affected also	Loss of attachment >3 mm. Lack of precise criteria. Generally agreed 1st molar(s) and incisor(s) must be affected, and up to one or two other teeth may be affected	Loss of attachment >3 mm. Distinct from and more generalized than localized early-onset periodontitis. Affects at least three teeth other than 1st molars and incisors
Radiographic features	Incipient horizontal crestal bone loss, affecting a few sites. May be detected on serial bitewing radiographs	Severe bone loss in 1st molars and incisors. Characteristic presentation as arc-shaped lesions and angular defects	Severe bone loss. More generalized than localized early-onset periodontitis
Prevalence, severity, extent, progression	Prevalent. Not very severe attachment loss. Variable extent, depends on factors such as age and ethnic group. Relatively slow rate of progression of attachment loss	Low prevalence. Severe attachment loss >3 mm. Some tooth loss may occur. Extent and rate of progression variable, but generally lower than generalized early-onset periodontitis. May progress to generalized early-onset periodontitis	Low prevalence. Severe attachment loss >3 mm. Some tooth loss may occur. Greater extent than localized early-onset periodontitis. Rate of progression variable but generally greater than for localized early-onset periodontitis or incidental attachment loss
Altered host function	No evidence	Some earlier reports of altered neutrophil function	Some earlier reports of altered neutrophil function
Microflora	As for adult periodontitis, including *Spirochetes, Porphyromonas gingivalis, Prevotella intermedia* and *Actinobacillus actinomycetemcomitans*	*A. actinomycetemcomitans* is key organism	Bacteroides forsythus, *P. gingivalis, P. intermedia,* *A. actinomycetemcomitans, Campylobacter rectus, Fusobacterium nucleatum*
Subgingival calculus, gingival inflammation	Significant association between plaque, subgingival calculus, gingival inflammation and subsequent development and progression of loss of attachment	Concept of little subgingival calculus, gingival inflammation has been challenged, Significant association between presence of subgingival calculus and gingival inflammation and subsequent attachment loss	As for localized early-onset periodontitis, but teeth with subgingival calculus and inflammation in generalized early-onset periodontitis group develop even more attachment loss than localized early-onset periodontitis group
Ethnic status	Increased prevalence in some ethnic groups, such as Indo-Pakistani	Increased prevalence in some ethnic groups, such as Blacks	As for localized early-onset periodontitis
Genetic basic	Not a key feature	Yes	Yes

Modifications made in 1999 classification

- The term prepubertal periodontitis has been replaced by "Periodontitis as a manifestation of systemic diseases. It was attributed to the fact that certain diseases were sufficient strong enough to cause periodontal destruction even in absence of plaque and calculus.
- Juvenile periodontitis was replaced by "aggressive periodontitis"
- Term "rapidly progressive periodontitis "has been discarded.

Generalized Early-onset Periodontitis

- Generalized early-onset periodontitis has its onset from puberty until 35 years of age.
- According to **Hart et al.**, clinical diagnosis is based on attachment loss of more than 5 mm on a minimum of eight permanent teeth (one of which must be a 1st molar), at least three of which should not be 1st molars or incisors. Individuals must be systemically healthy.

Recent developments in classification of the periodontal diseases relevant to children and adolescents

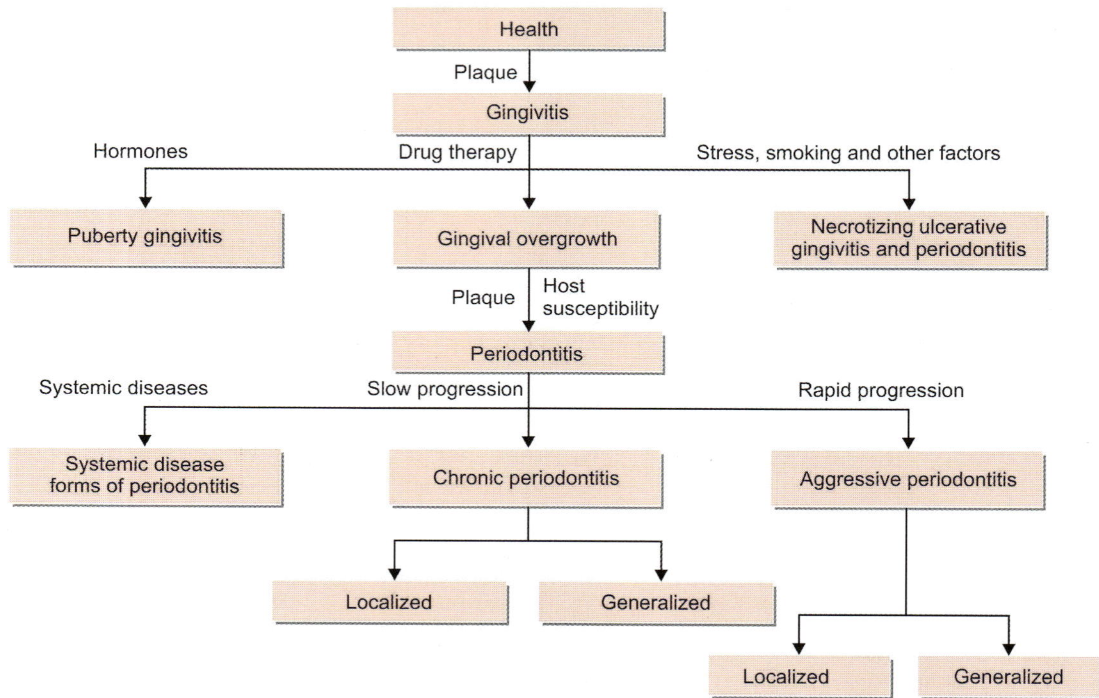

Adult Periodontitis

- Adult periodontitis is probably initiated at or soon after puberty, but does not manifest symptoms until the middle of the fourth decade.
- Adult periodontitis is a slowly progressing form of periodontitis.
- However, it may at any stage undergo an acute exacerbation with associated attachment loss.

Necrotizing Forms of Periodontal Disease

- Necrotizing ulcerative gingivitis is characterized by gingival necrosis presenting as "punched-out" papillae, with gingival bleeding and pain.
- Halitosis and pseudomembrane formation may be secondary diagnostic features.
- Fusiform bacteria, other anaerobic gram-negative bacteria and spirochetes have been associated with the gingival lesions.
- Related factors may include emotional stress, poor diet, cigarette smoking, seasonal changes, and HIV infection.
- Necrotizing ulcerative periodontitis is characterized by necrosis of gingival tissues, periodontal ligament, and alveolar bone. Lesions are commonly observed in individuals with systemic conditions including, but not limited to viral infections, severe malnutrition, and immunosuppression.
- Necrotizing ulcerative periodontitis is preceded by necrotizing ulcerative gingivitis, which is an acute inflammatory condition associated with a fusospirochetal microbiota.

MICROBIOLOGY OF PERIODONTITIS (TABLES 59.3 AND 59.4)

Table 59.3: Suspected pathogens in localized early-onset periodontitis.

Organism/species	Criteria
Aggregatibacter actinomy cetemcomitans	Increased prevalence in localized early-on periodontitis sites/patients Decrease in health or gingivitis Increase in active/progressing sites Elimination/reduction with treatment
Porphyromonas gingivalis	Increased prevalence Decrease in health/gingivitis Increase in active disease Elimination/reduction with treatment
Prevotella intermedia	Increased prevalence Decrease in health/gingivitis Increase in active disease Elimination/reduction with treatment
Capnocytophaga	Increased prevalence Decrease in health/gingivitis Elimination/reduction with treatment
Fusobacterium nucleatum	Increased prevalence Increase in active disease Elimination/reduction with treatment
Eikenella corrodens	Increased prevalence Increase in active disease Elimination/reduction with treatment
Campylobacter	Increased prevalence
Spirochetes	Increased prevalence Decrease health/gingivitis
Eubacterium	Increased prevalence
Bacteroides forsythus	Unaware of any studies
Black-pigmented anaerobic rods	Increased prevalence

Table 59.4: Other species investigated in localized early-onset periodontitis.

Species	***Suspected role in localized early- onset periodontitis***
Haemophilus	Associated with health
Enterococcus	Occur frequently and may contribute in high numbers
Streptococcus	Found in higher numbers but not associated with disease
Peptostreptococcus	More prevalent in adult periodontitis
Staphylococcus	Occur frequently and may contribute in high numbers
Kingella	No correlation with disease
Mycoplasma	Invade oral epithelial tissue, numbers increase in disease
Actinomyces	*Actinomyces naeslundii* associated with health
Yeasts	Associated with tissue invasion

ETIOPATHOGENESIS (FIGS. 59.1A AND B)

Host Response

The host defense system comprises a collection of tissues, cells, and molecules whose function is to protect the host against infectious agents.

Protective Mechanisms

- Physical barriers such as the skin and mucous membranes represent a component that infectious agents must breach to gain access to the host.
- The washing action of fluids such as tears, saliva, urine and gingival crevicular fluid keeps mucosal surfaces clear of invading organisms and also contain bactericidal agents.
- The intact epithelial barrier of the gingiva, sulcular, and junctional epithelium normally prevents bacterial invasion of the periodontal tissues. It is normally an effective physical barrier against bacterial products and components.
- The epithelial cell wall, secreted proteins, and fatty acids are toxic to many microbes.
- Salivary secretions provide a continuous flushing of the oral cavity as well as providing a continuing supply of agglutinins and specific antibodies.
- Furthermore, the gingival crevicular fluid flushes the gingival sulcus and delivers all the components of serum, including complement and specific antibodies.
- Macrophage produce cytokines (such as interleukin-1) induce fibroblasts and osteoblasts to produce proteases, which result in bone and tissue breakdown.

INFLUENCES OF SYSTEMIC DISEASES ON PERIODONTITIS IN CHILDREN AND ADOLESCENTS

There are various systemic conditions that may reduce the host response in children and adolescents, thus increasing their susceptibility to periodontal bone loss and ultimately loss of teeth.

Leukocyte Disorders

As far as neutrophils are concerned, inborn (genetic) defects leading to a depressed or to a complete loss of cellular chemotaxis are always accompanied by a severe prepubertal periodontitis.

Neutropenia

These diseases have periodontal manifestations and the group includes agranulocytosis, cyclic neutropenia, chronic benign neutropenia, chronic idiopathic neutropenia, and familial benign chronic neutropenia.

Dental Aspects

- The attached, papillary and marginal gingival are enlarged, edematous, and erythematous and bleed easily on a gentle probing.
- Extreme inflammation with proliferation of marginal gingiva is noticed.

Treatment

In patients with malignancies of the blood and blood-forming organs and other cancers, recombinant human granulocyte colony-stimulating factor is effective at correcting chemotherapy-induced neutropenia and is useful in the management of infections that complicate neutropenia.

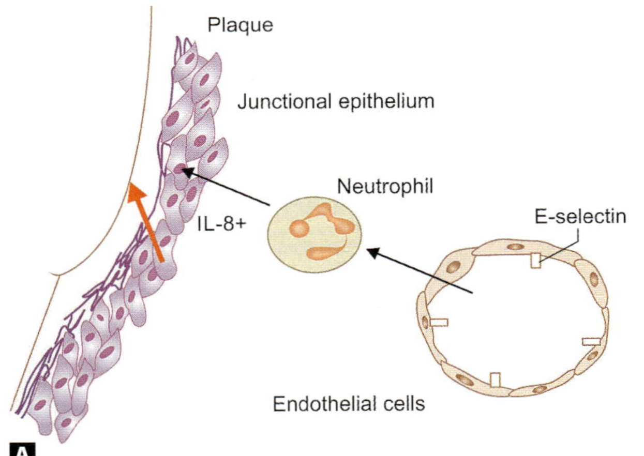

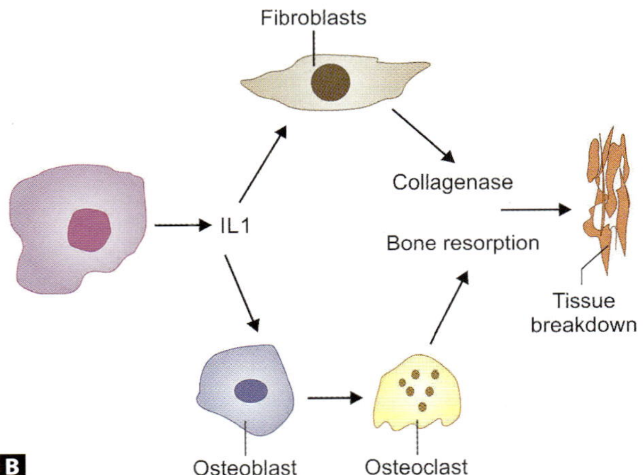

Figs. 59.1A and B: Etiopathogenesis of periodontitis. (IL: interleukin).

Other systemic condition that manifests as periodontal diseases
- Leukocyte adhesion deficiency syndrome
- Down's syndrome
- Histiocytosis syndromes
- Ehlers-Danlos syndrome
- Virus-associated hemophagocytic syndrome
- Hypophosphatasia
- Juvenile hyaline fibromatosis of gingiva
- Acquired immunodeficiency syndrome
- Malnutrition
- Diabetes mellitus

Chédiak-Higashi Syndrome

- Chédiak-Higashi syndrome has frequently been linked with severe periodontitis.
- It is a rare autosomal recessive immunodeficiency disorder characterized by large lysosomal granules in granulocytes, partial oculocutaneous infections, and intermittent febrile episodes.

Dental Aspects

Extreme periodontal manifestations along with mobility of teeth.

Treatment

- Functional defects in Chédiak-Higashi syndrome leukocytes are corrected by ascorbic acid.
- Other treatments consisted of management regimens such as vincristine–corticosteroids, etoposide–corticosteroids–intrathecal methotrexate, and high doses of intravenous globulin, inducing a transient remission.

Papillon-Lefèvre Syndrome

- In 1924, Papillon and Lefèvre first described a syndrome characterized by hyperkeratosis of palms and soles combined with precocious periodontal destruction and shedding of the deciduous and permanent dentitions.
- In most of the cases it has been found that cathepsin C is expressed in the areas of epithelium often affected by hyperkeratotic lesions such as palms, soles, knees and oral keratinized gingiva.

Dental Aspects

Swollen gingival, migration and mobility of teeth, periodontal pockets, fetor oris, and exfoliation of teeth.

Treatment

A combined approach including meticulous plaque control, administration of chlorhexidine in combination with a systemic antibiotic therapy for the eradication of known periodontal pathogens in conjunction with retinoids.

Genetic conditions associated with periodontal destruction in children and adolescents

Condition	*Nature of condition*	*Periodontal effects*
Leukocyte disorders • **Neutropenia** • **Chédiak-Higashi syndrome** • **Leukocyte adhesion deficiency syndrome**	• Reduction in number of granulocytes. • Rare autosomal recessive immunodeficiency disorder • Large lysosomal granules in granulocytes • Neutrophil and monocyte defects • Recurrent infections, may be severe • Defects in integrin receptors of leukocytes • Impaired adhesion and chemotaxis • Increased susceptibility to infection, including otitis media, septicemia, impaired pus formation, delayed wound healing.	• Severe gingivitis periodontitis. Tooth loss due to periodontal destruction. • Ulceration of mucosa, tongue, hard palate. • Early-onset prepubertal periodontitis. Rapid attachment loss and bone loss shortly after eruption of deciduous dentition. • Early exfoliation
Papillon-Lefèvre syndrome	• Autosomal recessive inheritance. Rare 1:3 or 4 million. Often history of consanguineous families palmoplantar hyperkeratosis • Impaired neutrophil chemotactic, phagocytic and bactericidal activities and decreased migration may play a role in the disease pathogenesis and defects in immune function have also been cited	• Early-onset prepubertal periodontitis. • Rapid attachment loss and bone loss affecting deciduous dentition. Early exfoliation or need for extraction. Therapy difficult. Permanent dentition may be affected resulting in tooth loss. • Bacterial associated include *Porphyromonas gingivalis, Fusobacterium nucleatum*, and *Eikenella corrodens*, but the etiological role of *Actinobacillus actinomycetemcomitans* seems pivotal. High antibody titers to *A. actinomycetemcomitans* have been reported in some cases
Down's syndrome	• Autosomal chromosomal anomaly associated with trisomy of chromosome 21. Affects 1 of 700 live births. • Mental handicap. • T-cell immunodeficiency and inappropriate enzyme regulation. • Functional defects in neutrophils and monocytes. Abnormal capillary morphology. • Connective tissue disorders. • Hyperinnervation of gingivae	• Periodontal disease very prevalent and more severe than in age-matched controls especially in lower anteriors. Differences not explained by plaque levels. • Rapid progression. Onset apparent in deciduous dentition
Hypophosphatasia	• Autosomal inherited trait. Inborn error of metabolism. • Deficiency serum alkaline phosphatase increased urinary excretion phosphoethanolamine, defective bone/tooth mineralization. • Three forms: lethal neonatal/perinatal, severe infantile, milder form in childhood/late adolescence	• Cementum hypoplasia or aplasia. • Periodontal destruction may affect deciduous dentition, resulting in premature exfoliation, tooth loss. • Variable effects on permanent dentition, not necessarily as severe

Contd...

Contd...

Condition	Nature of condition	Periodontal effects
Ehlers-Danlos syndrome	• Collagen disorder affecting joints (loose-joint-edness) and skin (fragile and hyperextensible). • The mucosa is easily traumatized. • Prolonged bleeding may be a feature, and therefore hematological investigations are warranted. • Ten types; type VIII has periodontal implications: autosomal dominant inheritance. • Distinguish by skin biopsy from type IV (autosomal dominant/ recessive) which has life-threatening potential complications.	• Type VIII: Aggressive early-onset periodontitis leading to premature loss of permanent teeth

Periodontal Screening

Periodontal screening in children and adolescents provides a simple and quick method of identifying periodontal problems which is comfortably tolerated and gives the dental practitioner an indication of the need for treatment or further assessment **(Fig. 59.2)**.

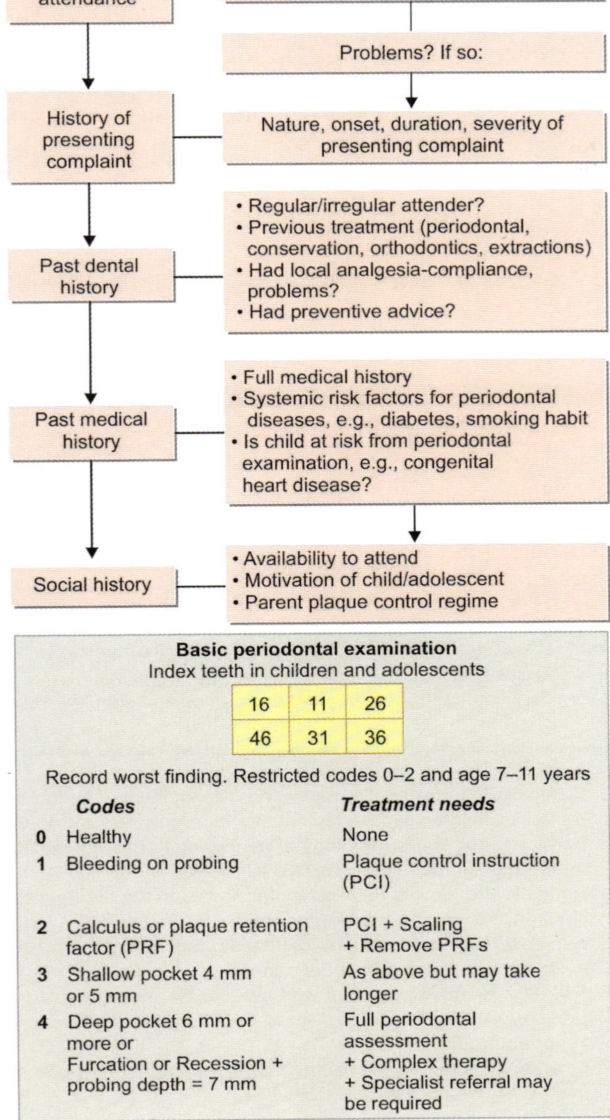

Fig. 59.2: Screening using the basic periodontal examination for the child/adolescent.

Diagnosis and Management

A number of different forms of periodontal disease can present in children and adolescents, ranging from reversible conditions limited to the gingival tissues to those characterized by destruction of the periodontal connective tissue attachment and alveolar bone, which may jeopardize the longevity of the deciduous or permanent dentition. The prevalence, extent, severity, and prognosis of periodontal disease in the younger age groups vary according to the disease in question. The diagnostic options are determined by an up-to-date classification of the periodontal diseases, and this has been an area of ongoing debate and review. Fundamental principles need to be applied to identify and manage periodontal problems in these patients together with an understanding of the causation and contributory risk factors and an appreciation of the different strategies inherent in working with a younger age group compared with the adult patient. The patient's history, in conjunction with the examination, forms the basis for the diagnosis of the periodontal condition and should involve both the child or adolescent and the parents or guardians of minors.

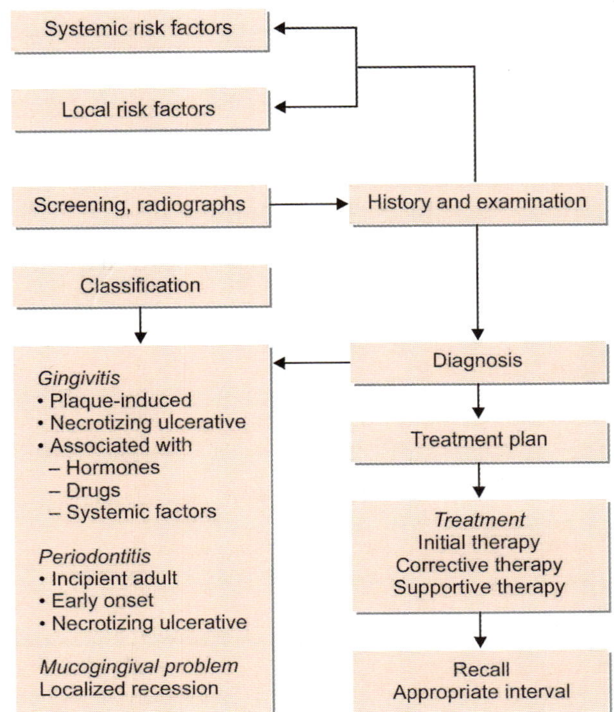

Health promotion and behavioral approaches in the prevention of periodontal disease in children and adolescents	
Chairside activities	***Societal activities***
Smoking cessation	**Smoking cessation**
• Remember the simple method of the four A's: ask, advise, assist, and arrange in smoking cessation • Make a note of smoking on a patient's dental chart and assess the level of nicotine dependence using, for example, Fageström test for nicotine dependence • An approached oriented towards family and peer group is preferable. At least remember their influence on your patient's smoking behavior • Assess the smoker's reasons for quitting and obstacles to doing so to assist in building up the smoker's motivation for change • Avoid victimizing your patient and his or her family or friends • Try to delay the age of smoking initiation rather than strictly banning it • Show your expertise in common risk-factor thinking • Supply your smoking patients with written information too	• Influence your local school authorities for a strict and supervised ban on smoking at schools • Collaborate with your partners and local colleagues in sharing knowledge and establishing practical plans of action • Collaborate with other health professionals in the spirit of common risk-factor thinking • Contact local coalitions for preventing tobacco use for possible collaboration
Oral health education	**Oral health education**
• An approach oriented towards the mother and father and peer group is preferable • Avoid victimizing your patient or his or her parents • Try to look for options in which the easy choice is the healthy choice, such as where to buy an electric toothbrush and how much it will cost • Keep it simple—self-assessment of bleeding approach could be useful for many people ***Recall and intensive prevention*** Prefer family checkups if alarming signs of early-onset periodontitis are evident. Behavioral and genetic factors dominate—siblings may need your help and you need good family support and collaboration to improve your patient's oral hygiene to the required exceptionally high level	• Check the availability and quality of oral health leaflets in your local area—schools, drug stories, etc. • Organize meetings with people responsible for general health education in schools and other institutions and upgrade their knowledge and motivation to bring the message to the children • Collaborate with your local dental association for backup support • Collaborate with your local toothpaste, toothbrush, and other related companies for material support

Clinical Significance

- Chronic periodontitis is rarely seen in children because the duration required for it to develop is too long (primary teeth stay for a shorter period of time)
- Aggressive periodontitis is also not seen in children under 12 years of age, however teenagers might develop due to long standing accumulation of plaque and calculus along with genetic predisposition .
- Early exfoliation of primary and permanent teeth in a child indicates an underlying systemic disease (Papillon Lefevre, Cyclic Neutropenia, etc.) and proper overall whole body assessment should be done.

POINTS TO REMEMBER

- The term "periodontal disease" may encompass all pathological conditions of the periodontal tissues. The classification of the periodontal diseases has undergone considerable iterations over the years.
- Physical barriers such as the skin and mucous membranes represent a component that infectious agents must breach to gain access to the host.
- Salivary secretions provide a continuous flushing of the oral cavity as well as providing a continuing supply of agglutinins and specific antibodies.
- There are various systemic conditions that may reduce the host response in children and adolescents, thus increasing their susceptibility to periodontal bone loss and ultimately loss of teeth.
- Periodontal screening in children and adolescents provides a simple and quick method of identifying periodontal problems which is comfortably tolerated gives the dental practitioner an indication of the need for treatment or further assessment.
- Periodontal diseases can present in children and adolescents, ranging from reversible conditions limited to the gingival tissues to those characterized by destruction of the periodontal connective tissue attachment and alveolar bone.
- The patient's history, in conjunction with the examination, forms the basis for the diagnosis of the periodontal condition and should involve both the child or adolescent and the parents or guardians of minors.

Questionnaire

1. Classify gingival and periodontal disease in children.
2. Enumerate the organisms causing gingival and periodontal disease in children.
3. Risk factors associated with gingival manifestations in children and adolescents.
4. Write a note on localized juvenile periodontitis.

FURTHER READING

1. American Academy of Periodontology. Proceedings from the 2017 World Workshop on the Classification of Periodontal and Peri-implant Diseases and Conditions. 2017. Available at: https://www.perio.org/2017wwdc (accessed September 2020).
2. Clerehugh V, Tugnait A. Diagnosis and management of periodontal disease in children and adolescents. Periodontol. 2001;26:146-68.
3. Darby I, Curtis M. Microbiology of periodontal disease in children and young adults. Periodontol. 2001;26:33-53.
4. Hodge P, Michalowicz B. Genetic predisposition to periodontitis in children and young adults. Periodontol. 2001;26:113-34.
5. Jenkins WMM, Papapanou PN. Epidemiology of periodontal disease in children and adolescents. Periodontol. 2001;26:16-32.
6. Kallio PJ. Health promotion and behavioral approaches in the prevention of periodontal disease in children and adolescents. Periodontol. 2001;26:135-45.
7. Kinane DF, Podmore M, Ebersole J. Etiopathogenesis of periodontitis in children. Periodontol. 2001;26:54-91.
8. Kinane DF. Periodontal disease in children and adolescents: introduction and classification. Periodontol. 2001;26:7-15.
9. Meyele J, Gonzales JR. Influences of systemic diseases in children and adolescents. Periodontol. 2001;26:92-112.

CHAPTER

Infection Control

Gurvanit Kaur Lehl, Ramanandvignesh P, Chaitanya P, Nikhil Marwah

Chapter Outline

- Personal Protective equipment
- Handwashing and Handcare
- Surface Barriers
- Chemical Disinfectants
- Spill Management
- Sterilization
- Protocol during Pandemic Period
- Management of Dental Biowaste
- Regulations by OSHA to be Followed to Prevent Cross infection

Microorganisms cause virtually all pathoses. It reminds about Florence Nightingale's favorite dictum "The first requirement of a hospital is that it should do the sick no harm". The scientific study of hospital or nosocomial cross infection began during the first-half of 18th century, and from that time until the start of the "Bacteriological Era" many notable contributions originated and remarkable among these early pioneers was the physician **Sir John Pringle**, who strongly believed that overcrowding and poor ventilation added greatly to the problem of hospital infection.[1,2] The understanding of hospital infection followed upon the discoveries of **Pasteur, Koch,** and **Lister**, it was the beginning of the "Bacteriological Era". With the opening of numerous hospitals in the 20th century, it was soon realized that infections occurred not only in obstetric, surgical, and medical patients, but in dental patients as well and air could be a source of such infection and that many viral, as well as bacterial, infections might spread via this route.[1,2] It was not until **Joseph Lister** 1867, in Scotland proposed his Germ Theory and put forward the idea of antisepsis to reduce infections in surgical patients. This was one of the major fundamental advances.

WD Miller who authored a book "*Microorganisms of the Human Mouth*" in 1890 associated the presence of bacteria with pulpal and periapical disease and is considered to be the father of oral microbiology. In 1910, a British physician, **William Hunter** presented a lecture on the role of sepsis and antisepsis to the faculty of McGill University condemned the practice of dentistry in United States, which emphasized restorations instead of tooth extraction.[3] **Hunter** stated that the restorations were "a veritable mausoleum of gold over a mass of sepsis" which he believed was the cause of illness. **Antony Van Leeuwenhoek**, the inventor of single lens microscope, was the first to observe oral flora and his descriptions of animalcules observed in microscope included those from dental plaque and from an exposed pulp cavity.

DEFINITIONS

Sterilization: *Defined as the process by which an article, surface or a medium freed of all microorganisms including viruses, bacteria, their spores and fungi both pathogenic and non-pathogenic.*

Disinfection: *The elimination of virtually all pathogenic microorganism on inanimate objects with the exception of large number of bacterial endospore reducing the level of microbial contamination to an acceptable safe level.*

Sanitization: *Used as a synonym for disinfection, particularly with reference to food processing and catering.*

Antisepsis: *It is used as to indicate the prevention of infection, usually by inhibiting the growth of bacteria in wounds or tissues.*

Antiseptics: *Chemical disinfectants, which can be safely applied to skin or mucous membrane and are used to prevent infection by inhibiting the growth of bacteria.*

Bactericidal agents: *The agents those are able to kill bacteria.*

Bacteriostatic agents: *Only prevent the multiplication of bacteria, which may however remain alive.*

Contamination: *It is any activity that reduces the microbial load to prevent inadvertent contamination or infection.*

Universal precautions: *It refers to the method of infection control in which all human blood and certain human body fluids (saliva in dentistry) are treated as infectious for human immunoglobin virus (HIV), hepatitis B virus (HBV), and other blood borne pathogens.*[4]

Standard precautions: *A set of combined precautions that include the major components of universal precautions (designed to reduce the risk of transmission of blood borne pathogens) and body substance isolation (designed to reduce the risk of transmission of pathogens from moist body substances).*

PERSONAL PROTECTIVE EQUIPMENT

The World Health Organization (WHO) has launched its global safety challenge promoting "clean care is safer care" which identifies the dangers of healthcare-associated infections. The WHO's "clean care is safer care" focuses on clean hands, clean equipment, clean clinical procedures, and clean environment. It is important to put on a barrier or personal protective equipment (PPE) whenever there is risk of coming in contact with mucous membranes or body fluids.[5]Dentists, other dental healthcare personnel (DHCP), and dental students have been categorized as high-risk groups for occupationally acquired infections as they are continually exposed to the potential risk of needle stick injuries, contact with blood and other body fluids from patients.[6,7]

Gloves

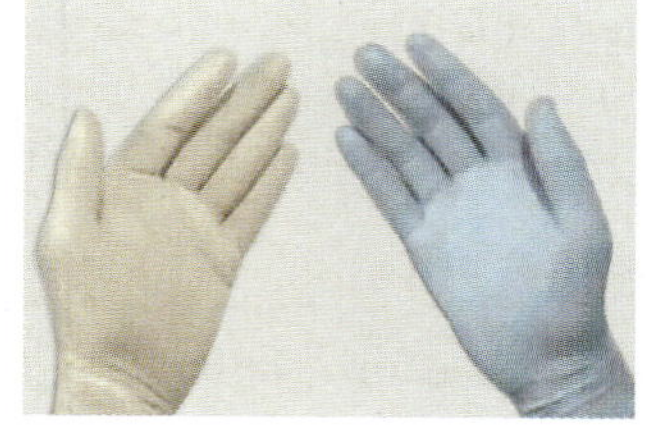

- The most important worn PPE is quality vinyl gloves.
- Remove gloves promptly after use and perform hand hygiene before touching clean items, environmental surfaces, your eyes, nose and mouth, and before going on to another client.
- Properly fitting gloves should be snug but not restrictive, and should cover the cuffs of a long sleeved gown. Care should be taken to avoid injury during procedures. If gloves are torn, cut or punctured they must be changed as soon as it is safely possible. Wash hands thoroughly and replace gloves before continuing with the procedure.
- Some healthcare workers have reported allergies to the latex or the powder used in gloves which may be as irritation contact dermatitis, delayed contact dermatitis (rash), and immediate allergic urticaria. Powdering of hand and cotton glove liners is available to provide a barrier between the skin and the latex.
- Nonlatex glove (vinyl or other nonsynthetic polymer) are also available for usage.

Masks (Surgical) for Face Protection

- These provide protection to nose and mouth from likely splashes and sprays of blood or body fluids. Splashes and sprays can be generated from a client's behavior (e.g., coughing or sneezing) or during procedures (e.g., suctioning, irrigation, cleaning equipment).
- Mask can be dome-shaped or surgical masks with/without a fluid resistant membrane layer.[8]
- Surgical masks with ear loops are the easiest to put on and remove. Wear within three to five feet of the coughing and sneezing client. This prevents transmission of microorganisms to the dentist.

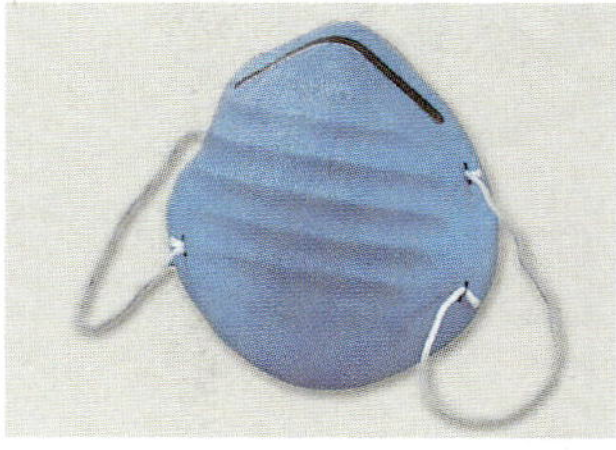

- Absence of an airtight fit around the periphery of the mask increases the chances of air to get inside the mask through the periphery and this phenomenon is called "blow-by".[2]
- Dental aerosols that are generated during patient care are usually smaller than 5 microns in diameter and are suspended in air. The passing of the liquids from the outer layer of the mask on to the inner surface is called "strike through" and this should be avoided by using masks that are impervious for liquid passage.
- The surgical mask may have three layers: (1) The outer (esthetic layer), (2) the middle (fluid shield layer), and (3) the inner layer (that is soft and compatible with the skin of the face). The mask may be shaped for a good fit such as being pleated or being duckbill shaped.

Respirators

- Respirator such as N95 masks is a particulate filtering face piece respirator that filters at least 95% of airborne particles. N series respirators are only effective in absence of oil particles such as lubricants/glycerine. N95 is most commonly used in health care settings.
- N95 respirator is flat folded and expands into convex shaped mask with polyamide elastic head loops to secure the mask to the user's face and malleable aluminium strip positioned above the nose for a tighter seal.
- It is composed of four layers; an outer layer consists of spun-bound polypropylene and coated with hydrophilic plastic, second layer of cellulose/polyester and coated with copper and zinc ions, third layer of melt-blown polypropylene filter and fourth (inner) layer of spun bound polypropylene.
- Dental care personnel are advised to wear N95 respirator when screening and performing treatment in suspected/confirmed COVID-19 patients.[9]

Gowns

- Put on the gown as first procedure, mask and eye protection as the second procedure **(Fig. 60.1)**.
- Wear long sleeved gowns to protect uncovered skin and clothing from likely splashes, sprays during procedures and client care activities.
- Gowns are to be changed between patients to control cross contamination between patients.[8]
- It is recommended that all dental students under- graduate and postgraduates wear hospital clinical attire while treating patients in the clinical areas based on the level of anticipated exposure. It is also recommended that dentists

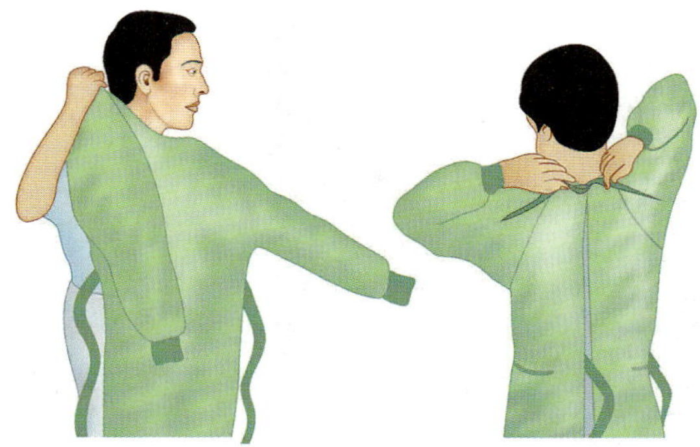

How to put on a gown?

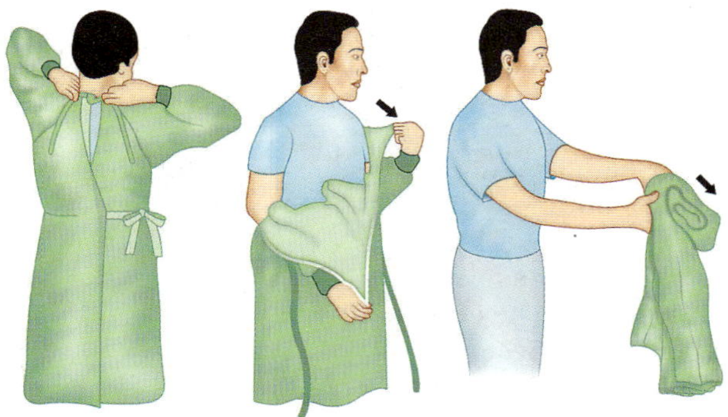

How to remove a gown?

Fig. 60.1: Procedure of wearing and removal of gown.

and faculty members who guide dental students in clinical area should routinely wear clinical attire while working on patients or in laboratories and while working chair side with students.[8]

- Practicing universal precautions in the form of personal barrier technique for all patients is considered one of the most efficient methods to minimize the risk of cross infection in the dental office.[7]

Glove types and indications

Glove	Indication	Comment	*Commercially available glove materials**	
			Material	***Attributes***†
Patient examination gloves§	Patient care, examinations other nonsurgical procedures involving contact with mucous membranes, and laboratory procedures	Medical device regulated by the Food and Drug Administration (FDA). Nonsterile and sterile single-use disposable. Use for one patient and discard appropriately.	Natural-rubber latex (NRL)	1,2
			Nitrile	2,3
			Nitrite and chloroprene (neoprene) blends	2,3
			Nitrile and nrl blends	1,2,3
			Butadiene methyl methacrylate	2,3
			Polyvinyl chloride (PVC or vinyl)	4
			Polyurethane	4
			Styrene-based copolymer	4,5
Surgeon's gloves§	Surgical procedures	Medical device regulated by the FDA. Sterile and single-use disposable use for one patient and discard appropriately.	NRL	1,2
			Nitrile	2,3
			Chloroprene (neoprene)	2,3
			NRl and nitrile or chloroprene blends	2,3
			Synthetic polyisoprene	2
			Styrene-based copolymer	4,5
			Polyurethane	4
Nonmedical gloves	• Housekeeping procedures (e.g., cleaning and disinfection) • Handling contaminated sharps or chemicals • Not for use during patient care	Not a medical device regulated by the FDA. Commonly referred to as utility, industrial, or general purpose gloves. Should be puncture- or chemical-resistant, depending on the task. Latex gloves do not provide adequate chemical protection. Sanitize after use.	NRl and nitrile or chloroprene blends	2,3
			Chloroprene (neoprene)	2,3
			Nitrile	2,3
			Butyl rubber	2,3
			Fluoroelastomer	3,4,6
			Polyethylene and ethylene vinyl alcohol copolymer	3,4,6

*Physical properties can vary by material, manufacturer, and protein and chemical composition.

†1. Contains allergenic NRL proteins.

2. Vulcanized rubber, contains allergenic rubber processing chemicals.

3. Likely to have enhanced chemical or puncture resistance.

4. Nonvulcanized and does not contain rubber processing chemicals.

5. Inappropriate for use with methacrylates.

6. Resistant to most methacrylates.

§Medical or dental gloves include patient examination gloves and surgeons (i.e., surgical) gloves and are medical devices regulated by the FDA. Only FDA cleared medical or dental patient examination gloves and surgical gloves can be used for patient care.

Protective Eyewear

- In dentistry, polycarbonate glasses with side-shields, face-shields and glasses with disposable side-shields are used.[5,8]
- While trimming models, dentures, cutting wires and doing lab work or during reprocessing of instruments, use of protective eyewear is a must to reduce the probability of exposure to hazardous materials and hard matter that may damage the eyes.[8] Eye injuries may occur from projectiles such as bits of calculus during scaling procedures and splatters from body fluids while using high speed hand pieces and another potential source of eye injury is the intense dental curing light.[9]

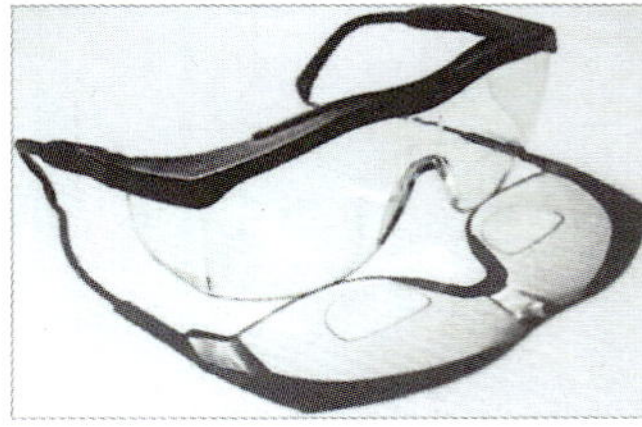

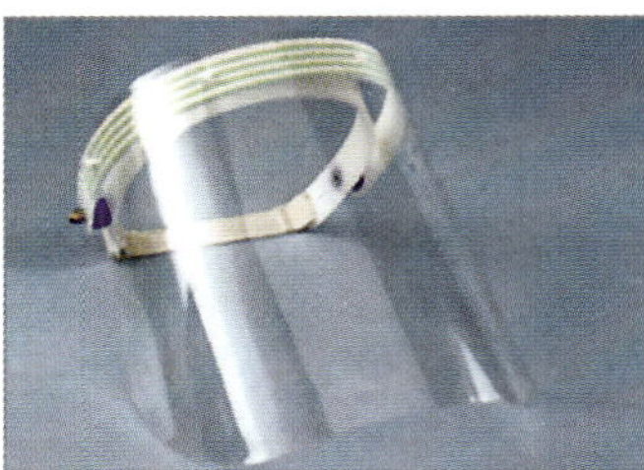

- Two types of products generally available are goggles or eye shields which cover only eyes and face shields that cover entire face.[5] Protective eyeglasses benefits as a barrier against physical and chemical injuries.[10]

HANDWASHING AND HANDCARE

- Patients notice most things in the clinic from cleanliness to personal hygiene and clinician's professionalism. Sometimes, they even take into notice whether the clinician and staff have clean finger nails, washed hands with soap before donning gloves, whether the hair is unkept, and also whether the clothes are clean and presentable as a clinic staff or dentist.[8]
- Hand hygiene is one of the simplest inexpensive and effective measures of infection control in the health care setting including dentistry.[10] Hands have been identified as important vectors in cross infection.
- It was reported that orthodontists have the highest incidence of hepatitis B among dental professionals.[11]
- While examining the indoor patient, we should follow the '5 moments of hand hygiene' **(Fig. 60.2)**.[4] Before wearing PPE, staffs need to remove jewellery, wrist watch, and examine their hands for cuts, bruises and nails. Cuts and bruises should be medicated and covered using band-aid/dressing to avoid coming in contact with patient material.

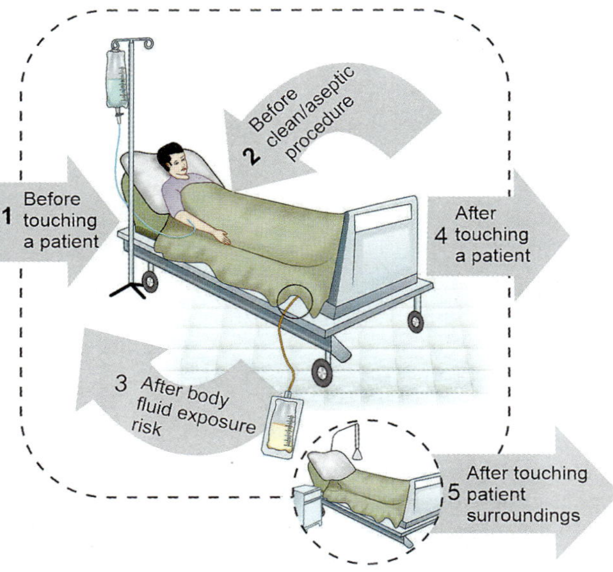

Fig. 60.2: WHO "5 moments of hand hygiene".

- Hands should be washed with water and antimicrobial soap, but use of solid soap without adequate drainage and of fabric towels may compromise its efficacy.[10]
- Handwashing with water and plain soaps is adequate for patient examination and nonsurgical procedures and for surgical procedures, an antimicrobial handrub should be used.[4]
- Surgical handwashing involves scrubbing hands all the way up to the elbow for about 2–6 minutes using a single use disposable sponge or a soft scrub brush and antimicrobial soap.

Sequence followed in handwash procedure (Fig. 60.3)

- Remove jewelry, wrist watch, and examine hands.
- Wet hands with warm water and dispense an adequate amount of soap.
- Thoroughly rub both surfaces of hands around the thumb and fingers for about 30–60 seconds.
- Wash hands with warm water to remove the soap and dry hands with paper towels.
- Examine hands for injuries such as nicks, cuts and bruises, and treat as needed. Wear single use disposable gloves.

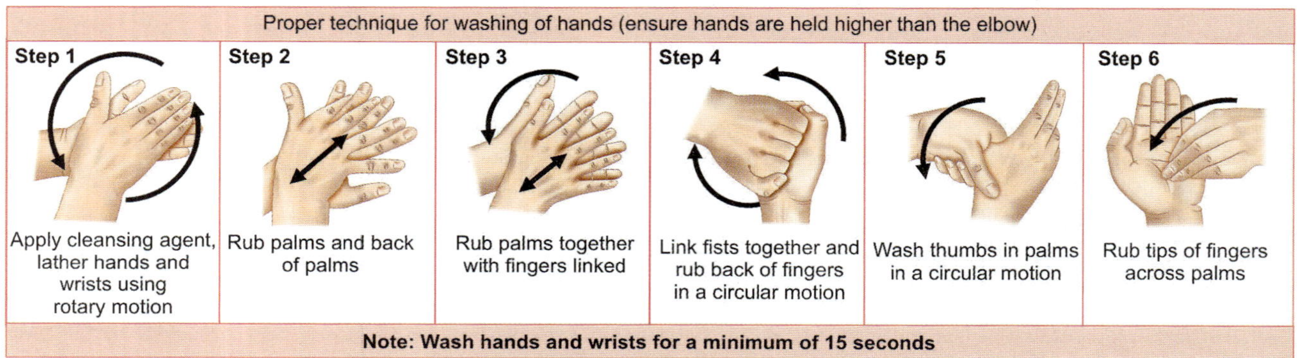

Proper technique for washing of hands (ensure hands are held higher than the elbow)
Step 1
Apply cleansing agent, lather hands and wrists using rotary motion
Step 2
Rub palms and back of palms
Step 3
Rub palms together with fingers linked
Step 4
Link fists together and rub back of fingers in a circular motion
Step 5
Wash thumbs in palms in a circular motion
Step 6
Rub tips of fingers across palms
Note: Wash hands and wrists for a minimum of 15 seconds

Fig. 60.3: Effective handwashing technique.

Hand hygiene methods and indications

Methods	Agents	Technique	Duration	Indications
Routine handwash	Water and nonmicrobial detergent (e.g., plain soap)	• Wet hands and rinse under cool running water • Dispense handwashing agent sufficient to cover hands and wrists	15 seconds	• When variably soiled • After barehanded touching of inanimate objects likely to be contaminated by blood or saliva
Antiseptic handwash	Water and antimicrobial agent/ detergent (e.g., chloriodine, iodine, and chloroxylenol triclosan)	• Rub the agent into all areas, with particular emphasis around nails and between fingers before running under cool water • Dry hands completely with disposable towels before wearing gloves • Use a towel to turn off the tap if automatic contacts are not available		• Before and after treating each patient • Before leaving patient care, laboratory, or instrument processing area • Before and after removing gloves that are torn out or punctured
Antiseptic handrub	Alcohol-based handrub	• Apply the product to palm of one hand • Rub hands together covering surfaces of hands and fingers until hands are dry • Follow manufacturer's recommendations regarding volume of product		
Surgical	Water and antimicrobial agent detergent (e.g., chlorodyne, iodine, iodophors, and chloroxylenol)	• Remove rings, watches, and bracelets • Remove debris from underwash fingernails using a nail cleaner under running water • Wet hands and wrists under cool running water	2–4 minutes	Before wearing sterile surgeon's gloves for surgical procedures
	Water and nonantimicrobial detergent (e.g., plain soap) followed by an alcohol- based surgical hand scrub product with persistent activity	• Using an antimicrobial agent, scrub hands and forearms for the length of time recommended by the manufacturer's instructions before rinsing with cool water • Dry hands completely using a sterile towel in idea before downing sterile surgeon's gloves • Follow manufacturer instructions for surgical hand scrub product	Follow manufacturer instructions for surgical hand scrub with persistent airway	

SURFACE BARRIERS

- Barriers can be sterile or nonsterile depending on whether they are used for a surgical or a nonsurgical routine dental care.
- Barriers need to be routinely changed between patients, disinfection of surfaces may be done at beginning of the clinic session and at the end of clinic session and when visibly soiled.[8]
- Air/water syringes, HVE and saliva ejector syringe may be covered to at least 6 inches below the couplings.
- Work surfaces that are in immediate proximity to the clinician and within hands reach are at a higher risk of contamination.
- Aluminum foils can be used as this type of barrier.
- Single use disposable barriers used over commonly or regularly touched surfaces are:
  - Dental unit light handles, electrical, or mechanical controls
  - Dental chair head and arm rest
  - Handpiece
  - Air/water syringe
  - Saliva ejector
  - Intraoral digital sensors and radiovisiography (RVG) equipment
  - Apex locators, endosonic ultrasonic units, and Ni-Ti torque control handpieces.[8]

CHEMICAL DISINFECTANTS

- Chemical disinfectants or germicides that are commonly used in dentistry can be classified into three main categories such as:
  1. *Liquid sterilants/high level disinfectants:*
     - Glutaraldehyde
     - Chlorine dioxide
     - Hydrogen peroxide
  2. *Intermediate and low level disinfectants surface:*
     - Hydrogen peroxide
     - Sodium hypochlorite
     - Chlorine dioxide
     - Iodophors
     - Synthetic phenols
     - Quaternary ammonia compounds
  3. *Antiseptics:*[2]
     - Active chlorine dioxide germicides
     - Essential oil compounds
     - Iodinated compounds
     - Chlorhexidine compounds
     - Cetylpyridinium compounds

- Sanguinarine-based compounds
- Parachlorometaxylenol compounds
- Other bacteriostatic/bactericidal compounds

❖ Surfaces that cannot be immersed such as bracket table, light handles, hoses, counter surfaces, chair controls, X-ray unit head/handles/controls, and other surfaces that have a tendency to get contaminated during patient care must be disinfected.[8]

❖ Certain surfaces such as electrical controls, the chair surfaces including the headrest, arm rest, and seat may be sanitized and disinfected by initially spraying the disinfectant on a disposable paper towel and wiping the surfaces thoroughly once to remove the bioburden.

❖ Reusable sponges or cloth towels must not be used, as they tend to harbor bioburden, bacterial debris, and hinder the efficacy of the disinfectant.

❖ Sodium hypochlorite is used as a traditional disinfectant. Formaldehyde is used as an antimicrobial bactericide and fungicide for maintenance of critical and semicritical dental equipment, floors, walls, and other areas.

❖ Most commonly used disinfectants methods are summarized in below table:

Disinfection methods							
Name	***Level of disinfection***	***Bacteria***	***Virus***	***Fungi***	***Uses***	***Advantages***	***Disadvantages***
Alcohol (ethyl and isopropyl 60–85%)	Intermediate	+	+/–	+	Antiseptics of skin, solution of choice 70%	Iodophors Broad spectrum Short biocidal activity Few reactions Residual biocidal action	• Unstable at high temperatures • Dilution and contact time critical Solution to be prepared daily Rust inhibitor needed Inactivated by hard water May discolor some surfaces
Phenol (4–5%), cresol, chloroxylenol (Dettol)	Intermediate	+	+/–	+	Disinfection of walls, floors, swab prior to use	Sodium hypochlorite (Bleach) Rapid antimicrobial action Broad spectrum kill • Effective in dilute solution • Economical	Very corrosive to metals Damages plastic and rubber, clothes To be prepared daily • Unpleasant odor • Toxic disinfection by-products
Glutaraldehyde (2–5%)	High	+	+	+	used on metal, plastics	Chlorine • Three minutes for disinfection • Six hours for sterilization • No trihalomethanes	• Highly corrosive to metals and certain plastics • To be mixed daily • Adequate ventilation needed
Quaternary ammonia compounds (Cetrimide, Savlon)	Low	+	–	+/–	0.5% for washing skin wound	Glutaraldehyde • Potent germicide, sporicidal • Active in the presence of bioburden • Prolonged shelf and active life, reusable • Good for use in dental laboratories	• Items must be rinsed with sterile water • Severe tissue/respiratory irritant • Must have good ventilation and evacuation • Can sensitize users
Iodophors (30–1,000 ppm i2, povidone-i2)	Intermediate	+	+	+/–	2% oral wounds, 5% skin	Synthetic phenols • Triphenols are better than dual phenols • Compatible with most materials • Residual biocidal action • Fast acting, long shelf life	• May affect some polymers • Some have film accumulation • May not be used in neonatal and pediatric practices due to possible adverse reaction
Chlorine 100–1,000 ppm (sodium hypochlorite)	Intermediate	+	+	+	Disinfecting instrument and linen after surgery	Hydrogen peroxide (7%) • Very potent germicide, sporicidal • Active in the presence of bioburden • Prolonged shelf and active life, reusable • Compatible with plastics and impressions • Good for use in dental labs	• Can be corrosive on metals • Can be dangerous to skin (burns) • Not tested widely
Hydrogen peroxide	High	+	+	+	Regular dental surfaces in dental labs	• Broad spectrum disinfectant • Can be easily stored and transported transparent	• Not effective against bacterial spores • Skin irritant • Inflammable

SPILL MANAGEMENT

Blood spillage occurs due to accidental laboratory sample breaks, during sample transportation or excessive bleeding during procedures. Standard operative procedures (SOP) should be initiated immediately using the following procedures.[10]

- Isolate the area and place the barrier around the spillage area.
- Wear a pair of gloves and appropriate PPE.
- Use pan and brush to sweep as much of broken glass/ container as possible and discard it in suitable bin.
- Cover the spill with blotting paper/paper towel and wipe the area with detergent until visibly clean.
- Pour freshly prepared 0.5% sodium hypochlorite solution (10000 ppm available chlorine) and wait for 30 minutes for contact.
- Wet mop the area and mop should be thoroughly cleaned after use and stored dry.
- Wash hand carefully with soap and water and dry thoroughly.
- Record the incident in the OSH (occupational safety and health) form, if the source of blood/body fluid was unknown or person exposed to blood and body fluids.

STERILIZATION

Instrument Reprocessing

- Instrument reprocessing is the most important aspect of dental infection control.
- The dental team must ensure the safety of both patients and personnel by adequately sterilizing dental instruments and other equipment before their use.[12] Any dental instrument that enters the oral cavity is classified as critical or semi critical surfaces as per Spaulding's classification and must be sterilized.

Instrument Processing Area

- Dental healthcare personnel should process all instruments in a designated central processing area to more easily control quality and ensure safety.
- The central processing area should be divided into sections for receiving, cleaning, and decontamination; preparation and packaging; sterilization; and storage. Ideally, walls or partitions should separate the sections to control traffic flow and contain contaminants generated during processing.
- When physical separation of these sections cannot be achieved, adequate spatial separation might be satisfactory if the DHCP who process instruments are trained in work practices to prevent contamination of clean areas.

Receiving, Cleaning, and Decontamination

- Reusable instruments, supplies, and equipment should be received, sorted, cleaned, and decontaminated in one section of the processing area.
- Prior to sterilization, instruments must be cleaned to reduce bioburden.[12,13]
- Cleaning should precede all disinfection and sterilization processes; it should involve removal of debris as well as organic and inorganic contamination. Removal of debris and contamination is achieved either by scrubbing with a surfactant, detergent, and water, or by ultrasonic cleaner. After cleaning, instruments should be rinsed with water to remove chemical or detergent residue.
- Ultrasonic cleaning (sonication) is very efficient process that helps tear away dirt and debris from instrument surfaces. Sometimes, even after an ultrasonic process patient material may still be on the surface of instruments that may need to be physically removed by using a long handle brush. Sonication of loose instruments should be carried out for 8–10 minutes.
- To avoid injury from sharp instruments, DHCP should wear puncture resistant, heavy-duty utility gloves when handling or manually cleaning contaminated instruments and devices along with a mask, protective eye wear or face shield, and gown or jacket to prevent effect of spillage.

Inspection of Cleaned Instruments

- After cleaning, the instruments should be pat dried using a small stack of paper towels and inspected for residual bioburden or debris. The inspected instruments can now be made into sets and bagged.[8]
- Safe and effective decontamination procedures must be carried out before instruments are put into the appropriate equipment for sterilization.[12]
- Packaged sterile instruments can be stored for as long as the integrity of the pouch/package is not broken, damaged or affected by moisture.
- If instruments are to be "cold sterilized" in glutaraldehyde or any approved immersion sterilant, they should be rinsed with sterile water to remove residual chemical sterilant from the surfaces of the instrument and used immediately.[8]

Preparation and Packaging

- In another section of the processing area, cleaned instruments and other dental supplies should be inspected, assembled into sets or trays, and wrapped, packaged, or placed into container systems for sterilization.
- Hinged instruments should be processed open and unlocked. An internal chemical indicator should be placed in every package. In addition, an external chemical indicator (e.g., chemical indicator tape) should be used when the internal indicator cannot be seen from outside the package.
- Cleaned instruments should be packed and sealed using Sealing device (**Fig 60.4**).
- Critical and semicritical instruments that will be stored should be wrapped or placed in containers designed to maintain sterility during storage.
- Materials for maintaining sterility of instruments during transport and storage include wrapped perforated instrument cassettes, peel pouches of plastic or paper, and sterilization wraps (i.e., woven and nonwoven).

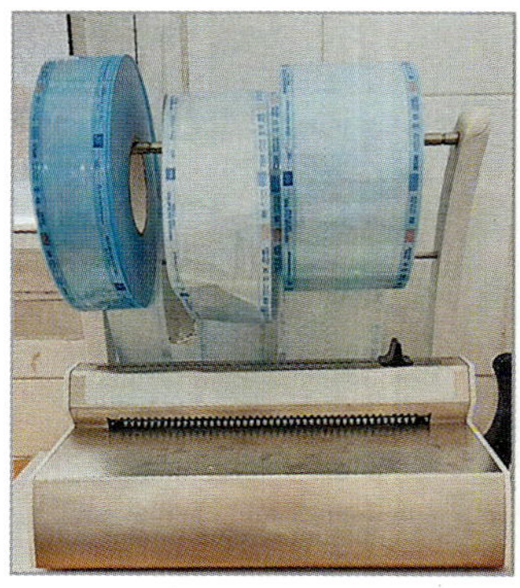
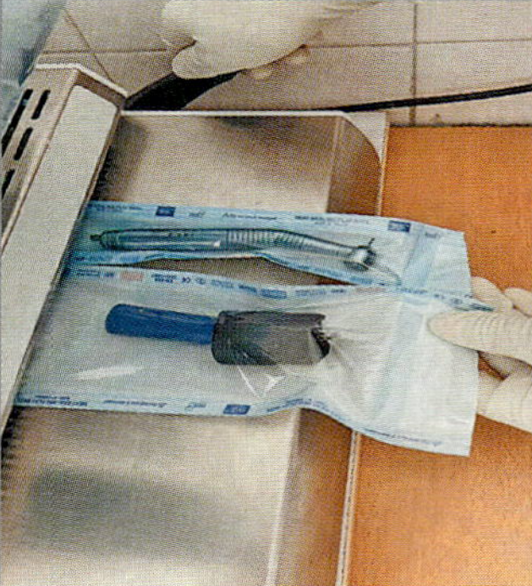

Fig. 60.4: Sealing machine.

Sterilization Procedures

- Heat-tolerant dental instruments usually are sterilized by:
  - Steam under pressure (autoclaving)
  - Dry heat
- Unsaturated chemical vapor.
- All sterilization should be performed by using medical sterilization equipment cleared by FDA. The sterilization times, temperatures, and other operating parameters recommended by the manufacturer of the equipment used, as well as instructions for correct use of containers, wraps, and chemical or biological indicators (BIs), should always be followed.

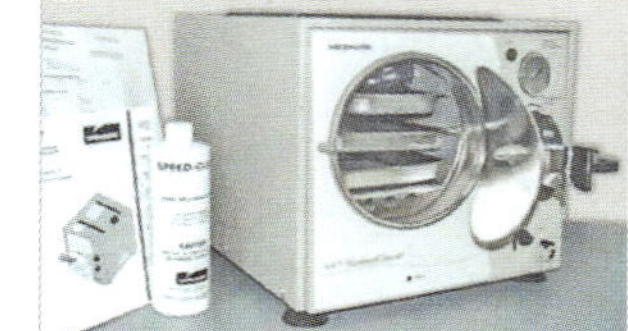

- Instrument packs should be allowed to dry inside the sterilizer chamber before removing and handling. Packs should not be touched until they are cool and dry because hot packs act as wicks, absorbing moisture, and hence, bacteria from hands.

Autoclave

- Autoclaving or sterilization using steam and pressure is the most common and reliable method of sterilization.[13]
- This method could be more corrosive for instruments that have a high content of carbon steel (especially if packages are not adequately dried).[8,13]

Parameters	*Standard cycle*	*Fast cycle*
Sterilization time	15–20 minutes	3–5 minutes
Temperature	121° C (250°F)	134° C (273°F)
Pressure	15 pounds per square inch (psi)	30 pounds per square inch

Chemiclave

- It is sterilization with chemical vapors.
- A combination of liquid chemicals (with <15% water) are introduced into the chamber, heat and pressure for a sterilization cycle. The parameters for sterilization are temperature of 131°C (270°F), 20 psi, and sterilization time of 30 minutes.[8]

Dry Heat

Parameter	*Slow cycle*	*Fast cycle*	*Rapid heat*
Temperature	160°C (320°F)	170°C (340°F)	190°C (375°F)
Sterilization	120 minutes	60 minutes	6–12 minutes

Storage of Sterilized Items

- The storage area should contain enclosed storage for sterile items and disposable (single use) items. Storage practices for wrapped sterilized instruments can be either date-or-event related.
- Packages containing sterile supplies should be inspected before use to verify barrier integrity and dryness.
- Even for event-related packaging, minimally, the date of sterilization should be placed on the package, and if multiple sterilizers are used in the facility, the sterilizer used should be indicated on the outside of the packaging material to facilitate the retrieval of processed items in the event of a sterilization failure.
- If packaging is compromised, the instruments should be recleaned, packaged in new wrap, and sterilized again.
- Clean supplies and instruments should be stored in closed or covered cabinets and should not be stored under sinks or in other locations where they might become wet.

Sterilization Monitoring

- Monitoring of sterilization procedures should include a combination of process parameters including mechanical, chemical, and biological.
- These parameters evaluate both the sterilizing conditions and the procedure's effectiveness.
- Mechanical techniques for monitoring sterilization include assessing cycle time, temperature, and pressure by observing the gauges or displays on the sterilizer and noting these parameters for each load. Correct readings do not ensure sterilization, but incorrect readings can be the first indication of a problem with the sterilization cycle.
- Chemical indicators, internal and external, use sensitive chemicals to assess physical conditions (e.g., time and temperature) during the sterilization process. Although chemical indicators do not prove sterilization has been achieved, they allow detection of certain equipment malfunctions, and they can help to identify procedural errors.
- External indicators applied to the outside of a package (e.g., chemical indicator tape or special markings) change color rapidly when a specific parameter is reached, and they verify that the package has been exposed to the sterilization process.
- Internal chemical indicators should be used inside each package to ensure the sterilizing agent has penetrated the packaging material and actually reached the instruments inside.
- Multiparameter internal indicators are available only for steam sterilizers (i.e., autoclaves).
- Biological indicators (i.e., spore tests) are the most accepted method for monitoring the sterilization process because they assess it directly by killing known highly

resistant microorganisms (e.g., *Geobacillus* or *Bacillus* species), rather than merely testing the physical and chemical conditions necessary for sterilization.

Flash Sterilization

- Sterilization of unwrapped instruments.
- The time required for unwrapped sterilization cycles depends on the type of sterilizer and the type of item (i.e., porous or nonporous) to be sterilized.
- Flash sterilization should be used only under certain conditions:
  - Thorough cleaning and drying of instruments precedes the unwrapped sterilization cycle.
  - Mechanical monitors are checked and chemical indicators used for each cycle.
  - Care is taken to avoid thermal injury to DHCP or patients.
  - Items are transported aseptically to the point of use to maintain sterility.

Low-temperature Sterilization

- Done with ethylene oxide (ETO) gas, which has been used extensively in larger healthcare facilities.
- Its primary advantage is the ability to sterilize heat and moisture-sensitive patient-care items with reduced deleterious effects.
- However, extended sterilization times of 10–48 hours and potential hazards to patients and DHCP requiring stringent health and safety requirements make this method impractical for private-practice settings.

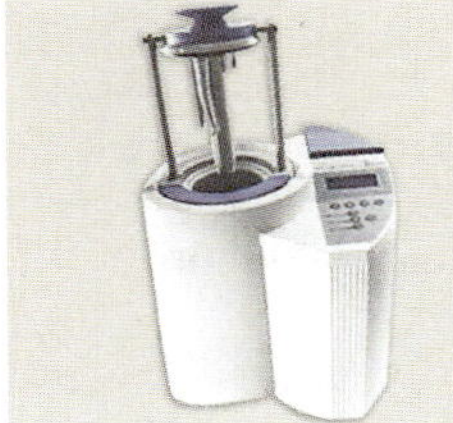

Sterilization of Handpieces

- Both, high-speed and slow-speed handpieces retract patient material and are difficult to clean and decontaminate using chemical germicides.
- The method of sterilization of handpieces is first to lubricate the handpiece with spray and then it is left vertical on shelf to drain out the excess. This is followed by insertion of handpiece in special autoclaves meant exclusively for them.

Sterilization of Dental Chair Water System

- Most modern dental unit water systems are made up of a complex maze of waterlines, control blocks, valves, barbs, and connectors that are of various sizes and composed of different metals, plastics, and rubbers. Water delivered from these devices is not sterile and has been shown to contain relatively high number of bacteria.[8,14]
- All disposables and reusable types of prophy angles have a vent or opening to reduce or eliminate excessive heat buildup which may allow internal contamination, therefore contributing to cross contamination between patients unless the handpiece motors, nose cones, and reusable angles are heat sterilized between uses.
- The design of all dental unit water systems allows settling of contaminants from water and air. These contaminants can be inorganic materials such as salts from the hardness of the source water that coat the lines and cause corrosion of metals and allow settling of microbes.[8] Bacterial cells accumulating and growing on the inner surface of the tubing as biofilm are responsible for high levels of contamination in dental unit water system.[14]
- The water coming out of the dental handpiece and air/water syringe may have more than a million microbes per millimeter.
- In 2003, Centers for Disease Control and Prevention (CDC) recommended that treatment water should contain less than 500 CFU/mL.[15,16]
- Most of the microbes found in the dental water system biofilms are Gram-negative[14-16] when they die, they release a toxin called bacterial endotoxins which in large amounts have potential to cause health problems in patients.[8]
- CDC have recommended flushing the waterline for several minutes prior to the first patient and for 20–30 seconds between patients. Flushing between patients has been shown to decrease the number of bacteria in the water phase. In addition to this, it has been demonstrated that flushing has a little or no effect on biofilm as the laminar flow will barely result in sloughing due to biofilm phenomenon.[14]
- The most widely tested product, household bleach used in 1:10 dilution in the waterlines has demonstrated efficacy.

PROTOCOL DURING PANDEMIC PERIOD

The infection control management is very challenging in pandemic times like coronavirus disease (COVID-19) due to high risk of transmission. Dental procedures require close contact with the patient's oral cavity, saliva, blood and respiratory tract infections. Many patients who are asymptomatic have a risk of shedding virus. Hence all patients visiting a dental clinic must be considered as potential source of infection and dental professional must follow appropriate infection prevention and control and occupational health and safety measures **(Fig. 60.5)**. Health care workers (HCW) should wear appropriate PPE when screening patients at the triage area. Medical masks should be provided to all patients presenting flu-like symptoms or possible COVID-19 infections.

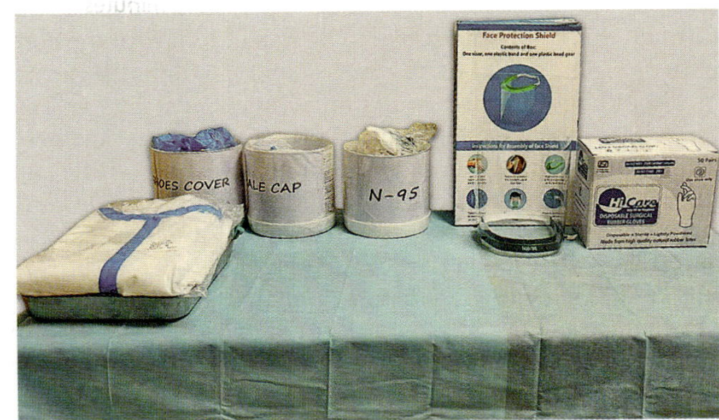

Fig. 60.5: COVID protocols.

Steps to Put on (Donning) PPE

- First, remove all personal items. (watches, jewelleries, etc.)
- Wear shoe cover and move on to isolation room.
- Select appropriate PPE size and perform hand hygiene **(Fig. 60.6)**.
- Wear gloves.
- Then, put on gown that is tested for resistance to body fluid/blood borne pathogens.
- Wear face mask.
- Wear face shield/goggles.
- Put on head and neck covering.
- Wear second pair of gloves.

Fig. 60.6: PPE.

Steps to Take Off (Doffing) PPE

- Ensure that appropriate disposable bin available nearby for doffing.
- Do hand hygiene on gloved hands.
- Remove apron by leaning forward and taking care to avoid contaminating your hands. When removing apron, tear it in the centre and rolling it down without touching the front area. Then untie the back and roll the apron forward.
- Perform hand hygiene again on gloved hands.
- Remove outer pair of gloves and perform hand hygiene on gloved hands.
- Remove head and neck covering by starting from bottom of hood in the back and rolling from back to front and from inside to outside and dispose in appropriate container.
- Perform hand hygiene again on gloved hands.
- Remove the gown by untying the knot first, pulling from back to front rolling it from inside to outside and safely dispose it. Perform hand hygiene again on gloved hands.
- Remove face shield/goggles by pulling the string from behind the head and do hand hygiene on gloved hands.
- Remove shoe cover and do hand hygiene on gloved hands.
- Remove gloves and dispose it safely.
- Perform hand hygiene.[17]

Control of Airborne Infections in Dental Offices

Preventing the spread of air borne infection is critical in dental set ups due to presence of bacteria and viruses are transmitted through this route and prove to be a health hazard for both patients and dental health care personnel. Dental clinic set up should have proper ventilation with exhaust fans and air filters. Air purifiers utilize different types of filtration such as carbon, high efficiency particulate arresting (HEPA) air filters, or a mixture such as a carbon/HEPA filtration unit. While a carbon filter is ideal for chemicals and odors in the air, HEPA is ideal for air particles. HEPA filters are constructed from paper such as glass fiber or polymer sheets, which are pleated many times in a "V" pattern to maximize the surface area within a small volume to enhance their effectiveness in removing particles. It protects from bio aerosols which may lead to adverse effects on respiratory function and maintain better indoor air quality in the dental clinics[18] **(Fig. 60.7)**.

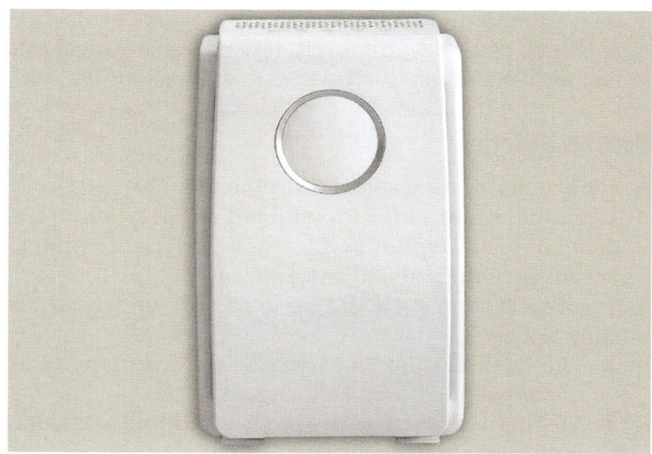

Fig. 60.7: HEPA filter.

MANAGEMENT OF DENTAL BIOWASTE

The present day dental clinics use a wide variety of drugs, antibiotics, cytotoxic, corrosives, chemicals, and radioactive substances which ultimately become a part of hospital waste. These clinics which provide relief can also create health hazards and other potential health concern to the general public of the surrounding areas.[17] Waste can be classified as:

Sterilization methods				
Method	***Temperature/ Pressure***	***Exposure time***	***Advantages***	***Precautions***
Steam autoclave	121°C (250°F) 115 kPa	13–30 min 3.5–12 min	Good penetration Nontoxic Time efficient	Non-stainless steel items corrode May damage rubber and plastics Do not use closed containers Unwrapped items quickly contaminated after cycle
			No corrosion	Long cycle time
Dry heat (oven-type)	134°C (273°F) 216 kPa	60–120 min	Nontoxic Items are dry after cycle Can use closed container	• May damage rubber and plastics • Door can be opened during cycle • Unwrapped items quickly contaminated after cycle
Dry heat	191° C (375° F)	12 min: wrapped 6 min	No corrosion Nontoxic Time efficient Items dry quickly	• May damage rubber and plastics • Door can be opened during cycle • Unwrapped items quickly contaminated after cycle

Contd...

Contd...

Method	Temperature/ Pressure	Exposure time	Advantages	Precautions
Unsaturated chemical	134° C (273° F) 216 kPa	20 min	No corrosion Time efficient	• May damage rubber and plastics • Do not use closed containers • Must use special solution • Uses hazardous chemical • Unwrapped items quickly contaminated after cycle

Emerging technologies for treatment of waste
- Molten salt technology
- Electric reactors
- Plasma system/plasma torch technology
- Molten glass technology
- Infrared system
- Detoxification technology (superheated steam sterilization)
- Wet oxidation technology
- Thermal dry heat technology (synonym: TAPS)
- Electrokinetic gasification technology[17]

Regulated Waste

- **Biological waste:** Gauze and cotton rolls (saturated/ soaked in saliva/blood), soft tissues (oral soft tissues including biopsy specimen) and hard tissues (bone and teeth).[8]
- **Disposable sharps:** Scalpel blades, needles, orthodontic wires, disposable matrix bands, single-use-disposable burs, contaminated broken glass, and wire sutures used for splinting and failed implants.[8]
- **Environmentally hazardous chemicals and metals:** Mercury, amalgam, beryllium, and chemicals used in processing radiographs (silver nitrate), formaldehydes, glutaraldehyde, and phenols.[8]

Nonregulated Wastes

Unsaturated cotton rolls, paper towels, gauze, nonsharp single-use disposable devices (saliva ejector tip), disposable syringe, plastics, disposable PPE, and other inanimate surface barriers.[9]

Safe Handling of Sharps

- Safe handling of sharps reduces exposure to blood borne pathogens.
- After procedures, needle should be burnt in the needle destroyer and disposed in puncture resistant container. Then the syringe should be cut and disposed in clearly labeled container **(Fig. 60.8)**.
- Do not bend or manipulate needles in any way for disposal.
- The container should be filled only to three-fourth full and have a tightly fitting lid that seals to prevent leakage thereby reducing risk to dentist, clients, and others in the environment (e.g., waste disposal handlers).

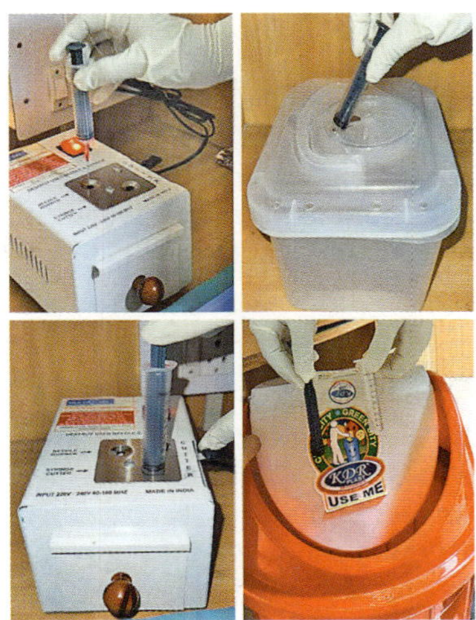

Fig. 60.8: Procedure for disposing needle and syringe.

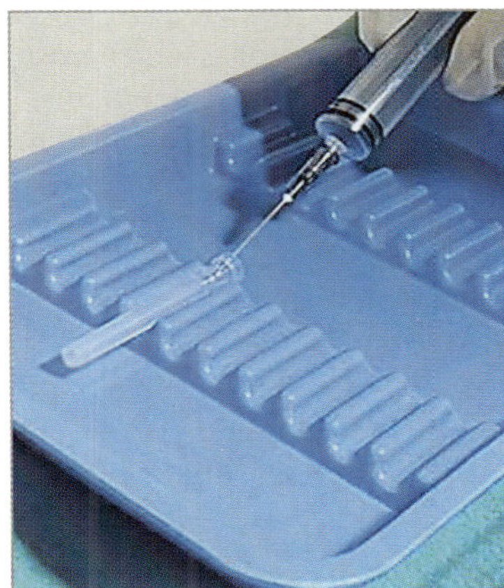

Fig. 60.9: One hand scoop technique.

- Used sharps are considered biomedical waste in healthcare offices and labs. Dispose of used sharp containers should be in accordance with regulations from municipal and provincial authorities.[5]
- Current guidelines state that used needles should never be recapped by using both hands. If this is necessary, it should be done only by one hand scoop technique or by using a mechanical device to hold the needle sheath[15] **(Fig. 60.9)**.

The incidence of sharp injuries estimates 38500 annually (>1000 injuries/day) among hospital based healthcare personnel. Injuries with sharp devices and contaminated needles are of critical concern due to increased risk of blood borne virus transmission to healthcare personnel. The pathogens that cause most serious health risks in our dental offices are HBV, HCV and HIV. Preventing needle stick injuries is the best way to protect oneself.

Prevent needle stick injuries:
- Use safe and effective alternatives instead of needles.
- Use devices with safety features provided as per manufacturer's instructions.
- Recapping needles can be avoided. Use scooping method if necessary.
- Plan for safe handling and disposal of needles before using them.
- Proper disposal of needles in the appropriate containers.
- Report all sharp related injuries.
- Hepatitis B vaccination is must for healthcare personnel.

Steps to manage immediately if exposed to sharp injuries or patient blood/body fluids:

1. Wash needle sticks and cuts with soap and water.
2. Flush splashes to the nose, mouth or skin with water.
3. Irrigate eyes with clean water and sterile irrigants.
4. Report the incident to the respective personnel.
5. Seek the medical treatment immediately.[19]

REGULATIONS BY OSHA TO BE FOLLOWED TO PREVENT CROSS INFECTION

Infection control guidelines for dentistry are issued in 1993 and updated in 2003 by the CDC, Atlanta are regarded as "Gold Standard". It can be summarized as:

- Hepatitis B immunization is a must for all.
- Universal precautions must be observed to prevent contact with blood and other potentially infectious material.
- Safe handling of needles and other sharp items.
  - Engineering controls to reduce protection of contaminated spatter, mists, and aerosols.
  - Work practice control precautions to minimize splashing, spatter, or contact of bare hands with contaminated surfaces.
  - Provide facility and instructions for washing hands after removing gloves and washing skin as soon as possible after contact with infectious material.
  - Flush eyes or mucosa after contact.
  - Prescribe the disposal of single use needles, vials carpules, and sharps as close to place of use as possible, in a hard walled, and leak-proof containers.
  - Contaminated reusable, sharp instruments must not be stored or processed in a manner that requires employees to reach hands into containers to retrieve them.
  - Provision of PPE to the employees at no cost.
  - Use biohazard labeled or red bags that are leak-proof and puncture resistant.
- Prohibit eating, drinking, handling contact lenses, and application of facial cosmetics in contaminated environment such as operatories and cleanup areas.
- Provide laundering of protective garments used for personal protection and universal precautions at no cost to employees.
- Schedule for cleaning and decontamination equipment, work surfaces, and contaminated floors.

Sterilization disinfection in dental office

Dry heat oven	***Autoclave***
Extraction forceps and elevator	Handpieces
Hand scalers U	Ultrasonic
Filling instruments T	Towels
Tray and tumbler	Sutures
Mouth mirror and probes	Gloves
Impression trays	Cotton and gauze
Chemical solution	***Formaldehyde***
Surgical burs	Plastic cheek retractor
Diamond burs	Acrylic obturators
Light cure tips	Splints

Biomedical waste disposal management.

Color coding	*Method of disposal*	*Items*	*Treatment*
Yellow	Plastic bag	Biopsy samples, extracted teeth, suction fluid, solid waste items contaminated with blood and fluid (gauze, cotton rolls, mouth mask, and disposable gowns), impression compound, dental waxes, gutta- percha, paper points, and mylar strip	Incineration and deep burial
Red	Disinfected container/plastic bag	*Autoclaving/microwaving:* Buff, towels, aprons, operation theater gown, metallic hand-filling instruments, and surgical instruments. *Chemical treatment:* Plastic spatula and hand piece	Autoclaving/microwaving/ chemical treatment
Blue/white	Plastic bag/puncture	Burs, handpiece, local anesthesia cartridges, endodontic instruments, implant set	Autoclaving/microwaving/ chemical
Translucent	Proof container	Orthodontic rubber bands, gloves, and plastic syringes	Treatment and destruction/shredding
Black	Plastic bag	Rubber base impression materials, pumice, acrylic, discarded medicines, alginate, old models and casts, mercury, orthodontic brackets and bands and wires, matrix band, old acrylic dentures and teeth	Disposal in secured landfill

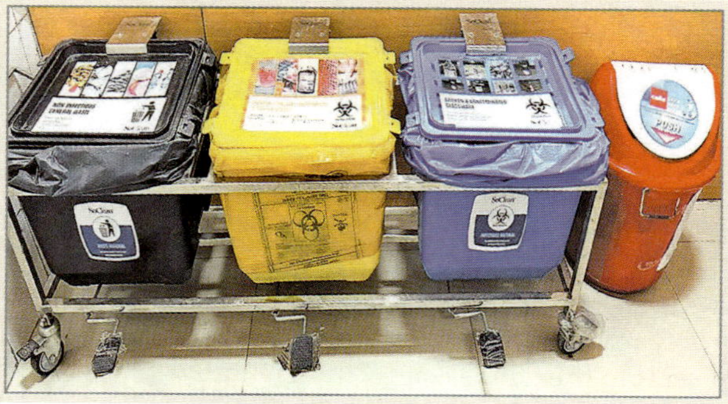

POINTS TO REMEMBER

- WD Miller is the father of oral microbiology.
- Antony Van Leeuwenhoek was the first to observe oral flora.
- Sterilization: Defined as the process by which an article, surface, or a medium freed of all microorganisms including viruses, bacteria, their spores, and fungi both pathogenic and non pathogenic.
- Disinfections the elimination of virtually all pathogenic microorganism on inanimate objects with the exception of large number of bacterial endospore reducing the level of microbial contamination to an acceptable safe level.
- Personal protection is accomplished by use of gloves, masks, gowns, and eyewear.
- Correct procedure of handwashing is remove jewellery and wrist watch; wet hands with warm water and dispense an adequate amount of soap; thoroughly rub both surfaces of hands around the thumb and fingers for about 30–60 seconds; and wash hands with warm water to remove the soap and dry hands with paper towels.
- The best methods of sterilization are steam autoclaving, dry heat, and chemiclave.
- Autoclave is done for 15–20 minutes at temperature of 121°C and pressure of 15 pounds psi.
- The standard operating procedures should be followed during spill management.
- Chemiclave is autoclaving with chemicals at 131°C (270° F), 20 psi for 30 minutes.
- Dry heat sterilization is done at 160°C for 120 minutes or 190°C for 6–10 minutes.
- During pandemic times, proper protocol for donning and doffing, well ventilated area with use of air filter should be followed.
- Biowaste disposal bag coding: Yellow bag—infectious waste must be incinerated and treated by alternative technology; Red bag—not to be incinerated, may be used for microwaving, autoclaving; Black bag—should be treated as household waste and can go with municipal solid waste; Blue bag—needle, etc. to be broken are packed in puncture proof bag. use services of contractor (agency to manage the sharp waste).

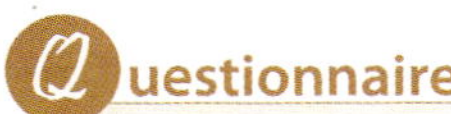

Questionnaire

1. Write a note on personal protective equipment.
2. Describe handwashing for infection control in detail.
3. What is disinfection and what are the agents used for it?
4. Describe standard operating procedures for spill management.
5. Explain the procedure of sterilization in detail.
6. Describe the working of as autoclave.
7. Write a note on management of biomedical waste in dental operatory.
8. What are the OSHA regulations?
9. Describe protocol for needle stick injury management.
10. What are the steps for donning and doffing of PPE?

REFERENCES

1. Forder AA. A brief history of infection controls past and present. S Afr Med J. 2007;97(11 Pt 3):1161-4.
2. http://findarticles.com/p/articles/mi_6869/is_11_97/ai_n28533881/
3. Baumgartner CJ, Bakland LK, Sugita EI. Microbiology of Endodontics and Asepsis in Endodontic Practice, 5th edition. London: BC Decker Inc.; 2002.
4. https://www.who.int/campaigns/worLd-hand-hygiene-day
5. De Souza RA, Namen FM, Galan J Jr, et al. Infection control measures among senior dental students in Rio de Janeiro state, Brazil. J Public Health Dent. 2006;66(4):282-4.
6. Williams HN, Singh R, Romberg E. Surface contamination in dental operatory: a comparison over two decades. J Am Dent Assoc. 2003;134:325-30.
7. DePaola LG. Managing the care of patients infected with blood borne diseases. J Am Dent Assoc. 2003;134:350-8.
8. Toxics Link Factsheet. (2005). Bio-medical waste. [online] Available from http://toxicslink.org/docs/06101_fs- formaldehyde.pdf [Accessed April 2018].
9. Ceratta R, Paula MM, Angioletto E, et al. Evaluation of the effectiveness of peracetic acid in the sterilization of dental equipment. Indian J Med Microbiol. 2008;26(2):117-22.
10. Bellissimo-Rodrigues WT, Bellissimo-Rodrigues F, Machado AA. Occupational exposure to biological fluids among a cohort of Brazilian dentists. Int Dent J. 2006;56:332-7.
11. Cleveland JL, Barker LK, Cuny EJ, et al. Preventing percutaneous injuries among dental health care personnel. J Am Dent Assoc. 2007;138(2):169-78.
12. Mukhopadhya A. Hepatitis C in India. J Biosci. 2008;33(4): 465-73.
13. Chopra SS, Pandey SS. Occupational hazards among dental surgeons. Med J Armed Forces India. 2007;63:23-5.
14. AlNegrish A, Al Momani AS. Al Sharafat F. Compliance of Jordanian dentists with infection control strategies. Int Dent J. 2008;58:231-6.
15. Kevin R, Manus Mc. Purchasing, installing and operating dental amalgam separators. J Am Dent Assoc. 2003;134:1054-65.
16. Hered S, Chin J, Palenik CJ, et al. The in vivo contamination of air driven low speed handpieces with prophylaxis angles. J Am Dent Assoc. 2007;138:1360-5.
17. Sudhakar V, Chandrashekar J. Dental health care waste disposal among private dental practices in Bengaluru city, India. Int Dent J. 2008;58(1):51-4.
18. Batchu S, Chou HN. The effect of disinfectants and line cleaners on the release of mercury from amalgam. J Am Dent Assoc. 2006;137(10):1419-25.

FURTHER READING

1. Acosta-Gio AE, Borges-Yáñez SA, Flores M, et al. Infection control attitudes and perceptions among dental students in Latin America: implications for dental education. Int Dent J. 2008;58(4):187-93.
2. Bellissimo-Rodrigues WT, Bellissimo-Rodrigues F, Machado AA. Infection control practices among a cohort of Brazilian dentists. Int Dent J. 2009;59:53-8.
3. CDC. Infection control routine for dental office. 2016.
4. CDC. National institute for occupational safety and health (NIOSH). 2021.
5. Chin JR, Miller CH, Palenik CJ. Internal contamination of air driven low speed handpieces and attached prophy angles. J Am Dent Assoc. 2006;137(9):1275-80.
6. Garge HG, Kumar M, Kalia D. Waste disposal in dental practice. J Dentistry Def Sec. 2008;3(2):38-41.
7. Kamma JJ, Bradshaw DJ. Attitudes of general dental practitioners in Europe to the microbial risk associated with dental unit water systems. Int Dent J. 2006;56(4): 187-95.
8. Katz AR, Nekorchuk DM, Holck PS, et al. Dentists' preparedness for responding to bioterrorism: A survey of Hawaii dentists. J Am Dent Assoc. 2006;137:461-7.
9. Kermode M, Holmes W, Langkham B, et al. HIV-related knowledge, attitudes and risk perception amongst nurses, doctors and other health care workers in rural India. Indian J Med Res. 2005;122:258-64.
10. Lee JJ, Nettey-Marbell A, Cook A Jr, et al. Using extracted teeth for research: the effect of storage medium and sterilization on dentin bond strengths. J Am Dent Assoc. 2007;138:1599-603.

11. Mahmood SU, Crimbly F, Khan S, Choudry E, Mehwish S. Strategies for Rational Use of Personal Protective Equipment (PPE) Among Healthcare Providers During the COVID-19 Crisis. Cureus. 2020 May 23;12(5):e8248.
12. Morrison A, Conrod S. Dental burs and endodontic files: are routine sterilization procedures effective? Tex Dent J. 2010;127(3):295:300.
13. Porteous NB, Redding SW, Thompson EH, et al. Isolation of an unusual fungus in treated dental unit waterlines. J Am Dent Assoc. 2003;134:853-8.
14. Qian Y, Willeke K, Grinshpun SA, Donnelly J, Coffey CC. Performance of N95 respirators: filtration efficiency for airborne microbial and inert particles. Am Ind Hyg Assoc J. 1998 Feb;59(2):128-32.
15. Ritter AV, Ghaname E, Leonard RH. The influence of dental unit waterline cleaners on composite to dentin bond strengths. J Am Dent Assoc. 2007;138(7):985-91.
16. Saglam AM, Sarikaya N. Evaluation of infection-control practices by orthodontists in Turkey. Quintessence Int. 2004;35(1):61-6.
17. WHO Guidelines on Drawing Blood: Best Practices in Phlebotomy. Geneva: World Health Organization; 2010. Annex H, Blood spillage.
18. Yadav N, Agrawal B, Maheshwari C. Role of high-efficiency particulate arrestor filters in control of air borne infections in dental clinics. SRM J Res Dent Sci 2015;6:240-2
19. Yilmaz H, Aydin C, Bal BT, et al. Effects of disinfectants on resilient denture-lining materials contaminated with *Staphylococcus aureus, Streptococcus sobrinus, and Candida albicans.* Quintessence Int. 2005;36(5):373-81.

CHAPTER

Local Anesthesia

Nikhil Marwah, Sunny Priyatham, Prateek Aggarwal

CHAPTER OUTLINE

Local anesthesia: *Local anesthesia is defined as a loss of sensation in a circumscribed area of the body caused by a depression of excitation in nerve endings or an inhibition of the conduction process in peripheral nerves.*

Local anesthetics (LAs) *are drugs which upon topical application or local injection cause reversible loss of sensory perception especially of pain, in a restricted area of the body. Not only sensory but also motor impulses are interrupted when applied to a mixed nerve, resulting in muscular paralysis and loss of autonomic control as well.*

IDEAL REQUIREMENTS OF ACCEPTABLE LOCAL ANESTHETIC

- It should have potency sufficient to give complete anesthesia.
- It should be relatively free from producing allergic reactions.
- It should be stable in solution and readily undergo biotransformation in the body.
- It should be sterile or capable of being sterilized by heat without deterioration.
- It should have low degree of local toxicity.
  - It should not be irritating to the tissue to which it is applied.
  - It should not cause any permanent alteration of nerve structure.
  - It should have low degree of systemic toxicity.
- It should possess versatility. It must be effective regardless of whether it is injected into the tissue or applied locally to mucous membranes.
- It should have a rapid onset and be of sufficient duration to be advantageous.

STRUCTURE OF LOCAL ANESTHETICS

The basic components of LA structure are **(Fig. 61.1)**:
- A lipophilic aromatic portion
- A hydrophilic amine portion
- An intermediate hydrocarbon chain containing either an ester or an amide linkage.

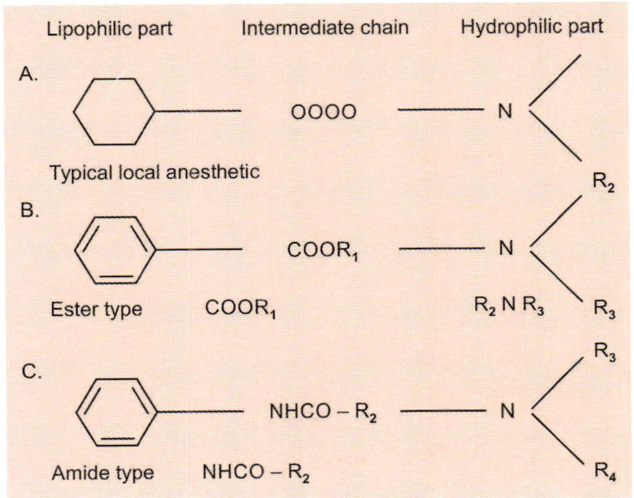

Fig. 61.1: Structure of local anesthetic.

Mechanism of action of local anesthesia
- Altering the basic resting potential of the nerve membrane
- Altering the threshold potential (firing level)
- Decreasing the rate of depolarization
- Prolonging the rate of repolarization.

Local anesthetic's classification		
According to the Salt		
I. *Esters*	*Amides*	*Quinoline*
	Lidocaine	Centbucridine
Esters of benzoic acid	Bupivacaine	
Cocaine	Mepivacaine	
Butacaine	Dibucaine	
Ethyl aminobenzoate (benzocaine)	Etiodocaine	
	Articaine	
Piperocaine	Prilocaine	
Isobucaine	Ropivacaine	
Meprylcaine	Parethoxycaine	
	Pyrrocaine	
Esters of PABA		
Chloroprocaine		
Procaine		
Propoxycaine		
Butethamine		
Tetracaine		
Esters of meta-aminobenzoic acid		
Meta-butethamine primacaine		
II. *Injectable*		
Low potency, short duration		
Procaine		
Chloroprocaine		
Intermediate potency and duration		
Lidocaine		
Prilocaine		
High potency, long duration		
Tetracaine		
Bupivacaine		
Ropivacaine		
Dibucaine		
III. *Surface anesthetic*		
Soluble		
Cocaine		
Lidocaine		
Tetracaine		
Insoluble		
Benzocaine		
Butyl aminobenzoate (butamben)		
Oxethazaine		

COMPOSITION OF LOCAL ANESTHETIC SOLUTION

- **Local anesthetic agent:** Lignocaine, etc.
- **Vasoconstrictor:**
  - Decrease blood flow to the site of injection
  - Absorption of the LA into the cardiovascular system is slowed
  - Decrease the risk of LA toxicity
  - Higher volume of the LA agent remains in and around the nerve for longer period, thereby increasing the duration of action
  - Vasoconstrictors decrease bleeding at the site of their administration.
- **Reducing agents:** Vasoconstrictors are unstable in solution and may oxidize, especially on a prolonged exposure to sunlight. Sodium metabisulfite which competes for the available oxygen is added in the concentration between 0.05% and 0.1%.
- **Preservative:** Stability of modern LA solution is maintained by adding caprylhydrocuprienotoxin and methylparaben.
- **Fungicide:** Thymol.
- **Vehicle:** All the earlier solutions and LA agent are dissolved in a modified Ringer's solution. This isotonic vehicle minimizes discomfort during injection.

THEORIES EXPLAINING THE MECHANISM OF ACTION

Acetylcholine Theory (Dettbarn, 1967)

Acetylcholine was involved in nerve conduction in addition to its role as neurotransmitter at nerve synapses.

Calcium Displacement Theory (Goldman, 1966)

- Stated that LA nerve block is produced by the displacement of calcium from some membrane site that controlled permeability to sodium.
- There is evidence that varying the concentration of Ca^{2+} ions bathing a nerve does not affect LA potency.

Surface Charge (Repulsion) Theory (Wei, 1969)

- Local anesthetics bind to the nerve membrane RNH^+ (cationic) drug molecules were aligned at the membrane—water interface and because some of the LA molecules, carried a net positive charge, they made the electric potential at the membrane surface more positive, thus decreasing the excitability of the nerve by increasing the threshold potential.
- Evidence indicates that resting potential is unaltered by LA, conventional LA act within the membrane channels rather than at the membrane surface.
- This theory cannot explain the activity of uncharged anesthetic molecules, e.g., benzocaine.

Membrane Expansion Theory (Lee, 1976)

- Local anesthetic molecules diffuse to hydrophobic regions of excitable membranes, producing a general disturbance of the bulk membrane structure, expanding some critical region(s) in the membrane and preventing an increase in permeability to Na^+ ions. LA that are highly lipid soluble can easily penetrate the lipid portion of the cell membrane, producing a change in configuration of the lipoprotein matrix of the nerve membrane.
- This theory explains the action of benzocaine which does not exist in cationic form, yet still exhibits potent topical anesthetic activity.
- It has been demonstrated that nerve membranes in fact, do expand and become more "fluid" when exposed to LA. However, there is no direct evidence that nerve conduction is entirely blocked by membrane expansion *per se*.

Specific Receptor Theory (Strichartz, 1987)

- Local anesthetic act by binding to specific receptors on the sodium channel either on its external surface or on the internal axoplasmic surface. Once access is gained to these receptors, permeability to Na^+ ions is decreased or eliminated and nerve conduction is interrupted.
- There are at least four sites within the sodium channel at which drugs can alter nerve conduction.

Contd...

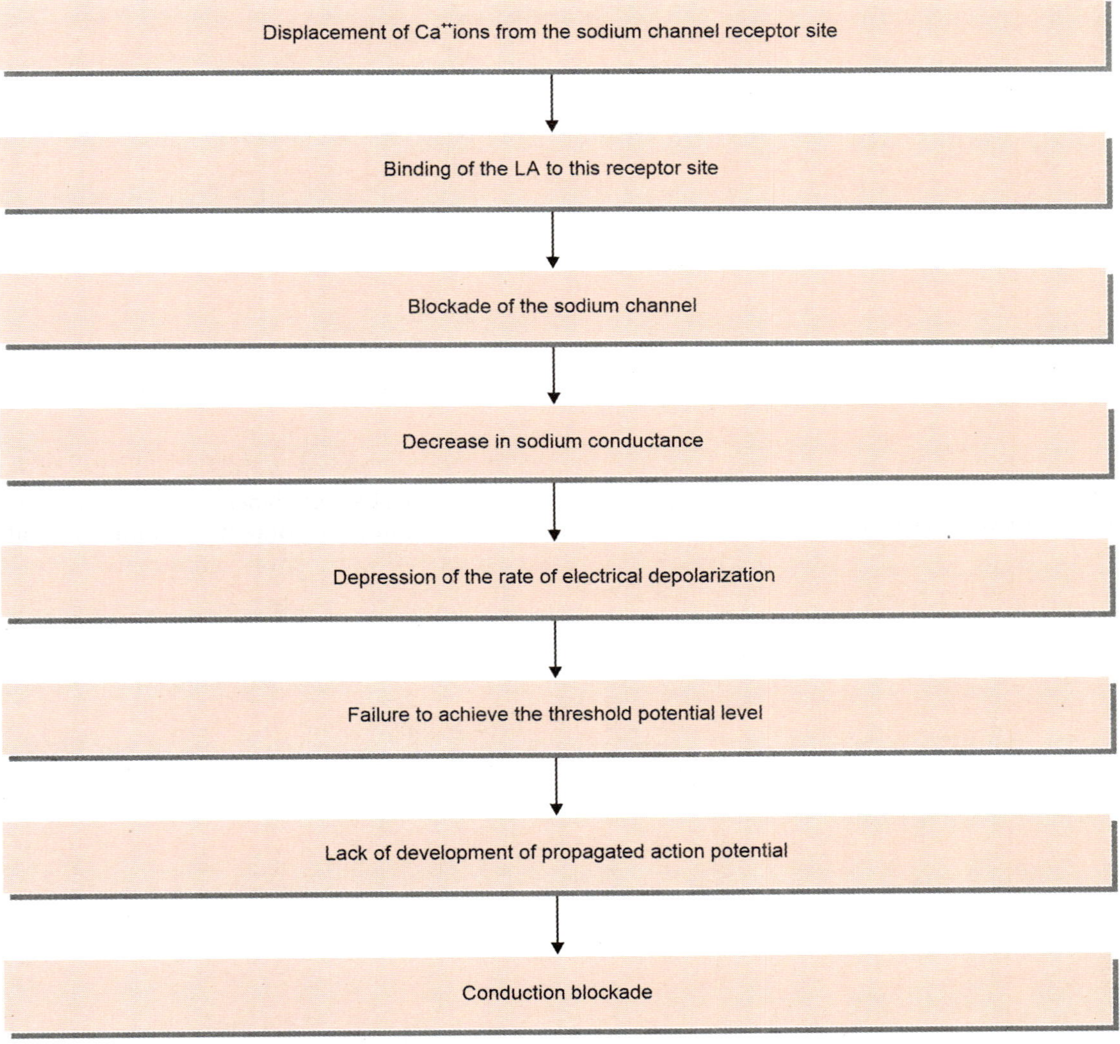
Displacement of Ca^{++} ions from the sodium channel receptor site
Binding of the LA to this receptor site
Blockade of the sodium channel
Decrease in sodium conductance
Depression of the rate of electrical depolarization
Failure to achieve the threshold potential level
Lack of development of propagated action potential
Conduction blockade

Local Anesthetic Agents

Local anesthetic	*Comments*	*Onset (minutes)*	*Duration*	*Effective dental concentration*	*Maximum received dose (mg/kg)*	*Topical effect*	*Maximum dose (mg)*
Procaine	• Most potent vasodilator—hence clean surgical field difficult to maintain • Allergic reactions are due to metabolic product—PABA • Reduces effectiveness of sulfonamides. Undergoes rapid hydrolysis—hence low degree of systemic toxicity • Used in the immediate management of inadvertent intra-arterial injection of a drug (e.g., thiopental) to break arteriospasm. It has slow onset, hence the reason for inclusion of propoxycaine	Slow 6–10	Short	2–4%	15–20	Not clinically acceptable concentration	
Chloroprocaine	• Greater potency and less toxicity than procaine • Greater potency and rapid hydrolysis provides favorable therapeutic index • Commonly used in obstetrics • Occasionally applicable to dentistry when anesthesia of very short duration is advantageous (in children who may inadvertently traumatize their lips, tongue, or cheek)	Fast	Short	2%	11		
Lidocaine	• Metabolized in the liver to monoethyl glycine and xylidide • Xylidide is a local anesthetic and potentially toxic • Allergy to lidocaine and other amides is virtually nonexistent. • Formulations: » 2% lidocaine without vasoconstrictor » Pulpal anesthesia 5–10 minutes » Few clinical indications because of vasodilation » 2% with epinephrine 1:50,000 » Pulpal anesthesia 60 minutes » Soft tissue 3–5 hours » Only recommended use is for hemostasis » 2% with epinephrine with 1:100,000 » Pulpal anesthesia 60 minutes » Soft tissue 3–5 hours. • 2% with 1:100,000 is preferred to 2% with 1:50,000 (1:100,000 has only half as much epinephrine as 1:50,000), especially in elderly patients and ASA III and ASA IV risks with histories of cardiovascular disease • Lidocaine has been used to control myocardial contractility. Antiarrhythmic effect produced by 300 mg as a deltoid IM or 50–100 mg as IV • For topical two forms: » *Lidocaine base—5%*: Poorly soluble in water » *Lidocaine hydrochloride—2%*: Water-soluble » Water-soluble form penetrates tissue more efficiently than base, but systemic absorption is greater providing greater risk of toxicity than base form	Rapid 2–3		2%	• 4.4 mg/kg for lidocaine without vasoconstrictor • 7 mg/kg for lidocaine with vasoconstrictor	Yes 5%	Not to exceed 300 mg for lidocaine without vasoconstrictor or not to exceed 500 mg for lidocaine with vasoconstrictor

Contd..

Contd..

Local anesthetic	Comments	Onset (minutes)	Duration	Effective dental concentration	Maximum received dose (mg/kg)	Topical effect	Maximum dose (mg)
	• Availability: » *Aerosol*—xylocaine 10 mg/ metered spray ointment » 50 mg/mL (octacaine) patch » 46.1 mg/patch (dentipatch) solution » 25, 50 mg/mL (xylocaine) • Lignocaine HCl: » Oral topical solution » 20 mg/mL (xylocaine viscous) » Solution 40 mg/mL (xylocaine)						
Bupivacaine	• Potency is four times that of lidocaine, mepivacaine, and prilocaine • *Toxicity*: Less than four times that of lidocaine, mepivacaine. Two primary indications are—lengthy dental procedures where pulpal anesthesia of more than 90 minutes is required, e.g., full mouth reconstruction, implant surgery • Extensive periodontal procedures: » Management of postoperative pain (e.g., endodontic, periodontal, and surgical) patients requirement for postoperative opioid analgesics is lessened » Not recommended in younger patients or those for whom the risk of soft tissue injury by self-mutilation is increased • Can relieve pain of labor at concentration 0.125% while permitting some motor activity of abdominal muscle to aid in expelling the fetus	Longer 6–10	• Longer *pulpal*: 3 hours • *Soft tissue after nerve block*: 12 hours	0.5%	1.3	Not clinically acceptable concentration	90
Mepivacaine	• Only dental cartridge not containing methylparaben 3% mepivacaine without vasoconstrictor » It is recommended for patients for whom vasoconstrictor is not indicated and for minor dental procedures—most used local anesthetic in pediatric patient » Appropriate for geriatric patients	Fast 1.5–2	Moderate without vasoconstrictor—Pulpal anesthesia 20–40 minutes	3% without vasoconstrictor and 2% with vasoconstrictor	4.4	Not clinically acceptable concentration	300
Articaine	• Originally known as carticaine • First and only local anesthetic of the amide type to possess a thiophene ring as its lipophilic moiety • It has many physicochemical properties of other local anesthetics with the exception of the aromatic moiety and degree of protein-binding • It is able to diffuse through soft tissues and hard tissues more reliably • Potency is 1.5 times that of lidocaine • Methemoglobinemia is a potential side effect • Contraindicated in the presence of a documented allergy to sulfur-containing drugs (only local anesthetic with this contraindication)	• *1:200,000 INFIL*: 1–2 minutes • *MANDBLK*: 2–3 minutes • *1:100,000 INFIL*: 1–2 minutes • *MANDBLK*: 2–2.5 minutes	With 1:100,000 epinephrine—75 minutes of pulpal anesthesia and with 1:200,000 epinephrine—45 minutes of pulpal anesthesia	4%	7.0 mg/kg—adult 5.0 mg/kg/child (for both 1:200,000 and 1:100,000 epinephrine concentrations)	Not clinically acceptable concentration	500 (for both 1:200,000 and 1:100,000 epinephrine)
Benzocaine (ethyl amino- benzoate)	• Not soluble in water—not soluble for injection • Poor absorption into cardiovascular system • Inhibit antibacterial actions of sulfonamides • Localized allergic reactions may occur after prolonged or repeated use • It can also induce methemoglobinemia, but only when administered in very large doses	Prolonged	10%, 15%, and 20%			Only topical application	

(ASA: American Society of Anesthesiologist; EMLA: eutectic mixture of local anesthetic; HCl: hydrochloric acid; IM: intramuscular; IV: intravenous)

TOPICAL ANESTHESIA

Topical anesthesia also called as topical local anesthesia or surface anesthesia, can induce loss of sensation of applied tissues or mucosa up to a depth of 2–3 mm. Efficacy of topical anesthetic is dependent upon factors such as composition, concentration, solubility, form in which it is given, site of application, duration of application.

Classification of Topical Anesthesia

- Based on composition: Chemical, herbal
- Based on preparation:
  - Simple (lignocaine, benzocaine, dyclonine hydrochloride)
  - Compounded (EMLA, precaine, TAC, TAC alternate, XAP, cetacaine)
- Based on delivery: Gel, patch, spray, cream

Simple topical anesthesia: Lignocaine (2–15%) and benzocaine (8-20%) are the most common topical anesthetic preparations used in pediatric dentistry. Benzocaine preparations are more commonly used. Gel formulations are more commonly used than other preparations such as spray, patch, cream.

Compounded topical preparations: Compounded topical preparations are combinations of two or more anesthetic agents for improved clinical efficacy and improved properties.

- **Eutectic mixture of local anesthesia (EMLA):** Eutectic mixture of local anesthetics (EMLA) is a eutectic combination of 2.5% lidocaine and 2.5% prilocaine. It consists of a mixture of two crystalline powders (2.5% lidocaine and 2.5% prilocaine), which has a melting point below room temperature and turns into a liquid oil emulsion phase. In this way, it would be able to penetrate intact skin or mucosa into a depth of 5 mm. Originally, EMLA is not indicated for the oral mucosa but several authors have reported it as the most effective topical agent in dentistry.

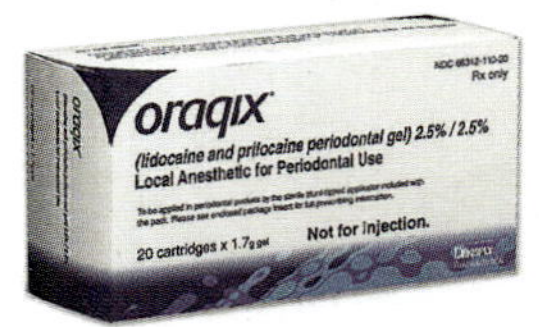

- **Precaine (8% lidocaine + 0.8% dibucaine):** Dibucaine is also called as cincain. Dibucaine is a quinoline derivative and amino amide with anesthetic activity. Dibucaine reversibly binds to and inactivates sodium channels in the neuronal cell membrane. Inhibition of sodium channels prevents the depolarization of nerve cell membranes and inhibits subsequent propagation of impulses along the course of the nerve, thereby limiting the excitation of nerve endings. This results in loss of sensation. Dibucaine is potent, toxic and long-acting local anesthetics, its parenteral use was restricted to spinal anesthesia. It is now generally only used (usually as the hydrochloride) in creams and ointments.

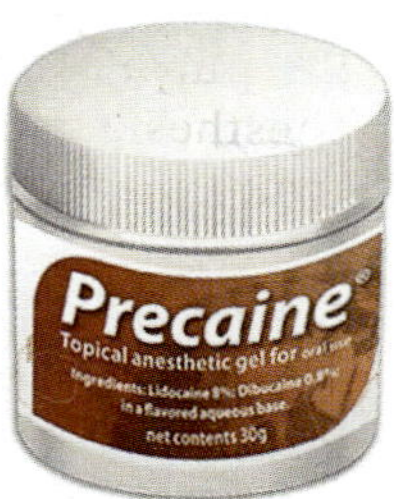

- **TAC:** TAC (0.5% tetracaine, 1:2,000 adrenaline, 11.8% cocaine) usually used as a topical analgesia for lacerations in emergency.
- **TAC 20% alternate:** TAC 20% alternate is a compound topical gel containing two anesthetic agents (20% lidocaine and 4% tetracaine), one vasoactive agent (2% phenylephrine) and seven inactive ingredients that provide structure and give taste to the gel. Tetracaine is a long-acting ester that is included in the anesthetic to provide more profound anesthesia. The product's name TAC 20% Alternate is a misnomer; although it is named after TAC gel, TAC 20% Alternate does not contain any cocaine.
- **LPT (profound and profound PET):** Profound is a compound topical gel containing three anesthetic agents: 10% lidocaine, 10% prilocaine and 4% tetracaine. This can be particularly used in soft tissue surgeries. Profound PET has additional ingredients such as 2% phenyl epinephrine, and various other ingredients such as methyl cellulose for increased viscosity.
- **Cetacaine:** Cetacaine is a combination of benzocaine 14%, butamben 2%, tetracaine HCl 2%. Cetacaine is available in liquid and spray forms.

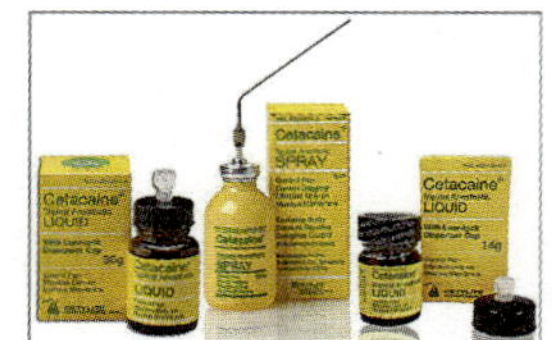

> *Risks associated with compounded topical preparations:* The maximum recommended dosage of the compounded preparations are poorly established as a result of which there is a higher probability of toxicity. Compounded preparations are usually a mixture of different classes of drugs (amides, esters, etc.), there are higher chances of hypersensitivity reactions. Compounded topical preparations containing phenylepinephrine are photosensitive hence prolonged exposure to light can result in the degradation of the product.

- **Herbal topical anesthetics:**
  - Herbal preparations such as clove, cinchona, datura, thymol, Jasmine has local anesthetic properties and are used in medicine and dentistry.
  - Piper betel leaf is an evergreen perineal creeper belonging to family piperaceace. The main constituents of leaf is betel oil, phenolic compounds chavibetol, chavicol and the analgesic efficacy of betel leaf is mainly due to alkaloid compounds arakene and eugenol.
  - Clove extract (Syzygium aromaticum) family myrtaceae, a common spice is basically a dried flower bud used in Asian countries. Clove flower buds contain up to 18% of essential oil which consists of eugenol, eugenol acetate and β-cariofileno. Analgesic efficacy of clove is conferred to eugenol which acts by activation of chloride and calcium channels in ganglional cells or by capascain antagonist activity. FDA classified clove as GRAS (generally recognized as safe) and the acceptable daily amount of clove in humans is 2.5 mg/kg body weight.
  - *Anacyclus pyrethrum (A. pyrethrum)* is a wild species belonging to the family Asteraceae, which is used in

traditional medicines to treat toothache. The root extract of this plant contains a compound pyrethrine or pellitorine, is believed to be the reason for analgesic action.

- Spilanthes acmella is commonly known as toothache plant. The main constituents, namely, "spilanthol" and "acmellonate", reduces the pain associated with toothaches and can induce saliva secretion.

SPECIFIC CLINICAL RECOMMENDATIONS

- **Needle prick pain:** Needle prick pain is one of the most feared procedures by children in clinical practice. Cetacaine and EMLA are shown to be more efficacious for providing palatal anesthesia.
- **Pediatric exodontia:** In conditions of pre-shedding mobility where there is advanced root resorption, and it is retained only by mucosal contact topical anaesthesia alone can provide analgesia sufficient for tooth extraction.
- **Oral ulcers:** Topical local anesthesia is commonly used for symptomatic pain relief in the oral ulcer conditions. Bio-adhesive pastes containing the active topical analgesia by forming protective coat can provide symptomatic relief.
- **Teething pain:** Traditionally topical anesthetic preparations (benzocaine and lignocaine) were used extensively to alleviate discomfort due to teething in babies. In 2011, FDA warned that, using over the counter (OTC) benzocaine gels for teething or mouth pain can cause a rare but serious condition called methemoglobinemia. Hence, FDA recommended benzocaine products should not be used on children less than two years of age, except under the advice and supervision of a healthcare professional. Later in 2014, FDA warned that, prescription of oral viscous lidocaine 2% solution should not be used to treat infants and children with teething pain.
- **Gingival anesthesia for rubber-dam clamp placement and stainless-steel crown try in and placement:** The discomfort associated with rubber-dam clamp placement can be reduced with the application of topical local anesthetics in children. Benzocaine 20%, lignocaine 2%, EMLA have shown better results for the same in children. Topical anesthesia preparations can reduce the discomfort associated with the repeated try-in and placement of stainless steel crowns in children.
- **Pediatric restorative dentistry and endodontics:** Certain topical preparations (EMLA, benzocaine) can induce partial anesthesia of the pulp after prolonged application to the buccal mucosa. This can make the restorative procedures more comfortable by reducing the dentinal sensitivity during cavity preparations in primary teeth.
- **Pediatric orthodontics:** Pain and mucosal irritation due to orthodontic bracket application can be reduced by application of topical anesthetics. Compounded preparations are better in reducing pain.
- **Pediatric oral maxillofacial surgery:** Compounded oral preparations such as LAT and LPT are used in pediatric maxilla-facial surgery for facial and oral laceration suturing. EMLA is also used to reduce pain during venipuncture in emergency pediatric department.

ALTERNATIVES TO CONVENTIONAL TOPICAL ANESTHESIA

- **Precooling:** Precooling is also called cryoanesthesia. It involves the application of cold to the surface of the oral mucosa. Unlike topical anesthesia, cryoanesthesia acts on all the cells. Many studies reported the use of precooling to be effective in reducing pain due to needle insertion in children. Precooling in conjunction with other techniques such as vibration is proved to be effective in reducing pain and discomfort associated with needle insertion in children.
- **Counter-irritation or counter-stimulation:** Vibration, pressure application will come under counter-irritation, where larger A-delta fibers are stimulated to block the transmission of nociception. Inhibitory neurons in the spinal cord are stimulated which reduces nociception by A-δ and C fibers. Many studies report the usage of vibration to be an effective counter stimulant to alleviate intraoral needle prick pain in children. Vibratory stimulus can be delivered directly at the injection site (intraorally) or indirectly (extraorally). Pressure application in the injection site is also an effective counter stimulation technique for pain reduction during needle prick especially for palatal injections.
- **Electronic dental anesthesia (EDA):** It is a modification of transcutaneous electrical nerve stimulation (TENS) for intraoral usage. It delivers a small current stimulus through the tissue to reduce pain sensation. Many studies reported the usage of EDA for the purpose of surface anesthesia in children. EDA is reported to have a beneficial effect with minor non-invasive procedures such as cavity preparation, rubber dam clamp placement in children.

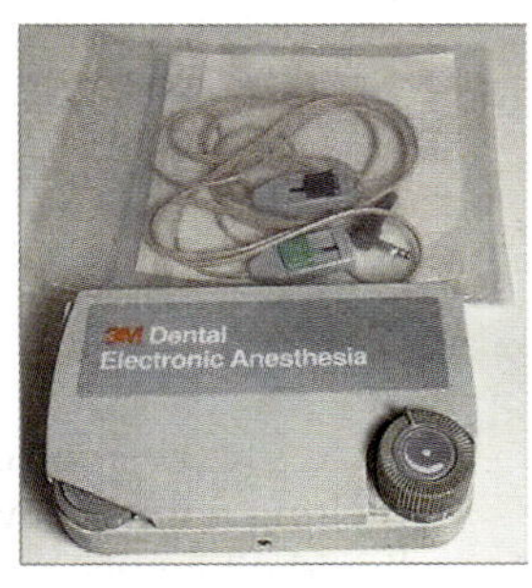

- **Iontophoresis:** Iontophoresis can serve the purpose of surface anesthesia in dentistry. Lignocaine and adrenaline which are positively charged molecules penetrate deeper into the tissues with the influence of constant low-intensity electrical charge. This process is called iontophoresis. It can be accomplished with a current of 0–3 mA and is facilitated by two electrodes. Few studies reported painless extraction of primary teeth with the help of iontophoresis alone. Nowadays, Iontophoresis is being tested on carious lesions to improve fluoride and calcium uptake.

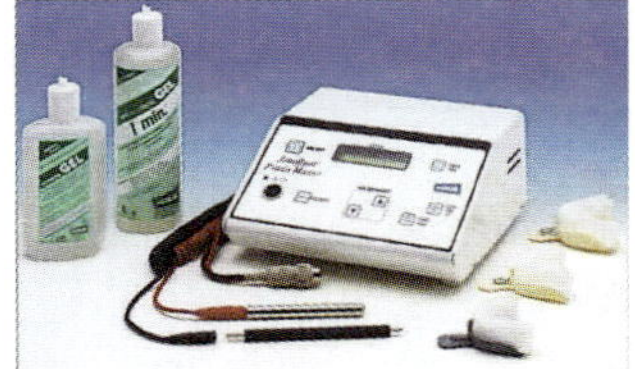

MAXILLARY INJECTION TECHNIQUES

Intraoral techniques	*Extraoral techniques*
Anterior, middle superior alveolar, and infraorbital nerve block	Anterior and middle superior alveolar nerve block (infraorbital)
Posterior superior alveolar nerve block (zygomatic)	Maxillary nerve block
Nasopalatine nerve block	
Anterior palatine nerve block	
Maxillary nerve block	

Anterior/Middle Superior Alveolar and Infraorbital Nerve Block (Figs. 61.2 to 61.4)

- **Nerves anesthetized:** Infraorbital, anterior and middle superior alveolar nerves, inferior palpebral, lateral nasal, and superior labial nerves.
- **Areas anesthetized:** Incisors, cuspids, bicuspids, and mesiobuccal root of the first molar on the side injected, including bone and soft tissue, upper lip, and a portion of nose on the same side.
- **Indications:** Anesthesia of five anterior maxillary teeth on the same side of the median line.

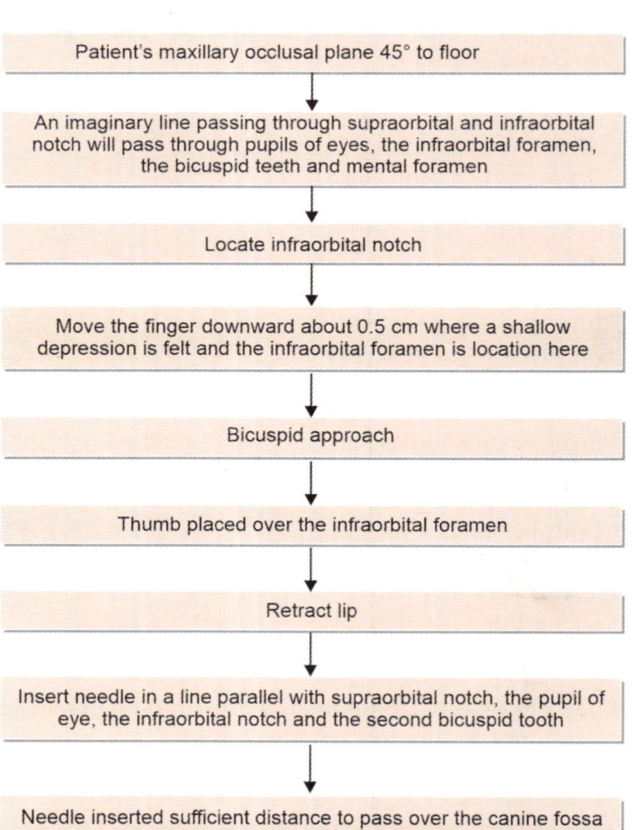
Patient's maxillary occlusal plane 45° to floor
An imaginary line passing through supraorbital and infraorbital notch will pass through pupils of eyes, the infraorbital foramen, the bicuspid teeth and mental foramen
Locate infraorbital notch
Move the finger downward about 0.5 cm where a shallow depression is felt and the infraorbital foramen is location here
Bicuspid approach
Thumb placed over the infraorbital foramen
Retract lip
Insert needle in a line parallel with supraorbital notch, the pupil of eye, the infraorbital notch and the second bicuspid tooth
Needle inserted sufficient distance to pass over the canine fossa while the thumb is used to maneuver the needle into a position so that it contacts the bone at the entrance to the foramen

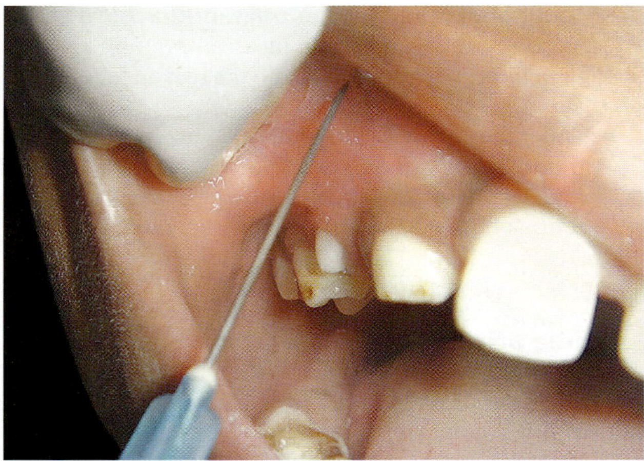

Fig. 61.2: Anterior superior alveolar nerve anesthesia.

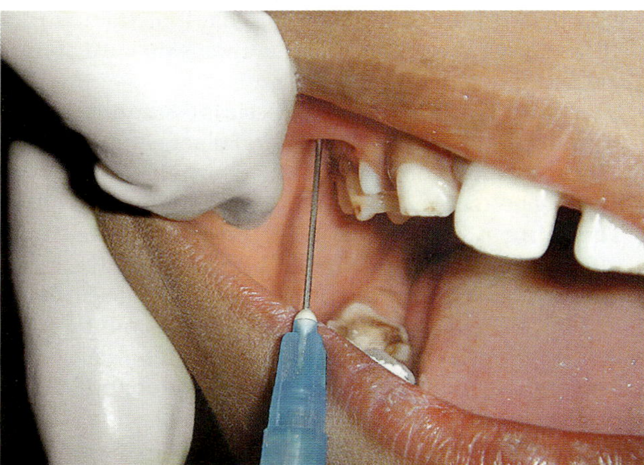

Fig. 61.3: Middle superior alveolar nerve anesthesia.

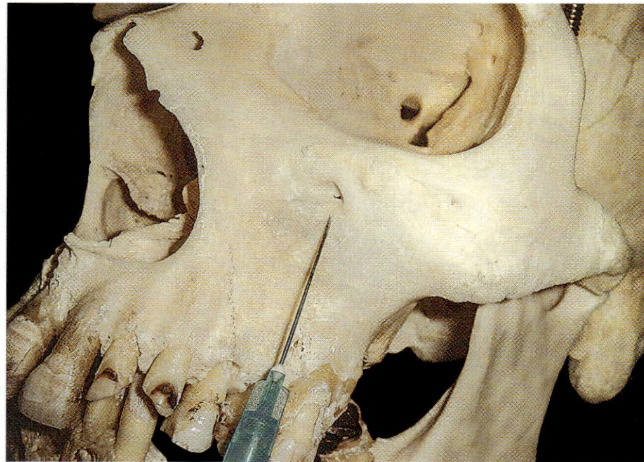

Fig. 61.4: Infraorbital nerve anesthesia.

Posterior Superior Alveolar Nerve Block (Figs. 61.5A and B)

- **Nerves anesthetized:** Posterior superior alveolar nerve.
- **Areas anesthetized:** Maxillary molars with the exception of mesiobuccal root of first molar, buccal alveolar processes

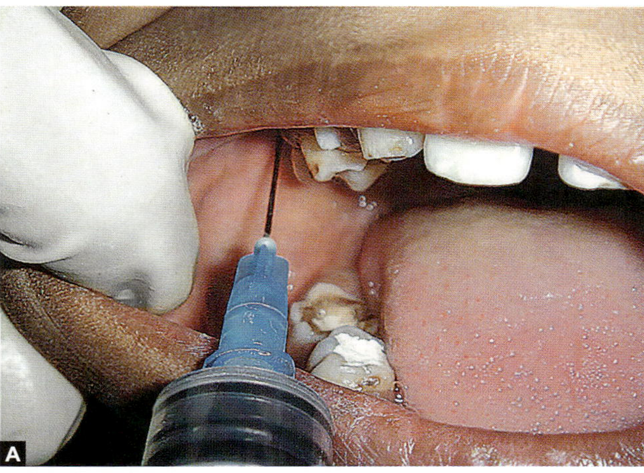

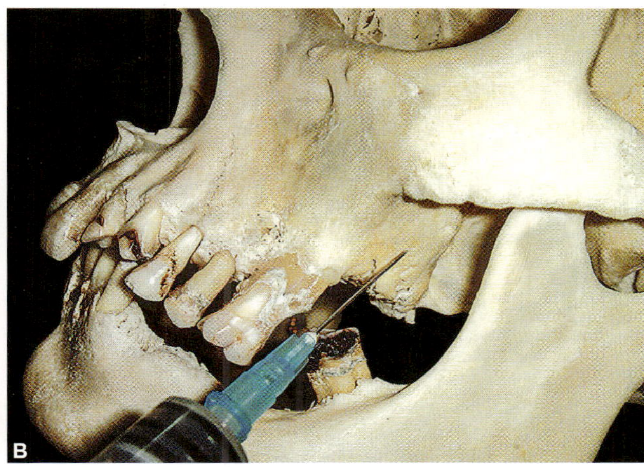

Figs. 61.5A and B: Posterior superior alveolar nerve anesthesia.

of the maxillary molars, periosteum, connective tissue, and mucous membrane.

- **Indications:** Operative procedures of molar teeth and supporting structures. This injection must be combined with palatal injection for extractions and instrumentation extending into this area.

Maxillary occlusal plane at 45° to the floor

↓

Move finger over mucobuccal fold in posterior direction from the bicuspid area until zygomatic process of maxilla is reached

↓

At its posterior aspect, the finger tip will rest in concavity in the mucobuccal fold

↓

At this point finger is rotated so that its bulbous portion is still in contact with the posterior surface of zygomatic process

↓

With the finger in the same position, the hand is lowered, so that the finger is in a plane at right angles to occlusal surfaces of the maxillary teeth and 45° to the patient's sagittal plane

↓

Index finger should be pointing in the same direction, the needle is to follow

↓

Needle is inserted in a line parallel with the index finger and bisecting the fingernail

↓

Insertion is made for distance of about ½ to ¾ inch going upward, inward and backward. Aspirate and inject

Nasopalatine Nerve Block (Figs. 61.6A and B)

- **Nerves anesthetized:** Nasopalatine nerve as it emerges from the anterior palatine foramen.
- **Areas anesthetized:** Anterior portion of the hard palate and overlying structures back to the bicuspid.
- **Indications:**
  - For palatal anesthesia
  - To supplement the block of the anterior and the middle superior alveolar nerves
  - To augment analgesia of the six maxillary incisors
  - To complete anesthesia of nasal septum.

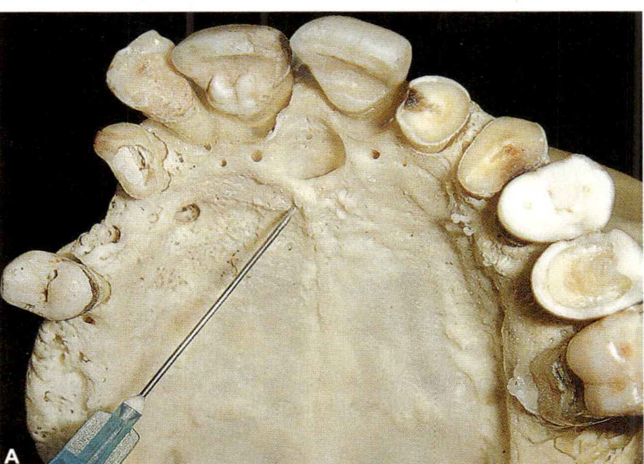

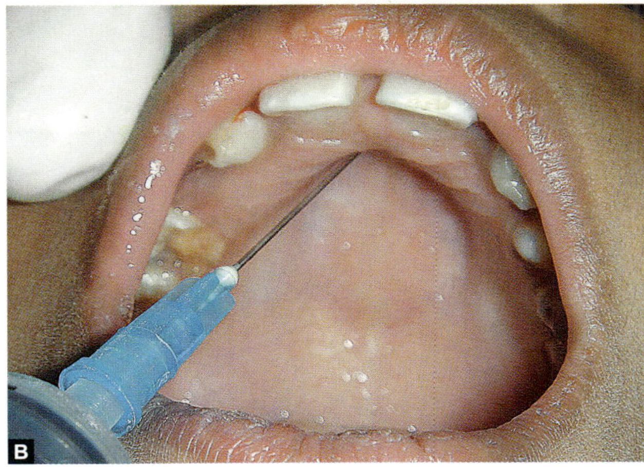

Figs. 61.6A and B: Nasopalatine nerve anesthesia.

A very painful injection, hence a preparatory injection is required

↓

Needle inserted into the labial interseptal tissue between the maxillary central incisors, at right angle to the labial plate and passed into tissues until resistance is met, 0.25 mL solution is then deposited

↓

Now the needle is inserted into the incisive papilla making certain that it is line with the labial alveolar plate

↓

Needle slowly advances into incisive foramen, about 0.5 cm into the canal. Inject 0.25–0.5 mL very slowly

Greater Palatine Nerve Block (Figs. 61.7A and B)

- **Nerves anesthetized:** Anterior palatine as it leaves the greater palatine foramen.
- **Areas anesthetized:** Posterior portion of the hard palate and overlying structures up to the first bicuspid area on the side injected.
- **Indications:**
  - For palatal anesthesia to be used in conjunction with posterior superior alveolar nerve block or middle superior alveolar nerve block .
  - For surgery of posterior portion of hard palate.

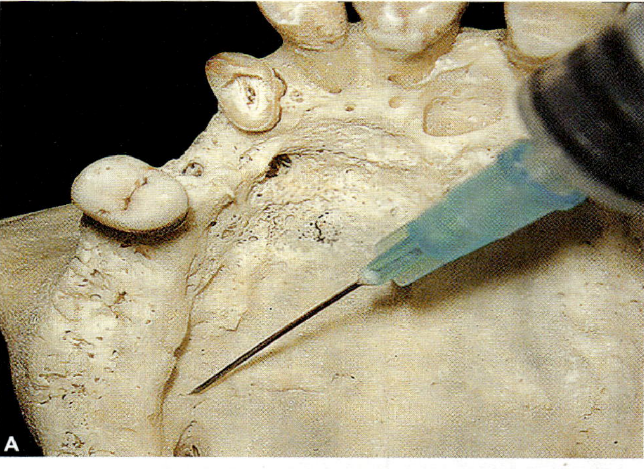

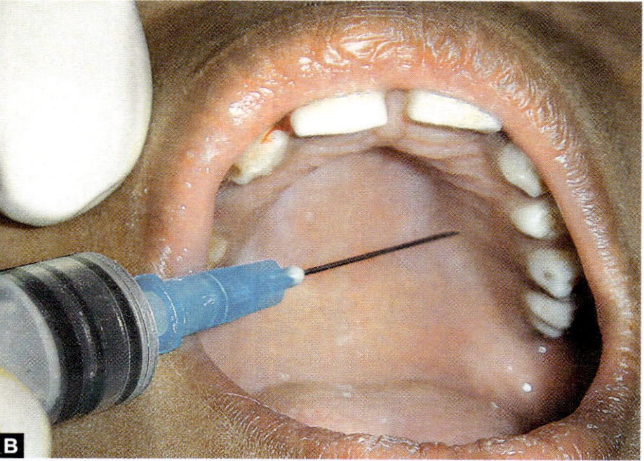

Figs. 61.7A and B: Greater palatine nerve anesthesia.

Greater palatine foraman is situated between the 2nd and 3rd molars about 1 cm from the palatal gingival margin towards the midline. This foramen is approached from the opposite side, with needle kept as near to a right angle as possible with the curvature of the palatal bone

↓

Needle inserted until palatal bone is contacted, injection done very slowly. This nerve can be blocked at any point along its course after emergence from the foramen

↓

When bicuspid area (which receives dual innervation from the anterior palatine nerve and nasopalatine nerve), is to be anesthetized inserted needle and deposit solution in the palatal curvature opposite the bicuspids also

Greater palatine canal approach

↓

The greater palatine foramen is located between the 2nd and 3rd molars about 1 cm to the midline of the palate from the palatal gingival margin a slight depression in this area may be palpated and used as a guide in locating the foramen

↓

First the tissue over this area should be anesthetized by local infiltration

↓

The needle is then inserted and it may be necessary to probe slightly to locate the foramen

↓

Once located the needle is passed very slowly into the canal at a marked depth not to exceed 1.5 inches. The 2 mL solution in injected very slowly

Maxillary Nerve Block

- **Nerves anesthetized:** Entire maxillary nerve and all its subdivisions peripheral to the site of injection.
- **Areas anesthetized:**
  - Maxillary teeth on the affected side
  - Alveolar bone and overlying structures
  - Hard palate and portions of soft palate
  - Upper lip, cheek, side of nose, and lower eyelid.
- **Indications:**
  - When anesthesia of entire distribution of maxillary nerve is required for extensive surgery
  - Local injection makes blocks of terminal branches unfeasible
  - For diagnostic or therapeutic purposes such as tics or neuralgias of the maxillary division of the fifth nerve.

MANDIBULAR INJECTION TECHNIQUES

Intraoral	*Extraoral*
Inferior alveolar nerve block: • Open mouth technique: » Indirect approach » Direct approach • Closed mouth technique: » Vazirani–Akinosi technique	• Inferior alveolar nerve block • Mental and incisive nerve block • Mandibular nerve block
Buccinator nerve block	
Mental nerve block	
Incisive nerve block	
Local infiltration	
Mandibular nerve block: Gow–Gates technique	

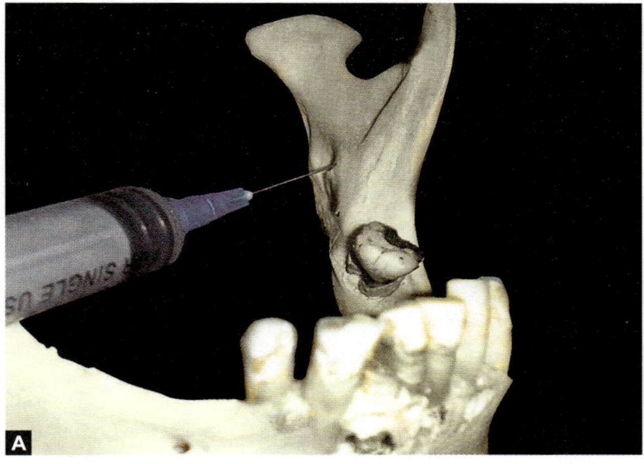

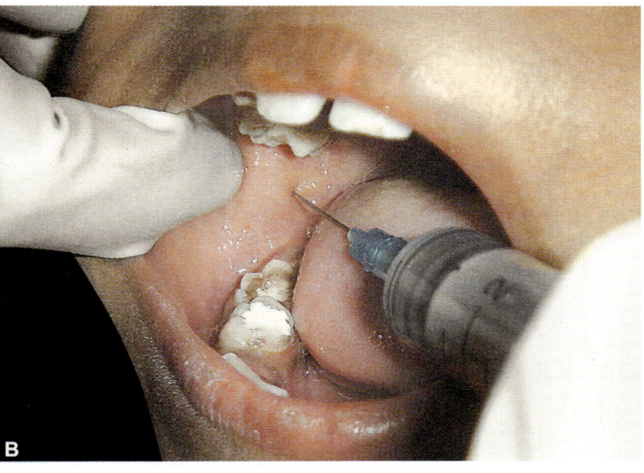

Figs. 61.8A and B: Inferior alveolar nerve block in children.

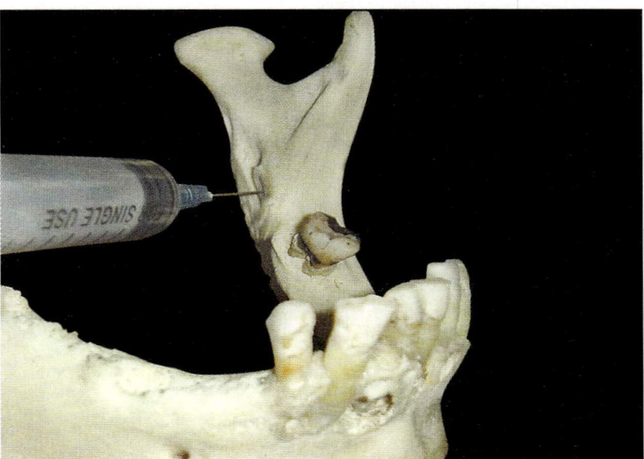

Fig. 61.9: Inferior alveolar nerve block in adults.

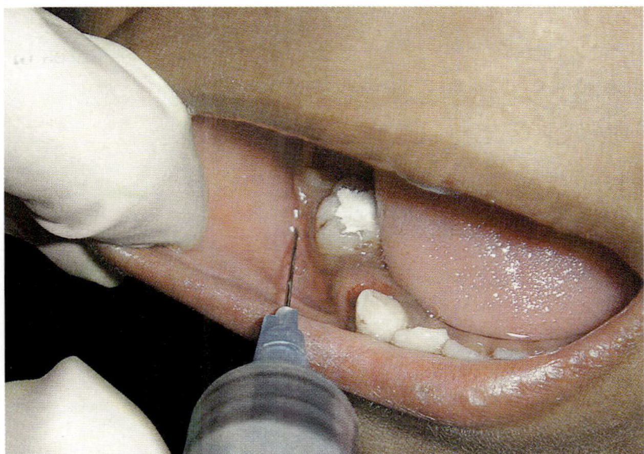

Fig. 61.10: Long buccal nerve anesthesia.

Inferior Alveolar Nerve Block (Figs. 61.8 and 61.9)

- **Nerves anesthetized:**
  - Inferior alveolar nerve
  - Mental nerve
  - Incisive nerve
  - *Occasionally*—lingual nerve, buccinator nerve.
- **Areas anesthetized:**
  - Mandibular teeth to midline
  - Body of mandible
  - *Inferior portion of ramus*—mucous membrane, buccal periosteum anterior to first molar (mental nerve)
  - Anterior two-thirds of tongue
  - Floor of mouth
  - Lingual soft tissues and periosteum.
- **Indications:**
  - Analgesia for operative dentistry in all mandibular teeth
  - Surgical procedures on mandibular teeth and supporting structures anterior to first molar when supplemented by lingual nerve anesthesia
  - When supplemented by long buccal **(Fig. 61.10)** and lingual nerve **(Fig. 61.11)**—surgical procedures on mandibular teeth posterior to second bicuspid
  - Diagnostic and therapeutic purposes.

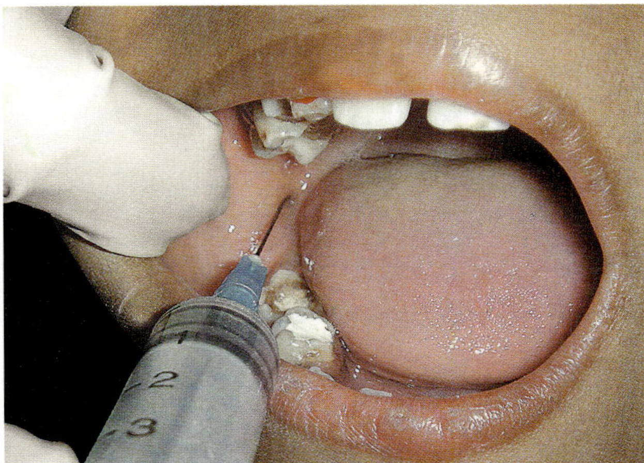

Fig. 61.11: Lingual nerve anesthesia.

- **Landmarks:**
  - Lingual, mandibular sulcus, anterior border of ramus, distal border of ramus, coronoid notch, external oblique ridge, internal oblique ridge, mucobuccal fold, and pterygomandibular ligament.

- **Open mouth/conventional technique**

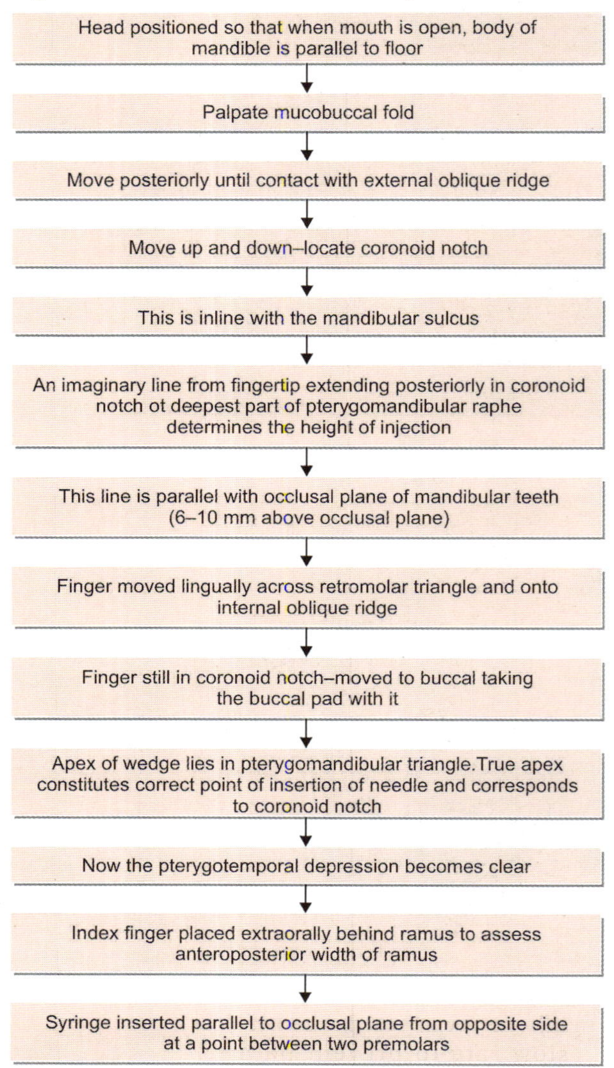

Head positioned so that when mouth is open, body of mandible is parallel to floor
Palpate mucobuccal fold
Move posteriorly until contact with external oblique ridge
Move up and down–locate coronoid notch
This is inline with the mandibular sulcus
An imaginary line from fingertip extending posteriorly in coronoid notch ot deepest part of pterygomandibular raphe determines the height of injection
This line is parallel with occlusal plane of mandibular teeth (6–10 mm above occlusal plane)
Finger moved lingually across retromolar triangle and onto internal oblique ridge
Finger still in coronoid notch–moved to buccal taking the buccal pad with it
Apex of wedge lies in pterygomandibular triangle.True apex constitutes correct point of insertion of needle and corresponds to coronoid notch
Now the pterygotemporal depression becomes clear
Index finger placed extraorally behind ramus to assess anteroposterior width of ramus
Syringe inserted parallel to occlusal plane from opposite side at a point between two premolars

In children mandibular foramen is situated at a level lower than the occlusal plane of primary teeth. So, injection is made at a lower level and posteriorly.
- Age 0–6 years: level of injection is below occlusal plane.
- Age 6–12 years: level of injection is at occlusal plane.
- Age 12 and above: level of injection is above occlusal plane.

- **Closed mouth/Vazirani-Akinosi technique**

Area of insertion is soft tissue over medial border of ramus directly adjacent to maxillary tuberosity at the height of mucogingival junction adjacent to maxillary 3rd molar

↓

Bevel of syringe away from bone of mandibular ramus

↓

Place finger on coronoid notch. Reflect tissues on medial aspect of ramus

↓

Ask patient to gently occlude cheek and muscles of mastication relaxed

↓

Syringe parallel to maxillary occlusal plane at level of mucogingival junction of maxillary 3rd molar

↓

Direct needle posteriorly, laterally advance to 25 mm, this distance is measured from tuberosity

↓

Aspirate and inject

Buccinator Nerve Block

- **Nerves anesthetized:** Buccinator nerve
- **Areas anesthetized:** Soft tissues and periosteum, buccal to mandibular molar teeth

Area of insertion is mucous membrane distal and buccal to most distal molar tooth

↓

Pull buccal soft tissues and make them taut

↓

Bevel towards bone, syringe parallel to occlusal plane, buccal to mandibular molar with depth of penetration 1–2 mm

↓

Aspirate and inject

Mental Nerve Block (Fig. 61.12)

- **Nerves anesthetized:** Mental nerve.
- **Area anesthetized:** Soft tissues of lower lip, chin, and buccal soft tissues anterior to mental foramen are anesthetized.

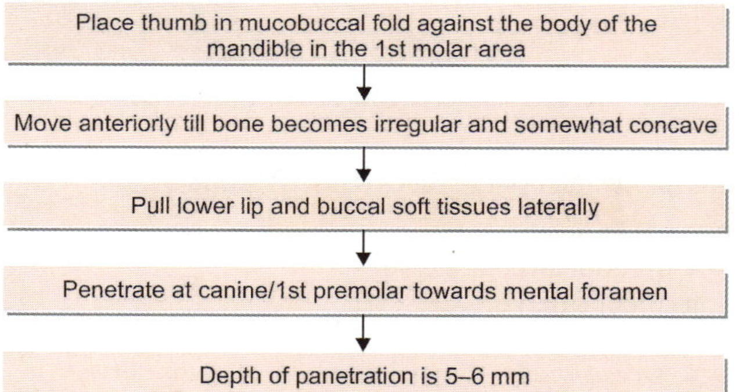

Place thumb in mucobuccal fold against the body of the mandible in the 1st molar area
Move anteriorly till bone becomes irregular and somewhat concave
Pull lower lip and buccal soft tissues laterally
Penetrate at canine/1st premolar towards mental foramen
Depth of panetration is 5–6 mm

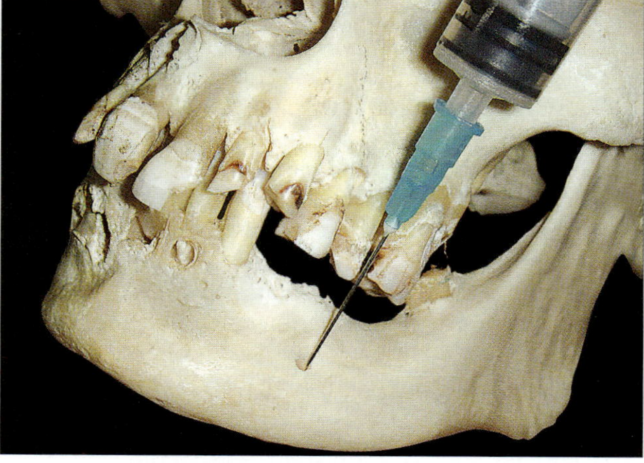

Fig. 61.12: Mental nerve anesthesia.

INFILTRATION ANESTHESIA (FIGS. 61.13A AND B)

Supraperiosteal Infiltration

- **Nerves anesthetized:** Large terminal branches of dental plexus.
- Areas anesthetized:
  - Pulp and root area of the tooth
  - Buccal periosteum
  - Connective tissue and mucous membrane.
- **Indications:**
  - Pulpal anesthesia of maxillary teeth when treatment limited to one or two teeth
  - Soft tissue anesthesia when indicated for surgical procedures in a circumscribed area.
- **Area of insertion:** Height of the mucobuccal fold above the apex of the tooth to be anesthetized.
- **Target area:** Apical region of tooth to be anesthetized.

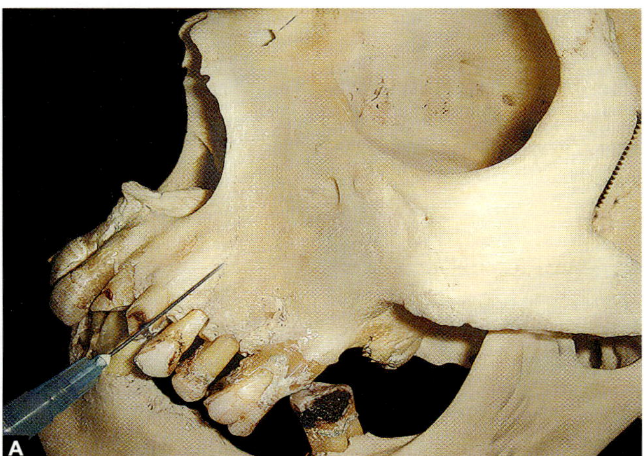

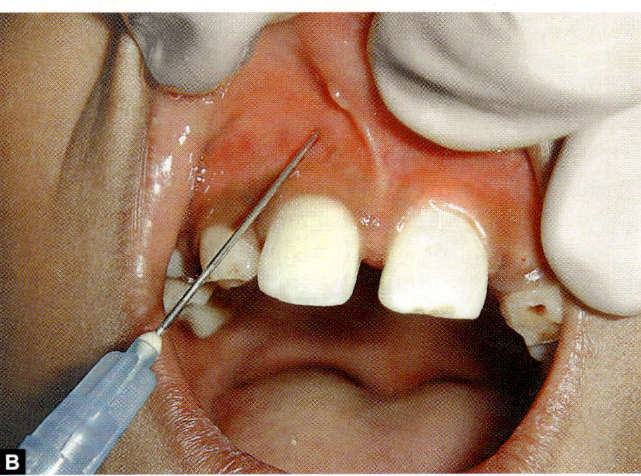

Figs. 61.13A and B: Infiltration nerve anesthesia.

RECENT TRENDS IN PAIN CONTROL

Safety Syringes

- They minimize the risk of accidental needlestick injury occurring with contaminated needle.
- They possess a sheath that locks over the needle when it is removed from patient's tissues.
- Advantages include disposable, single use, sterile until opened, and lightweight.
- Disadvantages are more costly and may be different to use for first timers.
- For example, UltraSafe syringe, Ultra Safety Plus XL syringe, Hypo Safety syringe, Safety Wand™, and Rev Vac™ Safety syringe.

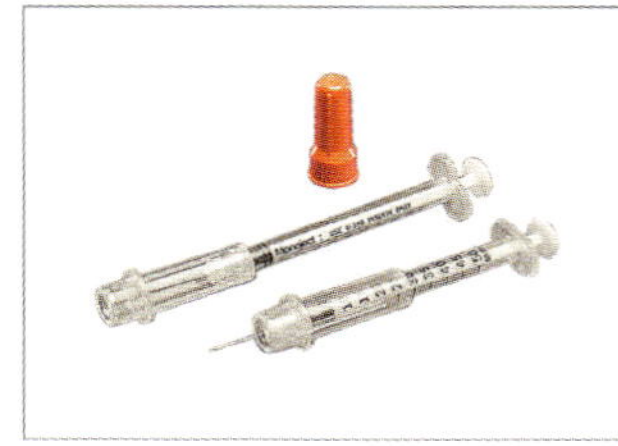

Computer Controlled Local Anesthetic Delivery System

- Introduced into dentistry in 1997.
- Also called as Wand system.
- Single use disposable safety handpiece.
- Luer-Lock needle.
- Pen-like grasp allows operator to rotate handpiece during penetration and insertion.
- This system administers local anesthetic solution at two specific rates:
  1. Slow rate 0.5 mL/min
  2. Fast rate 1.8 mL/min
- Advantages are precise control of flow rate and pressure, increased tactile sensation, and non threatening, automatic aspiration.

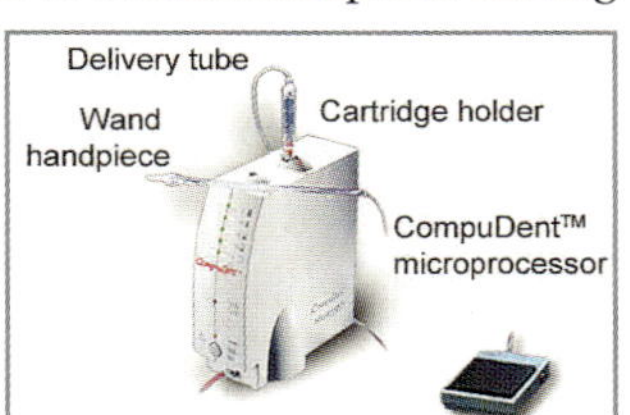

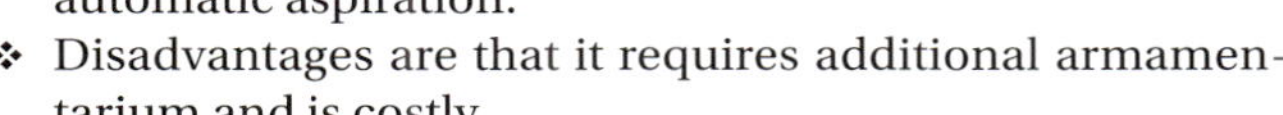

- Disadvantages are that it requires additional armamentarium and is costly.

Comfort Control Syringe

- Introduced after Wand.
- Electronic preprogrammed delivery device.
- Local anesthetic is deposited more slowly and consistently.
- It consists of a two stage delivery system:
  1. Injection begins at an extremely slow rate to prevent pain associated with quick delivery
  2. After 10 seconds, comfort control syringe automatically increases speed to the preprogrammed rate.

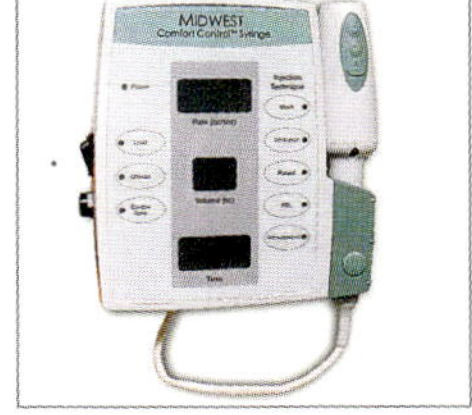

Local Anesthetics with New Additives

Like centbucridine, ropivacaine, and tetrodotoxin.

Eutectic Mixture of Local Anesthetic

- Eutectic mixture of local anesthetic (EMLA) is oil in water emulsion in which the oil phase is a eutectic mixture of lidocaine and prilocaine in a ratio of 1:1 by weight.
- It consists of a 5% cream containing 25 mg/g of lidocaine and 25 mg/g of prilocaine.

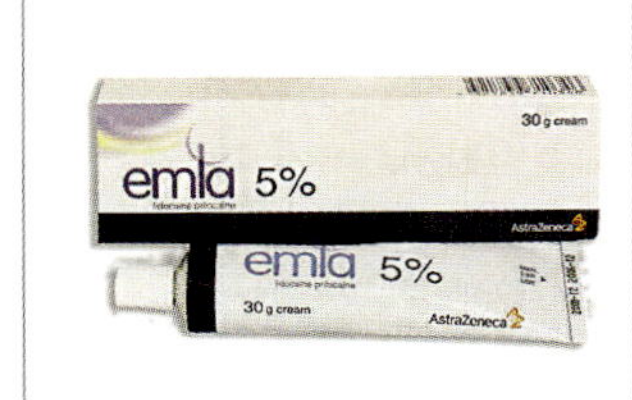

- Should be applied 1 hour before procedure and the cream is covered with an occlusive dressing. Numbing occurs

1 hour after application and lasts for 1–2 hours after removal.

- Its use is contraindicated in infants under 6 months of age because of the possibility of a metabolite of prilocaine inducing methemoglobinemia and in patients with known sensitivity to amides.
- **Adverse responses:** Transient and mild skin blanching and erythema.

Electronic Dental Anesthesia

- It provides pain control for administration of LA.
- It provides excellent soft tissue anesthesia.
- Effective for pain control in needle phobics.
- Aids in reversing local anesthetic effect. Electronic dental anesthesia (EDA) when applied at its low frequency setting for a period of 10–15 minutes removes a large volume of residual anesthetic solution and thereby partially/totally reverses the anesthetic effect.

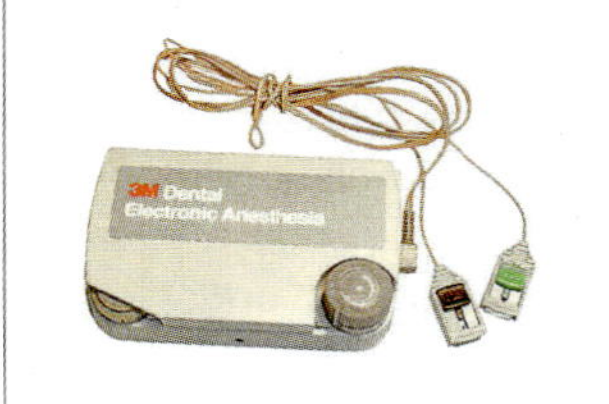

- Used in the management of chronic pain and acute pain.
- Contraindications are ASA IV patients, patients with cardiac pacemaker, neurological disorders, pregnancy, and very young pediatric patients.
- Advantages include no needle usage, no injection of drug, and no residual anesthetic effect at the end of the procedure.
- Disadvantages are cost of the unit, extensive training, and the presence of intraoral electrodes.

VibraJect

- VibraJect LLC (USA) was first introduced in 1995.
- It is a small vibrating dental injection attachment device.
- The device has a clip bracket with a small motor that gets easily attach to most kind of dental injections. The clip bracket is autoclavable, which prevent cross-contamination between patients.

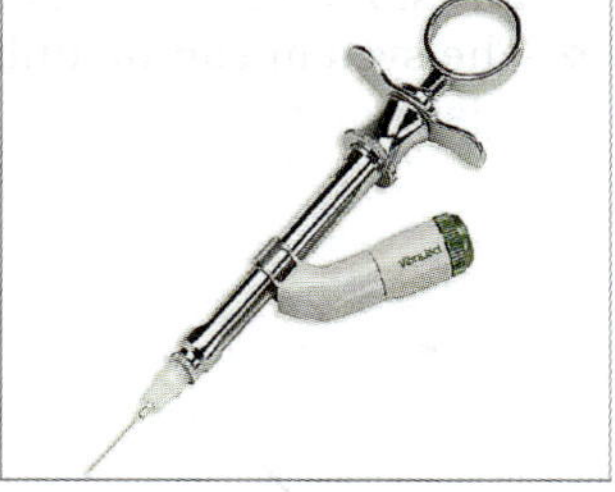

DentalVibe

- It is a cordless, rechargeable, and hand-held device that delivers soothing, pulsed, and percussive micro-oscillations to the site where an injection is being administered.
- Its U-shaped vibrating tip attached to a microprocessor- controlled Vibra-Pulse motor that gently stimulates the sensory receptors at the injection site, effectively closing the neural pain gate, and blocking the painful sensation of injections.

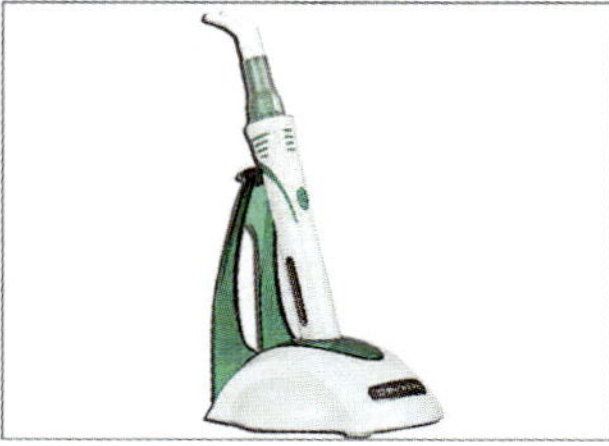

- It also lights the injection area and has an attachment to retract the lip or cheek.

Accupal

- The Accupal (Hot Springs, AR, USA) is a cordless device that uses both vibration and pressure to precondition the oral mucosa.

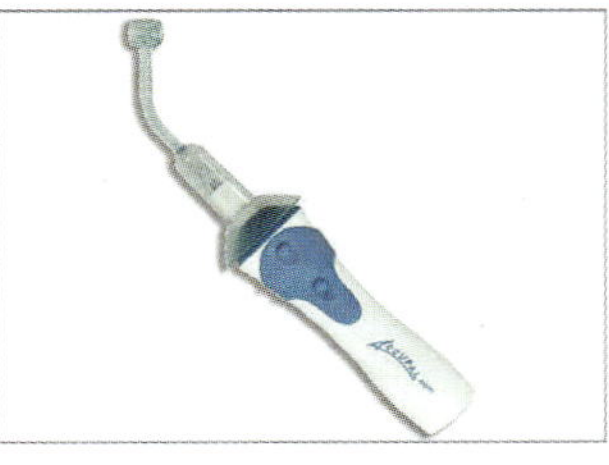

- Accupal provides pressure and vibrates the injection site 360° proximal to the needle penetration, which shuts the "pain gate", according to the manufacturer.
- After placing the device at the injection site and applying moderate pressure, the unit light up the area and begins to vibrate. The needle is placed through a hole in the head of the disposable tip, which is attached to the motor.

Jet Injectors

- Jet-injection technology is based on the principle of using a mechanical energy source to create a release of pressure sufficient to push a dose of liquid medication through a very small orifice, creating a thin column of fluid with enough force that it can penetrate soft tissue into the subcutaneous tissue without a needle.

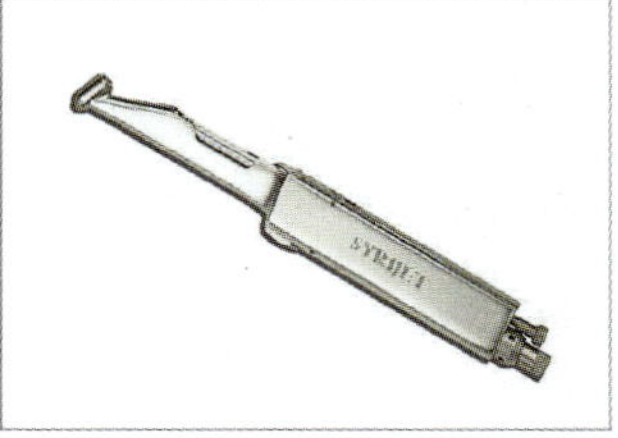

- Jet injectors are believed to offer advantages over traditional needle injectors by being fast and easy to use, with little or no pain, less tissue damage, and faster drug absorption at the injection site.

Syrijet

- The Syrijet Mark II (aka Mizzy), (Cherry Hill, NJ, USA) has been on the market for nearly 40 years and had some minor improvements over the years.
- It accepts the standard 1.8 mL cartridges of LA solution (thereby ensuring sterility of the solution).
- It permits the administration of a variable volume of solution from 0 mL to 0.2 mL.
- Completely autoclavable.

Med-Jet H III

- Med-Jet (Medical International Technologies, Montreal, QC, Canada) has been launched in 2011 with the manufacturer's claim that medication being injected with the device is directed through a small orifice seven times smaller than the smallest available needle in the world.
- This extremely small stream of liquid under pressure pierces and then the remain der of the dose will be dispersed into the desired layer of tissue.

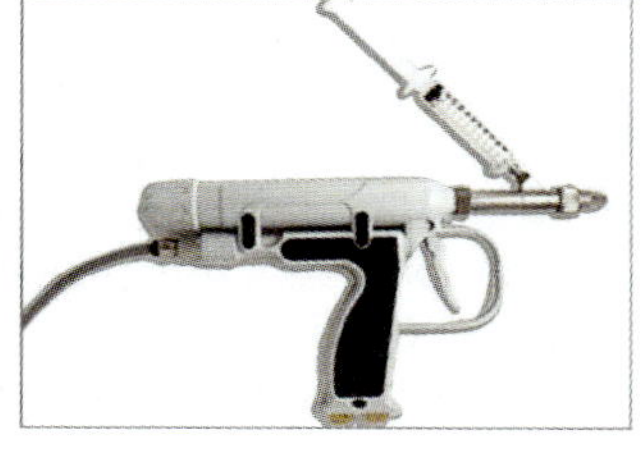

- The system's uniqueness is its ability to utilize low pressure delivery methods without compromising accuracy, convenience, and ease of use—while ensuring patient comfort, environmental safety, and user affordability.

Injex

- This jet of anesthetic solution painlessly or by causing only slight pain can penetrate the mucosal tissue.
- The degree of penetration in the tissue is a function of volume of anesthetic being used and the nozzle pressure.
- The shorter onset time also reduces the treatment- induced stress for children.

Devices for Intraosseous Anesthesia

Several systems have been developed to achieve intraosseous (IO) anesthesia. Although, significant differences exist among them, they all aim to inject local anesthetic solution into the cancellous bone adjacent to the apex of the tooth.

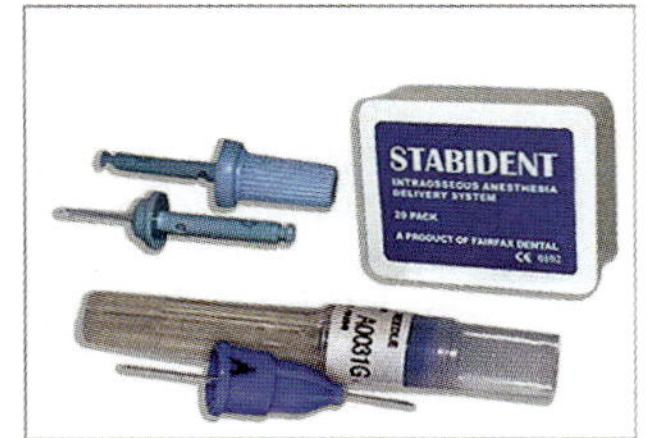

Stabident

- The advantages of the product are that it is relatively inexpensive and can be used with equipment already existing in a dental office. A slow-speed handpiece with a latch contra-angle for the perforator and a standard dental anesthetic syringe for the needle.
- The main disadvantage of the device is that the perforation needs to be made in a reasonably accessible and visible location in the attached gingiva distal to the tooth to be anesthetized. If the penetration zone is located in alveolar mucosa that moves once the perforator is withdrawn, it can be extremely difficult to locate the perforation site with the anesthetic needle.

IntraFlow

Single step method, which allows entry into the penetration zone, injection and withdrawal in one continuous step, without the need to relocate the perforation site.

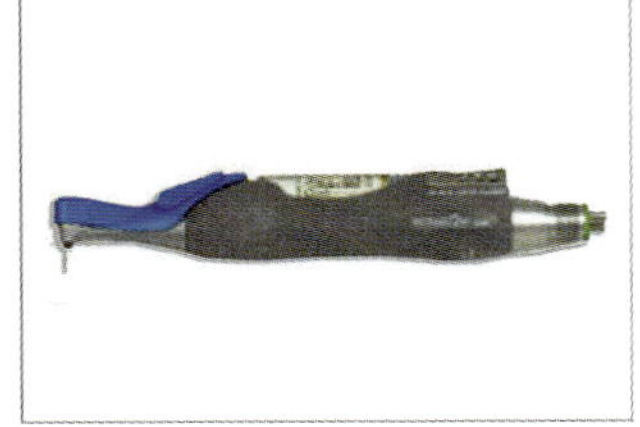

Nonconventional Local Anesthesia Techniques

The anterior middle superior alveolar (AMSA) and palatal approach—anterior superior alveolar nerve block.

- The AMSA nerve block provides pulpal anesthesia to the maxillary incisors, canines, and premolars on the side of injection. Soft tissue anesthesia is achieved for the entire hard palate on both that side and the intraoral mucosa of the five anesthetized teeth.
- The palatal approach-anterior superior alveolar nerve block provides pulpal anesthesia to the six anterior teeth—canine to canine bilaterally, as well as the palatal and labial gingiva and mucoperiosteum and bone overlying these teeth. As noted with the AMSA, there is no collateral anesthesia extraorally.

Periodontal Ligament Injection

- Another injection technique, the periodontal ligament injection (PDL), also known as the intraligamentary injection (ILI) has been extremely useful when anesthesia of a single tooth in the mandible is required.
- The PDL injection provides pulpal anesthesia to the tooth, with only localized soft tissue anesthesia.
- Advantage is that when administered in the mandible, there is no associated extraoral or lingual anesthesia like traditional inferior alveolar nerve block.
- Disadvantages are difficulty in locating the precise site for needle placement (within or at the entrance to the PDL), the chances of leakage of bitter-tasting LA solution into the patient's mouth.

Single Tooth Anesthesia

- In 2006, the manufacturers of the original computerized control local anesthesia delivery (CCLAD), the Wand, introduced a new device, Single Tooth Anesthesia (STA™).

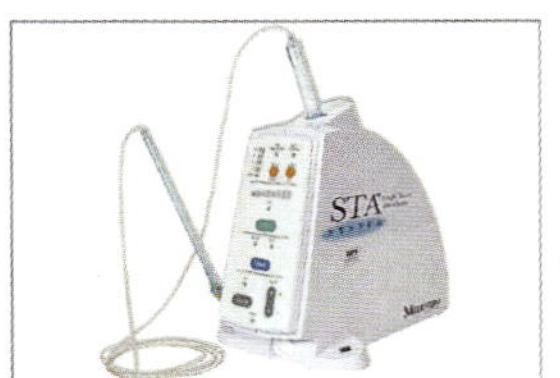

- Single tooth anesthesia incorporates dynamic pressure-sensing (DPS) technology that provides a constant monitoring of the exit pressure of the local anesthetic solution in real time during all phases of the drug's administration.
- Single tooth anesthesia utilizes an adaptation as a means of overcoming the problems associated with PDL injection and simplifies AMSA and P-ASA injections.
- The system can be utilized for all traditional intraoral injecttion techniques.
- Unlike earlier variants, the STA includes a training mode that verbally explains how to use the device, and multicartridge and autocartridge retraction features.
- Since the pressure of the LA is strictly regulated by the STA system, a greater volume of LA can be administered with increased comfort and less tissue damage than seen with traditional syringes or PDL pressure devices.

Buzzy System

- Buzzy® is a reusable 8 × 5 × 2.5 cm plastic bee containing a battery powered vibrating motor with an 18 g solidly frozen ice pack underneath.
- Designed specifically for pain control for children, it is shaped like a bumblebee whose wings contain freeze able gel packs, hence making it fun for children while also distracting them from the pain.

- Considered to be an effective combination of coldness and vibration.

Insulin Syringe

- Insulin syringe with its miniature needle, bright color, and slim look appears like a toy to the child patient.
- The use of insulin syringe for injecting LA solution helps in curtailment of dental appointments in child patients as less time is required for convincing them to receive the injection and gaining their confidence as the syringe looks less menacing.
- Calibrations in insulin syringe are marked at 0.025 mL intervals and so that there is controlled and fractionated administration of drug not requiring excessive force on the plunger.

COMPLICATIONS OF LOCAL ANESTHESIA

- **Local:** Complications occurring locally in the region of injection.
- **Systemic:** Complications which are impact on the general bodily health.
- **Primary:** Complications caused and manifested at the time of anesthesia.
- **Secondary:** Complications manifested later, even though caused at the time of insertion of needle and injection.
- **Mild:** Only slight changes produced which reverse without specific treatment.
- **Severe:** Pronounced deviation from normally expected pattern and requires definite plan of treatment.
- **Transient:** Complications may be severe but leaves no residual effect.
- **Permanent:** Complications may be mild but leave a residual effect.

Complications that are attributed to solution or insertion of needle

Solution	*Insertion of needle*
• Toxicity • Idiosyncrasy • Systemic drug reactions • Allergy and anaphylactoid reactions • Infection caused by contaminated solution • Local irritation/tissue reaction	• Syncope • Muscle trismus • Pain/hyperalgesia • Edema • Infection • Broken needle • Hematoma and sloughing of tissues • Facial nerve paralysis • Burning on injection

Research regarding pain control

- **Yoshikawa et al.**[1] (2003) found no significant pain reduction when VibraJect was applied with a conventional dental syringe.
- **Saijo et al.**[2] (2005) evaluated the effectiveness of VibraJect in combination with an electrical injection device. They found no statistically significant decrease in pain scores at needle insertion or anesthetic injection.
- **Nanitsos et al.**[3] (2009) recommended the use of VibraJect for painless injection.
- **Dabarakis NN et al.**[4] reported that 17.6% (patients) experienced pain during injection of the anesthetic, and 32.3% reported feeling dread or fear from the explosion of the injector as it released the anesthetic.
- **Nusstein et al.**[5] (1998) found supplemental mandibular IO injection using the Stabident system and 1.8 mL of 2% lidocaine with 1:100,000 epinephrine was 88% successful in gaining total pulpal anesthesia for posterior teeth diagnosed with irreversible pulpitis.
- **Remmers et al.**[6] (2008) reported that the IntraFlow system as a primary technique that provide reliable anesthesia of posterior mandibular teeth in 13 of 15 subjects, compared to 9 of 15 with an inferior alveolar nerve block.
- **Ghasemi et al.**[7] (2014) concluded a significant difference concerning pain when 27 and 30 gauge needles were used to give inferior alveolar nerve block in children.
- **Asokan et al.**[8] (2014) concluded that pain due to injection penetration may be controlled using thinner gauge needles.
- **Baxter et al.**[9] (2011) concluded that external cold and vibration stimulation via Buzzy® have been shown to be a quick-acting option for pain reduction.

POINTS TO REMEMBER

- Local anesthesia is defined as a loss of sensation in a circumscribed area of the body caused by a depression of excitation in nerve endings or an inhibition of the conduction process in peripheral nerves.
- Composition of LA agent: Lignocaine, vasoconstrictor: adrenaline, reducing agents: sodium metabisulfite, preservative: Caprylhydroxamic acid toxin, fungicide: thymol, and vehicle: modified Ringer's solution.
- Maxillary injection techniques are anterior, middle superior alveolar and infraorbital nerve block, posterior superior alveolar nerve block, nasopalatine nerve block, greater palatine nerve block, and maxillary nerve block.
- Mandibular injection techniques are inferior alveolar nerve block, buccinator nerve block, mental nerve block, incisive nerve block, and mandibular nerve block.
- Posterior superior alveolar nerve block anesthetizes maxillary molars with the exception of mesiobuccal root of first molar, buccal alveolar processes of the maxillary molar.
- Nasopalatine nerve block anesthetizes anterior portion of the hard palate and overlying structures back to the bicuspid. Greater palatine nerve block anesthetizes posterior portion of the hard palate and overlying structures up to the first bicuspid area on the side injected.
- Inferior alveolar nerve block anesthetizes mandibular teeth to midline, body of mandible, inferior portion of ramus, mucous membrane, buccal periosteum anterior to first molar, anterior two-thirds of tongue, floor of mouth, and lingual soft tissues.
- Infiltration anesthesia acts on large terminal branches of dental plexus and the area of insertion is height of the mucobuccal fold above the apex of the tooth to be anesthetized.
- Wand system is computer controlled local anesthetic delivery system.
- Complications due to solution are toxicity, idiosyncrasy, systemic drug reactions, allergy and anaphylactoid reactions, and local irritation/ tissue reaction.
- Complications due to insertion of needle are syncope, muscle trismus, infection, broken needle, nerve paralysis, and burning sensation.

Questionnaire

1. Define and classify local anesthetics.
2. What are the ideal requirements of local anesthetic (LA) solution?
3. What is the mechanism of action of local anesthesia?
4. Write a short note on lignocaine.
5. Explain anterior, middle, and posterior superior alveolar nerve blocks.
6. Write a note on infiltration anesthesia.
7. Describe in details the indications, area of activity, and technique of injection of inferior alveolar nerve block in children.
8. What are the recent modifications in the field of local anesthesia?
9. What is Wand?

REFERENCES

1. Yoshikawa F, Ushito D, Ohe D, et al. Vibrating dental local anesthesia attachment to reduce injection pain. J Japanese Dent Soc Anesthesiol. 2003; 31:194-5.
2. Saijo M, Ito E, Ichinohe T, et al. Lack of pain reduction by a vibrating local anesthetic attachment: a pilot study. Anesth Prog. 2005; 52:62-4.
3. Nanitsos E, Vartuli A, Forte A, et al. The effect of vibration on pain during local anesthesia injections. Aust Dent J. 2009; 54:94-100.
4. Dabarakis NN, Alexander V, Tsirlis AT, et al. Needle-less local anesthesia: clinical evaluation of the effectiveness of the jet anesthesia Injex in local anesthesia in dentistry. Quintessence Int. 2007;38: E572-6.
5. Nusstein J, Reader A, Nist R, et al. Anesthetic efficacy of the supplemental intraosseous injection of 2% lidocaine with 1:100,000 epinephrine in irreversible pulpitis. J Endod. 1998; 24:487-91.
6. Remmers T, Glickman G, Spears R, et al. The efficacy of IntraFlow intraosseous injection as a primary anesthesia technique. J Endod. 2008; 34:280-3.
7. Ghasemi D, Rajaei S, Aghasizadeh E. Comparison of inferior dental nerve block injections in child patients using 30-gauge and 27-gauge short needles. J Dent Mater Tech. 2014; 3:71-6.
8. Asokan A. A pain perception comparison of intraoral dental anesthesia with 26 and 30 gauge needles in 6-12 year old children. J Pediatr Dent. 2014; 2:56-60.
9. Baxter AL, Leong T, Matthew B. External thermomechanical stimulation versus vapocoolant for adult venipuncture pain: Pilot data on a novel device. Clin J Pain. 2009; 25:705-710.

FURTHER READING

1. Al-Melh MA, Andersson L. Comparison of topical anesthetics (EMLA/Oraqix vs. benzocaine) on pain experienced during palatal needle injection. Oral Surg Oral Med Oral Pathol Oral Radiol Endod. 2007;103(5):e16-20.
2. Bhardwaj I, Sharma M. Herbal anesthetic agents: An overview on sources, uses and future perspectives. Asian Journal of Pharmacy and Pharmacology. 2019;5(S1):21-7.
3. Chandrasekaran J, Prabu D, Silviya M, et al. Efficacy of painless injection technique – Vibraject – A clinical trial in Chennai, India. IJMDS. 2014; 3:250-6.
4. Clark TM, Yagiela JA. Advanced techniques and armamentarium for dental local anesthesia. Dent Clin North Am. 2010; 54:757-68.
5. Daubl M, Miller R, Lipp M. The incidence of complications associated with local anesthesia in dentistry. Anesth Prog. 1997; 44:132-41.
6. Donald MJ, Derbyshire S. Lignocaine toxicity: a complication of local anaesthesia administered in the community. Emerg Med J. 2004; 21:249-50.
7. Ferrari M, Cagidiaco MC, Vichi A, et al. Efficacy of the Computer-Controlled Injection System STATM, Ligmaject, and the dental syringe for intraligamentary anesthesia in restorative patients. Int Dentistry. 2008;11:4-12.
8. Inal S, Kelleci M. Relief of pain during blood specimen collection in pediatric patients. Lippincott: Williams and Wilkins; 2012. pp. 339-45.
9. Kaban L, Troulis M. Preoperative assessment of the pediatric patient. In: Kaban L (Ed). Pediatric Oral and Maxillofacial Surgery. Philadelphia: Saunders; 2004.
10. Malamed SF Handbook of Local Anesthesia, 5th edition. DDS(Ed); 2004.
11. Ogle OE, Mahjoubi G. Advances in local anesthesia in dentistry. Dent Clin North Am. 2011; 55:481-99.
12. Tirupathi S, Rajasekhar S. Topical Anesthesia in Pediatric Dentistry: An Update. Dent. 2022;15(2):240-5.
13. Tirupathi SP, Nanda N, Pallepagu S, Malothu S, Rathi N, Chauhan RS, et al. The combined effect of extraoral vibratory stimulus and external cooling on pain perception during intra-oral local anesthesia administration in children: a systematic review and meta-analysis. J Dent Anesth Pain Med. 2022;22(2):87-96.
14. Tirupathi SP, Rajasekhar S. Effect of precooling on pain during local anesthesia administration in children: a systematic review. J Dent Anesth Pain Med. 2020;20(3):119-27.
15. Tirupathi SP, Rajasekhar S. The effect of vibratory stimulus on pain perception during intraoral local anesthesia administration in children: a systematic review and meta-analysis. J Dent Anesth Pain Med. 2020;20(6):357-65.
16. Tsuchiya H. Anesthetic Agents of Plant Origin: A Review of Phytochemicals with Anesthetic Activity. Molecules. 2017;22(8):1369.

CHAPTER

Pediatric Exodontia

Nikhil Marwah, Neha Bhargava

CHAPTER OUTLINE

The horrifying experience associated with the tooth extraction in the past is still to overcome by the layman. Even today the removal of a tooth is still dreaded by the patient almost more than any other surgical procedure. Many patients have extraction phobia, despite modern methods of anesthesia. Today dentists often consider tooth extraction a minor and unimportant procedure and without proper training, attempt difficult cases, and land up in a mess. Before undertaking the extraction of a tooth, one should thoroughly evaluate the care involved. Further, consideration should be given to type of anesthesia used and a good radiograph should be secured to rule out any abnormalities that may make extraction difficult. So, in this way we can avoid the hasty use of forceps and the type of procedure can be selected that is most likely to yield the best results.

The ideal tooth extraction *is the procedure of painless removal of whole tooth, or root with minimum trauma to soft tissue and hard tissue so that the wound heals uneventfully and with no postoperative problem.*

INDICATIONS FOR EXTRACTION OF TEETH

The value of a tooth should not be underestimated as they are important not only from an esthetic point of view but also help in proper digestion of food. There are many reasons why both deciduous and permanent teeth have to be extracted. Sometimes, normal teeth occasionally must be sacrificed to improve mastication and prevent malocclusion. In most of the instances, teeth are extracted because they are affected by disease or can cause ill health due to spread of the infection. Following are the main indications:

- Teeth affected by advanced caries and its sequelae
- Teeth affected by periodontal disease
- Extraction of healthy teeth to correct malocclusion
- Over-retained teeth
- Trauma to the teeth or jaws may cause dislocation of a tooth from its socket (avulsion)
- Extraction of teeth for esthetic reasons
- Extraction of teeth for prosthodontic reasons
- Impacted and supernumerary teeth
- Extraction of decayed first or second molars to prevent impaction of third molars
- Teeth involved in fracture line
- Teeth involved in tumors or cysts
- Tooth as foci of infection
- Teeth affected by crown, abrasion, attrition, or hypoplasia
- Teeth affected by pulpal lesions, e.g., pulpitis, pink spot, or pulp polyp
- Teeth in the area of direct therapeutic irradiation.

CONTRAINDICATIONS FOR EXTRACTION

It is necessary for the well-being of the patient to delay extraction until certain local or systemic conditions can be corrected or modified. Analgesics and antibiotics can be used to keep the patient comfortable. It is sometimes best to treat the infection first and extract the tooth when the acute symptoms subside. There are few absolute contraindications to the removal of teeth when it is necessary for the well-being of the patient:

- Presence of acute oral infections such as necrotizing ulcerative gingivitis or herpetic gingival stomatitis.

- Pericoronitis (difficult surgical procedure involving bone removal is anticipated).
- Extraction of teeth in previously irradiated areas (at least 1 year should be allowed for maximal recovery of circulation to the bone).
- There are number of relative systemic contraindications to the tooth extraction, e.g.
  - Uncontrolled diabetes
  - Acute blood dyscrasias
  - Untreated coagulopathies
  - Adrenal insufficiency
  - General debilitation for any reason
  - Myocardial infarction (wait for 6 months period).

PREPARATION FOR EXTRACTION

Preoperative Assessment

- A history of general disease, nervousness, or previous difficulty with extractions, will govern both the choice of anesthesia and procedure of tooth extraction.
- The general cleanliness of the patient's mouth and oral hygiene are observed.
- Pre-extraction scaling should be performed, especially in neglected mouths, at least 1 week prior to surgery.
- Sick or fatigued should rest before operative procedures.
- Highly apprehensive patient should receive some form of sedation before the operation.
- Patient undergoing general anesthesia should be instructed to omit the previous meal and to take nothing by mouth for at least 6 hours before extraction.
- Patient with inflamed or infected gingival should use an antiseptic mouth rinse before the extraction.
- Removable prostheses must be taken out of the patient's mouth.
- The administration of antibiotics is recommended as a prophylactic measure in all medical compromised patients.

Pre-extraction Radiograph

The purpose of pre-extraction radiograph is to show the whole root structure and the alveolar bone investing the tooth with IOPA, lateral oblique view, OPG. The following are the main indications for preoperative radiographs:

- History of difficult or attempted extractions
- A tooth which is resistant to forceps extraction
- If a tooth is to be removed by dissection
- Close relationship of tooth or root with:
  - Maxillary sinus
  - Inferior alveolar canal
  - Mental nerves.
- All mandibular and maxillary third molars, in standing premolars, or misplaced canines
- Pulpless teeth with resorbed roots
- Teeth affected by periodontal disease
- Traumatic teeth
- An isolated tooth
- Any partially erupted or unerupted tooth or retained root
- Retained deciduous tooth
- Submerged tooth
- Conditions which predisposes to dental or alveolar abnormality, e.g.
  - *Cleidocranial dysostosis*: For pseudoanodontia
  - *Osteitis deformans*: For hypercementosed root
  - Patient with therapeutic irradiation
  - Osteopetrosis.

Choice of Anesthesia

- Teeth may be extracted under either local anesthesia or general anesthesia and one should assess the indication and contraindications of both before deciding which to use in a particular case. Most extraction of tooth can be done with local anesthesia alone.
- To decrease the nervousness, relieve tension, and control psychic behavior, sedation can be used in conjunction with the local anesthesia. In young children, general anesthesia rather than local anesthesia may be indicated to facilitate patient management.
- All patients with general anesthesia or local anesthesia should be observed in a recovery area until they are able to go home unaided or should be accompanied by adult and not permitted to drive.

PRINCIPLE OF EXTRACTION

In routine practice, the following three time mechanical principles of extraction should be followed for the well-being of the patients by doing atraumatic extraction.

Expansion of the Socket

The extraction of a tooth requires the separation of its attachment to the alveolar bone via the crestal and principal fibers of the periodontal ligament (PDL) injection which involves a process of expansion of alveolar socket. This is achieved by using the tooth as the dilating instrument with the help of forceps, to permit the removal of the tooth.

Use of a Lever and Fulcrum

This basic principle is used with elevators that force a tooth or root out of the socket along the path of least resistance.

The Insertion of a Wedge

This is done between the tooth root surface and the bony socket wall to help the tooth to rise in its socket.

EXODONTIA TECHNIQUES

The following techniques may be used for tooth removal:

- **The forceps technique**: Closed method
- **The elevator technique**: Open method
- **Transalveolar technique**: Open method
- Odontotomy.

Forceps Technique

It is the most commonly used method for the extraction of teeth. But, it should not be used in difficult cases, e.g., tooth with hypercementoid root or tooth with deformity of the roots.

This forceps technique gives least amount of trauma to soft tissues and hard tissue of judiciously used. In multiple extractions, the marginal gingival may have to be reflected to permit rounding and smoothing of the sharp prominences of the alveolar process. Care should be taken to preserve the height and breadth of the ridge for stability of a future denture. Proper use of this technique involves the application of several basic principles.

- The beaks of the selected forceps **(Figs. 62.1 and 62.2)** should be sealed as far apically as possible without compression of the soft tissues after reflecting the cervical gingival.
- The placement of the beaks of the forceps should be as parallel as possible to the long axis of the tooth.
- The application of excessive force should be avoided so that the fracture of the alveolar process or tooth itself does not occur.

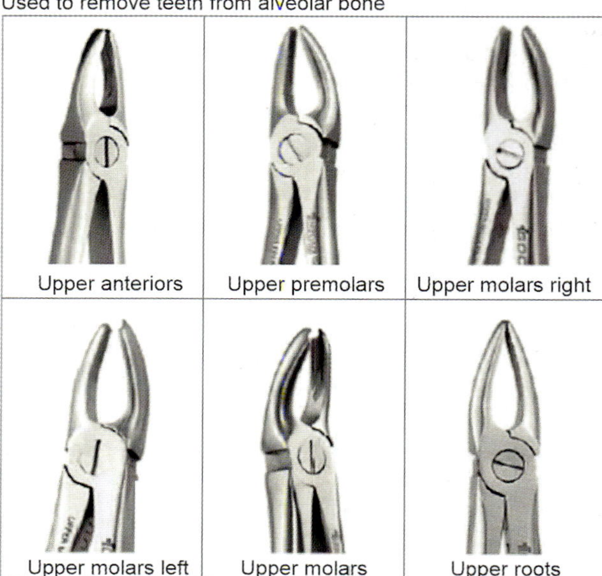

Fig. 62.1: Maxillary extraction forceps.

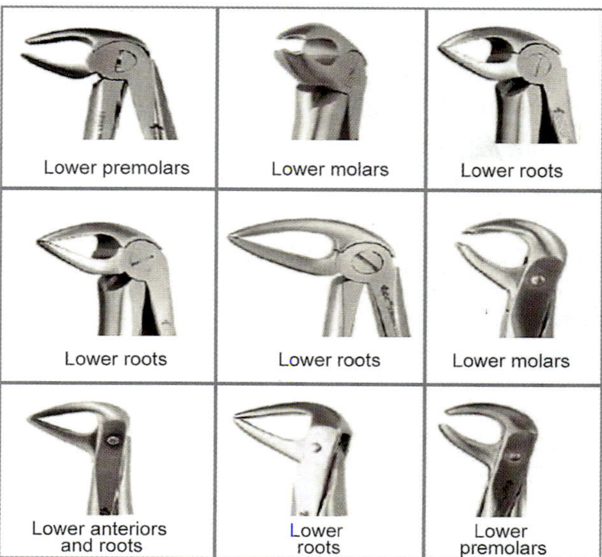

Fig. 62.2: Mandibular extraction forceps.

Elevator Technique

This technique is used in two ways:

1. **Elevator as a lever:** In this case, the alveolar crest serves as the fulcrum. The area of the compressed bone should be removed with a file or rongeur to reduce the postoperative pain and infection. With elevators **(Figs. 62.3A to D)**, one should avoid traumatizing the gingival and loosening of adjacent teeth. This method is used for the removal of whole or nearly whole roots.

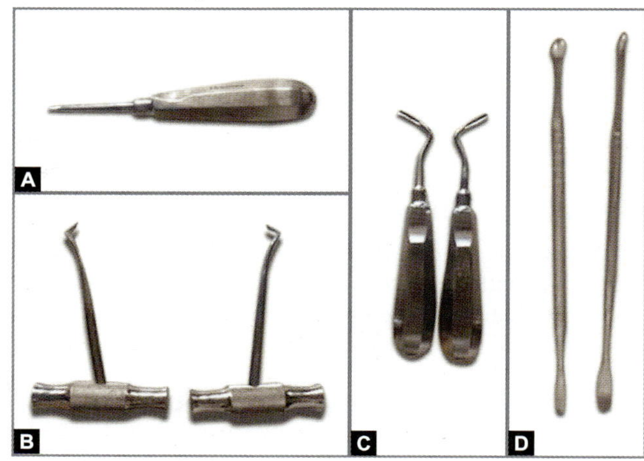

Figs. 62.3A to D: Elevators for tooth extraction: (A) Straight; (B) Cryers; (C) Millers; (D) Periosteal.

2. **Elevator as a wedge:** This principle is used for the removal of small root tips by way of displacement. If the root tip cannot be dislodged from the socket easily, an open view method should be used.

Transalveolar Method (Open View Technique)

This method is used where roots are inaccessible to routine removal by forceps or by an elevator, when they cannot be luxated with simple forces, or when the roots are covered by bone. This method is far less traumatic than when there is prolonged use of forceps or elevator attempted root removal.

Odontotomy

In this method, the extraction procedure may be simplified by cutting a tooth apart, e.g., in multirooted deciduous or permanent teeth with divergent roots, where crown is decayed.

PROCEDURE FOR EXTRACTION

Instrumentation and Positioning

- Instruments are selected and arranged according to the need and according to the surgeon's preference.
- **Position of the operator:**
  - When extracting any tooth except the right mandibular quadrant the operator stands on the right hand side of the patient.
  - For the removal of the teeth in right mandibular quadrant, the operator stands behind the patient.
  - For maxillary teeth, the chair should be adjusted so that the site of operation is about 8 cm below the shoulder level of the operator.

- During the extraction of mandibular tooth the chair height should be about 16 cm below the level of the operator's elbow.
- When the operator is standing behind the patient the chair should be adjusted to enable him to have a clear view of the field of extraction.

❖ All these aspects combined with good illumination of the operative field are an essential condition for the successful extraction of the teeth.

Technique

Administer local anesthesia

↓

Before attempts are made to extract a tooth the gingival tissue at the cervical region should be detached with the help of Moon's probe

↓

After this, insert the beaks of the forceps under the gingival as far on the outer and inner aspects of the tooth as possible

↓

The forceps are carefully adapted and the root is grasped firmly with the beaks parallel to the long axis of the tooth

↓

For maxillary teeth extraction, one hand is used to reflect the cheeks or lip and stabilize the patient's head in the head rest

↓

For mandibular teeth, one hand supports the mandible and retracts the cheek or lip

↓

To extract any tooth, the handles of the forceps are grasped with enough force to hold the tooth firming but not to crush it

↓

Then the tooth is rotated or carefully socked, depending upon its shape and until PDL attachment is broken and the socket is dilated and tooth is taken out of the socket

EXTRACTION OF MAXILLARY TEETH (FIGS. 62.4 TO 62.6)

❖ **Central incisors:** These often have a conical root and rarely deformed or curved. They are grasped with straight wide beaked forceps and can be safely rotated first in one direction and then in the other direction until PDL attachment is broken and it can be taken out with slight tractions.

❖ **Lateral incisors:** They have slender roots which are often flattened on the mesial and distal surfaces. A fine bladed forceps is used for the extraction of lateral incisors.

❖ **Canines:** These can be the most difficult upper teeth to remove because of the length and frequent apical curvature of their roots. Since great force is needed to dislodge these teeth, partial or total fracture of the labial wall of the alveolus is common. Forceps are placed as high as possible under the gingival margin, and the tooth is then rotated back and forth while upward pressure is maintained and traction is applied for its removal.

❖ **First premolar:** It has two fine roots which may be both curved and divergent and fracture occurs readily during extraction. Buccopalatal rocking with upper universal forceps or bayonet forceps is used to locate the tooth and tooth should be removed in the direction of least resistance.

❖ **Second premolar:** These are much easier to extract than the first premolars because they have only one root. Careful rotary motion with rocking to the buccal sides with gradual fraction will usually deliver the tooth.

❖ **First molar:** It usually has three divergent roots, strongest, and longest of which is the palatal root. The buccal roots are often curved distally. For the safe extraction of first molar, careful rocking of the tooth buccally with upper universal or bayonet forceps is used to loosen the palatal root, and buccopalatal traction aids in complete luxation of the tooth which is removed without rotation.

❖ **Second molars:** It can be removed by a technique similar to that used for first molar extraction. Buccopalatal rocking and traction may be used and even moderate torsion is permissible to detach and remove the tooth.

❖ **Third molars:** Third molars may be removed with the same forceps that are used for first and second molars. The long axis of the maxillary third molar is such that its crown is usually more posteriorly placed than its roots. As a rule, teeth that are buccally inclined can be removed easily, those distally inclined may fracture. No attempt should be made to apply forceps to either a semierupted maxillary third molar unless both buccal and lingual surfaces are visible. If more pressure is applied in an upward direction, the tooth or root may be displaced into the maxillary antrum.

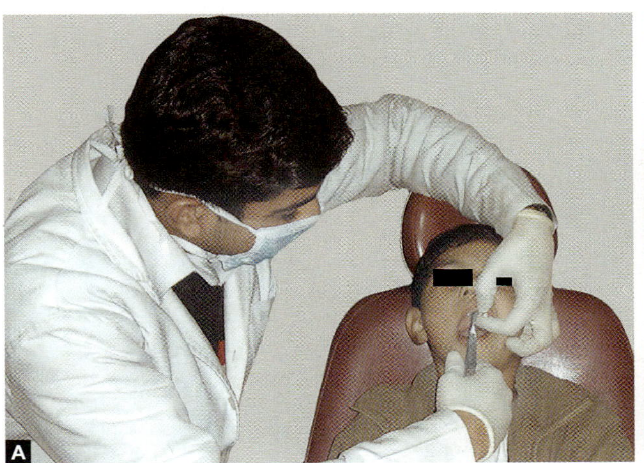

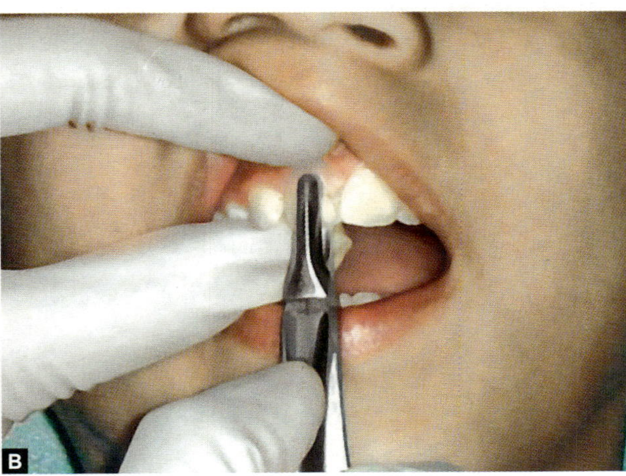

Figs. 62.4A and B: (A) Position of right handed dentist for performing extraction of teeth in maxillary anterior segment; (B) Position of forceps for maxillary anterior segment.

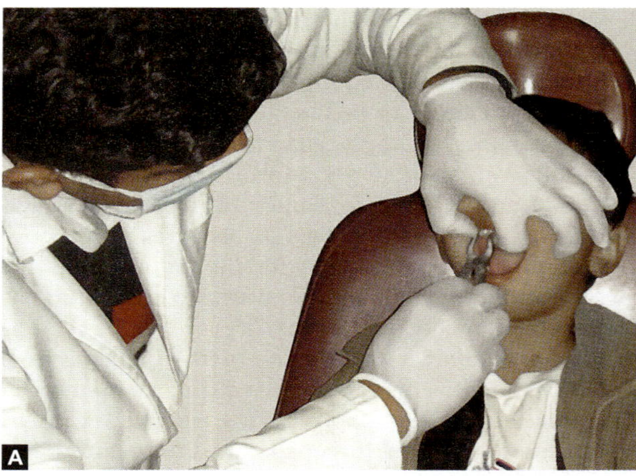
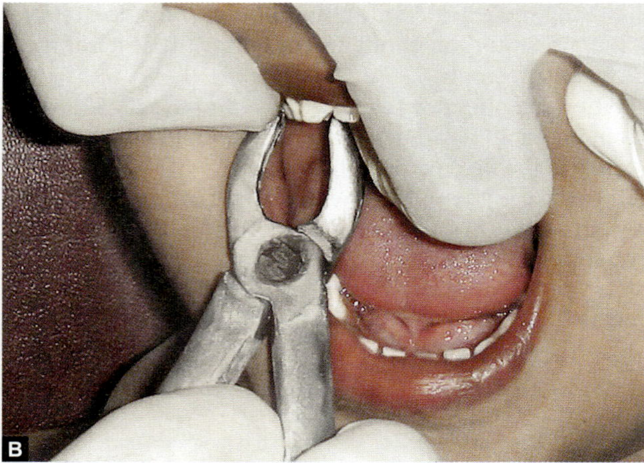

Figs. 62.5A and B: (A) Position of right handed dentist for performing extraction of teeth in maxillary first quadrant; (B) Position of forceps for maxillary first quadrant.

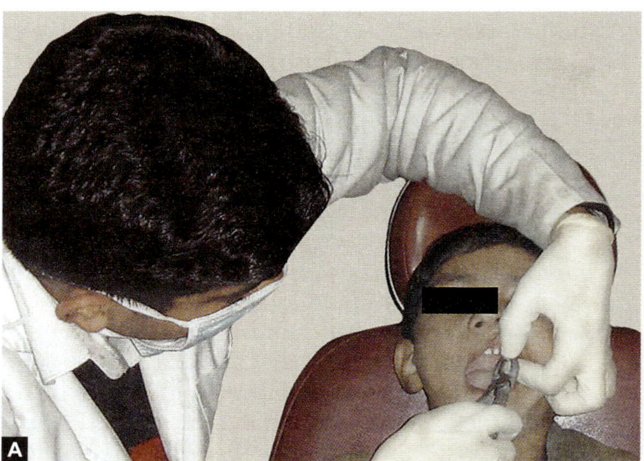
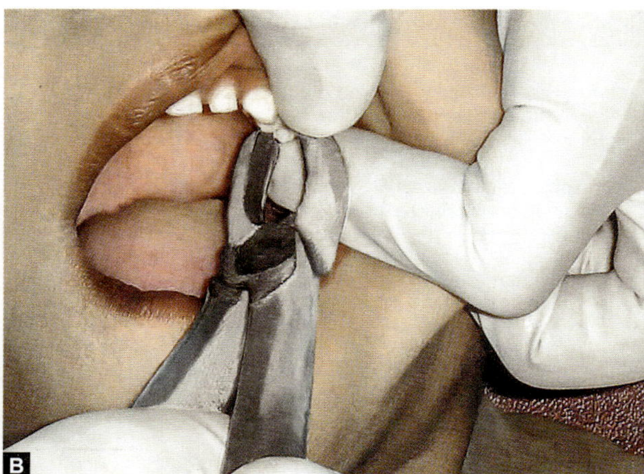

Figs. 62.6A and B: (A) Position of right handed dentist for performing extraction of teeth in maxillary second quadrant; (B) Position of forceps for maxillary second quadrant.

EXTRACTION OF MANDIBULAR TEETH (FIGS. 62.7 TO 62.9)

- **Incisors:** Lower incisors have fine roots with flattened sides. The supporting alveolar process is very thin, and it is easy to luxate the tooth when it is rocked labially. Fine bladed forceps should be used to grasp them, e.g., lower universal.
- **Canines:** It is long and bulky, firmly embedded, and difficult to extract the apex is often inclined distally. A heavier bladed forceps should be used and movement in a buccolingual direction is applied for extraction of this tooth.
- **Premolars:** They have tapering roots and their apices may be distally inclined and surrounded by thick compact bone.

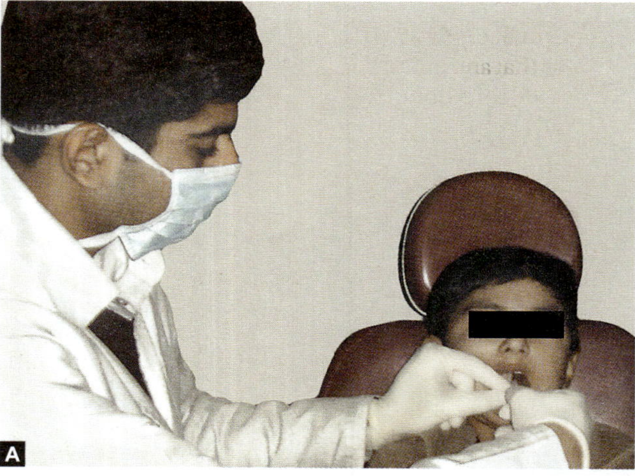
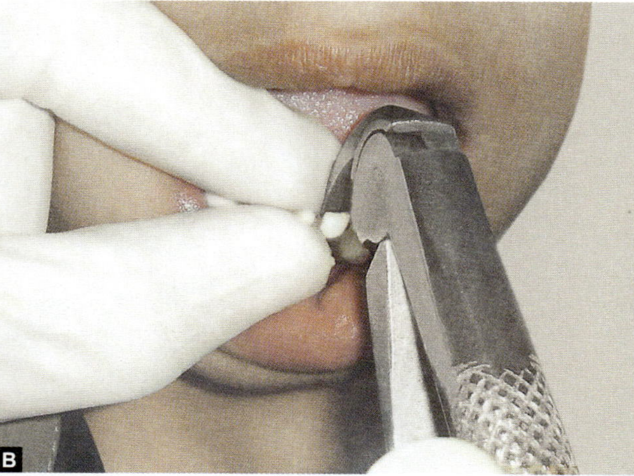

Figs. 62.7A and B: (A) Position of right handed dentist for performing extraction of teeth in mandibular anterior region; (B) Position of forceps in mandibular anterior region.

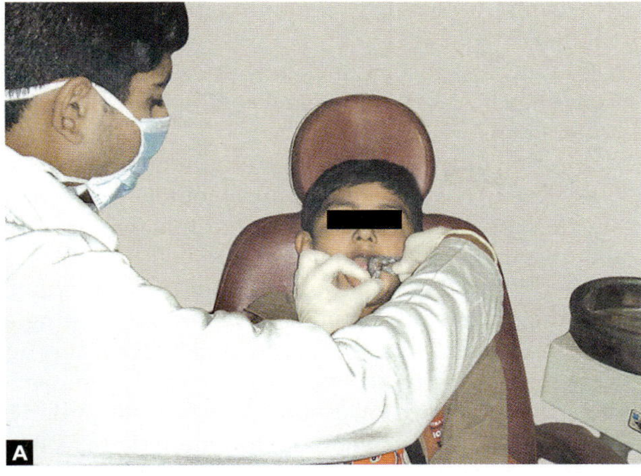
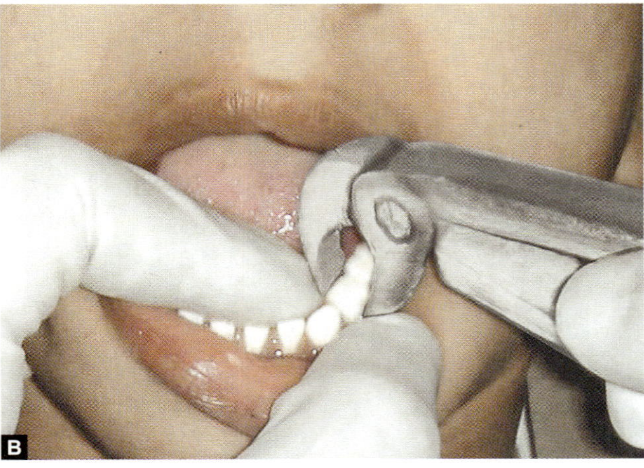

Figs. 62.8A and B: (A) Position of right handed dentist for performing extraction of teeth in mandibular third quadrant; (B) Position of forceps in mandibular third quadrant.

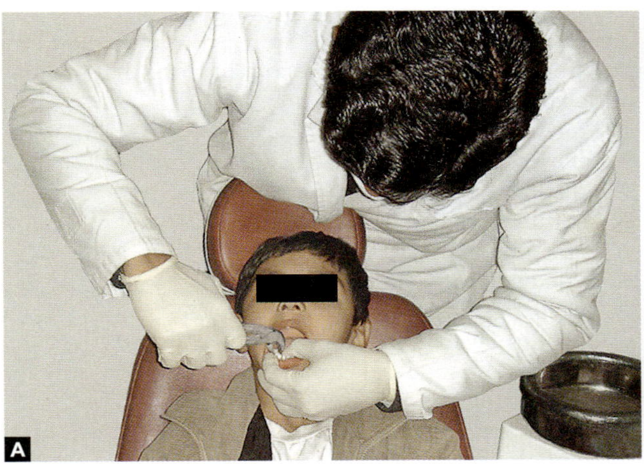
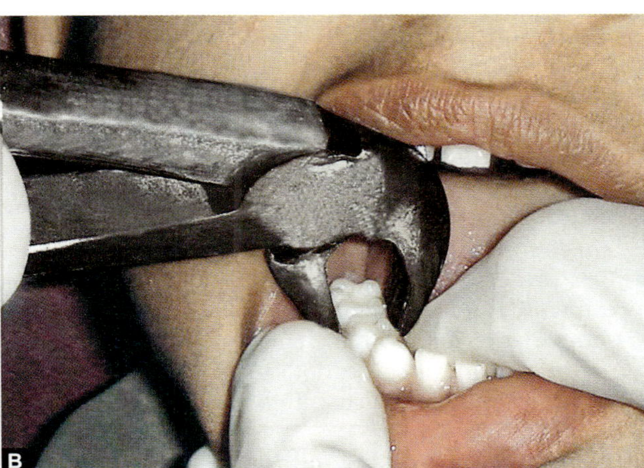

Figs. 62.9A and B: (A) Position of right handed dentist for performing extraction of teeth in mandibular fourth quadrant; (B) Position of forceps in mandibular fourth quadrant.

A forceps with blades fine enough to give "two-point contact" on the root should be applied to the tooth. The first movement should be firm but gentle and torsion may be employed freely, combined with buccolingual rocking as in the case of canines.

- **Lower molars:** These molars are best extracted with full molar forceps and often loosened by buccolingual pressure and are best delivered by secondary rotation. The extraction of second and third molars can often be facilitated by the mesial application of an elevator before the application of forceps if not malposed, impacted or unerupted, the mandibular third molars can be quite easily removed with the forceps technique.

EXTRACTION OF ROOTS

- **Roots may be extracted with forceps:** If they are not decayed. Bayonet or universal forceps are used for roots in the upper jaw and forceps such as those used for premolars are used in the mandible.
- If forceps cannot be applied directly to the roots, an elevator technique may be used.
- In open beak technique, alveolar bone rather than the root itself is grasped with the forceps and crushed bone should be carefully removed after removal of the root.
- Mandibular molar roots can be removed by placing a straight elevator or Cryer elevator between them and using the inter-radicular septum as a fulcrum to remove one root. If roots are attached, a bur is first used to separate them.
- Maxillary molar roots removed by simultaneously grasping the distobuccal and palatal roots with the forceps and mesiobuccal root can be removed separately with forceps or a small elevator.
- Roots that are under the gingival margin or roots completely embedded in bone are removed by the open view method of extraction.

EXTRACTION OF DECIDUOUS TEETH

- Before extraction of deciduous teeth, a thorough examination should be performed to minimize complications.
- As tooth crown and root structure differ from those of adult teeth, the use of specially designed pediatric instrument **(Fig. 62.10)** is recommended.
- The main consideration in the removal of deciduous teeth is to avoid injury to the developing permanent dentition.
- The most critical step in extraction of deciduous teeth is the administration of local anesthesia. If the child allows

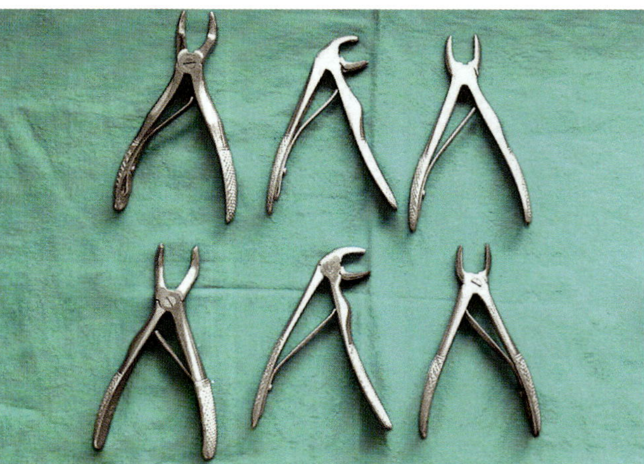

Fig. 62.10: Pediatric dental extraction forceps.

this step, then he will be definitely cooperative for the next step, the extraction. This is because most anxiety and fear is generated during this phase. Studies by most authors explain the rise of pulse rate and blood pressure during this time. So, it is critical to alleviate the fear of the child rather than increase it. It is most recommended to perform some behavior shaping of children prior to extraction and local anesthesia. Some methods are:

- ***The first step:*** This is to make the patient comfortable.
- It is imperative that we do not proceed with the extraction immediately. It is best if we first engage in some friendly talk with the child and explain him the merits of taking out his carious teeth in a language that he can comprehend according to the developmental status of the child.
- ***Tell-show-feel-do:*** This modification involves describing the procedure from the application of topical anesthetic to postoperative reward. The patient is then showed an empty syringe without needle and made to feel it to dispel any fears of injections that he may have. However, during the actual procedure it is best not to load anesthetic or bring the needle or syringe in front of child so as to avoid anxiety. It is best to cover the child's eye with one hand and perform the task with other.
- ***Use of euphemisms:*** Like comparing the pinch of needle to mosquito bite or comparing local anesthetic (LA) solution to water to flush out bacteria from teeth have proven to be useful.
- ***Audiovisual distraction:*** It is also a vital technique as it allows multisensory distraction.
- ***Use of bite blocks:*** These are recommended for difficult patients who have a tendency to close their mouth while the procedure as they are helpful in opening the mouth so as to avoid any injury during procedure.
- ***Modeling:*** This is especially useful in case of a close friend or a sibling who can be observed performing the desired behavior.
- ***Physical restraints:*** This is the last and least preferred option with the dentist and is used in highly uncooperative or special children.

- The technique of extraction is the same as that used in the removal of permanent teeth. But it is important to ensure before application of forceps that the blades are fine enough to pass down the periodontal membranes and applied to the roots.
- A firm lingual movement usually causes the tooth to rise in its socket and it can be delivered by moving buccally and rotated forward.
- The roots of the extracted deciduous teeth should be examined to ensure that they are complete. Fracture root surfaces are flat and shiny with sharp margins, resorbed roots are with irregular margins.
- In case of fracture of a root fragment the best option is to radiographically visualize it before attempting any kind of retrieval. In case it is located superficially away from underlying tooth bud it can be safely removed by reinstrumentation. However, if it is close to the underlying tooth bud it is advisable to let it remain there as it may undergo resorption or may appear with the erupting tooth.

OPERATIVE COMPLICATIONS

The most frequent operative complications that encounter during the extraction of teeth are:

- Fracture of the tooth
- Injuries to adjacent teeth
- Fracture of the alveolar bone
- Fracture of the tuberosity
- Extraction of the wrong tooth
- Root displaced in the sinus
- Maxillary sinus perforation
- Root displaced in the submandibular space
- Gingival and mucosal lacerations
- Injury to the inferior alveolar nerve
- Hemorrhage and hematoma
- Temporomandibular joint (TMJ) trauma
- Damage to permanent successor.

POSTOPERATIVE CARE

After care when the tooth has been extracted the socket should be inspected and any loose fragment of bone is removed or necessary socket irrigation is performed. The alveolar process then should be pressed together with the thumb and forefinger in order to reduce any distortion of the supporting tissues; suturing should always be done after multiple extractions and if the gingival flaps are loose enough to be approximated. After extraction, a gauze pack is placed over the socket and patient is directed to bite on the pack for 0.5 h, exerting firm even pressure. This will prevent bleeding while the patient returns home and it allows a blood clot to form. Some postoperative instructions are:

- The patient should be warned that sucking the wound, investigating the socket with tongue, and rinsing during the first day disturbs the blood clot and may cause dry socket.
- Patient should be directed to remain quiet for several hours, preferably sitting in a chair or if lying down, keeping the head elevated.
- Only liquids and soft solids should be advice on the first day. They may be warm or cold but not extremely hot.
- The teeth should be brushed as usual and on the day after surgery, rinsing of the mouth should begin. A warm saline solution is best for this purpose.

Additional advisory in case of children

- Parent is instructed to keep a check on the status of cotton so that the child does not swallow it inadvertently.
- Patient is instructed to keep the cotton for 30 minutes to 1 hour and avoid spitting out.
- It is best to give cold food stuff like ice cream to children to aid in clot formation.
- Explain the effect of anesthesia will keep the area numb for a specific time so as to avoid lip or cheek biting, especially in children.
- In case of pediatric exodontia it is best to allow the child to be seated in the dental chair for at least 10 min before discharging him so as to avoid any shock symptoms.
- Advise parents to keep children under close supervision that particular day and avoid sports of heavy nature.
- Parents should use alternate methods to distract the child so as to avoid his attention toward the wound.

- ❖ Some degree of postoperative pain accompanies many exodontia procedures and begins after the effects of the anesthetic have left. So, it is better to take some analgesic before the effect of anesthetic wears off.
- ❖ Prevention of swelling after extensive or difficult operation adds to the comfort of the patient. The degree of swelling that occurs postoperatively is generally in direct proportion to the degree of surgical trauma. The application of cold to the operated site is beneficial in reducing the amount of postoperative swelling. Pressure dressings are also beneficial in limiting the postoperative swelling.
- ❖ Smoking should be avoided after tooth extraction as it increases the incidence of alveolar osteitis and should be discontinued for 5 days.

POINTS TO REMEMBER

- The ideal tooth extraction is the procedure of painless removal of whole tooth, or root with minimum trauma to soft tissue and hard tissue so that the wound heals uneventfully and with no postoperative problem.
- Indications for extraction are teeth affected by advanced caries, periodontal disease, over-retained teeth, impacted and supernumerary teeth, teeth involved in tumors or cysts, teeth affected by pulpal lesions, and teeth in the area of direct therapeutic irradiation.
- Contraindications are presence of acute oral infections and systemic contraindications.
- Techniques used for tooth removal are forceps technique, elevator technique, transalveolar technique, and odontotomy.
- *Position of the operator*: When extracting any tooth except the right mandibular quadrant the operator stands on the right hand side of the patient. For the removal of the teeth in right mandibular quadrant, the operator stands behind the patient. For maxillary teeth, the chair should be adjusted so that the site of operation is about 8 cm below the shoulder level of the operator. During the extraction of mandibular tooth the chair height should be about 16 cm below the level of the operator's elbow.
- The most important behavior modification during extraction for pediatric patients are tell-show-feel-do, audiovisual distraction, and modeling.
- Operative complications during extraction of teeth are fracture of the tooth or bone, root displacement, sinus perforation, laceration, nerve injury, TMJ trauma, damage to succeeding tooth, and cheek biting.

Questionnaire

1. What are indications and contraindications for tooth extraction?
2. Describe the techniques of extraction.
3. Explain the principles of extraction.
4. What are the operating positions for extracting different teeth?
5. Write note on extraction of deciduous teeth.
6. Enumerate the postextraction instructions given to patient.
7. What are the complications associated with extraction in relation to children?

FURTHER READING

1. Berman SA. Basic principles of dentoalveolar surgery. In: Berman SA (Ed). Principles of Oral and Maxillofacial Surgery. Philadelphia: Saunders; 1992.
2. Blakey GH, Ruiz RL, Turvey TA. Oral trauma. In: Fonseca RJ, Walker RV (Eds). Oral and Maxillofacial Trauma. Philadelphia: Saunders; 1997. pp. 1003-41.
3. Byrd DL. Exodontia: modern concepts. Dent Clin North Am. 1971; 15:273-98.
4. Cerny R. Removing broken roots: a simple method. Aus Dent J. 1978; 23:357.
5. Kaban LB. Oral surgery. In: Kaban LB (Ed). Pediatric Oral and Maxillofacial Surgery. Philadelphia: Saunders; 1990. pp. 233-60.

CHAPTER

Traumatic Injuries to Anterior Teeth

Nikhil Marwah, Prabhadevi C Maganur, Bhavna Dave, Manojit Mahato

Chapter Outline

- Response of Oral Tissues to Trauma
- Etiology
- Mechanism of Dental Injuries
- Classification of Traumatic Injuries
- Examination and Diagnosis
- Management of Traumatic Injuries
- Reimplantation
- Storage Media for Avulsed Teeth
- Periodontal Healing Reactions
- Splinting
- Trauma to Primary Dentition
- Effect of Traumatic Injuries on Developing Dentition

Tooth trauma has been and continues to be the common occurrence that every dental professional must be prepared to assess and treat when necessary. It has no perspective method for occurring, possesses no significant predictable pattern of intensity or extensiveness and is occurring at times when dentists are least prepared or when the dental office is closed. The dynamic panorama of sporting activity worldwide and the significant increase in violence in our population, tooth trauma and its management loom as a major challenge to the dental practitioner.

RESPONSE OF ORAL TISSUES TO TRAUMA

An injury can be defined as an interruption in the continuity of tissues. The result of this process can either be tissue repair, where the continuity is restored but the healed tissue differs in anatomy and function or tissue regeneration, where both anatomy and function are restored. Dental tissues are unique in comparison to most other tissues in the body due to their ability to completely regenerate. Injury and its sequelae in some important structures of teeth are:

Dental Follicle

Traumatic injuries can be transmitted easily from the primary to permanent dentition. It has been shown in experiments that when parts of the dental follicle are removed an ankylosis is formed between the tooth surface and the crypt.

Cervical Loop

Cervical loop is highly resistant to trauma. Only profound contusion due to intrusion of primary incisor results in total arrest of odontogenesis.

Inner Enamel Epithelium

In case of total loss of ameloblasts in the secretory phase, no regenerative potential exists. In case of partial damage, enamel matrix formation and maturation may be affected. If there is total loss of the ameloblasts during the maturation stage hypomineralized enamel will develop.

Reduced Enamel Epithelium

Minor injury to the reduced enamel epithelium is repaired with a thin squamous epithelium whereas, larger area of destruction result in ankylosis and tooth retention.

Enamel and Enamel Matrix

Trauma to primary tooth may cause contusion of the permanent matrix. Ameloblasts will also be destroyed thereby arresting enamel maturation and resulting in a permanent hypomineralized enamel defect.

Hertwig's Epithelial Root Sheath

Chronic trauma to the Hertwig's epithelial root sheath (HERS), such as orthodontic intrusion of immature teeth often leads to fragmentation. An acute trauma to the epithelial root sheath transmitted indirectly for example by the intrusion of a primary tooth can damage HERS and lead to partial or complete arrest of root development.

Gingival and Periosteal Complex

The gingival attachments is often lacerated during luxation and displacement injuries. In injury to the underlying bone, firstly the cortical bone plate loses an important part of its vascular supply and secondly, the cellular cover of bone provided by the innermost layer of periosteum is partially or totally removed.

Periodontal Ligament: Cementum Complex

Following a severe dental injury, the periodontal ligament (PDL) must respond to a variety of insults, these include temporary compressive, tensile, or shearing stresses which result in hemorrhage, edema, rupture, or contusion of the PDL.

Dentin: Pulp Complex

Any deviation in the composition of the organic structure of dentin may lead to fracture. Thus patients suffering from dentinogenesis imperfecta have a high-risk of tooth fracture. Furthermore, the exposure of dentinal tubules during trauma leads to bacterial invasion with a resultant permanent or transitory inflammatory reaction in the pulp. Two basic responses determine pulpal wound healing response. General feature of the pulpal wound healing response is replacement of damaged tissue with newly formed pulpal tissue along the pulpodentinal border.

Incidence and prevalence of traumatic injuries

- Prevalence in primary dentition is 11–30% and permanent dentition is 5–29% **(Table 63.1)**
- For age groups less than or equal to 6 years, the prevalence of TDI is 15% and that of more than 6 years is 12%.[1]
- Boys show more frequency than girls in permanent teeth, no significant sex difference in primary teeth
- Peak incidence in boys is 2–4 years and 9–10 years and in girls is 2–3 years
- Facial injuries are more common in boys of 6–12 years of age, mandible is most affected
- Inadequate lip coverage or an overjet ranging between 3.5 and 5.5—more likely to have TDI[2]
- ***Teeth involved:***
  - 37% upper central incisor
  - 18% lower central incisor
  - 6% lower lateral incisor
  - 3% upper lateral incisor
- Most frequent injury in primary teeth is luxation and permanent teeth is uncomplicated crown fracture (**Figs. 63.2A to H**).

ETIOLOGY

Following factors can be attributed:

- Falls in infancy
- Child abuse—battered child syndrome
- Sports injuries
- Horse riding
- Automobile injury
- Assault torture
- Mental retardation and epilepsy
- Drug related injuries
- Developmental defects of enamel and dentin like dentinogenesis imperfecta.

MECHANISM OF DENTAL INJURIES

- **Direct trauma:** Occurs when tooth itself is struck, e.g., against table or chair.
- **Indirect trauma:** Seen when the lower dental arch is forcefully closed against upper, e.g., blow to chin. The extent of trauma can be assessed by four factors given by **Hallet** in 1954 **(Fig. 63.1)**.
  1. Energy of impact:
     - Energy = Mass × Velocity.
     - Hence, if the impacting object either has more mass or has high velocity, the impact will be more.
  2. Resilience of impacting object:
     - This can be either hard or soft.
     - More injury is bound to occur in the case of former and less in case of later.
  3. Shape of impacting object: The nature of wound depends on whether the object is sharp or blunt.
  4. Direction of impacting force: Type of fracture will directly depend on direction.

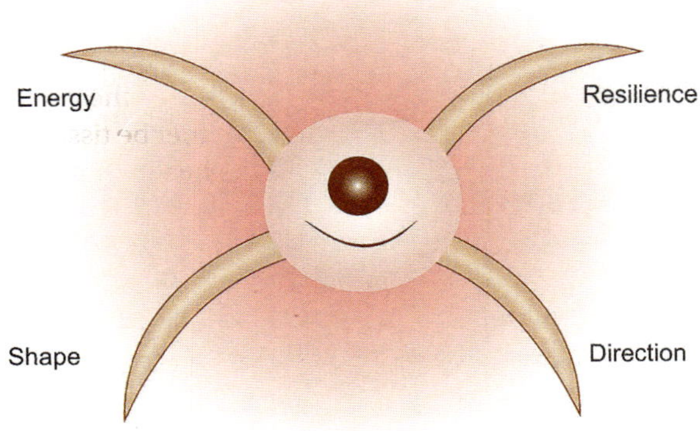

Fig. 63.1: Hallet's factors influencing trauma.

Table 63.1: Reported frequencies of traumatic dental injuries in various countries.

Examiner	Year	Country	Age groups	Sample size	No. with dental injuries	
					No.	%
Kessler	1922–37	Germany	—	40.203	1.857	4.6
Marcus	1951	USA	8–17	150	25	16.0
Kessler	1951–58	Germany	6–14 10–18	20.000	—	7–9.8 13.8
Grundy	1959	England	5–15	625	37	5.9
Ellis	1960	Canada	—	4.251	178	4.2
McEwen et al.	1967	England	13	2.905	239	8.2
Wallentin	1967	Germany	—	11.966	893	7.5
Beck	1968	New Zealand	15–21	2.145	201	9.4
Büttner	1968	Switzerland	—	1.000	81	8.1
Akpata	1969	Nigeria	6–25	2.819	410	14.5
Hargreaves and Craig	1970	England	4–18	17.831		5.9
Land et al.	1970	Sweden	0–7	702	88	12.5
Schützmannsky	1970	Germany	2–6 7–18	3.098 22.708	338 1.202	10.9 5.2
Gutz	1971	USA	6–13	1.166	236	20.2
O'Mullane	1972	Ireland	6–19	2.792	357	12.8
Andreasen and Ravn	1972	Denmark	3–7 7–16	487 487	147 109	30.2 22.3
Bergink	1972	Holland	11–16	943	142	15.1
Zadik et al.	1972	Israel	6–14	10.903	948	8.7
Clarkson et al.	1973	England	11–17 15–59	756 1.604	74 148	9.8 9.2
Holm and Arvidsson	1974	Sweden	3	208	50	24.0
Patkowska-Indyka and Plonka	1974	Poland	10–15	1.946	191	9.8
Ravn	1974	Denmark	14–15	75.000	9.665	12.9
Wieslander and Lind	1974	Sweden	6–16	2.065	180	8.7
Zadik	1976	Israel	6–14	965		11.1
York et al.	1978	New Zealand	11–13	430	72	16.7
Järvinen	1979	Finland	6–16	1.614	—	19.8
Sanchez et al.	1981	Dominican Republic	3–6	278	59	16.6
Baghadadi et al.	1981	Iraq	6–12	6.090	467	7.6
Baghadadi et al.	1981	Sudan	6–12	3.507	180	5.1
Garcia-Godoy et al.	1981	Dominican Republic	7–14	596	108	18.1
Garcia-Godoy et al.	1983	Dominican Republic	3–5	800	280	35.0
Garcia-Godoy	1984	Dominican Republic	5–14	1.633	81	10.0
Garcia-Godoy et al.	1985	Dominican Republic	6–17	1.200	146	12.2
Holland et al.	1988	Ireland	15	1.106	403	16.4
Uji and Teramoto	1988	Japan	6–18	15	822	21.8
Yagot et al.	1988	Iraq	1–4	2.389	584	24.4
Kaba and Marechaux	1989	Switzerland	6–18	262		10.8
Ravn	1989	Denmark	6	391	86	22.0
Hunter et al.	1990	UK	11–12	968		15.3
Forsberg and Tedestam	1990	Sweden	7–15	1.635	483	30.3
Sanchez and Garcia-Godoy	1990	Mexico	3–13	1.010	287	28.4
Bijella et al.	1990	Brazil	1–6	576	174	30.2

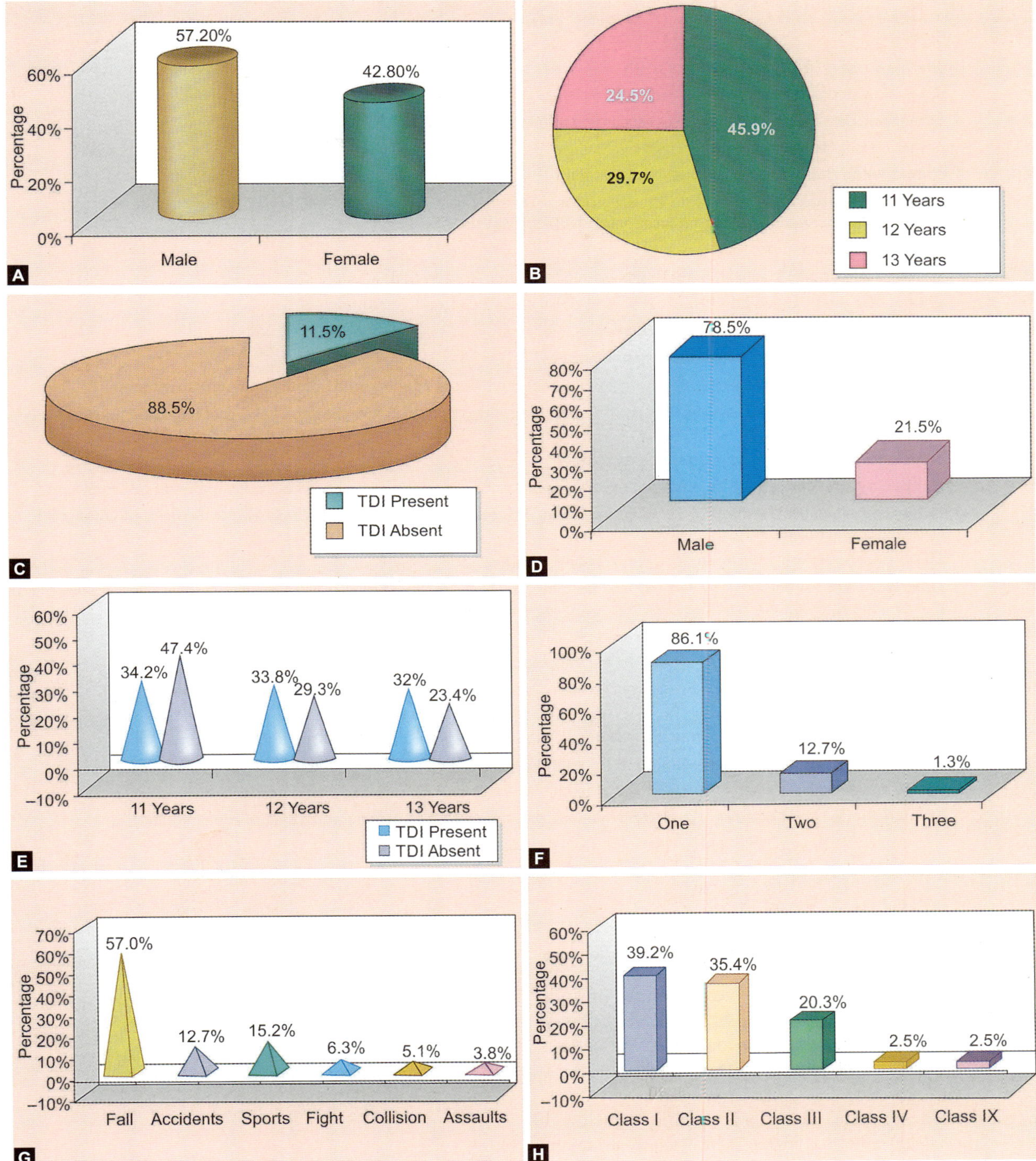

Figs. 63.2A to H: (A) Distribution of sample according to sex; (B) Distribution of sample according to age; (C) The prevalence of traumatic dental injury (TDI); (D) The prevalence of traumatic dental injury by gender; (E) The distribution of traumatic dental injury according to age; (F) Distribution according to the number of fractured teeth among children; (G) Distribution of patients according to cause of fracture; (H) Distribution of fractured teeth according to Ellis and Davey classification of injury.

Table 63.2: History of dental traumatic injuries.

Year	*Author*
1936	**Brauer** classified fractures of anterior teeth
1944	**Adams** divided traumatized young teeth into 6 classes
1946	**Hogeborn** classified fracture of incisors according to the degree of the break
1955	**Sweet** classified anterior teeth
1956	**Rabinowitch** classified injuries of the primary teeth
1961	**Ellis** classified anterior teeth fracture into six groups: (1) enamel fracture; (2) dentin fracture; (3) crown fracture with pulp exposure; (4) root fracture; (5) tooth luxation; and (6) tooth intrusion
1963	**Bennet** classified anterior teeth
1968	**Garcia-Godoy** gave classification for traumatic injuries to primary and permanent teeth
1970	**Ellis** and **Davey** modified **Ellis** classification and classified anterior teeth fracture
1970	**Hargreaves** and **Craig** modify **Ellis** and **Davey** classification
1978	**Silvestri** and **Singh** classified posterior teeth fractures
1978	WHO classified oral structures injuries using code numbers while considering both primary and permanent teeth
1981	**Andreasen** modified WHO classification by including terms uncomplicated complicated crown-root fracture and concussion/ subluxation/lateral luxation
1981	**Johnson** classified traumatic injuries to anterior teeth
1982	**Heithersay** and **Morile** gave classification of subgingival fracture in relation to various horizontal planes of periodontium
1982	**Pulver** combined the classifications of **Ellis** and **Davey**, **Andreasen**, **Hargreaves** and **Craig**, and **McDonald** and **Avery** and classified traumatized teeth
1983	**McDonald**, **Avery** and **Lynch** modified Ellis and Davey classification
1984	**Leubke** based on separation of fragments classified root fractures into two types, i.e., complete fracture and incomplete fracture or it can be supraosseous fractures and intraosseous fractures
1985	**Ulfohn** classified crown fractures into three simple classes
1986	**Dean et al** classified teeth fracture based on the orientation of the fracture plane to the long axis of the tooth
1992	Application of International Classification of Diseases of Dentistry and Stomatology (WHO) classified traumatic dental injuries and appointed codes
1995	**Feiglin** classified transverse root fracture into three zones
2001	Dentofacial injuries classification adopted by International Association of Dental Traumatology
2002	**Spinas** and **Altana** classified crown fractures of teeth
2007	**Berman**, **Blanco** and **Cohen** classified tooth injuries into crown fractures, root fractures and luxation injuries

CLASSIFICATION OF TRAUMATIC INJURIES

Although numerous classifications have been mentioned in literature about traumatic injury to anterior teeth **(Table 63.2)**, the focus will remain on some specific classifications which are explanatory and have stood the test of time.

Classification of Anterior Teeth Trauma by Sweets (1955)

- It is mainly based on the anatomy and morphology of the tooth structure
- The disadvantage of this classification is that no stress has been laid on injuries to supporting structures soft tissue and bone
- It indicates more towards the permanent teeth than primary teeth

Class I	A simple of crown exposing no dentition
Class II	A parallel of crown involving little dentin
Class III	Extensive fracture of crown involving more dentin, but no pulp exposure
Class IV	Extensive fracture of crown exposing pulp
Class V	Complete fracture of crown exposing pulp
Class VI	Fracture of root with or without loss of crown structure
Class VII	Tooth loss as a result of trauma

Ellis and Davey Classification (1960) (Figs. 63.3A to I)

Class I	Simple fracture of crown involving only enamel with little or no dentin
Class II	Extensive fracture of crown involving considerable dentin, but not exposing dental pulp
Class III	Extensive fracture of crown involving considerable dentin and exposing dental pulp
Class IV	The traumatized tooth that becomes nonvital with or without loss of crown structure
Class V	Total tooth loss—avulsion
Class VI	Fracture of the root with or without loss of crown structure
Class VII	Displacement of tooth with neither crown nor root fracture
Class VIII	Fracture of crown en masse and its displacement
Class IX	Traumatic injuries of primary teeth: According to Cohen—cracked tooth According to Mathewson—cyclic dislocation of tooth

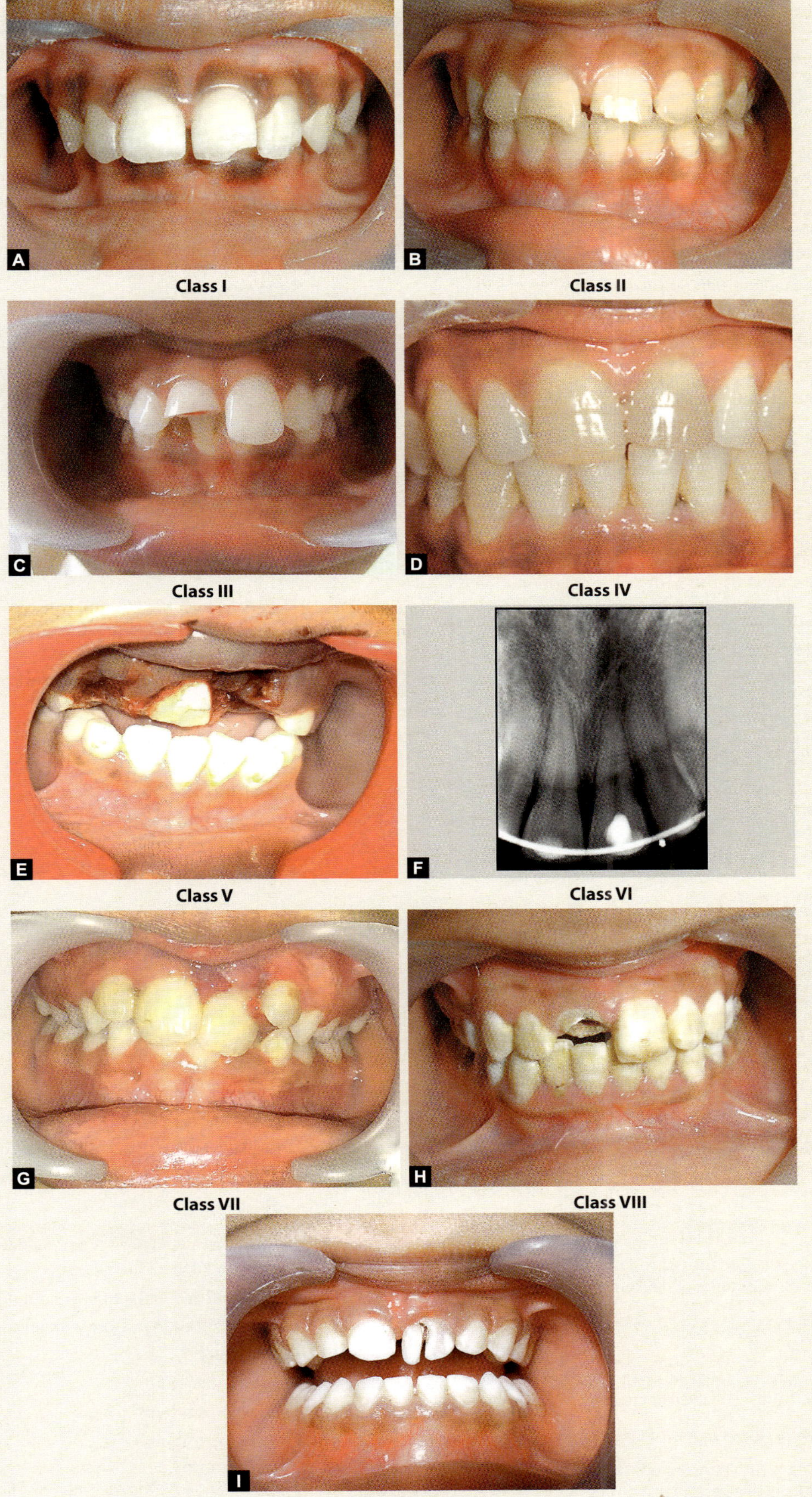

Figs. 63.3A to I: Ellis and Davey classification.

Bennett's Classification (1963)

Bennett's classification is according to injuries to periodontium and alveolus considering the anatomy and morphology of the teeth, which can be applied partially for primary and permanent teeth.

Class I Ia Ib	Traumatized tooth Tooth is firm in alveolus Tooth is subluxed in alveolus
Class II IIa IIb	Coronal fracture Fracture of enamel Fracture of enamel and dentin
Class III	Coronal fracture with pulp exposure
Class IV IVa IVb	Root fracture Without coronal fracture With coronal fracture
Class V	Avulsion of tooth

Zerman-Cavalleri G Classification (1995)

- Dental trauma was divided into the following categories based on the anatomic, morphological aspects and injuries to supporting tissue.
- It is indicated more towards the permanent dentition than the primary dentition.
  - Fracture of enamel, including enamel chipping
  - Fracture of enamel dentin without pulpal involvement
  - Fracture of enamel dentin with pulpal involvement
  - Fracture of root
  - Crown-root fracture without pulpal involvement
  - Crown-root fracture with pulpal involvement
  - Concussion
  - Subluxation
  - Intrusive luxation
  - Extrusive luxation
  - Lateral luxation
  - Avulsion.

Modified Ellis's Classification [By McDonald, Avery and Lynch (1983)]

Class I	Simple fracture of crown, involving little or no dentin
Class II	Extensive fracture of the crown involving considerable dentin, but not the dental pulp
Class III	Extensive fracture of the crown involving considerable dentin and exposing the pulp
Class IV	Loss of the entire crown

Subgingival Fracture Classification (By Heithersay and Morile)

They classified subgingival fractures based on the level of tooth fracture in relation to various horizontal planes of periodontium.

Class I	Fracture line does not extend below the level of attached gingiva
Class II	Fracture line below the level of attached gingiva, but not below the level of alveolar crest
Class III	Fracture line extends below the level of alveolar crest
Class IV	Fracture line is within the coronal third of root, but below the level of alveolar crest

Hargreaves and Craig Classification (1970)

Proposed a simplified classification of trauma to anterior teeth.

Class I	No fracture or fracture of enamel only, with or without loosening or displacement of the tooth
Class II	Fracture of the crown involving both enamel and dentin without exposure of the pulp and with or without loosening or displacement of the tooth
Class III	Fracture of the crown exposing the pulp, with or without loosening or displacement of the tooth
Class IV	Fracture of the root with or without coronal fracture, with or without loosening or displacement of the tooth
Class V	Total displacement of the tooth

Garcia-Godoy's Classification (1984)

- It is a numerically descriptive classification that holds good for the primary and permanent teeth
- It is based on Andreasen's modification of World Health Organization (WHO) classification

Class 0	Enamel crack
Class 1	Enamel fracture
Class 2	Enamel-dentin fracture without pulp exposure
Class 3	Enamel-dentin fracture with pulp exposure
Class 4	Enamel-dentin-cementum fracture without pulp exposure
Class 5	Enamel-dentin-cementum fracture with pulp exposure
Class 6	Root fracture
Class 7	Concussion
Class 8	Luxation
Class 9	Lateral displacement
Class 10	Intrusion
Class 11	Extrusion
Class 12	Avulsion

David Classification (1988)

- It is simple and clear classification
- Description of the incisal injuries to supporting tissue and soft tissue has not been given

Class I	Enamel chip off
Class II	Enamel + dentin involvement
Class III	Pulpal involvement
Class IV	Displacement

WHO Classification (1993)

873.60	Enamel fracture
873.61	Enamel and dentin fracture without pulp exposure
873.62	Enamel and dentin fracture with pulp exposure
873.63	Root fracture
873.64	Crown-root fracture
873.66	Concussion, luxation
873.67	Intrusion, extrusion
873.68	Avulsion
873.69	Soft tissue injuries

Classification by Hargreaves (1999)

- It is a classification on basis of the type of injury to individual tooth and injuries to the supporting tissues and alveolar bone.
- Trauma by type of injury to individual teeth.

Description

- Fracture of enamel only
- Fracture involving dentin
- Fracture involving dental pulp
- Displacement or excessive mobility no fracture
- Displacement or excessive mobility and fracture of enamel
- Displacement or excessive mobility and fracture of dentin
- Displacement or excessive mobility fracture to dental pulp
- Discoloration but no other sign of injury
- Tooth lost because of trauma (luxation)

Rocha MJC Classification (2001)

- This classification is based on the type of injury of the dentition and due consideration to the coronal fractures, radicular fractures, and the injuries to the supporting tissue have been laid.
- Types of crown fracture:
  - Enamel fracture
  - Radicular fracture
  - Crown fracture with pulp exposure
  - Crown fracture without pulp exposure
  - Coronoradicular fracture with pulp exposure
- Types of luxations:
  - Subluxation
  - Intrusive luxation
  - Avulsion
  - Concussion
  - Lateral luxation
  - Extrusive luxation

Al-Majed Classification (2001)

- Classified the maxillary incisors for dental trauma.
- This classification is applicable to both primary and permanent dentition.
- It is based on anatomic considerations with the therapeutic and prognostic considerations:
  - *Code 0:* No trauma
  - *Code 1:* Discoloration
  - *Code 2:* Fracture involving enamel
  - *Code 3:* Fracture involving enamel and dentin
  - *Code 4:* Fracture involving enamel, dentin, and pulp
  - *Code 5:* Missing due to trauma
  - *Code 6:* Acid etch composite restoration
  - *Code 7:* Permanent replacement including crown, denture, and bridge pontic
  - *Code 8:* Temporary restoration
  - *Code 9:* Assessment could not be made, when the tooth was either missing or badly broken by dental cases.

According to the International Classification of Diseases (1992).

Injuries to the hard dental tissues and pulp enamel infraction	N 502.50	An incomplete fracture (crack) of the enamel without loss of tooth substance
Enamel fracture (uncomplicated crown fracture)	N 502.50	A fracture with loss of tooth substance confined to the enamel
Enamel-dentin fracture (uncomplicated, crown fracture)	N 502.51	A fracture with loss of tooth substance confined to enamel and dentin but not involving the pulp
Complicated crown fracture	N 502.52	A fracture involving enamel and dentin and exposing the pulp
Complicated crown-root fracture	N 502.54	A fracture involving enamel-dentin and cementum and exposing the pulp
Root fracture	N 502.53	A fracture involving dentin, cementum, and the pulp
Injuries to the periodontal tissues concussion	N 503.20	An injury to the tooth-supporting structures without abnormal loosening or displacement of the tooth, but with marked reaction to percussion
Subluxation	N 503.20	An injury to the tooth supporting structures with abnormal loosening, but without displacement of the tooth
Extrusive luxation (peripheral dislocation, partial avulsion)	N 503.20	Partial displacement of the tooth out of its sockets
Lateral luxation	N 503.20	Displacement of the tooth in a direction other than axially. This is accompanied by communication or fracture of the alveolar socket
Intrusive luxation (central dislocation)	N 503.21	Displacement of the tooth into the alveolar bone. This injury is accompanied by comminution or fracture of the alveolar socket
Avulsion (exarticulation)	N 503.22	Complete displacement of the tooth out of its socket
Comminution of mandibular or maxillary	N 502.40 N 502.60	Alveolar socket crushing and compression of the alveolar socket. This condition is found concomitantly with intrusive and lateral luxations
Fracture of the mandibular or maxillary alveolar socket wall	N 502.40 N 502.60	A fracture confined to the facial or oral socket wall
Fracture of the mandibular or maxillary alveolar process	N 502.40 N 502.60	A fracture of the alveolar process which may or may not involve the alveolar socket
Fracture of the mandible or maxilla	N 502.61 N (502.42)	A fracture involving the base of mandible or maxilla and often the alveolar process (jaw fracture). The fracture may or may not involve the alveolar socket
Laceration of gingiva or oral mucosa	S 01.50	A shallow or deep wound in the mucosa resulting from a tear, and usually produced by a sharp object
Contusion of gingiva or oral mucosa	S 00.50	A bruise usually produced by impact with a blunt object and not accompanied by a break in the mucosa, usually causing submucosal hemorrhage
Abrasion of gingiva or oral mucosa	S 00.50	A superficial wound produced by rubbing or scraping of the mucosa leaving a raw and bleeding surface

Classification of Dental Trauma of Primary Teeth by Fried and Erickson (1995)

- Classification of hard tissue fractures:
  - Class I: Simple fracture of enamel only
  - Class II: Fracture involving enamel and dentin
  - Class III: Fracture extends farther into the tooth, with a small pulpal exposure
  - Class IV: Fracture involves significant amount of pulpal exposure
  - Class V: Complete loss of the tooth
  - Class VI: Fracture of the root
- Trauma affecting the periodontium:
  - Concussion: Sensitivity of the tooth to trauma without abnormal loosening or mobility
  - Subluxation: Loosening of the tooth without mobility
  - Luxation: Displacement of the traumatized teeth

Classification by Spinas (2002)

- It is an "easy to use" classification of dental crown lesions that helped to gather data easily, to choose the right materials, to improve communication among practitioners including by electronic means.
- It consist of 4 classes (A-B-C-D) and 3 subclasses (b1-c1-d1)
  - **Class A:** All the simple enamel lesions, which involve a mesial or distal crown angle, or only the incisal edge.
  - **Class B:** All the enamel dentin lesions, which involve a mesial or distal angle and the incisal edge. When a pulp exposition exists defined as a subclass b1.
  - **Class C:** All the enamel dentin lesions, which involve the incisal edge and at least a third of the crown surface. In case of pulp exposure defined as subclass c1.
  - **Class D:** All the enamel dentin lesions, which involve a mesial or distal crown angle and the incisal or palatal surface, with root cement involvement (crown-root fracture) in case of pulpal exposure exists defined as subclass d1.

Andreasen classification (1981) (Figs. 63.4A to R)

- Injuries to hard dental tissues and pulp
- Injuries to periodontal tissues
- Injuries to supporting bone
- Injuries to gingiva and oral mucosa

Injuries to hard dental tissues and pulp

- *Enamel infraction:* Incomplete fracture (crack) of enamel without loss of tooth substance.
- *Enamel fracture (uncomplicated crown fracture):* A fracture with loss of tooth substance confined to enamel only.
- *Enamel-dentin fracture (uncomplicated crown fracture):* A fracture with loss of tooth substance confined to enamel and dentin but not involving pulp.
- *Complicated crown fracture:* Fracture involving enamel and dentin and also exposing pulp.
- *Uncomplicated crown-root fracture:* Fracture involving enamel, dentin, and cementum but not exposing pulp.
- *Complicated crown-root-fracture:* Fracture involving enamel, dentin, and cementum and also exposing pulp.
- *Root fracture:* A fracture involving dentin, cementum, and pulp. They can also be classified according to displacement of coronal fragment.

Injuries to periodontal tissues

- *Concussion:* An injury to tooth supporting structures without abnormal loosening or displacement of tooth, but with marked reaction to percussion.

Contd...

Contd...

- *Subluxation:* An injury to the tooth supporting structures with abnormal loosening, but without displacement of tooth.
- *Extrusive luxation (peripheral dislocation and partial avulsion):* Partial displacement of tooth out of its socket.
- *Lateral luxation:* Displacement of tooth in any other direction other than axial. Accompanied by fracture of alveolar socket.
- *Intrusive luxation (central dislocation):* Displacement of tooth into alveolar socket accompanied by fracture of alveolar socket.
- *Avulsion (exarticulation):* Complete displacement of tooth out of its socket.

Injuries to supporting bone

- *Comminution of mandibular or maxillary alveolar socket:* Crushing and compression of the alveolar socket found mostly with intrusive and lateral luxation.
- *Fracture of maxillary or mandibular socket wall:* A fracture confined to facial or lingual socket wall.
- *Fracture of maxillary or mandibular alveolar process:* A fracture involving the base of the mandible or maxilla and often the alveolar process. May or may not involve alveolar socket.

Injury to gingiva or oral mucosa

- *Laceration of gingiva or oral mucosa:* Shallow or deep wound in the mucosa resulting from a tear usually produced by sharp object.
- *Contusion of gingiva or oral mucosa:* A bruise usually produced by impact with blunt object and not accompanied by a break in mucosa, but usually causing submucosal hemorrhage.
- *Abrasion of gingiva or oral mucosa:* Superficial wound produced by rubbing or scraping of mucosa leaving a raw bleeding surface.

EXAMINATION AND DIAGNOSIS

A dental injury should always be considered as an emergency and be treated immediately to relieve pain, facilitate reduction of displaced teeth and improve prognosis. Rational therapy depends upon a correct diagnosis, which can be achieved with the help of various examination techniques. While a dental injury can often present a complex picture, most injuries can be broken down into several smaller components. Information gained from the various examination procedures will assist the clinician in defining these trauma components and determining treatment priorities. During the examination several questions are asked and the implication of each answer is different, but all these together help in forming the correct diagnosis.

- **Patient's name, age, sex, address, and telephone number:** Apart from the obvious necessity of such information, the ability of the patient to provide the desired information might also provide clues to possible cerebral involvement or general mental status.
- **When did the injury occur:** The time interval between the injury and treatment significantly influences the result. For example, in reimplantation of avulsed teeth.
- **Where did the injury occur:** The place of accident may indicate a need for tetanus prophylaxis.
- **How did injury occur:** As already indicated, the nature of the accident can yield valuable information on the type of injury to be expected, i.e., a blow to the chin will result in crown-root fractures in the premolar and molar regions. Accidents, in which a child has fallen with an object in its mouth, tend to cause dislocation of teeth in a labial direction.

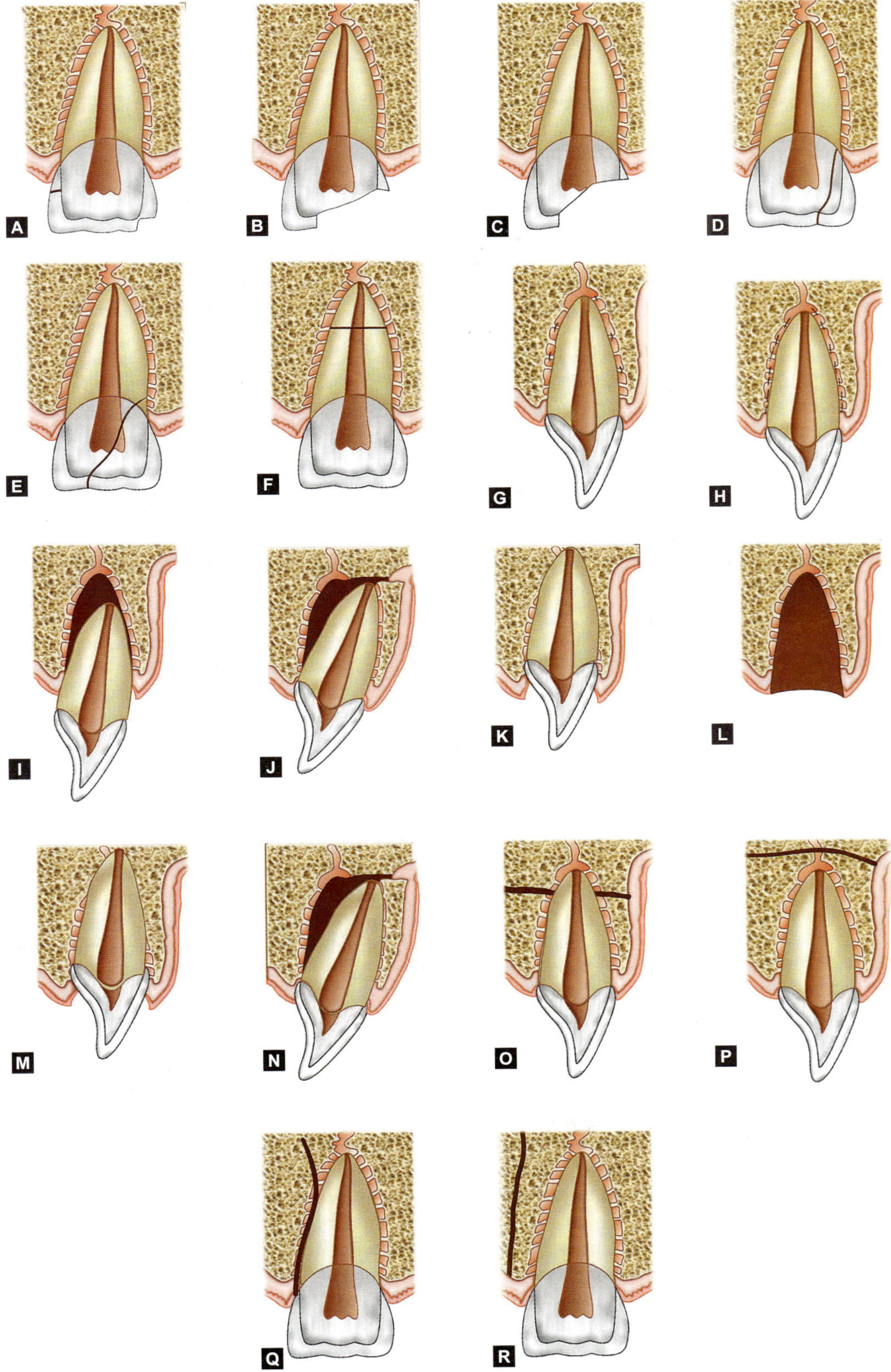

Figs. 63.4A to R: Andreasen classification: (A) Enamel fracture; (B) Enamel-dentin fracture; (C) Enamel-dentin fracture involving pulp; (D) Uncomplicated crown-root fracture; (E) Complicated crown-rot fracture; (F) Root fracture; (G) Concussion; (H) Subluxation; (I) Extrusion luxation; (J) Lateral luxation; (K) Intrusion; (L) Avulsion; (M) Comminution of mandibular or maxillary alveolar socket; (N) Fracture of maxillary or mandibular socket wall; (O) Fracture of maxillary or mandibular alveolar process; (P) Laceration of gingiva or oral mucosa; (Q) Contusion of gingiva or oral mucosa; (R) Abrasion of gingiva or oral mucosa.

- **Treatment elsewhere:** Previous treatment, such as immobilization, reduction, or reimplantation of teeth should be considered before further treatment is instituted. It is also important to ascertain how the avulsed tooth was stored, e.g., tap water, sterilizing solutions, or dry.
- **History of previous dental injuries:** A number of patients may have sustained repeated injuries to their teeth. This can influence pulpal sensibility test and the recuperative capacity of the pulp and periodontium.
- **General health:** A short medical history is essential for providing information about a number of disorders, such as allergic reactions, epilepsy, or bleeding disorders, like as hemophilia. These conditions can influence emergency as well as subsequent treatment.
- **Did the trauma cause drowsiness, vomiting or headache:** Episodes of amnesia, unconsciousness, drowsiness, vomiting, or headache indicate cerebral involvement. Amnesia can be disclosed by the patient's repetition of questions like "Where am I?"/"What happened?" and inability to recall events immediately before or after the injury.
- **Is there spontaneous pain from the teeth:** Spontaneous pain can indicate damage to the tooth supporting structures, e.g., hyperemia or extravasation of blood into the PDL. Damage to the pulp due to crown or crown-root fractures can also give rise to spontaneous pain.
- **Are the teeth tender to touch or during eating:** Reaction to thermal or other stimuli can indicate exposed dentin or pulp. This symptom is to some degree proportional to the area of exposure.
- **Is there any disturbance in the bite:** If the tooth is painful during mastication or if the occlusion is disturbed, injuries such as extrusive luxation, lateral luxation, or alveolar fractures should be suspected.
- **Recording of extraoral wounds and palpation of the facial skeleton:** Extraoral wounds are usually present in cases resulting from traffic accidents. The location of these wounds can indicate where and when dental injuries are to be suspected, e.g., a wound located under the chin suggests dental injuries in the premolar and molar regions and/or concomitant fracture of the mandibular condyle and/or symphysis. Palpation of the facial skeleton can disclose jaw fractures.
- **Recording of injuries to oral mucosa or gingival injuries:** Wounds penetrating the entire thickness of the lip can frequently be observed, often demarcated by two parallel wounds on the inner and outer labial surfaces. If present, the possibility of tooth fragments buried between the lacerations should be considered.
- **Examination of crowns of teeth:** For the presence and extent of fractures, pulp exposures or changes in color. Before examining traumatized teeth, the crowns should be cleaned of blood and debris. When examining crown fractures, it is important to note whether the fracture is confined to enamel or includes dentin. The fracture surface should be carefully examined for pulp exposures, if present, the size and location should be recorded.
- **Recording of displacement of teeth:** Displacement of teeth is usually evident by visual examination; however minor abnormalities can often be difficult to detect. In such cases, it is helpful to examine the occlusion as well as radiographs taken at various angulations.
- **Disturbances in occlusion:** Abnormalities in occlusion can indicate fractures of the jaw or alveolar process. All teeth should be tested for abnormal mobility, both horizontally and axially. Disruption of the vascular supply to the pulp should be expected in case of axial mobility. Abnormal mobility of teeth or alveolar fragments, uneven contours of the alveolar process usually indicate a bony fracture. Moreover, the direction of the dislocation can sometimes be determined by palpation.
- **Tenderness of teeth to percussion and change in percussion tone:** Reaction to percussion is indicative of damage to the PDL. The test may be performed by tapping the tooth lightly with the handle of a mouth mirror, in vertical as well as horizontal direction. Injuries to the PDL will result in pain. As with all examination techniques used at the time of injury, the percussion test should begin on a noninjured tooth to assure a reliable patient response. Recently, a calibrated percussion instrument has been introduced, a periotest. However, the force imparted by such an instrument might contribute to a new trauma, as in the case of root fractures. The sound elicited by percussion is also of diagnostic value. Thus, a hard, metallic sound elicited by percussion in a horizontal direction indicates that the tooth is locked into bone; while a dull sound indicates subluxation or extrusive luxation.
- **Reaction of teeth to pulpal testing:** Pulp testing following traumatic injuries is a controversial issue. These procedures require cooperation and a relaxed patient, in order to avoid false reactions. However, this is often not possible during initial treatment of injured patients, especially children. Pulpal sensibility testing at the time of reference for evaluating pulpal status at later follow-up examinations. A number of tests have been proposed. However, the value of these has recently been questioned. The principle of the test involves transmitting stimuli to the sensory receptors of the dental pulp and registering the reaction.

RADIOGRAPHIC EXAMINATION[3]

- The clinician should evaluate each case and determine which radiographs are required for the specific case involved. A clear justification for taking a radiograph is essential. There needs to be a strong likelihood that a radiograph will provide the information that will positively influence the selection of the treatment provided. Furthermore, initial radiographs are important as they provide a baseline for future comparisons at follow-up examinations.
- The use of film holders is highly recommended to allow standardization and reproducible radiographs.
- Since maxillary central incisors are the most frequently affected teeth, the radiographs listed below are recommended to thoroughly examine the injured area:
  - One parallel periapical radiograph aimed through the midline to show the two maxillary central incisors.
  - One parallel periapical radiograph aimed at the maxillary right lateral incisors (should also show the right canine and central incisor).

- One parallel periapical radiograph aimed at the maxillary left lateral incisor (should also show the left canine and central incisor).
- One maxillary occlusal radiograph.

- At least one parallel periapical radiograph of the lower incisors centered on the two mandibular centrals. However, other radiographs may be indicated if there are obvious injuries of the mandibular teeth (e.g., similar periapical radiographs as above for the maxillary teeth, mandibular occlusal radiograph).
- The radiographs aimed at the maxillary lateral incisors provide different horizontal (mesial and distal) views of each incisor, as well as showing the canine teeth. The occlusal radiograph provides a different vertical view of the injured teeth and the surrounding tissues, which is particularly helpful in the detection of lateral luxations, root fractures, and alveolar bone fractures.
- The above radiographic series is provided as an example. If other teeth are injured, then the series can be modified to focus on the relevant tooth/teeth. Some minor injuries, such as enamel infractions, may not require all of these radiographs.
- Radiographs are necessary to make a thorough diagnosis of dental injuries. Tooth root and bone fractures, for instance, may occur without any clinical signs or symptoms and are frequently undetected when only one radiographic view is used. Additionally, patients sometimes seek treatment several weeks after the trauma occurred when clinical signs of a more serious injury have subsided. Thus, dentists should use their clinical judgment and weigh the advantages and disadvantages of taking several radiographs.
- Cone beam computerized tomography (CBCT) provides enhanced visualization of traumatic dental injuries, particularly root fractures, crown/root fractures, and lateral luxations. CBCT helps to determine the location, extent, and direction of a fracture. In these specific injuries, 3D imaging can be useful and should be considered, if available. A guiding principle when considering exposing a patient to ionizing radiations (e.g., either 2D or 3D radiographs) is whether the image is likely to change the management of the injury.

PHOTOGRAPHIC DOCUMENTATION

The use of clinical photographs is strongly recommended for the initial documentation of the injury and for follow-up examinations. Photographic documentation allows monitoring of soft tissue healing, assessment of tooth discoloration, the re-eruption of an intruded tooth, and the development of infra-positioning of an ankylosed tooth. In addition, photographs provide medico-legal documentation that could be used in litigation cases.

PULP STATUS EVALUATION: SENSIBILITY AND VITALITY TESTING

Sensibility Tests[4-7]

- Sensibility testing refers to tests (cold test and electric pulp test) used to determine the condition of the pulp. It is important to understand that sensibility testing assesses neural activity and not vascular supply. Thus, this testing might be unreliable due to a transient lack of neural response or undifferentiation of A-delta nerve fibers in young teeth.
- The temporary loss of sensibility is a frequent finding during post-traumatic pulp healing, especially after luxation injuries.
- Thus, the lack of a response to pulp sensibility testing is not conclusive for pulp necrosis in traumatized teeth. Despite this limitation, pulp sensibility testing should be performed initially and at each follow-up appointment in order to determine if changes occur over time.
- It is generally accepted that pulp sensibility testing should be done as soon as practical to establish a baseline for future comparison testing and follow-up. Initial testing is also a good predictor for the long-term prognosis of the pulp.

Vitality Tests[5,8]

- The use of pulse oximetry, which measures actual blood flow rather than the neural response, has been shown to be a reliable non-invasive and accurate way of confirming the presence of a blood supply (vitality) in the pulp. The current use of pulse oximetry is limited due to the lack of sensors specifically designed to fit dental dimensions and the lack of power to penetrate through hard dental tissues.
- Laser and ultrasound Doppler flowmetry are promising technologies to monitor pulp vitality.

MANAGEMENT OF TRAUMATIC INJURIES

Enamel Infarctions

- These are very common but often overlooked.
- These fractures appear as crazing within the enamel substance which do not cross the dentinoenamel junction and appear with or without loss of tooth substance.
- Infarctions are caused by direct impact to the enamel (e.g., traffic accidents), which explains their frequent occurrence on the labial surface of upper incisors. Various patterns of infarctions lines can be seen depending on direction and location of trauma.
- Infarctions are easily visualized by seeing long axis of the tooth from the incisal edge; fiberoptic light sources and transillumination are also useful in detecting infarctions.
- Treatment is layering with composite.

Enamel Fractures

Clinical Features

- These occur more often than complicated crown fractures in both the permanent and primary dentitions.
- They are often confined to a single tooth and are usually seen in the maxillary region.
- Manifest as broken anterior teeth with loss of enamel only **(Fig. 63.5)**.

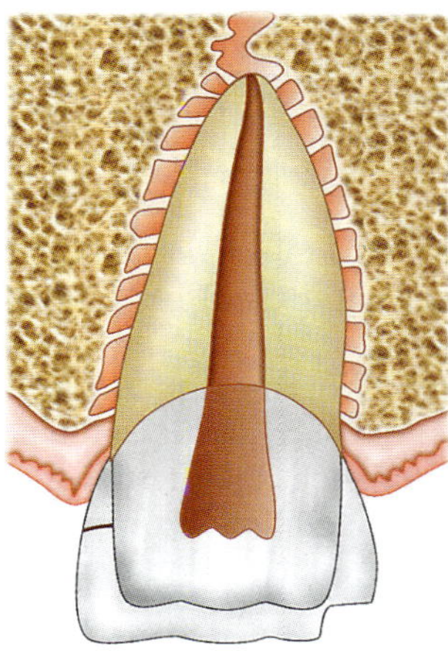

Fig. 63.5: Enamel fracture.

Treatment

The treatment of choice for this is restoration with composite resin, but corrective grinding and removal of sharp edges is also useful **(Figs. 63.6A and B)**.

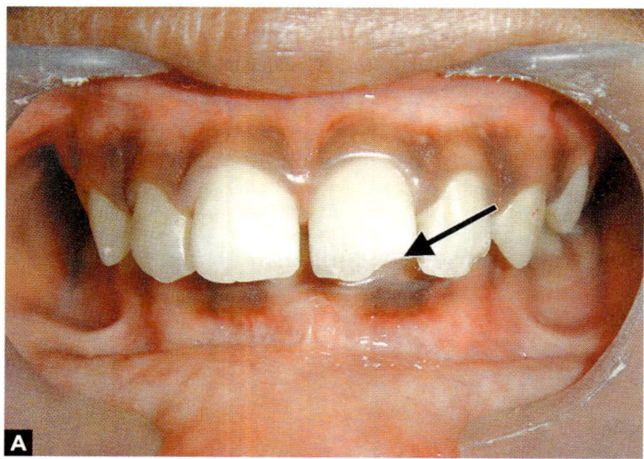

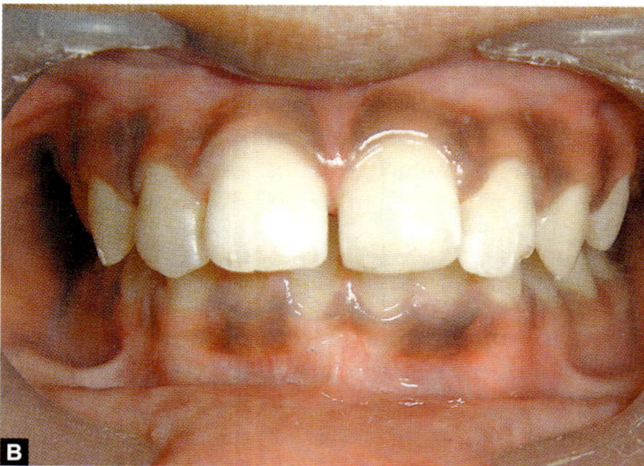

Figs. 63.6A and B: Enamel fracture and subsequent restoration with composite.

Uncomplicated Crown Fractures

Clinical Features

- This is characterized by fracture of crown involving enamel and dentin without pulp exposure **(Fig. 63.7)**.
- Thorough cleansing of the injured teeth with a water spray should precede examination of fractured teeth.
- This is followed by an assessment of the extent of exposed dentin as well as a careful search for minute pulp exposure.
- Dentin exposed after crown fractures usually give rise to symptoms such as sensitivity to thermal changes and mastication, which are to some degree proportional to the area of dentin exposed.

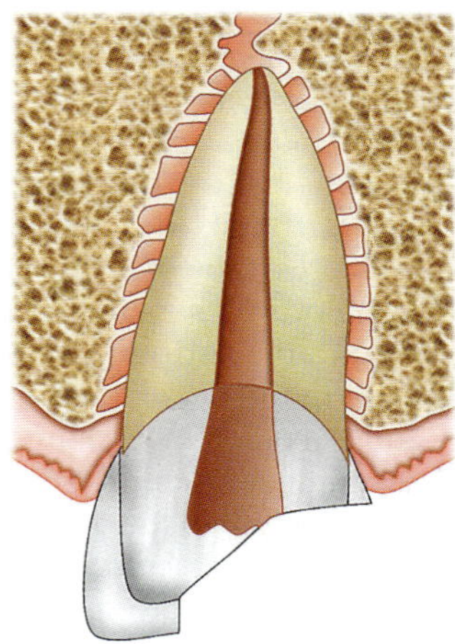

Fig. 63.7: Uncomplicated crown fracture.

Treatment

- **Immediate provisional treatment:** Place $Ca(OH)_2$ on the exposed dentin and restore.
- **Permanent treatment:** Reattachment of the crown fragment, restoration with composite resin or full coverage crown **(Figs. 63.8A and B)**.

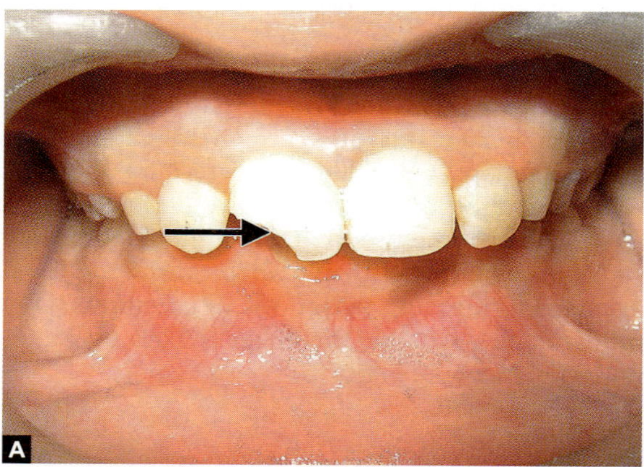

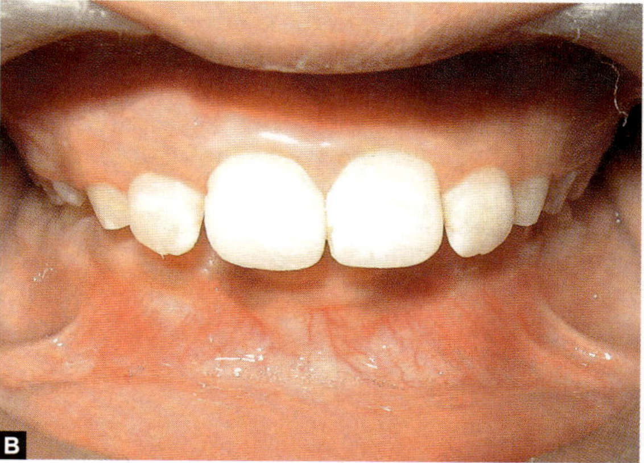

Figs. 63.8A and B: Uncomplicated crown fracture and its subsequent restoration.

Complicated Crown Fractures

Clinical Features

- This occurs when there is a fracture of enamel, dentin along with exposure of pulp **(Fig. 63.9)**.
- This usually presents as a fractured segment of tooth with frank bleeding from the exposed pulp.

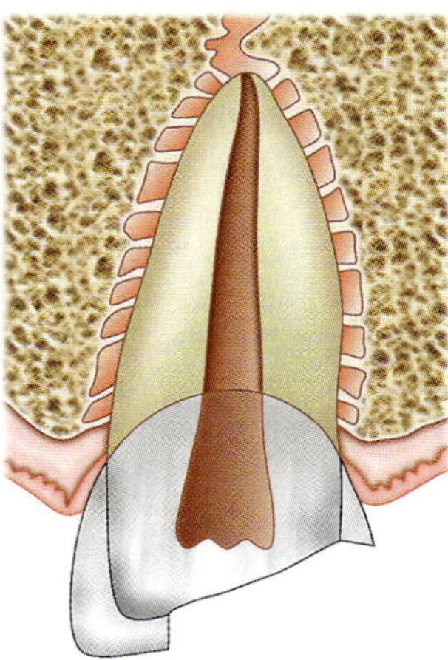

Fig. 63.9: Complicated crown fracture.

Treatment

The type of treatment will depend upon the extent and time of pulp exposure.

- When the exposure is small and pulp has not been exposed for more than 4–5 minutes then it is advisable to do pulp capping.
- When the exposure is large and pulp has been exposed for more than 5 minutes then it is ideal to do pulpotomy/root canal treatment (RCT) **(Figs. 63.10A to E)**.

Crown-root Fracture

- It is defined as a fracture involving enamel, dentin, and cementum **(Figs. 63.11A and B)**
- These fractures may be grouped according to pulpal involvement into uncomplicated and complicated
- Crown-root fractures in the anterior region are usually caused by direct trauma and in the posterior region fractures of the buccal or lingual cusps of premolars and molars may occur due to indirect trauma. The direction of the impacting force determines the type of fracture.

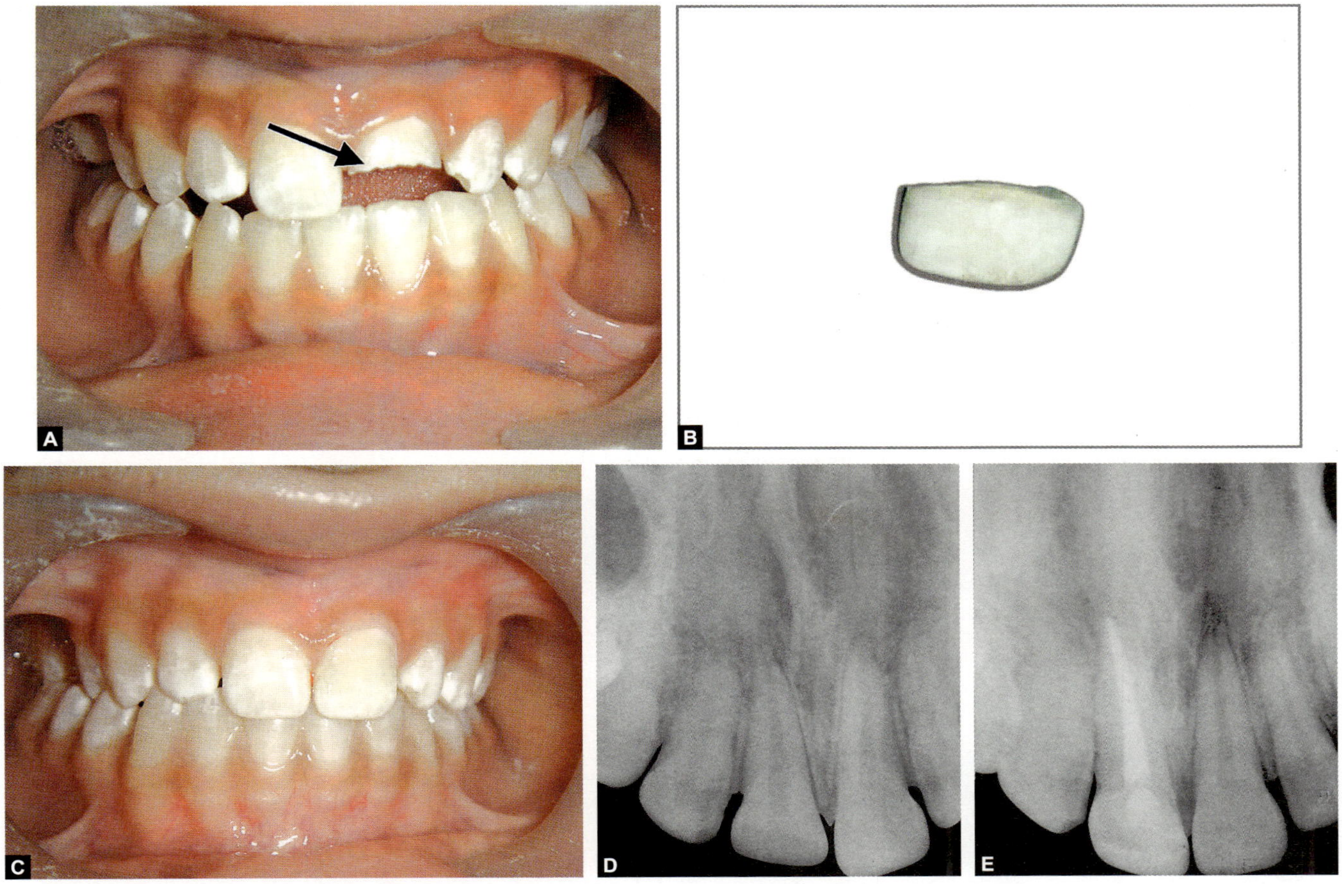

Figs. 63.10A to E: Treatment of complicated crown fracture: (A) Clinical presentation of complicated crown fracture: (B) Fractured fragment; (C) Reattachment of crown following root canal treatment (RCT); (D) Preoperative radiograph; (E) Postoperative radiograph showing RCT and attachment.

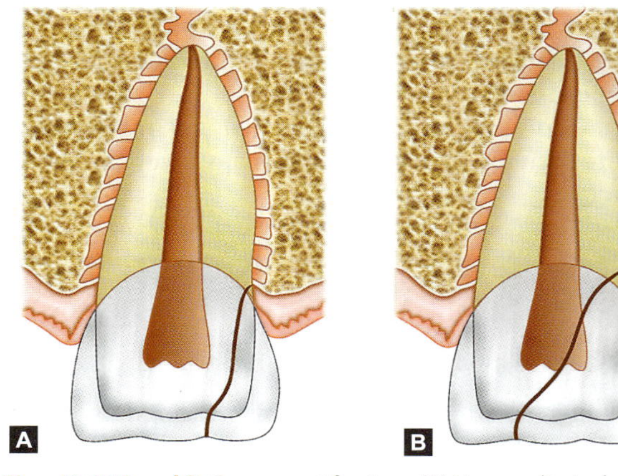

Figs. 63.11A and B: Crown-root fracture: (A) Uncomplicated crown-root fracture; (B) Complicated crown-root fracture.

Clinical Features

Most commonly the fracture line begins a few millimeters incisal to marginal gingiva or to facial aspect of the crown following an oblique course below the gingival crevice orally.

Radiographic Features

Radiographic examination of crown-root fractures following the usual course seldom contributes to the clinical diagnosis, as oblique fracture line is almost perpendicular to central beam.

Treatment

- Emergency treatment can include stabilization of coronal fragment with an acid etch splint to adjacent teeth. However, it is essential that definitive treatment begins within a few days after injury
- In case of uncomplicated crown-root fracture in the premolar and molar region immediate provisional treatment can include removal of loose fragment and coverage of exposed supragingival dentin with glass ionomer cement (GIC). In uncomplicated fracture in anterior teeth, the mobile segment is stabilized with adhesive bonding
- In case of vertical fractures of immature permanent incisors the fractures are usually seen slightly apical to the level of alveolar crest. These fractures are amenable to orthodontic extrusion whereby the level of the fracture is brought to level where pulp capping and restoration are possible
- In case of complicated crown-root fractures of anterior teeth, the mobile segment is first removed and preserved. The next step is to complete the RCT if access allows and if it is not possible then minor orthodontic extrusion or gingivectomy can be done to accomplish the access to do RCT. Following this the preserved segment is attached back and full coverage crown is given in due course of time **(Figs. 63.12A to D).**

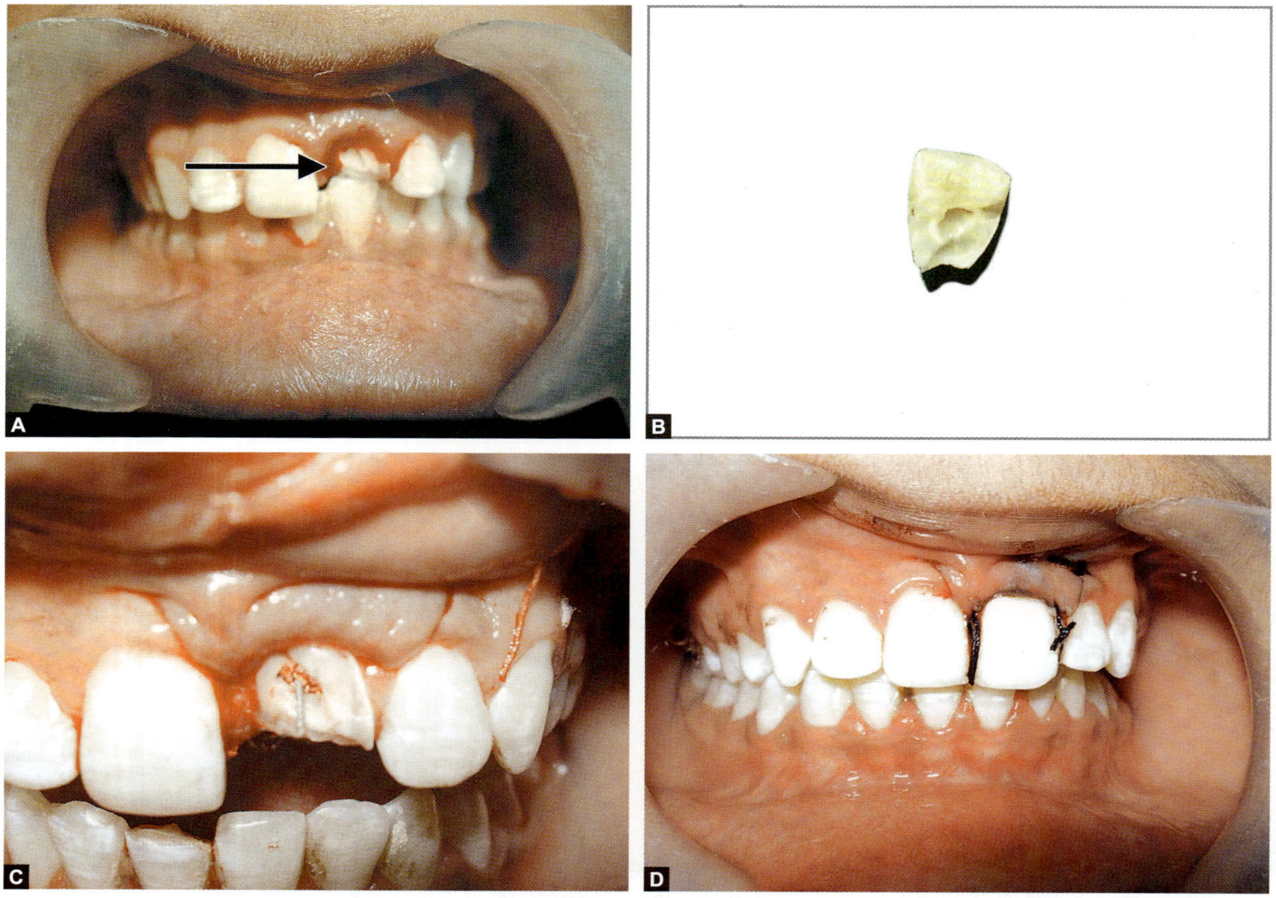

Figs. 63.12A to D: Treatment of crown-root fracture: (A) Clinical presentation of crown-root fracture; (B) Fractured fragment; (C) Root canal treatment of tooth with placement of post; (D) Reattachment of crown following raising of flap.

Root Fracture

- It is defined as fractures involving dentin, cementum, and pulp **(Fig. 63.13)**
- They are relatively uncommon ranging from 0.5 to 7% in permanent dentition and 2–4% in primary dentition
- The mechanism of root fractures is usually a frontal impact, which creates compression zones labially and lingually. The resulting shearing stress zone then dictates the plane of fracture.

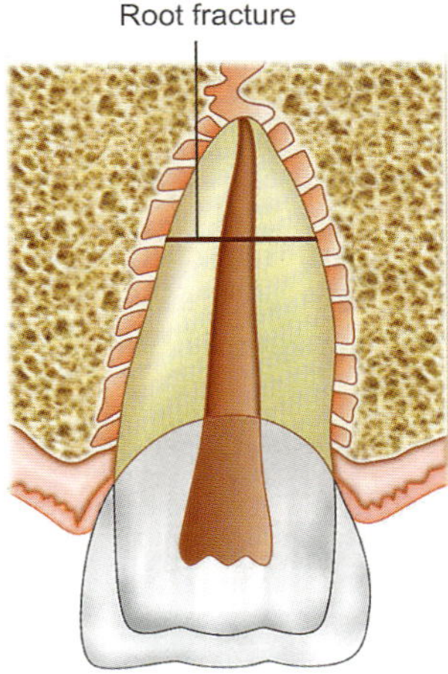

Fig. 63.13: Root fracture.

Clinical Features

- Root fractures involving the permanent dentition predominantly affect the maxillary central incisor region in age group of 11–20 years
- Coronal fragments are displaced lingually or slightly extruded
- Temporary loss of sensitivity.

Radiographic Features

Radiographic demonstration of root fractures is facilitated by the fact that the fracture line is most often oblique and at an optimal angle for radiographic disclosure. In this context it should be remembered that a root fracture would normally be visible only if the central beam is directed within a maximum range of 15–20° of fracture plane.

Classification of Root Fractures

- **Based on direction of fracture line with long axis of tooth:**
  - *Horizontal:* Fracture perpendicular to long axis of tooth
  - *Oblique:* Fracture is at an angle to long axis
  - *Vertical:* Fracture parallel to long axis.
- **Based on location:**
  - Cervical third
  - Middle third
  - Apical third.
- **According to number of fracture lines:**
  - *Simple:* Only one fracture line dividing root into two fragments
  - *Multiple:* When root is divided into more than two fragments
  - *Comminuted:* Multiple fracture lines.
- **According to extension of line of fracture:**
  - *Partial:* Fracture involves a portion of root
  - *Total:* Entire root is involved with fracture line
- **Position of root fragments:**
  - *Without displacement:* Segments face each other
  - *With displacement:* When fracture segments are not aligned.

Treatment

- The principle of treatment of permanent teeth is reduction of displaced coronal fragments and firm immobilization
- Immobilization of teeth with root fractures is achieved with rigid fixation with an acid-etch splint
- The fixation period should be 2–3 months to ensure sufficient hard tissue consolidation
- Following treatment modalities are recommended based on the fracture line:
  - When fracture is present in middle third **(Fig. 63.14A)**—extraction
  - When fracture is in apical third **(Fig. 63.14B)**—obturation till the possible working length and apical surgery to remove the fragment
  - When fracture is near to gingival margin **(Fig. 63.14C)**—orthodontic or surgical extrusion of the fragment followed by immobilization and later crown fabrication.

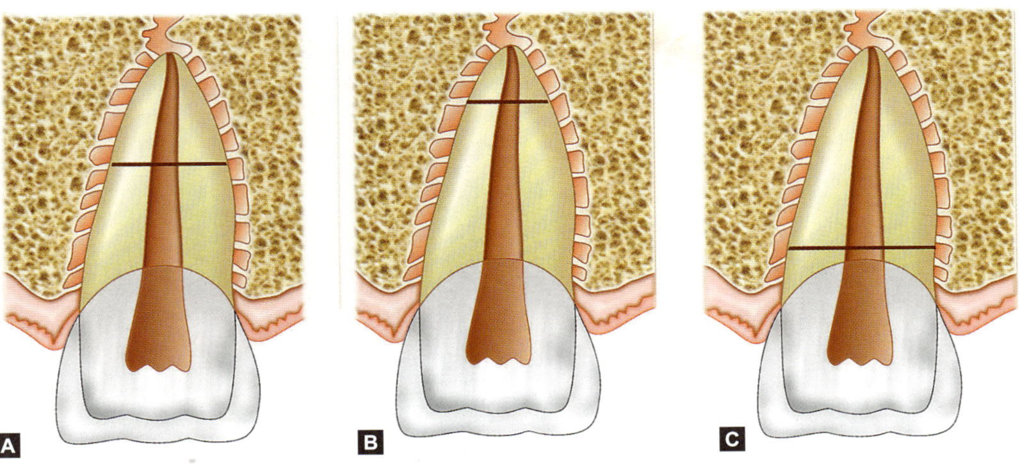

Figs. 63.14A to C: Treatment of root fracture depending on fracture line.

Vertical Root Fracture

- It is also called as cracked tooth syndrome
- It runs lengthwise from crown towards the apex **(Fig. 63.15)**
- It is mostly found in posterior teeth and its etiology is mostly iatrogenic like insertion of screws, after pulp therapy or due to traumatic occlusion.
- **Clinical features:**
  - Persistent dull pain of long-standing origin
  - Pain is elicited by applying pressure.
- **Radiographic features:**
  - If the central beam lies in the line of fracture it is visible as radiolucent line
  - Thickening of PDL is also seen.

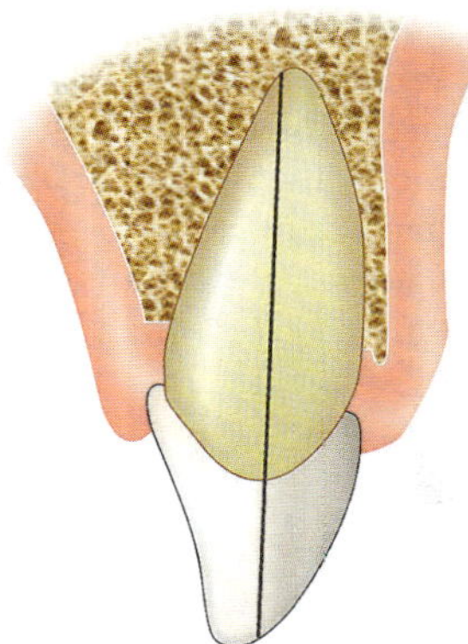

Fig. 63.15: Vertical root fracture.

- **Occlusal pressure test:** When asked to bite/chew on a cotton applicator or a rubber polishing wheel patient gets sharp pain.
- **Treatment:**
  - Single rooted teeth—extraction
  - Multi rooted teeth—hemisection and the remaining tooth is endodontically treated and restored with crown.

Concussion

An injury to tooth supporting structures, when there is some crushing injury to apical vasculature and PDL with resultant inflammatory edema with marked reaction to percussion but without abnormal loosening or displacement **(Fig. 63.16)**.

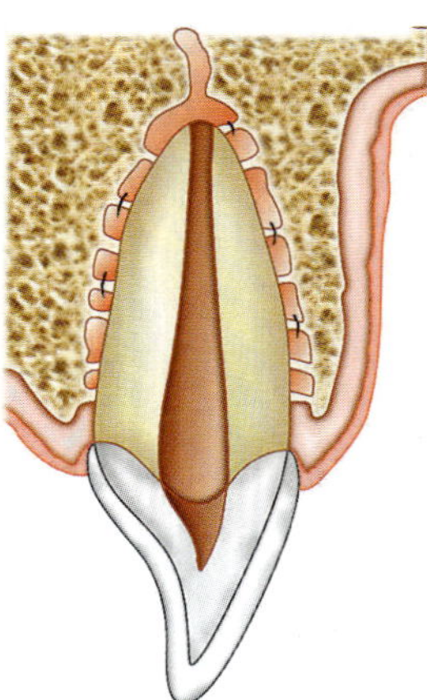

Fig. 63.16: Concussion.

Clinical Features

- Traumatized tooth is sore
- Tooth is tender to percussion
- Sensitive to biting forces.

Radiographic Features

- Widening of PDL space apically
- Reduction in size of pulp after few months.

Treatment

- Slight adjustment of opposing tooth to relieve occlusion
- Soft diet for 10–14 days.

Subluxation

An injury to tooth supporting structures with abnormal loosening but without clinically or radiographically demonstrable displacement of the tooth **(Fig. 63.17)**.

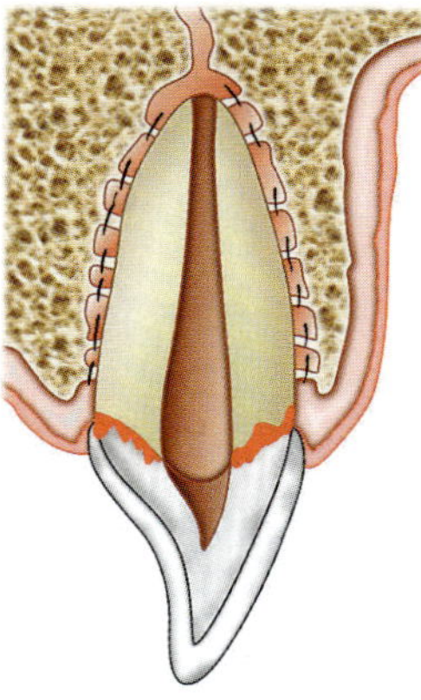

Fig. 63.17: Subluxation.

Clinical Features

- Tooth is tender on palpation
- Mobility
- Evidence of hemorrhage at gingival margin.

Radiographic Features

- Widening of PDL space
- Reduction in size of pulp after few months.

Treatment (Fig. 63.18)

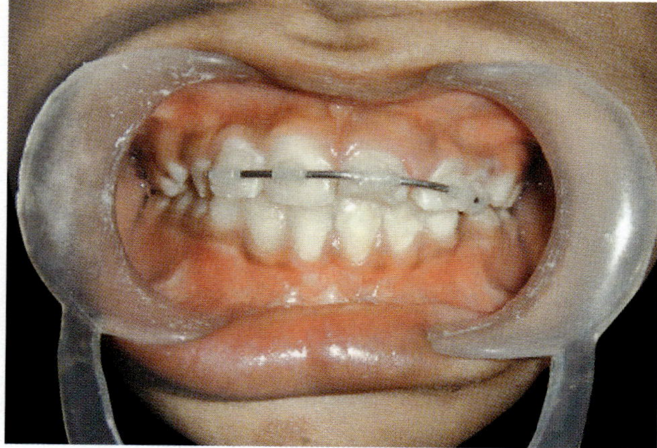

Fig. 63.18: Treatment of subluxation with splinting.

- ❖ Slight adjustment of opposing tooth to relieve occlusion
- ❖ Splinting for 10 days
- ❖ Soft diet for 10–14 days
- ❖ Follow-up the tooth clinically and radiographically.

Intrusive Luxation

Term used to describe displacement of tooth into alveolar bone **(Fig. 63.19)**.

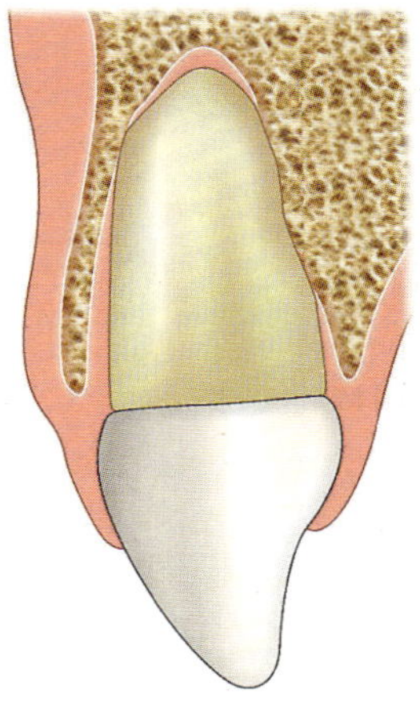

Fig. 63.19: Intrusive luxation.

Clinical Features

- ❖ Displacement is accompanied by fracture or crushing of alveolar bone **(Fig. 63.20)**
- ❖ Tooth is mobile
- ❖ Bleeding from gingival crevice
- ❖ Tooth is tender to percussion and masticatory forces
- ❖ Clinically crown appears shorter.

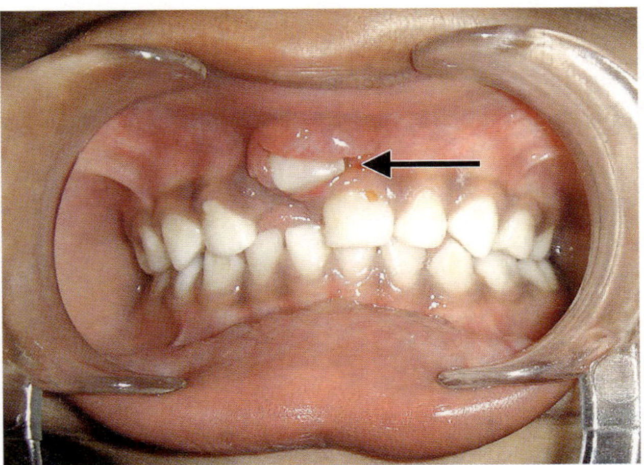

Fig. 63.20: Presentation of intrusion.

Radiographic Features

- ❖ Obliteration of apical portion of PDL space.
- ❖ Crushing of lamina dura.

Treatment

- ❖ Spontaneous eruption, orthodontic, or surgical repositioning of tooth **(Figs. 63.21 to 63.24)**. The treatment lines for the management of intrusion depend on the degree of intrusion which has taken place.
  - ■ In case of minor (1–2 mm) of intrusion it is best to wait up to 3 months for spontaneous eruption to occur before initiating any type of treatment.
  - ■ In case of severe intrusion the two best mentioned approaches are orthodontic and surgical extrusion. The former is more methodical and is mostly indicated when the traumatized tooth have incomplete root/apex formation. This approach would bring the tooth slowly into position without compromising the blood and nerve supply. However, the drawbacks of this technique are more time consuming, and can be used for isolated single teeth traumas.
  - ■ The surgical extrusion is more rigid method of repositioning and provides immediate results and is indicated in multiple trauma but can lead to nonvitalization of teeth due to severing of blood supply.
- ❖ Suture the gingival laceration
- ❖ Splint for 2 to 3 weeks after tooth has come to normal position
- ❖ Soft diet for 14 days
- ❖ Follow-up period of 1 year.

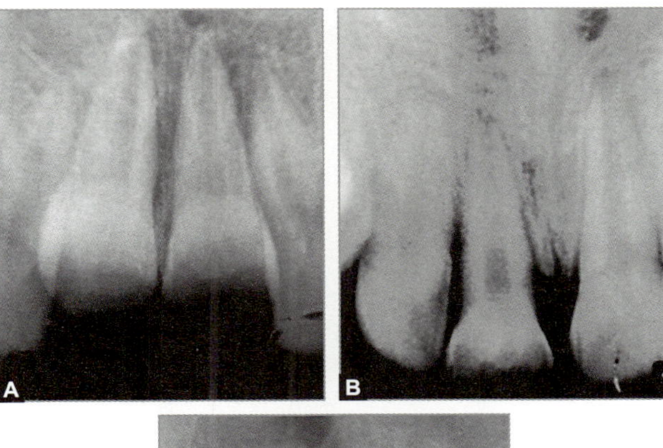

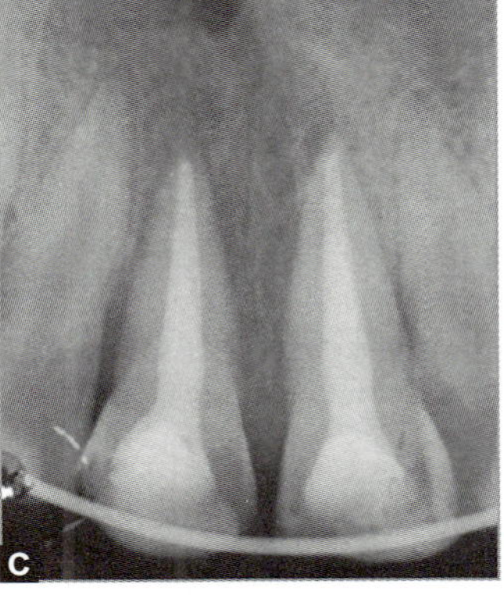

Figs. 63.21A to C: Radiographic presentation of intrusion and its treatment.

Extrusive Luxation

It is also called peripheral displacement or partial avulsion. It is partial displacement of tooth out of its socket **(Fig. 63.22)**.

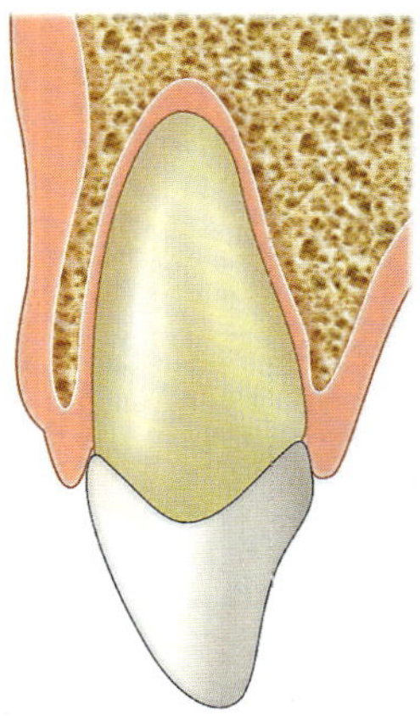

Fig. 63.22: Extrusive luxation.

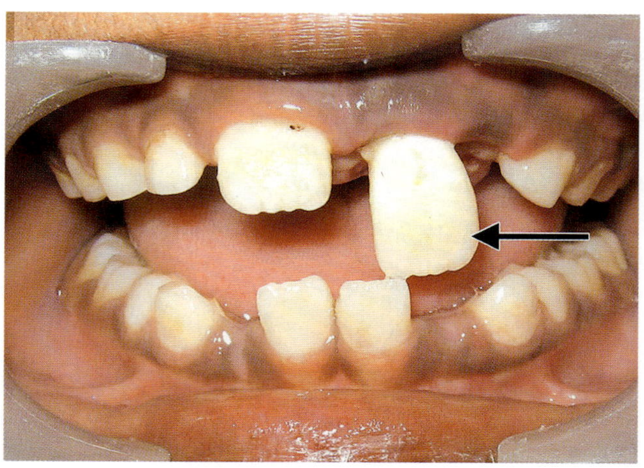

Fig. 63.23: Clinical presentation of extrusion.

Clinical Features

- Tooth is mobile
- Bleeding from gingival crevice
- Tooth is tender to percussion and masticatory forces
- Clinically crown appears longer **(Fig. 63.23)**.

Radiographic Features

- Widening of PDL space.

Treatment (Figs. 63.24A to M)

- Administer local anesthesia if forceful positioning is anticipated.
- Reposition the tooth in normal position using digital pressure
- Splint the tooth for 2–3 weeks
- Advice soft diet
- Follow-up period of 1 year.

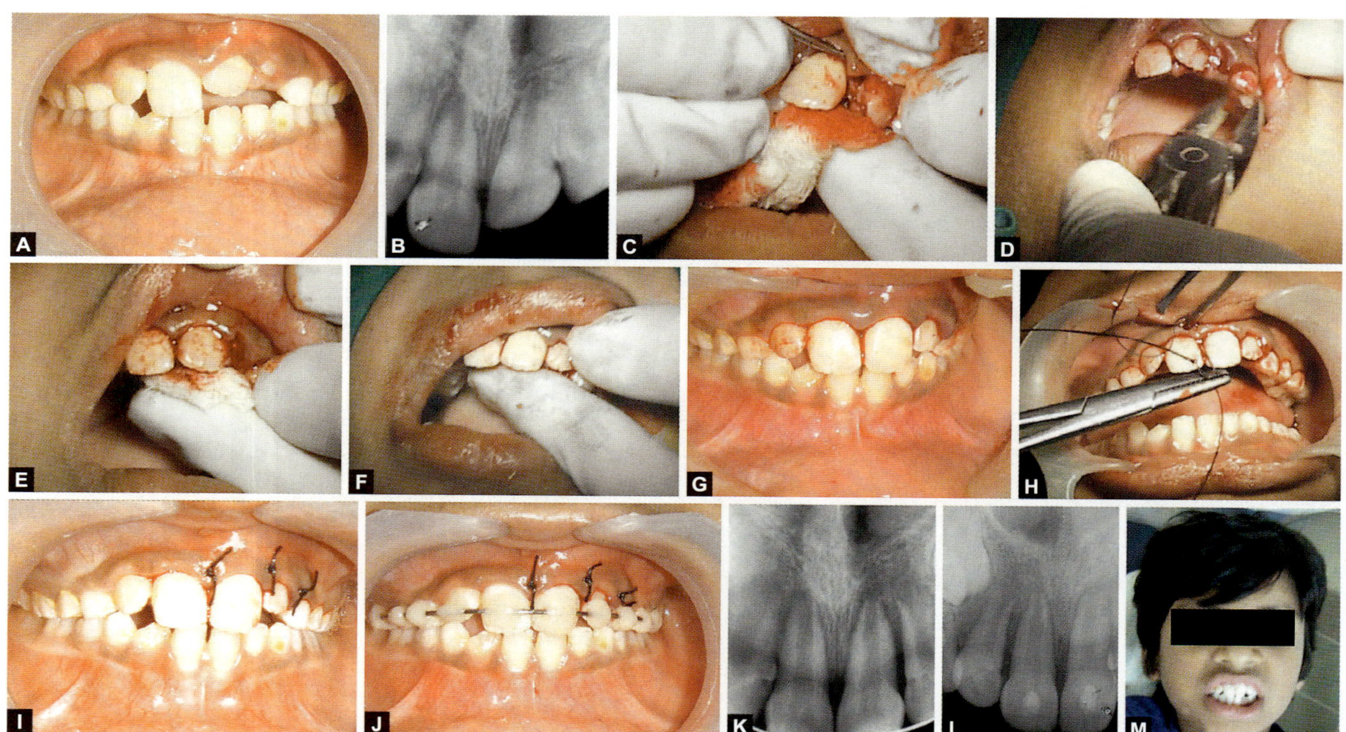

Figs. 63.24A to M: Traumatic injury to 21, 22 treated by surgical extrusion of 22 and intrusion of 21: (A) Preoperative view; (B) Pretreatment IOPA; (C) Flap being raised; (D) Extrusion of 22 with forceps; (E) Intrusion of extruded 21; (F) Stabilizing after extrusion of 22 and intrusion of 21; (G) Post stabilization; (H) Sutures being placed; (I) After suturing; (J) Wire composite acid etch resin splint placed; (K) IOPA after surgery and splinting; (L) IOPA after apexification with $Ca(OH)_2$; (M) Postoperative view.

Lateral Luxation

It is displacement of tooth in any direction other than axial **(Fig. 63.25)**.

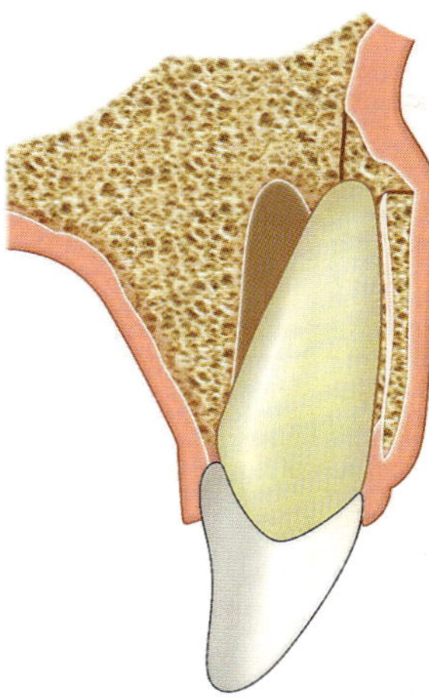

Fig. 63.25: Lateral luxation.

Clinical Features

- Tooth is mobile and displaced **(Fig. 63.26)**.
- Bleeding from gingival crevice.
- Tooth is tender to percussion and masticatory forces.

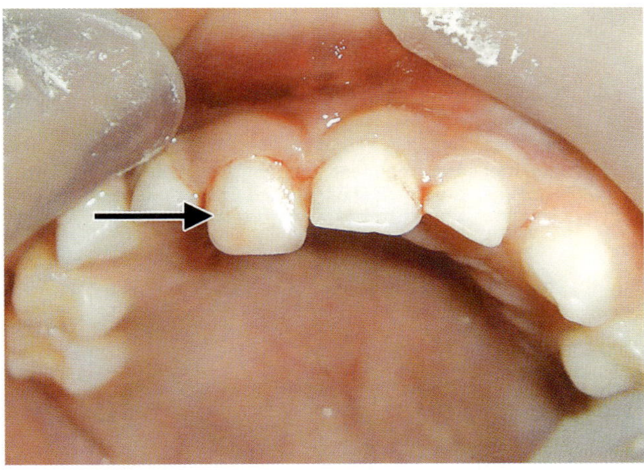

Fig. 63.26: Lateral luxation of maxillary central incisors.

Radiographic Features

- Widening of PDL space on one side and crushing of lamina dura on other side **(Fig. 63.27)**.

Treatment

- Administer local anesthesia if forceful positioning is anticipated.
- Reposition the tooth in normal position using digital pressure.
- Splint the tooth for 2 weeks and if there is marginal bone breakdown then splint for 6–8 weeks.
- Advice soft diet.
- Follow-up period of 1 year.

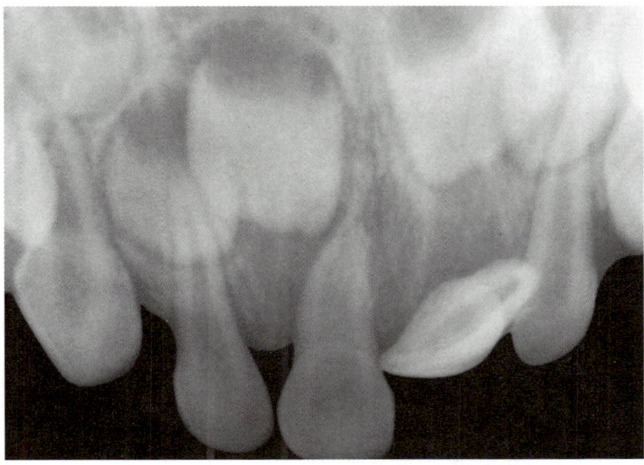

Fig. 63.27: Radiographic view of lateral luxation.

Avulsion

Term used to describe complete displacement of tooth from its alveolus. It is also called as exarticulation and most often involves the maxillary teeth **(Fig. 63.28)**.

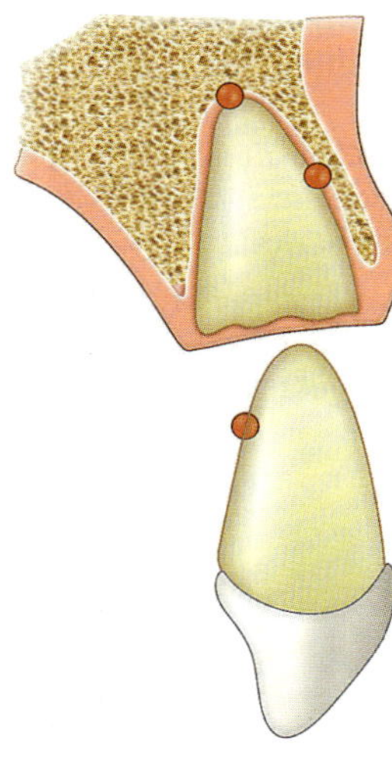

Fig. 63.28: Clinical presentation of avulsion.

Clinical Features

Bleeding socket with missing tooth **(Fig. 63.29)**.

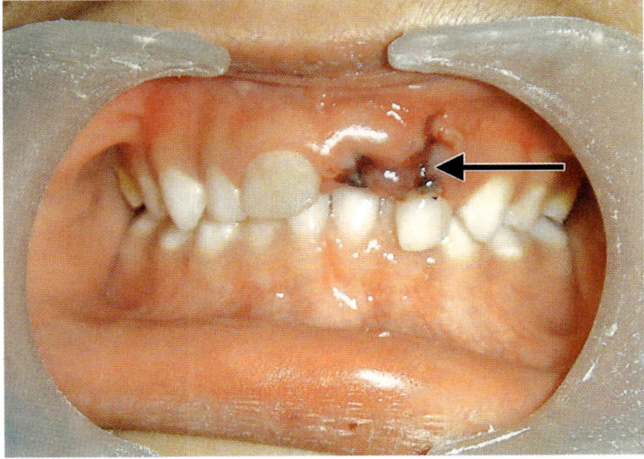

Fig. 63.29: Bleeding socket with missing tooth.

Radiographic Features

- Empty socket.
- Associated bone fractures.
- If the wound is recent then lamina dura is visible otherwise it is obliterated.

Treatment

- Reimplantation depends on extraoral time.
- If apical foramen is not closed—endodontic therapy is delayed till first signs of apical closure are seen.
- If apical foramen is closed—endodontic therapy is done after 1–2 weeks depending on type of reimplantation.

Prognosis

- **Tooth survival:** 51–89%
- **PDL healing:** 9–50%
- **Pulp healing:** 4–15%.

REIMPLANTATION

Case history should include exact information on the time interval between injury and reimplantation as well as conditions under which the tooth has been stored (e.g., saline, saliva, milk, tap water, or dry environment). The following conditions should be considered before replanting a permanent tooth:

- The alveolar socket should be reasonably intact in order to provide a seat for the avulsed tooth.
- The extra-alveolar period.

Short extra-alveolar storage: This is done if the tooth since the time of injury has been placed in a suitable medium and the extra-alveolar time elapsed is short.

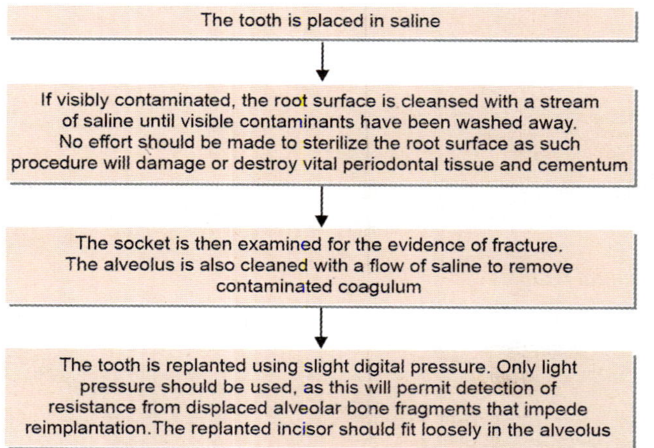

Contd..

Contd..

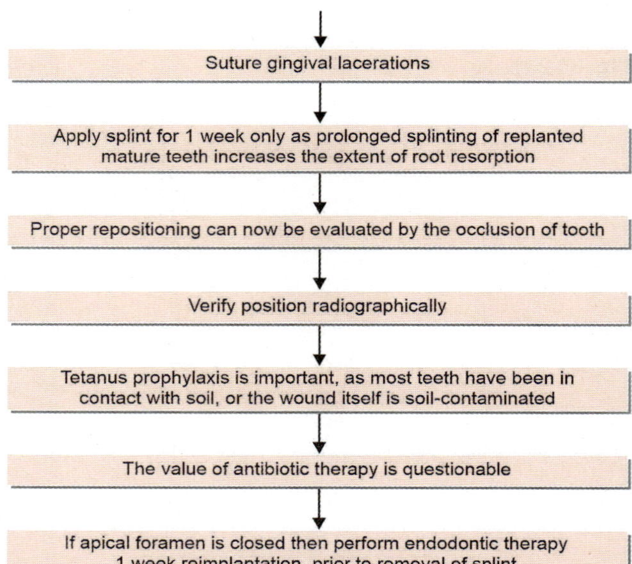

Long extra-alveolar storage: This is done in cases where the extraoral dry period of tooth is long **(Figs. 63.30 and 63.31)**.

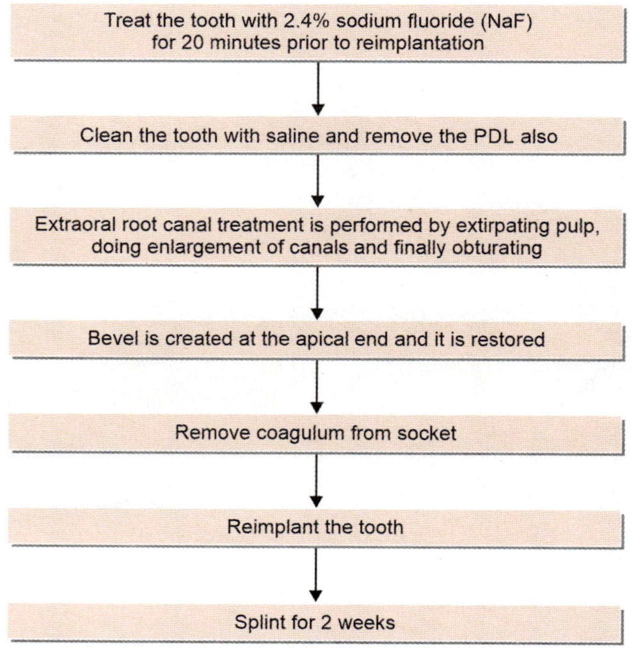

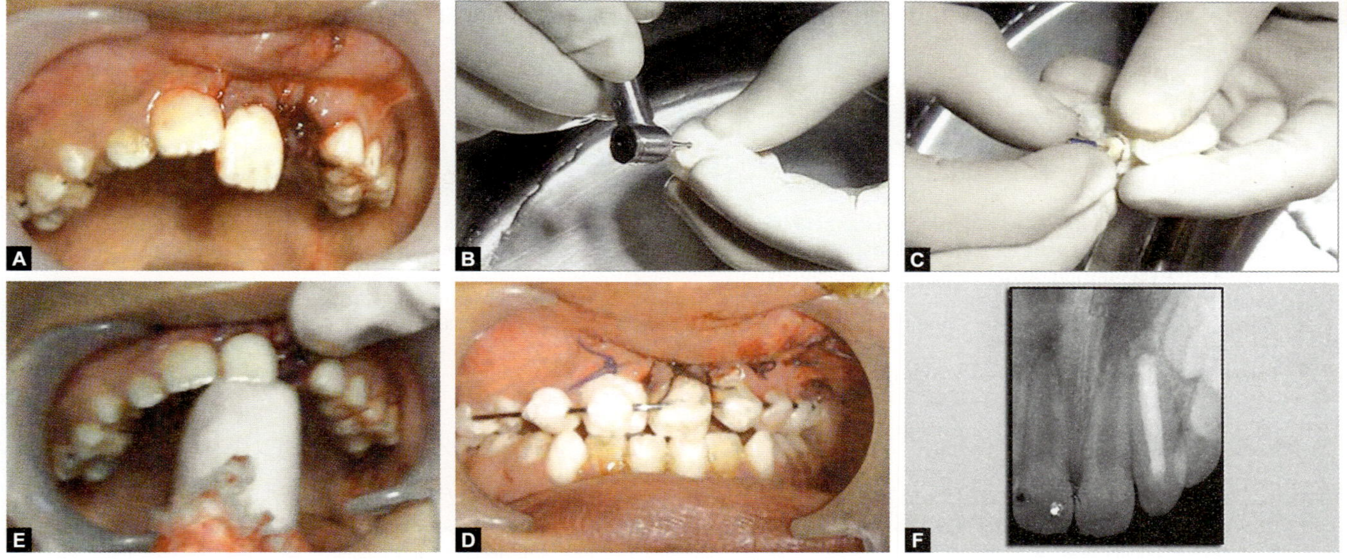

Figs. 63.30A to F: Reimplantation of avulsed tooth: (A) Clinical presentation of case with displacement of 21 and avulsion of 22; (B) Extraoral root canal treatment (RCT) of the avulsed tooth (access opening); (C) Extraoral RCT of the avulsed tooth; (D) Repositioning of 21; (E) Splinting and suturing after reimplantation of 22; (F) Radiographic presentation of tooth following reimplantation and RCT.

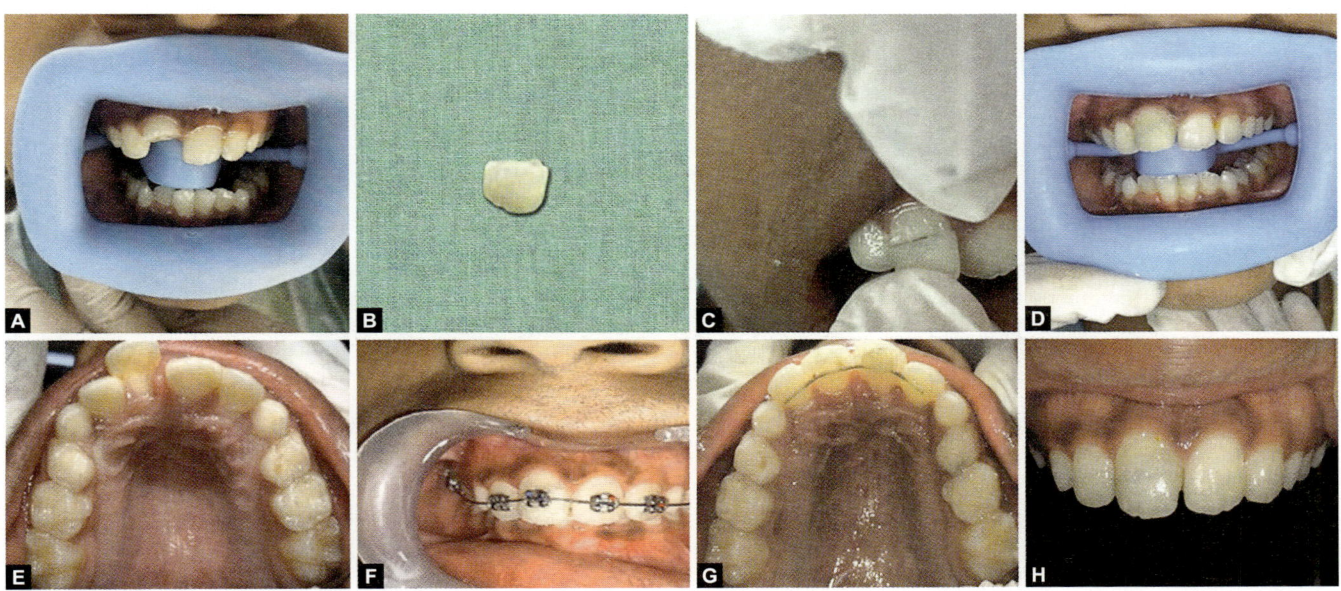

Figs. 63.31A to H: Reattachment of fractured segment irt 11: Patient reported to the Department 45 mins post trauma with the fractured segment irt 11 and pin-point pulpal exposure (A) Clinical presentation of case with class III Ellis fracture irt 11; (B) Fragment of the fractured tooth 11; (C) Repositioning of the fractured fragment irt 11; (D) Cveks pulpotomy followed by fragment reattachment irt 11; (E) Labial displacement of 11 due to trauma; (F and G) 2*4 appliance and lingual soft splint given to stabilize and reposition the traumatized 21. (H) Postoperative front view of maxillary arch.

Management of Avulsion in the Dental Office [According to Dental Clinics of North America (DCNA), 1995] Depending upon the Extraoral Time

- **Preparation of the root:**
  - Extraoral time less than 20 minutes

Open apex	*Closed apex*
• Revascularization of pulp as well as root development is possible • Soak the tooth in 1 mg of doxycycline in 20 mg of physiologic saline for 5 minutes. Doxycycline inhibits bacteria in the pulp lumen thus removing the major obstacle to revascularization • Rinse the root with saline or water without disturbing the PDL fibers and replant tooth gently into the socket • Follow-up visit every month till apex is closed	• Revitalization is not possible but because the tooth was dry less than 20 minutes chances of PDL attachment is excellent • Rinse the root with saline or water without disturbing the PDL fibers and replant tooth gently into the socket

  - Extraoral time 20–60 minutes

Open apex	*Closed apex*
• Soak the tooth in appropriate medium like saline or Hank's balanced salt solution (HBSS) solution for 30 minutes • This reduces the ankylosis. Survival of the remaining PDL cells get improved • Necrotic cells and debris including bacteria float off the root during the soaking period leaving less stimulus for inflammation when tooth is replanted • Additional soaking in doxycycline for 5 minutes also helpful • Follow-up every month • Endodontic treatment done in later stages if pain or swelling occurs	• Soak the tooth in appropriate medium like saline or HBSS solution for 30 minutes • This reduces the ankylosis. Survival of the remaining PDL cells get improved • Necrotic cells and debris including bacteria float off the root during the soaking period leaving less stimulus for inflammation when tooth is replanted • Additional soaking in doxycycline for 5 minutes also helpful • Follow-up every month

  - Extraoral time more than 60 minutes

Open apex	*Closed apex*
• When the root is dried more than 1 hour, soaking in the storage medium is not effective as almost all periodontal cells would have been died • In this condition, root should be prepared to be resistant to resorption • Soak the tooth in citric acid for 5 minutes followed by 2% stannous fluoride for 5 minutes and later in doxycycline for 5 minutes • Perform the endodontic treatment extraorally • After completing RCT seal the blunderbuss open apex extraorally and replant the tooth gently into the socket • Follow-up visit is must every month for the first 6 months later once in 6 months	• When the root is dried more than 1 hour, soaking in the storage medium is not effective as almost all periodontal cells would have been died • In this condition, root should be prepared to be resistant to resorption • Soak the tooth in citric acid for 5 minutes followed by 2% stannous fluoride for 5 minutes and later in doxycycline for 5 minutes • Perform the endodontic treatment extraorally • Follow-up visit is must every month for the first 6 months later once in 6 months

- Preparation of the socket:
  - Socket plays negligible role in onset of complication after avulsion and should be left undisturbed till replantation of the tooth
  - Just before replantation
- Socket should be slightly aspirated if blood clot is present
- If alveolar bone is collapsed a blunt instrument is inserted carefully into the socket and wall is repositioned followed by replantation of the tooth

FOLLOW-UPS AND DETECTION OF POST-TRAUMATIC COMPLICATIONS

Follow-ups are mandatory after traumatic injuries. Each follow-up should include questioning of the patient about any signs or symptoms, plus clinical and radiographic examinations and pulp sensibility testing. Photographic documentation is strongly recommended. The main post-traumatic complications are as follows: pulp necrosis and infection, pulp space obliteration, several types of root resorption, breakdown of marginal gingiva and bone. Early detection and management of complications improves prognosis.

CORE OUTCOME SET

The International Association for Dental Traumatology (IADT) recently developed a core outcome set (COS) for traumatic dental injuries (TDIs) in children and adults. This is one of the first COS developed in dentistry and is underpinned

Table 63.3: Core outcome set.

	2W	*4W*	*6–8 W*	*3M*	*4M*	*6M*	*1Y*	*Yearly upto atleast 5 Y*	*Generic outcomes to consider collecting as identified by the core outcome set*	*Injury-specific outcomes to consider collecting as identified by the core outcome set*
Infraction	No follow up									
Enamel fracture			*R				*R		Periodontal healing (including bone loss, gingival recession, mobility, and ankylosis/resorption)	Quality of restoration
Enamel/dentin fracture			*R				*R			Loss of restoration
Crown fracture			*R	*R		*R	*R		Pulp healing (including infection)[#]	
Crown/root fracture			*R	*R		*R	*R	*R	Pain Discoloration	Quality of restoration Loss of restoration
Root fracture (apical third, mid-third)		*S*R	*R		*R	*R	*R		Tooth loss Quality of life (days off work, school, and sport)	Root fracture repair
Root fracture (cervical third)		*R	*R		*S*R	*R	*R	*R	Esthetics (patient perception)	
Alveolar fracture		*S*R	*R		*R	*R	*R	*R	Number of clinic visits	Infra-occlusion
Concussion		*R					*R		Periodontal healing (including bone loss, gingival recession, mobility, and ankylosis/resorption)	
Subluxation	(*S) *R			*R		*R	*R		Pulp healing (including infection)[#]	
Extrusion	*S*R	*R	*R	*R		*R	*R	*R	Pain	Infra-occlusion
Lateral luxation	*R	*S*R	*R	*R		*R	*R	*R	Discoloration	
Intrusion	*R	(*S) *R	*R	*R		*R	*R	*R	Tooth loss Quality of life (days off work, school, and sport) Aesthetics (patient perception)	Infra-occlusion Realignment—where spontaneous repositioning undertaken
Avulsion (mature tooth)	*S*R	*R		*R		*R	*R	*R	Trauma-related dental anxiety	Infra-occlusion
Avulsion (immature tooth)	*S*R	*R	*R	*R		*R	*R	*R	Number of clinic visits	

Note: At these follow-up visits consider collecting the generic and injury-specific outcomes as identified by the Core Outcome Set—Kenny et al., Dent Traumatol 2018.

* = clinical review appointment

S = splint removal

R = radiograph advised even if no clinical signs or symptoms

[#] = for immature permanent teeth with necrotic and infected pulps, consider the following additional outcomes: root length, root width, and late stage crown fracture.

(*Source:* Levin L, Day PF, Hicks L, et al. International Association of Dental Traumatology guidelines for the management of traumatic dental injuries: General introduction. Dent Traumatol. 2020; 36: 309-13).

by a systematic review of the outcomes used in the trauma literature and follows a robust consensus methodology. Some outcomes were identified as recurring throughout the different injury types. These outcomes were then identified as "generic" (i.e., relevant to all TDIs). Injury-specific outcomes were also determined as those outcomes related only to one or more individual TDIs. Additionally, the study established what, how, when, and by whom these outcomes should be measured. The table below shows the generic and injury specific outcomes to be recorded at the follow-up review appointments recommended for the different traumatic injuries **(Table 63.3)**.

STORAGE MEDIA FOR AVULSED TEETH

A variety of factors such as age of the individual, width and length of the root canal, stage of root development≠--≠, mechanical damage during trauma and reimplantation, type of splinting, mastication, treatment of the socket, endodontic treatment, antibiotics, time of reimplantation, macroscopic contamination, storage media, and storage period are important and can influence the clinical success of reimplantation. To achieve a successful functional outcome, it is recommended to store the avulsed teeth in an interim storage medium, in cases of delayed reimplantation.

Effect of Storage Media on Periodontal Healing

Teeth are usually subjected to a period of desiccation between their avulsion and reimplantation. Therefore, it is desirable to reimplant the avulsed tooth as quickly as possible to ensure maximal viability of PDL cells attached to the root surface. As dry storage is detrimental to the preservation of the PDL, the avulsed tooth must be prevented from drying by the use of storage media of correct osmolarity and pH.

Andreasen (1981), observed that even 30 minutes of dry storage elicited greater inflammatory resorption compared with saline and saliva storage. **Hammarström** 1986, used logistic regression analysis and confirmed that the treatment of avulsed teeth stored in saliva, milk, or saline was more successful than those that were allowed to dry. **Patil** 1994, showed that extracted teeth stored dry for 120 minutes exhibited significantly lower viable PDL cells per tooth than teeth that were stored wet prior to PDL cell collection. Also with nonphysiological storage, the chances of pulpal revascularization are minimal. Therefore, in cases where an immediate reimplantation is not feasible, use of a storage medium is prudent to enhance and preserve the vitality of PDL fibroblasts of an avulsed tooth.

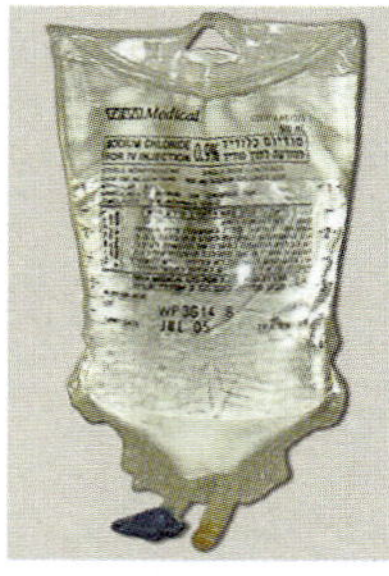

Types of Storage Media

- **Saline solution:**
  - The saline solution provides osmolality of 280 mOsm/kg and despite being compatible to the cells of the PDL, it lacks essential nutrients necessary to the normal metabolic needs of the cells of the PDL.
  - **Blomlöf** (1981), **Courts** 1983, and **Krasner** 1992 have stated that saline solution was harmful to the cells of the PDL in avulsed teeth if it is used for longer than two hours.

Ideal requirements of storage medium
- It should have antimicrobial characteristics.
- It should be able to maintain the viability of periodontal fibers for an acceptable period of time.
- It should favor proliferative capacity of the cells. It should have the same osmolarity as that of body fluids. It should not react with body fluids.
- It should not produce any antigen antibody reactions.
- It should reduce the risk of post-reimplantation root resorption or ankylosis.
- It should have a good shelf-life.
- It should be effective in different climate and under different conditions.
- It should wash off extraneous materials and toxic waste products.
- It should aid in reconstitution of depleted cellular metabolites.

- **Tap water:**
  - It is an unacceptable storage media for avulsed teeth.
  - **Blomlöf** (1981), found that storing cultured human PDL cells in tap water for 1 hour caused more PDL cell damage than the other physiological and nonphysiological storage media tested.
  - They attributed the increased cell damage to the cells lysis caused by the very low osmolarity of tap water.
  - Thus, tap water is not suitable interim storage medium for retaining the viability of PDL cells.

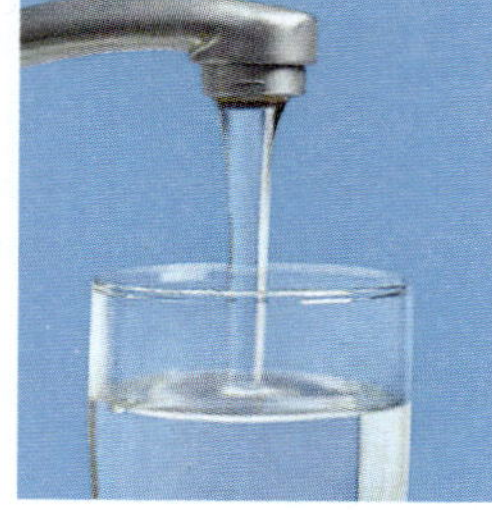

- **Saliva:**
  - It can be used as a storing medium for a short period of time, for it can damage the cells of the PDL if used for longer than an hour.
  - Its osmolality is much lower than the physiologic saline (60–70 mOsm/kg), thus it boosts the harming effects of bacterial contamination
  - Its only advantage is it availability.
- **Milk:**
  - The American Association of Endodontics indicates milk as a solution for avulsed teeth, for keeping the viability of the human cellular PDL
  - Milk is significantly better than other solutions for its physiological properties, including pH and osmolality compatible to those of the cells from the PDL; the easy way of obtaining it and for being free of bacteria, but it is important that it is used in the first 20 minutes after avulsion
  - The favorable results of milk probably occur due to the presence of nutritional substances, such as amino acids, carbohydrates, and vitamins
  - The pasteurization of milk is responsible for diminishing the number of bacteria and bacteriostatic substances, also for the inactive presence of enzymes, which could be potentially harmful to the fibroblasts of the PDL
  - **Blomlöf** (1983) and **Trope** and **Friedman** (1992) recommended milk as an excellent storing solution for 6 hours, however, milk cannot revive the degenerated cells.

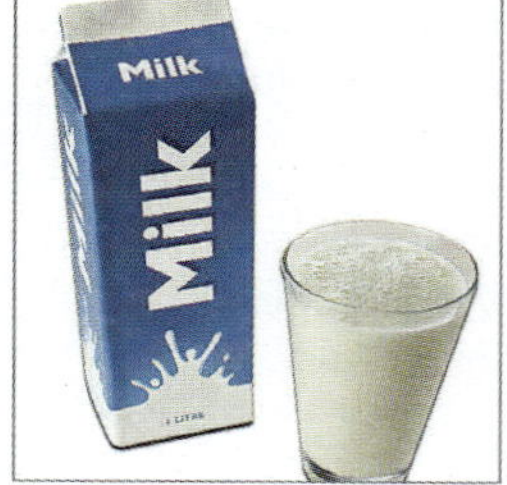

- **Hank's balanced salt solution:**
  - It is a standard saline solution that is widely used in biomedical research to support the growth of many cells types
  - This solution is nontoxic, it is biocompatible with PDL cells, pH balanced at 7.2 and has an osmolality of 320 mOsm/kg
  - It is composed of 8 g/L sodium chloride; 0.4 g/L of D-glucose; 0.4 g/L potassium chloride; 0.35 g/L sodium bicarbonate; 0.09 g/L sodium phosphate; 0.14 g/L potassium phosphate; 0.14 g/L calcium chloride, 0.1 g/L magnesium chloride, and 0.1 g/L magnesium sulfate. It contains ingredients, such as glucose, calcium, and magnesium ions which can sustain and reconstitute the depleted cellular components of the PDL cells.

- It is the best solution for storing avulsed teeth since it does not require refrigeration and it can be kept on the shelf for 2 years and it has been recommended and used successfully as a storage medium by clinicians and researchers.
- It is commercially available as Save-A-Tooth [Pottstown, PA], which has an inner net to receive the avulsed tooth and to minimize cell trauma during transport.

❖ **ViaSpan (DuPont, USA):**

- It is a cold transport organ storage medium that has been suggested for the storage of avulsed teeth.
- Its osmolarity is 320 mOsm/L, with a pH = 7.4, which is ideal for cell growth.
- **Hiltz** and **Trope** (1991), observed ViaSpan to be effective storage medium, with 33% vital cells at 144 hours. Trope reported that replanted dog incisors that were stored in ViaSpan for up to 12 hours showed no signs of replacement or inflammatory resorption. However, since this product is presumably even less available than HBSS, the practicality of using ViaSpan as a storage medium must be considered judiciously.

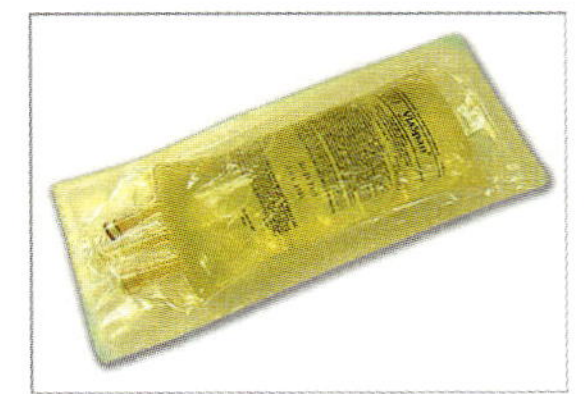

❖ **Gatorade (Quaker Oats Company, USA):**

- It is a transport medium commonly found at sporting events.
- It is a noncarbonated sports drink often consumed by nonathletes as a snack beverage. It contains water, sucrose and glucose, fructose syrups, citric acid, sodium chloride, sodium citrate, monopotassium phosphate, and flavoring/coloring agent.

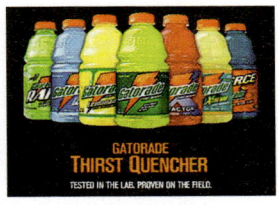

- It has a pH_3 and osmolarity ranging from 280 mOsm/L to 360 mOsm/L.
- Gatorade preserves more viable cells than tap water, but fewer than all other media, both at room temperature and on ice. Therefore, Gatorade can only serve as a storage medium if other more acceptable media are not available, rather than allowing the avulsed tooth to dry out.

❖ **Propolis:**

- It is a sticky resin that seeps from the buds or bark of trees, chiefly conifers. It consists of resin, waxes fatty acids, essential oils, pollen proteins, and other organic compounds and minerals.

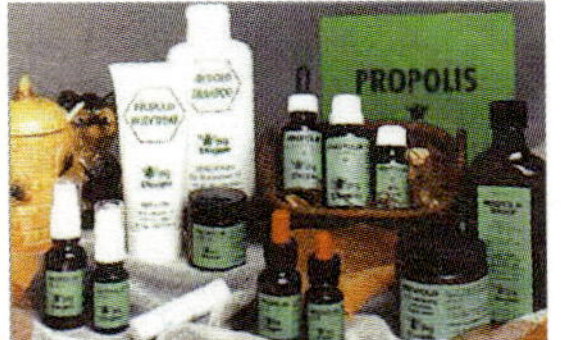

- It has antiseptic, antibiotic, antibacterial, antifungal, antiviral, antioxidant, anticarcinogenic, antithrombotic, and immunomodulatory properties.
- **Margaret** and **Pileggi** (2004), reported that teeth stored in propolis demonstrated the highest viability for PDL cells, when compared with HBSS, milk, and saline.
- **Shaher** (2004), observed that with propolis, the viability of PDL fibroblasts can be maintained for as long as 20 hours. Hence propolis can act as a good alternative natural storage medium for avulsed teeth.

❖ **Contact lens solution:**

- It is a convenient preservation medium for teeth after avulsion injuries as these solutions are available in school or athletic grounds and at home, where most injuries occur.

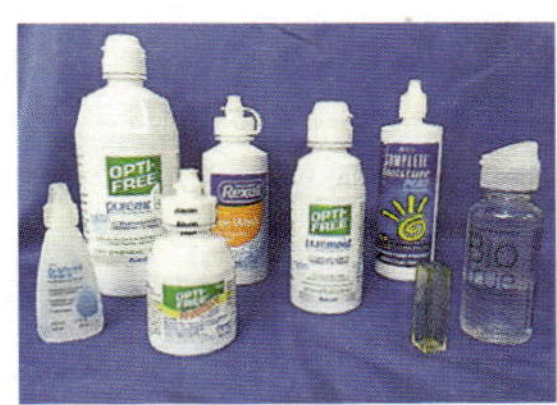

- They contain buffered, isotonic saline solutions with the addition of preservatives that may preserve the viability of PDL cells.
- These solutions preserve significantly more viable cells than tap water and Gatorade, but are not as effective as HBSS and milk.

❖ **Emdogain:**

- According to **Ashkenazi** and **Shaked** (2006), Emdogain diminishes the percentage of fibroblasts of the PDL with capability of forming colonies and that lowers the capability for the fibroblasts to repopulate the dental radicular surface after dental avulsion.

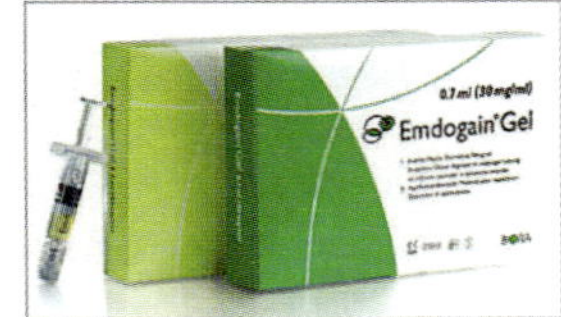

- It can delay, but not stop the development of replacement resorption, one of the worst complications of dental trauma.
- On its own, it is not efficient in the regeneration of injured periodontal tissues of the avulsed tooth.

❖ **Egg white: Khademi** (2008), had compared milk and egg white as solutions for storing avulsed teeth, and the results have shown that teeth stored in egg white for 6–10 hours had a better incidence of repair than those stored in milk for the same amount of time.

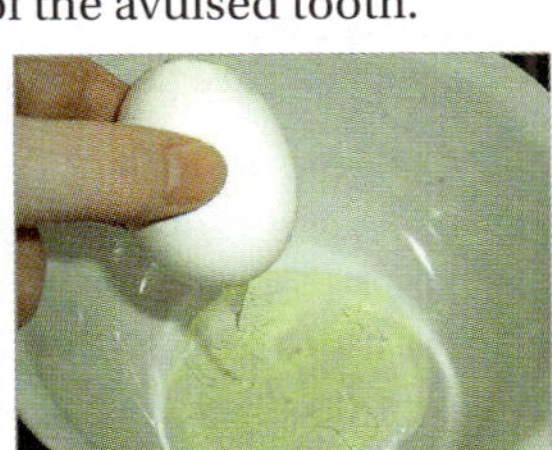

❖ **Eagle's medium:**

- It contains 4 mL of L-glutamine; 10^5 IU/L of penicillin; 100 µg/ mL of streptomycin, 10 µg/mL of nystatin and calf serum [10% v/v].

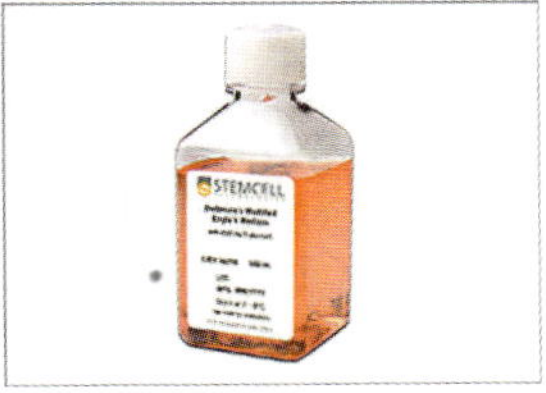

- It has high viability, mitogenic, and clonogenic capacity up to 8 hours of storage at 4°C.
- When the storage time was up to 24 hours, Eagle's medium was less effective than milk or HBSS, which could be attributed to the low temperature [4°C] which may have induced aggregation and thus lowered the cell's functional capacity.

❖ **L-Dopa (levodopa; Sigma chemicals, Perth, Australia):**

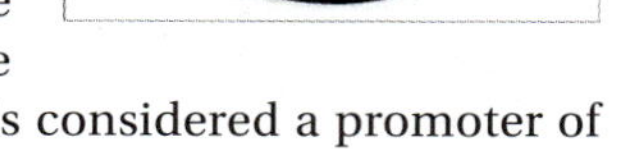

- It is a drug with possible mitogenic effects.
- Levodopa stimulates dopaminergic systems in the anterior portion of the pituitary gland to secrete growth hormone, which is considered a promoter of the healing process.
- Levodopa can also have a local effect on the growth of cells, including the PDL cells and can preserve as a preserving medium for avulsed teeth.

❖ **Coconut water:**

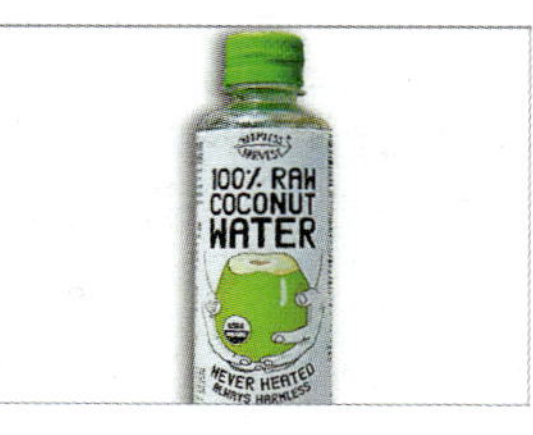

- Biologically pure tender coconut water, which aids in replenishing the fluids, electrolytes, and sugar lost from the body during heavy physical work, has been suggested as a promising storage medium for avulsed teeth.
- **Gopikrishna** (2008), observed coconut water to be superior to HBBS, milk, or propolis in maintaining the viability of PDL cells.

❖ **Green tea extract:** Epigallocatechin-3-gallate [EGCG] is a major polyphenol of green tea, having anti-oxidative, anti-carcinogenic, anti-mutagenic, anti-inflammatory, anti-microbial, and anti-viral activities. Hwang et al., and Jung et al., reported enthusiastic results with green tea, with the maintenance of 90% of cell viability for up to 24 h, similar to the HBSS control.[9] Jung et al. also observed that the higher the extract concentration the more efficient the medium.[10] In view of this, the use of green tea extract and its compounds may be an alternative for the conservation of avulsed teeth and its beneficial effect is enhanced by higher extract concentrations.

❖ **Aloe Vera:** In a study carried out by Badakhsh et al., it was revealed that *A. vera* at a concentration of 10%, 30%, and 50% performed similarly as supplemented culture media for up to 9 h. *A. vera* at this concentration maintained the cell viability over 90% and was superior to 100% *A. vera* and egg white. They recommended *A. vera* as suitable storage media for avulsed teeth.[11]

❖ **Red Mulberry:** Mulberry fruits are used medicinally as a deworming agent, as a remedy for dysentery, as laxative, odon-talgic, expectorant, hypoglycemic, and emetic. Ozan et al. compared four different concentrations of *Myrmica rubra* (4%, 2.5%, 1.5%, and 0.5%) with HBSS andtap water at 1h, 3h, 6h, 12h, and 24h to check the effect on PDL viability. They recommended mulberry as a storage media for the avulsed teeth. They concluded that the number of viable PDL cells was significantly high when an avulsed tooth stored in 4.0% concentrated solution of *M. rubra* as compared to other concentrations.[12]

Tooth Rescue Box[14]

Dentosafe (Miradent, Germany) is the commercial name of a tooth rescue box containing special cell culture medium which is a combination of amino acid, vitamins, and glucose. In the USA, it is marketed as EMT tooth saver (Phoenix, USA). It has demonstrated the maintenance of vitality of PDL cells for 48 h at room temperature. If unopened, this medium has a shelf life of 3 years. Avulsed teeth can be stored in the tooth rescue box for a longer duration, and its early availability can result in an excellent healing prognosis after replantation.

PERIODONTAL HEALING REACTIONS

Immediately after reimplantation a coagulum is formed between two parts of severed PDL. The line of separation is most often situated in the middle of PDL although separation can also occur at the insertion of Sharpey's fibers. Proliferation of connective tissue soon occurs and after 3–4 days, the gap in the PDL is obliterated by young connective tissue. After 1 week, the epithelium is reattached at the cementoenamel junction. This is of clinical importance because it reduces risk of gingival infection and reduced risk of bacterial invasion of root canal via the gingival pocket. After 2 weeks, the split line in the PDL is healed and collagen fibers are seen extending from the cemental surface to alveolar bone. Histologic examination of replanted human teeth has revealed four different healing modalities in PDL.

Healing with a Normal Periodontal Ligament (Fig. 63.32)

Histologically, this is characterized by complete regeneration of PDL, which usually takes place 2–4 weeks to complete. This type of healing will only occur if innermost cell layers along the root surface are vital.

Radiographically, there is normal PDL space without signs of root resorption and clinically tooth is in normal position and a normal percussion tone can be elicited. This type of healing will probably never take place, as tooth avulsion will result in at least minimal injury to innermost layer of PDL.

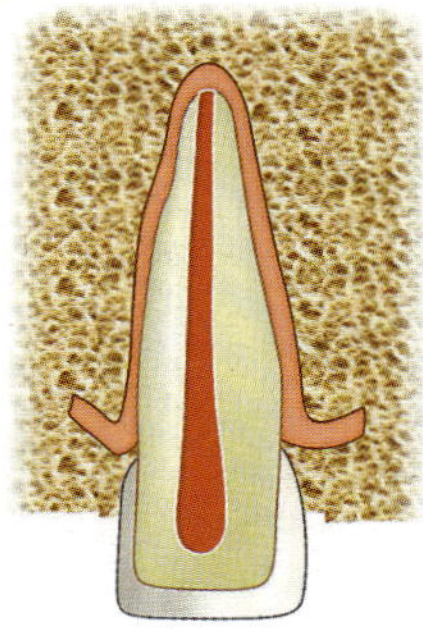

Fig. 63.32: Healing with a normal periodontal ligament.

Healing with Surface Resorption (Fig. 63.33)

Histologically, this type of healing is characterized by localized areas along the root surface, which shows superficial resorption lacunae repaired by new cementum. This surface resorption presumably represents localized areas of damage to PDL or cementum, which is healed by PDL, derived cells. Clinically, the tooth is in normal position and a normal percussion tone can be heard.

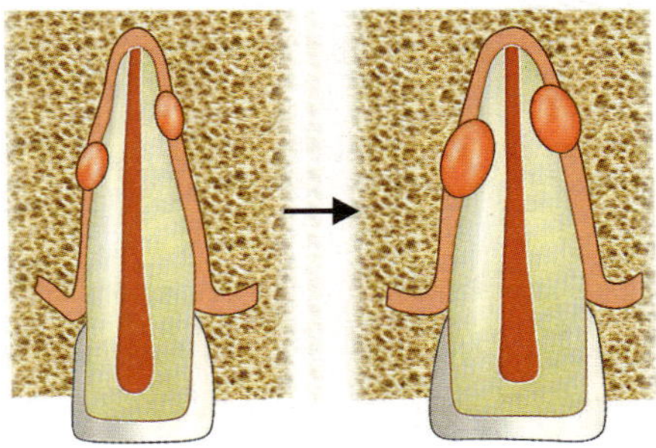

Fig. 63.33: Healing with surface resorption.

Healing with Ankylosis (Replacement Resorption) (Fig. 63.34)

Histologically ankylosis represents a fusion of the alveolar bone and the root surface and can be demonstrated 2 weeks after reimplantation. The etiology of replacement resorption appears to be related to the absence of vital PDL cover on the root surface. Replacement resorption develops in two different directions depending upon the extent of damage to the PDL surface of the root. Progressive replacement resorption, which gradually resorbs the entire root, is always elicited when the entire PDL is removed before reimplantation or after extensive drying of the tooth before reimplantation. It is assumed that the damaged PDL is repopulated from adjacent bone marrow cells, which have osteogenic potential and will consequently form ankylosis. Transient replacement resorption is possibly related to areas of minor damage to the root surface. In these cases, the ankylosis is formed initially and later resorbed by adjacent areas of vital PDL. The ankylosed root becomes part of the normal bone remodeling system and is gradually replaced by bone. After some time little of tooth substance remains, at this stage the resorptive process are usually intensified along the surface of the root canal filling a phenomenon known as tunneling resorption.

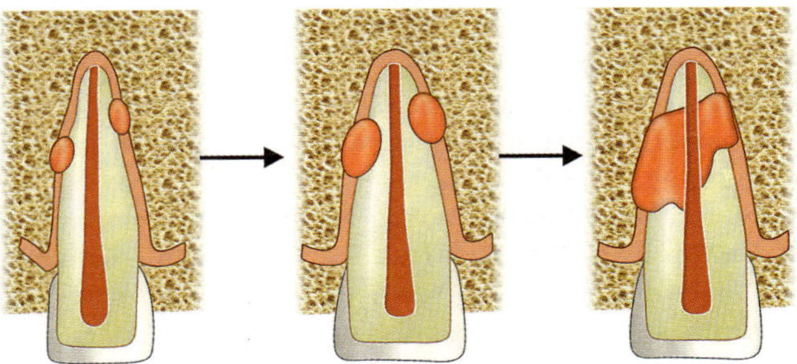

Fig. 63.34: Healing by replacement resorption.

Healing with Inflammatory Resorption (Fig. 63.35)

Histologically inflammatory resorption is characterized by bowl-shaped resorption cavities in cementum and dentin associated with inflammatory changes in the adjacent periodontal space. Pathogenesis is that minor injuries to PDL and cementum due to trauma or contamination with bacteria induce small resorption cavities on the root surface. If these resorption cavities expose dentinal tubules and root canal contains infected necrotic tissue, toxins from these areas will penetrate along dentinal tubules to lateral periodontal tissue and provoke an inflammatory response. This in turn will intensify the resorption process, which advances towards root canal, and within a few months entire root can be resorbed. Radiographically inflammatory resorption is characterized by radiolucent bowl-shaped cavitations along root surface with corresponding excavations in adjacent bone. Clinically, the replanted tooth is loose, extruded, and sensitive to percussion with dull tone.

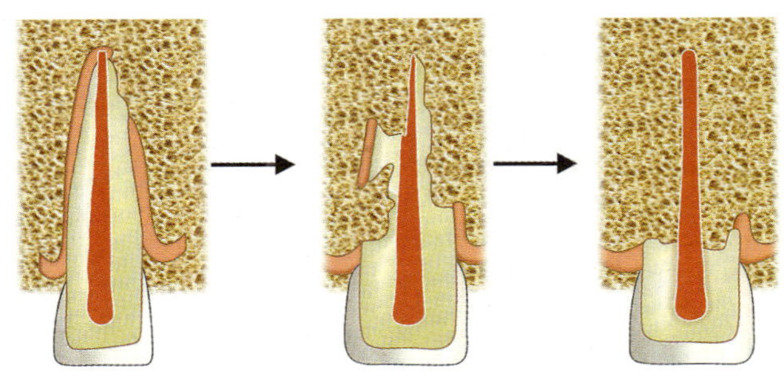

Fig. 63.35: Healing by inflammatory resorption.

SPLINTING

A splint has been defined as "a rigid or flexible device that maintains in position a displaced or movable part; also used to keep in place and protect an injured part".

Rationale for Tooth Stabilization and Splinting

Biologic rationale for splinting:

- Rest
- Redistribution of forces
- Preservation of arch integrity
- Restoration of functional stability
- Psychological well-being.

Clinical rationale for tooth stabilization and splinting:

- Occlusal therapy
- Effects of splinting
- Implant and treatment planning paradigm shift.

Indications for Splinting

- To stabilize moderate-to-advanced tooth mobility that cannot be treated by any other means.
- To stabilize teeth in secondary occlusal trauma
- To stabilize teeth when increased tooth mobility interferes with normal masticatory function and comfort of the patient
- To prevent tipping or drifting of teeth
- To stabilize teeth following orthodontic movement
- To create adequate occlusal stability when replacing missing teeth
- To prevent extrusion of unopposed teeth
- To stabilize teeth following acute trauma.

Contraindications for Splinting

- When there is moderate-to-severe increased tooth mobility in the presence of periodontal inflammation and/or primary occlusal trauma
- Prior occlusal adjustment has not been done on teeth with occlusal interference and occlusal trauma
- When there are insufficient numbers of immobile teeth to adequately stabilize the mobile teeth
- Oral hygiene maintenance is inadequate.

Classification of Splinting

According to Ross, Wiesgold and Wright (1968):

- **Temporary stabilization:**
  - Removable extracoronal splints
  - Fixed extracoronal splints
  - Intracoronal splints
  - Etched metal resin-bonded splints
- **Provisional stabilization:**
  - Acrylic splints
  - Metal-band-and-acrylic splints
- **Long-term stabilization:**
  - Removable splints
  - Fixed splints
  - Combination removable and fixed splints

According to Grant (1988):

- **Temporary:**
  - *External (extracoronal)*
    - Ligature splint
    - Enamel bonding material
    - Welded band splints
    - Continuous splints
    - Night guards
  - *Internal (intracoronal)*
    - Acrylic splints
    - Composite splints
    - Acrylic full crown.
- **Provisional splinting:** Serves to stabilize a permanently mobile dentition from the time of initial tooth preparation until the time the dentition is periodontally stable enough for permanent restorations.
- **Permanent splints:**
  - *Removable (external)*
    - Continuous clasp devices
    - Swing lock devices
    - Over denture
  - *Fixed internal*
    - Full coverage
    - 3/4 crowns and inlays
    - Posts in root canals
    - Horizontal pin splints
- **Cast metal resin bonded fixed partial denture (FPD) (Maryland splints):**
  - *Combined*
    - Partial dentures and splinted abutments
    - Removable fixed splints
    - Full or partial dentures on splinted roots
    - Fixed bridges incorporated in partial dentures seated on posts and copings.
  - Endodontic.

Procedure for Composite Splinting

The teeth to be splinted are repositioned together with crowns of adjacent teeth which act as a support for the splint

↓

Orthodontic wire of desired gauged is selected and required length is taken and fabricated so that it will include at least one abutment tooth on either side

↓

Middle 1/3rd of the crown is etched with 37% phosphoric acid for 30 seconds followed by application of bonding agent

↓

Small blob of composite resin is placed on the bonded area. Place the wire on the composite and cure it. Curing procedure should start from one end to other and the tooth to be splinted should be cured at the last

↓

Composite resin can be added to ensure that the wire is secured and is cured

TRAUMA TO PRIMARY DENTITION

Injuries to the primary dentition are estimated to affect 30% of preschool children. Trauma often occurs in this population because young children tend to be unstable on their feet as they first start to walk and then in running around with their newfound mobility. The roots of the primary teeth are in close relationship to the developing permanent successors and an acute impact can easily be transmitted to the developing permanent dentition. The most serious primary tooth injuries in term of damage to the permanent successor are intrusion, avulsions (52%), extrusions, and subluxation (each 34%). The treatment strategy following injury in the primary dentition is therefore dictated by concern for the safety of the permanent dentition.

Treatment should be organized in order, first to relieve the child of pain or discomfort and then restore the dentition, keeping the prognosis of the permanent successor foremost in the mind. As primary tooth trauma usually occurs in the very young child, cooperation is the main problem. It may be necessary after initial examination to advise the parents regarding analgesia, soft diet, and oral hygiene, and then arrange to review the child following week when he or she is less upset. This is particularly relevant if it is the child's first dental experience.

- **Enamel infraction:** No treatment
- **Enamel fracture:** Restoration with composite and selective grinding
- **Enamel and dentin fracture:** $Ca(OH)_2$ and restoration
- **Enamel and dentin fracture with pulp exposure:** Pulpotomy, if root resorption is advanced then extraction.
- **Concussion and luxation:** If the luxation injury is slight and the tooth is not at risk of coming out of the socket spontaneously, then it can be left and advice regarding soft diet and careful oral hygiene instruction given. If the tooth has been luxated palatally it might be possible to gently reposition and splint it manually, but only if the displacement is less than 2 mm. If the tooth has been displaced by more than 2 mm extraction may be more appropriate in such cases.

- **Intrusion:** If the intruded tooth is not obstructing the permanent successor then allow it to erupt on its own and if it is obstructing then it is best to extract. The approach to treatment for these teeth is largely to establish where they are in the alveolus and then to leave them alone. If less than three-quarters of the crown is intruded then the tooth can be allowed to re-erupt spontaneously. Normally, this occurs within 2–4 months after injury. If more than three-quarters of the crown has intruded, the tooth may cause symptoms such as pain and the tooth may require extraction.
- **Extrusion:** Extrusion injuries, which occur in the primary dentition, usually interfere with the occlusion; therefore extraction is often indicated.
- **Root fracture:** Because of short roots primary root fractures are unusual. The location of a root fracture in primary teeth usually determines the outcome. Fractures in the apical third of the root have best prognosis. If the incisal segment is stable the tooth is maintained. The tooth usually remains vital and resorbs normally. Fractures in the middle third of primary root are usually vey mobile and should be extracted. Exercise care when removing the root segment to avoid damaging the permanent developing tooth bud. If the fracture line is infrabony and the pulpal tissue is vital, the root tip does not always have to be removed; however, it has to be monitored radiographically to ensure proper resorption of root tip and eruption of permanent tooth.
- **Displacement:** According to many authors (**Andreason JO, Andreason FM, Camp JH,** and **Mc Tigue DJ**) displacement is most frequent injury to primary dentition. Displacement occurs more frequently than crown or root fractures because of the resiliency of the alveolar bone and the short tooth roots (Andreason JO). Because of fear of damage to the developing permanent teeth, some authors recommend the extraction of all displaced primary teeth (Mc Tigue), whereas some authors (Andreason and Andreason) advise retaining the displaced teeth until need indicates a need to remove them. It is suggested by Harding that teeth that cannot be repositioned or that interfere with the occlusion should probably be removed.
- **Avulsion:** The maxillary central incisors are more frequently avulsed than other primary teeth (Andreason JO). The first and most important step is to locate the entire exarticulated teeth to rule out intrusion or displacement into the soft tissues. The avulsed tooth should be examined to determine that the entire crown root is present. Avulsed primary teeth are not reimplanted. A high failure rate because of pulp necrosis, infection, and possible damage to the permanent dentition are given as reasons (Andreason JO and Andreason FM).

EFFECT OF TRAUMATIC INJURIES ON DEVELOPING DENTITION

Traumatic injuries to developing teeth can influence their growth and maturation, usually leaving a child with a permanent and often readily visible deformity. The close relationship between the apices of primary teeth and developing permanent successors explains why injuries to primary teeth are easily transmitted to the permanent dentition. Anatomic and histological deviations due to injuries to developing teeth can be classified as follows:

- White or yellow brown discoloration of enamel.
- White or yellow brown discoloration of enamel with circular enamel hypoplasia.
- Crown dilacerations.
- Odontoma like malformation.
- Root duplication.
- Vestibular root angulation.
- Lateral root angulation or dilacerations.
- Partial or complete arrest of root formation.
- Sequestration of permanent tooth germs.
- Disturbance in eruption.

White or Yellow Brown Discoloration of Enamel

These lesions appear as sharply demarcated stained enamel opacities most often located on the facial surface of the crown. Their extent varies from small spots to large fields. The frequency of these lesions has been reported to be 23% following injuries to primary dentition commonly affecting maxillary incisors. Radiographic examination prior to tooth eruption will usually not reveal defective mineralization; consequently these disturbances will be diagnosed clinically after tooth eruption.

White or Yellow Brown Discoloration of Enamel with Circular Enamel Hypoplasia

These lesions are a more severe manifestation of trauma sustained during the formative stages of permanent tooth germ. Typical finding in this group, which distinguishes these lesions from those in first group, is a narrow horizontal groove, which encircles the crown cervically to the discolored areas. The frequency of this type of change has been reported to be 12% following injuries to the primary dentition. It is assumed that the displaced primary tooth traumatize tissue adjacent to permanent tooth germ and possibly odontogenic epithelium therefore interfering with final mineralization of enamel.

Crown Dilaceration

These malformations are due to traumatic nonaxial displacement of already formed hard tissue in relation to the developing soft tissues.

Odontoma like Malformations

The type of injury affecting the primary dentition appears to be intrusive luxation or avulsion. These cases show a conglomerate of hard tissue having morphology of complex odontoma or separate tooth element.

Root Duplication

This is a rare occurrence seen after intrusive luxation of primary teeth. The pathology of these cases indicates that a traumatic division of the cervical loop occurs at the time of injury resulting in formation of two separate roots.

Vestibular Root Angulation

This developmental disturbance appears as a marked curvature confined to the root as the result of an injury. The malformed tooth is usually impacted and crown palpable in labial sulcus. Histopathologic findings in these cases consist of a thickening of cementum in the area of angulation, but with no sign of acute traumatic changes. Incisor can present an obstacle in the eruption of developing tooth forcing it to change its path of eruption in a labial direction and presumably HERS remains in the same position despite the impact and thereby creates a curvature of root.

Lateral Root Angulation

These changes appear as a mesial or distal bending confined to the root of the tooth. In contrast to vestibular angulation most teeth with lateral root angulation or dilacerations erupt spontaneously.

Partial or Complete Arrest of Root Formation

This is a rare complication among injuries in primary dentition affecting 2% of involved permanent teeth due to avulsion of primary incisors. A number of teeth with this type of root malformation remain impacted while others have inadequate periodontal support. In some instances, a typical calciotraumatic line separating hard tissue formed before and after injury is seen. In these cases, trauma directly injures HERS thus compromising normal root development.

Sequestration of Permanent Tooth Germs

In case of jaw fractures infection can complicate healing sometimes leading to spontaneous sequestration of involved tooth germs.

Disturbances in Eruption

Disturbances in permanent tooth eruption may occur after trauma to the primary dentition and this is related to abnormal changes in the connective tissue overlying the tooth germ. The eruption of succeeding permanent incisors is generally delayed after premature loss of primary incisor. Early loss of primary incisors causes ectopic eruption of permanent incisors due to lack of eruption guidance otherwise offered by primary dentition.

Research regarding dental traumatology

- **Oikarinen et al.** in 1987 conducted a survey and found that among all the reasons, falls (64.46%) was the most common one. Falls happened while playing sports, chasing each other, walking unguardedly, walking along swimming pool, and slipping under raining or snowing. Most injuries occurred outdoors (51.17%). Most indoor injuries happened at school.
- **Ge L et al.** in 2005 conducted a study and concluded that the most common type of injury was crown fracture without pulp exposure, composing 37.3% of total injuries. Next was crown fracture with pulp exposure, the proportion of which was 33.9%. No difference of patient distribution was observed in other trauma types.
- **Onetto JE et al.** in 1994 conducted a study and concluded that the highest occurrence of dental injury was found in the age interval of 9–10 years of age. This could be attributed to the fact that children are usually more active in this period of life and often lack motoric coordination because of their developmental stage, for this reason they cannot precisely evaluate velocity and danger.
- According to **Castro JC et al.** in 2005, the most frequently affected teeth were maxillary anterior teeth (97.07%), 54.49% of which had only one tooth involved, 31.45% had both central incisors injured.
- **Bhavya DP et al.** in 2013 conducted a cross-sectional survey on traumatic injuries in the primary teeth and concluded that enamel fracture (55.6%) was most prevalent type of dental trauma, followed by dentine fracture (9.6%), and least prevalent were fractures involving pulp (2%) and tooth discoloration (3.6%).
- In a study evaluating traumatized permanent incisors, Andreasen found that when intrusion occurred in teeth with closed apices, pulp necrosis was present in 100% of the cases, whereas for teeth with open apices this rate decreased to 62.5%. Thus, in cases of closed apices, endodontic intervention should be initiated as early as possible, to prevent inflammatory external root resorption.
- Luxative intrusion is a serious kind of injury of maxillary incisors and such an occurrence is found to be most frequent between 6 years and 12 years of age and generally affecting 1.9% of traumatic injuries involving permanent teeth.
- **Blomlof et al.** found that storing cultured human PDL cells in tap water for 1 hour caused more PDL cell damage than the other physiological and nonphysiological storage media tested. They attributed the increased cell damage to the cell lysis caused by the very low osmolarity of tap water.
- **Cvek et al.** found that avulsed teeth soaked in an isotonic saline for 30 minutes before replantation showed less resorption than those stored dry between 15 minutes and 40 minutes. They proposed that if an avulsed tooth has been kept dry for more than 15 minutes, it should be stored in an isotonic saline solution for about 30 minutes before replantation, presuming that PDL cells might be reconstituted or reconditioned by this procedure.
- **Gopikrishna et al.** observed that coconut water was superior to HBSS, milk, or propolis in maintaining the viability of PDL cells. Gopikrishna et al have recently reported that coconut water had a greater capacity to maintain cell viability when compared to propolis, HBSS, and milk.
- The ViaSpan (Belzer VW-CSS, Du Pont Pharmaceuticals, and Wilmington, DE, USA) is a medium used for the transportation of organs which are going to be transplanted and it has been very effective for storing avulsed teeth. ViaSpan has osmolality of 320 mOsm/kg and pH is around 7.4 at room temperature; ideal for the cellular growth. Hiltz and Trope have compared the vitality of lip fibroblasts, at room temperature which were stored in milk, HBSS, and ViaSpan. Hiltz and Trope observed ViaSpan to be an effective storage medium, with 33% vital cells at 144 hours. The ViaSpan was the best storage medium observed at all times, and after 18 hours, there was still 37.6% of living cells.
- **Mendonça DHDS et al.** in 2012 reported that esthetic and functional rehabilitation with direct composite resin is a viable option for the conservative treatment of fractured anterior teeth having an oblique crown fracture with extensive involvement of the incisal angle, without pulp exposure.

- **Fidel SR et al.** in 2011 presented a case report which describes the treatment of a complicated crown-root fracture in the maxillary left central incisor with a wide open apex of a 10-year-old male patient, due to fall from his own height by performing cervical pulpotomy and adhesive tooth fragment reattachment which showed pulp necrosis and an associated periapical lesion after 1 year. Endodontic therapy with calcium hydroxide base intracanal dressing, root canal filling, and orthodontic extrusion were performed and the tooth was restored with a post-core system and a prosthetic crown.
- **Sahebi S et al.** in 2011 reported the clinical management of crown-root fracture in maxillary central incisors, which was successfully treated by forceps eruption with 180° rotation to restore the biological width. Follow-up for 18 months showed normal function and no inflammatory root resorption of the replanted tooth.
- **Kambalimath et al.** in 2015 presented a case report in which management of an avulsed primary canine in a 7-year-old was done by extraoral intentional metapex pulpectomy and reimplantation followed by splinting. Follow-up of 7 and 21 days confirmed the immobilization.
- **Acharya et al.** in 2017 reported a case of 3-year-old child with an avulsed primary left lateral incisor and displacement of primary right lateral incisor, primary central incisor and fractured alveolar bone. Semirigid splinting was done in respect to the traumatic teeth after reimplantation.
- **Kapur et al** in 2014 presented a case report of a 3-year-old patient with avulsion of primary central incisor, which was managed by a multiflex wire and composite splint for stabilization. Reimplantation was done after pulpectomy was performed.
- **Prabhakar AR et al.** in 2016 compared the fracture resistance of incisor tooth fragments stored in four storage media: (1) dry air, (2) milk, (3) coconut water, or (4) egg white before reattaching them with G-aenial Universal Flo and concluded that along with milk, coconut water which is being tested for time can be considered a viable alternative.
- **Shanmugam HV et al.** in 2011 reported a case which provided a brief insight into surgical repositioning as an alternative treatment option for the management of intruded primary tooth in a 4-year-old girl.
- **Arikan V et al.** in 2010 reviewed that the majority of trauma occurred between the ages of 2 and 4. The most common type of injury was lateral luxation (33.3%). Most injuries (33.3%) presented during May. The most common form of treatment was follow-up only (39.4%), followed by extraction (29.3%) and RCT (12.1%).

POINTS TO REMEMBER

- Prevalence of trauma in primary dentition is 11–30% with more predilection for boys in ages 2–4 years and 9–10 years. Most frequent teeth involved are upper central incisors and the most common injury is luxation or displacement.
- The extent of trauma is governed by four factors: (1) energy of impact, (2) resilience of impacting object, (3) shape of impacting object, and (4) direction of impacting force.
- Type of fracture: Class I: Enamel fracture; Class II: Enamel and dentin fracture; Class III: Enamel and dentin fracture exposing dental pulp; Class IV: The traumatized tooth that becomes nonvital; Class V: Avulsion; Class VI: Fracture of the root; Class VII: Displacement of tooth; Class VIII: Fracture of crown en masse; and Class IX: Traumatic injuries of primary teeth.
- Uncomplicated crown fractures are characterized by fracture of crown involving enamel and dentin without pulp exposure. Immediate provisional treatment—place $Ca(OH)_2$ on the exposed dentin and restore and permanent treatment—reattachment of the crown fragment, restoration with composite resin or full coverage crown.
- Complicated crown fracture is when there is a fracture of enamel, dentin along with exposure of pulp. The type of treatment will depend upon the extent and time of pulp exposure. When the exposure is small and pulp has not been exposed for more than 4–5 minutes then it is advisable to do pulp capping. When the exposure is large and pulp has been exposed for more than 5 minutes then it is ideal to do pulpotomy/RCT.
- Root fractures are relatively uncommon in primary dentition. For radiographic diagnosis of root fracture the central beam is directed within a maximum range of 15–20° of fracture plane. When fracture is present in the middle third—extraction; when fracture is in apical third—obturation till the possible working length and apical surgery to remove the fragment and when fracture is near to gingival margin— orthodontic or surgical extrusion of the fragment followed by immobilization and later crown fabrication.
- Concussion is an injury to tooth supporting structures, when there is some crushing injury to apical vasculature and periodontal ligament with resultant inflammatory edema with marked reaction to percussion, but without abnormal loosening or displacement and subluxation is an injury to tooth supporting structures with abnormal loosening, but without clinically or radiographically demonstrable displacement of the tooth. Intrusion is the term used to describe displacement of tooth into alveolar bone, which is accompanied by fracture or crushing of alveolar bone so the crown appears shorter. The treatment lines for the management of intrusion depend on the degree of intrusion which has taken place. In case of minor (1–2 mm) of intrusion it is best to wait up to 3 months for spontaneous eruption to occur before initiating any type of treatment. In case of severe intrusion the two best mentioned approaches are orthodontic and surgical extrusion.
- Avulsion is the term used to describe complete displacement of tooth from its alveolus. Treatment is reimplantation which depends on extraoral time. If extra-alveolar storage time is short, the teeth is reimplanted back and then according to apical closure next step is performed (if apical foramen is not closed—endodontic therapy is delayed till first signs of apical closure are seen and if apical foramen is closed—endodontic therapy is done after 1–2 weeks depending on type of reimplantation). In case of long extra-alveolar storage time the teeth is cleaned, treated, and reimplanted after performing extraoral RCT.
- Different types of storage media are saline solution, tap water, saliva, milk, HBSS, ViaSpan, Gatorade, propolis, contact lens solution, Emdogain, egg white, Eagle's medium, L-Dopa, and coconut water.
- Effect of trauma on developing dentition is white or yellow brown discoloration of enamel, crown dilacerations, odontoma like malformation, root duplication, vestibular root angulation, lateral root angulation, arrest of root formation, sequestration of permanent tooth germs, and disturbance in eruption.
- In case of primary tooth if the displaced tooth is not obstructing the permanent successor then allow it to erupt on its own and if it is obstructing then it is best to extract. In case of avulsion reimplantation is contraindicated.

Questionnaire

1. Enumerate some of the classifications of traumatic injury and explain in detail Andreasen's classification.
2. Explain Ellis and Davey classification and give the management of Class IV injury.
3. Classify and explain the management of root fractures.
4. Give detailed management of luxation injuries.
5. What is avulsion? Give an explanation of its management in dental office with reference to reimplantation.
6. Explain the different types of available storage media.
7. Write a note on splinting.
8. What are the healing reactions after avulsion injury?
9. Describe trauma to primary dentition.

REFERENCES

1. Tewari N, Mathur VP, Siddiqui I, Morankar R, Verma AR, Pandey RM. Prevalence of traumatic dental injuries in India: A systematic review and meta-analysis. Indian J Dent Res. 2020;31(4):601-14.
2. Narayanan SP, Rath H, Panda A, Mahapatra S, Kader RH. Prevalence, Trends, and Associated Risk Factors of Traumatic Dental Injury among Children and Adolescents in India: A Systematic Review and Meta-analysis. J Contemp Dent Pract. 2021;22(10):1206-24.
3. Bourguignon, C, Cohenca, N, Lauridsen, E, et al. International Association of Dental Traumatology guidelines for the management of traumatic dental injuries: 1. Fractures and luxations. Dent Traumatol. 2020; 36: 314-30.
4. Fulling HJ, Andreasen JO. Influence of maturation status and tooth type of permanent teeth upon electrometric and thermal pulp testing. Scand J Dent Res. 1976; 84:286-90.
5. Gopikrishna V, Tinagupta K, Kandaswamy D. Comparison of electrical, thermal, and pulse oximetry methods for assessing pulp vitality in recently traumatized teeth. J Endod. 2007; 33:531-5.
6. Bastos JV, Goulart EM, de Souza Cortes MI. Pulpal response to sensibility tests after traumatic dental injuries in permanent teeth. Dent Traumatol. 2014; 30:188-92.
7. Alghaithy RA, Qualtrough AJ. Pulp sensibility and vitality tests for diagnosing pulpal health in permanent teeth: a critical review. Int Endod J. 2017; 50:135-42.
8. Gopikrishna V, Tinagupta K, Kandaswamy D. Evaluation of efficacy of a new custom-made pulse oximeter dental probe in comparison with the electrical and thermal tests for assessing pulp vitality. J Endod. 2007;33:411-4.
9. Hwang JY, Choi SC, Park JH, Kang SW. The use of green tea extract as a storage medium for the avulsed tooth. J Endod 2011;37:962-7.
10. Jung IH, Yun JH, Cho AR, Kim CS, Chung WG, Choi SH. Effect of epigallocatechin-3-gallate on maintaining the periodontal ligament cell viability of avulsed teeth: A pre-liminary study. J Periodontal Implant Sci 2011;41:10-6.
11. Badaksh S, Eksandarian T, Esmaeilpour T. The use of Aloe vera extract as novel storage media for the avulsed tooth. Iran J Med Sci 2014;39:327-32.
12. Ozan F, Tepe B, Polat ZA, Er K. Evaluation if in vitro effect if Morus rubra (Red Mulberry) on survival of periodontal ligament cells. Oral Surg Med Oral Pathol Oral Radiol Endod 2008;105:e66-9.
13. Pohi Y, Tekin U, Boll M, Fillipi A, Kirscher H. Investigations on a cell culture medium for storage and transportation of avulsed teeth. Aust Endod J 1999;25:70-5.
14. Filippi C, Krischner H, Filippi A, Pohl Y. Practicability of a tooth rescue concept- the use of a tooth rescue box. Dent Traumatol 2008;24:422-9.B

FURTHER READING

1. Acharya S. Avulsion and replantation of primary teeth—A feasible option. Dentist Case Rep. 2017;1(1):1-3.
2. Andreasen FM. Pulpal healing after luxation injuries and root fracture in the permanent dentition. Endod Dent Traumatol. 1989;5(3):111-31.
3. Andreasen JO, Andreasen FM. Textbook and Colour Atlas of Traumatic Injuries to Teeth, 3rd edition. Copenhagen: Munksgaard; 1994.
4. Andreasen JO, Andreasen SM. Essentials of Traumatic Injuries to the Teeth, 2nd edition. Copenhagen: Munksgaard; 1990.
5. Andreasen JO, Andreasen SM. Root resorption following traumatic dental injuries. Proc Finn Dent Soc. 1991; 88:95- 114.
6. Andreasen JO, Bakland LK, Matras RC, et al. Traumatic intrusion of permanent teeth—part 1. An epidemiological study of 216 intruded permanent teeth. Dent Traumatol. 2006;22(2):83-9.
7. Andreasen JO, Borum M, Jacobson H, et al. Reimpantation of 400 avulsed permanent incisors. 4 Factors related to periodontal ligament healing. Endod Dent Traumatol. 1995; 11:76-89.
8. Andreasen JO, Ravn JJ. The effect of traumatic injuries to the primary teeth on their permanent successors. II. A clinical and radiographic follow-up study of 213 injured teeth. Scand J Dent Res. 1971; 79:284-94.
9. Andreasen JO, Sundstrm B, Ravn JJ. The effect of traumatic injuries to primary teeth on their permanent successors. I. A clinical and histologic study of 117 injured permanent teeth. Scand J Dent Res. 1971; 79:279-83.
10. Andreasen JO. Effect of extra-alveolar period and storage media upon periodontal and pulpal healing after replantation of mature permanent incisors in monkeys. Int J Oral Surg. 1981; 10:43-53.
11. Andreasen JO. The influence of traumatic intrusion of primary teeth on their permanent successors. A radiographic and histologic study of monkeys. Int J Oral Surg. 1976; 5:207-19.
12. Arikan V, Sari S, Sonmez H. The Prevalence and Treatment Outcomes of Primary Tooth Injuries. Eur J Dent. 2010;4(4): 447-53.
13. Ashkenazi M, Marouni M, Sarnat H. In vitro viability, mitogenicity and clonogenic capacity of periodontal ligament cells after storage in four media at room temperature. Dent Traumatol. 2000; 16:63-70.
14. Ashkenazi M, Sarnat H, Keila S. In vitro viability, mitogenicity and clonogenic capacity of periodontal ligament cells after storage in six different media. Dent Traumatol. 1999; 15:149-56.
15. Barrett EJ, Kenny DJ. Avulsed permanent teeth: a review of the literature and treatment guidelines. Endod Dent Traumatol. 1997; 13:153-63.
16. Bhayya DP, Shyagali TR. Traumatic injuries in the primary teeth of 4-to 6-year-old school children in gulbarga city, India. A prevalence study. Oral Health Dent Manag. 2013;12(1): 17-23.
17. Blomlöf L, Lindskog S, Andersson L, et al. Storage of experimentally avulsed teeth in milk prior to replantation. J Dent Res. 1983; 62: 912-6.
18. Blomlöf L, Otteskog P, Hammarström L. Effect of storage in media with different ion strengths and osmolalities on human periodontal ligament cells. Scand J Dent Res. 1981; 89:180-7.
19. Castro JC, Poi WR, Manfrin TM, et al. Analysis of the crown fractures and crown-root fractures due to dental trauma assisted by the Integrated Clinic from 1992 to 2002. Dent Traumatol. 2005;21(3):121-6.
20. Clark J, Weatherford T, Mann W. The wire ligature acrylic resin splint. J Periodontol. 1969; 40:371.
21. Croll TP, Pascon EA, Langeland K. Traumatically injured primary incisors: a clinical and histological study. ASDC J Dent Child. 1987; 54:401-22.
22. Cvek M, Granath L, Holender L. Treatment of non-vital permanent incisors with calcium hydroxide. 3. Variation of occurrence of ankylosis of reimplanted teeth with duration of extra-alveolar period and storage environment. Odontol Revy. 1974; 25:43-56.
23. de Carvalho Rocha MJ, Cardoso M. Reimplantation of primary tooth—case report. Dent Traumatol. 2008;24(4):e4-10.
24. Diab M, elBadrawy HE. Intrusion injuries of primary incisors. Part I: Review and management. Quintessence Int. 2000; 31:327-34.
25. Fidel SR, Fidel junior RAS, Sassone LM, et al. Clinical Management of a Complicated Crown-Root Fracture: A Case Report. Braz Dent J. 2011;22(3):258-62.
26. Ge L, Chen J, Zhao Y, et al. Analysis of traumatic injury in 886 permanent anterior teeth. J Hard Tissue Biol. 2005;14(2):53-4.
27. Gopikrishna V, Baweja PS, Venkateshbabu N, et al. Comparison of coconut water, Propolis, HBSS, and milk on PDL cell survival. J Endod. 2008; 34:587-9.

28. Hiltz J, Trope M. Vitality of human lip fibroblast in milk, Hank's balanced Salt Solution and ViaSpan storage media. Endod Dent Traumatol. 1991; 7:69-72.
29. Huang SC, Remeikis NA, Daniel JC. Effects of long-term exposure of human periodontal ligament cells to milk and other solutions. J Endod. 1996; 22:30-3.
30. Iqbal MK, Bamaas NS. Effect of enamel matrix derivative (Emdogain) upon periodontal healing after replantation of permanent incisors in Beagle dogs. Dent Traumatol. 2001; 17:36-45.
31. Kapur A, Goyal A, Gauba K. Replantation of an Avulsed Primary Incisor: Report of a Case with Favorable Outcome. J Postgrad Med Edu Res. 2014;48(2):105-8.
32. Kenny DJ, Jacobi R. Management of trauma to the primary dentition. Ont Dent. 1988; 65:27-9.
33. Khademi AA, Atbaee A, Razavi SM, et al. Periodontal healing of replanted dog teeth stored in milk and egg albumen. Dent Traumatol. 2008; 24:510-4.
34. Kinoshita S, Kojima R, Taguchi Y, et al. Tooth replantation after traumatic avulsion: a report of 10 cases. Dent Traumatol. 2002; 18:153-6.
35. Krasner P, Person P. Preserving avulsed teeth for replantation. J Am Dent Assoc. 1992; 23:80-8.
36. Krasner P. Tooth avulsion in the school setting. J Sch Nurs. 1992; 8:20-6.
37. Laux M, Abbott PV, Pajarola G, et al. Apical inflammatory root resorption: a correlative radiographic and histological assessment. Int Endod J. 2000; 33:483-93.
38. Layug ML, Barret EJ, Kenny DJ. Interim storage of avulsed permanent teeth. J Can Dent Ass. 1998; 64:357-69.
39. Lehninger AL, Nelson DL, Cox MM. Princípios de bioquımica. SarvierEditora. São Paulo: Sarvier; 1995. p. 839.
40. Lemmerman K. Rationale for stabilization. J Periodontol. 1976; 47:405-11.
41. Mackie IC, Worthington HV. An investigation of replantation of traumatically avulsed permanent incisor teeth. Br Dent J. 1992; 172:17-20.
42. Marino TG, West LA, Liewehr FR, et al. Determination of periodontal ligament cell viability in long shelf-life milk. J Endod. 2000; 26:699-702.
43. Mendonça DHDS, Azevedo MLDC, Leandrini JCDS, et al. Functional-aesthetic treatment of crown fracture in anterior teeth with severe crowding. RSBO. 2012;9(3):328-33.
44. Oikarinen K, Kassila D. Causes and types of traumatic tooth injuries treated in a public dental health clinic. Dent Traumatol. 1987;3(4): 172-7.
45. Onetto JE, Flores MT, Garbarino ML. Dental trauma in children and adolescent in Valpariso, Chile. Endod Dent Traumatol. 1994; 10: 223-7.
46. Prabhakar AR, Yavagal CM, Limaye NS, et al. Effect of storage media on fracture resistance of reattached tooth fragments using G-aenial Universal Flo. J Conserv Dent. 2016;19(3):250-3.
47. Ravn JJ. Developmental disturbances in permanent teeth after intrusion of their primary predecessors. Scan J Dent Res. 1976; 84:137-41.
48. Ravn JJ. Sequelae of acute mechanical traumata in the deciduous dentition. J Dent Child. 1968; 35:281-9.
49. Roberts G, Longhurst P. Oral and Dental Trauma in Children and Adolescents. Oxford: Oxford University Press; 1996.
50. Sahebi S, Dolatkhah V, Shojaee NS. Management of a crown- root fracture in central incisors with 180° rotation: A case report. Iranian Endod J. 2011;6(4):183-7.
51. Schreiber CK. The effect of trauma on the anterior deciduous teeth. Br Dent J. 1959; 106:340-3.
52. Serio FG. Clinical rational for tooth stabilization and splinting. Dent Clin North Am. 1999; 43:1-6.
53. Shanmugam HV, Arangannal P, Vishnurekha C, et al. Management of intrusive luxation in the primary dentition by surgical repositioning: an alternative approach. Aust Dent J. 2011; 56:207-11.
54. Simiring M. Splinting-theory and practices. J Am Dent Assoc. 1952; 45:402-14.
55. Spinosa GM. Traumatic injuries to the primary and young permanent dentition. Univ Toronto Dent J. 1990; 3:34-6.
56. Stern IB. The status of temporary fixed splinting procedures in the treatment of periodontally involved teeth. J Periodontol. 1960; 31:217-23.
57. Wilson CFG. Management of trauma to primary and developing teeth. Dent Clin North Am. 1995; 39:133-67.

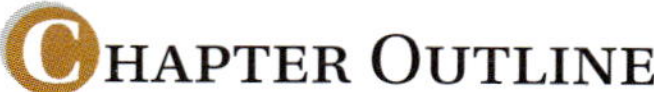

Pediatric Minor Oral Surgery

Amit Bhamboo, Sunil Sharma, Nikhil Marwah, Ahmad Faisal Ismail

Chapter Outline

- Lesions of the Newborn
- Lesions of Erupting Dentition
- Mucocele
- Ranula
- Maxillary Frenectomy
- Ankyloglossia
- Apicoectomy

Surgery performed on pediatric patients involves a number of special considerations unique to this population. It is important to perform a thorough clinical and radiographic pre-operative evaluation of the dentition as well as extra oral and intra oral radiographs. It includes intraoral films and extraoral imaging if the area of interest extends beyond the dentoalveolar complex. Behavioral guidance of children in the operative and perioperative periods presents a special challenge. Special attention should be given to the assessment of the social, emotional, and psychological status of the pediatric patient prior to surgery. Children have many unvoiced fears concerning the surgical experience, and their psychological management requires that the dentist be cognizant of their emotional status. Answering questions concerning the surgery is important and should be done in the presence of the parent.

The potential for adverse effects on growth from injuries and/or surgery in the oral and maxilla-facial region markedly increases the risks and complications in the pediatric population. Traumatic injuries involving the maxilla-facial region can affect growth, development, and function adversely. For example, injuries to the mandibular condyle result in restricted growth, but also limit mandibular function as a result of ankylosis. Surgery involving the maxilla and mandible of young patients is complicated by the presence of developing tooth follicles. Alteration or deviation from standard treatment modalities may be necessary to avoid injuring the follicles. To minimize the negative effects of surgery on the developing dentition, careful planning using radiographs, tomography, cone beam computed tomography, and/or 3-D imaging techniques is necessary to provide valuable information to assess the presence, absence, location, and/or quality of individual crown and root development.

LESIONS OF THE NEWBORN

- Oral pathologies occurring in newborn children include Epstein pearls, dental lamina cysts, Bohn's nodules, and congenital epulis.
- Epstein pearls are commonly found in about 75–80% of newborns. They occur in the median palatal raphe area as a result of trapped epithelial remnants along the line of fusion of the palatal halves. They are generally yellowish or whitish in color with diameter of 1-3 mm. Generally, they do not require treatment and resolve on its own. Breastfeeding, bottle feeding or use of pacifiers breaks down this bump and dissolve it quickly.
- Dental lamina cysts or gingival cyst or alveolar cysts found on the crests of the alveolar ridges, originates from remnants of dental lamina. These cyst generally rupture on their own or undergo degeneration. They can occur in varying numbers that ranges from solitary to multiple nodules. These can be often misdiagonosed with natal teeth. Generally these disapper on their own and do not cause any pain so just reassurance to parent is needed.
- Bohn's nodules are keratin filled cysts in new born. These are remnants of salivary gland epithelium and usually are found on the buccal and lingual aspects of the ridge, away from the midline.

- No treatment is required, as these cysts usually disappear during the first 3-months of life.

LESIONS OF ERUPTING DENTITION

- These include all eruption complications like eruption cyst, eruption hematoma, natal and neonatal teeth.
- Eruption cyst is a soft tissue benign cyst, which is associated with a primary or permanent tooth. Shortly occuring before eruption of teeth. Mostly occur between 6-9 years of age when pemanent molars and icisors erupt. They are dome shaped raised swelling on the alvelolar ridge with color ranging from transparent, bluish, purple.
- Small intraoral hemangiomas of the buccal mucosa and alveolar ridge that may appear in infants known as eruption haematomas. Generally these eruption cysts resolve on their own but may require surgery if they become infected, painful to patient or compromise esthetics **(Fig. 64.1)**.

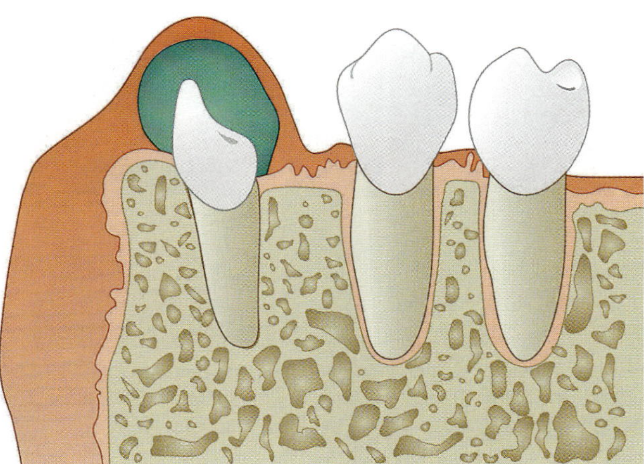

Fig. 64.1: Diagrammatic representation of eruption cyst.

- Natal teeth have been defined as those teeth present at birth, and neonatal teeth are those that erupt during the first 30 days of life.
- The other synonyms for these teeth are Dentitia praecox, dens connatalis, congenital teeth, fetal teeth, infancy teeth.
- The clinical manifestation and treatment for all these conditions has been dealt in detail earlier (teething).

MUCOCELE

- The term mucocele is derived from the Latin word muco meaning mucous and coele meaning cavity.
- An oral mucocele is a cavity of mucus that develops in association with the minor salivary glands. It may be a retention cyst or extravasation cyst. Most commonly occurring cyst in children is extravasation type.
- The most common benign salivary gland problem in childhood. The lesion is a pseudocyst and does not have an epithelial lining.
- Mucoceles are most frequently found on lowerlip. Mucoceles also can be found on the buccal mucosa, ventral surface of the tongue, retromolar region. If they occur on floor of mouth they are called as ranulas.

Etiology

- The main reason is usually trauma. The mucocele is a common lesion in children and adolescents resulting from the rupture of a minor salivary gland excretory duct, with subsequent leakage of mucin into the surrounding connective tissues that later may be surrounded in a fibrous capsule
- When the duct is totally or partially obstructed, and there is accumulation of saliva behind the obstruction, a retention cyst develops. This collection of mucus is surrounded by duct epithelium, and is therefore by definition a true cyst.

Clinical Features

- They are bluish, soft, and transparent cystic swelling. Blue color is due to vascular congestion, tissue cyanosis above, and accumulation of fluid below. They resolve on their own.
- Many lesions however require treatment to minimize the risk of recurrence.
- Though mucocele are generally asymptomatic but they may cause discomfort in speech, chewing and swallowing.

Treatment Options

- Surgical excision
- Marsupialization
- Micro-marsupialization
- Laser excision
- Cryosurgery

Technique of Removal

Surgical excision is most common technique of removal of mucocele. Elliptical incision is preferred so as to decrease the formation of fibrous scar and decrease the loss of mucosal tissue as well as to avoid spillage of cystic content, which may lead to reoccurrence. The lesion should be removed down to muscle layer as well as all glandular acini must be removed before placement of suture **(Figs. 64.2A to J)**. Laser can also be used effectively for the same with much less tissue damage, optimized bleeding control and excellent wound healing **(Figs. 64.3A to E)**.

Complications

- Recurrence is a common complication
- Excision in the lower lip may be harmful to the labial branches of the mental nerve.

RANULA

- Ranula is a mucocele in the floor of the mouth
- The name ranula is derived from the Latin, *Ranula Pipiens* meaning frog. Elevation of the tongue by fluid filled pseudocyst is reminiscent of the appearance of a frog's tongue.

Etiology

- These are most commonly pseudocysts originated in the deeper portion of the sublingual gland, but may be

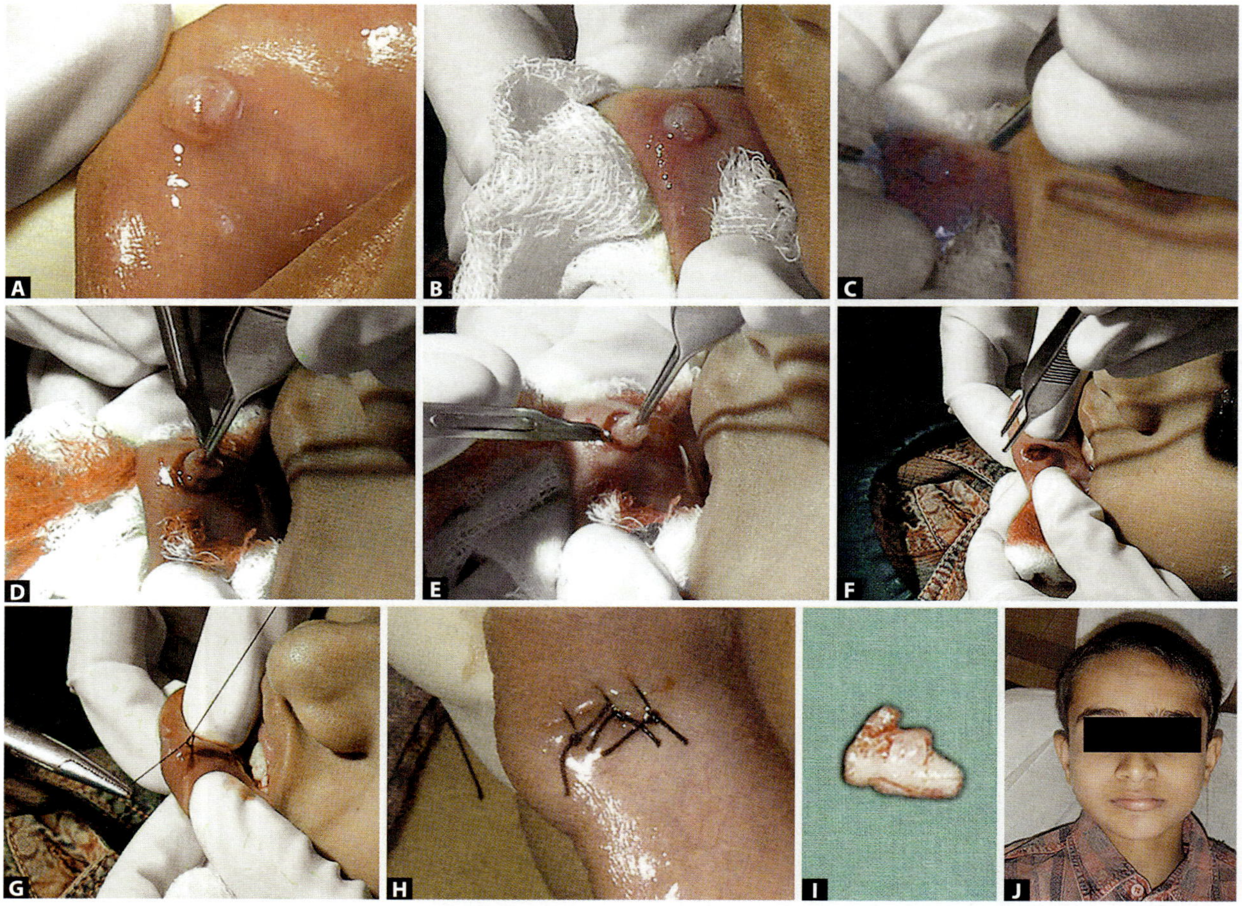

Fig. 64.2A to J: Surgical procedure of removal of mucocele; (A) Preoperative view; (B) Before excision; (C) Lower lip being help held; (D) Incision being placed; (E) Tissue being excised with scalpel; (F) After excision; (G) Sutures being placed; (H) After suturing; (I) Excised tissue; (J) Postoperative.

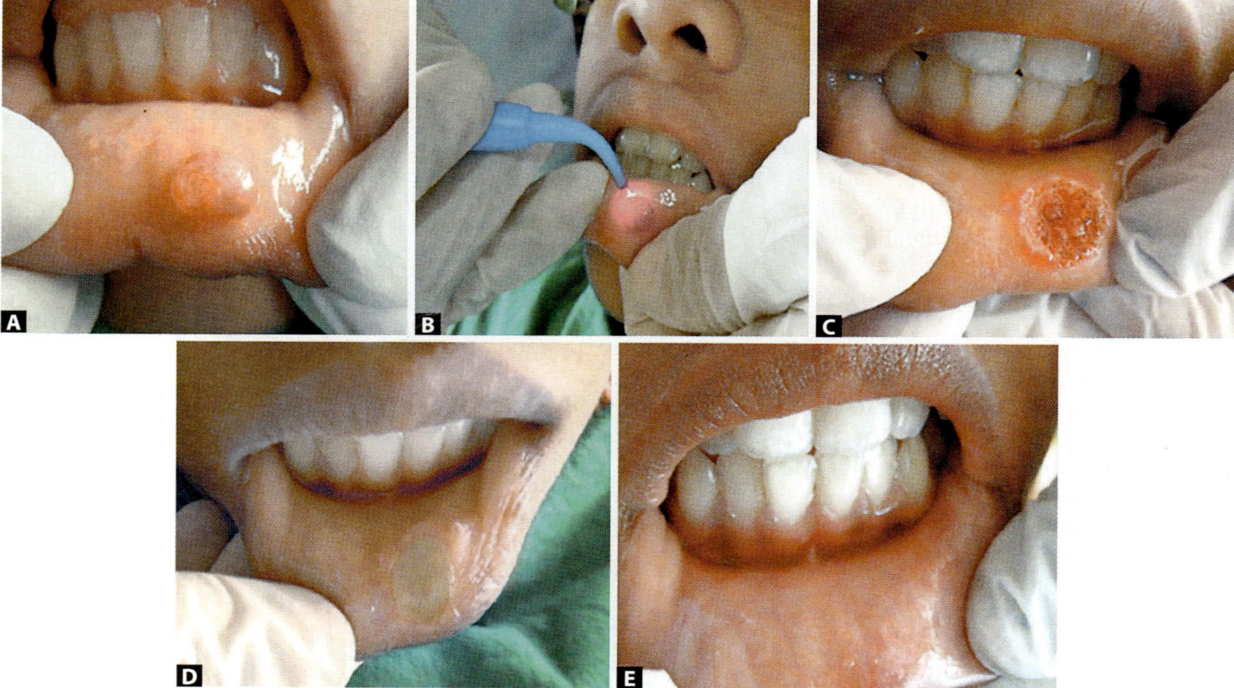

Figs. 64.3A to E: Laser excision of mucocele and subsequent healing: (A) Pre-operative presentattion; (B) Laser treatment; (C) Immidiate post operative; (D) Laser healing; (E) Post operative picture after 1 week.

retention cyst from the ducts of Rivini (of the superficial portion of the sublingual gland)

- To a lesser degree they also may be retention cysts from the Wharton's duct of the submandibular gland.

Clinical Features

- Ranulas appearing in infants and toddlers are congenital, a result of dilatation of sublingual or submaxillary gland ducts in the floor of the mouth whereas those appearing in older children are usually traumatic.
- Ranulas characteristically are located in the sublingual space between the mylohyoid muscle and the lingual mucosa.
- Plunging ranula often requires excision of the sublingual gland to prevent recurrence.
- They may occasionally extend into the submental or submandibular spaces by perforating through the mylohyoid muscle and are then called as "Plunging ranula".

Technique of Removal (Figs. 64.4A and B)

- Small ranulas can be excised, however, large ones should be observed for several months until the lining is mature before we undertake any treatment.

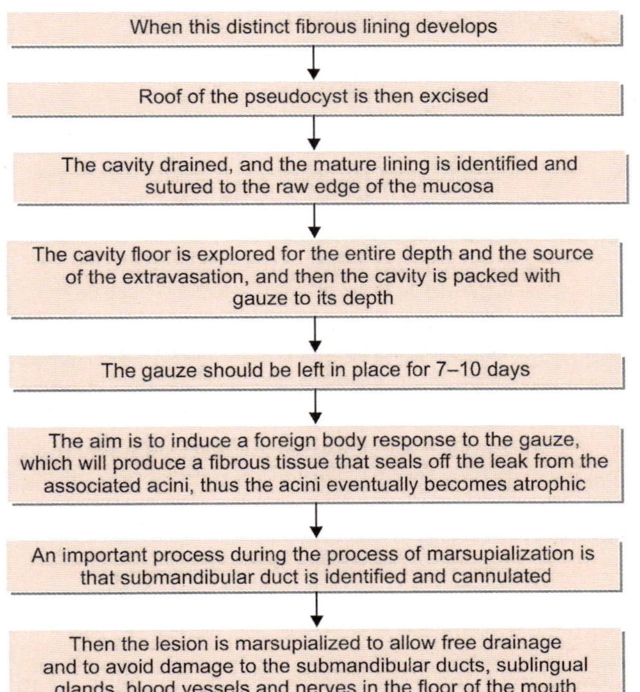

When this distinct fibrous lining develops
Roof of the pseudocyst is then excised
The cavity drained, and the mature lining is identified and sutured to the raw edge of the mucosa
The cavity floor is explored for the entire depth and the source of the extravasation, and then the cavity is packed with gauze to its depth
The gauze should be left in place for 7–10 days
The aim is to induce a foreign body response to the gauze, which will produce a fibrous tissue that seals off the leak from the associated acini, thus the acini eventually becomes atrophic
An important process during the process of marsupialization is that submandibular duct is identified and cannulated
Then the lesion is marsupialized to allow free drainage and to avoid damage to the submandibular ducts, sublingual glands, blood vessels and nerves in the floor of the mouth

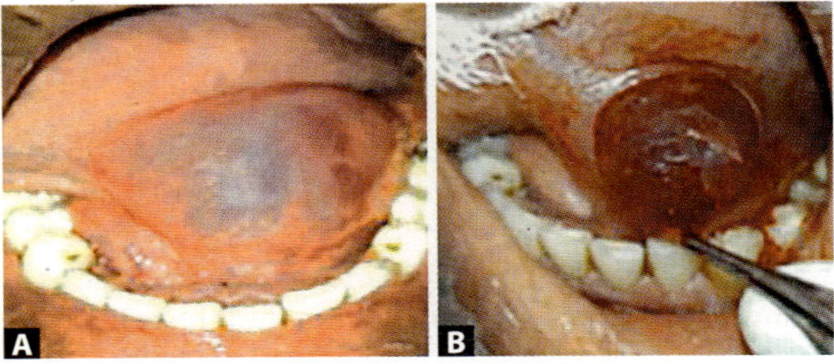

Figs. 64.4A and B: (A): Presentation of ranula; (B) Exposing of ranula. (*Pic courtesy:* Dr Prem Sasikumar).

MAXILLARY FRENECTOMY

- The superior labial frenum is a triangular fold of tissue that originates in the lip and inserts into the attached gingiva at the maxillary midline.
- It is a remnant of embryonal structures (the tectolabial bands).
- Frenectomy is the complete excision of the frenum and the term frenotomy indicates a partial removal (relocation).

Etiology

An apical relocation usually takes place during normal growth of the alveolar process, but an abnormal frenum attachment may be seen between the central incisors when this migration fails.

Clinical Features

- A prominent maxillary frenum in children, although a common finding, is often a concern, especially when associated with a diastema.
- Interference with oral hygiene measures, esthetics, and psychological reasons are contributing factors that relate to treatment of the maxillary frenum.

Diagnosis

- An abnormal frenum will appear excessively wide and/or attached especially close to the gingival margin.A lack of apparent zone of attached gingiva along the midline may be observed, and stretching of the upper lip and observing the movement and ischemia/blanching of interdental and/or palatal tissues may be helpful.
- When a hypertrophic frenum is associated with an incomplete fusion of the intermaxillary suture, the contour of the alveolar process between the central incisors is W-shaped or irregular ovoid instead of the normal V-shape.

Indications for Removal

- The main indications for removal are when the frenum restricts lip movement, a frenal attachment that prevents closure of a midline diastema.
- In cases when a frenum attachment prevents mechanical tooth cleansing, a frenectomy should be considered.

Timing

- The timing is dependent upon the indications for removal. In cases with a maxillary midline diastema there are different options for timing of the removal.
- The first alternative is initial diastema closure by orthodontic treatment, followed by removal of the frenum and retention appliances. Then the wound contraction will contribute to retention of the treatment result.
- Second option is to remove the frenum before the end of active orthodontic treatment.This is performed when the frenum may inhibit orthodontic closure.
- In both of these cases, the removal is usually done after the eruption of the permanent canines and lateral incisors.

Technique

- This can be done by two methods viz. simple frenectomy **(Figs. 64.5A and B)** and Z-plasty.
- The Z-plasty involves excision of the frenum and making two oblique incisions down to periosteum and the resulting triangular flaps are raised and sutured with interrupted sutures in a reverse position.

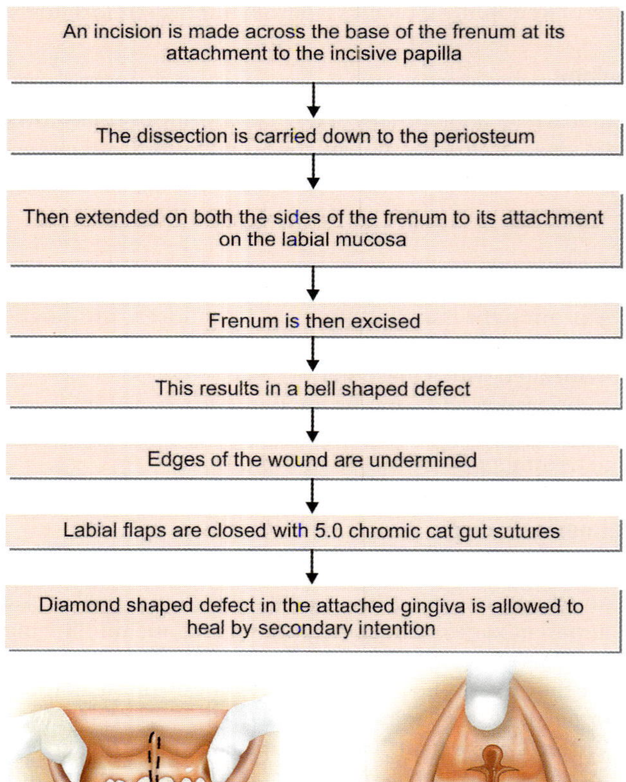

An incision is made across the base of the frenum at its attachment to the incisive papilla
The dissection is carried down to the periosteum
Then extended on both the sides of the frenum to its attachment on the labial mucosa
Frenum is then excised
This results in a bell shaped defect
Edges of the wound are undermined
Labial flaps are closed with 5.0 chromic cat gut sutures
Diamond shaped defect in the attached gingiva is allowed to heal by secondary intention
A

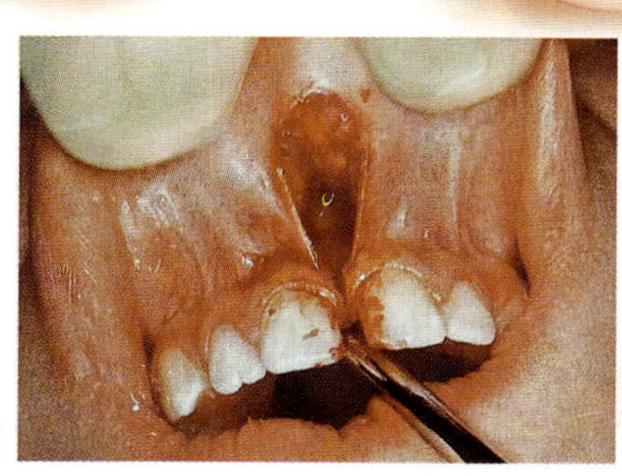

Figs. 64.5A and B: Frenectomy.

ANKYLOGLOSSIA

- Ankyloglossia is derived from the greek word agkilos means curved and glossa meaning tongue.
- Ankyloglossia is a developmental anomaly of the tongue characterized by a prominent lingual frenum attached high on the lingual alveolar ridge, the thick lingual frenum results in limitation of tongue movement (partial ankyloglossia) or by the tongue fused to the floor of the mouth (total ankyloglossia).
- It is also called as tongue-tie.
- The reported prevalence is 0.1–10.7% of the population.

Diagnosis

- The frenum is often abnormally short and thick and with decreased mobility.
- A heart-shaped tongue may be seen during protrusion.
- Inability to protrude the tongue past gum line.

Clinical Features

- There is a higher prevalence of nipple pain and nipple trauma in mothers feeding infants with ankyloglossia than in mothers feeding infants without ankyloglossia.
- Some difficulties in making sounds such as t, d, z, s, th, n and l.
- Other problems related to reduce tongue mobility might be discomfort, difficulties with licking the lips, keeping the teeth clean, increased frequency of dental caries.
- Because of intense pulling, ankyloglossia has been associated with gingival recessions.
- It has also been hypothesized that a tongue that is in low position may predispose for maxillary hypodevelopment and mandibular prognathism, typical features of class III malocclusions and that ankyloglossia indirectly can cause malocclusion.
- Frenal attachment may interfere with denture stability, dislodging the denture when the tongue is moved.

Surgical Technique

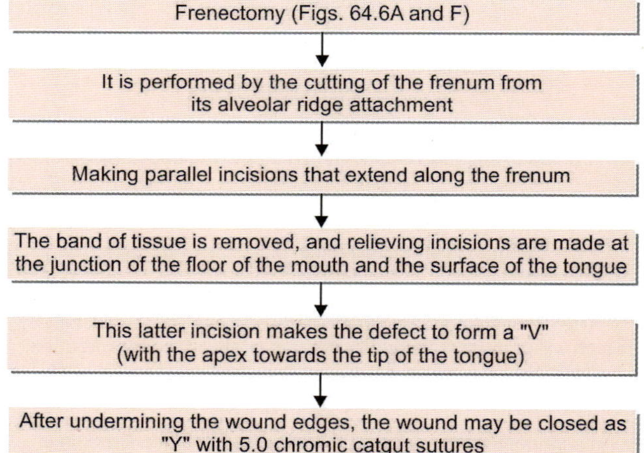

Frenectomy (Figs. 64.6A and F)
It is performed by the cutting of the frenum from its alveolar ridge attachment
Making parallel incisions that extend along the frenum
The band of tissue is removed, and relieving incisions are made at the junction of the floor of the mouth and the surface of the tongue
This latter incision makes the defect to form a "V" (with the apex towards the tip of the tongue)
After undermining the wound edges, the wound may be closed as "Y" with 5.0 chromic catgut sutures

APICOECTOMY

Apicoectomy is the term used for surgery involving the root apex to treat the apical infection. It is the removal of the apical portion of the root and curettage of periapical necrotic, granulomatous, inflammatory or cystic lesions.

Indications

- Apical anomaly of root apex-intracanal calcifications, dilacerations, open apex. Roots with broken instruments or overfillings.
- Fracture of apical- third of the root formation of periapical granuloma or cyst. Draining sinus tract unresponsive to RCT.
- Extension of root canal sealant cement or filling beyond the apex.

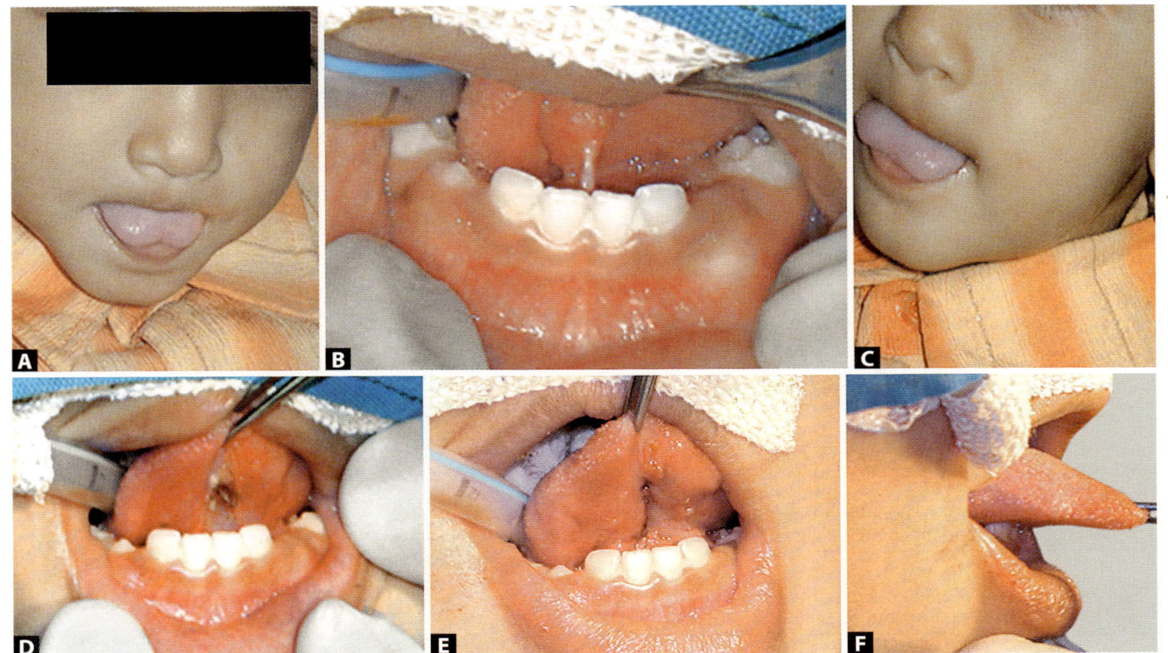

Figs. 64.6A to F: Management of ankyloglossia: (A) Heart-shaped tongue; (B) High frenal attachment on alveolar ridge and tip of tongue; (C) Restricted elevation; (D) Elliptical incision; (E) Relief of the frenal attachment; (F) Improved elevation and protrusion.

Contraindications

- Presence of systemic diseases.
- Teeth with deep periodontal pockets and grade III mobility. When traumatic occlusion cannot be corrected.
- Acute infection, which is nonresponsive to the treatment.

Technique (Figs. 64.7A to G)

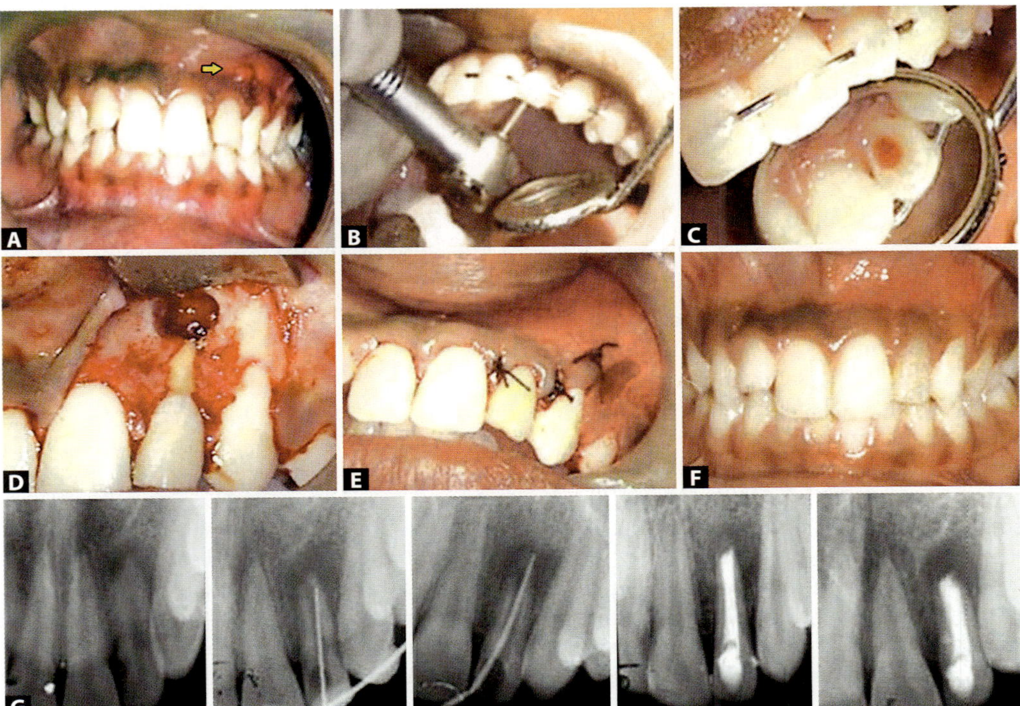

Figs. 64.7A to G: Procedure for apicoectomy: (A) Chronic periapical abscess and subluxation due to trauma in 21; Access cavity prepared; (C) Serosanguineous discharge from root canal; (D) Apicoectomy and periapical curettage done; (E) Immediate postoperative view; (F) Two-weeks post operative view; (G) Pretreatment working length, mastercones election, obturation, following apicoectomy.

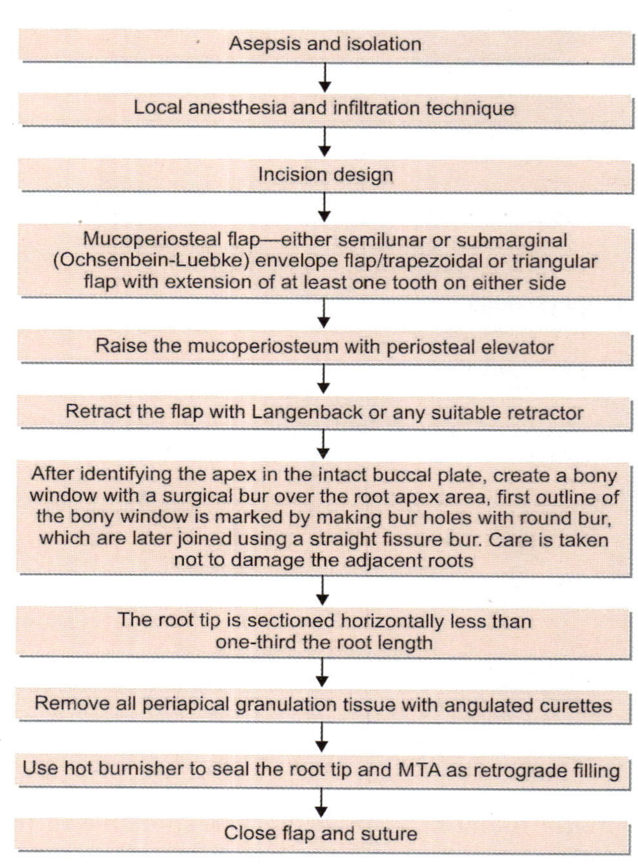

Asepsis and isolation
Local anesthesia and infiltration technique
Incision design
Mucoperiosteal flap—either semilunar or submarginal (Ochsenbein-Luebke) envelope flap/trapezoidal or triangular flap with extension of at least one tooth on either side
Raise the mucoperiosteum with periosteal elevator
Retract the flap with Langenback or any suitable retractor
After identifying the apex in the intact buccal plate, create a bony window with a surgical bur over the root apex area, first outline of the bony window is marked by making bur holes with round bur, which are later joined using a straight fissure bur. Care is taken not to damage the adjacent roots
The root tip is sectioned horizontally less than one-third the root length
Remove all periapical granulation tissue with angulated curettes
Use hot burnisher to seal the root tip and MTA as retrograde filling
Close flap and suture

UNERUPTED MAXILLARY INCISORS

Maxillary incisors usually erupted between ages of 7-9 years. Maxillary incisors can be considered unerupted when:

- Contralateral maxillary incisor has erupted 6 months earlier
- Maxillary incisors are still unerupted when lower incisors have erupted one year previously
- Deviation from the normal sequence of tooth eruption.

Assessment

- Clinical assessment and radiographic investigations should be conducted to determine the management plan and surgical access.
- Clinical assessment should be performed prior to any radiographic investigations.
- Clinician should check for presence of retained primary tooth, presence of labial or palatal swelling and availability of space for the maxillary incisor to erupt.
- Radiographic investigation should be performed to confirm the diagnosis of unerupted incisor, to identify and localized position of maxillary incisor, and to plan for surgical access.
- Basic requirements for radiographic assessment should have at least 2 different views (combination of 2 different angle of periapical radiographs or combination of periapical radiographs with upper occlusal view or dental panoramic tomogram).
- The 3D imaging can be used in complex cases should baseline radiographs are unable to provide confirmative information.

Management of Unerupted Maxillary Incisors

- There are three principal's management in managing unerupted maxillary incisors:
  1. Ensuring satisfactory space available for the incisor
  2. Removal of any obstruction
  3. Monitor eruption or active orthodontic traction of unerupted tooth
- Space should be created prior to surgical intervention
- Should space is available, maintenance of the space is very crucial
- Presence of retained primary incisor should be extracted
- Incision (Surgical or Laser) can be done if there is presence of thick mucosal tissue covering unerupted incisor **(Figs. 64.8A to D).**

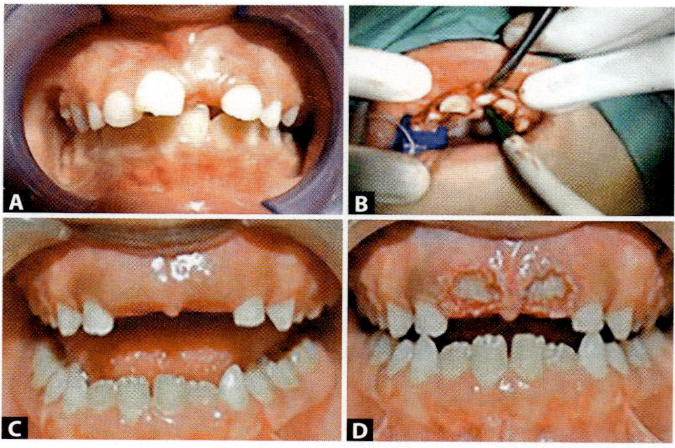

Figs. 64.8A to D: (A) Preoperative view of unerupted incisor; (B) Surgical excision of the overlying tissue; (C) Preoperative view of unerupted incisor; (D) Laser excision and subsequent eruption of teeth. (*Pic courtesy:* Dr Vidya Bhat S).

ORAL IMPALEMENT INJURIES IN CHILDREN

Injuries to the oropharynx and soft palate are relatively common in children. Children often walk with object in their mouth. Most of the injuries are manageable at primary care level and requires conservative treatment with minimal surgical intervention. The exact incidence of oral impalement injuries is unknown as most cases go unrecognized and unreported.

Clinical Presentations

- Most injuries occur without palatal perforation and commonly on hard and soft palate
- Wound are typically linear and superficial
- Typical presentation of wound is flat or v-shaped
- Common site of injuries:
  - Supratonsilar area
  - Soft/hard palate
  - Uvula
- Common etiologies are object such as pencil/pens, toothbrush, cylindrical toys, straws and sticks.

Management

- Management should always begin with identifying any life threatening injuries and complications.
- Neurological assessment of the child is recommended as a baseline assessment although some neurovascular complications may appear at later stage.
- Primary healing can be expected in most cases and is often uneventful. Therefore, it is recommended to treat the injuries conservatively **(Figs. 64.9A and B).**
- Most of the palatal injuries usually heal without surgical intervention.
- Suture placement is not required in most of the injuries, unless indicated for surgical intervention.
- Prophylactic antibiotic can be prescribed to prevent spread of infection to deep facial spaces and facial cellulitis.
- Soft diets and regular follow-up visit are highly recommended.

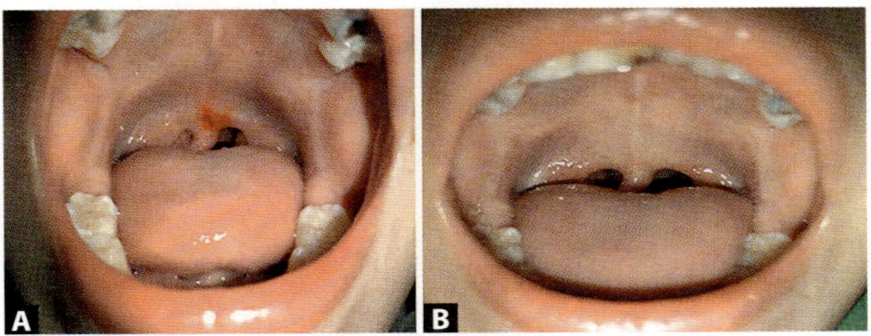

Figs. 64.9A and B: Injury and subsequent healing.

DENTIGEROUS CYST (FOLLICULAR CYST)

- Second most common odontogenic cyst after radicular cyst.
- Most common developmental odontogenic cyst
- Usually seen in teenagers/young adults, although can occur over a wide age range.
- By definition, a dentigerous cyst occurs in association with an unerupted tooth.
- Most commonly around permanent mandibular third molars (wisdom teeth).
- Rarely involves supernumerary teeth and odontomas.
- The eruption cyst is essentially a subtype of dentigerous cyst that is confined only by the overlying alveolar mucosa **(FIgs. 64.10A to C)**.

Pathophysiology

- Develops due to fluid accumulation between reduced enamel epithelium of dental follicle and crown of unerupted permanent tooth.
- Vast majority are developmental odontogenic cysts; may have inflammatory pathogenesis:
  - Inflammation progressing from root apex of carious or necrotic deciduous tooth brings about development of dentigerous cyst around underlying, unerupted permanent tooth.

Clinical Features

- May be small/asymptomatic, identified on routine radiographs taken for unrelated reasons or for imaging to investigate delayed tooth eruption.
- Can grow large enough to produce a painless bony expansion, can displace the involved tooth, cause resorption of adjacent teeth.
- If secondarily infected, may be associated with pain.

Radiology Description

- Typically, dentigerous cysts are asymptomatic and found on routine radiographic examination, appearing as a well-defined unilocular or multilocular radiolucent lesion.

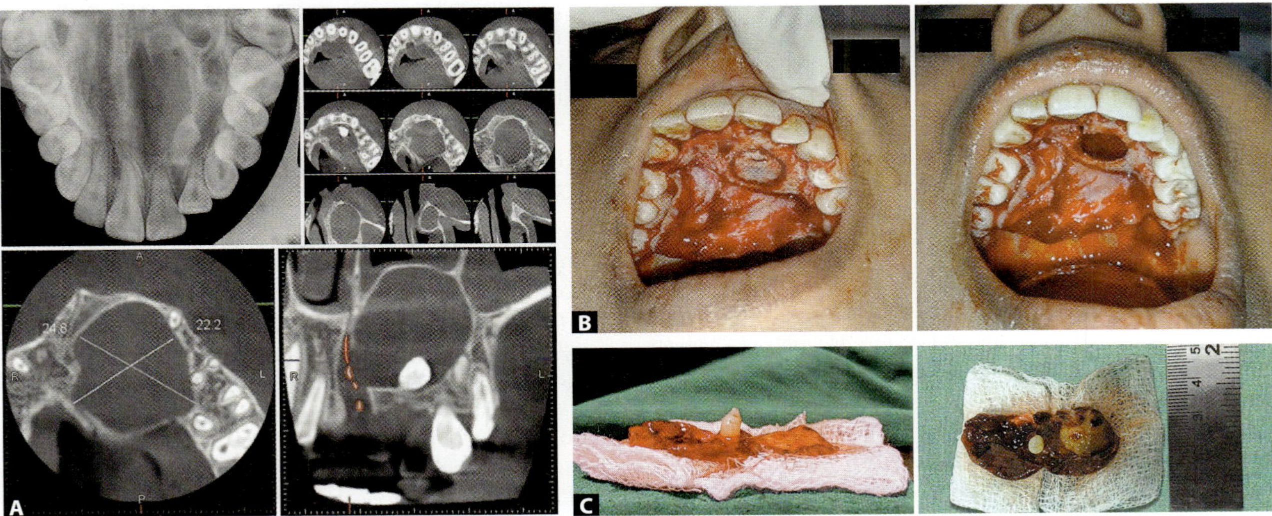

Figs. 64.10A to C: Cystic pathology associated with supernumerary tooth: (A) Preoperative maxillary occlusal radiograph and CBCT images sowing large radiolucent cystic lesion associated with supernumerary tooth; (B) Surgical exposure of maxillary cyst through palatal approach. Enucleation of the lining along with supernumerary tooth; (C) Enucleated specimen.

- Often has sclerotic rim.
- May resorb the roots of primary teeth, cause the divergence of or completely displace permanent teeth, and produce large areas of bone destruction in either the mandible or the maxilla.
- The lesion may vary in size from one in which the differentiation from an enlarged dental follicle is somewhat arbitrary to a large, bone-destructive lesion.
- According to Farah and Savage a pericoronal space of 2.5 mm on an intraoral radiograph and greater than 3 mm on a rotational panoramic radiograph should be investigated thoroughly.

Prognostic Factors

- Excellent prognosis and very rare recurrence with complete enucleation.
- Tooth sparing marsupialization procedures may have higher risk of cyst recurrence/persistence, therefore follow up radiographic studies recommended in this treatment modality.

Treatment

Varies based on age, maturity, anatomic position and relative importance of tooth involved, size of cyst, presence of additional neoplasms; also patient preference, including cosmetic and functional considerations.

Following treatment options:

- Enucleation of entire cyst with extraction of the associated tooth is most common approach
- If the cystic lesion is detected early and is associated with a permanent tooth with incomplete root formation then enucleation without extraction of associated tooth can be considered. In such cases after cyst removal root formation can provide normal eruption of the offending tooth **(Figs. 64.11 to 64.13).**

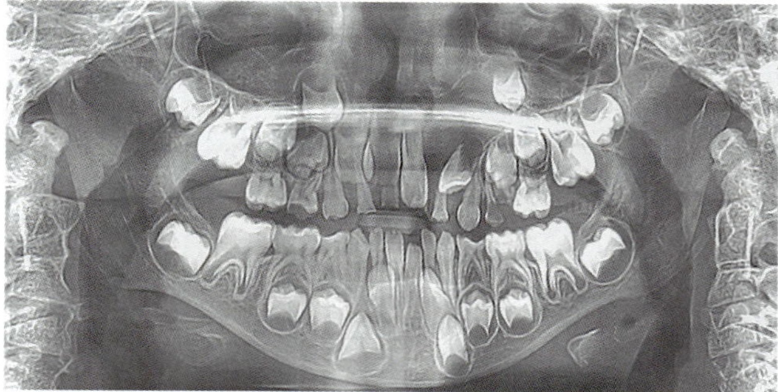

Fig. 64.11: Preoperative OPG showing incompletely roots of 23 along with a large radiolucency surrounding the crown and causing deviation adjacent tooth.

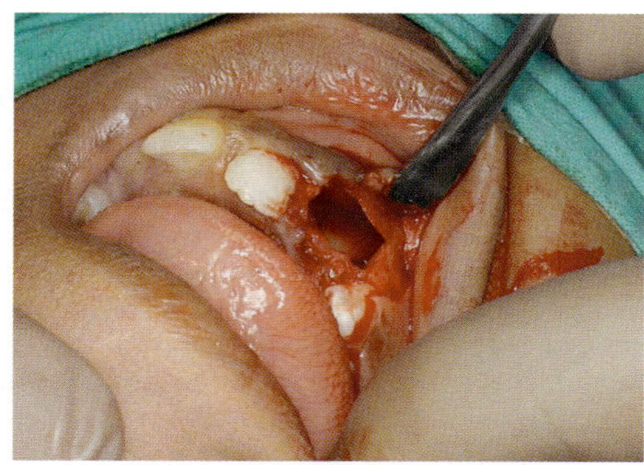

Fig. 64.12: Intraoperative picture: Exposure of underlying crown of 23 after extraction of deciduous root stumps and enucleation of cystic lining.

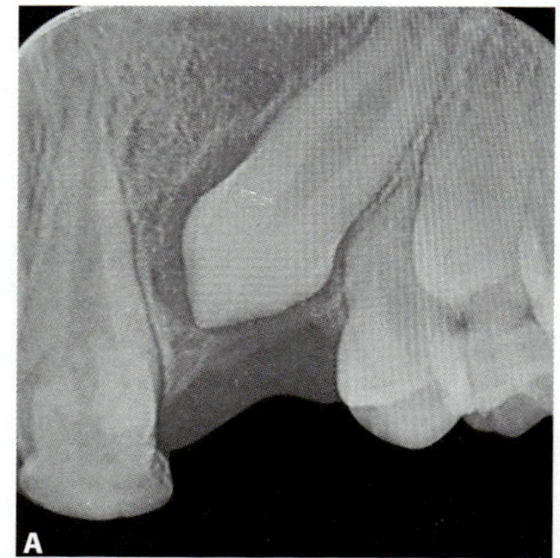

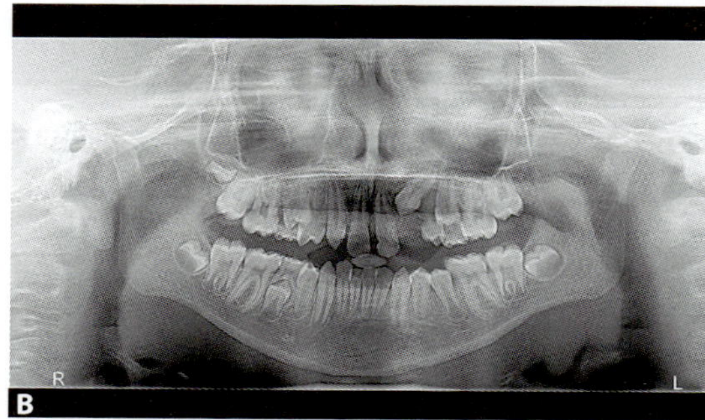

Figs. 64.13A and B: 9 month postoperative radiographs showing root formation of 23 along with natural bone formatio n in cystic space and favorable eruption movement of tooth.

- Marsupialization/enucleation with secondary healing **(Figs. 64.14A to D)**: As the cyst is less aggressive this treatment modality is useful as it will prevent extraction of an useful tooth as shown in case. This method uses natural healing process of bone so results in normal bone healing and prevents the need of any major reconstructive surgery, which otherwise becomes necessary in cases of resections. Requires close follow up to monitor for recurrence.

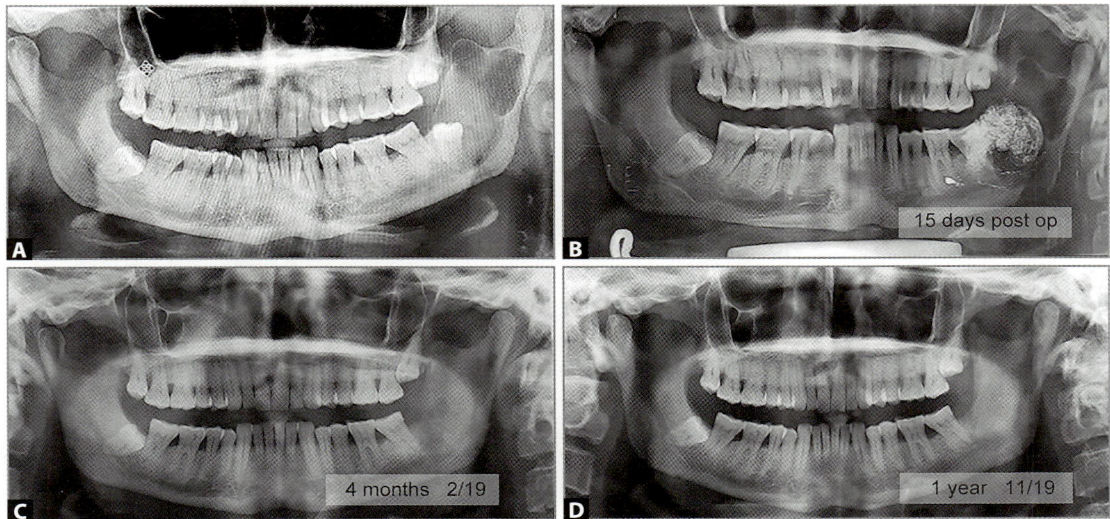

Figs. 64.14A to D: (A) Large cystic lesion shown as radiolucency involving entire left mandibular ramus angle region associated with distoangular impacted 38; (B) Treatment done—enucleation and extraction of 38 and secondary healing by using BIPP pack changed on monthly interval for 8 months. Pack visible in 15 days postoperative radiograph; (C) 4 month follow up image; (D) One year follow up with complete bone formation in defect site is seen in long-term radiographic follow up.

POINTS TO REMEMBER

- Epstein's pearls are common, found in about 75–80% of newborns. They occur in the median palatal raphe area as a result of trapped epithelial remnants along the line of fusion of the palatal halves.
- Dental lamina cysts, found on the crests of the dental ridges, most commonly are seen bilaterally in the region of the first primary molars. They result from remnants of the dental lamina.
- Bohn's nodules are remnants of salivary gland epithelium and usually are found on the buccal and lingual aspects of the ridge, away from the midline.
- An oral mucocele is a cavity of mucus that develops in association with the salivary glands. It may be a retention cyst or extravasation phenomena, depending on etiological and histopathological features and develops as a result of trauma.
- Ranula is a mucocele in the floor of the mouth and it originates in the deeper portion of the sublingual gland, but may also be retention cyst from the ducts of Rivini. These present as a big swelling in the floor of mouth usually causing obstructive symptoms.
- Frenectomy is the complete excision of the frenum. Frenotomy indicates a partial removal or relocation.
- Frenectomy is usually done after the eruption of the permanent canines and lateral incisors.
- Ankyloglossia is a developmental anomaly of the tongue characterized by a prominent lingual frenum attached high on the lingual alveolar ridge, the thick lingual frenum resulting in limitation of tongue movement (partial ankyloglossia) or by the tongue appearing to be fused to the floor of the mouth (total ankyloglossia).

Questionnaire

1. Write a short note on mucocele.
2. Discuss the clinical features and technique of removal of ranula.
3. Explain maxillary frenectomy.
4. Describe the clinical implications and management of ankyloglossia.

FURTHER READING

1. American Academy of Pediatric Dentistry. Guideline on Pediatric Oral Surgery. Pediatric Dent. 2009;34:264-71.
2. Baurmash HD. Marsupialization for treatment of oral ranula: a second look at the procedure. J Oral Maxillofac Surg. 1992;50(12):1274-9.
3. Baurmash HD. Mucoceles and ranulas. J Oral Maxillofac Surg. 2003;61(3):369-78.
4. Cunha RF, Boer FA, Torriani DD, Frossard WT. Natal and neonatal teeth: Review of the literature. Pediatr Dent. 2001;23(2):158-62.
5. Edwards JG. The diastema, the frenum, the frenectomy: a clinical study. Am J Orthod. 1977;71(5):489-508.
6. Ellis E. Principles of differential diagnosis and biopsy. In: Peterson LJ, Ellis E, Hupp JR, Tucker MR (Eds). Contemporary Oral and Maxillofacial Surgery, 4th Edition. Mosby: St.Louis; 2003.pp.458-78.
7. Esmeili T, Lozada-Nur F, Epstein J. Common benign oral soft tissue masses. Dent Clin North Am. 2005;49(1):223-40.
8. Farah CS, Savage NW. Pericoronal radiolucencies and the significance of early detection. Aust Dent J. 2002;47(3):262–266.
9. Kaban L, Troulis M. Infections of the maxillofacial region. In: Pediatric Oral and Maxillofacial Surgery. Philadelphia: Saunders;2004. pp.171-86.
10. Kaban L, Troulis M. Intraoral soft tissue abnormalities. In: Pediatric Oral and Maxillofacial Surgery. Philadelphia: Saunders;2004. pp.3-19.
11. Kaban L, Troulis M. Pediatric Oral and Maxillofacial Surgery. Philadelphia: Saunders; 2004.
12. Koora K, Muthu MS, Rathna PV. Spontaneous closure of midline diastema following frenectomy. J Indian Soc Pedod Prev Dent. 2007;25(1):23-6.
13. McGurk M.Management of the ranula. J Oral Maxillofac Surg. 2007;65(1):115-6.
14. Minguez-MartinezI, Bonet-Coloma C, Ata-Ali MahmudJ, et al. Clinical characteristics, treatment, and evolution of 89 mucoceles in children. J Oral Maxillofac Surg. 2010;68(10):2468-71.
15. Segal LM, Stephenson R, Dawes M, et al. Prevalence, diagnosis, and treatment of ankyloglossia: methodologic review. Can Fam Physician. 2007;53(6):1027-33.
16. Suter VG, Bornstein MM. Ankyloglossia: facts and myths in diagnosis and treatment. J Periodontol. 2009;80(8):1204-19.

CHAPTER

Maxillofacial Trauma in Children

Sunil Sharma, Nikhil Marwah, Prateek Aggarwal

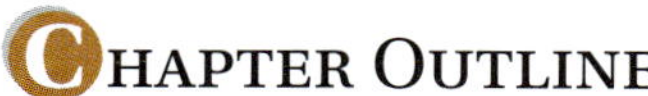

Facial injuries in children are considered separately because of special problems that arise in their treatment and management. Children, like adults are subject to similar types of injuries and trauma, but their capacity for healing in the shortest possible time with a minimum complications and the inherent ability to adapt to new situations are quite different from adults. However, facial injuries in children are much less common than in adults, particularly during the first five years of age. It is not until the age of puberty that the frequency and pattern of such injuries begin to parallel those seen in adults.

The principles for the treatment of children's facial fracture are basically the same as those utilized in adults. However, the techniques used are necessarily modified by certain anatomical, physiological and psychological factors specifically related to childhood. The process starts with kind patient handling, making sure that the child is engaged with dialogue and a trust is established, this trust is transferred to the parents, who will help during the more uncomfortable stages of examination and treatment. Further, this trust also helps deal with the psychological aftermath felt by the patient.

Soft tissue injuries and fractures may require special therapeutic techniques owing to difficulties in obtaining the cooperation of young children. Further, young bone possesses unique physical properties that coupled with the space occupying developing dentition which give rise to patterns of fracture that is not seen in adults and results in a need for different forms of fixation for shorter period of time. Another aspect of facial injuries in children is the potential for later effects upon facial development. A post-traumatic facial deformity in the child is a result of displacement of bony structures caused by the fracture and also of faulty or arrested development due to injury.

INCIDENCE

- Fractures of facial bones are less frequent in children than in adults. It is difficult to come to conclusion about the true incidence of these injuries because of variation in the patient population and variation of incidence from one country to another.
- It is clear that fracture of the facial bones in children occurs in frequently, i.e., 1.3–4.9% in younger than 11 years and 4.1–9.2% in those younger than 16 years. The middle third of the facial structure is rarely involved and **Rowe** (1969) concluded that such fractures in children comprise only 0.5% of the total fracture sustained.
- During their early stage of growth, children live in a more protected environment under close supervision of parents. The resilience of the developing bone and the thick overlying soft tissue enable the child to withstand the forces. The tooth to bone ratio in the developing mandible is comparatively high and the bone has a more elastic resistance.
- All the major studies show that facial fractures are most common in males than females. Below 5 years old, the incidence is almost equal, but the ratio of male-female increases with age.
- Fracture of the nasal bones and of the mandible account for the great majority of facial fracture in children.

History of Oral and Maxillofacial Surgery		
Ancient Egypt	**The Edwin Smith Treatise**	Written approximately 3000 BC in hieroglyphics, but "carpetbagged" by American **Edwin Smith** in approximately 1862, who bought it off an Egyptian peasant for mere trinkets.
Ancient Greece	**Hippocrates**	The first description of closed reduction with maxillary-mandibular fixation (MMF) was written in 460 BC "Displaced but incomplete fractures of the mandible where continuity of the bone is preserved should be reduced by pressing the lingual surface with the fingers while counter pressure is applied from the outside. Following reduction, teeth adjacent to fracture are fastened to each other by gold wire."
Modern Europe	1180 AD	The first European medical school, in Salerno, Italy, was established.
America	**Thomas Gunning**	A dentist during the civil war, during which time the therapy of mandibular fractures was greatly advanced. He designed the "Gunning splint" for **William Seward**, the Secretary of State to **Abraham Lincoln**, who suffered bilateral body fractures after falling out of a carriage. The splint was a single piece of vulcanite with a space for eating. Screws were used to stabilize the splint to the hard palate and the mandible.

- Although less frequent than in adults and second to nasal fractures, mandibular fractures are the most common facial fracture reported in pediatric trauma patients. Mandibular fractures are rare in children under 5 years. **MacLennan** has shown under 6 years at 1%, children aged 6–11 at 5% and under 16 years 7.7%.
- The distribution between the sexes is similar to a 2:1 male predominance for all mandibular fractures and an 8:1 predominance for condylar fractures.

Site and Pattern

- The site and pattern of a fracture depend on the interrelationship between etiology and force of the injury, and the unique anatomic features of the child's stage of development.
- While infants (below age 2 years) are more likely to sustain injuries of the frontal region, older children are more prone to injuries of the chin or lip region.
- Children below age 3 years usually sustain isolated, non-displaced fractures caused by low-impact or low-velocity forces.
- The condylar region is the most frequently fractured site, being affected bilaterally in about 20% of pediatric patients. Fractures of the condyle are more common in children than in adults because the highly vascularized pediatric condyle and thin neck are poorly resistant to impact forces during falls.
- Fractures in the condylar region are followed in number by symphysis, and angle and body fractures, respectively. While body fractures are less common than in adults, symphysis and parasymphysis fractures of the mandible occur more often.
- Mid-face fractures in children, usually resulting from high-impact and/or high velocity forces, are rare. Zygomatic complex fractures are the most frequent, after maxillary alveolar and nasal injuries.
- Le Fort fractures (at all levels) are uncommon and are almost never seen before age 2 years. The highest incidence of mid-face fractures occurs in children 13–15 years of age.
- Orbital injuries constitute approximately 20% of pediatric facial fractures. They result from transmission of forces directly from a blow to the bony orbital ring to the thin orbital walls and/or indirect forces from a hydraulic pressure effect of displaced orbital soft tissues. Orbital roof fractures occur in young children, in whom the frontal sinus is still underdeveloped whereas orbital floor fractures are more common in older children, in whom the maxillary sinus has expanded beyond the equator of the globe.

Associated Injuries

- A higher percentage of associated injuries are seen in the pediatric age group.
- Soft tissue injuries, particularly facial lacerations, are the most common in both adults and children, but children include a relatively high percentage of cranial injuries.
- **Morgan et al.** (1972) reported 94 cases of injuries in which 23% were soft tissue and dental injuries while 55% were associated cranial injuries.

MANAGEMENT OF MAXILLOFACIAL TRAUMA

Clinical Examination

- The history of the injury may indicate the mechanisms and direction of force of the injury and may provide clues for the clinical examination such symptoms may include swelling pain, numbness in a cranial nerve distribution.
- Nasal or oral bleeding, tooth displacement, difficulty in eating, malocclusion, decrease excursion of the jaw and ecchymosis point to a skeletal injury.
- A cerebrospinal fluid (CSF) leak may indicate involvement of the cranial base. Subcutaneous emphysema is seen in the periorbital area when air enters the tissue from fractures of the nose, orbit or sinuses.
- The clinical examination consists of an orderly inspection of all facial areas, including observation, palpation and a functional examination. An orderly palpation of all bony surfaces should be performed by beginning in the forehead area and by palpating the rims of the orbits bilaterally and the nose, in order to identify any tenderness, irregularity or step. The examination is continued over the zygomatic arches, cheeks and the surface of the mandible.

- An intraoral examination is performed to look for any loose teeth, a laceration or hematomas
- Lateral pressure on the mandibular and maxillary dental arches is necessary to determine instability or pain in fractures involving the midline of the mandible or maxilla.

Radiographic Examination

- The standard radiographic evaluation consists of plain films, PNS view, submentovertex, Towne's and lateral skull views with orthopantomogram (OPG). Failure to confirm a suspected fracture on radiography should not always delay the treatment. Clinical judgment should overrule other considerations
- The CT scanning has improved the radiographic diagnosis of midfacial and upper facial fractures

- Lateral oblique: View from the condyle to the mental foramen.
- Posteroanterior (PA): View of the ramus, angle and body.
- Reverse Towne's (PA): Medial/lateral displacement of condylar fractures.
- OPG is the choice for mandible fractures.
- CT scanning: It is especially useful for temporomandibular joint (TMJ) evaluation, midface and nasoethmoid fracture.
- Occlusal views: Used for evaluating symphyseal displacement.

Glasgow Coma Scale in Children

	Infant	*1–4 years*	*Age 4–adult*
Eyes			
4	Open	Open	Open
3	To voice	To voice	To voice
2	To pain	To pain	To pain
1	No response	No response	No response
Verbal			
5	Coos, babbles	Oriented, speaks, interacts, social	Oriented and alert
4	Irritable cry, consolable	Confused speech, disoriented, consolable	Disoriented
3	Cries persistently to pain	Inappropriate words, inconsolable	Nonsensical speech
2	Moans to pain	Incomprehensible, agitated	Moans unintelligible
1	No response	No response	No response
Motor			
6	Normal, spontaneous movement	Normal, spontaneous movement	Follows commands
5	Withdraws to touch	Localizes pain	Localizes pain
4	Withdraws to pain	Withdraws to pain	Withdraws to pain
3	Decorticate flexion	Decorticate flexion	Decorticate flexion
2	Decerebrate extension	Decerebrate extension	Decerebrate extension
1	No response	No response	No response

GENERAL PRINCIPLES OF TREATMENT

Emergency Care

- The provision of an adequate airway, prevention of aspiration, and control of hemorrhage are the major considerations in the emergency management along with to obtain baseline vital signs. In a multiple injured child, the cervical spine should be stabilizes during airway assessment
- The mouth and pharynx should be cleaned of blood, food and broken teeth and the child is ventilated and intubated. Because of the small size of the airway in a child, laryngeal edema or retroposition of the base of the tongue may produce sudden obstruction that needs emergency tracheostomy. The next priority is control of bleeding and establishment of venous access. Direct pressure should be applied to accessible bleeding points
- Almost all cases of shock in traumatized children are related to hemorrhage, tachycardia, cool extremities and a systolic blood pressure less than 70 mm Hg are clear indications of shock when shock is diagnosed and fluid bolus of 20 mL/kg of warm crystalloid should be given.

Soft Tissue Injuries in Infants and Children

- Maxillofacial soft tissue trauma and injuries range from contusions and abrasions to massive avulsive injuries. Soft tissue wounds in children heal rapidly and therefore require early primary sutures
- History of tetanus vaccination should be sought and tetanus immune globulin or toxoid should be administered. If the injury resulted from an animal bite, a careful history must be taken to assess the necessity for rabies prophylaxis
- The basic fundamentals of management of such injuries are similar to those pertaining to adults. Careful cleaning and irrigation of wounds should be carried out in order to remove dirt and any foreign bodies and should be closed within 12 hours of injury, if required
- If hematoma is present in its gelatinous phase, it should be incised and evacuated. After further liquefaction, aspiration may be performed, if teeth or fragments of teeth are unaccounted for and laceration which exist in lips, soft tissue radiographs of the wounds are indicated
- Lacerations of the tongue are sutured in several layers to lessen the chance of hematoma formation. Lacerations of the special region of the face, such as eyebrows, eyelids margin and the vermilion border of the lips require careful alignment
- Blunt trauma may result in extensive and prolonged tissue damage with subsequent deep scarring and poor esthetics.

Pediatric Dental and Skeletal Anatomy

- The dentition and mandible in children are very different from those in adults. Pediatric teeth have poor retentive qualities, the roots are short and narrow, and the crowns have reduced retention contours, making them poor candidates for circumdental wire fixation
- A child's condyle is the growth center for the mandible. Thus, trauma or iatrogenic injury may cause growth retardation, malocclusion and facial asymmetry
- Children have a higher surface-to-body volume ratio, metabolic rate, oxygen demand and cardiac output than adults. They also have lower total blood and stroke volumes than adults. Therefore, the risk for hypothermia, hypotension and hypoxia after blood loss is higher in

pediatric patients. Even mild airway swelling or mechanical airway obstruction can quickly compromise the airway. For these reasons, maintenance of the airway and breathing, control of hemorrhage and early resuscitation are even more critical and time dependent in children than in adults.

DENTOALVEOLAR FRACTURE

- These are common in children
- Dentoalveolar injuries range from 8 to 50% of pediatric mandibular fractures **(Fig. 65.1)**. The principle of their management in children differs little from those in adults
- If the fragment is small and mobile and only deciduous teeth are attached, the fragment is removed. If the fragment contains permanent teeth, it should be repositioned out of occlusion and fixed with a wire and composite splint
- Short-term (1–2 weeks) maxillomandibular fixation is sometimes necessary to maintain stability of the fragment. Owing to the greater vascularity and speed of healing, the prognosis of bone healing is better in children than in adults
- Depending on the stage of development, dentoalveolar injury may lead to a host of dental growth disturbances ranging from dilaceration to ankylosis with an altered eruption sequence.

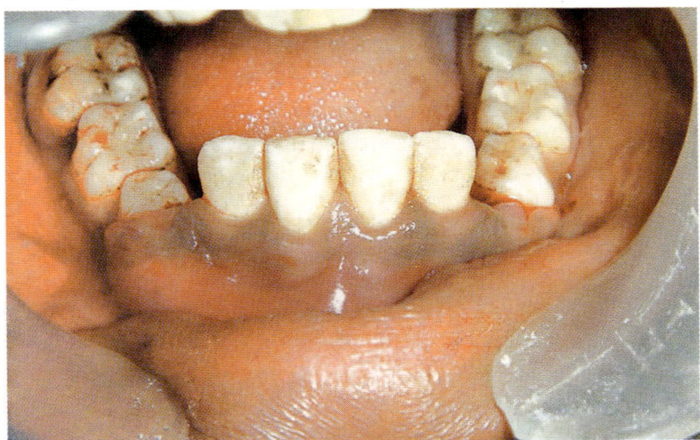

Fig. 65.1: Dentoalveolar fracture mandibular.

FRACTURES OF THE MANDIBLE

- Mandibular fractures are the second most common fractures after the nasal bones in children
- The OPG, combined with Towne's view, generally provide excellent imaging of the mandibular fractures
- However, there are often situations where more conservative management will be appropriate while considering different methods of immobilization of fractures of jaw, it is quite important to subdivide the patients depending upon the stages of the dentition at the time of injury.
- **Infancy to 2-year old**
  - When the fracture is in the tooth-bearing part of the mandible: The fracture should be treated as an edentulous problem. A prefabricated acrylic 'open-cap splint' **(Fig. 65.2)** lower splint is pressed down over the lower teeth and alveolus following manual disimpaction and reduction of any displacement of fragments. The splint is retained in place by two circumferential wires placed with the help of small-sized 'Awl' instrument, one on either side of the fracture line, 2 or 3 weeks is generally sufficient to ensure union

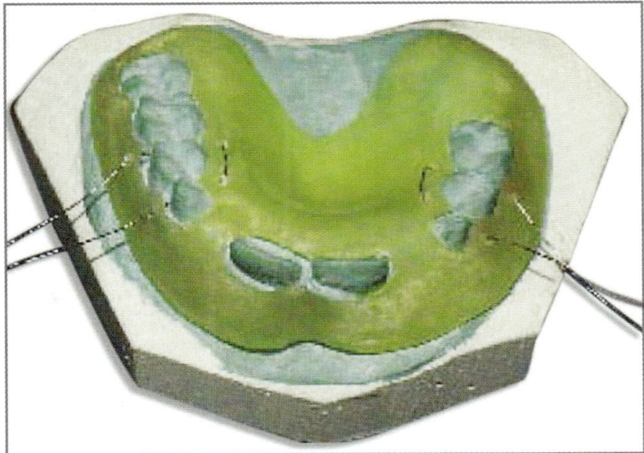

Fig. 65.2: Open cap splint.

  - When the fracture is proximal to the tooth-bearing area, i.e. through the angle: In order to immobilize the mandible, the prefabricated acrylic splint is adjusted over the mandibular arch to occlude with the maxillary teeth, thus stabilizing the bite. Other method of immobilization of mandible is by nasomandibular fixation in which wires from the margins of the piriform aperture of the nose pass beneath the circumferential wires that secure the lower splint to the mandible.
- **In 2–4 years old:** At this stage, provided sound sufficient primary teeth are present, interdental eyelet wiring **(Fig. 65.3)** can be used. If there are gaps in the primary dentition, arch bar may be used. If the fracture is within tooth bearing area of the mandible, a single one- piece lower cap splint, may be the best method since immobilization of the lower jaw is avoided

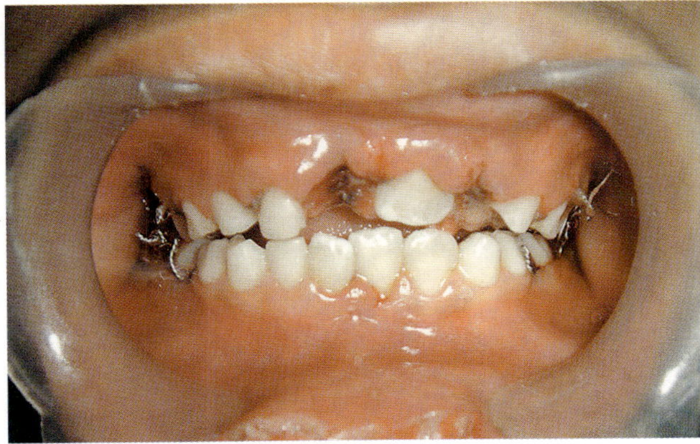

Fig. 65.3: Eyelet wiring.

- **In 5–8 years old:** It is between these ages that the greatest problems arise with regard to fixation of the mandible. The anterior teeth are of little or no use because of roots are resorbed in deciduous teeth or incompletely formed in the permanent teeth. These difficulties can be overcome by constructing partial maxillary and mandibular "Gunning type" splints with occlusal blocker. This mandibular splint

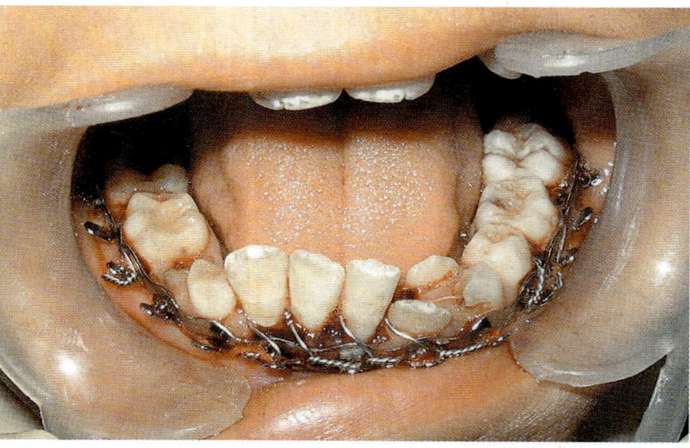

Fig. 65.4: Splinting with arch bar.

is secured by circumferential wires fixation of the upper splint to the maxilla is provided by the use of prenasal wires whereby the splint is suspended by two wires which rest on the floor of the nose, one either side of the septum

- **In 9–11 years old:** In patients of this age group, the permanent incisors and 1st molar teeth can safely be employed for fixation, either by means of cap splints or arch bars **(Fig. 65.4),** plating or transosseous wiring, arch bar elastics.

SYMPHYSEAL AND PARASYMPHYSEAL MANDIBULAR FRACTURES

- Pediatric mandibular fractures require thoughtful consideration in management to avoid further injury to the developing dentition and significant growth disturbance. Most pediatric mandible fractures are amenable to closed reduction with MMF and the use of splints with skeletal fixation **(Figs. 65.5A to D)**
- Bilateral fracture of the anterior mandible is common
- These fractures are frequently greenstick and require no active treatment. If mobile, they are well-managed with an acrylic splint and circummandibular wires **(Figs. 65.6A to D)**
- Undisplaced and immobile fractures of the anterior mandible can be treated with soft diet and careful follow-up.
- Displaced anterior fractures may be managed with closed manipulation and wiring of an acrylic splints or with open reduction and miniplate **(Figs. 65.7A and B)** and screw fixation and the splint needs to stay in place for only 2–3 weeks.

ANGLE FRACTURE

- Undisplaced fractures are common and may be treated with soft diet alone if the occlusion is not disturbed. If bilateral fractures are present, the patient should be treated with MMF **(Fig. 65.8).**
- Displaced fracture of angles requires open reduction, as the proximal fragment cannot be reduced or controlled with either MMF or a splint.
- The presence of developing teeth within the mandible requires transosseous wiring but these must be kept as close to the lower border as possible. This can be performed through either a transoral or extraoral approach. The patient is then placed in MMF for 2–3 weeks.

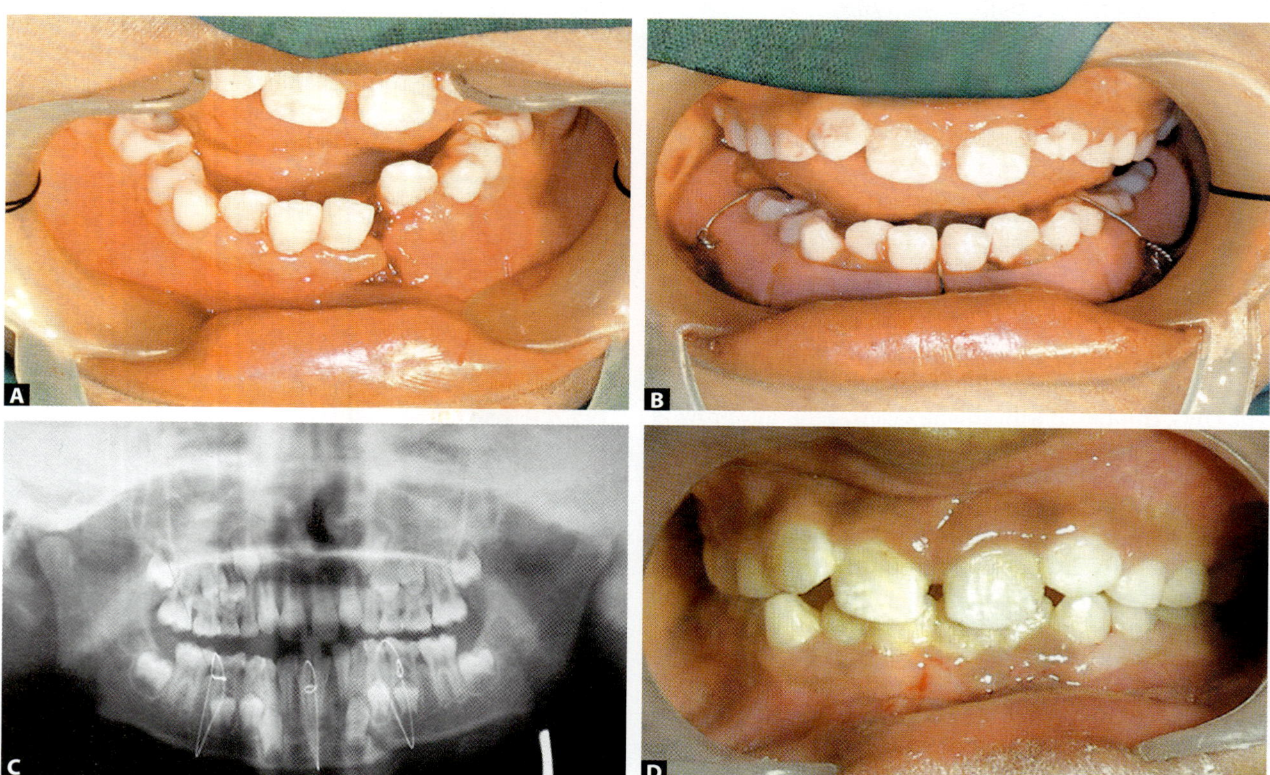

Figs. 65.5A to D: Management of parasymphyseal fracture with splint: (A) Preoperative view of parasymphyseal fracture; (B) Splint in place; (C) Radiographic view; (D) Postoperative occlusion.

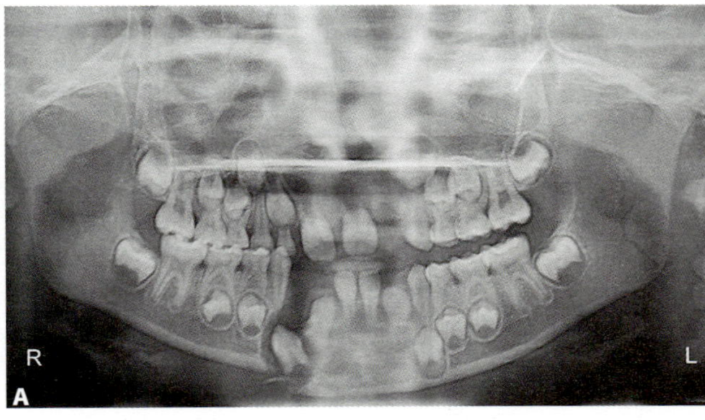

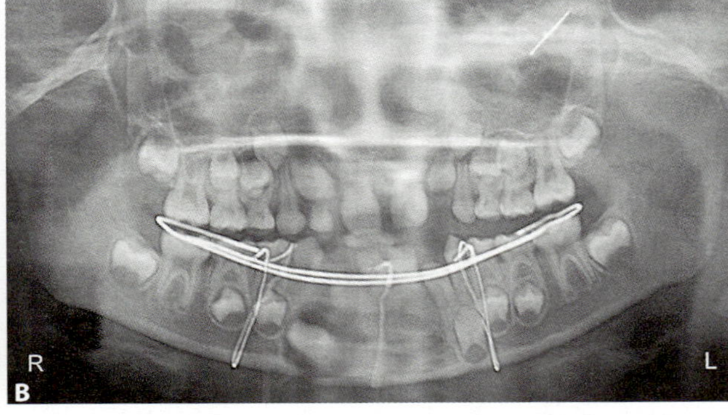

Figs. 65.6A and B: Management of parasymphyseal fracture using circummandibular wiring: (A) Preoperative view of parasymphyseal fracture; (B) Reduction using circummandibular wiring.

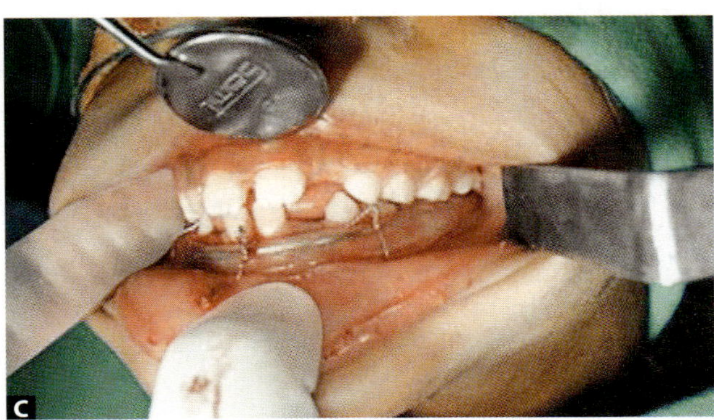

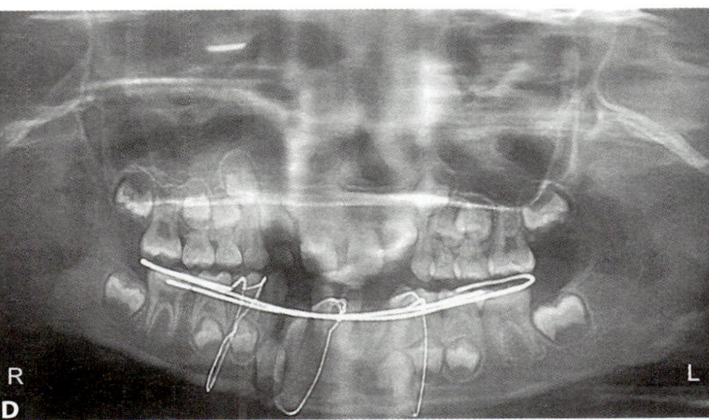

Figs. 65.6C and D: Management of parasymphyseal fracture using circummandibular wiring: (C) Intraoral view of circummandibular wiring; (D) Postoperative view showing alignment of bone and toothbud.

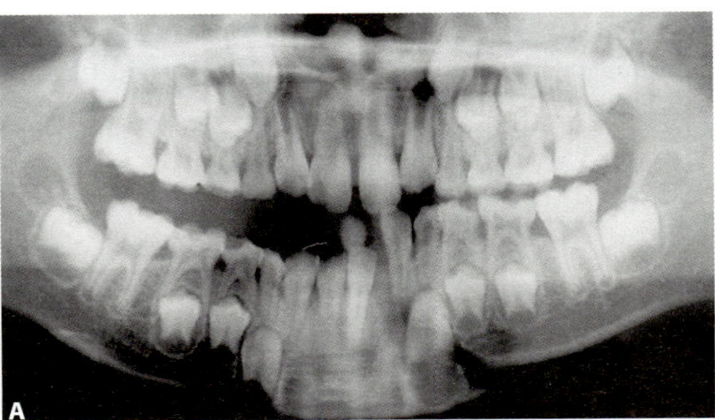

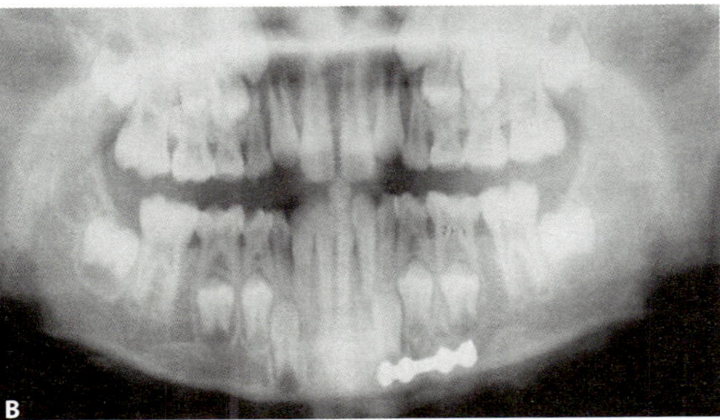

Figs. 65.7A and B: Management of parasymphysis fracture with miniplate: (A) Parasymphysis fracture; (B) Miniplate in place.

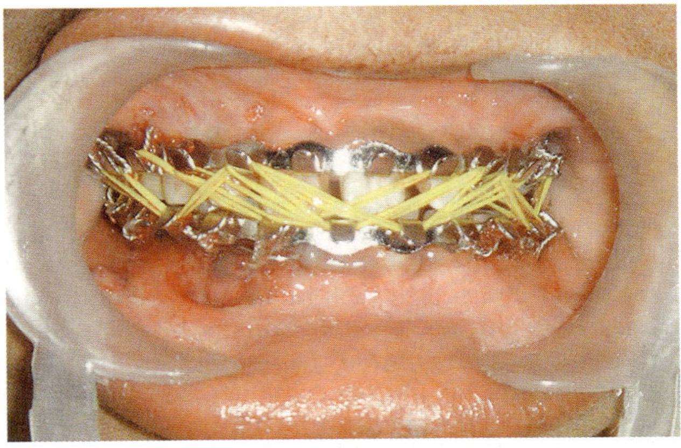

Fig. 65.8: Intermaxillary fixation.

CONDYLAR FRACTURES

The condylar fracture of the babies and infants are of intra-articular crush injury type. The condylar neck does not undergo any change in development until 2 years of age but grows to resemble adult anatomy by age 7 or 8 years.

In this group, most fractures of the condyles are extracapsular involving the condylar neck.

- Condyle fractures are characterized by shortening of the ramus on the affected side causing deviation of the chin to the affected side. On the unaffected side, open bite and flattening of the body of the mandible are seen. This is accompanied with preauricular tenderness or reduced mouth opening

- The treatment of condylar fractures differs from adult treatment owing to the increased healing and regeneration capacity. The younger the patient at the time of injury the greater the likelihood of complete or near complete condylar remodeling
- Closed treatment of the condyle fracture in children remains the standard for treatment today
- Treatment is directed toward the restoration of normal function, pain free jaw movement as early as possible after injury. Painful jaw movement can be relieved by rest and analgesics for the first few days, or by MMF (6–9 days) followed by active movement of jaw. The younger the patient the shorter should be the duration of MMF
- MMF should not be used in intracapsular fractures because of the increased potential for ankylosis. Exercise should continue for 3 months and followed by review every 2–3 months for one year
- In patients with fracture of condyles and other facial fractures, open reduction and plating of facial fractures may allow earlier mobilization of the mandible.

FRACTURES OF THE MIDDLE-THIRD OF THE FACIAL SKELETON

- Midfacial fractures in children up to the age of 12 years have account for less than 0.5% of all facial fractures (**Rowe**, 1968). This is presumably because:
  - Higher degree of elasticity of the facial bones
  - Poor pneumatization of paranasal sinuses
  - Lesser degree of development of the midfacial skeleton in relation to the cranial area
  - Attachment to the cartilaginous growth plates of the skull base
  - Presence of greater facial fat.
- The diagnosis of midfacial fractures is made difficult by fat and edema masking underlying contour deformities and lack of cooperation of the patient. Plain radiographs are difficult to obtain. But axial and coronal CT scan can be of choice
- The typical Le Fort line of fractures is rarely encountered in children's fractures. Low maxillary or Le Fort I types of fracture are not common until the age of 10 years. Pyramidal or Le Fort II is seen more commonly and sometimes unilaterally.

Le Fort I Fracture

- Horizontal fracture of the maxilla at the level of the nasal fossa. It is also known as a Guérin fracture or 'floating palate'
- The fracture extends from the nasal septum to the lateral pyriform rims, travels horizontally above the teeth apices, crosses below the zygomaticomaxillary junction, and traverses the pterygomaxillary junction to interrupt the pterygoid plates
  - Allows motion of the maxilla while the nasal bridge remains stable
  - Facial edema
  - Malocclusion of the teeth
  - Fracture line which involves nasal aperture, inferior maxilla and lateral wall of maxilla (**Figs. 65.9A and B**).

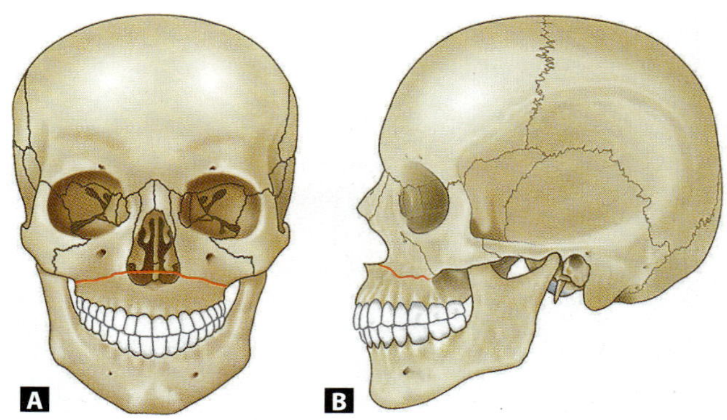

Figs. 65.9A and B: Le Fort I fracture.

Le Fort II Fracture

Pyramidal fracture through maxilla, nasal bones and medial aspect of the orbits.

Such a fracture has a pyramidal shape and extends from the nasal bridge at or below the nasofrontal suture through the frontal processes of the maxilla, inferolaterally through the lacrimal bones and inferior orbital floor and rim through or near the inferior orbital foramen, and inferiorly through the anterior wall of the maxillary sinus; it then travels under the zygoma, across the pterygomaxillary fissure, and through the pterygoid plates.

- Marked facial edema
- Nasal flattening
- Traumatic telecanthus
- Epistaxis
- Fracture line involves nasal bones, medial orbit, maxillary sinus and frontal process of the maxilla (**Figs. 65.10A and B**).

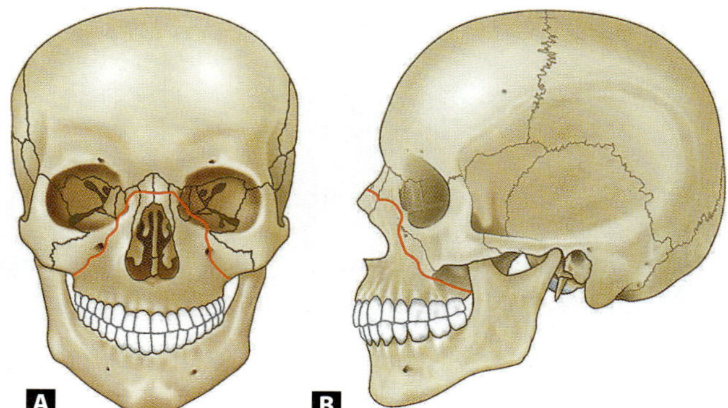

Figs. 65.10A and B: Le Fort II fracture.

Le Fort III Fracture

- Transverse fractures involving maxilla, zygoma, nasal bones, ethmoid bones, base of the skull (**Figs. 65.11A and B**)
- These fractures start at the nasofrontal and frontomaxillary sutures and extend posteriorly along the medial wall of the orbit through the nasolacrimal groove and ethmoid bones. The thicker sphenoid bone posteriorly usually prevents continuation of the fracture into the optic canal. Instead, the fracture continues along the floor of the orbit along the inferior orbital fissure and continues superolaterally through the lateral orbital wall, through the zygomaticofrontal junction and the zygomatic arch.

Intranasally, a branch of the fracture extends through the base of the perpendicular plate of the ethmoid, through the vomer, and through the interface of the pterygoid plates to the base of the sphenoid

- Dish faced deformity
- Epistaxis and CSF rhinorrhea
- Motion of the maxilla, nasal bones and zygoma
- Severe airway obstruction
- Fractures through zygomatic—frontal suture, zygoma, medial orbital wall and nasal bone **(Figs. 65.11A and B).**

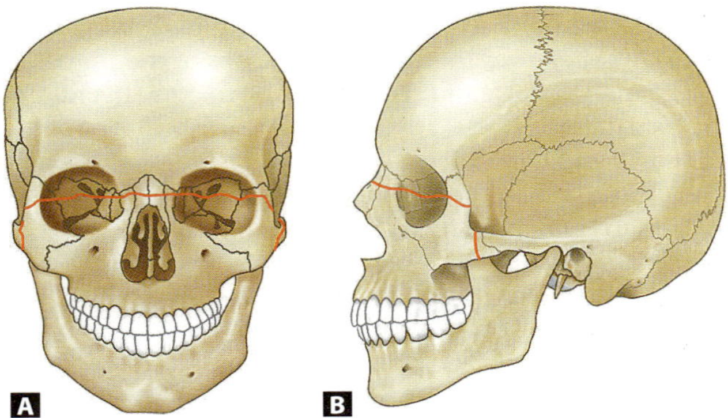

Figs. 65.11A and B: Le Fort III fracture.

Management of Le Fort Fractures

- Treatment techniques depend on the anatomic location of the fractures, their mobility and amount of displacement
- Minimally displaced fractures occurring during the period of tooth development and eruption require either no treatment or a short period of MMF
- In a child, 2 weeks of MMF are adequate
- The use of closed reduction or to wiring in conjunction with external fixators has given way to wide exposure, anatomic reduction and plate and screw fixation. The combinations of coronal, superior lid or subciliary or transconjunctival and maxillary vestibular incisions allow for exposure of the entire facial skeleton. The piriform rim is relatively thick in children and readily accepts plates and screws
- The zygomatic buttress must be used with caution in children younger than 12 because of the thinness of the bone and process of underlying teeth
- The use of plates and screws frequently obviates the need for MMF.

ZYGOMATIC AND ORBITAL FRACTURES

- Displaced fractures of zygomatic bone are rare in children and rarely occur before the age of 8 years but increase in frequency with age
- When fractures of the zygoma are sustained, displacement is due to weak and easily disrupted frontozygomatic (FZ) sutured ligament. Depressed malunited zygomatic fractures vary in their severity
- **Clinical features**
  - Residual hypoesthesia of the upper eye, nose and cheek
  - Flatness of the cheek
  - The lateral canthus may be displaced inferiorly, giving an antimongoloid slant to the palpebral fissure
  - The inferior displacement of the fracture may impinge the zygoma against the coronoid process, resulting in an open bite.
- **Radiographic evaluation**
  - Consists of Waters' and Caldwell's views to assess displacement
  - Posterior displacement of the malar eminence and the zygomatic arch is assessed through the submentovertex skull view or axial CT scans.
- **Treatment**
  - Undisplaced zygomatic fractures do not require treatment
  - Displaced fractures are treated by open reduction and interfragmentary wiring at the FZ suture and the infraorbital rim
  - The infraorbital rim and the zygomaticofrontal suture are exposed through a subciliary incision with a skin muscle flap. In patients with comminution of the zygomatic body or arch, the coronal flap provides the most satisfactory access
  - Unlike in adults, the zygomatic buttress in children is not useful for the placement of plates and screws owing to thin bone and the presence of unerupted teeth. The indications for open reduction are deformity, enophthalmos, vertical malposition of the globe, retrusion of the malar eminence, persistent diplopia and anesthesia or hypoesthesia in the infraorbital nerve distribution.
- **Zygomatic arch type fracture**
  - Palpable bony defect over the arch
  - Depressed cheek with tenderness
  - Pain in cheek and jaw movement
  - Submental view (jug handle view)
  - *Treatment:* Possible open elevation.
- **Zygomatic tripod fracture**
  - This includes zygomatic arch, zygomaticofrontal suture and inferior orbital rim and floor
  - Periorbital edema and ecchymosis
  - Hyperesthesia of the infraorbital nerve
  - Palpation may reveal step deformity
  - Concomitant globe injuries are common
  - Radiographic imaging by Water's, submental and Caldwell's views
  - *Treatment:* Displaced tripod fractures usually require admission for open reduction and internal fixation.

NASO-ETHMOIDAL-ORBITAL FRACTURE

- Fractures that extend into the nose through the ethmoid bones. Associated with lacrimal disruption and dural tears
- Suspect if there is trauma to the nose or medial orbit. Patients complain of pain on eye movement
- Flattened nasal bridge or a saddle-shaped deformity of the nose. Widening of the nasal bridge (pseudo-telecanthus)
- CSF rhinorrhea or epistaxis
- Tenderness, crepitus and mobility of the nasal complex. Intranasal palpation reveals movement of the medial canthus.

ORBITAL FRACTURES

- In children younger than 7 years of age, orbital fractures more frequently involve the roof than the floor and are associated with anterior cranial base injury
- Orbital fractures in children are observed after automobile accidents and are often characterized by a separation of FZ junction in the lateral orbital wall, with downward displacement of the floor. Blowout fractures are the most common of the orbital fractures. They occur when the globe sustains direct blunt force
- The first is a true blowout fracture, where all the energy is transmitted to the globe. Since the spherical globe is stronger than the thin orbital floor, the force is then transmitted to the thin orbital floor or medially through the ethmoid bones with the resultant fractures. The object causing the injury must be smaller than 5–6 cm; otherwise the globe is protected by the surrounding orbit. Fists or small balls are the typical causative agents
- The second mechanism occurs when the energy from the blow is transmitted to the infraorbital rim causing a buckling of the floor. Entrapment and globe injury are less likely with this injury

Clinical Features

- The diagnosis of an orbital fracture is suggested by the presence of periorbital and subconjunctival hematomas
- Orbital wall and floor fractures may occur with or without other fractures
- Depending upon the extent of the orbital floor involvement, there may be extraocular muscle dysfunction, which results in diplopia
- Periorbital tenderness, swelling, ecchymosis
- Enophthalmos or sunken eyes
- Impaired ocular motility
- Infraorbital anesthesia
- Step deformity.

Radiographs

These have hanging tear drop sign; open trap door appearance with change in air fluid levels.

Treatment

- Orbital fractures are approached in the same manner as in adults except that transantral techniques cannot be used until the premolar teeth are fully erupted and their roots are clear of the surgical field
- Despite the small size of the maxillary antrum, escape of orbital contents through the fractured floor may occur and this can give rise to enophthalmos and diplopia
- Since antral packing is contraindicated in children, open exploration of the orbital floor is the treatment of choice. Comminuted fragments should be conserved, as they consolidate rapidly when realigned.

NASAL FRACTURES

- The nose as the most projecting part of the face is particularly exposed to trauma
- Fractures of the nasal bones are more frequent than fractures of the maxilla and zygoma. In the early years of childhood, the nasal skeleton is proportionally more cartilaginous than bony and the diagnosis of nasal fracture is more difficult. It is of three types:
  1. Depressed
  2. Laterally displaced
  3. Nondisplaced

Clinical Features

- The 'open book' type of fracture, with overriding of the nasal bones over the frontal processes of the maxilla, is a characteristic feature of nasal bone fracture in children
- Nasal deformity
- Edema and tenderness
- Epistaxis
- Crepitus and mobility.

Treatment

- Direct pressure
- Topical vasoconstrictor such as phenylephrine 1% or cocaine
- Cauterize with silver nitrate
- Nasal packing
- *Draining septal hematomas:* Anesthetize the area and using a # 11 blade incise the inferior portion of the hematoma and allow it to drain. Then pack the nose with Vaseline gauze to prevent reaccumulation of blood. If there is no epistaxis or deformity, treat the patient with ice and analgesics.

MANDIBULAR DISLOCATION

Dislocation generally results from a direct blow to chin while the mouth is open, or more commonly in predisposed individuals after a vigorous yawn. Opening the mouth excessively wide while eating or laughing may also result in dislocation. It can also be seen in patients who have had a seizure, and in patients who have had a dystonic reaction from their neuroleptic medication.

The mandible can be dislocated in the anterior, posterior, lateral and superior plane. Anterior dislocation is the most common and occurs when the condyle is forced in front of the articular eminence. Anterior dislocation occurs in up to 70% of the normal individuals but can be spontaneously reduced by the patient. Once the jaw is dislocated, muscular spasm, particularly the temporalis and lateral pterygoid muscles tend to prevent reduction. Dislocations are most frequently bilateral, but they also can be unilateral.

Risk Factors

- Weakness of the temporal mandibular ligament. Overstretched joint capsule
- Shallow articular eminence. Neurologic diseases.

Types of Dislocations

- **Posterior dislocations**
  - Direct blow to the chin
  - Condylar head is pushed against the mastoid.

- ❖ **Lateral dislocations**
  - Associated with a jaw fracture
  - Condylar head is forced laterally and superiorly.
- ❖ **Superior dislocations**
  - Blow to a partially open mouth
  - Condylar head is force upward.

Clinical Features

- ❖ Inability to close mouth
- ❖ Pain
- ❖ Facial swelling
- ❖ Palpable depression
- ❖ Jaw will deviate away
- ❖ Jaw displaced anteriorly.

Recent advances

- Rapid IMF is an adjustable flexible plastic band that wraps around the tooth to create an anchorage point for temporary maxilla-mandibular fixation and immobilization
- Resorbable plates: These plates provide initial osseous fixation strength for direct bone healing and then they disappear over a period of time leaving behind no foreign body
- The blunt tips of the screws and their eventual resorption offer essentially no risk to developing teeth and nerve structures or ongoing facial growth and eliminate long-term foreign body retention
- The Sonic Weld Rx® process takes advantage of polymer characteristics instead of adapting titanium screw designs.

Treatment

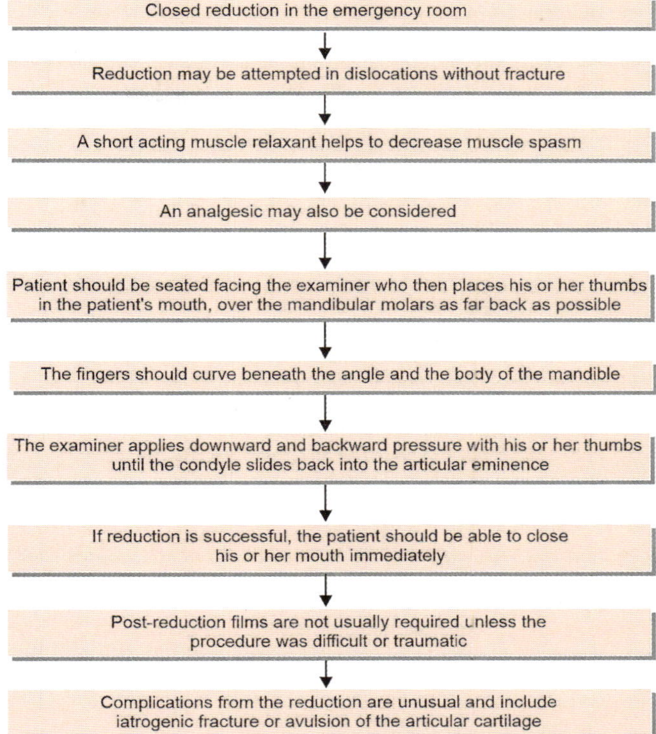

Closed reduction in the emergency room
Reduction may be attempted in dislocations without fracture
A short acting muscle relaxant helps to decrease muscle spasm
An analgesic may also be considered
Patient should be seated facing the examiner who then places his or her thumbs in the patient's mouth, over the mandibular molars as far back as possible
The fingers should curve beneath the angle and the body of the mandible
The examiner applies downward and backward pressure with his or her thumbs until the condyle slides back into the articular eminence
If reduction is successful, the patient should be able to close his or her mouth immediately
Post-reduction films are not usually required unless the procedure was difficult or traumatic
Complications from the reduction are unusual and include iatrogenic fracture or avulsion of the articular cartilage

POINTS TO REMEMBER

- Fractures of facial bones are less frequent in children than in adults.
- All the major studies show that facial fractures are most common in males than females.
- While infants (below age 2) are more likely to sustain injuries of the frontal region, older children are more prone to injuries of the chin or lip region. Children below age 3 usually sustain isolated, non-displaced fractures caused by low-impact or low-velocity forces.
- Le Fort fractures (at all levels) are uncommon and are almost never seen before age 2. The highest incidence of midface fractures occurs in children 13–15 years of age.
- Dentoalveolar fracture is found in 10–50% of children and managed by wire splints.
- Symphyseal and parasymphyseal mandibular fractures are the most complex fractures and are managed by miniplates, acrylic splint and circummandibular wires.
- Condylar fractures are characterized by shortening of the ramus on the affected side causing deviation of the chin to the affected side. On the unaffected side, open bite and flattening of the body of the mandible are seen. Closed treatment of the condyle fracture in children remains the standard for treatment today.
- Le Fort I fracture is horizontal fracture of the maxilla at the level of the nasal fossa.
- Le Fort II fracture is pyramidal fracture through maxilla, nasal bones and medial aspect of the orbit.
- Le Fort III fracture is transverse fractures involving maxilla, zygoma, nasal bones, ethmoid bones, base of the skull.
- The diagnosis of an orbital fracture is suggested by the presence of periorbital and subconjunctival hematomas and its classical features are diplopia, infraorbital anesthesia, and ecchymosis.
- Fractures of the nasal bones are more frequent than fractures of the maxilla and zygoma.

Questionnaire

1. Give the incidence and site prevalence of maxillofacial trauma.
2. Write a note on radiographic examination in trauma patients.
3. Describe the etiology, clinical features and management of mandibular fractures.
4. What are dentoalveolar fractures?
5. Explain the Le Fort fractures.
6. Give the clinical features and management of orbital fracture.
7. Write a note on mandibular dislocation.
8. Classify and describe zygomatic fracture.

FURTHER READING

1. Anderson PJ. Fractures of the facial skeleton in children. Injury. 1995;26(1):47-50.
2. Blakey GH III, Ruiz RL, Turvey TA. Management of facial fractures in growing patient. In: Fonseca RJ, Walker RV (Eds). Oral and Maxillofacial Trauma, 2nd Edition. Vol. 2. Philadelphia: WB Saunders; 1997. pp. 1003-41.
3. Carroll MJ, Hill CM, Mason DA. Facial fractures in children. Br Dent J. 1987;163(1):23-6.
4. Crockett DM, Funk GF. Management of complicated fractures involving the orbits and nasoethmoid complex in young children. Otolaryngol Clin North Am. 1991;24(1):119-37.

5. Demianczuk AN, Verchere C, Phillips JH. The effect on facial growth of pediatric mandibular fractures. J Craniofac Surg. 1999;10(4):323-8.
6. Dufresne CR, Manson PN. Pediatric facial trauma. In: McCarthy, et al (Eds). Plastic Surgery. Vol. 2. Philadelphia: WB Saunders; 1990.
7. Eppley BL. Use of resorbable plates and screws in pediatric facial fractures. J Oral Maxillofac Surg. 2005;63(3):385-91.
8. Hardt N, Gottsauner A. The treatment of mandibular fractures in children. J Craniomaxillofac Surg. 1993;21(5):214-9.
9. Haug RH, Foss J. Maxillofacial injuries in pediatric patient. Oral Surg Oral Med Oral Pathol Oral Radiol Endod. 2000;90(2): 126-34.
10. Jamerson RE, White JA. Management of pediatric mandibular fractures. J La State Med Soc. 1990;142(3):11-3.
11. Kaban LB, Mulliken JB, Murray JE. Facial fractures in children: an analysis of 122 fractures in 109 patients. Plast Reconstr Surg. 1977;59(1):15-20.
12. Kaban LB. Diagnosis and treatment of fractures of the facial bones in children 1943-1993. J Oral Maxillofac Surg. 1993;51(7):722-9.
13. Kaban LB. Facial trauma II. Dentoalveolar injuries and mandibular fractures. In: Kaban LB (Eds). Pediatric Oral and Maxillofacial Surgery.; Philadelphia: WB Saunders; 1990. pp. 233-60.
14. Koltai PJ, Amjad I, Meyer D, et al. Orbital fractures in children. Arch Otolaryngol Head Neck Surg. 1995;121(12):1375-9.
15. Koltai PJ, Rabkin D. Management of facial trauma in children. Pediatr Clin North Am. 1996;43(6):1253-75.
16. Koltai PJ. Maxillofacial injuries in children. In: Smith JD, Bumsted RM (Eds). Pediatric Facial Plastic and Reconstructive Surgery. New York: Lippincott-Raven; 1993.
17. Krausen AS, Samuel M. Pediatric jaw fractures: indications for open reduction. Otolaryngol Head Neck Surg. 1979;87(3): 318-22.
18. Kumar AV, Staffenberg DA, Petronio JA, et al. Bioabsorbable plates and screws in pediatric craniofacial surgery: a review of 22 cases. J Craniofac Surg. 1997;8(2):97-9.
19. MacLennan WD. Fractures of the mandible in children under the age of six years. Br J Plast Surg. 1956;9(2):125-8.
20. Maniglia AJ, Kline SN. Maxillofacial trauma in the pediatric age group. Otolaryngol Clin North Am. 1983;16(3):717-30.
21. McCoy FJ, Chandler RA, Crow ML. Facial fractures in children. Plast Reconstr Surg. 1966;37(3):209-15.
22. McGrath CJ, Egbert MA, Tong DC, et al. Unusual presentations of injuries associated with the mandibular condyle in children. Br J Oral Maxillofac Surg. 1996;34(4):311-4.
23. McGuirt WF, Salisbury PL 3d. Mandibular fractures. Their effect on growth and dentition. Arch Otolaryngol Head Neck Surg. 1987;113(3):257-61.
24. Morgan WC. Pediatric mandibular fractures. Oral Surg Oral Med Oral Pathol. 1975;40(3):320-6.
25. Pogrel MA, Kaban LB. Mandibular fracture. In: Haban MB, Ariyan S (Eds). Facial Fractures. Toronto: BC Decker; 1989.
26. Polayes IM. Facial fractures in the pediatric patient. In: Habal MB, Ariayn S (Eds). Facial Fractures. Toronto: BC Decker; 1989.
27. Posnick JC, Wells M, Pron GE. Pediatric facial fractures: evolving patterns of treatment. J Oral Maxillofac Surg. 1993;51(8):836-44.
28. Posnick JC. Craniomaxillofacial fractures in children. Atlas Oral Maxillofac Surg Clin North Am. 1994; 6:169-85.
29. Rowe NL. Fractures of the jaws in children. J Oral Surg. 1969;27(7):497.
30. Shapiro AM. Injuries of the nose, facial bones, and paranasal sinuses. In: Bluestone CD, Stool SE, Kenna MA (Eds). Pediatric Otolaryngology. Philadelphia: WB Saunders; 1966.
31. Siegel MB, Wetmore RF, Potsic WP, et al. Mandibular fractures in the pediatric patient. Arch Otolaryngol Head Neck Surg. 1991;117(5):533-6.
32. Spring PM, Cote DN. Pediatric maxillofacial fractures. J La State Med Soc. 1996;148(5):199-203.
33. Tanaka N, Uchide N, Suzuki K, et al. Maxillofacial fractures in children. J Craniomaxillofac Surg. 1993;21(7):289-93.
34. Thaller SR, Mabourakh S. Pediatric mandibular fractures. Ann Plast Surg. 1991;26(6):511-3.
35. Thoren H, Iizuka T, Hallikainen D, et al. Different patterns of mandibular fractures in children. An analysis of 220 fractures in 157 patients. J Craniomaxillofac Surg. 1992;20(7): 292-6.
36. Thoren H, Iizuka T, Hallikainen D, et al. Radiologic changes of the temporomandibular joint after condylar fractures in childhood. Oral Surg Oral Med Oral Pathol Oral Radiol Endod. 1998;86(6):738-45.
37. Waite DE. Pediatric fractures of jaw and facial bones. Pediatrics. 1973;51(3):551-9.
38. Winzenburg SM, Imola MJ. Internal fixation in pediatric maxillofacial fractures. Facial Plast Surg. 1998;14(1):45-58.

CHAPTER

Medical Emergencies in Dental Practice

Shilpa Ahuja, MK Jindal

Chapter Outline

Emergency is a condition that warrants for immediate attention by the doctor. This situation is an unexpected one under unforeseen circumstances and calls for an urgent treatment. Many emergency problems can be definitely avoided by simple preventive measures like a careful medical history, general physical examination regarding patient health status and proper preoperative preparation of the patient.

Emergency according to Dorland's Medical dictionary is defined as a sudden, urgent, usually unforeseen occurrence requiring immediate action.

Shock

It is a phenomenon marked by circulatory deficiency which is either cardiac or vasomotor in origin exhibiting marked hypotension.

Signs and symptoms

- The patient is unconscious with ashen gray face and cold, clammy skin
- Mucous membrane is pale whereas lips, nails, finger tips and lobules of the ear are grayish blue. Face is expression less with sunken eyes
- Pupils are dilated but react feebly to light
- Pulse is weak and thread
- Shallow and irregular respiration
- Temperature is subnormal

Treatment

- Position: Put the patients head at the lower level than feet 15°–Trendelenburg position
- Maintain the body heat by covering the patient with blanket and keep a hot water bottle between the thighs
- Check for any airway obstruction and patency of airway be maintained
- Control the loss of blood in hemorrhage shock by pressure packs
- Restore the lost body fluids. Infusion with plasma expanders or Ringer's lactate solution should be carried out to maintain the intravenous line and restore the volume loss
- Administer 100% oxygen
- The blood pressure, pulse rate and respiratory rate should be constantly monitored to assess the vitals
- Injection hydrocortisone sodium hemisuccinate 100 mg in 5 mL of water intravenously as stress bearing factor of the body
- Injection mephentermine to raise BP
- Injection atropine is given for bradycardia
- Broad-spectrum antibiotics
- Narcotic analgesic to relieve pain.

Allergic reaction

It is an unwanted response of the body to a complete dose of the drug. It is the result of immunological response of/in the individual

Gell and Coombs classification

- Type 1 (IgE—mediated hypersensitivity) most life-threatening few minutes
- Type 2 (cytotoxic/cytolytic antibody-mediated) IgM or IgG antibodies mediated
- Type 3 (immune complex mediated) 1–4 weeks, IgM or IgG soluble metabolite
- Type 4 (Delayed hypersensitivity) sensitized T-cell lymphocytes

Signs and symptoms

- Cutaneous reactions are the most common occurrence and include urticarial, exanthematous, and eczematoid reactions. Itching is common and can also find exfoliative dermatitis and bullous dermatosis
- Angioedema (swelling) this varies from localized slight swelling of the lips, eyelids, and face to more uncomfortable swelling of the mouth, throat, and extremities
- Respiratory (tightness in chest, sneezing, bronchospasm) bronchospasm is a generalized contraction of bronchial smooth muscles resulting in the restriction of airflow. This may also be accompanied by edema of the bronchiolar mucosa
- Bronchospasm is more common with preexisting pulmonary disease such as asthma or infection but can also be caused by the inhalation of a foreign substance
- Ocular reactions include conjunctivitis and watering of eyes
- Hypotension can occur with any allergic reaction

Anaphylaxis

This is a severe systemic type allergic reaction and is a medical emergency

Signs and symptoms

- *Cardiovascular shock including:* Pallor, syncope, palpitations, tachycardia, hypotension, arrhythmias, and convulsions
- Respiratory symptoms include: Sneezing, cough, wheezing, tightness in chest, bronchospasm, laryngospasm
- Skin is warm and flushed with itching, urticaria, and angioedema
- Nausea, vomiting, abdominal cramps, and diarrhea are also possible

Treatment

General treatment

- ABC's (is expansion required or removes the bullet from the next point)
- Maintain airway, administer oxygen, and determine possible need for intubation or surgical airway
- Monitor vital signs
- If in shock put patient in a horizontal or slight Trendelenburg position

Mild reactions

- Antihistamines usually effective. (Benadryl 50–100 mg or chlorpheniramine maleate 4–12 mg PO, IV, or IM)
- Identify and remove allergen
- Follow-up medications in 4–6 hours

Severe reactions

- If available start IV fluids
- Epinephrine is drug of choice. Usually prepackaged 1:1,000 in 1 mg vials or syringe
- If IV in place titrate 1:1,000 solution to effect
- If drop in blood pressure is minimal, start with 0.5 mL (0.5 mg)
- If drop in blood pressure is severe start with 2 mL (2 mg)
- Repeat after 2 minutes if needed
- If no IV use 1:1,000 (1 mg/cc), IM 0.3–0.5 mg (0.3–0.5 cc)
- For an adult repeat this dose in 10–20 minutes
- If the patient is intubated can give epinephrine endotracheally
- If asthma, edema or pruritus (itching) is present, can use corticosteroids. However, these drugs are too slow-acting to be used for an emergency situation
- Hydrocortisone sodium succinate (solu-cortef) 100–500 mg IV or IM. Dexamethasone (Decadron) 4–12 mg IV or IM
- Repeat dose at 1, 3, 6, and 10 hours as indicated by severity of symptoms

Respiratory emergencies

Airway obstruction

Acute airway obstruction is the major cause of non-traumatic cardiac arrest in infants and children

- Sit down dentistry (supine or semi-supine) → increased incidence of airway obstruction
- If swallowed → GI blockage, peritoneal abscess, perforations, peritonitis
- If aspirated → lung abscess, pneumonia, atelectasis

Prevention

- Rubber dam
- Oral packing (Pharyngeal curtain: 4 × 4 inch gauze pack usually used in sedated patients)
- Ligature (Dental floss tied to dental instruments such as rubber dam clamps, endodontic instruments, cotton rolls, gauze pads, etc.)

Management

- *If assistant is present*—patient placed into supine or Trendelenburg position, use Magill intubation forcep or suction to remove foreign body
- *If assistant not present*—instruct patient to bend over arm of chair with their head down and encourage patient to cough

Management of swallowed objects

- Consult radiologist—obtain radiographs to determine location of object and initiate medical consultation with appropriate specials

Management of aspirated foreign bodies

- Place patient in left lateral decubitus position—encourage patient to cough if foreign body is retrieved, initiate medical consultation before discharge
- If foreign body is not retrieved—consult with radiologist and obtain radiographs, perform bronchoscopy to visualize and retrieve foreign body.

Complete upper airway obstruction

Signs and symptoms

- *First phase (1–3 minutes):* Conscious, universal choking, struggling paradoxical respirations without air movement or voice, increased blood pressure and heart rate
- *Second phase (2–5 minutes):* Loss of consciousness, decreased respiration, blood pressure, heart rate
- *Third phase (>3–5 minutes):* coma, absent vital signs, dilated pupils.

Signs of partial airway obstruction

Individuals with good airflow

- Forceful cough
- Wheezing between coughs
- Ability to breath

Individuals with poor air exchange

- Weak, ineffectual cough "Crowing" sound on inspiration
- Absent or altered voice sounds
- Possible cyanosis
- Possible lethargy
- Possible disorientation

Management

Step 1: Position → supine with feet elevated.
Step 2: Head tilt-chin lift
Step 3: A + B (look, listen, feel)
Step 3a: Jaw-thrust maneuver if indicated.
Step 4: A + B repeat step 3
Step 5: Rescue breathing, if indicated establishing an emergency airway

- Non-invasive procedure:
  - Back blows
  - Manual thrust
  - Abdominal thrust (Heimlich maneuver)
  - Chest thrust
  - Finger sweep
- Procedure for obstructed airway in infants and children: Combination of back slaps and chest thrust is still recommends protocol for the infant under 1 year
- Surgical procedure: Invasive procedures are tracheostomy and cricothyrotomy.

Bronchospasm

Patients with a history of bronchial asthma may develop acute bronchospasm. It may be triggered by emotional stress and anxiety during the course of treatment

Types of asthma

- *Extrinsic:* Allergic asthma, younger patients, type 1 hypersensitivity reactions
- *Intrinsic:* Older patients, non-allergic factors, cold temperatures, exercise, stress

Signs and symptoms of an asthma attack

- Sense of suffocation, patient will sit-up like they are fighting for air
- Pressure or tightness in chest
- Nonproductive cough
- Expiratory and inspiratory wheezes
- Expiration is prolonged and harder than inspiration
- Chest is distended
- Thick, stringy mucous: At termination of a period of intense coughing the patient will expectorate this mucous

Severe asthma attack

- Cyanosis of the nail beds
- Perspiration and flushing of the skin
- *Use of accessory muscle of respiration:* Sternocleidomastoid and shoulder or abdominal muscles
- Patient may also appear confused and agitated

Management of an asthma attack

- Discontinue dental treatment
- Place patient in easiest position for them to breath. This is usually upright with arms outstretched
- Albuterol inhaler (Proventil) 2 puffs every 2 minutes
- Supplemental oxygen at 10 L/min
- Monitor vital signs
- If no improvement call emergency medical services (EMS)
- Start IV
- Consider epinephrine 1:1,000, 0.3 g every 20 minutes

Dental treatment considerations for the asthmatic patient

- Take a good medical history prior to treatment; determine how often the patient has an asthma attack and what precipitates it
- Consider scheduling morning appointments
- If patient uses an inhaler they should have it on hand during treatment. consider prophylactic use prior to treatment

Hyperventilation

It denotes the increase in alveolar ventilation disturbing the optimum levels of oxygen and carbon dioxide. It is caused by abnormally rapid and deep breathing leading to respiratory alkalosis. Hyperventilation syndrome in dental clinic is often precipitated by anxiety, fear, nervousness and emotional stress in a hysterical form at the conscious level. It is more commonly seen in females. It results in lower carbon dioxide level in the blood.

Signs and symptoms

- Dizziness
- Hard to breathe
- Shaking and trembling
- Cold clammy hands (diaphoresis)
- Tight feeling in chest, chest pain, and palpitations
- Lightheaded, giddy, impaired consciousness
- Uncontrolled over breathing. Respiration rate increase to 25–30/min
- *Globus hystericus:* Feeling of lump in throat and suffocating
- Tingling in hands, feet, and perioral areas
- Increase in blood pressure and increase heart rate

Treatment

- Discontinue treatment and remove any foreign objects from the patient's mouth
- Position patient upright
- Assess airway
- Reassure patient and try to calm them
- Have patient breath slowly and shallowly into a paper bag or mask 6–10 times/min
- Monitor vital signs
- If available it can use versed IV 1 mg/min up to 4–6 mg or IM 5 mg to calm the patient
- Determine what precipitated attack

Hypertension

When a patient exhibits blood pressure above 160/100 mm Hg is in the preoperative phase, he is labeled as hypertensive. Patient complains of headache, dizziness, nausea and even vomiting Fundus examination reveals hemorrhages or exhibits blood spots over the retina with increased intracranial tension

Treatment

- This can be avoided by proper premedication
- Should this emergency arise intraoperatively? The patient is allowed to take rest in a semi-sitting position
- Oxygen may be administered to bring down the blood pressure
- Injection diazepam may be administered. This normally settles the stress-related hypertension
- Injection furosemide IV and is maintained as a preparation to any serious emergency
- 10 mg capsule nifedipine sublingually to bring the blood pressure down

Hypotension

A fall in blood pressure or hypotension during oral surgical procedures can be due to a simple common fainting attack

Signs and symptoms

- There is associated weak pulse, bradycardia
- Confusion, restlessness, nausea, stupor

Treatment

- Put the patient in supine position with legs raised
- 100% oxygen should be administered
- IV line maintained with Ringer's lactate solution

- Atropine 0.6 mg in 5 mL of sterile water is given intravenously slowly if the pulse is less than 6/min. Atropine should be stopped when a good volume radial pulse with rate of 72/min appears
- Injection mephentermine 15 mg can be administered intramuscularly
- Injection hydrocortisone succinate 100 mg should be administered for combating stress

Ischemic heart disease

It denotes ischemia of the myocardium leading to arrhythmias, angina pectoris, myocardial infarction and sudden death. The condition is characterized by tightness in the chest, sensation of choking and a referred pain in the left arm and shoulder. The pain may be referred to jaw and neck. The attack may be precipitated on exertion or by the stress during the dental treatment.

Treatment

- In case of an acute attack of angina pectoris occurs in dental chair, the dental treatment should immediately be stopped, adjust the chair in semi-reclining position
- A tablet of nitroglycerin is placed sublingually and can be repeated after 5 times
- Oxygen administration
- Patient physician should be immediately called
- In case of myocardial infarction pain may be controlled with small amounts of morphine
- Injection atropine should be given if there is bradycardia
- In case of recent history of myocardial infarction, any elective surgery should not be undertaken for a period of 6 months

Cardiopulmonary arrest

There is sudden arrest of ventilation and circulation. It may occur in patients with already existing cardiovascular disease, anaphylaxis, toxic reactions of medicines, asphyxia, etc. Clinically it is characterized by absence of chest and abdominal movements; breath sounds, carotid and femoral pulse. the patient is unconscious with dilated pupils.

Treatment

Basic life support (BLS)

Airway: The airway must be patent. If foreign body is suspected, the patient must be rolled on one side and 4–5 forceful blows must be delivered rapidly between the shoulder blades with the heel of the hand. The patient is then put in supine position and abdominal thrust in the upward direction just below the sternum.

After the foreign body is excluded the patient should be kept in supine position as he requires external cardiac massage and artificial respiration. The patient head must be lifted with one hand under the neck and the other hand pressing the forehead so that the head is tilted backwards to keep the airway patent.

Breathing: once the airway patency is maintained and if breathing is inadequate, artificial ventilation must be given. With the above position patient nostrils must be sealed with thumb and index finger and mouth to mouth respiration must be given. This is done by taking a deep inspiration and exhaling it into the patient's mouth.

Circulation: With the patient in supine position, a sudden sharp thrust is given on the chest wall. this may restore the effective beating of the heart.

Cardiac massage: The heel of the hands, one above the other and the arms straight and extended and in kneeling position, the lower sternum should be compressed firmly to depress it for 1–1½ inch. This is carried out at the rate of 60–80/min.

Advanced cardiac life support (ACLS)

- Adrenalin: 1 mL of 1:1,000 IV followed by bolus of dextrose
- Calcium: 10 mL calcium gluconate 10% injected IV
- Sodium bicarbonate 1 mEq/kg should be given intravenously in order to overcome acidosis

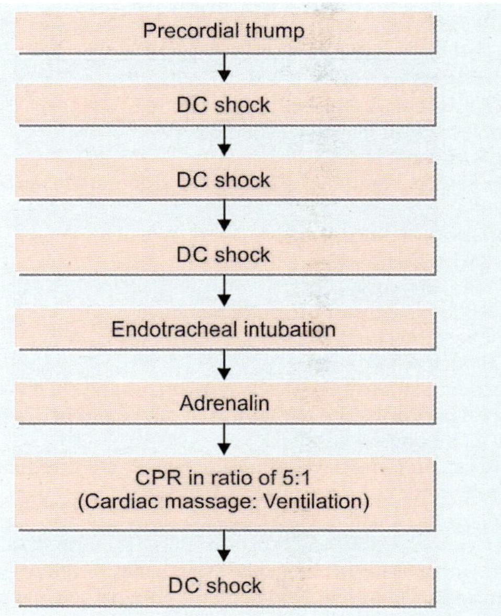

Chest pain/angina

The development of central chest discomfort frequently results from stressful situations in patients with coronary artery disease. In angina episodes, the coronary artery narrowed by atherosclerosis is unable to supply the heart muscle with adequate amounts of oxygenated blood, causing chest pain.

Signs and symptoms

- Central, substernal discomfort.
- May radiate to shoulder, neck and jaw or epigastric region. Dull heavy pressure sensation of short duration. Prompt relief with rest or nitroglycerin.

Treatment

- Position patient semi-upright or upright administer oxygen
- Administer nitroglycerin 0.5 mg SL every 5 minutes. Monitor, assess and record vital signs

Acute myocardial infarction

Signs and symptoms

- Central, substernal discomfort
- May radiate to shoulder, neck and jaw or epigastric region. Dull heavy pressure sensation of short duration
- Dyspnea, syncope, diaphoresis, sudden death
- Pain not relieved by rest or nitroglycerin and is of long duration
- Women may experience different signs—upper abdominal pain and fatigue

Treatment

- Position patient semi-upright or upright
- Administer oxygen
- Administer nitroglycerin 0.5 mg SL every 5 minutes
- *Initiate fibrinolysis:* if possible have the patient to chew 162–325 mg of aspirin. Calm and reassure the patient

Diabetic emergencies

- There are two types of problems associated with diabetes getting treatment in dental office
- Hypoglycemia or insulin shock
- Diabetic coma or ketoacidosis or hyperglycemia

Signs and symptoms

- Hypoglycemia is presented by pallor, sweating and tremors. There are palpitation, generalized weakness and hunger pains. Patient exhibit symptoms like tachycardia, headache, confusion, visual and disturbances of speech. Ultimately coma may develop

- Hyperglycemia is characterized by dry skin and hypotension. There is history of polydipsia, polyurea and polyphagia. Patient has typical acetone breath with a rapid deep breathing. Patient looks ill, dehydrated with dry skin, dry mouth and enophthalmos. Ultimately diabetic coma will develop

Management

Hypoglycemia

- In a conscious patient administer 20 g of oral glucose
- In an unconscious patient 50 cc 50% glucose given IV
- *Adrenalin:* 0.5 cc of 1:1,000 adrenalin is given subcutaneously. It stimulates hepatic gluconeogenesis and counteracts hypoglycemia
- *Glucocorticoid:* 100 mg of hydrocortisone sodium hemisuccinate IV
- *Glucagon:* 1–2 mg IM raises blood sugar

Hyperglycemia

- Circulating insulin present is ineffective because of poor tissue perfusion. Hence, tissue perfusion must be improved. One liter of fluid can be given in the first half hour and subsequently 1 L/h till dehydration is corrected
- Insulin therapy forms the mainstay of hyperglycemia. It not lowers the blood sugar but also prevents further lipolysis thereby preventing accumulation of ketones and hydrogen ions

Adrenal insufficiency

- The adrenal cortex produces over 25 different steroids. These steroids are broken into three groups: Sex steroids, mineralocorticoids, and glucocorticoids. Of primary concern in dentistry are the glucocorticoids. A physiologic dose of approximately 20 mg/day of cortisol is produced. This plays a key role in the body ability to adapt to stress. Cortisol provides a chemical link within the cells of the body allowing regulation of vital functions including blood pressure and glucose utilization.
- Cortisol production is triggered by real or threatened "stress" such as trauma, illness, fright, and anesthesia. In a patient with suppressed adrenal function a failure of this cortisol production eliminates the chemical link to regulate vital functions resulting in sudden shock and possibly death. Suppressed adrenal function or adrenal failure is classified as either primary (Addison's disease caused by disease states such as TB, bacteremia, carcinoma, and amyloidosis) or secondary (caused by pituitary disorder, hypothalamic disorders, or steroid therapy).
- Steroid therapy suppresses the function of the adrenal cortex reducing the production of natural cortisol. Because of this suppression patients who have been on long-term steroid therapy lose their ability to respond to stress. If these patients are stressed symptoms of acute adrenal insufficiency may result.

Signs and symptoms of acute adrenal insufficiency

- Mental confusion
- Muscle weakness
- Fatigue
- Nausea and vomiting
- Hypotension
- Intense pains in abdomen, lower back, and/or legs
- Mucocutaneous pigmentation
- Hypoglycemia
- Hyperkalemia
- Increase heart rate, decreased blood pressure

Management of suspected acute adrenal insufficiency

- Discontinue all treatment and remove foreign objects from the patient's mouth
- Initiate basic life support (BPS) and activate emergency response system (ERS)
- Place patient supine
- Monitor and record vital signs
- Oxygen at 5–10 L/min

Dental treatment considerations

- For patients with a history of glucocorticoid therapy use stress reduction protocols
- The following guidelines can be used to determine if replacement therapy is indicated. This is a change from the old rule of two's based on an article done at NNDC. It is always a good idea to get a medical consult in such cases
- If the patient has undergone supraphysiologic (more than 20 mg/day) glucocorticoid therapy that was discontinued more than 30 days prior to the planned dental treatment no supplementation is required
- If the patients have undergone supraphysiologic glucocorticoid therapy within 30 days of the planned dental procedure considered the patients suppressed and provide steroid supplementation equivalent to 100 mg of cortisol
- If the patient has undergone or is undergoing alternate day dosing schedule glucocorticoid therapy no supplementation is required but it is best to provide dental treatment on the off day of the patient's dose schedule
- If the patient is currently receiving daily glucocorticoid therapy at a supraphysiologic level (more than 20 mg) supplementation is required. If the daily dose is subphysiologic supplementation is not required

Hypochlorite accident

It is due to expelling of an irrigant such as NaoCl beyond the apex. This happens only by locking the needle of the irrigating syringe in the canal and forcefully injecting the irrigant

Signs and symptoms

- Within minutes the patient feels sudden extreme pain
- Swelling within minutes
- Profuse, prolonged bleeding through the root canal
- This bleeding is the body's reaction to the irrigant

Treatment

- Allow the bleeding to continue. If the body rids itself of toxic fluid healing may be faster
- If the treated tooth is pulpless consider prescribing an antibiotic and an analgesic for 5 and 3 days, respectively
- Since this may be hypersensitive reactions consider prescribing an antihistaminic

Toxic reaction due to drug (local anesthesia) over dosage

Local anesthetic and epinephrine toxicity

Signs and symptoms of epinephrine toxicity

- Agitation, weakness, and headache
- Pallor, tremor, palpitation
- Sharp rise in blood pressure and heart rate

Signs and symptoms of local anesthetic toxicity

- Agitation
- Muscular twitching and tremors
- Increased blood pressure and heart rate
- Lightheadedness
- Visual and auditory disturbances (tinnitus, difficulty focusing)
- If moderate to high overdose of local anesthetic can also have convulsions and depression of blood pressure, heart rate, and respiration

Management of toxic reactions to epinephrine: Toxic effect of epinephrine is transitory rarely lasting more than a few minutes

- Stop dental treatment
- Place patient in most comfortable position
- Monitor vital signs
- Consider administering oxygen
- Allow time for the patient to recover

Dental treatment considerations for use of epinephrine

- Due to its cardiovascular effects limit use in patients with history of heart disease or stroke
- Can cause uterine contractions in the pregnant female
- Possible drug interactions (especially monoamine oxidase inhibitors and cocaine)
- Remember the patient has endogenous epinephrine. Production of this is increased in stressful situations

Management of toxic reactions to local anesthetic: Treatment varies with the onset and severity of the reaction.
Mild reaction/rapid onset (example is an intravascular injection)

- Reassure patient
- Administer oxygen
- Monitor and record vital signs
- Allow for recovery; determine if patient can be allowed to leave unescorted

Mild reaction/slow onset

- Toxic reaction with a delayed onset is most likely a result of impaired biotransformation
- Evolves slowly, use caution
- Monitor patient, record vital signs

Severe overdose/rapid onset, severe overdose/slow onset

- ABC's
- Activate ERS
- Administer oxygen by mask at 10–15 L/min
- Start IV if available (18-gauge catheter with normal saline)
- If needed and available administer anticonvulsant, versed 2 mg, than 1 mg/min to effect (monitor respiration)
- Monitor and record vital signs
- Allow for recovery and discharge with appropriate escort or transport to hospital if required

Treatment considerations to avoid adverse drug reaction

- Prevention is the key. Take a complete medical history. Determine if there are any diseases present that affect the use of a drug
- Know what medications the patient is taking and possible drug interactions
- Careful injections make sure to aspirate to avoid an intravascular injection

Maximum recommended doses of local anesthetic	
Lidocaine "plain"	4.4 mg/kg
Lidocaine 2% with 1:100 k epinephrine	7.0 mg/kg
Mepivacaine "plain"	4.4 mg/kg
Mepivacaine with 1:20 k neocobefrin	6.6 mg/kg
Bupivacaine with 1:200 k epinephrine	3.2 mg/kg
Maximum recommended doses of epinephrine	
Healthy adult	0.2 mg/kg
Cardiac patient	0.04 mg/kg

Epilepsy

This is a central nervous system disturbance involving convulsions followed by loss of consciousness. Majority of the patients are conscious of their problem and should be warned about the importance of medicine which is generally recommended on long-term basis. An emergency can arise in the dental clinic when the epileptic seizures occur during treatment. When two or more seizures occur in succession, it is labeled as status epilepticus. And it is a serious emergency. Convulsions can also be seen in high grade fever, brain tumor, and head injury, hypoglycemia and drug toxicity. Therefore a careful history prior to treatment is important. The airway should be kept patent during an epileptic fit. Crush injury to the tongue should be avoided by holding a blunt object between the teeth.

Generalized seizures

- Tonic-clonic, clonic seizures, tonic seizures, atonic seizures myoclonic seizures
- Absence (petit mal) seizures

Partial seizures

- Simple partial seizures, complex partial seizures
- Partial seizures secondarily generalized

Treatment protocol

- Most seizures last <2 minutes
- Emergency medical services (EMS) activated
- Assure patient and staff safety
- Administer oxygen
- Manage airway
- Monitor vitals, pulse oximetry
- Suction available
- If seizure is lasting > 2 minutes, establish IV, administer medicines
- Diazepam
- *Adult:* 5–10 mg IV/IM
- *Pediatric:* 0.2–0.5 mg/kg IV/IM
- Midazolam 0.05–0.1 mg/kg IV 0.2 mg/kg IM (max 10 mg) pharmacologic management
- Emergency medical services not arrived >5 minutes
- *Adult:* Dextrose 50 mL bolus off 50% glucose
- *Pediatric:* 2 mL/kg 25% dextrose solution
- Evaluate airway maintenance
- Evaluate cardiac rhythm

Medical emergencies in the pediatric dental patient

Most of the recommendations for treating emergencies in the dental office are oriented towards the adult patient and recommendations for the management of medical emergencies in the child patient are not readily available. The pedodontist must have equipment specifically for the pediatric dental patient, "Basic emergency kit for the pedodontist." The dosages of emergency drugs as well as the techniques for providing supportive therapy for the pediatric dental patient need to be altered. Since consideration must be given to the persons in the reception room some of whom in a pedodontic practice approach the age and size where adult recommendations for emergency therapy may apply, the pedodontist must be capable of treating medical emergencies in adults as well as in children.

When confronted with a medical emergency, the pedodontist should remain calm and act swiftly and definitively in order to provide immediate therapy without causing undue panic in the patient or the auxiliary personnel. The pedodontist should be concerned with maintaining airway, breathing, and circulation and then should treat symptomatically. The pedodontist should never administer a drug without a definite indication for its use and should also avoid multiple drug therapy since it will complicate the diagnosis for medical personnel.

Pediatric dosage schedule

The dosage schedules presented for children in each of the following emergency situations are reported as a range. The first dose in the range corresponds to the approximate dose for a 30-pound child, and the second dose corresponds to a 60-pound child. The milligrams per kilogram dose are listed along with the maximum dose. The adult dose is based on a 150-pound adult. However, the author recommends that a concise reference chart and instructions in an emergency kit list the doses as a range to facilitate the estimation of the proper dose to be given during an emergency. If the dosages were listed as milligrams per kilogram, it would be too time-consuming and impractical to calculate the exact dose to be given during an emergency episode especially if the exact weight of the child is unknown or cannot be readily determined by the pedodontist.

Cerebrovascular accidents/transient ischemic attacks

A cerebrovascular accident (CVA or stroke) or a transient ischemic attack (TIA) is caused by an interruption of blood flow to the brain. These episodes are usually seen in older patients as a consequence of atherosclerosis or untreated hypertension. The interruption in flow may be due to a blood clot, spasm of the arteries, or even due to rupture of a blood vessel in the brain. Blood flow to the cerebral cortex is insufficient and the patient will exhibit symptoms within seconds. The signs and symptoms may be of short duration (TIA) which resolve spontaneously or persist for months or years. A transient ischemic attack is a forewarning of a major ischemic CVA; these patients must be evaluated by a physician to prevent such an occurrence.

Signs and symptoms

- Altered level of consciousness
- Aphasia
- Unilateral muscle weakness or paralysis

Treatment

- Maintain airway
- Position patient in semi-supine, position suction
- Monitor, assess and record vital signs

Syncope

It is a transient loss of consciousness due to cerebral anoxia. It is perhaps the most common untoward accident seen in the dental clinic.

Predisposing factors

These are anxiety, fear, and sight of blood, pain, fasting and hot environment. These emotional stresses lead to release of catecholamine. Resultantly, there is lower peripheral resistance and hence peripheral pooling of blood and fall in blood pressure leading to a sudden decrease in cerebral blood flow.

Signs and symptoms

Patient feels weakness, warmth, nausea and pain in the epigastrium and hunger, etc. Following this sweating, dizziness, pallor and light headedness and low pulse pressure develops. If the treatment is not instituted at this stage, unconsciousness develops with ashen gray color of the skin, shallow respiration, low blood pressure and weak pulse.

Clinical manifestations

Early

- Warmth
- Pallor
- Perspiration
- Nausea
- Blood pressure may be normal
- Significant tachycardia (80–120 beats/min)

Late

- Pupillary dilation
- Yawning
- Hyperapnea
- Cold peripheries
- Hypotension
- Bradycardia
- Visual disturbances
- Dizziness
- Finally syncope

Stages clinically

Presyncope presents as

(Precedes about 30 seconds)

Syncope presents as

- Jerky irregular/shallow imperceptible breathing/apnea
- Dilated pupils
- Convulsions
- Bradycardia
- Asystole
- Hypotension
- Weak pulse

Postsyncope presents as

- Regains consciousness
- Short period of disorientation
- BP begins to rise
- Heart rate comes to base line
- Pulse becomes stronger

Treatment

- *Position of the patient:* Made to lie down in supine position with legs raised to improve venous return
- In case the patient is sitting in the dental chair, the back of the chair should be immediately lowered so the head of the patient is at lower level than the feet. It helps in venous return to the heart and oxygenated blood to the brain
- *Loosening of the clothes:* Tight clothing should be loosened
- A patent airway should be maintained. Any foreign body should be removed manually or with suction apparatus
- Inhalation of the aromatic spirit of ammonia or application of cold sponges to the face helps in securing reflex stimulation
- 100% oxygen should be administered
- If bradycardia atropine injection 0.6 mg in 5 mL of water should be given slowly intravenously
- If hypotension persists, drugs like phenylephrine should be administered

Dental treatment considerations

- Delay further dental treatment 24 hours especially if the patient lost consciousness
- If the patient lost consciousness they must not be permitted to leave unescorted or drive a motor vehicle
- Determine the cause of the syncopal episode prior to completing further treatment
- Stress is the major cause of syncope in the dental practice. Prevention is the key to management of syncope. This includes taking a complete medical history and thorough evaluation of the patient
- Use stress management protocols, morning appointments, consider sedation
- Ensure that patients do not miss meals prior to treatment

Medical emergency—quick reference

Emergency	*Signs and symptoms*	*Treatment*
Anaphylaxis	Acute anxiety, rash, itching, respiratory distress, wheezing, cyanosis, severe drop in blood pressure	Epinephrine 1:1,000 IV or intralingual, 0.125–0.25 cc (child) 0.5 cc (adult), oxygen, Benadryl IM 25–50 mg (child), 50–100 mg (adult)—hospitalization
Allergic reaction	Itching, swelling of face, hands, and eyelids, rash	Mild—Benadryl orally 25–50 mg (child), 50–100 mg (adult)—physician Moderate—Benadryl IM 25–50 mg (child), 50–100 mg (adult),— physician
Acute asthmatic attack	Wheezing, rapid and full pulse, prolonged expirations	Mild—patient should carry and use his own inhaler, oxygen. Severe—epinephrine 1:1,000 subcutaneously 0.125–0.25 cc (child), 0.25–0.5 cc (adult), semi-erect position, oxygen—physician
Syncope	Slow, weak pulse, drop in blood pressure, cold, clammy skin, dilated pupils, loss of consciousness	Trendelenburg position, oxygen, loosen clothing, cold towel on forehead, ammonia stimulant
Respiratory obstruction	Choking, coughing, wheezing, violent attempts to breathe, cyanosis	Blows on back, Heimlich maneuver, suction, ventilate, attempt removal with forcep, cricothyrotomy
Epileptic seizure	Grand mal—clonic convulsions, frothing at mouth, unconsciousness	Patient on floor, protect from injury, loosen clothing—physician
Insulin shock	Hunger, weakness, dizziness, mental confusion, disorientation, irritability	Oral sugar if conscious. 50% dextrose, IV 20–30 cc (child), 50 cc (adult), if unconscious—physician
Diabetic acidosis	Thirst, frequent urination, loss of appetite, fruity (acetone) breath, vertigo, coma	Keep warm until hospitalized
Drug toxicity	Central nervous system excitement, than central nervous system depression–convulsions, unconsciousness	Supportive treatment until hospitalized
Cerebrovascular accident (CVA)	Hemiplegia, slow, deep breathing, eyes deviate to one side, speech impairment	Avoid unnecessary movement, keep warm, oxygen until hospitalized
Angina pectoris	Substernal and precordial pain radiating to arm, rapid pulse	Oxygen, sublingual nitroglycerin tablet, repeat 3 minutes (× 3), hospitalization
Myocardial infarction	Severe, persistent substernal gain radiating to left arm, possible cyanosis, cold clammy skin, no relief with nitroglycerin	Oxygen, supportive therapy and keep warm until hospitalized
Cardiac arrest	20–30 seconds of gasping respirations, respiratory arrest, no pulse, cyanosis, pupils dilated, centric and fixed	Place patient on floor, CPR until hospitalization
Adrenal crisis	Past history of episodes, weakness, pallor, perspiration, weak and rapid pulse	Oxygen and supportive therapy until hospitalized. Decadron IV or IM 1–4 mg (child) and 4–6 mg (adult)

The best form of emergency therapy is prevention. Thorough medical histories and follow-up consultations for underlying disease states can be invaluable in avoiding potential medical emergencies. There can be no argument against practicing defensively. A valuable adjunct toward preventing medical emergencies is a good rapport and proper consultation with the local medical personnel. It is important to have a manual on the treatment of potential medical emergencies which includes the duties required of the various members of the office staff available for periodic review. In addition, a quick reference on emergency therapy should be readily available.

Questionnaire

1. Describe the management of shock in dental setting.
2. How do you manage anaphylaxis in dental operator?
3. What is hypochlorite accident?
4. How do you manage syncope?

FURTHER READING

1. Alty CT. Coping with a Medical Crisis. RDH. 2002.
2. Anderson PE. Effectively handling medical emergencies. Dental Econ. 1989;79(11):54-61.
3. Being prepared for office emergencies. Dent Assist Update. 1994;3(3):3-8.
4. Bertold M. Florida mandates defibrillators in dental offices. http://www.ada.org/prof/resources/pubs/adanews/adanewsarticle.asp?articlesid=1371. Accessed 2/06.
5. Bird D, Robinson D. Modern Dental Assisting, 9th Edition. St. Louis, MO: Elsevier; 2009.
6. Braun RJ. The dental assistant's role in medical emergencies. Dent Assist. 1985;54(5):19-22.
7. Curriculum guidelines for management of medical emergencies in dental education. J Dent Educ. 1981;45(6):379-81.
8. Curriculum guidelines for management of medical emergencies in dental education. J Dent Educ. 1990;54(6):337-8.
9. Fast TB, Martin MD, Ellis TM. Emergency preparedness: A survey of dental practitioners. J Am Dent Assoc.1986;112(4):499-500.
10. Goepferd SJ. Medical emergencies in the pediatric dental patient. Pediatr Dent. 1979;1(2):115-21.

11. Grimes E. Medical Emergencies: Essentials for the Dental Professional. Upper Saddle River: Pearson Education; 2009.
12. Highlights of the 2010 American Heart Association CPR Guidelines. [Online] http://www.heart.org/idc/groups/ heart- public/@wcm/@ecc/documents/downloadable/ ucm_317350.pdf [Accessed on April, 2018].
13. Malamed S. Emergency Medicine. Dental Econ. 2010;38–43.
14. Malamed SF. Managing medical emergencies. J Am Dent Assoc. 1993;124(8):40-53.
15. Theisen FC, Feil PH, Schultz R. Self perceptions of skill in office medical emergencies. J Dental Educ. 1990;54:(10):623-5.
16. Wahl MJ. Myths of dental-induced endocarditis. Compend. Cont Educ Dent. Vol. XV, No. 9, 1100–19.
17. Wakeen LM. Dental office emergencies: Do you know your legal obligations? J Am Dent Assoc. 1993;124(8):54-8.
18. Wall HK, Beagan BM, O'Neill J, et al. Addressing stroke signs and symptoms through public education: the Stroke Heroes Act FAST campaign. Prev Chronic Dis. 2008;5(2): A49.
19. Weissman D. Emergency education. J Am Dent Assoc. 1993; 124:51–3.

CHAPTER 67

Cardiopulmonary Resuscitation

Saima Yunus Khan, Nikhil Marwah, MK Jindal

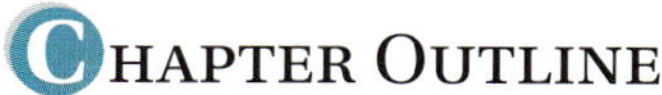

CHAPTER OUTLINE

- Cardiopulmonary Resuscitation Guidelines for Adults
- Cardiopulmonary Resuscitation Guidelines for Children
- Cardiopulmonary Resuscitation Guidelines for Infants

Cardiopulmonary resuscitation (CPR) is a life-saving procedure useful in many emergencies. Cardiopulmonary resuscitation involves a combination of mouth-to-mouth rescue breathing and chest compression that keeps oxygenated blood flowing to the brain and other vital organs. The 2010 American Heart Association Guidelines for CPR and Emergency Cardiovascular Care (ECC) had recommend a change in the BLS sequence of steps from A-B-C (Airway, Breathing, Chest compressions) to C-A-B (Chest compressions, Airway, Breathing) **(Fig. 67.1)**.

The reason for this change from A-B-C (Airway, Breathing, Chest compressions) to C-A-B (Chest compressions, Airway, Breathing) is that in vast majority of cardiac arrests, the highest survival rates from cardiac arrest are reported among patients who have a witnessed arrest and an initial rhythm of ventricular fibrillation (VF) or pulseless ventricular tachycardia (pVT). In these patients, the critical initial elements of BLS are chest compressions and early defibrillation. In the A-B-C sequence, chest compressions are often delayed while the responder opens the airway to give mouth-to-mouth breaths, retrieves a barrier device, or gathers and assembles ventilation equipment. By changing the sequence to C-A-B, chest compressions will be initiated sooner and the delay in ventilation should be minimal.

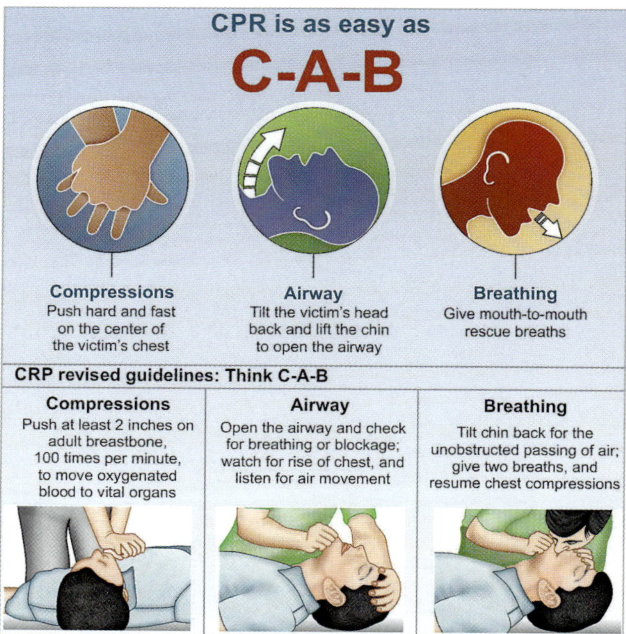

CPR is as easy as
C-A-B
Compressions
Push hard and fast on the center of the victim's chest
Airway
Tilt the victim's head back and lift the chin to open the airway
Breathing
Give mouth-to-mouth rescue breaths
CRP revised guidelines: Think C-A-B
Compressions
Push at least 2 inches on adult breastbone, 100 times per minute, to move oxygenated blood to vital organs
Airway
Open the airway and check for breathing or blockage; watch for rise of chest, and listen for air movement
Breathing
Tilt chin back for the unobstructed passing of air; give two breaths, and resume chest compressions

Fig. 67.1: New modified CPR approach of C-A-B. (*Source:* With permission from American Health Association, USA).

Cardiopulmonary resuscitation guidelines for adults (Fig. 67.2)

New 2020 guidelines

Stipulate that cpr should be initiated even if the patient is not in cardiac arrest.

New evidence supports that risk of harm is low to a victim who receives chest compressions when not in cardiac arrest

Check unresponsive: No breathing or no normal breathing (only gasping).
Call for help.

Compressions
- Push chest at least 2 inches, 30 times in the center of the chest
- Push 2-handed, with one hand on top of the other
- Push at a rate of at least 100-200 pushes per minute
- Allow complete chest recoil after each push
- Limit interruptions in chest pushes to less than 10 seconds

Airway
- Open the airway and check for breathing
- Watch the rise of chest
- Listen for air movement

Breathing
- *Head tilt-chin lift:* Tilt the head back and lift the chin
- Give 2 breaths. Give each breath over 1 second
- The victim's chest should rise with each breath

Continue
- Continue cycles of 30 pushes and 2 breaths
- Rotate compressors every 2 minutes

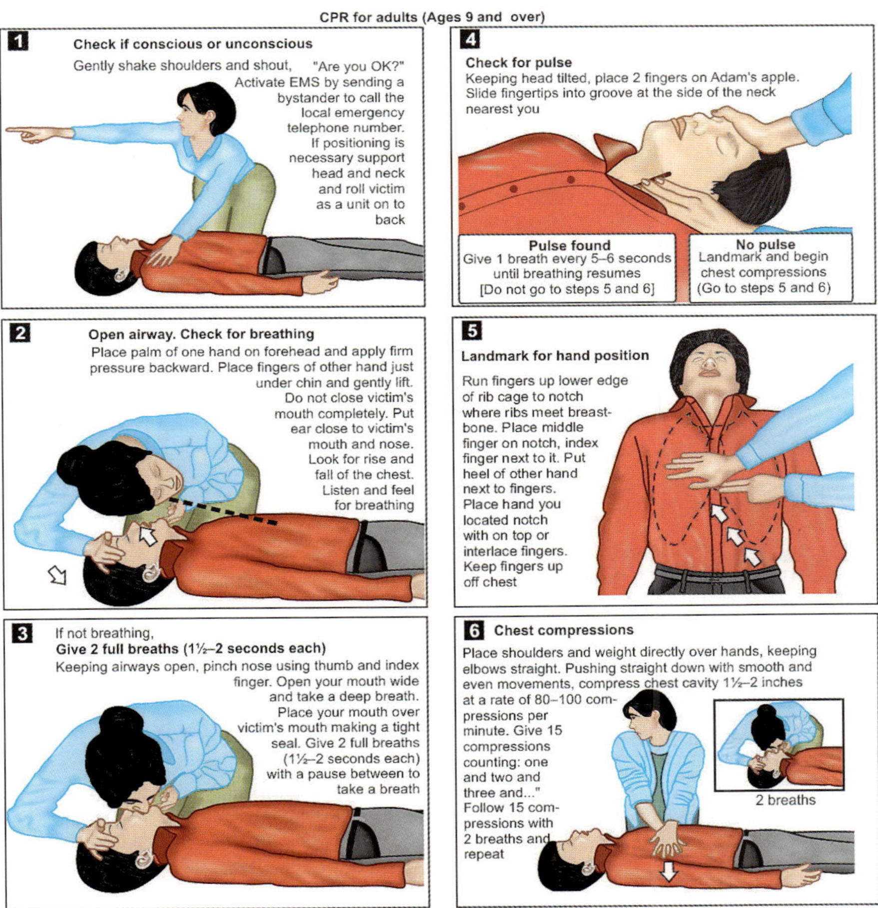

CPR for adults (Ages 9 and over)
1
Check if conscious or unconscious
Gently shake shoulders and shout, "Are you OK?" Activate EMS by sending a bystander to call the local emergency telephone number. If positioning is necessary support head and neck and roll victim as a unit on to back
2
Open airway. Check for breathing
Place palm of one hand on forehead and apply firm pressure backward. Place fingers of other hand just under chin and gently lift. Do not close victim's mouth completely. Put ear close to victim's mouth and nose. Look for rise and fall of the chest. Listen and feel for breathing
3
If not breathing,
Give 2 full breaths (1½–2 seconds each)
Keeping airways open, pinch nose using thumb and index finger. Open your mouth wide and take a deep breath. Place your mouth over victim's mouth making a tight seal. Give 2 full breaths (1½–2 seconds each) with a pause between to take a breath
4
Check for pulse
Keeping head tilted, place 2 fingers on Adam's apple. Slide fingertips into groove at the side of the neck nearest you
Pulse found
Give 1 breath every 5–6 seconds until breathing resumes
[Do not go to steps 5 and 6]
No pulse
Landmark and begin chest compressions
(Go to steps 5 and 6)
5
Landmark for hand position
Run fingers up lower edge of rib cage to notch where ribs meet breast-bone. Place middle finger on notch, index finger next to it. Put heel of other hand next to fingers. Place hand you located notch with on top or interlace fingers. Keep fingers up off chest
6
Chest compressions
Place shoulders and weight directly over hands, keeping elbows straight. Pushing straight down with smooth and even movements, compress chest cavity 1½–2 inches at a rate of 80–100 compressions per minute. Give 15 compressions counting: one and two and three and..." Follow 15 compressions with 2 breaths and repeat
2 breaths

Fig. 67.2: Conventional CPR by old method of A-B-C. (*Source:* With permission from American Health Association, USA).

Cardiopulmonary resuscitation guidelines for children (Fig. 67.3)

New 2020 guidelines
For infants and children with pulse, but absent or inadequate respiratory effort,
Give 1 breath every 2-3 seconds (20-30 breaths/minute)

Check unresponsive

- No breathing or no normal breathing (only gasping)
- Provide 2 minutes of CPR before calling for help

Cardiopulmonary resuscitation

- Push chest at about 2 inches, 30 times just below the nipple line
- You may use either 1 or 2 hands for chest pushes
- Push at a rate of at least 100 pushes per minute
- Allow complete chest recoil between each push
- Cardiopulmonary resuscitation ratio for two-person CPR is 15 pushes to 2 breaths
- In two-person CPR, the rescuers should change positions after every 2 minutes

Breathing

- *Head tilt-chin lift:* Tilt the head back and lift the chin
- Give 2 breaths. Give each breath over 1 second
- The victim's chest should rise with each breath

Continue

- Continue cycles of 30 pushes and 2 breaths
- Rotate compressors every 2 minutes

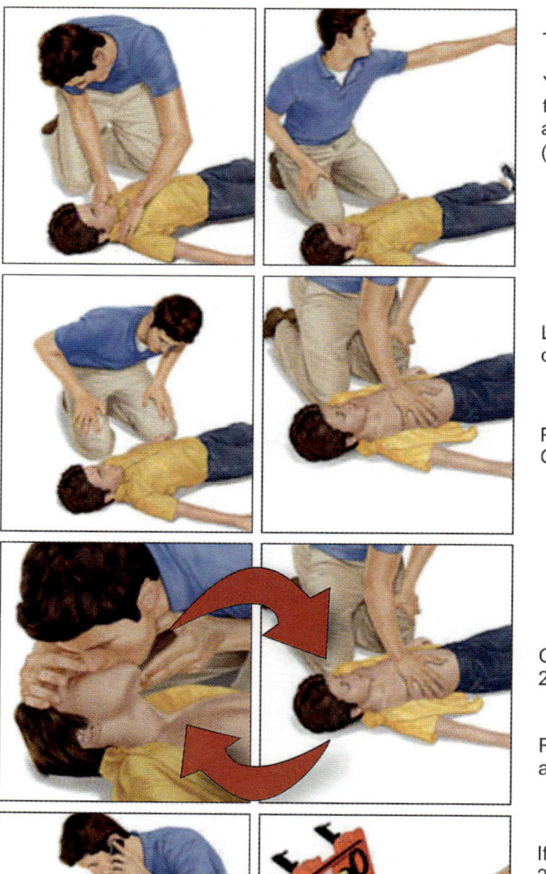

Tap and shout

Yell for help. Send someone to phone emergency and get an automated external defibrillator (AED)

Look for no breathing or only gasping

Push hard and fast. Give 30 compressions

Open the airway and give 2 breaths

Repeat sets of 30 compressions and 2 breaths

If you are alone after 5 sets of 30 compressions and 2 breaths, phone emergency, and then resume sets of 30:2

When the AED arrives, turn it ON and follow the prompts

Fig. 67.3: Cardiopulmonary resuscitation for children. (*Source:* With permission from American Health Association, USA).

Cardiopulmonary resuscitation guidelines for infants (Fig. 67.4)
Check unresponsive
• No breathing or no normal breathing (only gasping) • Provide 2 minutes of CPR before calling for help
Cardiopulmonary resuscitation
• Push chest about 1½ inch and 30 times just below the nipple line • Push with the two-finger push technique • Push at a rate of at least 100 pushes per minute • Allow complete chest recoil between each push • Cardiopulmonary resuscitation ratio for one-person CPR is 30 pushes to 2 breaths • Cardiopulmonary resuscitation ratio for two-person CPR is 15 pushes to 2 breaths • Use the two-thumb encircling technique for pushes
Breathing
• *Head tilt-chin lift:* Tilt the head back and lift the chin • Give 2 breaths. Give each breath over 1 second • The victim's chest should rise with each breath
Continue
• Continue cycles of 30 pushes and 2 breaths • Rotate compressors every 2 minutes

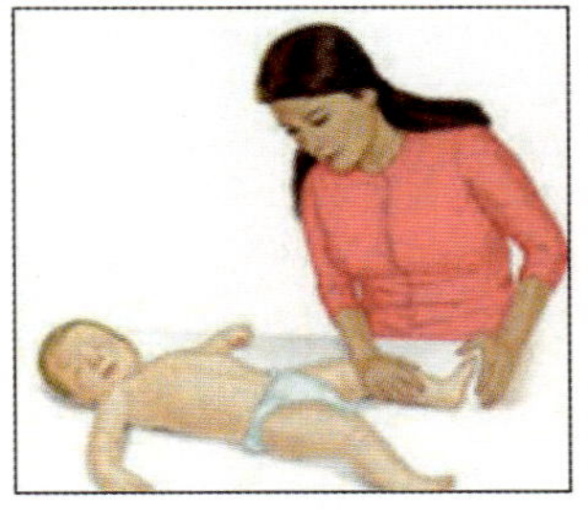
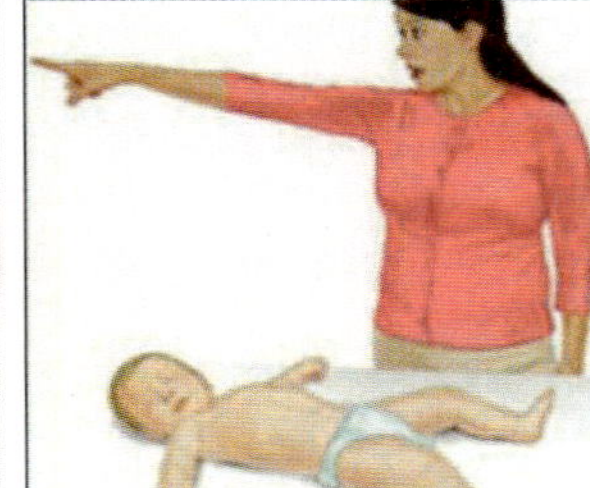

Tap and shout

Yell for help. Send someone to phone emergency

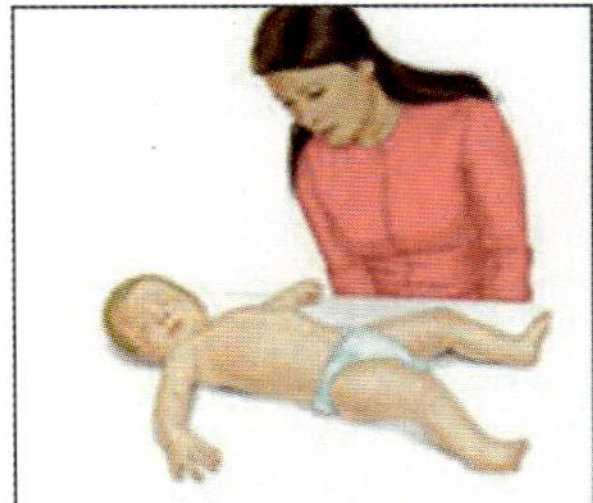
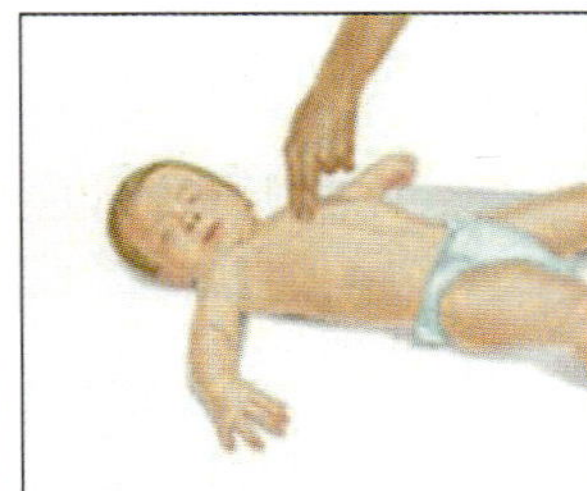

Look for no breathing or only gasping

Push hard and fast. Give 30 compressions

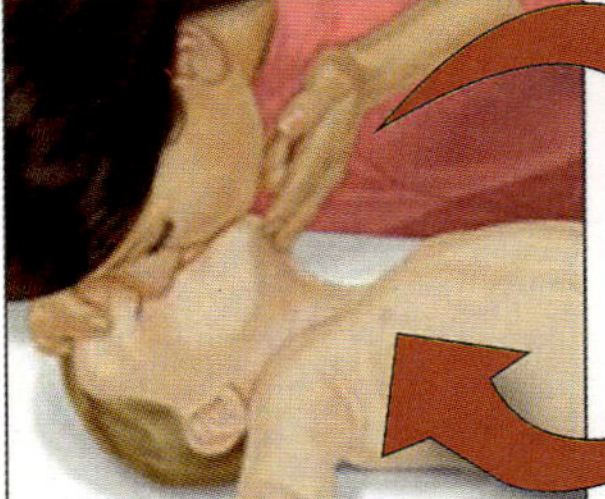
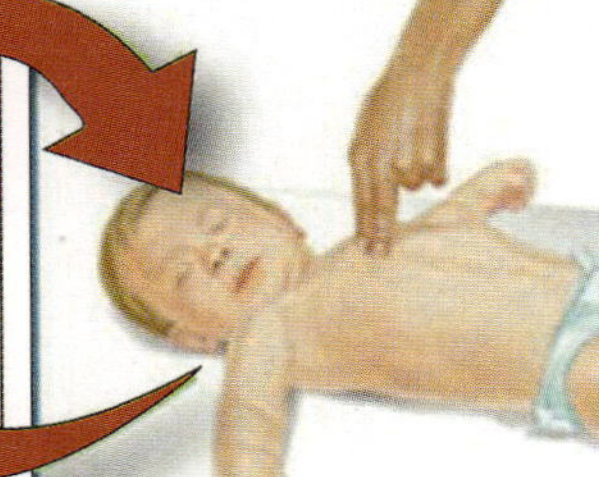

Open the airway and give 2 breaths

Repeat sets of 30 compressions and 2 breaths

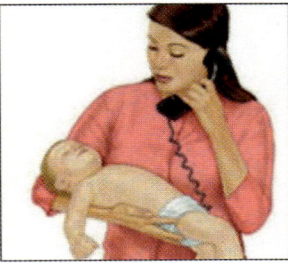

If you are alone after 5 sets of 30 compressions and 2 breaths, phone emergency, and then resume sets of 30:2

Fig. 67.4: Cardiopulmonary resuscitation for infants. (*Source:* With permission from American Health Association, USA).

Summary of key basic life support components for adults, children, and infants			
components	***Adults***	***Children***	***Infants***
Recognition	Unresponsive (for all ages)		
	No breathing or no normal breathing (i.e. only gasping)	No breathing or only gasping	
	Don't waste time on pulse palpation, directly initiate CPR		
CPR sequence	C-A-B		
Compression rate	At least 100-120/min		
Compression depth	At least 2 inches (5 cm)	At least ½ AP diameter About 2 inches (5 cm)	At least ½ AP diameter About 1½ inches (4 cm)
Chest wall recoil	Allow complete recoil between compressions HCPs rotate compressors every 2 minutes		
Compression interruptions	Minimize interruptions in chest compressions attempt to limit interruptions to <10 seconds		
Airway	Head tilt-chin lift (HCP suspected trauma: Jaw thrust)		
Compression-to-ventilation ratio (until advanced airway placed)	30:2 1 or 2 rescuers	15:2 Single rescuer 15:2 2 HCP rescuers	
***Ventilations:* When rescuer untrained or trained and not proficient**	Compressions only		
Ventilations with advanced airway (HCP)	1 breath every 6–8 seconds (8–10 breaths/min) asynchronous with chest compressions about 1 second per breath and visible chest rise		
Defibrillation	Attach and use AED as soon as available. Minimize interruptions in chest compressions before and after shock; resume CPR beginning with compressions immediately after each shock		
(AED: automated external defibrillator; AP: anterior-posterior; CPR: cardiopulmonary resuscitation; HCP: healthcare provider. Excluding the newly born, in whom the etiology of an arrest is nearly always asphyxia)			

POINTS TO REMEMBER

- The approach for CPR has changed from A-B-C to C-A-B.
- C-A-B is Compressions-Airway-Breathing.
- For compression push 2 inches for children and 1.5 inches for infants at the rate of 100/minute.
- For children press using 1 or 2 hands and for infants use 2 fingers technique.

Questionnaire

1. What is CPR?
2. Describe the process of C-A-B in children.

FURTHER READING

1. American Heart Association. CPR-ECC Guidelines; 2010.
2. Highlights of 2020 American Heart Association Guidelines for CPR and ECC.

CHAPTER

General Anesthesia in Pediatric Dentistry

Hind Pal Bhatia, Milind Shah, Deepa G, Mahesh Ramakrishnan

CHAPTER OUTLINE

- Preanesthetic Medication
- Aims and Objectives of providing General Anesthesia
- Stages of Anesthesia
- Drugs used in General Anesthesia
- Complications of General Anesthesia

It is important to ensure that children and adolescents receive safe and effective pain control. A range of techniques are available comprising four overlapping categories: (1) behavioral techniques, (2) local anesthesia (LA), (3) conscious sedation, and (4) general anesthesia (GA). The aim of this chapter is to focus on the use of GA in Pediatric Dentistry. Before the 19th century, a number of agents like alcohol, opium, cannabis, or even concussion and asphyxia were used to obtund surgical pain, but operations were horrible ordeals. **Horace Wells**, a dentist, picked up the idea of using nitrous oxide (N_2O) from a demonstration of laughing gas in 1844. However, he often failed to relieve dental pain completely and the use of GA had to wait till other advances were made. **Morton** was the first dentist to experiment with ether anesthesia in 1846. The first intravenous (IV) anesthetic thiopentone was introduced in 1935.

Most children and adolescents can receive effective dental care by traditional methods through the successful use of non-pharmacological behavioral management techniques in the dental clinic. However, Pediatric Dentists routinely treating children do come across patients who tend to exhibit reduced level of cooperation and cannot be managed by other behaior management techniques can be treated under general anesthesia. When the procedure cannot be performed in the dental clinic, hospitalization for dental treatment under general anesthesia (GA) can and should be considered. Active involvement in hospital-based dentistry has added a rewarding component to the practice of many pediatric dentists. Special children with reduced coping abilities such as autism, cerebral palsy, down syndrome and children with Frankl definitely negative scale are most commonly indicated for general anesthesia which facilitate a better treatment outcome and also reduced iatrogenic injuries when attempted in chair side.

PREANESTHETIC MEDICATION

It refers to the use of drugs before anesthesia to make it more pleasant and safe **(Table 68.1)**.

Aims and Objectives

- Relief of anxiety and apprehension preoperatively and to facilitate smooth induction
- Amnesia for pre- and postoperative events
- Supplement analgesic action of anesthetics
- Decrease secretions and vagal stimulation caused by anesthetics
- Antiemetic effect extending to the postoperative period
- Decrease acidity and volume of gastric juice so that it is less damaging if aspirated.

GENERAL ANESTHESIA

General anesthesia *is defined as a controlled state of unconsciousness accompanied by a loss of protective reflexes, including the ability to maintain an airway independently and respond purposefully to physical stimulation or verbal command.* The use of GA sometimes is necessary to provide

Table 68.1: Drugs used for preanesthetic medication.

Drugs	Dosage	Route of administration	Features
Opioids	Morphine (10 mg) Pethidine (50–100 mg)	Intramuscular	*Uses:* They allay anxiety and apprehension of the operation, produce preoperative and postoperative analgesia, smoothen induction, reduce the dose of anesthetic required and supplement poor analgesic, and to reduce postoperative restlessness. *Disadvantages:* Depressed respiration, fall in blood pressure during anesthesia, lack of amnesia, flushing, delayed gastric emptying, and biliary spasm.
Sedative antianxiety drugs	Diazepam (5–10 mg) Lorazepam (2 mg)	Oral and intramuscular	*Uses:* Produce tranquility and smooth induction *Disadvantages:* Loss of recall of preoperative events, accentuation of postoperative vomiting.
Anticholinergics	Atropine (0.6 mg)	Intramuscular and intravenous	*Use:* To reduce salivary and bronchial secretions *Disadvantages:* Dryness of mouth in the preoperative and postoperative period may be distressing disadvantage.
Neuroleptics	Chlorpromazine (25 mg) Haloperidol (2– 4 mg)	Intramuscular	*Uses:* They allay anxiety, smoothen induction, and have antiemetic action *Disadvantages:* Potentiate respiratory depression and hypotension.
H2 blockers	Ranitidine (150 mg)	Oral	*Uses:* In patients undergoing prolonged operations, cesarean section, and obese patients at increased risk of gastric regurgitation. It reduces the pH of gastric juice and may also reduce its volume.
Antiemetics	Metoclopramide (10–20 mg)	Intramuscular	*Use:* Effective in reducing postoperative vomiting *Disadvantages:* Extrapyramidal effects and motor restlessness.

quality dental care for the child. Depending on the patient, this can be done in a hospital or an ambulatory setting, including the dental office. The cardinal features of GA are:

- Loss of all sensations, especially pain.
- Sleep (unconsciousness) and amnesia.
- Immobility and muscle relaxation.
- Abolition of somatic and autonomic reflexes.

Properties of an ideal anesthetic

For the patient:

- Pleasant
- Nonirritating
- Should not cause nausea or vomiting.
- Induction and recovery should be fast with no after effects.

Objectives of general anesthesia

- Provide safe, efficient, and effective dental care
- Eliminate anxiety
- Reduce untoward movement and reaction to dental treatment
- Aid in treatment of the mentally, physically, or medically compromised patient
- Eliminate the patient's pain response.

- **For the surgeon:**
  - It should provide adequate analgesia, immobility, and muscle relaxation.
  - It should be noninflammable and nonexplosive so that electric cautery may be used.
- **For the anesthetist:**
  - Its administration should be easy, controllable, and versatile.
  - Margin of safety should be wide. Heart, liver, and other organs should not be affected.
  - It should be potent so that low concentrations are needed and oxygenation of the patient does not suffer.
  - Rapid adjustments in depth of anesthesia should be possible.
  - It should be cheap, stable, and easily stored.

Physical status classification

The American Society of Anesthesiologists (ASA) adopted what is now commonly referred to as the ASA physical status classification. It was last approved by the ASA House of Delegates on October 15, 2014. It is a method to determine the anesthetic risk.

ASA Class I: Normal healthy patient without systemic disease.

ASA Class II: Patient with mild systemic disease.

ASA Class III: Patient with severe systemic disease. These patients have at least some degree of restriction of daily physical activity but are not incapacitated.

ASA Class IV: Patient with severe systemic disease that is a constant threat to life.

ASA Class V: Moribund patient who is not expected to survive without operation.

ASA Class VI: A declared brain dead patient whose organs are being removed for donor purpose.

The addition of 'E' denotes emergency surgery.

Indications of General Anesthesia

The need to diagnose and treat, as well as the safety of the patient, practitioner, and staff, should be considered for the use of GA. The decision to use GA must be taken into consideration as an alternative behavioral guidance modalities, dental needs of the patient, and his emotional and medical status. Indications for GA are:

- Patients who cannot cooperate due to a lack of psychological or emotional maturity and/or mental, physical, or medical disability
- Patients for whom LA is ineffective because of acute infection, anatomic variations, or allergy.

- The extremely uncooperative, fearful, anxious, or uncommunicative child or adolescent.
- Patients requiring significant surgical procedures.
- Patients for whom the use of GA may protect the developing psyche and/or reduce medical risk.
- Patients requiring immediate, comprehensive oral/dental care.

Indications for Outpatient GA

- Children and adolescents with ASA class I or II rating and severe dental disease with reliable parents who will deliver proper pre- and postoperative care.
- Some children with well-controlled chronic systemic disease such as asthma, diabetes, and congenital heart disease can also be considered for outpatient anesthesia following prior consultation with an anesthetist.

Indications for Inpatient GA

- The child should be treated as an inpatient if a medical condition exists that requires close follow-up, or if even the slightest doubt exists in the dentist's mind regarding the ability and reliability of the parents or guardians to implement proper pre- and postoperative instructions.
- Patients categorized as class III ASA are generally considered for inpatient GA unless they are transferred to a facility with proper postoperative management.
- Patients with Class IV ASA and higher.

Contraindications for GA

- A healthy, cooperative patient with minimal dental needs.
- Predisposing medical conditions which would make GA inadvisable like upper respiratory tract infections, productive cough, rhinitis, or wheezing, uncompensated vascular heart lesions, and failure to comply with preoperative nil per os (NPO) instructions.

Attitude of Parents

Attitude of parents towards dental treatment for their children under general anaesthesia have changed over time in the favor of it. Nowadays, there is a shift toward increasing acceptability of GA in parental opinion. Parents perceive dental GA as a treatment method which positively influences children's quality of life. The level of child's cooperation ability, the risks of GA modality, the cost of anesthetic and dental procedures are the factors influencing parental decision to choose GA for their child.

ADVANTAGES OF GENERAL ANESTHESIA

- Under GA, all required treatments are performed in a single session in a hospital environment providing efficient services in a safe manner.
- Parents of children who received dental care under GA to treat early childhood caries have reported improved quality of life and improved health status for their children, mainly regarding improvements in pain levels, eating, sleeping, and behavior.
- Procedure under GA reduces intraoperative patient awareness by causing amnesia.
- Facilitates complete control of airway, breathing, and circulation.
- Can be administered rapidly and is reversible.

DISADVANTAGES OF GENERAL ANESTHESIA

- Requires increased complexity of care and associated costs.
- Requires high degree of preoperative patient preparation.
- Associated with less serious complications such as nausea or vomiting, sore throat, headache, and shivering.
- Can induce physiologic fluctuations that require active intervention.

Procedure of Anesthesia (According to American Dental Association, October 2012)

- **Explanation of risk:**
  - Once a decision has been made to use GA, it should be explained to the parents that the anesthetic is not administered by a dentist, but by an anesthetic consultant who has undergone specialist training in pediatric anesthesia.
  - The potentially serious nature of the procedure should be clearly explained to the parent(s), and where appropriate, the patient.
  - There is a small but real risk of a catastrophe during GA. Agreement should be reached between the dental and anesthetic teams concerning how and when anesthetic risk is explained and documented.
- **Treatment planning:**
  - Comprehensive planning aims at ensuring that all the treatment required is carried out under a single GA.
  - Extraction, restoration, and pulp therapies should all be done in one go rather than accomplishing only few most important tasks and leave the rest for subsequent visits. The practice of extracting the most grossly carious and/or symptomatic teeth and leaving restorable teeth for future visits as an outpatient using LA with or without sedation is to be deprecated.
- **Consent:**
  - Parents should be informed priorly change of treatment can take place on the operatory table depending on the extent of the lesions.
  - The parent should be well explained about the anesthetic and dental procedures to be performed along with the risk and benefit of general anesthesia.
  - This provides a suitable period of reflection for the parents and/or child.
  - Care should be taken to ensure that the parent understands whether primary teeth, permanent teeth, or both are included in the treatment plan.
  - A blanket consent such as "restorations and extractions as necessary" is inadequate, and it should be explained that the decision about the number of fillings and extractions can sometimes only be made when the child is anesthetized and that this decision is left to the judgment of the operating clinician.

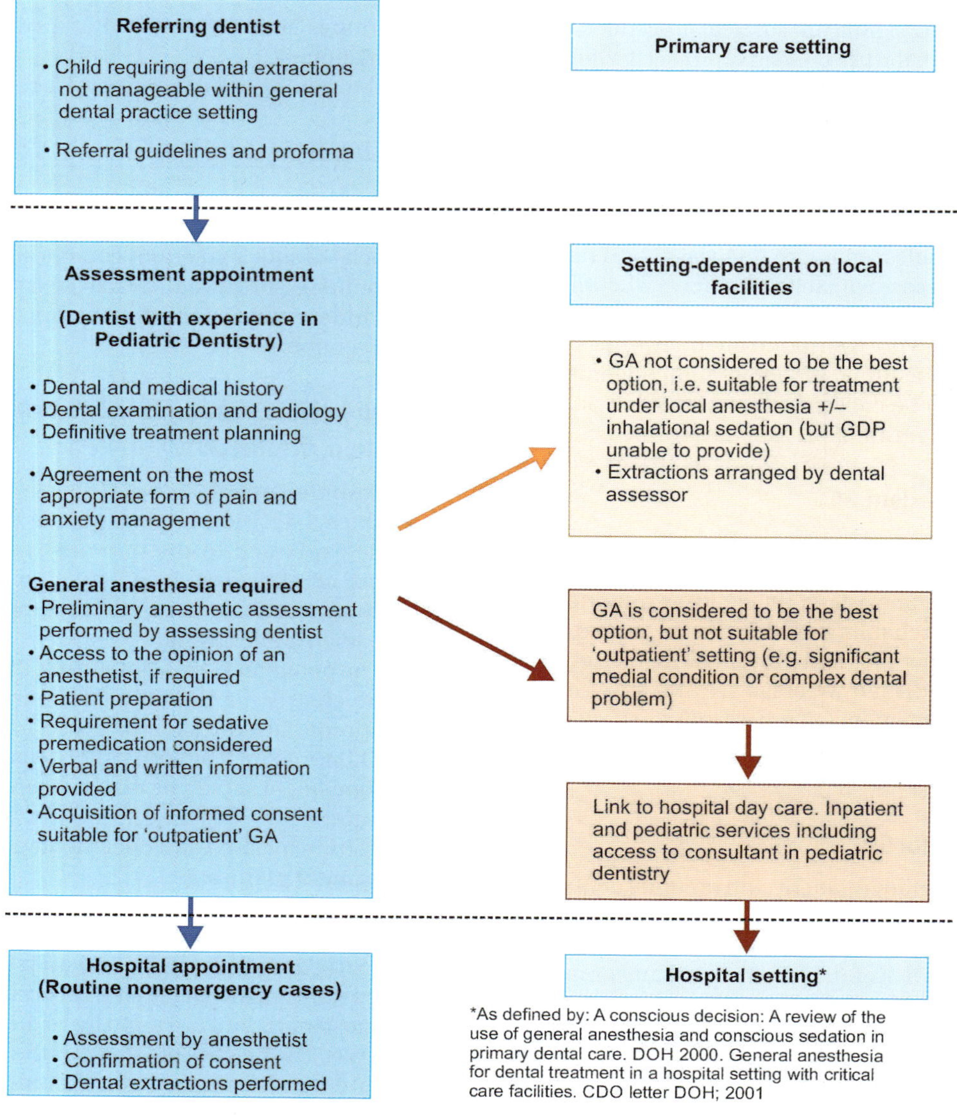

- **Preanesthetic clearance**
  - Now the child is referred to his/her pediatrician for a general evaluation and to obtain a fitness certificate for GA. An explanatory letter containing a professional request for consent to perform the dental procedure under general anesthesia is sent to the pediatrician. The letter should contain the dental diagnosis and the treatment planned for the child.
  - Generally, the following laboratory and diagnostic tests are recommended:
    - Complete blood count (CBC)
    - Bleeding time, clotting time, and platelet count
    - Posteroanterior chest X-ray
    - Electrolyte screening: sodium, potassium, chloride, glucose, and blood urea nitrogen (BUN)
    - Routine urine analysis
    - Other tests if indicated like ECG, prothrombin time, partial thromboplastin time, etc. depending on the patient's medical history.
  - A preanesthetic evaluation is scheduled now for anesthesiology. An anesthetist who is well-versed with pediatric dental cases is generally chosen for the procedure. The anesthesiologist will assess the child's past and present reports and hospital records (if any), focusing on prior exposures to GA and any complications that may have occurred. The decision regarding how long to keep the child off solid foods and liquids (NPO) before the procedure is also determined by the anesthetist. Generally, no oral intake (NPO) from midnight (minimum of 6 hrs NPO is mandatory), on the night before the procedure is advised.

- Parental compliance with pre- and postoperative diet instructions is the most important and critical factor to keep the child safe during GA and recovery to minimize the risk of intraoperative and postoperative complications. A printed instruction sheet regarding eating and drinking is given to the parents for this purpose.

❖ **Clinical setting for general anesthesia:**
- General anesthesia must be carried out in a "hospital setting" with adequate "critical care facilities"
- The facilities for anesthesia should be adequate along with monitoring devices and a good hospital for postoperative care **(Fig. 68.1)**.

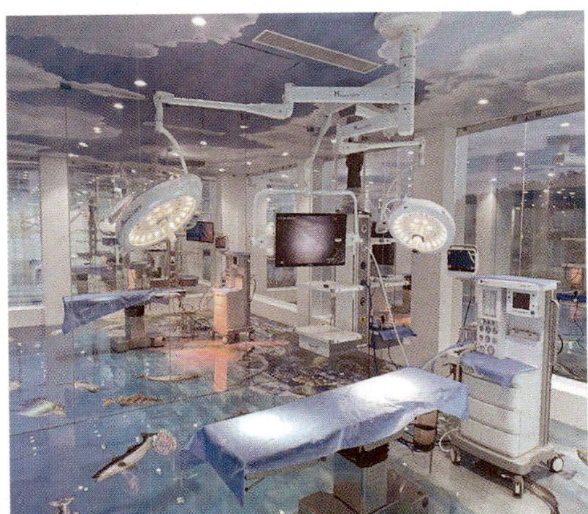

Fig. 68.1: Explicit general anesthesia unit. (*Pic courtesy:* Saveetha Dental College, Chennai).

❖ **Teamwork:**
- Issues of airway management, pain control, underlying medical conditions, management/extent of blood loss, and duration of the procedure are a shared responsibility.
- Effective communication with the anesthetist is the key to providing optimal care for the child under GA.

❖ **Personnel requirements:**
- A minimum of three individuals must be present.
- A dentist qualified in accordance with part III C of these guidelines to administer the deep sedation or GA.
- Two additional individuals who have current certification of successfully completing a basic life support (BLS) course for the healthcare provider.
- When the same individual administering the deep sedation or GA is performing the dental procedure, one of the additional appropriately trained team members must be designated for patient monitoring.

❖ **Dental team and preparation of equipment:**
- An effective teamwork is the key to carrying out optimal dental services. Performing a case under GA requires an efficient dental team comprising of a pediatric dentist, associate dental surgeon, and two well-trained dental assistants who help the operator in instrument transfer, preparing the materials, and so forth **(Fig. 68.2)**. Having a GA checklist helps to avoid missing out on important equipments and materials **(Fig. 68.3)**. The functioning of portable compressor or GA trolley is checked prior to the procedure. The dental assistants who are well-trained in hospital operating room procedures should arrange all the instruments in a sterile manner before the procedure.

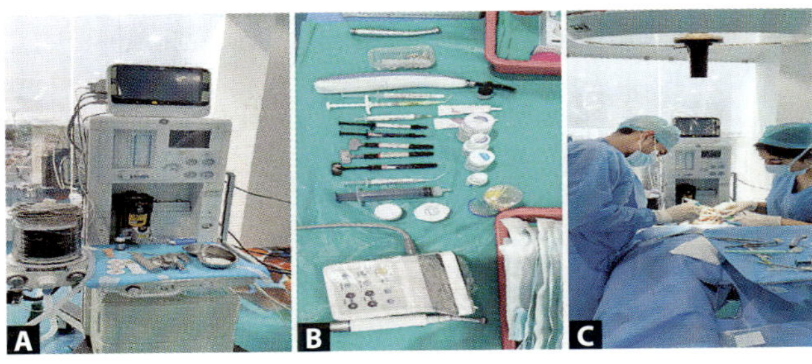

Figs. 68.2A to C: (A) Set up for general anesthesia procedure; (B) Tray arrangement for GA; (C) Treating patient under GA.

- Mouth mirror
- Straight probe
- Explorer
- Tweezer
- Gloves
- Mouth mask
- Head cap
- Spoon excavator
- Filling instrument
- Carvers
- Ball burnisher
- Instrument tray
- kidney trays
- Waste receiver
- Instrument bin
- Cotton rolls
- Latch type converter
- Mouth prop
- Bur box

Crowns
- Stainless steel crown kit
- Pliers (Crimping and contouring)
- Strip crown kit
- Crown cutting scissor
- GIC type 1 cement
- Scalpel blase and BP handle
- Composite kit including pit and Fissure sealant
- Light cure unit
- Composite finishing burs

Pulpectomy
- Endo box: k-files (15–40)
H-files (15–40)
Barbed broaches
- Micro-motor attachment
- Contra-angle and airotor hand piece
- Saline
- Syringe and needle
- Sodium hypochlorite
- Paper points
- Glass ionomer type 2 cement

Splinting
- 0.6 and 0.7 mm stainless steel wire
- Universal orthodontic plier
- Orthodontic wire cutter
- Composite kit

Extractions/minor surgery
- Periosteal elevator
- Extraction forceps
- Suture material
- Tissue holding forceps
- Rongeur
- Bone file

Fig. 68.3: Checklist for general anesthesia.

❖ **Anesthetic procedure:**
- It should be according to the prescribed standards and guidelines for GA for dentistry
- The anesthetic equipment should be pre-evaluated along with other monitoring facilities.

❖ **Preparation of children before bringing into OT:**
- Psychological management is highly helpful to permit patients to allay their distress before the procedure. Simple explanation, game playing and distraction are some methods to reduce patient fear. Parental presence upto the initiation of the procedure is found to be helpful to reduce the anxiety in children.

❖ **Induction of general anesthesia:**
- The choice of premedication and general anesthetic technique to be used is determined by the anesthetist. Most patients do not require heavy premedication.

- The anesthetist usually uses an agent or combination of agents providing rapid postoperative recovery. In children, because of the fear of needles, anesthesia is commonly induced by inhalation via face mask. Sevoflurane is the drug of choice for inhalational induction due to its lower blood/gas partition coefficient and it is associated with less myocardial depression and fewer and less significant respiratory problems. After mask induction, an intravenous line is started and maintained throughout the procedure.
- It is important for the pediatric dentist to request for a nasal intubation instead of oral intubation for maintenance of anesthetic state. This type of intubation does not interfere with the working space in the mouth and requires less airway manipulation. Therefore, the dental treatment can be performed in a shorter time.
- It is a common practice by anesthesiologists to administer an antisialagogue such as glycopyrolate which helps to reduce salivary flow and provides a dry field and prevents aspiration of oral secretions. It also helps to maintain the heart rate under GA. Some anesthetists place an ophthalmic ointment in the eyes and then tape them shut to prevent conjunctivitis and foreign bodies in the eyes. Usually steroid creams such as kenocort oral paste are applied in the lips to reduce the swelling in the lips postoperatively.

❖ **Operative procedures:**

- The dentist now prepares the child by cleaning the extraoral area with betadine using sterile sponge. The child is then draped, leaving only the mouth exposed. Next step is to place a throat pack carefully. This ensures an adequate seal against leakage of anesthetic gas and helps prevent debris from falling into the pharynx. A mouth prop is placed now and the operative work can begin.

❖ **Determining the duration of the procedure:**

- Because of the operation complexity, estimating operation time is really difficult and not exact. Most of the operations may take longer than estimated preoperatively. This depends upon the clinical expertise of the operator and the skill of the dental assistants. On an average, 1–3 hours is the routine treatment time for a dental rehabilitation. It is important to be fast and efficient without sacrificing quality.
- Few things to remember which helps in saving time in the operatory.
  - Use a portable compressor with airotor handpiece for fast and efficient work **(Fig. 68.4)**.
  - Due to unavailability of portable compressor in certain facilities and while using a micromotor with contra- angle handpiece; instead of repeatedly changing burs for different procedures keep extra handpieces (with different burs attached) and change the handpiece itself whenever required.
  - Prepare the crowns beforehand. Stainless steel crowns (SSCs) should be festooned, strip crown collar should be cut and vent holes prepared before the procedure.

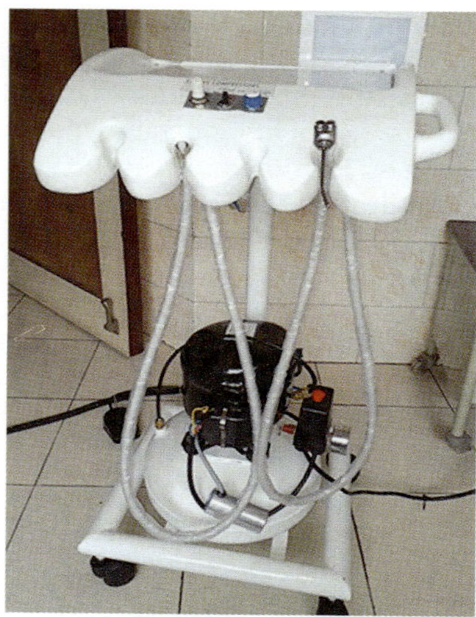

Fig. 68.4: Portable compressor used for general anesthesia.

  - Work quadrant wise. Extraction can be planned first, so that blood clot will be formed when all the remaining operative procedures are completed.
  - Use rotary files when there are multiple pulpectomies to be done. Use barbed broaches judiciously.
  - Having a portable X-ray unit and digital radiograph helps a lot.
  - Use a hemostatic agent containing aluminium chloride or ferric sulphate to control bleeding from gingiva after crown preparation.

❖ **Protocol for operative procedures under general anesthesia (Figs. 68.5A to F):**

The following points should be noted while performing any operative procedure under GA:

- While deciding the treatment plan, more definitive treatments should be selected.
- Teeth with doubtful or poor prognosis should be removed. This helps to reduce the likelihood of any failure or the possibility of another GA.
- Grossly unrestorable teeth are good candidates for extraction.
- Among restorative procedures, full coverage SSCs have higher success rate than multi-surface composite or GIC. SSCs are the most durable and functional restorations, which can decrease the need of retreatment in teeth with proximal caries or circumferential decay.
- Complex treatment such as pulp therapy for teeth with abscess or swelling should be avoided under GA.
- Operative and endodontic procedures are done first under rubber dam to minimize foreign body scatter in the oral cavity.
- Local anesthesia should be given if multiple extractions are planned to minimize bleeding and aids in postoperative pain control. Placement of resorbable sutures in multiple extraction site prevents drooling of blood in the recovery bed.
- Scaling can be planned at the end of the procedures, since it helps to remove the excess cement around the crowns and complete examination of all the teeth.

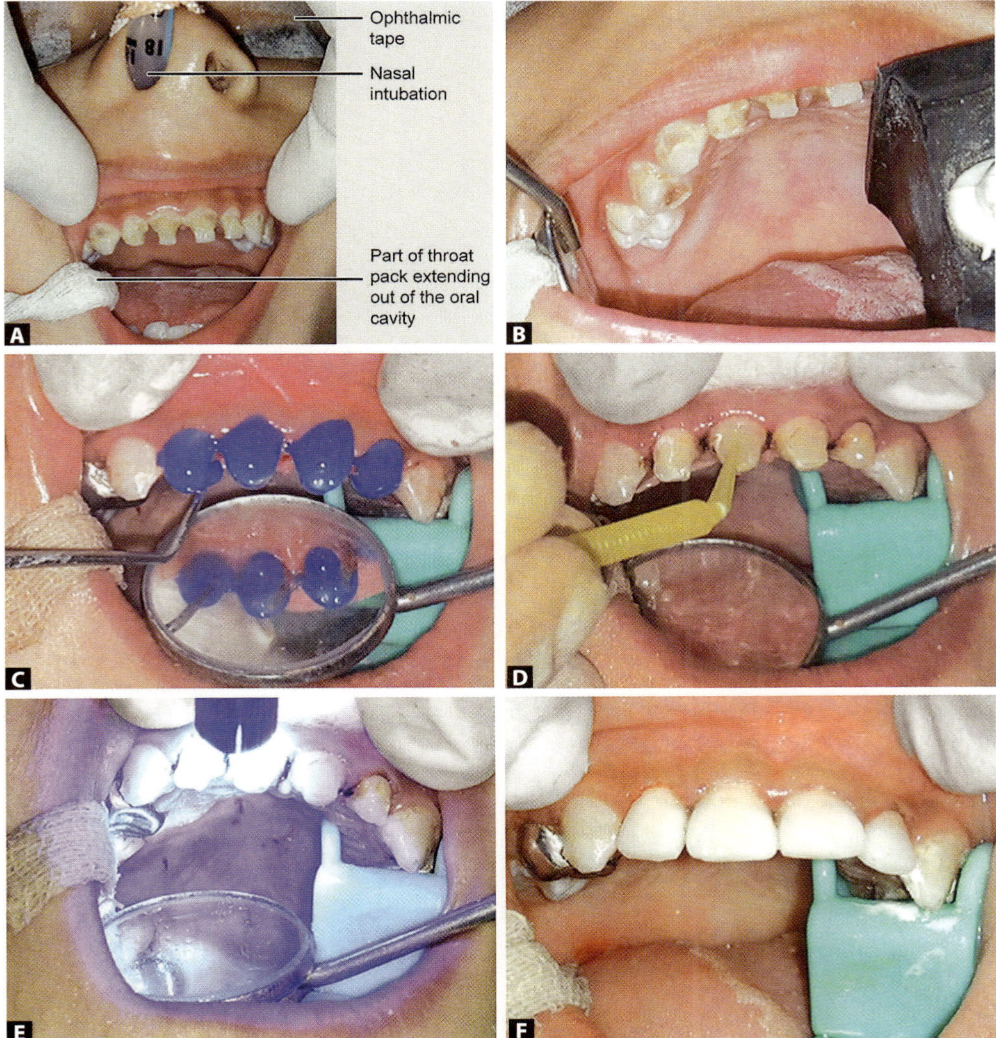

Figs. 68.5A to F: (A) Preoperative photo of 3-year-old child with severe early childhood caries; (B) Preoperative; (C) Etching; (D) Application of bonding agent; (E) Light curing; (F) Postoperative: Pulpectomy followed by strip crowns placed with 51, 52, 61, 62. Composite restorations with 63, 53.

- Preferable techniques of local anestheis are intraligamental and intrapulpal in consideration to Inferior alveolar nerve block. These techniques prevent postoperative lip or cheek biting.
- About 15 minutes before completing treatment, the anesthetist should be informed. The oral cavity is thoroughly cleansed, suctioned out, and examined to ensure that it is free of debris. The throat pack is carefully removed and oropharynx is inspected for any bleeding. The anesthetist will begin to extubate the patient now.

❖ **Safety of the patient:**
- There is a increased use of GA for dental procedures over the past two decades. Hence it is required to focus more on safety aspects during dental procedures performed in general anesthesia. Arrhythmias, disloged or obstructed endotracheal tube, IV infiltrates or disconnects, edema of the tongue or lips and nasal bleeding are intraoperative complications. Inexperienced staff and/or inadequate machines and equipment may lead to adverse events. To maintain skills and minimize the risk of adverse events or optimally eliminate it, it is needed to follow guidelines and participate in standard and regular training courses.

❖ **Clinical effectiveness:**
- The goal is to restrict to the planned treatment and finish it effectively within the stipulated time frame using four-handed dentistry.

❖ **Monitoring:**
- A qualified dentist administering deep sedation or GA must remain in the operatory room to monitor the patient continuously until the patient meets the criteria for recovery.
- The dentist must not leave the facility until the patient meets the criteria for discharge and is discharged from the facility.
- Monitoring must include checking for oxygenation, ventilation, circulation, and temperature.

Table 68.2: Dental care under general anesthesia—discharge advice for parents.

Discharge

You will be able to take your child home when you and the nurses feel confident that he/she:
- Can walk steadily around the ward
- Is reasonably comfortable
- Is not feeling sick
- Is drinking water/juice and able to hold it down.

Eating and drinking

Your child needs to have a soft, smooth diet and nothing which is too warm or too cold, to avoid discomfort, and further bleeding.

Oral hygiene

It is important to maintain good oral hygiene as this will promote healing.

Problems to look for
- *Pain:* Following dental extractions, a certain amount of discomfort is inevitable. Our aim is for your child to be as comfortable as possible after their operation. Your child may be discharged with pain relieving medication. Please follow the advice from the nursing staff on how to take this medication.
- *Swelling:* Your child may experience facial swelling. This is common and will disappear within a few days. You may find it helpful to wrap something cool (e.g. frozen peas) in a towel and rest it on the swollen area for a few minutes.
- *Bleeding:* Do not be alarmed if there is a small amount of blood from the extraction sockets. Roll up a clean handkerchief or gauze, moisten with warm water, place over the socket, and have your child bite firmly for at least 10 min. If this fails to control the bleeding after about 30 min, seek professional help.
- *Stitches:* Any dissolving stitches should be gone in a week. Non-dissolving stitches need to be removed and you should receive an appointment for this.

General instructions

Now that your child is going home, we wish to remind you that after a general anesthetic there is a period in which his/her judgment, performance, and reaction time are affected by the anesthetic, even though the child may feel quite normal again. It is therefore, very important in the 24 h after the operation that your child is not allowed to do anything potentially dangerous to her/ himself or others, such as playing in an adventure playground, riding a bicycle, climbing trees, swimming, or going out by themselves.

- **Oxygenation:**
  - Color of mucosa, skin, or blood must be continually evaluated.
  - Oxygenation saturation must be evaluated continuously by pulse oximetry.
- **Ventilation:**
  - *Intubated patient:* End-tidal carbon dioxide ($ETCO_2$) must be continuously monitored and evaluated.
  - *Non-intubated patient:* Breath sounds via auscultation and/or end-tidal CO_2 must be continually monitored and evaluated.
  - Respiration rate must be continually monitored and evaluated.
- **Circulation:**
  - The dentist must continuously evaluate heart rate and rhythm via electrocardiogram (ECG) through- out the procedure, as well as pulse rate via pulse oximetry.
  - The dentist must continually evaluate blood pressure.
- **Temperature:**
  - A device capable of measuring body temperature must be readily available during the administration of deep sedation or GA.
  - The equipment to continuously monitor body temperature should be available and must be performed whenever triggering agents associated with malignant hyperthermia are administered.
- **Postoperative care:**
  - Accompany the patient to the recovery room and do an immediate follow up oral examination. Write an operative summary and postoperative orders for the hospital staff. It is important to talk to the parents now and discuss the case with them and reassure them.
  - Prescriptions are written for pain control and antibiotics. The patient is observed frequently until fully recovered. The most common problems have been short episodes of nausea, vomiting, and mild discomfort. Lips may be dry and cracked and may require application of petroleum jelly.
  - Sometimes, if the operator has stretched the lips excessively when gaining access to the mouth, he will find the lips slightly swollen within few hours. This will cause only mild discomfort, which should be treated symptomatically with ice packs to reduce the swelling.
- **Discharge:**
  - Responsibility for the discharge process is shared between the dentist, the anesthetist, and the recovery nursing staff.
  - Usually, after 5 h small sips of plain water are given, followed sweet drinks. Aerated drinks should not be given during first 24 h.
  - Choice of analgesics/antibiotics should be prescribed.
  - Vital signs like pulse, blood pressure (BP), respiration, and saturation to be monitored.
  - Intravenous fluids maintenance.
  - Patients and parents should receive verbal and written postoperative instructions **(Table 68.2)**.

STAGES OF ANESTHESIA

General anesthetics cause an irregularly descending depression of central nervous system (CNS), i.e. the higher functions are lost first and progressively lower areas of the brain are involved. **Guedel** (1920) described four stages with ether anesthesia but the precise sequence of events differs among each anesthetic.

Stage	*Features*
Stage of analgesia	Starts from beginning of anesthetic inhalation and lasts up to the loss of consciousness. Pain is progressively abolished during this stage. Patient remains conscious, can hear and see, and feels a dream-like state. Reflexes and respiration remain normal. Though some minor and even major operations can be carried out during this stage, it is rather difficult to maintain so its use is limited to short procedures only.
Stage of delirium	From loss of consciousness to beginning of regular respiration. Apparent excitement is seen in many patients and he may shout, struggle, and hold his breath; muscle tone increase, jaws are tightly closed, and breathing is jerky; vomiting, involuntary micturition, or defecation may occur. Heart rate and blood pressure may rise and pupil dilates due to sympathetic stimulation. No stimulus should be applied or operative procedure carried out during this stage. This stage can be cut short by rapid induction and appropriate premedication. It is inconspicuous in modern anesthesia.
Surgical anesthesia	Extends from onset of regular respiration to cessation of spontaneous breathing. This has been divided into four planes which may be distinguished as: 1. *Plane 1:* Roving eyeballs. This plane ends when eyes become fixed. 2. *Plane 2:* Loss of corneal and laryngeal reflexes. 3. *Plane 3:* Pupils start dilating and light reflex is lost. 4. *Plane 4:* Intercostal paralysis, shallow abdominal respiration, and dilated pupil.
Medullary paralysis	Includes the stage from cessation of breathing to failure of circulation and death. Pupil is widely dilated, muscles are totally flabby, pulse is imperceptible, and blood pressure is very low.

COMPLICATIONS OF GENERAL ANESTHESIA

During anesthesia	*After anesthesia*
• Respiratory depression and hypercarbia • Salivation, respiratory secretions • Cardiac arrhythmias, asystole • Fall in blood pressure • *Aspiration of gastric contents:* Acid pneumonitis • Laryngospasm and asphyxia • Delirium, convulsions • *Fire and explosion:* Rare now due to use of noninflammable gases.	• Nausea and vomiting • *Persisting sedation:* Impaired psychomotor function • Pneumonia, atelectasis • *Organ toxicities:* Liver, kidney damage • Emergence delirium • *Cognitive defects*—Prolonged excess cognitive decline has been observed in some patients, especially the elderly who have undergone general anesthesia, particularly of long duration.

POINTS TO REMEMBER

- Wells was the first to use N_2O.
- Morton was the first dentist to experiment with ether anesthesia in 1846.
- Preanesthetic medication refers to the use of drugs before anesthesia to make it more pleasant and safe.
- General anesthesia is defined as a controlled state of unconsciousness accompanied by a loss of protective reflexes, including the ability to maintain an airway independently and respond purposefully to physical stimulation or verbal command.
- Objectives of GA are to provide safe, efficient, and effective dental care, eliminate anxiety, aid in treatment of the mentally, physically, or medically compromised patient.
- General anesthesia is indicated in patients who cannot cooperate due to a lack of psychological or emotional maturity and/or mental, physical, or medical disability; patients for whom LA is ineffective because of acute infection, anatomic variations, or allergy; extremely uncooperative, fearful, anxious, or uncommunicative child or adolescent; patients requiring immediate, comprehensive oral/dental care.
- Procedure of anesthesia includes explanation of risk, treatment planning, consent, preoperative assessment, clinical setup with required personal and equipment, starting of anesthesia, working, monitoring, and discharge.
- Inhalation agents for GA are N_2O, ether, halothane, isoflurane, desflurane, sevoflurane.
- Intravenous agents for GA are thiopentone sodium, methohexitone sodium, propofol, etomidate, diazepam, lorazepam, ketamine, and fentanyl.
- Side effects during procedure of anesthesia are respiratory depression and hypercarbia, salivation, respiratory secretions, cardiac arrhythmias, fall in BP, aspiration of gastric contents, laryngospasm, delirium, and fire and explosion. Side effects after procedure of anesthesia are nausea and vomiting, persisting sedation, pneumonia, atelectasis, organ toxicities, emergence delirium, and cognitive defects.
- The most important indication for GA is patients who cannot co-operate due to lack of physiological maturity or any disability.
- The advantage of GS is that all treatment can be finished in one appointment with minimal patient compliance.
- The increased rate of complexity and care and various complications are the obvious disadvantage.
- Factors that affect GA decision making are age, cooperation, risk assessment.

Questionnaire

1. What is preanesthetic medication?
2. Define general anesthesia and give its indications, contra-indications, and goals.
3. Explain in details the procedure for general anesthesia.
4. What are the stages of anesthesia?
5. Write a note on drugs used for general anesthesia.
6. Describe the complications of general anesthesia.
7. What are the indications and contraindications of general anesthesia?
8. What are the indications for inpatient and outpatient GA?
9. Write in detail about the step by step procedure for performing a dental procedure under GA.
10. Mention the protocol for operative procedures under GA.
11. Write about the factors affecting decision making under GA.

FURTHER READING

1. American Academy of Pediatric Dentistry. Clinical guideline on the elective use of minimal, moderate, and deep sedation and general anesthesia for pediatric dental patients. Pediatr Dent. 2004; 26:95-103.
2. American Academy on Pediatric Dentistry Ad Hoc Committee on Sedation and Anesthesia; American Academy on Pediatric Dentistry Council on Clinical Affairs. Policy on use of deep sedation and general anesthesia in pediatric dental office. Pediatr Dent. 2008-2009;30(7 Suppl):66-7.
3. American Dental Association (ADA). (2012). Guidelines for the Use of Sedation and General Anesthesia by Dentists. [online] Available from www.ada.org/~/media/ADA/Advocacy/Files/ anes_policy_statement.pdf?la=en. [Accessed April, 2018].
4. Camilleri A, Roberts G, Ashley P, et al. Analysis of paediatric dental care provided under general anaesthesia and levels of dental disease in two hospitals. Br Dent J. 2004; 196:219-23.
5. Davies C, Harrison M, Roberts G. (2008). UK National Clinical Guidelines in Paediatric Dentistry: Guideline for the Use of General Anaesthesia (GA) in Paediatric Dentistry. [online] Available from www.rcseng.ac.uk/-/media/files/rcs/fds/ publications/guideline-for-the-use-of-ga-in-paediatric- dentistry-may-2008-final.pdf?la=en. [Accessed April, 2018].
6. FDA Drug Safety Communication. (2017). FDA review results in new warnings about using general anesthetics and sedation drugs in young children and pregnant women.
7. Ferretti GA. Guidelines for outpatient general anesthesia to provide comprehensive dental treatment. Dent Clin North Am. 1984;28:107.
8. Forsyth AR, Seminario AL, Lee H, et al. General anesthesia time for pediatric dental cases. Pediatr Dent. 2012;34(5): 129-35.
9. Holt RD, Rule DC, Davenport ES, et al. The use of general anaesthesia for tooth extraction in children in London: a multi- centre study. Br Dent J. 1992; 173:333-9.
10. Landes DP, Clayton-Smith AJ. The role of pre-general anaesthetic assessment for patients referred by general dental practitioners to the Community Dental Service. Community Dent Health. 1996; 13:169-71.
11. Malhotra N. General anesthesia for dentistry. Indian J Anaesth. 2008;52 (suppl 5):725-37.s
12. O'Sullivan EA, Curzon ME. The efficacy of comprehensive dental care for children under general anesthesia. Br Dent J. 1991;171(2):56-8.
13. O'Sullivan EA, Curzon ME. The efficacy of comprehensive dental care for children under general anesthesia. Br Dent J. 1991; 171:56-8.
14. Pike D. A conscious decision. A review of the use of general anaesthesia and conscious sedation in primary dental care. SAAD Dig. 2000; 17:13-4.
15. Ramazani N. Different aspects of general anesthesia in pediatric dentistry: a review. Iran J Pediatr. 2016;26(2):e2613.
16. Simmons D. Sedation and patient safety. Crit Care Nurs Clin North Am. 2005; 17:279-85.
17. Smallridge JA, Al GN, Holt RD. The use of general anaesthesia for tooth extraction for child outpatients at a London dental hospital. Br Dent J. 1990;168:438-40.
18. Standards and Guidelines for General Anaesthesia for Dentistry. Royal College of Anaesthetists; 1999.
19. Tochel C, Hosey MT, Macpherson L, et al. Assessment of children prior to dental extractions under general anaesthesia in Scotland. Br Dent J. 2004;196:629-33.

CHAPTER

Pediatric Drug Therapy

Sangeetha P Venkatesh, Nikhil Marwah

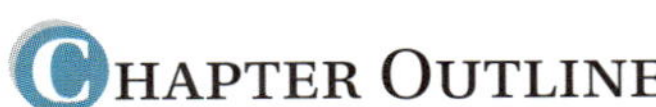

CHAPTER OUTLINE

The pediatric population represents a spectrum of different physiologies, it extends from the neonate, infant, toddler, and child to the adolescent. Their ability to process drugs (pharmacokinetics) is influenced by radical developmental changes of biological maturation. Drug prescribing to this cohort is dependent on understanding the pharmacokinetics (PK) and pharmacodynamics (PD) of that particular drug, as well as the clinical characteristics of the pediatric patient being treated with the drug. Pediatric dental patients are treated with medicines for oral conditions. Hence, it is vital to better understand the intricacies of medication use in children.

Pharmacology studies the effect of drugs on the organism, and pharmacokinetics study the effects suffered by the drug when in contact with the organism. Pharmacodynamics refers to the relationship between drug dosage and its effect on a certain organ or system.

The application of pharmacokinetic and pharmacodynamic knowledge to the pediatric field implies the understanding of the maturing process in a continuing changeable organism at every age, from preterm neonates to adolescence.

THE ABCDE OF PEDIATRIC PHARMACOTHERAPY

(ACRONYM ABCDE: *Absorption, bioavailability, clearance, distribution, and effects*)

Absorption

Oral administration	**Gastric pH** • Neonates have near-neutral pH in their first 1 to 2 weeks of life, with the exception of a low gastric pH during the first 24 to 48 hours after birth. Gastric pH gradually decreases as gastric acid production begins until around age 2 when it approaches adult levels of 1 to 3. **Gastric emptying time** • Until about 6 months of age, neonates and infants have significantly slower gastric emptying times. It varies depending on gestational age and disease status. **Intestinal motility** • Medication transit time is reduced in neonates and infants due to decreased motility and peristalsis. The increased absorption of penicillins is aided by the longer time that drugs spend in the stomach of a newborn. • Motility patterns differ not only between pediatric age groups but also between individual newborns. The rate and extent of absorption are also affected by these patterns, which are dependent on gestational age. Absorption is reduced due to reduced intestinal surface area and transit times. **Gastric enzymes** • Gastric and pancreatic enzymes, as well as biliary excretions, are lower in neonates. These compounds may be required for the solubilization, cleavage, protonation, and deprotonation of certain drug molecules in order for them to be absorbed.

Contd..

Contd..

Intramuscular administration	• Slow, erratic, delayed absorption due to low blood flow, less muscle mass, and a higher proportion of water during the first few days of life. • Intramuscular drug absorption is faster in early childhood than in neonates and adults.
Transdermal/percutaneous absorption	• An infant's stratum corneum is extremely thin. Infants have more blood flow in their skin than older patients. • Absorption is inversely related to the thickness of the epidermal stratum corneum, whereas skin hydration has a direct impact on absorption. • Infants' development is faster and more complete than that of older children and adults. • Topical drugs have a higher risk of toxicity in infants.
Rectal absorption	• The rectal area is small but well-vascularized, with absorption taking place through the superior, medial, and inferior hemorrhoidal veins. Maturation has little effect on the rectal route. • In adults, the local pH of the rectum is close to neutral, but in most children, it is alkaline. • The bioavailability of rectal doses may be affected by the first pass effect. Medications placed low in the rectum are distributed systemically before passing through the liver, whereas drugs administered high in the rectum are delivered directly to the liver and are thus prone to metabolism and enterohepatic circulation. • Bioavailability is highly variable amongst neonates, babies, children, and adults depending on the absorption site of the rectum.
Intrapulmonary administration (inhalation)	• Apart from general anesthetics, the primary objective of this mode of administration is to create a large local effect, however, systemic exposure can occur. • Developmental changes in the architecture of the lung and its ventilatory capacity affect drug absorption following intrapulmonary delivery.
Intranasal administration	• There are numerous advantages of administering medications intranasally, including ease of administration, speed of action, good tolerance, and the absence of a hepatic first-pass effect. • However, disadvantages include a limited volume of administration and poor absorption of hydrophilic medicines. • Midazolam, fentanyl, butorphanol, ketamine, sufentanil, corticosteroids, antihistamines, sumatriptan, and desmopressin are some medications that have been tried intranasally in children.

Bioavailability

Is a subcategory of absorption	• The extent to which the active ingredient of a drug dosage form becomes available at the site of drug action. • By definition, when a medication is administered intravenously, its BA is 100%. • However, when a medication is administered via other routes (such as orally), its BA generally decreases (due to incomplete absorption and first-pass metabolism) or may vary from patient to patient. • The route of administration (ROA) and the dose of a drug have a significant impact on both the rate and extent of bioavailability.

Distribution

Protein binding	• Drug binding to albumin and other plasma proteins is reduced in the newborn. • Serum albumin levels are relatively low.
Blood-brain barrier	• Not fully developed at birth. • Drugs and other chemicals have relatively easy access to the CNS. • Infants are especially sensitive to drugs that affect CNS function. • Dosage should also be reduced for drugs used for actions outside the CNS if those drugs are capable of producing CNS toxicity as a side effect.
Endogenous compounds compete with drugs for available binding sites	• Limited drug/protein binding in infants. • Reduced dosage needed. • Adult protein binding capacity by 10 to 12 months of age.

Metabolism

• The CYP450 enzyme system in the liver and small bowel is the most significant system for drug metabolism. • Enzyme systems mature at different phases of development, and they may be absent or present at low levels at birth.	• The rate of hepatic metabolism varies from 1 year to adolescence. • Beginning at the age of one year and continuing until the baby reaches the age of two years, the baby's metabolism is significantly faster than that of adults. • The rate of hepatic metabolism then gradually decreases. • At puberty, the rate of hepatic metabolism slows dramatically. • Because the rise in metabolic rate in children is generally greater than in adults, children may require higher milligram-per-kilogram doses or more frequent dosing than adults, or the gap between doses may be reduced correspondingly.

Clearance/Elimination

The bile and the kidney eliminate drug metabolites.	• Drugs are broken down and removed more slowly in neonates and infants than in older children and adults. • The rate of medication clearance in the kidney is determined by the glomerular filtration rate, renal blood flow, plasma protein binding, and tubular secretion. • These parameters are altered over the first two years of life. Renal plasma flow is low at birth and approaches adult values by the age of one year. • The glomerular filtration rate is low at birth and rises to adult levels by the time the infant is 3 to 5 months old.

PEDIATRIC DRUG DOSAGE

❖ ***When should you use it?***

- It is frequently uncertain when to transition from weight-based (pediatric) to fixed-dose (adult). Children 12 years of age and below, as well as those weighing less than 40 kg, can utilize standard pediatric-dose conversion formulas.

❖ ***Which one to use?***

- Drug dosage rules are based on age, weight, and body surface area. Almost all pediatric drug dosage rules use a percentage of adult dose to calculate an appropriate child's dose with the mg/kg regimen being the exception.
- For dosing in pediatrics, whether weight-based dosing is better than body surface-area-based dosing is dependent on the particular medication (e.g., methotrexate, prednisone, prednisolone, zidovudine, didanosine, growth hormone, and 13-*cis*-retinoic acid).
- Age-based dosing strategy is better than weight-based dosing in some cases (e.g., intravenous busulfan and dalteparin).
- It is necessary to compare different dosing methods from the perspectives of efficacy, safety, pharmacoeconomics, patient preference, and adherence to high-alert medications, expensive medications, and antibacterials.

Despite disadvantages mg/kg regimen has widespread popularity. It is more advisable to base one's calculation on the ideal weight for the child's height and age. Prescriptions based on the weight of the child is the most common method used in pediatric dental practice. Weight-adjusted medications should not be prescribed, dispensed, or administered (except in emergencies) unless patient's weight is available and considered by all relevant healthcare providers. Prescribers should confirm the accuracy of patient's weight and include the patient's weight on the prescription or physician order prior to weight-based dosing. The calculated dose and the dosing determination such as the dose per weight (e.g., mg/kg) should also be specified by the prescriber. Electronic weight-based order integrated with computer physician order entry could significantly increase the percentage of appropriate dosing.

SAFE DOSE RANGE

Many pediatric drugs have a therapeutic range, also known as a safe dose range (SDR). The drug manual specifies the "range" (e.g., Amoxicillin 25-50 mg/kg), i.e., "minimum" and "maximum." Many guidelines suggest a lower limit; nonetheless, the optimal dosage is determined by the clinical condition. Prescribers should use caution and adhere to this dose range while prescribing medications.

Based on age	Fried's Rule	Age in Months x Adult Dose ÷150
	Young's Rule	Age in Years x Adult Dose ÷ Age + 12
	Dilling's Formula	Age in Years x Adult Dose
	Augsberger's Rule	{[(4 × Age in Years) + 20]/100} × Adult Dose = Child's Dose
	Gabius'Rule	1 year–1/12th of adult dose
		2 years–1/8th of adult dose
		3 years–1/6th of adult dose
		4 years–1/4th of adult dose
		7 years–1/3rd of adult dose
		14 years–1/2nd of adult dose
		20 years–2/3rd of adult dose
		21 years–adult dose
	Catzel's Rule	1 year of age- 25 *Percentage (%) of adult dose*
		3 years of age-35 *Percentage (%) of adult dose*
		7 years of age-50 *Percentage (%) of adult dose*
		12 years of age-75 *Percentage (%) of adult dose*
Based on body weight	Clark's Rule	Weight in lbs or kg x Adult dose ÷ 150 lbs or 70 kg.
	Penna's Formula	Adult dosage x child's weight ÷ child's weight/2 + 30
	Augsberger's Rule	{[(1.5 × weight in kg) + 10]/100} × Adult dose = Child's dose
	Salisbury's Formula	Children weighing less than 30 kg = weight x 2 = % of the adult dosage. Children weighing more than 30 kg = weight + 30 = % of the adult dosage
	most commonly used mg/kg regimen	Ratio-proportion method: Multiply the means and the extremes (e.g., 3: 4 = x: 8)
		Formula method: D/H x Q = XD - dosage desired or ordered; H - what is on hand (available); Q-unit of measure that contains the available dose. X - The unknown dosage you need to administer.
Based on body surface area: **(BSA)**	A nomogram or formula can be used to determine BSA.	The body surface area (BSA) of an individual can also be calculated from the Dubois formula: BSA(m)^2 = BW (kg) 0.425 × Height (cm) 0.725 × 0.007184 BSA of the child x adult dose /1.73 m.

The 'd' confusion

- What are the difference between per dose(d), per day (d) [maximum single dose (MSD)], and the maximum dose per day (MDD)?
- Drug reference manuals express drug dosages per dose (d) or per day(d),e.g., Amoxicillin 15 mg/kg per dose or Amoxicillin 25-35 mg/kg per day.
- **Hence, vigilance is required.**
- Prescriptions should specify per day or per dose regimen.
- Maximum single dose (MSD) Maximum daily dose (MDD) 20-40 mg/kg/day in divided doses every 8 hours (maximum single dose 500 mg) OR 25–45 mg/kg/day in divided doses every 12 hours (maximum single dose 875 mg) a maximum daily dose of 2000 mg/day.

STANDARDIZATION OF PEDIATRIC DOSING GUIDELINES

A variety of dosing guidelines is published for pediatric use, with lack of standardized weight-based dosing range. Inconsistencies in the dosing guidelines make defining, under doses and overdoses problematic. Standardization of the various sources of pediatric dosing guidelines, with current and comprehensive dose information would resolve this problem. [24,2]

CHALLENGES IN PEDIATRIC FORMULATIONS OR DOSAGE FORMS

Dosage forms should be safely and effectively adapted to the needs of pediatric patients.

The magnitude of doses required through childhood can vary by 100-fold and the ability to cope with different dosage forms can also vary considerably. Thus, if a medicinal product is to be used in all age groups, a range of different dosage forms should be available providing different strengths or concentrations to allow simple, accurate, and safe dosing.

Pharmaceutical excipients are substances that are included in a pharmaceutical dosage form not for their direct therapeutic action, but to aid the manufacturing process, to protect, support or enhance stability, or for bioavailability or patient acceptability, e.g., arginine, ethanol, benzyl alcohol, saccharin, a spartame, propylene glycol, cyclodextrins, polyethylene glycol, parabens, etc. Pediatric medicaments usually contain excipeints which may be harmful when administered to children. The use of excipients can be harmful when given to children.

Important considerations for pediatric drug formualtions are:

- Minimal dosage frequency
- One dosage form fits all or a full range
- Minimal impact on lifestyle
- Minimum, nontoxic excipients
- Convenient, easy, reliable administration
- Easily produced, elegant, stable
- Cost and commercial viability

Tablets and capsules are more convenient for adolescents. Crushing or splitting some tablets, or opening capsules destroys their release properties and can cause dose inaccuracies. The resulting powder is often mixed with food or beverages, potentially affecting drug absorption. Many of the dosage forms designed for adults, such as granules, fast-dissolving 'melt' formulations, orodispersible tablets, buccal gels, and transdermal patches, would also benefit children if they contain an appropriate pediatric dose. Chewable tablets should be avoided during the transition from primary to permanent teeth.

Liquid medicaments are usually recommended for infants and younger children. Sugars like sucrose, glucose or fructose are added to increase the palatability of the drug.

These sugars and their endogenous low pH may initiate or potentiate erosive and carious lesions. Hence, long-term and/or frequent consumption (especially at night) requires appropriate oral hygiene and preventive strategies. Xylitol is a preferred sugar in pediatric oral preparations.

Commonly used antibiotics and analgesia in children

Sl. No.	Drugs	Adolescents and adults	Pediatric dose
1.	Amoxicillin	250–500 mg three times/day	Infants > 3 months, children, and adolescents < 40 kg: 20-40 mg/kg/day in divided doses every 8 hours (maximum single dose 500 mg) OR 25-45 mg/kg/day in divided doses every 12 hours (maximum single dose 875 mg)
2.	Amoxicillin + Clavulanic acid (Co-amoxiclav)	250–500 mg amoxicillin + 125–250 mg clavulanic acid three times a day	*Children >3 months of age up to 40 kg*: 25–45 mg/kg/day in doses divided every 12 hours *Children >40 kg and adults*: 500–875 mg every 12 hours
3.	Ciprofloxacin	250–500 mg every 12 hours	25 mg/kg/day divided into two doses (12 hours each). To be avoided in children below 18 years *Children ≥6 months up to 16 years*: 5–12 mg/kg one time/day (maximum 500 mg/day) or 30 mg/kg as a single dose (maximum 1,500 mg)
4.	Azithromycin	500 mg OD	*Children ≥16 years and adults*: 250–600 mg one time/day or 1–2 g as a single dose
5.	Cephalexin	Adults: 250–1,000 mg every 6 hours (maximum 4 g/day)	*Children >1 year:* 25–100 mg/kg/day in divided doses every 6–8 hours (maximum 4 g/day)
6.	Cefixime	200 mg two times a day for 7–10 days	8 mg/kg/day in two divided doses
7.	Erythromycin	250–500 mg (stearate or estolate salts) or 400 mg ethyl succinate salt every 6 hours	30–50 mg/kg/day in divided doses every 6 hours
8.	Doxycycline	200 mg on day 1 (100 mg every 12 hours) then 100 mg daily	*Age 8 years or older:* 4.4 mg/kg in two divided doses on day 1 then 2.2 mg/ kg/day
9.	Tetracycline	250–500 mg every 6 hours	*Age 8 years or older:* 25–50 mg/kg/day divided into 6 hourly doses

Contd..

Contd..

10.	Metronidazole	250–750 mg every 8 hours, not to exceed 4 g in 24 hours	For anaerobic skin and bone infections *Children*: 30/mg/day in divided doses every 6 hours *Adolescents and adults*: 7.5 mg/kg every 6 hours For periodontal disease, including necrotizing ulcerative gingivitis: *Adolescents and adults:* 250 mg every 6–8 hours for 10 days *For aggressive oral infections:* 250 mg three times/day with amoxicillin (250–375 mg three times/day) for 7–10 days
11.	Paracetamol	0.5–1 g every 4–6 hours, maximum dose 4 g/day	*Children <12 years*: 10–15 mg/kg/dose every 4–6 hours as needed (maximum 90 mg/kg/24 hours but not to exceed 2.6 g/24 hours) *Children ≥12 years and adults*: 325–650 mg every 4–6 hours or 1,000 mg 3–4 times/day as needed
12.	Nimesulide	100 mg/dose every 12 hours	5 mg/kg/day divided every 8–12 hours
13.	Diclofenac sodium	75–150 mg/day in 2–4 divided doses, maximum dose–150 mg/ day	2–3 mg/kg/day in 2–4 divided doses
14.	Mefenamic acid	500 mg TID	*Analgesic dose*: 10–25 mg/kg/day (divided into 6 hourly doses) *Antipyretic dose*: 3 mg/kg/dose every 6 hours
15.	Ibuprofen	400–600 mg/dose every 6–8 hours, maximum dose 2,400 mg/day	*Children <12 years*: 4–10 mg/kg/dose every 6–8 hours as needed (maximum 40 mg/kg/24 hours) *Children 12 years*: 200 mg every 4–6 hours as needed (maximum 1.2 g/24 hours)

Pediatric prescription mathematics

Almost every pediatric drug therapy necessitates a complex mathematical computation. The most common calculations involve fractions, percentages, decimals, and ratios. To prescribe drugs to a pediatric patient on an mg/kg regimen, the prescriber must complete several tasks. Accurate weight should be obtained and correctly transcribed. The weight in pounds may need to be converted to kilograms. Then the total daily dose may need to be divided into multiple doses to obtain the appropriate frequency for the medication. Thus, the prescriber has to compute, convert, conceptualize, and critically evaluate to ensure safe prescribing.

Example 1: Calculate the dose of amoxicillin suspension in mL for dentoalveolar abscess for a child weighing 22 lbs.
The dose required is 40 mg/kg/day divided by BID and the suspension comes in a concentration of 400 mg/5 mL.
Step 1: Convert pounds to kg: 22 lbs x 1 kg/2.2 lbs = 10 kg
Step 2: Calculate the dose in mg: 10 kg x 40 mg/kg/day = 400 mg/day
Step 3: Divide the dose by the 400 mg/day ÷ 2 (BID) = 200 mg/dose BID frequency
Step 4: Convert the mg dose to mL: 200 mg/dose ÷ 250 mg/5 mL = 4 mL BID

RECOMMENDATIONS FOR PRESCRIBERS TO ABATE DRUG DOSING ERRORS

- Drug orders must be legible and include all of prescription components.
- Spell clearly the official (generic) or trademarked drug name.
- Do not use abbreviations.
- Dosage strengths or concentrations and quantities to be written in exact metric units (e.g., mg, units).
- A leading zero should always precede decimal expressions less than one (e.g., 0.1 mg), but a trailing zero should never follow after a whole number (i.e., 1.0 mg)
- The calculations used to determine the dose should be included in the medicine order.
- If a patient's dose is modified, new prescriptions should be written and old ones canceled.
- Odd dosages should be rounded-off for more convenient and accurate measurement.
- Instruct to shake a drug product that is labeled "shake well."
- Appropriate measuring devices should be recommended for liquid medicaments. The use of household teaspoons and tablespoons should be discouraged because of the variability and resulting inaccuracies. The oral dosing syringe is the best device for delivering liquid medication of fewer than 5 mL.
- The prescriber should also counsel the patient and the caregiver, familiarizing them with the name, indication, route of administration, dose, dose frequency, potential adverse effects, and management of adverse effects for each medication the patient receives.
- Parents must be reminded to continue drug therapy for the entire period prescribed. Treatment should not be interrupted, even if the child seems to be completely well.

Future of Drug Prescribing

Precision medicine tailors' treatment to a patient's specific needs based on a genetic, biomarker, epigenetic, phenotypic, socioeconomic, and psychological factors that separate one person from others with comparable clinical symptoms. One of the essential aspects of customized or precision medicine is pharmacogenomics (PGx). Pharmacogenomics includes enzyme-guided dose, genotyping-guided dosing, and artificial intelligence. The use of genetic data to guide pharmaceutical decisions has the potential to improve therapeutic outcomes by increasing efficacy and lowering side effects. The one-dose-does not-fit-all approach to pediatric dental medication therapy may soon embrace with Genome-informed prescribing.

Questionnaire

1. What is the ABCDE of pediatric pharmacotherapy-enumerate?
2. Enumerate the various drug dosage formulas and explain in detail dosage calculation using mg/kg regimen.
3. Steps to minimize pediatric dosing errors?

FURTHER READING

1. Psych Central. (2016). RxList: The Internet Drug Index. [online] Available from www.psychcentral.com/weeklywebsite/2016/11/rxlisttheinternetdrugindex/. [Accessed April, 2018].
2. Venkatesh SP. Medicine use in children: a critical area. J Clin Pediatr Dent. 2010 Spring;34(3):207-11
3. Wilson W, Taubert KA, Gewitz M, et al. Prevention of infective endocarditis: guidelines from the American Heart Association: a guideline from the American Heart Association Rheumatic Fever, Endocarditis, and Kawasaki Disease Committee, Council on Cardiovascular Disease in the Young, and the Council on Clinical Cardiology, Council on Cardiovascular Surgery and Anesthesia, and the Quality of Care and Outcomes Research Interdisciplinary Working Group. Circulation. 2007;116:173654.
4. Wynn RL, Meiller TF, Crossley HL. Drug Information: Handbook for Dentistry, 13th edition. Ohio: Lexicomp; 2007.

CHAPTER

Dental Considerations in Children with Special Healthcare Needs

Priya Verma, Divya Prahlad, Nikhil Marwah, Umme Azher, Tabassum Tayab

Chapter Outline

- Definition
- Attitudes towards Children with SHCN
- Barriers to Dental Treatment
- Role of the Dental Team
- Classification of Children with SHCN
- Concerns of the Pediatric Dentist
- Intellectual Disability
- Cerebral Palsy
- Childhood Autism
- Visual Impairment
- Hearing Loss
- Treatment Considerations of Medically Compromised Children

Oral health of a differently-abled child has been one of the gray areas in the field of Pediatric Dentistry. There has been a general agreement that the disabled population has increased prevalence of poor oral hygiene, compromised gingival and periodontal health, and dental caries in comparison to the general population. In the past, the emphasis was on providing basic dental care but in recent years, the dental profession and parental groups have shown increased concern in providing complete oral healthcare to the intellectually or physically disabled children. This is attributed to the awareness that individuals with a disability, whether developmental or acquired, are entitled to the opportunity to achieve appropriate rehabilitation, to enable them to realize their maximal level of functioning and to assist them in not only "normalizing" their lives but also lengthening their lifespan. Unfortunately, the service provided to this unique population by both community-based dental care facilities and individual providers has been grossly inadequate. Historically, five basic reasons have been given to account for the inadequacy of dental care for this group by **Plummer**:

- On the part of the profession, there has been lack of knowledge, understanding, and actual experience in treating the differently abled patient.
- There has been inadequate literature on the oral hygiene status and dental needs of the differently abled population.
- The importance of dental care for the differently abled has been overlooked by health planners and administrators in establishing programs for the non-institutionalized population.
- Parents and guardians of differently-abled children have not been made aware of the importance of oral health and may lack knowledge of the healthcare system and financial resources available to them.
- Home care has been so neglected that most differently-abled patients need extensive dental treatment.

Furthermore, the lack of acceptance, and increased financial burden results from the need for special equipment and medical care thereby leading to less priority towards dental care. Therefore, to plan appropriate treatment for the differently abled individual and to deliver it effectively, it is necessary for the dental care provider to understand the total implications of his own attitudes toward the differently-abled.

Disability statistics show that 2.21% of India's population have at least one type of disability. About 69% of the overall disabled Indian population (1.86 crore) lives in rural areas. The percentage of persons with disability is highest in the 10–19 years age group at 17%. The United Nations Universal Declaration of Human Rights (1948) emphasizes equal rights to good health and well-being to all, including those with SHCN.

Caring for children with SHCN requires several modifications to conventional treatment approaches. Parental attitudes towards dental treatment vastly differ due to the physical and emotional burden of the condition. Children may present with more than one disability requiring excellent coordination among members of the medical and dental team, use of specialized equipment, psychological intervention and at times hospital dental services. To effectively cater to the oral needs of such individuals, the dental team must be trained and prepared to accommodate children with any type of disability.

DEFINITIONS

Disability *is any condition of the body or mind (impairment) that makes it more difficult for the person with the condition to do certain activities (activity limitation) and interact with the world around them (participation restrictions).* According to the World Health Organization, disability has three dimensions:

Impairment in a person's body structure or function, or mental functioning; examples of impairment includes loss of a limb, loss of vision or memory loss.

Activity limitation, such as difficulty in seeing, hearing, walking, or problem solving.

Participation restrictions in normal daily activities, such as working, engaging in social and recreational activities, and obtaining health care and preventive services.

- **Special healthcare** *needs [American Academy of Pediatric Dentistry (AAPD), 2013] defined as "any physical, developmental, mental, sensory, behavioral, cognitive, or emotional impairment or limiting condition that requires medical management, healthcare intervention, and/or use of specialized services or programs". The condition may be congenital, developmental, or acquired through disease, trauma, or environmental cause and may impose limitations in performing daily self-maintenance activities or substantial limitations in a major life activity. Healthcare for individuals with special needs requires specialized knowledge acquired by additional training, as well as increased awareness and attention, adaptation, and accommodative measures beyond what are considered routine.*
- **Differently-abled child** *(American Public Health Association): A child who cannot within limits play, learn, work, or do things other children of his age can do; he is hindered in achieving his full physical, mental, and social potentialities.*
- **Differently-abled child [World Health Organization (WHO)]**: *One who over an appreciable period of time is prevented by physical or mental conditions from full participation in the normal activities of their age group including those of social, recreational, educational, and vocational nature.*
- ***Dental handicap (AAPD, 1996)****: A person should be considered dentally differently abled if pain, infection, or lack of functional dentition which affects the following:*
  - *Restricts consumption of diet adequate to support normal growth and developmental needs.*
  - *Delays or alters growth and development.*
  - *Inhibits performance of any major life activity including work, learning communication, and recreation.*
- **Dental disability:** Dental caries, periodontal disease, dentoalveolar trauma, and other pathological orofacial conditions, left untreated, can limit substantially an individual's development and quality of life. Therefore, an individual should be considered to have a dental disability if orofacial pain, infection, or pathological condition and/or lack of functional dentition affect nutritional intake, growth and development, or participation in life activities.

ATTITUDES REGARDING CHILDREN WITH SPECIAL HEALTHCARE NEEDS

Parental Attitude

- Parenting a child with a SHCN poses stressors beyond those experienced while raising typically developing children, such as elevated medical expenses, time demands, physical care, and worry about the child's future. Provision of service may be directly interfered with by the inability of dentists to understand these attitudes, so it is important for the provider to realize the massive impact that a disability can have on a family.
- Parents seem to go through several emotional and psychologic stages after becoming aware that their child is differently abled. The initial feeling that parents experience is shock and depression and also likely to be negative during the early postpartum period. The reaction to this catastrophic event may be characterized by denial and by refusal to recognize symptoms that are present. Subsequent stages may include self-pity, depression, guilt, rejection, hostility, and overprotection.
- Parents also describe stress associated with social habits that includes staring, discomfort, inappropriate ignoring, or drawing attention of the child. Most parents also reported that they were able to adjust better with the difficulties of the child after knowing their clinical condition or diagnosis. However, it is not only the parents of the family who get affected but a family in totality.
- The intense effort that is required to take care of a differently-abled child is often at the expense of the normal child. The normal child is expected to behave like a mature child who he is unable to rationalize with. He might also have to face increased demands for the supervision of the child with disabilities that lead to frustration and eventual refusal of corporation.
- Basically, if a parent believes in good dental care and prevention of dental disease, he will provide this care to his child irrespective of his disability.
- An important variable in seeking dental care is the degree of disability. In children with higher degrees of disability, there may be many other physical difficulties to cope with and dental care low on the list of priorities. Dentists might not be able to understand the multiple reasons for the observed parental attitudes towards seeking timely dental care and might hesitate or even inadvertently obstruct provision of dental treatment. Therefore it is important for the dental healthcare provider to realize the massive impact that disability can have on a family and appropriately accommodate requests from the parent and offer practical advice.

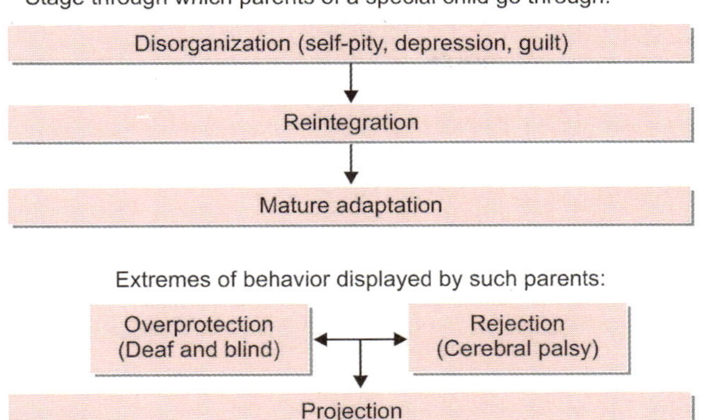
The family environment
Barsch (1968) has aptly phrased that, "no parent is ever prepared in advance to become the parent of a handicapped child"
Stage through which parents of a special child go through:
Disorganization (self-pity, depression, guilt)
Reintegration
Mature adaptation
Extremes of behavior displayed by such parents:
Overprotection (Deaf and blind)
Rejection (Cerebral palsy)
Projection

BARRIERS TO DENTAL TREATMENT

According to **Miller et al.** (1965) dental treatment for disabled children has usually been restricted to relief of painful emergency procedures; However, over a period of time a transient shift was observed in the attitude of the dentist. According to **Fenton et al.** (1993) there was particular number of lecture hours in predoctoral curriculum devoted to teaching dental management of child with disability ranging up to 40, 23 of dental schools reported 5 or few hours. This shows that the need of dental treatment for such children is considered less important thereby providing them limited services. Insufficient undergraduate and postgraduate education resulting in dentists who are not prepared or willing to manage and treat these patients in their private setup.

- **Parental attitude towards dental treatment:** Parental anxiety frequently delays dental care until significant oral disease has developed. Burden of the disability may be too high for parents to recognize oral problems as a significant health issue. 20.8% dental professionals quoted inadequately motivated caretakers to be a significant barrier to dental treatment, according to a study conducted in Kerala.
- **Inadequacy in training:** Insufficient dental education resulting in dentists who are not trained to manage patients with SHCN. 32.6% of dental professionals in Kerala stated lack of training and experience as a barrier to managing disabled children.
- Dental treatment in these children is time consuming, thus the need of multiple trained assistants becomes a necessity to reduce chair side time.
- **Dental access:** Most dental practices are not designed to accommodate needs of children with SHCN. Lack of wheelchair ramp, elevator, reserved car parking space, inadequate wheelchair turning space in the operatory, etc., can be barriers to seeking dental care.
- **Coexisting medical conditions:** Children with SCHN may have to visit multiple therapy units such as speech and occupational therapists, physiotherapists routinely. Lack of flexibility in scheduling appointments by either parents or dental office can hinder seeking timely dental care.
- **Psychosocial:** Children with SHCN are already sensitized to health care professionals as many develop in an environment of chronic care, painful procedures in aspects of health other than dentistry. This may affect their ability to cope with the stress of dental treatment.
- **Financial:** Repeated medical expenses may hinder parents from spending on dental care. Lack of reimbursing and insurance options is an issue for many parents.
- **Language and communication:** Communicating with children with SHCN is challenging and dentists should be prepared to learn new, unconventional ways of communication. Every child with SHCN requires an individualized approach. For example, effective communication with a patient with hearing impairment requires aids such as written materials, photographs, videos and lip-reading guided by an interpreter.

Design considerations in a dental practice for individuals with SHCN

External/internal building features	*Gradient*	*Length*	*Width*	*Surface, other specifies*
Parking space	1:50 maximum slope	Standard	Auto: 90 inches Van: 144 inches	Nonskid, paved, sign-posted, adjacent to walkway
Walkway	1:12 maximum slope	Not applicable	36 inches	Nonskid; no obstructions overhangs; smooth
Passenger loading zone	Flat	20 feet	36 inches	Same as above
Curb ramps	1:12 maximum slope	Standard	36 inches	Nonskid; side flair <1:10 slope
Door	5 foot entrance and exit platform area	Standard	32-inch minimum; preferably 36 inches	Away from prevailing winds, lever with 10-lb pull, auto-assisted door available, kick plate
Interior ramp	1:20 maximum slope	72-inch minimum length if rise >6 inches	36 inches	Nonskid, handrails

Contd...

Contd...

External/internal building features	*Gradient*	*Length*	*Width*	*Surface, other specifies*
Wheelchair lift	Bilevel	8-foot maximum drop	36 × 48 inches	Nonskid; dependent on specific chair
Corridor	Not applicable	Standard	48 inches/64 inches	New facility, no obstacles
Flooring	Flat, firm carpet	Not applicable	0.5 inch maximum thickness	No doormats, level thresholds
Signs	Braille, raised letters	Above 5 feet	Readable	Near latch of office door
Waiting room	Flat	Standard	36-inch aisle; one cleared area: 36 × 52 inches	No carpet pad, well-insulated, minimum low-frequency background noise
Restrooms	Flat	–	32 inch stall min., preferably 36 inches	Nonskid, magnetic catch door
Public telephone	No higher than 4 feet	3 feet above floor	26-inch clearance	Phone directory near phone, adjustable volume control
Elevator	Flat	–	54 × 68 inches	Nonskid, call and control box 48 inches high include Braille or incised letters
Operatory	Flat 8 × 10 feet	Standard	32–36 inch door	Nonskid, rotating or movable chair; drill and suction

ROLE OF THE DENTAL TEAM

A parent or caregiver's initial contact with the dental practice is usually through the front desk. The reception must be attentive, trained and prepared to get appropriate details regarding the type and nature of SHCN along with the child's name, age and chief complaint. The dental team must coordinate the appointment time slot with the pediatric dentist to allow ample time for examination and proposed treatment. Need for increased treatment time and additional auxiliaries must be discussed in advance. Considerations for time of appointment such as morning, post nap slot, or when there are limited patients in the waiting area, readiness with wheelchair assistance, etc., ensure a positive experience. A team member may be allocated the following duties

- Obtaining preliminary information which the dentist later reviews with the patient or family
- Instructing the patient or family on oral hygiene
- Assisting in the use of restraints and other methods of patient behavioral control
- Anticipating problems and preparing for emergencies and other contingencies
- Advising the dentist of any noteworthy or unusual patient, family, or guardian problems.

A good working relationship between the two requires effort, time, practice, and patience with the net result being "fourhanded and single-minded dentistry".

Wheelchair Transfer

Persons with severe physical disabilities who come to the office may employ wheelchairs as their principal means of mobility. Transferring most of these individuals from the wheelchair to the dental chair is not a difficult procedure. It can be characterized as self-transferal in which the patient accomplishes the procedure alone; partially assisted in which the patient requires assistance in movement, generally the lower half; and fully assisted in which the patient takes a relatively passive role and the transferring is done by others.

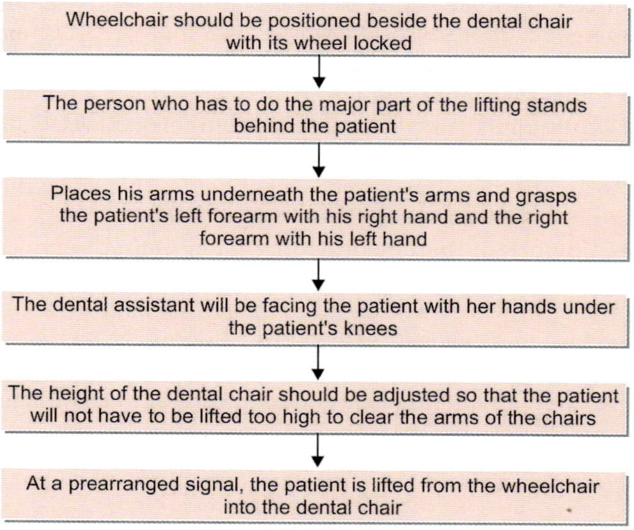

Wheelchair should be positioned beside the dental chair with its wheel locked

↓

The person who has to do the major part of the lifting stands behind the patient

↓

Places his arms underneath the patient's arms and grasps the patient's left forearm with his right hand and the right forearm with his left hand

↓

The dental assistant will be facing the patient with her hands under the patient's knees

↓

The height of the dental chair should be adjusted so that the patient will not have to be lifted too high to clear the arms of the chairs

↓

At a prearranged signal, the patient is lifted from the wheelchair into the dental chair

CLASSIFICATION OF DIFFERENTLY-ABLED CHILD

Frank and Winter (1974)

- Blind or partially sighted
- Deaf or partially deaf
- Educationally subnormal
- Epileptic
- Maladjusted
- Physically differently abled
- Defective of speech
- Senile.

Nowak (1976)

- Physically differently-abled—Polio
- Mentally differently-abled—Retardation
- Congenital—Cleft palate
- Convulsive—Epilepsy
- Communication—Deafness

- Systemic—Hemophilia
- Metabolic—Juvenile diabetes
- Osseous disorders—Rickets
- Malignant disorders—Leukemia.

CONCERNS OF THE PEDIATRIC DENTIST

- **Communication**: A pediatric dentist will need to modify his/her communication and behavior management approach and at times acquire new methods to enhance communication with a child with SHCN. For example, while communicating with a child with intellectual disability, nonverbal communication is more important than verbal; a child with visual impairment cannot appreciate facial expressions and hence a reassuring, gentle touch and calm tone are essential.
- **Coping mechanisms in children with SHCN:** These children may appear to be un-cooperative but the observed negative behavior is due to an underlying inability to cope with a particular stimulus at the dental office. Understanding the child's coping mechanisms and triggers for adverse response helps in dental management. For example some children with autism who are hypersensitive to noise may throw a temper tantrum at the sound of the high speed handpiece. Desensitizing the child by starting with a hand instrument or a slow speed drill and then slowly progressing to a high speed handpiece will equip them to handle the dental appointment better.
- **Child positioning and protective stabilization**: Protective stabilization may be required to diagnose and provide dental treatment in children with cerebral palsy (CP), poor neuromuscular control and combative patients. Aids such as soft foam rolls below knees, padded and wrapped tongue blades, papoose boards, Pedi-Wraps, beanbag inserts and head positioners are useful.
- **Planning the dental visit:** Need for additional auxiliaries, time of the appointment, allocating enough time for treatment are critical to successful completion of dental treatment in a child with SHCN.
- **Modifications in home oral care regimen:** Some children with SHCN may experience oral sensitivities and poor oral muscle coordination which directly affects their ability to brush, and chew and swallow food. These are areas which the dentist must discuss with parents and a referral to an occupational therapist and physiotherapist must be made when appropriate.

INTELLECTUAL DISABILITY (MENTAL RETARDATION)

In the *Diagnostic and Statistical Manual of Mental Disorders, 5th Edition* (DSM-5), the term 'mental retardation' was officially replaced by 'intellectual disability (intellectual developmental disorder)'. The term 'intellectual disability' is the equivalent of 'intellectual developmental disorders', which was adopted in the draft of **International Classification of Diseases 11th** Revision (ICD-11 WHO).

DSM-5 defines intellectual disability (ID) as a disorder with onset during the developmental period and characterized by intellectual and adaptive functioning deficits in conceptual, social, and practical domains. The DSM-5 diagnosis of ID requires the satisfaction of three criteria:

1. **Deficits in intellectual functioning:** "Reasoning, problem solving, planning, abstract thinking, judgment, academic learning, and learning from experience"—confirmed by clinical evaluation and individualized standard IQ testing.
2. Deficits in adaptive functioning that significantly hamper conforming to developmental and sociocultural standards for the individual's independence and ability to meet their social responsibility. Without ongoing support, the adaptive deficits limit functioning in one or more activities of daily life, such as communication, social participation, and independent living, across multiple environments, such as home, school, work, and community.
3. The onset of these deficits during childhood.

Intellectual disability (ID, previously termed "mental retardation") is a term used when an individual's intellectual development is significantly lower than average and his or her ability to adapt to the environment is consequently limited. IQ score is the standardized measure of intelligence and a score below 70 (two standard deviations below the mean of 100 in the population) is indicative of cognitive deficits.

Intellectual disability is characterized by significant limitation both in intellectual functioning and adaptive behavior. It should be clearly understood that while diagnosing infants and preschoolers, the utmost important thing is to distinguish between intellectual disability and developmental delay. In the absence of clear-cut evidence of intellectual disability it is appropriate to give the diagnosis of developmental delay. In clinical practice, a child under the age of 2 years should not be diagnosed as intellectually disabled unless the deficits are severe and is highly correlated with intellectual disability.

- Delayed motor, language, and social milestones may be identifiable within the first 2 years of life among those with more severe intellectual disability, while mild levels may not be identifiable until school age when difficulty with academic learning becomes apparent.
- When intellectual disability is associated with a genetic syndrome, there may be a characteristic physical appearance (as in, e.g., Down syndrome). Some syndromes have a behavioral phenotype, which refers to specific behaviors that are characteristic of particular genetic disorder (e.g., Lesch-Nyhan syndrome).
- In acquired forms, the onset may be abrupt following an illness such as meningitis or encephalitis or head trauma occurring during the developmental period.
- When intellectual disability results from a loss of previously acquired cognitive skills, as in severe traumatic brain injury, the diagnoses of intellectual disability and of a neurocognitive disorder may both be assigned.
- After early childhood, the disorder is generally life-long, although severity levels may change over time.
- Early and ongoing interventions may improve adaptive functioning throughout childhood and adulthood. In some cases, this result in significant improvement of intellectual functioning, such that the diagnosis of intellectual disability is no longer appropriate. Thus, it is common practice when assessing infants and young children to delay diagnosis of intellectual disability until after an appropriate course of intervention is provided.

For many years, the potential abilities of people with intellectual disabilities were poorly understood and were described using the terms idiot (IQ [intelligence quotient] <25), imbecile (IQ 25–50), and moron (IQ 50–70). Even though, a child who scores 2 standard deviations below the mean on the Stanford-Binet intelligence scale or the Wechsler intelligence scale for children may have some degree of mental limitations, a diagnosis of intellectual disability is not made based on IQ alone. Both inadequate adaptive functioning and intellectual deficiency are required to fulfill a diagnosis of intellectual disability.

Severity	*Percent distribution*	*Approximate IQ range*	*DSM-5 criteria classified based on daily skills*
Mild	85%	50–69	Can live independently with minimum levels of support
Moderate	10%	36–49	Independent living can be achieved with moderate levels of support
Severe	3.5%	20–35	Requires daily assistance with self-care activities and safety supervision
Profound	1.5%	<20	Requires 24 hour care

Intelligence Quotient Scales

Subaverage general intellectual functioning *is defined by* ***Capute*** *as a developmental or intelligence quotient (IQ) that is below 70 and represents two or more standard deviation from a mean of 100.* The tests used to determine the IQ are:

- **The *Cattell infant intelligence scale:*** Used in a child whose developmental age or mental age is estimated to be below 2 years.
- **The *Stanford–Binet intelligence scale:*** Used in children whose developmental or mental age is estimated to be at least 2 years.
- **The *Wechsler intelligence scale:*** Generally used in children with chronological ages from 6 years to 17 years.
- **The *Wechsler adult intelligence scale:*** It is used with individuals having 16 years and older.

The standard formula for computing a ratio of IQ is:

$$IQ = (MA/CA) \times 100$$

MA–mental age
CA–chronological age.

Etiology

Etiology of intellectual disability

Prenatal	*Natal*	*Postnatal*
Genetic disorders (e.g., sequence variations or copy number variants involving one or more genes; chromosomal disorders)	Birth injuries	Cerebral infections
Inborn errors of metabolism		Hypoxic ischemic injury
Maternal and fetal infections	Infection	Traumatic brain injury
Kernicterus	Cerebral trauma	Intoxications (e.g., lead, mercury)
Cretinism	Hemorrhage	Cerebrovascular accidents
Prenatal unknown	Hypoxia	Demyelinating disorders
	Anoxia	Seizure disorders (e.g., Infantile spasms)
Environmental influences (e.g., alcohol, other drugs, toxins, teratogens)	Hypoglycemia	Toxic metabolic syndromes

Clinical Features

Level of intellectual disability and clinical features

Level	*IQ (Intelligence quotient)*	*0–6 years*	*6–21 years*	*21 years and over*
Profound (lowest function level)	25	• Gross retardation • Needs nursing care	• Delay in all areas of development • Shows emotions • May respond to training in use of hand, legs, and jaws • Needs close supervision	• May walk • Needs care • Primitive speech • Incapable of self-maintenance
Severe (lowest functioning level)	25–40	• Significant delay in motor development • Little communication skill of speech • May respond to training	• Usually walks • Some understanding activities • Can profit from systematic habit training	• Can confirm to daily • Needs supervision • Protective environment
Moderate (trainable)	40–55	• Delay in motor development • Speech delay • Responds to training	• Can learn communication skills • Does not progress in arithmetic and reading	• Can perform simple tasks • Participates in recreation • Incapable of self-maintenance • Travels alone in known places

Contd...

Contd...

Level	*IQ (Intelligence quotient)*	*0–6 years*	*6–21 years*		*21 years and over*
Mild (educable)	55–70	• Often not noticed as retarded	• Educable class • Can progress in arithmetic and reading till 6th grade level		Can achieve social and vocational skills • May need support under stress
			• Slow walking	• Can be guided toward social conformity	
Borderline	70–80		• Not detected as slow until 1st grade • Physical developmental stages slightly below average	• Slow learners • Can acquire academic skills till 8th grade level • Can confirm socially	• Can achieve social and vocational skills • Less guidance

Classification of Intellectual Disability

Degree of intellectual disabilty	*SB-IV*	*WISC-III*	*Communication*	*Special requirements for dental care*
Mild	67–52	69–55	Should be able to speak well enough for most communication needs	Treat as normal child; mild sedation or nitrous oxide-oxygen analgesia may be beneficial
Moderate	51–36	54–40	Has vocabulary and language skills such that the child can communicate with others at a basic level	Mild to moderate sedation may be beneficial; use restraints and positive reinforcement; general anesthesia may be indicated in cases of severe generalized dental decay
Severe/Profound	35 and below	39 and below	Mute or communicates in grunts; little or no communication skills	Same as for moderately intellectually disabled

Oral Manifestations (Fig 70.1)

- Higher incidence of poor oral hygiene, gingivitis, malocclusion, and untreated caries.
- Increase in severity of intellectual disability is associated an increase in typical oral signs of clenching, bruxism, drooling, pica, trauma, and self-injurious behaviors.
- Due to poor oral hygiene and soft diet, periodontal condition is poor and, caries rate tends to be higher in children with ID than average.
- Early childhood caries induced by prescription medication
- Altered salivary flow induced by medications or the disease itself, increased plaque and calculus formation contribute to gingivitis and dental caries. Habits such as pouching of food or medicine between the cheek and teeth for a long period of time can also lead to dental caries.
- Other features may include congenitally missing permanent teeth, fractured anterior teeth, enamel hypoplasia and medication induced gingival hyperplasia, traumatic occlusion, and bruxism.
- Malocclusions can occur due to abnormal jaw growth, spacing or crowding.
- Self-injurious behavior such as lip biting or biting of buccal mucosa. More severe form of self-injurious behavior is seen in Lesch–Nyhan syndrome. With increasing severity of ID, oral signs such as clenching, drooling, trauma, pica and self-injurious behaviors also increase.

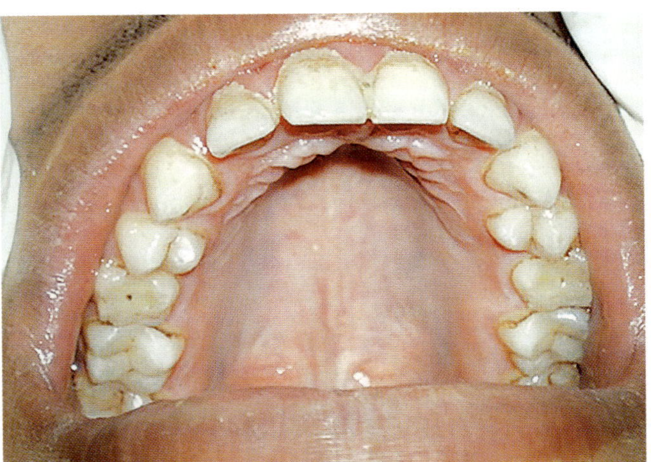

Fig. 70.1: Oral cavity of a mentally retarded child showing poor oral hygiene and gingival inflammation.

Dental Treatment of a Person with Intellectual Disability

Providing dental treatment for a person with intellectual disability requires adjusting to social, intellectual, and emotional delays. A short attention span, restlessness, hyperactivity, and erratic emotional behavior may characterize patients with intellectual disability undergoing dental care. The following procedures have proved beneficial in establishing dentist-patient rapport and reducing the patient's anxiety about dental care:

- **Appointment scheduling**
  - Make the first visit to the dentist as convenient and comfortable as possible to the patient and family.
  - Check for any specific preferences prior to treatment.
  - Advise parents to bring child's medical assessment records, medication list and test reports if any, to the dental office. Consult with the medical team and obtain medical fitness for undergoing dental treatment.

- Schedule the child's visit early on a lightly scheduled day, when the dentist, the staff, and patient will be less fatigued. Every member of the dental team must be aware of the needs of the child in advance.
- Enquire about anxiety levels of child and any specific coping mechanisms used, e.g., favorite toy, security blanket and advice parents to bring them along for the duration of the dental appointment.

❖ **First dental visit**
- Ensure any special requests made over phone are met.
- Provide a brief tour of the office before attempting any dental treatment.
- Introduce the patient and family to the office staff.

❖ **Communication**
- Be clear and repetitive; speak slowly and in simple terms.
- Ensure explanations are understood by asking the patient if there are any questions.
- If the individual has an alternative communication system, such as a picture board or electronic device, be sure it is available to assist with dental explanations and instructions.
- Be particularly sensitive and attentive to gestures and verbal requests throughout the treatment.

❖ **Dental considerations**
- Break down the dental procedure into many simple steps.
- Give only one instruction at a time.
- Use positive reinforcement with compliments after successful completion of every step.
- Keep the appointment short.
- Gradually progress to more difficult procedures such as those requiring local anesthesia after the patient has become accustomed to the dental environment.
- Some children with ID, such as those with CP may have a strong gag reflex—making it difficult to make dental radiographs.
- Use of glass ionomer restorations is preferred due to its fluoride release and caries inhibition properties.
- Use of 38% silver diamine fluoride (SDF) is recommended to arrest dentinal caries when patient cooperation is a challenge and general anesthesia poses significant risks. Stainless steel crowns must be considered in multi surface carious lesions.
- Single visit endodontics is preferred when possible over multi-visit root canal therapy. Extraction of infected deciduous teeth is recommended when pulp therapy is not feasible.
- Removable orthodontic appliances, prosthesis and fixed space maintainers are contraindicated.
- Preventive treatment such as biannual sodium fluoride varnish application and pit and fissure sealants must be stressed on to prevent caries in the permanent dentition.
- Children with moderate to severe ID requiring complex dental treatment would require management under general anesthesia.
- Reward the patient with compliments after the successful completion of each procedure.

CEREBRAL PALSY

Nelson *used the term Cerebral Palsy to describe a group of non-progressive disorders resulting from malfunctioning of the motor centers and pathways of the brain.* CP is a heterogeneous disorder that may result from congenital defects, mechanical or chemical injury, and infection. CP is a congenital neurological disorder due to cerebral damage that occurs around the time of birth (primarily due to hypoxia) manifesting with disordered movement and posture and about 50% of patients have associated problems such as learning disability, epilepsy, defects of vision, hearing or speech, or emotional disturbances. Patients may also experience swallowing problems, drooling, TMJ subluxation, malocclusion, poor manual dexterity and dental disease. There is no effective treatment and is generally a nonfatal, incurable, non-progressive condition that, in part, is amenable to education, therapy, and training.

The *American Academy for Cerebral Palsy and Developmental Medicine describes CP as a group of disorders of the development of movement and posture, causing activity limitations that are attributed to non-progressive disturbances that occurred in the developing fetal or infant brain.* The motor disorders of CP are often accompanied by disturbances of sensation, cognition, and communication perception and/or by a seizure disorder. October 6th is celebrated as the World Cerebral Palsy day.

Etiology

The etiology of CP can be thought of using the four Ps: (1) prenatal, (2) perinatal, (3) postnatal, and (4) prematurity. Common prenatal, perinatal, and postnatal causes of CP include:

❖ **Prenatal:**
- Congenital defects of the brain
- *In utero* stroke
- Congenital cytomegalovirus infection

❖ **Perinatal:**
- Complications of labor and delivery such as pre-term birth, hypoxic ischemic encephalopathy and any factor causing reduced oxygenation to the brain
- Toxemia of pregnancy
- Infections of the brain such as viral encephalitis and meningitis

❖ **Postnatal:**
- Accidental head trauma
- Anoxic insult
- Poisoning with certain drugs and heavy metals
- Child abuse.

Classification of Palsy (Fig. 70.2)

❖ **Spastic:**
- Occurs in more than 60–70% of the cases

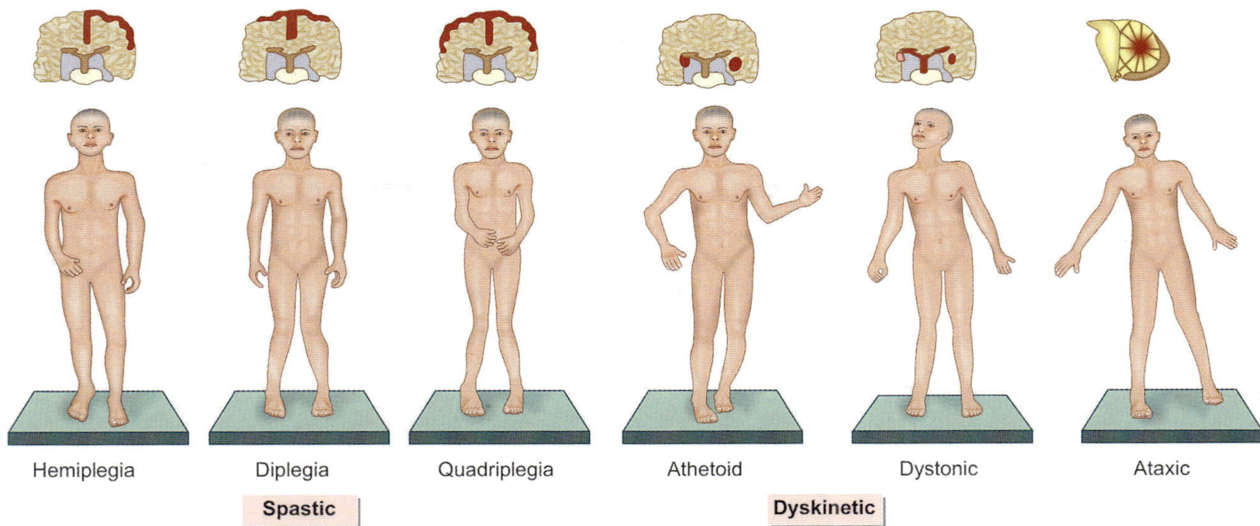

Fig. 70.2: Types of cerebral palsy.

- Caused by a lesion in the cerebral cortex
- Tendency for the antigravity muscles to maintain a state of contraction and for the antagonists to lengthen, producing the characteristic flexion deformities, particularly in the large joints
- Limited control of neck muscles, resulting in "head roll"
- Spastic quadriplegia frequently associated with convulsions and intellectual disability
- Increased motor tone resulting in stiffness
- Impaired chewing and swallowing
- Hypertonicity of facial muscles
- Slow jaw movement
- Hypertonic orbicular muscles
- Spastic tongue thrust
- Drooling of saliva
- Constricted mandibular and maxillary arches
- Class II, division II malocclusion (75%), usually with unilateral posterior crossbite.

❖ **Athetosis:**
- Occurs in about 25% of the cases
- Caused by a lesion in the basal ganglion
- Distinguishing characteristic is a slow, writhing, involuntary movement (athetosis) that occurs with violent jerky movements (choreoathetosis), and interferes with normal muscle action
- Excessive head movement or head drawn back with bull-type neck
- Involuntary movements either tremor or rotary
- Most often not associated with convulsions
- Perioral muscles hypotonic with mouth breathing
- Bruxism
- Grimacing and drooling
- Tongue protruding between teeth and lips
- High, narrow palatal vault
- Class II, division I malocclusion
- Poor swallowing, sucking, etc., because of impaired function of muscles of deglutition

❖ **Ataxia:**
- Occurs in 10% of CP patients
- Caused by a lesion of the cerebellum
- Distinguishing characteristic is a disturbance in equilibrium, lack of positional sensation
- Lack of balance leading to staggering gait, poor sense of balance, and uncoordinated voluntary movements, e.g., difficulty in grasping objects
- No muscular involvement
- Visual organs may be involved
- Poor proprioceptive response
- Slow, tremor-like head movement
- Hypotonic orbicular muscles
- Grimacing and drooling.

❖ **Rigidity:**
- Occurs in 5% of the cases
- Caused by a lesion of the basal ganglion
- Manifested by constant rigidity
- Voluntary movements are slow and stiff
- Patients resistant to flexor and extensor movements.

❖ **Tremors:**
- Present in about 5% of the cases
- Caused by a lesion of the cerebellum
- Distinguishing characteristic is repetitive, rhythmic, and involuntary contraction of flexor and extensor muscles.

❖ **Mixed:**
- Seen in approximately 10% of cases
- Combination of characteristics of more than one type of CP (e.g., mixed spastic-athetoid quadriplegia).

	Spastic	***Athetosis***	***Ataxia***	***Rigidity***	***Tremors***
Prevalence	60–70%	25%	10%	5%	5%
Etiology	Caused by a lesion in the cerebral cortex	Caused by a lesion in the basal ganglion	Caused by a lesion of the cerebellum	Caused by a lesion of the basal ganglion	Caused by a lesion of the cerebellum
Features	Flexion deformities, particularly in the large joints Limited control of neck muscles, resulting in "head roll" Spastic quadriplegia associated with convulsions and ID Increased motor tone resulting in stiffness Hypertonic orbicular muscles	Slow, writhing, involuntary movement (athetosis) that occurs with violent jerky movements (choreoathetosis), and interferes with normal muscle action Excessive head movement or head drawn back with bull-type neck Involuntary movements like tremors Most often not associated with convulsions or ID	Disturbance in equilibrium, lack of positional sensation Lack of balance leading to staggering gait, slow, tremor-like head movement, and uncoordinated voluntary movements, e.g., difficulty in grasping objects No muscular involvement Visual organs may be involved	Manifested by constant rigidity Voluntary movements are slow and stiff Patients resistant to flexor and extensor movements	Distinguishing characteristic is repetitive, rhythmic, and involuntary contraction of flexor and extensor muscles

Clinical Manifestations

In many patients with CP, certain neonatal reflexes may persist long after the age at which they normally disappear. This is because the subcortical dominance of the infant's behavior is suppressed by higher centers of nervous system. Three of the most common reactions, which a dentist should recognize, are: (1) asymmetric tonic neck reflex, (2) tonic labyrinthine reflex, and (3) startle reflex. Some of the common manifestations are:

- Abnormalities of muscle tone
- Delayed milestones
- Intellectual disability
- Seizure disorders
- Speech disorders—usually dysarthria, an inability to articulate well because of lack of control of the speech muscles.
- No control over movements
- Muscle weakness
- Spasticity and loss of coordination
- Retention of primitive reflexes
- Poor development of gross and fine motor control
- Apraxia
- Impaired cortical sensation
- Impaired sensation of movement
- Impaired proprioception
- Contractual deformities.
- **Motor abnormalities:** Abnormalities of muscle tone, gross and fine motor control, spasticity and loss of coordination and contractual deformities such as abnormal limb postures.
- Delayed milestones, with about 60% exhibiting varying degrees of ID.
- **Epilepsy:** Seizure disorders occur in about 30–50% of CP cases.
- **Sensory deficits:** Hearing and visual defects are higher than in the normal population. Speech disorders with the inability to articulate well because of lack of orofacial muscle coordination.
- **Retention of primitive reflexes:** Certain neonatal reflexes may persist long after the age at which they normally disappear.

Oral Manifestations

- Children with CP frequently have gastroesophageal reflux, as well as episodes of vomiting. Either problem can lead to dental erosion, or loss of tooth structure. Gingival overgrowth, due to seizure medications, is a frequent problem in children with CP.
- Orofacial findings in spastic CP: The head is tensely reclined. The mouth is open, and facial movements are tense. The tongue is hypertonic and cigar-shaped. There is tongue thrust during swallowing and speaking. Since the upper lip is underdeveloped, it does not produce enough pressure on the front teeth to align them correctly.
- Orofacial findings in athetotic CP: The tongue shows spontaneous wave-like movements. Abrupt and wide opening of the mouth, which can lead to jaw dislocation. Uncoordinated movements of tongue, jaw, and face muscles.
- Orofacial findings in hypotonic CP: The tongue is large, flat, and protruded. Facial movements are weak, and the upper lip is inactive.
- Increase in frequency of occurrence of periodontal disease and poor oral hygiene
- Patients with CP and who take phenytoin to control seizure activity may have a degree of gingival hyperplasia.

- Conflicting data regarding the incidence of dental caries in patients with CP compared with its incidence in the general population. Except among institutionalized patients, the incidence of caries does not seem to be considerably greater among persons with cerebral palsy.
- The prevalence of malocclusions in patients with CP is approximately twice that in the general population. Commonly observed conditions include proclination of the maxillary anterior teeth, excessive overbite and overjet, open bites, and unilateral cross-bites. A disharmonious relationship between intra-oral and perioral muscles has been attributed to the incidence of malocclusion. Uncoordinated and uncontrolled movements of the jaws, lips, and tongue are observed with greater frequency in patients with CP, thereby leading to impaired chewing and swallowing, excessive drooling, tongue thrust, and speech impairment.
- Bruxism is noticed commonly in patients with athetoid CP. Severe occlusal attrition of the primary and permanent dentition, with the resulting loss of vertical inter-arch dimension has been observed.
- Increased susceptibility to trauma, particularly to the maxillary anterior teeth. This is attributable to the increased tendency to fall, along with a diminished extensor reflex to cushion such falls.

Management

To an uninformed dentist, a person with CP might be perceived as an uncooperative and unmanageable patient. A clinician who is not knowledgeable about physically and mentally disabling conditions may feel uncomfortable about treating such patients and may refuse to do so. The following suggestions are offered to the clinician as being of practical significance in treating a patient with CP:

- *First dental visit*: Evaluate every patient thoroughly in terms of personal characteristics, behavior and medical condition. Record medical, dental and drug history. If associated with an underlying medical condition, e.g., epilepsy always consult with the patient's physician before treatment.
- For a wheelchair bound patient, lock the chair and consider examination and treatment in the wheelchair itself. If a patient is required to be transferred to the dental chair, check preference for the mode of transfer. If the patient has no preference, the two-person lift is recommended.
- *Patient positioning*: These children require assistive stabilization and postural maintenance which can be achieved by ensuring that the head, limbs, torso and mouth are correctly positioned:
  - Head position maintained in the midline by one of the dental staff over a head support (position device) located at the occipital level.
  - Maintenance of bent and juxtaposed upper members in the midline, with the help of Velcro straps.
  - Maintenance of bent lower members by decreasing the hip angle to 120° in relation to the trunk using soft foam rolls as positioning devices for support under the knees.
  - Maintain the child in the midline of the dental chair with arms and legs as close to the body as possible. Keep the patient's back slightly elevated to minimize difficulty in swallowing.
- Maintenance of an open mouth with the use of mouth props.
- With spastic and athetoid patients, sudden movement may precipitate the startle reflex so the child should be informed about procedure to help them to relax. This will not prevent the reflex but relaxing the child will prevent the child from going into another spasm. The treating facility should be prepared with papoose board, beanbag dental chair inserts, Pedi-Wrap and other aids in protective stabilization with parental consent.
- *Dental considerations*: In cases of involuntary jaw movements that manifest as hyperactive bite or gag reflex during instrumentation in the mouth use of mouth props or finger splints is absolutely essential. The patient can be desensitized by introducing intraoral stimuli slowly while placing the patient's chin in a neutral or downward position. Mouth props should not be left for considerable length of time as the child's muscles tire quickly hence frequent periods of rest are important. Mouth mirrors made of steel should be preferably used.
- Consider use of the rubber dam for restorative procedures to reduce the risk of aspiration.
- 38% SDF, atraumatic restorative treatment and full coverage restorations are preferred when traditional restorations are not feasible.
- Two modified radiographic techniques for use in children with CP are: (1) the 45° oblique head plate, and (2) the reverse bite wing (buccal technique).
- Preventive treatment methods such as pit and fissure sealants for permanent molars are strongly advocated.
- Definitive treatment such as extractions are preferred over pulp therapy.
- Removable orthodontic appliances are not well tolerated and breakages pose a risk of aspiration or accidental swallow; hence contraindicated. Fixed orthodontics and space maintainers are contraindicated since they severely compromise oral hygiene.
- Dental treatment under general anesthesia is the only option for more complex dental procedures for children with CP.

Home dental care for children with CP

- Home dental care should begin in infancy; the dentist should educate the parents to gently cleanse the incisors daily with a soft cloth or an infant toothbrush. In case of older children or children who are unwilling or physically unable to cooperate, the dentist should teach the parent or guardian the correct toothbrushing techniques that safely restrain the child when necessary.
- A well-lit location should be chosen to look into the child's mouth.
- Always support the head while toothbrushing, regardless of the position. Some of the positions most commonly used for children requiring oral care assistance are:
  - The standing or sitting child is placed in front of the adult so that the adult can cradle the child's head with one hand while using the other hand to brush the teeth.

- The child reclines on a sofa or bed with the head angled backward on the parent's lap. Again, the child's head is stabilized with one hand, while the teeth are brushed with the other hand.
- The parents sit facing each other with their knees touching. The child's buttocks are placed on one parent's lap, with the child facing that parent, while the child's head and shoulders lie on the other parent's knees; this allows the first parent to brush the teeth.
- The extremely difficult patient is isolated in an open area and reclined in the lap of the parent brushing the teeth. An extra attendant then immobilizes the patient, while the tooth brushing is being instituted. If one person cannot adequately immobilize a child, then both parents and perhaps siblings may be required to complete the home dental care procedures.

- Positive reinforcement while brushing child's teeth.
- Parents should help brush their children's teeth every day, after every meal. Clean the tongue, to help prevent halitosis.
- Parents can help make children's teeth more decay resistant by using an American Dental Association (ADA)-approved children's toothpaste. Place only a pea-sized amount of toothpaste on the toothbrush.
- Children taking oral medications should have their teeth cleansed after each dose of medication.
- Nearly 100% of children's medications contain sucrose, which can increase the risk of developing dental caries
- Children should have their first oral/dental health evaluation by the age of 12 months, or within 6 months of the eruption of the first tooth.

CHILDHOOD AUTISM

The word autism is derived from a Greek word "autos," which means self, and "ismos," which means a state of self-absorbed to the exclusion of everyone around them. In general, autism is the prototypical form of a spectrum of related, complex neurodevelopmental disorders referred to as the autistic spectrum disorders. Autism spectrum disorder (ASD) refers to a neurodevelopmental disorder that is characterized by difficulties in communication, social interaction, restricted and repetitive patterns in behavior, interests, and activities. Symptoms are present early on in development and affect daily functioning. The term 'spectrum' is used because of the heterogeneity in presentation, severity of symptoms, skills and level of functioning of individuals with ASD. It consists of five subtypes, which include: (1) autism disorder (AD), (2) Asperger's syndrome, (3) Rett's disorder, (4) childhood disintegrative disorder (CDD), and (5) pervasive developmental disorder not otherwise specified (PDD-NOS). Individuals with an ASD vary widely in abilities, intelligence, and behaviors. Recognition of the disorder called autism may have its origin in **Itard's** 1801 description of the "wild boy of Aveyron", a violent child with no language skills who related to other people as if they were objects. **Bleuler** used the expression "autism" for the first time in 1911, to assign the loss of the contact with the reality that was caused by difficulty or impossibility of communication. In 1944, American child psychologist **Leo Kanner** first described a clinical syndrome in children to which he gave the name early infantile autism. Though great variations in severity and manifestations of the disturbance were observed, the one symptom common to all children with the disease was inability to relate appropriately to people and situations.

Autistic disorder *is a pervasive developmental disorder defined behaviorally as a syndrome consisting of abnormal development of social skills (withdrawal, lack of interest in peers), limitations in the use of interactive language (speech as well as non-verbal communication), and sensorimotor deficits (inconsistent responses to environmental stimuli). Generic terms autism and autistic refer to the broad spectrum of pervasive developmental disorders that exhibit autistic features as their primary presenting behaviors.*

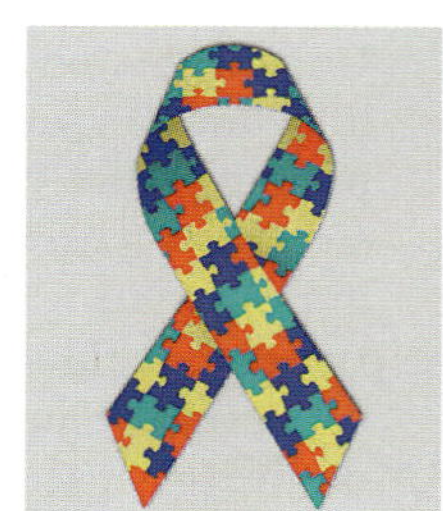

The United Nations General Assembly unanimously declared 2 April as World Autism Awareness Day to highlight the need to help improve the quality of life of those with autism so they can lead full and meaningful lives as an integral part of society. The puzzle ribbon was adopted in 1999 as the universal sign of autism awareness. The puzzle piece signifies the complexity of the autism spectrum. The ribbon represents the diversity of individuals with autism and their families.

Theories of Autism

- **Kanner** postulated that biological deficits are responsible for theories for autism.
- Refrigerator mother theory says that emotionless parenting style was the most common etiology of autism that has been completely discarded.
- Mind hypothesis of autism states that the autistic child fails to impute mental states to themselves and others and fails to gauge the mental state of others. This theory was supported by unexpected transfer test of false belief by **Wimmer** and **Perner** in 1983 where 80% of the autistic children failed the transfer task.
- *Executive dysfunction in autism:* Executive function is defined as the ability to maintain an appropriate problem-solving set for attainment of a future goal. It includes behaviors such as planning, impulse control, inhibition of prepotent but irrelevant responses, set maintenance, organized search, and flexibility of thought and action. In contrast to the theory of mind hypothesis of autism, the theory was not well understood.
- Weak central coherence theory suggests that autism is characterized by weak or absent drive for global coherence. That is, individuals with autism process things in a detail-focused or piecemeal way—processing the constituent parts, rather than—in totality.
- Cognitive complexity and control (CCC) theory is a hybrid theory that states that executive function theory and theory of mind in typical and atypical individuals are related to each other because both theory of mind and measures of executive ability involve the use of high order rule.

Etiology

Lotter postulates that the personalities, attitudes, and behavior of the child's parents contribute to the psychodynamics of autism but it is a widely held view that autism may be early manifestation of childhood schizophrenia. However, no single cause has been identified for the development of autism. The etiology is considered to implicate a combination of genetic and environmental factors.

- *Genetic:* There is a familial tendency for autism. There is a 3–8% recurrence risk if a family already has one autistic child. Recent research work has elucidated that parameters such as CNTNAP2 gene, de novo mutations, mitochondrial defects, cytokine dysregulation, high maternally derived intrauterine androgen concentrations may play a role in the pathophysiology of autism.
- *Syndromes:* Fragile-X, Rett syndrome
- *Medical conditions:* Tuberous sclerosis complex
- *Prenatal factors:* Intrauterine rubella, and cytomegalic inclusion disease
- *Postnatal factors:* Untreated phenylketonuria, infantile spasms, herpes simplex, and encephalitis.
- *Environmental:* Parental age, maternal nutritional and metabolic status, infection during pregnancy, prenatal stress, and exposure to certain toxins, heavy metals, or drugs. The etiology of non-syndromic ASD may be due to a combination of de novo mutations, prenatal and postnatal environmental factors.

The cause of autism is not known, though evidence from family and twin studies suggests that it is an inherited disorder involving up to 20 interacting genes. Genes located on chromosomes 2, 7, 15, 16, and 19 have been suggested. The preponderance of males with the disorder suggests an X-linked disorder. A recent study, however, has noted that the father's age at the time of an offspring's birth influences the child's risk of developing autism. Children whose fathers were 40 years or older at the time of their births are 5.75 times more likely to have autism than are children whose fathers were younger than 30 years at the time of their births.

Language

- Only two-thirds of autistic children achieve some functional speech while the rest remain without functional language throughout their lives.
- Even if speech is acquired, autistic children do not seem to enjoy this activity and speak infrequently.

Diagnosis

Diagnosis of ASD involves developmental screening, followed by a comprehensive diagnostic evaluation. General developmental screening is performed for children to evaluate; basic learning skills, such as behavior, speech, and movement are at appropriate time. Age intervals for this screening are 9, 18, 24, and 30 months. The screening is specifically designed for autistic child who are at the age of 18 and 24 months. This includes: Modified checklist for autism in toddlers (M-CHAT) and screening tool for autism in toddlers and young children (STAT).

Signs and Symptoms

The symptomatology of ASD initiates before the third year of age and generally undergoes a steady course without remission through ageing.

Feature of autistic child	
Early symptoms	***Young children***
• A baby who does not babble or gesture by the age of 12 months • A baby who lacks eye contact with its mother by the age of 12 months • A baby who resists being held or cuddled by its mother • A baby who does not respond when its mother says its name • A baby who appears to be deaf • An infant who does not say single words by 16 months of age • A toddler who does not say two-word phrases by 24 months of age.	• Do not engage themselves in group activity and seems to be in their own world • unable to share in another child's interest in an activity • unable to recognize intentions, desires, feelings, and beliefs of other people that can be different from their own • inability to interpret the behavior of others • Failure to use facial expression and body language to interact with others those results in social conflict.
First year of life	***Teenagers and young adults***
• Reduced social interaction, absence of social smile, and lack of facial expression • Abnormal muscle tone, posture, and movement patterns • Failure to orient to name, lack of pointing, and decreased orienting to faces • Lack of spontaneous imitation.	• Are usually remaining oblivious to the presence of parents • Are unable to empathize with and see the world from other people's perspectives • They also lack an interest in sharing their achievements with others; instead, they prefer to engage in solitary activities rather than form friendships.

General Clinical Features

- **Social:** Appear self-sufficient, introvert with poor eye contact, not responding to one's name. Unlike typically developing children, who when unhappy reach for a parent, children with autism remain detached.
- **Communication:** Children with milder forms of autism achieve some functional speech but those with severe autism are non-verbal.
- **Repetitive behaviors:** Include staring, floppy hands, preoccupation with moving or shiny inanimate objects, such as a string of keys or a spinning top for hours.

Dental Findings of an Autistic Child (Fig. 70.3)

Although there appears to be no known autism-specific oral manifestations, oral problems might arise because of autism-related behaviors.

- **Higher susceptibility to caries:** Due to soft and sweetened food, pouching due to poor tongue coordination and difficulties in brushing and teeth flossing.
- **Bruxism:** Forceful grinding of the teeth is one of the sleep disorders in autistic children.
- **Damaging oral habits:** Such as tongue thrusting, picking at the gingiva, lip biting, and pica.
- **Traumatic injuries:** Traumatic ulcerated lesions usually brought on by self-injury from head banging, picking, or face tapping.
- **Gingivitis and poor oral hygiene:** Occur due to heavy plaque accumulation and hormonal influences are the likely explanations for the dental concerns.

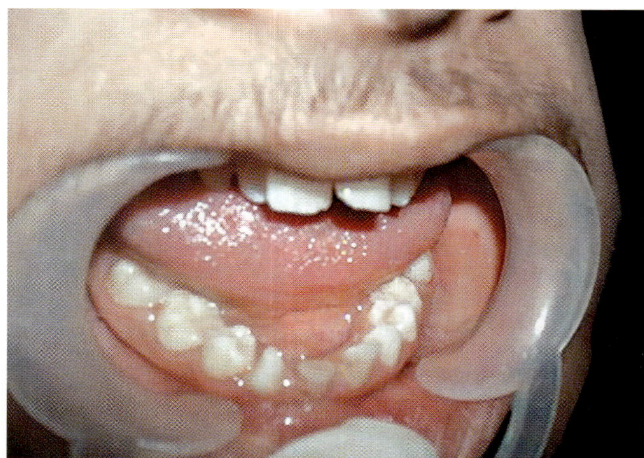

Fig. 70.3: Dental manifestation in autistic child—fracture of teeth and bruxism.

- **Texture sensitivities:** Food texture sensitivities leads to the consumption of refined and high-sugar diet.
- Children with ASD are known to possess unusual sensory processing. Sensory processing disorder (SPD)/Sensory integration dysfunction is a neurological disorder in which the individual finds it difficult to assimilate, process and respond to sensory information from the environment and also from within their own body. The senses are visual, auditory, tactile, olfaction, gustatory, vestibular and proprioception (kinesthetic, the sense of one's own limbs in space). Oral sensitivity issues in children with ASD can be of two different types: Oral hypersensitivity and oral hyposensitivity.
- Children with oral hypersensitivities/oral defensiveness have the following characteristic features:
  - Do not like their teeth to be brushed and/or face washed.
  - May avoid food of mixed textures.
  - Take the food from the fork or spoon by keeping their lips retracted and using only their teeth.
  - Have gag reflex, so each spoon of food will be swallowed taking a drink with it.
- Exhibit signs of tactile defensiveness—dislike being touched, avoid messy play with glue, mud, sand, finger paints, etc., and do not pick up things with a grasp involving the palm of their hand.
- The children with oral hyposensitivity exhibit:
  - Crave for intense flavors, i.e., sweet, sour, salty, spicy
  - Avoid mixed textures as they find it difficult to chew and swallow properly. This is because they cannot "feel" the food in their mouth correctly
  - Messy eaters—smear food all over their face and/or leaving bits of food in their mouths at the end of meals
  - Food pouching—take large bites and stuff their mouths or "pocket" food in their cheeks
  - At risk of choking as they do not chew the food thoroughly before swallowing
  - Excessive drooling is seen
  - Tend to put inedible things in their mouth

Treatment

- **Challenges in the dental office**
  - The abundant sensory stimuli encountered in the dental office, such as bright lights, vibration from dental instruments, touch in and around the mouth, taste and smell of dental materials can cause a sensory overload and may negatively impact children with autism, eliciting negative behavior to dental treatment. Thus, preparing children for the dental visit is important.
  - To accomplish this, social stories with pictures of the dental set up, dental team, dental exam tools should be used.
  - During appointment scheduling, ask parents for child's preferences with respect to particular sensitivities and history of previous dental visits.
  - Many children with ASD strictly adhere to routines, and thus may require several dental visits to acclimate them to the dental environment.
- **First dental visit**
  - At the office, offer parents and children a tour of the clinic.
  - Introduce them to the dental assistant that will be present during treatment.
  - Be gentle and reassuring, observing cues for the child's social behavior. Many children with autism are visual learners. A visual schedule may help to reduce apprehension by understanding the sequence of planned dental procedures.
  - Allow the child to bring comfort items, e.g., a toy or be accompanied by their primary caregiver.
  - Make the first appointment short and positive.
- **Communication**
  - Approach the child in a quiet, non-threatening manner. Speak in simple, direct and short sentences.
  - Since many children with autism are less verbal and more visual, alternate methods of communication such as picture exchange communication system (PECS) may be helpful. PECS consists of a book of word pictures to express desires, observations, and feelings and is very helpful for those who are less verbal.
  - Distraction techniques like watching a favorite cartoon, listening to music may work in some children.
  - Non-verbal communication that usually works with typical children might trigger unwanted responses from a child with autism.
  - Many children resist being touched or patted. Deep pressure might have a calming effect on some children. Inputs from parents may help avert adverse behavioral consequences.
- **Dental considerations**
  - Use the same office space, with the same dentist and dental team members. Be open to suggestions from the parent or caregiver on how best to deal with the child as minor changes in the environment or treatment plan may elicit extreme anxiety in children with autism.
  - Keep the light out of their eyes. Ear muffs to drown out noise from dental drills may be beneficial in children who are hyper responsive to auditory stimulus.

- Begin cursory examination by using only fingers and then slowly introduce dental tools.
- Show the child simple picture cards of dental procedures in the sequence in which it will be offered ahead of treatment. Use tell-show-feel-do before every step.
- A blanket or Pedi-Wrap may comfort some children during the procedure. Mild cases of children with autism can be managed well on the dental chair with adequate preparation and planning.
- Removable orthodontic appliances and prosthesis will not be tolerated well.
- Cements with strong flavors such as those with eugenol should be substituted with resin based cements or glass ionomer cement to avoid adverse behavior response.
- ART restorations, use of hand instruments, slow speed drill instead of high speed are some modifications to the conventional approach. 38% SDF can be used to arrest dentinal caries in less verbal children where traditional adhesive restorations are not feasible.
- Invite the child to sit alone in the dental chair to become familiar with the treatment setting
- Behavior modification techniques by **Lovaas** have proved to be effective in producing behavioral changes in autistic children.
- Visual Pedagogy was first used in 1999 by **Backman B and Pilebro C** in dentistry for increasing the cooperative levels of the children with ASD for dental treatment. At the time of pre-visit consultation of parents, the dentist can organize a home-centered preparation that includes custom-made photo books to familiarize the child with dental office and the dental instruments, teaching phrases required for the dental examination such as 'open your mouth' so that the child gets acquainted with the dental operatory room. Through visualization, the actual office set-up, the staff, the instruments and the procedure could be studied at home by the child before visiting the clinic which helps them to understand the scenario easily, thereby their cooperation level also increases.
- TEACCH (Treatment and Education of Autistic and related Communication-handicapped Children) is a pedagogic concept developed by **Schopler** in 1972, and comprises of structured teaching in which visual pedagogy is one part of the concept, and it is an effective technique to teach children with autism both at home and in school. Application of the TEACCH concept to desensitize the children to dental procedures and oral hygiene procedures has proven to be effective in training the children.
- The key to all behavior modification programs lies in the use of positive reinforcement to promote desirable behavior
- Applied behavior analysis (ABA) is based on the analysis and modification of human behavior and environment in order to modify behaviors so that the desired effects are achieved. American Academy of Pediatrics has accepted the ABA procedures in the management of children with ASD. Reinforcement forms the basis of behavioral concepts and it occurs when there is an increase in certain behaviour, due to a stimulus or event following that behavior and it can be either a 'positive' or 'negative' reinforcement.
- An appropriate reward is often difficult to find for autistic children. In the early stages of the program, sweet foods can serve as desirable rewards. In the latter stages of modifying behavior, such oral rewards should be changed to social rewards, such as a pat on the back or a hug.
- Complex dental treatment in nonverbal children should be performed under general anesthesia.

❖ **Toothbrushing**

- It is a challenge due to oral sensitivities in ASD. Sensitivity is usually the greatest in the morning on waking up and therefore brushing later in the day might be more comfortable. Brushing after a meal might help in reducing sensitivity as the mouth is already stimulated by food.
- Dipping the toothbrush in lukewarm water causes only a mild change in oral temperature and hence may be better accepted.
- Children with oral sensitivities may be unable to accept foam and certain flavors in toothpastes and may benefit from non-foaming and non-flavored toothpastes (e.g., OraNurse, Tom Maine).
- Some children prefer the vibrations from an electric toothbrush to a manual one, while others who are hypersensitive might dread the vibrations and accept the manual brush better.

VISUAL IMPAIRMENT

Visual impairment is the consequence of the functional loss of vision rather than an eye disorder itself; however, sensory disabilities alone do not require changes in treatment methods, just modifications in provisions. Blindness is not an all-or-none phenomenon; a person is considered to be affected by blindness if the visual acuity does not exceed 20/200 in the better eye, with correcting lenses or if the acuity is greater than 20/200 but accompanied by a visual field of no greater than 20°. Not all visual impairments carry the same degree of blindness. Some individuals who may be considered blind may not be totally without sight. They may be able to distinguish images, light, colors, and may even be able to read large print. Low vision is different than legal blindness and covers a wide range of conditions. Low vision can interfere with a person's ability to perform everyday activities like reading, walking unassisted and even tooth brushing.

Etiology of visual impairment	
Prenatal causes	***Postnatal causes***
Optic atrophy, microphthalmus, cataracts, dermoid and other tumors, toxoplasmosis, syphilis, rubella, and developmental abnormalities of the orbit.	Trauma, hypertension, premature birth, polycythemia vera, hemorrhagic disorders, leukemia, diabetes mellitus, and glaucoma.

Dental Management

- **First dental visit:** Visual impairment may be a part of other co-existing medical conditions and therefore a thorough medical history must be elicited. For example, a child with congenital rubella may have deafness, intellectual disability, dental defects and accompanying blindness. For practical purposes, the dentist must determine the extent and degree of visual impairment; e.g., can the patient tell light from dark, recognize shapes/faces at close distance. Some children may be photophobic. Ask parents about light sensitivity and keep sunglasses in the clinic for safety and comfort. Establish patient's need for assistance. If assistance is required hold the child's hand and guide them through the clinic to the operatory while describing exits from the entrances cheerfully. Keep distractions to a minimum and avoid unexpected loud noises. Establish rapport with the child and parents. Always give the child adequate descriptions before performing treatment procedures.
- **Communication:** Ask the patient how he or she prefers to communicate. Face the patient and speak slowly using simple sentences. Remember your patient cannot see your smile and hence the need to offer continuous physical and verbal reassurance. Appropriate holding of the child's hand often promotes relaxation. At times the child may want to feel your face and if the patient desires, allow them as it allays their fears. To communicate written matter use Braille dental pamphlets explaining specific dental procedures to supplement information and decrease chair time **(Fig. 70.4).** Use large print material with 16–18 point type size or larger with double-line spacing. In a school setting, presence of the child's teacher plays a vital role in the child's ability to cooperate towards dental treatment.
- **Dental considerations:** Children with visual impairments experience more falls while learning to walk in the early years and therefore fractured anterior teeth is a frequent finding. Plaque accumulation and gingivitis are common features due to inability to see and remove plaque while brushing. The dentist must make a distinction between children who at one time had sight and those who have not and thus cannot form visual concepts. More explanation is required for children who have never had vision to help them perceive the dental environment. Explanation is accomplished through touching and hearing, reinforcement takes place through smelling and tasting, all of which help the child develop coping mechanisms towards dental treatment. As visually impaired children rely a lot on their other senses to interact and communicate with their environment the tell-show-do approach needs to be modified to tell-touch-hear and tell-smell-taste techniques. Avoid references to sight. Demonstrate a rubber cup on the patient's fingernail. Strong tastes may be rejected; therefore, use smaller quantities of dental materials with such characteristics. Use the same office setting and the same dentist for each dental visit to allay patient fears. Indicate when you move from one place to another or leave the room and avoid sudden movements. Always maintain a relaxed atmosphere. To give children a sense of control in the dental operatory, ask the child to hold a handkerchief in the left hand and raise it if they wish to signal the dentist to stop. All elective procedures can be carried out, except orthodontic treatment. Demonstrate the process of tooth brushing by placing the patient's hand over yours as you slowly but deliberately guide the toothbrush.

HEARING LOSS

Hearing impairment or hard of hearing or deafness refers to conditions in which individuals are fully or partially unable to detect or perceive at least some frequencies of sound which are generally heard by normal people. This disability is often overlooked because it is not obvious. Many times, mild hearing losses are not diagnosed, leading to management problems because of understanding of instructions, whereas children with more severe hearing losses already possess psychological and social disturbances that make dental behavior management more complex. Early identification and correction of hearing loss is essential for normal development of communication skills. No abnormal dental findings are associated with hearing. In India, hearing loss (HL) among

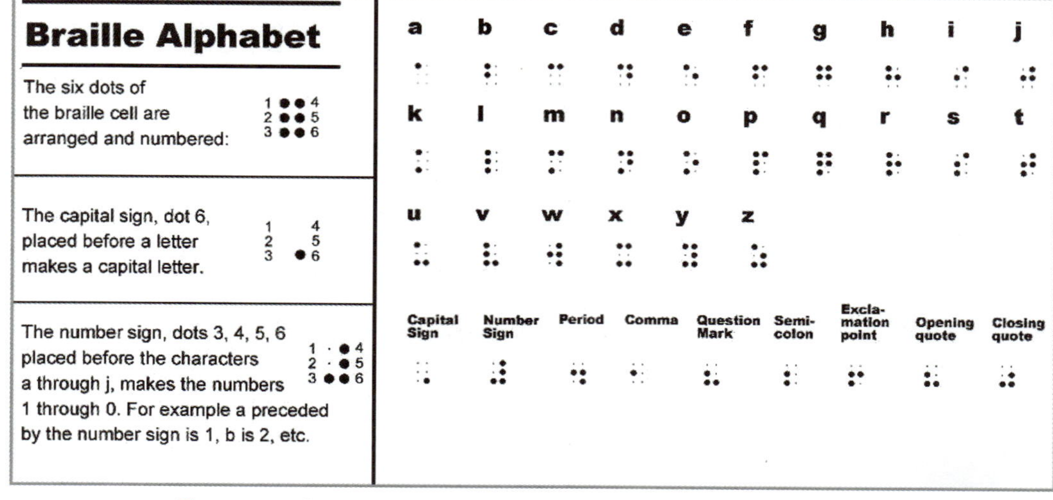

Fig. 70.4: Braille signboard. (*Pic courtesy:* National Braille Press copyright 2000).

children ranges between 6.6 and 16.47%. Almost inevitably children with HL also suffer speech difficulties. If the dentist and child cannot communicate verbally, then sight, taste, and touch should be used to communicate and to allow the child to learn about dental experiences.

Classification

- **Bowley** and **Gardner** have described four levels of deafness:
  1. *Mild hearing loss:* Hard of hearing
  2. *Partial hearing loss:* Hearing aid
  3. *Severe hearing loss:* Difficulty in learning language
  4. *Profound hearing loss:* Lip reading and manual method.
- **Conductive and sensorineural hearing impairments:**
  - A conductive hearing impairment is an impairment resulting from dysfunction in any of the mechanisms that normally conduct sound waves through the outer ear, the eardrum, or the bones of the middle ear.
  - A sensorineural hearing impairment is one resulting from dysfunction in the inner ear, especially the cochlea where sound vibrations are converted into neural signals, or in any part of the brain that subsequently processes these signals.
- **Age of onset:**
  - Prelingual deafness is hearing impairment that is sustained prior to the acquisition of language, which can occur as a result of a congenital condition or through hearing loss in early infancy. Prelingual deafness impairs an individual's ability to acquire a spoken language
  - Postlingual deafness is hearing impairment that is sustained after the acquisition of language, which can occur as a result of disease, trauma, or as a side effect of a medicine. Typically, hearing loss is gradual and often detected by family and friends of affected individuals long before the patients themselves will acknowledge the disability.

Etiology of hearing loss

Prenatal factors	*Perinatal factors*	*Postnatal factors*
• Viral infections such as rubella and influenza • Ototoxic drugs • Congenital syphilis • Heredity (e.g., Treacher Collins syndrome)	• Toxemia late in pregnancy • Birth injury • Anoxia • Erythroblastosis fetalis	• Viral infections such as mumps, influenza, and poliomyelitis • Ototoxic drugs
Genetic	***Diseases***	***Medications***
• Stickler syndrome • Waardenburg syndrome • Pierre Robin syndrome • Hemifacial microsomia • Congenital deformities	• Measles • Mumps • Meningitis • Autoimmune diseases • Enlarged adenoids • AIDS and HIV • Fetal alcohol syndrome	• Aminoglycosides, diuretics NSAIDs, and macrolide antibiotics • Extremely heavy hydrocodone (Vicodin or Lorcet) • Narcotic pain killers, in particular Vicodin and OxyContin

(AIDS: acquired immunodeficiency syndrome; HIV: human immunodeficiency virus; NSAIDs: nonsteroidal anti-inflammatory drugs)

- **Unilateral and bilateral impairment:**
  - People with unilateral hearing impairment [single-sided deafness (SSD)] have an impairment in only one ear. This can impair a person's ability to localize sounds (e.g., determining where traffic is coming from) and distinguish sounds from background noise in noisy environments.
  - A similar effect can result from King–Kopetzky syndrome (also known as *auditory disability with normal hearing* and *obscure auditory dysfunction*), which is characterized by an inability to process out background noise in noisy environments despite normal performance on traditional hearing tests. They are also known-as cocktail party effect.

Do's and Don'ts Conversing with Deaf Patients

- Do not have anything between your lips (cigarette, pen) or in your mouth (chewing gum, sweets).
- The face mask is a barrier for lip reading. Pronounce clearly, without exaggerating or shouting. Lip movements must be clear.
- Always speak using your voice.
- Speak naturally, neither very fast nor very slowly.
  - In order to facilitate the integration of the hearing impaired, it is important to explain what is going on and what is being said around him or her.
  - The dentist should teach hearing-impaired children new words relating to dental health.
  - Repeat your message if it has not been understood, use natural gestures, or some written words. Always have pencil and paper to hand. An alternative is to have some written sheets prepared in advance explaining the main dental procedures.
  - It is recommended that the doctor should know how to use his or her face and body to express feelings of happiness, sadness, anger, fear, interest, etc., to facilitate understanding for the deaf child.

Dental Management

- **First dental visit:** Prepare the patient and parent before the first visit with a welcome letter that states what is to be done and include a medical history form. Let the patient and parent determine how the child would like to communicate (i.e., interpreter, lip reading, sign language, writing notes, or a combination of these). Assess speech, language ability, and degree of hearing loss when taking the patient's complete medical history. Identify the age of onset, type and cause of hearing loss, whether any other family members are affected.
- **Communication:** Look for ways to improve communication. It is useful to learn some basic sign language **(Fig. 70.5)** Face the patient and speak slowly at a natural pace and directly to the patient without shouting. Enhance visibility for better communication. Remove face mask to facilitate lip reading. Write out and display information when appropriate for better clarity. It is good practice to have written sheets with pictures prepared in advance explaining the main dental procedures. Reassure the patient with appropriate gestures, physical contact and smiles to build confidence and reduce anxiety. You

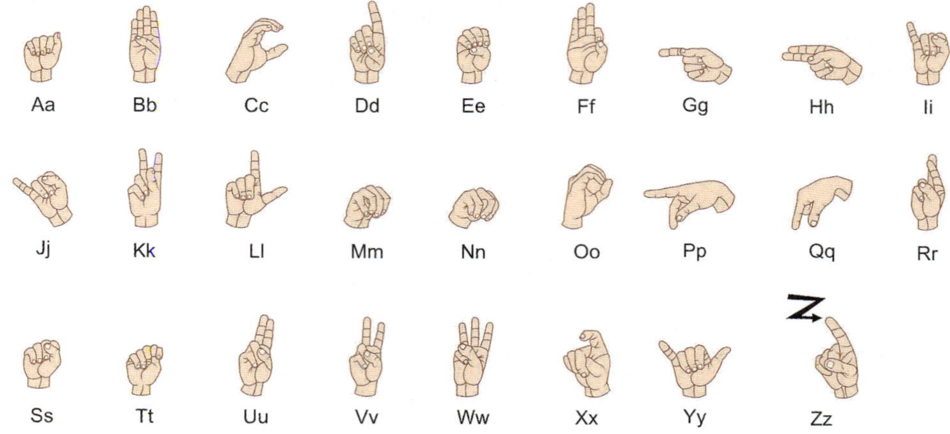

Fig. 70.5: Sign language.

may hold the patient's hand initially or place a hand reassuringly on the patient's shoulder while the patient maintains visual contact. Use of an interpreter in some cases may be extremely helpful.

- **Dental considerations:** Use tell-show-feel-do approach. Use visual aids and allow the patient to see and feel dental instruments and demonstrate how they work. Children with hearing loss may be excessively sensitive to vibration. Have the patient use hand gestures if they need to communicate in the middle of a procedure. Watch the patient's expression while performing dental treatment for any discomfort. Adjust the hearing aid (if the child has one) before the handpiece is in operation because a hearing aid amplifies all sounds. Many times the patient will prefer to have it turned off. There is no absolute contraindication to elective dental procedures in children with hearing loss.

Implications of auditory loss relative to International Standards Organizations Reference Levels

ISO (db)	*Disability*	*Speech comprehension*	*Psychologic problems in children*
0	Insignificant	Little or no difficulty	None
>25	Slight	Difficulty with faint speech; language and speech development within normal limits	May show a slight verbal deficit
>40	Mild-moderate	Frequent difficulty with normal speech at 3 feet; language skills are mildly affected	Psychologic problems can be recognized
>55	Marked	Frequent difficulty with loud speech at 3 feet; difficulty in understanding with hearing aid in school situation	Child is likely to be educationally retarded, with more pronounced emotional and social problems than in children with normal hearing
>70	Severe	Might understand only shouts or amplified speech at 1 foot from ear	The prelingually deaf show pronounced educational retardation and evident emotional and social problems
>90	Extreme	Usually no understanding of speech even when amplified; child does not rely on hearing for communication	The prelingually deaf usually show severe educational retardation and also emotional underdevelopment

TREATMENT CONSIDERATIONS OF MEDICALLY COMPROMISED CHILDREN

Cardiovascular System

- Diseases of heart can be divided into two general types—(1) congenital, and (2) acquired.
- The cause of congenital heart defect is obscure but may be related to aberrant embryonic development of a normal structure. These types of defects include aortic stenosis, tetralogy of Fallot.
- Acquired heart disease includes rheumatic fever and infective bacterial endocarditis. Rheumatic fever is a serious inflammatory disease that occurs as a sequel to pharyngeal fever and is commonly seen in patients less than 40 years of age.
- Infective endocarditis (IE) is an example of an uncommon but life-threatening complication resulting from bacteremia. It is characterized by microbial infection of heart valves. Both require special precautions during treatment so, a dentist should closely evaluate the medical history to ascertain the cardiovascular status.
- Viridans group streptococci, *Staphylococcus aureus*, and *Enterococcus* species are the main microorganisms implicated in IE. *Enterococcal* and other organisms such as *Haemophilus* species, *Aggregatibacter* species, *Cardiobacterium hominis, Eikenella corrodens*, and *Kingella* species are less common.
- In 2007, the American Heart Association (AHA) revised its guidelines for the prevention of IE and reducing the risk for producing resistant strains of bacteria. The significant reasons for the revision include that IE is much more likely to result from frequent exposure to random bacteremias associated with daily activities than from bacteremia caused by a dental procedure.
- Daily activities would include toothbrushing, flossing, chewing, using toothpicks, using water irrigation devices, and other activities. Prophylaxis may prevent an exceedingly small number of cases of IE if any, in individuals who undergo a dental procedure.
- The risk of antibiotic-associated adverse events exceeds the benefit, if any, from prophylactic antibiotic therapy.
- Children with cyanosis with specific periodontal concerns may have an increased risk of IE, which makes optimum oral hygiene very important.

- The AHA guidelines focus on antibiotic prophylaxis prior to certain dental procedures for patients in the highest risk group. The high risk cardiac conditions for which antibiotic prophylaxis is suggested is represented in **Box 70.1.**

Box 70.1: High risk cardiac conditions for which antibiotic prophylaxis is suggested

Prosthetic cardiac valve or material
- Presence of cardiac prosthetic valve
- Transcatheter implantation of prosthetic valves
- Cardiac valve repair with devices, including annuloplasty, rings, or clips
- Left ventricular assist devices or implantable heart.

Previous, relapse, or recurrent IE

Congenital heart disease (CHD)
- Unrepaired cyanotic congenital CHD, including palliative shunts and conduits.
- Completely repaired congenital heart defect with prosthetic material or device, whether placed by surgery or by transcatheter during the first 6 months after the procedure.
- Repaired CHD with residual defects at the site of or adjacent to the site of a prosthetic patch or prosthetic device.
- Surgical or transcatheter pulmonary artery valve or conduit placement such as Melody valve and Contegra conduit.

Cardiac transplant recipients who develop cardiac valvulopathy

Antibiotic prophylaxis for a dental procedure not suggested in case of:
- Implantable electronic devices such as a pacemaker or similar devices
- Septal defect closure devices when complete closure is achieved
- Peripheral vascular grafts and patches, including those used for hemodialysis
- Coronary artery stents or other vascular stents
- CNS ventriculoatrial shunts
- Vena cava filters
- Pledgets

Antibiotic Prophylaxis

- Previously, the 1997 guidelines recommended prophylactic antibiotics for patients in high-risk and moderate-risk categories
- The 2007 guidelines now recommend that only patients in this high-risk category require coverage
- Amoxicillin remains the first choice as the prophylactic antibiotic. In 1997, amoxicillin was to be administered 1 h before the procedure. The 2007 guidelines recommend administration of amoxicillin (and any other recommended antimicrobial) 30–60 min before the procedure.
- Clindamycin may cause more frequent and severe reactions than other antibiotics used for AP, and its use is no longer suggested.
- A study by Thornhill et al observed that a single dose of clindamycin may cause complications, including death, from *Clostridioides difficile* infection.
- Doxycycline is an alternative in patients who are unable to tolerate a penicillin, cephalosporin, or macrolide. A serious reaction from a single dose of doxycycline is extremely rare.
- According to the revised guidelines by AAPD (2019), minimal use of antibiotics is indicated to avoid the risk of developing resistance due to antibiotic usage; however, dentist should consider the use of antibiotics in patients with underlying cardiac conditions for all dental procedures that involve manipulation of gingival tissue, involvement of the periapical area, or breach of oral mucosa.

Antibiotic prophylaxis suggested	***Antibiotic prophylaxis not suggested***
• All dental procedures that involve manipulation of gingival tissue or the periapical region of teeth or perforation of the oral mucosa such as extraction, scaling, periodontal surgery, dental implants, etc.	• Anesthetic injections through non-infected tissue • Dental radiographs • Placement of removable prosthodontic or orthodontic appliances • Adjustment of orthodontic appliances, placement of orthodontic brackets • Bleeding from trauma to the lips or oral mucosa

Situation	***Agents***	***Adults***	***Children***
Oral	Amoxicillin	2 gm	50 mg/kg
Unable to take oral medication	Ampicillin OR	2 g IM or IV	50 mg/kg IM or IV
	Cefazolin or ceftriaxone	1 g IM or IV	50 mg/kg IM or IV
Allergic to penicillin or ampicillin—oral	Cephalexin* OR	2 g	50 mg/kg
	Azithromycin or Clarithromycin OR	500 mg	15 mg/kg
	Doxycycline	100 mg	<45 kg, 2.2 mg/kg >45 kg, 100 mg
Allergic to penicillin or ampicillin and unable to take oral medication	Cefazolin or ceftriaxone†	1 g IM or IV	50 mg/kg IM or IV

Clindamycin is no longer recommended for antibiotic prophylaxis for a dental procedure.
IM indicates intramuscular; and IV, intravenous.
*Or other first- or second-generation oral cephalosporin in equivalent adult or pediatric dosing.
†Cephalosporins should not be used in an individual with a history of anaphylaxis, angioedema, or urticaria with penicillin or ampicillin.

Dental Management

- The dentist should obtain a detailed medical and dental history, perform a thorough clinical examination and formulate a complete treatment plan.
- Careful dental evaluation of patients who are scheduled for cardiac surgery for the proper diagnosis and treatment of oral and dental infections.
- Obtain a written consent prior to the treatment from the child's physician or cardiologist. The cardiologist will indicate the specific desired antibiotic prophylaxis needed before the dental treatment.
- Conscious sedation and nitrous oxide–oxygen analgesia have been proven beneficial in reducing anxiety and behavior management of these patients. Conscious sedation monitoring and cardiopulmonary resuscitation equipment should be readily available during the appointment.
- In case of dental treatment under general anesthesia, the dental procedures should be completed in a hospital setting, with adequate supportive care.
- Pulp therapy is not recommended for primary teeth with a poor prognosis because of the high incidence of associated chronic infection. Extraction of such teeth with appropriate fixed-space maintenance is preferred.

- Endodontic therapy in the permanent dentition can usually be accomplished successfully if the teeth to be treated are carefully selected and the endodontic therapy is adequately performed.
- In case of patients who are to undergo cardiac surgery, implementation of preventive dental program, will decrease the incidence of postoperative IE from oral sources and also the improve surgical outcome and patient's overall health. The dental examination and preventive dental program should be implemented before the child reaches 6 months of age when possible. Ideally, dental treatment should be completed within 3 or 4 weeks of the planned surgery to allow for healing and the return of normal flora.
- It will also be worthwhile to mention that medically compromised patients with noncardiac factors may also have a compromised immune system and may not be able to tolerate transient bacteremia following any invasive dental procedure. This category may include diseases secondary to immunosuppression such as acquired immunodeficiency syndrome (AIDS), human immunodeficiency virus (HIV), autoimmune diseases, post-radiotherapy, prolong use of steroid, and metabolic disorders such as diabetes by American Heart Association (AHA) for prevention of infective endocarditis.

Diabetes Mellitus

Diabetes mellitus (DM) often simply referred to as diabetes—is a condition in which a person has high blood sugar levels because either the body does not produce sufficient amount of insulin or the patient does not respond to the insulin that is produced. This high blood sugar levels are classically manifested as polyuria (frequent urination), polydipsia (increased thirst), and polyphagia (increased hunger). There are three main types of diabetes:

1. **Insulin-dependent diabetes mellitus (type 1 diabetes):** Results from the body's failure to produce insulin due to deficient insulin production caused by the destruction of the beta cells of the islets of Langerhans (pancreas) and require the person to inject insulin.
2. **Noninsulin-dependent diabetes mellitus (type 2 diabetes):** Results from insulin resistance, a condition in which cells fail to use insulin properly, sometimes combined with an absolute insulin deficiency.
3. **Gestational diabetes mellitus:** When pregnant women, who have never had diabetes before, have a high blood glucose level during pregnancy. It may precede development of type 2 DM.

Oral Manifestations

- Altered salivary levels also known as xerostomia may act as a predisposing factor in the development of oral infections. Dry and damaged mucosa is more susceptible to opportunistic infections by *Candida albicans*.
- Concomitant diffuse, nontender bilateral enlargement of parotid glands (diabetic sialadenosis).
- Altered taste and burning mouth/tongue syndrome has been reported in poorly controlled diabetes.
- Higher incidence of dental caries in patients with poorly controlled diabetes is seen. This is attributed to increased glucose levels in the saliva and crevicular fluid.
- Poor healing, xerostomia with subsequent increased accumulation of plaque and food debris, higher susceptibility to infections, and pronounced hyperplasia of attached gingiva all contribute to the progressive periodontitis in diabetes.
- Delayed wound healing, pulpitis in noncarious tooth, acetone breath are few of the other oral manifestations of diabetes.

Dental management

It is aimed at implementation of a preventive protocol, symptomatic relief of any oral manifestations of the disease, and immediate provision of primary care.

- Dental appointments should be short, stress free, as atraumatic as possible
- Early morning appointments are preferred and the patient should eat a normal breakfast before the appointment to prevent hypoglycemia
- Use of pulp capping and pulpotomy procedures is questionable in the child with uncontrolled diabetes
- Vital pulp therapy may be preferred to a stressed extraction procedure under local anesthesia
- Prophylactic antibiotic may be recommended in use of surgical procedures
- Vasoconstrictor drugs with local anesthesia (LA) to ensure profound anesthesia are advocated, but excessive adrenalin dosage is contraindicated to prevent an increase in blood glucose levels and for this reason glucocorticosteroids should be avoided.
- Two critical steps involved in treating patients with diabetes: establishing the diagnosis (type 1 or type 2 diabetes, form of therapy) and the level of disease control (well controlled or poorly controlled)
- Acquire a thorough, updated medical history
- Understand potential complications that can be triggered by dental procedures in a diabetic patient and anticipate the need for pre or post-treatment medication or emergency care.
- The most common dental office complication is hypoglycemic episode. This occurs when insulin levels are high such as when a child takes his early morning insulin shot but skips breakfast to attend an appointment. Always ensure patients have eaten prior to their treatment. Decreased sugar levels also precipitate hypoglycemia and if uncorrected can rapidly result in unconsciousness. In a conscious patient administer 15 mg of simple carbohydrates and repeat finger-stick glucose test in 15 minutes. If blood glucose level is >60 mg/dL patient should be asked to eat or drink a sugar-sweetened beverage. If blood glucose level is <60 mg/dL, repeat treatment of 15 g of simple carbohydrates and check blood glucose every 15 minutes. Continue until blood glucose level >60mg/dL is attained and then ask patient to report to his/her physician
- Children with poorly controlled diabetes and acute oral infections are susceptible to development of ketoacidosis. In such situations children should be treated on an in-patient basis. Only after good glycemic control has been established, should any dental procedure under antibiotic cover be attempted.
- Early morning, short, stress-free dental appointments are preferred
- Since poor oral health in patients with poor glycemic control can have systemic repercussions, glucose levels should always be checked prior to the start of any dental procedure. Normal blood glucose range in children according to age: 0–5 years 100–180 mg/dL; 6–9 years 80–140 mg/dL; ≥10 years 70–120 mg/dL.

- Hb1Ac ≤7%: Restorations, removable orthodontic appliances, space maintainers, preventive procedures can be safely performed and do not require any precaution.
- Hb1Ac ≥8%: Caution advised, managed in a hospital setting under physician's supervision with prophylactic antibiotic cover and appropriate insulin dose adjustment. Avoid multiple extractions, surgical extractions, minor oral surgical procedures when possible.
- 1 or 2 dosage of local anesthesia with adrenaline can be safely given to ensure profound anesthesia but excessive dosage is contraindicated as it may increase blood glucose levels
- General anesthesia should never be considered on an out-patient basis for dental surgery in a diabetic child as the NPO protocol before operation could precipitate insulin shock. Hence general anesthesia is always arranged on an in-patient basis.
- Conscious sedation is not contraindicated and can be safely performed, provided insulin dose is modified in consultation with the patient's physician due to dietary alterations.
- Preventive care with periodic dental examinations and prophylaxis, oral hygiene instruction, dietary assessment and instruction, and fluoride application are essential ongoing services that need to be implemented in all diabetic children.

Diabetic Emergencies

- Hypoglycemic attack or insulin shock
  - Develops due to stress, insulin overdose and poor dietary control or glucose levels at or below 40 mg/dL
  - Condition develops quickly and treatment must begin rapidly
  - In severe cases if delayed is treatment, seizures can develop which may prove fatal
  - Signs and symptoms
    - Mood changes and irritability
    - Disorientation, blurred vision
    - Sweaty skin
    - Loss of consciousness
    - Lethargy, Slurred speech
    - Strong bounding pulse
    - Nausea, stomachache
    - Hunger, shaking, tingling around mouth
    - Hypothermia
  - Management
    - Administer oral carbohydrates
    - No recovery within 2–5 min: Administer IV dextrose (50 mL in 5% concentration)
    - Intramuscular glucagon (1 mg) followed by IM epinephrine (0.5 mg of 1:1000 conc)
    - Patient usually takes 5–10 min to recover, observe until stable and administer oral glucose when conscious to prevent recurrence of hypoglycemia
    - No response in 5 min: emergency procedures
- Hyperglycemic reaction/Diabetic coma
  - Develops more slowly than hypoglycemia
  - Diabetic coma occurs at glucose levels between 300 and 600 mg/dL, when ketones are present in urine and blood pH is below 7.36
  - Signs and symptoms
    - Weak pulse
    - Rapid and deep breathing
    - Dry skin
    - Acetone breath
    - Increased frequency of micturition
    - Thirst
    - Severe hypotension
    - Abdominal pain and vomiting
    - Loss of consciousness (Diabetic coma)
  - Management
    - Maintain open airway in hospital unit
    - Administer 100% oxygen
    - Determine blood glucose levels
    - Administer insulin
    - Recovery is usually slow than in insulin shock

Idiopathic Thrombocytopenic Purpura

Idiopathic thrombocytopenic purpura (ITP) is a common childhood disorder characterized by an abnormal reduction in the number of platelets in the blood. Platelets are cells in the blood that help stop bleeding. A decrease in platelets can result in easy bruising and an increased bleeding tendency.

Classification

- Acute ITP occurs in children below 10 years old, affecting both genders. It is usually associated with a history of viral infection before the development of clinical signs with an interval of 2–21 days from the viral infection and the beginning of an acute episode of IPT.
- Chronic ITP mostly affects teenagers with a predilection for female gender. A thrombocytopenia present for more than 6 months before the first signs and symptoms are observed is considered as chronic. The probability of patients with chronic ITP to develop autoimmune diseases is greater, and 1/3 of these patients present laboratorial and clinical symptoms of collagen vascular disease.

Etiology

- Thrombocytopenia could be due to reduction in platelet production due to bone marrow failure as seen in.
  - Megaloblastic anemia
  - Aplastic anemia due to drugs [e.g., cytotoxics, chloramphenicol], viruses (Epstein-Barr virus, varicella zoster and, particularly, after rubella vaccination), chemicals or irradiation
  - Tumors infiltrating the bone marrow including leukemias and multiple myeloma
- Thrombocytopenia could be due to platelet destruction as seen in
  - Autoimmune idiopathic thrombocytopenia and other immune-mediated thrombocytopenias, caused by drugs (e.g., heparin may cause a type III hypersensitivity reaction)
  - Viruses (e.g., HIV)
  - Systemic lupus erythematosus (SLE)
  - Post-transfusion purpura

General Manifestations

- Conjunctival and retinal hemorrhages
- Epistaxis
- Hemorrhages, bullae, and vesicles of mucous membrane often occur as a result of platelet count below 20,000/mm^3
- Ecchymoses and frank hemorrhages
- Profuse gingival hemorrhages.

Oral Manifestations

- Petechiae also occur in the mucosa, and commonly in palate that appear as numerous, tiny, and grouped clusters of reddish spot only a millimeter or less in diameter
- Bleeding gums
  - Elective dental treatment should be deferred until a platelet count is above 50,000/mm^3
  - Give steroids at a dose of 1–2 mg/kg to bring up the platelet level.

Assessment

A complete blood count should be done prior to starting dental treatment. Assessment and degree of severity of thrombocytopenia is based on the platelet count and dental management is planned accordingly. The coagulogram shows prolonged in bleeding time and coagulum retraction. Since the main dental consideration in ITP is postoperative bleeding the degree of severity of ITP helps in identifying those patients that need to undergo transfusion prior to oral surgical procedures. The white cell count is normal and anemia may be present in some cases.

Platelet count	Degree of severity of Purpura	Postoperative bleeding	Platelet transfusion needed
100,000–150,000 Mm^3	Mild	Increased	Only for major surgery
50,000–100,000 Mm^3	Moderate	Increased	Even for minor surgery
25,000–50,000 Mm^3	Severe	Increased even after venipuncture	Even for regional anesthetic block
<25,000 mm^3	Spontaneous	Increased maybe life threatening	Usually and avoid surgery if possible

General and Dental Management

- Elective dental procedures can be safely performed in patients with platelet counts above 50,000/mm^3.
- Transfusion with platelets when required is done immediately preoperatively, repeating if necessary, as sequestration is rapid.
- Antibiotic prophylaxis should be considered before restorations, endodontic and surgical treatment, to reduce risk of postoperative infections.
- Splenectomized patients do not usually need antimicrobial prophylaxis before dental procedures.
- Patients on long-term corticosteroids (autoimmune thrombocytopenia) may need corticosteroid cover and are prone to develop infections. 1–2 mg/kg of steroids are given to increase the platelet count.
- Control of dental biofilm is of the utmost importance to prevent gingival inflammation and infections
- Antiplatelet drugs, e.g., aspirin, beta-lactam antibiotics, cytotoxics, furosemide, diazepam and some antihistamines should be avoided.
- Local hemostatic measures e.g., absorbable oxidized regenerated cellulose surgicel, desmopressin or antifibrinolytics (tranexamic acid or epsilon amino caproic acid) can reduce the need for platelet transfusions.
- Regional or floor of mouth LA injections should be avoided due to the risk of bleeding into fascial spaces of the neck and obstruction of the airway.

Leukemia

Leukemia is a hematopoietic malignancy in which there is a proliferation of abnormal leukocytes in the bone marrow and dissemination of these cells into the peripheral blood. The abnormal leukocytes (blast cells) replace normal cells in bone marrow and accumulate in other tissues and organs of the body.

Classification

- Leukemia is clinically and pathologically subdivided into a variety of large groups
- Acute leukemia is characterized by the rapid increase of immature blood cells
- Chronic leukemia is distinguished by the excessive buildup of relatively mature, abnormal, white blood cells
- Four main categories of leukemia are:
  - Acute lymphoblastic leukemia (ALL)
  - Chronic lymphocytic leukemia (CLL)
  - Acute myelogenous leukemia (AML)
  - Chronic myelogenous leukemia (CML).

Etiology

Although the exact etiology of leukemia is unclear. Genetic alteration and susceptibility, environmental factors, such as: parental smoking and alcohol consumption, chemicals, infections, and exposure to ionizing radiation, non-ionizing electromagnetic and electric fields have been implicated in the development of childhood leukemia.

Childhood Leukemia

Acute leukemias account for 80–85 % of malignant disease in children with a peak incidence at 4 years of age. They are characterized by the presence of more than 25% primitive blast leukocytes. Clinically they present with weight loss, fatigue and anorexia, as well as features of leukemic infiltration into:

- Bone marrow
  - Anemia (weakness, tiredness, breathlessness, pallor)
  - Ineffective leukocytes (infections, recurrent fever)
  - Thrombocytopenia (bruising, petechiae, bleeding from mucosae)
- Lymphoreticular system (enlargement of lymph nodes, spleen and liver)

Diagnosis is confirmed by blood count with low RBC and platelet counts, unusually high WBC levels, film (blast cells), bone marrow biopsy and immunophenotyping (categorization of blast cells). Acute lymphoblastic leukemia (ALL) is the most common leukemia of childhood. Treatment of ALL is with cytotoxic drugs singly or in combination with stem cell transplantation and radiation therapy. Two thirds of patients respond well to chemotherapy (CT) and are cured. Remission is increasingly achieved with combination chemotherapy, but recurrences are common, especially in older patients.

Oral Manifestations of Hematological Malignancies and Chemotherapy

Oral manifestations of leukemia prior to chemotherapy are due to infiltration of leukemic cells into tissues while those occurring during chemotherapy are mainly adverse effects and complications of CT.

- **Pre-chemotherapy:** Due to leukemic cell infiltration
  - Anemia
  - Predisposition to infections including oral infections
  - Bleeding tendency in patients due to reduced platelet count
  - Carriers of blood-borne viruses due to multiple transfusions of blood products or bone marrow transplants
  - Localized or generalized gingival hyperplasia, mainly affecting interdental papillae and marginal gingiva caused by inflammation, or leukemic infiltration
  - Infiltration of leukemic cells into periapical tissues simulate periapical inflammatory lesions., both clinically and radiographically.
- **During chemotherapy:** most cytotoxic agents target rapidly dividing cells with an aim to kill cancer cells, but the process is not selective and there is a degree of damage to all tissues with a high cell turnover. Bone marrow, GI tract, skin, hair, oral mucosa and gonads are commonly damaged. A common side effect of CT is oral mucositis. Oral mucositis and ulceration may occur at any site in the mouth, especially the buccal mucosae and fauces. Although these ulcers heal within 2 to 3 weeks of discontinuation of chemotherapy, they can be so severe that an antidote may be needed to reverse the effects of the cytotoxic drug, e.g., leucovorin to prevent harmful effects of methotrexate.
  - Oral mucositis, bleeding, ulceration, gingival abscess, pain
  - Oral purpura and gingival bleeding may result from thrombocytopenia induced by CT
  - Eighth cranial nerve damage (e.g., Cisplatin)
  - Candidial (oral thrush), viral (recurrent herpetic stomatitis) and gram-negative bacterial infections are common in the mouth
  - Salivary gland dysfunction, xerostomia (e.g., Doxorubicin) and increased caries rate
  - Dysgeusia
- **Postchemotherapy:** Long term effects on developing bone and dentition manifested as:
  - Enamel hypoplasia
  - Blunt v-shaped roots observed on radiographs

Dental Management

Performing dental procedures can offer risk to the patient, depending on his/her state of health and phase of therapy. Furthermore, some procedures offer greater risk than others. Thus, noninvasive procedures can be performed at any stage of the disease or treatment in the clinic. However, invasive procedures that offer higher risk such as in acute oral infections, should be preferably treated in a hospital setting, as hematological indices need to be increased (transfusions) and antibiotic coverage given when required. The role of the dentist in the management of leukemic patients can be discussed at three different stages:

1. Pre-chemotherapy evaluation and preparation of patients
2. Oral healthcare during treatment
3. Post-treatment care

Prechemotherapy Evaluation and Preparation of Patients

- These patients are considered high-risk as they have active leukemia, with a high number of neoplastic cells in the bone marrow and peripheral blood; they are thrombocytopenic and neutropenic. Gather information about underlying disease, time of diagnosis, modalities of planned treatment by consulting with the oncologist.
- The dental examination should occur immediately after diagnosis and before initiation of chemotherapy. Dental treatment should be completed 1 week prior to start of chemotherapy after evaluating platelets, erythrocytes and neutrophil levels.
- Ascertain current hematological status by performing a baseline complete blood count (CBC):
  - Platelets 81,000/mm^3 (normal: 150,000–400,000)
  - WBC 4,100/mm^3 (5,000–15,000)
  - Absolute neutrophil count (ANC) 2,600/mm^3 (1,500–8,000)
  - Red blood cells 4.16 × 10^{12}/L (4–5.2)
  - Hematocrit 34% (34–40%)
  - Hemoglobin 11.2 g/dL (11.5–13.5)
- Since patients have neutropenia and thrombocytopenia, all sources of potential irritation such as sharp teeth, chipped or broken fillings or broken appliances must be removed.
- All potential sources of infection of dental origin e.g., teeth with deep periodontal pockets, pulpal pathology, partially erupted third molars and nonrestorable teeth must be extracted.
- Extractions should be done 10–14 days prior to chemotherapy.
- Restore multi-surface carious lesions with stainless steel crowns
- Apply sealants on discolored molar fissures and fluoride varnish on demineralized areas
- Consider general anesthesia to provide comprehensive dental treatment at one time to avoid delaying cancer therapy

Oral Health Care During Chemotherapy

- Patients undergoing chemotherapy are immunosuppressed and therefore susceptible to systemic infections. They are also classified as high-risk patients, due to the possibility of developing infections as well as the rapidity with which infections can become potentially fatal. Consult the oncologist for information on planned treatment protocol, drugs administered thus far, planned surgeries, anticipated complications of treatment, prognosis and allergies.

- Anemia, bleeding tendency and the effects of cytotoxic drugs on other organs can complicate dental management. Check CBC before starting any dental procedure. The most important is platelet count; if platelet count ≥75,000/mm^3 prolonged bleeding can be anticipated during extractions and hence the dentist should be prepared with local hemostatic measures. A platelet count ≤75,000 invasive dental procedures are contraindicated and should be managed by medication.
- Maintenance of oral health during cancer therapy is very important because oral complications develop in a significant proportion of patients who undergo cancer irradiation and chemotherapy. The main objectives of dental care at this stage are to treat side effects of chemotherapy and any emergency needs of patients.
- During the induction and consolidation phase of CT, the patient is immunosuppressed and extraction should be favored over pulpal therapy of primary teeth due to possible residual infection and treatment failure.
- Oral mucositis may be relieved by benzydamine, lidocaine or glutathione rinses. Chlorhexidine mouth rinses may also help by preventing secondary infections. Any infections that develop must be treated aggressively with medications.
- Caution must be exercised during administration of drugs to prevent cross reactivity and adverse drug reactions. Aspirin and other NSAIDs should be avoided in patients on methotrexate because they may increase drug toxicity.

Post-treatment Care

- Post-treatment patients are considered a low-risk category and have successfully completed treatment and present no evidence of malignancy or myelosuppression.
- However, children who received CT during the stage of tooth formation, require frequent reviews as tooth enamel may show hypoplastic areas and changes in the development of dental roots observed as short and V-shaped.
- For invasive dental procedures like surgical extractions, periodontal surgery, implant placement and multiple extractions, antibiotic prophylaxis is required until 6 months of completion of CT.
- There are no constraints in this phase and all elective dental procedures can be safely performed. If orthodontic treatment was interrupted during chemotherapy it can be restarted provided the patient has been disease free for 2 years.
- Aggressive preventive care with regards to oral hygiene, topical fluoride application, pit and fissure sealants needs to be instituted with emphasis on patient education and motivation.

Hemophilia

Hemophilia is a group of hereditary genetic disorders that impair the body's ability to control blood clotting or coagulation. It presents as impaired secondary hemostasis (stabilization of the platelet plug with fibrin) while primary hemostasis (platelet plug formation) is normal. Hemophilia patients are at high risk of secondary bleeding following oral surgery and hence present a significant challenge in dental management. They usually require management in a hospital setting under specialized care.

Classification

- Hemophilia A or classic hemophilia (inherited as X-linked recessive trait—gene located on the long arm of the X chromosome at Xq28) caused by deficiency of factor VIII (antihemophilic factor/antihemophilic globulin) is the most common form of the disorder, occurring at about 1 in 5,000–10,000 male births.
- Hemophilia B or Christmas disease (inherited as X-linked recessive trait) is caused by a deficiency in factor IX (plasma thromboplastin component) that occurs in about 1 in 20,000–34,000 male births.
- Hemophilia C/Rosenthal's disease inherited as an autosomal recessive trait is due to factor XI or plasma thromboplastin antecedent deficiency.
- Von Willebrand's disease is a hereditary bleeding disorder resulting from an abnormality of the Von Willebrand's factor (VWF).
- A fourth type of hemophilia was proposed by the Norwegian physician **Owren** in 1947, the Owren's disease or parahemophilia, caused by a deficient factor V, with an incidence of 1 case per 1 million children.
- Classification of hemophilia (Based on the level of procoagulant)
  - Severe-less than 1% (< 0.02 U/mL): Frequent bleeding episodes, often occurring 2 to 4 times per month. May be spontaneous without a specific history of trauma. Common sites: joints, muscles and skin. Hemarthoses (joint hemrrhages) are common and symptoms include pain, stiffness and limited motion. Repeated episodes of hemarthroses or muscle hemorrhage may culminate in debilitating painful arthritis. Commonly affected joints: knees, elbows, ankles, hips and shoulders. Pseudotumors (hemorrhagic pseudocysts) may occur in several locations including the jaw.
  - Moderate—levels b/w 1% and 5% (0.01–0.05 U/mL): Experience less frequent bleeding episodes ≃ 4 to 6 times per year. If target joint develops (joint with repeated episodes of bleeding) in a patient with moderate deficiency, spontaneous bleeding may occur.
  - Mild deficiency—levels greater than or equal to 5% to less than 50% (>0.05–0.4 U/mL): Bleed infrequently and only in association with surgery or injury. Diagnosis may occur when an abnormality is found during presurgical evaluation or when bleeding occurs in association with surgery or trauma.

General and Oral Features

Hemophilia is characterized by bleeding from multiple sites in the mouth such as the gingiva and extraction socket. Patients may report a history of multiple bleeding events over their lifetime, depending on the severity of hemophilia. Bleeding episodes are more in severe hemophilia, followed by moderate hemophilia. The most common sites of bleeding involving oral structures is labial frenum 60%; tongue 23%;

buccal mucosa 17%; gingiva and palate 0.5%. Hemarthroses are common and symptoms include pain, stiffness and limited motion. Individuals may develop debilitating painful arthritis and pseudotumors (hemorrhagic pseudocysts).

Principle agents for systemic management of patients with bleeding disorders are as follows:

- Hemophilia A:
  - Factor VIII concentrate is indicated in hemophilia A in active bleeding cases or presurgery. One unit raises factor VIII level by 2%
  - 1-Deamino-8-D-arginine vasopressin (DDVAP)
- Hemophilia B:
  - Purified coagulation factor IX concentrate in active bleeding cases or presurgery. One unit raises factor IX level by 1–1.5%
- Von Willebrand's disease:
  - 1-Deamino-8-D-arginine vasopressin.

Patient preparation during invasive oral surgical procedures:

- Replacement therapy for Hemophilia A with Factor VIII in dentoalveolar surgery—50% of normal, given preoperatively, for major surgery—100%, repeated twice daily for 7–10 days and in head and neck trauma—100%, repeated for 3 days
- Desmopressin (DDAVP) twice daily IV infusion, for up to 4 days
- Tranexamic acid 1 g orally qds × 10 days
- Local hemostatic measures such as resorbable sutures, Surgicel, collagen, oxycellulose, gelatin, fibrin glue or cyanoacrylate.
- Antibiotics such as oral penicillin V 250 mg qds × 5 days to reduce the risk of secondary hemorrhage from wound infection
- Careful postoperative care (soft diet, etc.) and in-hospital stay for up to 10 days

Dental Considerations in Hemophilia

- A detailed history of bleeding episodes, frequency and site is essential
- Type of hemophilia and severity of disease to determine if the patient can be managed in the clinic or hospital
- Prior to invasive dental procedures, the dentist needs to liaise with the hematologist outlining the treatment plan to manage episodes of bleeding and plan appropriate replacement therapy.
- Severe and moderate forms of hemophilia require the use of clotting factor replacement therapy for all invasive surgical dental procedures.
- **Pain management:** Pain of dental origin is controlled with codeine and acetaminophen. NSAID's and Aspirin should be avoided due to their inhibitory effect on platelet aggregation.
- **Use of local anesthetic agent:** There are no restrictions regarding the type of local anesthetic agent used although those with vasoconstrictors may provide additional local hemostasis, but LA technique requires extra care. A buccal infiltration can be given without any factor replacement. The inferior alveolar nerve block requires appropriate replacement therapy because of the risk of bleeding into the muscles along with potential airway compromise due to risk of hematoma formation in the retromolar or pterygoid space. Similarly lingual nerve block and also posterior superior alveolar nerve block requires appropriate factor replacement since the injection is into an area with a rich plexus of blood vessels.
- Endodontic treatment is usually safe if not instrumented beyond the apex. Persistent bleeding from canals during pulpectomy is indicative of pulp tissue remnants in the canal and can be managed by irrigation with sodium hypochlorite followed by use of calcium hydroxide or formaldehyde-derived substances.
- Incision and drainage of swelling to be done under coverage of antifibrinolytic agent (tranexamic acid) and pressure pack, to achieve hemostasis.
- Matrix bands and rubber dam are protective for the gingivae, but must be applied with care.
- Saliva ejectors must also be used with caution.
- Periodontal scaling can be carried out under antifibrinolytic cover.
- Surgical treatment, including dental extractions, periodontal surgeries, and implants must be planned under appropriate replacement therapy to minimize the risk of bleeding, excessive bruising, or hematoma formation. For simple extractions, a 30–40% factor is administered within 1 hour before dental treatment. After extractions are completed, the direct topical application of hemostatic agents, such as bovine thrombin may help with local hemostasis. The socket should be packed with an absorbable gelatin sponge (e.g., Gelfoam). Topical thrombin may then be sprinkled over the wound. Direct pressure with gauze should then be applied to the area. Stomahesive may be placed over the wound for further protection from the oral environment.
- **Antifibrinolytic therapy:** These agents include epsilon-aminocaproic acid (Amicar) or tranexamic acid (Cyklokapron) in children. Epsilon-aminocaproic acid is given immediately before dental treatment in an initial loading dose of 100–200 mg/kg by mouth. Subsequently, 50–100 mg/kg of epsilon-aminocaproic acid is administered orally every 6 hours for 5–7 days.
- In case of surgical extractions of impacted, partially erupted, or unerupted teeth, a higher factor activity level may be targeted before surgery due to the increased likelihood of surgical trauma and the extended healing period. Discussion with hematologist is essential as he/she may also elect to administer factor replacement to the patient postoperatively. Antifibrinolytic therapy should be started immediately before or following the procedure and continued for 7–10 days.

Acquired Immunodeficiency Syndrome

Acquired immunodeficiency syndrome is the condition diagnosed when there are a group of related symptoms that are caused by severe HIV infection. **Popovic** in 1983 made identification of human T-lymphotropic virus-III (HTLV-III) as the causative agent of AIDS.

Modes of Transmission

- Parenteral transmission
- Perinatal transmission

- Sexual transmission
- Body fluids transmission
- Dental transmission—**Michael Glick et al.** (1989) have detected HIV proviral deoxyribonucleic acid (DNA) in the dental pulp.

Oral Manifestations of Acquired Immunodeficiency Syndrome

- **Bacterial infections:** Gingivo-periodontal disease
- **Fungal infections:**
  - Candidiasis
  - Other fungi.
- **Viral infections:**
  - Epstein-Barr virus
  - Herpes simplex virus
  - Varicella-zoster virus
  - Human papilloma virus
  - Cytomegalovirus.
- **Neoplasms:**
  - Kaposi's sarcoma
  - Lymphoma
  - Other neoplasms.
- **Other oral lesions:**
  - Oral ulcers
  - Salivary gland enlargement.

General and Dental Management

Prevention

- Barrier techniques
- Proper sterilization:
  - Human immunodeficiency virus is sensitive to autoclaving at 121°C 15 utes at 1 atmospheric pressure
  - Dry heat of instruments up to 170°C
  - Virus can be inactivated by heating lyophilized factor at 68°C for 72 hours.
- Disinfectants for innate objects:
- Calcium hypochlorite
  - 0.2% sodium hypochlorite
  - 6% hydrogen peroxide for more than 30 min
  - 2% glutaraldehyde and 6% hydrogen peroxide
  - Sodium dichloroisocyanurate
  - Human immunodeficiency virus is inactivated by treatment for 10 min at room temperature with 10% household bleach, 50% ethanol, and 3% hydrogen peroxide
  - Gloves may be disinfected by immersing them in boiling water for 20 min and alternatively overnight soaking in 1% sodium hypochlorite.

Drugs used for acquired immunodeficiency syndrome

- Acyclovir 1–2 g daily orally or intravenous (IV)
- Zidovudine (AZ7), which attacks the virus through the enzyme reverse transcriptase
- Three other inhibitors are also in market, namely: (1) dideoxycytidine (ddC), (2) dideoxyinosine (ddi), and (3) stavudine (d4t)
- Use of protease inhibitors like saquinavir, indinavir, and ritonavir.

POINTS TO REMEMBER

- Special healthcare needs (AAPD, 2013) defined as any physical, developmental, mental, sensory, behavioral, cognitive, or emotional impairment or limiting condition that requires medical management, healthcare intervention, and/or use of specialized services or programs. The condition may be congenital, developmental, or acquired through disease, trauma, or environmental cause and may impose limitations in performing daily self-maintenance activities or substantial limitations in a major life activity.
- Differently-abled child is the one who over an appreciable period of time is prevented by physical or mental conditions from full participation in the normal activities of their age group including those of social, recreational, educational, and vocational nature.
- Barriers in care for differently-abled children are accessibility, psychosocial, financial, communication, mobility and stability, preventive, lack of trained personnel, and ignorance by parents.
- Dental assistant is helpful in obtaining preliminary information, instructing the patient assisting, and advising the dentist of any noteworthy or unusual patient, family, or guardian problems.
- In the *Diagnostic and Statistical Manual of Mental Disorders, 5th Edition* (DSM-5), the term 'mental retardation' was officially replaced by 'intellectual disability.
- Is defined as an overall IQ lower than 70, associated with functional deficit in adaptive behavior, such as daily-living skills, social skills, and communication. It can be due to genetic disorders, maternal and fetal infections, fetal alcohol syndrome, birth injuries, cerebral trauma, or hypoglycemia. Its oral manifestations include tooth decay, altered salivary flow, abnormal jaw development, marked alterations in mastication, poor esthetics, gingival overgrowth, and bruxism.
- Cerebral palsy is a group of disorders of the development of movement and posture, causing activity limitations that are attributed to nonprogressive disturbances that occurred in the developing fetal or infant brain. Spastic palsy is caused by a lesion in the cerebral cortex and has impaired chewing and swallowing, hypertonicity of facial muscles, spastic tongue thrust, drooling of saliva, and constricted mandibular and maxillary arches. Athetosis is caused by a lesion in the basal ganglion and its classical dental sign is perioral muscles hypotonic with mouth breathing. Ataxia is due to a lesion of the cerebellum and has lack of balance leading to staggering gait, poor sense of balance, and uncoordinated voluntary movements.
- The United Nations General Assembly unanimously declared 2 April as World Autism Awareness Day
- The puzzle ribbon was adopted in 1999 as the universal sign of autism awareness.
- Modified checklist for autism in toddlers (M-CHAT) and screening tool for autism in toddlers and young children (STAT) are used for screening of children for ASD.
- Autistic disorder is a pervasive developmental disorder defined behaviorally as a syndrome consisting of abnormal development of social skills (withdrawal, lack of interest in peers), limitations in the use of interactive language (speech as well as nonverbal communication), and sensorimotor deficits (inconsistent responses to environmental stimuli). Most often the cause is genetic. These children seem to be self-sufficient and introvert and want to be left alone and have no attachment to their parents and relate well to objects like moving or shiny inanimate objects.
- In case of prophylaxis for infective endocarditis and other heart ailments, amoxicillin remains the first choice as the prophylactic antibiotic. The 2007 guidelines recommend administration of amoxicillin 30–60 min before the procedure.
- According to the revised guidelines by AAPD (2011), minimal use of antibiotics is indicated to avoid the risk of developing resistance due to antibiotic usage; however, dentist should consider the use of antibiotics in patients with underlying cardiac conditions for all dental procedures that involve manipulation of gingival tissue, involvement of the periapical area, or breach of oral mucosa.

- Clindamycin may cause more frequent and severe reactions than other antibiotics used for antibiotic prophylaxis, and its use is no longer suggested. Doxycycline is an alternative in patients who are unable to tolerate a penicillin, cephalosporin, or macrolide.
- Pulp therapy in primary teeth is not usually recommended in leukemic patients. In case of patients with granulocyte suppression following chemotherapy, endodontic treatment for permanent teeth is not recommended.
- Laboratory diagnosis of hemophiliac patients demonstrates normal platelet count, normal bleeding time (BT), prolonged activated partial thromboplastin time (APTT), and normal prothrombin time (PT).
- Block anesthesia should be used with caution in hemophiliacs. Loose connective, fibrous and highly vascularized tissue at the site of Inferior alveolar nerve and posterior superior alveolar injections are predisposed to development of dissecting hematoma which potentially may cause airway obstruction and life threatening bleeding episode.
- High-speed vacuum and saliva ejectors must be used with caution to prevent sublingual hematomas in patients with bleeding and coagulation disorders.

Questionnaire

1. Define a child with special healthcare needs and list out its classification.
2. What are the barriers in providing care to children with SHCN?
3. Write a note on disability accessibility guidelines.
4. Explain the features, oral manifestations, and treatment implications in case of dental treatment of a child of intellectual disability.
5. What is cerebral palsy? How do you manage the dental treatment for such patients?
6. Write a note on autism.
7. Explain prophylactic antibiotic regimen.
8. Discuss the oral manifestation and management of hemophilic patient in dental operatory.

FURTHER READING

1. Agerholm M. Handicaps and the handicapped: a nomenclature and classification of intrinsic handicaps. R Soc Health J. 1975;95:3-8.
2. American Academy of Pediatric Dentistry. Antibiotic prophylaxis for dental patients at risk for infection. The Reference Manual of Pediatric Dentistry. Chicago, Ill.: American Academy of Pediatric Dentistry;2021:465-70.
3. American Academy of Pediatric Dentistry. Dental management of pediatric patients receiving immunosuppressive therapy and/or radiation therapy. The Reference Manual of Pediatric Dentistry. Chicago, Ill.: American Academy of Pediatric Dentistry;2021:471-9.
4. American Heart Association. Prevention of bacterial endocarditis; recommendation by the American Heart Association by the committee on rheumatic fever and endocarditis. J Am Med Assoc. 1997;277:1794-801.
5. American Psychiatric Association: Diagnostic and Statistical Manual of Mental Disorders, 5th edition. Arlington, VA, American Psychiatric Association, 2013.
6. Bill D, Weddell JA. Dental office access for the disabled. Spec Care Dentist. 1987;7:246-52.
7. Chandrashekhar S, Bommangoudar JS. Management of Autistic Patients in Dental Office: A Clinical Update. Int J Clin Pediatr Dent. 2018;11(3):219-27.
8. Council on Clinical Affairs. (2004). Guideline on Management of Dental Patients with Special Health Care Needs. [online] Available from www.aapd.org/media/policies_guidelines/g_shcn.pdf. [Accessed April 2018].
9. Delli K, Reichart PA, Bornstein MM, Livas C. Management of children with autism spectrum disorder in the dental setting: concerns, behavioural approaches and recommendations. Med Oral Patol Oral Cir Bucal. 2013;18(6):e862-8. doi: 10.4317/medoral.19084. PMID: 23986012;PMCID: PMC3854078.
10. Eswari R, Prathima GS, Sanguida A, Harikrishnan E. "Dental Care of Children with Autism Spectrum Disorder: An Overview". Acta Scientific Dental Sciences. 2019;3(7): 52-56.
11. Franks AS, Winter GB. Management of the handicapped and chronic sick patient in dental practice. Brit Dent J. 1974;13:107-10.
12. Hassan Abed BD, Abdalrahman Ainousa BD. Dental management of patients with inherited bleeding disorders: a multidisciplinary approach. Gen Dent. 2017.
13. McDonald RE, Avery DR, Dean, JA. McDonald and Avery's Dentistry for the child and adolescent, 10th edition. St. Louis, Missouri. 2016.
14. Mink JR. Dental care for the handicapped child. In: Goldman HM (Ed). Current Therapy in Dentistry. St. Louis: Mosby;1966. p. 2.
15. Nirmala SVSG, Saikrishna D, Nivvula S. Dental concerns of children with intellectual disability: A narrative review. Dent Oral Craniofac Res. 2008;4(5):1-4.
16. Nirmala SVSG, Saikrishna D. Dental Care and Treatment of Children with Diabetes Mellitus: An Overview. J Pediatr Neonatal Care. 2016;4(2):00134. DOI: 10.15406/jpnc.2016.04.00134.
17. Nunn JH. The dental health of mentally and physically handicapped children: a review of the literature. Comm Dent Health. 1987;4: 157-68.
18. Ohmori I, Awaya S, Ishikawa F. Dental care for severely handicapped children. Int Dent J. 1981;31:177-84.
19. Padmini C, Bai KY. Oral and Dental Considerations in Pediatric Leukemic Patient. ISRN Hematology; 2014. Article ID 895721. http://dx.doi.org/10.1155/2014/895721.
20. Rossier VF, Campos Vieira SMCPA, Ana Lídia Ciamponi AL, Guare RO. Dental considerations on the management of Idiopathic Thrombocytopenic Purpura in children: case report. RGO, Rev Gaúch Odontol, Porto Alegre. 2015;3(4):472-76.
21. Scully, Crispian;Kalantzis, Athanasios. Oxford Handbook of Dental Patient Care, 2nd edition; 2005.
22. Sehrawat N, Marwaha M, Bansal K, Chopra R. Cerebral Palsy: A Dental Update. Int J Clin Pediatr Dent 2014;7(2):109-18.
23. Thornhill MH, Dayer MJ, Forde JM, Corey GR, Chu VH, Couper DJ, et al. Impact of the NICE guideline recommending cessation of antibiotic prophylaxis for prevention of infective endocarditis: before and after study. BMJ. 2011;342: d2392. doi: 10.1136/bmj.d2392.
24. Vernillo AT. Dental considerations for the treatment of patients with diabetes mellitus. J Am Den Ass. 2003;134:24S-33S.
25. Walker BR, Colledge NR, Ralston S, Penman ID, Britton R. Davidson's principles and practice of medicine, 22nd edition. London, England. Elsivier Health Sciences.
26. Wilson WR, Gewitz M, Lockhart PB, Bolger AF, Desimine DC, Kazi DS, et al. American Heart Association Young Hearts Rheumatic fever, Endocarditis and Kawasaki Disease Committee of the Council on lifelong congenital heart disease and heart health in the young;council on cardiovascular and stroke Nursing;and the council on quality care and outcomes research. Prevention of Viridans Group Streptococcal Infective Endocarditis: A scientific statement from the American Heart Association. Circulation. 2021;143(20):e963-78. DOI: 10.1161/CIR.0000000000000969. Epub 2021 Apr 15. Erratum in: Circulation. 2021;144(9):e192. Erratum in: Circulation. 2022;145(17):e868.

Cleft Lip and Palate

Prabhadevi C Maganur, Ruchi Singhal, Amrish Bhagol

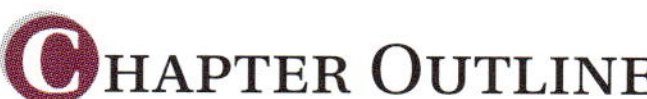

- Historical Perspective
- Development of Palate
- Pathogenesis of Clefting
- Incidence of Cleft
- Etiology of Cleft Lip and Palate
- Classification of Cleft
- Clinical Features of the Cleft
- Parental Attitudes
- Cleft Palate Team
- Multidisciplinary Sequencing of Treatment in Clefts
- Speech-language Therapy
- Fabrication of Prosthesis
- Role of Pedodontist

Cleft lip and palate are one of the most common congenital deformities seen at birth. It can be defined as congenital abnormal gap in the palate that may occur alone or in conjunction with lip and alveolus cleft. In historical times there were numerous theories and misbelieves that were associated with clefting. Some thought that it was due to effect of solar eclipse, while other thought it to be a bad omen and message of anger from the God and so such children were killed or they and their families were banished from the tribe. However, now the concept has changed with the scientific knowledge of embryology of cleft. But the etiology of cleft lip and palate still remains a mystery although various reasons and postulations have been put forward.

HISTORICAL PERSPECTIVE

AD 1000	Ancient Egyptian writings	Indicated the speech difficulties due to cleft palate, and the condition thought to have been not uncommon among primitive people
1561	**Pare**	Described the making of obturators to fill the cavity of palate. There are records of attempts to repair a hair lip
1764	**Le Monnier**	First operated a cleft of the palate surgically, mainly to facilitate eating and drinking
1826	**Dieffen Bach**	Suggested separation of the soft tissues of the palate from the underlying bone, when attempting to repair the hard palate
1844	**Fergusson**	Advancement of cleft palate
1862	**Von Langenbeck**	Using median suture, were among those surgeons who contributed notably to the surgery at that time
1923	**Brophy**	Suggested that midline suture would be simplified if the palatal gap were first narrowed by compression
1930	**Victor Veau**	Used various methods to elongate the soft palate, sometimes described as pushback operations

Contd...

Contd...

1942	**Anderson**	Conducted extensive studies of genetic pattern, found two different hereditary genes
1943	American Cleft Palate Association	To bring together members of all various professions to contribute to the knowledge of cleft palate and its treatment
1950	**R Millard**	Comprehensive cleft lip repair procedure identified

DEFINITIONS

Cleft: *Split or divided; refers to muscle, skin, and bone.*
Cleft lip (Cheiloschisis): *Congenital deformity of the upper lip that varies from a notching to a complete division of the lip; any degree of clefting can exist.*
Cleft palate (Palatoschisis): *A congenital split of the palate that may extend through the uvula, soft palate, and into the hard palate; the lip may or may not be involved in the cleft of the palate.*
Submucous cleft palate: *A cleft of the muscle layer of the soft palate with an intact layer of mucosa lying over the defect.*
Velopharyngeal insufficiency (VPI): *Inadequate velopharyngeal closure resulting in hypernasality (excessive flow of air through the nose); also called velopharyngeal incompetence.*
Fistula: *Abnormal opening from the mouth to the nasal cavity remaining after surgical closure of the original cleft.*
Cheiloplasty: *Surgical repair of cleft lip.*
Cleft palate–craniofacial team: *Group of professionals involved in the care and treatment of patients having cleft lip/palate and other craniofacial malformations; consists of representatives from some of the following specialties: pediatrics, plastic surgery, otolaryngology, audiology, speech-language pathology, pedodontics, psychiatry, orthodontics, prosthodontics, psychology, social service, nursing, radiology, genetics, and oral surgery.*
Maxillary orthopedics: *The movement of palatal segments by the use of appliances (also called dentofacial orthopedics).*
Obturator: *A plastic (acrylic) appliance, usually removable, used to cover a cleft or a fistula in the hard palate, or to help achieve velopharyngeal closure in order to promote clear speech.*
Presurgical infant orthopedic (PSIO) appliances: *Appliances or techniques that aim at bringing the alveolar segment closer, reducing the amount of initial cleft and improving the morphology and alignment of the nasolabial complex before the surgery.*

DEVELOPMENT OF PALATE

Primary Palate

At the end of the 5th week of intrauterine life as a result of the medial growth of the maxillary process and the medial nasal process forms the intermaxillary component/single globular process **(Fig. 71.1)**. This contains three components **(Fig. 71.2)**:

1. Labial component includes philtrum of upper lip, tip of nose, and columella.

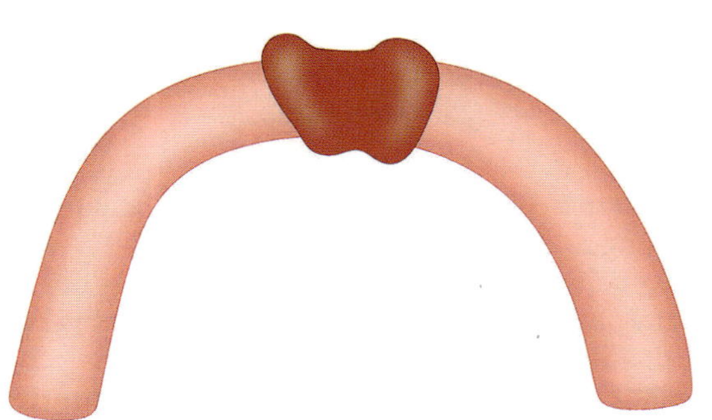

Fig. 71.1: Development of primary palate.

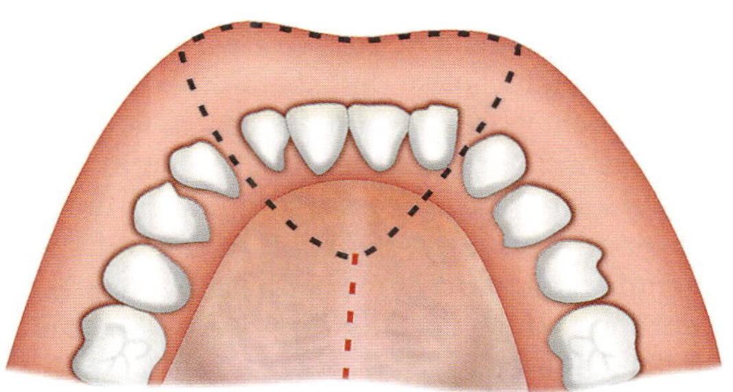

Fig. 71.2: Three components of palate.

2. Upper jaw component contains four incisors.
3. Palatal component includes triangular primary palate.

Secondary Palate

- By the 6th week of development, primitive nasal cavities are separated by a primary nasal septum and are partitioned from the primitive oral cavity by the primary palate **(Fig. 71.3)**. The primary palate and primary nasal septum are derived by the frontonasal process. At this stage the stomatodeal chamber is divided into:
  - Small primitive oral cavity beneath primary palate
  - Relatively large oronasal cavity behind the primary palate.
- During the 6th week two lateral palatal shelves develop behind the primary palate from the maxillary process, a secondary nasal septum grows down from the roof of the stomodeum behind the primary nasal septum, thus dividing the nasal part of the oronasal cavity into two **(Fig. 71.4)**.
- During the 7th week of development the oral part of the oronasal cavity becomes completely filled by the developing tongue. Growth of the palatal shelves continues such that they come to lie vertically.
  1. During initial shelf outgrowth
  2. During vertical shelf elongation.

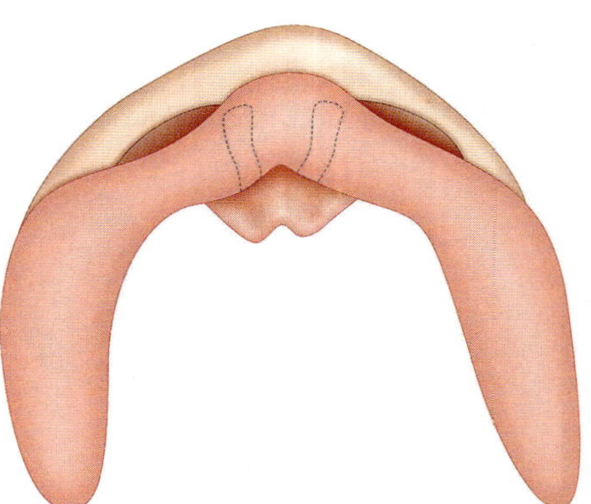

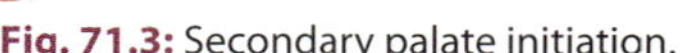

Fig. 71.3: Secondary palate initiation.

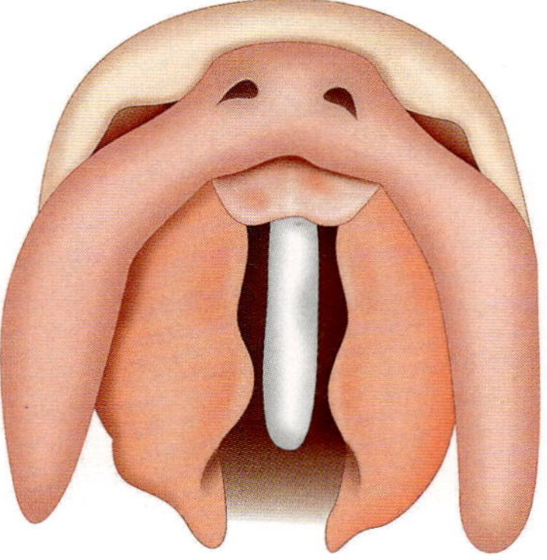

Fig. 71.4: Fusion of palatal shelf.

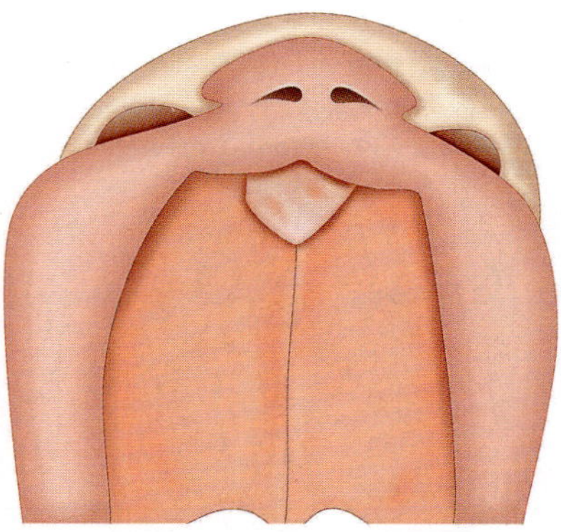

Fig. 71.5: Secondary palate formation.

- During 8th week of development, the stomodeum enlarges, the tongue drops down and vertically inclined palatal shelves become horizontal. On becoming horizontal, palatal shelves contact each other in the midline to form the definitive or secondary palate **(Fig. 71.5)**.
- The shelves contact the primary palate anteriorly so that the oronasal cavities become subdivided into its constituent oral and nasal cavities. After the contact the medial edge epithelia of the two shelves fuse to form the midline epithelial seam. Subsequently this degenerates so that mesenchymal continuity is established across the now intact and horizontal secondary palate.
- Fusion of the palatal process is complete by the 12th week of development. After elevation of the palatal shelves they contact each other and adhere by means of sticky glycoprotein which coats the surface of the medial edge epithelia of the shelves.
- Several mechanisms have been proposed to account for the rapid movement of the palatal shelves from the vertical to the horizontal position.
  - Biochemical transformation in the physical consistency of the connective tissue matrix of the shelves
  - Variations in the vasculature and blood flow to these structure
  - Sudden increase in their tissue turgor
  - Rapid differential mitotic growth
  - Muscular movements, jaw movements, forces derived from the tongue
  - Intrinsic factors
    - Role of glycosaminoglycans
    - Role of matrix components
    - Role of collagen
    - Role of mesenchymal cells.

Palatal Ossification

- Once the fusion is complete, hard palate ossifies intramembraneously from four centers of ossification, one in each developing maxilla and one in each developing palatine bone.
- Maxillary ossification centers lies above the developing deciduous canine tooth germ and appears in 8th week of development.
- Palatine centers of ossification are situated in region forming the future perpendicular plate; appear in 8th week of development.

PATHOGENESIS OF CLEFTING

Various Theories of Clefting

- *Dursy-His hypothesis:* Failure of fusion between median nasal and maxillary process
- *Veau's hypothesis:* Failure of in-growth of mesoderm between the two palatal shelves
- Alternations in intrinsic palatal forces
- Excessive head width or diminutive palatal shelves
- Excessive tongue resistance
- Nonfusion of shelves
- Fusion of shelves with subsequent breakdown
- Failure of tongue to drop down as in case of Pierre Robin syndrome
- Inclusion cyst pathology.

The theory of mesodermal reinforcement of epithelial membranes was given by **Victor Veau** and later developed by **Stark** in 1954. According to this theory, the upper lip and jaw are formed by the penetration of mesoderm between the layers of pre-existing epithelial membrane formed by the invagination of the oral pit **(Fig. 71.6)**. The mesenchyme may originate from neuroectoderm at the neural crest and migrate from the back of the head by three routes. The first route is over the top of the developing head and down into the central part of the face, which is called as the frontal prominence. The two routes are around the sides of the head into the areas of developing cheeks. As the mesoderm penetrates between the layers of epithelium it gives to the surface swelling known as medial and lateral nasal process and maxillary process. A

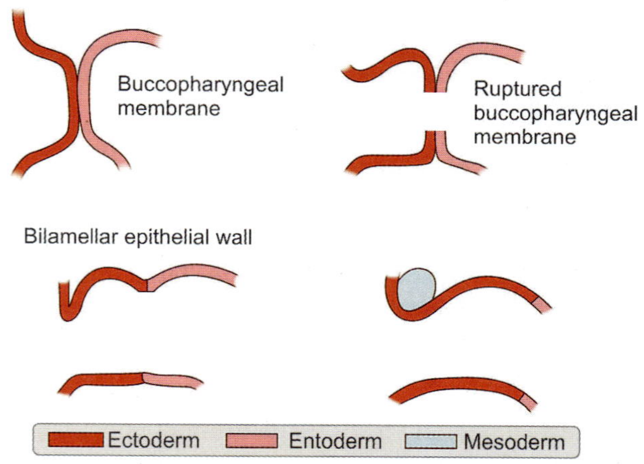

Fig. 71.6: Victor Veau's theory.

congenital cleft of the lip, alveolus, or anterior palate is due to failure of mesoderm and the subsequent breakdown of the unsupported epithelial membrane and not to the failure of fusion of separate process **(Fig. 71.7)**.

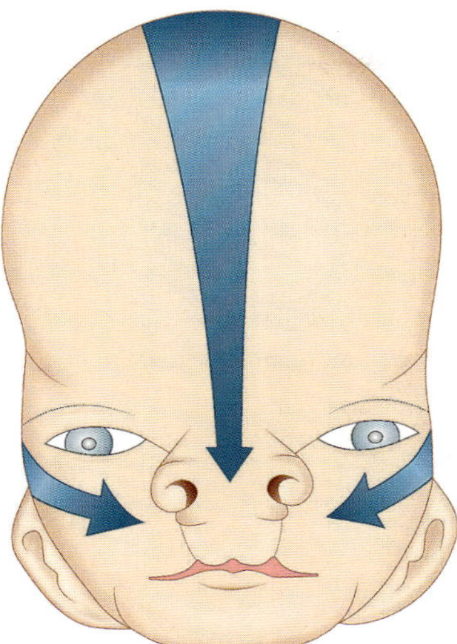

Fig. 71.7: Pathogenesis of clefting.

Cleft palate may result from conditions, which interfere with normal growth, elevation, adherence and fusion of the secondary palatal shelves and/or which interfere with fusion between primary and secondary palates. At 7th week of intrauterine development, the tongue lies between the 2 palatal shelves which hang vertically down on either side, but as the neck begins to extend during the 8th week, the tongue moves downwards and the palatal shelves spring upwards above it to the horizontal position where they can grow towards each other. Failure of the tongue to descent keeps the 2 palatal shelves apart. It may be due to the failure of mesodermal migration into the palatal shelves so that they fail to reach the midline resulting in a wide cleft with deficiency of tissue.

Factors Affecting Development of Palate

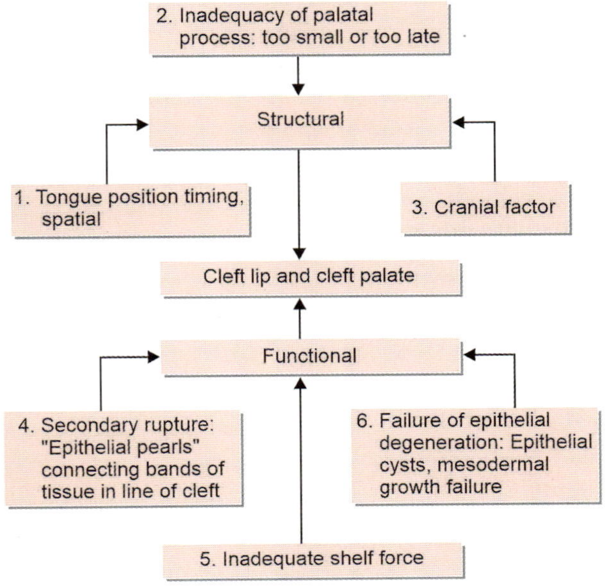

INCIDENCE OF CLEFT

Cleft lip and palate affects approximately 1:1,000 Caucasian, 1:500 Asians, and 1:2,000 African Americans.

- Overall incidence varies from 0.3 to 6.5 per 1,000 live births
- Negroid race has least incidence while mongoloid have the maximum
- Cleft lip is more common in males
- Cleft palate is more in females (fusion of palatal shelves occurs 1 week late in females, exposing the female's palate longer to teratogenic influences. Hence, incidence of cleft palate is more in females)
- Unilateral clefts are more common (80%) as compared to bilateral (20%)
- Left side has more predisposition for clefts
- Incidence is increased with increase in parental age
- More chances of cleft in patients with family history of the same and in consanguineous marriages.

Although the majority of patients with cleft lip and palate are otherwise healthy, approximately 25% have associated birth defects/chromosomal abnormality, or a genetic syndrome. There are more than 400 syndromes reported in association with cleft lip or cleft palate. Syndromes commonly associated with cleft lip and palates are:

- Stickler's syndrome
- Loeys-Ditz syndrome
- Patau syndrome (Trisomy 13)
- Velocardiofacial syndrome
- Vander Woude syndrome.

Cleft lip may be associated with following syndromes:

- Down's syndrome (Trisomy 21)
- Wardenburg's syndrome
- Vander Woude syndrome
- Orofacial digital syndrome
- Treacher Collins syndrome
- Pierre-Robin syndrome
- Klippel-Feil syndrome.

ETIOLOGY OF CLEFT LIP AND PALATE

Some of the postulated reasons are:

- **Heredity:** It is presumed that every individual carries some genetic liability for clefting, but if this is less than the threshold level, there is no cleft. When the individual liabilities of the two parents are added together in their offspring, a cleft occurs if the threshold value is exceeded.
- **Environment:** Teratogens like exposure of mother to infections (rubella virus, influenza, toxoplasmosis etc.), drugs (thalidomide, all cytotoxic anticancer drugs, cortisone, diphenyl hydantoin, hormonal pills, LSD, quinine, antimitotic drugs, etc.) during pregnancy
- Acute hypoxia produced by carbon monoxide or morphine overdose
- Aminopterin, an antifolic drug is occasionally used as an abortifacient. Surviving fetuses of such abortion attempts are grossly malformed
- **Mutant genes:** Some syndromes follow Mendelian inheritance, e.g., lobster defect-cleft with ectodermal dysplasia

- **Chromosomal aberrations:** Cleft can occur with many chromosomal defects like trisomy 21
- Increased maternal age
- Decreased blood supply in nasomaxillary region
- Deficiency of folic acid, riboflavin and hypervitaminosis A
- **Multifactorial inheritance:** Recent studies have shown that cleft cannot be attributed to one single factor and is a conglamation of multiple genetic and environmental factors.
- Alcoholic mother may give birth to a child with fetal alcoholic syndrome which maybe associated with cleft palate.
- Children from consanguineous marriage show increased incidence of clefts.

CLASSIFICATION OF CLEFT

Historical classification	*Based on embryology*	*Graphic methods of recording clefts*
• Davis and Ritchie's classification • Veau's classification	• Fogh-Anderson classification • Kernahan's and Stark's classification • American Cleft Palate Association	• Pfeiffer classification • Kernahan's striped Y classification • Millard's modification of striped Y classification • Tessier system of classification of orofacial clefts

Davis and Ritchie's Classification (1922)

- **Group 1—prealveolar clefts:** Lip clefts only with subdivision, unilateral, medial, and bilateral.
- **Group 2—postalveolar clefts:** Clefts involving the soft or hard palate or both, submucous clefts also included.
- **Group 3—alveolar cleft:** Complete clefts of palate, alveolar ridge, with subdivision of unilateral, medial, and bilateral.

Veau's Classification (1931)

For cleft palate:

- **Group 1:** Cleft of the soft palate only
- **Group 2:** Cleft of the hard and soft palate to the incisive foramen
- **Group 3:** Complete unilateral cleft of the soft and hard palate and lip and alveolar ridge on one side
- **Group 4:** Complete bilateral cleft of the soft hard palate and lip and alveolar ridge on both sides.

For cleft lip:

- **Class I:** *A unilateral notching of the vermilion not extending into the lip.*
- **Class II:** *A unilateral notching of the vermilion border, with the cleft extending into the lip but not including the floor of the nose.*
- **Class III:** *A unilateral clefting of the vermilion border of the lip extending into the floor of the nose.*
- **Class IV:** *Any bilateral clefting of the lip, whether it be incomplete notching or complete clefting.*

Kernahan's and Stark's Classification of Clefts

1. **Clefts of primary palate:**
   - Unilateral (r/l)
     - Complete
     - Incomplete.
   - Median
     - Complete (premaxilla absent)
     - Incomplete (premaxilla rudimentary).
   - Bilateral
     - Complete
     - Incomplete.
2. **Clefts of secondary palate only:**
   - Complete
   - Incomplete
   - Submucous
3. **Clefts of primary and secondary palate:**
   - Unilateral (r/l)
     - Complete
     - Incomplete
   - Median
     - Complete
     - Incomplete
   - Bilateral
     - Complete
     - Incomplete.

American Cleft Palate Association's Classification

Clefts of prepalate

- Cleft lip
  - Unilateral
  - Bilateral
  - Median
  - Prolabium
  - Congenital scar
- Cleft of alveolar process
  - Unilateral
    - Bilateral
    - Median
  - Any combination of foregoing types
- Cleft of prepalate
  - Prepalate protrusion
    - Prepalate rotation
    - Prepalate arrest (median cleft)

Clefts of palate

- Cleft soft palate
  - Extent
    - Palatal shortness
    - Submucous cleft
- Cleft hard palate
  - Extent
    - Vomer attachment
    - Submucous cleft
  - Cleft of soft and hard palate.

Clefts of prepalate and palate

- Any combination of clefts described under clefts of prepalate and clefts of palate.

Schuchardt and Pfeiffer's Classification (Fig. 71.8)

This is symbolic classification in which different regions depicted and then shaded according to type of cleft depending on whether it is total or partial.

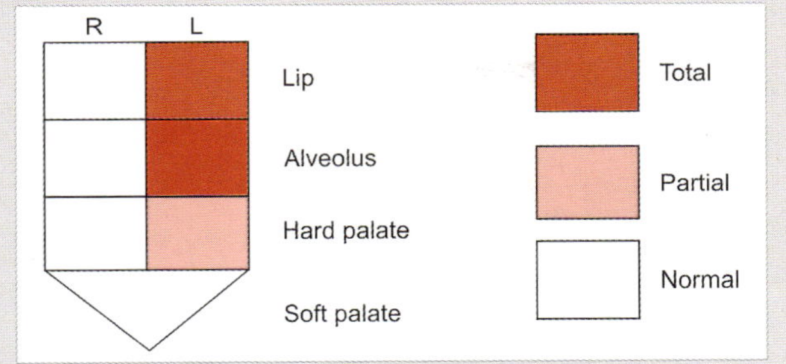

Fig. 71.8: Schuchardt and Pfeiffer's classification.

Kernahan's Striped "Y" Classification (Fig. 71.9)

This is a symbolic classification in which numbering is given to each site representing the oral cavity. The shaded area denotes presence of cleft in the particular area.

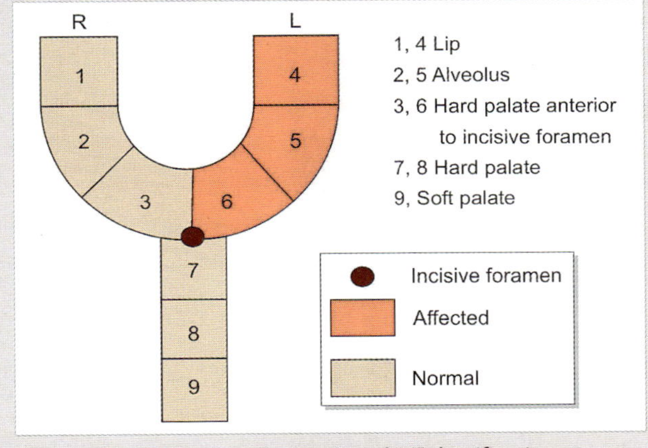

Fig. 71.9: Kernahan's striped "Y" classification.

Millard's Modification of Striped "Y" (Fig. 71.10)

He added another parameter to the Kernahan's classification and that was the addition of nasal floor.

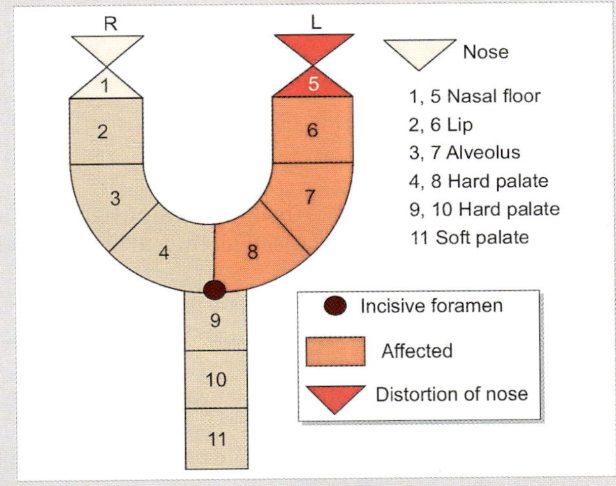

Fig. 71.10: Millard's modification of striped "Y".

LAHSHAL's Classification

This was given by **Okrein's** in 1987. He developed a paraphrase for each area and the cleft could be denoted as such:

L = Lip	H = Hard palate
A = Alveolus	A = Alveolus
H = Hard palate	L = Lip
S = Soft palate	

A cross-sectional survey among cleft providers around the world, recommend the usage of the LAHSHAL classification, due to its comprehensiveness, relatively high implementation rate globally, convenience of usage. (Houkes et al. Classification Systems of Cleft Lip, Alveolus and Palate: Results of an International Survey. The Cleft Palate-Craniofacial Journal)

V Tessier System of Classification of Orofacial Clefts (Fig. 71.11)

- All clefts are numbered from 0–14
- Midline clefts are numbered 0
- Facial clefts are numbered out laterally from 1–7 inferior to the orbit
- Cranial clefts are numbered in medially from 8–14 superior to the orbit
- Facial and cranial clefts can be connected

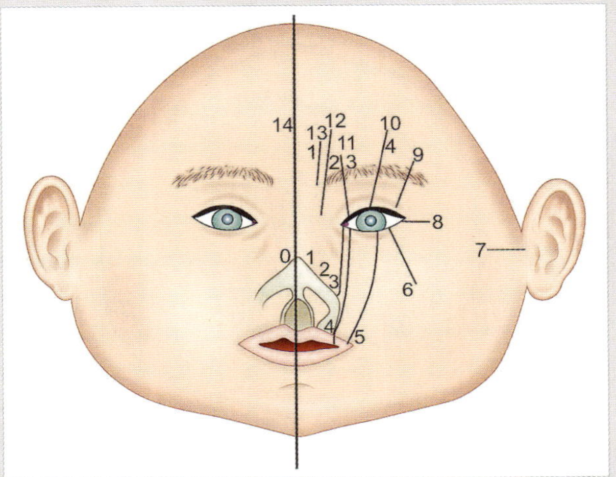

Fig. 71.11: V Tessier system of classification of orofacial clefts.

CLINICAL FEATURES OF THE CLEFT

Easy way to examine a cleft lip/palate baby is with its head gently lowered on to the dentist lap and the parent sitting facing the dentist, supporting and controlling arms and legs. Use of small dental mirrors—No. 2, 18 mm diameter (Busch and Co Engelskirchen, Germany) is very useful. Careful examination of cleft area especially on the hard palate and alveolus should be done to evaluate type of cleft **(Figs. 71.12A to C)** and to note down the:

- Number of teeth
- Eruption patterns
- Morphology
- Position
- Missing teeth
- Enamel hypoplasia
- Supernumerary teeth.

Any one of the following features should be looked out for as these can occur in greater incidence in cleft than in normal population:

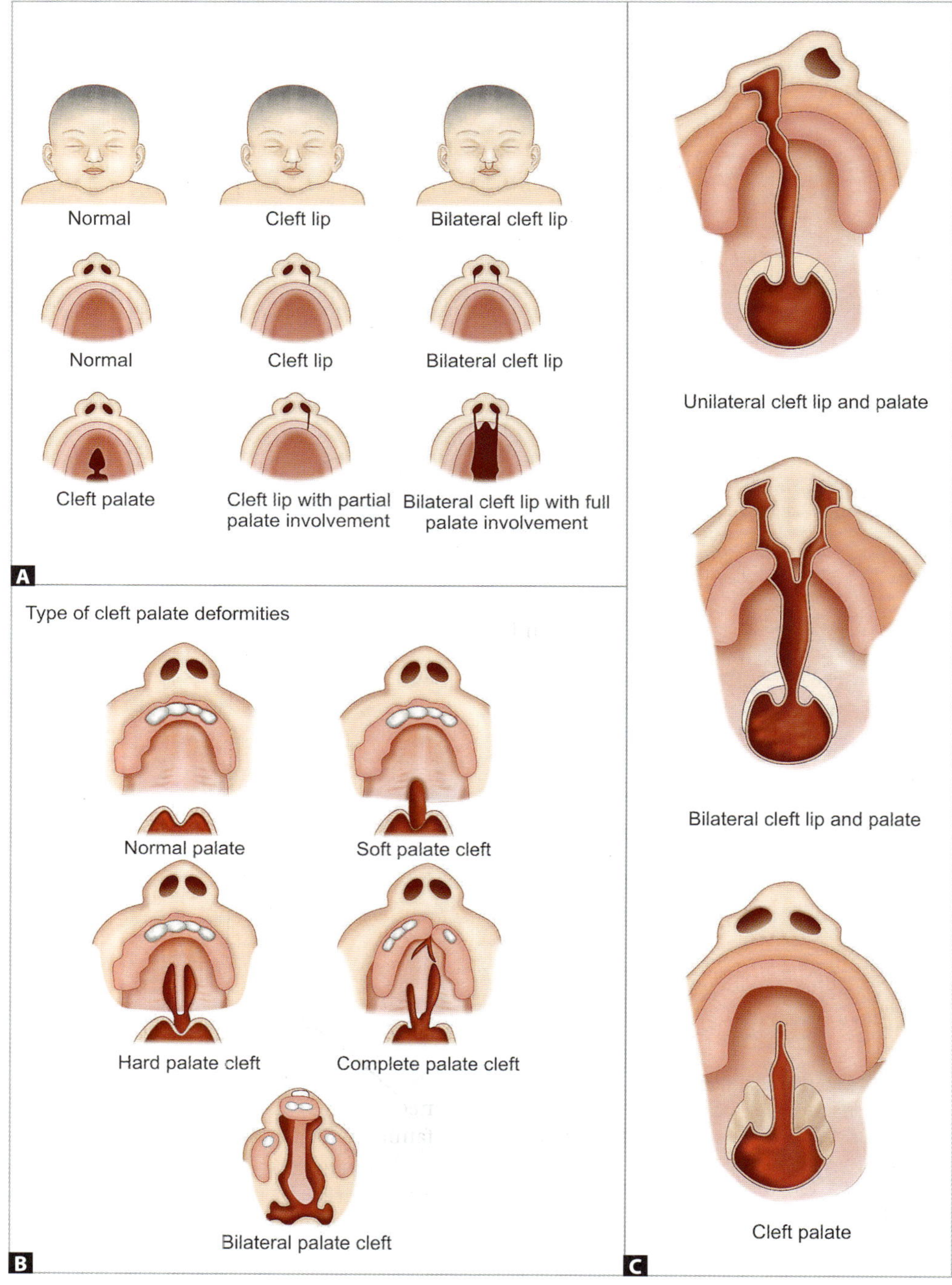

Figs. 71.12A to C: Different types of cleft lip and palate.

- Natal or neonatal teeth usually observed in maxillary central incisor is common finding in complete unilateral/bilateral cleft palate
- Increase incidence of congenital absent lateral incisor—primary/permanent adjacent to cleft alveolar teeth
- Increase incidence of congenital missing of premolar
- Increase frequency of supernumerary teeth is another finding complete unilateral/bilateral cleft
- Presence of ectopic primary LI—palatally adjacent to or within cleft side
- Permanent canines on side of alveolar clefts may erupt palatally into the clefts
- Various anomalies of tooth like enamel hypoplasia, microdontia, macrodontia, fused teeth, and aberration in crown shape primary
- Presence of increased overbite leads to stripping of labial attached gingiva overlying mandibular incisor which causes traumatic anterior deep bite
- Lateral facial profile is noticeably convex in complete U/B clefts, which increases as child grows
- Presence of protuberant and mobile premaxilla in infants with complete bilateral cleft lip
- Presence of posterior crossbite in patients with U/B cleft palate

Major syndromes associated with cleft lip/palate

Autosomal dominant
- Van der Woude syndrome (lip pits with cleft lip/palate)
- EEC syndrome (ectrodactyly, ectodermal dysplasia and clefting)
- Larsen syndrome (originally thought to be recessive)

Autosomal recessive
- Chondrodysplasia punctata (Conradi syndrome)
- Meckel syndrome
- Orofaciodigital syndrome, type II
- Fryns syndrome

X-linked
- Orofaciodigital syndrome, type I (dominant, lethal in male)
- Isolated X-linked cleft palate with ankyloglossia

Chromosomal
- Trisomy 13
- Trisomy 18

Non-Mendelian
- Pierre Robin sequence
- Clefting with congenital heart disease.

- Increase incidence of rotated permanent central incisor adjacent to the alveolar cleft area
- Premature loss, deficiency of alveolar bone is seen in permanent teeth adjacent to cleft of alveolar ridge.

Associated Conditions

- Presence of middle ear disease with attendant hearing loss in children.
- Otitis media develops quite early in most, if not all infants with cleft palate and it probably develops within the 1st month of life. Speech problems are usually created by cleft lip and palate. Retardation of consonant sound (p, b, t, d, k, and g) is most common finding.
- Language activity is compromised because consonant sounds are necessary for the development of early vocabulary which leads to good sound discrimination.
- If the clefts extend into the floor of the nose, alar cartilage on that side is flared; columella of the nose is pulled to the noncleft side.
- Surgical correction of the nasal deformities should not be done until all cleft deformities and associated problems have been corrected, as the correction of alveolar cleft defect and maxillary skeletal retrusion will alter osseous foundation of nose.

Chief complaints	• Deformity of face • Unable to feed • Nasal regurgitation of fluids
Dental problems	• Congenital missing teeth • Neonatal teeth • Ectopic eruption • Supernumerary teeth • Anomalies of tooth size and shapes • Micro- and macrodontia • Fused teeth • Enamel hypoplasia • Deep bite • Crossbite • Crowding or spacing of teeth
Esthetic concerns	• Loss of facial morphology • Missing structure
Hearing and speech pathology	• Disorders of middle ear • Nasal twang in voice • Difficulty in articulation
Psychological effects	• Due to the defect the patients are object of curiosity, pity and are often separated from their normal counterparts in society. This can result in life long trauma be it social, mental, or recreational

PARENTAL ATTITUDES

- Psychosocial issues are a critical part of the assessment and management of the child with cleft lip/palate, and must be addressed from the onset of care.
- The birth of a child is always a time of great family adjustment, and it is especially stressful when the child is born with a birth defect such as cleft lip/palate. Parents often experience feelings of sadness, guilt, anger and fear for their child's future social acceptance.
- In addition, the feeding difficulties these infants experience can be threatening to new parents, who may doubt their own ability to feed and nurture an infant with such differences. The loss of the ability to breastfeed is especially traumatic for some mothers.
- In part, through good psychosocial support and proper instructions, most families are able to work through their own emotional turmoil and effectively master the skills needed to feed and nurture these babies.
- As the child grows, the family will have other concerns, often relating to teasing, peer acceptance, speech difficulties, and learning and behavior problems. For many families, securing appropriate community and financial resources remain important issues.
- During adolescence there are new challenges, as the maturing teen strives for independence and copes with being different in a highly appearance-conscious culture. Adolescents and pre-teens should be given an opportunity to confidentially share feelings and concerns with a qualified professional.
- Psychosocial assessment and support may also become necessary when a high level of patient compliance and family commitment are required for certain interventions, such as obturator therapy. Other important circumstances that are often addressed by a psychosocial professional include child abuse/neglect, substance abuse, domestic violence and other family dysfunction.
- There is research to suggest that unless such emotional issues are addressed prior to surgery, such interventions alone are less likely to change self-image and improve quality of life. A detailed and specific psychosocial assessment is appropriate for all families presenting to a cleft palate team, regardless of socioeconomic status and perceived stability.
- **Weachter** (1959) reported 10 parental attitudes of the parents towards the cleft lip and palate.
  - Child appearance
  - Request for immediate surgery
  - Speech development
  - Feeding
  - Reaction of the spouse
  - Action of the siblings

- Reaction of family and friends
- Intellectual development
- Financial problems
- Recurrence of the defect in other unborn children.

CLEFT PALATE TEAM

Patient care coordinator	He who arranges the appointment, maintain the records of the patient
Obstetrician	First to observe the child and sends for referral
Pediatrician	Provides routine care and contacts other team members. Often is family doctor, perform complete physical evaluation and helps to assess the patient physiological status and developmental milestones
Plastic surgeon	Carries out esthetic repair. He plans out the timing of surgery, will be responsible for obtaining alveolar bone grafts and examines nasopharyngeal for speech. Pharyngoplasty—improve velopharyngeal function and correct internal nasal deformities
Surgeon	Helps during surgery
Oral surgeon	Carries out lip and palate repair. Plans the treatment along with other team members. Surgically alter skeletal relationship of maxillomandibular complex and repair cleft lip and palate
Neurologist	Identifies syndromes
Pedodontist	Helpful during all steps like presurgical orthopedics, obturator fabrication, and maintenance of growth
Orthodontist	Carries out all types of orthodontic interventions during the treatment and also after it. Plays a major role in the diagnosis and treatment of the cleft condition. Maintain records, orthopantomogram (OPG), study model and diagnostic photographs. He also works with surgeon to plan and to render an appropriate treatment to the child
Speech therapist	Monitors speech development and prevents any mishap
Psychologist	Prevents stress for the child and family
Prosthodontist	Helps in appliance fabrication. Replaces, restores, or rehabilitates orofacial structure that may be congenitally missing or malformed
Ear-nose-throat (ENT) specialist	For any associated defects
Social worker	Important part in today's changing world and helps with the social component
Parents	Since the child is small so the parents are required to provide consent on his behalf
Genetic counselor	Examines the patient to find characteristics of syndromes associated with cleft lip and palate
Audiologist	Performs test for hearing difficulties and also performs middle ear surgery if needed
Nurse	Advisor, support family during time of anxiety/ daily care of infant/teaches mother to take care of nose, facial skin, cleaning of splints at each feeding time/actively communicate with team members.

MULTIDISCIPLINARY SEQUENCING OF TREATMENT IN CLEFTS

The comprehensive treatment of cleft patients can be divided into four stages:

Stage I: Maxillary Orthopedic Stage (Birth to 18 Months)

It begins with immediate attention to the needs of newborn. The treatment modalities in this stage are management of feeding problems, fabrication of feeding obturators, presurgical orthopedics, surgical management of cleft lip, and surgical management of cleft palate. The feeding problems can be effectively dealt with using appliances like plates, pumps, and nipples as explained earlier.

Management of Feeding Problems

Feeding problems are often associated with cleft anamolies which lead to inadequate nutrition. The purpose of the palate is to separate the mouth from the nose. Normally, the soft palate at the back of the mouth moves up to close the passage to the nose during feeding. This creates a closed system, and the sucking motions create negative pressure which pulls the milk out of the breast or bottle. A cleft palate prevents the infant from creating a closed system in his/ her mouth, and makes it impossible for the milk to be pulled out. The infant will look like he/she is sucking, but he/she will be using up precious calories in a futile attempt to gain adequate nutrition.

The problems are:
- Insufficient suction to pull milk from the nipple
- Excessive air intake during feeding
- Choking
- Nasal discharge/regurgitation
- Excessive time required to take nourishment.

Various methods have been advocated to overcome these problems:

1. **For babies with cleft lip only**
   - Breastfeeding can be possible as the soft tissue of the mother's breast might fill in the gap and help the infant to form a seal.
     - Close monitoring should be done, if the baby is making noises during the feeding such as clicking or kissing noises, it means they are not able to form proper seal and suction
     - In such cases special cleft bottles and nipples with a wider base must be used.
2. **For babies with cleft lip and palate**
   - In these cases, special cleft lip/palate bottle's use should be advocated as these infant fails to feed directly from the breast. If mother want to breastfeed, she can pump breast milk and then feed it to the baby through a bottle.
   - Feeding by bottle rather than spoon is much more natural for the baby and encourages the biting action of lower lip and jaw function and development.
   - Relax the baby before starting to feed
   - Place the baby in an upright, sitting position as it helps to prevent the flow of the milk through the nose.

- Place the nipple or rub it against the lower lip of the baby so as to initiate the sucking reflex.
- Keep the bottle tilted in such a way that the nipple is pointing downwards, away from the cleft. Gravity will help to prevent milk from coming through the baby's nose. This limits choking and gas. It also helps to decrease the risk of ear infections.
- Watch the baby closely during the feeding to make sure baby is actively engaged in feeding
- Burp the baby often during the feed as the baby may swallow air during feeding
- Feeds should be completed in 30 min (2–3 ounces milk) excluding the time spent in burping, so that baby does not get too tired while doing so.
- Baby should regain his or her birth weight by the age of 2 weeks and should ideally gain 5-7 ounces per week.
- Nostril must be cleaned. Lips should be well lubricated with Vaseline. When the feeding is finished, small amount of two to three teaspoonful of sterile water is used to clean the mouth and palate.
- Area around the folds of the neck should also be carefully washed and dried as the baby often dribbles excessive saliva.

3. **Nursing bottles and teats for CLP babies**
   - **Feeding bottles:** *The proper bottle is the key to a successful feeding plan. There are three options currently widely used all of which work without the infant needing to create intraoral suction in order to pull milk out of the nipple.*
   - **Cleft palate nurser** (Mead-Johnson Company): It is a soft-sided bottle that is squeezed in coordination with the infant's sucking efforts, and thus milk is delivered into the mouth.

Cleft palate nurser

   - **Haberman™ and Mini-Haberman feeder** (Medela Company): This feeder consists of a large, compressible nipple with a one-way valve at its base that keeps the nipple full of milk. The infant's effort to compress the soft nipple is often sufficient to dispense the milk into the infant's mouth, but this can also be assisted by squeezing the nipple to increase the flow.

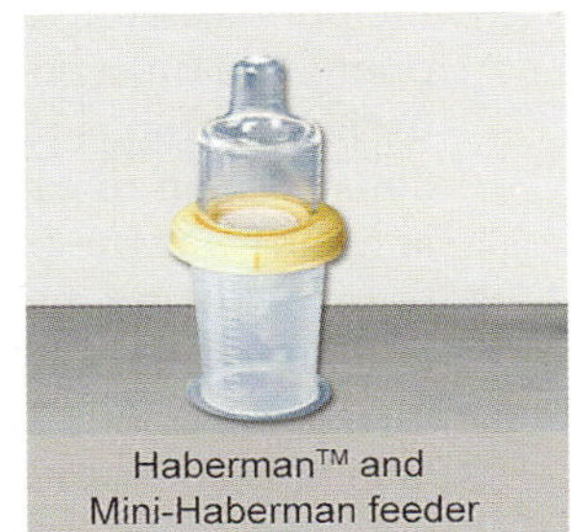
Haberman™ and Mini-Haberman feeder

   - **One-way valve** (children's medical ventures): This system also makes use of one-way valve at the base of the nipple. In addition, the nipple is constructed with a thinner, more compressible side so that the infant's tongue is effective in compressing the nipple to produce the flow.

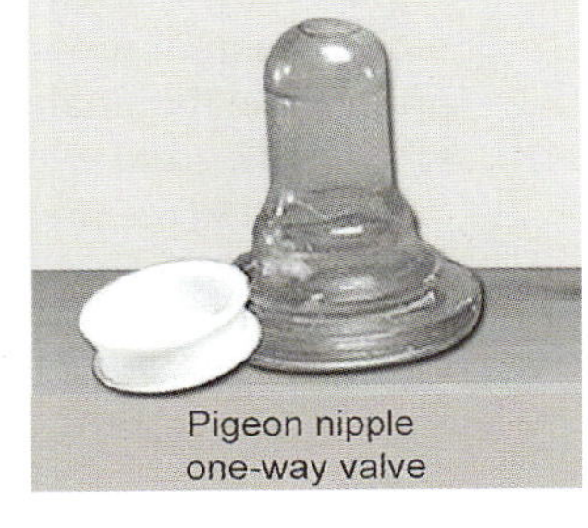
Pigeon nipple one-way valve

   - The regular bottles can also be supplemented with special teats namely Newborn Teat, Orthodontic shaped teat, MAM soft sipper spout, NUK cleft palate teat, MAM vented teat size 2, tapered teat.

Fabrication of feeding obturators

Initial obturator therapy: This is done from birth to 3 months. It is generally indicated for child born with complete cleft lip and palate. The appliance is fabricated after taking impression and is made of acrylic. Appliance should be cleaned before and after each feed.

Advantages:

- Provides a false palate, against which the infant can suck, reduces the incidence of feeding difficulties in newborns and helps maintain adequate nutrition.
- Provides maxillary cross-arch stability and prevents arch collapse after definitive cheiloplasty (surgical closure of lip).
- Provides maxillary orthopedic molding of the cleft segments into approximation before primary alveolar cleft bone grafting.

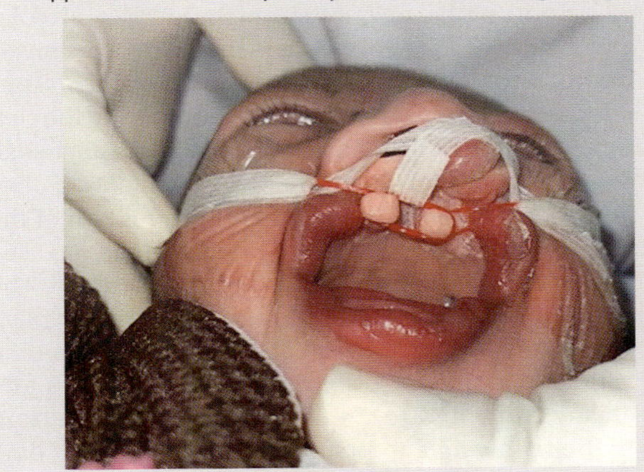

Presurgical Orthopedics (Birth to 4 or 5 Months)

- In some cases of bilateral CLP, the infant has a premaxillary segment positioned severely anterior to the maxillary arch segments or deviated laterally to one side of the cleft defect. If lip surgery is undertaken with the premaxilla in such an abnormal position, the chances of lip dehiscence (lip separation caused by increased pressure at the suture lines) are increased.
- Nasoalveolar moulding (NAM) is a very effective procedure opted worldwide with the basic principle of sculpturing and moulding the alveolus as well as the nasolabial complex. It aims at bringing the alveolar segment closer, reducing the amount of initial cleft and improving the morphology and alignment of the nasolabial complex before the surgery. This helps the surgeon to operate the patient less invasively, producing better aesthetics as well as finer scar after the surgery. In the literature several presurgical infant orthopedic (PSIO) appliances have been introduced to facilitate this reform. Beginning in 1950, when **McNeil** introduced active moulding appliances for presurgical orthopaedic treatment in cleft patients. However, a paramount transition in thinking from the traditional methods occurred in 1993 when **Grayson** and **Cutting** introduced a concept combining an intraoral moulding

device along with a nasal moulding stent named as PNAM. This concept was based on the increased hyaluronic acid in the infant cartilage, causing the cartilaginous structure to temporarily lack elasticity and have increased pliability and plasticity. More recently in 2009, the concept of DynaCleft® came into being which is basically a premade topical approximation device which has been successfully used to mold the upper lip and alveolus and support the developing nasal tissues prior to cleft lip repair.

- Although all these PSIO appliances aim at one single goal of achieving a reduced deformity before surgical correction, yet they have not always been proven to bring out the best results in all the CLP scenarios. Selection of an appropriate treatment option depending upon the type and situation of each CLP patient is very essential to bring out the best results. Commonly used PSIO appliances used in clinical practice are mentioned below:
  - **Grayson's NAM technique:** It is a versatile appliance which not only narrows the size of the intraoral alveolar cleft by molding the bony segments, but also actively molds and positions the surrounding soft tissues affected by the cleft, including the deformity in the cleft nose through the use of a nasal stent that is attached to the labial flange of a conventional oral molding plate and enters the nasal aperture. An impression of the cleft is made using a polyvinylsiloxane material. The impression is poured and the model is obtained. The cleft is filled with wax and an intra-oral molding plate is fabricated using the self cure acrylic resin material which is retained extraorally using facial tapes and elastics attached to the external retentive button. In the following appointments at a gap of 7-10 days the appliance is sequentially modified to mold the alveolar cleft segments. Adjustment is done in such a way that acrylic is removed from the area where the alveolar bone is to move and at the same time, a soft reliner material is added to the area from where bone is to be moved. When the cleft gap has been reduced to approximately 5 mm a nasal stent is added for active nasal cartilage molding. It is a wire and acrylic projection that is placed inside the nasal dome on the cleft side of the nose producing slight blanching of the tissue overlying the tip of the nasal stent. In the patients with unilateral cleft lip and palate, the nasal stent straightens the deviated columella towards the noncleft side and in the patients with bilateral cleft lip and palate, it lengthens the columella.

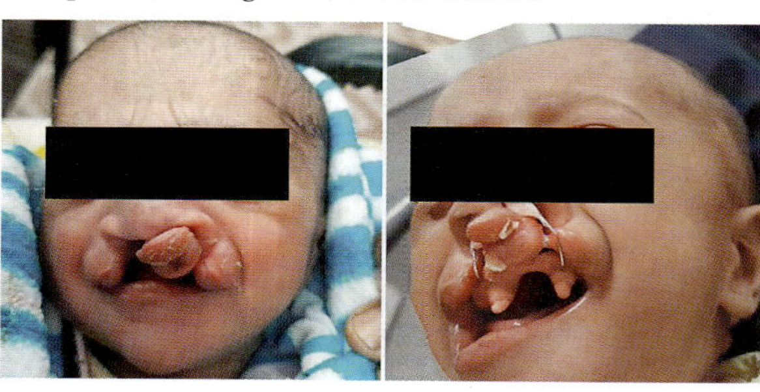

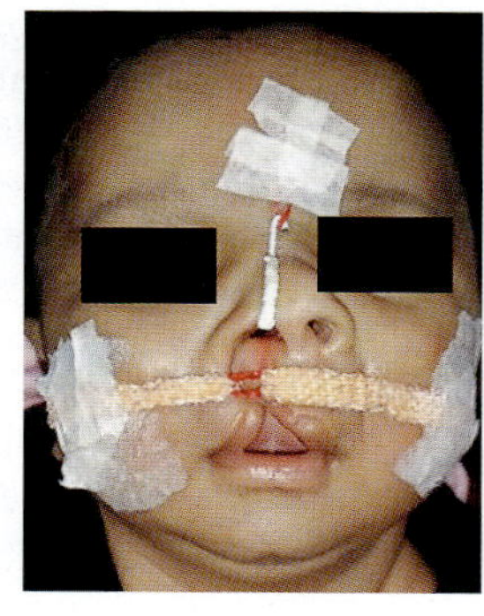

  - **Customized lip taping with nasal elevator:** Originally introduced as DynaCleft system (Canica Design Inc., Almente, Ontario, Canada), it consists of a tape called the Dynacleft tape to approximate the lips and alveolar ridges and Nasal elevator that comes with a hook, adhesive tether and paper template, to elevate the nose. It can be easily fabricated chairside using readily available material in dentist's office and at a cheaper price. Lip taping can be customized using Dynaplast and micropore. Dynaplast is attached to orthodontic elastic which on other end is connected to the micropore. This assembly is then attached to the infant's cheeks with Dynaplast on one side which is stretched in the region of elastic attachment and attached to the other cheek with micropore. The force should be as such that the elastic is stretched to twice its original size. The Nasal elevator system can be made from a plastic-coated paper clip that is bent in the desired shape with the tip being covered with Teflon tape. The device is connected with an orthodontic elastic band and fixed to the frontal area with sticky tape. Tension can be measured with a dynamometer; one ounce of tension is enough, and slight blanching of the skin can be observed.
  - **Elastic tape (Microfoam tape):** A soft elastic tape can be used to retract the premaxillary segment in a simpler manner. Its advantage is its ease of fabrication. But it does not afford same control of force direction and therefore cannot be used in all instances.
  - **Bulb prosthesis:** In cases of laterally deviated premaxilla, a straight extraoral force would not place the premaxilla in the frontal midline. Therefore, the premaxilla must be centralized using Bulb prosthesis. An impression is made of the infant's premaxilla for construction of external acrylic bulb prosthesis. It is fitted over the protruding and laterally deviated premaxilla and anchored to the infant's head with a bonnet appliance. By application of sequentially increasing differential forces to the premaxilla with elastic straps attached to the bulb prosthesis, the premaxilla is brought into the facial midline. It is worn for 24 hours a day for 3–4 weeks. Once the premaxilla is moved into central midline, the bulb appliance is replaced by a single elastic strap. Over the next 1–2 months, equal pressure is applied to reposition the premaxilla. Rationale for use of bulb prosthesis:
    - Affords greater control over differential forces applied to the premaxilla.
    - Movement of premaxilla into midline decreases the risk of distorting the vomer stalk.
    - Need for surgical premaxillary setback is eliminated.

- Optimum premaxillary positioning eliminates the need for a staged lip closure and thereby decrease total hospitalization time and cost.
- Appearance of nose and lip is improved because lip can be closed surgically under less tension and alveolar segments have an underlying symmetric alignment.

Surgical Management of Cleft Lip (Cheiloplasty)

- Appearance of unrepaired cleft lip can be distressing. Lip surgery will significantly improve the infant's appearance and may thereby relieve parental apprehension and enhance acceptance. Surgical closure is usually accomplished at 10 weeks of age. When repairing the cleft lip, the following aspects must be taken into consideration.
  - The esthetic appearance of the lip, including the lip skin with the philtrum edges, the lip white-red junction, the lip red-dry wet junction and the nasal sill with alar base rotation.
  - The function of the lip with the correct muscle alignment; which automatically improve aesthetics.
  - The long-term mid-facial growth.
- Optimum time for repair- generally "rule of ten" is followed, according to which the operation is carried out when
  - Weight of the baby is 10 lbs
  - Age–10 weeks old
  - TLC 10000/cmm (i.e no infection)
  - Hemoglobin–10 g%
- The operation is preferred to carry out at the age of 3 months as:
  - The lip is larger and thick at this age, so that technically repair will be easier.
  - The baby has sufficiently developed to accept GA and operative assault
  - Feeding with dropper in post operative period is not difficult
  - However few surgeons prefer to carry out immediate repair of the cleft lip in newly born infant
- Advantages of lip closure
  - It facilitates sucking
  - It helps in development of alveolus. In case of cleft alveolus, early operation helps in closure of alveolar gap.
  - Defective speech is avoided.
  - When cleft lip is associated with cleft palate, early reconstruction of lip will reduce the gap in the palate.

Lip surgery is always performed before time for primary dentition to avoid defective dentition. If patient reports late, operation should be performed, but the final results may not be satisfactory. If there is any protruded tooth which may cause pressure on the suture line, it should be extracted.

Various types of lip repair are: Millard's rotation advancement flap—most commonly used **(Figs. 71.13A to E)**, Tennison-Randall triangular flap method **(Figs. 71.14A to C)**. Other rarely used methods are- Rose—Thompson straightline repair, Skoog's procedure and Rectangular flap method of Hagedorn-Le Mesurier. For bilateral cleft lip repair: Veau's III procedure **(Figs. 71.15A and B)**, Black procedure and Millard's single stage procedure are done.

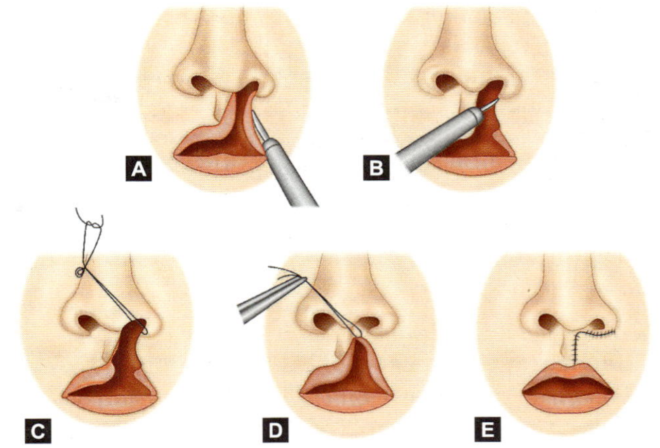

Figs. 71.13A to E: Millard's repair.

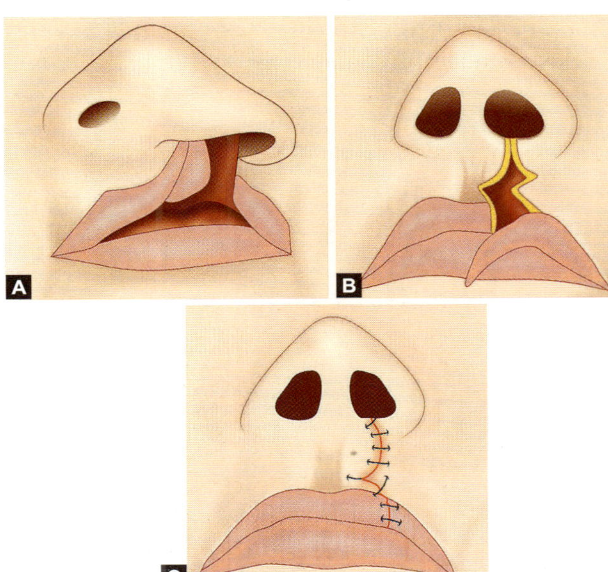

Figs. 71.14A to C: Tennison-Randall repair.

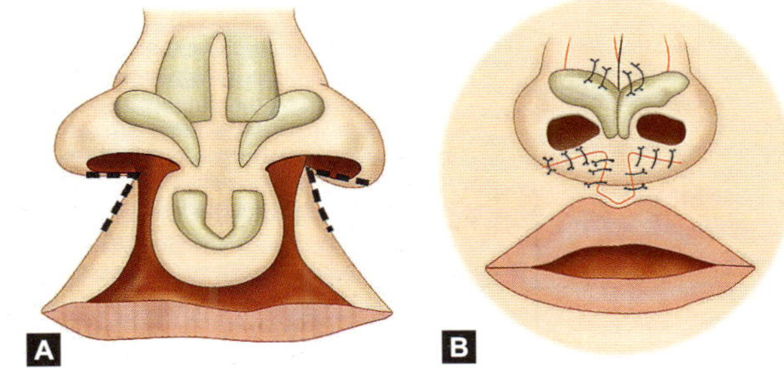

Figs. 71.15A and B: Veau's repair.

Surgical management of cleft palate—Palatoplasty (10–18 months)

Closure of palate is accomplished between 12 months and 2 years of age. The primary purpose of completing palate closure by 2 years of age is to facilitate the acquisition of normal speech, because this correlates with the age at which most children begin to talk. The procedure may improve hearing and swallowing by aligning the cleft palatal musculature. The time of palatal repair is very vital for further growth and aesthetics. If repair is done too early, then good aesthetics and speech development will be established but growth will be hampered and if repair is too late, facial growth will be better but aesthetics and speech will be compromised.

After primary closure of cleft palate, approximately 25% of patients demonstrate some velopharyngeal insufficiency. This results in unsatisfactory speech, regurgitation of fluids from nose and facial grimacing. It can be corrected by pharyngeal flap surgery.

There are two types of palatal repair:

1. **Single stage:** Von Langenbeck repair **(Figs. 71.16A to D)** and V-Y pushback palatoplasty **(Figs. 71.17A to D)**. This is carried out at 1½ year. The disadvantages include midfacial growth retardation.
2. **Two-stage repair:** Soft palate is repaired around 18 months and then hard palate is repaired at 4 years by Schweckendiek procedure **(Figs. 71.18A to E)**.

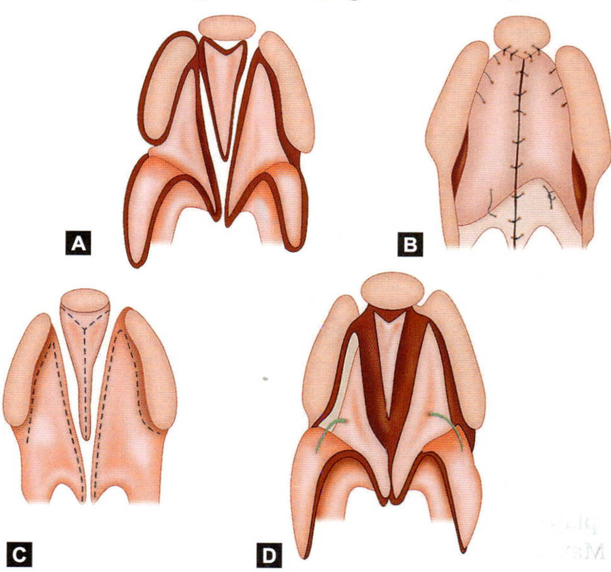

Figs. 71.16A to D: Von Langenbeck repair.

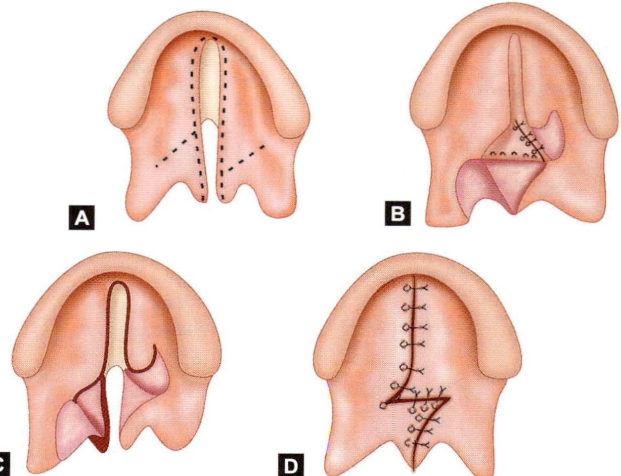

Figs. 71.17A to D: V-Y pushback palatoplasty.

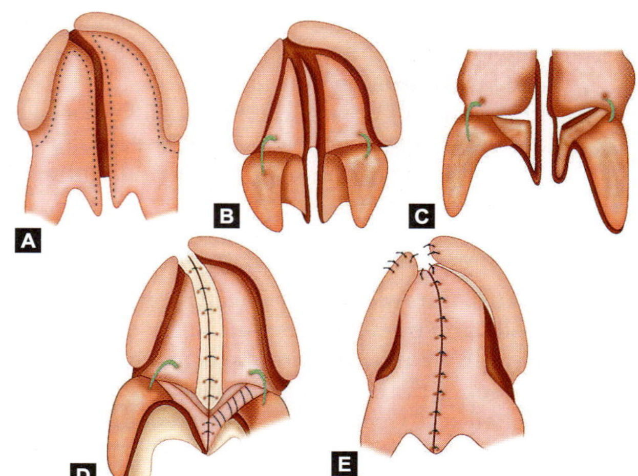

Figs. 71.18A to E: Two-stage repair by Schweckendiek procedure.

Pre- and Post-operative Care of Cleft Patient

- If any sign of an upper respiratory tract infection is seen, then postpone the surgery.
- Because the oral mucosa cannot be properly cleaned preoperatively in the way that the skin can be prepared, it is important to ensure that there are no pathogenic bacteria in the mouth or nasopharynx before embarking on surgery. Bacterial swabs are taken. If group-A hemolytic *Streptococcus* is found, operation is postponed, for there is risk of wound breakdown.
- If presurgical orthopedic appliance is being worn there may be some superficial mucosal ulceration, in which case the appliance should be removed a few days preoperatively.
- The lips should be well massaged with Vaseline after feeds, especially at the angles of the mouth, as this helps to reduce the splitting of mucosa when the mouth is stretched by the gag.
- On admission the child should be weighed and his Hb checked (weight—10 lbs, Hb—10 g, and age 10 weeks.)
- If a baby is breastfed there is no need to change the regime before lip surgery, as it can be safely continued post-operatively. Bottle feeding in post-operative period can damage the lip and it is safer to use a spoon or cup.
- After surgery to palate, a spoon or a cup with short sprout should always be used and it is wise to get the child used to feeding from these preoperatively.
- The last feed before the operation should be given 4 hours beforehand and be followed by sterile water.
- Elbow splints are applied for 3 weeks post-operatively to prevent thumb or finger sucking and other interferences with operation site.
- After palate repair, breast or bottle feeding are contraindicated because the sucking action can cause breakdown of repair.
- Plentiful drinks, with feeds followed by sterile water are adequate to keep the mouth clean and care must be taken to prevent dehydration.

Bone Grafting of Alveolar Cleft Defects

- **Primary bone grafting** refers to bone grafting procedures involving alveolar defects in children younger than 2 years of age.

- **Early secondary bone grafting**—between 2–4 years of age
- **Secondary bone grafting**—between 4–15 years of age
- **Late secondary bone grafting**–in adults

Stage II: Primary Dentiton Stage (18 Months to 5 Years of Age)

Problems of dental occlusion and position of teeth and jaw segments are less marked in the primary than in the secondary dentition. Defects of growth seem to have a progressive effect, the discrepancies between upper and lower jaws becoming more marked throughout the growth period.

The common aberrations seen are:

- **Medial displacement of the maxillary segments**: It occurs soon after repair of cleft of lip and palate, it often is differential displacement, being more marked at the anterior end of the segment, in the region of the primary canine teeth. The posterior end of the segment is often in correct relationship with lower arch
- **Displacement of the premaxillary element:** Premaxillary displacement at this early stage is related to the preoperative position of the premaxilla. Maxillary growth deficiency which positions premaxilla behind the arch of the lower teeth is often not so marked in primary dentition as it is in older child. If premaxilla is not adequately reduced by strapping before lip repair, protrusion tends to persist, particularly if associated with medial displacement of maxillary segment. If there has been severe retraction of premaxilla, there may be vertical discrepancy between premaxilla and maxillary segment because premaxilla rotates backwards and downwards.
- **Alveolar defects**: It is usually limited to aberrations in tooth position, the most common at this stage being palatal eruption of primary upper lateral incisors. There may be space in alveolar arch.
- **Treatment in the primary dentition:** The defects outlined above can cause speech problems. Since these defects are present at an important time during speech development, it would be reasonable to correct them as early as possible. Since the primary teeth roots are small and undergoing progressive resorption, it is more reasonable to attempt segment realignment than tooth repositioning. The maxillary segments can be expanded using fixed splints (W-arch or Arnold expander). If there is sufficient vertical development of the segment to establish positive locking of the occlusion of buccal teeth, particularly of primary canine teeth, the expansion of jaws will be self-retaining, otherwise a mechanical retention is needed. Treatment is mainly focused on establishing and maintaining oral health. Meticulous oral hygiene should be emphasized to reduce development of dental caries. Periodic recalls enable the dentist to intercept areas of decalcification. Adjustments to obturators are also done.

Stage III: Late Primary or Mixed Dentition Stage

The occlusal problems at this stage can be considered under three categories: Problems of dentition, problems of segment alignment and problems of jaw relationship.

- **Problem of dentition:** The most noticeable effects of cleft malformation on teeth are seen with eruption of permanent maxillary incisor teeth. The discrepancies affecting the dentition are:
  - **Malformation of teeth:** Usually affect teeth in immediate vicinity of the cleft, viz. central and lateral incisors. They are usually small, mis-shaped and hypoplastic.
  - **Malposition of teeth:** Central incisor is frequently rotated or tilted and lateral incisors is often high in the cleft.
  - **Anomalies in the number of teeth:** Supernumerary and congenitally missing teeth. Lateral incisor is most usually affected.
- **Segment alignment:** It shows little change in mixed dentition when compared to the primary dentition. The only change at this stage is addition of 1st permanent molars.
- **Jaw relationship:** The relationship between upper and lower jaws in the sagittal plane usually shows relative mandibular prognathism in cleft patients. If jaw growth is defective the condition is usually evident at mixed dentition stage and may be progressive. The first clinical sign is often that permanent upper central incisor erupts into a lingual relationship with lower incisors.

Treatment in the Mixed Dentition Period

This is the stage, which is most often neglected by dentist, as it is believed that since the child has to undergo the main orthodontic treatment in any case, why should the child be treated now?

Repositioning of the anterior dentition in anterior cross bites, as soon as permanent incisors have erupted, may lead to a successful overjet relationship with a normal functional dentoalveolar arch alignment. This may reduce pseudoclass-III dental and mandibular prognathic skeletal dentoalveolar arch growth. Removable appliance with Z spring or antero-posterior expansion screw or a functional appliance such as bite plane or even Frankel's appliance can also be used.

Maxillary expansion to correct posterior segmental collapse is accomplished by quad helix or fixed palatal expander or a removable appliance with midline screw. A retainer for maintaining the expansion must be worn for six months after surgical intervention on a full-time wear basis. After arch expansion has occurred, the bone graft can be placed in defect to maintain a good arch form. Pregraft expansion also widens the clefts site, which allows better access for nasal floor closure.

Secondary alveolar cleft bone graft: Several objectives—

- **Providing bone support to teeth adjacent to cleft site**: Bone should be grafted into the cleft before orthodontic tooth alignment is began. When the cleft is filled with normal viable bone, the orthodontist can proceed with tooth alignment without fear of exposing tooth surface into the cleft site.
- **Providing bone through which tooth can erupt**: When canines and in some cases central incisors are allowed to erupt before bone grating, they often lack adequate periodontal bone support. Eldeeb et al have recommended

that the graft be placed between 9 and 12 years of age when the canine root is one quarter to half formed. They reported that canine subsequently has normal root development and that morphologic conditions will be unaffected by the surgical procedures.

- **Restoring the maxillary arch continuity:** Alveolar ridge contour is restored so that the ability to provide a stable esthetic prosthesis is enhanced.
- **Closure of oronasal fistula:** Often most significant result of bone graft surgery according to patients. Fluid regurgitation and speech problems can be corrected.
- **Supports alar base of nose:** The alar base on cleft side is often depressed because of lack of underlying bone support. Bone grafting can provide support that elevates the alar base.
- Secondary alveolar clefts bone grafting is an important procedure that greatly facilitates total rehabilitation. Not only is speech improved but dental, esthetic and psychological benefits are to be gained

Stage IV: Permanent Dentition Stage (12 to 13 Years of Age)

- **Orthodontic correction**: Some cleft patients require a combined orthodontic surgical approach in the permanent dentition to achieve optimal outcome. Extensive orthodontic correction is needed prior to surgery as good alignment of both arches leads to a stable occlusion post surgery. This allows the supporting bone to recover and the surrounding tissues such as lips, cheeks and tongue to readapt.
- **Surgical correction**: Most surgical procedures involving maxilla and mandible are deferred until teenage years, when maximum growth of jaws has been attained and all permanent teeth except the 3rd molars have erupted. In boys, surgery is delayed until approximately 17–18 years of age; in girls, because of early maturation, surgery sometime after 15 years of age is possible.
  The manner in which maxilla and mandible relate to each other spatially after growth is frequently difficult to predict based on patients appearance as a child, e.g., patient which bilateral cleft lip and palate that has protuberant maxilla and convex profile during childhood may assume a concave facial profile with time. Thus, early treatment with premaxillary segment surgical setback could be potentially deleterious. In patient with severely retrusive maxilla, surgery must be deferred until permanent dentition has erupted since horizontal cuts to free the maxilla must be made above the apices of permanent dentition.
- **Removable prosthesis:** May be required to replace missing teeth. These have to be adjusted to allow eruption of the developing dentition.
- **Fixed prosthesis:** May be required such as Porcelain veneer for malformed or hypoplastic tooth, Maryland bridge, Crown, Fixed bridge with abutment crowns, implants.

SPEECH-LANGUAGE THERAPY

Production of speech is a very complex process. The smooth development of speech depends on the structural and functional adequacy of the relevant anatomical structures. The airstream passes through the glottal opening in the larynx, enters the pharynx and is divided and directed through the oral and nasal cavities. The opening or closing of the nasal cavity is controlled by the velopharyngeal valve. The buildup and release of air within the oral cavity produces the consonant sounds of the language. In case of a cleft palate, where no repair has been done or where air leaks under pressure into the nasal cavity, the child will communicate with a distorted, functionally compromised speech pattern known as 'cleft palate speech'.

Velopharyngeal competence is sealing off of the nasal cavity from the oral cavity, by means of contact between the soft palate and the pharyngeal wall. Hypernasality is a typical sign of velopharyngeal incompetence. Hypernasality mainly affects (p, b, t, d, k, g, f and s) whereas problem of a blocked nasal cavity (denasality will be noticed) mainly affects m, n and g. Hypernasality and denasality has to be differentiated.

Speech is produced with the first cry of the infant. The obturator temporarily closes the cleft hard palate, so that the nasal cavity is separated from the oral cavity. The positioning of the tongue is therefore normalized as it is kept out of the cleft. Suction and drinking are then relatively functional, and these functions stimulate the use of the soft palate muscles.

Recognizable phonetic sounds are produced at the age of 4–6 months. The infant babbles or plays with sounds from this age onwards. It is therefore important that the cleft soft palate should be repaired at about this age. Vocalization control and training in the production of words, immediately preoperatively as well as directly postoperatively after closure of the soft palate is essential.

Functional versus Organic Disorder

Organic disorders are due to velopharyngeal insufficiency whereas functional disorders may originate from a structural disorder, e.g., deviant articulation associated with cleft palate. Articulation is correct development of consonant and vowel sounds. Deviant articulation results from deviant tongue movements or inappropriate constriction of the glottis or pharynx, in an effort to compensate for the lack of adequate intraoral air pressure. Organic disorders (such as nasal escape or nasal resonance) of velopharyngeal insufficiency should be treated surgically, whilst functional disorder should be treated with speech therapy.

The speech therapy consists of 5 stages

1. The correct production of consonants in isolation.
2. Consonants + vowel combination
3. Single words
4. Sentences
5. Everyday speech

Stages 1 and 5 are most difficult to achieve and helped by intensive therapy. Unlike children who have a phonological speech problem, the speech problems of cleft palate children are usually at the basic level of consonants in isolation.

A technique which should produce success with children who direct the air string nasally rather than orally for 's' and 'z' is to work from a pressure consonant they can produce orally, e.g., /t/ and ask them to move their tongue forward from a 'S' (pronounced 'sh') or backwards from a 'ø' 'ø' (pronounced 'th').

If production of a consonant in isolation, e.g., 't' is proving difficult, proprioception neuromuscular facilitation techniques (PNF), e.g., contrasting heat with cold on tongue tip as it comes into contact with the alveolar ridge, or a dental plate with a ridge made where the tongue should touch for 't' (or possibly myofunctional therapy), may solve the problem. Two-point discrimination tasks with toothpicks are also used.

Feedback

A number of therapies/techniques are based on strategies of feedback; palatal training device is one of them. The palatal training appliance consists of an acrylic plate, the posterior edge of which has a loop of orthodontic wire attached to it. This touches the soft palate at rest. The patient is encouraged by this sensation to lift the soft palate. Another aid which consists of acrylic base plate into which is embedded 2 electrodes at the point of contact with the soft palate. When the palate is at rest the current passes through, and a light shows in the control box. When the palate is elevated, the circuit is broken, and the light is extinguished.

Velopharyngeal incompetence due to anatomic disproportion between palate and posterior pharynx: When repaired soft palate is short or the pharynx is too deep to ensure adequate valving, a prosthesis which employs the principle of soft palate lift combined with obturation of the residual velopharyngeal lumen is employed.

Velopharyngeal incompetence due to an immobile palate without disproportion: The objective is to elevate the soft palate to a position approximating that of normal retraction, thereby narrowing the nasopharyngeal orifice. It is also used in treating patients with neuromuscular difficulties and depends on retentive and stabilizing qualities of maxillary part of prosthesis design.

FABRICATION OF PROSTHESIS

The speech prosthesis consists of three parts:

1. Maxillary section
2. Palatal extension
3. Pharyngeal section

Maxillary section: The construction is similar as for partial or complete dentures. It can be made either in acrylic resin or metal.

Palatal extension: This part connects maxillary and pharyngeal section. It is a metal bar which extends beyond the soft palate into the nasopharynx.

Pharyngeal section: This area is developed in a wax or modeling compound or functional impression material and confounds to pharyngeal muscle activity. The so-called muscle trimming or moulding results from patients swallowing and head rotation, flexion and extension which will reproduce an accurate recording of contact with the surrounding musculature during function. The speech bulb is adjusted until the patient can produce a clear 'p', a sustained 'f' or 's' without nasal emission (easily determined by the patient to produce the required sounds, while holding a mirror under the patient's nose), as well as produce adequate nasal sound 'm'.

The design of this bulb should be minimal in size, therefore the span of soft palatal tissue contacting the posterior pharyngeal wall during velopharyngeal closure is not great and also it helps relieve muscular strain and torque on the prosthesis.

ROLE OF PEDODONTIST

- A key member who sees the baby and the parent at the time of repair of the lip.
- Provides presurgical orthopedic treatment for the baby
- Monitors growth and development
- To maintain perfect oral health
- To guide the occlusion and facial growth
- Motivates the parent and child to cooperate with the treatment.

Prenatal and Genetic Counseling

- In the past, prenatal diagnosis of a cleft lip was almost always made in association with other abnormalities in the fetus. With improvements in ultrasound technology, the prenatal diagnosis of isolated cleft lip is increasingly common. However, it is easy to miss cleft lip on diagnostic ultrasounds, particularly those performed for routine indications in the physician's office.
- In the United Kingdom, routine views of the face and lips were added to antenatal ultrasound guidelines in 2000 and detection rates of cleft lip in low-risk populations increased from 16 to 75% with two-dimensional (2D) ultrasound between week 18–23 gestation.
- The use of 3D ultrasound of the face improves detection rate significantly.
- Thus, if there is a family history of clefting or if there is a concern about a possible cleft for other reasons, a referral should be made for a complete diagnostic ultrasound (including 3D images, if possible) and genetic counseling.
- Ultrasound can often establish whether a cleft lip is unilateral or bilateral.
- It is still very difficult to make the diagnosis of a cleft palate antenatally, unless it is detected in association with a large cleft lip.
- Recently, fetal magnetic resonance imaging (MRI) has been used to detect fetal abnormalities including cleft palate, but experience and availability of fetal MRI, however, is extremely limited at this time.
- Once a cleft lip/palate is identified, the family should be referred for genetic counseling to discuss other testing, including amniocentesis. During the genetic counseling session, a complete pregnancy and family history should be performed. This should include information on any teratogenic exposures, and the presence of family members with clefts or other birth defects, developmental problems and genetic syndromes. Even if genetic tests are negative, parents should be informed that an accurate diagnosis and complete discussion of prognosis and recurrence risks can only take place after the baby is born.

- When a cleft lip/palate is detected prenatally, the family should be referred to a cleft lip/palate team to learn about the care and management of children with clefts. At the family's first visit with the cleft lip/palate team, feeding instructions should be provided, and a clear plan for the newborn period should be formulated. Additional medical information provided at this visit should include a general description of the types of problems the baby may encounter. This opportunity to formulate a feeding plan, learn about the future care the child will receive, and meet the providers involved in this care can greatly increase a parent's sense of control and preparedness in the face of this unanticipated diagnosis.
- A dysmorphology or genetics assessment is part of the complete evaluation of every child with a cleft. Parents typically have many questions about the etiology of clefts to be addressed by the cleft lip/palate team. There is considerable cultural and social variability in family attitudes towards birth defects and their causation. These issues should be explored and, when appropriate, correct information supplied, recognizing that western medical information will not necessarily supplant other cultural and ethnic beliefs.
- Since genetic factors play a role in clefting conditions even in the nonsyndromic child, information on causation and empirical recurrence risks should be provided to all families with clefts based upon the family history. For parents with one affected child, the recurrence risk for future pregnancies is 2–5%. This risk increases if there are additional family members with clefts.
- Condition-specific recurrence risks and prenatal testing options should be provided to families of a child with syndromic clefting condition. Parents should be informed of the option of ultrasonography for future pregnancies. Similarly, a discussion regarding the potential preventive role of preconception/prenatal folate supplementation and avoidance of environmental risk factors (tobacco smoke, alcohol, and isotretinoin) should be considered.
- The advantage of dealing with the child in these separate stages, with distinct targets in mind, within set time scales is to avoid the parent and the child making frequent visits throughout the child's developing years. All clinicians involved in the treatment of cleft palate child should recognize that above all he or she is a developing child who should be allowed and encouraged to live life as normally as possible.

POINTS TO REMEMBER

- Le Monnier in 1764 operated a cleft of the palate surgically, mainly to facilitate eating and drinking.
- *Cleft lip:* Congenital deformity of the upper lip that varies from a notching to a complete division of the lip; any degree of clefting can exist.
- *Cleft palate:* A congenital split of the palate that may extend through the uvula, soft palate, and into the hard palate; the lip may or may not be involved in the cleft of the palate.
- Theories of clefting are Dursy—failure of fusion between median nasal and maxillary process; Veau's hypothesis—failure of ingrowth of mesoderm between the two palatal shelves, alternations in intrinsic palatal forces, excessive tongue resistance, fusion of shelves with subsequent breakdown, failure of tongue to drop down, and inclusion cyst pathology.
- Etiology of clefting is due to heredity, teratogens, chromosomal aberrations, increased maternal age, decreased blood supply in nasomaxillary region and deficiency of folic acid and vitamin A.
- Classification of cleft lip/cleft palate are Davis and Ritchie's classification; Veau's classification; based on embryology (Fogh-Anderson classification, Kernahan's and Starks classification, American Cleft Palate Association); and based on graphic methods of recording clefts (Pfeiffer classification, Kernahan's striped Y classification, Millard's modification of stripped Y classification, Tessier system of classification of orofacial clefts).
- Dental problems with cleft patients are congenital missing teeth, neonatal teeth, ectopic eruption, supernumerary teeth, enamel hypoplasia, deep bite, crossbite, crowding or spacing of teeth.
- Management of clefting firstly includes taking care of the neonate which is mainly dealing with feeding. Special bottles and teats are available for accomplishing this task. The next step is the maxillary orthopedic stage in which treatment modalities are feeding obturators, presurgical orthopedics, surgical management of cleft lip and surgical management of cleft palate. The next stage is primary dentition stage in which essence is on restoration and maintenance. Subsequent to this is mixed dentition stage which deals with malalignments and the last stage is permanent dentition stage where fixed orthodontic treatments are done.
- "Rule of Ten" is an important criterion for lip repair. It states that at the time of surgery the age of the child should not be less than 10 weeks of age, have no less than 10 g% of hemoglobin, and should weigh at least 10 pounds.
- Surgical lip closure (3–9 months): Millard's repair, Tennison-Randall repair, Veau's repair, and Rose-Thompson repair.
- Surgical plate repair (10–18 months): Single stage by Von Langenbeck repair and V-Y pushback palatoplasty and two-stage repair by soft palate repair at 18 months and hard palate repair at 4 years by Schweckendiek procedure.

Questionnaire

1. Discuss the development of palate.
2. Describe the etiopathogenesis of clefting.
3. Classify the clefts.
4. What are the dental features of cleft patients?
5. Describe the cleft management team.
6. Write a note on feeding management of a cleft neonate.
7. What is the age specific management of cleft child?
8. Explain the treatment plan of managing a child with cleft lip and palate with special reference to the cleft lip surgery.
9. Write a note on prenatal genetic counseling of clefts.
10. What are the different techniques of Presurgical Infant Orthopedics (PSIO)?

FURTHER READING

1. American Cleft Palate-Craniofacial Association. Parameters for the evaluation and treatment of patients with cleft lip/ palate or other craniofacial anomalies. Cleft Palate Craniofac J. 1993;30 Suppl:S1-16.
2. American Cleft Palate-Craniofacial Association. Team Standards Self-Assessment Instrument; 1996.
3. Batra P, Duggal R, Prakash H. Genetics of cleft lip and palate revisited. J Clin Pediatr Dent. 2003;27(4):311-20.
4. Berkowitz S. Standards of care for cleft lip and palate. The Cleft Palate Story. Chicago: Quintessence Publishing Co. Inc; 1994.
5. Chakravati A. Finding needles in haystacks—IRF6 gene variants in isolated cleft lip and palate. N Engl J Med. 2004; 351:822-4.
6. Cleft Palate Foundation. As You Get Older: Information for teens born with cleft lip and palate; 2002.

7. Cleft Palate Foundation. Cleft lip and cleft palate: The First Four Years; 2001.
8. Cleft Palate Foundation. Cleft Lip and Palate: The school-aged child; 1998.
9. Cleft Palate Foundation. Feeding an infant with a cleft; 2002.
10. Cleft Palate Foundation. The Genetics of cleft lip and palate: Information for families; 2001.
11. Cohen MM. Etiology and pathogenesis of clefting. Oral Maxillofac Surg Clin North Am. 2000;12(3):379-96.
12. CRANE. The Annual Report of the Cleft Lip and Palate Register for England and Wales from the Cleft Development Group; 2005.
13. Ghi T, Tani G, Savelli L, et al. Prenatal imaging of facial clefts by magnetic resonance imaging with emphasis on the posterior palate. Prenat Diagn. 2003; 23:970-5.
14. Hanikeri M, Savundra J, Gillett D, et al. Antenatal transabdominal ultrasound detection of cleft lip and palate in Western Australia from 1996 to 2003. Cleft Palate Craniofac J. 2006; 43:61-5.
15. Johnson N, Sandy J. Prenatal diagnosis of cleft lip and palate. Cleft Palate Craniofac J. 2003; 40:186-9.
16. LaRossa D. The state of the art in cleft palate surgery. Cleft Palate Craniofac J. 2000;37(3):225-8.
17. Millard D, Latham R. Improved primary surgical and dental treatment of clefts. Plast Reconstr Surg. 1990; 86:856-71.
18. Moller KT, Starr CD. Cleft Palate: Interdisciplinary Issues and Treatment. Austin, TX: Office of Maternal and Child Health US Department of Health and Human Services; 1987.
19. Mulliken JB. Primary repair of bilateral cleft lip and nasal deformity. Plast Reconstr Surg. 2001;108(1):181-94.
20. Redford-Badwal DA, Mabry K, Frassinelli JD. Impact of cleft lip and palate on nutritional health and oral motor development. Dent Clin North Am. 2003; 47:305-17.
21. Rivkin CJ, Keith O, Crawford PJ, et al. Dental care of patients with cleft lip and palate from birth to mixed dentition stage. Br Dent J. 2000;188(2):78-83.
22. Schendel SA. Unilateral cleft lip repair—state of the art. Cleft Palate Craniofac J. 2000;37(4):335-41.
23. Sloan GM. Posterior pharyngeal flap and sphincter pharyngoplasty: the state of the art. Cleft Palate Craniofac J. 2000;37(2):112-22.
24. Sphrintzen RJ, Bardach J. Cleft palate speech management: a multidisciplinary approach. St Louis: Mosby; 1995.
25. The Center for Children with Special Health Needs Children's Hospital and Regional Medical Center. Cleft Lip and Palate Elements of Critical Care, 4th edition. Seattle, WA; 2006.
26. Turner SR, Rumsey N, Sandy JR. Psychological aspect of cleft lip and plate. Euro J Orthod. 1998; 20:407-15.
27. Wilcox AJ, Lie RT, Solvoll K, et al. Folic acid supplements and risk of facial clefts: national population-based case-control study. BMJ. 2007; 334:464.
28. Wyszynski D. Cleft Lip and Palate: From origin to treatment. New York: Oxford University Press; 2002.

Prosthodontic Management of Pediatric Patient and Implants in Pediatric Dentistry

Pragati Kaurani, Vivek Lath, Nilesh Rathi

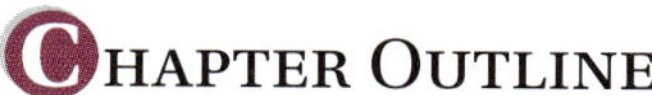

Chapter Outline

- Prosthodontic Rehabilitation with Crowns
- Fixed Partial Denture
- Resin-bonded Retainers
- Removable Partial Denture
- Complete Denture Rehabilitation in Ectodermal Dysplasia Patients
- Overdentures in Children
- Obturators
- Maxillofacial Prosthesis
- Implants in Pediatric Dentistry

The current status of caries may be decreasing all over the world, but there are many issues which still affect and cause loss of teeth in children such as trauma, neoplasm, systemic disorders, infection, congenital abnormalities such as clefts or inborn defects such as ectodermal dysplasia. Some of the esthetic treatment needs resulting from these conditions can be managed with resin bonding procedures and porcelain laminate veneers, and whenever possible they should be considered as the treatment of first choice. When these procedures have not been able to provide a satisfactory result or when there are missing teeth, then prosthodontic procedures such as single crowns, fixed partial dentures (FPDs), implant prostheses, or removable prosthesis are indicated.

Because children are often affected psychologically by the unacceptable appearance of diseased, damaged, or missing teeth, one should not allow chronologic age to preclude performing whatever treatment is necessary to provide proper function and esthetics. If the teeth involved are fully erupted, have achieved complete root formation, and may be prepared without causing irreversible damage to the pulp, successful prosthodontic treatment can often be provided for patients as young as 12–14 years of age.

Prosthodontic treatment options

A. *Fixed prosthesis:*
   - Single crowns:
     - Anterior crowns
     - Posterior crowns
   - Fixed partial dentures:
     - Full veneer retainers
     - Partial veneer retainers
     - Resin-bonded retainers
   - *Radicular retained prosthesis (post and core):* Implant prosthesis

B. *Removable prosthesis:*
   - Overdentures
   - Removable partial dentures
   - Implant retained prosthesis

C. *Maxillofacial prosthesis*:
   - Obturators
   - Rehabilitation prosthesis

D. *Prosthesis in special case considerations.*

Prosthodontics in children is more challenging because of the anatomy, erupting teeth, growth patterns, patient cooperation, and understanding. Pediatric patients may be required to follow-up more often than adult patients needing procedures like relines or refits of removable prosthesis because of growth patterns. There are various prosthodontic treatment options that can be rendered to a patient with missing teeth. However, careful diagnosis and understanding of the clinical findings is essential for the success of the treatment.

PROSTHODONTIC REHABILITATION WITH CROWNS

All-ceramic Crowns

- These are the most esthetic complete coverage restorations currently available in dentistry.
- Optimal longevity with all-ceramic crowns requires normal tooth preparation form because the prepared tooth must provide support for the restoration. Therefore, if a large portion of tooth structure is missing because of trauma, caries, or if previous restorations become dislodged during tooth reduction, then a separate restoration that is well-retained in remaining tooth structure should be placed to establish an ideal preparation form.
- All ceramic crowns are able to achieve superior esthetics.
- Patients with heavy occlusal forces, parafunctional habits are a definite contraindication to receive all ceramic crowns.
- It is essential that the centric occlusal contacts are located over the cingulum concavity.

Tooth Preparation for an All-ceramic Crown

A well-defined shoulder margin with 0.8 mm depth is recommended to provide the marginal integrity of the restoration. The finish line should be smooth and uniform around the entire tooth with uniform reduction of the axial walls of 0.8 mm. The lingual reduction is recommended of about 1 mm with 1.5–2 mm reduction on the incisal edges **(Fig. 72.1)**. The margin placement should be equigingival. Subgingival placement of the margins should be avoided in adolescent patients as it can lead to accelerated recession of the gingiva or interfere with the normal relocation of the gingiva as the patient matures **(Figs. 72.2A to C)**.

- Possess a well-defined smooth shoulder finish line that is 0.8 mm deep.
- Axial surfaces reduced to a depth of 0.8 mm.

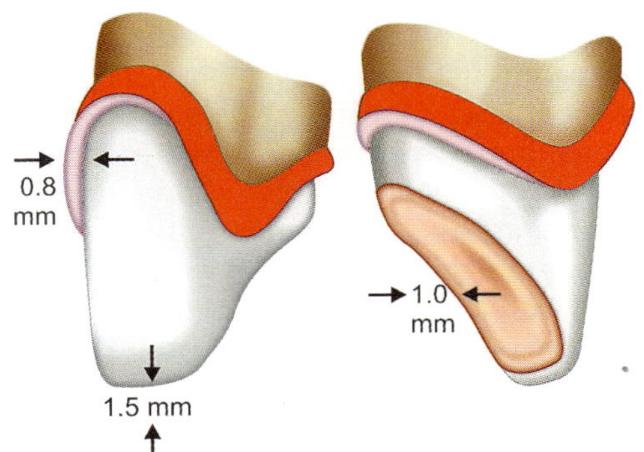

Fig. 72.1: Two views of all-ceramic (porcelain jacket crown) preparation showing recommended reduction depths and shoulder finish line.

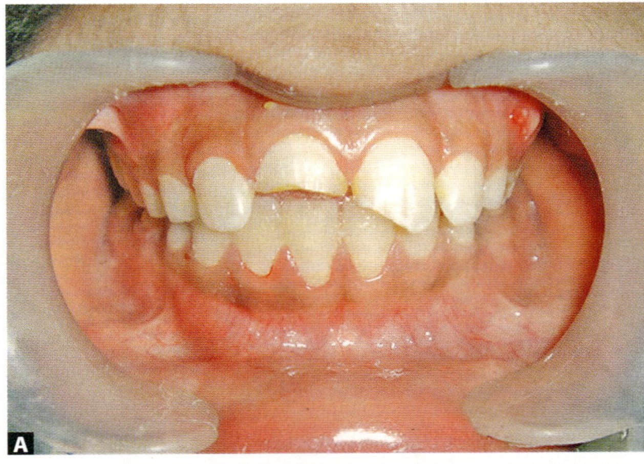

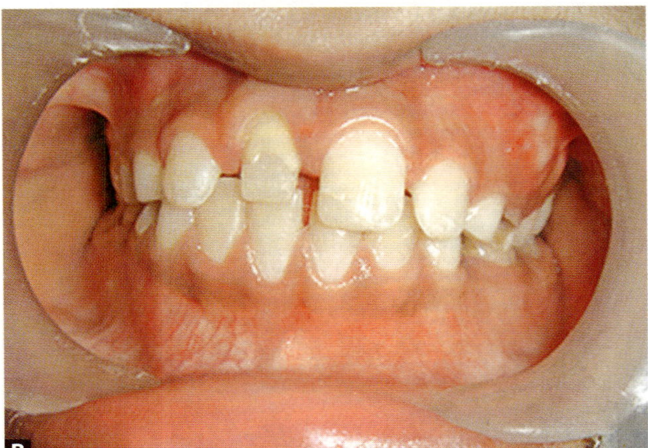

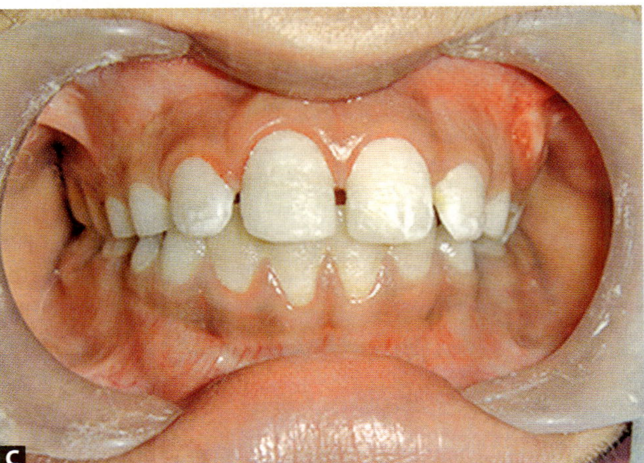

Figs. 72.2A to C: All-ceramic crown fabrication.

- The lingual reduction for occlusal clearance should be 1.0 mm.
- An incisal edge reduction of 1.5–2.0 mm.

Metal Ceramic Crowns

When the ideal tooth preparation form is compromised or the magnitude of occlusal forces contraindicates an all-ceramic crown, stronger metal ceramic crown is indicated **(Figs. 72.3A to C)**.

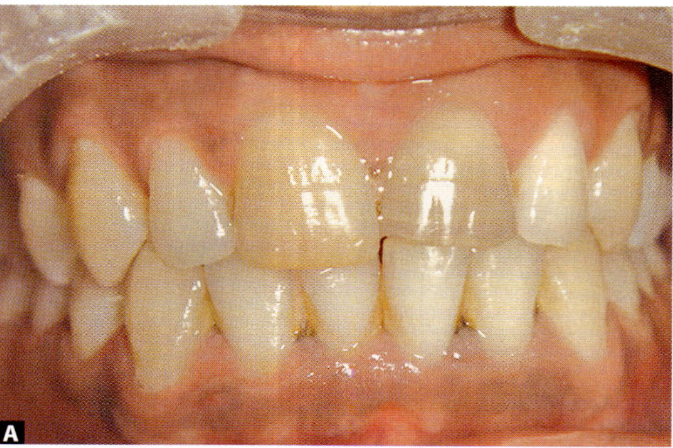

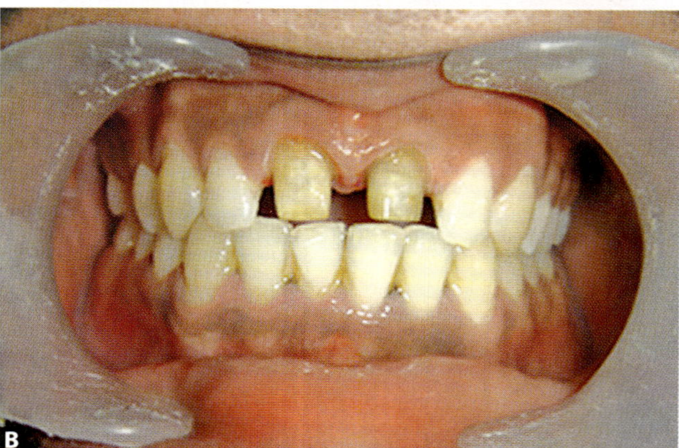

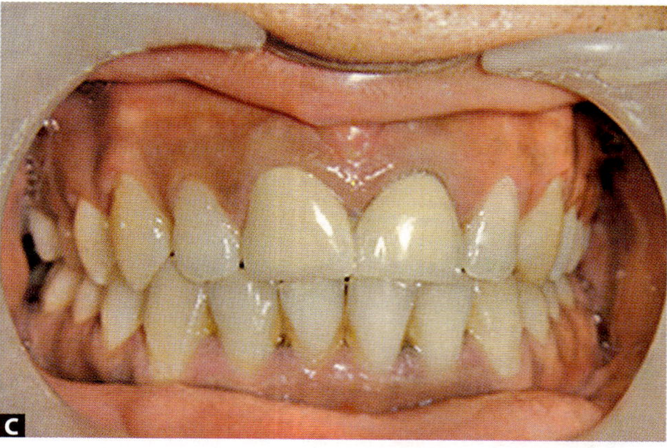

Figs. 72.3A to C: Porcelain fused metal (PFM) crown fabrication.

Tooth Preparation Design for Metal Ceramic Crown

This restoration consists of a ceramic layer bonded to a thin cast metal coping that fits over the tooth preparation. These restorations combine the strength and accurate fit of a cast crown with the cosmetic effect of a ceramic crown. The labial surface is prepared with over all 1.2 mm reduction using planar reduction.

The palatal surface is reduced maintaining the tooth anatomy. A uniform reduction of 1.5 mm is done and sufficient clearance from the opposing teeth is maintained. 2 mm of incisal reduction is desirable to achieve optimum esthetics **(Fig. 72.4)**.

- Possess a well-defined smooth chamfer finish line that is 1 mm deep
- Lingually finish line should not be more than 0.5 mm
- The lingual reduction for occlusal clearance should be 1.0 mm
- An incisal edge reduction of 2.0 mm.

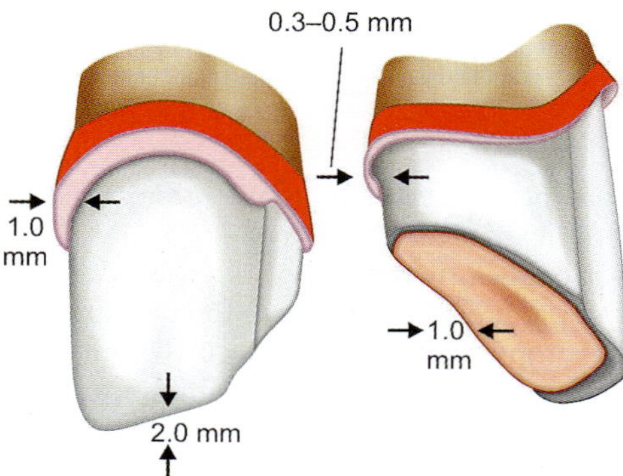

Fig. 72.4: Two views of metal ceramic crown preparation showing minimal facial reduction and shoulder finish line, minimal incisal reduction, lingual axial reduction depth and chamfer finish line, and lingual reduction for occlusal clearance.

Crown in Single Posterior Tooth

- When all or most of the axial surfaces of a posterior tooth have been affected by caries, or they have been restored or endodontically treated, the tooth requires a full crown.
- The preparation is started by the occlusal reduction of about 1.5 mm on the functional cusps and 1.0 mm on the nonfunctional cusps. The axial reduction of the buccal and the lingual walls is done to obtain a uniform chamfer finish line. Functional cusp bevel is placed on the buccal inclines of the mandibular buccal cusps and lingual inclines of the maxillary lingual cusps. All sharp angles in the preparation are rounded **(Figs. 72.5A to D)**.

Crowns with Post and Core Build-up

- For the teeth that do not have sufficient coronal structure for the support of the crown, radicular retained restorations with core build-ups should be done.
- Used in teeth with pulpal involvement when remaining coronal tooth structure does not provide adequate retention for the definitive restoration.
- The posts are primarily used to retain a core in the tooth with extensive loss of tooth structure.
- The post can be of a variety of materials like metal, fiber, glass fiber or preformed depending on the requirement of the operating dentist. Any type of post can be used anywhere, however glass fiber posts are more indicated in anterior region where esthetics is of prime importance and metal posts are used in posterior teeth where load bearing capacity is of significance.
- After the endodontic treatment of the tooth, up to 2/3rd obturative material is removed (only apical 3–6 mm for maintaining the apical seal). The canal is prepared to receive a post of appropriate length and width. The post is then cemented, and core build-up is done with a restorative material like composite. Once sufficient coronal structure is restored, it is prepared to receive a crown **(Figs. 72.6A to I)**.

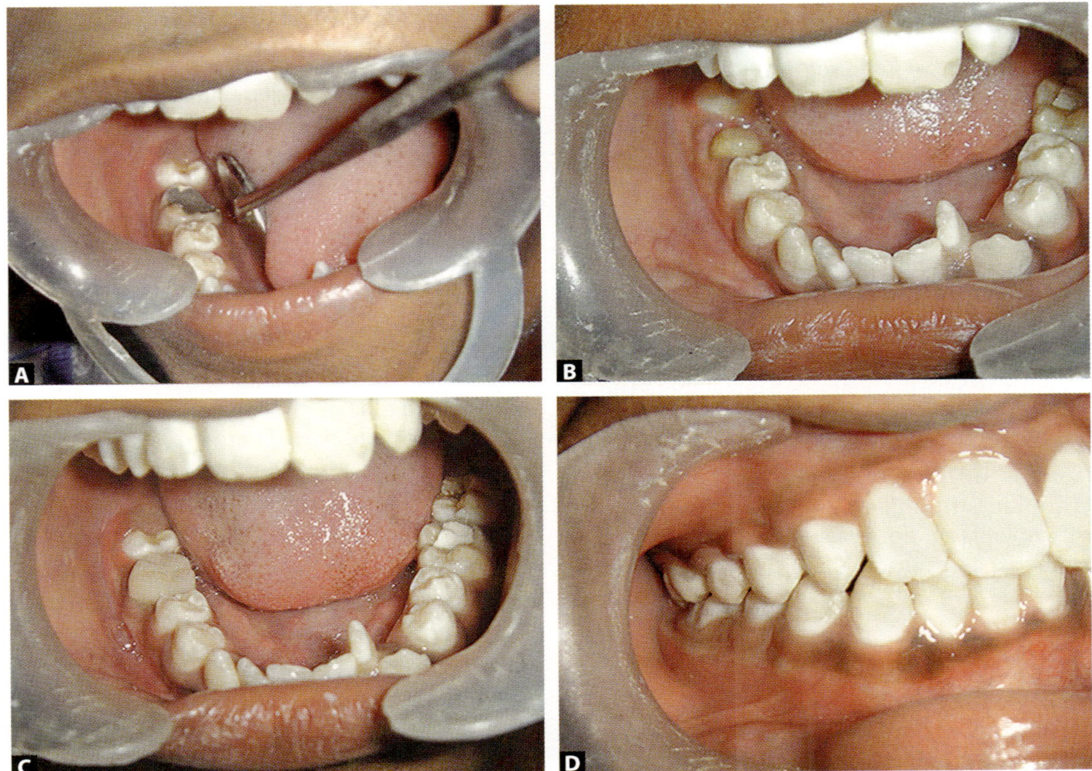

Figs. 72.5A to D: Posterior ceramic crown placement.

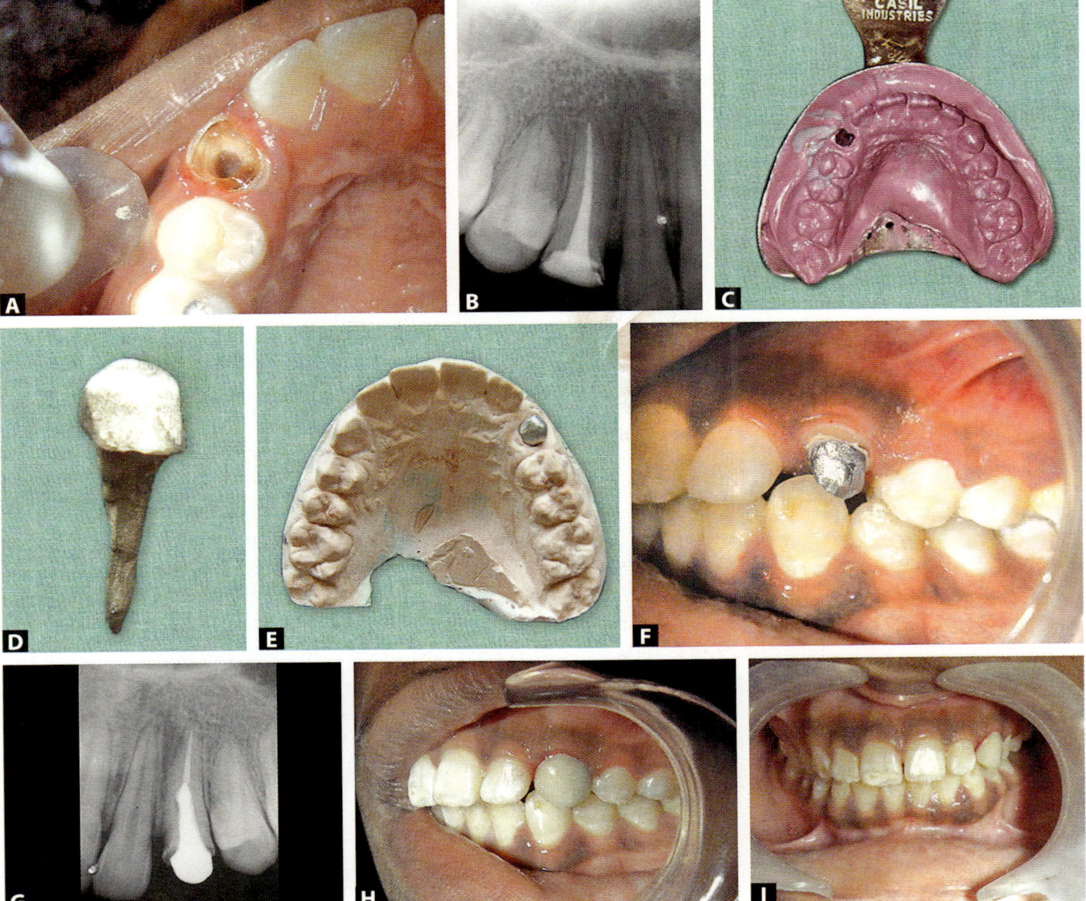

Figs. 72.6A to I: Post and core with crown.

FIXED PARTIAL DENTURE

- *Fixed partial dentures is a tooth-borne partial denture that is intended to be permanently attached to teeth or roots that furnish support to the restorations* **(Figs. 72.7A and B)**.
- Fixed partial denture can be defined as a partial denture that is lasted or securely retained to natural teeth, roots, or dental implant abutment that furnishes primary support for prosthesis glossary of prosthodontic term (GPT).
- In a child, when a tooth is lost the space maintenance should be provided immediately to prevent tipping or rotation of the abutment teeth or eruption of the opposite teeth. A FPD usually requires complete coronal preparations of the abutment teeth to receive the retainers. Thus, it should not be given in teeth with high pulp horns. In case of children, it is now advisable to place an interim prosthesis like removable partial denture (RPD), wait till the growth is completed and then replace the missing teeth using implants. However, if implants cannot be given or are not indicated, FPD becomes an appropriate definitive treatment plan.

Indications

- Missing teeth
- Endodontically treated teeth
- Congenital malformed or missing teeth
- For obtaining proper function and esthetics.

Contraindications

- Age of patient (young or advanced age)
- Great length of edentulous span
- Excessive bone loss in area of missing teeth.

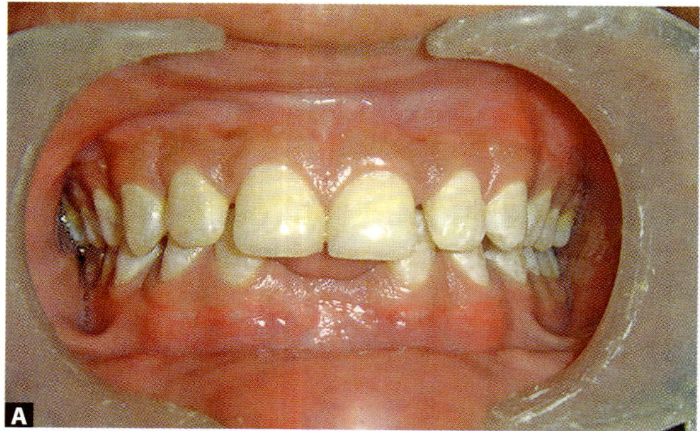

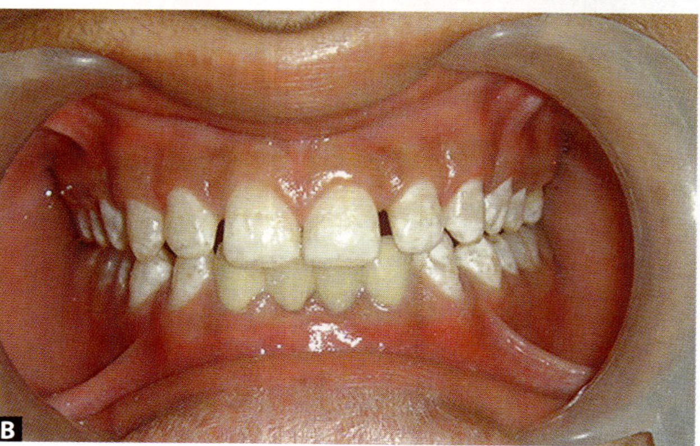

Figs. 72.7A and B: Missing teeth and fixed denture rehabilitation.

Components of a Fixed Partial Denture

- **Retainers:** The retainers used can be full veneer crowns or can be resin-bonded retainers.
- **Connectors:** It is the portion of a fixed partial prosthesis that unites the retainer and pontic.
- **Pontics:** It is an artificial tooth on a fixed dental prosthesis that replaces a missing natural tooth, restores function, and usually fills the space previously occupied by the clinical crown.

Treatment Options for Single or Multiple Missing Teeth

- Porcelain fused to metal FPD
- All metal FPD
- Resin-bonded partial denture
- All ceramic partial denture
- Cantilever prosthesis.

Technique

Clinical and Laboratory Steps in Fixed Partial Denture (Metal Crown)

Clinical steps	*Laboratory steps*
• Examination, diagnosis, and treatment planning	• Die preparation
• Tooth preparation	• Articulation of dies and casts
• Impression of the prepared tooth	• Wax pattern fabrication and casting
• Temporization	• Finishing and polishing
• Cementation	

Clinical and Laboratory Steps in Fixed Partial Denture (Porcelain Fused to Metal Crown)

Clinical steps	*Laboratory steps*
• Examination, diagnosis, and treatment planning	• Die preparation
• Tooth preparation	• Articulation of dies and casts
• Impression of the prepared tooth	• Wax pattern fabrication and casting of coping
• Temporization	• Ceramic builds up
• Coping trial and shade matching	• Finishing
• Bisque trial	
• Cementation	

RESIN-BONDED RETAINERS

Recent advances in bonding techniques have encouraged the use of more conservative approach towards replacing missing teeth, i.e., using resin-bonded retainers. They were first introduced by **Rochette** in 1973. These prostheses are most ideal to be given in a young patient as the preparation of the teeth is minimal reducing any damage to the pulp. However, case selection is extremely important as these bridges cannot withstand stronger occlusal forces or cannot replace more number of teeth. **Dunne** and **Millar** found higher success rates with single pontics than long span prosthesis.

Indications

- Most common indication is congenitally missing single anterior teeth, e.g., lateral incisor.
- Missing mandibular incisors.

Contraindications

- Patients with affected enamel like enamel hypoplasia as bonding is poor.
- Replacement of posterior teeth. Replacements in cases with parafunctional activity.
- It cannot be given where there is crowding in the abutment teeth.

Advantages

- Minimal tooth preparation thereby preventing any trauma to the pulp. Ideal for large pulp horns.
- Excellent esthetics as the labial surface of the teeth is not prepared.
- Local anesthesia need not be administered as the preparation is minimal.

Disadvantages

- Most common failure noted is frequent debonding of the prosthesis.
- The laboratory techniques for fabrication have to be very exacting for a perfect fit of the restoration.

REMOVABLE PARTIAL DENTURE

- Removable partial denture *is defined as any prosthesis that replaces some teeth in a partial dentate arch. It can be removed from mouth and replaced at will (GPT)* **(Figs. 72.8A to D)**.
- When treatment is planned for an adolescent patient who needs a RPD, there are three major objectives:
  1. The restoration of the functions of mastication and speech.
  2. The restoration of dental and facial esthetics.
  3. The preservation of the remaining teeth and their supportive tissues.

Indications

- Long edentulous span contraindicated for FPD
- Distal extension cases
- Compromised periodontal support of remaining teeth
- Purpose of achieving cross arch stabilization
- Excessive bone loss
- Replacement of teeth immediately after extraction.

Contraindications

- When FPD is possible
- Esthetics a primary concern in replacing less number of anterior teeth.
- Disabled patients who cannot maintain RPD.

Design of the Partial Denture

The RPD is made of acrylic resin that could be either heat cured or self cured. These resins provide advantages like ease of fabrication, biocompatibility, and adequate strength to with stand occlusal forces. As the patient is a growing child, refabrication, relines, repairs, or minor adjustments of the partial denture can be easily done with an acrylic denture as compared to a cast partial denture. An acrylic RPD consists of:

- Denture base
- Retentive clasps
- Artificial teeth.

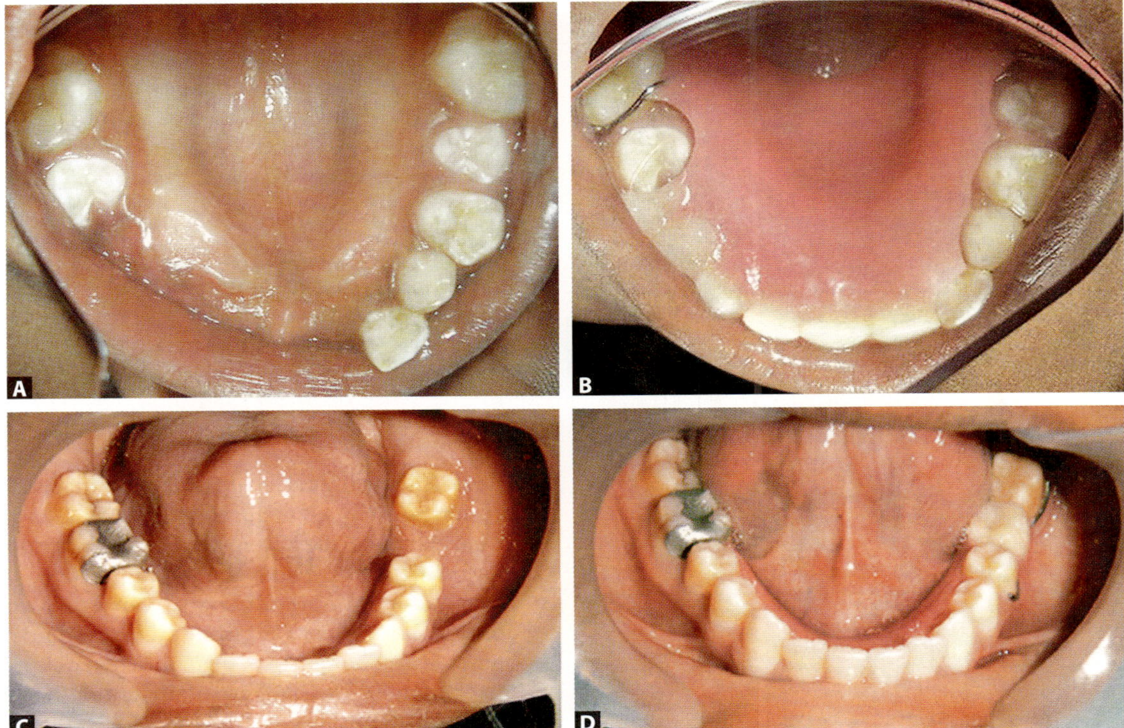

Figs. 72.8A to D: Removable partial denture.

Advantages

- Removable prosthesis can be easily relined and refitted.
- Removable prosthesis can be used as space maintainers.
- They are easy to fabricate and economical option for the patient.
- Maintenance of oral hygiene is easy as it is a removable prosthesis.

Disadvantages

- Patient cooperation is essential as it is a removable prosthesis.
- The patient has to be motivated to wear the prosthesis.
- It may be uncomfortable for the patient due to palatal coverage.
- Accidental aspirations of the prosthesis may occur.

Steps for Construction of Removable Partial Denture

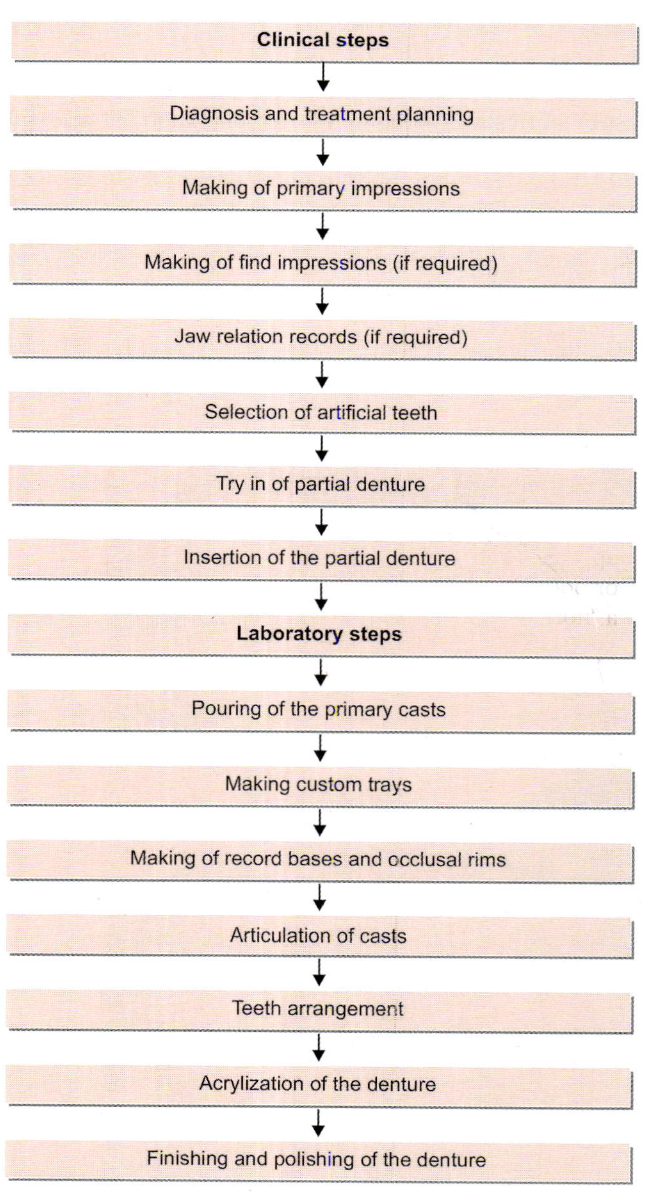

COMPLETE DENTURE REHABILITATION IN ECTODERMAL DYSPLASIA PATIENTS

There are a lot of conditions which cause anodontia in patients and warrant the need of complete denture rehabilitation in pedodontics. The most important and commonly encountered condition is ectodermal dysplasia.

The term "ectodermal dysplasias" indicates a heterogeneous group of hereditary diseases involving the epidermis and its appendages. Freire-Maia-Pinheiro have described 154 patterns of ectodermal dysplasias, divided them into 11 subgroups, and then classified them according to the involved structures (the hair, the teeth, and some or all of the sweat glands). The most frequent form is the Christ-Siemens-Touraine syndrome, a recessive autosomal disorder characterized by an anomalous development of the ectodermal structures and depending on the severity of clinical manifestations; it can be classified as hypohidrotic ectodermal dysplasia or as anhidrotic ectodermal dysplasia.

The hypohidrotic-anhidrotic type or Christ-Siemens-Touraine syndrome was first described in 1848 by **Thurman**, and is characterized by the triad of hypotrichosis (skin, hair, and nail anomalies), either hypodontia, or anodontia and hypohidrosis (partial or total absence of exocrine sweat glands) and other features such as frontal bossing, saddle-shaped nose, everted lips, etc. The hidrotic type was first defined in 1929 by **Clouston** and is distinguished by hypotrichosis, lingual dystrophy and hyperkeratosis of the palms and soles.

The etiology of this disease is unknown; nevertheless, genetic studies showed ectodermal dysplasia is due to a mutation of the gene "*EDA*" (ectodermal dysplasias anhidrotic). This gene is located in position q12 to q13 of the chromosome X. The *EDA* gene encodes a predicted transmembrane protein of 135 amino acids found to be expressed in keratinocytes, hair follicles, and sweat glands. The mutation responsible for ectodermal dysplasia has been thought to be attributed to a change in the histidine/tyrosine in position 54 of the protein. Another mutation (A1270G) has also been revealed to be responsible for Tyr343Cys substitution in a patient with anhidrotic ectodermal dysplasia.

Clinical Signs

- Tri chondrodysplasia (abnormal hair)
- Abnormal dentition
- Onchondysplasia (abnormal nails)
- Dyshidrosis (abnormal or missing sweat glands).

Manifestations

- The skin is usually dry, scaly, and easily irritated as a result of poorly developed or absent oil glands.
- Sweat glands can be absent, few, or nonfunctioning which may result in a high body temperature.
- Scalp hair may be absent, sparse, very fine pigmented, or abnormal in texture. Eyebrows, eyelashes, and other body hair may also be sparse or absent. When hair is present, it may be fragile, dry, and generally unruly because of the lack of oil glands.
- Recurrent ocular infections

- Chronic rhinitis
- Dystrophic nails
- Epistaxis
- Dysphagia
- Dysphonia
- Alopecia
- Extramedullary hematopoiesis of cranial dura
- Diminished resistance to respiratory infections
- Nasopharyngeal rhabdomyosarcoma
- Supraorbital ridges, frontal bossing, and a saddle nose
- The nose may appear pinched and the ala hypoplastic
- **Dental features include:** Complete or partial anodontia of the primary and permanent dentition, malformation of teeth, peg-shaped incisors and canines, primary second molar tooth, if present, is mostly affected by taurodontism, absence or deficiency of alveolar ridges, reduced vertical dimension, vermilion border disappears, maxilla may be underdeveloped and the lips thick and prominent.

The oral rehabilitation of these cases is often difficult, and patients must be attentively followed by a multidisciplinary team involving pediatric dentistry, orthodontics, prosthodontics, and oral-maxillofacial surgery. The patient's age, the pattern of dysplasia, and the morphology of the alveolar ridges influence dental treatment. Following factors should be considered when constructing complete dentures in a child:

- Patients using dentures during growth years must be examined periodically (at least once a year, to assess the need to reline/rebase or remake depending on the fit). It has been observed that the dentures need to be relined every 2–4 years, while they need replacement every 4–6 years. The number of reline procedures necessary is directly related to the growth patterns of the child.
- As permanent teeth erupt, the dentures must be relieved internally to accommodate them.
- Once full growth of the patient takes place, it has been noticed that the dentures function well for about 10 years.
- It has been seen that mandibular dentures fracture at the midline due to its shape to accommodate the narrow anterior mandibular ridge. Thus, the acrylic resin in this region needs to be thick enough to resist fractures.
- It can be very challenging to make a preliminary diagnostic impression in a child due to limited mouth opening and developing swallowing mechanisms. It has been recommended to make the mandibular impression and then the maxillary impression in order to decrease anxiety in a child. The usage of higher viscosity and fast setting irreversible hydrocolloid material is helpful in preventing aspiration of the impression material. The impression of the mandibular arch is recommended before the maxillary to avoid gagging.
- Various impression materials such as irreversible hydrocolloid, polysulfide rubber base, and vinyl polysiloxane have been described in the literature. Some clinicians have used border molding techniques, using a warm green stick compound prior to making the final impression. However, this technique has limited advantages for a child because of the requisite time, patient discomfort related to the procedure, and potential risk of thermal injury.

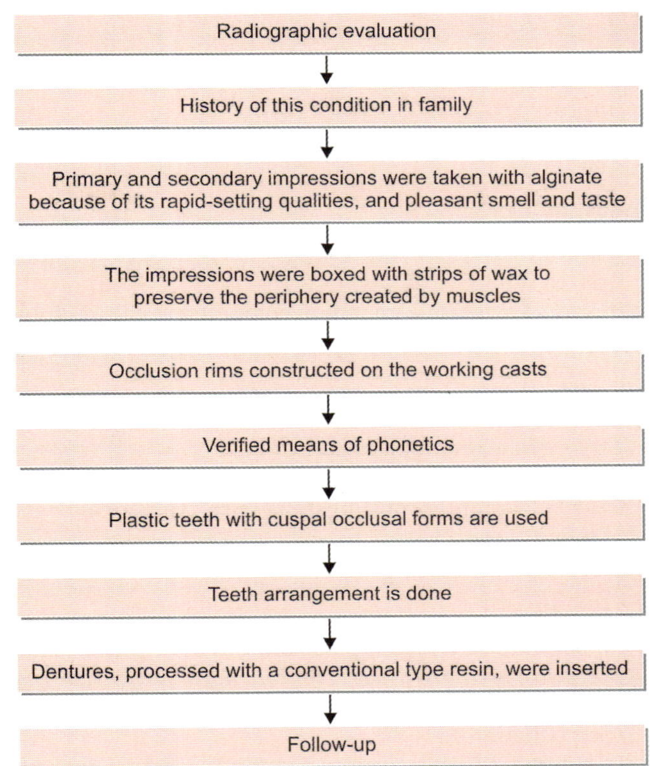

- **Jaw relations:** In case of young children, recording jaw relations may be difficult as neuromuscular development is completed only by seven years.
- **Teeth selection and arrangement:** Sometimes adult incisor teeth can be incorporated to simulate a mixed dentition. Selection of posterior teeth molds is done based on the arch size and space availability. It has been recommended to use monoplane occlusion due to its simplicity and freedom of mandibular movement for the growing child. Attention must be paid to incorporating this spacing to make the prosthesis look natural and age appropriate. It has also been advocated to incorporate an orthodontic arch wire in the denture prosthesis to simulate a "normal" appearance.

OVERDENTURES IN CHILDREN

- *Overdenture is defined as any removable dental prosthesis that covers and rests on one or more remaining natural teeth, roots of natural teeth, and/or implants.*
- It is a complete or a partial removable denture supported by retained roots to provide support, stability, tactile, and proprioceptive sensation.
- The retained roots or teeth are called an abutments and are treated to receive the overdenture. The abutments usually require intentional endodontics as the coronal structure is reduced to receive the denture.

Advantages

- Presence of abutments preserves bone and improves proprioception.
- As the support is derived from the abutments and the denture bearing mucosa, the stability and retention

of the dentures is superior compared to conventional dentures.
- Masticatory efficiency is markedly increased.
- Improved speech
- Increased psychological support for the patient.

Disadvantages

- It requires more clinical settings thus greater cooperation from the child.
- It is more expensive treatment compared to conventional dentures as abutments need to be treated.

Complications

- Abutment teeth prone to decay
- Patient compliance is must
- Recall of 6 months must be done to re-evaluate the need of reline or refit.

OBTURATORS

- *An obturator is a disk or plate, natural or artificial, which closes an opening or defect of the maxilla as a result of a cleft palate or partial or total removal of maxilla for a tumor mass* (**Chalian** 1971).
- It is derived from a Latin word "Obturare" meaning to stop up.

Indications

- To act as a framework over which tissues may be shaped by the surgeon.
- To serve as a temporary prosthesis during the period of surgical correction.
- To restore a patient's cosmetic appearance rapidly for social contacts.
- When surgical primary closure is contraindicated as the patient's age contraindicates surgery.
- When the local avascular condition of the tissues contraindicates surgery.
- When the patient is susceptible to recurrence of the original lesion which produced the deformity.

Uses

- For feeding purposes.
- It may be used to keep the wound or defective area clean and may enhance the healing of traumatic or postsurgical defects.
- It may help to reshape and reconstruct the palatal contour and/or soft palate.
- It improves speech or, in some instances makes speech possible. In the impression area of esthetics, the obturator can be used to correct lip and cheek contour.
- It can benefit the morale of patients with maxillary defects.
- When deglutition and mastication are impaired, it can be used to improve function.
- It reduces the flow of exudates into the mouth.
- The obturator may be used as a stent to hold dressings or packs postsurgically in maxillary resections. It reduces the possibility of postoperative hemorrhage and maintains pressure either directly or indirectly on split thickness skin grafts, thus causing close adaptation of the graft to the wound which prevents the formation of a hematoma and ultimate failure of the graft.

Types of Obturators

- **Feeding obturator:** Used to cover maxillary defects in newborns to aid in feeding and suckling.
- **Surgical obturator:** Given after surgery to aid in wound healing, hold dressings, maintain pressure on split thickness skin grafts.
- **Functional obturator:** To help in deglutition.
- Speech obturator (speech aid prosthesis, nasopharyngeal obturator, speech appliance, prosthetic speech aid, and speech bulb): A temporary or interim prosthesis used to close a defect in the hard and/or soft palate to replace tissue lost due to developmental or surgical alterations, which is necessary for the production of intelligible speech.

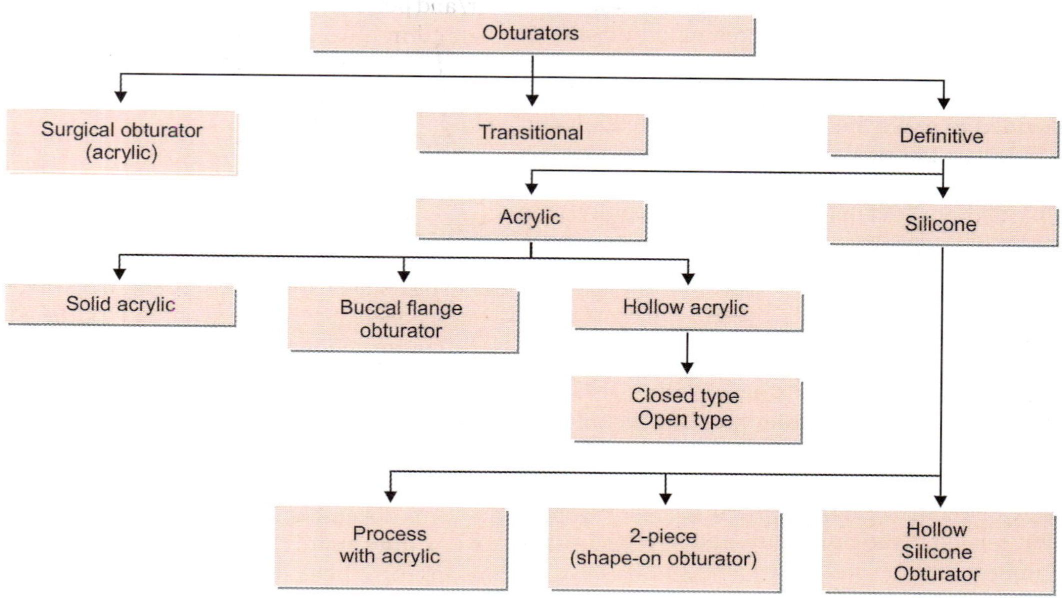

MAXILLOFACIAL PROSTHESIS

It is God given right of every human being to appear human. Few areas of dentistry offer more challenges to the technical skills or greater satisfaction for the successful rehabilitation of function and esthetics in the patient with gross anatomic defects and deformities of the maxillofacial region. Although remarkable advances in surgical management of oral and facial defects, but cannot be satisfactorily required by plastic surgery alone so. The demand for maxillofacial prosthetic devices for the rehabilitation of patients with congenital or acquired defects has intensified in recent years.

Maxillofacial prosthetics *is the art and science of anatomic, functional, or cosmetic reconstruction by means of nonliving substitutes of those regions in the maxilla, mandible, and face that are missing or defective because of surgical intervention, trauma, pathology, or development or congenital malformation.*

History of Maxillofacial Prosthetics

- Early records indicate that artificial eyes, ears, and nose were found on Egyptian mummies.
- The Chinese also made facial restoration with waxes and resins of various types.
- Tycho-Brahe, a Danish astronomer in 16th century lost his nose in a duel and replaced it with an artificial nose made of silver and gold.
- The London Medical Gazette of 1832 describes the case of the "Gunner with silver mask" French soldier whose face was seriously injured in battle.

Objectives of Maxillofacial Prosthetics

The most important objectives of maxillofacial prosthetics and rehabilitation include:
- Restoration of esthetics or cosmetic appearance of the patient.
- Restoration of function
- Protection of tissues
- Therapeutic or healing effect
- Psychological therapy.

Types of Maxillofacial Prosthetics

- **Nasal prosthesis:** A removable prosthesis which artificially restores a missing nose.
- **Orbital prosthesis:** A removable replacement of the contents and surrounding structures of the eye socket.
- **Ocular prosthesis:** An artificial replacement for a missing or damaged eyeball.
- **Auricular prosthesis:** A removable prosthesis which artificially restores a missing ear.
- **Midfacial prosthesis:** A large removable prosthesis which restores a defect in the middle third of the face which may include upper jaw, lip, nose, and orbit.
- **Somato prosthesis:** A prosthesis that replaces external parts of the body such as fingers, breasts, and soft tissue defects.
- **Implant craniofacial prosthesis:** Also known as a skull plate, it is a permanently implanted replacement for a portion of the skull (auricular, nasal, orbital, etc.).
- **Obturators for hard and soft palate defects:** A prosthesis used to replace a missing portion of the hard palate or the soft palate.
- **Mandibular resection prosthesis:** A prosthesis that replaces a missing portion of the jaw and teeth.
- **Cleft palate prosthesis:** A prosthesis which can improve speech and eating ability by obturating a palatal cleft or fistula.
- **Palatal augmentation prosthesis:** A prosthesis used for patients with a partially removed tongue or lower jaw and who have difficulty lifting the tongue to positions that would allow for more normal speech and swallowing.
- **Speech aid prosthesis:** A prosthesis used to improve speech in neurologic impairment.
- **Trismus appliance:** Prosthesis that assist in increasing the mouth opening.

Advantages of Maxillofacial Prosthetics

The maxillofacial prosthetic approach has three main advantages:
1. It requires little surgery or no surgery.
2. The patient spends less time away from home and job.
3. Reconstruction is often more natural looking.

Disadvantages of Maxillofacial Prosthetics

- The necessity of fastening the appliance to the skin and removing it everyday.
- The occasional need of constructing a new prosthesis.

DENTAL IMPLANTS IN CHILDREN

Dental implants for children are a new treatment modality. The use of implants in children or in individuals where growth is not completed is a controversial one. Before placement of an implant, it is essential to understand growth, development and the dynamics of a placed implant in a biologic environment of a growing patient. Dental implants have been defined as a prosthetic device made of alloplastic material implanted into the oral tissues beneath the mucosa or/and periosteal layer, and on/or within the bone to provide retention and support for a fixed or a removable partial denture. From a physiologic standpoint, the conservation of bone may be the most important reason for the use of dental implants in growing patients and it even may be beneficial in some cases to stimulate alveolar bone development in cases of congenital partial anodontia and traumatic tooth loss where oral rehabilitation is required even before skeletal and dental maturation has occurred. Other factors that favor implant placement in children are their excellent local blood supply, positive immunobiologic resistance, and uncomplicated osseous healing. However, in spite of these positives, the issue of timing of placement of implant in children is still under critical evaluation as there are two major concerns:
- First, if implants are present during several years of facial growth, there is a danger of them becoming embedded, relocated, or displaced as the jaw grows.
- Second area of concern is the effect of prosthesis on growth.

Review of the literature

- **Bjork** implanted pins in the jaws of children for longitudinal cephalometric studies and reported that those in the path of erupting teeth were displaced and those placed in resorptive areas were lost.
- **Thilander et al.** concluded that osseointegrated implants in pigs remained stable in space.
- **Ledermann et al.** in their 7-year follow-up with a mean length of 35.5 months, reported a 90% success rate on 42 endosseous dental implants placed in 34 patients aged 9–18 years. There was a positive soft and osseous tissue reaction to the implants. The major complication reported was the failure of dental implants to respond to the vertical growth of adjacent teeth and alveolus due to ankylosis.
- According to **Smith et al.** implant use in children with ectodermal dysplasia is a treatment of choice, since its placement in the mandibular anterior region of a 5-year-old patient did not affect adjacent tooth buds.
- **Guckes et al.** described a case of a 3-year-old patient with ectodermal dysplasia in which dental implants located in the mandible and maxilla have not moved despite growth. During the 5-year follow-up, the prosthesis was remodeled to accommodate eruption of the maxillary teeth and facial growth.

Growth and Implant Placement

The most crucial aspect to be considered in implant placement in children is the effect of growth. As they are rigid fixations, any incorrect placement can have serious consequences on the growth and development of the arches, trauma to the developing tooth buds or a deviation of the path of an erupting tooth. Therefore, it is important that clinicians understand the impact of growth and the potential risks involved in implant placement in a growing child.

Vertical Craniofacial Growth

- Placement of implant is influenced by the great amount of growth in the vertical direction along with the eruption of maxillary teeth. Increase in anterior facial height due to vertical growth of the craniofacial skeleton is especially rapid during the early teenage years.
- If an implant is placed too early (before growth and eruption are complete), the implant crown will become submerged.
- **Brugnolo et al.** described 3 patients (11.5–13 years of age) who received implants in the anterior regions of the maxilla. After 2.5–4.5 years, all patients had implant crowns in infraocclusion.
- **Ödman** showed that implants placed in young patients may show implant infraposition after several years due to craniofacial growth, which may continue in the young adult patient.

Transverse Craniofacial Growth

- **Moorrees et al.** suggested that a decrease of incisor-canine circumference noted from 13–18 years of age was associated with a decrease in arch length, rather than a narrowing in arch width. Overall, the changes are those that would contribute to crowding in the dental arches.
- **Bishara et al.** observed that tooth size arch length discrepancy increases significantly from early adolescence to mid adulthood in both maxillary and mandibular arches. The decrease was calculated to be 1.9 mm in males and 2.0 mm in females in the maxillary arch, 2.7 and 3.5 mm in the mandibular arch respectively.
- Increased crowding and changes in arch form could have a significant effect on a single-tooth implant in a patient who undergoes maximum growth changes, resulting in an implant crown that is out of alignment with adjacent natural teeth.

Sagittal Growth

The sagittal growth of the mandible has no impact on the implant placement in children. Only the rotation of the mandible in the sagittal plane has to be considered.

Growth Spurt

In a study carried out by **Iseri** and **Solow**, the average velocity of eruption of maxillary incisors in girls 9–25 years of age was 1.2–1.5 mm per year during active growth and 0.1–0.2 mm per year after age 17–18. Changes of this magnitude are difficult to compensate for if an implant is placed in a 9–10-year-old girl. The change in boys is even more.

Maxillary Growth

- The midpalatal suture is an important growth site that must be allowed to grow undisturbed, and any interference during its growth can result in dental crossbite. A fixed prosthesis that crosses the midpalatal suture and is attached to implants may restrict transverse growth, and the restriction becomes greater as the implants are placed more and more posterior.
- When the maxilla widens at its midline suture, the central incisor teeth change their position in the bone to compensate and are prevented from separating by the periodontal fibers. Implants are not subject to this compensatory system, and if located in the anterior on opposite sides of the midpalatal suture of a child, they will be carried apart for a significant distance by transverse growth, creating esthetic and functional problems.

Timing and Placement of Implant

Replacing a permanent tooth lost from trauma with an implant poses a challenging dilemma because of the implant's lack of eruption potential can lead to discrepancies in the occlusal plane, esthetic problems and possible disruption of the normal development of the jaw.

- **Op Heij et al.** summarized the growth patterns of each jaw, noting their implications and giving treatment recommendations **(Table 72.1)**.
- The key to implant placement in these patients appears to be the determination of cessation of growth. The average age of growth spurts in girls is 12 years, while the average age in boys is 14 years. However, growth changes occur beyond the time of the growth spurt and may vary by as much as 6 years.
- **Shaw** reported that the dramatic growth changes occurring in infancy and early childhood were not conducive to the maintenance of implants.
- According to **Dietschl** and **Schatz** implant placement in children younger than 16–18 years must be avoided, or

Table 72.1: Implication of early implant placement by location and type of growth.

	Transverse growth	*Sagittal growth*	*Vertical growth*	*Recommendation*
Maxilla Implication	• Anterior region completed prior to adolescent growth spurt • Sutural widening greater in posterior can lead to diastema and shifting of midline to the implant side	Closely associated with skeletal growth: When it follows the mandibular growth, loss of sutural growth via resorption results • Anterior resorption could result in loss of bone on labial side of implant	Maxilla displaced downward via sutural growth, remodeling and eruption; adult levels of vertical growth usually reached at age 17–18 in girls and later in boys • Leads to infraocclusion; unfavorable • Endosseous-supraosseous ratio	Delay implant placement until skeletal growth complete • In anodontic child, implant placement in the posterior could be considered under well planned conditions
Mandible	• Anterior growth ceases early; limited remodeling causes least problems • Posterior growth continues longer through remodeling and bone apposition	Endochondral growth at condyle and remodeling of ramus	• Height increase by condylar growth and bone apposition • Facial types develop in different ways: » Normal; minor rotation. » Short; horizontal growth, forward rotation, deep bite » Long; vertical growth posterior rotation, skeletal open bite	Delay implant placement until skeletal growth complete • In a severe anodontic or oligodontic child, implants may be placed in the anterior mandible • Lack of reports with regard to implantsin posterior mandible
Implication	Premolar or molar implant could be shifted into a lingual position	• No impact on implant placement • Rotation in sagittal plane must be considered	• Affects anteroposterior and vertical eruption patterns • Affects relationship between implant and adjacent tooth in vertical and labiolingual direction	

they will remain in infraocclusion due to adjacent alveolar bone growth.

- **Bergendal et al.** stated that implants must be placed when growth is almost complete, except for rare cases of total aplasia, as in ectodermal dysplasia.
- According to **Guckes et al.** bone volume in children may not be sufficient for the placement of implants.
- Osseointegrated implants behave like ankylosed teeth, arresting both eruption and alveolar bone growth and not adapting to changes secondary to alveolar bone growth.
- Therefore, an implant placed in growing patient can become embedded in bone hence changes in growth, disturbances in alignment and occlusion occur.
- The timing of implant placement in growing patients was discussed at a *Scandinavian Consensus Conference* in Jönköping, Sweden where there was a general agreement that implant placement should be postponed until skeletal growth is completed or nearly completed in normal adolescents. In the individual with oligodontia or anodontia, however, earlier intervention could be indicated, especially in the mandible. Anodontia and severe oligodontia were mentioned as exceptions to the rule.

Factors to be Considered for Implant Placement in Growing Patients

Skeletal Maturity Level/Age of the Patient

Implants placed after 15-years in girls and 18-years in boys or when two annual cephalograms show no change in position of adjacent teeth and alveolus are said to be most predictable prognosis.

Sex of the Patient

As males grow for a longer time period than females, implants in adolescent boys must be delayed longer than adolescent girls to allow growth completion.

Number and Location of Missing Teeth

In patients with complete anodontia, implants can be planned in the maxilla and anterior mandible as early as 7 years. However, it must be kept in mind that the implants may have to be replaced, or prosthesis may have to be modified. It is advisable to restore a larger edentulous area with implants than to place a single implant supported crown.

Recommendation for Implant Placement by Quadrant

- Maxillary anterior quadrant is an important area for consideration due to traumatic tooth loss and frequent congenital tooth absence. The vertical growth of the maxilla exceeds all other dimensions of the growth in this quadrant; therefore, premature implant placement can result in the repetitive need to lengthen the transmucosal implant connection which leads to poor implant-to-prosthesis ratios. According to **Krant**, the placement of implants in the anterior maxillary quadrant before the age of 15 in female patients and 17 in male patients should be attempted to achieve unique treatment planning goals and with particular emphasis on the only determination of skeletal age, informed consent, and the possibility of future implant replacement.
- Maxillary posterior quadrant is subjected to same general growth factors described for the maxillary anteroposterior area. An additional growth factor is transverse maxillary growth at midpalatal suture. Placement of osseointegrated dental implants in the maxillary posterior quadrant is best

delayed until the age of 15-years in females and 17-years in males.

- Mandibular anterior quadrant is the best site for the placement of an osseointegrated implant before skeletal maturation as mandibular anterior quadrant presents fewer growth variables and closure of the mandibular symphyseal suture occurs during the first 2-years of life. Reports were published by **Cronin et al.** and **Smith et al.** documenting the placement of endosseous implants in the anterior mandibular region as early as 5-years of age with positive treatment results.

According to the 1988 *National Institute of Health Consensus Development Conference* on Dental Implants at Bethesda, it was agreed that oral implants in young patients, should not be placed until growth and skeletal development is completed or nearly completed; the area best suited for implants in children was anterior mandible and least indicated was maxillary anterior segment.

Suggestions for Implant Placement in Unaffected Patients

- Whenever possible, implant placement must be delayed until the age of 15-years for girls and 18-years for boys. Growing patient treated with dental implant should have adequate follow-up.
- Further research is needed in the areas of implants in growing children.
- Implant location, the sex of the patient, and the skeletal maturation level are the most important factors in the final decision of when to place implant.
- It is still recommended to wait for the completion of dental and skeletal growth, except for severe cases of ED.

Advantages of the Implant Placement in Early Age in Pediatric Dentistry

- **Esthetics:** The prosthesis on implants provides acceptable esthetics as compared to the conventional treatment options like removable partial denture, Andrews bridge, dentures and overdentures. They provide multiple options of material and morphology of the teeth.
- **Functions:** The prosthesis over the implant are stable, fixed and ensures reproduction of the required occlusion.
- **Maintenance of the soft and hard tissue architecture:** The loss of the tooth results into the atropic changes in the bone and soft tissue in both vertical and horizontal plane. The rehabilitation with fixed partial denture also cannot meet the optimal esthetic demands. This condition may require bone augmentation surgical procedures like guided bone regeneration, ridge split technique, sinus lift procedures. Vertical bone augmentation is complex and unpredictable. The biomechanical forces acting on the bone under influence of mastication may maintain the hard and soft tissue architecture. (Escobar et al.) Therefore an early implant placement is the best option for maintaining the current as well future treatment requirements to avail the morphology of bone and overlying soft tissue.

Indications of Placing Dental Implants in Pediatric Dental Patients

- Pediatric patients with ectodermal dysplasia (1988 National Institute of Health Consensus Development Conference on Dental Implants at Bethesda).
- Implant combined with bone grafting in patients with cleft of the alveolus and palate.
- children and adolescents having anodontia, partial anodontia, congenitally missing teeth, teeth lost as a result of trauma.

Contraindications for the use of Dental Implants

- Pre-pubertal age group.
- Individual With Pubertal growth spurt.
- Inadequate mesiodistal space.

Implant and Prosthesis for Hypodontia Used in Children and Adolescent

Type of edentulous space	Prosthesis	Type of implants
Hypodontia	Fixed partial denture crowns	• Single piece implants • Provisional implants • Bioactive implants • Metallic implants without bioactive surface coating
Oligodontia/ anodontia	• Implant supported overdenture • Fixed partial denture	• OnPlants • Single piece implants • Provisional implants • Bioactive implants • Metallic implants without bioactive surface coating

Types of Implants Indicated in Children and Adolescents

Types	Types of the implant	Bone implant contact
Bioactive metal implants	Acid etched and/ or ossteoinductive material coating	Formation of the osseous tissue adjacent to the implant
Bioinert metal implant	Provisional implants	Formation of the fibrous and osseous tissue—fibrosseous integraiton
Non-metallic implants	PEEK implants, carbon implants, zirconia implants	

Alternative Implants Used in Pediatric Dentistry

The reluctance for the placement of the implant due to growth of bones, alteration in occlusion and submergence of the implant can be addressed with early placement of the implant with gradual loading and its removal as and when required. This treatment option gives liberty to harness the benefit of implant and remove it whenever required. This can be achieved by using provisional implants, OnPlants.

Provisional implants: Provisional Implants or Transitional implants are the grade 4 or grade 5 solid titanium implants

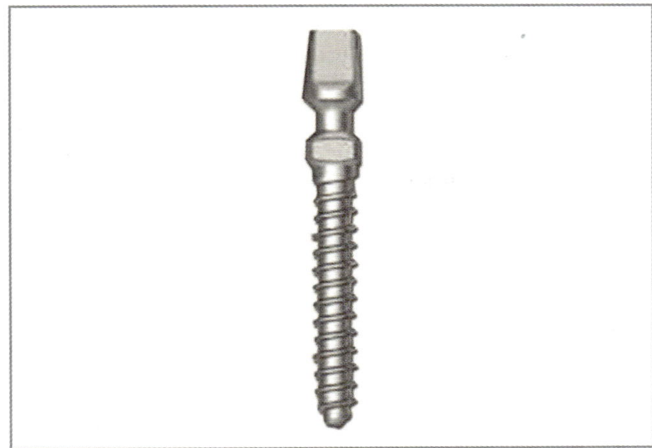

Fig. 72.9: Provisional implants.

which are prepared by grinding on CNC machine followed by polishing. This implant possesses any coating for early osseointegration. They have upper abutment portion and a lower fixture attached by a neck, supposed to be at gingival level. These implants are bendable to the required prosthesis of the crown **(Fig. 72.9)**. They are attached by fibro-osseous integration and reduced bone implant contact which facilitate its retrievability even after few years. (**Stuart J Froum et al.**, 2005) The implants are indicated for restoring missing permanent teeth. The stability provided by provisional implant is nearly equivalent to bioactive implant. (**Dhaliwal JS et al.**, 2017). They are suitable for individual during and after growth spurt and even after completion of the growth. (**Rathi N et al.,** 2022). Cope et al found that temporary anchorage device (TAD) can also be used for the replacement of the tooth. The provisional implant has advantage of possessing the suitable abutment for loading and the bending tool to adjust it to the required occlusion form unlike TADS.

OnPlants: It is short subperiosteal disk implant utilized in the palatal region by **Block and Hoffman** in 1995, marketed by Nobel Biocare. This implant is indicated in case of oligodontia/anodontia in maxillary teeth with reduced bone volume. It has a wider titanium disc covered by the hydroxyapatite plate for osseointegration with palatal bone. This titanium disc

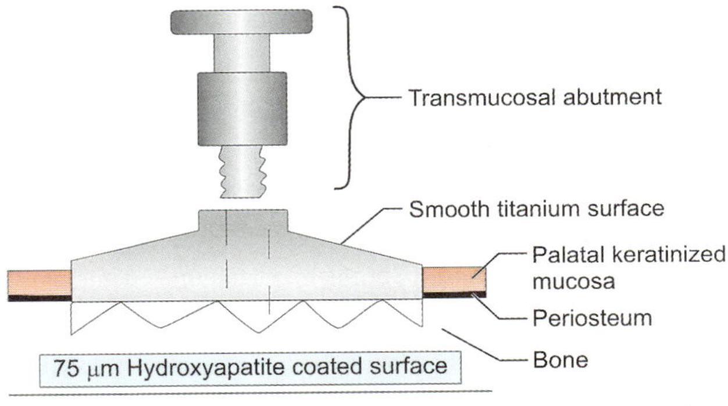

Fig. 72.10: OnPlants.

is attached by the titanium screw inserted in the bone. This anchor device is meant to hold the cast bar in the oral cavity **(Fig. 72.10).** The attaching clips are acrylised in the denture or the overdenture. The bar will engage with the clip of the acrylic prosthesis to provide retention to the removable device. (**Simone Heuberer et al.,** 2011) The remodeling of the bone may continue gradually without damaging the ossteointegrated plate.

Mini Impalnts an Alternative to Conventional Implant

Mini implant is a miniature sized titanium implant that acts like the root a of tooth which were first developed by **Dr Victor I Sendax** of New York in the early 1985. **Bulard** added single one-piece O-ball design. They have a diameter of 1.8 mm to 2.7, they are available in multiple tips, thread, body and head **(Fig. 72.11).**

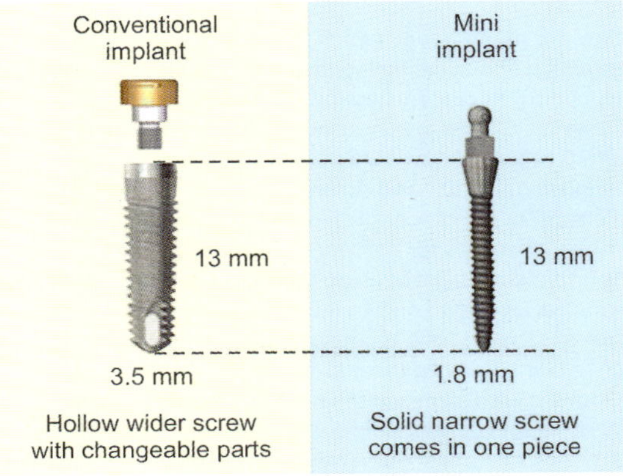

Fig. 72.11: Comparison of conventional and mini implant.

Drawbacks of Conventional Implants in Children

- **Balut et al.** and **Kramer et al**. had found that the insertion of conventional implants during jaw development may lead to trauma of dental follicles, impaired tooth eruption and delayed development of orofacial structures.
- **Mishra et al**. explore the possibilities of successful prosthesis with implants in adolescents and summarize as implantation should be performed after completion of the skeletal growth; The only possible site for prosthesis before reaching the skeletal maturation is the lower frontal area, due to the lowest number of registered changes in this area.

Comparison between Mini Implant and Conventional Implant

Properties	*Mini Implant*	*Conventional implant*
Size	Smaller	Normal
Use	Smaller teeth Limited spaces	Larger teeth or bridge
Component	1 piece titanium system with a ball shaped head for denture stabilization	Two parts: 1. Implant 2. Abutment
Diameter	Narrower 1.8–2.7 mm	Wider

Research on implants in children

- **Tanner** states ectodermal dysplasia with an abnormal appearance may affect normal social and psychological development in young patients.
- **Alcon et al** conducted a study in a 4-year-old ED patient. Mandibular endosseous implants were paced. Follow-up of 6.3 years was done. After loading, vertical growth pattern changed to low angle due to lack of alveolar growth in time. Correction by changing the vertical heights of the abutment and prosthesis was done. They concluded that early implant placement and fixed prosthesis could be a good treatment option for ED patient.
- **Bonvin et al.** reported the clinical course and follow-up of a child with ED treated with implant surgery very early. Different possibilities for prosthetic restoration were reviewed. Good cover of the implant was achieved at 4 years.
- **Bergendal et al.** Surveyed dental implant in children with ED up to age 16 years in Sweden between 1985 and 2005. He concluded that the failure rate in children treated because of tooth agenesis was only slightly higher than that reported for adult individuals The small jaw size and preoperative conditions, rather than ED, were thought to be the main risk factors.
- **Guckes et al** conducted a prospective clinical trial. The effect of endosseous dental implants on the mandible of children with ED was studied in twenty-three adolescents (12–17 years) and 12 preadolescents (7–11 years). 225 implants were placed in all. Twenty-two implants failed with a success rate of 91.3% (preadolescent group 88% and adolescent group 90%). They concluded that Osseointegrated implants in children with ED seem to be a feasible treatment.

POINTS TO REMEMBER

- There are many issues which still affect and cause loss of teeth in children such as trauma, neoplasm, systemic disorders, infection, and congenital abnormalities such as clefts or inborn defects such as ectodermal dysplasia.
- Resin bonding procedures and porcelain laminate veneers, whenever possible should be considered as the treatment of first choice.
- All ceramic crowns are the most esthetic complete coverage restorations currently available in dentistry.
- Teeth that do not have sufficient coronal structure, post with core build-ups should be done.
- The most important and commonly encountered condition is ectodermal dysplasia, which causes anodontia in patients.
- An obturator is a disk or plate, natural or artificial, which closes an opening or defect of the maxilla as a result of a cleft palate or partial or total removal of maxilla for a tumor mass (Chalian 1971).
- Dental implants have been defined as a prosthetic device made of alloplastic material implanted into the oral tissues beneath the mucosaor/and periosteal layer, and on/or within the bone to provide retention and support for a fixed or a removable partial denture.
- Bjork was the first one to implant pins as implants.
- If an implant is placed too early (before growth and eruption are complete) the implant crown will become submerged. Increased crowding and changes in arch form could have a significant effect on a single-tooth implant in a patient who undergoes maximum growth changes,resulting in an implant crown that is out of alignment with adjacent natural teeth.
- The timing of implant placement in growing patients was discussed at a Scandinavian Consensus Conference in Jönköping, Sweden wherethere was a general agreement that implant placement should be postponed until skeletal growth is completed or nearly completed in normal adolescents.
- Factors to be considered for implant placement in growing patients are skeletal maturity level, age of the patient, sex of patient and number and location of missing teeth.
- The area best suited for implants in children was anterior mandible and least indicated was maxillary anterior segment. Whenever possible,implant placement must be delayed until the age of 15-years for girls and 18-years for boys.

Questionnaire

1. Explain the crowns used for permanent anterior teeth rehabilitation.
2. Describe post and core fabrication in detail.
3. Write a note on removable partial denture.
4. What is the indication, advantage and techniques for fixed partial denture?
5. What is the rationale for use of overdentures in children?
6. Explain the dental rehabilitation of a child with ectodermal dysplasia.
7. Describe obturators.
8. Classify the various types of maxillofacial prosthesis
9. Discuss growth and implant placement.
10. Explain the implications of timing on implant.
11. What are the factors to be kept in consideration while placement of implants in children?
12. Enumerate the implant and prosthesis planned for rehabilitation of the oligodontia.
13. Differentiate between ossteointegration vs fibro-osseointe-gration.
14. What the advantages of provisional implants over bio-active implants.
15. What are OnPlants? Describe its construction.

FURTHER READING

1. Agarwal N, Godhi BS, Verma P. Pediatric implants: a clinical dilemma. JOHCD. 2012;6(3).
2. Bergendal B, Koch G, Karol J, et al. (Eds). Consensus conference on ectodermal dysplasia with special reference to dental treatment. Stockholm: Forlagshuset Gothia AB; 1998.
3. Bergendal B. When should we extract deciduous teeth and place implants in young individuals with tooth agenesis. J Oral Rehabil. 2008;35(suppl 1):55-63.
4. Beumer J III, Curtis TA, Firtell DN. Maxillofacial Rehabilitation Prosthodontic and Surgical Consideration. St Louis: Mosby; 1979. pp. 286-7.
5. Bishara SE, Jakobsen JR, Treder JE, et al. Changes in the maxillary and mandibular tooth size or arch length relationship from early adolescence to early adulthood. Am J Orthod Dentofacial Orthop. 1989;95(1):46-59.
6. Björk A, Skieller V. Growth of the maxilla in three dimensions as revealed radiographicaily by the implant method. Br J Orthod. 1977;4(2):53-64.
7. Björk A. Variations in the growth pattern of the human mandible: A longitudinal radiographic study by the implant method. J Dent Res. 1963;42(1)Pt2:400-11.
8. Brahmin JS. Dental implants in children. Oral Maxillofacial Surg Clin N Am. 2005;17(4):375-81.

9. Brugnolo E, Mazzocco C, Cardioll G, et al. Clinical and radiographic findings following placement of single tooth implants in young patients— case reports. Int J Periodonts Restorative Dent. 1996;16(5):421-33.
10. Consensus statement. In: Koch G, Bergendal T, Kvint S, et al. (Eds). Consensus conference on Oral Implants in young patients. Stockholm: Forlagshuset Gothia AB; 1996. pp. 125- 33.
11. Cronin RJ Jr, Oesterle LJ. Implant use in growing patients. Dent Clin North Am. 1998;42(1):1-35.
12. Guckes AD, McCarthy GR, Brahim J. Use of endosseous implants in a 3-year-old child with ectodermal dysplasia: case report and 5-year follow-up. Pediatr Dent. 1997;19(4): 282-5.
13. Heij DG, Opdebeeck H, van Steenberghe D, et al. Facial development, continuous tooth eruption, and mesial drift as compromising factors for implant placement. Int J Oral Maxillofac Implants. 2006;21(6):867-78.
14. Hickey AJ, Vergo JT. Prosthetic treatments for patients with ectodermal dysplasia. J Prosthet Dent. 2001; 8:364-8.
15. Itthagarun A, King NM. Ectodermal dysplasia: a review and case report. Quintessence Int. 1997; 28:595-602.
16. Kraut RA. Dental implants for children: creating smiles for children without teeth. Pract Periodontics Aesthet Dent. 1996;8(9): 909-13.
17. Mackie IC, Quayle AA. Implants in children: a case report. Endod Dent Traumatol. 1993;9(3):124-6.
18. Mishra SK, Chowdhary N, Chowdhary R. Dental implants in growing children. J Indian Soc Pedod Prev Dent. 2013;31(1):3-9.
19. Moorrees CFA, Lebret LML, Kent RL. Changes in the natural dentition after second molar emergence 13–18 years. IADR. 1979:276.
20. Oesterle LJ, Cronin RJ Jr, Ranly DM. Maxillary implants and the growing patient. Int J Oral Maxillofac Implants. 1993;8(4):377- 87.
21. Percinoto C, Vieira AE, Barbieri CM, Melhado FL, Moreira KS. Use of dental implants in children: A literature review. Quintessence Int. 2001; 32:381–3.
22. Pigno MA, Blackman RB, Cronin RJ, et al. Prosthodontic management of ectodermal dysplasia: a review of literature. J Prosthet Dent. 76;541-5.
23. Quintessence Int. 2001;32(5):381-3.
24. Rahn AO, Boucher LJ. Maxillofacial Prosthetics Principles and Concepts. Toronto: WB Saunders; 1970. pp. 215-7.
25. Shobha Tandon. Pediatric prosthodontics. Textbook of Pedodontics, 2nd edition. Hyderabad: Paras Publication; 2008. pp. 704-20.
26. Smith RA, Vargervik K, Kearns G, et al. Placement of an endosseous implants in a growing child with ectodermal dysplasia. Oral Surg Oral Med Oral Pathol. 1993;75(6):669-73.
27. Taylor TD. Clinical Maxillofacial Prosthetics. Chicago: Quintessence Publishing Co Inc; 2000. pp. 129-31.

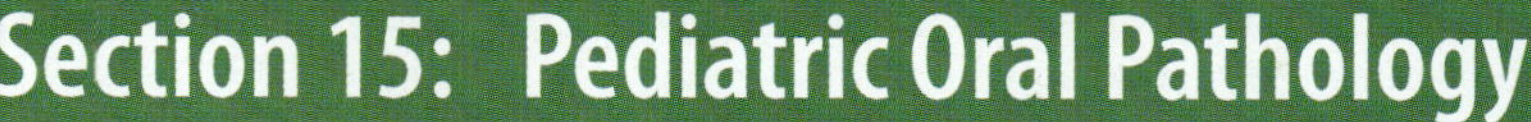

CHAPTER

Developmental Anomalies of Dentition

Nikhil Marwah, Parvind Gumber

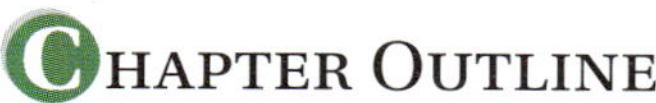

- Types of Developmental Anomalies

Malformations or defects resulting from disturbance of growth and development are known as developmental anomalies. A large number of such developmental anomalies, which involve the body in general and oral structure in particular can occur during the embryonic life.

TYPES OF DEVELOPMENTAL ANOMALIES

Congenital anomalies: *The defects, which are present at or before birth during the intrauterine life.*

Hereditary developmental anomalies: *When certain defects are inherited by the offspring from either of the parent, it is called hereditary developmental anomalies. Such types of anomalies are always transmitted by genes.*

Acquired anomalies: *Developed during intrauterine life due to some pathological environmental conditions. They are not transmitted through genes.*

Hamartomatous anomalies: *A hamartoma can be defined as an excessive, focal overgrowth of mature, normal cells and tissues, which are native to that particular anatomic location.*

Idiopathic anomalies: *Developmental anomalies of unknown cause.*

Developmental anomalies of dentition	
Number	• Anodontia • Hypodontia • Hyperdontia
Size	• Microdontia • Macrodontia
Position	Transposition
Shape	• Gemination fusion • Concrescence • Accessory cusps • Dens invaginatus • Ectopic enamel • Taurodontism • Hypercementosis • Accessory roots • Dilaceration
Structure	• Amelogenesis imperfecta (AI) • Dentinogenesis imperfecta • Regional odontodysplasia

Anomalies of number

Name of anomaly	*Definition*	*Etiology*	*Clinical features*	*Treatment*
Anodontia (**Fig. 73.1**) **Fig. 73.1:** Anodontia. (*Source:* HxBenefit.com).	Total lack of tooth development	• Genetic	• No teeth are present • Lack of alveolar growth • Associated with ectodermal dysplasia	Prosthetic rehabilitation

Contd...

Contd...

Name of anomaly	***Definition***	***Etiology***	***Clinical features***	***Treatment***
Hypodontia **(Fig. 73.2)** **Fig. 73.2:** Hypodontia.	Lack of development of one or more teeth	• Genetic • Hereditary • Associated with syndromes	• Prevalence is 3–8% • Female dominance • Less than 1% in deciduous dentition • Predominance is 3rd molars > 2nd premolars > lateral incisors	Prosthetic and orthodontic rehabilitation
Oligodontia **(Fig. 73.3)** 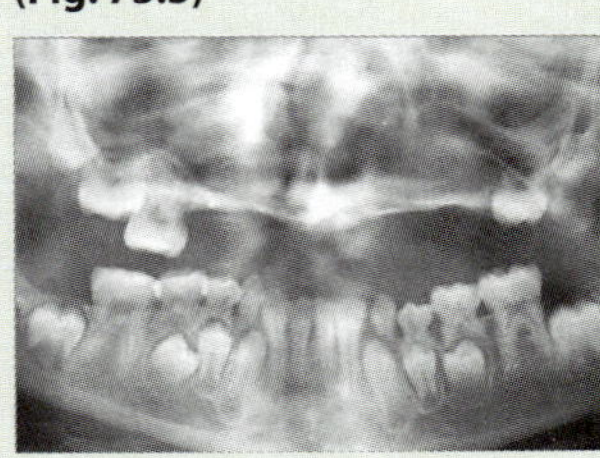 **Fig. 73.3:** Oligodontia. 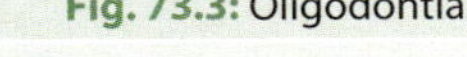	More than 6 teeth are missing	• Genetic • Hereditary	• Rare in primary dentition • Multiple missing teeth from either arch • It can result in collapse of arch and drifting due to excess space	Prosthetic and orthodontic rehabilitation
Hyperdontia (Supernumerary teeth) **(Figs. 73.4 to 73.8)**	Development of additional teeth in addition to normal dentition	• Genetic • Hereditary • Associated with syndromes • Develop as a consequence of proliferation of epithelial cells from dental lamina	• Prevalence is 1–3% • 80% associated with single tooth hyperdontia • Occurs mostly in permanent dentition in maxillary anterior region • Male predominance • Supernumerary in maxillary anterior region is called as mesiodens, in 4th molar region it is distomolar and if it is buccal to molars it is called as paramolar • Frequent cause of crowding type of malocclusion	Extraction of supernumerary tooth followed by orthodontic rehabilitation

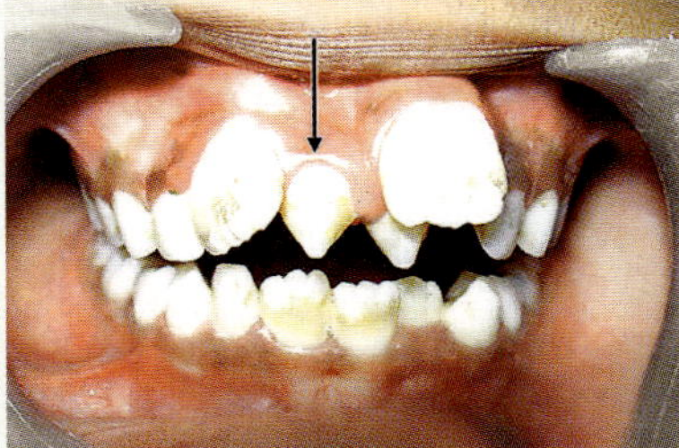

Fig. 73.4: Supernumerary teeth.

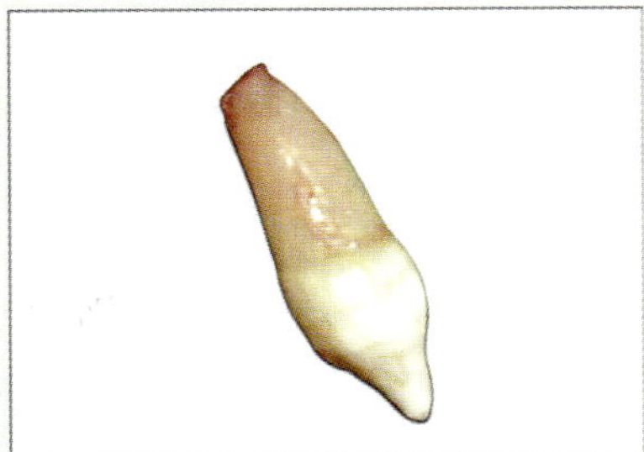

Fig. 73.5: Extracted supernumerary teeth.

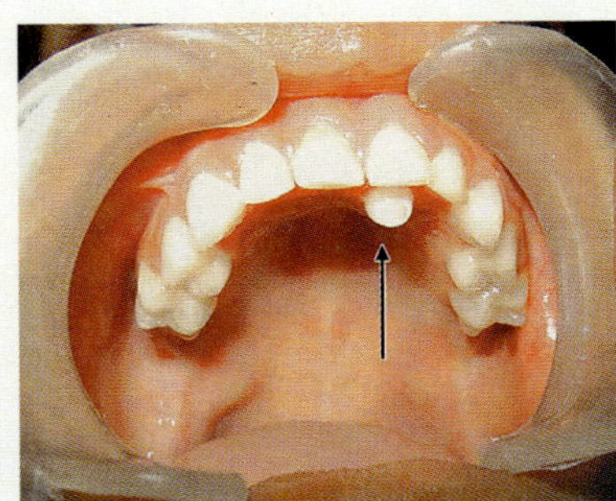

Fig. 73.6: Supernumerary teeth in primary dentition.

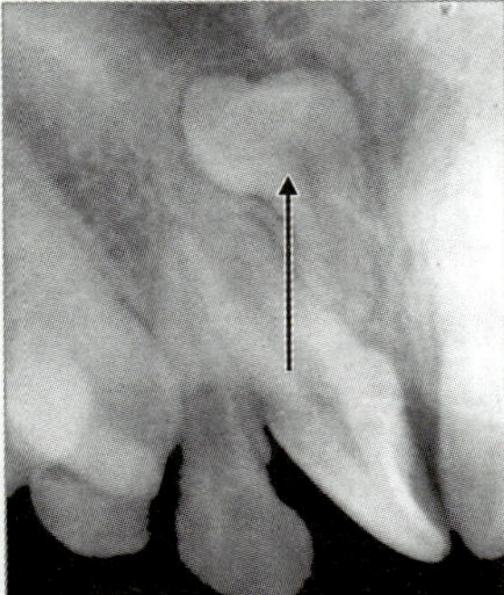

Fig. 73.7: Inverted mesiodens.

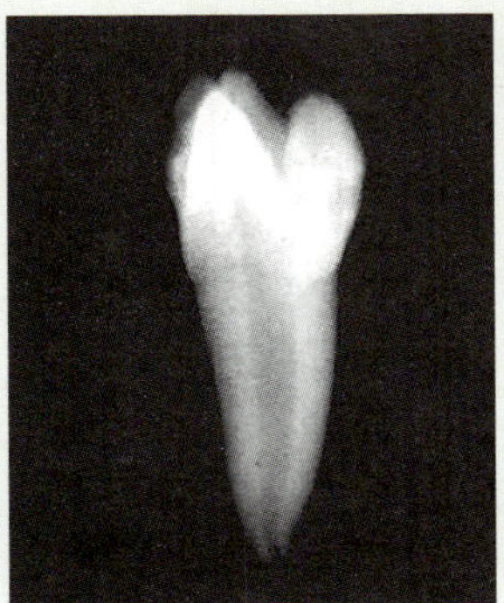

Fig. 73.8: Multilobed supernumerary teeth.

Contd...

Types of supernumerary teeth	Syndromes associated with hypodontia	Syndrome associated with hyperdontia
According to the site: • Mesiodens • Distomolar • Paramolar • Extralateral incisor *According to morphology:* • Conical type • Tuberculate type • Supplemental type • Odontoma associated	• Down's syndrome • Ectodermal dysplasia • Turner's syndrome • Robinson syndrome • Octodental dysplasia • Focal dermal hypoplasia • Sturge-Weber syndrome • Oral facial digital types I	• Cleidocranial dysplasia • Down syndrome • Ehlers-Danlos syndrome • Oral facial digital types I and III • Nance-Horan syndrome

Anomalies of position

Name of anomaly	Definition	Etiology	Clinical features	Treatment
Transposition **(Fig. 73.9)** 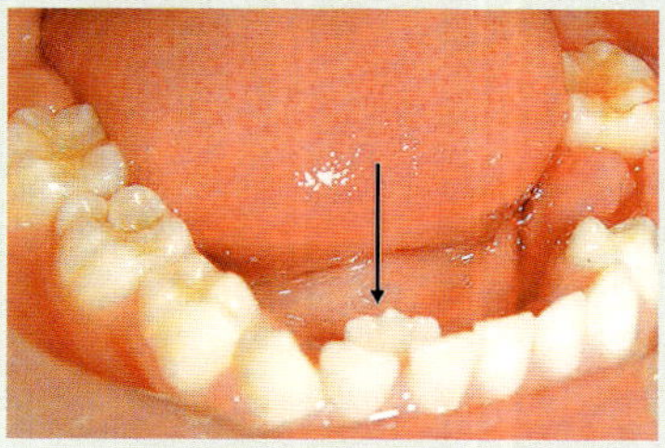 Fig. 73.9: Transposition.	Eruption of normal teeth in an inappropriate positions	Retained deciduous teeth or loss of space	• Maxillary canine and premolars are involved it may cause crowding	Orthodontic rehabilitation

Anomalies of size

Name of anomaly	Definition	Etiology	Clinical features	Treatment
Microdontia **(Fig. 73.10)** 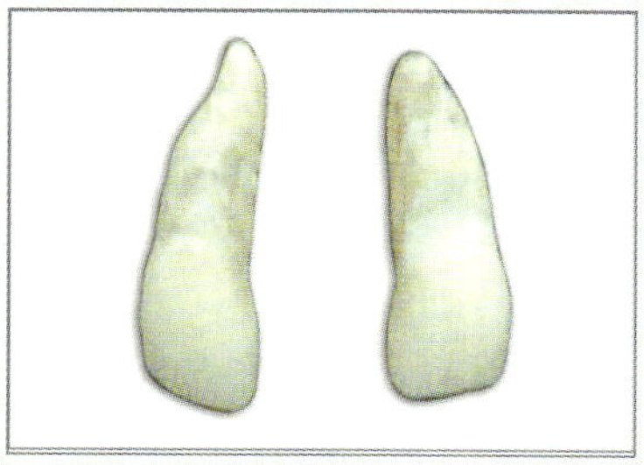 Fig. 73.10: Microdontia.	Teeth that are usually smaller than normal	• Genetic • Hereditary • Environmental	• Associated with hypodontia, Down's syndrome • Prevalence is 0.8–8% • Maxillary lateral incisor called as peg lateral is most affected • Mesiodistal diameter is reduced	Porcelain crowns can be provided
Macrodontia **(Fig. 73.11)** 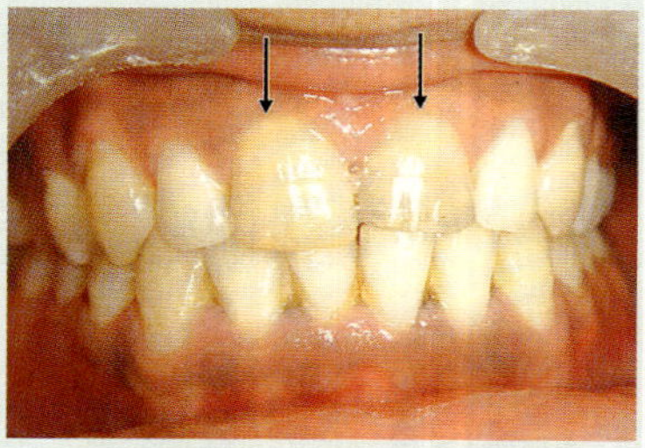 Fig. 73.11: Macrodontia.	Teeth that are bigger than average size for the specific age	• Genetic • Hereditary • Environmental	• Associated with hyperdontia • Usually incisors are involved • Frequent cause of crowding	Prosthetic and orthodontic rehabilitation

Contd...

Contd...

Name of anomaly	*Definition*	*Etiology*	*Clinical features*	*Treatment*
Fusion **(Figs. 73.12 to 73.14)**	Tooth fusion is defined as union between the dentin and/or enamel of two or more separate developing teeth	• Shafer—pressure produced by physical force prolongs the contact of the developing teeth causing fusion • Lowell and Soloman physical action causes the tooth germs to come into contact, thus producing necrosis of the intervening tissue, allowing the enamel organ and dental papilla to fuse together	• The fusion may be partial or total depending upon the stage of tooth development at the time of union: fusio-totalis, partialis-coronaries and partialis-radicularis • If the contact occurs before the calcification stage, the teeth unite completely and form one large tooth • Incomplete fusion may be at root level if the contact and union occur after formation of crown • Prevalence of 0.5–2.5% • Most commonly occurs in primary teeth with more predilections for anterior teeth • Radiographically, the dentin of fused teeth always appears to be joined • In some region with separate pulp chambers and canals	• It may cause malocclusion • Restorative, periodontal and endodontic considerations are needed before proceeding with any type of treatment

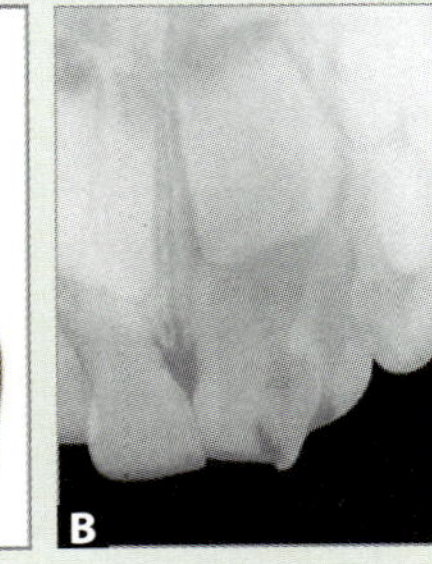

Figs. 73.12A and B: Fusion of triple teeth.

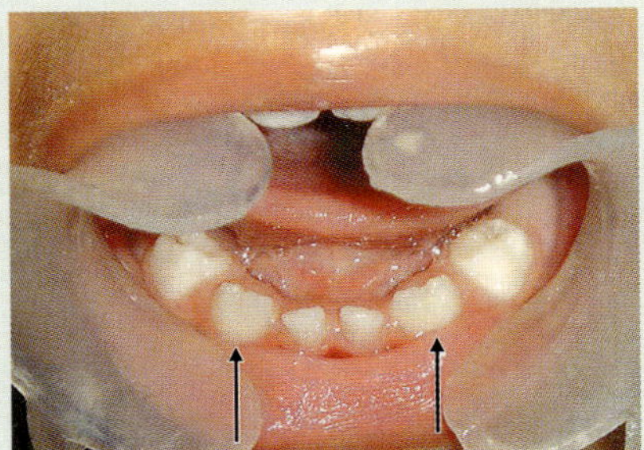

Fig. 73.13: Bilateral fusion of teeth.

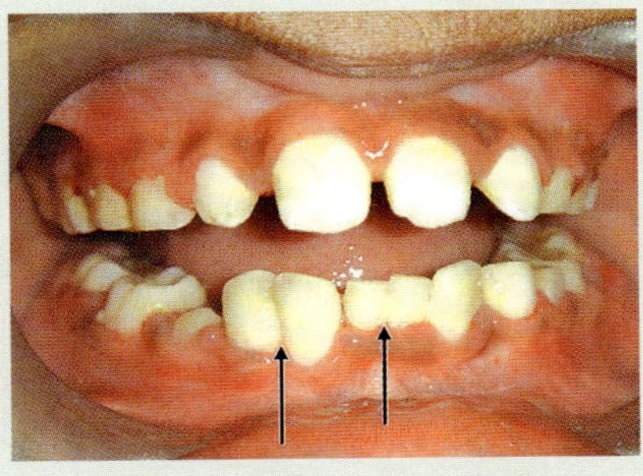

Fig. 73.14: Fusion in primary and permanent teeth.

Name of anomaly	*Definition*	*Etiology*	*Clinical features*	*Treatment*
Gemination **(Figs. 73.15 and 73.16)**	Abortive attempt by the single tooth bud to divide, with the resultant formation of bifid crown and common root	• Genetic • Hereditary Environmental	• More frequently in the primary dentition • Prevalence of 1% • Predilection in maxillary primary incisors and canine • Two teeth joined in coronal aspect but with single root and single root canal	• It may cause malocclusion • Restorative, periodontal, and endodontic considerations are needed before proceeding with any type of treatment

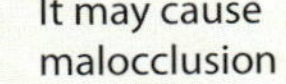

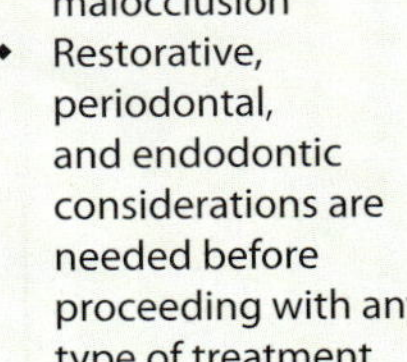

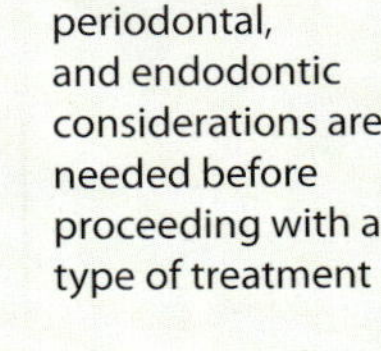

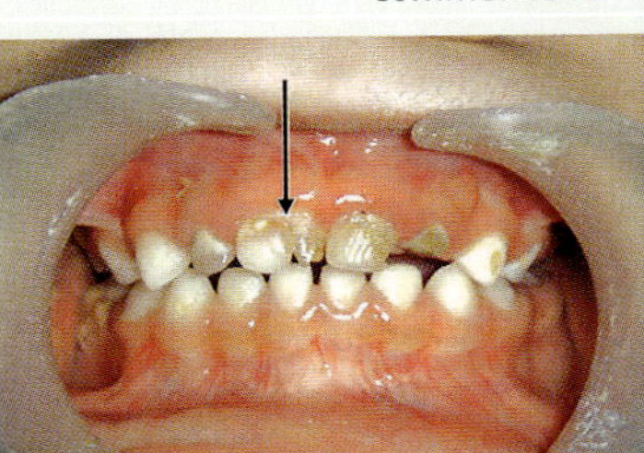

Fig. 73.15: Gemination in primary teeth.

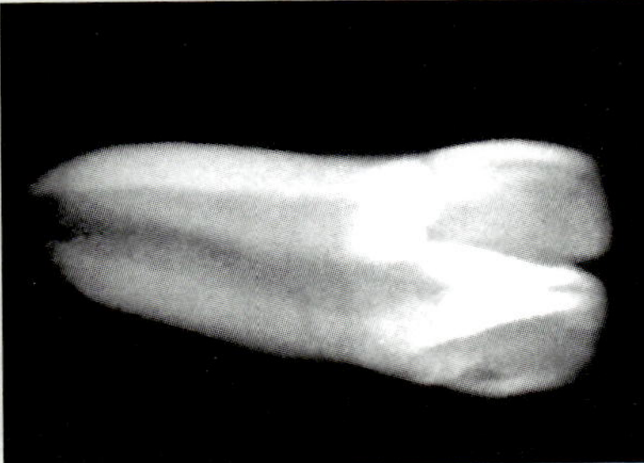

Fig. 73.16: Extracted geminated teeth.

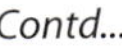

Contd...

Contd...

Name of anomaly	Definition	Etiology	Clinical features	Treatment
Concrescence **(Fig. 73.17)**	Union of teeth by cementum alone without confluence of dentin	Environmental	• Two separate teeth joined by cementum • Posterior maxillary region is favored	• No treatment required if patient is asymptomatic • Extraction if it interferes with eruption of succeeding tooth
Fig. 73.17: Concrescence.				
Accessory cusp **(Fig. 73.18)**	Cuspal morphology of teeth exhibit minor variations among different populations	Unknown	Extra cusp like structure seen on palatal cusp in maxillary and on lingual cusp in mandibular	• No treatment
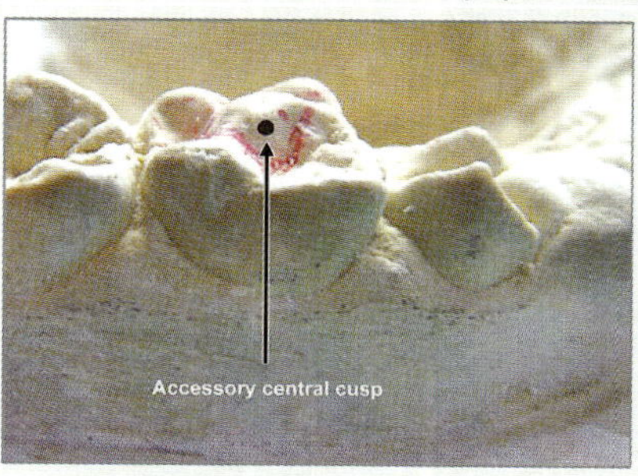 **Fig. 73.18:** Accessory central cusp.				

Anomalies of shape

Name of anomaly	Definition	Etiology	Clinical features	Treatment
Talon's cusp **(Figs. 73.19 and 73.20)**	Presence of an accessory cusp like structure projecting from cingulum area of cementoenamel junction (CEJ)	During the morpho-differentiation stage of tooth development as an outward folding of inner enamel epithelial (IEE) cells and transient focal hyperplasia of peripheral cells of mesenchymal dental papilla	• Prevalence is 0.06–7.7% • The anomaly also appears to be more prevalent in patients with Rubinstein-Taybi syndrome, Mohr syndrome and Sturge-Weber syndrome • Lateral incisors followed by central incisors and canines are affected • Pulp horn may project from the cusp • Compromised esthetics, occlusal interference, carious developmental grooves, displacement of teeth, periodontal problems, irritation of the tongue and diagnostic problems	• Gradual reduction with fluoride application as desensitizing agent • Single appointment reduction with or without pulp therapy • Sealant application in the dental grooves • Partial reduction with composite camouflage
Fig. 73.19: Talon's cusp. **Fig. 73.20:** Talon's cusp on supernumerary teeth.				

Contd...

Contd...

Name of anomaly	*Definition*	*Etiology*	*Clinical features*	*Treatment*
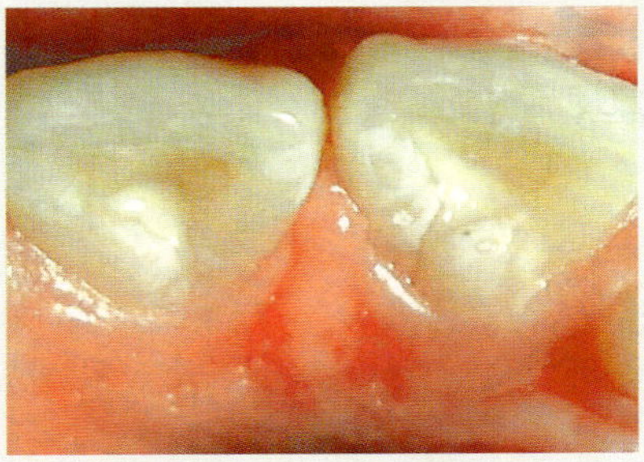 *Dens evaginatus* **(Fig. 73.21)**	Cusp like elevation of enamel in central groove	Proliferation and evagination of an area of IEE and adjacent mesenchyme into the enamel organ during tooth development	• This may contain enamel, dentin, pulp- like normal tooth • Radiographically pulp extension can be seen • Mostly on molars or maxillary incisors • May cause occlusal problems	Selective reduction with subsequent pulp therapy to remove the cusp and keep the teeth on position
Fig. 73.21: Dens evaginatus.				
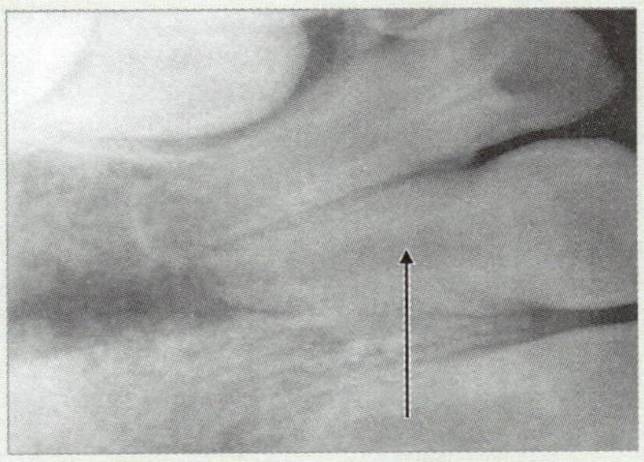 *Dens invaginatus (Dens in dente)* **(Fig. 73.22)**	Deep surface invagination of crown lined by enamel	Invagination of crown filled with soft tissue like dental follicle and on eruption this loses its blood supply and turns necrotic	• 1–10% • Predominance is lateral incisor > central incisors > premolars > molars • It can be of coronal or radicular type • Type 1 confined to crown • Type 2 extends below CEJ • Type 3 extends till root extends inside tooth giving it tooth in a tooth (dens in dente) appearance	Depending on type of dens invaginatus treatment can be restorative or pulp therapy
Fig. 73.22: Dens invaginatus.				
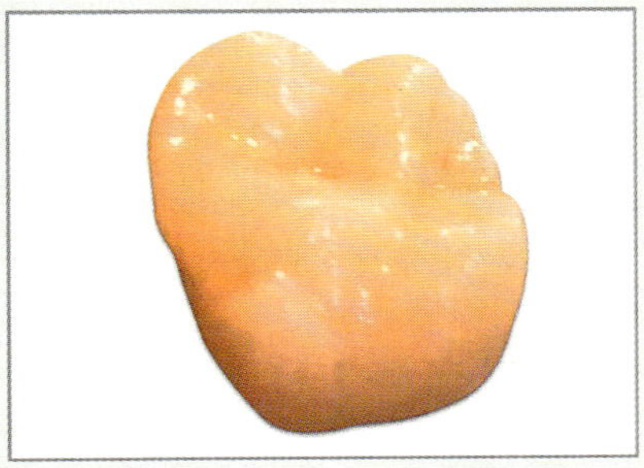 *Cusp of Carabelli* **(Fig. 73.23)**	Accessory cusp located on palatal surface of mesiolingual cusp of maxillary molar	Unknown	• 1st molar • Deep groove may predispose to caries	No treatment until groove is deep, may need restorative intervention
Fig. 73.23: cusp of carabelli.				
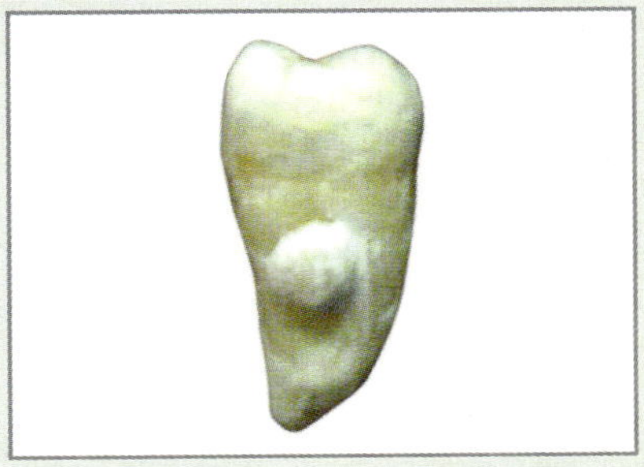 *Ectopicenamel (enamelpearl)* **(Fig. 73.24)**	Presence of enamel in unusual location	Localized bulging of odontoblastic layer that provides excess contact between Hertwig's epithelial root sheath (HeRS) and dentin triggering induction of enamel formation	• It may contain only enamel or may even have pulp • Mostly seen on roots of maxillary molars • Prevalence of 1–9% • Seen in furcation or CEJ area • Radiographically appear as circular well-defined area of radiodensity • Plaque retentive area	Meticulous hygiene and periodontal prevention is must
Fig. 73.24: Enamel pearl.				

Contd...

Contd...

Name of anomaly	***Definition***	***Etiology***	***Clinical features***	***Treatment***
Taurodontism **(Fig. 73.25)**	Enlargement of body and pulp chamber of multirooted teeth with apical displacement of pulpal floor	It may be as result of chromosomal abnormality or associated with a syndrome	• Tauro-bull, do not-teeth • Pulp chambers are large with decreased bifurcation of roots • Mostly in molars • Radiographic identification • It can be of three types: 1. Mild—hypotaurodontism 2. Moderate—mesotaurodontism 3. Severe—hypertaurodontism	Endodontic therapy has to be done carefully because of the dimensions of the chamber
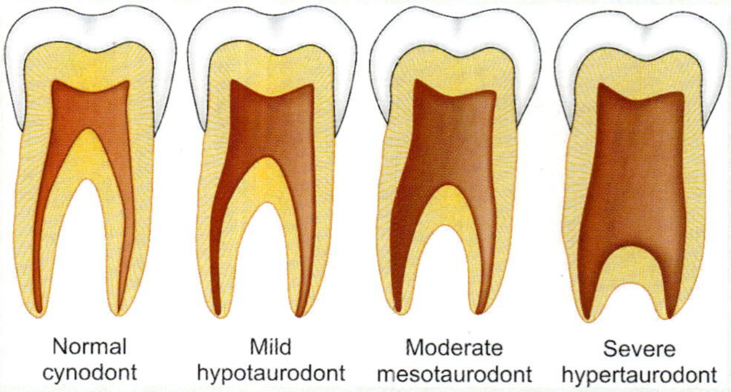**Fig. 73.25:** Taurodontism.				
Hypercementosis **(Fig. 73.26)**	Non-neoplastic deposition of excessive cementum	• Hereditary factor • Abnormal occlusal trauma • Nonantagonist teeth	• Thickening of root • Localized or generalized • Increases with age • Associated with Paget's disease, • acromegaly and calcinosis	No treatment is needed but such teeth may have to be sectioned during exodontia
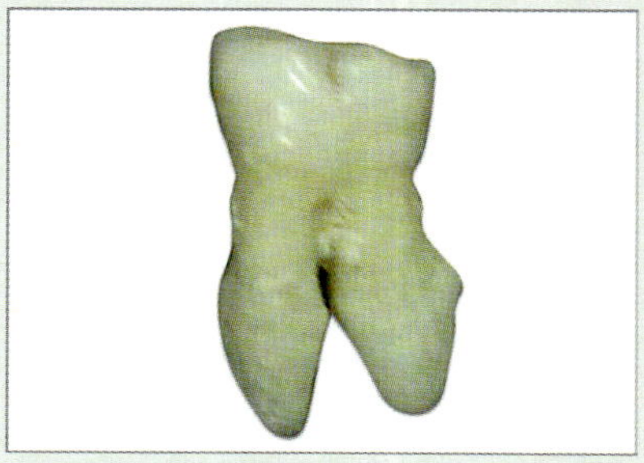**Fig. 73.26:** Hypercementosis.				
Dilaceration **(Fig. 73.27)**	Abnormal angulation of root or crown of a tooth	Injury to calcified portion of tooth germ during development	• Maxillary incisors are most affected • Rare in primary teeth • Teeth may have altered path of eruption, can be associated with periapical lesions or may be impacted	• Treatment depends upon the degree of dilacerations • Small deviation needs no treatment • Larger deviation may indicate the need for hemisection or even extraction
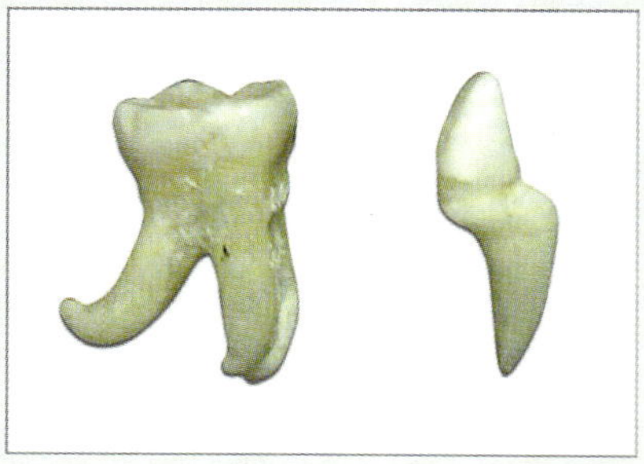**Fig. 73.27:** Dilaceration.				
Supernumerary roots **(Fig. 73.28)**	Development of increased number of roots compared to normal	unknown	Permanent dentition and molars are most affected	No treatment is required, but during endodontic therapy due consideration has to be given to the presence of such roots
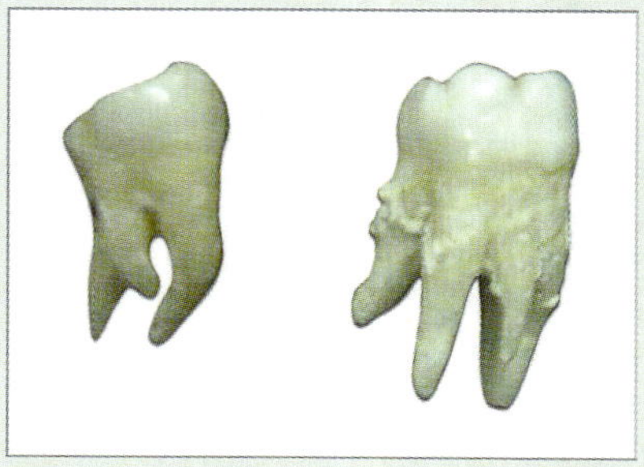**Fig. 73.28:** Supernumerary roots.				

Anomalies of structure (dentin)

Name of anomaly	***Definition***	***Etiology***	***Clinical features***	***Treatment***
Dentinogenesis imperfecta (Cap De Pont's teeth) **(Fig. 73.29)** Fig. 73.29: Dentinogenesis imperfecta.	Defective dentin formation in the absence of any systemic disease	Autosomal dominant	• More in whites • More in deciduous teeth • Molars and incisors are most affected • Blue to brown discoloration with translucence • Accelerated attrition • Thin and early obliterated pulp chamber and canals • Type 1 osteogenesis imperfecta with opalescent teeth • Type 2 hereditary isolated opalescent teeth • Type 3 Brandywine isolated opalescent teeth • Altered dentin, which may be due to anomaly of matrix or structure or mineralization	Full coverage crowns, overlays are best option because of enhanced attrition, thin dentin and more chances of pulp exposure and tooth fracture
Dentin dysplasia (DD) (rootless teeth) **(Fig. 73.30)** Fig. 73.30: Dentin dysplasia.	Loss of organization of root dentin	Autosomal dominant	• Enamel and coronal dentin is formed normally, but radicular dentin loses its organization and shortens • No detectable roots or pulp • Mobility is a feature • Permanent teeth are affected	Preventive strategy is of most importance owing to the structure of these teeth. in case of endodontic therapy it can only be done in short roots but the rootless teeth have to undergo extraction due to loss of support
Regional odontodysplasia (ghost teeth) **(Fig. 73.31)** 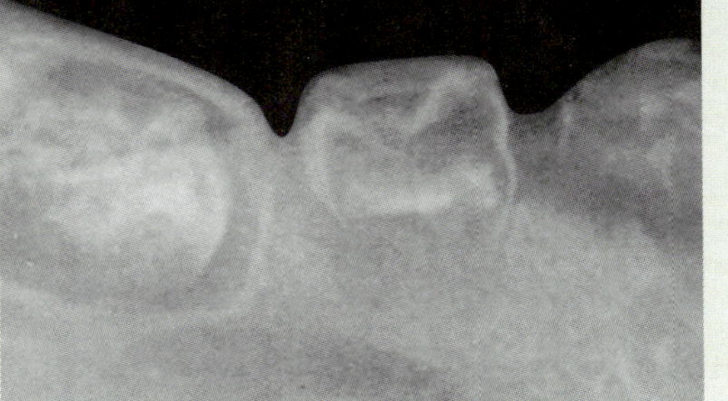 Fig. 73.31: Regional odontodysplasia.	Localized, hereditary developmental anomaly with adverse effects on enamel, dentin and pulp	• Abnormal migration of neural crest cells • Local circulatory deficiency • Local trauma or infection • Hyperpyrexia • Malnutrition • Medication during pregnancy	• Occurs in both dentition • Bimodal peak at 2–4 years and 7–11 years • More in anterior teeth • Teeth fail to erupt or erupt with yellow to brown discoloration and other enamel defects • Dentinal cleft and long pulp horns are present • Radiographically tooth shows as thin enamel and dentin with large pulp thereby giving it a floating appearance called ghost tooth • Associated with syndromes like nevi, ectodermal dysplasia and neurofibromatosis	• Therapy is to retain the altered teeth and to allow for development of arch • Unerupted teeth are not touched • Crowns can be given • Endodontic therapy in exposed teeth

Classification of dentinogenesis imperfecta		
Shields	***Clinical presentation***	***Witkop***
Dentinogenesis imperfecta I	Osteogenesis imperfecta with opalescent	Dentinogenesis imperfecta
Dentinogenesis imperfecta II	Isolated opalescent teeth	Hereditary opalescent teeth
Dentinogenesis imperfecta III	Isolated opalescent teeth	Brandywine isolate

Modified classification of hereditary disorders affecting dentin		
Disorder	***Inheritance***	***Involved Gene or Genes***
Osteogenesis imperfecta with opalescent teeth	Autosomal dominant or recessive	cOl 1A1, cOl1A2
Dentinogenesis imperfecta	Autosomal dominant	DSPP
DD type *i*	Autosomal dominant	
DD type II	Autosomal dominant	DSPP

Subclassification of dentin dysplasia type I	
DDIa	No pulp chambers, no root formation, and frequent periapical radiolucencies
DDIb	A single small horizontally oriented and crescent-shaped pulp, roots only a few millimeters in length and frequent periapical radiolucencies
DDIc	Two horizontally oriented and crescent-shaped pulpal remnants surrounding central islands of dentin, significant but shortened root length and variable periapical radiolucencies
DDId	Visible pulp chambers and canals, near normal root length, enlarged pulp stones that are located in the coronal portion of the canal and create a localized bulging of the canal and root, constriction of the pulp canal apical to the stone, and few periapical radiolucencies

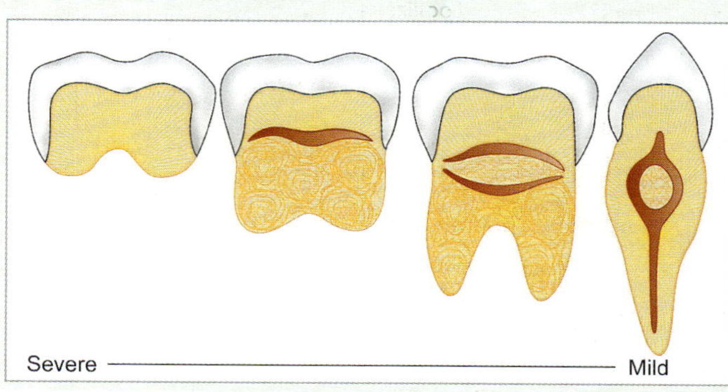

Anomalies of structure (enamel)				
Name of anomaly	***Definition***	***Etiology***	***Clinical features***	***Treatment***
Amelogenesis imperfecta (AI) **(Fig. 73.32)**	Complicated group of conditions that demonstrate developmental alterations in structure of enamel in absence of systemic disease	Autosomal dominant or recessive depending on subtype	**Hypoplastic** • **Generalized pattern:** » Inadequate deposition of enamel matrix » Pits are present on teeth » Buccal surfaces are affected and enamel is normal • **Localized pattern:** » Large area of hypoplastic enamel surrounded by zone of hypocalcification » Only middle third of buccal surface is involved » Mostly primary teeth are affected • **Smooth pattern:** » Enamel is smooth surfaced, thin, hard and glossy » Teeth are small like post crown preparation • **Rough pattern:** » Enamel is thin hard and rough surfaced » Yellow to white color » Open contacts present **Hypomaturation AI** • **General:** » Enamel matrix is laid down normally and begins mineralization, but fails to mature » Teeth exhibit mottled brown discoloration » Enamel is soft and chips away	Treatment varies according to the type of AI, but focus is on loss of vertical dimension, endodontic therapy and esthetics

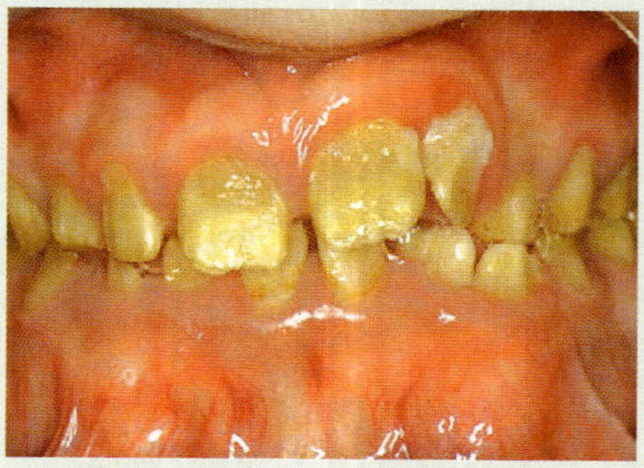

Fig. 73.32: Amelogenesis imperfecta.

Contd...

Contd...

Name of anomaly	Definition	Etiology	Clinical features	Treatment
			• **Pigmented pattern:** » Surface enamel is mottled and deep brown » Excessive calculus deposition » Enamel chips away and dentin is soft and can be punctured • **X-linked pattern:** » Deciduous teeth are opaque white with translucent mottling » Permanent teeth are yellow but darken with age » Enamel is chipped away leaving brown discoloration • **Snow capped pattern:** » Exhibit zone of opaque enamel on incisal third » Both dentitions are affected **Hypocalcified AI** • Enamel matrix is laid down but mineralization does not occur • On eruption enamel is yellow to orange and is gradually discolored • Teeth usually erupt as in normal shape but tend to fracture as they are soft • Over a period of time only cervical aspect of enamel of tooth remains	

Classification of amelogenesis imperfecta

Type	Pattern	Specific features	Inheritance
IA	Hypoplastic	Generalized pitted	Autosomal dominant
IB	Hypoplastic	Localized pitted	Autosomal dominant
IC	Hypoplastic	Localized pitted	Autosomal recessive
ID	Hypoplastic	Diffuse smooth	Autosomal dominant
IE	Hypoplastic	Diffuse smooth	X-linked dominant
IF	Hypoplastic	Diffuse rough	Autosomal dominant
IG	Hypoplastic	Enamel agenesis	Autosomal recessive
IIA	Hypomaturation	Diffuse pigmented	Autosomal recessive
IIB	Hypomaturation	Diffuse	X-linked recessive
IIC	Hypomaturation	Snow capped	X-linked
IID	Hypomaturation	Snow capped	Autosomal dominant
IIIA	Hypocalcified	Diffuse	Autosomal dominant
IIIB	Hypocalcified	Diffuse	Autosomal recessive
IVA	Hypomaturation-hypoplastic	Taurodontism present	Autosomal dominant
IVB	Hypoplastic-hypomaturation	Taurodontism present	Autosomal dominant

Modified classification of amelogenesis imperfecta

Inheritance	Phenotype	Related Genes
Autosomal dominant	Generalized pitted	
Autosomal dominant	Localized hypoplastic	*ENAM*
Autosomal dominant	Generalized thin	*ENAM*
Autosomal dominant	Hypocalcification	
Autosomal dominant	With taurodontism	*DIX3*
Autosomal recessive	Localized hypoplastic	
Autosomal recessive	Generalized thin	
Autosomal recessive	Pigmented hypomaturation	*MMP20, KIK4*
Autosomal recessive	Hypocalcification	
X-linked	Generalized thin	*AMEIX*
X-linked	Diffuse hypomaturation	*AMEIX*
X-linked	Snow-capped hypomaturation	

POINTS TO REMEMBER

- Anomalies of number: Anodontia, hypodontia, hyperdontia; Size: Microdontia, macrodontia; Position: transposition; Shape: Gemination, fusion, concrescence, accessory cusps, dens invaginatus, ectopic enamel, taurodontism, hypercementosis, accessory roots, dilaceration; Structure: Amelogenesis imperfecta, dentinogenesis imperfecta, regional odontodysplasia.
- Fusion is joining of two tooth buds, germination is attempt of tooth bud to split into two and concrescence is joining of two teeth by cementum.
- Talon's cusp is an accessory cusp like structure projecting from cingulum area of cementoenamel junction. Lateral incisors followed by central incisors and canines are most affected. Treatment is gradual reduction with fluoride application as desensitizing agent.
- Taurodontism is enlargement of body and pulp chamber of multirooted teeth with apical displacement of pulpal floor. Dentinogenesis imperfecta is defective dentin formation in the absence of any systemic disease. it is an autosomal dominant trait and is found more in white, primary teeth, molars, and incisors. Clinical picture of these teeth ranges from blue to brown discoloration with translucence.
- Dentin dysplasia is characterized as rootless teeth as enamel and coronal dentin are formed normally, but radicular dentin loses its organization and shortens.
- Amelogenesis imperfecta is a complicated group of conditions that demonstrate developmental alterations in structure of enamel in absence of systemic disease. It is of three types: (1) hypoplastic (inadequate deposition of enamel matrix), (2) hypomaturation (enamel matrix is laid down normally and begins mineralization but fails to mature), and (3) hypocalcified (enamel matrix is laid down but mineralization does not occur).

Questionnaire

1. Classify developmental anomalies of dentition and explain anomalies of number.
2. Write a note on supernumerary teeth.
3. Differentiate between fusion, gemination and concrescence.
4. Describe the developmental anomalies of shape. Explain taurodontism.
5. What are the developmental anomalies of dentinal structure?
6. Give the classification, etiology, and clinical features of amelogenesis imperfecta.

FURTHER READING

1. Andreason JO, Sundström B, Ravn JJ. The effect of traumatic injuries to primary teeth on their permanent successor. Scand J Dent Res. 1971; 145:229-83.
2. Chosack A, Edelmann E, Wisotski I, et al. Amelogenesis imperfecta among Israel Jews and the description of a new type of local hypoplastic autosomal recessive amelogenesis imperfecta. Oral Surg. 1979; 47:148-56.
3. Chow MH. Natal and neonatal teeth. J Am Dent Assoc. 1980;100(2): 215-6.
4. Mena CA. Taurodontism. Oral Surg Oral Pathol Oral Med. 1971; 32:812-23.
5. Thomas JG. A study of Dens in dente. Oral Surg Oral Pathol Oral Med. 1974; 38:653-5.
6. Thérèse Garvey M, Hugh J Barry, Marielle Blake. Supernumerary teeth: an overview of classification, diagnosis and management. J Can Dent Assoc. 1999;65: 612-6.
7. Witkop CJ Jr. Amelogenesis imperfect, dentinogenesis imperfecta and dentinal dysplasia revisited: problems in classification. J Oral Pathol. 1988; 17:547-53.

Common Orofacial Syndromes in Children

Kshitij Rohilla, Swati Karkare

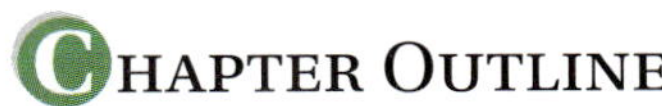

Chapter Outline

A syndrome is a group of signs and symptoms that occur together and characterize a particular abnormality or condition. The number of syndromes affecting the human race is virtually countless. One subset of this group includes the syndromes which manifest primarily in the pediatric age group. Another subset includes those syndromes in which oral manifestations form a significant component of the clinical spectrum. The overlap zone of these two subsets includes the entities which this chapter deals with. This chapter outlines the important features of more commonly occurring syndromes and also those syndromes with some peculiar and/or characteristic features which hold historic/ academic relevance.

An arbitrary categorization of syndromes of the oral and maxillofacial region, aimed at a better understanding of the disease process is as follows:

- **Chromosomal syndromes:**
  - Trisomy 21 syndrome (Down syndrome)
  - Trisomy 13 (Patau syndrome)
  - Trisomy 18 (Edwards syndrome)
  - Turner syndrome
  - Klinefelter syndrome.
- **Syndromes affecting bone:**
  - Osteogenesis imperfecta
  - *Skeletal dysplasias:*
    - Cleidocranial dysplasia
    - Infantile cortical hyperostosis (Caffey-Silverman syndrome)
    - Marfan syndrome
    - McCune-Albright syndrome.
  - *Craniotubular bone disorders:*
    - Osteopetrosis
  - *Chondrodysplasias and chondrodystrophies:*
    - Achondrogenesis
    - Achondroplasia
    - Ellis-van Creveld syndrome (chondroectodermal dysplasia).
- **Proportionate short stature syndromes:**
  - Bloom syndrome
  - Rubinstein-Taybi syndrome.
- **Overgrowth syndromes and postnatal onset obesity syndromes:**
  - Beckwith-Wiedemann syndrome [exomphalos-macroglossia-gigantism (EMG) syndrome]
  - Hemihyperplasia (hemihypertrophy).
- **Syndromes with craniosynostosis:**
  - Apert syndrome (acrocephalosyndactyly)
  - Crouzon syndrome (craniofacial dysostosis)
  - Carpenter syndrome (acrocephalopolysyndactyly)
  - Pfeiffer syndrome.
- **Branchial arch and oral-acral disorders:** Mandibulofacial dysostosis (Treacher Collins syndrome, Franceschetti-Zwahlen-Klein syndrome).
- **Orofacial clefting syndromes:**
  - Van der Woude syndrome
  - Pierre Robin syndrome.
- **Syndromes with unusual facies:**
  - Noonan syndrome
  - Parry—Romberg syndrome (progressive hemifacial atrophy).
- **Syndromes with gingival/periodontal components:**
  - Hyperkeratosis palmoplantaris and periodontoclasia in childhood (Papillon-Lefèvre syndrome).

Trisomy 21 (Down syndrome)

- Described by **John Langdon Down** in 1866 as a condition that he named "Mongolian idiocy".
- Most common and best known of all malformation syndromes.
- Occurs in offspring of mothers of all ages, but the risk increases with increasing maternal age.
- Three cytogenetics variants have been recognized:
  1. *Nondisjunction*—95%
  2. *Unbalanced chromosomal translocation (arising de novo or being transmitted from one of the parents)*—4.8%
  3. *Mosaicism*—3%.

Clinical features: Fetal brain growth is delayed (infants commonly are microcephalic at birth). Newborn infants are frequently described as being "good babies" because they are not easily disturbed and cause their mothers very little trouble. Such traits probably reflect reduced response to external stimuli and marked hypotonia.

- Mental retardation is considered to be a hallmark [intelligence quotient (IQ) varies between 30 and 50].
- Very few patients are judged to be aggressive or hostile or to display other varieties of maladaptive behavior.

Growth and skeletal abnormalities: Prenatal and postnatal growth deficiency; also a tendency toward premature birth. Osseous maturation is significantly delayed.

Craniofacial features: Brachycephaly and flat occiput [cephalic index is usually more than 0.80 and may exceed 1.00 (normal value is 0.75–0.80)].

- Large fontanels exhibiting delayed closure.
- Frontal and sphenoidal sinuses may be absent and maxillary sinuses may be hypoplastic.
- Bony midface hypoplasia produces ocular hypotelorism, a small nose with flattening of the nasal bridge, and relative mandibular prognathism.
- Upward slanting of palpebral fissures, epicanthic folds, Brushfield spots, fine lens opacities, convergent strabismus, nystagmus, keratoconus, and cataract.
- The ears tend to be small and misshapen.
- The lips are broad, irregular, fissured, and dry. An open mouth with a protruding tongue is observed. Relative macroglossia is observed, so it is fissured tongue.
- The palate is narrower and shorter but palatal height is not higher than that observed in the general population; it "appears" high because it is narrow.
- Articulation defects (pronunciation is often slurred, making speech incomprehensible).
- The voice is often hoarse, raucous, and low pitched.
- Periodontal disease has been observed in over 90% of cases. Severe involvement even below the age of 6 years is particularly common in the mandibular anterior and maxillary molar regions. Exfoliation of the lower central incisors from periodontal bone loss occurs frequently.
- The prevalence of dental caries has been stated to be low by several authors, although these findings have been challenged by others.
- Eruption of both deciduous and permanent teeth is delayed. An irregular sequence of eruption is common. Third molars, second premolars, and lateral incisors are most frequently absent in the permanent dentition.
- Malalignment of teeth is common. Posterior crossbite, mandibular overjet, mesio-occlusion, anterior open bite, crowded teeth, and widely spaced teeth.

Other findings: Broad, short neck, umbilical hernia, hypogenitalia, cryptorchidism, short broad hands showing brachydactyly, single palmar crease, clinodactyly, and hyperflexibility of joints.

Immune system: Immunodeficiency in Down syndrome is related to an increased susceptibility to infection, an increased risk for developing neoplasia, particularly leukemia, an increased frequency of autoantibodies, and early aging.

Trisomy 13 (Patau syndrome)

- Identified by **Patau et al.** in 1960, this syndrome is characterized by microcephaly, scalp defects, frequent holoprosencephaly, microphthalmia, orofacial clefting, congenital heart defects, polydactyly, severe developmental retardation, and early demise.
- Mean life expectancy is 130 days. Approximately 45% die during the 1st month, 70% during the first 6 months, and 86% during the 1st year. Survival beyond 3 years is exceptional.

Growth: Failure to thrive.

Central nervous system: Microcephaly, holoprosencephaly, apneic episodes, seizures, hypotonia, hypertonia, severe developmental retardation, and presumptive deafness.

Craniofacial features: Scalp defects, sloping forehead, capillary hemangiomas, ocular hypotelorism, epicanthic folds, microphthalmia, iris coloboma, cleft lip, cleft palate, micrognathia, and malformed ears.

Neck: Short neck, loose skin on the nape, nuchal translucency, and fetal cystic hygroma.

Cardiovascular anomalies: Patent ductus arteriosus, ventricular septal defect, atrial septal defect, dextrocardia, and coarctation of aorta.

Other findings: Inguinal/umbilical hernia, cryptorchidism, bicornuate uterus, and polydactyly.

Trisomy 18 (Edwards syndrome)

- Identified by **Edwards et al.** in 1960; features included growth deficiency, developmental retardation, prominent occiput, low-set malformed ears, micrognathia, short sternum, congenital heart defects, overlapped flexed fingers, dorsiflexed halluces, and prominent calcaneus.
- The median life expectancy for liveborn infants with trisomy 18 is 4 days with a range of 1 hour to 18 months.

Growth: Growth deficiency.

Central nervous system: Severe developmental retardation, hypertonia.

Craniofacial features: Microcephaly, dolichocephaly, prominent occiput, narrow palpebral fissures, small mouth, micrognathia, and low-set and malformed ears.

Neck: Short neck and loose skin on the nape.

Other findings: Inguinal/umbilical hernia, cryptorchidism, short sternum, small pelvis, limited hip abduction, overlapped, flexible fingers, hypoplastic nails, and syndactyly.

Turner syndrome

- In 1938, **Turner** recognized the syndrome that consists of short stature, streak gonads, webbed neck, shield chest, peripheral lymphedema at birth, coarctation of the aorta, hypoplastic nails, short metacarpals, and multiple pigmented nevi.
- Approximately, 98–99% of Turner syndrome fetuses are spontaneously aborted.
- Minimal diagnostic criterion is an abnormal karyotype in which all or part of one of the X-chromosomes is absent. Most patients have gonadal dysgenesis and short stature.

Growth: Growth pattern could be divided into four phases:
1. Intrauterine growth retardation
2. Height development which is normal up to a bone age of 2 years
3. Bone age of 2–11 years, when growth is markedly stunted
4. Bone age after 11 years when the growth phase is prolonged but total height gain is below normal.

Central nervous system: Intelligence quotient may be reduced or even normal. Intelligence is normal. Several psychiatric disturbances have been reported, especially depression, low self-esteem, and anorexia nervosa.

Head and neck abnormalities:
- Epicanthic folds, ptosis of the eyelids, prominent abnormal ears, and low hairline.
- Visual abnormalities, particularly strabismus, and myopia.
- Chronic suppurative otitis with resultant hearing loss.
- Webbed neck. Excess skin on the nape of the neck in infants. Neck blebs or cystic hygromas during embryonic life.
- High-arched palate with higher than normal frequency of cleft palate.
- Premature eruption of teeth (first permanent molars appearing between 1.5 and 4 years of age).
- Increased molarization of premolars.
- Reduced cusp height as well as crown size.
- Micrognathia. Short cranial base, so the face is retrognathic.
- Short mandible, maxilla being of normal length.
- Midfacial hypoplasia, deepening of posterior cranial fossa, and widely spaced mandibular rami.

Other findings: Gonadal dysgenesis, coarctation of the aorta, ventricular septal defect, hypoplastic nails, and multiple pigmented nevi.

Klinefelter syndrome

Klinefelter et al. in 1942 reported postpubertal males with small testes, azoospermia, and gynecomastia. Classic Klinefelter syndrome is diagnosed most commonly at puberty, although rarely clinical clues may be evident in childhood.

Growth: Until 3 years of age, height distribution is unremarkable. In adulthood, typical Klinefelter individuals are of average or somewhat above-average height. Tall stature is primarily the result of increase in leg length, which is present before puberty but not particularly obvious.

Central nervous system and performance: Delayed speech, delays in emotional development, school maladjustment, and poor gross motor coordination.
- Average IQ is approximately 90 (individuals are usually neither highly intelligent nor severely retarded).
- In adults, there may be disturbances of behavior, deviations in personality, neurotic and psychotic reactions, antisocial behavior, alcoholism, aggressiveness, depression, and periods of mania. Many Klinefelter individuals lead normal married lives.

Hormones: Leydig cells are defective; plasma testosterone is low in the presence of normal or high follicle-stimulating hormone (FSH) and luteinizing hormone (LH). Typically, patients have 50% or less of normal levels of plasma testosterone and a fourfold increase in urinary excretion of pituitary gonadotropin.

Craniofacial features: Cephalometric investigation shows smaller calvarial size, smaller cranial base angle, and larger gonial angle than normal. Both maxillary and mandibular prognathisms tend to occur. Permanent tooth crowns tend to be larger. Taurodontism has been reported in some instances.

Other findings may include microcephaly, cleft palate, "third" fontanel, nerve deafness, ear anomalies, downslanting palpebral fissures, corneal opacity, and strabismus.

Cleidocranial dysostosis

- First descriptions were those by **Martin** in 1765 and **Meckel** in 1760. **Marie** and **Sainton**, in 1897 named the syndrome "cleidocranial dysostosis" reporting the combination of aplasia or hypoplasia of one or both clavicles, exaggerated development of the transverse diameter of the cranium, and delayed ossification of fontanels.
- The syndrome has autosomal dominant inheritance and occurs due to mutations were found in the *core-binding factor A1 (CBFA1)* gene which controls differentiation of precursor cells into osteoblasts.

Facies and general appearance:
- The appearance is generally pathognomonic. Affected individuals are usually short. Brachycephalic skull, pronounced frontal and parietal bossing, hypoplastic maxilla, and zygomas, these features make the face appear small. The nose is broad at the base with the bridge depressed. There is hypertelorism.
- Neck appears long, and the shoulders are narrow and droop markedly.
- Increased mandibular length, vertically short maxilla.

Cranium: Large and short skull with biparietal bossing, cephalic index more than 80, delayed closure of the anterior fontanel and sagittal and metopic sutures, segmental calvarial thickening in the supraorbital portion of the frontal bone, the squama of the temporal bones, and the occipital bone above the inion.
- Presence of many wormian bones. Parietal bones may be absent at birth. Paranasal sinuses and mastoids often underdeveloped or absent.
- Cranial base has short sagittal diameter. Large foramen magnum with defects in the posterior wall.

Clavicle: Clavicles are absent unilaterally or bilaterally in about 10; more frequently, they are defective at the acromial end. Ability of the patient to approximate the shoulders in front of the chest is remarkable.

Contd...

Contd...

Oral manifestations:

- High-arched palate, submucous cleft palate, and complete cleft of the hard and soft palates.
- Delayed union at the mandibular symphysis is characteristic. Deficient ossification of the hyoid bone. Underdeveloped premaxilla along with normal mandibular growth causes relative prognathism. Newborns may have prolonged feeding problems.
- Multiple supernumerary teeth, multiple crown and root abnormalities, crypt formation around impacted teeth, ectopic localization of teeth, and lack of tooth eruption. The extra teeth are most often in the mandibular premolar and maxillary incisor areas. It is known that extraction of deciduous teeth does not promote eruption of permanent teeth. Roots lack a layer of cellular cementum.
- Deciduous root resorption is extremely delayed or arrested, and can probably be explained by diminished bone resorption. Abnormalities of root morphology in the permanent dentition appear secondary to arrested eruption.

Infantile cortical hyperostosis (Caffey–Silverman syndrome)

- Originally, described by **Roske** in 1930, but detailed by the clinical and radiographic studies of **Caffey** and **Silverman** in 1945–1946.
- Affects infants under 6 months of age; generally a benign and self-limited disorder.

Most constant features: Bilateral swelling over the mandible or other bones, radiographic evidence of new bone formation in the area, hyperirritability, and mild fever.

Facies: Because of the swelling, the facies is so striking that the condition may be diagnosed with considerable assurance even prior to confirmatory X-ray evidence. The swelling is symmetric and located over the body and ramus of the mandible, often with pallor.

Soft tissues: Tender, soft-tissue swelling over the face, around the orbits, thorax, or extremities which undergoes remission and exacerbation. It is firm, brawny, and often so painful as to cause pseudoparalysis of an extremity; not accompanied by redness or increased heat.

Fever and irritability: Pain, fever of mild degree, and hyperirritability commonly seen; one or all may, however, be absent. Anemia, leukocytosis, and elevation of erythrocyte sedimentation rate (ESR) may also occur.

Skeletal system: The most frequently affected bone is the mandible; less commonly involved are the clavicle, tibia, ulna, femur, rib, humerus, maxilla, and fibula.

- New periosteal bone formation appearing most often during the 9th week undergoes resolution slowly. Though complete clinical resolution takes place within 3–30 months, radiographic evidence may persist for many years.
- Leg length inequality and forward bowing of the tibia are common.

Oral manifestations: Jaw swelling is the most common presenting sign. Fever seems to have no effect on the enamel or on the eruption sequence, although radiographic evidence of residual bony asymmetry of the mandible (angle and ramus) and severe malocclusion in some patients may be seen. Dysphagia has also been reported.

Marfan syndrome

- French pediatrician **Antoine-Bernard Marfan** described a 5-year-old girl with skeletal manifestations of the disorder whose main features included disproportionate skeletal growth with dolichostenomelia, ectopia lentis, and fusiform and dissecting aneurysms of the aorta. It has been suggested that **Abraham Lincoln** had Marfan syndrome.
- Mutations in *fibrillin type I* gene; autosomal dominant pattern of inheritance.

Craniofacial features: Dolichocephaly with prominent supraorbital ridges resulting in a characteristic long face with deeply set eyes, prominent brows, downslanting palpebral fissures, hypoplastic malar eminences, and retrognathia.

- Cleft palate or bifid uvula.
- *Teeth:* Long and narrow and frequently maloccluded.
- Mandibular prognathism is common and temporomandibular joint disease is found with increased frequency. Large maxillary sinuses noted radiographically.

Musculoskeletal system: Dolichostenomelia, arachnodactyly, pectus excavatum, and hyperextensibility of joints with recurrent dislocation.

- In later life, secondary arthritic changes occur commonly.
- Scoliosis may develop in childhood and worsen during periods of rapid growth such as puberty, and can be accompanied by a thoracic or thoracolumbar kyphosis.
- The skull shows often dolichocephaly.

Ocular changes: Ectopia lentis, increased tendency to myopia, and megalocornea.

Cardiovascular abnormalities: Aorta aneurysm, mitral valve prolapse.

Pulmonary pathology: Thoracic cage deformities, increased risk for spontaneous pneumothorax, pulmonary infections, chronic emphysematous changes, and reduced pulmonary vital capacity.

Miscellaneous findings: Abnormalities of central nervous system (CNS) include dural ectasia, sacral meningocele, and dilated cisterna magna, but neurological manifestations are rare. Other symptoms in Marfan syndrome are nephrotic syndrome, hematologic abnormalities, hypogonadism, myopathic symptoms due to a diminished amount of skeletal muscles, sleep apnea, diminished amount of subcutaneous fat, biliary tract anomalies, and alopecia.

McCune–Albright syndrome

The **McCune–Albright** syndrome is characterized by: (a) Polyostotic fibrous dysplasia, (b) Multiple areas of cutaneous light brown pigmentation or café au lait spots, and (c) Autonomous hyperfunction of one or more endocrine glands especially gonads and thyroid.

Skeletal manifestations: Long bones are most frequently affected.

Bowing resembling a hockey stick may be produced, resulting in leg-length discrepancy. Limp, leg pain, or fracture is the presenting complaint. Fractures may be multiple and recurrent.

Contd...

Contd...

Histopathology: Bone is replaced by a yellowish to red-brown fibrous tissue, the stroma may vary from a finely fibrillar one with a loose whorled arrangement to one that is densely collagenous. Some areas appear edematous, with numerous small cystic spaces. Foci of hemorrhage and multinucleated giant cells may be observed. The trabeculae are irregular in form, and occasionally a few fragments of cartilage are present.

Craniofacial findings: Facial asymmetry, accompanied by protrusion of an eye with associated visual disturbances. The skull base becomes thickened and dense, bulging upward into the cranial cavity. The calvaria may also become thickened, with marked occipital and frontal bulging. Bossing may be asymmetric, with unilateral and occasionally bilateral, obliteration of the sinuses and nasal passages. Overgrowth of bone around foramina may result in deafness and blindness.

The jaws may be enlarged, expanded, and distorted. Radiographic examination may show a dense mass, especially in the maxilla, extending into and obliterating the sinuses and expanding the buccal plate in the tuberosity areas, or there may be a radiolucent area, more common in the mandible, similar to that seen in long bones. Often there is loss of trabeculae and a "ground-glass" appearance on radiographic examination.

Cutaneous manifestations: Café-au-lait type of pigmentation; well-defined, generally unilateral, irregular macular spots scattered over the forehead, nuchal area, and buttocks. Face, lips, or mucosa is rarely involved.

Endocrine manifestations: Sexual precocity occurs in both males and females. Precocious puberty in males may be accompanied by gynecomastia. Hyperthyroidism, Cushing's syndrome, hypersomatotropinism, hyperprolactinemia, hyperparathyroidism, X-linked dominant hypophosphatemic vitamin D-resistant rickets or osteomalacia without hypercalcemia have been reported.

Central nervous system: Most patients have normal intelligence, mental deficiency is rare, and may be secondary to factors such as prematurity, hypercorticalism, or grossly malformed skull.

Severe autosomal dominant osteopetrosis (Albers–Schönberg disease)

This disorder is characterized by increased density of nearly all bones and the following complications that occur from failure of resorption of the primary spongiosa and its resultant persistence: Anemia, hepatosplenomegaly, blindness, deafness, facial paralysis, and osteomyelitis.

Clinical findings: All tubular bones may be involved, but growth is usually normal. The skull is thickened and dense mainly at its base, but the calvaria, mastoid bones, and paranasal sinuses are poorly aerated, and the facial bones appear denser than normal. Facial paralysis results from the pressure of dense bone on the foramen of the 7th cranial nerve. The ossicles lack medullary cavities. Intracerebral calcifications at birth have been described.

Musculoskeletal findings: The bones are extremely uniformly dense but not distorted in form. The epiphyses, metaphyses, and diaphyses are similarly affected. The cortical and cancellous bones are indistinguishable radiographically. Fractures are common. Older children may show a "hair-on-end" phenomenon in the calvaria.

Hematopoietic findings: Although the liver and spleen are normal at birth, they enlarge in childhood because of extramedullary hematopoiesis. Hemolytic anemia, thrombocytopenia, and generalized lymphadenopathy can occur.

Oral manifestations: Osteomyelitis of the jaws, presumably the result of deficient blood supply, seems to be a significant complication of dental extraction; may lead to extraoral fistulas.

- Primary molars and all permanent teeth are greatly distorted and remain totally or partially embedded in basal bone. The teeth appear to be secondarily affected by failure of bone resorption and/or osteomyelitis.
- Ankylosis of cementum to bone, and higher incidence of dental caries.

Achondrogenesis

The term "achondrogenesis" was coined by **Fraccaro** in 1952. It is a type of lethal chondrodysplasia; half of the infants being stillborn and the rest succumbing within the first few hours.

Facies: The (usually normocephalic) head is disproportionately large relative to reduced neck, trunk, and limb length, causing the infant to be erroneously considered to have hydrocephaly. In type 1A, the forehead slopes and the face appears puffy. The nose is small with anteverted nares and long philtrum, and there is retrognathia with double chin. Type 1B and 2 infants have a large prominent forehead, flat face, depressed nose with marked anteversion of nostrils, normal philtrum, and more normal chin. The neck is short in all types. Cleft palate is common.

Skeletal alterations: The extremities are bowed, rarely exceeding 10 cm in length. The fingers and toes are similarly short and stubby. Polydactyly may be found. The belly is greatly enlarged, partly from the short chest cavity and partly from hydrops. The genitalia are normal. Marked underossification of vertebral bodies, sternum, ilia, ischia pubic bones, talus, and calcaneus. The ribs are short and cupped with flared ends.

Histopathology: The cartilage is hypercellular with clustered chondrocytes within a diffuse matrix. The resting chondrocytes contain periodic acid-Schiff (PAS)-positive, diastase-resistant, and round to oval intracytoplasmic inclusions. The lacunae are dilated.

Achondroplasia

- The term "achondroplasia" was first used by **Parrot** in 1878 to describe a rhizomelic form of short-limbed dwarfism associated with enlarged head, depressed nasal bridge, short stubby trident hands, lordotic lumbar spine, prominent buttocks, and protuberant abdomen.
- One of the most common of the nonlethal bone dysplasias.
- Homozygous achondroplastic infants are more severely affected, clinically and radiologically, than are infants heterozygous for the disorder, and the condition is lethal during infancy.

Molecular findings: The basic defect is a mutation in fibroblast growth factor receptor 3 (FGFR3).

Growth and development: There is a tendency toward obesity. Motor milestones are slow, possibly because acquisition of motor skills is influenced by the large head and short extremities. Head control may not occur until 3–4 months and affected children may not walk until 24–36 months. Ultimately, however, development falls within the population-based normal range and most individuals with achondroplasia are able to lead an independent and productive life.

- Reproductive fitness is considerably reduced among those with achondroplasia because of social difficulties in finding mates and because of obstetrical problems of achondroplastic women (prematurity and the necessity for cesarean deliveries due to cephalopelvic disproportion).
- Furthermore, premature menopause and an increased incidence of leiomyomata have been reported.

Contd...

Contd...

Facies and skull: The head is enlarged with frontal bossing and low nasal bridge. Occasionally, these features are not present at birth, but disproportionate growth of the head occurs during the 1st year of life.

Central nervous system: Mild ventricular dilatation, significant hydrocephaly, obstructive sleep apnea due to brainstem compression, and neurologic complications with age due to narrow spinal canal.

Skeletal system: Enlarged calvaria, basilar kyphosis, and small foramen magnum.

- The anterior cranial base length is normal and posterior cranial base length is shorter.
- Hypoplastic maxilla resulting in midface deficiency and relative mandibular prognathism. The frontal, occipital bones, and in some cases, the temporal bones may be prominent.
- The sacrum is narrow and horizontally oriented; pelvis is broad and short.
- The thoracic cage is relatively small in anteroposterior diameter.
- Legs are frequently bowed because of lax knee ligaments; limb bones are shortened in a rhizomelic pattern which is more prominent in the upper extremities; there is incomplete extension at the elbows.

Otolaryngologic findings: Otitis media is likely common during the first 6 years of life. History of ear infections; significant hearing loss.

Ellis–van Creveld syndrome (Chondroectodermal dysplasia)

- The disorder consists of bilateral postaxial polydactyly of the hands, chondrodysplasia of long bones resulting in acromesomelic dwarfism, ectodermal dysplasia affecting nails and teeth, and congenital heart anomalies.
- Autosomal recessive inheritance.
- Ellis–van Creveld syndrome is the most common type of dwarfism among the Amish.
- The life expectancy is mainly determined by the congenital heart defect and the respiratory problems due to the thoracic cage deformity.

Facies: The facies is not especially characteristic except for a mild defect in the middle of the upper lip which although often present, is usually not striking. Some patients have been noted to have hypertelorism.

Skeletal anomalies: Extremities are plump and markedly shortened progressively distalward, that is, from the trunk to the phalanges.

- Frequently, the patient cannot make a tight fist.
- Radiographically, the tubular bones are short and thickened. The diaphyseal ends of the humerus and the femur are plump. Fibula is most severely shortened, syncarpalism (hamate and capitate), synmetacarpalism, and polymetacarpalism are frequent.
- Histopathologic studies in three fetuses showed chondrocytic disorganization in the physeal growth zone, both in the long bones and vertebrae.

Hair and nails: The hair, particularly the eyebrows and pubic hair, is thin and sparse. Severe dystrophy of the fingernails which are markedly hypoplastic, thin, and often wrinkled or spoon-shaped.

Oral manifestations: The most striking and constant finding is fusion of the middle portion of the upper lip to the maxillary gingival margin so that no mucobuccal fold or sulcus is present anteriorly.

- The middle portion of the upper lip appears to have a notch.
- Natal teeth commonly observed, so are congenitally missing teeth, particularly in the mandibular anterior region. Supernumerary teeth have also been noted.
- Erupted teeth are usually small, have conical crowns, and are irregularly spaced.

Bloom syndrome

Bloom syndrome consists of intrauterine growth retardation, sunlight sensitivity leading to telangiectatic erythema, immunologic deficiency, hypogonadism and infertility in males, and an increased risk of neoplasia.

Clinical features: Light sensitivity is noticed early in infancy and leads to development of telangiectatic erythema, appearing by 2 years of age. Erythema involves light-exposed areas of the face; superficially it resembles lupus erythematosus because of the butterfly distribution across the nose. Severe lesions also may occur on the lower eyelids, lips, ears, and neck. A chronic fissure or ulcer of the lower lip is a bothersome complication and chronic cheilitis is a prominent feature. The eyelashes may be lost. Exposure to sunlight may cause bullae and vesicles.

Rubinstein–Taybi syndrome

In 1963, **Rubinstein** and **Taybi** observed a combination of broad thumbs and halluces, characteristic facial dysmorphism, growth retardation, and mental deficiency.

Growth: Length, weight, and head circumference at birth are below normal.

Craniofacial features: The facial appearance is striking with microcephaly, prominent forehead, downslanting palpebral fissures, epicanthal folds, strabismus, broad nasal bridge, beaked nose with the nasal septum extending below the alae, high-arched palate, and mild micrognathia. The features are recognizable in the newborn. Other findings may include long eyelashes, nasolacrimal duct obstruction, ptosis of eyelids, congenital or juvenile glaucoma, refractive error, and minor abnormalities in shape, position, and degree of rotation of ears.

- Low-frequency abnormalities have included bifid uvula, submucous palatal cleft, bifid tongue, macroglossia, short lingual frenum, natal teeth, and thin upper lip.
- Talon cusps have been observed in over 90% of subjects.

Beckwith–Wiedemann syndrome [exomphalos-macroglossia-gigantism (EMG) syndrome]

This syndrome includes macroglossia, omphalocele, cytomegaly of adrenal cortex, hyperplasia of gonadal interstitial cells, renal medullary dysplasia, hyperplastic visceromegaly, postnatal somatic gigantism, mild microcephaly, and severe hypoglycemia. Early diagnosis of this striking condition alerts the clinician to the dual threat of hypoglycemia and possible neoplasia.

Contd...

Contd...

Craniofacial features: Macroglossia is very common at birth but is not an obligatory feature of the syndrome, and it may not present until the first few months of life. Chronic alveolar hypoventilation has been reported secondary to macroglossia on occasion.

- Tongue biopsies have been normal.
- In some cases, macroglossia tends to regress with gradual accommodation of the tongue to the oral cavity. At present, it is not known whether this is caused by enlargement of the oral cavity relative to the tongue, shrinkage of the tongue relative to the oral cavity, or a combination of both processes. Persistent macroglossia seen in almost 100% leads to anterior open bite, and requires surgical intervention.
- Patients with the syndrome have also been observed to be prognathic; prognathism may reflect the generalized somatic gigantism that occurs in the syndrome.
- Facial nevus flammeus, mild microcephaly, persistent anterior fontanel, malformed cerebellum, preauricular pits, cleft palate, and conductive hearing loss from fixation of the stapes are some of the other features.

Hemihyperplasia (Hemihypertrophy)

Although the term hemihypertrophy has been used conventionally and frequently in the medical literature, it is inappropriate, as the condition so obviously refers to hemihyperplasia. In hemihyperplasia, the enlarged area may vary from a single digit, a single limb, or unilateral facial enlargement to involvement of half the body. Hemihyperplasia may be segmental, unilateral, or crossed. In some cases, the defect is limited to a single system, for example, muscular, vascular, skeletal, or nervous system, but it may frequently involve multiple systems. The etiology and pathogenesis are poorly understood.

Clinical manifestations: Asymmetry is usually evident at birth and may become accentuated with age, especially at puberty. Occasionally, asymmetry has been stated not to be present at birth, but to develop later. However, such observations are valid only when measurements are taken at birth. A variety of non-neoplastic abnormalities have been observed to affect the limbs, teeth, skin, CNS, cardiovascular system, liver, kidneys, and genitalia. Cutaneous anomalies include telangiectasia, nevus flammeus, and hirsutism. Various neoplasms have been reported in association with hemihyperplasia.

Oral and dental anomalies include enlarged hemitongue, enlarged teeth on affected side with early eruption, abnormal tooth roots, and an enlarged alveolar ridge on affected side.

Apert syndrome (Acrocephalosyndactyly)

Apert syndrome is characterized by craniosynostosis, midfacial malformations and symmetric syndactyly of the hands and feet, minimally involving digits 2, 3, and 4. Although most cases are sporadic, representing new mutations, autosomal dominant transmission with complete penetrance has also been reported.

Craniofacial features: During infancy, there is a wide midline calvarial defect that extends from the glabella to the posterior fontanel that gradually fills in with bony islands that coalesce.

- Hyperacrobrachycephaly, flat occiput, steep forehead, supraorbital groove, bulging at the bregma or malformed and asymmetric cranial base, and short anterior cranial base are observed. The cranial base angle is variable, but platybasia occurs most commonly. Cloverleaf skull may be observed.
- The middle third of the face is retruded and commonly hypoplastic resulting in relative mandibular prognathism.
- Depressed nasal bridge, beaked nose, and deviated nasal septum.
- Hypertelorism, shallow orbits, proptosis, downslanting palpebral fissures, and strabismus are seen. The absence of the superior rectus muscle has been noted.
- The ears may appear lowest. Minor anomalies are frequent. Otitis media is common related to the high frequency of cleft palate and to eustachian tube dysfunction.
- In the relaxed state, the lips frequently assume a trapezoidal configuration.
- The palate is highly arched, constricted, and usually has a median furrow. Lateral palatal swellings are present which increase in size with age. Cleft soft palate, or bifid uvula may be observed. The hard palate is shorter than normal, but the soft palate is both longer and thicker than normal.
- Alterations in the nasopharyngeal architecture consist of reduction in pharyngeal height, width, and depth. The combination of reduced nasopharyngeal dimensions and decreased patency of the posterior nasal choanae poses the possible threat of respiratory embarrassment and cor-pulmonale especially in the young child.
- The maxillary dental arch is V-shaped (due to maxillary hypoplasia) with severely crowded teeth and bulging alveolar ridges. Class III malocclusion, irregular positioning of teeth, anterior open bite, anterior and posterior crossbite, and delayed eruption of teeth are common findings.

Growth: The growth pattern in infancy and childhood consists of a gradual decrease in height. A significant proportion of patients are mentally retarded.

Hands and feet: Syndactyly, some degree of brachydactyly, and associated synonychia are common. Synostosis of adjacent distal phalanges occurs with age, so does stiffening of interphalangeal joints. Progressive calcification and fusion of the bones of the hands, feet, and cervical spine also becomes visible radiographically with age.

Crouzon syndrome (Craniofacial dysostosis)

- Crouzon syndrome, first described by **Crouzon** in 1912 is characterized by craniosynostosis, maxillary hypoplasia, shallow orbits, and ocular proptosis.
- Autosomal dominant transmission.

Craniofacial features: Cranial malformation depends on the order and rate or progression of sutural synostosis. Brachycephaly is most commonly observed, but scaphocephaly, trigonocephaly, and cloverleaf skull may be observed. Craniosynostosis commonly begins during the 1st year of life and is usually complete by 2–3 years of age; may be evident at birth in some cases.

- Shallow orbits and ocular proptosis are diagnostic features; may be evident at birth or during the 1st year of life. This proptosis predisposes to exposure conjunctivitis or keratitis, luxation of the eyeglobes, exotropia, poor vision, and blindness.

Contd...

- Various sutures may be prematurely synostosed, and multiple sutural involvement is found eventually in most cases.
- Lateral palatal swellings, sometimes large enough to produce the median pseudocleft palate appearance may be found.
- Cleft lip and cleft palate are anomalies of low frequency.
- Maxillary hypoplasia shortens the anteroposterior dimension of the maxillary dental arch. Dental arch width is also reduced, and the constricted arch gives the appearance of high-arched palate, although palatal height is normal by measurement. Crowding of maxillary teeth and ectopic eruption of maxillary first molars also occur.
- Unilateral or bilateral posterior crossbite may be evident. Anterior open bite, mandibular overjet, and crowding of mandibular anterior teeth are also commonly observed.

Carpenter syndrome (Acrocephalopolysyndactyly)

- Carpenter syndrome is characterized by craniosynostosis, commonly but not always preaxial polysyndactyly of the feet, short fingers with clinodactyly, and variable soft tissue syndactyly, sometimes postaxial polydactyly, and other abnormalities such as congenital heart defects, short stature, obesity, and mental deficiency.
- Autosomal recessive inheritance.
- Height is below normal, weight is often above average. Obesity of the trunk, proximal limbs, face, and neck is common.

Craniofacial features: Craniosynostosis usually involves the sagittal and lambdoid sutures first, the coronal being last to close. The calvaria may be grossly malformed in some instances, but variable in shape.

- Unilateral involvement of the coronal or lambdoid suture produces marked cranial asymmetry. The cloverleaf skull anomaly may also be observed.
- Downslanting palpebral fissures, epicanthic folds, microcornea, corneal opacity, slight optic atrophy, and blurring of the disc margins have been reported.
- Low set ears, short neck, preauricular fistulas, small mandible, and narrow or high-arched palate.

Hands and feet: The hands are short and the stubby fingers. Marked soft tissue syndactyly may be present. Clinodactyly of the fingers, single flexion crease, and sometimes postaxial polydactyly may be observed.

Pfeiffer syndrome

In 1964, **Pfeiffer** described a syndrome consisting of craniosynostosis, broad thumbs, broad great toes, and a variable feature, partial soft tissue syndactyly of the hands.

Craniofacial features: Maxillary hypoplasia and relative mandibular prognathism seen. Depressed nasal bridge, beaked nose, hypertelorism, downslanting palpebral fissures, ocular proptosis, and strabismus are common. High-arched palate, broad alveolar ridges, crowded teeth, and sometimes even natal teeth are found.

Hands and feet: Mild soft tissue syndactyly, brachydactyly, and clinodactyly are common. Symphalangism of both hands and feet has been reported.

Mandibulofacial dysostosis (Treacher Collins syndrome; Franceschetti–Zwahlen–Klein syndrome)

- Mandibulofacial dysostosis involves structures derived from the first and second pharyngeal arches, grooves, and pouches.
- Treacher Collins described the essential components of the syndrome; **Franceschetti et al.** coined the term mandibulofacial dysostosis.
- Autosomal dominant inheritance. The gene for the syndrome (Treacle or *TCOF1*) has been mapped to 5q32-33.1 and it encodes a putative nucleolar phosphoprotein.

Facies: The facial appearance is characteristic. Abnormalities are bilateral and usually symmetric. The nose appears large but this appearance is secondary to hypoplastic supraorbital rims and hypoplastic zygomas. The face is narrow. Downward-slanting palpebral fissures, depressed cheekbones, malformed pinnae, receding chin, and large downturned mouth are characteristic. Few patients manifest a tongue-shaped process of hair that extends toward the cheek.

Skull: The calvaria are essentially normal, but supraorbital ridges are poorly developed. Malar bones may be totally absent but more often are grossly and symmetrically underdeveloped with nonfusion of the zygomatic arches.

- Zygomatic process of the frontal bone, as well as lateral pterygoid plates and muscles show hypoplasia.
- Mastoids are not pneumatized and are frequently sclerotic.
- The paranasal sinuses are often small and may be completely absent.
- The orbits are hyperteloric, lower margin may be defective, and the infraorbital foramen is usually absent.
- Mandibular condyle and coronoid process are severely hypoplastic, flat, or even aplastic. The undersurface of the body of the mandible is quite concave. The angle is more obtuse than normal, and the ramus is deficient. The condyle is covered with hyaline cartilage rather than fibrocartilage. The condylar neck is short. There is no articular eminence, and the articular area is atypically medial.

Eyes: The palpebral fissures are short and slope laterally downward; there is a coloboma in the outer third of the lower lid.

Ears: The pinnae are often malformed, crumpled forward, or misplaced toward the angle of the mandible. Agenesis or hypoplasia of the mastoid, absence of the external auditory canal, narrowing or agenesis of the middle ear cleft, agenesis or malformation of the malleus and/or incus, absence of stapes and oval window, ankylosis of stapes in the oval window, deformed suprastructure of stapes, complete absence of middle ear, and epitympanic space have been seen. The inner ears are normal. Extra ear tags and blind fistulas may occur.

Nose: Obliterated nasofrontal angle, raised bridge of the nose, narrow nares, and hypoplastic alar cartilages. Nose appears large because of the lack of malar development and hypoplastic supraorbital ridges.

Oral findings: Cleft palate, congenital palatopharyngeal incompetence (agenesis of soft palate, foreshortened soft palate, submucous palatal cleft, and immobile soft palate), macrostomia (unilateral or bilateral), deficient elevator muscles of the upper lip, absent or hypoplastic parotid salivary glands, and pharyngeal hypoplasia (main cause of neonatal death).

Van der Woude syndrome (Cleft lip-palate and paramedian sinuses of the lower lip)

- Autosomal dominant inheritance with variable expressivity.
- Manifestations of the syndrome in other than the oral or facial areas are unusual.

Oral manifestations: Usually bilateral, often symmetrically placed depressions are observed on the vermilion portion of the lower lip, one on each side of the midline. The depressions represent blind sinuses that descend through the orbicularis oris muscle to a depth of 1 mm to 2.5 cm and communicate with the underlying minor salivary glands through their excretory ducts.

Adhesions between maxilla and mandible (syngnathia) have been noted. Absence of maxillary and mandibular second premolars and natal teeth has been described.

Pierre Robin syndrome (Robin sequence)

The well-recognized combination of micrognathia, cleft palate, and glossoptosis, was first reported in 1923 by **Pierre Robin**.

Clinical manifestations: The facies is striking at birth (small mandible which is symmetrically receded flattened base of nose, and U-shaped or V-shaped palatal cleft).

- Difficulty in respiration is apparent with periodic cyanotic attacks, labored breathing, and recession of the sternum and ribs. Although there is no complete agreement concerning the exact mechanism by which respiratory and feeding difficulties are produced, the classic explanation suggests that the micrognathia makes for little support of the tongue musculature allowing the tongue to fall downward and backward (glossoptosis) into the lower postpharyngeal space obstructing the epiglottis.
- Feeding problems are because of inadequate control of the tongue; nursing is difficult.

Musculoskeletal abnormalities: Syndactyly, hypoplastic digits, polydactyly, clinodactyly, oligodactyly, Poland anomaly, hyperextensible joints, congenital hip dislocation, as well as rib and sternal anomalies have been reported.

Central nervous system defects: Language delay, epilepsy, hypotonia, and hydrocephalus.

Other findings: Microphthalmia, glaucoma, low-set and malformed ears, otitis media, hearing loss, nasal deformity, and philtrum malformation.

Noonan syndrome

- Noonan syndrome is characterized by short stature, various congenital heart defects, broad or webbed neck, chest deformity, hypertelorism with characteristic facial appearance, and in some cases mild mental deficiency.
- Autosomal dominant inheritance.

Craniofacial features: Facial characteristics change with age.

- In the newborn, features include tall forehead, hypertelorism, downslanting palpebral fissures, epicanthal folds, depressed nasal root with upturned nasal tip, deeply grooved philtrum with high, wide peaks of the vermilion border, high-arched palate, micrognathia, low-set and posteriorly angulated ears with thick helices, and excessive nuchal skin with low posterior hairline.
- During infancy, the head is relatively large. Hypertelorism, prominent eyes, and thick hooded eyelids are characteristic. The nasal bridge is low and the nose has a wide base with bulbous tip.
- During childhood, the face may appear coarse or myopathic. Facial contour becomes more triangular with age.
- During adolescence and young adulthood, the eyes become less prominent and the nose has a thin, high bridge, and a wide base. The neck appears longer with accentuated webbing or prominent trapezius.
- In older adults, the nasolabial folds are prominent, the anterior hairline is high, and the skin appears wrinkled and transparent.
- Features present regardless of age include blue-green irides, halo iris, arched eyebrows, and low-set posteriorly angulated ears with thick helices.

Romberg syndrome (Parry–Romberg syndrome; progressive hemifacial atrophy)

Parry-Romberg syndrome consists of slowly progressive atrophy of the soft tissues of essentially half the face accompanied most frequently by contralateral Jacksonian epilepsy, trigeminal neuralgia, and changes in the eyes and hair.

Face, skin, and hair: In advanced cases, the face is quite distinct. The ear may become misshapen and smaller than normal, or because of lack of supporting tissues may project from the head. Early facial change usually appearing during the 1st decade involves the paramedian area of the face and slowly spreads, resulting in atrophy of underlying muscle, bone, and cartilage. First to be involved is usually the area covered by the temporal or buccinator muscles. The process extends to involve the brow, angle of the mouth, neck, or even half the body. The overlying skin often becomes darkly pigmented. The condition slowly progresses for several years (about 9 years) and then usually becomes stationary for life.

Oral manifestations: Atrophy of half of the upper lip and tongue are characteristic. Maxillary teeth on the involved side are exposed. Spontaneous fracture on the affected side of the mandible has also been noted. Other dental anomalies include delayed tooth eruption, abnormal root morphology, and in rare cases, root resorption.

Radiographically the body and ramus of the mandible are shorter on the involved side, and delayed development of the mandibular angle may be observed, resulting in malocclusion. Teeth on the affected side occasionally are delayed in eruption or have atrophic roots.

Hyperkeratosis palmoplantaris and periodontoclasia in childhood (Papillon–Lefèvre syndrome)

- **Papillon** and **Lefèvre**, in 1924 described a syndrome consisting of hyperkeratosis of palms and soles and destruction of the supporting tissues of both primary and secondary dentitions.
- Autosomal recessive inheritance.

Skin: Sometime between the 2nd years and 4th years of life, or on rare occasions even earlier, the palms and soles become diffusely red and scaly. The degree of hyperkeratosis is not severe, but normal skin markings become accentuated and involved skin may assume a parchment-like quality. The degree of involvement seems to fluctuate, possibly becoming worse during winter. The skin apparently improves somewhat with age but some degree of palmoplantar hyperkeratosis remains throughout life.

Other findings: Increased susceptibility to infection with *A. actinomycetemcomitans* has been suggested, but its specificity is dubious.

Contd...

Oral manifestations: The development and eruption of the deciduous teeth proceeds normally, but almost simultaneously with the appearance of palmar and plantar hyperkeratosis, the gingiva swell, bleed, and become boggy. Marked halitosis develops.

Destruction of the periodontium follows almost immediately the eruption of the last primary molar tooth. The teeth are involved in roughly the same order in which they erupt. Deep periodontal pocket formation precedes the exfoliation of teeth. By the age of 4 years, nearly all primary teeth are lost. After exfoliation, the inflammation subsides and the gingiva resumes its normal appearance. The mouth then appears normal until the permanent dentition erupts, when the process is repeated in essentially the same manner. Most teeth are lost by 14 years. The alveolar process is often completely destroyed. Even during active periodontal breakdown, the rest of the oral tissues appear perfectly normal.

Questionnaire

1. Write in details the clinical features of Down syndrome.
2. Write a note on Oral manifestations of cleidocranial dysostosis.
3. Write a note on Apert's syndrome.
4. Explain Rubinstein–Taybi syndrome.
5. Short note on Turner syndrome.

FURTHER READING

1. Beighton P. McKusick's Heritable Disorder of Connective Tissue, 5th edition. St. Louis: Mosby; 1991.
2. Cahuana A, Palma C, Gonzáles W, et al. Oral manifestations in Ellis-van Creveld syndrome: report of five cases. Pediatr Dent. 2004;26:277-82.
3. Cole WG. Etiology and pathogenesis of heritable connective tissue diseases. J Pediatr Orthop. 1993;13:392-403.
4. Gorlin RJ, Cohen MM, Levi LS. Syndrome of the head and neck, 3rd edition. Oxford: Oxford University Press; 1990.
5. Hennequin M, Faulks D, Veyrune JL, et al. Significance of oral health in persons with Down syndrome: a literature review. Dev Med Child Neurol. 1999;41:275-83.
6. Welbury RR. Ehlers-Danlos syndrome: historical review, report of two cases in one family and treatment needs. ASDC J Dent Child. 1989;56:220-4.

CHAPTER

Common Oral Pathologic Conditions Associated with Pediatric Dentistry

Shital Kiran DP, Parvind Gumber, Asmita Sharma

CHAPTER OUTLINE

- Dentigerous Cyst
- Odontogenic Keratocyst
- Radicular Cyst
- Pleomorphic Adenoma (Mixed Tumor)
- Sjögren's Syndrome
- Odontoma
- Ameloblastoma
- Cherubism

Cyst is a pathological cavity containing fluid, semifluid, or gas, which is usually lined by epithelium and is not formed by the accumulation of pus. Pathological cavity means any cystic lesion in the body must arise as a result of some pathologic processes and these cavities are filled with a variety of materials like fluid, keratin, blood, or gases. A cyst may be designated as true cyst if the lining epithelium is present in a cyst and pseudocyst if the lining epithelium is absent.

DENTIGEROUS CYST

- A dentigerous cyst is a cyst that forms around the crown of an unerupted tooth.
- Despite the fact that the dentigerous cyst is a form of odontogenic cyst that develops over time, it has been suggested that some may have an inflammatory origin, such as periapical inflammation from a nonvital primary tooth.
- Dentigerous cysts account for 49% of intraosseous cystic lesions in children aged 2–14.
- **Browne** and **Smith** changed the name from follicular cyst to dentigerous cyst.

Etiopathogenesis

- The epithelial lining of this cyst is derived from the reduced enamel epithelium or by the enamel organ remnant.
- The cyst arises around the crown of an erupted tooth, lying impacted within in the bone.
- Mechanical disturbance in the eruptive process may lead to fluid accumulation either within the reduced enamel epithelium or between it and the enamel surface resulting in cyst formation.
- The initiation of this cyst formation can be explained by the pressure created in the follicle surrounding the crown of the interrupted tooth as consequence of fluid transudation. It has been suggested that thin-walled venous channels are constricted by the impacted tooth, so leading to extravasation of fluid.
- In addition to physical mechanisms, cellular mechanisms are also involved. It has been demonstrated that large numbers of mast cells and immunoglobulin E (IgE) staining cells are present in the tissues surrounding the crown of erupting tooth. Interaction of IgE with mast cells results in histamine release and thus vasodilation and exudation.

Clinical Features

- Dentigerous cysts may grow to a large size before they are diagnosed.
- Dentigerous cysts are typically asymptomatic and can be detected on routine radiography examination as a well-defined unilocular or multilocular radiolucent lesion.
- Many patients first become aware of the cysts because of slowly enlarging swelling **(Fig. 75.1)**, and this is the common form of presentation with edentulous patients in whose jaws unerupted teeth have inadvertently been retained.
- Dentigerous cysts may occasionally be painful particularly if infected and due to its multipotential nature, it has the possibility to trigger bone damage.

Decision tree for oral mucosa lesions (Revised 3/08)

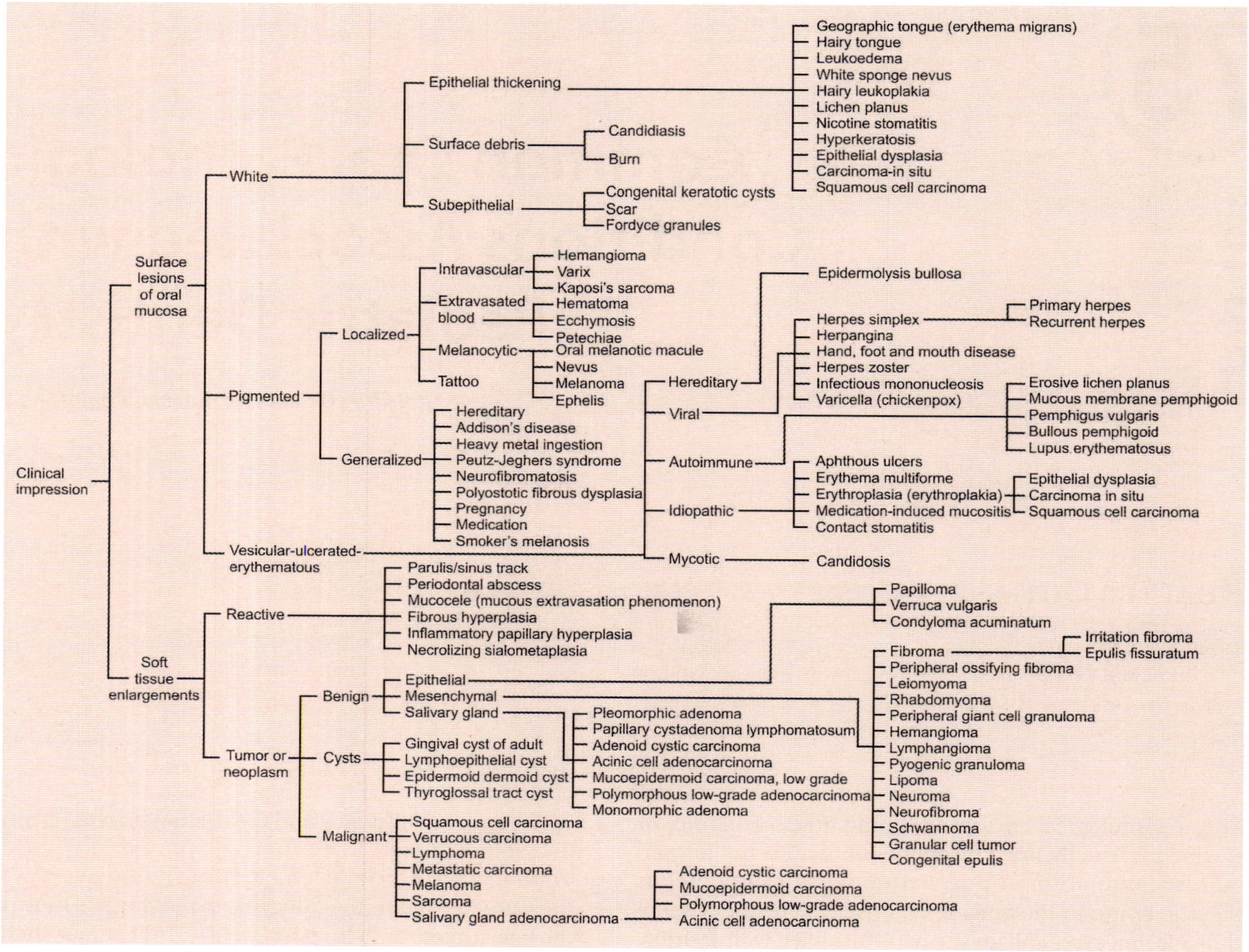

- Clinical impression
  - Surface lesions of oral mucosa
    - White
      - Epithelial thickening
        - Geographic tongue (erythema migrans)
        - Hairy tongue
        - Leukoedema
        - White sponge nevus
        - Hairy leukoplakia
        - Lichen planus
        - Nicotine stomatitis
        - Hyperkeratosis
        - Epithelial dysplasia
        - Carcinoma-in situ
        - Squamous cell carcinoma
      - Surface debris
        - Candidiasis
        - Burn
      - Subepithelial
        - Congenital keratotic cysts
        - Scar
        - Fordyce granules
    - Pigmented
      - Localized
        - Intravascular
          - Hemangioma
          - Varix
          - Kaposi's sarcoma
        - Extravasated blood
          - Hematoma
          - Ecchymosis
          - Petechiae
        - Melanocytic
          - Oral melanotic macule
          - Nevus
          - Melanoma
          - Ephelis
        - Tattoo
      - Generalized
        - Hereditary
        - Addison's disease
        - Heavy metal ingestion
        - Peutz-Jeghers syndrome
        - Neurofibromatosis
        - Polyostotic fibrous dysplasia
        - Pregnancy
        - Medication
        - Smoker's melanosis
    - Vesicular-ulcerated-erythematous
      - Hereditary
        - Epidermolysis bullosa
      - Viral
        - Herpes simplex
          - Primary herpes
          - Recurrent herpes
        - Herpangina
        - Hand, foot and mouth disease
        - Herpes zoster
        - Infectious mononucleosis
        - Varicella (chickenpox)
      - Autoimmune
        - Erosive lichen planus
        - Mucous membrane pemphigoid
        - Pemphigus vulgaris
        - Bullous pemphigoid
        - Lupus erythematosus
      - Idiopathic
        - Aphthous ulcers
        - Erythema multiforme
        - Erythroplasia (erythroplakia)
          - Epithelial dysplasia
          - Carcinoma in situ
          - Squamous cell carcinoma
        - Medication-induced mucositis
        - Contact stomatitis
      - Mycotic
        - Candidosis
  - Soft tissue enlargements
    - Reactive
      - Parulis/sinus track
      - Periodontal abscess
      - Mucocele (mucous extravasation phenomenon)
      - Fibrous hyperplasia
      - Inflammatory papillary hyperplasia
      - Necrolizing sialometaplasia
    - Tumor or neoplasm
      - Benign
        - Epithelial
          - Papilloma
          - Verruca vulgaris
          - Condyloma acuminatum
        - Mesenchymal
          - Fibroma
            - Irritation fibroma
            - Epulis fissuratum
          - Peripheral ossifying fibroma
          - Leiomyoma
          - Rhabdomyoma
          - Peripheral giant cell granuloma
          - Hemangioma
          - Lymphangioma
          - Pyogenic granuloma
          - Lipoma
          - Neuroma
          - Neurofibroma
          - Schwannoma
          - Granular cell tumor
          - Congenital epulis
        - Salivary gland
          - Pleomorphic adenoma
          - Papillary cystadenoma lymphomatosum
          - Adenoid cystic carcinoma
          - Acinic cell adenocarcinoma
          - Mucoepidermoid carcinoma, low grade
          - Polymorphous low-grade adenocarcinoma
          - Monomorphic adenoma
      - Cysts
        - Gingival cyst of adult
        - Lymphoepithelial cyst
        - Epidermoid dermoid cyst
        - Thyroglossal tract cyst
      - Malignant
        - Squamous cell carcinoma
        - Verrucous carcinoma
        - Lymphoma
        - Metastatic carcinoma
        - Melanoma
        - Sarcoma
        - Salivary gland adenocarcinoma
          - Adenoid cystic carcinoma
          - Mucoepidermoid carcinoma
          - Polymorphous low-grade adenocarcinoma
          - Acinic cell adenocarcinoma

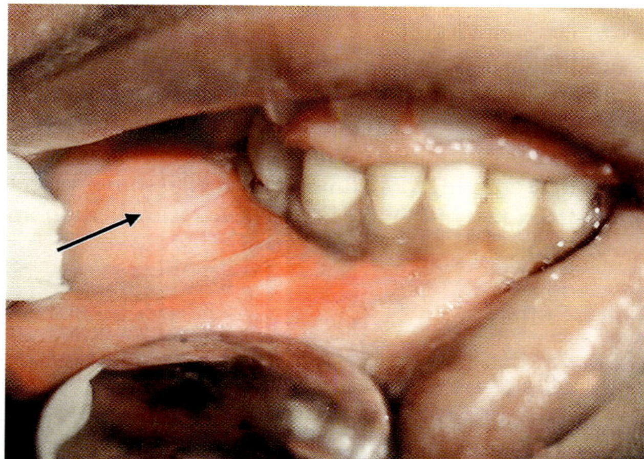

Fig. 75.1: Clinical presentation of dentigerous cyst.

Prevalence

- ❖ More frequency in whites than black race.
- ❖ They are most commonly found in people between the ages of 10 and 30.
- ❖ Most common region is mandibular third molar and maxillary permanent canine region.
- ❖ Significantly greater in men than women, i.e., 1.8:1.

Radiographic Features

- ❖ Radiographs show unilocular radiolucent areas associated with the crowns of unerupted teeth **(Figs. 75.2 and 75.3)**.
- ❖ The cysts have well-defined sclerotic margins unless they become infected.
- ❖ Occasionally, trabeculations may be seen and this may give an erroneous impression of multilocularity.

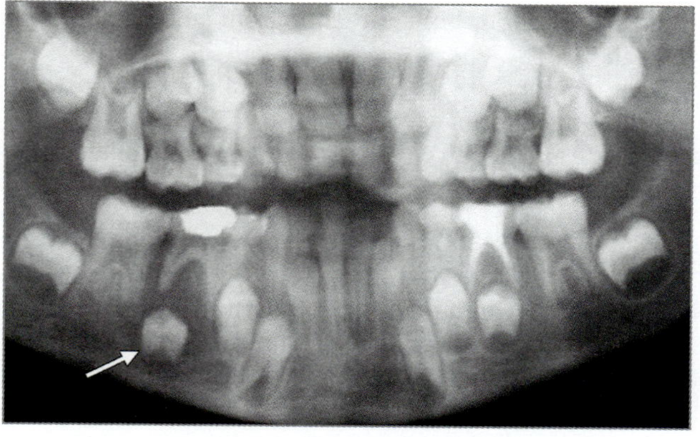

Fig. 75.2: Orthopantomogram (OPG) showing radiographic picture of cyst.

- This cyst attaches at the cementoenamel junction, which is an important diagnostic feature.
- The unerupted teeth may be impacted because of inadequate space in the dental arch or as a result of malpositioning such as by a horizontally impacted of the crown.

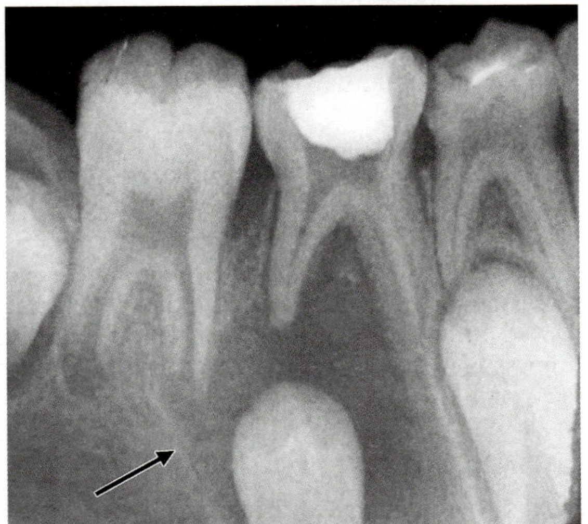

Fig. 75.3: Intraoral periapical radiograph (IOPA) showing well-defined margins.

Histopathological Features (Figs. 75.4 and 75.5)

- It is composed of thin cystic wall.

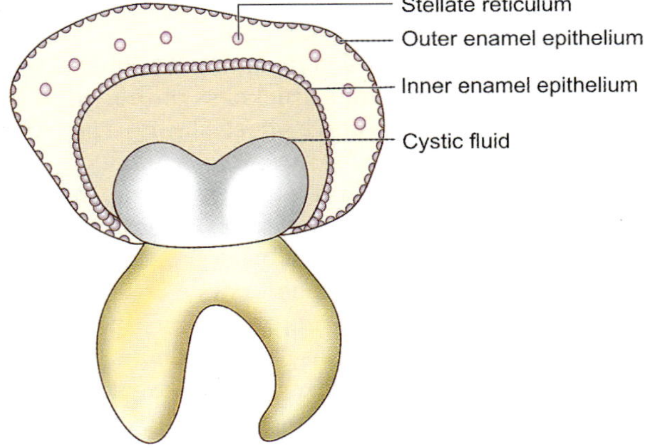

Fig. 75.4: Histological appearance of dentigerous cyst.

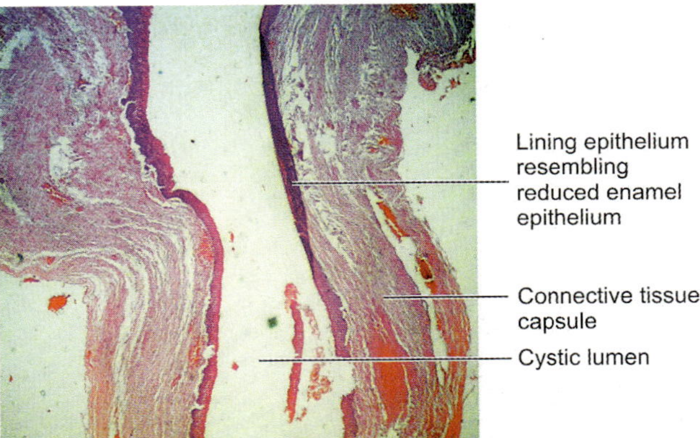

Fig. 75.5: Histological picture of dentigerous cyst.

- The lining is a thin layer of nonkeratinized stratified squamous epithelium.
- In very few instances, the lining may be keratinized and it may be mistaken as keratocyst or keratin may be produced rarely as due to metaplastic changes.
- The epithelial lining of a noninflamed dentigerous cyst is made up of two to four layers of flattened nonkeratinizing cells, with the epithelium and connective tissue interface being flat.
- The fibrous wall of an inflamed dentigerous cyst is highly collagenized, with a variable amount of chronic inflammatory cells infiltrating.
- The cells are cuboidal or low columnar.
- Rete pegs formation is absent.

ODONTOGENIC KERATOCYST

- Odontogenic keratocyst (OKC) is a developmental odontogenic cyst of epithelial origin which arises from cell rests of the dental lamina.
- Previously termed primordial cyst by **Robinson** (1945).
- According to **Pindborg** and **Hansen**, the designation keratocyst was used to describe any jaw cyst exhibiting keratinization in their lining which may occur in follicular, residual, and very rarely in a radicular cyst.
- Odontogenic keratocysts should be considered benign cystic neoplasms that is why World Health Organization (WHO) in its classification of odontogenic tumor has given name of keratocystic odontogenic tumor.

Pathogenesis

- Odontogenic keratocyst arises mainly from the:
  - Dental lamina or its remnants
  - Primordium of the developing tooth germ or enamel organs
  - Sometimes from the basal layer of the oral epithelium.
- It is mostly believed that the keratocyst develops due to the cystic degeneration of the cells of the stellate reticulum in a developing tooth germ (before its calcification starts). Daughter cysts are a common finding in this lesion.

Prevalence

- 1% among all types of jaw cysts.
- Between the ages of 10 and 40, 60% of all odontogenic keratocysts are detected.
- Slight male predilection compared to females.
- Involves the ascending ramus and posterior body of mandible.
- Maxillary lesions more frequently involve anterior part of the jaw, however, some can develop from the posterior region lesions that can even develop in relation to maxillary air sinus.
- On rare occasions, this cyst may occur in gingiva.

Clinical Features

- In the initial stages, OKC does not produce signs or symptoms and the lesion may be discovered only during routine radiographic examinations.

- ❖ Demonstrate a well-defined radiolucent area with smooth and often corticated margins.
- ❖ Grows in an anteroposterior orientation within the bone's medullary cavity without creating visible bone enlargement.
- ❖ Larger lesions often produce pain and swelling.
- ❖ Pain and mobility and displacement of involved teeth seen.
- ❖ Buccal expansion of bone.
- ❖ Odontogenic keratocysts in children are frequently the result of numerous cysts as part of the necessitated basal cell carcinoma syndrome.
- ❖ Paresthesia of the lower lip and teeth may be present occasionally.
- ❖ Excessive expansion and thinning of bone may result in pathological fracture in some cases.
- ❖ Discharge of pus may be seen in case the cyst is secondarily infected.
- ❖ Multiple OKC are found in Gorlin–Goltz syndrome, Marfan syndrome, Ehlers–Danlos syndrome, and Noonan's syndrome.

Radiographic Features (Fig. 75.6)

- ❖ Majority of lesions are unilocular with smooth borders but some unilocular lesions are large with irregular borders.
- ❖ Radiolucency is usually hazy due to keratin filled cavity and it is surrounded by thin sclerotic rim due to reactive osteocytes.
- ❖ Bone can expand in anterior-posterior direction and perforate the buccal and lingual cortical plates of bone and involve the adjacent soft tissue.

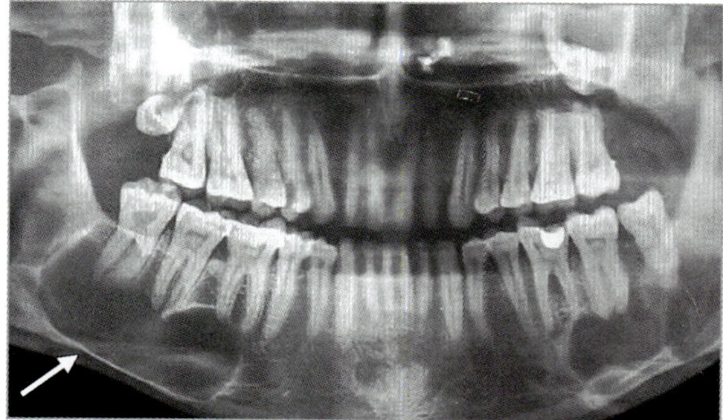

Fig. 75.6: Radiographic presentation of odontogenic keratocyst (OKC).

- ❖ Keratocysts often radiographically present multilocular radiolucent areas, with a typical "soap-bubble" appearance.

Radiological types of keratocysts	
Replacement type	When a keratocyst develops in place of a developing normal tooth, it is called the replacement type. In such cases, there will be absence of a normal tooth in the dental arch
Envelopmental type	When a cyst entirely encloses an impacted tooth within the bone, it is called the envelopmental type of keratocyst
Extraneous type	When a keratocyst develops away from the tooth bearing areas of the jaws, it is called extraneous type of keratocyst
Collateral type	When a cyst develops between the roots of a tooth, it is called collateral type of keratocyst.

- ❖ The histopathologic features of odontogenic keratocyst are used to make the diagnosis. Even though radiographic findings are frequently extremely suggestive, they are not diagnostic.

Histopathological Features (Figs. 75.7A and B)

- ❖ The OKC shows two types of linings, i.e., (1) parakeratinized stratified squamous epithelium and (2) orthokeratinized.
- ❖ The parakeratinized epithelium is more common, (80–90%) cases. The orthokeratinized OKC shows less common occurrence.
- ❖ The parakeratinized luminal surface may vanish in the presence of inflammatory alterations, and the epithelium may proliferate to produce rete ridges with the absence of the distinctive palisaded basal layer.
- ❖ The characteristic feature of the lining is pathognomonic corrugated, with a regular thickness of the epithelium between five cell layers and eight cell layers. The lining is without rete ridges.
- ❖ The nuclei of the basal cells are darkly staining, show basal cell hyperplasia, this is not present in other keratocyst.
- ❖ Connective tissue shows islands of odontogenic epithelium forming small duplicate daughter cysts or small satellite cysts. The satellite cysts are more common in patients with multiple cysts and nevoid basal cell carcinoma syndrome.
- ❖ Another notable aspect of this cyst is a weak epithelial-connective tissue attachment, which leads to epithelial separation and subsequent recurrences as evacuation of the cyst becomes more difficult.

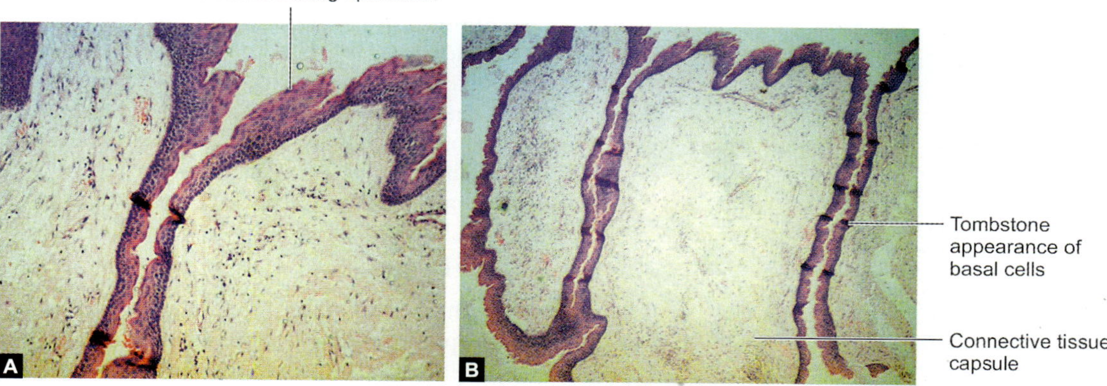

Figs. 75.7A and B: Histologic appearance of odontogenic keratocyst (OKC).

RADICULAR CYST

- Radicular or periapical cyst is the most common odontogenic cystic lesion of inflammatory origin, which occurs in relation to the apex of a nonvital tooth due to chronic pulpal inflammatory stimulated by rests of Malassez.
- In a radicular cyst, if the involved tooth is exfoliated or extracted and the cystic lesion remains within the bone, the condition is known as residual cyst.

Prevalence

- Radicular cyst constitutes about 50% or more among all types of jaw cysts.
- Radicular cysts are more common in the third to sixth decades, with a slight male predominance.
- The cyst can occur in relation to any of either jaw, but maxilla (60%) is usually commonly affected than mandible (40%).

Clinical Presentations

- The involved tooth is always nonvital that can be easily detected by the presence of fractures or discolorations, etc.
- Radicular cyst may occur rarely in association with nonvital deciduous tooth.
- The smaller cystic lesions are usually as symptomatic and are detected only with radiograph is taken.
- The larger lesions on the other hand, often produce a slow enlarging, bony hard swelling of the jaw with expansion and distortion of the cortical plates, or disturbance in occlusion mostly of the regional teeth.
- Severe bone destruction by the cystic lesion results in thinning of the cortical plates and it may produce a "springiness" of the jawbone when digital pressure is applied.
- Periapical inflammatory tissue which is not curetted at the stage of tooth extraction can result in a residual periapical cyst, which is an inflammatory cyst.

Radiographic Features

- Radicular cysts present well-defined corticated, unilocular, and round-shaped radiolucent areas of variable size (few millimeters to several centimeters in diameter).
- The cyst is always found in contact with the root apex of a nonvital tooth and it is bordered on the periphery by a well-corticated margin.
- The infected cysts often have hazy or an ill-defined border.

Histopathology (Figs. 75.8A to C)

- Histologically, radicular cyst shows presence of a cystic cavity, which is lined by nonkeratinized, stratified squamous epithelium of about 6–20 cell layers thickness.

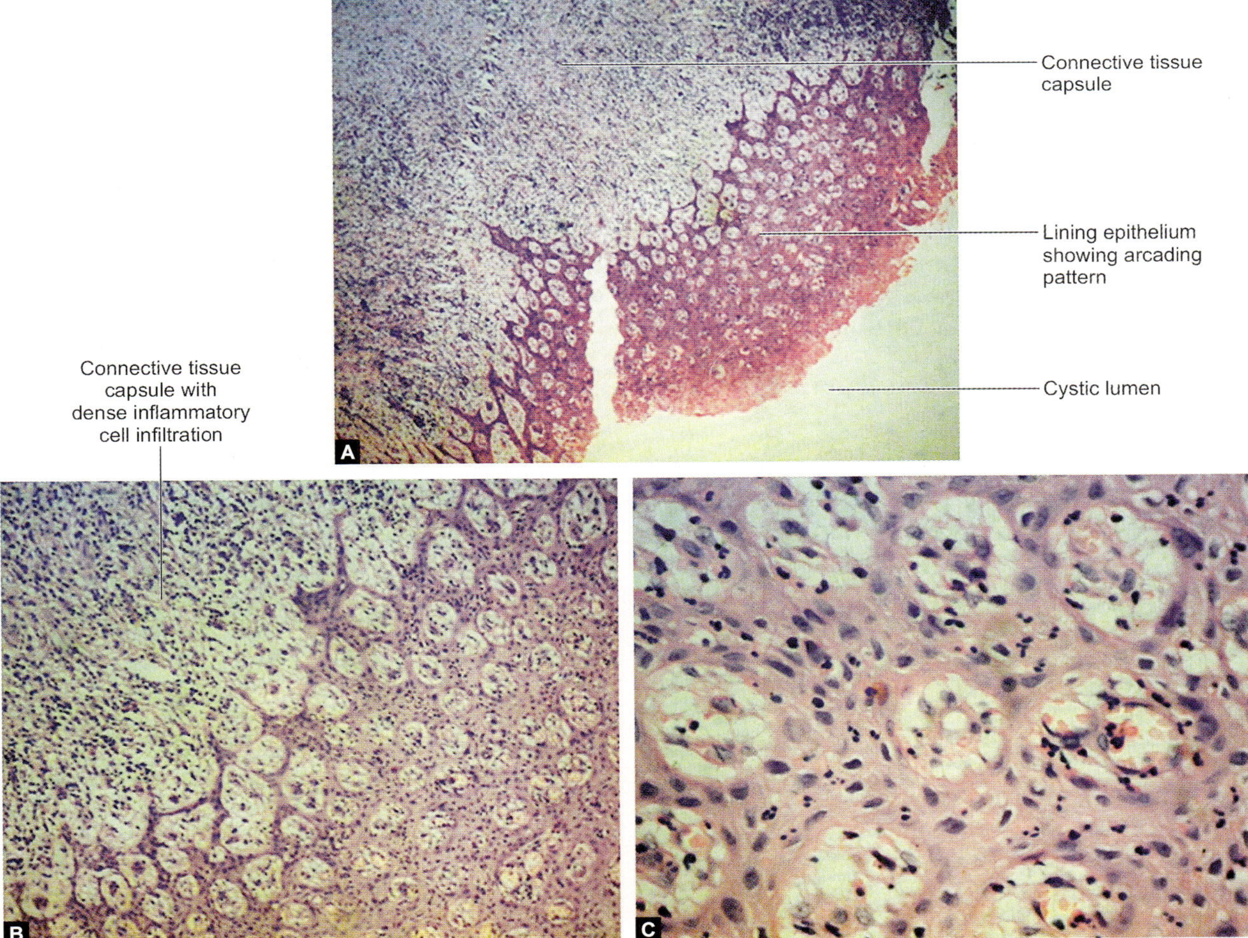

Figs. 75.8A to C: Histologic appearance of radicular cyst under 4X, 10X, and 40X magnification.

- ❖ Epithelium is nonkeratinized and it often shows localized areas of increased cell proliferation and edema.
- ❖ The proliferating cystic epithelium may sometimes grow in a peculiar fashion, by enclosing or encircling a mass of connective tissue capsule from all sides. This pattern of growth is called "arcading pattern".
- ❖ Presence of inflammatory cell infiltration and edema is often seen the cystic lining.
- ❖ The cyst capsule is made up of vascular connective tissue, which is often infiltrated by chronic inflammatory cells.
- ❖ Hyaline bodies, also known as Rushton bodies, can be found in a small percentage of periapical cysts.

PLEOMORPHIC ADENOMA (MIXED TUMOR)

- ❖ Pleomorphic adenoma and mixed tumor are two terms used to describe this tumor's unusual histopathologic characteristics, but neither is completely accurate.
- ❖ It is also called enclavoma, branchioma, endothelioma, and enchondroma.
- ❖ It is a benign neoplasm consisting of cells exhibiting the ability to differentiate to epithelial (ductal and nonductal) and mesenchymal (chondroid, myxoid, and osseous) cells.
- ❖ The complexity and diversity of appearance of this neoplasm account for the term "pleomorphic".
- ❖ According to the multicellular theory, these tumors originate from intercalated duct cells and myoepithelial cells of the salivary glands.

Prevalence

- ❖ The tumor can occur anyone at any age, but it is most common in young and middle-aged adults aged 30–60.
- ❖ 10% cases occur in children.
- ❖ Pleomorphic adenomas account for roughly 90% of all salivary gland tumors in children.
- ❖ More common among females than males (60:40).
- ❖ It accounts for 60–65% of all neoplasms of the parotid, 50% of submandibular, and 25% of sublingual gland.
- ❖ Approximately 45% of minor gland lesions are pleomorphic adenomas.

Clinical Features

- ❖ 80% of tumors that occur in the parotid gland are benign. Of these, 75% are pleomorphic adenomas and 5% are Warthin's tumors.
- ❖ The sites are palate followed by upper lip and then the buccal mucosa.
- ❖ Pleomorphic adenomas can occur in any location where minor salivary glands exist.
- ❖ The two most common clinical presentations are: (1) a painless firm mass in the superficial lobe of the parotid gland and (2) a painless firm mass in the posterior palatal mucosa.
- ❖ Small, painless, and quiescent nodule which slowly begins to increase in size, sometimes intermittently.
- ❖ It appears as firm, painless swellings that do not cause ulceration of the overlying mucosa in many cases.
- ❖ The growth is a slow growing firm mass and the patient will be usually aware of the lesion for months and years before seeking professional help in diagnosis and treatment.
- ❖ The tumor tends to be round or oval when it is small, as it grows bigger it becomes lobulated, not more than 1–2 cm in diameter.
- ❖ The minor gland neoplasms in the oral cavity frequently exhibit smooth surfaced, soft, or slightly firm, dome-shaped.
- ❖ Nodular swellings on the hard or soft palate without any ulceration on the surface.
- ❖ The palatal neoplasms are usually firm in consistency and are less movable due to the tough nature of the palatal mucosa, these lesions sometimes exhibits surface ulceration especially when traumatized.
- ❖ Large intraoral lesions are often associated with disturbance in speech and mastication.
- ❖ Malignant transformation is uncommon in pleomorphic adenomas but may occur on rare occasions.

Histopathological Features (Figs. 75.9A and B)

- ❖ **Foote** and **Frazewell** (1954) categorized the tumor histologically in following types:
  - Principally myxoid
  - Myxoid and cellular components present in equal proportion
  - Predominantly cellular
  - Extremely cellular.
- ❖ The epithelial component consists of epithelial duct-like cells, polygonal cells, cuboidal cells, and spindle cells arranged in different patterns. The epithelial cells may be arranged in sheets, clumps, islands, or interlace strands. Cuboidal cells show duct-like arrangement.
- ❖ These ducts like spaces may contain eosinophilic coagulum and mucoid material. Epithelial cells resembling squamous cells have distinct intercellular bridges.
- ❖ Cystic spaces are also uncommonly seen.
- ❖ Few stellate cells or spindle cells called myoepithelial cells are also seen with variable morphology. These cells have rounded eccentric nucleus and eosinophilic hyalinized cytoplasm resembling plasma cells. These cells are called plasmacytoid cells.
- ❖ Hyaline cells are also seen with dense eosinophilic cytoplasm.
- ❖ Squamous cells and keratin pearls may be present. Occasionally, there may be cribriform areas, suggesting the pattern of adenoid cystic carcinoma.
- ❖ Glandular epithelium is mainly found. A neoplastic altered cell with the potential for multidirectional differentiation is histogenetically responsible for pleomorphic adenoma.
- ❖ Malignant degeneration is possible within pleomorphic adenomas, and the incidence increases with tumor duration and size.
- ❖ Histologic features suggestive of malignant transformation include extensive hyalinization, cellular atypism, necrosis, calcification, and invasion.
- ❖ Plasmacytoid cells are highly indicative of mixed tumors and are rarely seen in other salivary gland tumors.

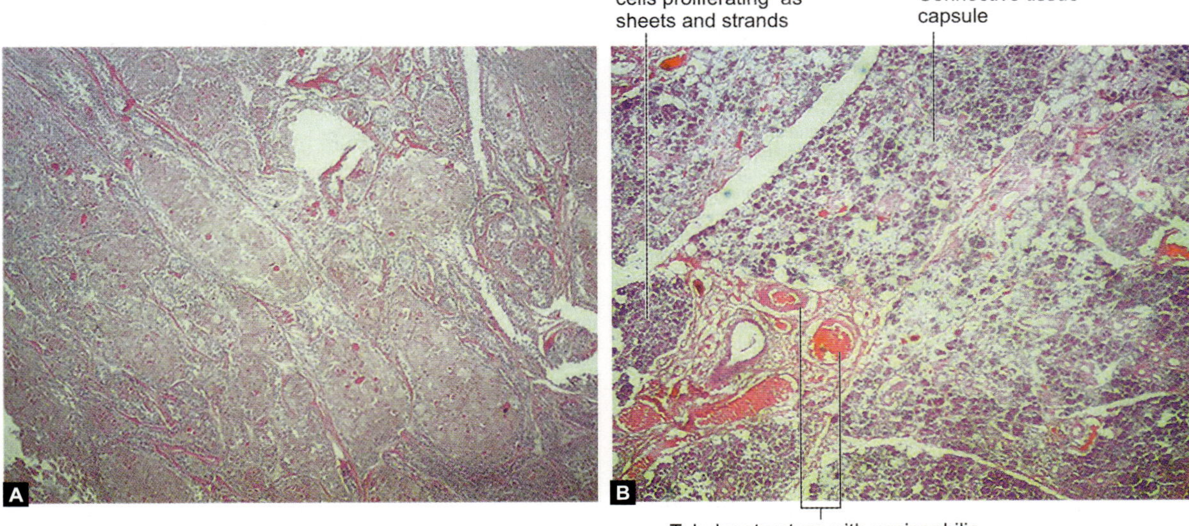

Figs. 75.9A and B: Histologic appearance of pleomorphic adenoma under 4X, 10X magnification.

SJÖGREN'S SYNDROME

- It is the second most common chronic autoimmune rheumatic disease, with a high illness burden.
- It is a chronic inflammatory disease that predominately affects salivary, lacrimal, and other exocrine glands.
- It was first described by **Henrik Sjögren** in 1933 as a triad consisting of keratoconjunctivitis sicca, xerostomia, and rheumatoid arthritis.
- It predominately affects middle-aged and elderly women.

Types

- **Primary Sjögren's syndrome:**
  - It is also called sicca syndrome
  - It consists a triad of dry eyes (xerophthalmia) and dry mouth (xerostomia). Eye lesion is called keratoconjunctivitis sicca.
- **Secondary Sjögren's syndrome:** It consists of dry eyes, dry mouth, and collagen disorders usually rheumatoid arthritis or systemic lupus erythematous.

Etiology

- Genetic
- Hormonal
- Infectious
- Immunologic.

Clinical Features

- Clinically, the mouth may appear moist in early stages of Sjögren's syndrome but later, there may be a lack of the usual pooling of saliva in the floor of the mouth and frothy saliva may form along the lines of contact with oral soft tissue. In advanced cases, the mucosa is glazed, dry, and tends to form fine wrinkles.
- The tongue typically develops a characteristic lobulated, usually red surface with partial or complete depapillation. There is also decrease in number of taste buds, which leads to an abnormal and impaired sense of taste.
- Female:Male ratio is 10:1.
- Painful burning sensation of oral mucosa.
- Dryness of nose, larynx, pharynx, and tracheobronchial tree is seen.
- Some patients will present with fatigue and mild arthralgia, but most will be active and tolerant of their disease.
- Many patients will have tooth loss secondary to caries.
- The constant polyclonal B-cell overactivity selects a single clone (usually of B cells) that overtakes the population, resulting in a lymphoma.
- Difficulty in eating dry food, soreness, or difficulty in controlling dentures.
- Pus may be emitted from the duct. Angular stomatitis and denture stomatitis also occur.
- Dry mouth may be accompanied by unilateral or bilateral enlargement of parotid gland, which occurs in about one-third of the patients and may be intermittent.
- Xerostomia may be linked to a higher risk of periodontal disease including a higher prevalence of plaque and gingival bleeding.
- Enlargement of submandibular gland may also occur.
- Soreness and redness of mucosa is usually the result of candidal infection.

Histopathology

- There may be intense infiltration of the glands by lymphocyte cells replacing all acinar structure.
- In some cases, there may be proliferation of ductal epithelium and myoepithelium to form epimyoepithelial islands.
- Lymphocytic infiltration of exocrine glands is the hallmark of Sjögren's syndrome. In major salivary glands, the

previously described benign lymphoepithelial lesion is considered typical. However, it is not consistently seen in minor salivary glands.

- The parotid gland will show an early lymphocytic infiltration, acinar atrophy, and epimyoepithelial islands. Proliferation of ductal epithelium and myoepithelium to form "myoepithelial islands" are seen in some cases.

Diagnostic Tests

- **Rose Bengal staining test:** Keratoconjunctivitis sicca is characterized by corneal keratotic lesion, which stains pink when rose Bengal dye is used.
- **Schirmer test:** The reduced lacrimal flow rate is measured by this test. A strip of filter paper is placed in between the eye and the eyelid to determine the degree of tears which is measured in millimeter. When the flow is reduced to less than 5 mm in a 5 min sample, patient should be considered positive for Sjögren's syndrome.
- **Sialometry:** Salivary flow rate estimation is a sensitive indicator of salivary gland function. Parotid glands make the major contribution to total salivary flow and are the most consistently affected glands in patients with Sjögren's syndrome. Stimulated flow rate in symptomatic primary and secondary Sjögren's syndrome is usually below 0.5–1.0 mL/min (normal 1–1.5 mL/min).
- **Sialochemistry:** Parotid saliva in Sjögren's syndrome contains twice as much total lipid and has elevated content of phospholipids and glycolipids than the normal saliva. The sodium chloride and phospholipids levels are higher in saliva of Sjögren's syndrome patient.

ODONTOMA

Odontomas are hamartomas, not true neoplasms, because they are made up of enamel and dentin with varying amounts of pulp and cementum when fully developed.

Types

World Health Organization has classified odontomas into two types depending on their degree of morphodifferentiation:

- **Compound odontome:** It consists of a completely disorganized and diffuse mass of odontogenic tissue with haphazardly arranged enamel, dentin, and cementum.
- **Complex odontome:** Compound odontome presents collections of numerous small, discrete, and tooth-like structures. Odontogenic tissues in compound odontome bear superficial anatomical resemblance to normal teeth.

Pathogenesis

Hamartomatous proliferation of odontogenic origin. It is thought that local trauma, infection, and genetic mutations cause this proliferation of odontogenic epithelium. These result in unsuccessful or altered ectomesenchyme interaction during early or later phases of tooth development leading to haphazard formation of enamel, dentin, and cementum. Both the epithelial and mesenchymal cells exhibit complete differentiation with the result that functional ameloblasts and odontoblasts form enamel and dentin. It is laid down in an abnormal pattern because of failure of cells to reach the morphodifferentiation stage.

Clinical Features

- Seen mostly in 1st and 2nd decades of life.
- There is slight predilection for occurrence in males.
- The maxilla has a higher incidence of odontomas than the mandible.
- Compound occurs in incisor, canine area of maxilla, and complex occurs in mandibular first and second molar area.
- Slow growing, expanding, and mostly painless lesions. Pain and inflammation associated with odontomas occur only in 4% of cases.
- In few cases, they may produce large, bony hard swellings of the jaw, with expansion of the cortical plates, and displacement of the regional teeth.
- Multiple odontomes can occur in the jaw simultaneously in some patients.

Radiographic Features

- Complex odontome appears as an irregular mass of calcified material surrounded by narrow radiolucent bands with a small outer periphery **(Fig. 75.10)**.
- The compound odontome appear as numerous, small, miniature teeth, or tooth-like structures, which are projecting from the roots of the erupted permanent teeth or above the crown of an impacted tooth **(Fig. 75.11)**.
- The complex odontome radiographically appears as round or oval or sunburst-like, conglomerated radiopaque mass within the jawbone.

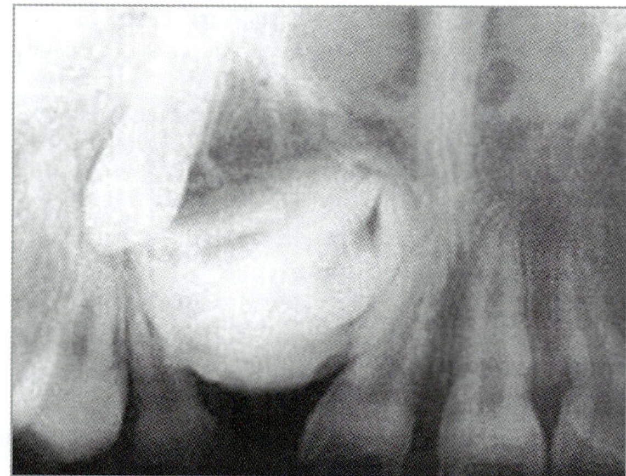

Fig. 75.10: Complex odontome.

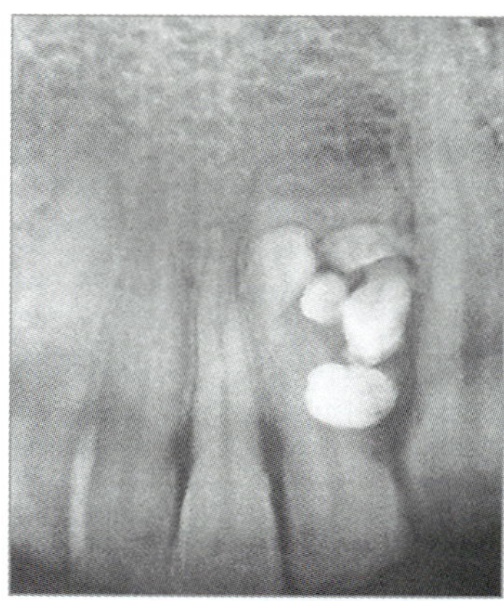

Fig. 75.11: Compound odontome.

Histopathology

- Fully developed compound odontome histologically reveals the presence of an encapsulated mass of multiple separate denticles, embedded in a fibrous tissue stroma.
- A thin layer of cementum may be present about the periphery of the tumor.
- Small islands of epithelial ghost cells are seen in the tumor, which are remnants of the odontogenic epithelium.
- There is presence of enamel, dentin, cementum, and pulp tissues, which are arranged in a similar fashion as seen in a normal tooth.
- The presence of ghost cell keratinization in the enamel-forming cells of some odontomas has no significance other than to show that these epithelial cells can keratinize.

AMELOBLASTOMA

- **World Health Organization definition:** Solid multicystic ameloblastoma is polymorphic neoplasm consisting of proliferating odontogenic epithelium, which usually has a follicular or plexiform pattern, lying in a fibrous stroma.
- **Broca** in 1868 was the first to report to ameloblastoma.
- Ameloblastoma is a benign, locally invasive, polymorphic neoplasm, and presumably derived from intraosseous remnants of odontogenic epithelium.
- The ameloblastoma, a true neoplasm of the odontogenic epithelium, is a locally invasive and persistent tumor with aggressive but benign growth characteristics.
- Tumor may be derived from cell rests of enamel organ either remnants of dental lamina or remnants of Hertwig's sheath the epithelial rest of **Malassez**.

Etiology

- Trauma
- Infection
- Previous inflammation
- Extraction of tooth
- Dietary factors
- Viral infection.

Clinical Features

- Commonly seen between 2nd and 5th decades of life.
- More commonly in blacks than whites.
- No gender predilection.
- Ameloblastoma in most of the cases involve the mandible (80%), especially in the molar-ramus area (70%).
- Clinically ameloblastoma presents a slow enlarging, painless, ovoid or fusiform, and bony hard swelling of the jaw.
- Larger lesions of ameloblastoma often cause severe expansion, destruction, and thinning of the cortical plates, which often result in "fluctuations" in the affected area. This thin shell of bone cracks under digital pressure and the phenomenon is called "eggshell crackling". "Pathological fractures", may occur in many such affected bones.
- It occur in three different clinico-radiographic situations:
  1. Conventional solid or multicystic (86%)
  2. Unicystic (13%)
  3. Peripheral (extraosseous) (1%)
- The mucosa surrounding the mass is normal, but teeth in the affected area may become displaced and mobile.
- Ameloblastoma patients rarely experience pain, paresthesia, fistula, ulcer formation, or tooth mobility.
- Many untreated lesions may reach to an enormous size with time and cause extensive deformity of the jaws and face, thereby leading to pressure sensation in the eyeball or nasal obstruction, etc.
- Most of the patients report with a typical long time history of presence of an "abscess" or a "cyst" in the jawbone that was operated on several occasions but has recurred after each attempt.

Radiological Findings (Fig. 75.12)

- **Multilocular type:** Bone is replaced by a number of small, well-defined radiolucent areas giving honeycomb or larger soap-bubble appearance.
- **Unilocular type:** Well-defined area of radiolucency that forms single compartment.

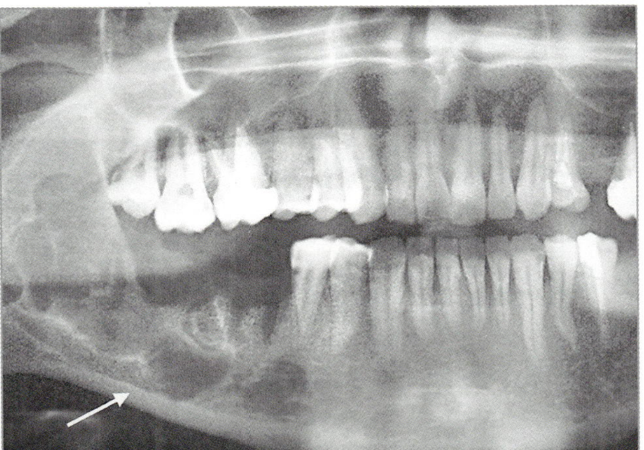

Fig. 75.12: Ameloblastoma.

Imaging

- CT imaging's ability to detect perforation of the outer cortex and invasion into the surrounding soft tissues is critical.
- Magnetic resonance imaging will provide superior images of the nature and extent of soft tissue invasion if it is extensive.

Histological Variants

- **Follicular type:**
  - Most common and constitutes about 32% among all ameloblastomas.
  - In a mature fibrous connective tissue stroma, islands of epithelium resemble enamel organ epithelium.
  - Follicular islands consist of central mass of polyhedral cells or loosely connected angular cells resembling stellate reticulum. Surrounded by peripherally arranged cuboidal or columnar cells resembling inner enamel epithelium or preameloblasts **(Figs. 75.13A and B)**.
- **Plexiform type:**
  - Second most common—28% among ameloblastoma.

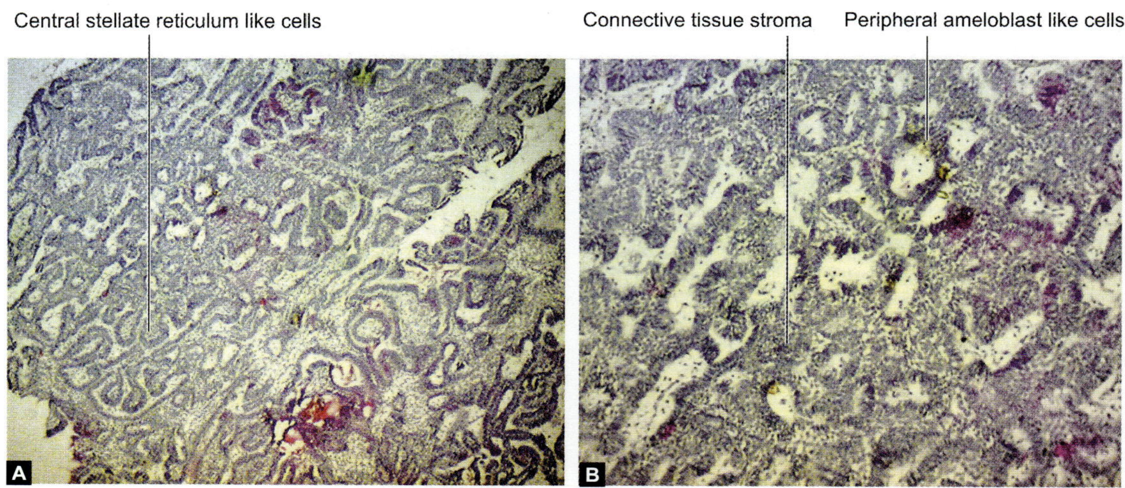

Figs. 75.13A and B: Follicular ameloblastoma on 4X, 10X magnification.

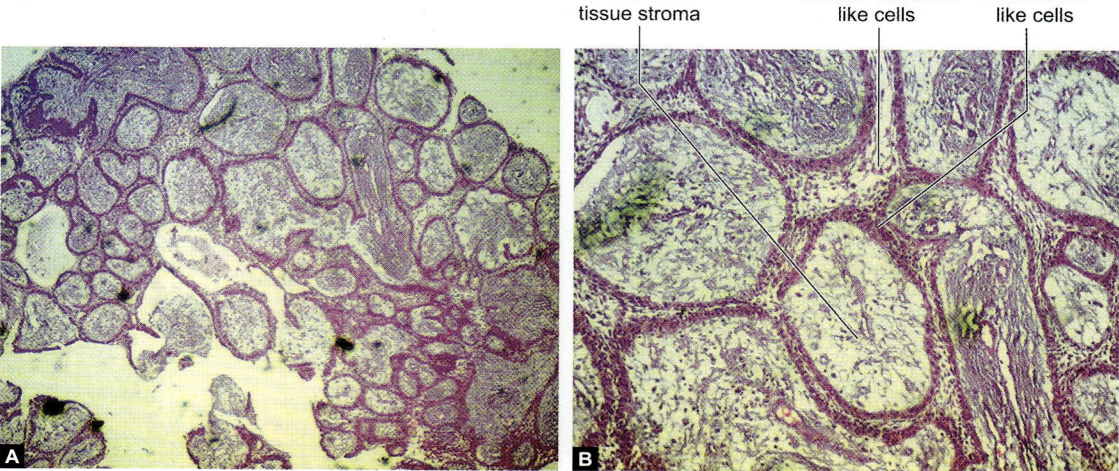

Figs. 75.14A and B: Plexiform ameloblastoma on 4X, 10X magnification.

- Tumor epithelium is arranged as a network which is bound by a layer of cuboidal to columnar cells and includes cells resembling stellate reticulum **(Figs. 75.14A and B)**.
- Long, anastomosing cords or larger sheets of odontogenic epithelium make up the plexiform type of ameloblastoma.
- Cyst formations occur due to stromal degeneration rather than cystic changes within epithelium.

❖ **Ameloblastoma acanthomatous type:**
- Third most common—12% among ameloblastoma.
- Usually in follicular type, there is extensive squamous metaplasia, sometimes with keratin formation within islands of tumor cells **(Fig. 75.15)**.

❖ **Desmoplastic type:** It occurs mostly in old age **(Fig. 75.16)**.

❖ **Granular cell pattern:**
- Ameloblastomas can sometimes show granular cell transformation of groups of lesional epithelial cells.
- These cells have a lot of cytoplasm filled with eosinophilic granules that are ultrastructurally and histochemically like lysosomes.

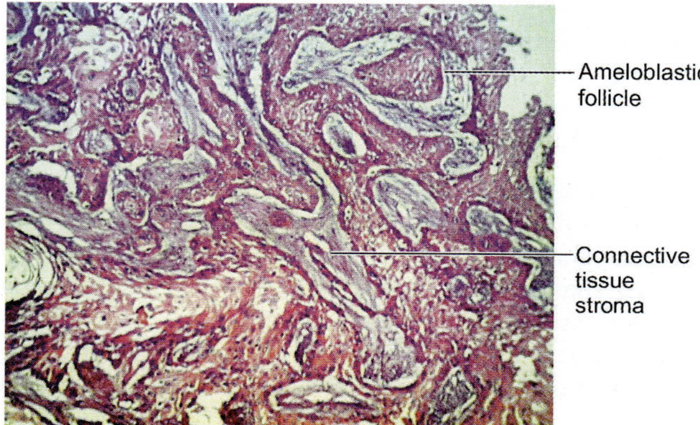

Fig. 75.15: Ameloblastoma acanthomatous type on 10X magnification.

❖ **Basal cell pattern:**
- These lesions are made up of nests of uniform basaloid cells and histopathologically look a lot like skin basal cell carcinoma.
- The central portions of the nests have no stellate reticulum.

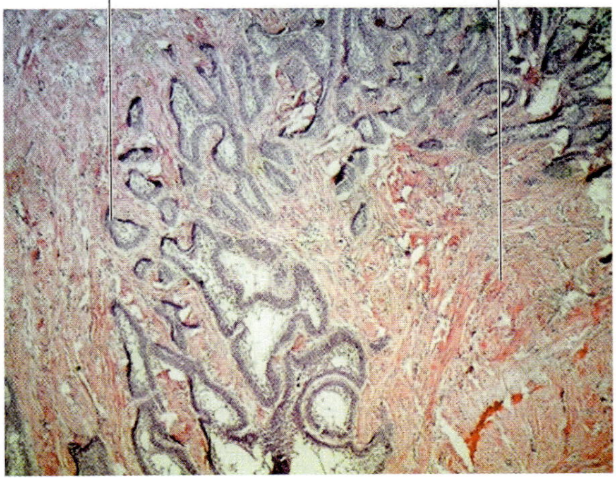

Fig. 75.16: Desmoplastic type.

CHERUBISM

- Cherubism is a rare benign hereditary condition/being inherited as an autosomal dominant which affects only the jawbones of children bilaterally and symmetrically, usually producing the so-called cherubic look **(Figs. 75.17A and B)**.
- Cherubism, a nonneoplastic hereditary bone lesion.

Types

According to **Ramon** and **Engelberg**:

- **Grade I:** Involving ascending ramus on both sides.
- **Grade II:** Involving ramus with maxillary tuberosities bilaterally.
- **Grade III:** Involvement of whole maxilla and mandible except for condylar process.
- **Grade IV:** Same as grade III along with involvement of floor of orbit.

Clinical Presentations

- The disease commonly affect between 1 year and 5 years of age.

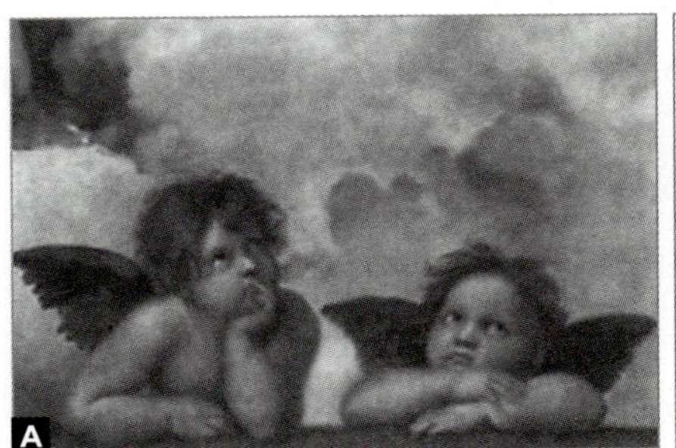

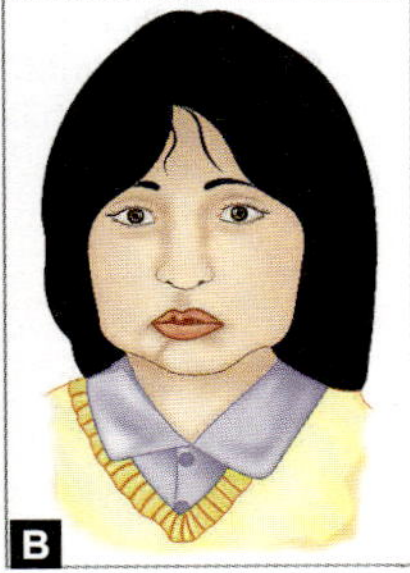

Figs. 75.17A and B: Cherub facial features: (A) Detailed painting of cherubs by Raphael's Sistine Madonna; (B) Illustration of a young girl with bilateral full cheeks (cherubism). Cherubism is a team used to describe bible drawings of children with full cheeks.

- More common among males than females.
- Cherubism does not occur in any other bone and will not cross a bony suture to an adjacent bone.
- There may be enlargement of the submandibular lymph nodes, but no systemic abnormalities are present.
- At birth the appearance of the patient is absolutely normal. However, between the age of 1 year and 5 years a bilateral, painless, symmetric swelling develops in mandible, or sometimes in maxilla in severe cases.
- Swelling of the maxilla can cause the skin on the cheeks to stretch, depressing the lower eyelids and exposing a thin line of sclera, giving the appearance of "eyes raised to heaven." Hence, the name cherubism is given as *cherub* means angel.
- The child will present with nasal obstruction, lymphadenopathy, dry mouth, drooling, missing teeth, multiple diastemas, and misplaced teeth.
- The enlargements may cause tooth displacement or failure of eruption, impair mastication, cause speech difficulties, or, in rare cases, lead to loss of normal vision or hearing, in addition to the aesthetic and psychologic effects.

Radiographic Features

- "Cyst-like" radiolucent areas or cavities on both sides of mandible.
- The initial destruction of bone starts at angle of the mandible, which can be detected by X-rays even before the clinical manifestation of the disease.
- Cherubism in later stages causes severe bilateral expansion of the jaw with thinning of the cortical plates. In few cases, there may be presence of tin classic "ground-glass" appearance in cherubism.
- Sometimes, multiple unerupted and displaced teeth appear to be floating within the cyst-like spaces and the condition is often referred to as "floating tooth syndrome".
- Cherubism lesions appear on radiographs as multilocular radiolucencies, which are often described as having a soap-bubble appearance.

Histopathology Features

- The lesions of cherubism consist of a vascular fibrous stroma, extravasated erythrocytes, and scattered multinucleated giant cell.
- The eosinophilic cuffing appears to be a cherubism-specific feature.
- An increase in the amount of fibrous tissue and a corresponding decrease in the number of giant cells is probably associated with regressing lesions.
- Clinical and radiographic correlation is necessary, as the histologic features strongly resemble those seen in central giant cell tumors and the lesions of hyperparathyroidism.
- A distinctive feature of the disease is the presence of an "eosinophilic perivascular cuffing" of collagen fibers, which often surrounds the blood capillaries.

POINTS TO REMEMBER

- Cyst is a pathological cavity containing fluid, semifluid, or gas, which is usually lined by epithelium and is not formed by the accumulation of pus.
- Dentigerous cyst is the developmental odontogenic cyst of epithelial origin which encloses the crown of an unerupted tooth by expansion of its follicle and is attached to the neck. Most of them are discovered on radiographs when these are taken because a tooth has failed to erupt or a tooth is missing. It is composed of thin cystic wall of nonkeratinized stratified squamous epithelium.
- Odontogenic keratocyst is a developmental odontogenic cyst of epithelial origin developed from cystic degeneration of the cells of the stellate reticulum in a developing tooth germ. Keratocysts often radiographically present as multilocular radiolucent areas, with a typical "soap-bubble" appearance. Histologically they have both orthokeratinized and parakeratinized epithelium. Characteristic feature of the lining of epithelium between five cell layers and eight cell layers without rete ridges.
- Radicular or periapical cyst is the most common odontogenic cystic lesion of inflammatory origin, which occurs in relation to the apex of a nonvital tooth. Radicular cysts present well-defined, unilocular, and round-shaped radiolucent areas of variable size and histologically epithelium is nonkeratinized and it often show localized areas of increased cell proliferation by enclosing or encircling a mass of connective tissue capsule from all sides called "arcading pattern".
- Pleomorphic adenoma is a benign neoplasm consisting of cells exhibiting the ability to differentiate to epithelial (ductal and nonductal) and mesenchymal (chondroid, myxoid, and osseous) cells. It presents as small, painless, and quiescent nodule which slowly begins to increase in size, sometimes intermittently. It can be myxoid or cellular. Compound odontome is a diffuse mass of odontogenic tissue and complex odontome is collection of small tooth-like structures.
- World Health Organization defines ameloblastoma as polymorphic neoplasm consisting of proliferating odontogenic epithelium, which usually has a follicular or plexiform pattern, lying in a fibrous stroma. Ameloblastoma is a benign, locally invasive, and polymorphic neoplasm, presumably derived from intraosseous remnants of odontogenic epithelium. It may be derived from cell rests of enamel organ either remnants of dental lamina or remnants of Hertwig's sheath and epithelial rests of Malassez. Mandibular molar ramus is most favored. Starts as slow growing bony hard swelling whereas large lesions of ameloblastoma often cause severe expansion, destruction, and thinning of the cortical plates called "eggshell crackling". Radiographically presents as well-defined radiolucent areas giving honeycomb or larger soap-bubble appearance. Its histological variants are follicular, plexiform, acanthomatous, and desmoplastic type.
- Cherubism is a rare benign hereditary condition/being inherited as an autosomal dominant which affects only the jawbones of children bilaterally and symmetrically, usually producing the so-called cherubic look.

Questionnaire

1. Define cysts and classify the oral mucosal lesions.
2. Describe the etiopathogenesis, clinical features, radiographic, and histologic picture of dentigerous cyst.
3. Explain the radiographic and histological features of odontogenic keratocyst (OKC).
4. What is radicular cyst?
5. Describe pleomorphic adenoma in detail.
6. What are the clinical features and diagnostic tests for Sjögren's syndrome?
7. Write a note on odontome.
8. What is ameloblastoma? Classify its histological variants.
9. Write a note on cherubism.

FURTHER READING

1. Aldred MJ, Cameron AC. Pediatric oral medicine and pathology. In: Cameron AC, Widmer RP (Eds). Handbook of Pediatric Dentistry, 3rd edition. St. Louis: Mosby; 2008. pp. 169-216.
2. Bezzera S, Costa I. Oral conditions in children from birth to 5 years: the findings of a children's dental program. J Clin Pediatr Dent. 2000;25:79-81.
3. Finkelstein MW, Lanzel E, Hellstein JW. (2013). A Guide to Clinical Differential Diagnosis of Oral Mucosal Lesions. [online] Available from www.dentalcare.com/en-us/ professional-education/ce-courses/ce110. [Accessed April, 2018].
4. Langlais RP, Miller CS. Color Atlas of Common Oral Diseases. Philadelphia: Lea & Febiger; 1992.
5. McDonald and Avery's Dentistry for the Child and Adolescent, 11th Edition, Mosby; 2021.
6. Neville BW, Damm DD, Allen CM, et al. Oral and Maxillofacial Pathology, 3rd edition. Philadelphia: Saunders; 2009.
7. Neville BW, Damm DD, White DK. Color Atlas of Clinical Oral Pathology, 2nd edition. Lippincott: Williams & Wilkins; 1999.
8. Regezi JA, Sciubba J. Oral Pathology: Clinical-Pathologic Correlations, 2nd edition. Philadelphia: Saunders; 1993.

CHAPTER

Child Abuse and Neglect

Nikhil Marwah, Shabnab Zahir

CHAPTER OUTLINE

- Historical Background
- Definitions
- Incidence of Child Abuse
- Characteristics of Child Abuse
- Types of Child Abuse and Neglect
- Physical Child Abuse
- Child Sexual Abuse
- Child Neglect
- Munchausen Syndrome by Proxy
- Role of Pedodontist in Child Abuse and Neglect
- Management of a Child Abuse Patient

Childhood should be a carefree time of life filled with love, new world to explore, and with joy of mastery of oneself and the environment. However, for many children, this is only a dream, not reality. Child abuse and neglect (CA/CN) is an increasing social problem not limited to medical, legal, or social service professions. The dentist treating the children must also be able to detect, document, report, and often help to manage these needy patients and their families.

HISTORICAL BACKGROUND

- Early civilizations regularly abandoned deformed or unwanted children, and the ritual sacrifice of children to appease the gods took place in the Egyptian, Carthaginian, Roman, Greek, and Aztec societies.
- During the Middle Ages (c. 350–c. 1450) in Europe, healthy but unwanted children were apprenticed to work or offered to convents and monasteries. Infanticide, or the murder of babies, was also common.
- A review by **Radbill** (1973) indicated that historically, children were considered to be their parent's property, having a few rights of their own. It was taken for granted that parents and guardians had every right to treat their children as they wished.
- With the coming of industrialization in Europe and the United States, the implied right of abuse was transferred to the factory, where orphaned or abandoned children as young as five worked sixteen hours a day. In many cases irons were riveted around their ankles to bind the children to the machines, while overseers with whips ensured productivity.
- During the nineteenth century, child labor laws were passed in most industrialized countries to limit the kinds of jobs children could do and the number of hours they could work.
- The first documented and reported case of CA/CN occurred in 1874 with a child named **Mary Ellen**.
- In 1946, in a classic article by **Caffey**, some common features of CA/CN were first described, and it reported the common association of subdural hematomas and long bone pathosis.
- In1974, Child Abuse Prevention and Treatment Act was signed into law. For the first time, it established within the federal government—National Center on Child Abuse and Neglect.
- In India the National Commission for Protection of Child Rights, set up in 2007, enquires, investigates, and recommends about child abuse and neglect and its prevention.
- The Indian Government has assigned focal responsibility for child rights and development to the Ministry of Women and Child Development (MWCD).
- The Indian Parliament had passed an Act in 2012 and made stringent laws to control sexual offences against young girls in India by introducing the Protection of Children against Sexual Offences Act **(POCSO).**
- The contribution of dentists to recognition of CA/CN emerged during late 1960s. Initially, dentistry focused on the forensic aspects of battered child syndrome and homicide. Only recently has the dental profession seriously considered its role in detecting and reporting CA/CN.

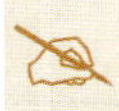

*In1962, the term battered child syndrome was coined by **Henry Kempe** in his milestone article. It was further elaborated by **Kempe** and **Helfer** in 1972.*

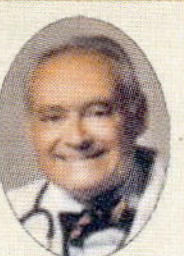

DEFINITIONS

- **Child abuse:** *According to* ***Gill*** *1968, it is defined as the non-accidental physical injury, minimal, or fatal, inflicted upon children by persons caring for them. It is an overt Act of Commission of a caretaker—physical, emotional, or sexual.*
- The most comprehensive and expanded definition of child abuse was proposed by **World Health Organization (WHO)** in 1999 in its report of the Consultation on Child Abuse Prevention which states that '*Child abuse and maltreatment constitutes all the forms of physical and/or emotional ill-treatment, sexual abuse, neglect or negligent treatment or commercial or other exploitation, resulting in actual or potential harm to the child's health, survival, development or dignity in the context of a relationship of responsibility, trust or power.*'
- **Battered baby:** *A child who shows clinical or radiographic evidence of lesions.*
- **PITS(Caffey)***or parent-infant traumatic stress syndrome that are frequently multiple and involve mainly the head, soft tissues, long bones, and the thoracic cage, and that cannot be unequivocally explained* (**Selwyn**,1985).
- **Neglected child:** *It is one who shows evidence of physical or mental health primarily due to failure on the part of the parent or caretakers to provide adequately for child's needs.*
- Child neglect: *An act of 'inattention or omission by the caregiver to provide for the child: health, education, emotional development, nutrition, shelter and safe living conditions'* (WHO, 1999).
- **Persecuted child:** *It is one who shows evidence of mental ill health caused by a deliberate infliction of physical or psychological injury that is often continuous in nature.*
- **Forensic science:** *It refers to areas of endeavor that can be used in a judicial setting and is accepted by the court and the general scientific community to separate truth form untruth. It deals with the study of collection of information connected with the crime.*
- **Forensic odontology:** *It is defined as the branch of odontology, which deals with the proper handling and examination of dental evidence and with the proper examination of dental evidence and with the proper evaluation, a presentation of dental findings in the interest of justice* (**Pederson**,1969).
- **Sexual abuse:** *Child sexual abuse to include contacts or interactions between a child and an adult when the child is being used for the sexual stimulation of the perpetrator or another person.*
- **Dental neglect:** *The failure by a parent or guardian to seek treatment for visually untreated caries, oral infections and/or oral pain, or failure of the parent or guardian to follow through with treatment once informed that the earlier condition(s) exists.*

INCIDENCE OF CHILD ABUSE

- The WHO (2017) reports that worldwide, child maltreatment is widespread with one in four adults reporting being physically abused as children.
- The National Commission for Protection of Child Rights (NCPCR), the Government of India's ombudsman of children's rights, published a report in 2012 based on the survey conducted in 2009–10 in seven states in which it was stated that 99.7% of children reported one or other form of punishment. 81.2% of children reported an outward rejection when on the ground of learning experience.
- Survey conducted by the National Crime Records Bureau (NCRB) reported an increase in the number of child abuse cases registered under POCSO Act from 8,904 in the year 2014 to 14,913 in 2015. In 94.8 % of POCSO cases, girls were raped by someone who were known to them.

CHARACTERISTICS OF CHILD ABUSE

The Abused Child	*The Abuser*
When all forms of child abuse are considered, the distribution between male and female is nearly equal. Some of the identifying features of the abused child are: • Unduly afraid or passive child • Evidence of prolonged confinement like delay in speech • Evidence of repeated skin or other injuries • Child is undernourished and is given in appropriate food or drink • Evidence of poor overall care • Child is cranky irritable or cries easily • Physically abused children were more aggressive than neglected.	Child abuse can occur in any cultural, occupational, socio-economic and ethnic group but a higher incidence is found in minority and low-income families. One parent is the active batterer, whereas the other passively approves of this maltreatment. The parent often has a history of being abused personally, so this practice is passed down for one generation to the other. Parents may have following characteristics, which may indicate abusive behavior: • Poor self-esteem • Violent temper or outbursts • Overly critical behavior toward the child • Embarrassment when discussing child's trauma • Avoidance of looking at or touching the child.

TYPES OF CHILD ABUSE AND NEGLECT (FIG. 76.1)

1.	Physical abuse
	Sexual abuse
	Failure to thrive
2.	Intentional drugging or poisoning
	Munchausen syndrome by proxy
	Health (medical) care neglect
	Dental neglect
	Safety neglect
3.	Emotional abuse and neglect
	Physical neglect
4.	Fabricated or induced illnesses
	Societal abuse
	Abuse by witnessing intimate partner violence (IPV)

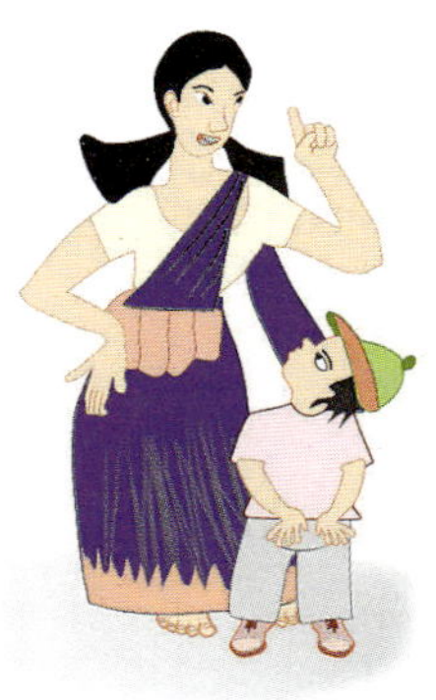
Verbally abusing a child

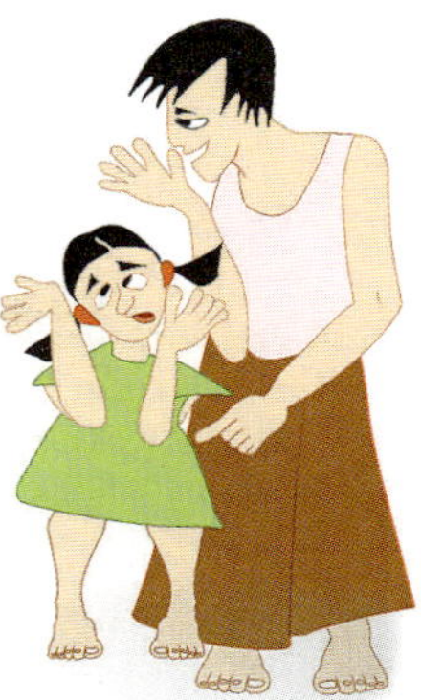
Teasing a child unnecessarily

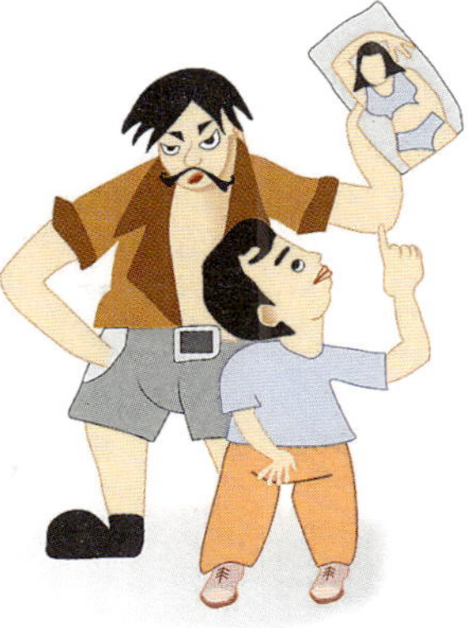
Exposing a child to porngraphics acts or literature

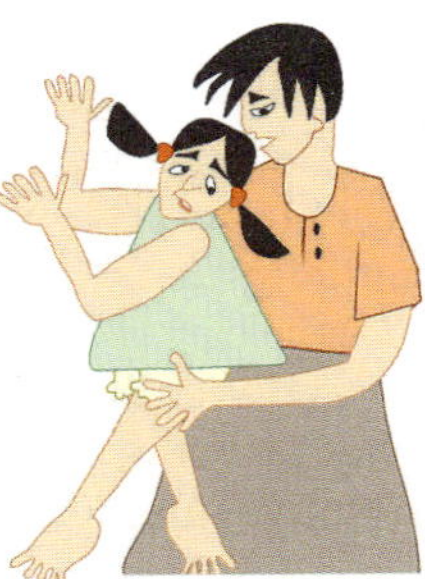
Touching a child where he/she does not want to be touched

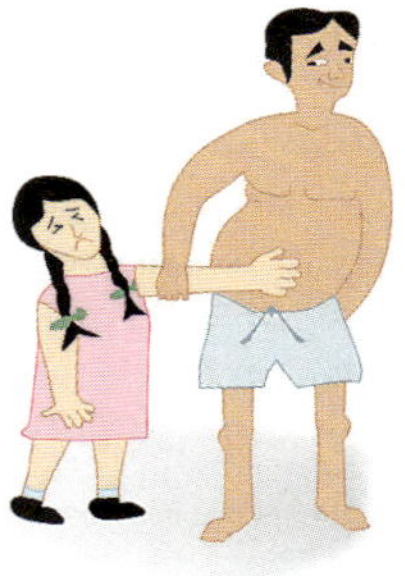
Forcing a child to touch you

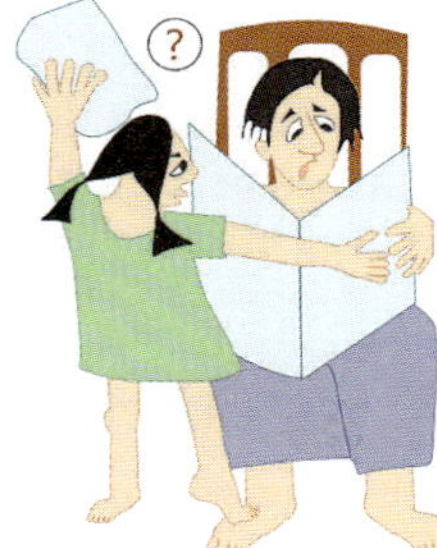

Breaking down the self-confidence of a child

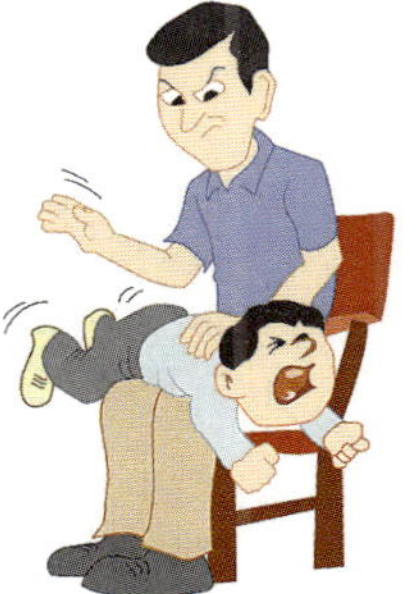
Hitting or hurting a child often to relieve your own frustration

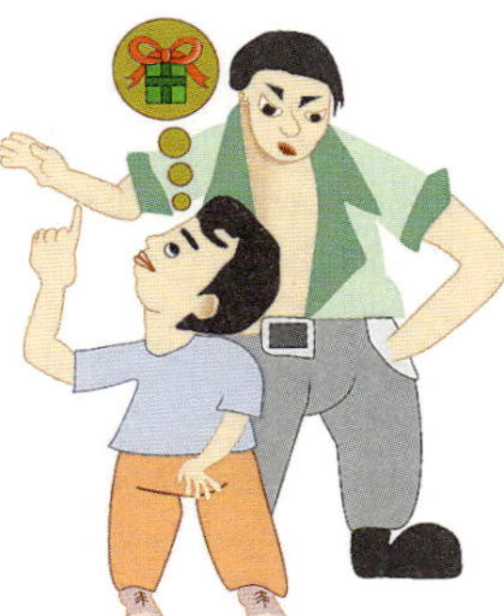
Manipulating a child

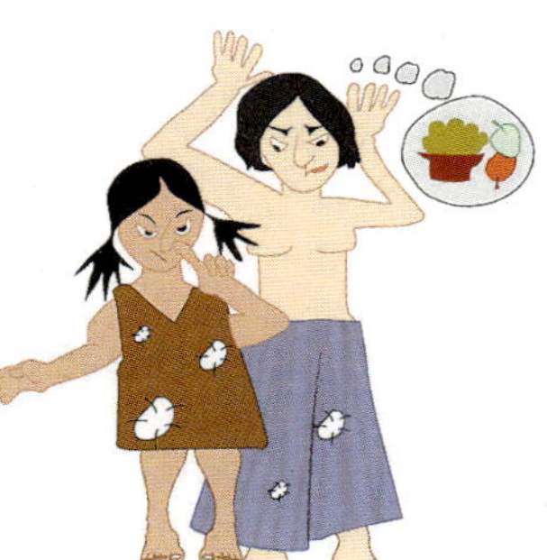
Not taking care of child for example: Unclean, unclothed, unfed child

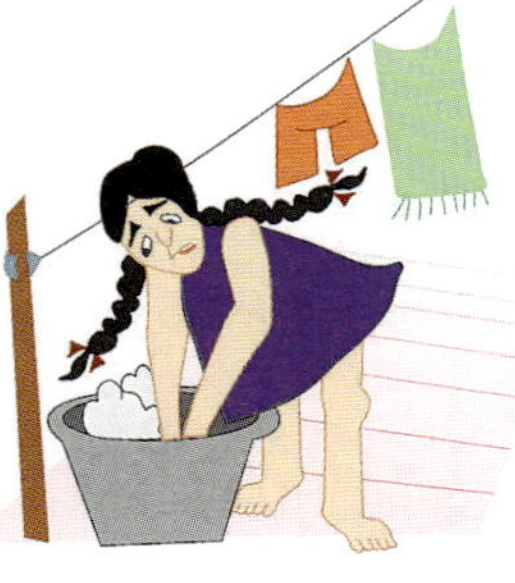
Using a child as a servant

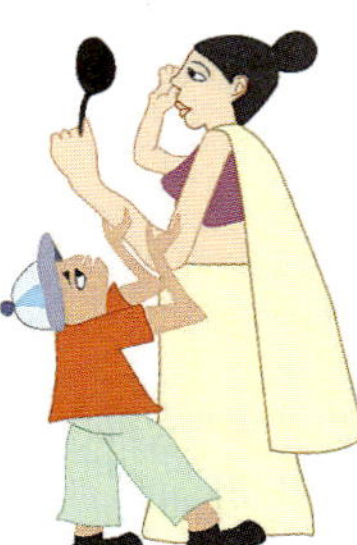
Not listening to a child

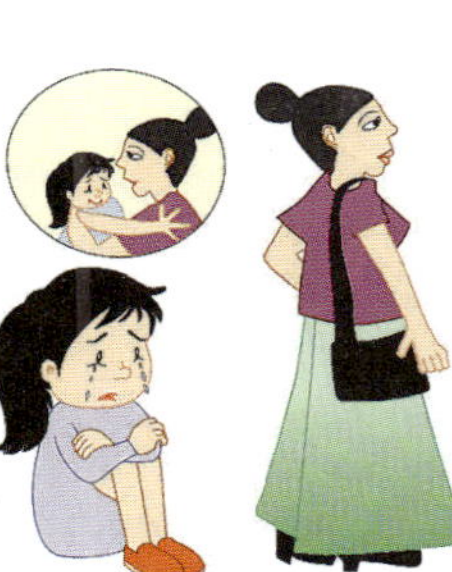
Neglecting emotional needs of a child

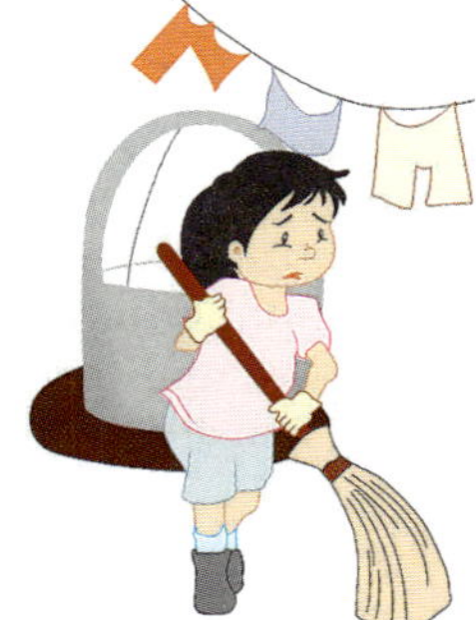
Making your own child a servant depriving of time for education/leisure

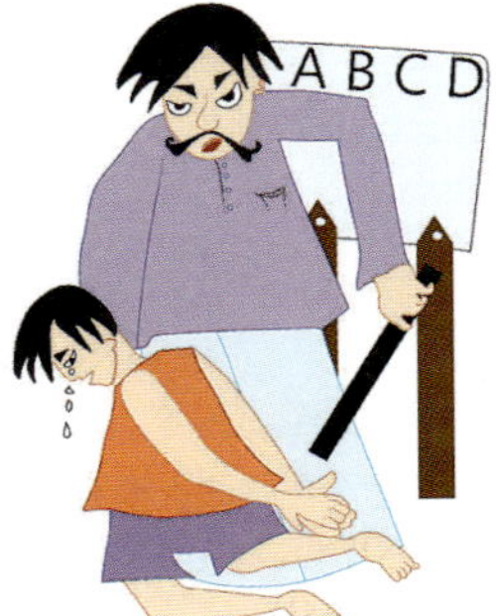

Hitting and redialing a child at school

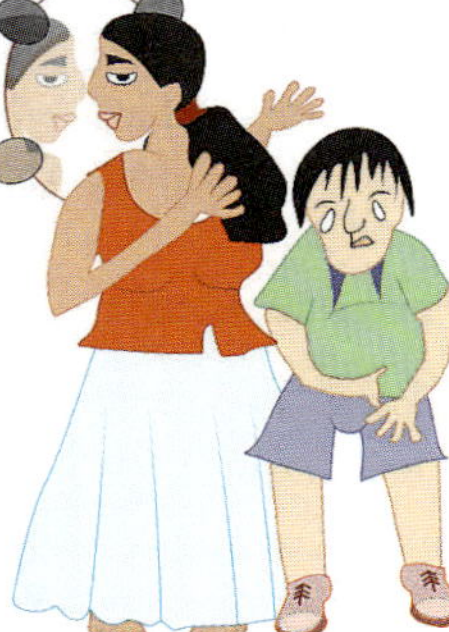
Neglecting a child's medical needs

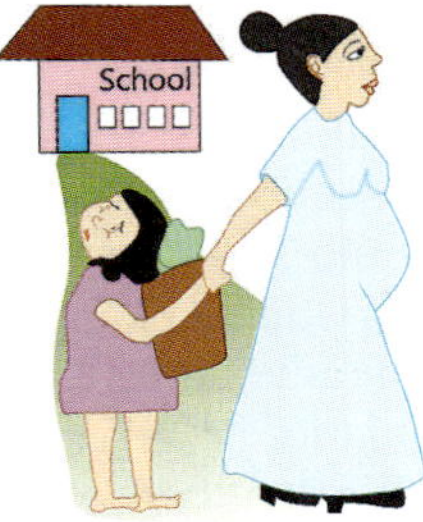

Neglecting a child's educational needs

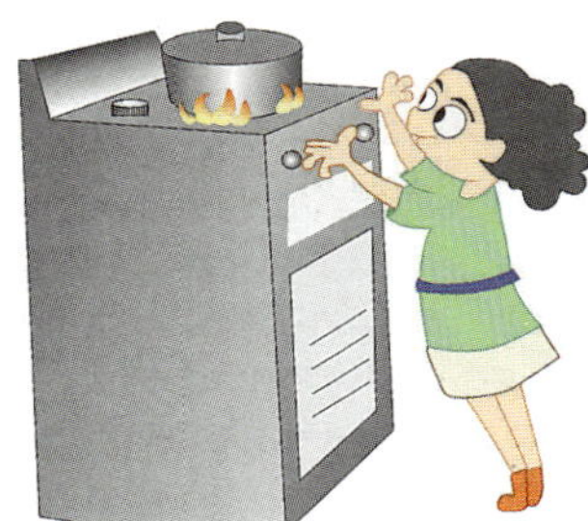
Leaving a child without supervision

Fig.76.1: Types of child abuse.

PHYSICAL CHILD ABUSE

Non-accidental trauma is one of the most common types of child abuse with the incidence being more than 10%. Physical abuse is probably the most important subtype of child maltreatment, because without intervention and services, it is potentially fatal. Often the injury stems from an angry response of the caretaker to punish the child form is behavior. Although many child abuse cases are based on physical findings but history is a helpful tool when child reports with non-descriptive findings.

History

- **Eyewitness history:** This usually has three aspects:
  1. Child himself states that injury is caused by parent
  2. One parent accuses the other about the injury
  3. Parent accepts that one of the many injuries is caused by him but not all.
- **Unexplained injury:** Some parents or caretakers deny knowledge of the injury; others can tell about the injury but can offer no explanation as to how the injury happened. They hope others believe that the injury was spontaneous. When pressed, they may become evasive or offer a vague explanation. These explanations are self-incriminating. As most parents know exactly how, where, and when their child was hurt.
- **Implausible history:** Many parents offer an explanation for the injury, but one which is implausible and in consistent with common sense like describing a minor injury whereas the marks on the child prove otherwise.
- **Alleged self-inflicted injury:** An alleged self-inflicted injury in a small baby is most serious. In general, if a child cannot crawl, he cannot cause self-injury.
- **Delay in seeking medical care:** Most non abusive parents seek immediate care when their child is injured. In contrast, some abused children are not presented for care for a considerable length of time even in major injury. Another feature of abusive parent will be that he will not accompany the child to the health care facility.

Bruises in Physical Child Abuse

- **Inflicted bruises:** Occur at typical sites or fit in recognizable patterns.
- **Accidental bruises:** A thorough knowledge of common and unusual accidental bruising will help in recognizing inflicted injuries. Understanding unusual customs or practices that leave bruises is also helpful. Lastly, it is important to remember that all bluish discolorations of the skin are not bruises. Most children acquire one or two bruises in daily activity like on knee and legs while walking and on forehead while jumping. The characteristics of these are similar to grab marks or abuse marks, however, the accidental bruises mostly lie over bony prominences whereas the abuse marks are on soft tissues.
- **Unusual bruises:** Some common ethnic practices can result in bruises that should not be confused with child abuse. The Vietnamese can induce symmetrical, linear bruises, from coin rubbing (Caogió). For symptoms of fever, chills, or headaches, the back and chest are covered with oil and then massaged in downward strokes with the edge of a coin.
- **Pseudo bruises:** Some skin conditions like Mongolian spot or allergic periorbital discolorations, *Haemophilus influenzae* may give appearance abusive marks.

Typical sites for inflicted bruises
- Buttocks and lower back (patting)
- Genitals and inner thighs
- Cheek (slap marks)
- Earlobe (pinch marks)
- Upper lip and frenum (forced feeding)
- Neck (choke marks).

Variables Affecting the Appearance of Bruises

- **Vascularity of the tissue injured:** Bruising in the loose and highly vascularized tissues around the eyes is more pronounced than skin in areas such as the palm of the hand or the soles of the feet.
- **Age:** Children and the elderly bruise more easily because of loose delicate skin.
- **Metabolic rate:** Women bruise more easily than men.
- **Medications:** Such as aspirin can increase bleeding.

Dating bruises

Age	*Color*
0–2 days	*Swollen, tender*
0–5 days	*Red, blue, and purple*
5–7 days	*Green*
7–10 days	*Yellow*
10–14 days	*Brown*
2–4 weeks	*Cleared*

- **Normal skin color:** The pigmentations on stain may affect the observation of a bruise.
- **Mass and velocity of the impact:** It may have an influence on the depth and surface of the injury, as well as the rate of healing. For example, deep subcutaneous injury can prolong bleeding time or previous bruising at the same site may affect subsequent bruising by increasing the rate of resolution.
- **Time of injury:** The time of appearance of bruise is related to the time required for the extravasated blood to reach the surface. This lag time will allow antemortem bruises to appear postmortem.
- **Other factors that affect bruising:** Rapidity of death after injury and environmental conditions.

Types of Physical Abuse

Location of bruise	*Indicative of bruise*
Genital or inner thigh	Toilet mishaps or sexual abuse
Cheeks	Slapping of child
Earlobes	Pinching or pulling
Upper lip/labial frenum	Impatient or forceful feeding
Neck	Strangulation
Circumferential bruises on ankles/wrists	Placement of restraints
Corners of mouth	Gagging of child

Marks in Physical Child Abuse

- **Human hand marks:** These are classified here. The most common type is grab marks which is oval-shaped bruise that resemble fingerprints due to holding of child in violent shaking. Some of the non-abusive grab marks are when the parent holds the child's legs to help him walk or on the cheeks, if an adult squeeze it in an attempt to get food or medicine into his mouth leaving a thumb mark bruise on one cheek and two to four finger mark bruises on the other cheek.
- **Strap marks:** These are 1–2 inches wide, sharp-bordered, rectangular bruises of various lengths, and sometimes covering a curved body surface often caused by a belt.
- **Lash marks:** These are narrow, straight, edges bruises, or scratches caused by thrashing with tree branch or switch.
- **Loop marks:** These are secondary to being struck with a doubled-over lamp cord, rope, or fan belt. The distal end of the loop strikes with the most force, commonly breaking the skin and leaving loop-shaped scars.
- **Bizarre marks:** These are always inflicted when a blunt instrument is used in punishment with the resulting bruise that will resemble it in shape.
- **Circumferential tie marks:** These are present on the ankles or wrists and are caused, when a child is restrained. If a narrow rope or cord is used, the child will be left with circumferential cut. If a strap or piece of sheet is used to restrain a child about the wrists or ankles, a friction burn or rope burn may result, usually presenting as a large blister that encircles the extremity.
- **Gag marks:** Seen as abrasions that appear near the corner of the mouth. Children may be gagged because of screaming or yelling.

CHILD SEXUAL ABUSE

This has increased dramatically over the last decade. An estimate of the incidence of the number of sexual assaults on children at 3 lakhs annually but authorities agree that these estimates are probably low, due to under reporting as a result of a number of factors:

- Cultural morals make sexual abuse a stigma for victim, perpetrator, and family.
- Victims are often young children whose fear, lack of awareness, or lack of language skills make them easy prey and victims who may not be ready or believable witnesses.
- Health professionals may be unaware of the signs or symptoms of child sexual abuse.
- Child sexual abuse often is hidden with no visible physical manifestations.
- Health professionals may be unwilling to report cases of sexual abuse where clear physical evidence is lacking for fear of error, reprisal, or loss of patients.
- Verification of sexual abuse by physical examination may be beyond the legal extent of practice of many professionals.
- Lack an accepted definition of sexual abuse.

Federal statues *define sexual abuse in the context of child abuse and include such acts like child pornography, rape, molestation, incest, and child prostitution.* **National Center on Child Abuse and Neglect** offers a more general definition of *child sexual abuse to include contacts or interactions between a child and an adult when the child is being used for the sexual stimulation of the perpetrator or another person. It can also be defined as any sexual activity with a child under age 18 by an adult.*

Victim

- The sexually abused child is most often a female, with the ratio of victimized females to males of 9:1.
- Children of all ages are abused sexually but those in the early teens seem to be most at risk.
- Most offenders are family-related, some are family acquaintances, and the least common are strangers. This close relationship between victim and perpetrator compounds the problem of reporting which leads to a victim who maybe abused repeatedly.
- The psychological profiles of sexually abused children vary widely and appear to have some relation to age, closeness to perpetuator, and the type of abuse. Young children often do not suffer long-term effects of sexual abuse as they do not identify the act with society's concepts of right and wrong.
- Some of the features that are noted are:
  - Emotional effects
  - Functional disturbances such as retention of feces
  - Frequent masturbation
  - Preoccupation with the genital area
  - Regression in behavior
  - Guilt and anxiety.

Perpetrator

- The perpetrator of sexual abuse is no longer considered to be the impersonal stranger who victimizes an unknown child. The numbers of sexual assaults by those familiar to the child have increased dramatically.
- The type of abuse may characterize the perpetrator. Incest most often is committed by a male parent against a female child.
- The father may have one of several profiles like, he maybe abusive or shy or withdrawn: sexual problems with spouse or alcoholism. Mother-son, or father-son incest is less common, but indicates psychological pathosis.

Act

- Types include molestation (fondling or masturbation), intercourse (vaginal, anal, or oral intercourse on a non-assaultive basis), or family-related rape. Pregnancy or venereal disease may be the sequelae of repeated sexual abuse.
- Forms of sexual abuse may include the act of sexual abuse is rarely a singular event, if perpetrated by someone familiar to victim. In many cases, abuse may involve repeated fondling of genitals or other body parts.

CHILD NEGLECT

Child neglect is a form of abuse, an act of caregivers (e.g., parents) that results in depriving a child of their basic needs, such as the failure to provide adequate supervision, health care, clothing, or housing, as well as other physical, emotional, social, educational, and safety needs.

Types of Child Neglect

- Physical neglect
- Nutritional neglect
- Educational neglect
- Healthcare neglect
- Dental neglect
- Emotional neglect
- Supervisory neglect
- Environmental neglect
- Educational neglect

Physical Neglect or Deprivation of Needs Neglect

- This type of neglect occurs when children's basic physical needs (e.g., food, shelter, and clothing) are not being met and often occurs in a persistent pattern.
- Examples of physical deprivation include being denied food and/or water and being left out in the elements.
- This is usually coaxial with physical abuse and involves presentation of child with dirty hair, dirty or insufficient clothing, inadequate lunches, incomplete immunization, unsanitary home environment, and inadequate after school supervision.

Nutritional Neglect

- Failure to thrive can be defined as an underweight, malnourished condition who has a weight that is below the third percentile and a height and head circumference that are above third percentiles on growth curves.
- On physical examination, the infants have gaunt faces, prominent ribs, wasted buttocks, and spindly extremities and is expressed in first 2 years of life.
- The causes of failure to thrive are estimated as 30% organic, 20% underfeeding due to understandable error, and 50% underfeeding from parental neglect. The mother may neglect to feed her baby because she feels overwhelmed with responsibilities or is chronically depressed and hostile toward the baby.

Healthcare Neglect

- When a child with a treatable chronic disease has serious deterioration of the condition because the parents or caretakers repeatedly ignore healthcare recommendations, healthcare neglect occurs.
- Healthcare neglect may occur in situations where an emergency exists, and the parents or caretakers will not acknowledge it as much.
- Refusals because of religious beliefs also lead to healthcare neglect.
- The child's right, however, to life and health must override the parents or caretakers constitutional right to religious freedom. If the disease is incurable, the parents or caretakers wishes regarding non-intervention; be they religious or philosophical, often are respected.

Dental Neglect

- The problem of dental neglect is ubiquitous; yet only recently has been defined apart from the broader category of child abuse and neglect. Consequently, the recognition and report of dental neglect by professionals has been difficult.
- Child neglect occurs when a parent or caretaker deliberately or unintentionally permits the child to experience suffering or falls to provide the necessities for the child's physical, emotional, and intellectual developments.
- Ad Hoc Committee on Child Abuse and Neglect of the American Academy of Pediatric Dentistry defined dental neglect as: The failure by a parent or guardian to seek treatment for visually untreated caries, oral infections and/or oral pain, or failure of the parent or guardian to follow through with treatment once informed that the earlier condition(s)exists.

Safety Neglect

- Although most accidents are due to a breach in safety and theoretically could have been prevented, the interruption of the fateful event would have required unusual prediction and timing on the part of the parent or caretaker. These are legitimate accidents, and every child has some.
- Safety neglect, however, has occurred when injury results from lack of supervision. These situations usually involve children younger than 4 years of age, when it is important that parents directly supervise them. This leads to injuries like burns, poisonings, and falls because children are not being watched.

Emotional Neglect

- Emotional abuse can be defined as the continual scapegoating and rejection of child by parent or caretaker.
- Severe verbal abuses are also apart of emotional abuse and so is the neglect of student by teacher.
- Emotional abuse is often difficult to detect and involves:
  - Severe psychopathology and disturbed behavior in child of a degree making it unlikely that he will be able to function and cope as an adult.
  - Abnormal child rearing practices of the parent that has caused behavior disturbances in child.
  - Refusal by the parent to get the treatment for the child.

Supervisory Neglect

- Supervisory neglect occurs when the adult responsible for a child either fails to supervise and keep the child from being harmed or fails to have someone else supervise the child and keep him or her from harm.
- This type of neglect can occur continually or only happen one time.
- Two examples of supervisory neglect include failing to supervise a child around weapons and other dangerous

Effects on children of neglect (Skuse,1993)				
	Infant	*Preschool*	*School child*	*Young person*
Physical	• Failure to thrive (FTT), dirty infect skin, and nappy rash	• Short/thin • Dirty, unkempt thin hair	• Short/thin • Dirty, unkempt thin hair	• Short/thin/obese • Dirty, unkempt delayed puberty
Developmental	• Generalized delay quiet	• Language delay • Poor attention immature	• Learning difficulties • Lacks confidence immature	• School failure
Behavioral	• Anxious • Avoidant unresponsive	• Overactive • Aggressive overfriendly	• Overactive • Aggressive withdrawn • No peer or friends • Wet, soils the bed	• School truancy • Smoking, drinking, and substance misuse • Runs away • Sexual precocity • Stealing, lying, and self-harm

circumstances and leaving a child with an impaired caregiver.

Environmental Neglect

This is related to both physical neglect and supervisory neglect, but it occurs when children's home environments are filthy. Rotting food may be left out, there may be infestations of rats or cockroaches, and children may regularly come to school in dirty clothing. Some professionals group environmental neglect with physical neglect.

Educational Neglect

- Educational neglect is when children are not given access to education.
- Examples of educational neglect include parents failing to register children for school or parents making children stay home from school to ensure that they don't report the abuse they experience at home.

MUNCHAUSEN SYNDROME BY PROXY (MSBP)

Munchausen syndrome was first described by **Dr Richard Asher** in 1951.

- He reported adults who fabricated symptoms about themselves and produced signs of illnesses. They presented themselves for medical care but did not inform the medical professional about the deception.
- On the other hand, in cases of Munchausen syndrome by proxy, a parent or caretaker attempts to bring medical attention to themselves by injuring or inducing illness in their children. It's another name is Factitious disorder imposed on another (FDIA).
- **Dr Roy Meadow** first coined the term "Munchausen syndrome by proxy" to describe the preservation of the deception in regard to the child.
- This describes children who are victims of parentally fabricated or induced illness. The fabricated symptoms and signs lead to unnecessary medical investigations, hospital admissions, and treatment. The mother often is a nurse or has a similar illness herself. Factitious symptoms are often of bleeding from various sites. If specimens are requested, the mother adds her own blood to the material. Factitious signs include recurrent sepsis from injecting contaminated fluids, chronic diarrhea from laxatives, fever from rubbing thermometers, or rashes from rubbing the skin or applying caustic substances.
- MSBP cases are very rare with incidence 0.4/100,000 in children below 16 years and 2–2.8 per 100,000 in children below 1 year.
- Death rate has been reported to be 6–10% for MSBP cases
- The mother is usually the perpetrator.
- Affected mothers are either 'Active inducers' who exaggerate the illnesses of their children or 'help seekers' who use their children to avoid social problems such as domestic violence or 'doctor addicts' who are more suspicious type.

Battered child syndrome

It was **Dr C Henry Kempe** monumental work published in 1962 in the Journal of the American Medical Association which brought the full impact of physical maltreatment to the medical community and subsequently, to the attention of the general public. His article was entitled, "the battered child syndrome". The impact of Dr Kempe's publication led to the passage of laws (1963–1968) in all states requiring health professionals to report to welfare departments and/or police departments. However, it is important to realize that the "battered child syndrome" is only one small, even though severe, portion of the physical abuse of children.

- Battered child syndrome can be seen in infants through adolescents but is most common in children younger than 3 years.
- More prevalent among stepchildren, handicapped, and first-born children.
- The victims are mostly younger than 2 years of age, with a average age of 16 months.
- Fractures are second only to soft tissue injuries as the most common finding in battered child syndrome.
- Multiple fractures in various stages of healing, Corner and bucket-handle metaphyseal fractures may be a classic finding of battered child syndrome.

ROLE OF PEDODONTIST IN CHILD ABUSE AND NEGLECT

If the initial examination reveals trauma including oral cavity and it is within the scope of the attending dentist, the definitive treatment should begin. In suspected cases of child abuse, follow-up dental care may not be possible because of lack of familial compliance or delay in disposition of the case by the investigating agency. The dentist's role in identifying and preventing child abuse is as follows:

- To observe and examine any suspicious evidence that can be ascertained in office.
- To record according to the law, any evidence which may be helpful in the case.
- To it any dental injuries. Dentist should be acquainted with management of injuries to both primary and permanent dentitions.
- To establish and maintain a professional therapeutic relationship with the family.
- To transfer the child to a physician or hospital for proper care.

Intervention and Prevention

Once a case of child abuse is suspected and reported, the multidisciplinary team of the institution initiates the screening process. A pedodontist can contribute toward prevention of this criminal act by understanding various issues related to child abuse and applying them at different levels.

- **Primary level:** Dentist should follow approaches, which are applicable to a population in general, without targeting a particular high-risk group.
  - Greater attention should be given toward screening children at a higher risk of maltreatment.
  - Parents at risk for abusing children are frequently very needy themselves, so they need to be screened and counseled.
  - Comprehensive evaluation of child and family situation should be done assisted by a social worker and mental health professional.
- **Secondary level:** Concerns and effects directed to those who are known to be especially at high-risk.
  - The pedodontist must recognize his limitation and assume responsibilities for applying an interdisciplinary approach.
  - Goal of intervention should be to enhance parenting capabilities to enable them to a more adequate care for their children and avoid possible maltreatment.
- **Tertiary level:** It refers to intervention after the condition is already identified. Prevention is considered, as the goal is to prevent recurrence of the condition.
  - Pedodontist should ensure that child is referred toa designated child protection agency.
  - He should not make the report and disengage, as he often has valuable information, which might help in treatment and monitoring the situation.

Legal Aspects

A dentist should be well versed with current legal system for child protection. A separate doctrine "Parens Patriae" is important in understanding laws developed to protect children.

Dentists should know the definitions of child abuse and existing related laws proposed under the Draft Model Child Protection Act 1977, to protect himself and apply it correctly in such cases. The same laws that mandate dentists to report suspected abuse often also protect them from legal litigation, often brought by angry or vengeful parents. This law also makes the dentist liable for any damage to child caused by the failure to report abuse. Although the laws vary from state-to-state, generally the dentist who fails to report such case is considered guilty of sample misdemeanor and is subject to affine or jail sentence, usually 30 days in length. In most situations, parents can be informed as follows: "Based on my training, I am concerned that this injury could not have happened this way. Because of this, I am required by law to make a report to child protective services". The principles that a dentist must remember in forensic pedodontics:

- Should be fully aware of legal standards of care and legal responsibilities.

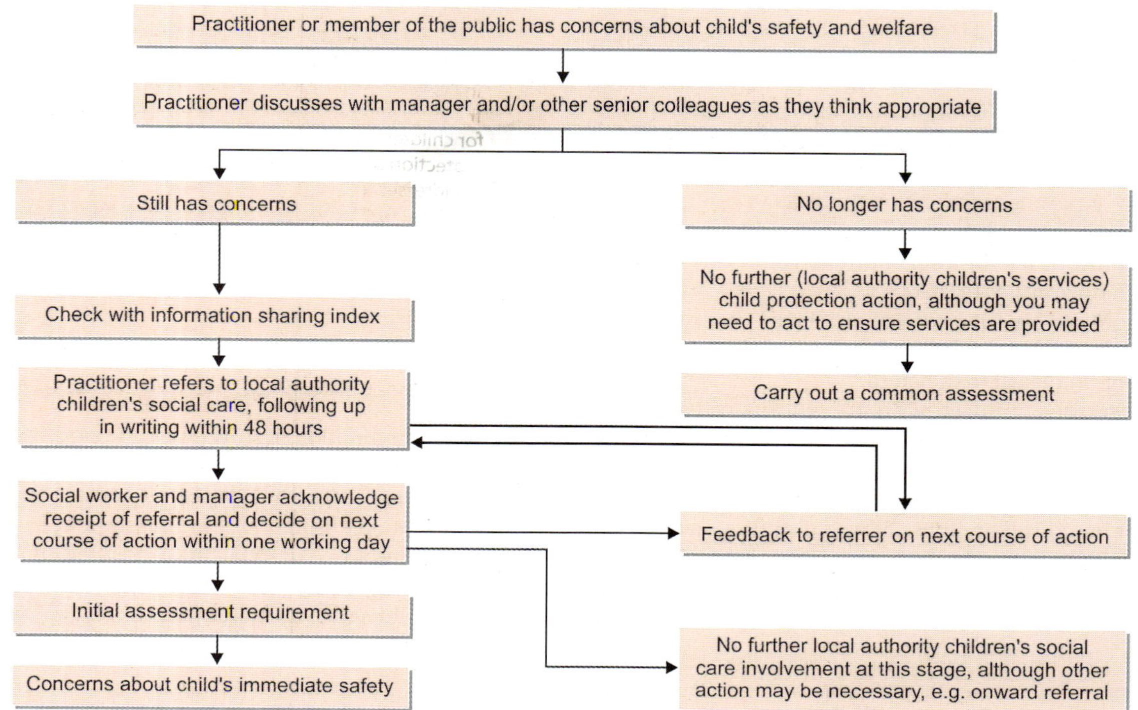

- Records should be made in presence of patients.
- Should keep legibly written, accurate case records.
- Should keep update knowledge.
- Diagnostic tools like radiographs should always be used.
- Should always consult a legal or medicolegal expert to review insurance policies or any financial or legal matter.

MANAGEMENT OF A CHILD ABUSE PATIENT

- Many institutions, especially schools and hospitals, teams have been set up to discuss management to cases and whether or not a report to the state agency ought to be filed. Ideally, such teams consist of representatives of different disciplines and different ethnic groups. A team offers the ideal approach to deal with the complex and frequently painful situations. They offer a shared responsibility and remove some of the burden placed on the individual. When a report is made then it goes through a screening process in the state agency. Depending on the state of urgency of the circumstances, the agency then investigates the case immediately or within a set time frame. This evaluation generally includes meeting with key family members, a home visit, and contact with professionals involved with the family such as a physician, dentist, or teacher. The investigation determines whether or not the report is substantiated. If not, there still remains the possibility that services can be offered on a voluntary basis, which the family can choose to accept or reject. When the case is substantiated a service plan is developed.
- Once a report has been substantiated, the social worker needs to assess the degree of the child's immediate risk so as to determine the appropriate placement. In the majority of cases, the child will remain in the home, but when there is serious concern about the child's safety, he will be removed. This is avoided because removing the child will cause deleterious psychological impact when an abused child when taken out of the home and placed away from the security of loved family members. For example, this could exacerbate the guilt felt by a child for "provoking"family problems.In such cases, it is best for the adult perpetrator to move out. When children are placed out of the home, reunion of the family is always the ultimate goal. Visits of the family are arranged. At first, these are supervised by a social worker in an office. Should these contacts go satisfactorily, visits gradually might be increased in frequency, length, and become unsupervised. In contrast, if visits present major difficulties for the child, they might be shortened, and become less frequent.
- A comprehensive social service plan should be developed as soon as possible that identifies the needs of the family and implements the appropriate services to meet these needs. In addition, clear goals should be articulated to the family in a supportive but for the right manner. It is critical that difficulties be addressed, both for individuals and the family as a whole. Frequently, a graduated stepwise approach is necessary. The social worker can be valuable in helping the family to obtain services and welfare benefits that they might be entitled to. These include payments for disabled children, or nutrition supplements for pregnant women, infants, and young children. Guidance in securing reasonable housing, help with transportation to important intervention programs, and information on work opportunities might be needed. Social worker can facilitate the development and learning of abused children by placing the intervention programs, therapeutic day care, or advocating a suitable school program. It is valuable to include the parent in plan, to support, and improve their parental skills. Social isolation is known to be an important, relate of child abuse, so it is important to facilitate supportive relationships within the extended neighborhood, and community. Monitoring the family situation and coordinating services are the crucial functions of the social worker as he must be empathic and supportive, persistent in pursuing needed services, and astute and sensitive in working with families.

- 1098 is a toll-free single helpline across India for reporting any form of child abuse
- NGO working for child rights
  - Save the children
  - Salaam Baalak Trust
  - World Vision India
  - SOS Children's village
- Important national legislation for child protection
  - The Juvenile Justice (Care and Protection) Act 2000 (amended in 2006) is a very important national legislation. It provides a framework for both children in need of care and protection and for children in conflict with the law.
  - Protection of Children from Sexual Offences (POCSO) Act 2012 It addresses the problem of sexual offences committed against children.

POINTS TO REMEMBER

- The first documented and reported case of CA/CN occurred in1874 with a child named Maryellen. In1962, the term battered child syndrome was coined by Henry Kempe.
- Child abuse is defined as the "non accidental physical injury, minimal or fatal, and inflicted upon children by person scaring for them". It is an overt act of commission of a caretaker—physical, emotional, or sexual.
- *Neglected child*: It is one who shows evidence of physical or mental health primarily due to failure on the part of the parent or caretakers to provide adequately for child's needs.
- Forensic odontology is defined as the branch of odontology, which deals with the proper handling and examination of dental evidence and with the proper examination of dental evidence and with the proper evaluation presentation of dental findings in the interest of justice.
- Dental neglect is the failure by a parent or guardian to seek treatment for visually untreated caries, oral infections and/or oral pain, or failure of the parent or guardian to follow through with treatment once informed that the earlier discussed condition(s) exists.
- Identifying features of the abused child are unduly afraid or passive child, delay in speech, repeated skin injuries, undernourishment, and poor overall care.

- Various types of child abuse are physical and sexual abuse and various types of neglect are emotional, physical, mental, dental, safety, and nutritional.
- Location of bruise is a significant indicator of type of abuse, e.g. bruise on genitals or thighs indicate sexual abuse; cheeks—physical abuse; circumferential marks on legs and hands—placement of restraints.
- Marks in physical child abuse are human hand marks, strap marks, lash marks, bizarre marks, circumferential tie marks, and gag marks.
- Role of a pediatric dentist in identification and reporting of abused child is to observe, examine and record any suspicious evidence, to maintain a professional therapeutic relationship with the family, and to transfer the child to a physician or hospital for proper care.
- Toll free helpline number to report child abuse–1098

Questionnaire

1. Define child abuse and give the characteristics of the abused and abuser.
2. Describe physical abuse with special reference to the bruises.
3. Write a note on child sexual abuse.
4. Explain the phenomenon of child neglect and its various implications.
5. What is battered child syndrome?
6. Describe the role of pedodontist in child abuse and neglect.
7. Write short note on Munchausen syndrome by proxy
8. Write short note on child abuse and neglect.
9. Role of pedodontists in child abuse and neglect.
10. Management of child abuse patient.

FURTHER READING

1. Casamassimo PS. Child sexual abuse and pediatric dentist. Pediatr Dent. 1986; 8:102-5.
2. Chandra V. Child Abuse and Neglect in India- Locating Child Abuse in Fractured Indian Families through Children's Lenses in Global Childhoods in International Perspective: Universality, Diversity and Inequality. Sage Publication Limited London. 2021:146-169.
3. Child abuse reporting laws. J Am Dent Assoc. 1967;75:1070.
4. DeFrancis Y, Lucht C. Child Abuse Legislation in the 1970s. Denver: The American Humane Association Children's Division;1974.
5. Fernandes G, Fernandes M, Vaidya N, et al. Prevalence of child maltreatment in India and its association with gender, urbanisation and policy: a rapid review and meta-analysis protocol. BMJ Open. 2021;11.
6. GammonJA. Ophthalmic manifestations of child abuse. In: Ejerstein NS (Ed). Child Abuse and Neglect: A Medical Reference. NewYork : John Wiley and Sons;1981.pp.121-39.
7. Hampton RL. National Study of the Incidence and Severity of Child Abuse and Neglect: May 1, 1979 to April 30, 1980. Denver: American Humane Association;1981.
8. Hazelwood AI. Child abuse: the dentist's role. New York Stat Dent J. 1970; 36:289-91.
9. Jaffe AC, Dynneson L, Ten Bensel RW. Sexual abuse of children: an epidemiologic study. Am J Dis Child. 1975; 129:689-92.
10. Johnson CF, Showers J. Injury variables in child abuse. Child Abuse Negl. 1985; 9:207-15.
11. Kempe CH, Silverman FN, Steele BF, et al. The battered child syndrome. J Am Med Assoc. 1962;181:17-20.
12. Krugman RD, Krugman MK. Emotional abuse in the classroom. The pediatrician's role in diagnosis and treatment. Am J Dis Child. 1984; 138:284-6.
13. Laskin DM. The battered-child syndrome. J Oral Surg.1973;31:903.
14. Laskin DM.The recognition of child abuse. J Oral Surg. 1978;36:349.
15. Luther SL, Price JH. Child sexual abuse: a review. Sch Health.1980;50:1-5.
16. Merten OF, Radkowki MA, Leonidas JC. The abused child: a radiological reappraisal. Radiology. 1983; 146:377-81.
17. Paul V, Rathaur VK, Bhat NK, Sananganba R, Ittoop AL, Pathania M. Child abuse: A social evil in Indian perspective. J Family Med Prim Care. 2021; 10:110-5.
18. Saini N. Child abuse and neglect in India: Time to act. jmaj. 2013;56(5):302-308
19. Schmitt BD. The child with nonaccidental trauma. In: Kempe CH, Helfer RE (Eds). The Battered Child. Chicago: University of Chicago Press; 1980. pp. 128-46.
20. Schwartz S, Woolridge E, Stege D. Oral manifestations and legal aspects of child abuse. J Am Dent Assoc. 1977;95:586-91.
21. Shamroy JA. A perspective on childhood sexual abuse. Soc Work. 1980;25:128-31.
22. Simley DO. Abused and neglected. J Wisc Dent Assoc.1975;51:377.
23. TeuscherCW.The battered child: a social enigma. J Dent Child.1974;41:335-6.
24. Unal EO, Unal V, Gul A, Celtek M, Dıken B, Balcıoglu İ. A serial Munchausen syndrome by proxy. Indian J Psychol Med 2017; 39:671-4.
25. Wilson EF. Estimation of the age of cutaneous contusions in child abuse. Pediatrics. 1977; 60:750-2.
26. "The First Six Years (2007-2013) – National Commission for Protection of Child Rights (NCPCR), Ministry of Women and Child Development, Government of India.

CHAPTER 77

Forensic Odontology and Bite Marks

Nikhil Marwah, Avantika Tuli

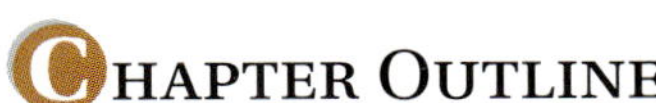

Chapter Outline

- Branches of Forensic Odontology
- Role of Dentists in Forensics
- Dental Identification
- Bite Marks
- Recent Advancements

Forensic is derived from a Latin word "forensis" which means "before the forum," a place where legal matters are discussed. According to FDI, *Forensic Dentistry is defined as a branch of dentistry which, in the interest of justice, deals with the proper handling and examination of dental evidence, and with proper evaluation and representation of dental findings.* (**Dr Oscar Amoedo** is called as father of forensic odontology. He wrote first dissertation entitled "L'Art Dentaire en Legale" in 1898). Today forensic odontology has evolved as separate specialty which relies on knowledge of teeth and jaws, dental anatomy, histology, radiography, pathology, dental materials, and developmental anomalies. Forensic identification is multidisciplinary team work that involves law enforcement officials, forensic anthropologists, forensic dentists, forensic pathologists, criminalists, serologists, and other specialists. Forensic odontology utilizes dentistry to identify human remains and bite marks, using both physical and biological dental evidence. Pedodontist can play important role in identification of bite marks. Dental trauma is a common finding in children which may be caused due to sports, accidents, or abuse. Thus, proper knowledge and its application is utmost important. Pediatric dentist can help in the investigations of legal officers by implementing his expertise in recognition of signs and symptoms of child abuse and identification of such victims.

Application of science and technology to the detection and investigation of crimes in order to bring justice is the essence of Forensic Science. According to the Fédération Dentaire Internationale, forensic odontology is a branch of dentistry that deals with the proper handling of dental evidence in the interest of justice and with the proper evaluation and presentation of dental findings. Dental identification has played a vital role in identifying deceased individuals since 66 AD. Ever since, this science has developed in leaps and bounds. The field of forensic odontology sees evolving trends in identification of human dental remains as we speak. Nevertheless, all the advancements are futile if not utilized in the right manner by the right people in the right situations. Currently, the dearth of trained personnel, paucity of training facilities, inadequate introduction to the subject during undergraduate years, are the major hurdles in the expansion of the use of forensic odontology for the day-to-day benefit of society. Forensic odontology is one of the most advanced branches of forensic medicine and forensic science. This is because of the key role of dental evidence in identification of victims of mass disaster, abuse or organized crime. Since victims of mass disaster abuse of organized crimes century also involved children; Pedodontist should have adept knowledge of all the subject if helping the forensic experts in identifying the affected victims therby contributing significantly in supporting families to enable them to care for children more adequately. (**Keiser-Neilson** *defined forensic dentistry as "that branch of forensic dentistry that in the interest of justice deals with the proper handling and examination of dental evidence and the proper evaluation and presentation of dental findings)".* Forensic odontology can be defined as the branch of dentistry which deals with the proper handling and examination of dental evidence and proper evaluation and presentation of dental findings in the interest of justice.

BRANCHES OF FORENSIC ODONTOLOGY

1. **Civil (non-criminal)**
   a. Identification of individual remains, where death is not due to any suspicious circumstances.
   b. Mass disaster identification of victims of hotel fires, aircraft disasters, earthquakes and other natural calamities.
   c. Craniofacial superimposition for individual recognition and identification.
2. **Criminal:**
   a. Identification of living or dead persons from their dentition or teeth.
   b. Dealing with mark identification on the assailant, perpetrators or victim or inanimate objects.
3. **Research:** (a) Forensic odontology should be a part of the curriculum for BDS as well as MBBS students and should also be included postgraduate training (MDS/PhD-Forensic medicine).Research in this field would be beneficial to the society.

ROLE OF DENTISTS IN FORENSICS

The positive identification of living or deceased persons using the unique traits and characteristics of the teeth and jaws is a cornerstone of forensic science. The teeth are the hardest substances in the human body and may be the only method available to identify the insults and consequences encountered at death and during decomposition. Currently, there are three types of personal identification circumstances that use the teeth, jaws, and orofacial characteristics. They are:

1. **Comparative dental identification:** It involves comparison of antemortem and postmortem dental records to identify the body. Congenital (anatomic) and acquired (treatment) characteristics of the teeth are compared between the antemortem and postmortem records. Discrepancies may exist because it is possible that the person may have additional dental treatments completed in the time interval between the dates represented by the antemortem and postmortem dental records. These discrepancies are explainable, however, still can provide an opportunity for a positive identification.
2. **Reconstructive postmortem dental printing:** The circumstantial evidence required to establish a putative identification is not always present. To determine who the deceased person may have been, it is often necessary to assess personal features such as age at death, sex, and other associated findings.
3. **Deoxyribonucleic acid profiling of oral tissues:** Used when dental treatments or other traits from dental records are not available for comparison. The DNA is the same in all the cells of the body and it does not change from birth to death and hence can be used to discriminate one individual from another. Forensic DNA profiling methods uses the PCR techniques to amplify small amounts of recovered DNA. The dental DNA comes from two potential sites:
   - The pulp tissue including fibroblasts, odontoblasts, and blood cells.
   - Developmental cells that are trapped during mineralization of the tooth can be liberated from the predentin and dentin layers to provide additional sources of DNA evidence.
4. **DVI analysis using dental evidence:**
   - Forensic odontology plays a key role in mass disaster victim identification (DVI) when good-quality ante-mortem (AM) dental records are available. Dental identification plays an important role when identification of remains of deceased person is skeletonized, decomposed, burned or dismembered and is invalid by visual or fingerprint methods. The identification of remains by dental evidence is possible because, the hard tissues are preserved after death and can even withstand a temperature of 1600 degree C when heated without appreciable loss of microstructure, and the status of a person's teeth change throughout the life and the combination of decay, missing, filling can be obtained from any fixed time.
   - In times of natural calamities such as earthquakes, fires, accidents, floods victim identification can be done with the help of dental records. DVI identification teams have identified large number of Victims of Indian Ocean Tsunami (2004), Bali Bombings (2002) and Christ church Earth Quake (2011) using dental evidence. It depends on adequate dental remains surviving the disaster and on the availability of dental records to be successful.
   - Most pediatric dentists nowadays use digital records for their pediatric patients therefore they can be of immense help in identification of any particular child in mass disaster, transport tragedy or criminal activity where children are being are not identifiable by physical remains. During a mass disaster number of victims who are burnt decomposed for mutilated can be identified and thereby claimed by their families the identification rates with the dental records are highly accurate.

   According to American board of forensic odontology dental identification can be divided into four types:
   i. *Positive identification:* The ante-mortem and post-mortem data match to establish that it is from same individual.
   ii. *Possible identification:* The ante-mortem and post-mortem data have few consistent features, but because of quality of the records it is difficulty to establish the identity.
   iii. *Insufficient evidence:* The data is not enough to from the conclusion.
   iv. *Exclusion:* The ante-mortem and post-mortem data clearly inconsistent.
5. **Accidental and non-accidental oral trauma:** Pediatric dentist play an important role in children who have sustained accidental or non-accidental trauma involving the orofacial structures via accidents, negligence, parents sign of neglect child abuse or malpractice. The patients radiographs and photographs can help the pediatric dentist to reach a correct diagnosis and treatment plan and can also be of benefit in the court of law.
6. **Dental and medical fraud**: Dental and medical fraud is a common place for litigation today. Due to the right to information dentists are required to examine patients

carefully and their records should be maintained in terms of radiographs and photographs so he /she can defend himself or herself when needed. Also all record should be maintained treatment and the mode of payments.

7. **Forensic age estimation:** Forensic age estimation is a scientific process that estimates an individual's true chronologic age by assessing skeletal and dental development and maturation. Dental maturity has an essential role in children's and adolescents' age estimations.
   - Age estimation plays an essential role in the identification process of victims of natural disasters and airplane accidents.
   - To identify an individual who has been subjected to a crime how to identify the criminal whose body is in stages of decomposition age determination is vital since teeth are the only tissue in the body which can sustain the highest temperature and also other decomposition changes.
   - Sex determination is very important subdivision of forensic odontology, which plays a major role in identification of the unknown individuals in natural disasters; chemical and bomb explosion scenarios.
8. **Bite mark identification:** Bite mark injuries are not often unintentional and indicates genuine child abuse. In most cases, the person inflicting the bite mark is the person responsible for abusing the child. Bite marks in children represent child abuse until proven differently. Bite marks are identified by their shape and size. They have a key role in identifying child abuse cases as bite marks are unique to each person therefore they cannot be forged, they can help to bring the accused to justice. This is dealt in detail in the next section.
9. **Lip print identification:** Cheiloscopy is a forensic investigation that deals with identification of human based on lip traces. Lip print wrinkle pattern has individual characteristics same as finger prints. The wrinkles and grooves on the labial mucosa form a characteristic pattern called lip prints. The presence or absence of a person from the crime can be verified based on lip prints since the lip prints being uniform throughout the life. The role of lip prints is a marker of evidence in identification of victims and suspects and no two individuals have same pattern of skin on the lips. It is a highly specialised field that can be used in forensic odontology for identification victims in crimes.

DENTAL IDENTIFICATION

Role of Radiographs and Photographs

- No matter how thorough the visual investigation of any forensic dental evidence is, it is of little or no value unless it is recorded permanently and accurately.
- Radiographs and photographs are necessary for proper evaluation, detailed comparison at a later date, and subsequent preparation of evidence.
- An accurate and reliable source for identification is a comparison of antemortem and postmortem radiographs.
- Photographs, if properly taken, are one of the most reliable and useful tools in forensic dentistry. These must be clear to show the precise size and shape measurements of the area of concern.

Role of Craniofacial Characteristics

- A proper knowledge of time of eruption and root completion of all deciduous and permanent teeth is important to determine the age of the deceased from the teeth present.
- Knowledge of time of suture closure of the skull is also an important parameter to determine the age.

Role of Blood Group Determination

- The use of saliva in forensic science is based on the presence of ABH blood group substances, which is in fairly high concentrations in saliva and bones of secretors.
- This finding is used in identification with the absorption-elution technique.

Computer-assisted Dental Identification

- The computerized identification system for comparison process of postmortem and antemortem records is called as computer-assisted postmortem identification (CAPMI) system.
- Computer can be used to process large numbers of dental records, such as would be encountered in mass fatality incidents or in the creation of central rewards repository for missing person investigations.

Role of Dental Team in Mass Fatality Incidents

- The very nature of a mass disaster implies the presence of an enormously destructive force, but it is surprising that only the most durable structure of the human body, i.e., the teeth, remains intact.
- Since dental evidence may be the principal method of resolving vital questions of identification, progressive agencies responsible for investigating disasters now recognize the forensic dentist as a key member of the investigating team. The dental identification team can be divided into several different sections based on its mission including recovery, postmortem examination, antemortem records, and comparison.

BITE MARKS

One of the most intriguing, complex, and sometimes controversial challenges in forensic dentistry is the recognition, recovery, and analysis of bite marks. These can be defined as marks caused by teeth alone or in combination with other oral parts. These can be on the skin or on inanimate objects like foods, cigarette, etc. and can also be differentiated as human or animal bite marks. The term "bite mark" is used in reference to human bite marks only and more specifically in relation to bite marks found on skin. **Sorup**, 1924 was the first to publish an analysis of bite marks. The markings found on the skin of the victim are more than just bite marks. The musculature of the lips, tongue, cheeks, and the mental state of the biter, each seen to play a role in infliction of tooth mark pattern on the skin and this is identified as a bite mark.

Bite marks in children represent child abuse until proven differently. The majority of child abuse patients are brought, to hospital emergency rooms, pediatric clinics, or emergency centers with a history of accidental trauma supplied by the parents or adult guardian. They are rarely accidental and are good indicators of genuine child abuse.

Classification of bite marks		
According to causative agent		
Human	***Animals***	***Mechanical***
• Children • Adults	• Mammals • Reptiles • Fish	• Full denture • Saw blade tooth marks • Electric cords, belt marks
According to the material bitten		
Skin	***Perishable items***	***Nonperishable items***
• Human • Animal	• Food items like cheese, apple, etc.	• Unanimated objects like pipes, pens, pencils, etc.
According to the degree of biting		
Definite marks	***Amorous marks***	***Aggressive marks***
Tissue damage due to direct application of pressure by the biting edge	These are made in amorous circumstances, slowly with the absence of movement between teeth and tissue	These show evidence of scraping tearing or avulsion of tissues and may be difficult to interpret

Factors Influencing Appearance of Bite Marks

- **Vascularity of the tissue:** Bruising of the loose and highly vascularized tissues around the eyes is more pronounced than skin in areas such as the palm of the hand or the soles of the feet.
- **Age:** Children and the elderly bruise more easily because of loose delicate skin.
- **Metabolic rate:** Women bruise more easily than men.
- **Medications:** Such as aspirin can increase bleeding.
- **Normal skin color:** The pigmentations on stain may affect the observation of a bruise.
- Mass and velocity of the impact.
- **Time of injury:** The time of appearance of bruise is related to the time required for the extravasated blood to reach the surface. This lag will allow the antemortem bruises to appear postmortem.
- **Other factors that affect bruising:** Rapidity of death after injury and environmental conditions.

Bite Mechanisms

- **Tooth pressure:** It is caused by direct application of incisal edges of anterior teeth or occlusal surfaces of posterior teeth. Most commonly seen in battered child syndrome.
- **Tongue pressure:** It is caused when the material is taken into mouth and pressed by tongue against teeth or palatal surface. They exhibit a central ecchymotic or "suck" mark with radiating pattern surrounding a central area. Most commonly seen in sexually abused cases.
- **Tooth scrape:** By scraping of teeth across the surfaces of skin.

Identification of Bite Marks

- Bite marks are found in a significant number of child abuse victims. Most reported cases are the result of attack bites and are recognized and documented only when the victim is examined by a medical examiner. In this environment, the bite mark is recognized early, a forensic odontologist is called as a consultant, and the evidence is preserved for future prosecution.
- The nature and location of the bite is likely to change with increasing age of the child. Bite marks in infants occur in body locations and under circumstances different from these of the preschooler, school age child, or adolescent. In infants, bite marks tend to be punitive and are often a response to crying or soiling. As a result, bite marks may appear anywhere, but tend to be concentrated on the cheek, arm, shoulder, buttocks, or genitalia. In childhood-bite marks tend to be less punitive and more a function of assault or defense. Sexually-oriented bite marks occur more frequently in adolescents and adults.

American Society of Forensic Odontology Protocol for Bite Mark Analysis, 1993

- *Description of the bite mark*
- *Collection of evidence from victim:*
  - Photography
  - Saliva swab
  - Impression
  - Tissue samples
- *Collection of evidence from the suspect:*
  - Dental records
  - Photography
  - Clinical examination
  - Impression
- *Comparing the bite marks.*

- Bite marks resulting from sexual attack may be present on the victim or assailant. The marks on assailant usually are caused by the anterior teeth of victim biting in self-defense. These bites are found frequently on the hand of the assailant and may be severe, resulting in laceration or avulsion of tissue. The most common bite marks are caused by the assailant which feature bites on either neck, cheek, arms, thighs, or nipples. Such marks are well-defined and show area of contusion of dental arch, which is a result of sucking which brings the tissue in apposition to palate.
- Human bite marks characteristics include an elliptical or ovoid pattern containing tooth and arch marks. Tooth mark is the bite mark produced by antagonist teeth. Arch mark is when four to five adjacent marks of teeth are present. The duration of bite mark is dependent upon force applied and the extent of tissue damage. Thin bite marks will remain for longer time. Tooth marks that do not break skin last from 7 h to 24 h, whereas if skin is broken it may last for several days depending upon thickness of tissue.

Characteristics of Human Bite Marks for Identification

- A human bite mark is usually of elliptical or ovoid pattern.
- Simplest form of bite mark consists of tooth marks produced by antagonist teeth.

- An arch mark may indicate presence of four to five teeth marks reflecting the shape of their incisal or occlusal surfaces.
- The puncture marks of incisors are narrow rectangular in shape.
- Canines leave triangular-shaped lesions, which tend to be more defined in adult than child bites.
- Premolars leave ovoid marks.
- Bite marks left by maxillary teeth tend to be more diffuse, while those left by mandibular teeth are more distinct.
- It is important to distinguish human bite from animal bite marks. Animal bite marks can be distinguished from human bites on the basis of arch width (animals tend to have longer, narrower bites), the width of individual teeth (animals have narrower teeth), and type of bite (animal bites usually result in deep tissue penetration with accompanying tearing and lacerations, whereas human bite marks tend to leave more superficial lesions, like bruising or abrasions).
- **Class characteristics:** These are commonly referred to as the measurable features and shapes that allow the forensic dentist to ascertain the biter and to determine which teeth are present in the pattern.
- **Individual characteristics:** These are deviations from standard class characteristics. For example, rotated tooth or a fractured tooth.

Analysis of Bite Marks

- The first method of analysis of bite marks was reported in 1968 by **Furness**.
- To maintain uniformity in the bite mark applications and to standardize the analysis of bite marks the American Board of Forensic Odontology (ABFO) established the following guidelines in 1986.

Guidelines for Bite Marks Analysis

- **History:** Obtain a thorough history of any dental treatment carried out after the suspected date of the bite mark.
- **Photography:** Extraoral photographs including full face and profile views, intraorals should include frontal views, two lateral views, and an occlusal view of each arch. Often it is useful to include a photograph of maximal mouth opening. If inaniate materials, such as food stuffs, are used for test bites the results should be preserved photographically.
- **Extraoral examination:** Record and observe soft and hard tissue factors that may influence biting dynamics.
- Measurements of maximal opening and any deviations on opening or closing should be made.
- **Intraoral examination:** Salivary swabs should be taken. The tongue should be examined to assess size and function. The periodontal status should be noted with particular reference to mobility. Prepare a dental chart if possible.
- **Impressions:** Take two impressions of each arch using material that meet the American Dental Association specifications. The occlusal relationship should be recorded.
- **Sample bites:** Whenever possible, sample bites should be made into an appropriate material, simulating the type of bite under study.
- **Study casts:** Casts should be prepared using type II stone.

Procedure for Bite Mark Analysis

It is the comparison of bite evidence to the suspect evidence to determine if a correlation exists. Analysis involves visualization, comparison, formation of the opinion, and often court testimony.

- **Description of bite marks:**
  - Demographic description
  - Anatomic location including surface, contour, color, size, and shape.
- **Collection of evidence from victim:**
  - Photography is essential to document bite marks and it should be initiated early and sequentially.
  - The photographs should be in color and black and white with and without scale.
  - Stains for elastic and collagen fibers and standard hematoxylin and eosin stain are useful.
  - Using absorption elution techniques and electrophoresis, a serological "fingerprint" can be developed to help individualize the assailant.
  - The suspect bite mark, after being photographed is swabbed with cotton moistened in saline, bottled, labeled, and refrigerated for processing by a forensic serologist.
- **Collection of evidence from suspect:**
  - Only after the legal consent has been obtained.
  - Includes photographs, casts, and saliva samples.
- **Analysis of all evidence:**
  - If adequate photographs have been obtained then the bite marks can be digitalized and viewed three-dimensionally.
  - The same is true with any impressions that might be relative to the case. These tool marks can be compared in detail.
  - The addition of computer manipulation to tool mark identification has added greatly to the possibilities of bite mark analysis.
  - Recent advances for collecting and analyzing evidence are xeroradiography, transillumination, videotape analysis, superimposition technique, scanning microscopy, and deoxyribonucleic acid (DNA) fingerprinting.

RECENT ADVANCEMENTS

- A recent advancement in documenting the bite mark records is the epiluminescence microscopy. It is a dermatological technique developed for evaluation of pigmented skin lesions. This technique, through rendering the stratum corneum translucent, aids is the visualization and photographic documentation.
- The recently developed imaging software CAPMI and WinID and other image capturing devices, such as scanners and digital cameras have further created an opportunity to better control the human errors.

- Use of ABFO scale number 2 and alternate light imaging (ALI) helps in reducing the errors of bite mark analysis. ABFO scale number 2 helps us get 1:1 life like size of the photograph, 18% gray color, and three circles help to rule out photographic distortion. With the help of ALI photography the marks, which are not visible, fluoresce, and become distinct. Fibers which are not easily located under normal light can become like beacons as they fluoresce under alternate light.
- Forensic DNA profiling methods uses the polymerase chain reaction (PCR) techniques to amplify small amounts of recovered DNA.

Above all, the forensic dentist must be knowledgeable and appreciate the constraints that may be imposed by the judicial process. Attention to dental, conscientious application of knowledge to the problem at hand, and most importantly, good common sense would appear to be the most important attributes of those, who by intent or by obligation to society enter this challenging field.

POINTS TO REMEMBER

- Bite marks can be defined as marks caused by teeth alone or in combination with other oral parts.
- Sorup, 1924 was the first to publish an analysis of bite marks.
- The first method of analysis of bite marks was reported in 1968 by Furness.
- Factors influencing appearance of bite marks are vascularity of the tissue, age, metabolic rate, skin color, time of injury, and type of impact.
- Characteristics of human bite: A human bitemark is usually of elliptical or ovoid pattern; consists of tooth marks produced by antagonist teeth; arch mark may indicate the shape of their incisal or occlusal surfaces.
- The puncture marks of incisors are narrow rectangular in shape, canines leave triangular-shaped lesions, and premolars leave ovoid marks.
- Bite marks left by maxillary teeth tend to be more diffuse, while those left by mandibular teeth are more distinct.
- Procedure for bite mark analysis involves visualization, description of bite marks, collection of evidence from victim and suspect, comparison and analysis of evidence, formation of the opinion, and often court testimony.
- Role of dentist in forensic is comparative dental identification, reconstructive postmortem dental printing, and DNA profiling of oral tissues.
- Dr Oscar Amoedo is called as father of Forensic Odontology. He wrote first dissertation entitled "L'Art Dentaire en Legale" in 1898.
- Keiser Neilson defined forensic dentistry as" that branch of forensic dentistry that in the interest of justice deals with the proper handling and examination of dental evidence and the proper evaluation and presentation of dental findings".

Questionnaire

1. Define and classify bite marks.
2. What are the factors influencing bite marks?
3. Write a note on human bite marks.
4. Describe the analysis of bite marks and guidelines.
5. What is the role of the dentist in forensic?
6. Explain dental identification.
7. What do you understand by forensic odontology according to Federation Dentaire International?
8. Define and classify the branch of forensic odontology.
9. Classify forensic odontology dental identification according to American Board.
10. Write a short note on recent advancements in documenting the bite mark records.

FURTHER READING

1. Aboshi H, Taylor JA, Takei T, et al. Comparison of bitemarks in foodstuffs by computer imaging: a case report. J Forensic Odontostomatol. 1994; 12:41-4.
2. Alastair J Sloan. Forensic Odontology: An Essential Guide. First Edition. John Wiley & Sons, Ltd; Development of the dentition.
3. American Board of Forensic Odontology, Inc. ABFO bite mark analysis guidelines. In: Bowers CM, Bell GL (Eds). Manual of Forensic Odontology, 3rd edition. Saratoga: American Society of Forensic Odontology; 1997. pp. 299-357.
4. Barbenel JC, Evans JH. Bite marks in skin–mechanical factors. J Soc For Sci. 1974; 14:235-8.
5. Catherine Adams. Forensic Odontology: An Essential Guide. First Edition. John Wiley & Sons, Ltd; 2014.Disaster victim identification.
6. Dongre PJ, Patil RU, Patil SS. Applications of forensic odontology in pediatric dentistry: A brief communication. J Dent Allied Sci. 2017; 6:17-21.
7. Furness J. Teeth marks and their significance in cases of homicide. J Soc For Sci. 1969; 9:169.
8. Guidelines for bite mark analysis. American Board of Forensic Odontology, Inc. J Am Dent Assoc. 1986;112:383-6.
9. Levine LJ. Bitemark evidence. Dent Clin North Am. 1977; 21:1- 58.
10. Limdiwala P, Shah J. Age estimation by using dental radiographs. Journal of Forensic Dental Sciences. 2013; 5(2):118-21.
11. Pooja Malik Puri, et al. DVI through dental evidence in Indian scenario. Forensic Sci Sem. 2015;5:39-42.
12. Rai B, Kaur J. Evidence-Based Forensic Dentistry. Springer-Verlag Berlin Heidelberg; 2013. DNA technology and Forensic Odontology.
13. Shah P, .Velani P, Lakade L, Dukle S. Teeth in forensics: a review. Indian Journal of Dental Research. 2019;30: 2291-299.
14. Shashikala K. Human bitemarks: The fingerprints of the mouth. JIAOMR. 2003; 15:165-71.
15. Sorup A. Odontoskopie. Ein Zahnirzhlicher Beitrag Zur gerichtillichen. Medicine. 1924; 40:385.
16. Sydney Levine. Forensic odontology-identification by dental means. Australian Dental Journal. 1977;22(6):481-487.
17. Uma Maheshwari TN, Krishnan M. Forensic pediatric dentistry. Int J Forensic Odontol. 2020;5:1-2.
18. Wagner GN, Bitemark identification in child abuse cases, Pediatric Dentistry. 1986;8 Special Issue 1,96-100
19. Wagner GN. Bitemark identification in child abuse cases. Pediatr Dent. 1986; 8:96-100.
20. Wald M. Child abuse in Wisconsin. The dentist's responsibility in reporting. Great Milwaukee Dent Bull. 1968; 34:113-6.
21. Wright FD, Golden GS. Forensic Photography. In: Stimson PG, Mertz CA (Eds). Forensic Dentistry, 1st edition. USA: Stern Robert; 1997. pp. 101-36.

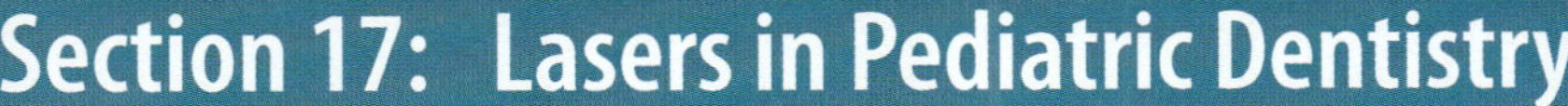

CHAPTER 78

Lasers in Pediatric Dentistry: Principle, Tissue Interactions and Types of Laser

Chandrashekar Yavagal, Sham S Bhat

Chapter Outline

- Basic Laser Science
- Principle of Laser Radiation
- Laser Delivery Systems
- Components of Laser
- Laser Tissue Interaction
- Photobiological Effects of Laser
- Photobiomodulation and Photodynamic Therapy
- Types of Lasers

The instant images that leap to one's mind at the mention of the word "Laser" are of star wars and light sabers. The word has a connotation of power almost akin to magic. The term laser is an acronym that stands for Light Amplification by Stimulated Emission of Radiation. A laser is not a device; it is a phenomenon that has been applied for specific uses in a wide variety of fields. Lasers are light sources composed of specific wavelengths that allow them to be focused into powerful beams, powerful enough that NASA used them to measure the distance between the Earth and the Moon. In medicine, laser therapy allows medical professionals to work on specific tissues with higher precision and less or no pain, scarring, or swelling for the patient.

Historical review

- ***Goldman, Stem*** and ***Segnnaes*** carried out the original research in the 1960s.
- **Vahl** used a ruby laser and reported extensive deep destruction of carious areas along with crater formation and melting of dentin.
- ***Kantola*** experimented with a CO_2 laser.
- ***Paghdiwala*** (1988) in the united States tested for the first time the ability of the erbium: Yttrium-aluminum-garnet (Er: YAG) laser to ablate dental hard tissues.
- In May 1997, the Er: YAG (2.94 um) laser was cleared for marketing by the US Food and Drug Administration (FDA).

BASIC LASER SCIENCE

Light

Light is a form of electromagnetic energy that exists as a particle, and travels in waves, at a constant velocity. Laser light is distinguished from ordinary light by two properties.

Laser light is monochromatic (it only generates a laser beam of a single collar), collimated and coherent in nature **(Fig. 78.1)**.

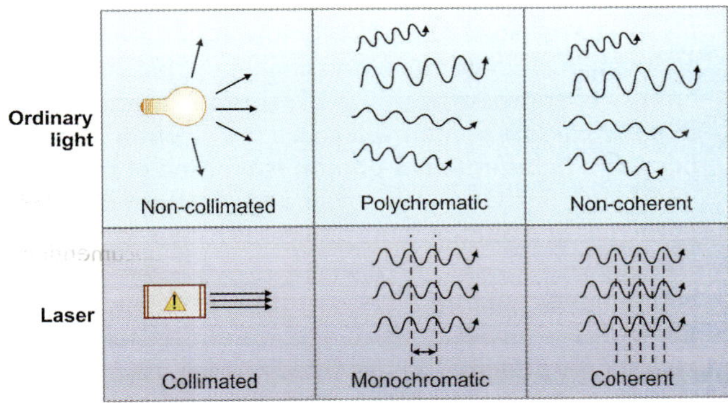

Fig. 78.1: Features of ordinary and laser light.

Spontaneous Emission

- The principle of spontaneous emission—when an atom or molecule absorbs energy, electrons or molecules move into higher orbits and fall back almost immediately into lower orbits letting out a spark of surplus energy-the "photon"—which is the basic unit of light.
- The photon emitted is in a random direction and a random phase.

Stimulated Emission

- The principle of stimulated emission is if an electron is in a high energy state (E2), and its decay path is to a

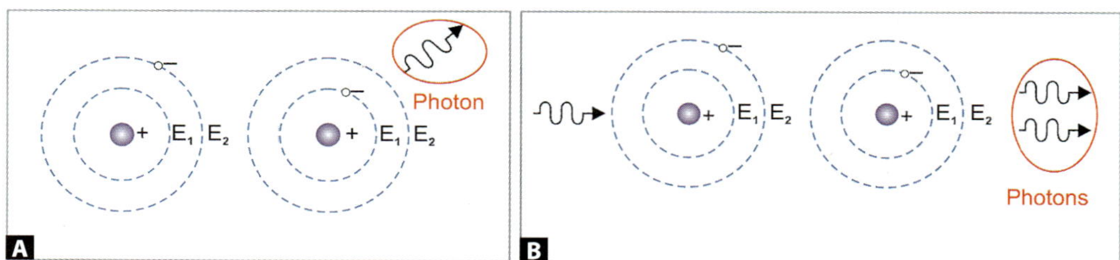

Figs. 78.2A and B: Schematic representation of spontaneous and stimulated emission.

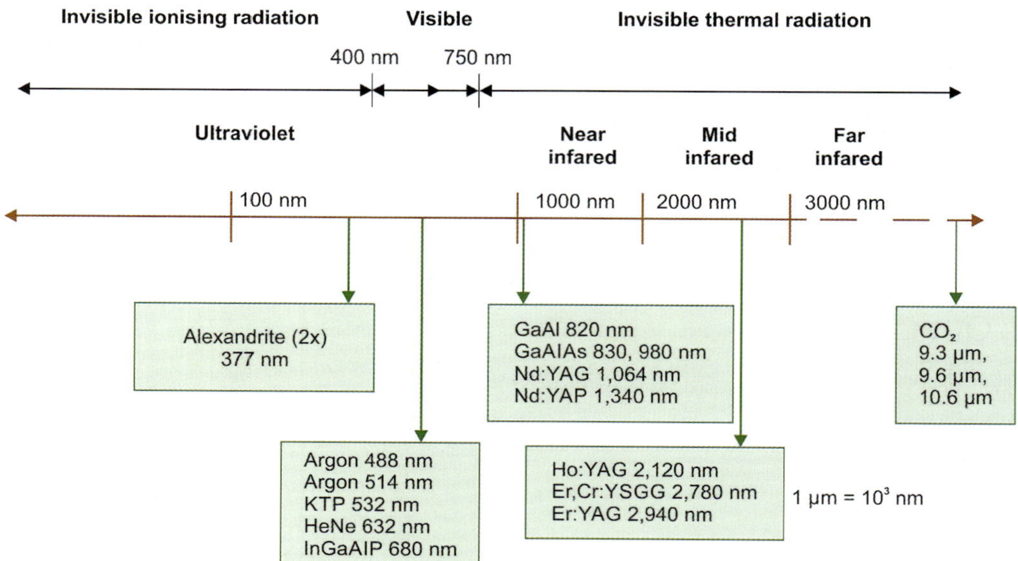

Fig. 78.3: Location of laser on the electromagnetic spectrum.

lower energy state (E1), but, before it has a chance to spontaneously decay, a photon happens to pass by whose energy is approximately E2-E1, there is a probability that the passing photon will cause the electron to decay in such a manner that a photon is emitted at the same wavelength, in the same direction, and with the same phase as the passing photon. This process is called "stimulated emission."

- Spontaneous emission is a quantum-mechanical effect and a direct physical manifestation of the Heisenberg uncertainty principle. The emitted photon has a random direction, but its wavelength matches the absorption wavelength of the transition. This is the mechanism of fluorescence and thermal emission. **(Figs. 78.2A and B).**

Radiation

The light waves produced by the laser are a specific form of radiation or electromagnetic energy. The electromagnetic spectrum is the entire collection of wave energy ranging from gamma rays, whose wavelength is about 10–12 m, to radio waves, whose wavelength can be thousands of meters. All available dental laser devices have emission wavelengths of approximately 0.5 µ or 500 nm to 10.6 µ or 10,600 nm. That places them in either the visible or the invisible portion nonionizing portion of the electromagnetic spectrum **(Fig. 78.3)**.

PRINCIPLE OF LASER RADIATION

The process of lasing occurs when an excited atom can be stimulated to emit a photon before the process occurs spontaneously. When a photon of exactly the right energy (wavelength) enters the electromagnetic field of an excited atom, the incident photon triggers the decay of the excited electron to the lower energy state. This is accompanied by the release of the stored energy in the form of a second photon. The first photon is not absorbed but continues to encounter another excited atom. Stimulated emission can only occur when the incident photon has the same energy as the released photon. Thus, the result of stimulated emission is two photons of identical wavelength traveling in the same direction. The release of the second photon is time linked to the oscillations of the first photon, so that the 2 photons oscillate together in the phase of a collection of atoms including more that are pumped up into the excited state that remains in the resting state, a population inversion exists. This is a necessary condition for lasing. Now, the spontaneous emission of a photon by one atom will stimulate the release of a second photon in a second atom, and these two photons will trigger the release of two more photons, these 4 photons then yield 8, 8 photons yield 16, and so on. In a small space at the speed of light, this photon chain reaction produces a brief, intense flash of monochromatic (same wavelength) and coherent (same phase) light **(Fig. 78.4)**.

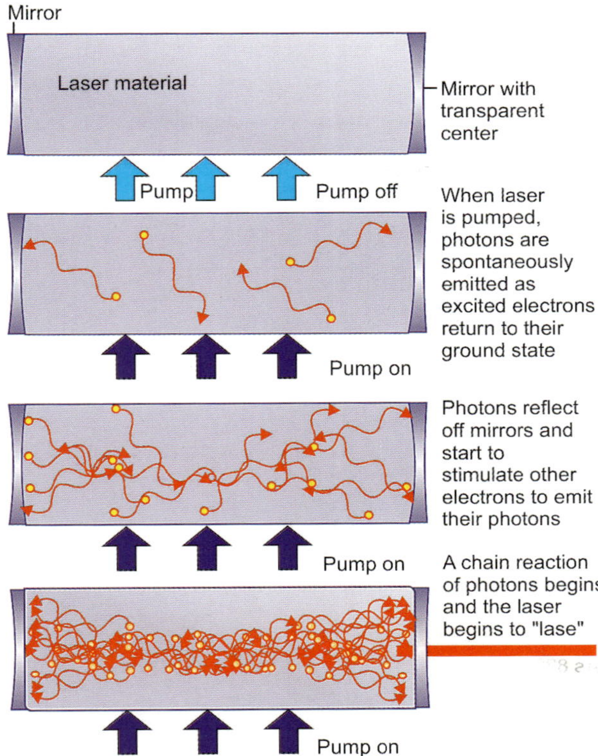

Mirror
Laser material
Mirror with transparent center
Pump
Pump off
When laser is pumped, photons are spontaneously emitted as excited electrons return to their ground state
Pump on
Photons reflect off mirrors and start to stimulate other electrons to emit their photons
Pump on
A chain reaction of photons begins and the laser begins to "lase"
Pump on

Fig. 78.4: Principle of laser radiation.

Photon of exact energy (wavelength) enters the electromagnetic field of an excited atom

↓

The incident photon triggers the decay of the excited electron to the lower energy state

↓

This is accompanied by the release of the stored energy in the form of a second photon

↓

The first photon is not absorbed but continues on to encounter another excited atom

↓

Stimulated emission can only occur when the incident photon has exactly the same energy as released photon. Thus, the result of stimulated emission is two photons of identical wavelength traveling in the same direction

↓

The release of the second photon is time linked to the oscillations of the first photon, so that the two photons oscillate together in phase of a collection of atoms. Hence, more photons are pumped up into the excited state, thereby causing a population inversion. This is a necessary condition for lasing

↓

Now, the spontaneous emission of a photon by one atom will stimulate the release of a second photon in a second atom, and these two photons will trigger the release of two more photons, these 4 then yield 8, 8 yield 16 and so on

↓

In a small space at the speed of light this photon chain reaction produces a brief, intense flash of monochromatic (one specific color/same wavelength), collimated (beam having specific spatial boundaries) and coherent (have identical amplitude and identical frequency) light

COMPONENTS OF LASER

There are three main parts of a laser delivery system **(Fig. 78.5)**:

- Lasing or active medium
- Energy or pumping source
- The optical or resonating chamber

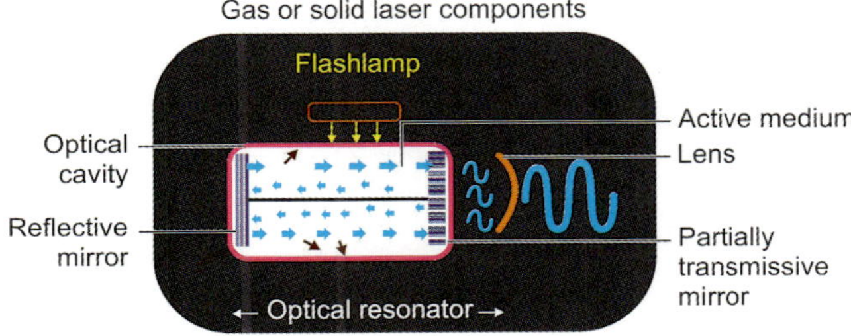

Gas or solid laser components
Flashlamp
Optical cavity
Reflective mirror
Active medium
Lens
Partially transmissive mirror
← Optical resonator →

Fig. 78.5: Components of laser system (Nd:YAG).

Lasing or Active Medium

A lasing medium is a material, which is capable of absorbing the energy, produced by an external source through the subatomic configuration of its component molecules and subsequently giving off this excess energy as photons of light. Lasing media can be solid (crystal or semiconductor), liquid or gas.

Energy or Pumping Source

An energy source is used to excite or pump the atoms in the lasing medium to their higher energy levels that are necessary for the production of laser radiation. The pumping source can be electrical, chemical, thermal, or optical energy.

Optical or Resonating Chamber

The lasing medium is located within resonating chamber, which has a cylindrical structure with a fully reflecting mirror on one side, and a partially reflecting mirror on another. They are precisely mounted so that they are exactly parallel to one another. This arrangement allows for the reflection of photons of light back and forth across the chamber, eventually resulting in the production of an intense photo resonance within the medium.

LASER EMISSION MODES

Dental laser devices can emit light energy in two modalities as a function of time constant or pulsed on and off. The pulsed lasers can be further divided into gated and free-running modes for delivering energy to the target tissue. Thus three different emission modes are described, as follows:

- **Continuous-wave mode,** in which the beam is emitted at only one power level for as long as the operator depresses the foot switch.
- **Gated-pulse mode** is characterized by periodic alternations of the laser energy, similar to a blinking light. This mode is achieved by the opening and closing of a mechanical shutter in front of the beam path of a continuous-wave emission.
- **Free-running pulsed mode** is sometimes referred to as *true pulsed* mode. This emission is unique in that large

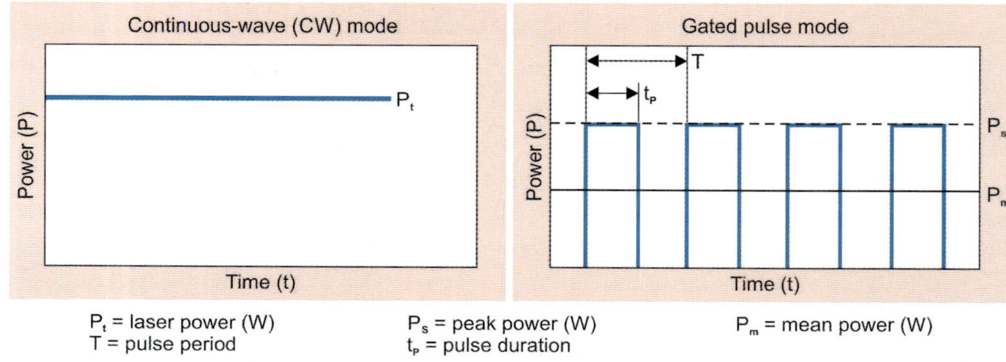

Fig. 78.6: Laser emission modes.

peak energy of laser light is emitted usually for microseconds, followed by a relatively long time in which the laser is off **(Fig. 78.6).**

LASER DELIVERY SYSTEMS

The coherent, collimated beam of laser light must be able to be delivered to the target tissue in a manner that is ergonomic and precise. Two delivery systems are used in dental lasers.

Flexible Hollow Waveguide

- Flexible hollow waveguide or tube that has an interior mirror finish.
- The laser energy is reflected along this tube and exits through a handpiece at the surgical end, with the beam striking the tissue in a non-contact fashion (i.e., without directly touching the tissue).

Glass Fiberoptic Cable

- This cable is pliant and comes in various diameters, with sizes ranging from 200 to 1,000 m.
- Although the glass fiber is encased in a resilient sheath, it can be somewhat fragile and cannot be bent at a sharp angle. The fiber fits snugly into a handpiece with the bare end protruding or, in some cases, with an attached glass-like tip.
- This fiber system can be used in contact or non-contact mode; however, most of the time, it is used in a contact fashion, touching the surgical site directly.
- For lasers using the optic fiber, the focal point is at or near the tip of the fiber. When the handpiece is moved away from the tissue and away from the focal point, the beam is defocused (or out of focus) and becomes more divergent.
- At a small divergent distance, the beam can cover a wider area, which is useful in achieving hemostasis. At a greater distance away, the beam loses its effectiveness because the energy dissipates.

LASER TISSUE INTERACTION (RATS PRINCIPLE)

The light energy from a laser can have four different interactions with the target tissue, and these interactions depend on the optical properties of that tissue and the wavelength used **(Fig. 78.7)**.

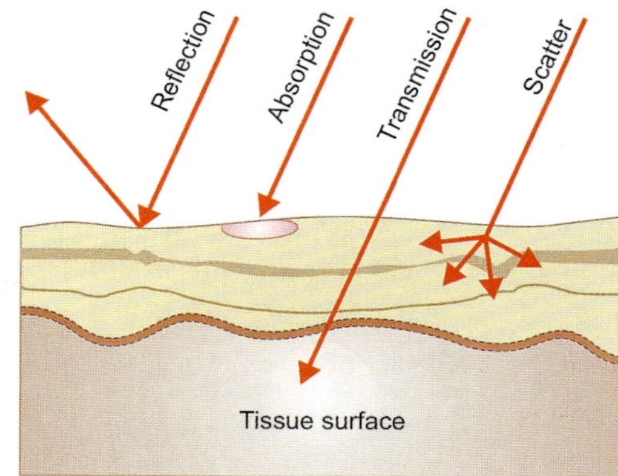

Fig. 78.7: Possible tissue interactions.

Reflection

- It is simply the beam redirecting itself off the tissue surface, having no effect on the target tissue. The reflected light could maintain its collimation in a narrow beam or become more diffuse.
- As stated previously, the laser beam generally becomes more divergent as the distance from the handpiece increases. The beam from some lasers can still have adequate energy at distances greater than 3 m.
- However, this reflection can be dangerous because the energy would be directed to an unintentional target, such as the eyes. This is a major safety concern for laser operation.

Absorption

- Absorption of the laser energy by the intended target tissue.
- This effect is the usual desirable effect, and the amount of energy that is absorbed by the tissue depends on the tissue characteristics, such as pigmentation and water content, and the laser wavelength and emission mode.
- Certain wavelengths are absorbed preferentially by certain tissue components and by water. In general, the shorter wavelengths, from about 500 nm to 1,000 nm, are absorbed readily in pigmented tissue.
- Argon has a high affinity for melanin and hemoglobin in soft tissue. Diode and Neodymium: Yttrium-aluminium-garnet (Nd:YAG) have a high affinity for melanin and less interaction with hemoglobin. The longer wavelengths are

more interactive with water and hydroxyapatite. Erbium is well-absorbed by hydroxyapatite and water. CO_2 is well-absorbed by water and has the greatest affinity for tooth structure.

Transmission

- Transmission of the laser energy directly through the tissue, with no effect on the target tissue.
- This interaction also is highly dependent on the wavelength of laser light. Water, for example, is relatively transparent to the Nd:YAG wavelength, whereas tissue fluids readily absorb CO_2 at the outer surface so that there is little energy transmitted to adjacent tissues. An Nd: YAG laser would work better in an environment difficult to keep dry, whereas a CO_2 laser would be less effective because of its absorption by saliva, water, and tissue fluids.

Scattering

- This weakens the energy and possibly produces no useful biologic effect.
- Scattering of the laser beam could cause heat transfer to the tissues adjacent to the surgical site, and unwanted thermal damage could occur. A beam deflected in different directions would be useful in facilitating the curing of composite resins.

Thermal Interaction of Tissue

The thermal effect of laser energy on tissue primarily revolves around the water content of tissue and the temperature rise of the tissue **(Fig. 78.8)**.

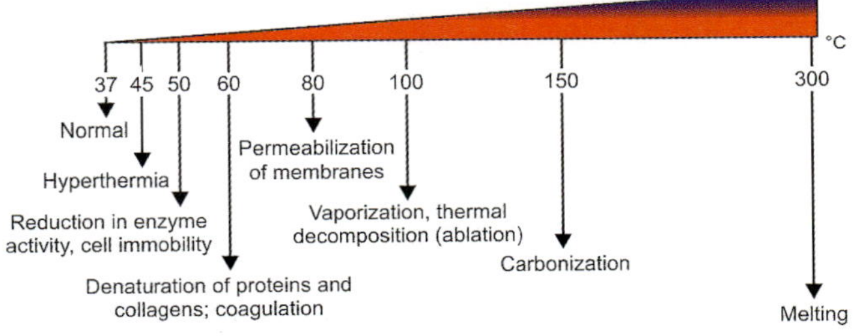

Fig. 78.8: Thermal interactions.

PHOTO-BIOLOGICAL EFFECTS OF LASER

When laser photonic energy is delivered and interacts with a tissue medium, three possible pathways exist to account for what arises from the delivered light energy:

Photo-thermal Effect

- The most common pathway when light is absorbed by living tissue is the internal conversion from incident photonic to thermal energy.
- With oral soft tissues and visible/near-IR laser wavelengths, the absorption by tissue chromophores gives rise to protein denaturation and secondary vaporization of interstitial water. Through this, a visible ablation and vaporization of target tissue occur.
- With longer mid- and far-IR laser wavelengths, the ablation of tissue is achieved through the near-instantaneous vaporization of interstitial water, leading to 'explosive' fragmentation of tissue structure.

Fluorescence

- Laser photonic energy values below target tissue ablation levels result in fluorescence. Fluorescence is a luminescence (re-emission) of light in which the absorption of a photon by a molecule triggers the emission of another photon with a longer wavelength from that molecule.
- This action provides the basis for optical scanning techniques employed for caries detection in enamel and dentine, and tomographic techniques utilized in scanning soft tissues for neoplastic change.

Photochemistry

- Photonic energy forms the first excited singlet state and this eventually undergoes intersystem crossing to the long-lived triplet state of the scavenger., The adjacent diatomic interstitial tissue oxygen (O_2) molecules undergo redox interconversions through energy transfer to form reactive oxygen species (ROS, such as superoxide anion) or singlet oxygen (O_2).
- Singlet oxygen is an ultra-short-lived product of the parent molecule that causes cell apoptosis through oxidative stress.

Photobiomodulation

- Photobiomodulation therapy is defined as a form of light therapy that utilizes non-ionizing light sources, including lasers, light-emitting diodes, and/or broadband light, in the visible (400–700 nm) and near-infrared (700–1100 nm) electromagnetic spectrum. It is a non-thermal process involving endogenous chromophores eliciting photo-physical (i.e., linear and nonlinear) and photochemical events at various biological scales. This process results in beneficial therapeutic outcomes including but not limited to the alleviation of pain, immunomodulation, and promotion of wound healing and tissue regeneration.
- It stimulates cytochrome C, increases the production of ATP (energy), NO, and ROS activity and restores cellular energy balance.

Photodynamic Therapy

Photodynamic therapy (PDT) can be defined as the administration of a nontoxic drug or dye known as a PS either systemically, locally, or topically to a patient bearing a lesion (frequently but not always cancer), followed after some time by the illumination of the lesion with visible light (usually long-wavelength red light), which, in the presence of oxygen, leads to the generation of cytotoxic species and consequently to cell death and tissue destruction.

- **Based on wavelength**
  - **Soft lasers or low-level lasers:** Provide cold thermal low-energy wavelengths of less than about 450 nm. These wavelengths are believed to stimulate circulation and cellular activity and cause various effects such as anti-inflammatory, vascular, muscle relaxation, analgesia, and tissue healing.
  - **Hard lasers:** Longer wavelength lasers produce the thermal effect, which cuts the tissue by coagulation, vaporization, and carbonization. These lasers have been used for surgical soft tissue application.
- **Based on active lasing medium**
  - Carbon dioxide laser
  - Argon laser
  - Nd:YAG
  - Potassium titanyl phosphate (KTP)
  - Helium-neon (He-Ne)
  - Ruby laser
  - Er:YAG laser
  - Erbium-chromium (Er-Cr): Yttrium-selenium-gallium-garnet (YSGG) laser.
- **Based on emission**
  - **Emit visible light:**
    - *Argon laser:* Blue wavelength of 488 nm.
    - *Argon laser:* Blue-green wavelength of 514 nm.
    - Nd:YAG
    - Potassium-titanyl-phosphate (KTP) lasers wavelength of 532 nm.
    - Red nonsurgical wavelengths of 635 nm.
  - **Emit invisible laser light in the near, middle, and far-infrared portion of the electromagnetic spectrum:**
    - Diode laser
    - Er-Cr:YSGG laser: 2,780 nm
    - Er:YAG laser: 2,940 nm
    - Carbon dioxide (CO_2) laser: 10,600 nm.

TYPES OF LASERS

Carbon Dioxide Laser

- In the United States, Stern at UCLA and Lobene the Forsyth Dental Center in Boston shifted their attention to the carbon dioxide laser because its wavelength of 10.6 um is well absorbed by enamel.
- In a series of studies employing scanning electron microscopy, X-ray diffraction, and electron probe microanalysis techniques, they determined the chemical and physical transformation that resulted from exposure of enamel and dentin by this wavelength **(Kantola 1972)**.
- While these studies confirmed the ability of the carbon dioxide laser to induce resistance to acid penetration of enamel, attempts to use this laser for the sealing of pits and fissures and the welding or fusion of materials such as hydroxyapatite to enamel were unsuccessful due to the excessively high surface temperatures generated during the process.
- During this same period, Melcer and others were actively involved in the clinical application of the carbon dioxide laser for the vaporization of caries. They reported the successful treatment of over 1,000 human patients in clinical trials of caries removal. The CO_2 laser is a gas-active medium laser that must be delivered through a hollow tube-like waveguide in continuous or gated-pulse mode. The wavelength of 10,600 nm, places it at the end of the mid-infrared invisible nonionizing portion of the spectrum. It is well-absorbed by water.
- It is a rapid soft tissue remover and has a shallow depth of penetration into tissue, which is essential when treating mucosal lesions. It is especially useful in cutting dense fibrous tissue. It has the highest absorption in hydroxyapatite of any dental laser, about 1,000 times greater than the erbium series of lasers.
- The CO_2 laser is delivered in a hollow waveguide with a handpiece. The laser energy is conducted through the waveguide and is focused onto the surgical site in a non-contact fashion. The loss of tactile sensation is a disadvantage for the surgeon, but the tissue ablation can be precise with careful technique. Large lesions can be treated easily using a simple back-and-forth motion.

Argon Laser

The argon laser is one of the rare gas ion lasers capable of outputs of several watts continuous till the visible green and blue portion of the spectrum.

- These systems have found applications in the excitation of tissue fluorescence, in making diagnostic measurements, and in materials processing, such as polymerization and stereolithography. The surgical argon laser is most useful for the treatment of vascular disorders due to the selective absorption of hemoglobin in the green portion of the spectrum.
- This laser has two emission wavelengths, and both are visible to the human eye: 488 nm, which is blue in color, and 514 nm, which is blue-green.
- Argon lasers have an active medium of argon gas that is fiber optically, delivered in continuous-wave and gated-pulse modes. Because of the short wavelength of green and blue light, it is possible to focus the argon beam on an extremely small spot.
- The 488 nm emission is exactly the wavelength needed to activate camphorquinone, the most commonly used photoinitiator that causes polymerization of the resin in light-cured composite restorative materials.
- The 514 nm wavelength has its peak absorption in red pigment. Tissues containing hemoglobin, hemosiderin, and melanin readily interact with this laser. It is a useful surgical laser with excellent hemostatic capabilities used in contact with the tissue, treatment of acute inflammatory periodontal disease, and highly vascularized lesions, such as a hemangioma.

Neodymium Laser

- The first report of the dental application of the neodymium laser to vital oral tissue in experimental animals was that by the Yamamoto School of Dentistry in Japan in 1974.
- In a series of experiments, Yamamoto determined that the Nd:YAG laser was effective for inhibiting the formation of incipient caries both *in vitro* and *in vivo*.
- Nd:YAG has a solid active medium, a crystal of yttrium-aluminum-garnet doped with neodymium, and is fiber

Lasers and their properties

Laser type	Wavelength	Waveform	Applications
Carbon dioxide	10.6 µm	Gated (or interrupted) or continuous	Soft-tissue incisions and ablation; de-epithelialization of gingiva during periodontal regenerative procedures
Neodymium: yttrium- aluminum-garnet	1.064 µm	Pulsed	Soft-tissue incision and ablation; incipient caries removal
Erbium: yttrium-aluminum- garnet	2.94 µm	Pulsed	Caries removal; cavity preparation in enamel and dentin; US food and drug administration clearance for use on cementum and bone; root canal preparation
Erbium-chromium: yttrium- selenium-gallium-garnet	2.78 µm	Pulsed	Enamel etching; caries removal; cavity preparation; cutting bone *in vitro* with no burning, melting or alteration of the calcium: phosphorus ratio; root canal preparation
Argon	457–502 nm	Pulsed or continuous	Curing resins; soft-tissue incisions and ablation; bleaching
Holmium: yttrium-aluminum- garnet	2.1 µm	Pulsed	Soft-tissue incisions and ablation
Gallium-arsenide (or diode)	904 nm	Pulsed or continuous	Soft-tissue incisions and ablation

optically delivered in a free-running pulsed mode, used most often in contact with the tissue. It was the first laser designed exclusively for dentistry, and it is the laser with the largest market share.

- The emission wavelength is 1,064 nm, in the near-infrared invisible nonionizing part of the spectrum. It is highly absorbed by pigmented tissue and is about 10,000 times more absorbed by water than an argon laser.

Potassium Titanyl Phosphate Laser

- The potassium titanyl phosphate laser is a frequency-doubled Nd: YAG laser, producing a 532 nm visible green beam by passing the Nd:YAG laser's output through a potassium-titanyl-phosphate crystal.
- It is absorbed by hemoglobin and melanin pigment. The tissue penetration is 1–3 mm.

Ruby Laser

- The first laser was developed by Maiman in 1960.
- A solid-state optically pumped laser that emits in the visible range.
- Taylor first reported the histologic effects of the ruby laser on the dental pulp.

Excimer Laser

An excimer is a molecule consisting of a halogen atom combined with an atom of a noble gas, existing only when the constituent atoms are in excited and ionized states. After this transient molecule exits radiation, it decomposes into its atomic parts, which are, then in their ground states. Because the excimer molecule has a lifetime measure in ns, and the excimers are 2-level energy systems, the XeCI laser can deliver 180 mJ of radiant energy in a 30-ns pulse.

Holmium: YAG Laser

- The lasing medium in this laser is a man-made, holmium-doped crystal rod of yttrium, aluminum, and garnet (Ho:YAG) and is fiber optically delivered in contact with the tissue in free-running pulsed mode.
- The wavelength produced by this laser is 2,120 nm, also in the infrared invisible nonionizing part of the spectrum. In conjunction with erbium and thulium, which enhance the efficiency of optical pumping of holmium.
- It emits radiation in the mid-infrared band of the electromagnetic spectrum; with a wavelength of 2.1 um. Its energy source that excites the crystal is a high-intensity flash lamp. This laser emits pulsed radiation of 250-µs duration. This wavelength can be transmitted through an optical fiber (quartz) and the radiation is delivered to the tissues in a non-contact free beam mode.

Erbium: YAG Laser and ER-CR:YAG Laser

- The lasing medium is an erbium-doped with a yttrium aluminum garnet.
- This material emits laser radiation at a 2,940 nm wavelength. It is a 4-level energy system but the lower laser level has a long lifetime, causing the erbium ions to accumulate in this lower level after emitting radiation. This accumulation interrupts the population inversion and limits the laser to pulsed operation.
- Er-Cr:YSGG (2,790 nm) has an active medium of a solid crystal of yttrium-scandium-gallium-garnet that is doped with erbium and chromium.
- Both of these lasers are delivered fiber optically in the free-running pulsed mode. The fibers are air-cooled and have a larger diameter than the other lasers mentioned, making the delivery system somewhat less flexible. At the end of the fiber, a handpiece and small-diameter glass tips concentrate the laser energy down to a convenient surgical size, approximately 0.5 m. These lasers are ideal for caries removal and tooth preparation when used with a water spray. The sound tooth structure can be preserved better when the carious material is being ablated; the increased water content of dental caries allows the laser to interact preferentially with that diseased tissue.
- The advantage of these lasers for restorative dentistry is that carious lesions close to the gingiva can be treated, and the soft tissue is re-contoured with the same instrumentation.

Diode Laser

- These have a solid active medium; it is a solid-state semiconductor laser that uses some combination of aluminum, gallium, and arsenide to change electric energy into light energy.
- The available wavelengths for dental use range from about 800 nm to 980 nm, placing them at the beginning of the near-infrared invisible nonionizing part of the spectrum.
- Each machine delivers laser energy fiber optically in continuous-wave and gated-pulse modes used ordinarily in contact with the tissue.
- These lasers are relatively poorly absorbed by tooth structure so that soft tissue surgery can be performed safely near the enamel, dentin, and cementum.
- The diode is an excellent soft tissue surgical laser indicated for cutting and coagulating gingiva and mucosa and for soft tissue curettage and sulcular debridement.
- The chief advantage of the diode lasers is the use of a smaller size instrument. The units are portable and compact, are easily moved with minimum setup time, and are the lowest-priced lasers currently available.

POINTS TO REMEMBER

- LASER is an acronym for Light Amplification by Stimulated Emission of Radiation. Bohr was the first to talk about the concept of lasers.
- In 1958, Schawlow and Townes discovered laser.
- First working laser, a pulsed ruby instrument, was built by Maiman.
- Laser light is monochromatic, coherent and collimated in nature.
- Delivery systems for lasers are flexible hollow waveguide and glass fiberoptic cable.
- Components of laser are laser medium, energy source and resonating chamber.
- Laser tissue interaction is reflection (it is simply the beam redirecting itself off the tissue surface, having no effect on the target tissue); absorption (by the intended target tissue); transmission (onto the target tissue without affecting the medium tissue) and scattering.
- Photo-biological effects of lasers comprises of photo thermal, fluorescence and photochemistry.
- Hard lasers have longer wavelength lasers producing thermal effect.
- Soft lasers provide cold thermal low energy wavelengths of less than about 450 nm.
- Carbon dioxide and Nd:YAG are used for soft tissue; Er:YAG for caries removal; argon for curing resins; diode can be used both for hard and soft tissues.
- The first report of the dental application of the neodymium laser to vital oral tissue in expermental animal was that by the Yamamoto School of Dentistry in Japan in 1974.

Questionnaire

1. Define laser and give the principle of laser radiation.
2. What are laser delivery systems?
3. Write a note on the components of the laser.
4. Explain laser-tissue interactions.
5. Describe photobiomodulation and photodynamic therapy.
6. Classify and compare lasers.

FURTHER READING

1. Boj JR, Poirier C, Hernandez M, et al. Review: laser soft tissue treatments for pediatric dental patients. Eur Arch Pediatr Dent. 2011;12(2):100-5.
2. Fried D, Radagio J, Akrivou M, et al. Dental hard tissue modification and removal using sealed transverse excited atmospheric-pressure lasers operating at 9.6 and 10.6 micrometer. J Biomed Optics. 2001;6:231-8.
3. Gutnecht N, Franzen R, Vanweersch L, et al. Lasers in Pediatric Dentistry --A Review. J Oral Laser Appl. 2005;4(5):207-18.
4. Hecht J. A short history of laser development. Appl Opt. 2010;49(25):F99-122.
5. Hibst R, Gall R. Development of a diode laser-based fluorescent caries detector. Caries Res. 1998;32:294.
6. Martens LC. Laser physics and a review of laser applications in dentistry for children. Eur Arch Pediatr Dent. 2011;12(2):61-7.
7. Martens LC. Laser-assisted Pediatric Dentistry: Review and Outlook. J Oral Laser Appl. 2003;3(4):203-9.
8. Parker S, Cronshaw M, Anagnostaki E, Mylona V, Lynch E, Grootveld M. Current Concepts of Laser-Oral Tissue Interaction. Dent J (Basel). 2020;8(3):61.
9. Sun G, Turnér J. Low-level laser therapy in dentistry. Dent Clin North Am. 2004;48(4):1061-76.
10. Walsh LJ. The current status of low-level laser therapy in dentistry. Part 1 Soft tissue application. Aust Dent J. 1997;42(4):247-54.

Contemporary Laser Application in Pediatric Dentistry and Recent Advances

Chandrashekar Yavagal, Sham S Bhat, Sundeep Hegde K

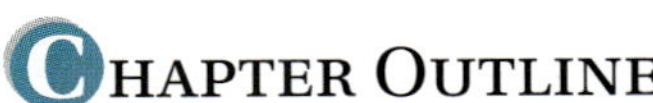

- Applications of Lasers in Pediatric Dentistry
- Lasers in Pediatric Endodontics
- Photobiomodulation Applications
- Lasers and their Application in Skin Lesions
- Pre-emptive Analgesia
- Reversal of Soft Tissue Anesthesia
- Advantages of Laser
- Disadvantages of Laser
- Laser Hazards

In medicine and surgery, laser energy has almost always been associated with its surgical usage. Medical professionals have always looked towards this technology as a means to work on specific tissues with higher precision and lower pain, scarring, and swelling for the patient. Dentistry is no exception to this rule. Since their inception, dental lasers have always been dabbled around as alternatives to the drill or the scalpel. Contrary to popular belief, Lasers and Light-based strategies can also be used at lower power settings to stimulate biological tissues rather than cutting them. This science of using low dose biophotonics for therapeutic applications is called **photobiomodulation.** It has many exciting applications from hair follicle stimulation to Alzheimer's and Parkinsonism. The influence of lower power laser irradiation on any organism has several clinical and biological effects including anti-inflammatory, immunostimulatory, neurotrophic, analgesic, desensitizing, bactericidal, antiedemic, and normalizing the blood rheology and hemodynamics effects as well.

APPLICATIONS OF LASERS IN PEDIATRIC DENTISTRY

- **Hard tissue applications**
  - Diagnosis of dental caries
  - Prevention of enamel and dental caries.
  - Caries removal
  - Cavity preparation
  - Pit and fissure sealants.
  - Bleaching
  - Curing light-activated resins.
- **Soft tissue surgical applications**
  - Tethered oral tissue surgery
  - Treatment of pericoronal problems in erupting teeth
  - Tooth exposure for orthodontic treatment
  - Lesion removal and biopsy
- **Lasers in pediatric endodontics**
  - Pulp vitality
  - Pulp capping
  - Pulpotomy
  - Laser-assisted endodontic disinfection
- **Photobiomodulation (PBM) applications**
  - PBM pulpotomy
  - Management of Steven-Johnson syndrome
  - Treatment of radiation-induced oral mucositis
  - Pre-emptive analgesia
  - Reversal of soft tissue anesthesia.

Diagnosis of Dental Caries

- **Laser-induced fluorescence: Kutsch** (1992) reported clinical findings comparing carious and non-carious tissue illuminated with an argon laser with dark-field photography. When illuminated with *argon laser* light, carious tissue has a clinical appearance of a dark, fiery, orange-red color and is easily differentiated from sound tooth structure.
- **Tetrahertz pulse imaging:** Tetrahertz-waves or millimeter-waves are located just below the infrared band in the electromagnetic spectrum and are generated by lasing semiconductors with ultrafast pulses of visible laser light.

- **Quantitative laser fluorescence:** A hardware and software system was developed in the Netherlands and Sweden that collects images of lesions based on excitation at 488 nm with an argon laser. The blue light is used to irradiate the surface of the tooth by a specially constructed handpiece, and the computer captures the fluorescent image.
- **Fluorescence resulting from red-light excitation of occlusal surfaces: Hibst** and **Gall** systematically studied this phenomenon and used a 655 nm laser as the excitation source and measured the fluorescent signal at higher wavelengths. This work culminated in the development of a commercial device (DIAGNOdent, KaVo, Germany) that is in use in several countries for the diagnosis of caries. The red laser diode light is directed to the occlusal surface by a specially designed probe tip and the fluorescent signal is filtered from the incident light and feedback to the detector through the same device. The signal comes out as a number on the instrument on a scale of 0–99.
- **Optical coherence tomography (OCT):** An imaging technique that is capable of two-dimensional or three-dimensional images of subsurface tissue. The differences in scattering or polarization between sound and carious enamel can be exploited.

Prevention of Dental Caries

- The role of lasers in the prevention of caries has been explored since the 1960s by using different types of lasers based on increasing the resistance to caries by reducing the rate of demineralization of the subsurface of enamel and dentin.
- The laser irradiation of enamel has been shown to increase the Ca/P ratio, decrease the amount of carbonate and protein, and facilitates the formation of tri and tetra calcium phosphate. (**Ana et al. 2006**).
- According to the organic blocking theory, the retarded enamel demineralization is attributed to partial denaturation of the organic matrix, which blocks the diffusion pathway in enamel (**Hsu et al. 2000**).
- The lased enamel shows a high positive birefringence suggesting the formation of micro-spaces within the enamel. These micro-spaces would impart an increased acid resistance to the enamel by trapping ions formed during acid demineralization (**Westerman et al.1991**).
- **Ralph H Stern** and **Reidan F Sognnaes (1972)** reported intact tooth enamel exposed to a super-pulsed CO_2 laser at an energy density of 10–15 J/cm^2. They observed that lased enamel showed much more resistance than unlased control enamel to the oral environment.
- **S Tagomori** and **T Morioka (1989)** demonstrated the combined effects of laser and fluoride on acid resistance of human dental enamel applied with a solution of sodium fluoride of APF solution before and after laser irradiation with normal pulsed Nd:YAG. They concluded that APF application after laser irradiation caused a remarkable increase in acid resistance of the enamel while before irradiation showed lesser effect and APF application after laser irradiation produced a greater fluoride uptake in the enamel than before irradiation.

Removal of Caries

- **Goldman, Sogannaes, Stern,** and **Gordon** were the first scientists to investigate the use of laser technology to remove dental caries. They used a pulsed *ruby laser* with high densities. They found extensive deep destruction of carious areas with sharply demarcated areas of affected enamel and dentin.
- The use of lasers for cavity preparation and caries removal is based on the ablation mechanism, in which dental hard tissue can be removed by thermal and/or mechanical effect during laser irradiation **(Seka et al., 1996).** Er: YAG and Er, Cr: YSGG can selectively remove dental caries due to the higher amount of water and organic content when compared to sound tissues **(Eberhard et al., 2008; Tachibana et al., 2008)** in this way, it is possible to obtain a conservative therapy, with no removal of sound tissue and lack of thermal damages.
- **T O Myers** and **W O Myers (1985) investigated** the effect of a pulsed *YAG laser* on enamel fissures. Around 30 recently extracted human teeth with pit and fissure, incipient lesions were used for the study Nd: YAG laser with a wavelength of 1600 A and pulse duration of 30 ps. They found that Nd: YAG laser has the potential to remove organic and inorganic debris from pits and fissures without causing pulpal or enamel injury due to the minimal laser energy.

Cavity Preparation

- The United States Food and Drug Administration approved the Er: YAG laser for cavity preparation in 1997. It is one of two types of lasers currently approved for cavity preparation, the other type being the Er, Cr: YSGG (Erbium, chromium-doped yttrium, scandium, gallium, and garnet).
- According to **Baraba and colleagues,** the high temperatures caused during laser irradiation, in other words, the photo-thermal effect, might also play a role in killing bacteria during laser irradiation, such as through the denaturation of proteins, damage to nucleic acid, and alterations to the cell wall and cell membrane of the bacterium, as well as through micro-explosions when the water in the bacterial cell absorbs the laser energy.
- **Shamsudeen and colleagues** prepared cavities with the Er:YAG laser at 600 W power and 300 mJ energy with water cooling and air spray, they found that the structure of enamel and dentin appeared normal in both groups, with both groups showing dead tracts in dentin below the cavity.

Pit and Fissure Sealant

- The laser can be used for fissurotomy, cleaning, and conditioning of pits and fissures before sealant application.
- Erbium laser is mostly used for fissurotomy procedures, but it does not eliminate the need for acid etching before sealant application.
- The formation of enamel cracks and resulting micro-leakage at the sealant enamel interface are the disadvantages of this technique, which can be prevented by curing the sealant material using an argon laser.

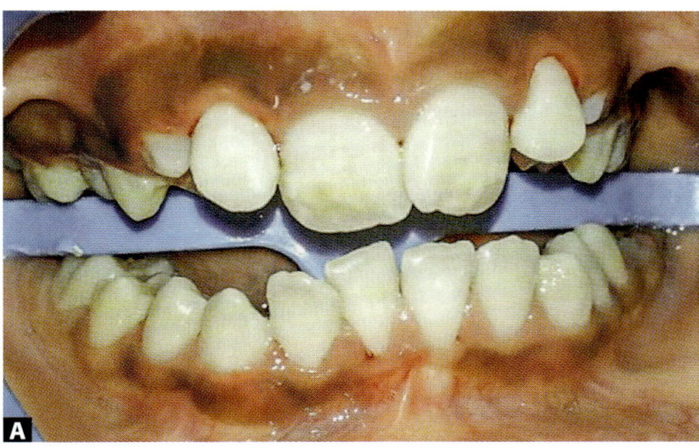

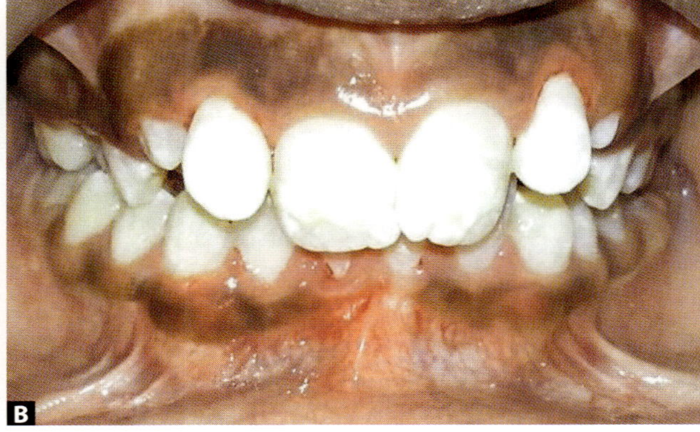

Figs. 79.1A and B: Pre and immediate postoperative photographs of laser bleaching.

Bleaching

- Thelaser light is converted to heat as it strikes the bleaching gel and accelerates the oxidation of the peroxide contained in the substance.
- **Figures 79.1A and B** depicts a case of laser bleaching done using an 810 nm diode laser with 4 W power using a teeth whitening prism.
- **Pleffkin PR et al (2012)** concluded in a study that low power laser increased the efficacy of bleaching gel with a minimum increase in pulpal temperature, much below the deleterious level at which pulpal damage could even be anticipated.
- **CM Yavagal et al (2014)** carried out a study to comparatively analyze the resistance to enamel solubility and demineralization with laser bleaching and the impact of CPP-ACP pre and post-laser bleaching. Post-laser bleaching, application of CPP-ACP followed by short bursts of laser provided exceptional resistance to enamel solubility.

Argon Laser Photopolymerization of Composite Resins

For polymerization of camphorquinone-activated composite resins, the argon laser increases the depth of cure, increases the diametric tensile strength, increases the adhesive bond strength, increases the degree of polymerization of the material, reduces the acid solubility of the surrounding enamel, and decreases the time of activation significantly.

Lasers in Soft Tissue Surgery

Lasers have been employed as surgical tools in many branches of medicine for nearly two decades. Dental surgical applications have also been reported primarily for soft-tissue incisions and the controlled destruction of several oral pathogens.

Tethered Oral Tissue Surgery (TOTS)

- A new term was coined by **Kevin Boyd**, DDS at the International Association of Tongue-tie Professionals at their annual conference in Quebec, Montreal Canada in October of 2014.
- Tethered oral tissues (TOTs) as a term are more inclusive of tissue restriction of the tongue, lips, and buccal frena (**Boyd**, 2014).

Frenum Revisions

- Indications of frenum revision in the infant, child, or adolescent patients range from an inability to nurse in newborns to speech pathologies in children to orthodontic problems in the preadolescent and adolescent patients.
- Patients with bleeding and clotting disorders who require hemostasis during soft tissue surgery benefit from diode, CO_2, or Nd: YAG laser.
- **Figures 79.2 A to C** show the management of ankyloglossia with 810 nm diode in CW mode with 2W in contact mode. **Figures 79.3 and 79.4** depicts the comparison of

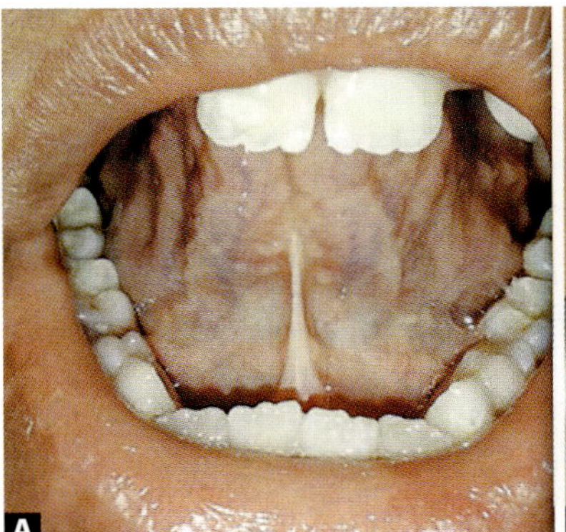

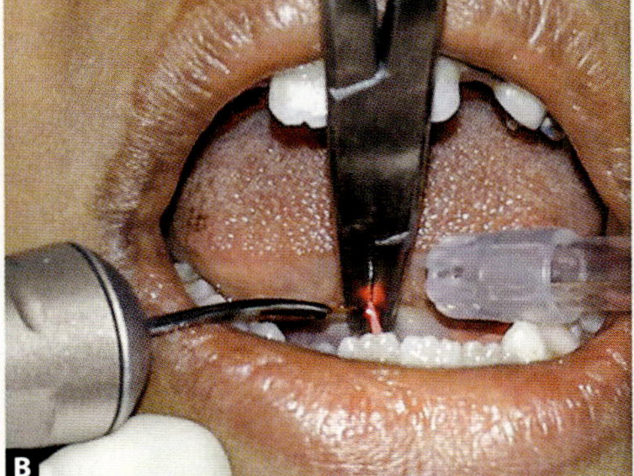

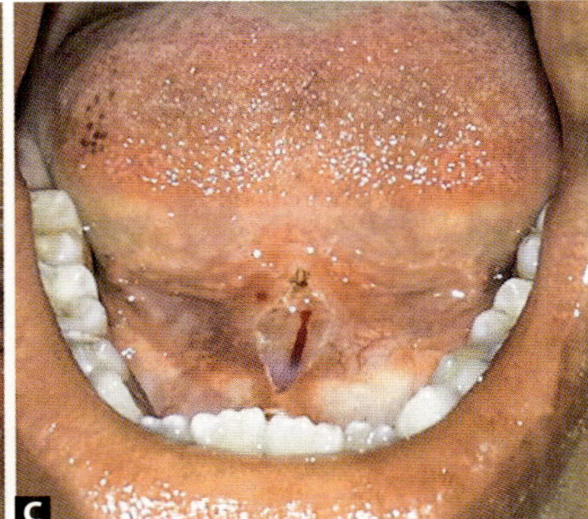

Figs. 79.2A to C: Pre, Intra, and immediate postoperative photographs. Treatment of ankyloglossia by laser lingual frenectomy.

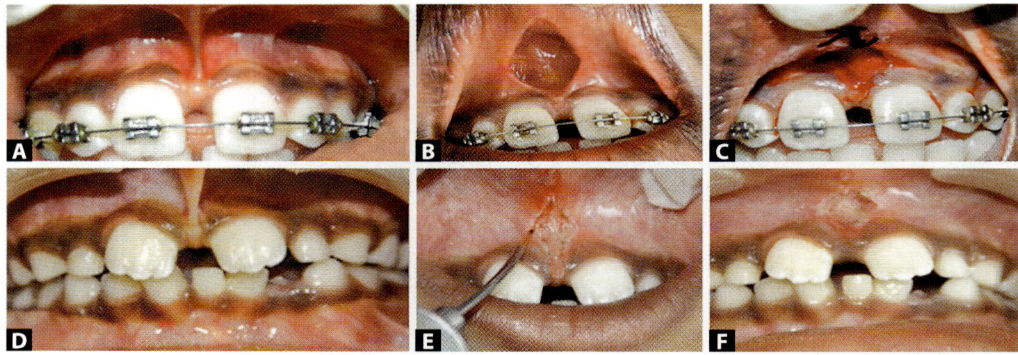

Figs. 79.3A to F: Comparison of surgical (A to C) and laser (D to F) maxillary labial frenectomy.

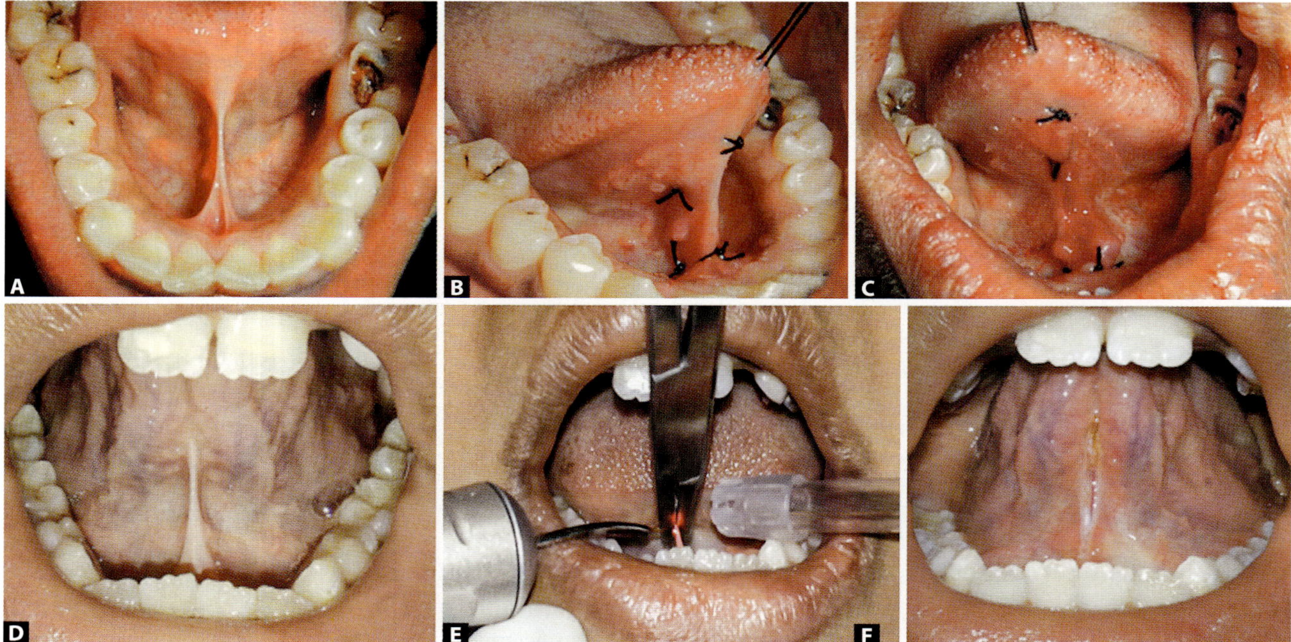

Figs. 79.4A to F: Comparison of surgical (A to C) and laser (D to F) lingual frenectomy.

surgical and laser maxillary labial and lingual frenectomy respectively.

Management of Soft Tissue Growth

Figures 79.5A and B depicts the management of soft tissue growth on mandibular gum pads in a 3-months-old infant with 810 nm surgical as well as photobiomodulation mode.

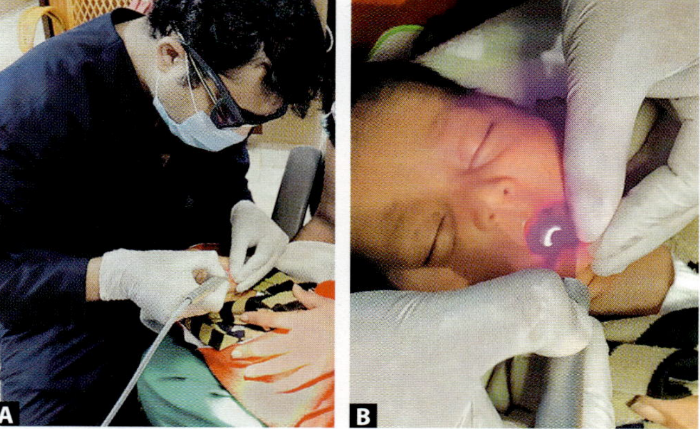

Figs. 79.5A and B: (A) Intraoperative photographs; (B) Management of soft tissue growth.

Treatment of Pericoronal Problems in Erupting Teeth

- Children whose first permanent molars are erupting to develop often experience discomfort, swelling, or infection in the tissue overlying the emerging tooth.
- Lasers can be used to ablate the involved tissue and expose the clinical crown of the involved tooth.

Tooth Exposure for Orthodontic Treatment

- The use of the laser in the disinclusion of impacted teeth offers several advantages when compared with conventional methods, including precision, minimal intraoperative hemorrhage, sterilization of the surgical area, healing with minimal scarring, and decreased postoperative pain and swelling.
- **Figures 79.6A to C** depict a 13-year-old patient for whom exposure of canines for orthodontic banding was done with

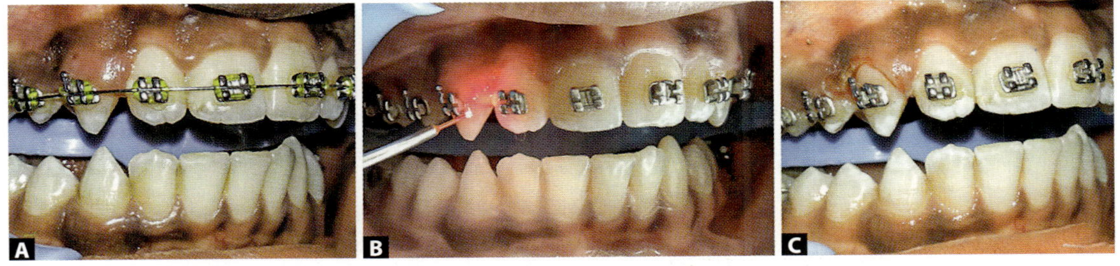

Figs. 79.6A to C: Pre, intra, and immediate postoperative photographs. Canine exposure with diode laser for orthodontic treatment.

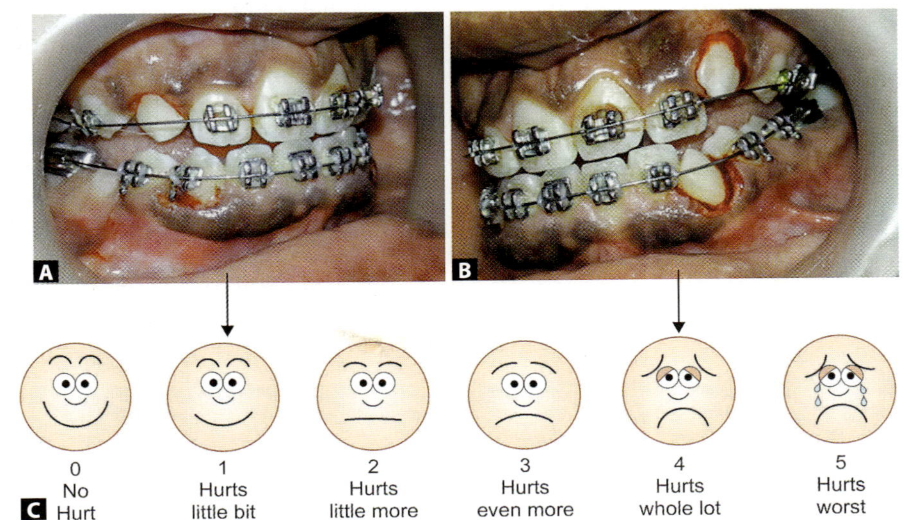

Figs. 79.7A to C: (A and B) Postoperative photographs of laser-assisted and surgical exposure of impacted canine respectively; (C) The intensity of perceived pain on the visual analogue scale.

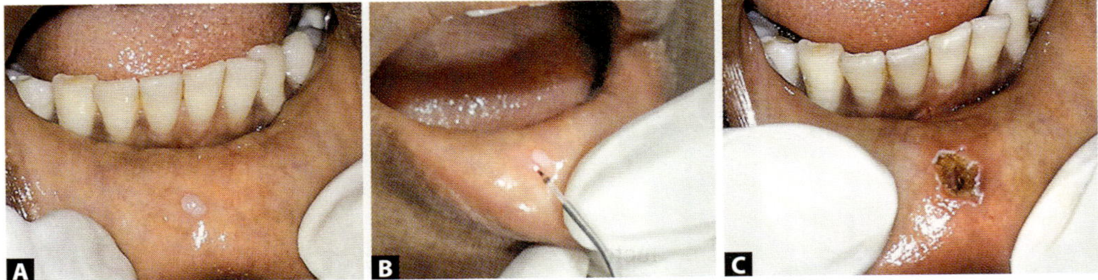

Figs. 79.8A to C: Pre, intra, and immediate postoperative photographs. Excision of fibroma using diode laser.

810 nm diode in pulsed mode with 2W using a laser tip of 400 microns diameter and 5 mm length. **Figures 79.7A and B** shows the comparison of surgical and laser-assisted disinclusion of impacted teeth with a representation of pain intensity on a visual analogue scale.

- In a case series published by **Impellizzeri** et al, the patient did not complains of any postoperative pain or discomfort and postoperative wound healing was rapid. Furthermore, an increase in compliance of these young patients occurred, because they were subjected to a minimally invasive surgery that did not require the application of uncomfortable orthodontic devices on the palate.

Lesion Removal and Biopsy

- Diode laser radiation is an excellent, simple, and safe form of treatment of oral lesions like fibrotic lesions, gingival growths, and other types of lesions. This procedure is virtually bloodless, and postoperative edema and discomforts are minimal. With laser irradiation, there is less damage to adjacent tissues and better visibility.
- Dental lasers offer several clinical advantages (especially for soft tissues), including hemostasis (the sealing of local vasculature), the ability to seal nerve endings and lymphatic vessels, reduced postoperative pain and swelling (thus reducing the need for postoperative analgesics/narcotics), reduced bacterial counts, and a minimized need for sutures in most surgical procedures.
- **Figures 79.8A to C** show a solitary sessile lesion on the lower lip. Excisional biopsy was performed with 810 nm diode in CW mode with 1.5 W using a laser tip of 400 microns diameter and 5mm length without local anesthesia.

LASERS IN PEDIATRIC ENDODONTICS

Diagnosis of Pulpal Vitality

- Laser light is transmitted to the pulp using a fibre optic probe. Scattered light from moving red blood cells will be frequency-shifted whilst that from the static tissue remains unshifted. The reflected light, composed of Doppler-shifted and unshifted light, is returned by afferent fibres and a signal is produced.
- The photodetectors convert the interference pattern arising from the mixing of shifted and unshifted light into a semi-quantitative measurement of blood flow, termed the Flux signal, which is measured in arbitrary units. The received signal is calculated with a preset algorithm in the LDF machine.
- The LDF output signal or Flux can be simplified as a function of the product of red blood cells' concentration as well as their mean velocity.
- To assess the vitality of teeth, the size of the flux signal obtained from a healthy vital control tooth can be compared with that of the suspected non-vital tooth. The Flux signal from a tooth with a vital pulp should be greater than from a tooth with a non-vital pulp. **(Roebuck et al. 2000).**

Pulp Capping

- Laser treatment has advantages concerning control of hemorrhage and sterilization and so it has attracted dentist's attention for pulp capping.
- In 1985, **Melcer et al.** reported a CO_2 laser-produced newly mineralized dentin formation without cellular modification of the pulpal tissue when tooth cavities were irradiated in beagles and primates.
- While using the CO_2 laser for this treatment, laser irradiation of the exposed dental pulp must be performed to stop bleeding and sterilize the area around the exposure. Laser irradiation should be performed at 1 or 2 W after irrigating alternatively with 8% sodium hypochlorite and 3% hydrogen peroxide for more than 5 min. Calcium hydroxide paste must be used to dress the exposed pulp after the laser treatment, after which the cavity should be tightly sealed with cement such as carboxylate cement.

Lasers used for direct pulp capping.

	Wavelength	*Power*	*Time*	*Indication*	*Waveform*	*Advantages*	*Disadvantages*
Co_2	10,600 nm	0.5–1 W Continuous wave and pulsed	0.5–3 s	Soft tissue	Continuous and/or gated pulsed mode	• Strong hemostasis • Decontamination • Photobiomodulation • Less expensive	• Major thermal change • (carbonization and strong • coagulation) • Not able to be guided by • optical fibers • Large-sized device
Nd:YAG	1,064 nm	1.75–2 W 20 pps	0.5–20 s	Soft tissue	Free-running pulsed mode	• Strong hemostasis Decontamination • Photobiomodulation • Fiber-optic or hollow-wave- • guiding delivery	• Major thermal change (carbonization and strong • coagulation) • Expensive and large-sized • device
Er:YAG	2,936 nm	25–200 mJ/ pulse 2–20 pps	5–15 s	Soft and hard tissue	Free-running pulsed mode	• Low to moderate hemostasis • Decontamination • Photobiomodulation • Minimal thermal change (slight coagulation) • Fiber-optic delivery	Expensive and large-sized device
Er,Cr:YSGG	2,780 nm	0.25–0.5 W (25 mJ/ pulse, 10–20 pps)	5–15 s	Soft and hard tissue	Free-running pulsed mode	• Low to moderate hemostasis Decontamination • Photobiomodulation • Minimal thermal change (slight coagulation) • Fiber-optic delivery	Expensive and large-sized device
Diode	810–980 nm	0.7–5 W Continuous wave	1–2 s	Soft tissue	Continuous and/or gated pulsed mode	• Strong hemostasis • Decontamination • Photobiomodulation • Wide selections of optical fibers • Less expensive and small-sized device • Fiber-optic delivery	Major thermal change (carbonization and strong coagulation)

Pulpotomy

- The diode laser has been described as being one of the most suitably fitted laser wavelengths to be applied to the pulp for completion of the pulpotomy procedure due to its high absorbance rate. Its conductivity through fiber optic helps its clinical application in dentistry while its small size and relatively low cost make it more affordable and convenient. On the other hand, diode laser has appeared to offer a series of benefits, including minimal or no bleeding, quick healing, reduced postoperative infection, and minimal or no need for anesthesia.
- In1989, **Ehihara** reported the effects of Nd: YAG laser on the wound healing of amputated pulps. He reported better wound healing in pulps, exposed to laser than in controls during the first week, and facilitation of dentinal bridge formation in the 4th and 12th postoperative weeks.
- **Wilkerson et al (1996)** evaluated the clinical, radiographic, and histological effects of argon laser on vital pulpotomy of swine teeth. The results showed normal soft tissue with some reparative dentin formation in histological assessment.
- **Liu et al (2006)**, investigated the success rate of Nd: YAG laser (2 W, 20 Hz, 100 mJ, and 320 nm optical fiber) pulpotomy to formocresol in human primary molars. The clinical and radiographic success rates of Nd: YAG pulpotomy was 97% and 94.1%, respectively.

Laser-assisted Endodontic Disinfection

- Lasers have become the latest choice to eradicate microorganisms in the root canal, especially in the lateral dentinal tubules as they can reach the areas of the root canal that are impossible to reach by the conventional techniques of irrigation. Different techniques involving lasers have been proposed to improve the efficacy of irrigating solutions, like laser-activated irrigation, photodynamic therapy, and photon-induced photoacoustic streaming.
- **Figures 79.9A to C** depicts the different laser-assisted endodontic disinfection techniques.

Laser-activated Irrigation

- Laser-activated irrigation (LAI) is based on the creation of specific cavitation phenomena and acoustic streaming in intracanal fluids as a result of photothermal and photomechanical effects. The strong absorption of the Erbium laser energy (at low settings of 50–75 mJ) in water and NaOCl causes vaporization and the formation of large elliptical vapor bubbles. The vapor bubbles cause a volumetric expansion of up to 1,600 times the original volume of an irrigant with high intracanal pressure which drives the fluid out of the canal. The bubbles implode after 100 to 200 microseconds, creating pressure that sucks fluid back into the canal: inducing a cavitation effect. This technique has been demonstrated to be effective in the removal of intracanal dentine debris and smear layer **(Ivona Bago 2014).**

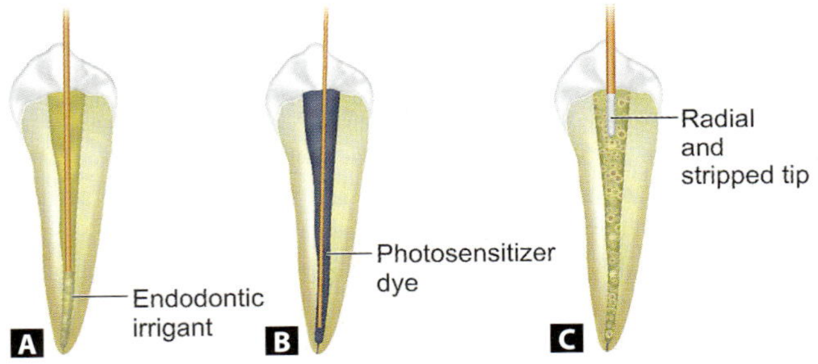

Figs. 79.9A to C: Different laser-assisted endodontic disinfection techniques: (A) Laser activated Irrigation (LAI); (B) Photodynamic therapy (PDT/aPDT); (C) Photon-induced photoacoustic streaming (PIPS).

- **De Moor et al.** and **De Groot et al.** showed higher efficiency of LAI with Er, Cr: YSGG, and Er: YAG (75 mJ, 20 Hz, 1.5 W, 4 x 5 s) and 2.5% NaOCl in the removal of dentine debris from the apical part of the root canal compared to conventional irrigation.
- In a study by **RG Naik et al**, The mean reduction in colony-forming units post diode laser application was seen to be 100% when compared to 98.46% reduction after CMD with 3% NaOCl.

Photodynamic Therapy

- Laser energy is used to activate a nontoxic photosensitizer in presence of oxygen, and free oxygen radicals released from these dyes cause damage to the membrane and DNA of microorganisms without affecting host cell viability in photo-activated disinfection.
- **Agarwal S et al (2013)** conducted a study to compare the disinfection of deciduous root canal by conventional chemomechanical debridement (CMD) with sodium hypochlorite (0.5%) *vs* laser-assisted photodynamic therapy (PDT) with 660 nm diode laser using methylene blue dye. In this study, Laser-treated canals showed a reduction in bacterial load by 99.99% as against 83.9% obtained after the use of conventional CMD with sodium hypochlorite. It was concluded that Laser-assisted PDT can be used as an excellent adjunct to CMD to obtain near-perfect disinfection of deciduous root canals. **Figures 79.10A and B** depicts the procedural illustration from the study.
- The results of a study by **Nagayoshi M et al.** suggest that the use of a diode laser in combination with photosensitizer dye like, indocyanine green may be useful for clinical treatment of periapical lesions. Likewise, Bago I et al, have found that PDT and endo activator systems were more successful in disinfection of root canals than the diode laser and NaOCl syringe irrigation alone.
- A study by **Tewani KK et al.** compared various disinfection strategies using a high-power diode laser by techniques like direct laser irradiation, laser-activated irrigation, or photoactivated disinfection. The study gave significant results in eliminating *E. faecalis*. Also, laser-activated irrigation and photoactivated disinfection were found to be similar in their effectiveness.

Photon-induced Photoacoustic Streaming

- The basis of PIPS is attributed to the photomechanical effect seen when light energy is pulsed in liquid. When activated in a limited volume of fluid, the high absorption of the Er: YAG wavelength in water, combined with the high peak power derived from the short pulse duration

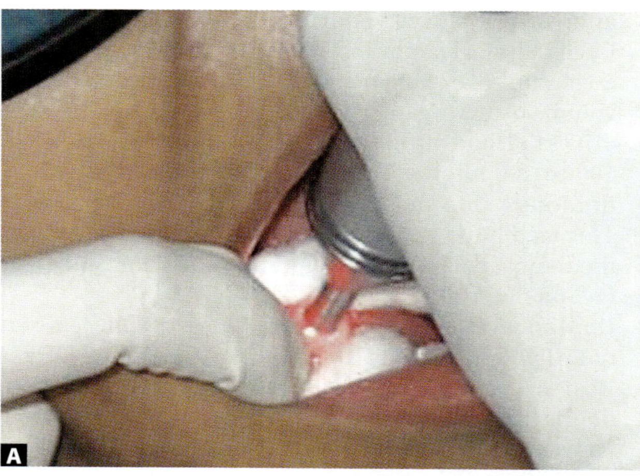

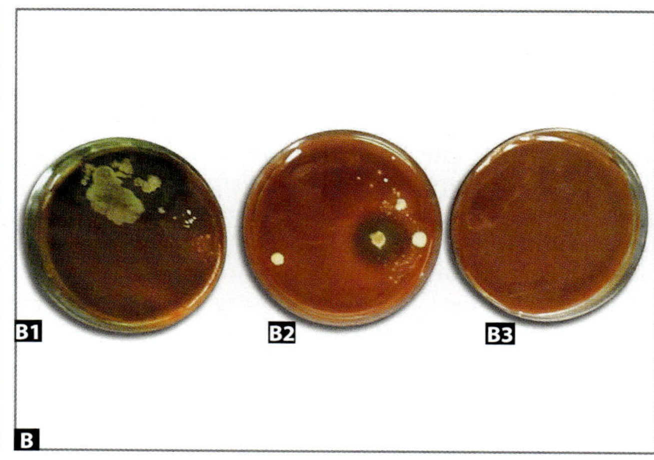

Figs. 79.10A to B: (A) Intraoperative photograph of photodynamic therapy; (B) The microbiological growth on blood agar plates: (B1) Before chemomechanical debridement; (B2) After chemomechanical debridement; (B3) After PDT.

that was used (50 μs), resulted in a photomechanical phenomenon.

- **Divot et al (2012)** described this light energy phenomenon noticed in their study as photon-induced photoacoustic streaming (PIPS). The effect of irradiation with the Er: YAG laser equipped with a novel 400 μm diameter radial and stripped tip at sub ablative power settings (0.3 W, 20 mJ) is synergistically enhanced by the presence of EDTA. This showed a profound "shockwave-like" effect when radial and stripped tips were submerged in a liquid-filled root canal. The study showed that standardized instrumentation, followed by a final Er: YAG laser irradiation in wet canals with EDTA irrigation resulted in more cleaning of the root canal walls and a higher quantity of open tubules in comparison with the traditional irrigation method.
- In a study done by **CM Yavgal et al (2021)**, total elimination of *E. faecalis* counts was obtained by the use of laser activated NaOCl irrigation in the infected root canals. It concluded by considering PIPS as a revolutionary attempt in achieving complete disinfection of the primary root canals, in spite of the morphological complexities.

PHOTOBIOMODULATION APPLICATIONS

PBM Pulpotomy

- In an effort to find a more biologically acceptable and effective alternative to formocresol, lasers pulpotomy with carbon dioxide, diode, neodymium-doped yttrium aluminum garnet (YAG), erbium-doped YAG, and erbium-doped yttrium-scandium-gallium-garnet have been tried. However, photobiomodulation/Low-level laser therapy (LLLT) has gained popularity with its potential to reduce pulpal inflammation, preserve dental pulp vitality, and improve healing.
- LLLT has a bio-modulatory effect on pulp cells and the expression of collagen, fibronectin, and tenascin. **Pretel et al.** reported that LLLT also accelerates dentin barrier formation and repair process after traumatic pulp exposure in monkeys. It has shown noble histopathological results in many studies where the pulp exhibited increased neovascularization, regenerative tissue formation, and also the proliferation of dental reparative cells like osteoblasts and fibroblasts.
- **C Yavagal et al.** conducted a randomized animal trial to evaluate the histological changes in dental pulp tissue after a pulpotomy procedure using a low-level diode laser in comparison with the gold standard formocresol. On histologic evaluation, the least amount of inflammation and maximal healing was evident in the LLLT group and the formocresol group showed severe inflammation **(Figs. 79.11A to C).** The study concluded by considering LLLT appears a safe, minimally invasive, yet a maximally effective modality for pulpotomy.
- **Uloopi KS** and co-authors compared the effectiveness of Low-Level Laser Therapy to Mineral Trioxide Aggregate (MTA) as a pulpotomy agent in vital human primary molars. The MTA showed a 94.7% success rate at all three intervals, whereas LLLT showed a success of 95% at three months, which decreased gradually to 85% at six months and 80% at 12 months.
- A histological study comparing LLLT, Pulpotec, and MTA by **AR Prabhakar et al.,** reported the least pulpal inflammation in LLLT followed by pulpotec and severe inflammation in the MTA group.
- A systematic review and meta-analysis done by **Nematollahi and co-authors (2018)** showed that clinical and radiographic success rates of laser pulpotomy at 1, 3, 6, 9, 12, and ≥18 months were comparable to other pulpotomy techniques, including MTA and FC. Moreover, the clinical and radiographic success of laser and other pulpotomy modalities were similar irrespective of time.
- In 2021, **CM Yavagal et al** conducted a clinical trial to evaluate and compare the efficacy of photobiomodulation pulpotomy with formocresol. There was no statistically significant difference in the clinical success rates between the formocresol group (97.05%) and the photobiomodulation group (94.1%) (χ^2 = 0.34, P = 0.55); however, the radiographic success rate was significantly high in the laser group (94.1%) compared to the formocresol group **(Figs. 79.12A and B)**.

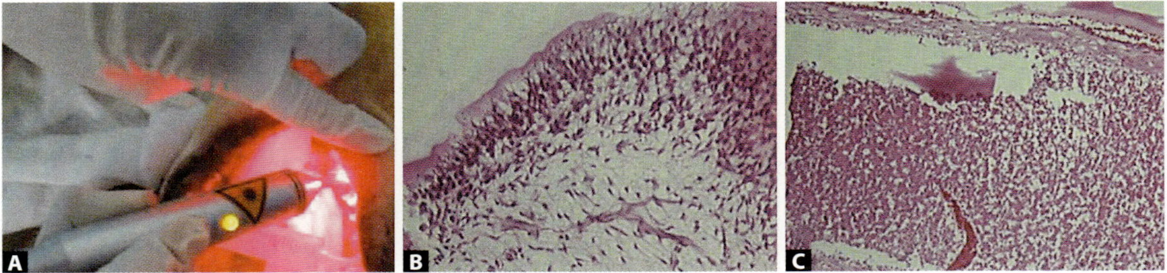

Figs. 79.11A to C: (A) Application of low-level diode laser; (B) Histological picture showing least inflammation in PBM pulpotomy; (C) Histological picture showing severe inflammation in formocresol pulpotomy.

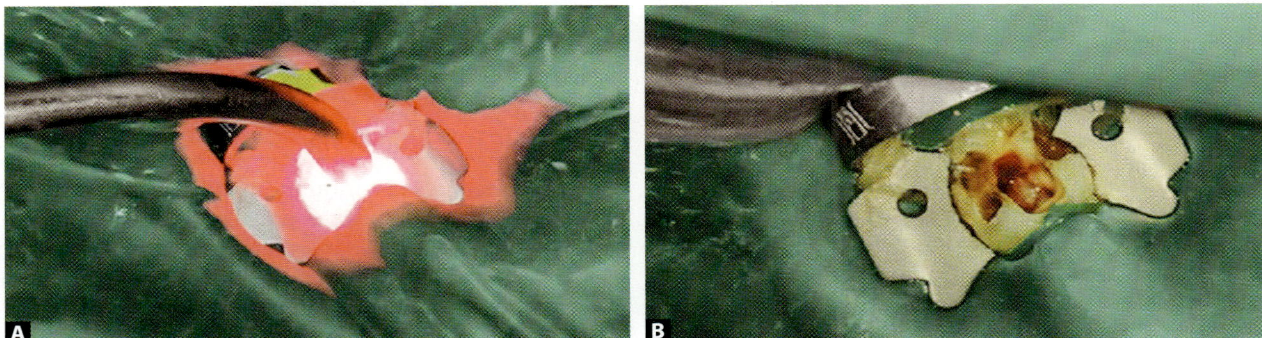

Figs. 79.12A and B: (A) Laser photobiomodulation using 660 nm GaAIAs diode laser; (B) Hemostasis at the site of laser photobiomodulation over pulp stumps.

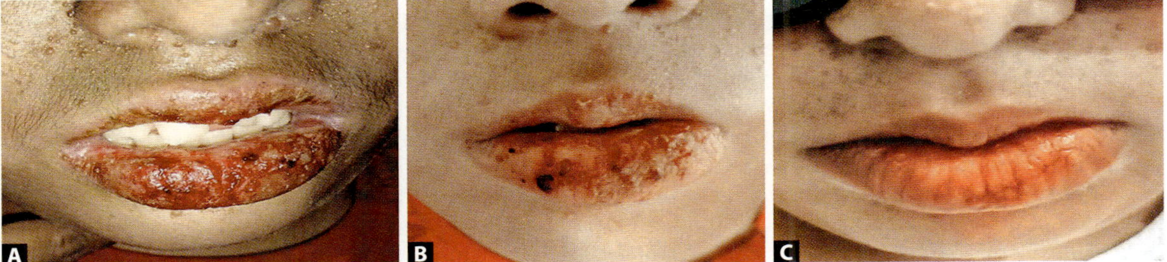

Figs. 79.13A to C: (A and B) Preoperative photographs showing lesions on the hand foot and mouth; (C) Postoperative healing intraoral lesion.

LASERS AND THEIR APPLICATION IN SKIN LESIONS

Management of Hand Foot and Mouth Disease

HFMD is usually caused by Coxsackie virus A16 (CA16) and often by enterovirus 71 (EV71). Most commonly affects children under 5 years of age, and it usually presents with acute stomatitis and a mild fever. Although the prognosis of HFMD is usually good, the intraoral sores often interfere with proper feeding, presenting a risk of dehydration and fluid imbalance, especially in infants. Thus, controlling the painful stomatitis becomes an important issue.

- LLLT in such cases is beneficial due to its analgesic, anti-inflammatory, and healing effects. **Toida et al (2003)** conducted a study to evaluate the usefulness of low-level laser therapy (LLLT) for the control of painful stomatitis in patients with hand-foot-and-mouth disease (HFMD) using an 830 nm semiconductor laser. The painful period was shorter in the LLLT group (4.0 ± 1.3 days) than in the placebo LLLT one (6.7 ± 1.6 days) with a statistically significant difference ($p < 0.005$). The treatment was judged acceptable for 90.0% (18 of 20) of patients. It was concluded that LLLT is a useful method to control HFMD stomatitis by shortening the painful period, with its high acceptability and lack of adverse events.
- **Figures 79.13A to C** shows the management of hand foot and mouth disease of a 4-year-old patient with a 660nm diode laser with an energy output of 4J/cm^2.

Management of Steven-Johnson syndrome

- Stevens-Johnson syndrome (SJS) is a delayed-type hypersensitivity reaction that typically involves the skin and the mucous membranes with high morbidity and mortality rates. Photobiomodulation therapy (PBMT) stands out as an alternative treatment for SJS since it improves tissue repair and helps pain control.
- In a case report documented by **Zinet et al 2020**, the patient had several ulcerated lesions throughout the oral mucosa and lips. PBMT (660 and 808 nm, 100 mW, 2 J/cm^2) was performed on oral mucosa and lips lesions, 3 sessions total. Healing of all ulcerated lesions and pain relief was observed, as well as a return to oral feeding.

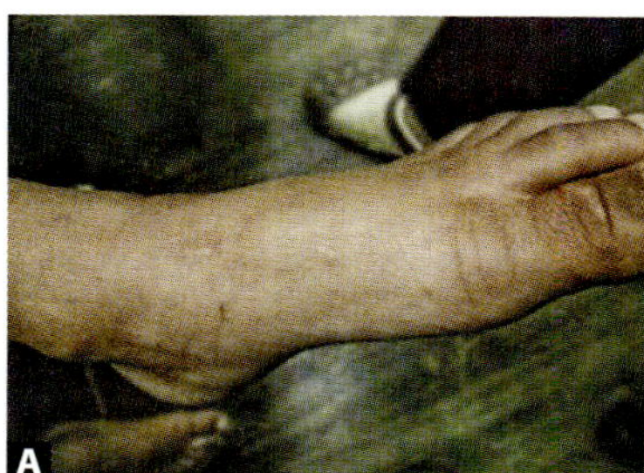
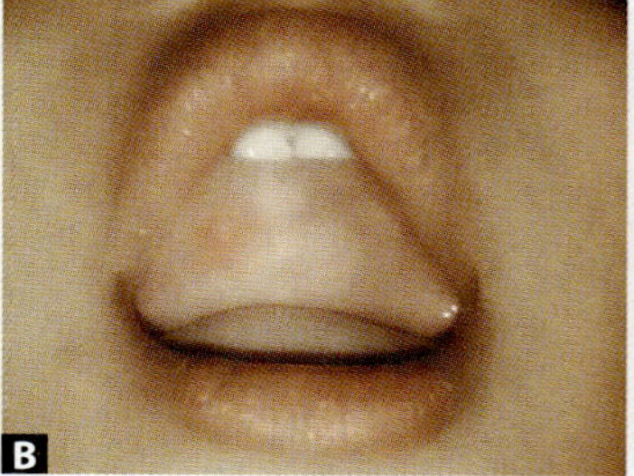
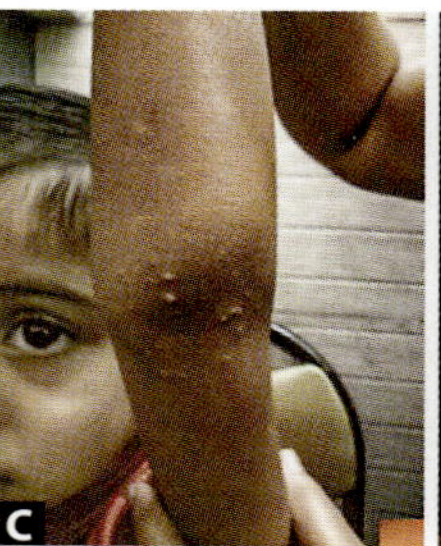
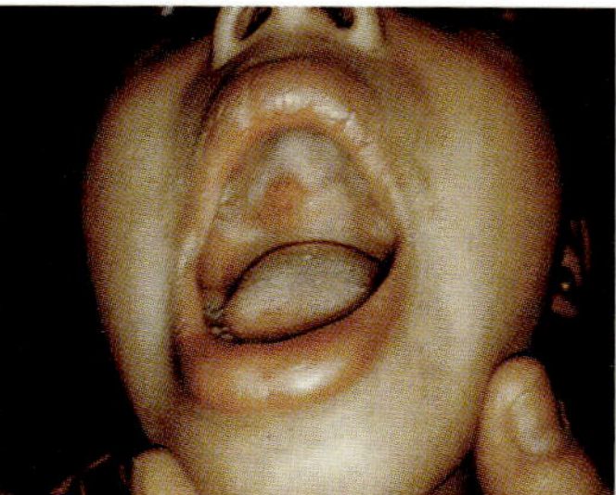

Figs. 79.14A to C: (A) Preoperative ulcerative lesions seen with bloody crusting involving upper and lower lips along with yellow exudate; (B) Postoperative after 48 hours of photobiomodulation therapy; (C) Postoperative after 5 days of photobiomodulation therapy.

- **Figures 79.14A to C** depicts the management of Steven Johnson syndrome in a 9-year-old patient using a 660 nm diode laser with an energy output of 6J/cm².

Management of Radiation-induced Oral Mucositis

- According to the existing literature, low-level laser therapy aims to treat or prevent OM by promoting healing, reducing inflammation, decreasing pain intensity and increasing cell metabolism.
- The results of the systematic review and meta-analysis by **Campos et al (2020)** showed that the laser therapy presented good results in clinical improvement and pain reduction, decreasing the patients' likelihood of developing oral mucositis, with degrees of debilitating lesions to 64%.
- **Multinational association of supportive care in cancer (MASCC) (2022)** identified high-level evidence studies that supported the clinical use of PBM to prevent or treat radiation-induced acute oral mucositis. Consistent findings across these randomized trials were a decrease in the incidence of acute mucositis, a decrease in pain intensity and opioid consumption, and an improvement in quality of life. It endorsed the clinical use of PBM for the prevention of radiation-induced acute mucositis.
- **Figures 79.15A and B** shows the management of radiation-induced oral mucositis in a patient suffering from nasopharyngeal carcinoma using a 660 nm diode laser with a power output of 100 mW and energy of 4–6 J/cm².

PRE-EMPTIVE ANALGESIA

- Fear of needles is common in childhood, especially in dentally anxious ones the prevalence may be as high as 91%. Fear of needles, and therefore intra-oral injections can have negative impacts on children's quality of life and dental treatment experiences including a requirement for pharmacological methods to facilitate dental treatment.
- In recent times, the analgesic effect of photobiomodulation has gained much attention hence the researchers have tried pre-emptive analgesia using the laser photobiomodulation technique. The intention of the technique of "pre-emptive laser analgesia" is to reduce sensation in that small percentage of patients who may experience unpleasant sensations during needle insertion.
- Recently **Fatemeh Shekarchi et al (2022)** conducted a clinical trial to evaluate the impact of photobiomodulation therapy (PBMT) on local anesthesia injection pain perception and compared it with a topical oral anesthetic gel. The low-level laser (diode laser, 808 nm, 250 mW; 16.25 J; 32.5 J cm²) was irradiated upon the buccal gingiva (site of needle insertion), while a benzocaine 20% topical anesthetic gel was applied on the other side. Results

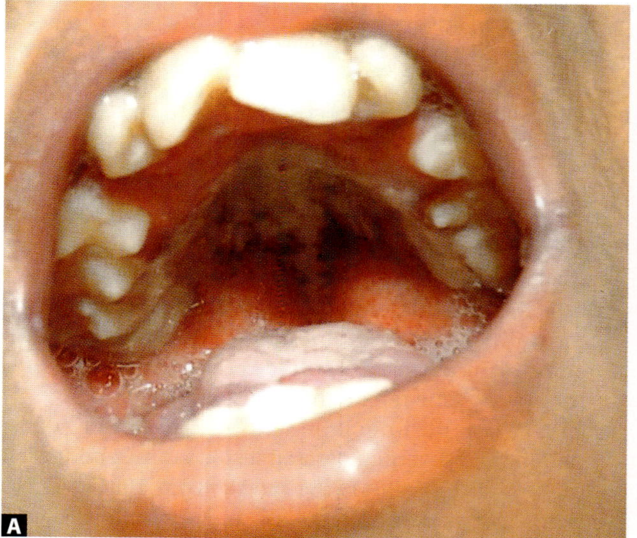
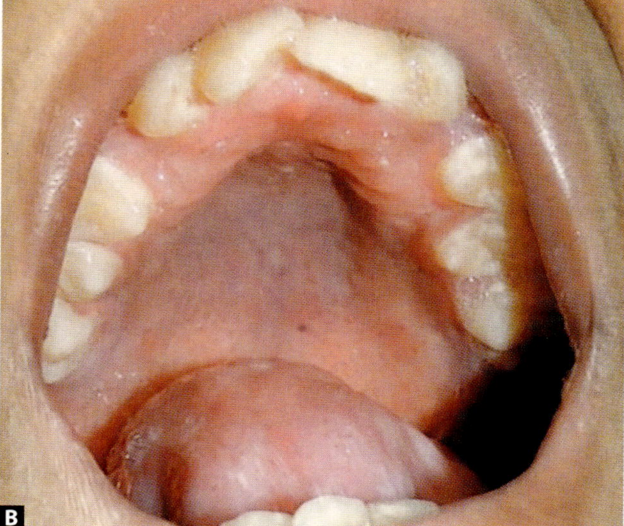

Figs. 79.15A and B: (A) Preoperative and immediate postoperative photobiomodulation photographs; (B) Management of oral mucositis in nasopharyngeal carcinoma.

demonstrated that PBMT could significantly decrease the injection pain perception and heart rate alternations compared to the topical anesthetic gels.

REVERSAL OF SOFT TISSUE ANESTHESIA

- Pain control via local anesthetics has become a major component of pediatric dental clinics. From the injection time until the elimination of anesthesia, children experience several unpleasant feelings such as speech impairment, biting of lips due to numbness as well as problems in swallowing, eating, drinking, and chewing.
- To reduce the level of these injuries, several methods have already been developed by the researchers, one of which in recent times is the reversal of soft-tissue local anesthesia by photobiomodulation.
- First-ever study in this regard was carried out by **Bahman Seraj et al (2019)**, to investigate the clinical effect of photobiomodulation therapy on the reversal of soft tissue anesthesia in children. After 45 min of injection, 810 nm wavelength laser irradiation was done with a power output of 200 mW, in continuous mode with 6.3 J/cm^2 of laser at each point and a total energy density of 37.8 J/cm^2 for 6 points. The mean duration of anesthesia expressed in minutes was equal to 145.15 ± 23.27 and 188.82 ± 12.31 for the laser group and sham laser group, respectively. There was a significant difference in the duration of anesthesia between the two groups ($P < 0.001$). Considering the results and limitations of the present study, photobiomodulation therapy by 810-nm diode laser can be proposed as a non-invasive method to reduce the duration of anesthesia in pediatric patients.

ADVANTAGES OF LASER

Conventional Advantages

- Minimal damage to surrounding tissues.
- A laser beam exerts a hemostatic effect by sealing blood vessels.
- Precision in tissue destruction because of good visualization of tissue planes using an operating microscope. Reduction of postoperative inflammation and edema due to sealing of lymphatic vessels.
- There is little postoperative scarring.
- Reduced postoperative pain sensation since nerve endings are sealed and closed. Dressing or suturing is not required for wound closing.
- Operating time is reduced.
- Sterilization of the wound due to a reduction in the number of microorganisms exposed to laser radiation. Excellent wound healing.
- Laser exposure to tooth enamel causes a reduction in caries activity.

Advantages of the Laser Over Conventional Surgery

- **Analgesia:** The use of lasers reduces the amount of local analgesia required and can reduce the perception of pain in some cases.
- **Hemostatic properties:** These properties are significant, due to the high vascularity of the oral cavity. They are extremely useful in vascular lesions and areas with a rich blood supply, such as the sublingual region, in the case of frenectomies. The carbon dioxide laser provides the best intraoperative control of bleeding, which enables precise surgery to be performed, as it is easier to identify anatomical structures when there is no bleeding in the surgical field. Erbium lasers have less of a hemostatic effect than CO and Nd: YAG lasers.
- **Sutures:** The need for sutures is eliminated, as hemostasis enables wounds to heal by secondary intention.
- **Lasers are cicatrizants:** They improve wound healing, which occurs faster and with less scarring than after conventional treatments. Lasers are good treatment options for ulcers and mucositis. Healing is fastest after the application of erbium lasers, as they have a low thermal effect. In addition, the defocused use of a CO laser at the base of a lesion completes hemostasis and enables immediate contraction of the surgical site, with a 30–40% reduction in wound size. As no mucosal tissue is lost, unesthetic scar formation caused by wound tension is avoided.
- **Antibacterial/disinfectant properties:** These properties enhance postoperative recovery and reduce the required dose of antibiotics (**Türkün et al.** 2006). According to **Kato et al.** 2007, lasers are very useful in developing countries where patients have high postoperative morbidity and mortality, as infections are prevented.
- **Anti-inflammatory properties:** Treatments that are undertaken with CO and Er,Cr: YSGG lasers cause less edema and postoperative pain, which reduces the required doses of analgesics and anti-inflammatory drugs. As the CO_2 laser cuts soft tissue, it seals nerve endings, blood, and lymph vessels, which reduces the inflammatory reaction. The anti-inflammatory properties of low-level lasers can be used to treat muscle contractures and traumas.
- **Operating time:** Lasers reduce the operating time needed for soft-tissue management.
- **Vibration:** The patient does not feel any vibration, pressure, or contact of the optical fiber on the tooth, as occurs with a rotary instrument. This increases a patient's collaboration and acceptance of the procedure.
- **Postoperative care:** Lasers improve postoperative comfort, due to hemostasis, the lack of sutures, and pain reduction. This is very useful in young patients (**Fornaini et al.** 2007).

DISADVANTAGES OF LASER

General Disadvantages

- A laser beam could injure the patient or operator by direct beam or reflected light causing a retinal burn. General anesthesia is usually required for patients undergoing laser treatment in the mouth.
- Combustion hazards.
- Loss of tactile feedback incising the laser instrument.
- Removal of soft tissue overlying the bone can damage the underlying bone. It is available only in hospitals.
- Specially trained person needed for operation. High cost of the equipment.

Limitations of Lasers Over Conventional Surgery

- Requires training: This introduction to the use of dental lasers discussed their scientific basis and tissue effects. It is most important for the dental practitioner to become very familiar with those principles, have clinical experience, and receive proper laser training.
- No single wavelength will optimally treat all dental diseases: Dentists can choose the proper laser(s)for the intended clinical application. Although there is some overlap in the type of tissue interaction, each wavelength has specific qualities that will accomplish a specific treatment objective.
- High cost of dental laser equipment.
- Lasers are the end-cutting instrument. Because a majority of dental instruments are both side and end-cutting, a modification of clinical technique will be required.
- Accessibility to the surgical area can sometimes be a problem with the existing delivery system and the clinician must prevent overheating the tissue and guard against the possibility of surgically produced embolism that could be produced by excessive pressure of the air and water spray used during the procedure.

LASER HAZARDS

The types of hazards that may be encountered within the clinical practice of dentistry maybe grouped as follows:

- Ocular hazard
- Tissue damage
- Respiratory hazards
- Fire and explosion
- Electrical shock

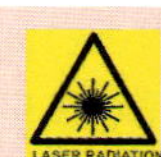

Laser radiation

Eye: Corneal and, or retinal burns, lens damage, cataracts
Skin: Burns, accelerated aging, cancer

Electrical hazards

High current: Power supplies (large capacitors)

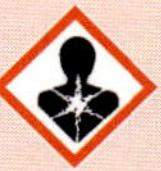

Chemical hazards

Material emissions: Particulate and gaseous materials (vaporised targets, reaction products)

Secondary hazards

Explosion: High gas pressure arc lamps
Fire: Combustible material in vicinity of beam

They can also be classified according to ANSI and OSHA standards as:

Class	*Description*
I	Low-powered lasers that is safe to view
II a	Low-powered visible lasers that is hazardous only when viewed directly for longer than 1,000 s
II	Low-powered visible lasers that are hazardous when viewed for longer than 0.25 s
III b	Medium-powered lasers (0.5 W max) that can be hazardous if viewed directly
IV	High-powered lasers (>0.5W) that produce ocular, skin and fire hazards

Ocular Hazard

- Potential injury to the eye can occur either by direct emission from the laser or by reflecting from a mirror-like surface. Dental instruments have been capable of producing reflections that may result in tissue damage to both operator and patient.
- Direct and specular reflections of relatively low intensity are capable of causing retinal damage because of the focusing effect of the lens and cornea.
- Energy from the CO_2 laser is absorbed in the cornea and can cause denaturation and coagulation of the proteins in the epithelial layers of the corne a, resulting in corneal calcification, resulting in permanent blindness.
- The maximum permissible exposure limit for visible lasers is less than 0.003 watts/cm fora 0.25 s exposure.
- The light produced by lasers presents a potential hazard for ocular damage by either direct viewing or reflection of the beam. Therefore, operators, staff, and patients must wear adequate eye protection. This can be provided by either safety goggles or screening devices. This eye protector is designed specifically for use with a particular wavelength of laser radiation **(Fig. 79.16)**. CO_2 laser protection can be afforded with clean safety glasses; for Nd: YAG laser energy, both the doctor and the staff need to wear green safety glasses; for argon laser orange safety glasses. To protect the patient's eyes, cover with moist swabs taped into places.

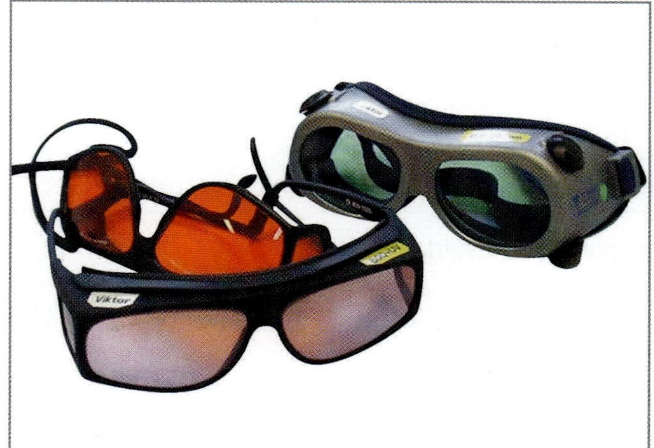

Fig. 79.16: Eye protection for lasers

Tissue Hazard

- Laser-induced damage to the skin and other non-target tissue can result from the thermal interaction of radiant energy with tissue proteins.
- Temperature elevations above the normal temperature (37°C) can produce cell destruction by denaturation of cellular enzymes and structural proteins, which interrupt basic metabolic processes.

Environmental Hazards

- Inhalation of air-borne biohazardous materials maybe released as a result of the surgical application of lasers. Inhaled airborne contaminants can be emitted in the form of smoke or plume generated through the thermal interaction of surgical lasers with tissue or through the accidental escape of toxic chemicals and gases from the laser itself.

- Inhalation of toxic or infectious matter in the form of aerosols and particles is potentially damaging to the respiratory system following both long-term and short-term exposure.
- Adequate suction must be available to collect the entire carbon plume from the operating field to prevent the plume from being inhaled by operating room personnel.
- Air borne contaminants may be controlled by ventilation, evacuation, or other methods of respiratory protection. Surgical staff should wear masks that remove particles as small as 0.3 μm.

Combustion Hazards

- In the presence of flammable materials, the laser may produce other significant hazards.
- Flammable solids, liquids, and gases used within the surgical room can easily ignite if exposed to the laser beam.
- Combustion of flammable gases and endotracheal tubes used during general anesthesia due to their proximity during head and neck procedures, when the anesthetic tube lies within the operative field. It must be protected by covering aluminum tape over it, which reflects the beam away from the tube.
- The use of explosives or flammable anesthetic agents such as cyclopropane or ether is contraindicated when the argon laser is in operation.
- Surgical drapes can be ignited by the laser resulting in burns to the patient, surgeon, or other personnel. So, to prevent this surgical drape should be fire retardant and should be wet to absorb the laser energy, use of flame-resistant material and other precautions are recommended.

Flammable Materials

- **Solids:** Clothing, paper products, plastics, waxes, and resins.
- **Liquids:** Ethanol, acetone, methyl methacrylate, solvents.
- **Gases:** O_2, N_2O, general anesthetics, aromatic vapors.

Electrical Hazards

- Surgical lasers often use very high currents and high-voltage power supplies. Electrical hazards of lasers can be grouped as electrical shock hazards, electric fire hazards, or explosion hazards. High voltages in the main power box can cause pain, burns, ventricular fibrillation, and death.
- Insulated circuits, shielding, grounding, and housing of high-voltage electrical components provide adequate protection from electrical injury.

Equipment Hazard

- The mechanical shutters of the laser are kept closed until the laser is ready to use. When the laser is in use, the shutter of the aiming beam is kept open at all times.
- Room lights should be positioned so that they will not interfere with the motion of a rigid laser arm.
- Interference has the potential for damaging either the laser in arm mirrors or the room light. This damage could interfere with the proper function of the unit or contaminate the operative field.
- Pedals for the laser and any auxiliary equipment should be on different sides of the surgical table to prevent unintended activation of the laser.

The effective use of lasers also requires strict adherence to safety protocols. The clinicians especially those dealing with young patients (pediatric specialists) need to be properly trained and certified. There has to be a designated "LSO - Laser Safety officer" for each facility to handle the operations. Wavelength-specific eyewear with verified optical densities is a must for the operator, the patient as well as the clinical assistant. Laser operatories should be adequately ventilated and must have respiratory protection against airborne contaminants. Fire safety precautions are mandatory, especially in the presence of flammable materials as well as electrical hazards.

The future of healthcare may as well be dominated by "photo" ceuticals as much as the previous era was dominated by pharmaceuticals. This challenging statement has been met with enthusiasm as well as with incredulity. Taking command of the cells by the use of light is still not part of mainstream medicine, despite growing scientific evidence. It is now obvious that we can indeed talk to the cells even though we are still rather poor at understanding their language. Further long-term in vitro and in vivo research trials are needed for us to better understand the nuances of these amazing sciences as well as to build stronger protocols from which we could derive accurate dosimetry and predictable treatment interventions.

POINTS TO REMEMBER

- Diagnosis of dental caries is by laser-induced fluorescence, tetra hertz pulse imaging, quantitative laser fluorescence, fluorescence resulting from red light excitation of occlusal surfaces, optical coherence tomography.
- The best instrument associated with laser for caries diagnosis is the DIAGNOdent.
- Argon laser is best used for prevention of caries as it alters the surface characteristics of enamel to make it more caries resistant.
- Er:YAG laser is the best for caries hard tissue removal.
- Mostly all lasers can be used in soft-tissue treatments. Some of the common laser assisted treatments are frenum revisions, exposure of teeth, removal of lesions and biopsies, treatment of pericoronal problems in erupting teeth, treatment of aphthous ulcers and herpes labialis, removal of hyperplastic tissue.
- Laser can be used for direct or indirect pulp capping even in primary teeth and CO_2 laser is used for this. Laser pulpotomy with Nd: YAG laser has successful results.

- Er: YAG laser is used for pulpectomy.
- Advantages of laser are minimal damage to surrounding tissues, precision in tissue destruction and reduction of postoperative inflammation, reduced postoperative pain; operating time is reduced and wound healing.
- Disadvantages are injury to operator or patient, combustion hazards, loss of tactile feedback, specialized training required to use and high cost of the equipment.
- Laser hazards include ocular hazard, tissue damage, respiratory hazards, fire and explosion and electrical shock.

Questionnaire

1. Describe the applications of laser in pediatric dentistry.
2. Explain the role of lasers in dental caries.
3. What are the uses of lasers in soft tissue treatments?
4. Uses of lasers in endodontics.
5. Explain photobiomodulatory applications in pediatric dentistry
6. Classify the lasers according to their uses.
7. Enumerate the advantages and disadvantages of laser.
8. Classify lasers according to OSHA standards.
9. Describe the hazards of dental laser.

FURTHER READING

1. Bjelkhajen H, Sundström F, Angmar-Mansson B, et al. Early detection of enamel caries by the luminescence excited by visible laser light. Swed Dent J.1982;6(1):1-7.
2. Boj JR,Poirier C,Hernandez M,Espasa E,Espanya A. Review: laser soft tissue treatments for pediatric dental patients. Eur Arch Pediatr Dent. 2011;12(2):100-5.
3. Boj JR, Poirier C,Hernandez M, et al. Case series: laser treatments for soft tissue problems in children. Eur Arch Pediatr Dent. 2011;12(2):113-7.
4. ConvissarRA. The Dental Clinics of North America. WB Saunders: Philadelphia; 2000.
5. Disinfection efficacy of Laser-induced photoacoustic streaming on primary root canals infected with Enterococcus faecalis: An ex-vivo study. International Journal of Dental Science and Innovative Research. Volume – 3, Issue – 2, Page No: 280 - 287 April-2020.
6. Donald J. Coluzzi. Lasers in Dentistry: From Fundamentals to Clinical Procedures. Seminar Series. American Dental Association.
7. Efficacy of laser photobiomodulation pulpotomy in human primary teeth: A randomized controlled trial. Journal of Indian Society of Pedodontics and Preventive Dentistry, Volume 39 Issue 4, 2021, Page 436.
8. Eggertsson H, Analoui M, van der Veen M, et al. Detection of early inter proximal caries in vitro using laser fluorescence, dye-enhanced laser fluorescence and direct visual examination. Caries Res. 1999:33(3):227-33.
9. Ferreira-Zandona AG, Analoui M, Beiswanger BB, et al. An in vitro comparison between laser fluorescence and visual examination for detection of demineralization in occlusal pits and fissures. Caries Res.1998;32(3):210-8.
10. Fred S Margolis. Clinical Uses of the Erbium Laser. Clinical Instructor, Loyola University's Oral Health Center Maywood, Illinois.
11. Fried D, Radagio J, Akrivou M Dental hard tissue modification and removal using sealed transverse excited atmospheric-pressure lasers operating at 9.6 and 10.6 micrometer. J Biomed Optics. 2001;6:231-8.
12. HibstR,GallR. Development of a diode laser-based fluorescent caries detector. Caries Res.1998;32:294.
13. Hicks MJ, Flaitz CM, Westerman GH, et al. Enamel caries initiation and progression following low fluence(energy)argon laser and fluoride treatment. J Clin Pediatr Dent. 1995;20(1):9-13.
14. Kotlow L. Diagnosis and treatment of ankyloglossia and tied maxillary frenum in infants using Er: YAG and 1064 diode lasers.Eur Arch Pediatr Dent. 2011;12(2):106-12.
15. Lawrence A Kotlow. Pediatric Dentistry: The New Standard of Care. US Dentistry; 2006.
16. Luc C Martens. Laser-assisted Pediatric Dentistry: Review and Outlook. J Oral Laser Appl. 2003;3(4):203-9.
17. Lussi A, Megert B, Longbottom C, et al. Clinical performance of a laser fluorescence device for detection of occlusal caries lesions. Eur J Oral Sci. 2001;109(1):14-9.
18. Martens LC. Laser physics and a review of laser applications in dentistry for children. Eur Arch Pediatr Dent. 2011;12(2):61-7.
19. Norbert Gutnecht, Rene Franzen, Leon Vanweersch, et al. Lasers in Pediatric Dentistry: a Review. J Oral Laser Appl.2005;4(5):207-18.
20. Panagiotis Kafas, Christos Stavrianos, Waseem Jerjes, et al. Upper-lip laser frenectomy without infiltrated anesthesia in a pediatric patient: a case report. Cases J. 2009;2:7138.
21. Pedronl G, Gatetta VC, Azeveda LH, et al. Treatment of mucocele of the lower lip with diode laser in pediatric patients: presentation of 2 clinical cases. Pediatr Dent. 2010;32(7):539-41.
22. Photobiomodulation: A Novel Treatment Approach for the Management of Radiation Induced Oral Mucositis-A Case Report. Journal of Advanced Medical and Dental Sciences Research. Volume 10, Issue 4, April 2022.
23. Roeykens H, De Moor R. The use of laser Doppler flowmetry in paediatric dentistry. Eur Archives Pediatr Dent. 2011;12(2):85-9.
24. Stookey GK,Jackson RD,Ferreira-Zandona, et al. Dental caries diagnosis. Den Clin North Amer. 2000;43(4):665-77.
25. Sun G, Tunér J. Low-level laser therapy in dentistry. Dent Clin North Am. 2004;48(4):1061-76.
26. Van As G. Erbium lasers in dentistry. Dent Clin North Am. 2004;48(4):1017-59.
27. Walsh LJ. The current status of low-level laser therapy in dentistry. Part 1 Soft tissue application. Aust Dent J. 1997;42(4):247-54.

CHAPTER 80

Sleep-disordered Breathing in Children: Role of Pediatric Dentist

Mihir Shah, Isha Angne

CHAPTER OUTLINE

- Sleep-disordered Breathing
- Spectrum of Sleep-disorderedBreathing
- Diagnosis of Sleep-disordered Breathing
- Role of Dentist in Management of Pediatric Sleep-disordered Breathing

SLEEP-DISORDERED BREATHING

According to American Thoracic Society Sleep-disordered breathing (SDB) *refers to a wide spectrum of sleep-related conditions including increased resistance to airflow through the upper airway, heavy snoring, marked reduction in airflow (hypopnea), and complete cessation of breathing (apnea)*. This can cause serious metabolic, cardiovascular, and neurocognitive morbidity in children. Increased upper airway resistance is an essential component of sleep-disordered breathing, this compromises breathing during sleep which then affects sleep homeostasis.

Causes of Increased Airway Resistance

Katz et al. summarized the various causes of increased airway resistance as follow:

Abnormal Craniofacial Morphology

- Narrow and retropositioned maxilla and/or retrognathic mandible:
- Retrusion of the maxilla and/or mandible is often associated with reduced airway size which contributes to airway resistance

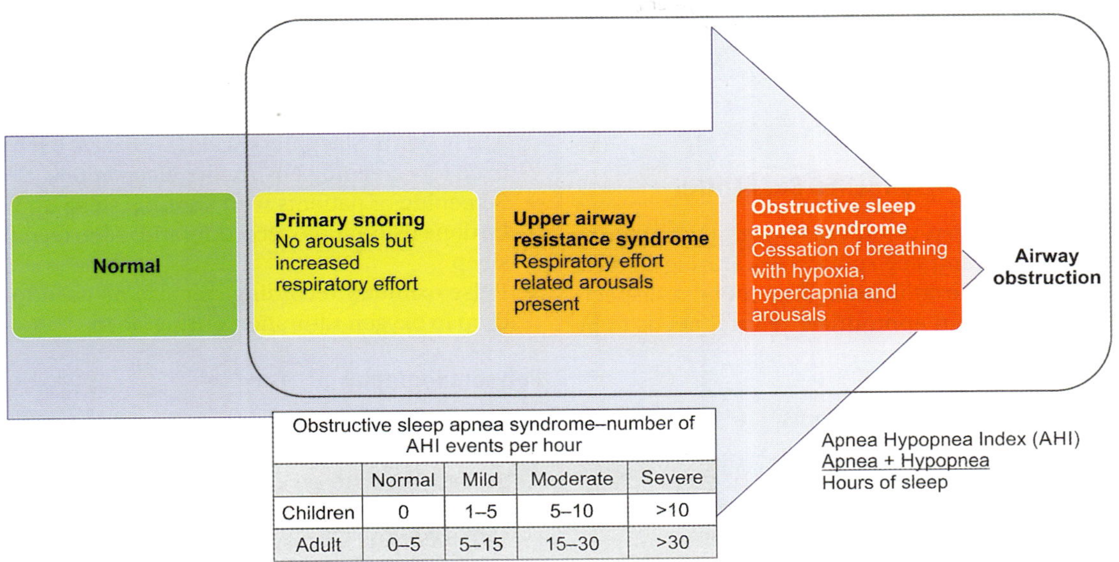

Obstructive sleep apnea syndrome–number of AHI events per hour				
	Normal	Mild	Moderate	Severe
Children	0	1–5	5–10	>10
Adult	0–5	5–15	15–30	>30

Fig. 80.1: Spectrum of sleep-disordered breathing.

- Longer lower facial height
- Caudal placement of hyoid bone

Pharyngeal Soft Tissue and Size of Upper Airway

Enlarged tonsils, adenoids and soft palate are associated with reduced pharyngeal lumen size and increased airway resistance contributing to SDB.

Childhood Obesity

It is often associated with adenotonsillar hypertrophy and removal of it often improves the symptoms.

SPECTRUM OF SLEEP-DISORDERED BREATHING (FIG. 80.1)

The spectrum of sleep-disordered breathing ranges from primary snoring, upper airway resistance syndrome (UARS), obstructive hypoventilation and obstructive sleep apnea (OSA).

AASM DEFINITIONS FOR SCORING FOR ADULTS American Association of Sleep Medicine, 2007 guidelines	
Obstructive Apnea	Decrease in the peak airflow signal excursion by 90% of the pre-event baseline for 10 sec (up to 2 breaths in children) with continued or increased respiratory effort throughout the entire period of absent airflow
Hypopnea	Decrease in the peak airflow signal excursion by 30% of the pre-event baseline for 10s with associated arousal or 3% oxygen desaturation with any one of the following: snoring, increased inspiratory flattening of the airflow signal, or associated thoracoabdominal paradox
Central apnea	Decrease in the peak airflow signal excursion by 90% of the pre-event baseline for 10s with absent respiratory effort throughout the entire period of absent airflow
Hypoventilation	Increase in the arterial PCO_2 to a value of 55 mm Hg for 10 min or an increase in arterial PCO_2 by 10 mm Hg from the awake baseline to a value >50 mm Hg for 10 min. In children, this is defined as hypercapnia, or increased PCO_2 >50 mm Hg for at least 25% of the total sleep time.
	Children from 13–18 years are scored according to adults
(*Source:* Sleep disorder GPD-Edmund Liem)	

DIAGNOSIS OF SLEEP-DISORDERED BREATHING

Primarily diagnosis of sleep-disordered breathing is made by otorhinolaryngologists and sleep physicians. During medical history assessment and examination if the dentist suspects symptoms of SDB then an appropriate referral needs to be made **(Mazumdar et al.)**.

History of Night and Daytime Symptoms

Daytime symptoms	*Night time symptoms*
Dry mouth	Abnormal sleeping position
Mouth breathing	Bruxism or teeth grinding
Excessive fatigue	Heavy snoring
Abnormal shyness and behavioral issues	Mouth breathing during sleep
Aggressiveness and irritability	Delayed sleep onset, and difficulty breathing during sleep
Poor concentration and learning difficulties	Drooling
Memory impairment and poor academic performance	Restless sleep and sleep arousals
Attention deficit/hyperactivity disorder (ADHD) pattern	Sleep talking or somniloquy, sleep walking
Morning headaches	• Enuresis (Bed wetting) • Sleep apnea-stoppage of breathing during sleep

Contd...

Contd...

Physical Evaluation

- A child with SDB/OSA may have various characteristics. The child may often demonstrate significant adenotonsillar hypertrophy which reduces the airway size. The orofacial characteristics of sleep-disordered breathing are often associated with mouth breathing habits and low tongue posture.
- Forward head posture
- Adenoid facies and dolichocephalic cranial pattern
- Narrow maxillary arch, deep palate and Class II growth
- SDB is often also associated with maxillary retrognathism and Class III pattern
- Downward rotation of mandible leading to vertical growth
- Dental crowding and posterior crossbites
- Short lingual frenulum or tongue tie is often associated with sleep-disordered breathing

Airway Evaluation

- Radiographic examination: lateral cephalographs/lateral nasopharynx help in the assessment of enlarged adenoids
- Computed tomography& magnetic resonance imaging helps to evaluate any obstruction in the airway
- Endoscopy: This helps to localize the obstruction in the airway.

Screening Studies

- Questionnaires like the Berlin questionnaire (BQ), STOP-BANG Questionnaire (SBQ), STOP Questionnaire (SQ), and Epworth Sleepiness Scale (ESS) have been commonly used for screening obstructive sleep apnea
- Screening of patients with snoring, sleep apnea can also be done using audio recording and video recording during sleep
- Pulse oximetry recording can also be used to screen the drop in oxygen saturation during sleep.

Polysomnography

- According to the American Association of Pediatrics, polysomnography is the gold standard for diagnosis and gradation of the severity of sleep-disordered breathing. It is often performed after the child is suspected to have SDB following History, Examination and Questionnaires.

- Polysomnography, also called sleep study, is a comprehensive test used to diagnose sleep disorders. Polysomnography records brain waves (EEG activity), heart rate and ECG, breathing and respiratory effort, oxygen saturation and end tidal CO_2, EMG for submental and masseter activity, nasal and/or oral airflow, snoring and vibrations, as well as eye and leg movements using audio-videography.

ROLE OF DENTIST FOR SCREENING OF CHILDREN WITH SLEEP-DISORDERED BREATHING

According to AAPD, pediatric dentists are in a unique position to identify children at risk of sleep-disordered breathing. Thorough history and comprehensive examination may help in the evaluation of signs and symptoms of SDB. According to AAPD dentists are encouraged to:

- Screen patients for sleep-related breathing disorders such as Obstructive sleep apnea (OSA) and primary snoring
- Assessment of the tonsils hypertrophy and tongue positioning as it may contribute to obstruction
- Recognize craniofacial anomalies and/or obesity which may contribute to OSA.
- Refer to an appropriate medical provider (e.g., otolaryngologist, sleep medicine physician, pulmonologist) for diagnosis and treatment of any patient suspected of having OSA.
- Consider non-surgical intraoral appliances only after a complete orthodontic/craniofacial assessment of the patient's growth and development as part of a multi-disciplinary approach.
- After comprehensive evaluation and diagnosis for sleep-disordered breathing by the primary physician, medical management of sleep-disordered breathing may be started which may include the use of nasal sprays to improve upper airway congestion. Adenotonsillectomy is also commonly performed by the surgeon in these kids with enlarged and inflamed pharyngeal tissues. This has often shown significant improvement in the apnea-hypopnea index (AHI) and symptoms of Sleep-disordered breathing
- Depending on the level of airway narrowing, dental management is often prescribed as a part of the multidisciplinary approach.
- Apart from medical management, dentists trained in this field may be able to provide:
  1. Maxillary expansion
  2. Mandibular advancement
  3. Breathing re-education
  4. Orofacial myotherapy

Role of Maxillary Expansion in Sleep-disordered Breathing

- The oral cavity and the nasal cavity share a common wall-the roof of the mouth or the floor of the nose. Often narrow maxillary palate may contribute to airway resistance.
- In such cases, rapid or semi rapid expansion may help to improve the width of the maxilla. The linear increase in the width of the maxilla brings about a volumetric increase in the nasomaxillary complex. This increase in the volume of the nasomaxillary complex not only improves the symptoms of sleep-disordered breathing but also helps in the correction of crossbite, and crowding and relieves malocclusion **(Fig. 80.2)**.
- Rapid maxillary expansion produces significant width increases in the maxilla and nasal cavity. This improves the stability of respiratory function and craniofacial development.

Role of Mandibular Advancement

- Just as maxillary expansion brings about sagittal improvement of the airway, mandibular advancement helps in anteroposterior improvement of the airway.

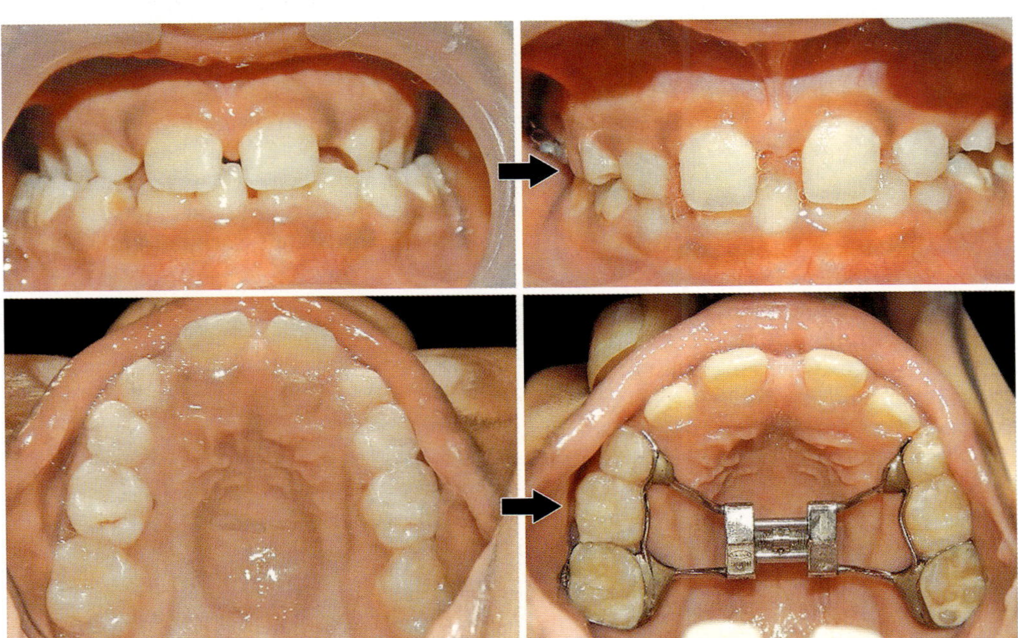

Fig. 80.2: Rapid palatal expansion brings about skeletal expansion of maxilla through mid-palatine suture, this brings about volumetric expansion of the nasal cavity. Rate of expansion 0.5–1 mm per day.

- Mandibular advancement appliances can also bring about improvement in symptoms of SDB **(Figs. 80.3A and B)**.
- Children with Class II malocclusion often suffer from symptoms of SDB. When mandibular advancement devices like twin block or mandibular anterior repositioning appliance are used, they not only improve symptoms of sleep-disordered breathing but also improve mandibular growth, improve the dental profile and dental alignment as well.

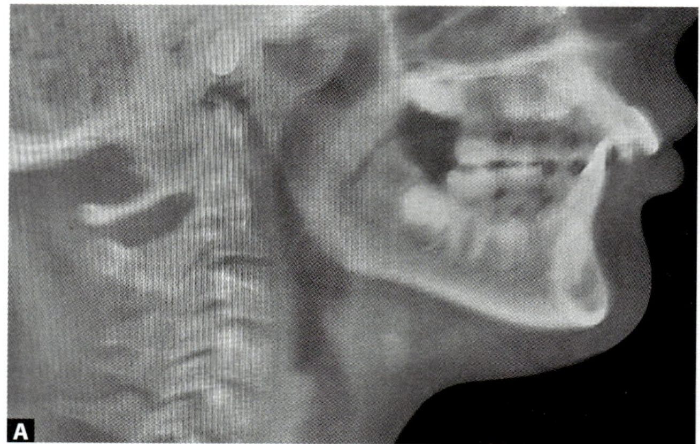

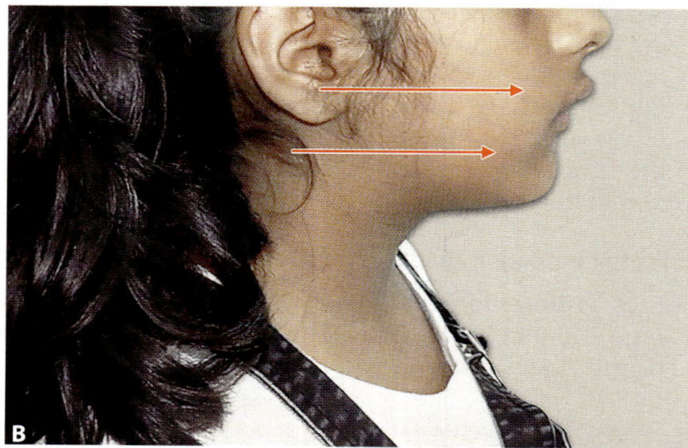

Figs. 80.3A and B: Mandibular retrognathism is often associated with compromised airway and SDB, mandibular advancement devices not only improves the airway but also improves facial profile and dental occlusion.

Breathing Re-education

- According to **Guilleminault**, nasal breathing is imperative for optimum craniofacial growth and airway development in children, Majority of the kids with SDB have a habit of chronic mouth breathing due to increased airway resistance in their upper airway. This habit of chronic mouth breathing is often associated with vertical growth of the face, narrow palate, respiratory congestion, worsening the SDB which worsens the mouth breathing as well, thus leading to a vicious cycle.
- Mouth breathing children usually have high sympathetic stress and low heart rate variability.
- According to **Patrick McKeown**, the fundamentals of breathing re-education involve three components, if performed correctly it helps in all four phenotypes of OSA.
- Breathe light—to reduce tidal volume and reduce chemosensitivity to CO_2.
- Breathe low—to engage diaphragm and lower lateral ribs. Mouth breathers tend to have upper chest breathing which increases the sympathetic stress, diaphragmatic breathing improves the parasympathetic nervous system tone.
- Breathe slow—ideally 6–10 breaths per min. Breathing slow improves the heart rate variability.

Use of Oral Appliances

Habit correction devices such as a vestibular screen or oral screen can be used which are customized according to the patient. Preformed appliances such as Myobrace, Myo Munchee, etc., can also be used as an adjunct to correct mouth breathing and associated orofacial myofunctional disorders.

Orofacial Myotherapy

- Orofacial myofunctional disorders (OMDs) are disorders of the muscles and functions of the face and mouth. It may affect, directly and/or indirectly breastfeeding, facial skeletal growth and development, chewing, swallowing, speech, occlusion, temporomandibular joint movement, oral hygiene, stability of orthodontic treatment, etc.
- Sleep-disordered breathing and dental malocclusions are often associated with orofacial myofunctional disorders.
- In normal human physiology, the posture of the tongue is usually on the maxillary palate, however, due to multiple causes like mouth breathing, hypotonia, etc., the posture of the tongue is affected leading to low tongue posture. Often this leads to an imbalance of oral and facial musculature leading to OMDs.
- Most OMDs are associated with mouth breathing and subsequent adaptation of orofacial muscles to disordered breathing patterns.
- Correction of these OMDs imperative to improve sleep-disordered breathing.
- Non-correction of OMD is associated with failure of surgery or orthodontic expansion for SDB as well.

Scales for Evaluation of OMDs

Orofacial myofunctional evaluations (OMEs) scale was developed by *CM De Felicio* et al. Another scale "Short evaluation of orofacial myofunctional protocol" was developed by *CC Correa et al.* These scales help in diagnosis of OMD component associated with OSA.

ShOM Scale CC Correa et al.	***Score—0: No alteration Score—1: Alteration***
Breathing mode	0 or 1
Breathing type	0 or 1
Lip competence	0 or 1
Lip tonus	0 or 1
Tongue resting position	0 or 1
Tongue deglutition position	0 or 1
Tonus of nose wing dilator	0 or 1
Occlusion	0 or 1
Glatzel test	0 or 1
Rosenthal test	0 or 1

(ShOM: short orofacial myofunctional protocol)

Management of Oromotor Dysfunction

- Correction of OMD involves orofacial myotherapy which includes multiple exercises for body posture, lip posture and function, and tongue posture and function.
- Various isotonic exercises and isometric exercises are used to correct OMDs.
- Isometric exercises help to improve posture while isotonic exercises help to improve strength.
- A child is prescribed various breathing, postural, and strengthening exercises for their body, lips and tongue. These are to be performed two-three times every day for 4–6 months for correction of OMD **(Figs. 80.4A to D)**.
- Parent counseling and the enthusiasm and motivation of the child towards the therapy are vital for the success of this therapy.
- Since these are compliance based therapies, lack of parental motivation and child discipline may lead to attrition during treatment.

Body Posture Exercises

Children with mouth breathing tend to have a forward head posture, it is very important to have correct body posture for optimum correction of breathing and oromotor dysfunction. To keep the body in good alignment one has to maintain the spine's natural curvature straight neck and shoulders parallel with the hips.

Lip Exercises

Lip pops: Perform 20 times	Roll your lips onto your teeth, press your lips together. Pop your lips apart, perform 20 times
Old Granny surprise face: Hold 20 counts	Roll your lips in over your teeth, Make an "O" shape with your lips, raise your eyebrows, and hold for 20 counts
Button pull: Pull 20 counts in three directions	Position the button in front of your teeth, close your lips over the button, and pull in all three directions. Keep your back teeth closed, (Perform the exercise with a strong thread no 20s with adequate safety taught to the parents and child)
Straw drink: 50 mL water	Close your back teeth, place the straw against your front teeth, and pucker your lips around the straw. Suck in water
Bottle hold: Hold for 20 counts	Put 200–300 mL water in a bottle, attach the button to the neck of the bottle, position the button in front of your teeth, close your lips around the button, bend over at a 90% angle, place your hands on your knees and hold for 20 counts. Add water gradually

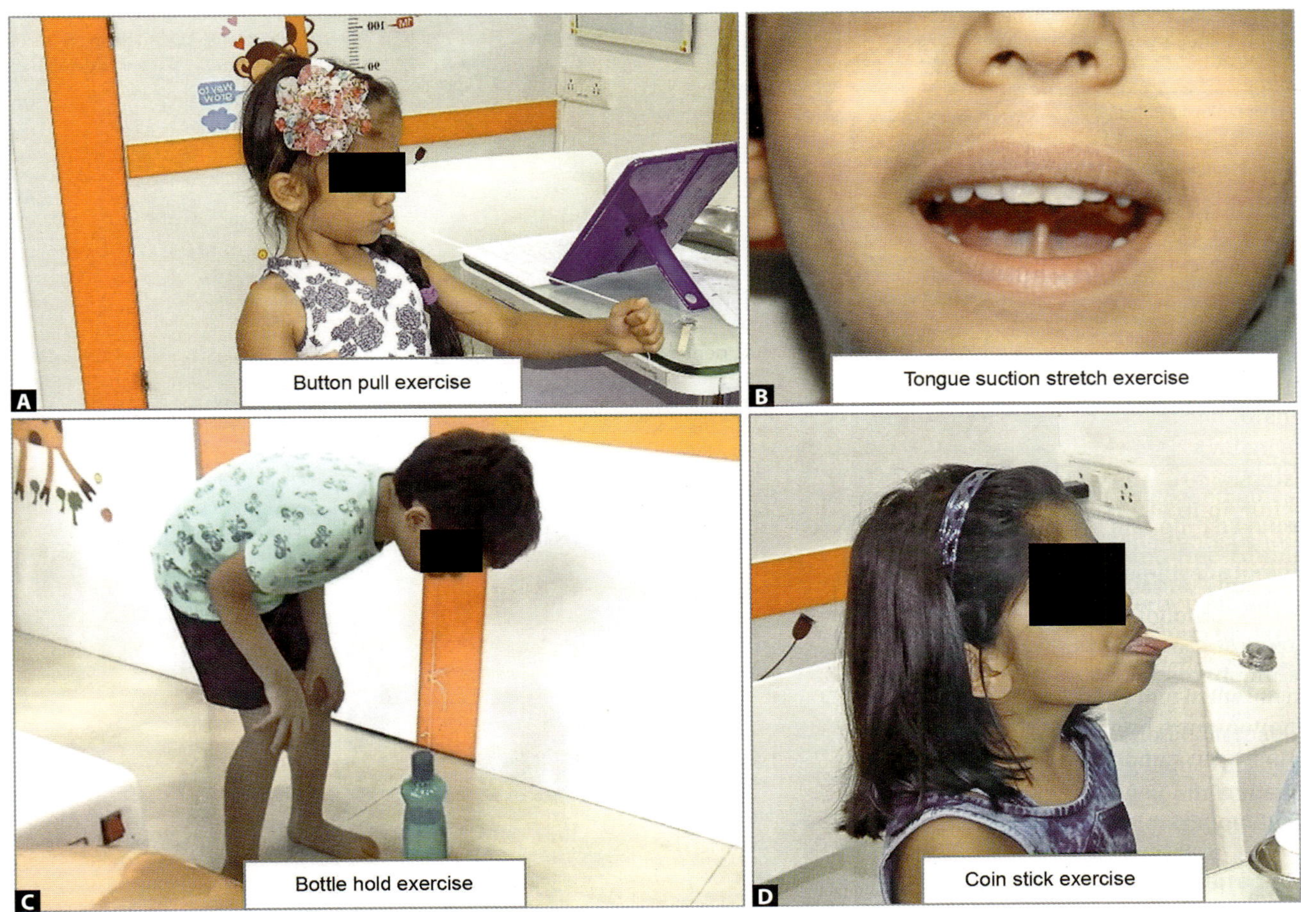

Figs. 80.4A to D: Children performing various orofacial myofunctional exercise with lip.

Tongue Exercises

Tongue clicks, perform 20 times	Suck/place your tongue tip on the palate, smile, pop, avoid touching tongue tip to the floor of the mouth
Tongue sit-ups	Stretch your tongue out, perform sit ups with your tongue
Palatal scrapes	Open wide: Place the tip of your tongue on spot, scrape the tongue back and forth towards the throat
Coin stick hold	Hold a popsicle stick with your upper lip and tongue, place coins at the other end, hold the stick straight, and add coins gradually
Tongue suctions stretch hold	Suck/place your tongue on the palate, open your mouth wide with tongue suction and hold for 20 counts

Reminder Therapy

Coloplast resin can also be placed 5 mm behind the incisive papilla which can serve as a reminder therapy.

Dentists play a vital role in identification and multidisciplinary management of children with SDB. along with medical management, correction of the abnormal craniofacial morphology with help of various orthopedic appliances along with breathing re-education & optimum oromotor function shall help to achieve good general and oral health and reduce the burden of developing malocclusion.

FURTHER READING

1. Camacho M, Certal V, Abdullatif J, Zaghi S, Ruoff CM, Capasso R, et al. Myofunctional therapy to treat obstructive sleep apnea: A Systematic review and meta-analysis. Sleep 2015 May;38(5):669–75.
2. Camacho M, Liu SY, Certal V, Capasso R, Powell NB, Riley RW. Large maxillomandibular advancements for obstructive sleep apnea: An operative technique evolved over 30 years. J Cranio-Maxillofacial Surg. 2015;43(7):1113-8.
3. Corrêa C de C, Weber SAT, Evangelisti M, Villa MP. The short evaluation of orofacial myofunctional protocol (ShOM) and the sleep clinical record in pediatric obstructive sleep apnea. Int J Pediatr Otorhinolaryngol. 2020;137:110240
4. D'Onofrio L. Oral dysfunction as a cause of malocclusion. Orthod Craniofac Res [Internet]. 2019;22(Suppl 1):43.
5. Katz ES, D' Ambuso CM. Pathophysiology of pediatric obstructive sleep apnea. Proc Am. Thorac Soc. 2008;5(2): 253-62.
6. Manfredini D, Guarda-Nardini L, Marchese-Ragona R, Lobbezoo F. Theories on possible temporal relationships between sleep bruxism and obstructive sleep apnea events. An expert opinion. Sleep Breath. 2015;19(4):1459-65.
7. McKeown P, O'Connor-Reina C, Plaza G. Breathing Re-education and Phenotypes of Sleep Apnea: A Review. J Clin Med. 2021;10(3): 1-22.
8. Muzumdar H, Arens R. Diagnostic issues in pediatric obstructive sleep apnea. Proc Am Thorac Soc. 2008;5(2):263-73.
9. Pediatric Sleep Medicine—David Gozal, 2021.
10. Sleep Disorders in Pediatric Dentistry—Edmund Liem, 2019.
11. Torre C, Guilleminault C. Establishment of nasal breathing should be the ultimate goal to secure adequate craniofacial and airway development in children. J Pediatr (Rio J), 2018;94(2):101-3.
12. Vale F, Albergaria M, Carrilho E, Francisco I, Guimarães A, Caramelo F, et al. Efficacy of rapid maxillary expansion in the treatment of obstructive sleep apnea syndrome: A systematic review with meta-analysis. J Evid Based Dent Pract. 2017;17(3):159-68.
13. Yoon A, Abdelwahab M, Bockow R, Vakili A, Lovell K, Chang I, et al. Impact of rapid palatal expansion on the size of adenoids and tonsils in children. Sleep Med. 2022;92:96-102.
14. Zaghi S, Valcu-Pinkerton S, Jabara M, Norouz-Knutsen L, Govardhan C, Moeller J, et al. Lingual frenuloplasty with myofunctional therapy: Exploring safety and efficacy in 348 cases. Laryngoscope Investig Otolaryngol. 2019;4(5):489-96.
15. Zhang C, He H, Ngan P. Effects of twin block appliance on obstructive sleep apnea in children: a preliminary study. Sleep Breath 2013;17(4):1309-14.

CHAPTER

Teledentistry

Mousumi Goswami

CHAPTER OUTLINE

This chapter gives an insight into the evolving role of Teledentistry in the current dental practice. The various types of Teledentistry modes and its aspects have been described. The applicability and the role of teledentistry in Pediatric Dentistry has also been discussed.

Advancements in the field of technology and communication have paved the way for extensive transformations in the field of dentistry, as seen with digital diagnostic imaging services, devices and appropriate software for their analysis. With the use of such advanced information and technology, dental science has come a long way.[1] Not only has new information technology improved the administration of treatment to dental patients, but it has also made it feasible for them to be partially or entirely managed by medical facilities, specialists or skilled dentists from thousands of kilometers away.[1,2]

Teledentistry, as defined by Cook in 1997 is "the practice of using video conferencing technologies to diagnose and advise about treatment over a distance". It is a branch of telemedicine that deals with dentistry that handles the full process of networking, sharing digital information, remote consultations, workup, and analysis.[2,3] With the re-emergence of teledentistry as a field of study that acts as an alternative way to provide dental treatments, it is crucial to determine the value of teledentistry in distant, isolated regions where there is a lack of access to specialized consultations.[3-5]

ORIGIN OF TELEDENTISTRY

The primary vision for tele dentistry was included as part of the dental informatics blueprint, created at a conference in Baltimore, Maryland, in 1989, with funding from the Westinghouse Electronics Systems Group. It focussed onfinding ways to effectively use dental informatics in dental practice to influence oral healthcare delivery.[1] U.S. Army's Total Dental Access Project, a military initiative launched in 1994 to enhance patient care, dental education, and the effectiveness of communication between dentists and dental laboratories, can be attributed to the origin of teledentistry as a subspecialty of telemedicine.[1] It proved that teledentistry lowers overall patient care expenses while extending dental treatment to remote and rural locations while providing comprehensive data needed for more in-depth analysis.[1]

TYPES OF TELEDENTISTRY

- Initially, telemedicine entailed only videoconferencing and its function in long-distance consultation and diagnosis.
- With rapidly developing technology in the twenty-first century, the term teledentistry broadened its scope to cover subdomains such as telediagnosis, teleconsultation, teletriage, and telemonitoring.[6-11]
- The various methods of teleconsultation through teledentistry include Two-Way Interactive or Real-Time Consultation/Synchronous Real-time consultation, Store-and-Forward Teledentistry/Asynchronous Information, Remote Monitoring of Patient, and Mobile Health (mHealth).[6-11]

Two-way Interactive or Real-time Consultation or Synchronous Real-time Teledentistry

- It comprises consultations that enable simultaneous information exchange, medical history collection, and

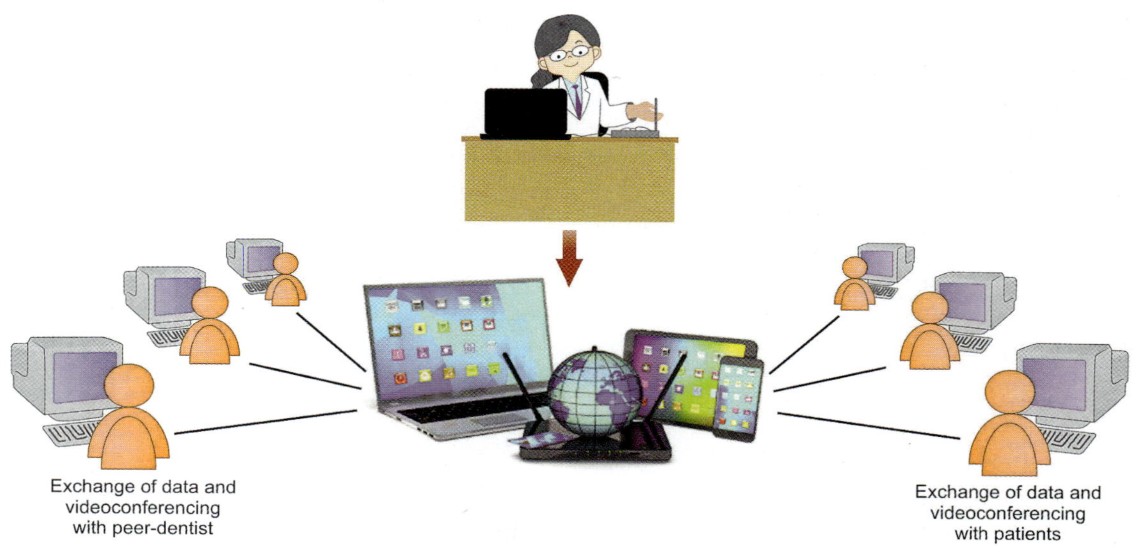
Exchange of data and
videoconferencing
with peer-dentist
Exchange of data and
videoconferencing
with patients
Two-way interaction/real time consultation

Fig. 81.1: Pictorial representation of synchronous real time dentistry.

exchange between a dentist and patient through video conference to arrive at a diagnosis in the same session **(Fig. 81.1)**.

- It also facilitates rapid information sharing and reporting with other specialists.
- Additionally, users in remote or distant sites can obtain real-time visuals or audio from an originating site using two-way interactive technology.[6-11]

Store-and-Forward Teledentistry/Asynchronous Information

- It enables the treating consultant to receive the information from one site, store it, and then transfer it to another location.
- After being reviewed or saved in the system, pertinent data in the form of X-rays, pictures, and scanned images can be uploaded and sent to the consultant. Before referring or monitoring the patient, this system aids in consulting an expert or team from a separate location, city, or country. After getting previous authorization, the data may be used to inform other colleagues **(Fig. 81.2)**.
- Many websites also offer a pattern of asynchronous consultation for retrieving a potential diagnosis by entering serology or pathology results.[9,10]
- Store-and-forward technology offers good outcomes for the majority of dental applications without incurring exorbitant fees for connection or equipment. A computer, an intraoral video camera, and a digital camera for taking photos are the main components of a standard store-and-forward teledentistry system along with a modem and an internet connection.[12-13]

Remote Monitoring of Patient Type of Telemedicine

It encompasses the health information and other medical data to be communicated from one place to another using electronic means.[11,12]

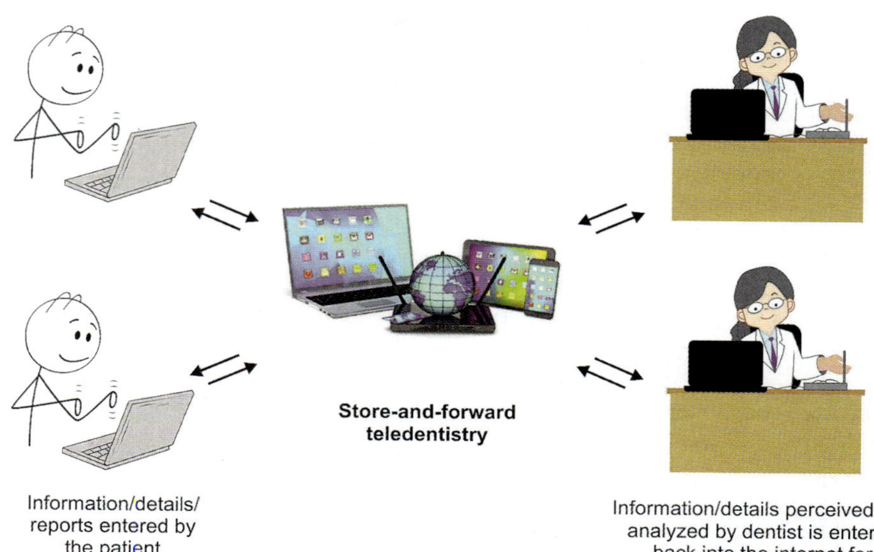

reports entered by

Information/details perceived and
analyzed by dentist is entered
back into the internet for

Fig. 81.2: Pictorial representation of disseminating asynchronous information.

Mobile Health (mHealth)

- It is another type of teledentistry practice in today's era, where mobile communication devices are used to support public health practice and education by using devices such as cell phones, tablets, computers, and personal digital assistants (PDAs).[12,13]
- Modern teleconsultations between the dentist and the patient are conducted using smartphones with built-in video conferencing tools which can be attributable to improvements in telecommunications technologies.[13]

TELEHEALTHCARE MODEL

Teletriaging

- Teletriage can be used to manage patients by categorization according to the urgency of the treatment required. Whether a patient's condition is elective or emergent can be determined by the dental team or the front office.[14]
- Emergency cases may be given priority whereas elective cases can be booked for teleconsultation at a convenient time thus ensuring suitable appointment placements and timings.[11,12]
- By addressing non-emergent patients before they arrive at a hospital, "forward triage" lessens the labour of a caregiver.[11,12]

Teleconsultation

- The core of the telehealth approach lies in the interactive consultation with a clinician through telephone or video conference.
- A teleconsultation is a virtual appointment that includes the exchange of chief complaint, medical history, recent and previous laboratory reports, extraoral photographs, intraoral photographs, dental cast photographs, radiographs, and other relevant examinations.

Telediagnosis

- A diagnosis is developed once the information gathered during the teleconsultation is analyzed. The patient is presented with the proper diagnosis and a complete treatment plan.
- **Haron et al**. designed the "Mobile Mouth Screening Anywhere (MeMoSAR)" for the detection of oral cancer. To improve oral cancer screening, a tablet-based mobile microscope (Cellscope Device) was developed to battle the problem of limited access to specialists.[13,15]

Telemonitoring

- Follow-ups and periodic checks in dentistry have traditionally shown to have multiple barriers such as being a low priority for patients.
- Telecommunication allows for the efficient monitoring of postoperative situations and follow-ups.
- The use of prearranged phone conversations, video conferences, or even just completing online forms about the resolution of symptoms inevitably lead to good oral health and allows the dental professionals to anticipate any treatment failure which may occur **(Fig. 81.3).**[16]

CURRENT TELEDENTISTRY PRACTICES IN INDIA

In India, dental diseases and the after-effects of those diseases continue to be a huge societal, healthcare and financial burden. In 1999, the All India Institute of Medical Sciences in New Delhi and the Centre for Dental Education and Research collaborated to develop the first National Oral Health Care Programme with the goal of raising public awareness through oral health education by using information and communication resources, ultimately aiming to lessen the suffering and morbidity caused by oral health problems.[17]

Through the Indian Space Research Organisation (ISRO), the Department of Information Technology and the Ministry

Telehealth model

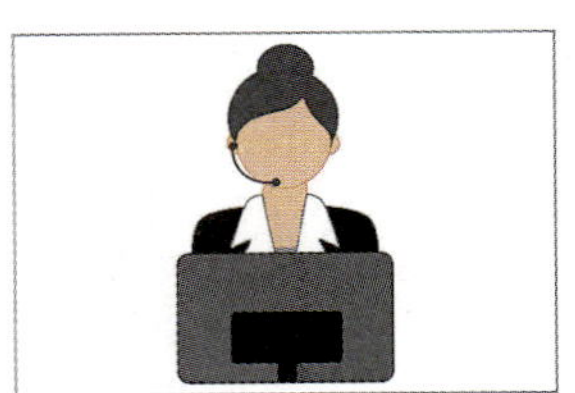

Teletriaging:
Emergent and nonemergent consultations

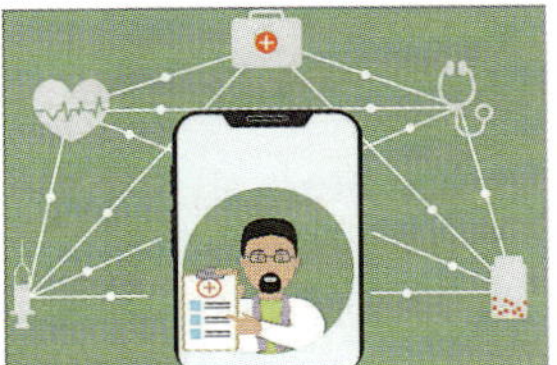

Telemonitoring:
Vitals, medication, sign and symptoms

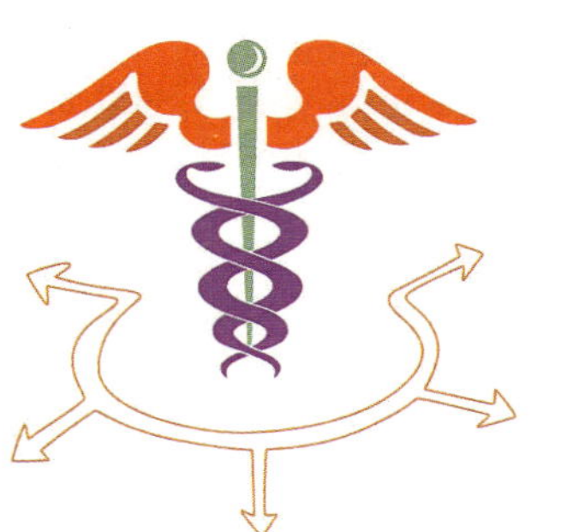

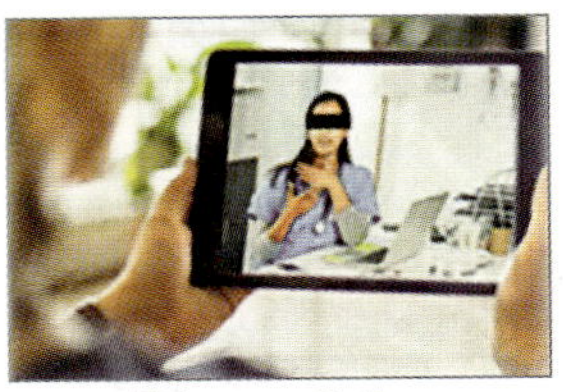

Teleconsultation

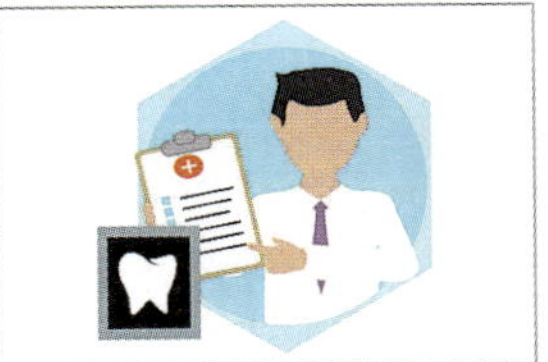

Telediagnosis

Fig. 81.3: Aspects of telehealthcare model.

of Communications and Information Technology began a prototype telemedicine initiative in 1999 where around 1,000 telemedicine nodes were set up nationwide by government, private, and charitable trust organizations, out of which 414 nodes were donated by ISRO. 384 of these nodes were situated in outlying medical care facilities connected to 60 speciality hospitals.

Collaborative Digital Diagnosis System (CollabDDS), is a special software designed to handle the logistical problems of providing high-quality healthcare and education in rural and distant places and has helped to set in motion, the present practice of teledentistry to carry out teleconsultations, diagnoses, and teaching in India.[18]

Telemedicine/Teledentistry Projects in India

- Another web-based interactive platform and mobile application by the national oral health program of the Indian Ministry of Health and Family Welfare is e-DANT SEVA. One of the many distinctive features of "eDantSeva" is "Find a Dental Facility," which helps to locate and map dental facilities near a particular place. India's 313 dentistry schools and 1,000 hospitals, along with basic and community health centers, have all been mapped and accessible.[19]
- Pan African e-Network Project (2009–2017) is an e-Network linking tele-education, telemedicine, video conferencing and voice-over-Internet protocol e-Network to make the facilities and expertise of some of the best universities and super-speciality hospitals in India available to 48 countries in Africa.[20]
- Maharashtra state extended teleconsultation facilities to 23 district hospitals and 39 sub-district/rural hospitals in 2014–2015 with the hub being Sir J.J. Hospital, Mumbai and provided expert opinion to 3767 patients with dental problems.[21]
- "Odi-telecon" in the state of Odisha has delivered successful teleconsultations, teleefollow-ups and online teaching courses.[22]
- The Tele-oncology Network and ONCONET-Kerala.[23]

APPLICATIONS OF TELEDENTISTRY

- **Dental education:** Students can select the location, timing, and manner of learning through internet-based teledentistry instruction. Modern Internet technologies also provide online video conferencing, streaming surgeries and treatments, and online training courses for continuing dental education.
- **Screening for triage:** Teledentistry can be used as a screening technique to assess a patient's dental needs. Dentists can determine if the condition of the patient is emergent or can be categorized under elective therapy. During pandemics and epidemics, urgent cases are rigorously given priority. With the help of teledentistry, patients can be screened beforehand and elective procedures can be deferred for later in turn reducing unnecessary movements and exposure.[24]
- **Diagnostic:** Different software features that allow dentists to know the state of the dental patient help in the diagnostic process while using teledentistry. Extraoral, intraoral, and dental cast pictures that were previously taken for clinical purposes can all be exchanged via these software tools. The original photos that were taken within a dental clinic can be used as diagnostic evidence for a correct diagnosis. The most effective approach to delivering healthcare, especially oral health, depends on a complete set of diagnostic tools. Teledentistry is made more effective as a diagnostic tool because of the excellent software support and telecommunications technology advancements in the present-day scenario.[25,26]
- **Treatment planning:** The dentist can determine the treatment that corresponds to each diagnosis. The use of advanced software which can give a graphic list of treatments and discuss the treatment plan with the patient can allow dentists to choose the appropriate treatment befitting the condition of the dental patient. Consultation with a specialist is also made possible if the software permits multiple participants in the video conference. This allows for real-time discussion by the dental health team.[26]
- **Specialist and interprofessional consultations:** The oral health team, which consists of a variety of specialists, can communicate to address issues about the patient. It is possible to hold meetings with the dental patient to develop active engagement from all sides. Teledentistry is ideal in times of crisis or epidemics or pandemics in addition to providing care to areas with limited access as it provides immediate feedback and produces cost-effective results.[27,28]

APPLICABILITY IN PEDIATRIC DENTISTRY

- Pediatric patients may have a range of treatment needs that require definitive operative, endodontic, orthodontic, or surgical intervention in a dental clinic/hospital.
- To reduce the requirement for dental clinic visits, a model of teledentistry-assisted management of children's dental issues during certain situations such as the COVID-19 pandemic may be incorporated with video-based and live teleconsultation demonstrations.
- It also provides at-home suggestions for non-emergent issues which may be communicated to the parents and caregivers via teleconsultation mode.[29]
- This specific problem-oriented management model provides suggested guidance and potential management changes based on accepted standards and has been described in the following tables.
- However, it must not take the place of the final care a patient needs at a dental clinic, which includes a careful clinical examination and other testing for a precise diagnosis and treatment strategy.

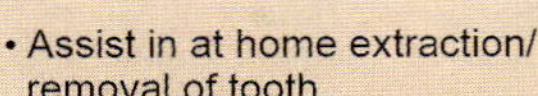

Exfoliating/mobile tooth

- Assist in at home extraction/ removal of tooth
- Apply topical anesthetic gel (over the counter/available online)
- Hold the tooth with clean guaze piece/sterile cotton, twist and pull out
- Arrest bleeding by pressure gauze
- Advise postextraction instructions: Biting down on guaze for at least 30–40 mins, avoid hard or hot foods and avoid spitting for 24 hours
- Prescribe analgesics (over the counter/available online)
- Use of orthodontic elastic/elastic module (available online) around the tooth* may be considered to stimulate exfoliation in over-retained teeth[16]

Teething problems

- Maintain oral hygiene
- Clean gums regularly after each meal using moistened cotton guaze/clean cotton cloth
- Advise using cold—non-sweetened teething rings/ pacifiers
- Use of topical benzyl alcohol/ lignocaine hydrochloride gel over gums

Oral ulcers

- Identify the cause of ulcer virtual diagnosis by dentist
- Avoid spicy and hot foods
- Application of lignocaine based topical anaesthetic gel or glycerin over the area
- Maintain oral hygiene by brushing twice daily and mouthrinsing after every meal

Decementation/accidental swallowing of crown

- Do not attempt to fix the dislodged crown
- If swallowed, usually crowns go into the gastrointestinal tract and pass out eventually
- In case of choking: Induce coughing or attempt Hemlich maneuver*
- Visit emergency service if choking persists

* Video based consultation and assistance can be more effective.

Initial cavity/ Blackspot/ discoloration

Advise non-restorative cavity control (NRCC) which involves:

- Proper brushing twice daily with fluoridated toothpaste*
- Dietary modification
- Flouride mouth rinse/Self applied topical fluoride gels (available online)

Considerably deep cavitated lesion

Asymptomatic:

- Maintain oral hygiene with effective cleaning of cavitated tooth using intraoral aids such as regular flossing and interdental brushes to avoid food lodgement
- Follow NRCC protocol of topical fluoride use at home
- Dietary modification

Symptomatic cavities (pain/ sensitivity):

- Dietary modification and maintainence of oral hygiene
- Mild-moderate and intermittent:
  - Small cotton pellet soaked in clove oil may give temporary pain relief in cavities
  - Analgesic coverage as and when required till dental visit is feasible.
- Severe and continous:
  - Analgesics for immediate relief but schedule dental visit as soon as possible

Dislodged restoration:

- Maintain oral hygiene
- Pack teflon tape into the cavity or a clean cotton pellet soaked in clove oil (in case of pain or sensitivity) using a clean toothpick/ tweezer and change daily till dental visit is feasible

Dental abscess:

- Teleconsultation for appropriate antibiotic and analgesic coverage
- Advise warm saline rinses for swollen gums and soft tissue
- Abstinence from any extraoral hot/ cold fomentation
- Maintain stringent oral hygiene
- Follow-up on teleconsultation and accordingly decide if emergency visit needs to be scheduled
- Cellulitis/Facial swelling/difficulty in swallowing: Emergency dental visit

Ongoing endodontic treatment

If intermediate restorative material is dislodged and root canals are exposed:

- Irrigate with chlorhexidine mouthwash/clean water using a syringe/water flosser
- Pack teflon tape or clean cotton pellet into the cavity and change daily till dental visit is feasible

* Video based consultation and assistance can be more effective.

Minor soft tissue injury

Control bleeding:

- Apply pressure with clean cotton/guaze peice
- If bleeding persists: Use moist tea bag to apply pressure
- Analgesic for pain relief (over the counter/available online)

Tooth fracture

Very small fractured segment Nonpainful:

- No emergency treatment required

Considerable fracture of tooth crown:

- Use densensitizing paste regularly
- Cover tooth with paraffin wax/ orthodontic wax (available online)
- Wrap tooth and cover edges with Teflon tape (PTFE) and change it regularly till the time dental visit is possible.*

Excessively mobile tooth fragment:

- Apply topical anesthetic gel (over the counter/ available online)
- If possible remove the mobile fragment with the help of clean gauze/cloth

Displaced tooth/ Luxation Injury:

- *Displacement without mobility:* Teleconsultation and regular follow-up required

  Consider analgesics in case of pain and visit dental clinic when possible for a definitive treatment
- *Displacement with mobility:*
  - Repositioning of permanent tooth can be attempted using finger pressure*
  - Consider soft diet and analgesics till dental clinic visit is feasible (as soon as possible)

Knocked out tooth/ Avulsion:

- Assess whether tooth is milk tooth or permanent tooth via teleconsultation
- Attempt to reimplant permanent tooth only
- Wash tooth under clean running water
- Try to put the tooth back in socket*
- Ask the child to bite down on the clean cloth.
- Seek simultaneous tele-help from dentist
- Store in cold milk/ coconut water if unable to replant tooth. Do not let it dry!
- Visit dentist immediately

Jaw fracture/bone fracture

- Teleconsultation for immediate help
- Try to control bleeding by pressure pack
- Emergency dental visit

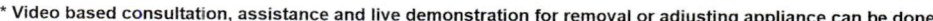

*** Video based consultation, assistance and live demonstration for tooth repositioning and reimplantation can be provided. Advise maintenance of strict oral hygiene.**

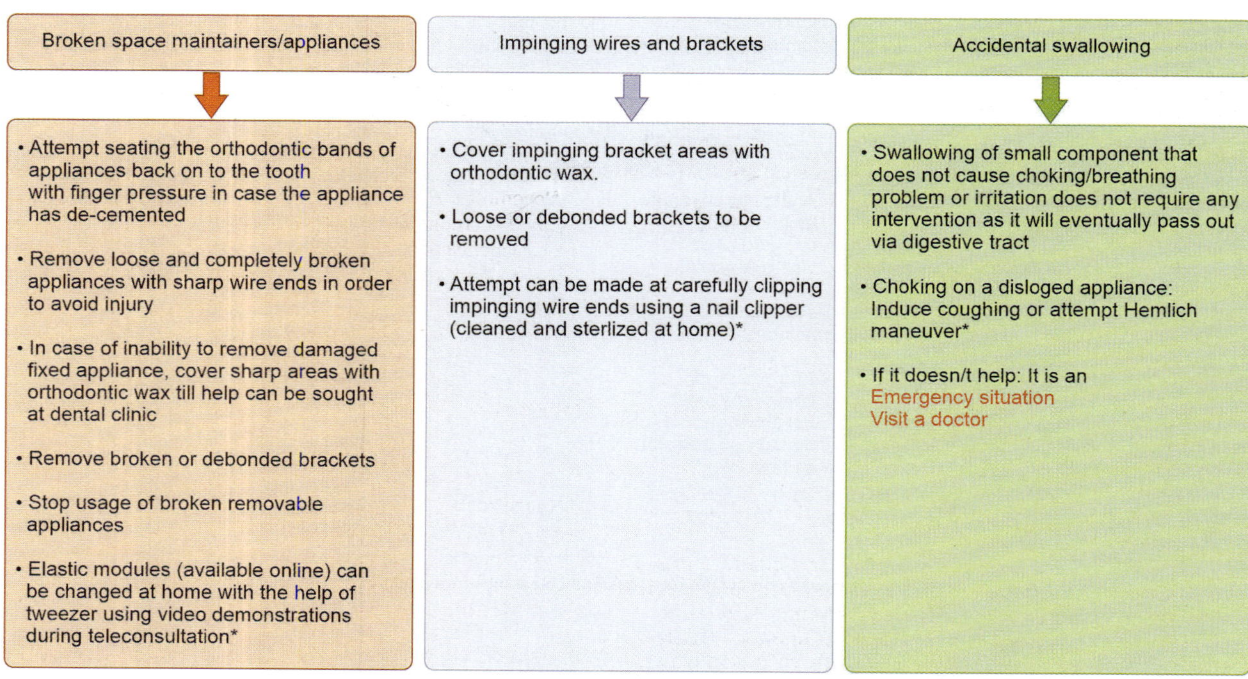

Broken space maintainers/appliances
• Attempt seating the orthodontic bands of appliances back on to the tooth with finger pressure in case the appliance has de-cemented
• Remove loose and completely broken appliances with sharp wire ends in order to avoid injury
• In case of inability to remove damaged fixed appliance, cover sharp areas with orthodontic wax till help can be sought at dental clinic
• Remove broken or debonded brackets
• Stop usage of broken removable appliances
• Elastic modules (available online) can be changed at home with the help of tweezer using video demonstrations during teleconsultation*
Impinging wires and brackets
• Cover impinging bracket areas with orthodontic wax.
• Loose or debonded brackets to be removed
• Attempt can be made at carefully clipping impinging wire ends using a nail clipper (cleaned and sterlized at home)*
Accidental swallowing
• Swallowing of small component that does not cause choking/breathing problem or irritation does not require any intervention as it will eventually pass out via digestive tract
• Choking on a disloged appliance: Induce coughing or attempt Hemlich maneuver*
• If it doesn/t help: It is an
Emergency situation
Visit a doctor

*** Video based consultation, assistance and live demonstration for removal or adjusting appliance can be done.**

BARRIERS TO THE USE OF TELEDENTISTRY

- **Technology**: Clinicians may find it challenging to accept teledentistry due to the complexity of technology since they may be reluctant to acquire and use a new skill.[25]
- **Practical implications**: Improper assessment of interproximal contact and posterior-most teeth as well as the inability to perform a tactile examination of the lesion/oral cavity and the use of two-dimensional images may restrict the accuracy of diagnosis. This may lead to clinicians being anxious about providing a possibly inaccurate diagnosis and thus an improper treatment plan.[26]
- **Communication**: Even though several polls show that teledentistry is becoming increasingly popular, patient acceptance due to a lack of in-person communication may prevent the establishment of an accurate treatment plan.[30-31]
- **Rural setting**: Inadequate infrastructure in remote and rural areas, such as internet access, a computer or smartphone, an X-ray machine, and an advanced armamentarium that aids in identifying the tooth/ lesion, presenting it to the patient, or transporting it to a professional at a distant area presents as a barrier to the acceptance and implementation of teledentistry.[32]
- **Privacy**: Although there are harsh penalties for violating a patient's privacy without their consent, the insufficiency of privacy in transmitted information may make it difficult to establish the trust of the patients. Hence all healthcare professionals and telehealth portals are urged to adhere to the Health Insurance Portability and Accountability Act (HIPAA).[33]

With the dynamic changes in the field of dentistry, the advancements are not limited to armamentarium and instruments but also encompass the various ways to reach patients that are denied care due to various factors like access to facilities and specialists, connectivity, financial barriers and socioeconomic status. This can be achieved through the developments in the telecommunication sector along with the establishment of internet-based social media platforms. Teledentistry has proven to act as a vital patient management strategy which not only aids in triaging and providing emergent care in times of crisis but is also a safer means of consultation and a platform to raise awareness and disseminate important information to patients.

REFERENCES

1. Jampani ND, Nutalapati R, Dontula BS., Boyapati, R. Applications of teledentistry: A literature review and update. Journal of International Society of Preventive & Community Dentistry. 2011; 1(2): 37-44. https://doi.org/10.4103/2231-0762.97695
2. Goswami M, Nangia T, Saxena A, Chawla S, Mushtaq A, Singh SR, Jain P. Practical applicability of teledentistry in pediatric patients amidst pandemic: A narrative review. Frontiers in Dental Medicine. 2021;2:748089.
3. Kharbanda OP, Priya H, Balachandran R, Khurana C. Current scenario of teledentistry in public healthcare in India. Journal of the International Society for Telemedicine and eHealth. 2019;7:e10-1.
4. Macapagal J. Applications of teledentistry during the COVID-19 Pandemic Outbreak. Applied Medical Informatics. 2020;42(3):133-41.
5. Deshpande S, Patil D, Dhokar A, Bhanushali P, Katge F. Teledentistry: A boon amidst COVID-19 lockdown—a narrative review. International Journal of Telemedicine and Applications. 2021;2021.
6. Clark GT. Teledentistry: What is it now, and what will it be tomorrow? J Calif Dent Assoc. 2000;28:121-7.
7. Folke LE. Teledentistry. An overview. Tex Dent J. 2001;118:10-8.
8. Farman AG, Farag AA. Teleradiology for dentistry. Dent Clin North Am. 1993;37:669-81.
9. Bhambal A, Saxena S, Balsaraf SV. Teledentistry: potentials unexplored. J Int Oral Health. 2010;2:1–6. doi: 10.1177/2229411220110105
10. Golder DT, Brennan KA. Practicing dentistry in the age of telemedicine. J Am Dent Assoc. 2000;31:734-44. doi: 10.14219/jada.archive.2000.0272
11. Daniel SJ, Wu L, Kumar S. Teledentistry: a systematic review of clinical outcomes, utilization and costs. J Dent Hyg. 2013;87:345-52.
12. Estai M, Kanagasingam Y, Tennant M, Bunt S. A systematic review of the research evidence for the benefits of teledentistry. J Telemed Telecare. 2018;24:147-56. doi: 10.1177/1357633X16689433.
13. Haron N, Zain RB, Ramanathan A, Abraham MT, Liew CS, Ng KG. mmHealth for early detection of oral cancer in low- and middle-income countries. Telemed J e-Health. 2020;26:278–85. doi: 10.1089/tmj.2018.0285
14. Goswami, M. Chawla S. Time to restart: a comparative compilation of triage recommendations in dentistry during the COVID-19 pandemic. J Oral Biol Craniofac Res. 2020;10:374-84. doi: 10.1016/j.jobcr.2020.06.014.
15. Skandarajah A, Sunny SP, Gurpur P, Reber CD, D'Ambrosio MV, Raghavan N, et al. Mobile microscopy as a screening tool for oral cancer in India: a pilot study. PLoS ONE. 2017;12:e0188440. doi: 10.1371/journal.pone.0188440
16. Mariño R, Ghanim A. Teledentistry: a systematic review of the literature. J Telemed Telecare. 2013;19:179-83. doi: 10.1177/1357633x13479704 37.
17. Census Report 2011. Available at: http://www.censusindia.gov.in accessed 4 November 2018.
18. Project ECHO-India. 2018. Available at: https://www.echoindia.in/ accessed 8 November 2018.
19. Collaborative Digital Diagnosis System (CollabDDS). Available at: https://www.collabdds.gov.in accessed 8 November 2018.
20. Pan African e-Network Project (PAENP). 2013. Available at: https://www.mea.gov.in/Portal/ForeignRelation/Pan_A frican_e_docx_for_xp.pdf accessed 20 November 2018.
21. Maharashtra State Telemedicine Network. Available at: https://www.nrhm.maharashtra.gov.in/telemed.htm
22. Telemedicine for Rural Mass- Current Initiatives and Future Scope. Available at: http://nmcn.in/nrc/ppt/Telemedicine%20for%20Rural%20Masses%20current%20initiative%20and%20futur e%20scope%20Oditelecon.pdf.
23. Sudhamony S, Nandakumar K, Binu PJ, Niwas SI. Telemedicine and tele-health services for cancer-care delivery in India. IET Commun. 2008;2(2):231-6. DOI:10.1049/iet-com:20060701.
24. eDantSeva. Available at: http://14.143.90.243/edent/ accessed 12 November 2018.
25. Smith AC, Thomas E, Snoswell CL, Haydon H, Mehrotra A, Clemensen J, et al. Telehealth for global emergencies: Implications for coronavirus disease 2019 (COVID-19). J Telemed Telecare. 2020;26(5):309-313. Doi:10.1177/1357633X20916567.
26. Portnoy J, Waller M, Elliott T. Telemedicine in the Era of COVID-19. J Allergy Clin Immunol Pract. 2020;8(5):1489-91. Doi:10.1016/j.jaip.2020.03.008
27. Morosini Ide A, de Oliveira DC, Ferreira F, Fraiz FC, Torres-Pereira CC. Performance of distant diagnosis of dental caries by teledentistry in juvenile offenders. Telemed J E Health. 2014;20(6):584-9. Doi:10.1089/tmj.2013.020
28. Greenhalgh T, Wherton J, Shaw S, Morrison C. Video consultations for COVID-19. BMJ. 2020;368:m998. Doi:10.1136/bmj.m998
29. Martignon S, Cortes A, Douglas GV, Newton JT, Pitts NB, Avila V, et al. CariesCare International adapted for the pandemic in children: Caries OUT multicentre single-group interventional study protocol. BMC Oral Health. 2021;21(1):1-3.
30. Ueda M, Martins R, Hendrie PC. Managing cancer care during the COVID-19 pandemic: Agility and collaboration toward a common goal. J Natl Compr Canc Netw. 2020;18(4):366-9. Doi:10.6004/jnccn.2020.7560

31. Dusseja SH, Rao D, Panwar S, Ameen S. Patients' views regarding dental concerns and tele dentistry during COVID-19 pandemic. Int J Sci Healthc Res. 2020;5:423-9. Available online at: https://ijshr.com/IJSHR_Vol.5_Issue.4_ Oct2020/IJSHR_Abstract.0056.html
32. Nuvvula S, Mallineni SK. Remote management of dental problems in children during and post the COVID-19 pandemic outbreak: a teledentistry approach. Dent Med Probl. 2021;58:237-41. doi: 10.17219/dmp/133182.
33. Peng X, Xu X, Li Y, Cheng L, Zhou X, Ren B. Transmission routes of 2019-nCoV and controls in dental practice. Int J Oral Sci. 2020;12:9. doi: 10.1038/s41368-020-0075-9.

FURTHER READING

1. American Dental Association. Summary of ADA Guidance During the COVID-19 Crisis [Internet]. 2020 [cited 2020 May 5].
2. Mandall NA, O'Brien KD, Brady J, Worthington HV, Harvey L. Teledentistry for screening new patient orthodontic referrals. Part 1: A randomised controlled trial. Br Dent J. 2005;199(10):659-62. Doi:10.1038/sj.bdj.4812930
3. Estai M, Kanagasingam Y, Huang B, Checker H, Steele L, Kruger E, et al. The efficacy of remote screening for dental caries by mid-level dental providers using a mobile teledentistry model. Community Dent Oral Epidemiol. 2016;44(5):435-41. Doi:10.1111/cdoe.12232
4. Hollander JE, Carr BG. Virtually Perfect? Telemedicine for Covid-19. N Engl J Med. 2020;382:1679-1681. Doi: 10.1056/NEJMp2003539
5. Patterson S, Botchway C. Dental screenings using telehealth technology: a pilot study. J Can Dent Assoc. 1998;64(11):806-10.
6. Torres-Pereira C, Possebon RS, Simões A, Bortoluzzi MC, Leão JC, Giovanini AF, et al. Email for distance diagnosis of oral diseases: a preliminary study of teledentistry. J Telemed Telecare. 2008;14(8):435-8. Doi:10.1258/jtt.2008.080510
7. Greenhalgh T. COVID-19: a remote assessment in primary care. BMJ. 2020;368:m1182. Doi:10.1136/bmj.m1182.
8. Davies A, Howells R, Lee SMG, Sweet CJ, Dominguez-Gonzalez S. Implementation of photographic triage in a paediatric dental, orthodontic, and maxillofacial department during COVID-19. Int J Paediatr Dent. 2020;31:547–53. doi: 10.1111/ipd.12773 19.
9. Rahman N, Nathwani S, Kandiah T. Teledentistry from a patient perspective during the coronavirus pandemic. Br Dent J. 2020; 229:1-4. doi: 10.1038/s41415-020-1919-6.
10. National Health Programs in India. Available at: https://www.nhp.gov.in/healthprogramme/national-health-programmes accessed 8 November 2018.
11. Life Expectancy in India; World Life Expectancy - WHO Data 2018. Available at: https://www.worldlifeexpectancy.com/india-life-expectancy accessed 24 November 2018.
12. Shah N, Pandey R, Duggal R, Mathur U, Kumar R. Oral health survey in India: A report of multicentric study, WHO – Oral health survey 2004. Geneva, Switzerland: World Health Organization; 2007. Available from: http://www.whoindia.org/en/section20/section30_1525.htm.

CHAPTER 82

Patents and Innovations in Pediatric Dentistry

Vaibhav Kumar, Suneet Sable

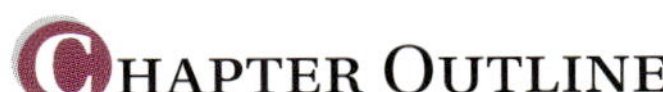

CHAPTER OUTLINE

- Patent
- Patenting in Pediatric Dentistry
- Patent Resource Triad
- Steps for Getting a Patent

Today, patents mostly protect inventions in the field of health research and intellectual property. If you are reading this book and if you are interested in Pediatric Dentistry and its use in the industry or any other innovative idea related to dentistry that you may come up with, then you should file a patent to protect your invention. It is interesting to note that in 2003, the toothbrush was chosen as the number one invention Americans could not live without, beating out the automobile, computer, cell phone, and microwave oven, according to the Lemelson-MIT Invention Index.

Patents are essentially granted for the new inventions, worldwide, inventions that are not an obvious modification to a Person Skilled In The Art (PHOSITA), and must have tangible use, not abstract ideas that cannot be brought into practice. Patent rights are negative rights, as they prevent others from using the patented inventions. Basically, a patent provides a monopoly to its owner. A patent is crucial for commercialization of the invention and to protect the monopoly. Starting off, protecting your intellectual property (IP) can be a daunting task, but do you know what's even worse? If you do not secure your intellectual property, you risk losing all of your amazing ideas and hard work to a competitor. Most of the patents filed in the 18th century were for:

- Artificial teeth/tooth replacement procedures
- Oral hygiene apparatus
- Jaw, tooth models, dental equipment
- Compositions for tooth replacing materials
- Dental floss

All these patents were in the US and China, mostly by individuals. In the first half of the 19th century, 3-D printing in dental industry, dental lasers, and dental education models are some areas of the domain that are popular. The dental equipment market is a very lucrative industry and the intellectual property (IP) landscape is very complex and overcrowded in the area of dental equipment.

PATENT

- *A patent is a grant of exclusive monopoly of rights granted to an 'inventor' (individual/company or organization) by the government (of India) to exclude other to prevent duplication, make use, offer to sell, sell/import, in a particulate jurisdiction (country), for a limited period of time* (In India, it is 20 years from the date of filing the patent application).
- *A patent is a techno-legal document that establishes intellectual property/ownership for a patentee (inventor) over their idea. The idea needs to be novel, enabling and practically amenable to be reduced to practice—displaying potential and extrapolation for industrial applicability.*

PATENTING IN PEDIATRIC DENTISTRY

Due to intensive research in universities, dentistry has acquired an interest in the realm of intellectual property, such as patents, in recent years. As it is a category that is constantly evolving and innovating, manufacturers and industries must pay close attention to stay competitive and satisfy the expectations of the domestic and international markets for dental products.

Why you should consider patenting your invention?

- You own the invention for a given time (20 years).
- Rent/license it to existing businesses.
- You can use it to build, bootstrap and augment a business venture.
- You can completely sell the patent to other company.

How much does it cost to get a patent in India?

- There are two elements for cost of getting patent
  1. The government fees for forms, requests and renewals. (fixed)
  2. Professional charges for patent professional, patent agency/attorney (variable-based on expertise and experience).

PATENT RESOURCE TRIAD

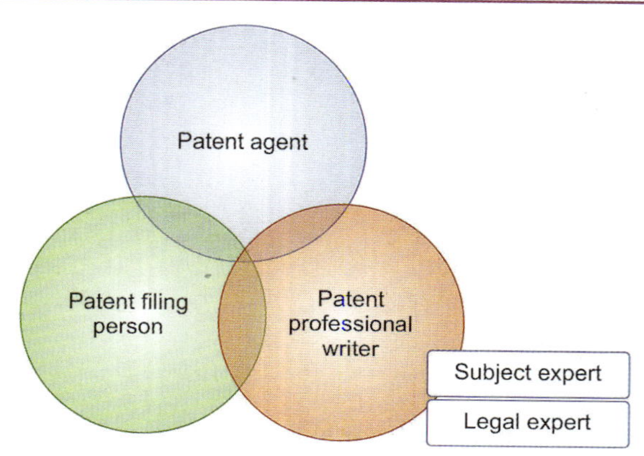

Types of Patents Granted in India

- Ordinary/non-provisional application
- Convetional application
- PCT international application
- PCT national phase application
- Patent of addition
- Divisional application

STEPS FOR GETTING A PATENT

Step 1: Invention disclosure
Step 2: Non-disclosure agreement
Step 3: Is my invention patentable?
Step 4: Writing and filling patent application
Step 5: Publication of the article
Step 6: Request for examination
Step 7: Response to objections in examination report
Step 8: Grant of patent

Step 1: Invention Disclosure

- Write down the invention with as much detail as possible.
- Area and nature of the invention.
- Description of the invention—what it does?
- How does it work?
- Similar existing solutions/products like your invention
- Advantages of your invention over existing solutions
- Include diagrams or sketches explaining the working of invention.

Step 2: Non-disclosure Agreement

When discussing with patent professionals, supervisors, partners, technical assistants, etc. You need to protect the confidentiality of it by the way of signing a non-disclosure agreement (NDA) by the parties to whom you are disclosing the invention.

Step 3: Is My Invention Patentable?

The patentability (Novelty search): Finds out whether your invention meets all patentability criteria as per Indian Patent Act.

1. Novelty means that the invention comprising of a product or a process should not have been anticipated by publication in any document or should not have been used in the country or anywhere in the world before filing of the patent application.
2. A patent should be non-obvious, means a person of ordinary skill should not be able to replicate the invention based on prior skill set.
3. The patent should have industrial applicability.

What cannot be patented?
Inventions with regard to:
- Atomic energy
- Inventions against public morality and decency
- Agricultural and horticultural methods
- Medical and surgical phenomenon
- Method of treatment cannot get a patent

Step 4: Writing and Filling Patent Application

Two ways to proceed about patent filing:

1. **Provisional Patent filing:** In case you are at a very early stage in the research and development of your invention, it gives you the following benefits:
   - Secures filing date, priority date
   - 12 months of time to file complete specification
   - Low cost
2. **Complete patent application:** The complete patent application includes entire description of the invention, diagrams, embodiments and claims. PCT is an ideal route when you want to file your application for multiple countries, but you are not sure in which countries your patent application will have commercial value, precisely where you can manufacture and sell or export your product, and where there is a good number of buyers. This 30-month time can be utilized to evaluate all these possibilities. A PCT (Patent Cooperation Treaty) application provides three advantages:
   - International priority—which means, if someone fires the same invention for patenting before your patents application is published, you will get priority in the signatory country.
   - Patentability report—this will validate the possibility of getting a patent. Government authorities issue this report.
     - Extending time to file a patent application in multiple countries approximately—you get 30 months to file the same patent application in other

countries. Whereas in the conventional route, you get only 12 months to file the same patent application in multiple countries.

- Filing of patent—file according to jurisdiction in 4 Patent Offices in India viz. Mumbai, Chennai, New Delhi, Kolkata (Head Office)
- Application scrutiny
  - Appropriate jurisdiction.
  - Proof or right to file
  - Relevant document submission
  - Preparation of examination report by the examiner for the approval of the Controller General.
  - Application is published after 18 months from the filing date. (To speed up this process optionally an early publication request can be made if you do not wish to wait till the expiry of 18 months from the date of filing for publishing your patent application.)
  - In the event of absence of an opposition and successfully substantiating the objection raised in the examination report, the patent is granted and published in the official journal.

Step 5: Publication of the Application (in the Patent Journal)

- Once the complete specifications are filed, the application is considered for publication after 18 months from the date of filing.
- This step does not require any special prerequisites from the applicant. Early publication requests can also be made by paying a prescribed fee and filling 'From 9'. Such applications get published within one month of the request, reducing the wait time of 18 months.

Step 6: Request for Examination

- Only upon receiving this request the controller gives your application to a patent examiner who examines the patent application with different patentability criteria.
- The first examination report submitted to controller by examiner generally contains objections raised to the patent application.

Step 7: Respond to Objections in Examination Report

- Majority of the patent applicants will receive some type of objections based in examination report.
- The best thing to do is to analyze the examination report with patent professional (patent agent) and creating a response to the objections raised in the report.

Step 8: Grant of Patient

- The application would be places in order for grant once it is found to be meeting all patentability.
- Despite the havoc caused in the global economy by the COVID-19 pandemic, innovators around the world managed to file what, given the circumstances, is an impressive 3.3 million patent applications in 2020. This represents an increase of 1.6% on 2019. With favorable government initiatives and policies in place, the entire world is seeking 'The East'. The future is not near, it is here!

POINTS TO REMEMBER

- In india, a patent is valid only for up to 20 years from the date of filing the application.
- Medical or surgical phenomena and methods of treatment cannot be patented.
- Patent filing is of two types:
  1. Provisional patent filing
  2. Complete patent filing
- A Patent Cooperation Treaty (PCT) provides an international priority and patentability report, hence validating the possibility of getting a patent

Questionnaire

1. Why are patents important?
2. What comprises the patent resource triad?
3. What are the procedures that are barrad from being granted a patent?

FURTHER READING

1. Sampat BN, Shadle KC. Patent watch: Drug patenting in India: looking back and looking forward. Nat Rev Drug Discov. 2015;14(8):519-20; doi:10.1038/nrd4681.
2. Tulasi GK, Rao BS. A detailed study of patent system for protection of inventions. Indian J Pharm Sci. 2008;70(5):547-54. doi:10.4103/0250-474X.45390.
3. Patents I intellectual Property India/Government of India. Accessed December 5, 2022. https://ipindia.gov.in/patents.htm
4. Rupinder Tewari, Mamta Bhardwaj. Intellectual Property- A Primer for Academia, 2021st edition. Publication Bureau Punjab University, Chandigarh.
5. India-Protecting Intellectual Property. Accessed December 5, 2022. https://www.trade.gov/country-commercal guides/india-protecting-intellectual-property.
6. Official website of Intellectual Property India. Accessed December 5, 2022. https://ipindia.gov.in/
7. Bagade OM, Pujari RR, Vanave MD, Shete AM, Kharat PP, Nemlekar NA. Evolving Pace of Patent in India and its Corollary in Past, Present and Future. AJADD. 2014;2(4);503-21.
8. Rupinder Tewari, Mamta Bhardwaj. Mapping Patents and Research Publications of Higher Education Institutes and National R&D Laboratories of India, 2018th edition.

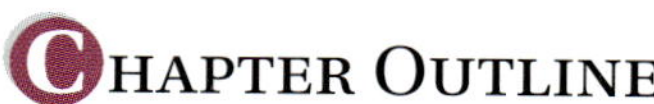

Stem Cells in Pediatric Dentistry

Viral Maru

Chapter Outline

It is said that human cells possess an extraordinary ability to reform or regenerate. Even though most of the cells found in animal tissues can reform uninterruptedly, certain inequalities lie with regard to the proliferation process. Some of these cells can develop into other cell lines and not just into cells pertaining to their original tissues. Such types of undifferentiated cells are called stem cells or progenitor cells that have the capability to specialize into multiple cell forms and ability to self-renew. By utilizing stem cells inherent propensity to specialize into specific cell types, regenerative medicine is able to substitute and help restore cellular functions. Adult stem cells (ASCs) are present in great number within the teeth, and human dental pulp stem cells (hDPSCs) are a significant source of them. hDPSCs have been employed in tissue reconstruction because of their excellent proliferation, capability to undergo multilineage differentiation and self-renew.

Russian histologist named **Alexander Maksimov** recommended the term 'stem cell' in 1908. It took many years until researchers were finally able to discover the applications of these stem cells to regenerate human cells that were previously damaged due to illnesses, accidents and congenital defects.

- *Stem cells (SCs) are defined as clonogenic, self-renewing, progenitor cells that can generate one or more specialized cell types (**Suchanek J**, 2007).*
- *Stem cells (SCs) are defined as cells that have the ability to continuously divide and produce progeny cells that differentiate into various other types of cells or tissues (**Rao**, 2004).*
- *Stem cells are defined as clonogenic cells that are capable of both self-renewal and multilineage differentiation (**Weissman**, 2000).*

FEATURES OF STEM CELLS

- **Ability of self-renewal**: This characteristic is uniformly present in all varieties of SCs. One daughter cell will be an identical clone of the parent and will remain a stem cell, whereas the other daughter cell may be similar (symmetrical division) or may differentiate, as asymmetrical division. Self-renewal guarantees that SCs population do not deplete during the course of an organism's lifetime.
- **Pluripotency**: It refers to having multiple possible outcomes. It denotes the capacity to generate cells/tissues from either mesoderm or endoderm or ectoderm germ layer, with the exception of extraembryonic tissues.
- **Clonality**: If a cell is produced through the division of a single cell and is genetically identical to that cell, it is clonally derived. Human pluripotent stem cells are clonally produced from embryos and fetal tissue.
- **Plasticity**: this refers to the capability of stem cells to undergo differentiation from one lineage to another. SCs can be genetically designed to convert into specialized cells of various tissues in a controlled condition.

CLASSIFICATION OF STEM CELLS

1. **Based on maturation**
   a. Embryonic stem cells
   b. Adult stem cells
      i. Mesenchymal stem cell
         1. Alveolar bone-derived mesenchymal stem cells (ABMSCs)
         2. Stem cell derived from human exfoliated deciduous teeth (SHED)
            » Mesenchymal
            » Adipocytes
            » Chondrocytes and osteoblasts
         3. Gingival MSC (GMSC)
         4. Dental pulp stem cells (DPSCs)
         5. Tooth germ progenitor cells (TGPCs)
         6. Dental follicle stem cells (DFSCs)
         7. Stem cells derived from apical papilla (SCAP)
         8. Periodontal ligament stem cells (PDLSCs)
      ii. Hematopoietic stem cell
      iii. Neural stem cell
      iv. Skin stem cell
      v. Epithelial stem cell
2. **Based on potency**
   a. Totipotent stem cell
   b. Pluripotent stem cell
   c. Multipotent stem cell
   d. Unipotent stem cell
   e. Precursor stem cell

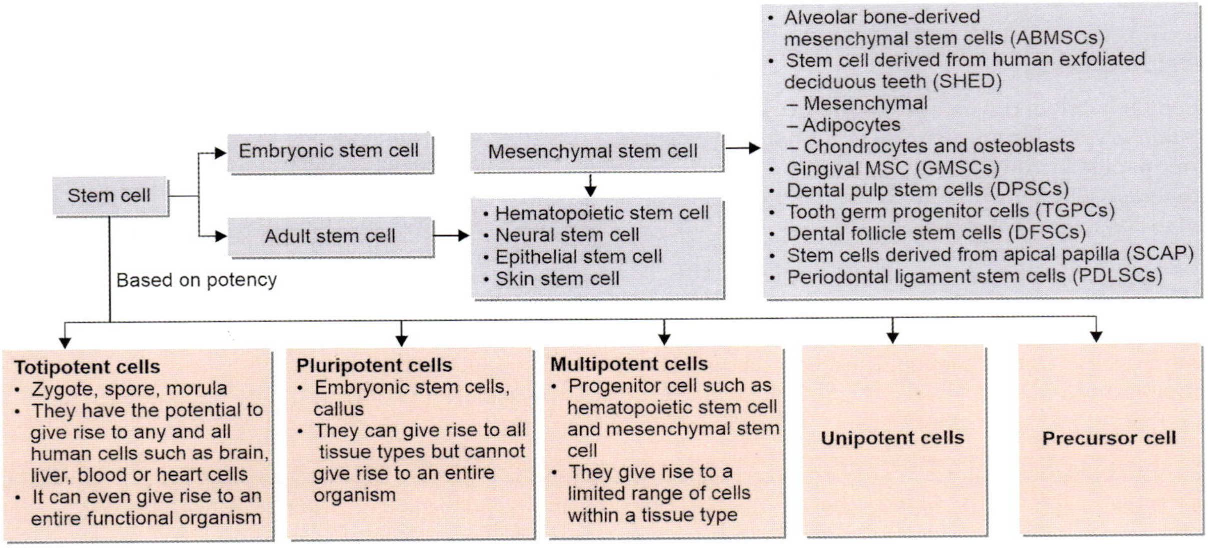

Stem cell
→ Embryonic stem cell
→ Adult stem cell → • Hematopoietic stem cell • Neural stem cell • Epithelial stem cell • Skin stem cell
Mesenchymal stem cell → • Alveolar bone-derived mesenchymal stem cells (ABMSCs) • Stem cell derived from human exfoliated deciduous teeth (SHED) – Mesenchymal – Adipocytes – Chondrocytes and osteoblasts • Gingival MSC (GMSCs) • Dental pulp stem cells (DPSCs) • Tooth germ progenitor cells (TGPCs) • Dental follicle stem cells (DFSCs) • Stem cells derived from apical papilla (SCAP) • Periodontal ligament stem cells (PDLSCs)

Based on potency

Totipotent cells
- Zygote, spore, morula
- They have the potential to give rise to any and all human cells such as brain, liver, blood or heart cells
- It can even give rise to an entire functional organism

Pluripotent cells
- Embryonic stem cells, callus
- They can give rise to all tissue types but cannot give rise to an entire organism

Multipotent cells
- Progenitor cell such as hematopoietic stem cell and mesenchymal stem cell
- They give rise to a limited range of cells within a tissue type

Unipotent cells

Precursor cell

EMBRYONIC STEM CELLS

- **Martin** in 1981 coined the term 'Embryonic stem cell.'
- Cleavage of the early embryo produces the fertilized oocyte, zygote, two-cell, four-cell, eight-cell, and morula. After numerous rounds of cellular division, the morula cells specialize within 5 to 6 days after conception, resulting in formation of blastocyst.
- A 5 to 6 days old human blastocyst's inner cell mass (ICM) is used to produce pluripotent human embryonic stem cells (hESCs).
- Using or harvesting these cells, results in damage of the embryo, thus making the use of these cells morally questionable.

ADULT STEM CELLS

- Somatic or adult stem cells contain all non-embryonic stem cells and are referred to as undifferentiated cells that can be found in the body alongside differentiated cells.
- They function to help in healing, growth as well as to generate new cells to substitute the damaged or dead cells.
- These cells are present in tissues like the umbilical cord, muscle, bone marrow, gut, placenta, brain, skin, fat tissue and other tissues.
- They have limited differentiation potential with regards to the cells from the native tissue.

Differences between embryonic and adult stem cells.

	Embryonic stem cells	*Adult stem cells*
1.	They originate from inner cell mass of blastocyst	They have no definite origin
2.	They have no capacity to undergo replicative senescence	They do undergo replicative senescence
3.	Possibility of host rejection is high	Possibility of host rejection is minimal
4.	Easy to isolate from blastocyst	Difficult to isolate in adult tissues
5.	Highly stable	Comparatively less stable
6.	High capacity for self-renewal	Limited capacity for self-renewal
7.	Pluripotent in nature	Multipotent in nature

Hematopoietic Stem Cells (HSCs)

- HSCs are deemed as architects of definitive hematopoiesis, i.e., blood cell production, which keeps occurring during an organism's lifetime.
- These cells can be defined based on their capabilities such as pluripotential—a single HSC's capacity to generate all of the different mature functional hematopoietic cell types.

Neural Stem Cells

- These cells are referred to as a subtype of progenitor cells of the nervous system and these can self-renew and produce both glia and neurons.
- These cells are present in the subventricular zone, hippocampus and in certain non-neurogenic regions that include the spinal cord.

Epithelial Stem Cells

- The epithelial stem cell niches are primarily regional, e.g., intestinal crypt being the niche for intestinal stem cells and kidney papilla for kidney stem cells.
- To maintain a lifelong mature cell production, these cells need to constantly self-renew.

Skin Stem Cells

- These cells are concerned with the continual regeneration of skin as well as wound healing. The epidermis basal layer includes skin stem cells.
- Currently, in clinics, these cells are employed to heal, the skin for patients faced with serious genetic disorders and burn injuries.

Mesenchymal Stem Cells (MSCs)

- These cells are usually associated with numerous tissues in the body.
- These are non-hematopoietic multipotent cells that are potential of differentiating into adipocytes, osteocytes, and chondrocytes, as well as endodermal (hepatocytes) and ectodermal (neurocytes) cell lines.
- Dental tissues, adipose tissue, endometrial, menstrual blood, limb bud, placenta, synovial fluid, salivary gland, skin and foreskin, peripheral blood, and the umbilical cord lining membrane are also good sources of mesenchymal cells.
- MSCs can self-renew and also possess in vitro capacity that allows them to differentiate into all the three lineages, i.e., mesoderm, ectoderm and endoderm, along with potency when used with suitable media and growth supplements to initiate lineage differentiation.
- They also have immunosuppressive attributes.
- Types of MSCs (named after the tissue they are extracted from):
  - Alveolar bone-derived mesenchymal stem cells (ABMSCs)
  - Stem cell derived from human exfoliated deciduous teeth (SHED)
  - Gingival MSC (GMSC)

Characteristics of different dental tissues derived MSCs (Fig. 83.1).

Type of dental stem cells	*Surface antigens*	*Immunomodulatory functions*	*Differentiation potential*
Dental pulp stem cells (DPSCs)	CD13, CD29, CD44, CD59, CD73, CD90, CD105, CD146, STRO-1	Release of transforming growth factor beta (TGF-β), prostaglandin E2 (PGE2) and interleukin-6 (IL-6); stimulation of T cells to release TGF-β	Odontogenic, angiogenic, myogenic, adipogenic, osteogenic, and neurogenic
Stem cell from apical papilla (SCAP)	CD146, CD90, CD44, CD24, STRO-1	Suppression of T cell proliferation	Osteogenic, odontogenic, neurogenic, adipogenic, and chondrogenic
Periodontal ligament stem cell (PDLSC)	CD105, CD73, CD44, CD29, CD10	Suppression of IL-1β production; suppression of peripheral blood mononuclear cells (PBMNCs) proliferation; down regulation of tumor necrosis factor-α (TNF-α).	Chondrogenic, osteogenic, neurogenic, and adipogenic
Gingival derived mesenchymal stem cell (GMSC)	CD73, CD90, CD105	Upregulation of interleukin-10 (IL-10); suppression of mast cell degranulation; suppression of PBMNCs proliferation	Chondrogenic, osteogenic, adipogenic, angiogenic, and neurogenic
Alveolar bone derived mesenchymal stem cell (ABMSC)	CD73, CD90, CD105, STRO-1	Immunosuppressive effects on monocyte and T cell activation; secretion of interleukin (IL)-6 and monocyte chemoattractant protein (MCP)-1	Osteogenic and adipogenic
Dental follicle stem cell (DFSC)	CD13, CD29, CD44, CD49d, CD56, CD59, CD90, CD105, CD106, CD166, STRO-1	Upregulation of TGF- and IL-6 secretion; suppression of PBMNCs proliferation	Odontogenic, cementogenic, and osteogenic
Tooth germ stem cell (TGSC)	CD73, CD90, CD105, CD166	-	Osteogenic, adipogenic, chondrogenic, and neurogenic
Stem cell derived from human exfoliated deciduous teeth (SHED)	CD166, CD146, CD90, CD73, CD29	Repression of T helper 17 (Th17) lymphocytes; upregulation of CD206+ M2 macrophages	Osteogenic, chondrogenic, adipogenic, odontogenic, angiogenic, and neurogenic

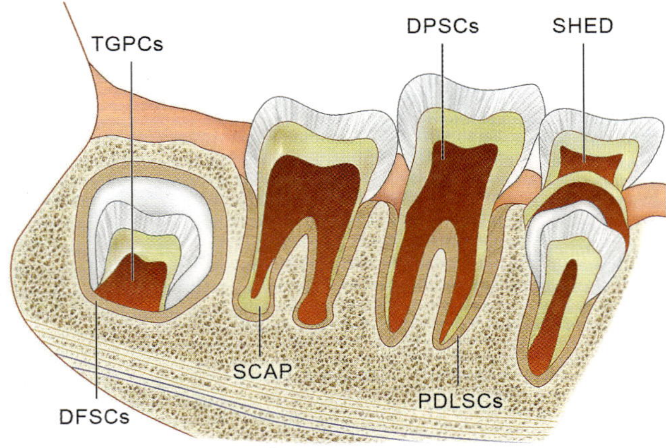

Fig. 83.1: Different types of dental mesenchymal stem cell population.

- Dental pulp stem cells (DPSCs)
- Tooth germ progenitor cells (TGPCs)
- Dental follicle stem cells (DFSCs)
- Stem cells derived from apical papilla (SCAP)
- Periodontal ligament stem cells (PDLSCs).

Dental Pulp Stem Cells (DPSCs)

- **Yamamura** was the first to discover dental pulp stem cells in 1985. It was the first form of dental stem cell to be identified.
- In 2002, **Gronthos et al**., isolated DPSCs from a patient's caries-free permanent molar. The pulp tissue of an impacted human third molar was enzymatically digested to obtain these cells.
- The appearance of DPSCs is similar to that of fibroblasts. They are clonogenic, and even after prolonged sub-culturing, they can sustain a high rate of multiplication. Even after freezing or cryopreservation, DPSCs are able to preserve stem cell characteristics. Certain studies indicate that a subtype of DPSCs known as "immature dental pulp stem cells" (IDPSCs) has significant prospects for future research. IDPSCs have been isolated from both permanent and primary dental pulp tissue.

Periodontal Ligament Stem Cells (PDLSCs)

- In addition to anchoring the teeth, the PDL aids to its nutrition, homeostasis, and healing. The tissue's heterogeneity and constant remodeling confirmed the existence of stem cells, that can be cultivated to differentiated cells. This observation led to the development of cells known as Periodontal Ligament Stem Cells in 2004. PDLSCs were first introduced by **Seo et al.,** 2004.
- They have a multilineage differentiation potential when cultured with the appropriate inductive medium.

Stem Cells from Apical Papilla (SCAP)

- The connective tissue found at the apex of the root of developing permanent teeth, which differs from the pulp, is known as the apical papilla. The apical papilla contains a richer source of mesenchymal stem cells when compared to the dental pulp. These cells were first identified and characterized by **Sonoyama et al.,** 2008, in human permanent immature teeth.
- SCAPs are clonogenic fibroblast-like cells, but have a higher proliferation rate than DPSCs.
- SCAPs have the capacity to undergo osteogenic, adipogenic, chondrogenic and neurogenic differentiation, when they are cultured in the appropriate inductive media.

Dental Follicle Precursor Cells (DFPCs)

- The dental follicle is a loose connective tissue of an ectomesenchymal origin and it is present as a sac surrounding the unerupted tooth. During tooth development it has been found that dental follicle plays an important role in the eruption process by controlling the osteoclastogenesis and osteogenesis needed for eruption.
- In 2005, **Morsczeck et al.,** isolated stem cells from the dental follicle of the human impacted third molar. The potential of DFPCs to undergo osteogenic, adipogenic and neurogenic differentiation was demonstrated in, in-vitro studies. In vivo transplantation of DFPCs with ceramic discs showed no evidence of dentine like structure but on the other hand there was presence of cement/immature bone-like structures with the osteocytes/cementocytes.

Stem Cells from Inflamed Dental Pulp

- Inflamed pulp, discarded during pulp therapy procedures were observed to be potential source for harvesting adult stem cells.
- According to **Saha et al**., adult MSCs derived from inflammatory dental pulp have evolved into multiple lineages, including osteoblasts, adipocytes, and chondrocytes.

Stem Cells Derived from Human Exfoliated Deciduous Teeth (SHEDs)

- **Songtao Shi et al**. [National Institutes of Health, USA] discovered multipotent progenitor cells in human exfoliated deciduous tooth, which they referred to as SHED, in 2003.
- SHED can also be referred to as a type of MSCs originally derived from the cranial neural crest ectomesenchyme. SHEDs are also referred as "immature DPSCs" due to the presence of immature cells in exfoliating primary teeth.
- Almost all of the SHEDs are fibroblast-like and spindle-shaped, while few may be cuboidal, polygonal or oval and remain adhered to the plastic tissue culture surface.
- The legal and ethical implications can be regarded as being negligible, since SHEDs have been derived from an exfoliating deciduous tooth.
- Types of SHEDs:
  - Adipocytes: The use of adipocytes to restore cardiac muscle damage following a serious heart attack has proved successful. It appears that they may be effective in the treatment of neurological and orthopedic conditions as well as coronary heart disease.
  - Chondrocytes and osteoblasts: Bone and cartilage may now be grown from these cells and utilized in transplants. Additionally, a complete set of animal teeth was created using them.
  - Mesenchymal: Using MSCs, paraplegic patients have been able to regain sensation and motion. Since MSCs

may form neuronal groups, they have the capacity to manage various types of neurodegenerative disorders such as Parkinsonism, Alzheimerism and many others.

- **Nakajima K et al**. 2019, examined the success rate as well as influencing factors of isolation of DPSCs and SHEDs and concluded that successful isolation of SHEDs was related to root condition, patient's age, mechanical stress to the teeth and length of the remaining root.
- **Werle SB et al.** 2016, reported identical capacity for tissue differentiation with regards to the stem cells derived from both sound and decayed primary teeth.
- **Tsai and co-workers** 2017, investigated the predictors pertaining to success rate defining the cultivation of SHEDs. Successful isolation of MSCs could be achieved in 63.3% of teeth lacking any caries versus only 12.5% in teeth that had severe caries.

Totipotent Stem Cells

- They have the potential to give rise to any and all human cells like brain, liver, blood or heart cells.
- It can give rise to an entire functional organism

Pluripotent Stem Cells

They can give rise to all tissue types but can't give rise to an organism, e.g., Ectoderm, endoderm.

Multipotent Stem Cells

They give rise to limited range of cell within a tissue type, e.g., Neural stem cells.

Unipotent Stem Cell

These stem cells can produce only one cell type but have the property of self-renewal that distinguishes them from non-stem cells, e.g., Epidermal stem cell producing skin.

Precursor Stem Cells

They are stem cells that have developed to the stage where they are committed to forming a particular kind of new blood cell.

STEM CELL BANKING

While stem cell banks that isolate cells from umbilical cord blood and bone marrow have been around for decade at least, but banks that isolate stem cells from teeth are newer. Particularly in United Kingdom, North America and India, the number of such banks is increasing. In 2004, Hiroshima University in Japan developed one of the first dental stem cells banks dedicated on stem cell preservation **(Table 83.1)**.

Table 83.1: Stem cell banking services available worldwide.

Dental pulp stem cell banking services	*Location of company*	*Collection of sample by (website)*	*Website*
Mothercell	India	Dentist	https://www.mothercell.com
ReeLabs	India	Unspecified	https://www.reelabs.com
Stemade	India	Dentist	http://www.stemade.com/
Store your cells	India	Dentist	https://www.storeyourcells.com
Dentcell	Mexico	Patient or dentist	https://dentcell.com.mx/
Future Health Biobank	UK	Patient	https://futurehealthbiobank.com
Stem Protect	UK	Patient	https://www.stemprotect.co.uk/
National Dental Pulp Laboratory	USA	Dentist	https://ndpl.net
Oothy	USA	Patient or dentist	https://www.oothy.com
Stemodontics	USA	Dentist	https://stemodontics.com/
Store-A-Tooth/ Provia Labs	USA	Dentist	http://www.store-a-tooth.com/
Tooth Bank/ Cryopoint	USA	Patient or dentist	https://www.toothbank.com/
Stem Save	USA	Dentist	https://www.stemsave.com/
BioEden	USA	Patient or dentist	https://www.bioeden.com/us/

Collection of Exfoliating Deciduous Teeth

- In order to isolate SHEDs, it is desirable to choose vital anterior deciduous teeth either from the maxilla or the mandible.
- Because of anatomical concerns, teeth distal to the primary canine are deemed undesirable, due to difficulty in the extirpation of the pulp tissue. Eruption of the subsequent underlying teeth typically necessitates a longer period to resorb the roots of primary molars, leading to an obliterated pulp chamber and thus possessing a very small amount of pulp tissue.
- Primary teeth that have been extracted for orthodontic procedures can also be deemed as good candidates, as these possess optimum sufficient pulp tissue.
- When compared with other teeth, the total numbers of cells isolated from the canines are found to be much more in numbers. More amount of pulp tissue could be associated with longer, unresorbed roots of the canines that were extracted in order to manage crowding of the anterior teeth.

Steps Followed for Tooth Collection

The first step is to instruct the parents/guardians to place the exfoliating primary teeth in sterile normal saline solution and contact the stem cell bank or the bank's resident dentist.

↓

The presence of red pulp tissue in an exfoliating primary tooth implies that the pulp had some amount of blood flow until the time of extraction, indicating good viability of cells. The pulp's blood supply is considered to be compromised, if the pulp is gray in color and as a result, the stem cells would have probably become necrotic and won't be capable of regeneration

Contd...

Contd...

↓

Extremely mobile teeth, whether caused by trauma or carious infection, are frequently associated with a disrupted blood flow and are therefore ineligible for isolation of pulp stem cells. After an extraction, it is preferable to harvest stem cells from primary teeth rather than a tooth with mobility that is "hanging on by a thread." **(Fig. 83.2).**

↓

Teeth with tumors, cysts or dentoalveolar abscesses are not the optimal sources for obtaining pulpal stem cells.

↓

In case of a planned extraction, the resident dentist examines the freshly extracted primary tooth to identify the likelihood of vital pulpal tissue. This specimen is then placed in a vial or centrifuge tube containing phosphate buffered saline (hypotonic solution), that provides nourishment and avoids the drying of tissue during transport (maximum of 4 teeth in the 1 vial) **(Fig. 83.3).**

↓

Storing this specimen in the vial at 37°C (room temperature) causes hypothermia. This vial is sealed and put in a thermette, which acts as a temperature phase change vehicle, before being placed in a metal transport insulated container. The thermette and the insulated container keep the specimen hypothermic throughout transport. This process is called as sustentation **(Fig. 83.4).**

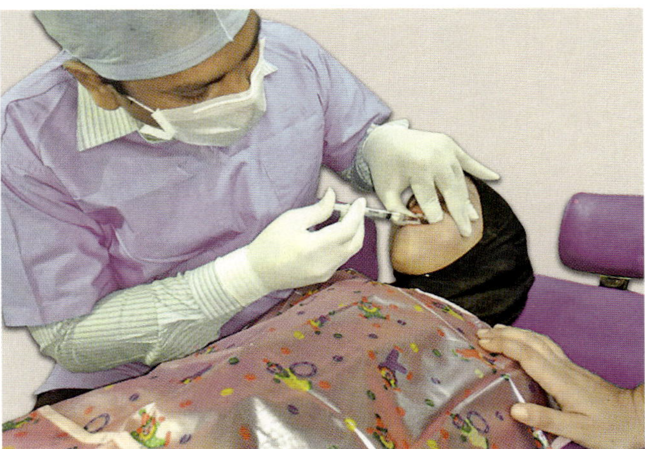

Fig. 83.2: Extraction of specimens (exfoliating deciduous teeth) by dentist from stem cell bank.

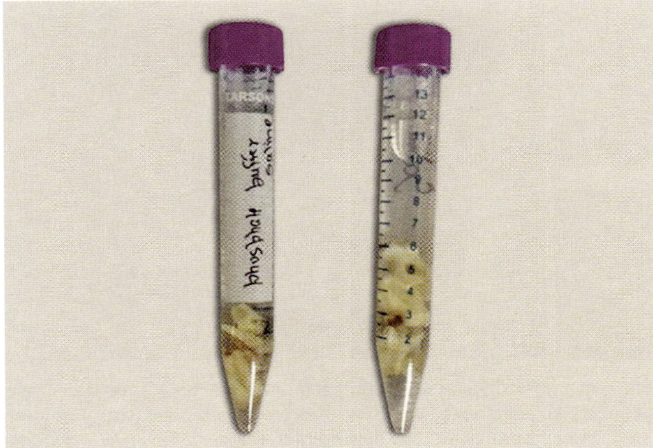

Fig. 83.3: Storage of specimens in centrifuge tubes containing buffer saline.

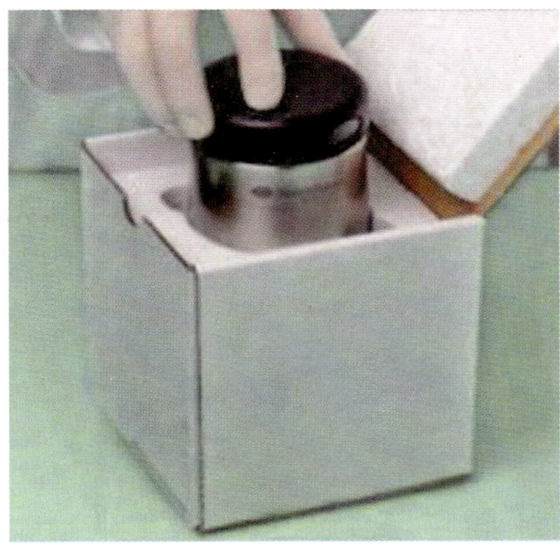

Fig. 83.4: Transport of specimens in thermette and insulate metal container.

Transport

- Numerous researches have assessed the efficacy of various dental preservation mediums.
- Balanced salt solutions such as phosphate buffered saline (PBS) and hanks buffered saline solution (HBSS) are most preferred among tooth banking companies. BioEden prefers bovine milk as transport medium.
- A number of practical needs are met by bovine milk like it is non-toxic, has a neutral pH, and is physiologically buffered.
- 'Store-A-Tooth', a well-known tooth bank transports the pulp stem cells from the dental clinic to the research lab using the same 'Save-A-Tooth' equipment used for transferring avulsed teeth.
- Stem cell viability is sensitive to both time and temperature, necessitating meticulous monitoring to guarantee that the sample remains viable. The time between collection of sample and arrival at the processing facility should not be more than 40 hours.

Isolation of SHEDs

- Typically, SHEDs isolation is carried out based on two methods, namely a tissue explant and an enzymatic digestion.
- The enzymatic digestion method normally employs type I collagenase and 4 mg/mL dispase that is mixed with the enzyme solution for 1 hour at 37°C to digest the minced pulp tissues from deciduous teeth.
- The tissue explant method involves keeping divided pulp tissues on tissue culture dishes to allow cells to grow from the tissues. When compared with the tissue outgrowth technique, the enzymatic digestion method yields a more diverse group of isolated cells.

- **Bakopoulou A et al.** 2011, showed that non-identical cultivation techniques would yield various cell lines corresponding to their differentiation and phenotypic characteristics. The study also demonstrated that higher mineralization ability in vitro was associated with enzymatic digestion - resulting SHEDs.
- **Jeon M** 2014, demonstrated that higher colony forming unit capacity, cell proliferation and adipogenic differentiation potential were associated with the isolation of SHEDs that employed enzymatic digestion.

Procedure for Isolation and Cultivation of SHEDs (Figs. 83.5 A to I)

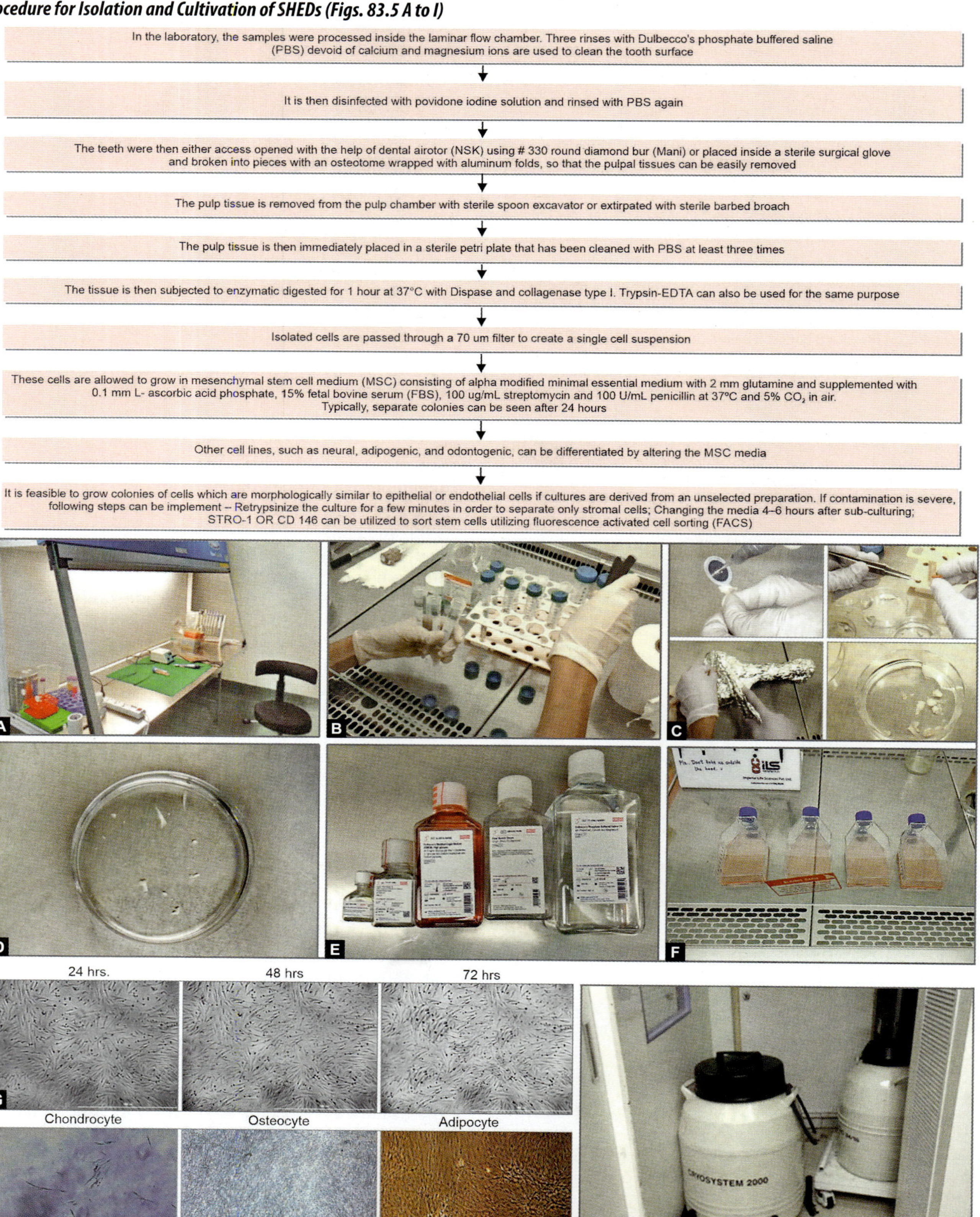

In the laboratory, the samples were processed inside the laminar flow chamber. Three rinses with Dulbecco's phosphate buffered saline (PBS) devoid of calcium and magnesium ions are used to clean the tooth surface
↓
It is then disinfected with povidone iodine solution and rinsed with PBS again
↓
The teeth were then either access opened with the help of dental airotor (NSK) using # 330 round diamond bur (Mani) or placed inside a sterile surgical glove and broken into pieces with an osteotome wrapped with aluminum folds, so that the pulpal tissues can be easily removed
↓
The pulp tissue is removed from the pulp chamber with sterile spoon excavator or extirpated with sterile barbed broach
↓
The pulp tissue is then immediately placed in a sterile petri plate that has been cleaned with PBS at least three times
↓
The tissue is then subjected to enzymatic digested for 1 hour at 37°C with Dispase and collagenase type I. Trypsin-EDTA can also be used for the same purpose
↓
Isolated cells are passed through a 70 um filter to create a single cell suspension
↓
These cells are allowed to grow in mesenchymal stem cell medium (MSC) consisting of alpha modified minimal essential medium with 2 mm glutamine and supplemented with 0.1 mm L- ascorbic acid phosphate, 15% fetal bovine serum (FBS), 100 ug/mL streptomycin and 100 U/mL penicillin at 37°C and 5% CO_2 in air. Typically, separate colonies can be seen after 24 hours
↓
Other cell lines, such as neural, adipogenic, and odontogenic, can be differentiated by altering the MSC media
↓
It is feasible to grow colonies of cells which are morphologically similar to epithelial or endothelial cells if cultures are derived from an unselected preparation. If contamination is severe, following steps can be implement – Retrypsinize the culture for a few minutes in order to separate only stromal cells; Changing the media 4–6 hours after sub-culturing; STRO-1 OR CD 146 can be utilized to sort stem cells utilizing fluorescence activated cell sorting (FACS)
A
B
C
D
E
F
24 hrs.
48 hrs
72 hrs
G
Chondrocyte
Osteocyte
Adipocyte
H
CRYOSYSTEM 2000
I

Figs. 83.5A to I: Isolation of SHEDs. (A) Processing of specimens inside lamina flow chamber; (B) Specimens rinsed thrice with PBS; (C) The specimens are access opened with the help of airotor, or placed inside a streile surgical glove and broken into pieces with an ostemtome wrapped with aluminum flods or cut at cervical line through slow speed contra angle handpiece and sterilized carborundum disc; (D) The pulp tissues are placed in a sterile petri plate; (E) Medias used for isolation and growth of SHEDs; (F) SHEDs cultured in culture flasks; (G) Morphology of SHEDs under inverted phase contrast microscope (20X), after 24, 48 and 72 hours incubation; (H) Trilineage differentiation of SHEDs into chondrocyte, osteocyte and adipocyte; (I) Storage of SHEDs in liquid nitrogen.

Cultivation of SHEDs

Post isolation of stem cells and dental tissue explants, the cell mass is made to pass via a 40–70 µm pore size filter and then cultivated in the growth medium to obtain single-cell suspensions. Two diverse media are usually utilized:

1. α-Modification of Eagle medium (α-MEM) augmented with 20% fetal calf serum (FCS),100 µmol/L l-ascorbic acid 2-phosphate, 2 mmol/L l-glutamine, 100 µg/mL streptomycin and 100 units/mL penicillin at 37°C in 5% CO_2.
2. Dulbecco modified Eagle medium (D-MEM) augmented with 10–20% fetal bovine serum (FBS), 100 µg/mL streptomycin, 100 U/mL penicillin, and, 0.25 µg/mL amphotericin at 37°C in 10% CO_2.

Preservation of SHEDs

- **Cryopreservation:** It is termed as an extremely effective technique for preserving the vitality of the transported stem cells by cooling to subzero temperatures, usually –196°C. The process encompasses slow cooling at 1 to 2°C/min in the presence of dimethyl sulphoxide (DMSO), a cryoprotectant, to evade the harmful response of intracellular ice formation. The tester that is taken is segmented into four different cryotubes, wherein each cryotube is placed in a distinct location under a cryogenic setting. This is performed to make sure that there will be one more sample available for usage in case there is an issue with any of the storage units. These cells are stored under a temperature of less than –150°C along with liquid nitrogen vapor. The temperature aids in conserving the cells and preserving their power and dormancy. Having 10,00,000–20,00,000 cells in 1.5 mL of medium is advisable.
- **Magnetic freezing:** In this method, a low magnetic area is introduced to the water and tissues, which results in decreasing in the chilling point up to 6°–7°C. It warrants minimum temperature minus any harm to the cell wall owing to nutrient drainage and ice expansion on account of the capillary action, as observed in traditional freezing approaches. Magnetic freezing is termed as more dependable as well as comparatively inexpensive as against cryopreservation.

Benefits of Banking SHEDs

- It ensures a lifelong donor match (autologous transplant).
- Protects cells against natural injury.
- It is comfortable and relatively pain free for the child and the parent.
- It costs less than the expense of cord blood storage.
- Adult stem cells do not face the same moral dilemmas as embryonic stem cells.
- SHED cells collaborate with cord blood stem cells to achieve their goals. SHED can repair solid tissues that cord blood cannot, such as bone, neurological tissue, dental tissues, and connective tissues.
- SHEDs may benefit the donor's close family relatives, such as parents, grandparents, siblings, and uncles.

DENTAL PULP STEM CELL APPLICATIONS IN PEDIATRIC DENTISTRY

- **Revascularization**: Trauma or infection that causes damage to the tooth results in loss of pulp vitality and arrests of the root growth in the young permanent teeth. In some cases, it is possible to maintain vitality of radicular pulp tissue to allow further root growth. The seeding of scaffolds with stem cells and growth factors is required for regenerating the tissue in the apical part of permanent tooth with open apex.
  Stem cells can be found in perivascular regions and locations near blood arteries and peripheral nerve endings, in addition to vital pulp tissue, the apical papilla, PDL, and alveolar bone. The Hertwig's epithelial root sheath (HERS) plays a crucial role in growth and rejuvenation of apical 1/3rd of the root by stimulating SCAP to form new dentin. The SCAP, which is found in the apical region of the permanent tooth with open apex, is more resistant than the DPSCs. As a result, they are able to withstand the infection better and preserve their capacity to specialize into odontoblasts.
- **Apexogenesis**: It is emphasized that stem cell-based strategies are a viable option for the effective regeneration of injured dental tissues. Therefore, it is vital to comprehend the biological mechanism of the diverse dental stem cell populations and their behavior following transplantation to ectopic sites. Innervation and vascularization play

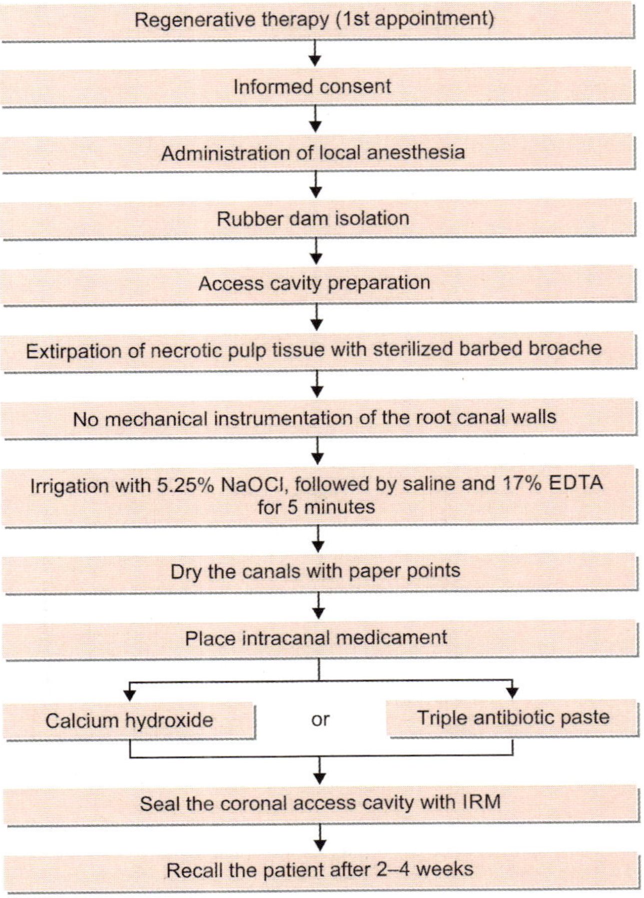

Regenerative therapy (1st appointment)
Informed consent
Administration of local anesthesia
Rubber dam isolation
Access cavity preparation
Extirpation of necrotic pulp tissue with sterilized barbed broache
No mechanical instrumentation of the root canal walls
Irrigation with 5.25% NaOCl, followed by saline and 17% EDTA for 5 minutes
Dry the canals with paper points
Place intracanal medicament
Calcium hydroxide
or
Triple antibiotic paste
Seal the coronal access cavity with IRM
Recall the patient after 2–4 weeks

crucial roles in regulating the homeostasis of stem cell niches, hence influencing the fate and behavior of stem cells.

- **Periodontitis**: Periodontitis is an inflammation of the tooth's supporting components, specifically the periodontal ligament and alveolar bone. In a research by Gao, multiple doses of SHEDs induced regeneration of periodontal tissue. Application of SHEDs to a rat model altered the cytokine expression profile in gingival crevicular fluid, promoted fresh attachment of periodontal ligament, and reduced osteoclast development. In a separate investigation, injection of SHEDs lowered the expression of inflammatory markers, prevented osteoclast development, and encouraged regeneration of periodontal tissues.
- **Entire tooth and bio-root regeneration**: Multiple studies have demonstrated that SHED is an appropriate source for bio-root regeneration due to its angiogenesis, odontogenic, and neurotization potential. In the work by Yang et al., these cells were subcutaneously transplanted into mice. It resulted in the formation of fibrous structures resembling dentin and periodontal ligament. In addition, SHEDs demonstrated exceptional neurogenesis and angiogenesis capacity. Also observed was regeneration of the complete periodontal ligament alveolar bone complex. Specifically, root regeneration appears to be a more realistic and practical strategy for tooth restoration than complete tooth regeneration.

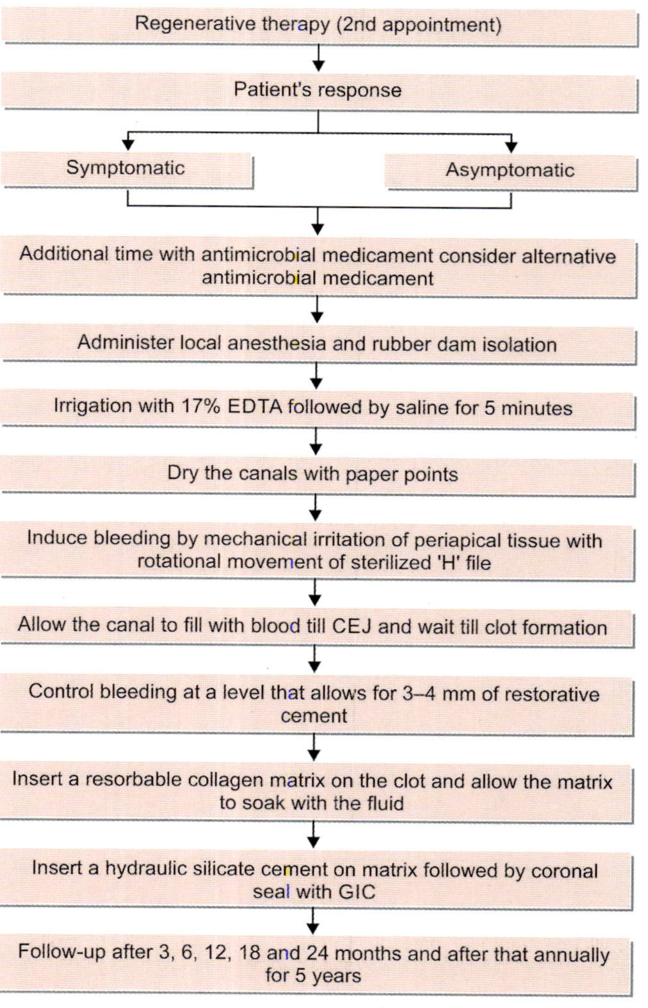
Regenerative therapy (2nd appointment)
Patient's response
Symptomatic
Asymptomatic
Additional time with antimicrobial medicament consider alternative antimicrobial medicament
Administer local anesthesia and rubber dam isolation
Irrigation with 17% EDTA followed by saline for 5 minutes
Dry the canals with paper points
Induce bleeding by mechanical irritation of periapical tissue with rotational movement of sterilized 'H' file
Allow the canal to fill with blood till CEJ and wait till clot formation
Control bleeding at a level that allows for 3–4 mm of restorative cement
Insert a resorbable collagen matrix on the clot and allow the matrix to soak with the fluid
Insert a hydraulic silicate cement on matrix followed by coronal seal with GIC
Follow-up after 3, 6, 12, 18 and 24 months and after that annually for 5 years

- **Restoration of cleft lip and cleft palate defects**: Management of craniofacial deformities, such as cleft palate, requires multiple surgical treatments employing bone grafting techniques, spanning at least a decade. In addition to obtaining a normal facial look, cleft lip and palate treatment tries to restore the child's ability to eat, speak, and hear without impeding his or her face and psychological development. Advances in developmental biology, stem cell biology, and the material sciences have increased the possibility of non-surgical treatments for certain congenital abnormalities.
- **Orofacial skeletal defects**: Maxillary and mandibular deformities may result from trauma, osteomyelitis, or malignancy. Not only is the prosthetic replacement of teeth on missing sections of the jaw difficult, but the results have not been particularly satisfactory. Several studies have demonstrated the efficacy of SHEDs implantation in the restoration of mandibular abnormalities. For instance, Zheng et al. transplanted stem cells from pig deciduous teeth into bony defects in swine mandible models. In their investigation, they observed complete bone repair within six months after surgery.
- **3D Cell printing**: This approach can be used to place cells so that they have the ability to form tooth pulp-like tissue. Following the apical and coronal anatomy, the pulp tissue in the cleaned and prepared root canal systems must be carefully adapted. This method is the most important requirement for the success of the therapeutic procedures. However, significant proof that three-dimensional cell printing may build functioning tissue in vivo has yet to be found.
- **Temporomandibular joint (TMJ) osteoarthritis**: This condition is an inflammation of the TMJ. Exosomes of SHEDs have been shown to reduce TMJ inflammation. The treatment with SHED-Exosomes inhibited the expression of interleukin-8 (IL-8), interleukin-6 (IL-6), matrix metalloproteinase 1, and other inflammatory mediators.
- **Post-traumatic injuries with facial nerve transection**: Following neurotmesis, the mandibular branch of the facial nerve of rats recovered by autograft and SHEDs in a polyglycolic acid tube in an experiment performed by Pereira and colleagues in 2019. The outcome of the investigation indicated that the transplanted stem cells agglomerated into the brain tissue, remained alive, and commenced differentiation in vivo.
- **Dysphagia associated with superior laryngeal nerve damage**: Dysphagia can be caused by a nerve injury sustained during trauma and surgery. In a trial by Tsuruta (2018), injection of SHEDs-conditioned medium (SHED-CM) led to functional rehabilitation and axonal healing of the nerve. Additionally, this enhanced the formation of new blood vessels at the injured region.

Reconstruction of the oral structures is a viable and advantageous substitute to more conventional therapeutic techniques, as damaged tissue is replaced with healthy tissue.

It is possible to usher in a modern age of restorative dentistry by promoting tissue regeneration. To fully comprehend the potential and behavior of dental pulp stem cells in various therapeutic strategies, additional research is required. Nevertheless, the prospects for their application in tooth tissue reconstruction can result in significant benefits for Pediatric Dentistry.

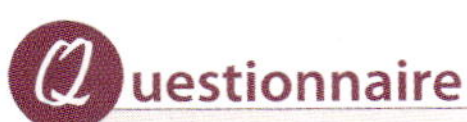

1. Write a note on stem cells in pediatric dentistry.
2. What is stem cell banking?

FURTHER READING

1. Alipour R, Adib M, Masoumi Karimi M, Hashemi-Beni B, Sereshki N. Comparingthe Immunoregulatory Effects of Stem Cells from Human Exfoliated Deciduous Teeth and Bone Marrow-derived Mesenchymal Stem Cells. Iran J Allergy Asthma Immunol. 2013; 12: 331-44.
2. Alongi D, Yamaza T, Song Y, Fouad A, Romberg E, Sao S.et al. Stem/progenitor cells from inflamed human dental pulp retain tissue regeneration potential. Regen Med. 2010; 5(4): 617-31.
3. Arora V, Arora P, Munshi AK. Banking stem cells from human exfoliated deciduous teeth (SHED): Saving for the future. J Clin Pediatr Dent. 2009;33(4):289-94.
4. Bakopoulou A, Leyhausen G, Volk J, Tsiftsoglou A, Garefis P, Koidis P et al. Assessment of the impact of two different isolation methods on the osteo/odontogenic differentiation potential of human dental stem cells derived from deciduous teeth. Calcif Tissue Int. 2011;88:130-41.
5. Casagrande L, Demarco FF, Zhang Z, Araujo FB, Shi S, Nor JE. Dentin-derived BMP-2 and odontoblast differentiation. J Dent Res. 2010; 89: 603-08.
6. Cordeiro MM, Dong Z, Kaneko T, Zhang Z, Miyazawa M, Shi S et al. Dental pulp tissue engineering with stem cells from exfoliated deciduous teeth. J Endod. 2008;34:962-9.
7. Eslaminejad MB, Vahabi S, Shariati M, Nazarian H. In vitro growth and characterization of stem cells from human dental pulp of deciduous versus permanent teeth. J Dent. (Tehran) 2010; 7:185-95.
8. Freshney I R, Stacy G N, Auerbach J M. 2007.Culture of Human Stem Cells. Wiley. USA. 193-203.
9. Gao X, Shen Z, Guan M, Huang Q, Chen L, Qinet W, et al. Immunomodulatory role of stem cells from human exfoliated deciduous teeth on periodontal regeneration. Tissue Eng Part A. 2018;24(17-18):1341-53.
10. Gao X, Shen Z, Guan M, Huang Q, Chen L, Qinet W et al. Immunomodulatory role of stem cells from human exfoliated deciduous teeth on periodontal regeneration. Tissue Eng Part A. 2018;24(17-18):1341-53.
11. Gronthos S, Brahim J, Li W, Fisher LW, Cherman N, Boyde A, et al. Stem cell properties of human dental pulp stem cells. J Dent Res. 2002;81:531-35.
12. Gronthos S, Mankani M, Brahim J, Robey PG, Shi S. Postnatal human dental pulp stem cells (DPSCs) in vitro and in vivo. Proc Natl Acad Sci. 2000; 97(25):13625-30.
13. Heng BC, Lim LW, Wu W, Zhang C. An overview of protocols for the neural induction of dental and oral stem cells in vitro. Tissue Eng Part B Rev. 2016; 22:220-50.
14. Hirata TM, Ishkitiev N, Yaegaki K, Calenic B, Ishikawa H, Nakahara T et al. Expression of multiple stem cell markers in dental pulp cells cultured in serum-free media. J Endod. 2010; 36: 1139-44.
15. Inoue T, Sugiyama M, Hattori H, Wakita H, Wakabayashi T, Ueda M. Stem cells from human exfoliated deciduous tooth-derived conditioned medium enhance recovery of focal cerebral ischemia in rats. Tissue Eng Part A. 2013;19(1-2):24-9.
16. Ivanova NB, Dimos JT, Schaniel C, Hackney JA, Moore KA, Lemischka et al. A stem cell molecular signature. Sci. 2002;298:601-4.
17. Jeon M, Song JS, Choi BJ, Choi HJ, Shin DM, Jung HS, et al. In vitro and in vivo characteristics of stem cells from human exfoliated deciduous teeth obtained by enzymatic disaggregation and outgrowth. Arch Oral Biol. 2014;59:1013-23.
18. Kanafi MM, Pal R, Gupta PK. Phenotypic and functional comparison of optimum culture conditions for upscaling of dental pulp stem cells. Cell Biol Int. 2013; 37: 126-36.
19. Kitase Y, Sato Y, Ueda K, Suzuki T,Mikrogeorgiou A, sugiyama Y et al. A Novel treatment with stem cells from human exfoliated deciduous teeth for hypoxic-ischemic encephalopathy in neonatal rats. Stem Cells Dev. 2020;29(2):63-74.
20. Konstantinov IE. In Search of Alexander A. Maximow. The Man behind the Unitarian Theory of Hematopoiesis. Perspect Biol Med. 2000;43:269-76.
21. Li X, Xie J, Zhai Y, Fang T, Rao N. Differentiation of stem cells from human exfoliated deciduous teeth into retinal photoreceptor-like cells and their sustainability in vivo. Stem Cells Int. 2019;2562981.
22. Li XX, Yuan XJ, Zhai Y, Rao N. Treatment with stem cells from human exfoliated deciduous teeth and their derived conditioned medium improves retinal visual function and delays the degeneration of photoreceptors. Stem Cells Dev. 2019;28(22):1514-26.
23. Li Y, Yang YY, Ren JL, Xu F, Chen FM, Li A. Exosomes secreted by stem cells from human exfoliated deciduous teeth contribute to functional recovery after traumatic brain injury by shifting microglia M1/M2 polarization in rats. Stem Cell Res Ther. 2017;8(1):198.
24. Matsushita Y, Ishigami M, Matsubara K, Kondo M, Wakayama H, Goto H, et al. Multifaceted therapeutic benefits of factors derived from stem cells from human exfoliated deciduous teeth for acute liver failure in rats. J Tissue Eng Regen Med. 2017;11(6):1888-96.
25. Miura M, Gronthos S, Zhao M, Lu B, Fisher LW, Robey PG et al. SHED: Stem cells from human exfoliated deciduous teeth. Proc Natl Acad Sci. 2003;100(10):5807-12.
26. Miura M, Gronthos S, Zhao M, Lu B., Fisher LW, Robey PG, Sh, S. SHED: stem cells from human exfoliated deciduous teeth. Proc Natl Acad Sci. 2003;100(10):5807-12.
27. Moreau, J. L., Caccamese, J. F., Coletti, D. P., Sauk, J. J. Fisher, J. P. Tissue engineering solutions for cleft palates. J Oral Maxillofac Surg 2007; 65(12):2503-2511.
28. Morsczeck C, Götz W, Schierholz J, Zeilhofe F, Kühn U, Möh, C, Hoffmann KH. Isolation of precursor cells (PCs) from human dental follicle of wisdom teeth. Matrix Biology. 2005;24(2):155-65.
29. Nakajima K, Kunimatsu R, Ando K, Ando T, Hayashi Y, Kihara T et al. Comparison of the bone regeneration ability between stem cells from human exfoliated deciduous teeth, human dental pulp stem cells and human bone marrow mesenchymal stem cells. Biochem Biophys Res Commun. 2018;497(3):876-82.
30. Nakajima K, Kunimatsu R, Ando K, Hirali T, Rikitake K, Tsuka Y et al. Success rates in isolating mesenchymal stem cells from permanent and deciduous teeth. Sci Rep. 2019;9:16764.
31. Nakamura S, Yamada Y, Katagiri W, Sugito T, Ito K, Ueda M. Stem cell proliferation pathways comparison between human exfoliated deciduous teeth and dental pulp stem cells by gene expression profile from promising dental pulp. J Endod. 2009;35:1536-42.
32. Nicola F, Marques MR, Odorcyk F. Stem cells from human exfoliated deciduous teeth modulate early astrocyte response after spinal cord contusion [published correction appears in Mol. Neurobiol. 2019;56(1):748-60.
33. Paschalidou M, Athanasiadou E, Arapostathis K, Kotsanos N, Koidis PT, Bakopoulou A, et al. Biological effects of low-level laser irradiation (LLLI) on stem cells from human exfoliated deciduous teeth (SHED). Clin Oral Investig. 2020;24(1):167–80.
34. Pereira LV, Bento RF, Cruz DB, Marchi C, Salomone R, Oiticicca J et al. Stem cells from human exfoliated deciduous teeth (SHED) differentiate in vivo and promote facial nerve regeneration. Cell Transplant. 2019;28(1):55-64.
35. Phuc VP. Mesenchymal stem cells: isolation, characteristics and applications. Croatia. In Tech, 2017.
36. Rao N, Wang X, Xie J, Jingzhi Li, Yue Zhai, Xiaoxia Li, et al. Stem cells from human exfoliated deciduous teeth ameliorate diabetic nephropathy in vivo and in vitro by inhibiting advanced glycation end product-activated epithelial-mesenchymal transition. Stem Cells Int. 2019;2019:2751475.

37. Rao N, Wang X, Zhai Y, ingzhi Li, Xie J, Zhao Y et al. Stem cells from human exfoliated deciduous teeth ameliorate type II diabetic mellitus in Goto-Kakizaki rats. Diabetol Metab Syndr. 2019;11:22.
38. Reddy BY, Xu DS, Hantash BM. Mesenchymal stem cells as immunomodulator therapies for immune-mediated systemic dermatoses. Stem Cells Dev. 2012;21:352-62.
39. Sabbagh J, Ghassibe –Sabbagh M, Fayya Kazan M, Al Nemer F, Fahed JC, Berberi A et al. Differences in osteogenic and odontogenic differentiation potential of DPSCs and SHED. J Dent. 2020;103413.
40. Sakai VT, Zhang Z, Dong Z, Neiva KG, Machado MAAM, Shi S, et al. SHED differentiate into functional odontoblasts and endothelium. J Dent Res. 2010;89:791-6.
41. Salmon B, Bardet C, Khaddam M, Naji J, Coyac BR, Baroukh B et al. MEPE- derived ASARM peptide inhibits odontogenic differentiation of dental pulp stem cells and impairs mineralization in tooth models of X- linked hypophosphatemia. PLoS ONE. 2013;8(2):e56749.
42. Seo, B. M., Miura, M., Gronthos, S., Bartold, P. M., Batouli, S., Brahim, J.,Shi, S. Investigation of multipotent postnatal stem cells from human periodontal ligament. The Lancet. 2004; 364(9429):149-155.
43. Seo BM, Sonoyama W, Yamaza T, Coppe C, Kikuiri T, Akiyama K, et al. SHED repair critical-size calvarial defects in mice. Oral Dis. 2008;14:428-34.
44. Shimojima C, Takeuchi H, Jin S, Parajuli B, Hattori H, Suzumura A et al. Conditioned medium from the stem cells of human exfoliated deciduous teeth ameliorates experimental autoimmune encephalomyelitis. J Immunol. 2016;196(10):4164-71.
45. Sonoyama W, Liu Y, Fang, D, Yamaza T, Seo BM, Zhang C,Wang S. Mesenchymal stem cell-mediated functional tooth regeneration in swine. PloS One 2006;1(1): e79.
46. Sonoyama W, Yi Liu, Yamaza T, Tuan R, Songlin Wang, Songtao Shi, George T-J Huang. Characterization of the apical papilla and its residing stem cells from human immature permanent teeth: a pilot study. J Endod 2008;34(2):166-71.
47. Stemple DL, Anderson DJ. Isolation of a stem cell for neurons and glia from the mammalian neural crest. Cell 1992;71:973-85.
48. Takahashi Y, Yuniartha R, Yamaza T. Sonoda S, Yamaza H, Kirino K, et al. Therapeutic potential of spheroids of stem cells from human exfoliated deciduous teeth for chronic liver fibrosis and hemophilia A. Pediatr Surg Int. 2019;35:1379-88.
49. Tsai AI, Hong HH, Lin WR, Fu JF, Chang CC, Wang IK, et al. Isolation of mesenchymal stem cells from human deciduous teeth pulp. BioMed Res Int. 2017:2851906.
50. Tsuruta T, Sakai K, Watanabe J, Katagiri W, Hibi H. Dental pulp-derived stem cell conditioned medium to regenerate peripheral nerves in a novel animal model of dysphagia. PLoS One. 2018;13(12):e0208938.
51. Wagner W, Horn P, Castoldi M, Diehlmann A, Bork S, Saffrich R, et al. Replicative senescence of mesenchymal stem cells: A continuous and organized process. PLoS One. 2008;3(5):e2213.
52. Wang H, Zhong Qi, Yang T, Qi Y, Fu M, Yang Xi et al. Comparative characterization of SHED and DPSCs during extended cultivation in vitro. Mol Med Rep.2018;17(5):6551-9.
53. Wang J, Wang X, Sun Z, Wang X, Yang H, Shi S, et al. Stem cells from human-exfoliated deciduous teeth can differentiate into dopaminergic neuron-like cells. Stem Cells Dev. 2010;19:1375-83.
54. Wang J, Wei X, Ling J, Huang Y, Huo Y, Zhou Y. The presence of a side population and its marker ABCG2 in human deciduous dental pulp cells. Biochem Biophys Res Community. 2010; 400: 334-9.
55. Wang X, Sha XJ, Li GH, Yang FS, Ji K, Wen, LY et al. Comparative characterization of stem cells from human exfoliated deciduous teeth and dental pulp stem cells. Arch Oral Biol. 2012; 57:1231-40.
56. Werle SB, Lindemann D, Steffens D, Demarco FF, de Araujo FB, Pranke P et al. Carious deciduous teeth are a potential source for dental pulp stem cells. Clin Oral Invest. 2016;20:75-81.
57. Yamada Y, Nakamura S, Ito K, Sugito T, Yoshimi R, Nagasaka T, et al. A feasibility of useful cell-based therapy by bone regeneration with deciduous tooth stem cells, dental pulp stem cells, or bone-marrow-derived mesenchymal stem cells for clinical study using tissue engineering technology. Tissue Eng Part A. 2010;16:1891-900.
58. Yamaza T, Alatas FS, Yuniartha R. In vivo hepatogenic capacity and therapeutic potential of stem cells from human exfoliated deciduous teeth in liver fibrosis in mice. Stem Cell Res Ther. 2015;6(1):171.
59. Yamaza T, Kentaro A, Chen C, Liu Y, Shi Y, Gronthos S, et al. Immunomodulatory properties of stem cells from human exfoliated deciduous teeth. Stem Cell Res Ther. 2010;1:5.
60. Zhang, W., Walboomers, X. F., Shi, S., Fan, M., Jansen, J. A. (2006). Multilineage differentiation potential of stem cells derived from human dental pulp after cryopreservation. Tissue Eng. 2006;12(10):2813-23.
61. Zhang N, Chen B, Wang W, Chen C, Kang J, Deng SQ, et al. Isolation, characterization and multi-lineage differentiation of stem cells from human exfoliated deciduous teeth. Mol Med Rep. 2016;14:95-102.
62. Zhang N, Lu X, Wu S. Intra striatal transplantation of stem cells from human exfoliated deciduous teeth reduces motor defects in Parkinsonian rats. Cytotherapy. 2018;20(5):670-86.
63. Zhang QZ, Nguyen AL, Yu WH., Le AD. Human oral mucosa and gingiva: a unique reservoir for mesenchymal stem cells. J Dent Res. 2012;91(11):1011-8.
64. Zhang Z, Nor F, Oh M, Cucco C, Shi S, Nor JE. Wnt/beta-catenin signalling determines the vasculogenic fate of postnatal mesenchymal stem cells. Stem Cells. 2016;34:1576-87.
65. Zheng Y, Liu Y, Zhang CM, Zhang HY, Li WH, Shi S, et al. Stem cells from deciduous tooth repair mandibular defect in swine. J Dent Res. 2009;88:249-54.
66. Zheng Y, Liu Y, Zhang CM, Zhang HY, W H Li, S Shi, et al. Stem cells from deciduous tooth repair mandibular defect in swine. J Dent Res. 2009;88(3):249-54
67. Zuk PA. Tissue engineering craniofacial defects with adult stem cells? Are we ready yet? Pediatr Res 2008; 63(5), 478-86.

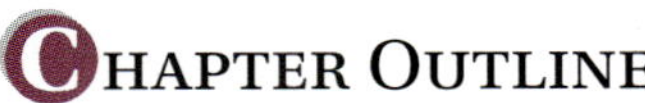

Digital Pediatric Dentistry

Gaurav Gupta, Shoba Fernandes, Bhaggyashri A Pawar, Suhani Khanna, Yash Bajna, Dimpal Parmar

CHAPTER OUTLINE

- Digital Radiography
- Digital Impressions
- Three-dimensionally Printed Space Maintainers in Pediatric Dentistry
- Digital Occlusion Scan
- Customized Digital Restorations
- Digital Photography
- 3D Printing

Digital Dentistry is the technology which incorporates digital applications almost exclusively. This practice helps itself of computerized radiographs, a computerized database, and an ability to scan all the documents for making digital records. Digital dentistry provides better efficiency, is much more precise, easy, quick, convenient, interactive, accurate and motivational for patient. Digital dentistry is the advancement in dental technology that enables patients to receive modern solutions to their dental problems. It provides digital equipment available to cosmetic as well as implants dentistry. The digital technologies that are available include digital radio video radiography (RVG), CBCT (cone-beam computed tomography), electronic prescriptions, CAD-CAM (computer aided designing and manufacturing) restorations and digital impressions. Digital dentistry provides quick, precise, easy and aesthetic treatment approach.

Advancements in technology have led medicine towards a new era. Digital dentistry is no more a concept, but it's a full hands-on reality today, enabling patients to receive modern solutions to old traditional dental problems. Among the digital technologies available in dentistry, there are some which have already proven to be useful in Pediatric Dentistry, as well. Digital radiography, along with a modern non-invasive caries detection tools, helps the practitioner in diagnosis, CAD/CAM restorations, and digitally-based surgical guides for the enhancement of treatment possibilities. Digital photography and virtual reality are specifically useful in patient management, especially in pediatric patients, as growth monitoring and behavioural management are two of the main concerns in Pediatric Dentistry. All above mentioned techniques incorporate the latest digital dental technological findings and aid practitioners to provide their patients a leading-edge dental treatment, with improved efficiency, precision and comfort.

DIGITAL RADIOGRAPHY

Early detection and diagnosis of the caries is a primary consideration of the Minimal Intervention Dentistry (MID) concept, which is particularly important in pediatric patients, due to the rapid caries progression in deciduous teeth.[1,2] When dealing with children, it is possible to improve images using image enhancement facilities; this could prove interesting for use with impatient children.[3] RVG is one of the digital radiography being most commonly used; CBCT and OPG orthopantamography are the most exciting advancement in oral radiology. The strength of CBCT is its ability to view any mineralized anatomic structure within the field of view from any angle, these images have zero magnification, and unless there are patient motion artefacts or patients have a plethora of dental restorations, and these anatomic structure can be visualized without distortions. But, the most significant limitation of CBCT is higher radiation dose. Lately, digital radiography has taken over the conventional radiographic techniques.

A digital sensor is used instead of the conventional film and the radiographic image is stored in a computer data base. The two types of digital receptors can be used in image acquisition—charge-coupled device (CCD) or photostimulable phosphor (PSP). A digital radiograph permits the use of computer facilities, such as image enhancement and processing, and also the possibility of sending images to other colleagues.[4-6] Advantages of digital intraoral radiography systems are—fewer errors in the image and environmental problems, since they use no chemicals. They also are quick, save time and reduce the dose to the patient.

DIGITAL IMPRESSIONS

- Nowadays, pediatric patients are also being treated by CAD-CAM systems with great success, especially molars utilizing the chair side CAD/CAM technology and CEREC (chairside economical restoration of esthetic ceramics) workflow.
- CAD-CAM is a process where non-digital data is captured, then converted into a digital format, edited where necessary, and converted back into a physical form with the exact dimensions and specific materials during the digital design process, usually by either 3D printing or milling, this set of stages is known as a "digital workflow".[7]
- Preparing the tooth, taking the optical impression, milling the restoration using a CAD/CAM technique, and then final cementation can be accomplished in about 20 minutes. Generally, these pediatric restorations mill in just about 2 minutes, due to their small size.[8,9]
- This technology helps in fabrication of fixed space maintainers, such as the band and the loop,[10] and metallic orthodontic appliances.[11]
- The space maintainer scan be obtained without making the classical impression, using digital technology. The entire procedure consists of—a digital impression taken using an intraoral scanner with artificial intelligence (AI) technology, information processing by specialized software, a 3D print of the model, which can be checked in the mouth of the patient for proper adaptation, and sent to the lab for obtaining an analogous metal appliance. The final metallic space maintainer is then fixed intraorally using resin cement. The final outcome shows excellent adaptation of the appliance and points out that the digital approach has definitely proved to be an efficient, quick and predictable method for manufacturing of fixed space maintainers.[10]

Digital Impression in Fabrication of Band and Loop Space Maintainer

Using CEREC Omnicam scanner (Densply Sirona): **(Figs. 84.1A and B)**

- Only desired side arch impression is made, these scanners can scan in presence of blood and saliva
- Scanning is done immediately after extraction **(Fig. 84.2 A)**.
- Within 30 seconds.
- Resulting file can be transferred to dental laboratory for 3D model printing **(Fig. 84.2B)**.
- Basic protocol to fabricate a cast metal band and loop is followed.
- After try-in final cementation done with modified glass ionomer resin cement (GIC) **(Fig. 84.2C)**.

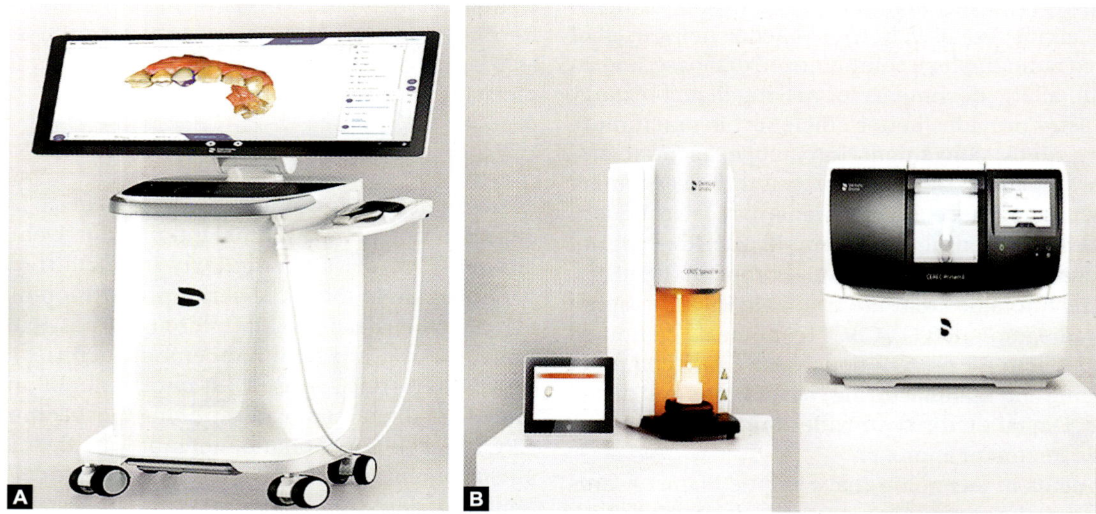

Figs. 84.1A and B: (A) CEREC Omnicam scanner; (B) Milling unit. (*Pic courtesy:* Wisdom Dental Clinic).

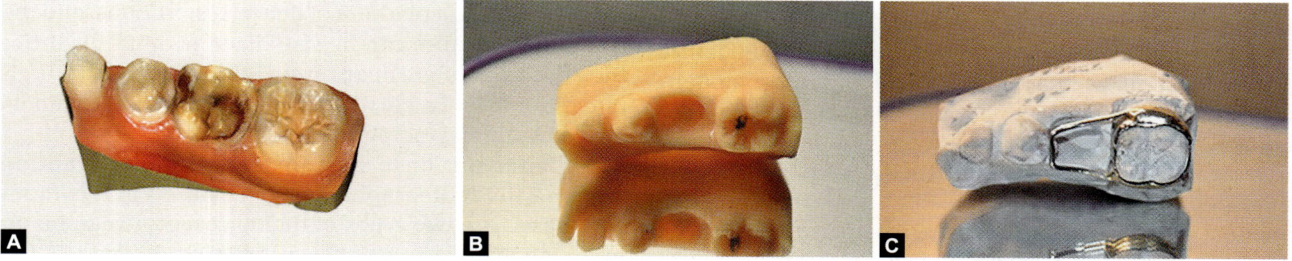

Figs. 84.2A to C: (A) Digital impression; (B) 3D model; (C) Band and loop space maintainer. (*Pic courtesy:* Wisdom Dental Clinic).

THREE-DIMENSIONALLY PRINTED SPACE MAINTAINERS IN PEDIATRIC DENTISTRY

The primary dentition is extremely important for a child's growth and development of the jaw. This is intended not only at improving speaking, chewing, attractiveness, and avoiding negative habits, but also at guiding and erupting permanent teeth. Exfoliation of primary teeth is a normal physiological process that enables the developed permanent teeth beneath to erupt. When this process is compromised, such as by the loss of primary teeth or a proximal carious lesion, the subsequent permanent teeth may migrate mesially, resulting in malocclusion in the form of crowding, impaction, and super-eruption of opposing teeth. The best approach to avoid these issues is to keep primary teeth in the arch until they reach their normal exfoliation time. Be a result, primary teeth are sometimes referred to as the best space maintainers (SMs) for the permanent dentition. Conversely, if an early extraction or loss of a primary tooth is unavoidable, the safest way to keep arch space is to use an space maintainer.

A novel innovative approach towards digitalization is the application of three-dimensional printing technology in Pediatric Dentistry by fabricating a space maintainer.

Three-dimensional (3D) printing, also popularly known as additive manufacturing or digital fabrication, is a novel technique recently pioneered by Pawar et al.,[12] in 2019 **(Fig. 84.3)** and reinforced by Khanna et al.,[13] in 2021 **(Fig. 84.4)**. It is a method for creating three-dimensional solid objects from a digital source. The stereolithography (STL) format is used to preserve the digital 3D model, which is then uploaded to a 3D printer to generate a layer by layer structure of a complete 3D task. Additive methods are used to create the 3D printed object. Each of these layers are visible as a thinly sliced horizontal cross-section of the completed product.

Advantages of 3D Printed Space Maintainers

- Precision work with minimum human error
- Less chances of breakage as it is one single unit
- Lessens the extensive laboratory work time
- No sign of plaque accumulation and gingival inflammation
- Reduced chair-side time
- Increased patient acceptability.

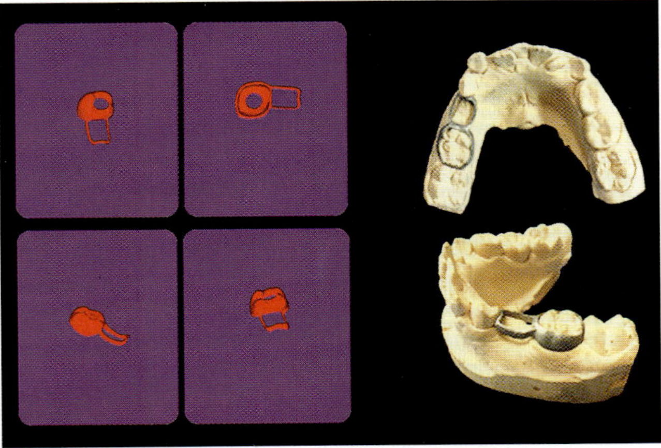

Fig. 84.3: Three-dimensionally designed and printed space maintainer. (*Source:* Pawar BA, JISCPD, 2019).[12]

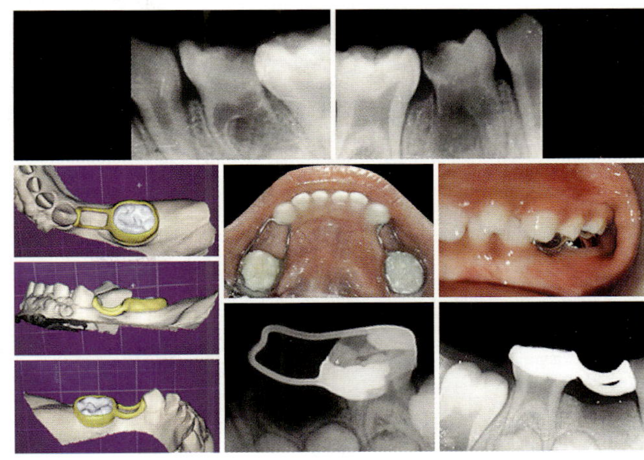

Fig. 84.4: A case of 3-D printed space maintainer. (*Source:* Reported by Khanna et al. JCPD, 2021).[13]

Fabrication Procedure

Single-step rubber base impression of the arch with the missing primary molar

↓

Retrieval of a cast from the impression.

↓

Scanning of the retrieved cast using a digital scanner (for example: Medit T500, Medit Corp., Seongbuk-gu, South Korea) **(Fig. 84.3)**

↓

Designing the space maintainer similar to conventional using a computer application (for example: Dental CAD 2.2 Valletta Exocad GmbH, Darmstadt, Germany) **(Fig. 84.4)**

↓

Selection of the material to be used for printing the final SM
1. Titanium based powdered metal material
2. Clear or colored photopolymer resin

↓

Printing of the SM using 3D printer that employs additive manufacturing **(Fig. 84.5)**

Newer alternatives

Scanning of the cast using a digital lab scanner (AutoScan-DS-EX– Shining 3D). The scanner takes a total of 12 seconds for scanning a single complete cast. The scanner has the ability to fill the gaps automatically by computing an improved scan path. Users don't need to manually rescan. The scanner also captures the textures and marks on the plaster model clearly, allowing technicians to complete the digital partial framework design.

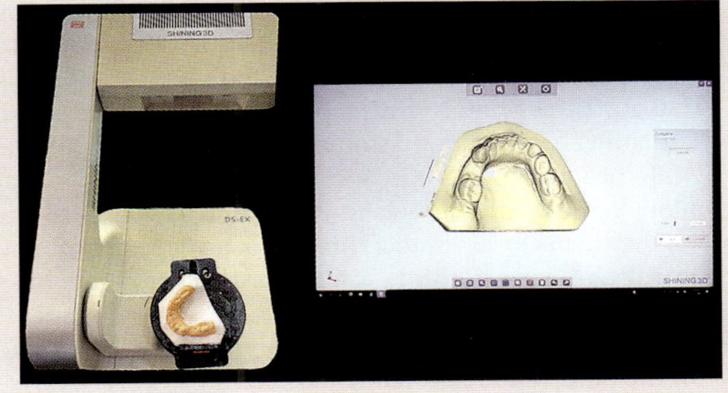

Three-dimensional designing of the band and loop space maintainer using Partial CAD 3.0 Galway. In this software with each movement, the anatomy of the teeth adjusts in real time, aiding in revolutionising our design process. The color coding was activated so that the design of the space maintainer loops and bad could be differentiated from the edentulous space.

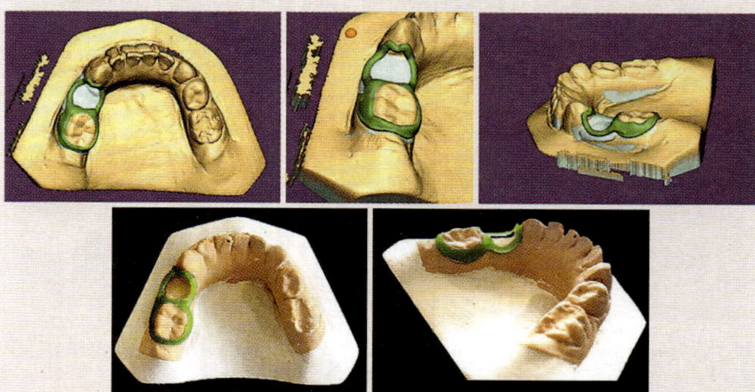

The placement and adaptation of 3-D printed space maintainer (*Pic courtesy:* Dr Tej Joshi, CeraLife Dental Lab, Mumbai).

NextDent® 5100 3D Printer and the printed space maintainer using coloured resin. The revolutionary (**Fig 84.4**) technology combined with NextDent's broad portfolio of dental materials addresses multiple indications, resulting in unparalleled speed, accuracy, repeatability, and productivity. This printer enables high-speed 3D printing for the manufacture of dental appliances.

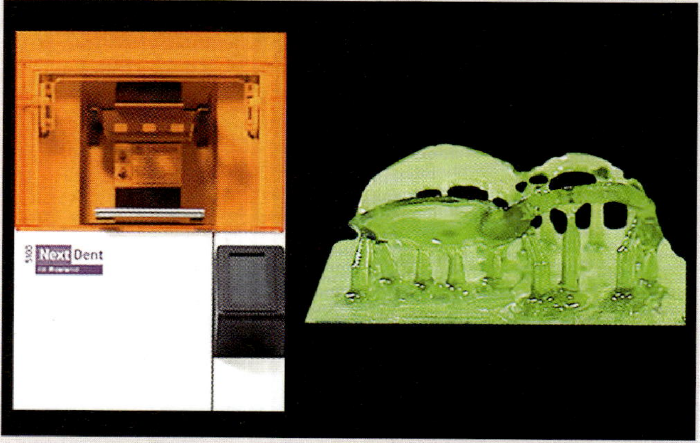

DIGITAL OCCLUSION SCAN

- The Digital System is designed to measure and record relative biting forces over time, being successfully used in orthodontics,[14] prosthodontics,[15] and in Pediatric Dentistry.
- The 3rd generation system includes intraoral sensors, scanning electronics (handle) and intuitive software having artificial intelligence (AI). The sensor fits into a sensor support that inserts into the sensor handle connected to the USB port of a PC and is easily movable among the scan field.
- The software records and stores data in a patient database, while providing with the occlusal analytic features that allow dental professionals to determine the contact, the balance of occlusal contacts present at any given moment, as well as to view multiple scans in order to compare bites **(Fig. 84.5).**[16]
- Graphic displays on computer's monitor are also an aid for the patient education and interaction[17,18] **(Fig. 84.6)**.

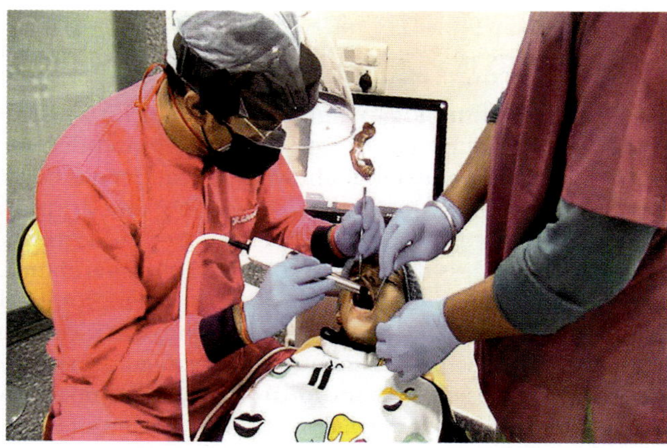

Fig. 84.5: Digital bite scan. (*Pic courtesy:* Wisdom Dental Clinic).

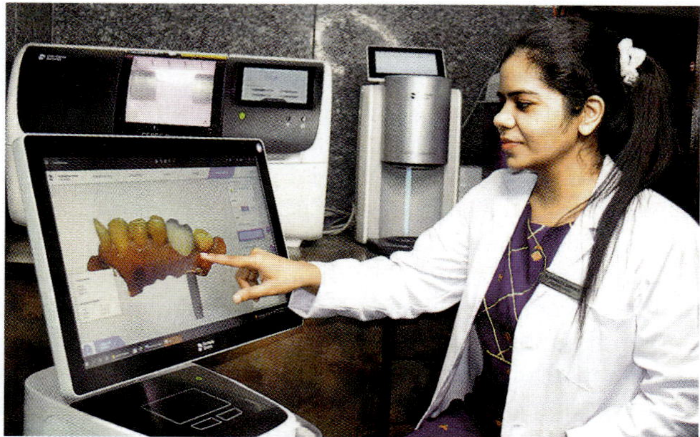

Fig. 84.6: Digital scan for educating parent. (*Pic courtesy:* Wisdom Dental Clinic).

CUSTOMIZED DIGITAL RESTORATIONS

- Crowns are being provided for teeth that have extensive caries, developmental defects or are decalcified following pulpectomy/root canal treatment. Until now, prefabricated crowns have been available of different sizes to match molars which require replacement after adolescence. Nowadays, CAD-CAM technology for fabrication of customized zirconium/inlay/onlay/endocrown is available in dental clinics, which is precise, quick, minimally invasive and single sitting alternative via its software/Artificial intelligence (AI)[19] with use of CAD-CAM for the fabrication of customized restoration can be given for grossly decayed young permanent molars.
- This approach has the advantage of customization along with definitive restoration in contrast to the prefabricated, un-aesthetic and provisional options.
- In children and adolescents, restoring endodontically-treated young permanent molars with an aesthetic and long-term option is extremely difficult. This is basically due to the challenge of obtaining the patient's cooperation, during the impression-taking, which is highly technique sensitive and also establishing margins of crown which should not interfere with eruption of succedaneous teeth. Till now, prefabricated zirconia crowns were available only for deciduous molars, and SSC's need replacement after adolescence but with digital workflow customized aesthetic restoration can be provided in single sitting.

- The overall method involve following phases with follow-up:
  - *Diagnosis:* Careful examination, medical and dental history and amount of tooth structure left.
  - Treatment planning
  - Child behavior
  - *Local anesthesia with/without nitrous oxide inhalation sedation:* Endodontic treatment and removal of caries from tooth
  - *Digital workflow:* Digital impression making, bite scan and digital transfer of files to in-house prime mill followed with—designing, milling and fabrication **(Fig. 84.7)**
  - *Final restoration:* Intraoral evaluation of restoration—cementation with resin cement and follow-up **(Figs. 84.8A to C)**

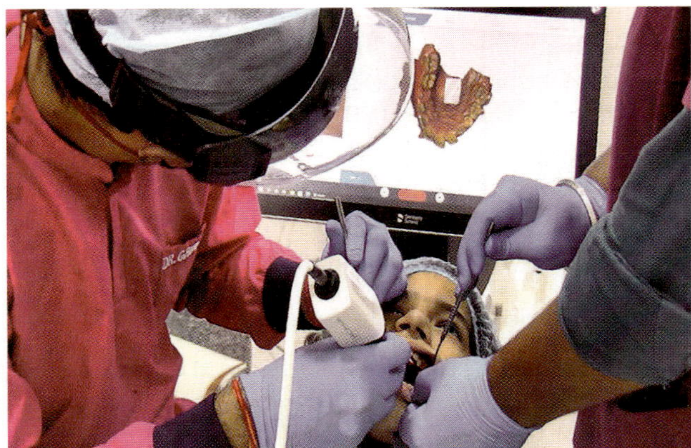

Fig. 84.7: Digital scan. (*Pic courtesy:* Wisdom Dental Clinic).

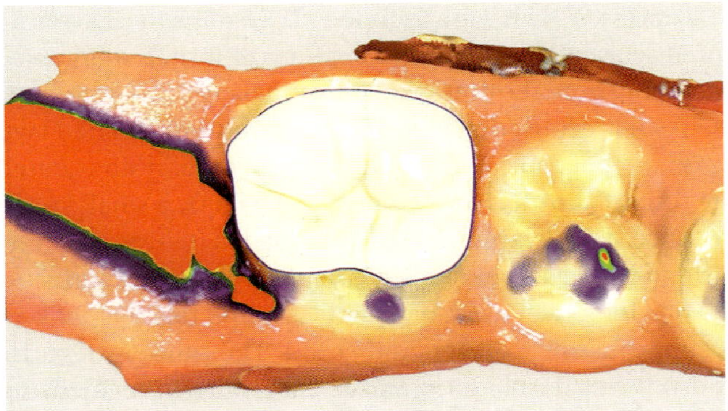

Fig. 84.8A: Digital designing of customized restoration. (*Pic courtesy:* Wisdom Dental Clinic).

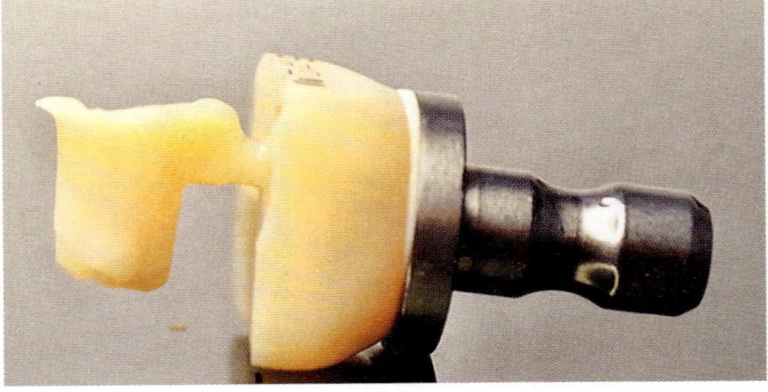

Fig. 84.8B: Customized restoration from single Hybrid zirconia CAD/CAM block. (*Pic courtesy:* Wisdom Dental Clinic).

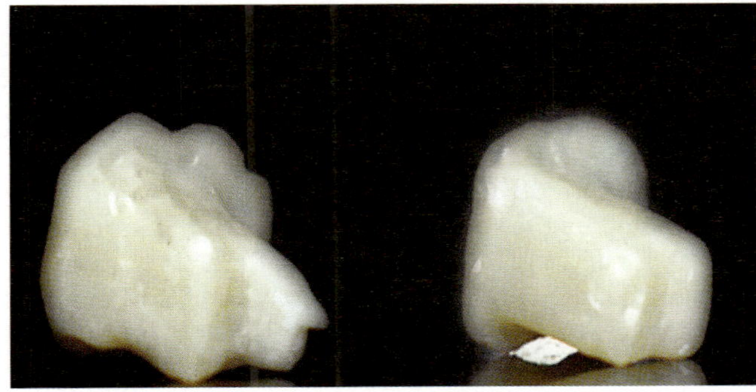

Fig. 84.8C: Customized zirconia restoration. (*Pic courtesy:* Wisdom Dental Clinic).

Advantages of digitally customized restoration over the previous prefabricated options especially in case of young permanent molars.

Restorative considerations	*Stainless steel crowns (SSC's)*	*Laboratory made zirconia crowns*	*Customized zirconia restorations (CAD/CAM)*
Tooth reduction	Both proximal and occlusal reduction	Proximal, occlusal and labio-lingual reduction	Only occlusal reduction
Aesthetics	Poor aesthetics	Good aesthetics	Excellent aesthetics
Precision	Less precised	Less precised	Highly precised
Cost	Low costing	High costing	High costing
Restoration longevity	Has to be replaced later when succedaneous teeth get in occlusion	Might have to be replaced later when succedaneous teeth get in occlusion	No need for replacement/ long-term restoration
Chair side	Single sitting	Multiple sittings	Single sitting
Fabrication and milling	Pre-fabricated/ pre- made	Laboratory made	Made in-house/ chair-side
Armamentarium	Minimal inventory needed (all sizes)	Minimal inventory needed	Intraoral scanner/milling unit/blocks are needed

DIGITAL PHOTOGRAPHY

- Photography has become an easy and accessible way for educating and documenting patients. Digital technology has changed the perspective of a dentist toward the data collection, academics and on treatment aspects.
- Digital photography is described as images stored in form of file format referred to as a digital image file. Digital images are usually taken by a DSLR (Digital Single Lens Reflex) camera, through a CCD (Charge-Coupled Device) sensor, and it can be easily stored and kept for future use and also for legal or academic purposes.[20]
- Digital facial photography used for facial growth assessment has significant advantages as when compared to other techniques. It is non-invasive, bi-dimensional, and quick and it can be subsequently re-evaluated each time

when needed. In order to obtain precise photographic measurements, the technique has to be standardized.[21]

- A very useful feature of this software for Pediatric Dentistry is the possibility to determine the dental age on a digital radiograph and stages of dental eruption can be followed. Based on a prediction table, the dental age can be directly calculated by the software. All information is stored in a database and can be revisited at any time.[21,22]
- The use of digital photography and virtual study models could allow a durable storage of a fully electronic patient record. This is particularly useful when patients are being treated in interdisciplinary teams, with many dental specialists that need to access to the whole documentation.[23]

3D PRINTING

3D printing is a phrase used to describe the process of creating three objects from digital file using a material—printer, in a manner similar to printing images on paper.[24]

Technology has become an integral part of dentistry in recent years that led to the development of devices and tools to improve treatment methods and teaching in the fields of endodontics, implant, craniofacial, maxillofacial, orthognathic, and periodontal treatments. The increased use of technology or "digital workflow" in dentistry comprise of three elements.

- Acquisition of data through scanning
- Processing of data using Computer Aided Design software (CAD)
- Use the information to build objects using computer aided manufacturing.[25]

The term 3D printing is generally used to describe a manufacturing approach that builds objects one layer at a time, adding multiple layers to form an object. This process is more correctly described as additive manufacturing, and is also referred to as rapid prototyping. 3D printing technologies are not all new; many modalities in use today were first developed and used in the late 1980s and 1990s. The first patient treated with the help of 3D printing was in 1999.[26] Early Additive Manufacturing (or AM) equipment and materials were developed in the 1980s. Very first patent application for RP technology was filed by a Dr Kodama, in Japan, in May 1980.[24]

Process of 3D Printing (from Design to Printing)[26] (Fig 84.9)

- Very first step to 3D print an object is to make a model of the object using CAD software. The model describes the geometrical properties of the object.
- The CAD file is then converted to STL file format. This file format defines the external closed surfaces of the original CAD model. The STL file also includes the data for each single layer and can make calculations for the layers.
- The STL file is sent to the 3D printer and the printer is setup before build process, where settings include build parameters, like energy source, layer thickness, etc. The part is then printed by an automated process without any supervision.
- When printing is done, the printed part is removed and sent for post processing. After that, the object is ready for application.

Different 3D Printing Technologies/Methods[26]

- Stereolithography (SLA)
- Fused deposition modelling (FDM)
- Selective laser sintering (SLS)
- Selective heat sintering (SHS)
- Selective laser melting (SLM)
- Electron beam melting
- Binder Jetting (BJG)
- Photo polymerization
- DLP projecting
- Laminated object manufacturing (LOM).

Stereolithography (SLA): As the oldest AM technology, SLA was first developed by **Dr Hideo Kodama** in 1981. He saw it as a fast and low-cost method of reconstructing models in 3D space as an alternative to holographic techniques. The first commercially available SLA printer was patented in 1986 by **Charles W Hull**, who founded 3D Systems Inc. Layers are cured sequentially and bond together to form a solid object beginning from the bottom of the models and building up. As the resin is exposed to the UV light, a thin well defined layer thickness becomes hardened. After a layer of resin is cured, the resin platform is lower within the bath by a small known distance. A new layer of resin is wipped across small known distance. A new layer of resin is wipped across the surface of the previous layer using a wiper blade, and this second layer is subsequently exposed and cured. The process of curing and lowering the platform into the resin bath is repeated until the full model is complete. The self adhesive property of the material causes the layers to bond to each other and eventually form a complete en bloc 3D object **(Fig. 84.10)**. The model is then removed from the bath and cured for a further period of time in a UV cabinet.[24]

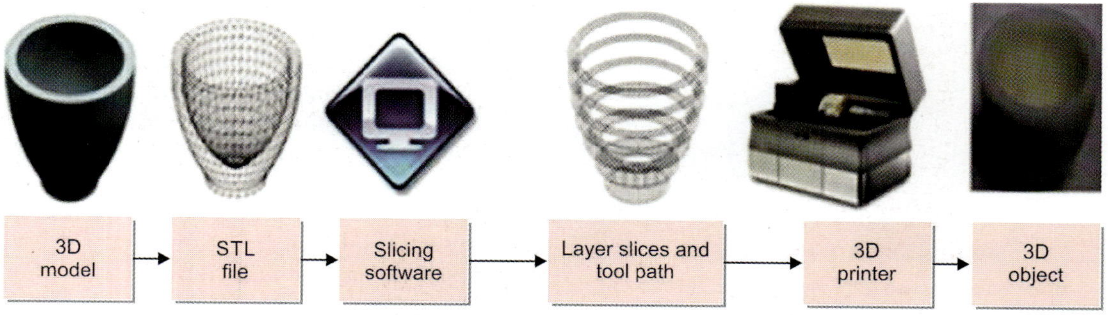

Fig. 84.9: Process of 3D printing (from design to printing).

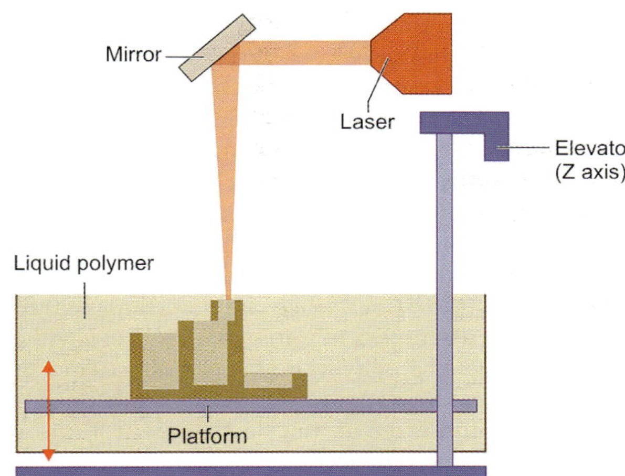

Fig. 84.10: Stereolithography.

Fused deposition modelling (FDM): Fused Deposition Modelling developed by **Schott Crump**. This is the process that is used by most low cost 'home' 3D printers. It allows for the printing of crude anatomical models without too much complexity, for example, printing an edentulous mandible.[27] FDM is the second most widely used 3D printing technology, after stereolithography.[24] In the FDM machine, usually two types of materials namely support material and model material are used for construction of physical model. Both the materials are supplied in the form of wires which are wound on the spools and these are fed in to the head of the machine. The head is temperature-control led and the material is fed into the head where it is heated to a semi-liquid state and deposited to produce the component. The material is extruded from the head and gets deposited on the fixtureless base of the FDM machine.

A plastic/wax filament is unwound from a coil and supplies material to an extrusion nozzle. The nozzle is heated to melt the plastic and has a mechanism which allows the flow of the melted plastic to be turned on and off. The nozzle is mounted to a mechanical stage which can be moved in both horizontal and vertical directions. As the nozzle is moved over the table in the required geometry, it deposits a thin bead of extruded plastic/wax to form each layer. The plastic/wax hardens immediately after being squirted from the nozzle and bonds to the layer below. The entire system is contained within a chamber which is held at a temperature just below the melting point of the material **(Fig. 84.11).**

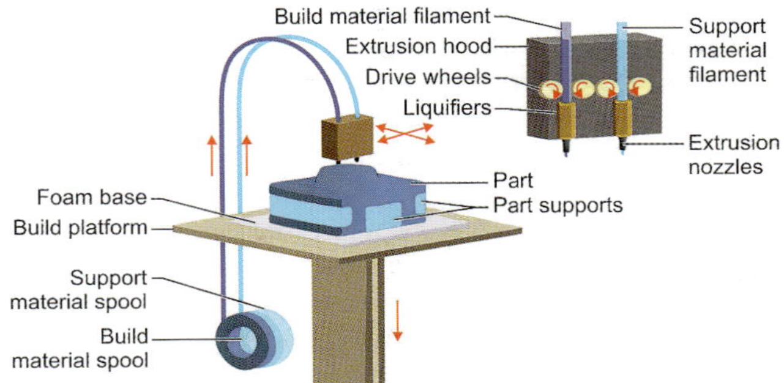

Fig. 84.11: Fused deposition modeling.

Selective laser sintering (SLS): It was developed and patented by **Dr Carl Dackard** and **Dr Joe Beaman** in 1980s.[24] The laser selectively fuses powdered material by scanning cross-sections generated from a 3D digital description of the part on surface of a powder bed. After each cross-section is scanned, powder bed is lowered by top, and the process is repeated until the part is completed. SLS machine preheats the bulk powder material in powder bed below its melting point by infrared heating in order to minimize thermal distortion (curling) and facilitate fusion to the previous layer. Various materials can be used such as fine polymeric powder – polysterene, polycarbonate or polyamide, etc. within the range of 20 to 100 micrometer diameter. The laser is modulated in such a way that only those grains, which are in direct contact with the beam are affected **(Fig. 84.12).**

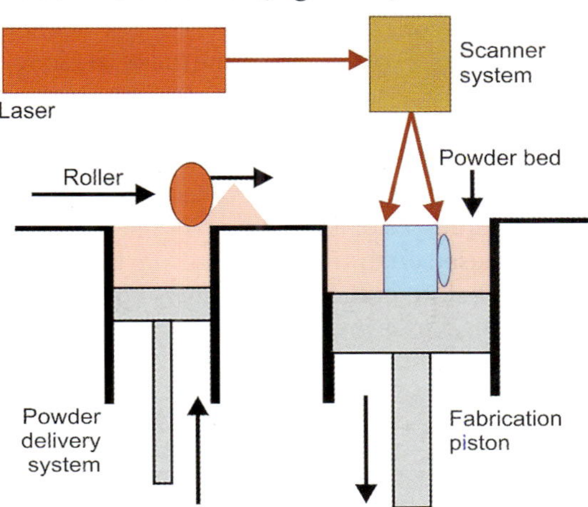

Fig. 84.12: Selective laser sintering.

DLP projecting: DLP (Digital Light Processing) is one kind of stereo lithographic procedure. It utilizes a projector to solidify a layer of photopolymer at once, as opposed to utilizing a laser for the following of distinctive layers.[28] A projector light source is curing the liquid resin layer by layer. The object is constructed on an elevating platform. The layer is created upside down. A mirror was most normally used to position and size the replication precisely onto layer of photopolymer. **(Fig. 84.13).**

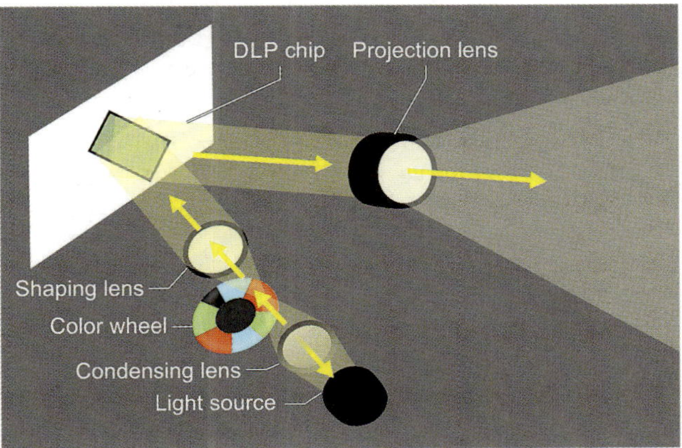

Fig. 84.13: DLP projecting.

Laminated object manufacturing (LOM): With LOM process, three-dimensional objects are manufactured by sequentially laminating and cutting two-dimensional cross-sections. The medium used in LOM process is adhesive-coated sheet

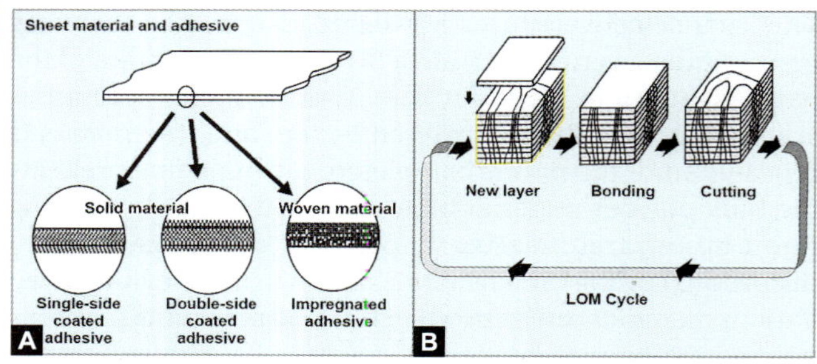

Figs. 84.14A and B: Laminated object manufacturing: (A) Material combination; (B) LOM cycle.

materials. As seen in **Figure 84.14A**, the sheet material carries the adhesive either on one side or both sides, or it contains the adhesive in itself, like woven composite material impregnated with bonding agent. The adhesive which can be pre coated on to material or be deposited prior to bonding, enables layers of sheet material to be attached to each other so as to construct a three-dimensional object. After one layer is deposited, peripheries of this layer's cross-section are cut by a laser beam based on the information from the CAD model. This bonding-before-cutting procedure is repeated until the full height of the part is reached **(Fig. 84.14).**[29]

Dental Application of 3D Printing

Digitalization through 3D printing is a remarkable advancement in the field of dentistry which allows precision in treating patients. The type of 3D printer, material used for printing, and build thickness are known to influence the accuracy of printed models.[30]

Its various applications in dentistry include: Fabrication of 3D printed tooth, implant-supported restorations, composite and ceramic esthetic inlays and onlays, guided endodontic interventions, customized myofunctional appliances, maxillofacial customised prosthesis like eye or nose prosthesis, obturator for maxillectomy, complete dentures, digital impressions, invisaligners orthodontic braces, bioprinting tissue or organs and also customised 3D printed dosage delivery system. Thus, 3D printing has revolutionized dentistry while able to produce high-quality dental prosthesis with precision.[30]

- **Mankovich et al. (1994)** first applied 3D technology for skull reconstruction. Because autogenous bone grafting would be the ideal standard for skull reconstruction, donor bone should be harvested. The ideal curvature should be researched in advance because the bone is so rigid that bending is quite difficult and risky.
- **Shahbazian M et al (2013)** evaluated the outcome of a new approach for tooth autotransplantation by using a CBCT-based surgical planning and stereolithographic transfer, compared to the outcome of a conventional autotransplantation protocol. They concluded that CBCT-based surgical planning of tooth autotransplantation may benefit from a shorter surgical time, while being a less invasive technique, causing fewer failures than a conventional approach.[31]
- **Bratosin C et al (2014)** presented a comparative study of the mechanical behavior of the deciduous molar restorative material bone assembly subjected to the loads occurring during the activity of mastication. A finite element analysis was performed using 3D models for two dental restorations : composite resin and Gic Fuji IX material. They concluded that finite element study of the 3D models led to the determination of the stress and displacement distributions in any point on the surface and in the sections of the structural assembly primary molar – restoration material, emphasizing the most stressed areas which occur during the activity of mastication.[32]
- **Strbac et al. (2016)** described the autotransplantation of immature premolars in a maxillary incisor avulsion scenario using a completely digital workflow. They used CAD to select the appropriate donor teeth based on dimensions and stage of root development. Prototype teeth were modified to accommodate the dimensions of Hertwig's epithelial root sheath and to minimize damage to the apical papilla. The CAD modified prototype teeth were virtually auto-transplanted into the donor sites to create successively larger osteotomy guides that allowed for a more precise and efficient surgical phase.
- **De Souza N (2018)** reported a case of 12 year old female patient which highlights the effective usage of 3D printed model as a surgical aid in the removal of a compound odontome and impacted incisors from the mandibular anterior region.[33]
- **Pawar et al. (2019)** reported the use of 3D printed band and loop space maintainer with successful outcomes. 3D printed space maintainers are advantageous in that they are customizable, can be printed in single units which is cost effective and they also eliminate the need for prolonged laboratory and chair side times.[12]
- **Zheng J et al (2019)** presented case report that described the treatment of 8 day old neonate with unilateral CLP by molding the nasolabial morphology and alveolar arch with the use of 3D printing of the PNAM device. By the end of PNAM treatment, the cleft gap was reduced with the 2 alveolar segments nearly contacted with a proper maxillary alveolar arch form.[34]
- **Swennen GR et al (2020)** developed custom-made 3D protective face mask, consisting of two reusable 3D-printed components (a face mask and a filter membrane support) and two disposable components (a head fixation band and a filter membrane).[35]
- **Amin D et al (2020)** described method of using a 3D printer to print face shields. They used FDM printer with additive manufacturing technology and a nozzle to make frame for the shield.[36]
- **Hakim MA et al (2020)** compared the stress distribution and displacement that resulted from the use of a Gerber space regainer and sagittal distalizer using three-dimensional finite element analysis. They found that Gerber space regainer showed greater displacement than that produced by the sagittal distalizer at the first permanent molar. However, such displacement was less at the other tested points when compared with that delivered by sagittal distalizer. The stresses created by Gerber appliance were higher in the crown and PDL of the deciduous canine than the crown of the first permanent molar crown.[37]
- **Guided non-surgical endodontics:** 3D printed directional guides can be useful for canal location during non-surgical

endodontic treatment where there are significant risks of procedural errors, including root perforation, which can severely compromise treatment outcome. CBCT scans, optical scans of intra-oral anatomy or plaster models are match and implant planning/CAD software are used to virtually design the directional guides and select the depth calibrated implant drills/dental burs.[38]

- **Guided surgical endodontics**, like other guided procedures, is reliant on meticulous treatment planning that includes finalising the design of the 3D printed surgical guide, using implant planning software loaded with the matched CBCT and optical scan data sets.[38]
- **Cranioplasty for the correction of syndromic craniosynostosis:** Similar to skull reconstruction with bone grafting, extensive bone grafting is needed to correct craniosynostosis. Current 3D printing technology can provide an osteotomy guide that is very useful for the reconstruction process. Moreover, surgeons can simulate the surgery in advance using the 3D printed tactile model. 3D printed prototype models are a particularly effective tool for simulating LeFort I, II, or III midface osteotomy, which require delicate blind osteotomy.
- **Orthognathic surgery:** 3D printing technology provides an additional osteotomy guide and occlusal splint. However, the 3D printing model generally shows some errors in terms of accuracy, which is problematic for ideal dental occlusion. Therefore, especially for dentition, scanning devices should be used to obtain ideal dental occlusal splints for orthognathic surgery.
- **Maxillary reconstruction:** Recent advances in 3D printing technology now enable fibular osteotomy and fixation guides to be provided, which enable the dental implant to be inserted in the ideal position.
- **Orthodontic 3D-printed models:** Invisalign system realigns the patient teeth digitally to make a series of 3D printed models for construction of aligners, where the patient will be receiving a new set of aligners every 2 weeks and reposition the teeth over a period of time. This technology will be time saving, patient data set can be digitally saved, printed when needed and minimises the physical storage requirement.
- **Three-dimensional printed bioresorbable scaffold for guided bone and tissue regeneration:** Recent advancement in the field of tissue engineering has led to the development of "3D printed" scaffolds. These multiphasic scaffolds consisting of both hard (bone and cementum) and soft tissues (gingiva and PDL) components of the periodontium, are not only specific for the particular tissue but are also competent mechanically. With the increasing demand for tissue regeneration, these scaffolds have been investigated in different periodontal procedures such as socket preservation, guided tissue and bone regeneration, sinus, and vertical bone augmentation.[25]
- **Goh et al.** reported the use of 3D-printed bioresorbable scaffold in socket preservation and reported normal bone healing and significantly better alveolar ridge preservation when compared to extraction socket without scaffold after 6 months.[25]
- **3D printing for implants placement:** Implant placement is a routine procedure done by dental professionals to replace missing teeth due to its predictable outcomes. Implant placement is a technically demanding procedure and if not done properly, can lead to various complications such as poor esthetics, damage to anatomically important structures, infections, and implant failure. Guided implant placement can prevent these complications by fabrication of surgical guides with the help of 3D printing. It helps in accurate 3D placement of implant thus preventing unwanted damage to anatomic structures and reduce time.[25]
- **3D drug delivery system:** It can print a biocompatible, patient specific morphological micro and macroscopic pore arrangement can incorporate drugs and proteins. The unexplored field of lipid based drug delivery system can enhance drug absorption, bioavailability of lipophilic drugs and high membrane permeability. Lipid has low temperature melting point and therefore is used in 3D print based thermolabile compounds. These compounds can be processed into local drug delivery system.
- **Mold (shell) for metal casting:** Compared to conventional methods of casting production (including the construction of tooling and the pouring of a casting), ceramic molds can be produced for metal parts directly by CAD models. These molds are created on a computer screen by using RP techniques. Three-dimensional printing, such as the direct shell production casting process, produces ceramic casting molds for metal casting using a layer-by-layer printing process.[39]
- **Mold for facial prosthesis :** Over the past decade, RP techniques have been applied successfully to the fabrication of a facial prosthesis. Pattern fabrication via RP has been effective; however, conventional flasking and investing procedures were still needed to make the actual prosthesis. An innovative design and production method (of the negative mold of the facial prosthesis) for casting the actual prosthesis with silicon directly (by using CAD and RP techniques) has been proposed. Instead of fabricating a positive RP pattern of the prosthesis (after the design and fitting stages), the prosthesis computer model is referenced to generate a CAD model of a mold.[39]
- **Mold for complete denture :** Researchers at Peking University developed a novel CAD and RP system to make individualized flasks (molds) for a complete denture. The process includes establishing a 3D graphic database of artificial teeth for parameterization positioning, getting 3D data of edentulous models and rims in centric relation, exploring a CAD route and developing software for complete dentures, fabricating physical flasks (molds) by 3DP, and finishing the complete denture using a traditional laboratory procedure.[39]
- **Fabrication of wax patterns for prosthetic constructions:** The manufacturing of wax pattern is the first step in the process of fabrication of a dental prosthesis. The RP technologies had made possible automatic build-up of numbers of wax patterns for different dental constructions by structuring them up layer by layer. The next step remains the traditional lost wax procedure.

- **Forensic odontology:** Forensic sciences are multidisciplinary in nature and typically require cooperation and coordination between the law enforcement officials, forensic pathologists, forensic odontologists, forensic anthropologists' etc. Although biting is a dynamic process and relies on multiple variables like the jaws position, teeth, the substrate, the force of biting etc., bite marks can provide valuable evidence to identify the criminal. After scanning the entire bite mark can be recreated in an appropriate material using 3D printing. This can then be utilized to match with the casts of the suspect's teeth, create overlays and can also be presented in court as evidence. The scans themselves can be uses for digitally matching the suspect's teeth using new software. Thus 3D printing can curtail the rapid loss of information that occurs in the bite marks and helps preserve maximum information in all the three dimensions.[40]

Limitations of 3D Printing[41,42]

- Rapid prototyping includes the restriction of material choice to substances amenable to additive fabrication, which can limit choice of color and product durability/ strength.
- The additive layering process can compromise surface finish and also pose difficulties for the creation of a working machine, whereby constituent parts work together to achieve a particular function.
- The size of objects produced is also limited by the size of the 3D printer, which can prevent large structures such as whole body models from being produced.
- The cost is an additional limitation, with the rapid prototyping machines costing in the tens to hundreds of thousands of dollars, not including the cost of the plastic and resin based materials.
- It can also take hours to days to produce a final product, depending on the machine used and the complexity of the product.
- An inherent weakness is built into the design due to its staircase effect. This effect is created by successive deposition of material on top of the first layer.
- Requires support materials, which are difficult to remove later.
- It is technique sensitive; a trained professional is required.
- Resin causes inflammation, irritation on contact or inhalation.
- Resin cannot be heat sterilized.
- Stereolithography can be done if only light-curable polymers are available.
- Depending on materials, additional treatment like sintering might be required for additional strength.
- Ethical and legal clearance is low.

Digital technology has become indispensable to modern dentistry. In terms of two universal values—saving time and money—digitalization sh.ows both advantages and setbacks. To the modern dentists, eliminating time-consuming processes from their work with the aid of technology is a step forward that might enable them to be more work efficient. On the other hand, a limitation of digital dentistry is its high cost. Going digital implies a significant investment, not only into devices, but also in their updates and trainings for the medical staff too who works with them. Digitalization in Pediatric Dentistry helps specialists to provide a complex, qualitative and most importantly patient friendly treatment, to reduce anxiety and pain, shorten the lengthy time taking procedures and enhance children's trust and enthusiasm regarding their dental visits.

POINTS TO REMEMBER

- 3D printing, also popularly known as additive manufacturing is a novel technique recently pioneered by Pawar et al (2019) and reinforced by Khanna et al (2021).
- STL format is used to preserve digital 3D model.
- First patent application for RP technology was filed by Dr Kodama in Japan, in May 1980.
- The first commercially available SLA printer was patented in 1986 by Charles W Hull.
- SLA was first developed by Dr Hideo Kodama in 1981.

Questionnaire

1. Digital Dentistry: What it is? What it is for? What are the benefits and limitations?
2. What is digitalization in dentisry? What are the steps for fabrication of space maintainer through digital impression?
3. Describe 3D printed space mainter, fabrication procedure and its advantages.
4. Describe briefly: Customized digital restoration and overall method. What are the advantages of customized restoration over previous prefabricated options?
5. What is 3D printing? What are its methods, application in dentistry and limitations?

REFERENCES

1. Tassery H, Manton DJ. Detection and Diagnosis of Carious Lesions. In Ece Eden (Ed). Evidence-Based Caries Prevention. Switzerland: Springer International Publishing; 2016. pp. 13-20.
2. Ellenbogen H. Minimally Invasive Dentistry for the Pediatric Patient [Internet]. California:Dentalacade myofce;2016 [cited 2018 May12]. Available from: https://www.dentalacademyofce.com/ courses/3174%2FPDF%2F1609cei_Ellenbogen_web. pdf.
3. Dias da Silva PR, Martins Marques M, Steagall W. Medeiros Mendes F, Lascala CA. Accuracy of direct digital radiography for detecting occlusal caries in primary teeth compared with conventional radiography and visual inspection: an in vitro study. Dentomaxillofac Radiol. 2010;39(6):362-7.

4. Braga M, Mendes F, Ekstrand K. Detection Activity Assessment and Diagnosis of Dental Caries Lesions. Dent Clin North Am. 2010;54(3):479-93.
5. Bahrami G, Hagstrøm C, Wenzel A. Bitewing examination with four digital receptors. Dentomaxillofacial Radiology. 2003;32:317-321.
6. Wenzel A. Bitewing and digital bitewing radiography for detection of caries lesions. J Dent Res. 2004;83 Spec No C:C72-5.
7. Ahmed KE. "We're Going Digital: The Current State of CAD/CAM Dentistry in Prosthodontics". Primary Dental Journal. 2018;7 (2): 30-5. doi:10.1177/205016841800700205. ISSN 2050-1684.PMID 30095879. S2CID 51957826.
8. Graf S, Cornelis MA, Hauber Gameiro G, Cattaneo PM. Computer-aided design and manufacture of hyrax devices: Can we really go digital? Am J Orthod Dentofacial Orthop. 2017;152(6):870-74.
9. Burde AV, Baciu S, Popa D, Constantiniuc M, Manole M, Kallay E, Campian RC. Highlighting knowledge, attitude and practices regarding CAD/CAM technology among oral healthcare providers in Cluj-NapocAInternational Journal of Medical Dentistry. 2016;20(4):293-300.
10. Lee SM, Lee JW. Computerized occlusal analysis: correlation with occlusal indexes to assess the outcome of orthodontic treatment or the severity of malocculusion. Korean J Orthod. 2016;46(1):27-35.
11. Mizui M, Nabeshima F, Tosa J, Tanaka M, Kawazoe T. Quantitative analysis of occlusal balance in intercuspal position using the T-Scan system. Int J Prosthodont. 1994;7(1):62-71.
12. Pawar BA. Maintenance of space by innovative three-dimensional-printed band and loop space maintainer. Journal of Indian Society of Pedodontics and Preventive Dentistry. 2019;37(2):205.
13. Khanna S, Rao D, Panwar S, Pawar BA, Ameen S. 3D printed band and loop space maintainer: A digital game changer in preventive orthodontics. Journal of Clinical Pediatric Dentistry. 2021;45(3):147-5110.17796/1053-4625-45.3.1
14. Kerstein RB, Thumati P, Padmaja S. Force finishing and centering to balance a removable complete denture prosthesis using the t-scan III computerized occlusal analysis system. J Indian Prosthodont Soc. 2013;13(3):184
15. Popşor S. Occlusion time in craniomandibular disfunction vs usual prosthetic patients. International Journal of Medical Dentistry. 2017;7(1):57-61.
16. Hosamuddin H. Computer-assisted technique for surgical tooth extraction. Int J Dent. 2016.http://dx.doi.org/10.1155/2016/7484159.
17. Jo C, Bae D, Choi B, Kim J. Removal of supernumerary teeth utilizing a computer-aided design/computer aided manufacturing surgical guide. J Oral Maxillofac Surg. 2017;75(5):924.e1-924.e9.
18. Collares K, Correa MB, et al. A practice-based research network on the survival of ceramic inlay/onlay restorations. Dent Mater. 2016 ;32(5):687-94. doi: 10.1016/j.dental.2016.02.006.
19. Kau CH, Kamel SG, Wilson J, Wong ME. New method for analysis of facial growth in a pediatric reconstructed mandible. Am J Orthod Dentofacial Orthop. 2011;139(4):e285-90.
20. Ogodescu EA, Bratu E, Tudor A. et al. Estimation of child's biological age based on tooth development.RomJ Leg Mede. 2011;19(2):115-24.
21. Wiederhold BK, Gao K, Sulea C, Wiederhold MD. Virtual reality as a distraction technique in chronic pain patients. Cyberpsychol Behav Soc Netw. 2014;17(6):346-52.
22. Ram D, Shapira J, Holan G, Magora F, Cohen S, DavidovichE. Audiovisual video eyeglass distraction during dental treatment in children. Quintessence Int. 2010;41(8):673-9.
23. Pandey A, Tiwari L. 3D-Printing-The New Frontier in Prosthodontics-A Review. Journal of Advanced Medical and Dental Sciences Research. 2019;7(11):69-73.
24. Gul M, Arif A, Ghafoor R. Role of three-dimensional printing in periodontal regeneration and repair: Literature review. Journal of Indian Society of Periodontology. 2019;23(6):504.
25. Dawood A, Marti BM, Sauret-Jackson V, Darwood A. 3D printing in dentistry. British Dental Journal. 2015;219(11):521.
26. Jasveer S, Jianbin X. Comparison of different types of 3D printing technologies. International Journal of Scientific and Research Publications (IJSRP). 2018;8(4):1-9.
27. Singh R, Garg HK. Fused deposition modeling–a state of art review and future applications. Reference Module in Materials Science and Materials Engineering. 2016 Jan.
28. Kumar S. Selective laser sintering: Recent advances. In Pacific International Conference on Applications of Lasers and Optics . 2010; 2010 (1):607. Laser Institute of America.
29. Feygin M, Hsieh B. Laminated object manufacturing (LOM): a simpler process. In1991 International Solid Freeform Fabrication Symposium 1991.
30. Vallabhaneni S, Saraf P, Khasnis S. Augmenting realm of 3D printing in restorative dentistry and endodontics-A review. International Journal of Dental Materials. 2020;2(1):24-9.
31. Shahbazian M, Jacobs R, Wyatt J, Denys D, Lambrichts I, Vinckier F, Willems G. Validation of the cone beam computed tomography–based stereolithographic surgical guide aiding autotransplantation of teeth: clinical case–control study. Oral Surgery, Oral Medicine, Oral Pathology and Oral Radiology. 2013;115(5):667-75.
32. Bratosin C, Baciu F, Rusu-Casandra A. Comparative study of the biomechanical behavior of the deciduous molar-restorative material-bone assembly. Procedia Engineering. 2014;69:1251-7.
33. De Souza N, Kamat S, Chalakkal P, Khandeparker RV. Use of 3D printed model as an aid in surgical removal of a rare occurrence of a compound odontome in the anterior mandible associated with impacted teeth. Journal of Clinical and Experimental Dentistry. 2018;(7):e721.
34. Zheng J, He H, Kuang W, Yuan W. Presurgical nasoalveolar molding with 3D printing for a patient with unilateral cleft lip, alveolus, and palate. American Journal of Orthodontics and Dentofacial Orthopedics. 2019;156(3):412-9.
35. Swennen GR, Pottel L, Haers PE. Custom-made 3D-printed face masks in case of pandemic crisis situations with a lack of commercially available FFP2/3 masks. International Journal of Oral and Maxillofacial Surgery. 2020 Apr 2.
36. Amin D, Nguyen N, Roser SM, Abramowicz S. 3D Printing of Face Shields During COVID-19 Pandemic: A Technical Note. Journal of Oral and Maxillofacial Surgery. 2020 May 1.
37. Hakim MA, Khatab NM, Mohamed KM, Elheeny AA. A comparative three-dimensional finite element study of two space regainers in the mixed dentition stage. European Journal of Dentistry. 2020;14(1):107 .
38. Shah P, Chong BS. 3D imaging, 3D printing and 3D virtual planning in endodontics. Clinical Oral Investigations. 2018 Mar 1;22(2):641-54.
39. Jawahar A, Maragathavalli G. Applications of 3D Printing in Dentistry–A Review. Journal of Pharmaceutical Sciences and Research. 2019;11(5):1670-5.
40. Katreva I, Dikova T, Abadzhiev M, Tonchev T, Dzhendov D, Simov M, et al. 3D-printing in contemporary prosthodontic treatment. Scripta Scientifica Medicinae Dentalis. 2016;2(1):7-11.
41. Khanna S, Dhaimade. Exploring the 3rd dimension: Application of 3D printing in forensic odontology. J Forensic Sci Criminal Inves. 2017;3:1-3.
42. Baskaran V, Štrkalj G, Štrkalj M, Di Ieva A. Current applications and future perspectives of the use of 3D printing in anatomical training and neurosurgery. Frontiers in Neuroanatomy. 2016;10:69.

CHAPTER

Infant Cleft Care

Saranya Mony

CHAPTER OUTLINE

Cleft lip (CL) and cleft palate (CP) are two of the most prevalent oral congenital defects in Indian children. Congenital oral cleft is estimated to affect one out of every 1,000 live births. The male to female ratio is thought to be around 1.8:1. Unilateral clefts are more common than bilateral defects. Oral clefts are occasionally linked to syndromes. For their basic survival in their early days and ongoing interdisciplinary care, infants born with congenital clefts require excellent support from a team of healthcare specialists.

An infant is defined as a child under the age of one year, which includes the neonatal phase, which lasts the first 28 days of life.

GOAL OF INFANT CLEFT CARE

- A healthcare provider's primary goal is to help the infant thrive, with a secondary focus on nutrition, fostering healthy growth and development, and assisting the family in coping.
- A pediatric dentist is a crucial member of a multidisciplinary team that plays a significant role in the holistic care of children with cleft deformities. They help with nursing care, feeding assistance, family psychological support, preventive care, and rehabilitation.
- It is critical to establish breastfeeding in the early days since the baby quickly adapts and imprints to the feeding methods introduced early on. Early intervention measures established by the pediatric dentist will serve as the foundation for the family's feeding practices.
- As neonatal care facilities improve every day in our country, with an emphasis on early intervention and rehabilitation of congenital problems, a dentist's inclusion in the early intervention team is imperative. Understanding our responsibility and acquiring the ability to intervene early in cleft babies would thus go a long way toward ensuring their healthy survival

CHALLENGES IN INFANT CLEFT CARE

Taking care of infants born with cleft lip and palate is challenging for a variety of reasons. The parental shock comes first, especially if the child was not diagnosed with a cleft during pregnancy scans. The parents are not mentally prepared to accept the fact that their child has a congenital abnormality. Many mothers are oblivious to the problem. The guilt of having given birth to a child with a disability, as well as superstitious beliefs in some Indian households that the family is cursed, make it even more difficult.

Keeping an Airway Open

- If there is an aspiration, infants may display signs of respiratory distress or cyanosis.
- There is a risk of airway blockage in infants who are born with a posterior tongue position and a smaller jaw, as in the Pierre Robin sequence. In such cases, anchoring the tongue anteriorly with a nasogastric tube or suture put into the tongue and taped to the mandible can help. Jaw surgery or a tracheostomy may also be necessary in severe cases.

Difficulty in Nursing

- The most crucial responsibility for parents is to provide nursing care, which includes feeding cleft babies without choking or aspiration.
- Nursing goals include not only ensuring appropriate nutrition for a healthy weight gain, but also assisting parents in coping with their concerns about feeding their newborn. The mother, as well as any family members who will be supporting them in their nursing journey, should also get psychoeducation on the condition.
- Nasal regurgitation, poor suction, excessive air intake, frequent burping, and longer feeding durations are all common feeding challenges that make it difficult to provide appropriate nutritional intake to infants with clefts.[1]

Psychological Concerns for the Mother

- The fear of handling a baby who is at danger of aspiration can cause anxiety or panic attacks, which can be avoided if a well-informed healthcare practitioner can handhold and educate the family on the first day after the baby is delivered. Facilitating the mother's ability to cope with anxiety related to feeding and providing reassurance go a long way in preventing postpartum depression. The mother-infant relationship is a dyad, and for the baby to thrive, the mother must be nurtured emotionally and psychologically.
- Emotional attachment and feeding: Attachment theory states that the emotional relationship that develops between the newborn and the primary caregiver throughout the first year of life is known as attachment. After seeing children who were deprived of maternal care, John Bowlby, a British psychoanalyst and psychiatrist, developed the attachment hypothesis. Early bonds, he discovered, lay the groundwork for healthy emotional development and can influence adult relationships.[2]
- Natural selection resulted in the newborn displaying five distinct behaviors: sucking, clinging, following, crying, and smiling. By having a responsive caregiver to address their requirements, these behaviors mechanisms allow immature offspring have a chance for a healthy survival. Early emotional relationships are crucial in developing distinct types of attachment between a child and the primary caregiver, according to attachment theory.[3] The emotional attachment that results becomes the child's internal working model, impacting their own emotions and personal interactions throughout their lives.
- In order for an infant born with an oral cleft to survive the first few months of life, the primary caregiver, who is usually the mother, must be in good physical and mental health. It aids in the establishment of attachment with the newborn when the healthcare practitioner can provide adequate information about the condition, current facts, and advice the parents on nursing. It is an important first step that is frequently delayed in many contexts, preventing a good mother-child attachment. The hormones that facilitate milk secretion are controlled by the mother's psychological state to be calm and feel pleased, hence a healthy mother-child attachment is vital for lactation.

EXAMINATION AND IDENTIFICATION OF AN ORAL CLEFT

- To rule out any congenital malformations, every baby should be screened shortly after birth. The Neonatologist, Pediatrician, Midwife, or Nurse who attends to the newborn soon after birth does delivery point screening. Following the delivery of the baby, an extraoral and intraoral examination is conducted.
- **Extraoral examination:** These are helpful in identifying clefts in the lip and the position of the mandible. Baby's mandibular retrognathia has been linked to Pierre Robin sequelae. When a baby cries, his or her ability to move the mandible downward and backward. In a very small percentage of cases, ankylosis of the jaw, oral cleft deformity. Any other clefts, growth in facial region or deformities in lips should be documented.
- **Intraoral examination:** To do the visual and tactile assessments, the examiner stands behind the newborn at 12 o'clock with his/her eyes directly above the infant's head. The first aspect is by visual examination under theater torch lighting of the oral cavity, compressing the tongue with a depressor to rule out any posterior uvular cleft; Tactile examination of the gum pads and palate surfaces with a gloved finger to rule out submucosal deficiencies; check for the sucking reflex and tongue posture.
- Document your findings in a casebook and photograph the defect to aid in treatment planning and discussion with the interdisciplinary team.
- After the infant has been checked and any other anomalies have been ruled out, a feeding plan must be devised. The first 24 hours are considered critical in establishing the mother-child relationship and beginning oral feeding.

STEPS IN INTERVENTION

- **Forming a therapeutic relationship:** As caregivers, the first priority is to build a positive relationship with the parents and family. This will serve as the foundation for assisting the baby's development. Regardless of the family's crises or emotional trauma, we strive to strengthen the link between mother and infant.
  - Help them comprehend the science and address the likely etiology of the problem
  - Talk about taboo and superstitious beliefs attached
  - Validate their humiliation, shock, guilt, sorrow, grief
  - Holding a non-judgmental space for venting out the disappointment
  - Letting them know we are there to help them take care of the baby
  - Inform the mother and her family about possibility of postpartum depression and encourage them to seek care.
- **Familiarizing mother with lactation concepts:** Assisting the mother in gaining confidence in her ability to lift, handle, and hold the infant is the first step in instilling confidence and gaining the family trust. Even if there is no milk flow, mother is taught to allow suckling, with the baby's head in an upright position. This aids in bonding because skin-to-skin contact makes the infant

feel secure, and the mother's brain generates oxytocin, which help the brain remember the experience of feeding the baby as positive one. Mother is taught the early signs of hunger, such as an infant sucking his lips, closing his fist, and shifting his face from side to side. This allows the mother to be ready to feed the baby before it begins to wail uncontrollably.

- **Promoting breast milk feeding:** WHO and UNICEF advise[4] that Breastfeeding should begin within one hour of birth, continue exclusively during the first 6 months and could be supplemented with nutritionally appropriate and safe complementary foods at 6 months of age, with continued nursing after 6 months and extended to 2 years and beyond.
- **Advantages of breastfeeding:** Infants with cleft defects should be assisted to feed on the breast whenever possible, and various positions of modified breastfeeding should be encouraged. Breastfeeding the infant from an early age helps to normalize the infant in the family. Unfortunately, the parents are misled due to the attitudes of many healthcare personnel and a lack of information. It aids in the normal development of facial musculature, teaches the infant to swallow, and protects them from upper respiratory infections and otitis media.[5]
- **Uses of breastfeeding:** The goal in the first 2–3 days of a baby's existence is to feed the baby colostrum, which is rich in antibodies and secreted 40–50 mL every day. Following days, milk secretion increases to 400–800 mL per day, depending on the baby's demands. In the first week, a feed of 20–30 mL every 2 hours is recommended. Later, as the appetite increases, the amount of milk per feed can be increased. To avoid mother-baby tiredness, each feed should be no longer than half an hour. It is important to empty one breast before moving on to the next. The baby's activity level, healthy appearance, regular intake, lack of dehydration, weight gain, and 4–6 diaper changes per day show that the supply is adequate.

MODIFIED BREASTFEEDING METHODS[6]

- Milk ejection can be facilitated by the mother placing four fingers below and thumb above the breast and squeezing whilst timing it to the baby's sucking rhythm and breathing.
- Breastfeeding can be initiated and sustained successfully in children born with an isolated cleft lip.
- A football or cross-cradle hold can provide a comfortable breastfeeding position **(Fig. 85.1)**. To close the defect in newborns born with unilateral cleft lip, either mother's finger or thumb can be placed alongside the nipple. Attempting to put the baby's head at a 30-degree upright angle helps in positioning the baby comfortably, and the swallowing reflex prevents milk from entering the nasal cavity. If the cleft palate is unilateral, the breast is directed towards a larger segment to prevent the nipple from entering the nasal cavity, which can help with better breast compression and milk ejection.
- A face on straddle position is ideal in an infant with bilateral cleft lip **(Fig. 85.2)**. In a baby with bilateral cleft palate, the nipple is pointed downwards, and milk is pumped into the baby's mouth while two fingers support the chin.

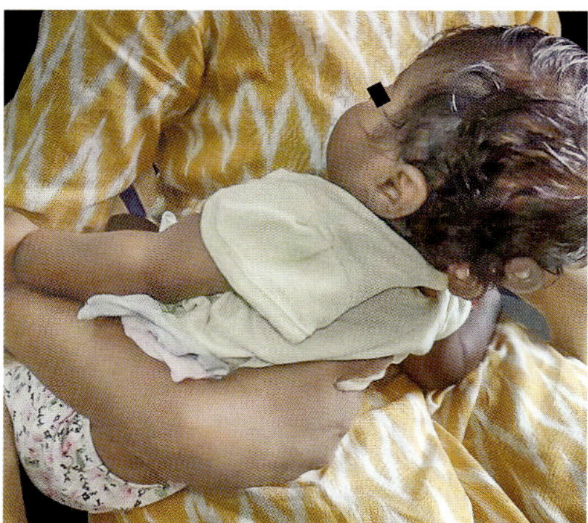

Fig. 85.1: Football or cross-cradle hold feeding position.

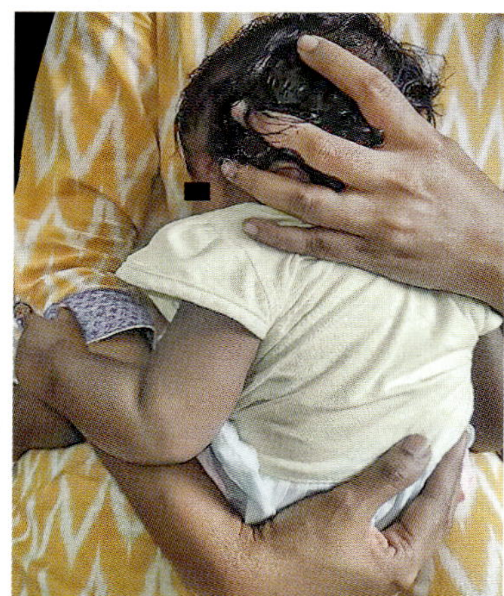

Fig. 85.2: Straddle feeding position.

Feeding with Assisted Methods

- Because of the various factors and challenges linked with oral cleft abnormalities, breastmilk/formula feeding with assisted methods is an alternative when direct nursing is not possible. Assisted feeding attempts to promote milk intake without aspiration or spilling, and to reduce feeding time so that both mother and baby get enough rest in between feeds.
- It comprises the use of over-the-counter modified feeding bottles and teats specifically designed to feed babies born with cleft.
- It may be beneficial to utilize a traditional palada or spoon-feeding.
- To feed the newborns without spillage, a syringe can also be utilized.

Use of Feeding Plate

- A feeding plate that is customized for the baby's anatomy resembles an artificial palate in neonates, allowing for unobstructed feeds and lowering the risk of milk aspiration. The fabrication of a feeding plate can help young mothers overcome their fear of aspiration while feeding. This, in turn, can help the mother bond with her baby better and raise the chances of having a longer breastfeeding journey.
- Fabrication of feeding plate **(Figs. 85.3A to H)**.

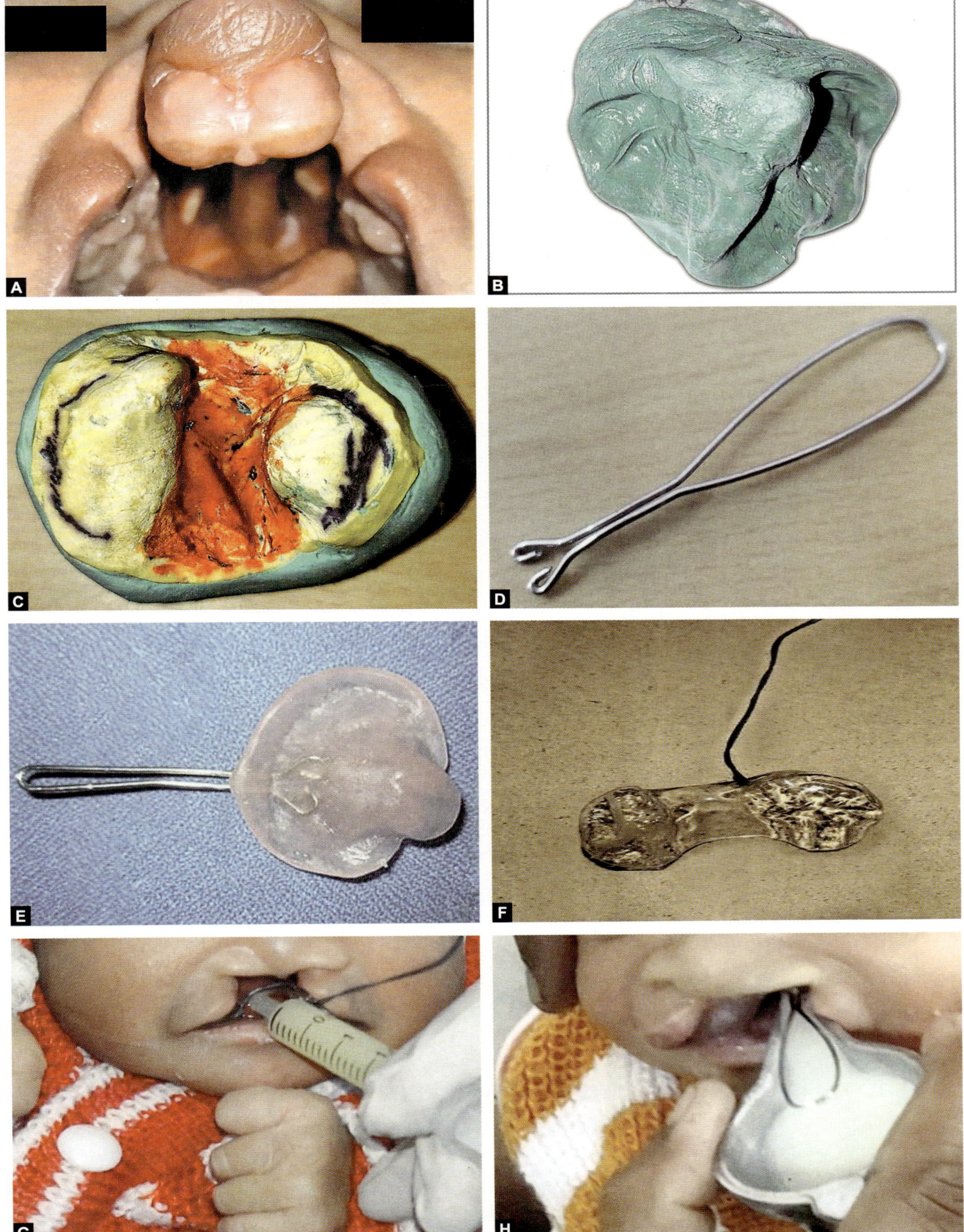

Figs. 85.3A to H: Fabrication of feeding appliance: (A) Cleft; (B) Impression made with greenstick compound; (C) Cast with markings of border in black and defect in red; (D) Handle for feeding plate; (E) Acrylic feeding plate with handle; (F) Vacuum formed thermoplastic feeding plate with suture thread; (G) Feeding plate used with palada feeding; (H) Feeding plate used with syringe feeding.

Impression is obtained using a stainless steel spoon head of suitable size, fingers, or the handle of an impression tray

↓

Hard putty or a low-fusing impression compound are recommended materials before placing the impression compound in the oral cavity, check the temperature with a non-gloved finger

↓

Use gauze over the impression material to prevent it from entering the nasal cavity or nasopharyngeal tube and inducing aspiration

↓

After impression is made, suction the oral cavity and visually examine for any remnants

↓

Cast is poured

↓

The borders of the cleft is marked and a wax is used to block the defect

↓

Handle made with stainless steel 19 gauge wire can be attached to help with easy handling, alternatively a suture thread or floss can be used to secure the feeding plate to jaws

↓

Heat cure acrylic or thermoplastic sheet used with vacuum press method can be used for fabrication of feeding plate. Two or three holes are drilled into the plate with a straight bur to allow airflow

Caregiver Training in Assisted Feeding

- It is critical to ensure that the baby is held upright when being fed using aided methods. Caregivers are instructed to hold the baby in the proper position when feeding. While using a feeding plate, caregivers are taught to perform hand hygiene before handling the appliance, inserting, removing, and maintaining it. After each feed, the plate is washed in running water and stored in drinking water. Cleaning with water and mild soap on a routine basis is advised. To prevent contamination, only the primary caregiver/mother should handle the appliance. After 24 hours, the infant is evaluated for any signs of discomfort, pain, gum redness, and pressure spots.
- The baby's oral hygiene is maintained by wiping gum pads with a washcloth, the neck with a soft cloth, and nose hygiene with cotton buds if drying or crusting is observed.
- The use of a palatal obturator when combined with lactation education, reduced feeding time and boosted volume intake, and was linked to proper development, resulting in timely surgical repair. Mothers who wanted to breastfeed chose to utilize the obturator to support high-volume intake, reduce infant tiredness, and provide breast milk for nutrition.

FOLLOW UP

- Follow-up visits are required every two weeks for the next three months to check weight gain and growth.
- During the first and subsequent visits, the height, weight, and head circumference are measured and plotted on a graph to ensure the infant is healthy and receiving adequate nutrition. An expected weight gain for a healthy infant is 30 g per day.
- Parents are counseled on the importance of good weight gain so that their child is ready for lip repair surgery at 3 months and palate repair surgery at 10 months.

PRESURGICAL CLEFT ORTHODONTICS

Presurgical cleft orthodontics may be commenced following a discussion with the surgeon for a infant with extensive bilateral cleft defects, as it has been found to improve surgery outcomes. Many cleft specialty centers use nasoalveolar moulding NAM to guide the growth of premaxilla and defective segments.

CARIES PREVENTION

- Early childhood caries prevention in children with cleft is gaining traction since it is one of the few instances where a pediatric dentist can treat a child before the teeth have erupted.
- A dental home can be established.
- Parents are given practical guidance on how to clean their gum pads, clean their teeth, and adopt a caries-preventive diet.
- The CAMBRA protocol is followed for caries prevention. Regular follow-up visits are ensured.

POINTS TO REMEMBER

- Cleft lip and palate are congenital oral defects that affect one in every 1,000 live births.
- The primary goal of infant cleft care is to enable the baby to thrive, which is accomplished by assisting the family in coping with the condition, establishing a good bond between the baby and caregiver, and ensuring proper nutrition and growth.
- Early intervention is critical for a cleft baby's proper development.
- The team faces a variety of challenges including maintaining an open airway, nursing difficulties, and psychological barriers encountered by the family.
- A thorough oral examination and documentation aids in the effective planning of interdisciplinary care.
- Early intervention steps include establishing a therapeutic relationship with the family, educating the mother about lactation and breastfeeding, discussing and demonstrating various feeding methods.
- Importance of establishing a dental home, caries prevention and providing anticipatory guidance to such parents.

Questionnaire

1. What are the goals of infant cleft care?
2. Elaborate the challenges faced by the cleft team while aiding in nursing.
3. How will you do an oral examination for an infant to rule out congenital oral defect?
4. What is attachment theory and explain its significance in a child's development?
5. Mention the early intervention strategies used in infant cleft care. What are the various methods of feeding an infant with a cleft defect?

REFERENCES

1. Goswami M, Jangra B, Bhushan U. Management of feeding Problem in a Patient with Cleft Lip/Palate. Int J Clin Pediatr Dent. 2016;9(2):143-5. doi: 10.5005/jp-journals-10005-1351. Epub 2016 Jun 15. PMID: 27365936; PMCID: PMC4921884.
2. Bretherton I. The origins of attachment theory: John Bowlby and Mary Ainsworth. Developmental Psychology. 1992;18(5):759.
3. Bowlby J, May DS, Solomon M. Attachment Theory. Lifespan Learning Institute; 1989.
4. Victora, Cesar G, et al. Breastfeeding in the 21st century: epidemiology, mechanisms, and lifelong effect. The Lancet. 2016;387(10017): 475-90.
5. Danner SC. Breastfeeding the infant with a cleft defect. NAACOGS Clin Issu Perinat Womens Health Nurs. 1992;3(4):634-9. PMID: 1476842.
6. Reilly S, Reid J, Skeat J, et al. ABM clinical protocol #18: guidelines for breastfeeding infants with cleft lip, cleft palate, or cleft lip and palate, revised 2013 [published correction appears in Breastfeed Med. 2013;8(6):519]. Breastfeed Med. 2013;8(4):349-353. doi:10.1089/bfm.2013.9988.

CHAPTER 86

Presurgical Nasoalveolar Molding in Management of Cleft Lip and Palate

Shrirang Sevekar, AR Prabhakar

CHAPTER OUTLINE

INTRODUCTION

Cleft lip and cleft palate (CLCP) is one of the most common congenital craniofacial disorders caused by incomplete fusion of maxillary, mandibular processes at embryonic stage. Patients born with a cleft deformity generally experience problems with feeding, speech, and hearing. The psychological stresses and social well-being secondary to their aesthetic deformity needs to be considered in the well-being of such patients. A multidisciplinary team approach is always desired to fully address the needs of such patient.[1] High incidence of one in every 1,000 newborn suffers from cleft lip and palate, highest among the Asians followed by Caucasians and Africans.[2]

The severity and form of cleft lip and palate can vary considerably among the patients. The unilateral cleft deformity is characterized by a wide nostril base and separated lip segments on the cleft side. The condition also features ill-defined philtral ridge and cupid bows, depressed nasal dome, apparently increased alar rim, an oblique columella and an overhanging nostril apex due to the displacement of the affected lower lateral nasal cartilage laterally and inferiorly. If there is associated cleft palate, the nasal septum deviates to the non-cleft side with an associated shift of the nasal base **(Figs. 86.1A and B)**. The bilateral cleft lip deformity typically presents with a procumbent or rotated premaxilla, deficient cupid bow and philtral ridge,

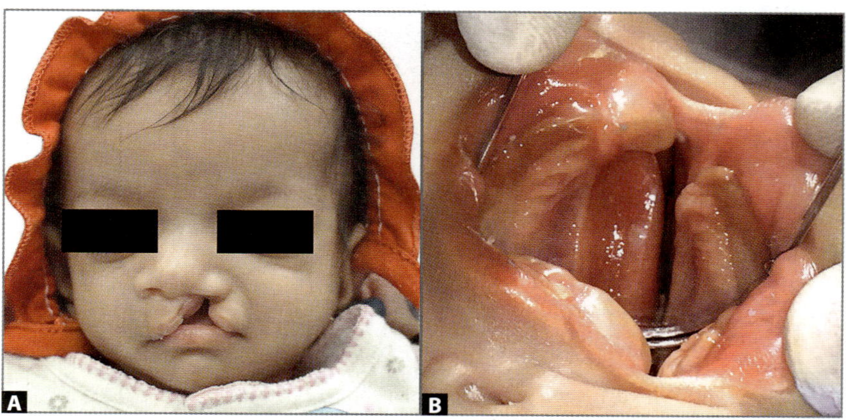

Figs. 86.1A and B: Unilateral cleft.

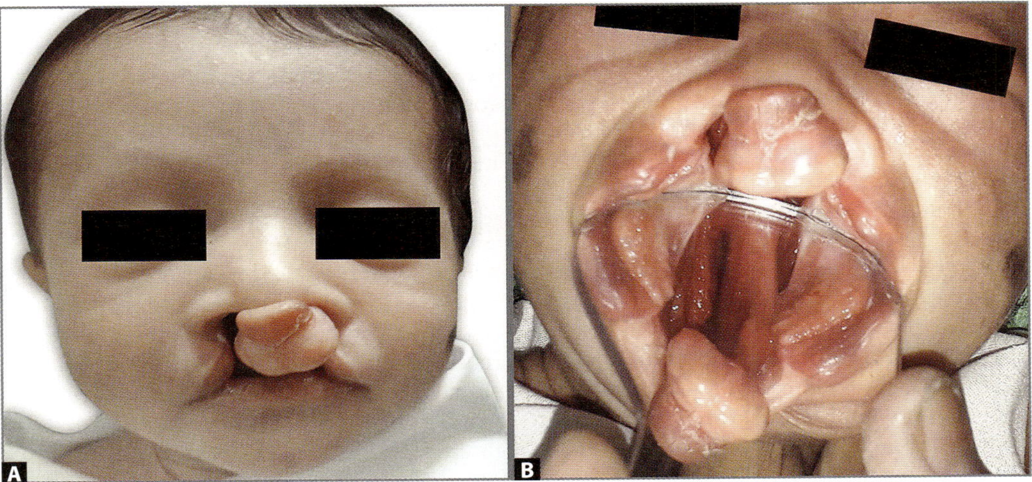

Figs. 86.2A and B: Bilateral cleft.

significantly increased alar width, widely separated lip segments and flared concave lower lateral alar cartilages. The prolabium is usually devoid of the well-developed muscles and flattened nasal tip is attached directly to it by a severely deficient or absent columella **(Figs. 86.2A and B)**. Complete care of the cleft patient is continuously evolving process with newer techniques developing all the time. This Chapter focuses on presurgical nasoalvelor moulding (PNAM), a newer technique in management of cleft lip and palate patients and the controversies sorrounding this technique.

BACKGROUND

Presurgical infant orthopedics (PSIO) is one of the initial line of treatment in comprehensive management of cleft lip and palate patients since many centuries. The early techniques were more focused on simple retraction and stabilization of protruded premaxilla before surgical intervention. Researchers like **Hoffmann** (1689), **Desault** (1790) in as early as 18th century demonstrated the use of facial binding to narrow the cleft and retract the maxilla before surgical repair in cleft lip palate patients. While **Hullihen** (1844) successfully used adhesive tape binding for presurgical cleft preparation. **Esmarch and Kowalzig** utilized Bonnet and strapping to stabilize the premaxilla. **Brophy** (1927) demonstrated cleft narrowing by passing a silver wire through the cleft alveolus and progressively tightening the wire to approximate the alveolus just before the lip repair. Recently, **McNeil** (1950) in his progressive approach towards the treatment of cleft lip palate patients used a series of plates to actively mould the alveolar segments into the desired position. **Georgiad and Lantham** (1975) used pin retained active appliance to simultaneously retract the premaxilla and expand the posterior segments over a period of several days. **Hotz** (1987) used passive orthopedic plate to slowly align the cleft segments. **Matsuo** (1991) employed silicon tubes to mold the nostrils. **Greyson et al** (1993) described presurgical nasoalveolar molding (PNAM) appliance developed at the institute of reconstructive plastic surgery at New York university medical center for molding the alveolar ridge and nasal cartilage concomitantly.[3]

NEED OF PNAM

In the management cleft lip palate repair, the basic approach is towards the restoration of the normal anatomy of the face. This includes the deficient tissue needs to be expanded. Reorganization of malpositioned structures through pressure appliances prior to surgery for better outcome. This offers higher possibility for lesser invasive surgical repair. In conventional surgical approaches the repaired clefted lip, columella and philtrum often result into severe scarring with lesser than ideal esthetic results. Multiple future additional surgeries are expected to be performed to correct the deficiencies of previous surgeries. The new approach of PNAM therapy describes the reduction of the size of the intraoral alveolar cleft through the active molding of the palatine segments through selective modifications in acrylic plate. Consequently, repositioning of surrounding soft tissue and cartilage of the overtly stretched cleft nose through lip tapping and nasal stent. This nasal stent provides support and gives shape to the nasal dome and alar cartilage. In bilateral cleft condition, PNM with columellar elongation can minimizes the extent and number of overall surgical procedures. When there is a close coordination of presurgical phase and surgical phase method employed in close proximity, this technique can greatly improve esthetic results of cleft conditions.[4]

Expectations from PNAM[5]

- Reduce the severity of cleft deformity
- Repositioning of the deformed nasal cartilages and alveolar processes
- Elongation of the columella to create neocolumella and improving the nasal esthetics.
- Approximation of lip segments to reduce tension at the surgical site after lip repair
- Reduce scarring.
- Reduces the need for secondary alveolar bone grafts.
- Reduce multiple surgeries to improve esthetics.

RATIONALE

Cartilage in newborn is soft. It lacks the elasticity. High maternal level of estrogen which passes from mother to newborn at the time of birth correlates with an increased hyaluronic acid level. This hyaluronic acid can alter the cartilage, ligament, and connective tissue elasticity by breaking down intercellular matrix. It inhibits the linking of the cartilage intercellular matrix necessary to relax the cartilages, ligaments and connective tissue. This enables the fetus to pass through the birth canal. The concept of nasoalveolar molding is based on this concept of mouldability of alveolar arches with considerable plastic changes that are retained. Maximum level of hyaluronic acid in infant is seen in first 6-8 weeks after birth. As the maternal estrogen level depletes the hyaluronic acid level in infant also depletes. Therefore, maximum molding of alveolar arches is seen in initial 2–3 months.

It is also suggested that PNAM stimulates immature nasal chondroblasts, producing an interstitial expansion that is associated with improvement in the nasal morphology. Alar cartilage is the same kind of elastic cartilage as auricular cartilage. Thus, alar cartilage is also malleable in the early neonate, with fair possibility for success in the nonsurgical correction of cleft lip nasal deformity.[6]

CLINICAL STEPS

The newborn CLCP infant should be always evaluated by interdisciplinary cleft palate team as soon as possible. The presence natal teeth, unusual undercuts, a Simonart bands or any other tissue abnormalities should be examined in cleft defects **(Figs. 86.3A and B)**. Natal teeth should be extracted with administration of minimal local anesthsia. Status of Vitamin K injection immediately post birth needs to be confirmed. It is always prudent to provide vitamin K injection prior to extraction of natal tooth to prevent post-extraction hemorrhage.

IMPRESSION TAKING

An impression of the intraoral cleft defects is made using an elastomeric material in a customized impression tray plate. Usually, this plate works as a template for the impression material. This plate can be obtained from the study cast of similar cleft babies treated previously. Various other methods can be utilized for primary impression, if the study models of cleft patients are not available, using 2 fingers, small coin or back of the small spoon are few templates used for primary impression **(Figs. 86.4A to D)**. It becomes essential to make secondary impression by acrylic plate prepared on the primary impression study model to get more precise anatomical landmarks.

The advantage of elastomeric material is the modifiability of its setting time. A fast-setting time with adequate working time can be achieved with 2:1 ratio of base and catalyst paste. Another advantage of this material is excellent tear resistance strength without significant distortion making it possible to make 2–3 study models. The wash of light body material is generally not necessary to record minute details. Irreversible hydrocolloids (Alginate material) are generally avoided as flow of this material cannot be completely controlled during impression taking. An excess loading of

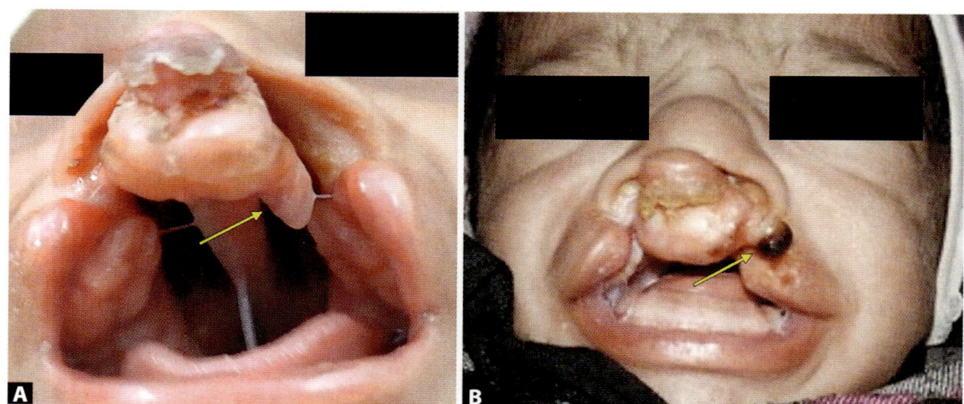

Figs. 86.3A and B: Presence tissue abnormalities.

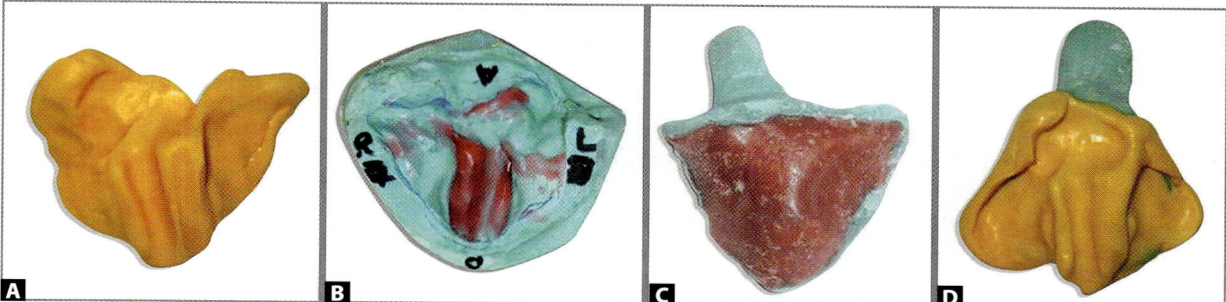

Figs. 86.4A to D: Preparation of template: (A) Impression with 2 fingers: (B) Primary cast preparation; (C) Primary tray/template; (D) Final impression.

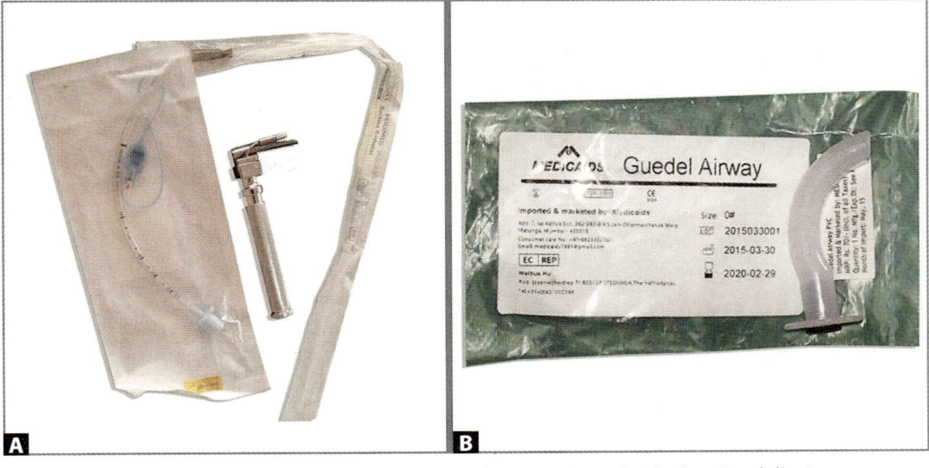

Figs. 86.5A and B: Laryngoscope, suction catheter, endotracheal tube, Guedel's airway.

this material can cause catastrophic flow beyond soft palate into the nasopharynx leading to blockade of nasal passages. The possibility of tearing of small chunks of material breaking free from the impression and blocking the airway can be extremely distressing emergency situation needing immediate medical attention. Moreover, this material does not show distortion resistance for multiple study models from single impression.

The impression is generally obtained in fully awake infant without any anesthesia. It is advised to take impression in hospital set up or clinical setting that is prepared to handle airway emergency. It is preferable to have anesthetist standby with availability of emergency equipment (laryngoscope, suction catheter, endotracheal tube, Guedel's airway) to negotiate airway accessibility. A high vacuum suction to remove any torn impression material from main impression should be kept handy **(Figs. 86.5A and B)**. There are various positions to take the impression of infant.

- **Infant upside-down position:** Witnessing an impression taking of newborn baby can be emotionally traumatic to the parents. Therefore, a seasoned nurse/pediatrician can be is given the task of holding the infant with appropriate support to fragile neck during impression taking. Mature, confident parent who understand the proper position and care in holding the baby during impression taking can be tasked. The clinician and nurse/parents position themselves of facing each other. The infant is held in an inverted upside down by nurse/parent with good support to neck and head by surgeon. Parents/assistant can help by holding the legs of infant lightly to prevent sudden movement of infant **(Fig. 86.6)**. An appropriately sized impression tray with adequate impression material is inserted by clinician into the oral cavity. The tray is seated until the impression material adequately covers the upper gum pads. Emphasis is given to have good impression of outer borders of alveolar arches with good depth of buccal and labial vestibule. Once the impression material is set, the tray is removed and mouth is thoroughly examined for any remnants of torn impression material. High vacuum suction should always be available chair side for use. The impression is then poured with dental stone to obtain the cast. The advantage of this technique is in its position. The inverted position of infant prevents the tongue from falling back and blocking the airway. It also allows the excess salivation to get drained out of oral cavity.[4]

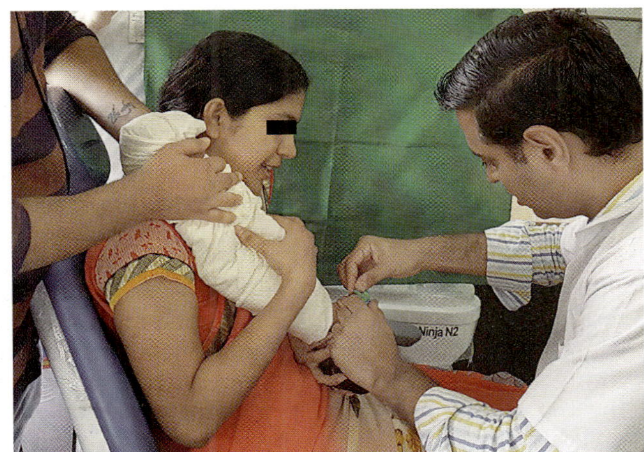

Fig. 86.6: Impression taking—infant upside-down position.

- **Infant face-down position:** In this position, the infant is held face down to prevent any possible aspiration of stomach content if baby vomits. As positioning of infant, itself is not very difficult, the help of nurse/pediatrician is not greatly necessary. Infant is positioned face down in Parent/trained clinical assistant's lap carefully. Parent can cradle the infant securely around the chest and torso with good support to head and neck of the infant. Clinician can take the impression by inserting the impression tray inside the oral cavity **(Fig. 86.7)**. Once the impression material is set, the tray is removed and mouth is thoroughly examined for any remnants of torn impression material. The head is gently held slightly upright position during impression taking. Special attention is given to proper fitting tray for better fit. The material must register the borders of maxilla and premaxilla with good depth of vestibule as well as cleft region. It is not necessary to get deeper impression of cleft region. Undue pressure in cleft region may unnecessarily traumatize the nasal tissues. Excess impression material in posterior region of tray must be avoided to reduce the risk of airway blockage. It is always prudent to let

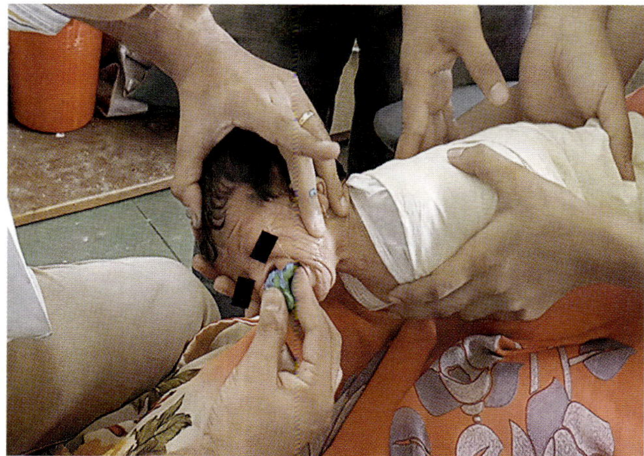

Fig. 86.7: Impression taking—infant face-down position.

the infant cry while impression taking, which will be an indicator of maintenance of airway patency. If no crying is heard during impression taking, it can be assumed that airway is compromised. It is better to keep one finger gently between the impression tray and tongue of infant without any pressure. Infant might suck the finger softly. The process of sucking itself will give good impression of cleft region.[5]

- **Infant face up position:** This position is recommended for experienced operator. Infant is placed on mother's/caregiver's lap. Mother should hold the infant's hand firmly. Clinician can take the impression by inserting the impression tray with impression material inside the oral cavity. A good support to head and neck is given by clinician to prevent any jerky movement by infant **(Fig. 86.8)**. Impression tray handle is held constantly at cleft region by clinician at all the time with a continuous finger motion in vestibule to get better impression of outer border of palatine shelves as well as to clear the excess material posterior to tray. Once the impression material is set, the tray is removed, and mouth is thoroughly examined for any remnants of torn impression material.

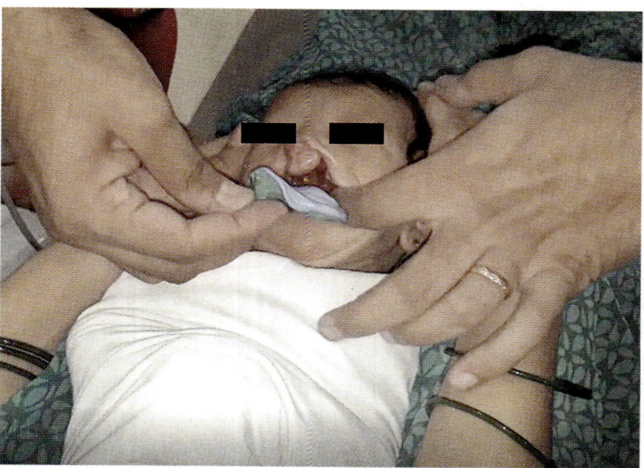

Fig. 86.8: Impression taking—infant face-up position.

NASAL CLEFT IMPRESSION

Any impression of nasal region is not essential but desirable in comparing the pre- and post-molding outcomes pragmatically. For nasal impression, the impression tray with the impression of the cleft palate region taken earlier should be placed back in the mouth and small amount of elastomeric impression material should be placed over nasal region extending over the handle of impression tray. Operator can prepare a basic template/plate with putty beforehand for ease of impression taking also should be made for placement of impression material. Once the impression is set, the impression tray along with nasal impression should be taken out in single swift movement to prevent dislodgement of nasal impression from oral impression **(Figs. 86.9A and B)**. The impression is then carefully poured in dental stone. One cast can serve as working model on which intraoral molding plate can be fabricated. Another cast (study cast) should always be made to maintain the record for the progress of molding. The undercut on cast is filled with wax. This modified cast is lubricated with any separating media available.

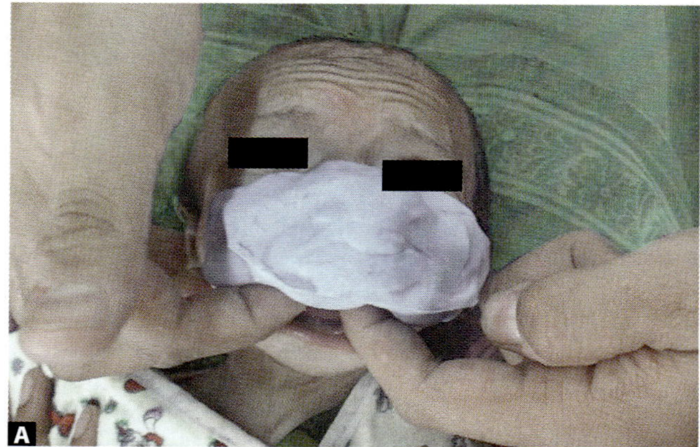

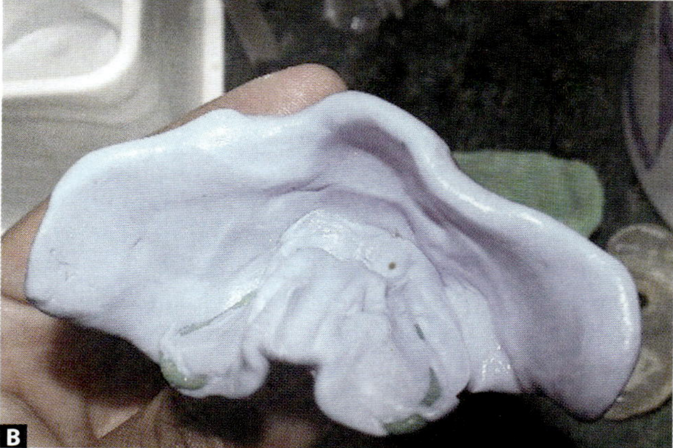

Figs. 86.9A and B: Nasal cleft impression.

PNAM PLATE FABRICATION

The plate is fabricated using clear acrylic resin using any convenient technique **(Figs. 86.10A to D)**. A heat cured method for preparing the acrylic plate is desired due to superior strength and lesser chances of porosities. In the scarcity of time, a simple sprinkle method of incremental addition of powder and monomer to the cast is also

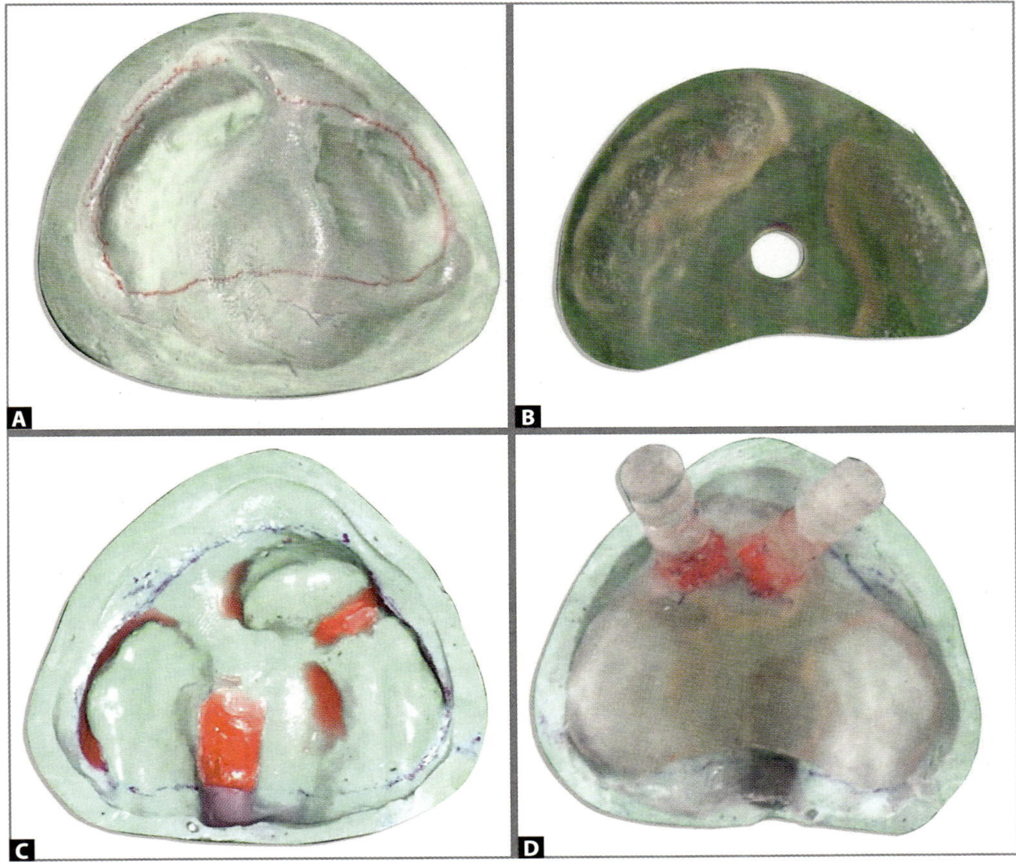

Figs. 86.10A to D: Unilateral and bilateral acrylic plate.

acceptable technique. This method can sometimes exhibit cloudy appearance. Another method of preparing a thicker consistency mix from the powder and monomer is directly expressed onto the entire cast. A care should be taken to ensure uniform coverage of entire cast with same thickness of acrylic (approximately 1- 1.5 mm). Higher thickness plate may compromise available tongue space in turn jeopardizing suckling. The cast is placed in pressure chamber for few minutes for acrylic to get fully cured. This method provides porosity free, uniform thickness clear acrylic plate. It also minimizes residual free monomer in acrylic plate.

The acrylic plate is trimmed with good polish. A special care is taken to ensure smooth borders to prevent any untoward injury in oral cavity. A good impression will give good molding appliance which will be fairly retentive. Infant will usually start sucking on the plate almost immediately after placement which will be the clear sign of good adaptation and self-retention of the plate. If the appliance shows less retention, the border region of vestibule should be trimmed and adjusted. An extra consideration to be given of relieving frenal attachments for better retention of plate. If the infant shows the gag reflex, the posterior region of the plate needs trimming and adjustments. In addition, this appliance is retained in the oral cavity by tapes and elastics. A care should be taken of prevention of any extra acrylic in the cleft area, as this can lead to hindrance in the desired movement of alveolar segments into projected positions. Thickness of the plate will determine the availability of tongue space. Extra thick appliance will illustrate less retention and compromised tongue space leading to compromised suckling. Therefore, care should be taken to reduce the thickness of appliance for good tongue movement.

STEPS IN UNILATERAL CLEFT ALVEOLAR MOLDING

After taking the impression of unilateral cleft with elastomeric impression, the plate is fabricated with clear acrylic as mentioned above.

Armamentarium (Figs. 86.11A to D):

- Small scissors
- Tegaderm (3M)/Duoderm
- Elastics 1/4" or 5/16"
- 3M Steri-strip R1547, ½ × 4 inches/Micropore (½ inch thickness)
- 3M Steri-strip R1541, ¼ × 3 inches/Micropore (¼ inch thickness)
- Anti-rash cream
- Storage box for the appliance
- Sterile ear buds (to clean the palate after feeding)

Lip taping: Lip taping should be initiated immediately after impression taking. Lip taping is relatively easy step to achieve by parents. As a first step in PNAM, teaching the parent about lip taping can go a long way in boosting the confidence in parents to continue this treatment. Two 0.25 × 3-inch Steri-strips/micropore are connected with red elastic is place across the lips after approximating both the lips as close as possible separated by cleft. The elastic should be pulled to double

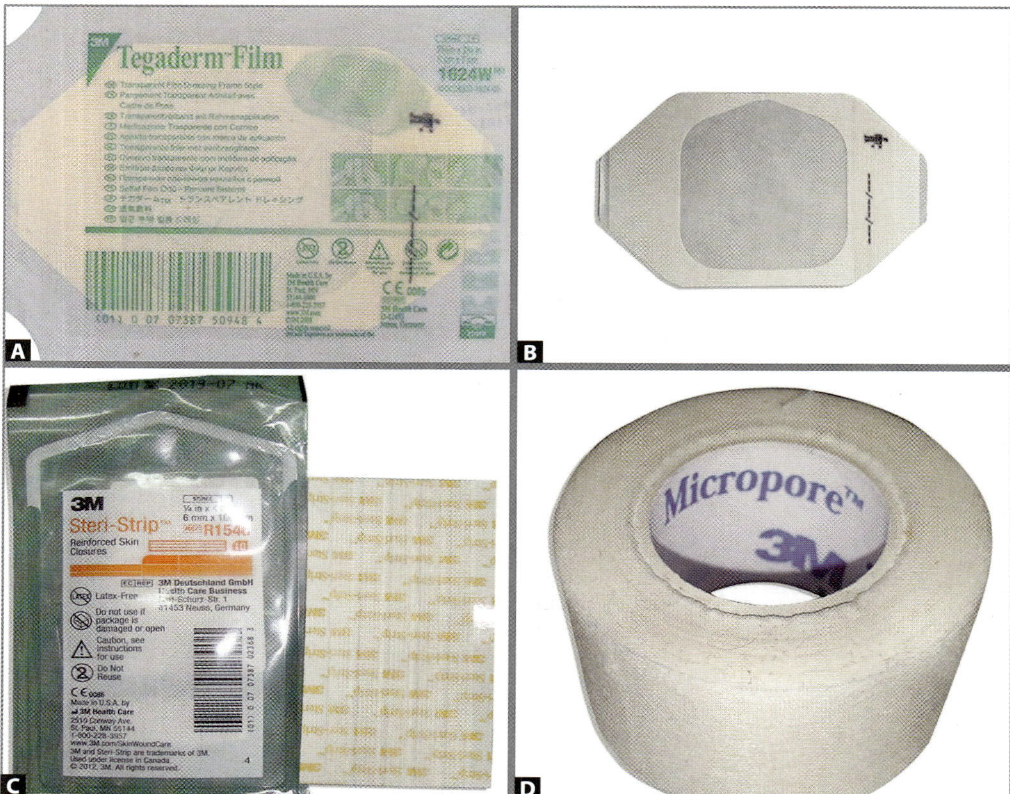

Figs. 86.11A to D: Armamentarium.

its diameter and the Steri-strips should be secured over the philtrum and cheek region to create a reciprocal force over lips. This will create instant pressure on alveolar segments inwardly leading to initiation of molding **(Fig. 86.12)**. Lip taping without NAM appliance alone can sometimes lead to uncontrolled force on alveolar segments. This uncontrolled orthopedic forces on alveolar segments can even lead to unfavorable molding. Lip taping along with appliance in situ capitulate a good controlled movement of alveolar segments. Joining the cleft lip with lip taping improves the alignment of nasal base by bringing the columella towards the center in the midsagittal plane. It can improve the nostril symmetry. Lip taping is critical first step in PNAM therapy. Sometimes, double lip taping is also advised for larger clefts with delayed initiation of treatment to achieve faster results **(Fig. 86.13)**.

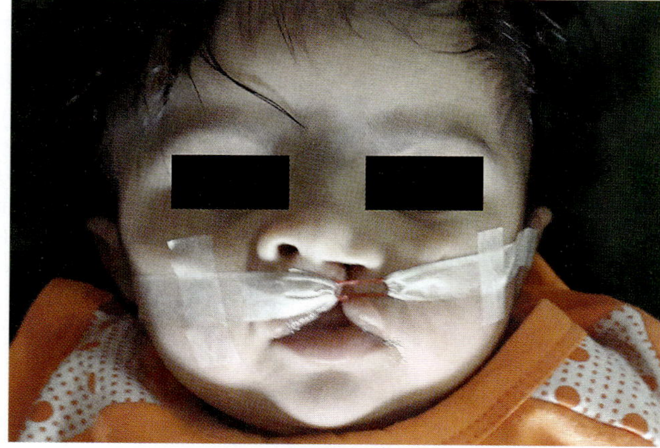

Fig. 86.12: Unilateral lip taping.

Handle position for unilateral cleft patient: An acrylic handle of around 8–10 mm should be made with clear orthodontic resin attached to the appliance at the site of cleft in lip. This handle or button facilitates the easy insertion of the plate in the oral cavity and attaching the elastics and retentive lip tapes to the appliance. The handle should be facing downwards and outwards making 45° angulation to the occlusal plane of the appliance allowing easy closure of upper and lower lip without any hindrance **(Fig. 86.14)**. The length of the handle must not cause any discomfort for mother during feeding. Two separate grooves (retention and activation grooves) are made on handle to receive the elastics. The depth of the groove should be adequate to prevent slipping of the elastics from grooves. Around 1–2 mm distance should be kept between the grooves. The elastics should be placed in same groove at any given time to prevent unequal forces on the plate.

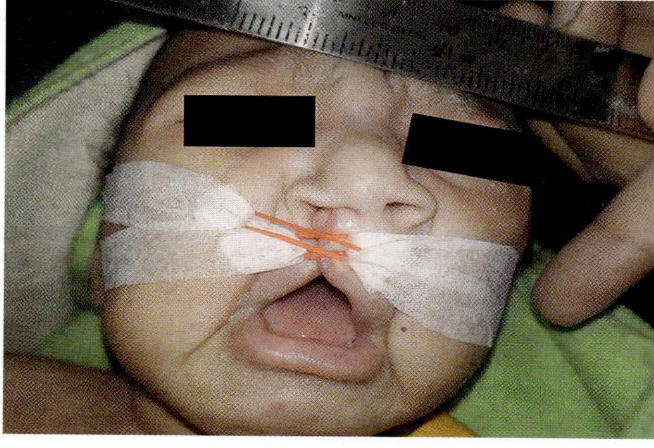

Fig. 86.13: Double lip taping.

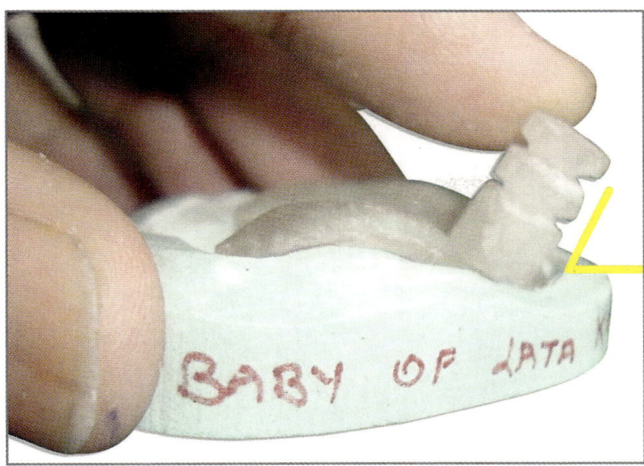

Fig. 86.14: Unilateral plate handle placement.

Selective trimming and addition: Alveolar molding can be achieved by selective removal of the acrylic from the region into which the alveolar bone needs to be moved. At the same time, a soft liner must be added in the region from where the bone needs to be moved or reduced. To achieve this task, with every appointment, the appliance is selectively trimmed in such a fashion that greater segment (premaxilla attached to palatine shelves) moves towards lesser segment (smaller palatine shelve without premaxilla). At the same time, lesser segment moves little outwards to create space for greater segment to move in. This greater segment movement inwardly towards cleft region is accomplished by adding soft liner to the inner side of labial surface of alveolar portion of appliance whereas reducing the hard acrylic from the opposite palatal aspect of the appliance. The addition of soft liner must not be exceed 1–1.5 mm. Likewise, the hard acrylic trimming should be approximately 1–1.5 mm. At the same time, the acrylic is strategically removed from inner vestibular part of lesser segment of plate with equal amount of addition of soft liner on opposite inner palatal part of plate approximating the lesser segment. At the site of acrylic trimming, an addition of hard acrylic must be done on the outer side of the appliance (outer portion of plate facing tongue intraorally) to prevent the perforation of the plate. The final goal is to achieve reduction of cleft between both the segments with approximation of greater and lesser segment towards each other making it near normal. A small hole should be made in the centre of the plate as a safety feature. In case the appliance slips in the oral cavity and gets stuck in the oropharynx, it can lead sudden airway obstruction. This simple modification can go a long way in prevention of emergency as well as easy retrieval of appliance by clinician/caregiver **(Fig. 86.15)**.

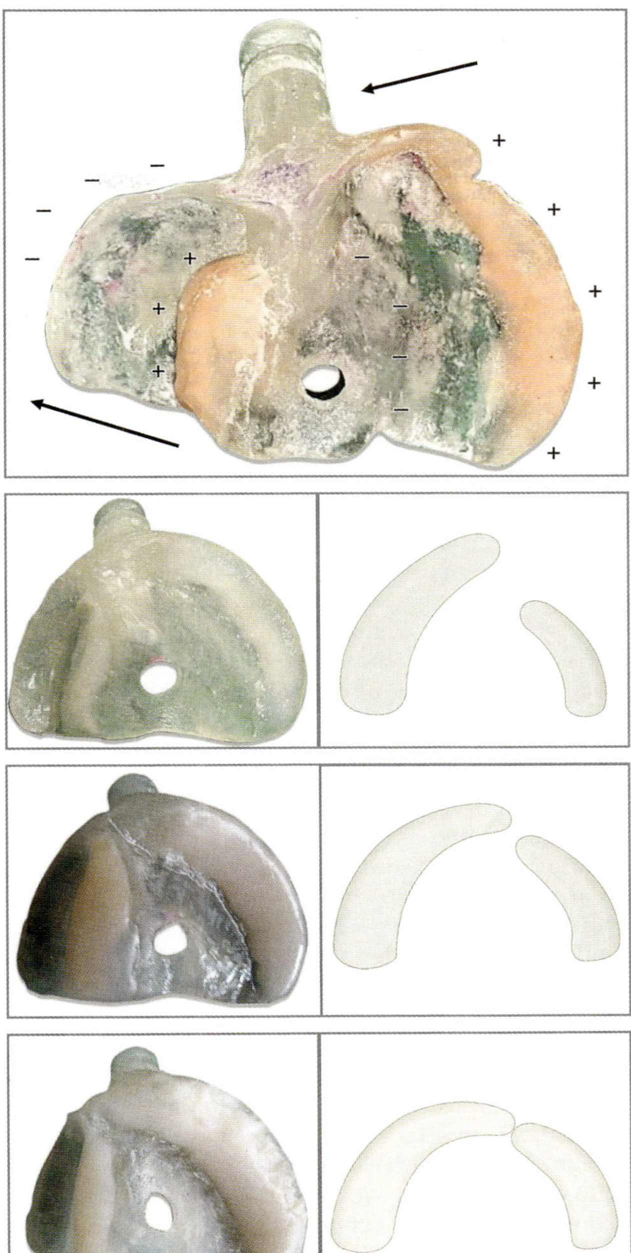

Fig. 86.15: Selective trimming and addition cleft case.

Retentive taping: A proper retentive taping between appointments is important for the appliance to be effective. A broader base tape of Steri-strip (0.5 × 1.5 inch) is first applied to the infant's cheeks lateral and superior to the commissures. These base tapes serve as an anchor to the thinner Steri-strips (0.25 × 4 inch) that are attached to the appliance by elastics. Red orthodontic elastics (0.25-inch diameter) are incorporated into the loops of Steri-strips that are folded over themselves. The elastics with Steri-strips are attached to the handle of the appliance. A special groove prepared on the handle prevent the slipping of the elastics. The elastic should be pulled to double its diameter and the steri strips should be secured over the base tapes. The retentive tapes should be placed on base tapes in such way that force on the plate will directed posteriorly and superiorly. The elastics and Steri-strips should be changed depending on the loss of adhesiveness. These tapes should always provide continuous retention of the appliance. The base plates generally remain for longer time. Whilst the retentive tapes need frequent changing. If there is excessive irritation due to base tapes, use of Tegaderm (3M) is advised though it works out little expensive. Sometimes adhesive tapes (Micropore) are also used instead of Steri-strips **(Figs. 86.16A and B)**. But they need much more frequent changing than Steri-strips. Parents

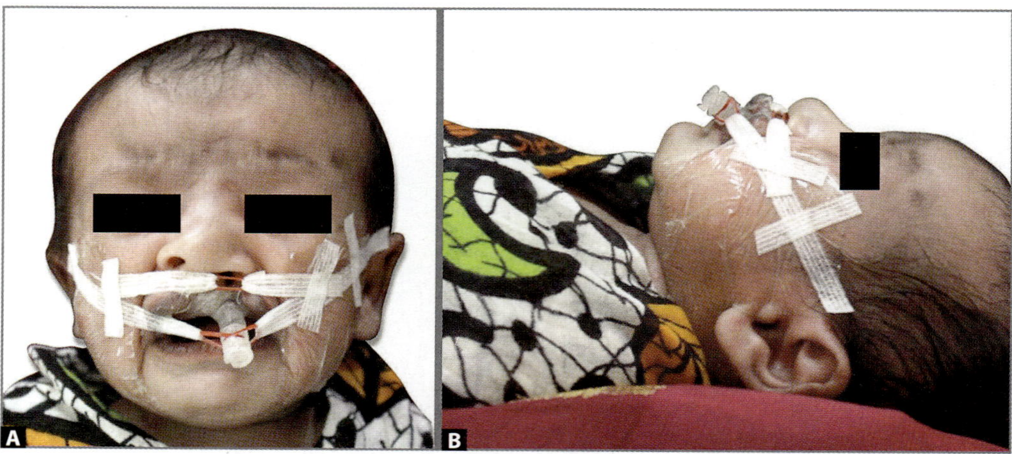

Figs. 86.16A and B: Unilateral PNAM appliance in situ.

are taught insertion and removal of appliance, attachment of elastics to retentive tapes and sticking of base tape and retentive tape on cheeks in right position. The infants are seen weekly once for modification in appliance. The removal of retentive/base tapes is done slowly by continuous wetting the tapes with lukewarm soap water. Rapid removal of dry tape can sometimes unfortunately peel the delicate skin of infant's cheek. Therefore, special care should be taken during removal. Every appointment, the progress of molding should be evaluated. Oral cavity should be thoroughly examined to check any possible sore spots ulcerations. Decrease in the cleft size can be measured by placing the soft wax into the cleft and later measuring this wax thickness. In subsequent appointments, the wax thickness will reduce if the alveolar molding is progressing in right direction. It is prudent to maintain all the interappointment records of soft wax to monitor the progress of cleft closure. The parents are provided with enough supply of tapes, adhesives and elastics with detailed instructions on proper method of taping and appliance insertion. If the appliance is properly modified at each visit, the alveolar segments (greater and lesser) show great movement towards each other sometimes even touching within 4–6 weeks. This will be an ideal achievement of oral molding. The movement of ridges needs a good monitoring. If the greater segment is directed inwardly more aggressively before lesser segment movement laterally, "locking out" of lesser segment can be seen. This situation needs to be avoided at all cost to prevent compromised arch form. A gap of 1 week is maintained between two appointments. During each follow up, an emphasis is given on building a good rapport with parents. A review of minutest problem, discomfort for infants should be done regularly to build a trust and camaraderie. A gap of around 5–6 mm between alveolar segments is considered acceptable time to start nasal molding.

Nasal molding: The nasal molding should start once alveolar molding has achieved reduction in cleft by 5–6 mm. This protocol allows avoidance of extreme stretching of alar rim circumference on clefted side. The nasal stent is the projection from the labial surface of the appliance extending inside the nasal dome on the cleft side of the nose. It can be created by hard acrylic or with combination of 0.036-inch stainless steel wire and hard acrylic. When the wire is used for stent, it is made into the curvature like swan neck and is carefully bent to end passively into the nostrils. The nasal end is made into alphabet R with close end progressing into the nostril and open end holds the nostril rim. The nasal end of the stent is covered in hard acrylic for stable form and support. The hard acrylic is then covered with soft liner to provide adequate pressure for columellar elongation and nasal tissue expansion. This addition of soft liner is done weekly/fortnightly once depending on the progress of the case. An appropriate addition should reveal a blanching of nasal tissue over the stent during infant suckling. This will be a good sign of positive pressure on nasal tissues. The base of the stent should be located on labial flange of the appliance above the acrylic handle **(Fig. 86.17)**. Especially, the superior aspect of the nasal stent is covered with soft liner for positive flexible pressure on the internal tissues of the nasal dome. The orientation of the nasal stent should project outward (not upward) and towards the cleft away from normal side, so that the columella is pulled towards the midline position. This will also help in correcting the flattened cleft lip. As the nasal molding progresses, the nasal tip and dome of cleft side appears more upright and visible symmetry can be noted in comparison to noncleft side. The nasal stent also exerts some intraoral force on alveolar segments for further molding. With nasal tissues getting pushed actively, the intraoral cleft width also decreases. The parents are educated about keeping the appliance in the oral cavity continuously except for cleaning.

With subsequent appointments, the continuous soft liner addition on the tip, the enlarged nasal stent will become unstable under pressure from nasal cartilage. In these cases, if further molding is still expected from the appliance, the soft liner should be removed. A fresh coat of hard acrylic followed by thin layer of soft liner is covered on nasal stent. The stent is readjusted in nasal dome to get good positive blanching on the nasal tissue. The purpose of continued modifications in nasal stent in subsequent appointments is to make sure that lip segments are approximated closely. The shape of nostril is moulded to resemble the teardrop appearance of unaffected nostril. The columella is elongated and drawn towards midline or even overcorrected **(Figs. 86.18A and B)**. The successful alveolar and nasal molding should provide aligned alveolar segments, repositioned nasal cartilages, columella and

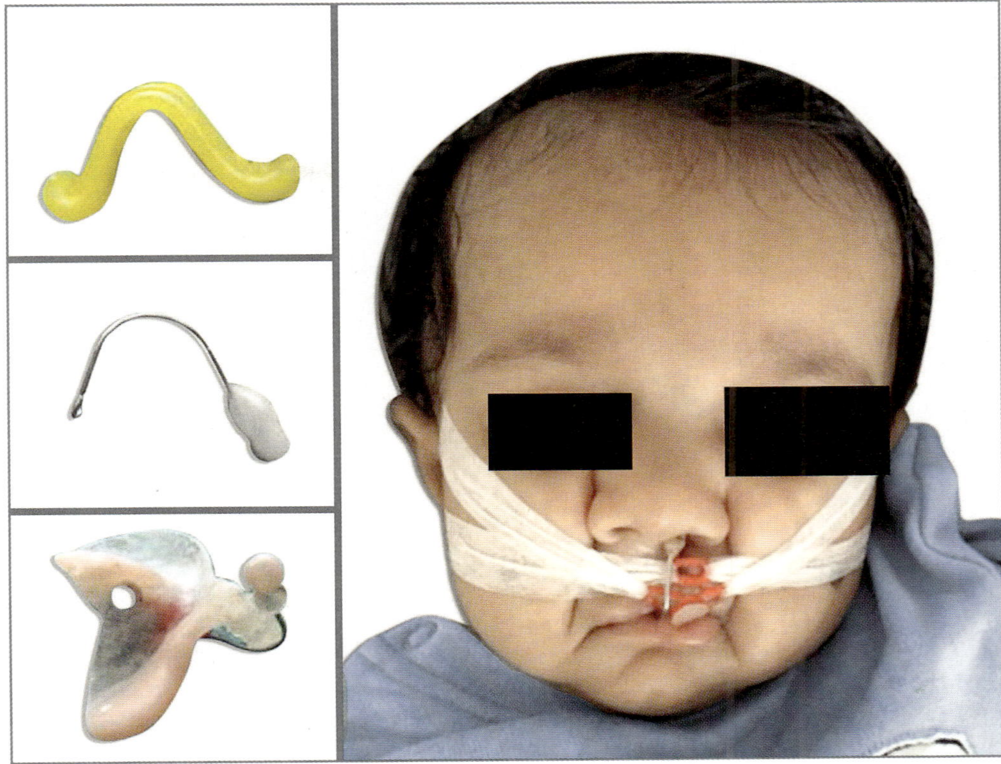

Fig. 86.17: Nasal stent design and appliance in situ.

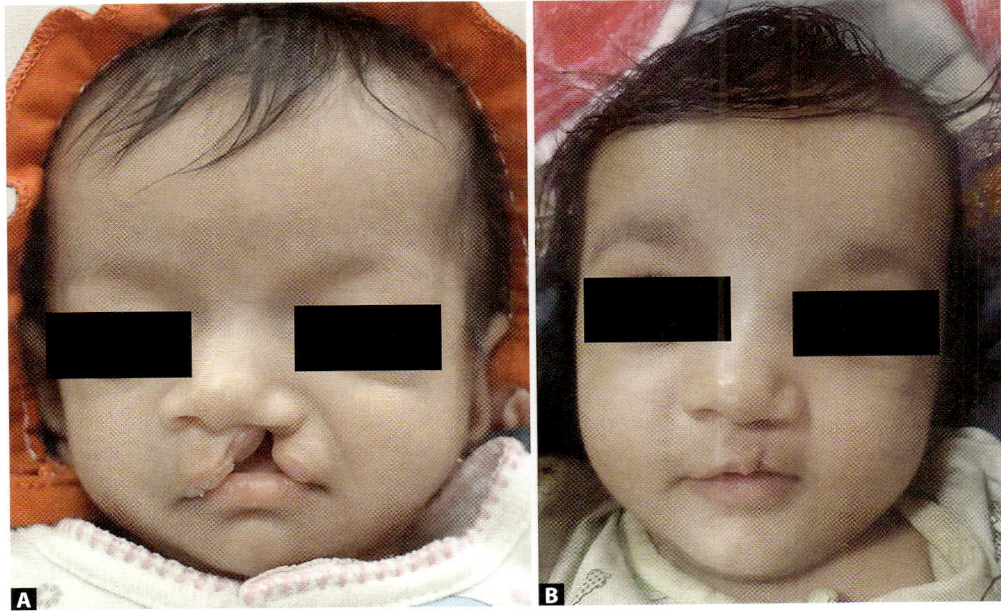

Figs. 86.18A and B: Preoperative and postoperative unilateral case.

philtrum. The appliance should ideally worn by infant till the time of surgery. Post-surgery, appliance need not be worn. Lip taping for few weeks is recommended.

BILATERAL ALVEOLAR CLEFT MOLDING

PNAM for bilateral CLCP cases is much more difficult than unilateral cases. The characteristic feature of short or absent columella with excessively wide prolabium. The purpose of PNAM is to elongate columella and nasal lining tissues nonsurgically. The nasal cartilages are moulded/adapted with retraction of premaxilla into its usual position. This should help in producing a symmetrical lip and nose without any severe scar formation after lip surgery. The entire nasoaveolar molding in bilateral deformity has three phase-wise objectives to achieve.

- To retract/derotate the premaxilla and align it with posterior lateral palatine shelve (segments)
- To mold the nasal cartilages through repositioning of alar cartilages
- Elongation of columella

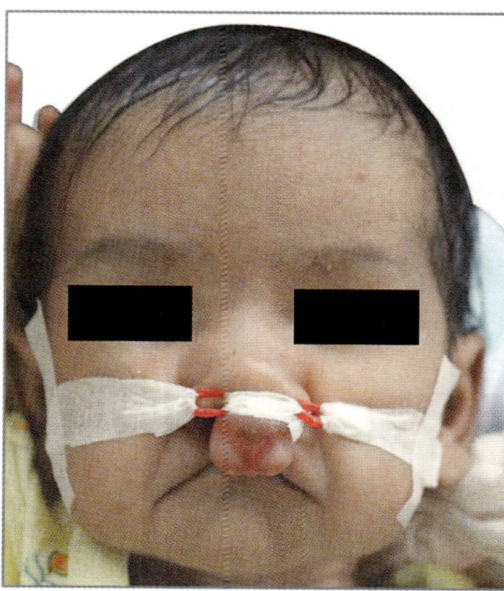

Fig. 86.19: Bilateral lip taping.

Similar to unilateral cases, the bilateral CLCP infants should be always evaluated by interdisciplinary cleft palate team as soon as possible. The presence natal teeth, unusual undercuts or any other tissue abnormalities should be examined in cleft defects to evaluate immediate intervention. After taking the impression of bilateral cleft with elastomeric impression, the plate is fabricated with clear acrylic.

Lip taping: Lip taping should be initiated immediately after impression taking. One 0.25-inch small piece of Steri-strips/micropore covering the lips over the premaxilla is connected with two red elastic to two 0.25 × 3 inch Steri-strips/micropore is place across the remaining two segments lips as close as possible separated by the clefts. The elastics should be pulled to double their diameter and the Steri-strips should be secured over the philtrum and cheek region to create a reciprocal force over lips **(Fig. 86.19)**. This will create instant pressure on alveolar segments (especially on premaxilla) inwardly leading to initiation of molding. Sometimes, double lip taping is also advised for delayed initiation of treatment to achieve faster results.

Handle position: In bilateral cases two acrylic handles/buttons are used. For accurate position of handle, two lines 'mid-anteroposterior and transverse' are drawn on the most convex part of the premaxilla. Two other lines equidistant from the mid-anteroposterior line and lateral borders of premaxilla are drawn. The two points coinciding with transverse line should be considered for handle position. These two handles should be parallel to the long axis of the clefts. The handles are positioned at 45° angle to the long axis of occlusal plane facing downwards and outwards are placed in premaxilla region for appropriate seating and retention of appliance. The length of the handle must not cause any discomfort for mother during feeding. Two separate retention and activation grooves (retention groove near the acrylic plate) are made on handle to receive the elastics. The depth of the groove should be adequate enough to prevent slippage of the elastics from grooves. Around 1–2 mm distance should be kept between the grooves. The elastics should be placed in same groove at any given time to prevent unequal forces on the plate. Two separate elastics with tapes are used to retain the appliance **(Figs. 86.20A and B)**.

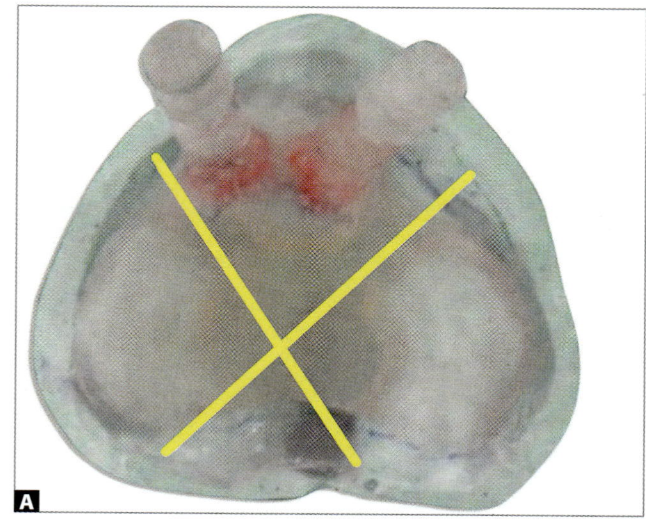

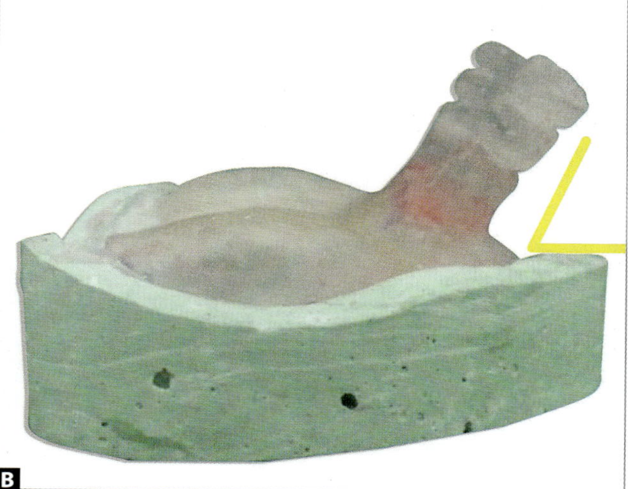

Figs. 86.20A and B: Handle position for bilateral cleft.

SELECTIVE TRIMMING

Expectations from bilateral alveolar molding needs to be dealt with two intentions.

- Alignment of posterior lateral alveolar segment
- Retraction and derotation of premaxilla

The posterior lateral alveolar segments are directed outwards to accommodate the premaxilla. This is made possible by selectively trimming hard acrylic on the lateral borders of appliance from inside to create space for lateral movement of alveolar segments. Simultaneously, addition of hard acrylic from outer (opposite) side of appliance is done to prevent the thinning and perforation of the plate. At the same time, the soft liner is added in the cleft region to put the force on palatine shelves to move laterally. The hard acrylic trimming and soft liner addition should not be more than 1–1.5 mm thickness to prevent excessive force during molding. The adjustments are done weekly once. The retraction/derotation of premaxilla is achieved by adding soft liner anterior to premaxilla. Simultaneously, reducing the hard acrylic posterior to premaxilla near the posterior lateral alveolar segments (palatine shelves). An addition of hard acrylic on outer side of the plate against the selective trimming is done to prevent perforation of plate **(Fig. 86.21)**. Again, the

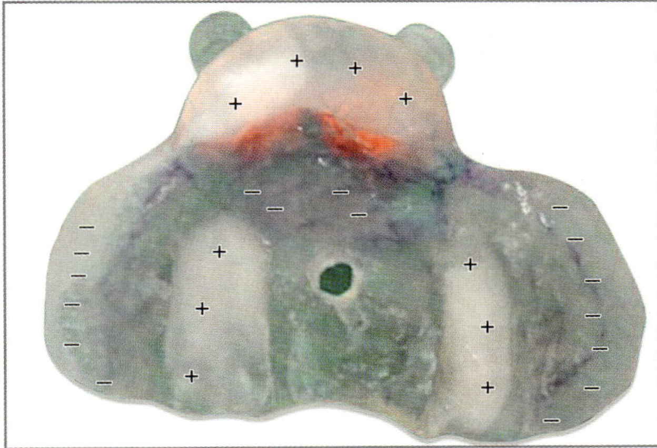

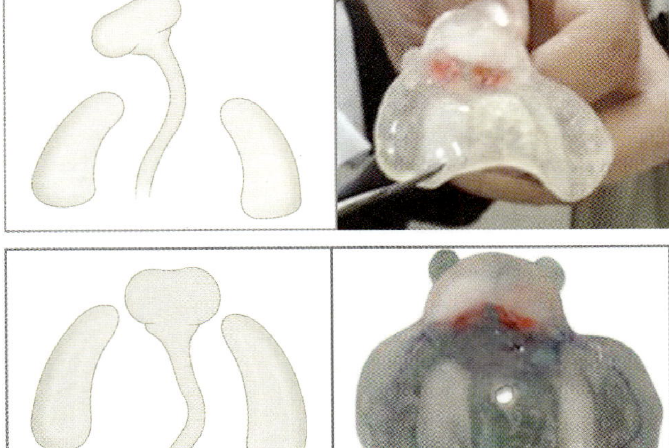

Figs. 86.21A to C: Selective trimming and addition for cleft case.

addition and reduction of the plate should not exceed more than 1–1.5 mm to prevent undue force on premaxilla.

The retraction of premaxilla can sometimes show bending of nasal septum to one side, which should be considered normal in these circumstances **(Figs. 86.22A to C)**. This is inevitable outcome of posterior and inferior movement of premaxilla. In our experience, sometimes the premaxilla fails to move/retract due to incomplete trimming of hard acrylic in posterior region of premaxilla which restricts the lateral bending of septum. Therefore, an extra care should be taken during trimming of this region. Once the premaxilla is retracted close enough to lateral segments (in around 3–4 weeks), the nasal molding is started.

Nasal molding: The main focus of nasal molding in bilateral cleft is elongation of the columella. Unlike unilateral cleft, in bilateral case, two nasal stents are utilized for nasal molding. The proper configuration of the nasal stent in approximation to nasolabial fold is difficult to achieve sometimes. A modelling/boxing wax can be used as a guide or template to create the swan neck pattern of the stent **(Fig. 86.23)**. The wax is positioned on the labial surface of molding plate and moulded into the desired shape entering in the nose of baby. This wax template is removed and kept handy for bending of wire into the desired curvature. The nasal stent should always have a swan neck pattern progressing into the nostril. The swan neck curvature is convenient for lip taping after stent incorporation. The stents can be created by either hard acrylic or with combination of 0.036-inch stainless steel wire and hard acrylic with the preserved wax template as a guide. The tip of nasal stent should have two lobes (closed and open ends of alphabet R). The superior lobe (upper part of R) should enter the nostril pressing anteriorly and outwardly on the nasal lining behind the dome of the alar cartilage. The nasal end of the stent is covered in hard acrylic for stable form and support. The hard acrylic is then covered with soft liner to provide adequate pressure for columellar elongation and nasal tissue expansion. The lower lobe (lower end of alphabet R) is located under the tip of the nostril sill. This open ended inferior lobes of both the nasal stents are first covered by hard acrylic followed by soft acrylic. The nasal lobes should be kept as close together as possible to reduce the space between the crus of the nasal tip cartilages and to create an appropriate width of collumella. The nasal lobes positioned away from each other can lead to unnecessary unesthetic increase in the width of columella. It is advisable to place the active tissue expansion force directed anteriorly at nasal tips.

Prolabial band: The lower lobe of both the nasal stents are attached to each other across the nasal columella by orthodontic E-chain covered with soft liner (A precaution to prevent contact tissue ulceration) to make a bridge at the level of lip-columella junction around the tip of nose (called as Prolabial band/saddle). This prolabial band pushes against the base of the columella and directs the expansion forces to preserve the nasolabial angle. A Steri-strip tape is placed

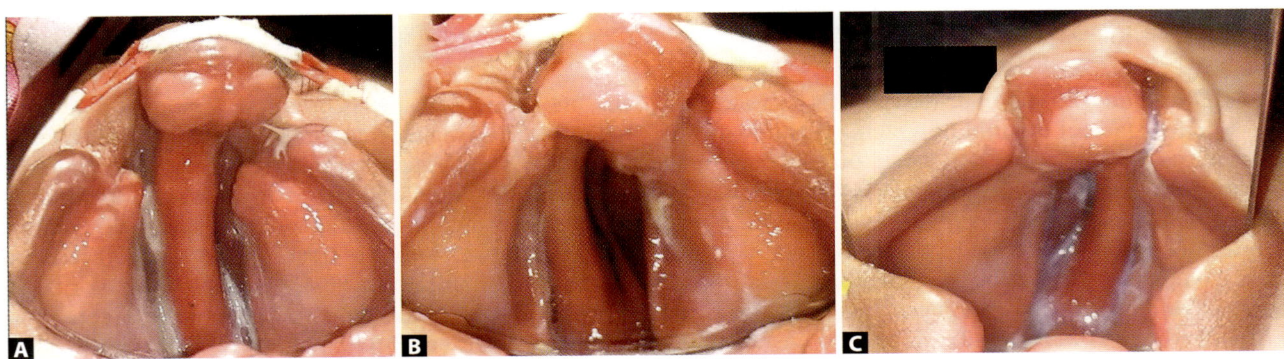

Figs. 86.22A to C: Bending of nasal septum in bilateral cleft during alveolar molding.

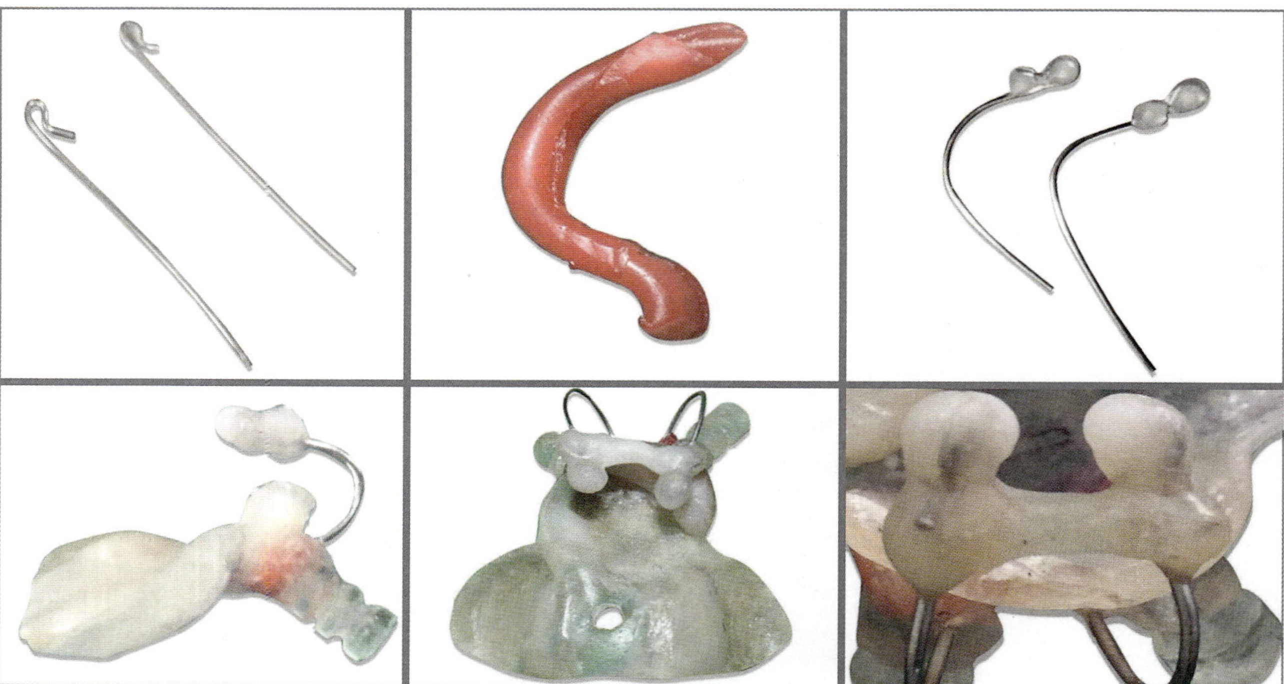

Fig. 86.23: Swan neck nasal stent with prolabial band in cleft case.

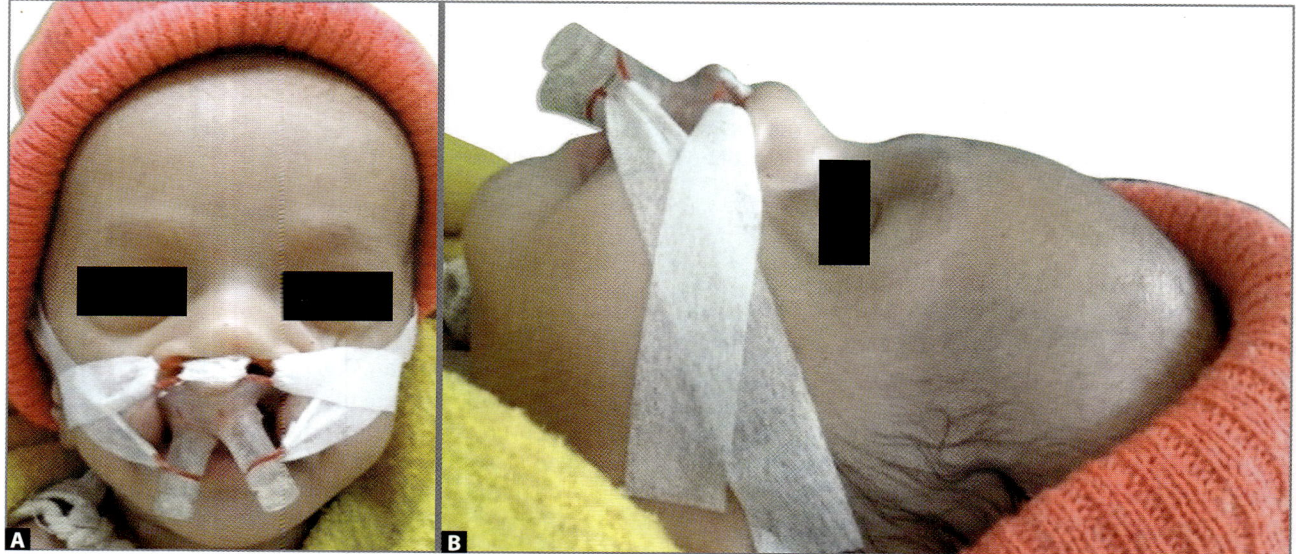

Figs. 86.24A and B: Bilateral PNAM appliance in situ.

on prolabium should be stretched downwards and attached to the labial surface of the molding plate. This downward pull combined with posteriorly directed force by horizontal bands at the nasolabial fold and anterior force applied by the superior bulge of nasal stent to the tip of the nose results in stretching and lengthening of the columella. Without prolabial band, the force vector on columella is less directed towards stretching and elongation and more towards tip of the nose leading to unfavorable pronounced nasal tips. As the stent is modified at each appointment with addition of soft liner, the nasal apex is projected forward while inferior lobe preserves the natural form of the nostril **(Figs. 86.24A and B)**. It is suggested that this technique can lengthen the columella between 4 mm and 7 mm nonsurgically.[7] The nasoalveolar molding with columellar elongation generally needs 5–6 months of active treatment before surgery. Similar to unilateral molding, the PNAM plate has to be worn till the day of surgery. No intraoral appliance or nasal stent is used postsurgically except for lip tapping for few weeks while the infant heals **(Figs. 86.25A to C)**.

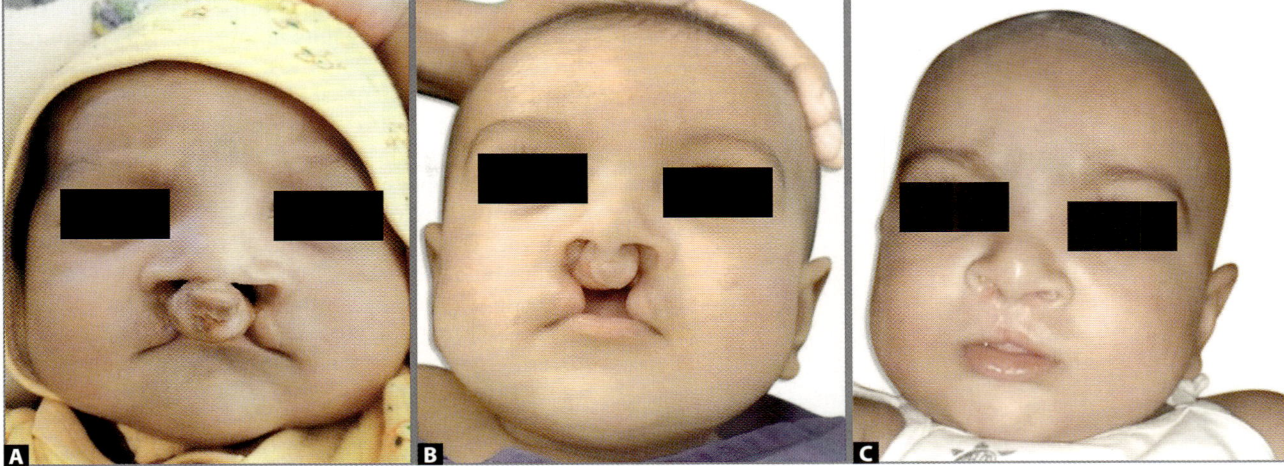

Figs. 86.25A to C: Preoperative and postoperative bilateral case.

COMPLICATIONS ASSOCIATED WITH NAM TECHNIQUE

1. **Tissue ulceration:** Perhaps most common complication of PNAM is ulceration. On occasion, it can occur intraorally on vestibular mucosa or extraorally in cheek region or in nasal region. Intraoral ulceration is generally results from ill-fitting, sharp-edged appliance or from addition of excess material during active molding. Accordingly, smoothening of appliance, coating of tissue lubricant on appliance or reducing excess material in subsequent appointment can be done. These ulcerations can be resolved mostly without much intervention. Ulceration in nasal region at the apex of nasal tip may result from tight contact of stent to nasolabial fold with excessive force. A certain minor correction in angulation of stent can reduce the ulceration. Cheek skin ulceration is commonly seen with excess pressure applied while taping. A slight change in the position of taping can help in healing of the ulcer. A care should be taken of wetting the tape with warm water while removing the tape gently from cheek to eradicate the chances of sloughing of the skin. Skin care ointment containing Aloe vera base can help in healing the ulcers quickly **(Fig. 86.26)**.
2. **Lack of retention of appliance:** Failure of retention of appliance lies on clinician as well as on parents. Unsatisfactory, inadequate impression of the vestibular extensions as well as cleft region by clinician will lead to the preparation of ill-fitting appliance resulting in lack of retention. Therefore, a good impression with all anatomical landmarks can go a long way for good retention of appliance. If the parents do not learn the proper application of tapes, elastics during molding, it can lead to lack of retention of appliance as well. If the appliance is lost, not worn regularly, the molded (closed) cleft can go back to original widened position due to constant position of tongue in the cleft during suckling by infant. Therefore, it is mandatory to have motivated parents who are actively involved in the treatment. A good education, demonstration, continuous encouragement with emotional support to parents by cleft team members is extremely important in success of the treatment.

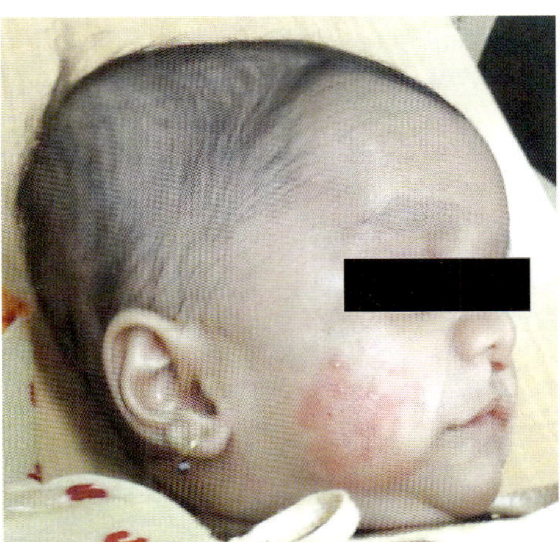

Fig. 86.26: Complications of PNAM—tissue ulcerations.

3. **Improper lip taping:** Incorrect or less aggressive taping will not culminate into maximum soft tissue expansion as expected. Inappropriate taping leads to non-retentive appliance and minimum closure of the clefts. A firm lip taping helps to support the appliance along with good expansion of lip segments.
4. **Premature eruption of primary teeth:** Ectopically situated primary tooth buds sometimes show early eruption during active molding pressures. It becomes necessary to remove the primary/natal tooth after checking the status of vitamin K injection at the time of birth. Generally, the removal of the primary tooth is advisable to continue with active molding. A small amount of surface anesthetics with local anesthetics infiltration is more than sufficient before extraction. A good hemostatic agent (optional) with pressure pack will give good hemostasis at extraction site within minutes. The appliance need not be worn for few days for uneventful healing **(Fig. 86.27)**.
5. **Locking of the segments:** The movement of alveolar ridges during active molding should be monitored carefully. Excessive or misdirected molding of the alveolar segments can lead to locking out of the smaller segments. If the greater segment or premaxilla is directed posteriorly

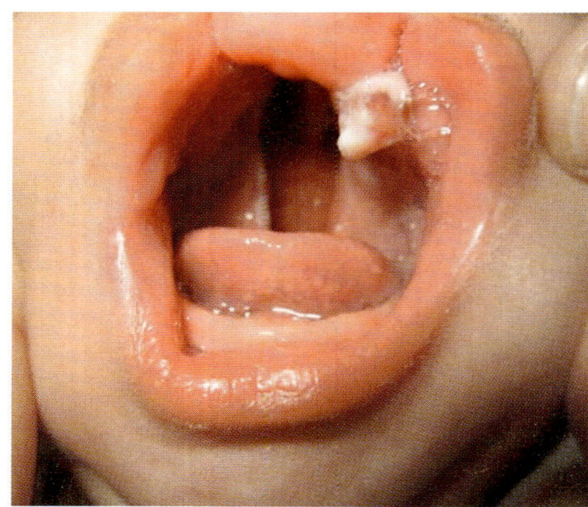

Fig. 86.27: Premature eruption of primary tooth.

more aggressively prior to the outward advancement the lesser segment/palatine shelves, the locking out of the lesser segment will result. This will create compromised arch form. This may result from poor molding process. If the segments get locked, it may be corrected through the remolding of the segments if recognized early. If not corrected, the locked-out segment will fail to provide a good soft tissue support. This compromised maxillary arch will have multiple undesired effects on occlusion to be corrected orthodontically later **(Figs. 86.28A and B)**.

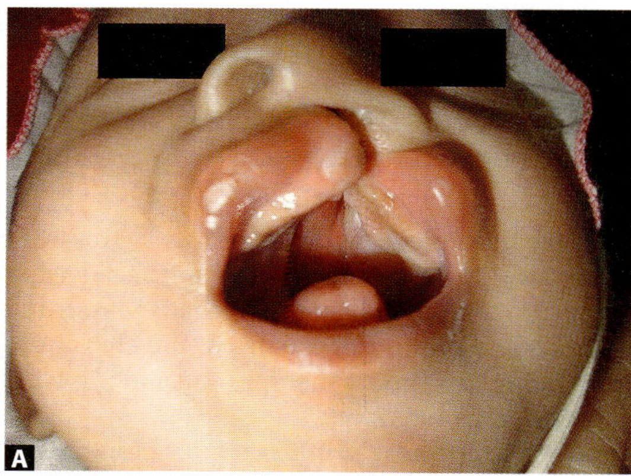

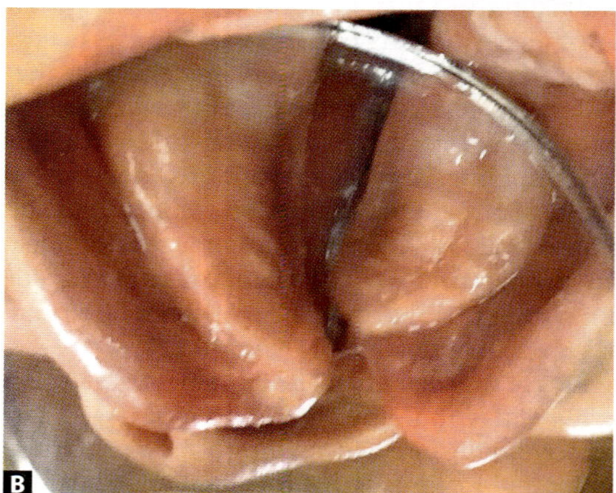

Figs. 86.28A and B: Locking of alveolar segments.

6. **Mega-nostrils:** Overexpansion of the alar rim in the unilateral cleft nose results in large nostril compared to the unaffected side. The most common cause of mega-nostril is addition of nasal stent before the size of the cleft gap is reduced sufficiently. Premature nasal molding develops undue force against the nasal tissues leading to excessive expansion. Hence, the direction of the molding force should be closely monitored weekly to prevent such outcome. There should be adequate material on the tip of the nasal stent extending into the nostril so that the radius of the tip will be large enough to exert gentle expansion force. The force trajectory should be directed anteriorly, not superiorly. Nonetheless, mega-nostril may settle in future as there is always a chance of tissue shrinkage post-surgery **(Fig. 86.29)**.

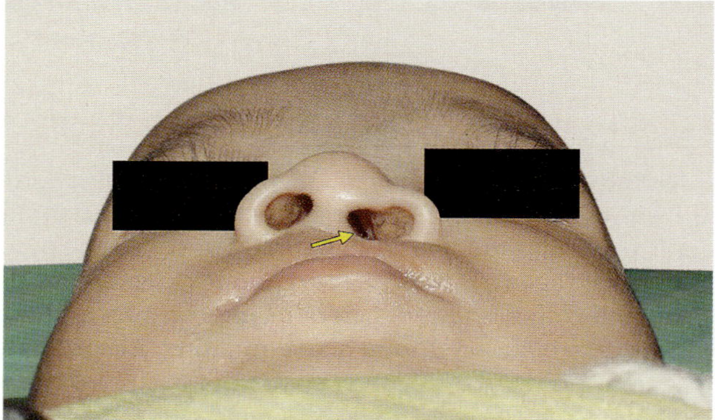

Fig. 86.29: Mega-nostril.

NAM CONTROVERSIES

- A recent survey of all surgeons in American Cleft Palate-Craniofacial Association and Canadian Society of Plastic Surgeons suggests that almost 71% cleft surgeons use some form of presurgical orthopedics with PNAM therapy most predominantly amongst others.[1,8] Nonetheless, PNAM has become a point of debate between proponents and opponents of this therapy. The proponents claim several advantages like improved aesthetic post-surgery, reduced overall cost, and psychosocial benefits to parents. The qualitative research on caregivers of PNAM treated infants indicate rapid decline in anxiety and depression symptoms and better coping skills with time. These positive changes are attributed to support and counseling from weekly visits to the cleft team.[9,10]
- Clinical benefits of PNAM in reducing the severity of cleft deformity mainly at anterior portion of maxillary arch are well documented. When compared to PNAM, the primary shortfall of other presurgical intraoral orthopedics (PSIO) is their neglect to address the nasal cartilage deformity during the duration of cartilage plasticity.[1,9] The nasal symmetry, ala projections, dome height, nasal bridge deviation have shown improvement greatly with PNAM when compared to Non PNAM groups.[11]
- The opponents of NAM argue that it is highly complex and expensive treatment therapy, which offers no great clinical benefit. One of biggest drawbacks of this therapy is parent compliance. The weekly visit to cleft team for

appliance adjustments; the responsibility of daily care of appliance, taping, appliance insertion, removal can be a burdensome task for already psychologically distressed parents. It is estimated of almost 30% missed appointments by parents as one of the indicators of noncompliance from caregivers.[1,12,13]

- Another substantial issue of dropout of almost 32% due to lack of parental support as another sign of higher variability of outcome based on parental compliance. A sort-term cost analysis suggests higher direct and indirect cost has to be born by parents when compared to non-PNAM group prior to surgery.[14]
- Opponents of NAM argue that no significant effects on maxillary growth, dentition or occlusion in long-term studies. They further argue of higher chances of relapse after short duration.

Nasal Conformers

Sometimes, it is advisable to keep preformed silicon nasal conformers/nasal stent immediately after surgery to prevent collapse of nose and collumella. This can transpire as an outcome from contraction of soft tissue post-surgery.[15-17] One of the Preformed Silicon Conformers (Manufacturer Koken Co. Ltd) are available commercially in different sizes. It should be placed straightaway after surgery preferably on OT table itself to prevent even minor collapse. The conformer consists of two hollow cylinders joined together over columella to support and retain the conformers in the nostrils. The conformer can be retained through micropore/Steri-strip. It is advisable to maintain nasal conformer six months after the surgery.

Ideal requisites for nasal conformer/retainer

- It is critical that the conformer is semi-rigid to prevent the collapse of nasal dome and columella.
- It should be easy and comfortable to wear.
- Baby should be able to breath comfortably through the conformer.
- It should be easy to wash
- It should be resistant to shrinkage over time.
- The retainer should be economical.

A customized nasal stent is an economically viable option to commercially available nasal conformers. Many different nasal conformers are also attempted by various researchers. Any customised conformer which fulfils the prerequisites of nasal conformer can be used for the benefits to the patients **(Figs. 86.30 to 86.32)**.

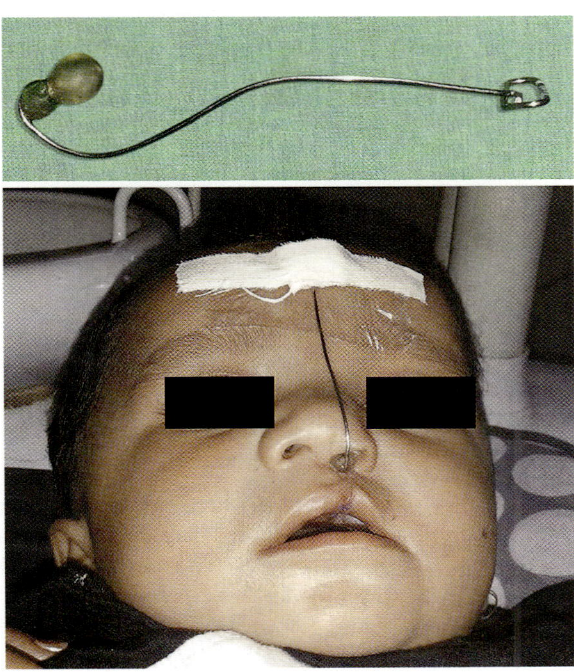

Fig. 86.30: Customised nasal conformer with SS wire, hard acrylic and soft liner.

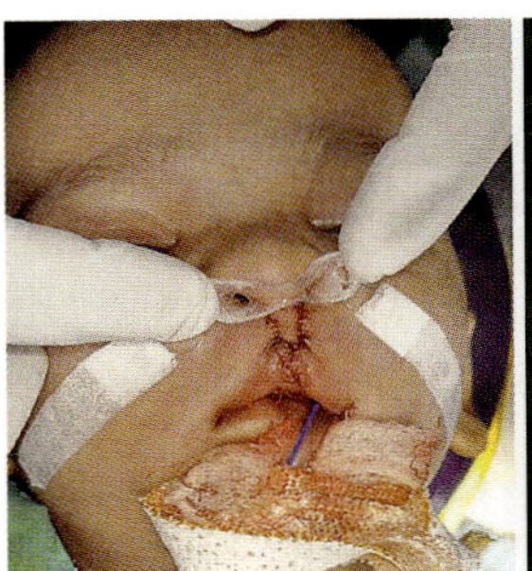

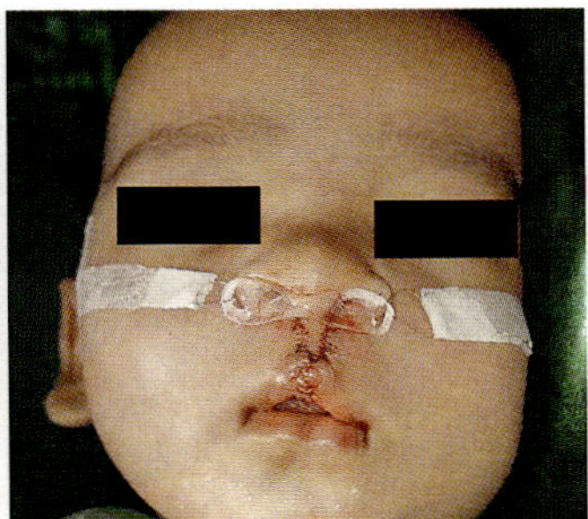

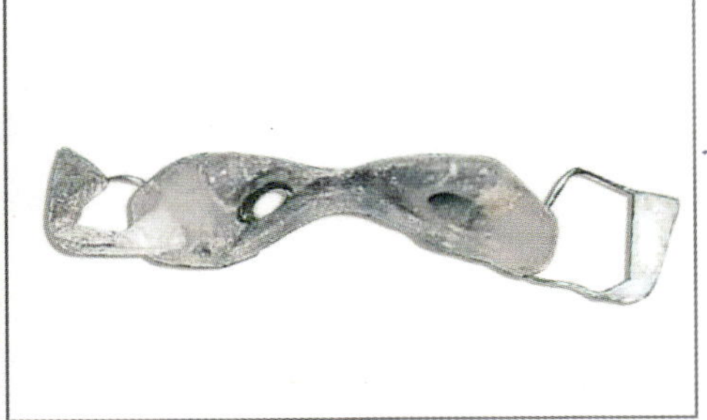

Fig. 86.31: Customised nasal conformer with thermoforming pressure moulding material.

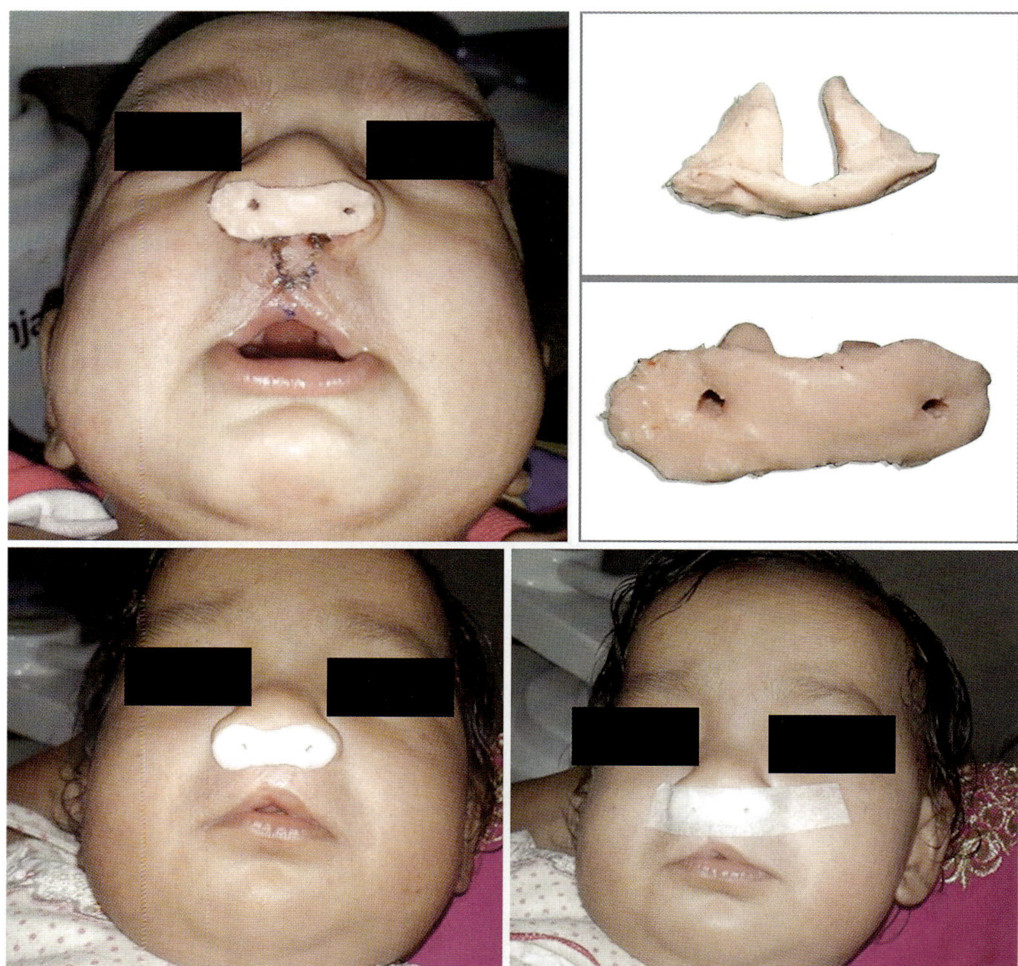

Fig. 86.32: Silicon nasal conformers.

RECENT ADVANCES

Modifications: Various modifications are being made in the appliance design by many clinicians depending on the individual case requirements. Few of them include split molding plate to bring out derotation of the rotated premaxilla (predirectional appliance), use of an acrylic button with an elastic chain as nasal bridge to carry out aggressive nasal molding with an increased range, use of a large nasal stent to decrease the chances of ulceration (Figueroa's technique). Few clinicians even have used a preformed extraoral appliance which does not contain a molding plate.[5]

CAD NAM: This includes the use of CAD technique for treatment planning and appliance designing, thereby enabling the accurate analysis of the required movement in multiple planes. XOR3 software is used to formulate the treatment objective. The guiding principle is the application of constant low-grade pressure to reshape and reposition the anatomic structures.[18]

Presurgical vacuum form NAM aligners: Al Khateeb et al. utilized a 3Shape D250 scanner to obtain the digital 3D model which was used to assess the changes in maxillary arch using a 3Shape software program. The cast was used for fabrication of the presurgical VF NAM aligners. Serial sequences of VF NAM aligners were fabricated on modified dental casts obtained through selective grinding and addition of contrasted stone on the same working cast gradually to achieve the desirable movements of the cleft alveolar segments.[19]

POINTS TO REMEMBER

- Cleft lip and palate is one of the most common congenital craniofacial disorders caused by incomplete fusion of maxillary, mandibular processes at embryonic stage.
- Maximum moulding of alveolar arches is seen in initial 2–3 months.
- PNAM for bilateral CLCP cases is more difficult than unilateral cases.
- CAD-NAM includes the use of CAD technique for treatment planning and appliance designing thereby enabling the accurate analysis of required movement in multiple places.
- Infant face up position is recommended for experienced operator.

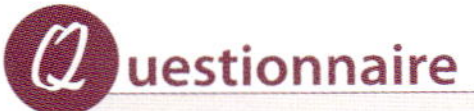

Questionnaire

1. Explain the role of presurgical nasoalveolar molding (PNAM) in movement of cleft lip and palate .
2. What are the various positions to take impressions of infant?
3. What are the steps involved in unilateral cleft alveolar molding?
4. What are the complications associated with NAM technique?

REFERENCES

1. Rodman RE, Tatum S. Controversies in the Management of Patients with Cleft Lip and Palate. Facial Plast Surg Clin North Am. 2016;24(3):255-64. doi: 10.1016/j.fsc.2016.03.004. PMID: 27400840.
2. Oner DA, Tastan H. Cleft lip and palate: Epidemiology and etiology. Otorhinolaryngol Head Neck Surg. 2020;5: doi: 10.15761/OHNS.1000246
3. Grayson BH, Shetye PR. Presurgical nasoalveolar moulding treatment in cleft lip and palate patients. Indian J Plast Surg. 2009;42(Suppl):S56-61. doi: 10.4103/0970-0358.57188. PMID: 19884682; PMCID: PMC2825057.
4. Brecht LE, Grayson BR, Cutting CB. Nasoalveolar Moulding in early management of Cleft lip and palate. In: Taylor TD (Ed). 1st edition. Clinical Maxillofacial Prosthesis. Illionis: Quintessence Publishing; 2000. p. 63-83.
5. Retnakumari N, Divya S, Meenakumari S, Ajith PS. Nasoalveolar molding treatment in presurgical infant orthopedics in cleft lip and cleft palate patients. Archives of Medicine and Health Sciences. 2014:2(1):36-47.
6. Hamrick MW. A chondral modeling theory revisited. J Theor Biol. 1999;201(3):201-8.
7. Grayson BH, Santiago PE, Brecht LE, Cutting CB. Presurgical nasoalveolar molding in infants with cleft lip and palate. Cleft Palate Craniofac J. 1999;36(6):486-98. doi: 10.1597/1545-1569_1999_036_0486_pnmiiw_2.3.co_2. PMID: 10574667.
8. Sitzman TJ, Girotto JA, Marcus JR. Current surgical practices in cleft care: unilateral cleft lip repair. Plast Reconstr Surg. 2008;121(5):261e-270e. doi: 10.1097/PRS.0b013e31816a9feb. PMID: 18453938.
9. Grayson BH, Garfinkle JS. Early cleft management: the case for nasoalveolar molding. Am J Orthod Dentofacial Orthop. 2014;145(2):134-42. doi: 10.1016/j.ajodo.2013.11.011. PMID: 24485726.
10. Sischo L, Clouston SA, Phillips C, Broder HL. Caregiver responses to early cleft palate care: A mixed method approach. Health Psychol. 2016;35(5):474-82. doi: 10.1037/hea0000262. Epub 2015 Aug 17. PMID: 26280177; PMCID: PMC4757521.
11. Barillas I, Dec W, Warren SM, Cutting CB, Grayson BH. Nasoalveolar molding improves long-term nasal symmetry in complete unilateral cleft lip-cleft palate patients. Plast Reconstr Surg. 2009;123(3):1002-6. doi: 10.1097/PRS.0b013e318199f46e. PMID: 19319066.
12. Tollefson TT, Gere RR. Presurgical cleft lip management: nasal alveolar molding. Facial Plast Surg. 2007;23(2):113-22. doi: 10.1055/s-2007-979280. PMID: 17516338.
13. Levy-Bercowski D, Abreu A, DeLeon E, Looney S, Stockstill J, Weiler M, et al. Complications and solutions in presurgical nasoalveolar molding therapy. Cleft Palate Craniofac J. 2009;46(5):521-8. doi: 10.1597/07-236.1. Epub 2008 Dec 24. PMID: 19929090.
14. Severens JL, Prahl C, Kuijpers-Jagtman AM, Prahl-Andersen B. Short-term cost-effectiveness analysis of presurgical orthopedic treatment in children with complete unilateral cleft lip and palate. Cleft Palate Craniofac J. 1998;35(3):222-6. doi: 10.1597/1545-1569_1998_035_0222_stceao_2.3.co_2. PMID: 9603556.
15. Chang CS, Liao YF, Wallace CG, Chan FC, Liou EJ, Chen PK, et al. Long-term comparison of the results of four techniques used for bilateral cleft nose repair: a single surgeon's experience. Plast Reconstr Surg. 2014;134(6):926e-936e. doi: 10.1097/PRS.0000000000000715. PMID: 25415115.
16. Kuo SCH, Lai JP, Hsieh CH, Chen TY, Chang YJ, Huang F. Use of Nasal Conformer After Birth Effectively Improves Nostril Symmetry in Patients with Unilateral Incomplete Cleft Lip. J Oral Maxillofac Surg. 2018;76(12):2612-7. doi: 10.1016/j.joms.2018.05.003. Epub 2018 May 10. PMID: 29864433.
17. Joshi K, Joshi D, Gurrala P, Amlani G. Design and Manufacturing of Nasal Conformer. Materials Science Forum 2018:939. DOI:10.4028/www.scientific.net/MSF.939.89
18. Yu Q , Gong X, Shen G. CAD PNAM effects on maxillary morphology in infants with UCLP. Oral Surg Oral Med Oral Path Oral Radiol. 2013;116(4):418-26.
19. Al Khateeb KA, Fotouh MA, Abdelsayed F, Fahim F. Short-term Efficacy of Presurgical Vacuum Formed Nasoalveolar Molding Aligners on Nose, Lip, and Maxillary Arch Morphology in Infants With Unilateral Cleft Lip and Palate: A Prospective Clinical Trial. Cleft Palate Craniofac J. 2021;58(7):815-823. doi: 10.1177/1055665620966189. Epub 2020 Oct 27. PMID: 33107321.

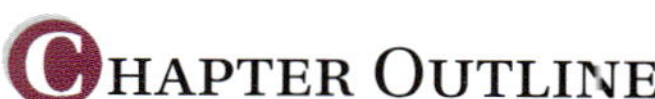

CHAPTER 87

Hypnosis in Pediatric Dentistry

Anup Panda

Chapter Outline

Hypnosis is art and science masquerading as conversation.
—***James Warnke***

Effective verbal communication is essential in the dental office because all behavior is modified by communication. The most challenging aspect of Pediatric Dentistry is persuading a child to readily accept the treatment. A child's responses are affected to a large extent by a language a clinician chooses to use. The choice of effective words and language patterns is very important in promoting a healthy relationship and a positive cooperation of the child. The art of influencing the child's mind in a normal conversation by selecting the use of correct words and language patterns is considered as conversational hypnosis (CH). CH is persuasion to accept a suggestion and could be easily comparable to a linguistic art and science that is accidentally practiced by clinicians all the time. This chapter would provide an overview of a newly recognized behavioral guidance technique in Pediatric Dentistry.

"Hypnosis started when the first mother kissed it and made it better" (**F Bauman**). There's something about hypnosis that captivates us—an unexplained phenomenon, an enigma, an entertainment, the fact that it works and may be because we just do not understand it. Although hypnosis has over 200 years of formal study, practice and development, it remains surrounded by a mystique that obscures its scientific framework. Research has progressed much slower than expected over this period of time. Many questions are still unanswered, especially concerning Children and Hypnosis. Part of the problem is that contemporary researchers have made greater use of adult rather than child subjects. The practice continues even though there is reason to believe that hypnosis with children is different from hypnosis with adults. (**Hilgard and LeBaron**,1982).

Hypno that means dream comes from Greek mythology *Hypnos* that was the personification of sleep and coined by the Scottish surgeon, **James Braid** in the year 1843, who carried out a great number of surgical procedures including dental extractions with hypnotized patients. He brought about the concept by focus of attention and heightened suggestibility, which became the basis of modern thinking and opened doors to clinical hypnosis for augmenting the treatment of a wide range of psychological and medical problems. Since then, hypnosis has been practiced, researched, investigated and many theories have evolved. One of the most well known contributors to the science of hypnosis and the acceptance of hypnosis and hypnotherapy in the 20th century was **Dr Milton Erickson**.

Hypnosis *is a state of consciousness involving focused attention and reduced peripheral awareness characterised by an enhanced capacity for response to suggestion* (The American Psychological Association,2014).

DEMYSTIFYING MISCONCEPTIONS

Hypnosis, the word that has some really strong negative connotations. Most people are ill informed about hypnosis. The first thing to realize is that hypnosis isn't any magical or mystical state. In fact, hypnosis is a completely natural state.

We actually go in and out of this hypnotic state several times a day. Ever since the inception of hypnosis many hypnosis myths have been in circulation. These myths serve to stop us from understanding what really hypnosis is. Some common fears and misconceptions are that hypnosis is sleep, it is dangerous, it will reveal your darkest secrets, works on certain people, you'll forget what happened during hypnosis and one of the biggest myth is that only weak minded people can be hypnotized. But the reality is that everyone is hypnotizable to a lesser or greater degree and the ease at which someone can hypnotized is dependent upon their ability to relax and simply listen. Hypnosis is persuasion to accept a suggestion. That is a very insightful, well thought out and accurate explanation by **Kreskin**. In other words when a person is hypnotized, they are simply following your suggestions. Hypnosis is an altered state of consciousness in which your ability to accept suggestions for psychological, physical and spiritual change is heightened. This hypnotic state automatically occurs anytime when one become deeply relaxed or highly focused.

RATIONALE OF HYPNOSIS

It is no secret that scientists have studied hypnosis and trance phenomenon for more than a century and failed to conclude a detectable pattern in the brain until the breakthrough research carried out by the legendary **Dr David Spiegel** at the Stanford school of medicine got their results published in the journal-Cerebral Cortex causing quite the buzz in the hypnosis world. They noticed neural changes associated with hypnosis were:

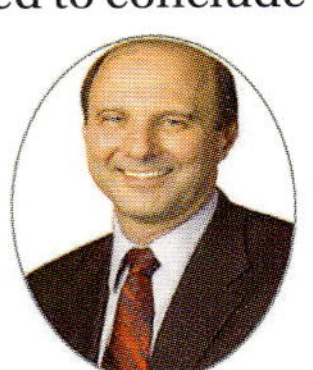

- **A drop in activity in the dorsal anterior cingulated:** This is a part of the brain that's stimulated when you're worried, but tends to be less active during hypnosis. Under hypnosis, highly hypnotizable people are more relaxed and more worry free.
- **An increase in connectivity between certain areas of the brain:** The dorsolateral prefrontal cortex, a part of the brain responsible for planning and organization and the insula (a part designed to help regulate body functions). This shows under hypnosis there is stronger connection being established between brain and the body.
- A decrease in connectivity between the dorsolateral prefrontal cortex and part of the brain concerned with self-reflection. David Spiegel explains during hypnosis self-reflection seems less important. People are less inhibited and will do silly things (stage hypnosis) without thinking about it.

These changes help to demonstrate how it is possible to feel less stress, less pain and less anxiety under hypnosis.

Conscious versus Subconscious

- **When it comes to hypnosis, the human mind function on two separate levels:** Conscious mind (logical thinking) and subconscious mind (automatic functioning).
- Conscious mind is our awareness at the present moment and Subconscious, which is about 90%, registers all accessible information and we become aware only when we direct our attention to it. It is the part of our brain that runs all our automatic functions. It operates all of our behavioral strategies, habitual patterns, emotions and memories. It works automatically without any conscious help and can handle millions of pieces of data all at the same time.
- The subconscious mind records all 1001 little details what the conscious mind neglects. The conscious mind can only deal with between 7 and 9 bits of information at any given time (Miller's Law).
- Our thoughts are mainly controlled by our subconscious, which is largely formed before the age of seven, and you cannot change the subconscious mind by just thinking about it.
- When communicating with the subconscious we do better with stories, metaphors, images, fantasy and suggestions.
- Hypnosis is a technique that helps to communicate with subconscious by bypassing the conscious mind.

CONVERSATIONAL HYPNOSIS

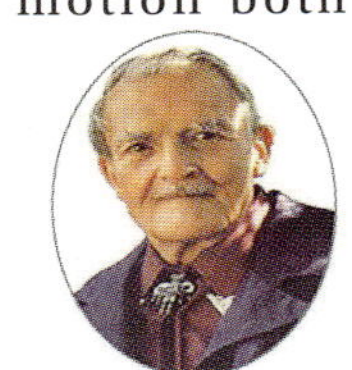

- Children are developmentally in motion both physiologically and psychologically. They are always in a creative and imaginative trance like state. We believe that kids are going in and out of hypnotic states countless times a day. Children are willing to receive ideas and enjoy responding to ideas. But the ideas should be presented to them in a manner comprehensible to them. The main aim therefore, is to get the child so involved in the process that they use their vivid imagination to maximum effect.
- Asking a young child to close his eyes, sit quietly and imagine something internally is rarely successful. Suggestions that ask a child to pretend to dream or imagine that you are dreaming are too cognitively complex. So, the effective way of hypnosis is through words and patterns usually carried out in a conversation that is covert or conversational hypnosis, which is process of inducing a trance during regular conversation. Conversational Hypnosis is a collection of techniques and strategies to change person's thoughts, emotions, decisions and behavior in a completely unconscious way. When you put these principles into practice, everything you do and say will enable you to communicate with the child's mind. Conversational Hypnosis relies on your thoughts, words, body language and tonality working together in harmony.
- Piaget's stages of development provide us an insight into the various characteristics a child attains at different ages. For example, children are incapable of abstract reasoning until they reach the age of eleven. The perception of precognitive children towards the external world is entirely based on how it presents to him/her. The child does so without any categorization. Children over 4 years have the necessary verbal understanding and their blind trust and vivid imaginations making them susceptible to suggestion dental office. This particular trait makes children as desirable hypnotic subjects.

- Pediatric dentists use a form of hypnosis and suggestion throughout the working day that manifests itself primarily in the mannerisms, what we call as the Chair-side Manner (**JH Wooley**, Hypnotism,1896). It is a latent form of hypnosis, which displays its best effect on children.
- The art of influencing the child's mind in a normal conversation by selecting the use of correct words and language patterns is considered as conversational hypnosis. It primarily is a distinctive style of hypnotism inspired and introduced by **Milton H. Erickson** (1901–1980). He was a widely influential hypnotherapist and is regarded as the father of modern clinical hypnosis.
- It is operationally defined by two concomitant, observable variables: first is the intentional use of verbal suggestion designed to elicit automatic, dissociated, or subconscious responding—the universal hallmark of hypnosis and secondly an increase in trance behaviour without the subject having been subjected to a formal induction ritual. Conversational hypnosis is a collection of techniques and strategies a Pediatric Dentist can use to change thoughts, emotions, decisions and behaviour of children in a completely unconscious way in the dental operatory.
- Erickson stated, "There is a need, to work primarily with and not on the children." There should not be talking down to the children, but rather a utilization of language, concepts, ideas, and word pictures meaningful to the children in terms of their learning. Our thoughts are the nidus of all our interaction and communication with the world. These thoughts are represented to us by five main senses: Visual, auditory, kinesthetic, olfactory, gustatory. Children solve the jigsaw puzzle of their own reality by using all of the pieces called "senses." However, one uses a favorite sense more often than the others. Determine what is the child's dominant sensory channel by listening to the words they use to describe experiences. While in conversation begin speaking to them using their favoured sensory channel.
- Five basic elements of CH are relatable,understandable, confidence, executable, manageable:
    1. *Relatable:* If you can be relatable, the child would respond to you better.
    2. *Understandable:* If they cannot understand what you are saying, they will not be able to respond the way you want.
    3. *Confidence:* You have to believe in what you say and you have to exude confidence.
    4. *Executable:* The more people realize you mean what you say and that you execute it according to your own words, the more they will follow you.
    5. *Manageable:* Communication is partially what you say and partially how you say it. Suddenly you would start to notice that you are doing CH without even trying.
- The covert model
    - The key to conversational hypnosis is how well we use language and words to increase influence throughout the course of a normal conversation.
    - Conversational model CH procedure begins with a normal conversation
    - Organize multiple stories that are simple anecdotes that have hidden meaning, e.g., childhood experiences, funny experiences at work, etc.
    - *Verbal breathing synchronization:* Match the pace of your verbalizations with the child's breathing.
    - *Encrypted instructions:* Encrypted instructions let you direct the behaviour of others without doing any of that. The most basic form of an encrypted instruction is a statement to do which is hidden inside a question.
    - *Repackaging sensory input:* Determine their dominant sensory channel and stimulate others.
    - *Triggering post-hypnotic instructions:* If the child performs your suggestion as soon as he comes out, it means you have successfully hypnotised him.

Traditional hypnosis	*Conversational hypnosis*
Traditional hypnosis (TH) is the description given to the sort of hypnosis that can occur when a person is aware of being hypnotized. For example, you tell them to close eyes after which a hypnotic induction paves the way for you to make them feel relaxed	In conversational hypnosis (CH), you communicate with the subconscious without them getting to know
TH is used mainly as a therapy	CH is used for persuasion
TH would be increased in the total minutes of dental consultation with the child	CH is carried out faster
The time spent looking for and adapting scripts or writing or rearranging or editing scripts in preparation for patient is time consuming	CH has its own magic when practiced and is interacting, creative and flexibly with children

TRANCE

Trance is a word used to identify the conditions under which someone responds to hypnotic suggestions. Therefore, being able to identify a trance or the signs of trance can help you know when a hypnotic relationship has been established. It gives you a green light to proceed. The child would exhibit the following changes:

- Dilated pupils
- The pulse rate would slow down when you are talking to them.
- Changing breathing patterns-altered breathing speed up or slow down, both are equally valid trance signals
- Relaxed facial expression
- Less blinking but slightly unfocused, they are probably paying close attention to what you are saying
- If you see them begin to make subconscious responses to what you are saying, that means they are in trance and in harmony with you. These are called as passive responses.
- Reduction in swallow reflex.

Conversational Hypnosis Techniques to Induce Trance

- Verbal description is the fundamental technique of inducing trance. Through this you can bring the child's mind to the setting desired by you.
- **Technique 1:** Inducing trance using natural trance state:
    - One among the methods of inducing trance is to use situations or words to evoke a way of trance which the child has already experienced before. When emotion provoking words fall into a child's ear, then the corresponding emotion will occur automatically and unconsciously.

Trance formations

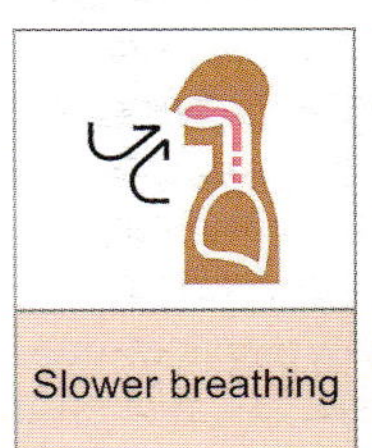
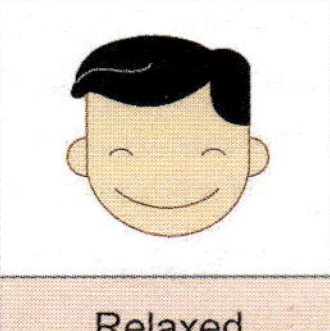

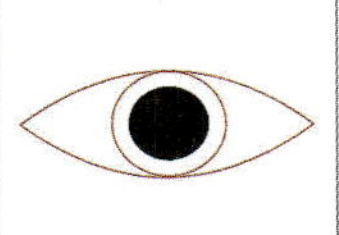
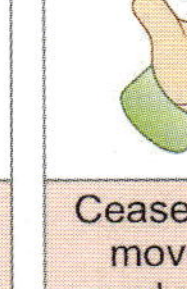

Slower breathing	Relaxed facial expression	Less blinking	Dilated pupils	Ceases making movements and gestures

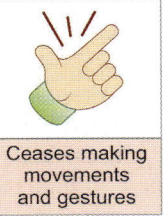

- "I wonder if you have ever been playing in the snow and may be you lost a glove, or your gloves got over so cold and wet...and your hand was so cold that you could move your fingers, and just couldn't feel anything at all..." (on receiving a positive response this can be extended into transferring the resultant numbness to the area of the dental work).

❖ **Technique 2:** Inducing trance with overlapping realities:
- Constantly weaving unrelated multiple stories with each other by smartly using conjunctions. A spiral illusion of entangled stories. This confusion wearies the mind and eschews a speaker from the content of the speech. Consciousness is not able to handle the obfuscation of the stories.
- "Once upon a time there were three little wolves and a big bad pig and then there was a wolf who cried boy, boy. The neighbor's mother's cousin brother's daughter heard. The boy was the fifth son of the fifth son and the wee foxy-woxy started chasing the little bunny rabbit (and can start your slow hand-piece) and you will open your mouth."
- While the child's mind tries to decode the tales, all of your hidden commands go to his/her subconscious.

❖ **Technique 3:** Verbal confusion:
- The confusion technique is employed to make mild confusion or shock in the child's mind. Verbal confusion means accumulated behaviour pattern is interrupted with game of words or information during a conversation, which creates confusion. This results in heightened suggestibility, which will induce trance rapidly.
- "I am asking you to listen to what I am saying, and you want to listen to what I am saying to sit still. Because you know what to do I bet you will open your mouth."

❖ **Technique 4:** Artificial and non-existent words.
- Consciousness is extremely rational and curious. Conscious mind tries to know the vague and put everything on the logical order. You can use this principle to distract it and make contact directly with subconscious.
- There is a certain way in which our speech leads to pronunciation of certain sounds. Any hindrance to this pattern, ceases the process of the conscious mind to figure out what is heard. The words used could be vernacular, gibberish or neologisms.
- "Mandy just like the little animals and your best doll and your toys go to bed every night...and there's this lovely feeling in your mouth, lips and tongue...just like when its so lovely and hot and sunny...and everything is so dry (controlling salivation). It is such a lovely feeling."

❖ **Technique 5:** Sensory overload.

❖ The influx of data that a human brain receives is processed at a certain velocity. It can store very limited and particular information in the short-term memory. Hence, when the brain is loaded with information more than it could handle, it goes into a trance state.

❖ Conscious mind cannot understand a phrase that is uttered without an interruption for more than 5–6 seconds.

❖ "That chair is there and that chair (pointing to another chair) is there. And where is there is there and if that chair isn't there and that chair isn't there. It hurts and it might hurt a while longer. It will probably keep left and right until it stops (The child hears it stops). A child who goes into hypnosis may experience reduced tension even reduced tension related pain."

If you could communicate directly with the subconscious mind-you could communicate anything to anyone at anytime and the outcome of the communication would be exactly what you had aimed for, each time.

THE ABS FORMULA

This is a powerful three-step model that in fact is one of the master keys for understanding any hypnotic process.

A-Absorb Attention

❖ Absorb and focus their attention. You need to draw the child's attention from the external environment to the subconscious.

❖ Maintain eye contact in a similar way that you would focus on a particular spot, this will eliminate distractions to help them focus and relax.

❖ Tell a story or use pictures that would hold attention. Use details of the conversation to steer in a hypnotic direction.

❖ **Revivification technique:** This technique consists of asking the child questions about an experience, and the more detailed the questions get, the more experience the child gets into which produces an altered state. This technique induces no pressure.

B-Bypass the Critical Factor

❖ Critical factor is the part of your mind that tells you "This is not possible, this cannot happen." Since the goal is to reach the subconscious, you need to bypass this critical factor and stop it from interfering.

❖ You can do this by telling engaging stories, using hot words that elicit emotional response, using power words that trigger the subconscious. The five most important power words are: and, because, which means, imagine and remember. Each of these techniques works by engaging the mind in such a way that the information is being enjoyed rather than analyzed.

- Children respond to emotions in a powerful way. Emotions are an unconscious response, so when you take someone on an emotional rollercoaster, you are activating unconscious responses. All you have to do is select an emotion and theme to match. For example, if you want someone to laugh, tell a funny story. If you want them to relax, tell a relaxing story where you are sitting by a lake or walking by a beach.

S-Stimulate the Unconscious Mind

- Achieving A and B automatically paves the way to accomplish S. You might get to see the mind getting into the hypnotic state. As you can imagine, this is a fluidic process. It can happen in a matter of minutes or even seconds.
- Once you have successfully engaged them in a hypnotic state, you have the power to plant whatever ideas you choose, within their subconscious.
- If you could communicate directly with the subconscious mind, you could communicate anything to anyone at anytime and the outcome would be exactly what you had aimed for, each time. Hence, in order to reach the rendezvous named "Relationship," it is important to have a car named "Trust" and the engine called "Rapport."

RAPPORT BUILDING SKILLS

Rapport is a term used to express the relationship of two or more people who are in complete sync or on the same wavelength as each other. Rapport dwells in the subconscious. It is one of the foundations of effective influencing. Your subconscious mind often notices another person's demonstration of a similar gesture, facial expression, tone of voice or even a shared opinion. The subconscious strata will now automatically acknowledge a similarity and create a link.

Establishing Rapport Using Mirroring and Matching

- The important thing to remember is the word "Subtle." You don't want to appear to be mimicking the other person. The idea is to either match what they are doing and saying or mirror it.
- **Mirror their gestures:** You must look at yourself as the mirror image of that person. Your gesture only has to be similar within about 30 seconds for the subconscious to pick up. This sends the signal that you are like them and they would feel closer to you. It is critical that you do not mimic them or make your movements exaggerated. This might lead to your mannerisms exposing your objectives.
- **Breathe with the child:** The breathing and the rhythm of the child's breath is another way in which you can get into their world. If you want to pace their breathing, pay attention to their breathing and breathe the way they do. When you are matching the child's breath, it sends the subconscious signal that you are on the same wavelength.
- **Verbal breathing synchronization:** Pace your verbalizations to match the child's inhalations or exhalations. Stay consistent. Begin by simply noticing your breath. Do not speak while doing so. Equalize the length of inhalations and exhalations. We modify our breathing in a way that we speak while we exhale. Therefore, inhalations would be shorter than exhalations. It is only when we pace our voice to the natural rhythm of our breathing that the attention of the listener is altered. A PACE (Perceive A Common Experience) is an instantly verifiable true statement, while a LEAD (Let them Enter A new Direction) is a plausible suggestion. PACE-ing is where you closely replicate parts of the child's communication so that they begin to recognise parts of themselves in you. LEAD-ing refers to doing something new when you are in rapport with another person. This will cause the other person to replicate you.

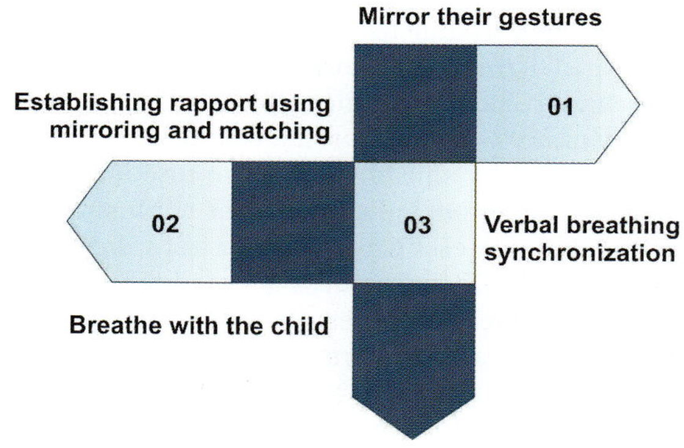

Eye Accessing Cues

- Eye accessing cues are actions that could help the clinicians to recognize how a child is processing a situation at any point of time.
- **Visual remembered (Vr):** Remembering visuals or images from the past. What is the color of your first bike (up and left).
- **Visual constructed (Vc):** Constructing or creating visuals or images. What would your house look like if it were painted violet with red circles (up and right).
- **Auditory remembered (Ar):** What does his voice sounds like when he was 10 years old (centre and left).
- **Auditory constructed (Ac):** What would your voice sound like in 20years from now (centre and right).
- **Kinesthetic (K):** Its both emotional feeling and sensations. What does it feel like walking barefoot on the ice (down and right).
- **Auditory digital (Ad):** Internal dialogues. Eye movement will be down to the left side.
- The brain is a made up of a right sphere and a left sphere. The former manages the more creative and conscious side, while the latter is responsible for the analytical and subconscious. In any conversation, watch the child's eyes. Are they looking to the right, accessing the conscious or to the left to access the subconscious. If they are accessing the subconscious, you can make a suggestion that their conscious awareness is not there. It is easy to know if a child is thinking in pictures, sounds or feelings. The idea is a very useful way of understanding how different people think and would be an invaluable skill for those who want to communicate better.

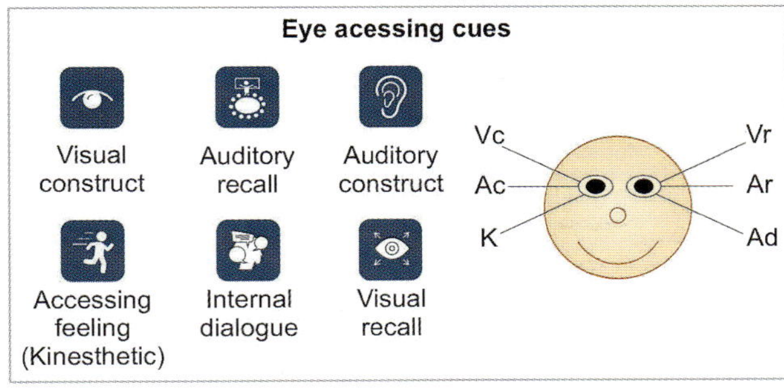

Hypnotic Voice

- Its not what you said, its the way you said it. A voice with variety contains a combination of pitch, pace, pause, volume and word emphasis.
- **The flat tone:** Consider the words *"You Will Open Your Mouth."* A flat monotone would simply describe the event, as if reading from a to-do list.
- **The rising tone:** It begins to sound like a question with a rising tone. A question is proclaimed to be agnostic. So even if spoken like a statement, it sounds feeble. "You Will Open Your Mouth?"
- **The downward tone:** It becomes an order, command or imperative. Project from down low, not up high, to have a persuasive voice. When you want to make a suggestion but don't want to give it a strong impact.

Structuring Suggestion

- Suggestions are an invitation to experience the world in a different way. They are commands you give to someone else. A successful suggestion delivers only if it is said with the apt words at the appropriate time in a fitting demeanor.
- You have to be utterly convincing, firm and soothing. Care should be taken that the suggestion does not take the pat of being pleading, pushy and frail. A lot of this depends on the content of your speech.
- A direct suggestion appeals directly to the conscious mind, which has the opportunity to evaluate:

  "Close your eyes. (Please, you can)."
  "I would like you to close your eyes now."

- An indirect suggestion goes directly to the unconscious mind and is not evaluated as much.

  "I am wondering if you can close your eyes."
  "Can you allow your eyes to close."
  "Isn't it nice not to have to listen with your eyes open"

- The only difference you could see is that it presents the suggestion more as an option rather than an ultimatum. Softening a suggestion means taking a direct suggestion and making it indirect.

Behavioral dentistry is an ever-evolving discipline. The successful practice of CH requires greater methodological clarity and its important to note that further research is needed to develop and implement such promising intervention and provide the evidence base that is needed.

Points to Remember

- Hypnosis is a state of consciousness involving focused attention and reduced peripheral awareness. This technique helps to communicate with subconscious by passing the conscious mind.
- Conversational hypnosis is a collection of techniques and strategies to change persons thoughts, emotions, decisions and behavior in a complete unconscious way.
- Children over 4 years have the necessary verbal understanding and their blind trust and vivid imaginations make them suscepitble to suggestions.
- Conversational hypnosis is persuasion to accept a suggestion. It is not about getting children to do things they do not want to do, it's about getting children to want to do things that you want.
- Traditional hypnosis is overt and conversational hypnosis is covert.
- Trance is used to identify the conditions under which someone responds to hypnotic suggestions.
- Absorb attention, bypass the critical factor and stimulate the unconscious mind (ABS) is a model for understanding hypnotic process.
- "People like people who are like them" By becoming "like" the other person(subtly mirroring their posture and voice qualities) you unconsciously induce support, a sense of trust and liking.
- Accessing memory is typically associated with a shift of the eyes to the left: constructing new content, with a shift to the right.
- Visual strategies are typically associated with upward gaze, auditory with horizontal and kinesthetic with downward gaze.
- Children will more likely to do what you want them to do if the request is made with the descending pitch. Descending pitch opens up command module in the brain.
- A direct suggestion appeals directly to the conscious mind whereas an indirect suggestion goes directly to the unconscious and is not evaluated.

Questionnaire

1. Define hypnosis. Write the difference between traditional hypnosis and conversational hypnosis.
2. What is trance and the signs to identify the trance?
3. What are the rapport building skills used while carrying out conversational hypnosis?
4. Describe the importance of eye accessing cues and hypnotic voice in conversational hypnosis.

FURTHER READING

1. Battino R, South TL. Ericksonian Approaches: A Comprehensive Manual. 2nd ed. Norfolk: Crown house Publishing Ltd; 2005.
2. Berberich FR. Pediatric suggestions: using hypnosis in the routine examination of children. Am J Clin Hypn. 2007;50(2):121-9.
3. Campbell C. Dental Fear and Anxiety in Pediatric Patients. 1st Ed. Cham: Springer publication; 2017.
4. Jay Michael N. Mastering Conversational hypnosis. Book Baby Publication, 2014.

5. Kaplowitz GJ. Communicating with patients. GenDent 1999Jul-Aug:399-403.
6. Kiff M. Conversational Hypnosis-A practical guide. Define Success Publication, 2012.
7. Kohen DP, Kaiser P. Clinical hypnosis with Children and adolescents-What? Why? How? Origins, Applications and Efficacy. Children (Basel). 2014;1(2):74-98.
8. Lyons L. Using hypnosis with children: Creating and delivering effective intervention. 1st Ed. London: WW Norton and Company Ltd; 2015.
9. Olness K, Kohen D. Hypnosis and hypnotherapy with children. 3rd Ed. New York: The Guilford Press; 1996.
10. Paul Adler S. Ericksonian Hypnosis: Strategies for effective communication. Telemachus Press, 2016.
11. Pendergrast RA. Incorporating hypnosis into pediatric clinical encounters. Children (Basel). 2017;4(3):18.
12. Santos SA, Gleiser R, Ardenghi TM. Hypnosis in the control of pain and anxiety in Pediatric Dentistry: a literature review. RGO, Rev Gauch Odontol.2019;67.
13. Short D. Conversational hypnosis: Conceptual and technical differences relative to traditional hypnosis. Am J Clin Hypn. 2018;61(2):125-39.
14. Simons D, Potter C, Temple G. Hypnosis and communication in Dental Practice. London: Quintessence Publishing Co Ltd; 2007.
15. Teleska J, Roffman A. A continuum of hypnotherapeutic interactions: from formal hypnosis to hypnotic conversation. Am J Clin Hypn. 2004;47(2):103-15.

CHAPTER 88

Applications of Nanoscience in Pediatric Dentistry

Arun Bhupathi

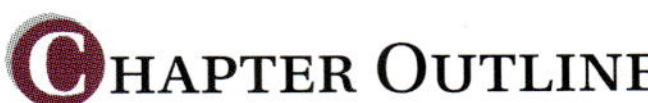

Chapter Outline

- Nanomaterials Synthesis
- Nanomaterials in Pediatric Dentistry

The concept of miniaturization was first put forth at an annual meeting held at the California Institute of Technology by the American Physical Society by **Dr Richard Phillips Feynman** on December 29, 1959. In his seminar lecture, "There's plenty of room at the bottom" the concept of miniaturization was exclusively presented, i.e., data storage on minute devices, atomic scale script engraving and interpretation, reduction in computer size, fabrication of atomic electronic circuits, etc. However, the term nanotechnology was not used by Feynman but was proposed by **Taniguchi** in his paper "On the basic concept of nanotechnology", which was published in 1974. In a book published in 1986, "Engines of creation: The coming era of nanotechnology", by **Dr Eric Drexler** considered Feynman's concept of numerous tiny factories and expressed his idea that a huge number of one's own copies can be made with the aid of computer control instead of human operator control.

With the advent of science and technology, the futuristic concept has turned into reality and nanotechnology has expanded its horizons to every aspect of the scientific world including dentistry. The incorporation of nanotechnology has changed the properties of certain materials used in dentistry and research is still on to overcome the challenges faced by the clinician. This chapter highlights the applications of nanosciences in pediatric dentistry.

According to the US government, "Nanotechnology is research and technology development at the atomic, molecular or macromolecular level in the length scale of approximately 1–100 nm range, to provide a fundamental understanding of phenomena and materials at the nanoscale and to create and use structures, devices and systems that have novel properties and functions because of their small and/or intermediate size".

With the alteration in size, the quantum mechanical properties of the nanomaterials or particles change and exhibit various adaptable physical, chemical and biological properties which are drastically different from their bulk counterparts of the same material **(Fig. 88.1)**.

NANOMATERIALS SYNTHESIS

For the fabrication of nanomaterials, two approaches are developed which include bottom-up and top-down procedures. However, a hybrid approach can also be used which has both the above-mentioned procedures to develop a complete nanostructure, e.g., lithography. With these approaches, zero, one, two-dimensional and special nanostructures can be developed.

- The Bottom-Up approach is typically the construction of the material atom by atom, molecule by molecule.
- The bio-physiological molecules often follow this synthesis procedure to develop into a complete stable and functional nanostructure, e.g., protein molecules, haemoglobin, etc. The various procedures included in this approach are the sol-gel method, electrospinning, electrochemical deposition, co-precipitation method, etc. The particles developed by this procedure will be smaller than the top-down synthesis procedures.
- The top-down approach is the procedural reduction in the dimensions of the bulk material till they attain a stable nano dimension structure. The nanostructures formed through this approach will have more structural imperfections. The nanofabrication procedures included in this approach are milling or attrition and quenching repeatedly.

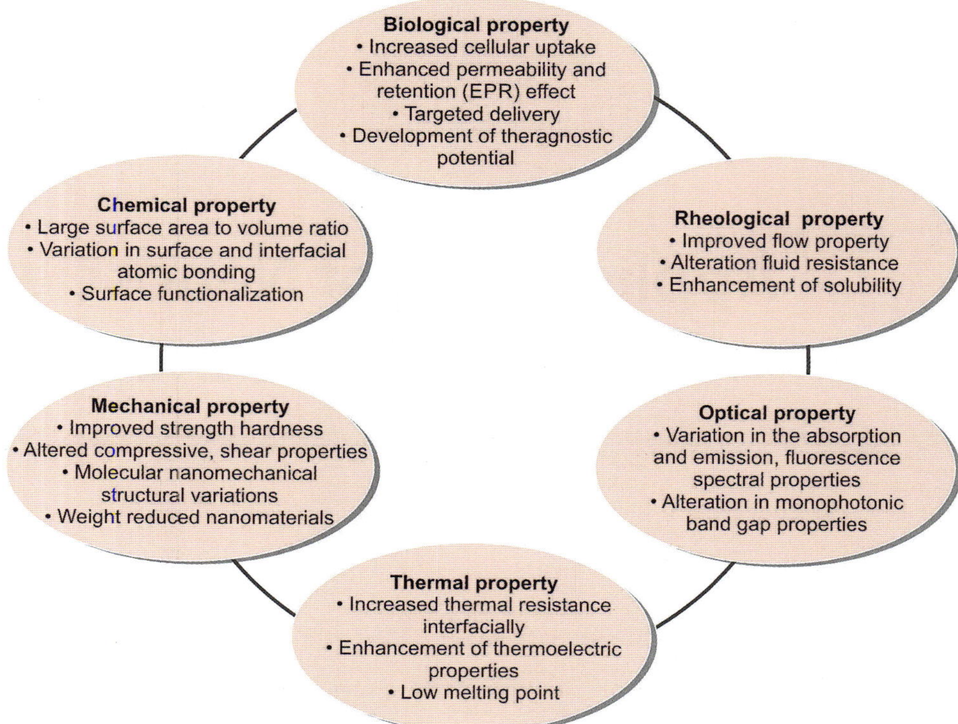

Biological property
• Increased cellular uptake
• Enhanced permeability and retention (EPR) effect
• Targeted delivery
• Development of theragnostic potential
Chemical property
• Large surface area to volume ratio
• Variation in surface and interfacial atomic bonding
• Surface functionalization
Rheological property
• Improved flow property
• Alteration fluid resistance
• Enhancement of solubility
Mechanical property
• Improved strength hardness
• Altered compressive, shear properties
• Molecular nanomechanical structural variations
• Weight reduced nanomaterials
Optical property
• Variation in the absorption and emission, fluorescence spectral properties
• Alteration in monophotonic band gap properties
Thermal property
• Increased thermal resistance interfacially
• Enhancement of thermoelectric properties
• Low melting point

Fig. 88.1: Depicting size-dependent altered properties.

- In the synthesis and processing of nanostructure materials the following challenges must be encountered:
  - Due to the large surface area to volume ratio, the high surface energy has to overcome.
  - Certainty in the development of desired uniform size and shape distribution, chemical structure and composition which together show the impact on physical properties.
  - Coarsening with time through agglomeration or Ostwald ripening should be prevented.
- After the fabrication of nanomaterials successfully, a thorough screening will be performed at *in vitro* (cellular level), *in vivo* (preclinical/animal model) and clinical analysis (human volunteers) levels. Due to the increased activity of the nanosystems with the biological system their retention in the body and toxic effect has been noticed and is still under research investigation. Nanoscience is still a developing research field, so long-term toxicological screening methods have to be developed yet.

NANOMATERIALS IN PEDIATRIC DENTISTRY

The existence of nano-dimensioned hydroxyapatite crystallites and collagen fibrils in the dentoalveolar structures led to the introduction of nanotechnology into dentistry which today we term nanodentistry. With the advent of nano precision equipment like scanning electron microscope (SEM), probe-based atomic force microscope (AFM), positron-resolved small angle X-ray scattering (SAXS), transmission electron microscopy (TEM), X-ray photoelectron spectroscopy (XPS), etc., the nanoscopic awareness over the macroscopic dentoalveolar structures were revealed and studied. This nano-dimension knowledge could furnish a basis for handling the physiological and pathological variants of the dentoalveolar structures. The description regarding the clinically implemented nanoscience products such as the nanocomposite restorative materials, nano-bonding adhesives, nano-glass ionomer restorative materials and nano-implants are discussed in the following:

Nanocomposite Restorations

- In the 1950s the research and development of resin-based composites were initiated in the field of restorative dentistry which underwent various innovations and the recent advancements over the last decade were nanoparticle and or nanocluster embedded conventional composite resins. With the advent of nanotechnology in dentistry, the addition of nanoparticle as filler contents such as ceramic, silica glass, quartz, metal, pre-polymerized particles in various shapes and sizes incorporated into dental materials have evolved.
- The color-based dental filling material consisted of an organic matrix phase, an inorganic filler phase and an activator system. The size of the nanoparticles governs the optical properties, i.e., the nanoparticle size (~20 nm) is lesser than the visible light wavelength of 400–800 nm thus the nanocomposites developed with these nanoparticles have exceedingly less opaque properties.
- Along with optical properties, an increase in the content of the inorganic filler phase and their shape also become significant in imparting enhanced physical and mechanical properties like elastic modulus, hardness, etc.
- The filler particle's size defines the type of composite either microfilled, nanofilled or nanohybrids. The microfilled composite restorative materials consisting of micron-sized

filler particles have been used for anterior restorations due to their esthetic properties such as high initial gloss and lustre retention. But unfortunately, as their strength parameters are compromising, they are not the material of choice in high load-bearing areas (e.g., Class I, II and IV restorations).

- The nanofilled composites consist of filler particles in the range of 1–100 nm in size, and a blend of both the larger-sized particles (0.4–5 µm) and nanosized particles constitute the nanohybrids. The incorporation of nanoparticles imparts high mechanical strength and long-term polish retention to the nanocomposite restorative materials. The addition of heavy metal fillers in nanofilled composites such as barium, aluminium, silicates, etc., increases the radio-opacity. Even though the nanocomposites have excellent wear resistance they form smoother wear facets when compared to the other conventional composites. Due to the increased contact surface area of nanofillers, the exclusive nanocomposite resins are more susceptible to solubility and water sorption.
- The commercially available minifilled composites in 1970 comprised silicon dioxide filler particles of 0.04 µm size (i.e., 40 nm), but the recently available nanofilled composites differ in the route of synthesis of the silica filler particles. However, the variation between the filler particles of minifilled composites and nanofilled composites is the route of synthesis in which the former was by pyrogenic method and the latter is by ordered growth of filler particles. The maximum allowable load for minifilled composites is 55 wt% and that of nanofilled is 87%. The nanofilled composites were synthesized by incorporation of silane functionalized spherical silica nanoparticles of 5–40 nm, where the bifunctional silane coupling agents (e.g., 3-methacryloxypropyl–trimethoxysilane (MPTS)) act as a surfactant in the pre-cured resin matrix and during curing as a bonding agent to resin matrix. One terminal functional group of the bifunctional coupling agent is a silica ester group which aids in bonding to the inorganic surface and another terminal functional group is the methacrylate group which prevents the aggregation of nanofiller particles and maintains the compatibility in the pre-cured resin matrix system.
- At the beginning of this century, nanotechnology has laid a commercial milestone by the inclusion of aggregated zirconia or silica nanoclusters into the composite resin with an average particle size of 20 nm for silica and 5–20 nm in the agglomerated cluster form. In the recently combined microhybrid and nanofilled composites, the filler weight percentage is increased from 75.75–87% by filling the lacunae between the bigger particles with the tiny ones.
- Irrespective of the storage and environmental conditions the nanoclusters possess a distinct reinforcing mechanism and thus exhibit improved strength and reliability which may be due to the infiltration of silane within the lacunae of the nanoclusters, thereby heightening the scathe allowance.
- Fluoride containing nanoparticles co-incorporated with cationic quaternary ammonium group has reduced the initial burst release and sustained the fluoride ion release along with long-term antibacterial activity. [18]

Nano-adhesive Bonding Agents

- Due to the effect of gravity, the larger filler particles which are meant to increase the cohesive strength of moderately viscous adhesives settle out during storage, thereby causing inconsistency in the performance of the dental adhesive.
- To overcome this problem, with the coordination of nanotechnology, nanofiller particle embedded dental adhesives were developed. The nanofiller particles were silica or zirconia within the range of 5–7 nm which remained stable and unaggregated under the gravitational forces. The zirconia nanoparticle-embedded adhesive systems exhibit radiopaque properties.

Nano-Glass Ionomer Cement

- The recent innovation in resin-modified glass ionomer cement is the incorporation of silica-zirconia nanofillers and nanoclusters and silica nanofillers in 2007, which has enhanced esthetic properties and retained the conventional properties of resin-modified glass ionomer cement.
- The silane functionalized nanofillers (5–25 nm) and loosely bound aggregates of nanoclusters (1 µm–1.6 µm) addition enhanced the optical property, i.e., tooth shade toning potential, less visual opacity, low surface roughness, high polishability and gloss reflectance, low wear rate and few other physical properties clinically.
- The filler loading was nearly 69% of fluoroaluminosilicate glass content and did not affect the cumulative fluoride release pattern suggesting that incorporation of nanofiller particles into the resin matrix does not interfere with cumulative fluoride release.
- The inclusion of metal oxide nanoparticles such as Al_2O_3, TiO_2, ZrO_2, has increased the compressive strength and the addition of nanoparticles is beneficial as it leads to reduction in the microscopic voids in the set glass ionomer cement.
- The antimicrobial efficacy of the glass ionomer cement is enhanced by the addition of silver, copper nanoparticles derived from plants extracts against dental caries microbes along with conventional antiobiotics.

Nano-Pit and Fissure Sealants

- The silver nanoparticle-added sealant reduced the demineralization and likely increased remineralization, compared to the conventional sealant.
- The bioactive fluoride-releasing and antibacterial sealant with nano CaF2 and dimethylaminohexadecyl methacrylate (DMAHDM) is promising to inhibit caries and promote the remineralizaton of enamel and dentin. The hardness of the nanoparticle incorporated sealant was significantly higher than the sealer.
- The application of nano silver fluoride (NSF) formulation is effective to arrest active dentine caries and not stain teeth in children compared to silver diamine fluoride.
- The combination of nano-hydroxyapatite gel and ozone therapy treatment procedures have remineralized the initial approximal enamel and dentine subsurface lesions of premolar and molar and it should be continued for a

long time in order to achieve the effect of nonrestorative treatment of caries.

- Silver nanoparticles incorporated in root canal sealer has better antibacterial efficacy compared to the conventional root canal sealer

Nano-Pulp Capping Agents

- In direct pulp capping the calcium hydroxide, mineral trioxide aggregate (MTA) materials containing calcium ions and high pH stimulates the dental pulp to form a reparative dentin bridge with minimum damage. Literature indicates that hydroxyapatite (HA) used as a pulp capping agent has caused inflammation and necrosis of the dental pulp. To overcome this limitation, the unique advantages of nanotechnology bioinspired and biomimetic nano hydroxyapatite (Nano-HA) similar to molecules of enamel and dentin was developed. It was observed that Nano-HA can produce a continuous dentin bridge similar to MTA. A regular pattern of dentinal tubules was formed by MTA whereas osteodentin formation occurred with nano-HA without any tunnel defects and cellular inclusions. The tissue reaction with nano-HA was an initial inflammatory response, necrosis which reduced over time and finally, a favourable cellular and vascular response were evoked.
- Chlorhexidine gluconate loaded polymer nanofiber scaffold was used in vital pulp therapy to manage caries exposed primary teeth. The biodegradable polymeric scaffold provides the temporal and spatial environment for cellular adhesion, tissue formation and local drug delivery to protect from the caries microbes.

Nano-implants

- One of the recent advances in clinical prosthetic replacement therapy is the dental implant system, which is providing a successful clinical solution.
- One of the main features of a dental implant is its surface topography. The host cellular response towards the dental implant determines the biocompatibility, ability to osseointegrate and functional retentivity.
- To enable these features the topography of dental implants has transformed from micron scale to nanoscale level. The natural nanoscale features such as the surface roughness of bone of nearly 32 nm and the epithelial basement membrane pore size of approximately 70–100 nm biomimics the implant nanotopography.
- Nanoscale surface-modified dental implants possess unique features that alter the cell attachment by the following mechanisms:
    - *Plasma protein or surface interactions:* The protein such as plasma fibronectin or vitronectin adsorption which occurs immediately to implant placement will mediate the subsequent cellular adhesion and behaviour. The conformational changes in these RGD proteins can be achieved by nanoscaled features, which affect cellular activity.
    - *Contact angle or wettability:* The change in the contact angle influences the wettability or surface energy which determines the adsorption of extracellular matrix proteins.
    - *Cell adhesion and motility:* These two cell traits are affected by nanoscaled surfaces. Integrins and adherent proteins influence these traits directly and indirectly respectively. The establishment of an interface between the nanoscaled dental implant– alveolar bone and oral mucosa is attributed to the cellular spreading and motility.
    - *Cell proliferation:* The outcome of the nanoscaled implant surface to the adhered cell signalling, determines the cellular proliferation rate. Even though the osteoblast proliferation is increased, the underlying mechanism of cellular (osteoblast) response to the nanoscaled surface remains unclear.
    - *Cell differentiation:* The mesenchymal cells adhered to the nanoscaled implant differentiate along the bone cell lineage, i.e., osteoblast lineage. An elevated level of alkaline phosphatase and calcium mineral content was noticed in the cell layers formed on nanoscaled materials which promote the osteoblastic activity and osseoinduction process. Up-regulation of gene expression responsible for osteoblastic differentiation occurs in nanoscaled implants.
    - *Cell adhesion selectivity:* The selectivity in cellular adhesion especially the fibroblast or osteoblast depends on the topographic features of the implant. The nanoscaled implants have shown a higher affinity towards osteoblasts than fibroblasts in the ratio of 3:1, whereas in the conventional systems it is 1:1. Similar response was noticed even with smooth muscle cells and chondrocytes which facilitate the adaptability of the implant to the mucosal surfaces. Reduced bacterial adhesion, colonization and proliferation further implicate the exploration of biofilm formation and peri-implantitis.

Nanoparticle Incorporated Oral Hygiene Aids

- The silver-coated toothbrushes can be recommended in various age groups of children because of potential effects on oral hygiene procedures, such as eliminating the remaining bacteria on the bristles and/or in an oral environment.[20]
- Long-term use of medical nano-hydroxyapatite toothpaste helps to increase the acid resistance and caries resistance of the enamel, which is very important for the prevention of caries. It effectively reduces tooth sensitivity in patients of different age groups.[21]
- The dentifrice containing nano- carbonate apatite (n-CAP) and Er, Cr: YSGG laser were effective in reducing dentin hypersensitivity. Initially the laser had a superior desensitizing effect, whereas the dentifrice maintained the effect for a longer duration.

Nanoparticle Incorporated Orthodontic Appliances

Polymethyl-methacrylate (PMMA) commonly used in orthodontic appliances baseplates incorporated with NanoAg *in situ* in PMMA have been inhibiting the planktonic growth and biofilm formation of the cariogenic bacteria. Wearing of NanoAg into baseplate has the potential to minimize dental plaque formation and caries during orthodontic treatment.[22]

Nanoscience is progressing rapidly in the development of new materials in dentistry. Nanobots are in the process of designing for various applications in dentistry which include dentin hypersensitivity, dental caries, orthodontic tooth repositioning, periodontal management, anesthesia, dental fluorosis, etc. Apart from it, extensive research is focused on cancer nanodiagnostics and nanotherapeutics. Polymer encapsulated nanoparticles to reduce immune rejection and perform multifunctional activities in biological systems are under research.

POINTS TO REMEMBER

- Dr Richard Phillips Feynman was the first to describe the use of nanotechnology. Term nanotechnology was proposed by Taniguchi.
- Nanotechnology is research and technology development at the atomic, molecular or macromolecular level in the length scale of approximately 1–100 nm range, to provide a fundamental understanding of phenomena and materials at the nanoscale and to create and use structures, devices and systems that have novel properties and functions because of their small and/or intermediate size.
- Nanosystems used in pediatric dentistry are nanocomposite restorations, nano adhesive bonding agents, nano glass ionomer cement and nano implants.

Questionnaire

1. Enumerate the various nanosystems used in pedodontics.
2. Briefly describe the nanoadhesive systems used in pediatric dentistry.
3. Elaborate on the features of nano implant, which is one of the prosthetic replacement choices for the missing dentition.
4. What are size-dependent properties of a nanosystem?
5. Write a note on nano GIC.

FURTHER READING

1. Amal Adnan Ashour, Mohammed Fareed Felemban, Nayef H Felemban, Enas T Enan, Sakeenabi Basha, Mohamed M. Hassan and Sanaa MF Gad El-Rab. Comparison and Advanced Antimicrobial Strategies of Silver and Copper Nanodrug-Loaded Glass Ionomer Cement against Dental Caries Microbes. Antibiotics, 2022, 11, 756.
2. Bayne SC. Dental biomaterials: where are we and where are we going? J Dent Educ. 2005;69(5):571-85.
3. Boone ME, Kafrawy AH. Pulp reaction to a tricalcium phosphate ceramic capping agent. Oral Surg Oral Med Oral Pathol. 1979; 47(4):369-71.
4. Bushan B. Handbook of Nanotechnology. 2010; Springer pp.147–80.
5. Chacko V, Kurikose S. Human pulpal response to mineral trioxide aggregate (MTA): a histologic study. J Clin Pediatr Dent. 2006; 30(3):203-209.
6. Daixing Zhang, Shuangting Li, Hongyang Zhao, Ke Li, Yiwei Zhang, Yingjie Yu, et al. Improving antibacterial performance of dental resin adhesive via co-incorporating fluoride and quaternary ammonium. Journal of Dentistry, Volume 122, 2022, 104156.
7. Elizabeta Gjorgievska, John W. Nicholson, Dragana Gabric, Zeynep Asli Guclu, Ivana Miletic, Nichola J. Coleman. Assessment of the Impact of the Addition of Nanoparticles on the Properties of Glass–Ionomer Cements. Materials. 2020, 13, 276; doi:10.3390/ma13020276
8. Feynman RP. There is plenty of room at the bottom. Eng Sci. 1960;23(5):22-36.
9. Ford P, Seymour G, Beeley JA, et al. Adapting to changes in molecular biosciences and technologies. Eur J Dent Educ. 2008;12(Suppl 1):40-7.
10. Gaiser S, Deyhle H, Bunk O, et al. Understanding nano- anatomy of healthy and carious human teeth: a Prerequisite for nanodentistry. Biointerphase. 2012;7(4):1-14.
11. Ghorbanzadeh R, Pourakbari B, Bahador A. Effects of Baseplates of Orthodontic Appliances with in situ generated Silver Nanoparticles on Cariogenic Bacteria: A Randomized, Double-blind Cross-over Clinical Trial. J Contemp Dent Pract. 2015;16(4):291-8.
12. Katarzyna Grocholewicz, Grażyna Matkowska-Cichocka, Piotr Makowiecki, Agnieszka Droździk, Halina Ey-Chmielewska, Anna Dziewulska, Małgorzata Tomasik, Grzegorz Trybek, Joanna Janiszewska-Olszowska. Effect of nano-hydroxyapatite and ozone on approximal initial caries: a randomized clinical trial. Scientific Reports. 2020;10:11192.
13. K S D Ravi Kalyan, C Vinay, Arun Bhupathi, K S Uloopi, R Chandrasekhar, K S RojaRamya. Preclinical Evaluation and Clinical Trial of Chlorhexidine Polymer Scaffold for Vital Pulp Therapy. The Journal of Clinical Pediatric Dentistry. 2019; 43(2).
14. Makeeva IM, Polyakova MA, Avdeenko OE, Paramonov YO, Kondrat'ev SA, Pilyagina AA. Effect of long-term application of toothpaste Apadent Total Care Medical nano-hydroxyapatite. Stomatologiia. 2016;95(4):34-36.
15. Mendonça G, Mendonça DB, Aragao FJ, Cooper LF. Advancing dental implant surface technology-from micron to nanotopography. Biomaterials. 2008;29(28): 3822-35.
16. Mitra SB, Wu D, Holmes BN. An application of nanotechnology in advanced dental materials. J Am Dent Assoc. 2003;134(10):1382-90.
17. Ozgul Baygin, Tamer Tuzuner, Nagehan Yilmaz, Simge Aksoy. Short-term antibacterial efficacy of a new silver nanoparticle-containing toothbrush. J Pak Med Assoc. Vol. 67, No. 5, May 2017.
18. Saunders SA. Current practicality of nanotechnology in dentistry. Part 1: Focus on nanocomposite restoratives and biomimetics. Clin Cosmet Investig Dent. 2009;1: 47-61.
19. Sharma S, Cross SE, Hsueh C, et al. Nanocharacterization in dentistry. Int J Mol Sci. 2010;11(6):2523-45.
20. Su-Young Lee, Hoi-In Jung, DDS, Bock-Young Jung, Young-Sik Cho, Ho-Keun Kwon, and Baek-Il Kim. Desensitizing Efficacy of Nano-Carbonate Apatite Dentifrice and Er, Cr:YSGG Laser: A Randomized Clinical Trial. Photomedicine and Laser Surgery. 2015;33(1):9-14.
21. Swarup SJ, Rao A, Boaz K, Srikant N, Shenoy R. Pulpal Response to Nano Hydroxyapatite, Mineral Trioxide Aggregate and Calcium Hydroxide when Used as a Direct Pulp Capping Agent: An in Vivo study. The Journal of Clinical Pediatric Dentistry. 2014;38(3): pp201-206.
22. Taniguchi N. On the basic concept of nanotechnology, Proc. ICPE; 1974. pp. 18-23.
23. Tomisa AP, Launey ME, Lee JS, et al. Nanotechnology approaches to improve dental implants. Int J Oral Maxillofac Implants. 2011;26(Suppl):25-44.
24. Valdeci Elias dos Santos Jr., Arnoldo Vasconcelos Filho, Andrea Gadelha Ribeiro Targino, Miguel Angel Pelagio Flores, Andre' Galembeck, Arnaldo de França Caldas Jr, Aronita Rosenblatt. A New "Silver-Bullet" to treat caries in children – Nano Silver Fluoride: A randomised clinical trial. Journal of Dentistry. 2014;42: 945-51
25. Xiuzhi Fei, Yuncong Li, Michael D. Weir, Bashayer H. Baras, Haohao Wang, Suping Wang. Novel pit and fissure sealant containing nano-CaF2 and dimethylaminohexadecyl methacrylate with double benefits of fluoride release and antibacterial function. Dental Materials. 2020;36(9):1241-53.

CHAPTER 89

Clinical Epidemiology and Biostatistics

Anupama Sharma, Rajesh Sharma, Suresh S

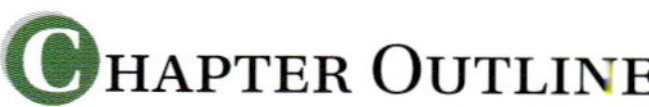

CHAPTER OUTLINE

- Uses of Biostatistics in Dentistry
- Data
- Sample and Sampling
- Measures of Central Tendency
- Measures of Variability
- Tests of Significance
- Errors in Biostatistics

Diseases vary in different populations or subgroups of persons within a population, in different places or at different times. This observation led to the assumption that diseases do not occur at random in human population, therefore their causes must lie in the environment. **Hippocrates** first suggested in fifth century BC that development of disease might be related to environment. He wrote in his treatise "Air, Waters and Places". Efforts to quantify disease and deaths in population began in 1662 when **John Grant** published analysis of births and deaths in London. He provided numerical impact of plague on the population of London and examined characteristics of the years in which plague outbreak occurred. His recognition of the value of routinely collected data in providing information on human illness forms the basis of epidemiology, which literally means "study (logos) of what is among (epi) the people (demos).

Later in 1839, **William Farr**, a Physician systematized the collection, analysis, and reporting of medical statistics in the office of the Registrar General for England and Wales. He compared the mortality and patterns of the causes of deaths in population according to characteristics of individuals and places of residence, etc. The availability of vital statistics enabled **John Snow**, a British Physician, to formulate and test hypothesis concerning the origins of an epidemic of cholera in London. On the basis the description of disease pattern provided by Farr, he postulated that cholera was associated with water. Snow walked from house to house and from every dwelling, in which a cholera death had occurred, to determine which of the two companies supplied the water. Thus he charted not only the distribution of cholera deaths but also determined the cause of the outbreak. A systematic comparison of the populations was at the core of this investigation. This quantitative approach for study of distribution and determinants of disease in human population, epidemiology, was applied to the study of epidemics of infectious disease in nineteenth century. Thus, the dictionary of epidemiology defines it as "the study of the distribution and determinants of health related states or events in specifies populations, and the application of this study to the control of health problems." **John Graunt** (1620–1674) is the Father of Health Statistics.

DEFINITIONS

Study: Epidemiology is a scientific discipline with sound methods of scientific inquiry at its foundation. It is data driven and relies on a systematic and unbiased approach to the collection, analysis, and interpretation of data.

Distribution: Epidemiology is concerned with frequency and pattern of health events in a population. Frequency refers to the number of health events in a population and the relationship of this number to the size of the population. Pattern refers to the occurrence of health related events by time, place and person.

Determinants: These are the causes and other factors that influence the occurrence of disease and other health related events.

Health related states or events: Anything that affects the well-being of a population. Epidemiology was originally focused exclusively on epidemics of communicable disease but was subsequently expanded to address endemic communicable diseases and noncommunicable infectious diseases. By the middle of the 20th century, additional epidemiological methods are applied to injuries, occupational diseases, maternal and child health, environmental health.

Application: It means not only study of health in a population but applying the knowledge to community based practice.

Epidemiology: It can be defined as "quantitative study of the distribution and determinants of disease in human population." Since quantification and comparison occupy a central place in epidemiology, it has strong links to statistics, which helps not only in organization of quantitative data but also in evaluation of role of chance in interpretation of data. Thus, it is important to know which of the observed variations are true or which are by chance.

Statistics: Science of collecting, summarizing, presenting data, and interpreting data to see whether sampling variations and associations are due to chance.

Biostatistics: Tool of statistics applied to the data that is derived from biological sciences.

Need for biostatistics
- To define normalcy.
- To test the difference between two population.
- To study the correlation or association between two or more attributes.
- To evaluate the efficacy of vaccines, sera, etc., by control studies.
- To locate, define and measure extent of a disease.
- To evaluate achievements in health program.
- To fix priorities in achieving health related benefits.

USES OF BIOSTATISTICS IN DENTISTRY

- **In physiology and anatomy**
  - To define the limits of normality for physical variable such as height or weight or blood pressure, etc., in a population.
  - Variation from natural/normal limits may be pathological, i.e., abnormal due to play of certain external factors.
  - To find correlation between two variables like height and weight.
- **In pharmacology**
  - To find the action of certain drugs
  - To compare the action of two drugs or two successive dosages of same drug
  - To find the comparative or relative potency of a new drug with respect to a standard drug
- **In medicine**
  - To compare the efficiency of a particular drug, operation or line of treatment
  - To find association between two attributes such as cancer and smoking
  - To identify signs and symptoms of disease
- **In community medicine and public health**
  - To test usefulness of sera or vaccine in the field
  - In epidemiologic studies the role of causative factors is statistically tested
- **In research**
  - It helps in compilation, analysis and interpretation of the data and making further recommendations.
- **For students**
  - It helps the students and research scholars to evaluate scientific studies and facilitates understanding of the subject.

DATA

A collective recording of observations either numeric or otherwise is called data.

Types of Data

I. *Stephen's classification:*
- Nominal data
- Ordinal data
- Interval
- Ratio

↓

II. *Qualitative data:*
- Nominal data
- Ordinal data
- Dichotomous data

Quantitative data:
- Interval
- Ratio

↓

III. Primary data—directly from the source (First hand information)
Secondary data—from pre-existing records (Second-hand data)

Qualitative or discrete data
- In such data there is no notion of magnitude or size of an attribute as the same cannot be measured.
- The number of person having the same attribute are variable and are measured, e.g., like out of 100 people 75 have class I occlusion, 15 have class II occlusion and 10 have class III occlusion.
- Class I, II and III are attributes, which cannot be measured in figures, only no of people having it can be determined.
- Types:
  - *Nominal data:* Naming or categorical variables that have no measurement scales, e.g., Recording blood groups, Reasons for extraction of teeth
  - *Ordinal (ranked) data:* Characterized in terms of more than two variables and have a clearly implied direction but the data are not measured on a measurement scale, e.g., Severity of patient perceived pain
  - *Dichotomous data (binary variables):* The variable can have only two values, e.g., Sex of the respondents

- Nominal, ordinal, and dichotomous data can together be called *categorical data.*

Quantitative or continuous data

- In this the attribute has a magnitude and both the attribute and the number of persons having the attribute may vary, e.g., Freeway space. It varies for every patient. It is a quantity with a different value for each individual and is measurable.
- Types:
  - Interval scale: No absolute zero, e.g., centigrade scale of temperature
  - Ratio scale: Has a true or absolute zero, e.g., Kelvin temperature scale.

Methods of Collecting Data

Statistical data can be majorly obtained by "The census registry of India".

1. **Census:** It is the total process of collecting, compiling, and publishing demographic, economic, and social data pertaining at a specified time or times, to all persons in a country or delimited territory
   - The first regular census in India—1881
   - Census Act—1948
   - *Functions are* demographics, social, and economic conditions of people.
   - Advantages include provision of complete information
   - Disadvantages are that it is expensive, time consuming, needs more manpower, and lesser accuracy.
2. **Sampling:** Sample is a portion of a population, selected from the population in some manner.

Presentation of Data

- Statistical data once collected should be systematically arranged and presented:
  - To arouse interest of readers
  - For data reduction
  - To bring out important points clearly and strikingly
  - For easy grasp and meaningful conclusions
  - To facilitate further analysis
  - To facilitate communication.
- Two main types of data presentation are:
  - Tabulation
  - Graphic representation with charts and diagrams.

Tabulation of Data

- It is the most common method
- Data presentation is in the form of columns and rows
- It can be of the following types:
  - Simple tables
  - Frequency distribution tables.

1. **Simple table**

Months	*Number of patients at MGDCH, Jaipur*
Jan 06	2,800
Feb 06	1,900
March 06	1,750

2. **Frequency distribution table**
   - In a frequency distribution table, the data is first split into convenient groups (class interval) and the number of items (frequency), which occurs in each group, is shown in adjacent column.

Number of cavities	*Number of patients*
0 to 3	78
3 to 6	67
6 to 9	32
9 and above	16

Graphic Representation with Charts and Diagrams

- Useful method of presenting statistical data.
- Powerful impact on imagination of the people.
- *Can be classified as:*
  - Bar chart
  - Histogram
  - Frequency polygon
  - Frequency curve
  - Line diagram
  - Cumulative frequency diagram
  - Scatter diagram
  - Pie chart
  - Pictogram
  - Spot map or map diagram.

Bar Chart

- Length of bars drawn vertical or horizontal is proportional to frequency of variable
- Suitable scale is chosen
- Bars usually equally spaced
- *They are of three types: Simple bar chart* **(Fig. 89.1)**; *Multiple bar chart:* Two or more variables are grouped together **(Fig. 89.2)**; *Component bar chart:* Bars are divided into two parts, each part representing certain item and proportional to magnitude of that item **(Fig. 89.3)**.

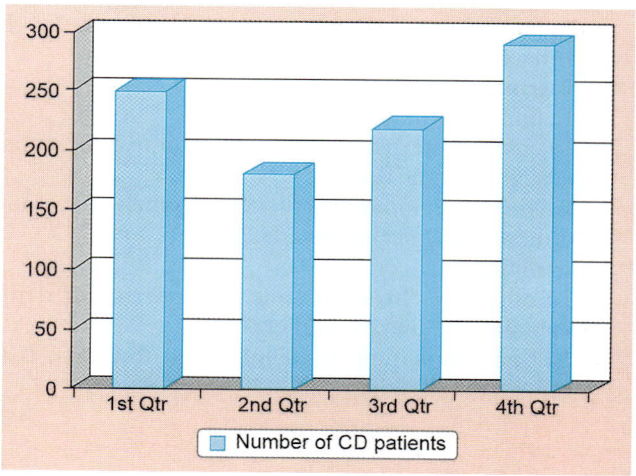

Fig. 89.1: Simple bar chart.

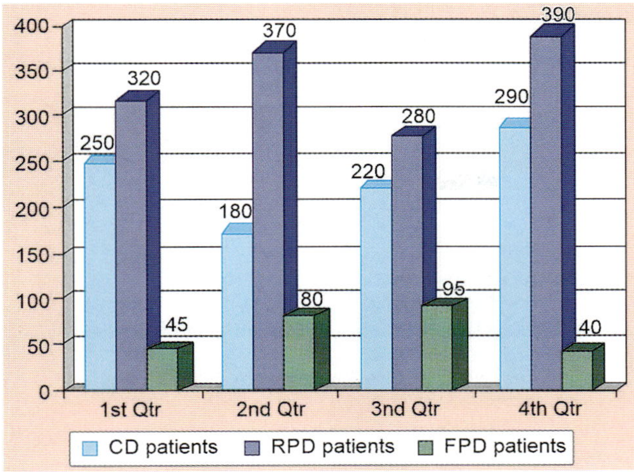

Fig. 89.2: Multiple bar chart.

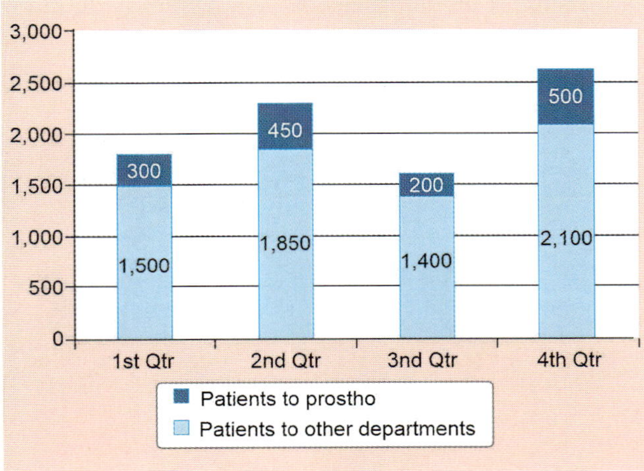

Fig. 89.3: Component bar chart.

Histogram (Fig. 89.4)

- Pictorial presentation of frequency distribution.
- Consists of series of rectangles.
- Class interval given on vertical axis.
- Area of rectangle is proportional to the frequency.

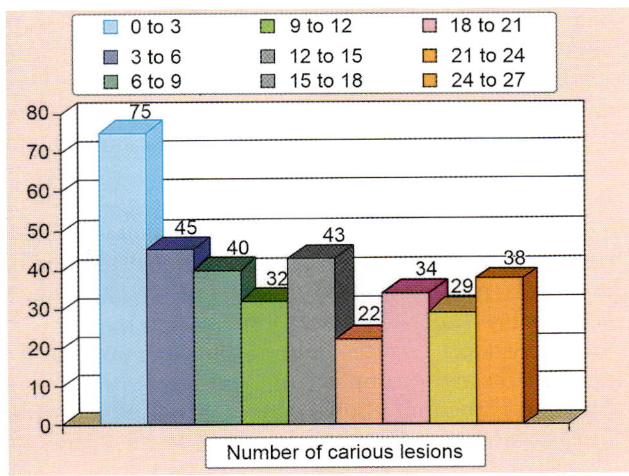

Fig. 89.4: Histogram.

Frequency Polygon (Fig. 89.5)

Obtained by joining midpoints of histogram blocks at the height of frequency by straight lines usually forming a polygon.

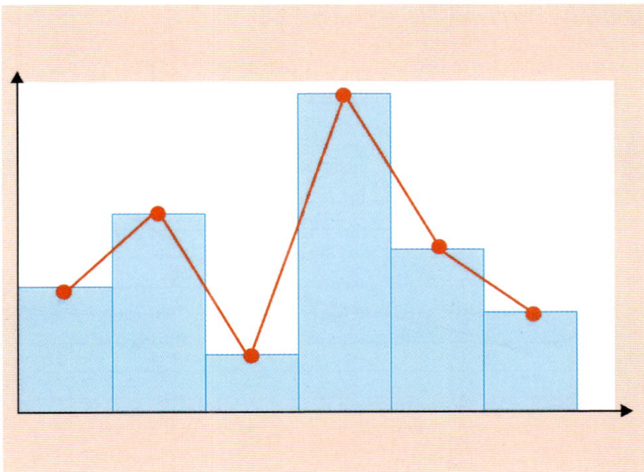

Fig. 89.5: Frequency polygon.

Frequency Curve (Fig. 89.6)

When number of observations is very large and class interval is reduced, the frequency polygon loses its angulations becoming a smooth curve known as frequency curve.

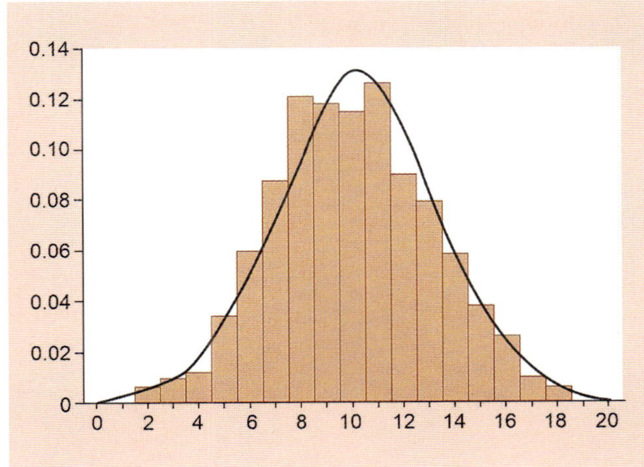

Fig. 89.6: Frequency curve.

Line Diagram (Fig. 89.7)

Line diagram are used to show the trends of events with the passage of time.

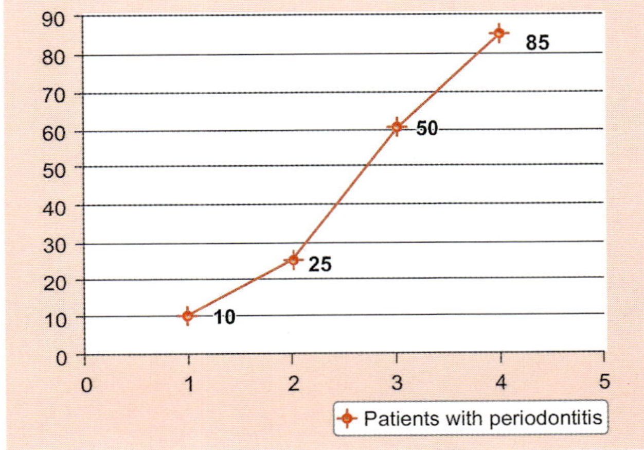

Fig. 89.7: Line diagram.

Cumulative Frequency Diagram (Fig. 89.8)

- Graphical representation of cumulative frequency.
- It is obtained by adding the frequency of previous class.

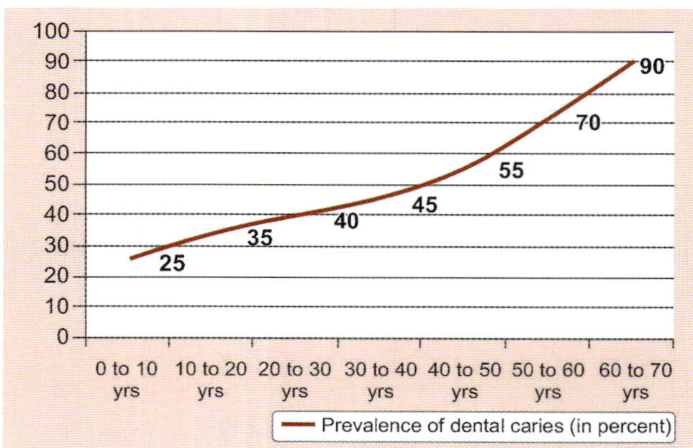

Fig. 89.8: Cumulative frequency diagram.

Scatter or Dot Diagram (Fig. 89.9)

- Shows relationship between two variables.
- If the dots are clustered showing a straight line, it shows a relationship of linear nature.

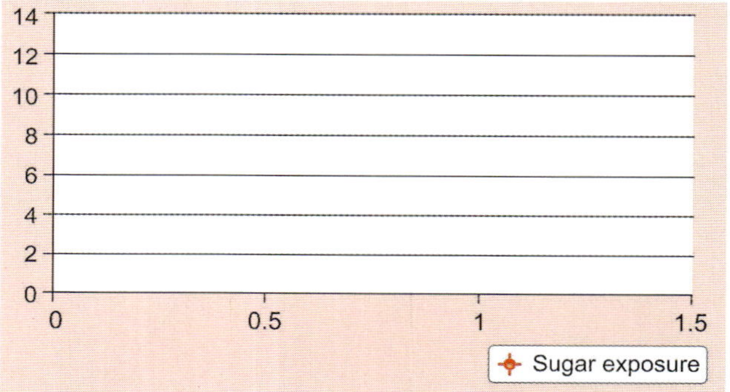

Fig. 89.9: Dot diagram.

Pie Chart (Fig. 89.10)

- In this frequencies of the group are shown as segment of circle.
- Degree of angle denotes the frequency.

$$\text{Angle is calculated by } \frac{\text{Class frequency} \times 360}{\text{Total observations}}$$

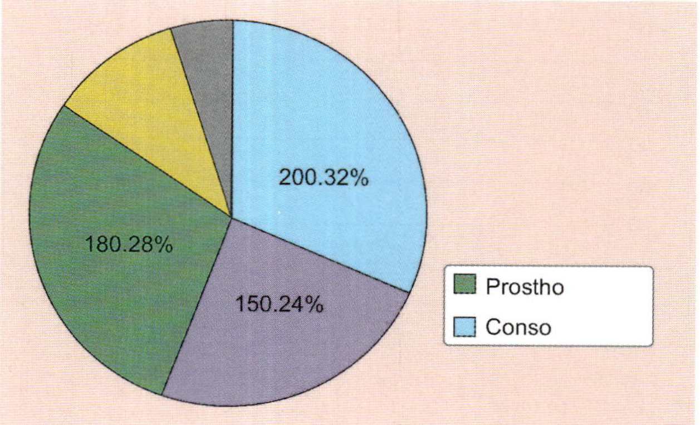

Fig. 89.10: Pie chart.

Pictogram (Fig. 89.11)

- Popular method of presenting data to the common man.

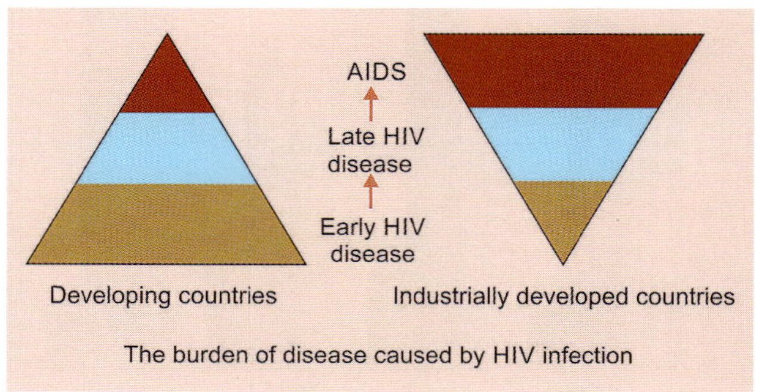

Fig. 89.11: Pictogram.

Spot Map or Map Diagram (Fig. 89.12)

These maps are prepared to show geographic distribution of frequencies of characteristics.

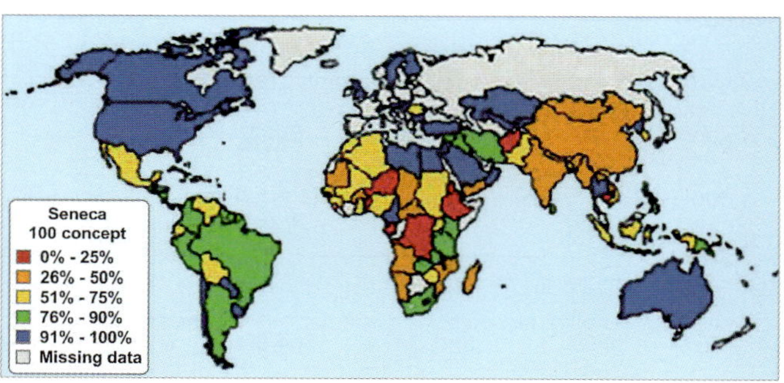

Fig. 89.12: Spot diagram.

SAMPLE AND SAMPLING

- In order to use the data for assessment process sampling is commonly used in statistical analysis.
- **Sample** is defined as a part of a population generally selected so as to be representative of the population whose variables are under study. A sample is a part of a population. Sampling is the process or technique of selecting a sample of appropriate characteristics and adequate size.
- It is the cornerstone of research design, which is set up to carry out the research.
- The reference population may be a population of people who are healthy or sick, clients of a clinic, acceptors of a certain program, having a set of problems, or people exposed to a certain stimulus. The population may not be people at all, as in the case of vital events (births, deaths) or records (medical or vital) or sampling may be of time as Wednesday clinics, February births, etc.
- The individuals, records, units or time are considered to be elements in the sample.
- **Element** is the unit of observation or unit about which information is collected and which is the subject of analysis.
- **Sampling frame** are the total of the elements of the population under the survey
- **Population** is group of all individuals who are the focus of investigation.

- ❖ The sample is drawn from this survey population and is subset of the sampling frame.

Classification of Sampling

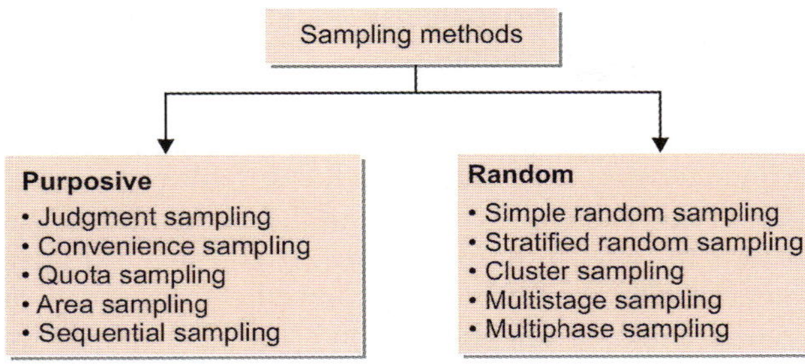

Purposive Sampling

- ❖ **Judgment sampling**
  - Selection of samples is left to the judgment of investigator
  - In this sampling accuracy of results depends upon investigator
  - *Indications:*
    - Employed mainly when population is small
    - Employed to conduct pilot study
  - *Limitations:*
    - Accuracy of results depends upon the knowledge of the investigator
    - If investigator is biased it affects the acceptance or rejection of a hypothesis
- ❖ **Convenience sampling**
  - Chunk is a fraction of population, which is selected for investigator because it is conveniently available
  - For example, in order to estimate oral hygiene status in the city, the investigator may select a few areas near by his house
  - Results of this sampling are rarely representative because they are generally biased
- ❖ **Quota sampling**
  - Each investigator is allotted quota of persons which are to be interviewed
  - Investigators are given instructions to interview persons within the quota with some specified characteristics
  - For example, persons within the quota of 10 housewives, 6 professionals
- ❖ **Area sampling**
  - It is a type of random sampling in which maps rather than lists are used
  - The area to be covered in a study is divided into smaller areas and a random sample is selected from the smaller areas
- ❖ **Sequential sampling**
  - Here a small sample is tested in order to answer certain questions about the population
  - If the questions are not answered, the number of subjects or units in the sample is increased gradually until conclusions may be drawn.

Random Sampling

- ❖ **Simple random sampling** (Unrestricted random sampling)
  - The procedure of selecting a sample in which, every item in a population has an equal chance of being included in the sample
  - Applicable when population is very small, homogeneous, and readily available
  - Selection methods are—Lottery method and Table of random numbers
  - Advantage is that it eliminates selection bias
  - Disadvantage is that selection of sample is costly and time consuming
  - *Limitation:* Difficult to collect data for large samples
- ❖ **Systematic random sampling**
  - By selecting one unit at random and then selecting additional units at evenly spaced intervals (sample interval) till the sample of required size has been formed
  - It is applied to field studies when the population is large, scattered, and homogenous
  - Sample interval is calculated by the following formula:

    $$K = N/n$$

    where, K: sample interval or sample ratio; N = Population size; n = Sample size
    For example, if 150 patients are to be included in the sample from a population of 3,000, K = 3000/150 = 20.
  - *Advantages:*
    - Systematic design is simple
    - Convenient to adopt
    - Time and labor in collection of sample is relatively small
    - It gives accurate results when population is large
  - Limitation is that it requires a preformed list
- ❖ **Stratified random sampling**
  - If population is heterogeneous, simple random sampling is not useful
  - Purpose of this sampling is to increase the efficiency of sampling by dividing heterogeneous sample population into homogenous groups. These homogenous groups are termed as strata like areas, classes, age groups, sexes, etc.
  - Indicated when the population is heterogeneous with regard to the characteristic under study
  - For example, an epidemiological study on prevalence of dental caries
  - *Advantages:*
    - There is a greater precision of results
    - It gives better results when population is scattered
    - More representativeness and accuracy
  - Disadvantage is that it is too technical method and time consuming

Cluster Sampling

- ❖ In this sampling, the required numbers of groups or clusters are selected by simple random sampling. Then all the individuals present in those clusters are included in the sample
- ❖ Indicated when population is vast and scattered over a wide area and the population forms natural groups, cluster sampling is applicable
- ❖ *Advantages:*
  - Simpler.
  - Involves less time and cost.

- For example, city is divided into wards, required number of wards are selected randomly. Then all the people residing in those selected wards are included in the sample.

Multistage Sampling

- As the name implies, this method refers to the sampling procedures carried out in several stages using random sampling technique
- Indicated when the study involves very large population, like nationwide surveys
- For example, a state level epidemiologic study—first stage: few of the districts are selected randomly; second stage: few of the revenue divisions are selected, randomly from each selected district; third stage: few of the towns or villages are selected, randomly from each selected division; fourth stage: few of the residents are selected randomly from each selected town or village.

Multiphase Sampling

- In this method, part of the information is collected from the whole sample and part from the subsample
- For example, a survey to identify the children who require RCT—first phase: identify children with clinically visible caries; second phase: isolate children with positive history for pulp necrosis; third phase: conduct pulp vitality tests; fourth phase: IOPA radiographs
- *Advantages:*
  - Economic
  - Purposeful
  - Saves time and manpower

Sample Size

Factors influencing	*Structure*
Degree of difference expected	Determine difference
Degree of variation among subjects	Determine standard deviation (SD) of groups
Level of significance desired	Set alpha error
Power of the study	Decide power of the study
Dropout rate	Select appropriate formula
Noncompliance to treatment	Calculate sample size, give allowance to dropout and noncompliance

Sample Size Formulae

$n = [2SD/SE]^2$; SD and SE from previous studies with 95% CI

$n = z^2 \sigma p^2/e^2$

z = constant; σ = SD of population; e = acceptable error

$n = Z^2 pq/e^2$: p = Sample proportion

Requisites for a Reliable Sample

- **Efficiency:** It means the ability of the sample to yield the desired information
- **Representativeness:** A sample should be representative of the parent population so that inferences drawn from the population can be generalized to that population with measurable precision and confidence
- **Measurability:** The design of the sample should be such that valid estimates of its variability can be made. In other words, the investigator should be able to estimate the extent to which the findings from the sample are likely to differ from what we would have found had we studied the entire parent population
- **Size:** A sample should be large enough to minimize sample variability to allow estimates of the population characteristics to be made with measurable precision
- **Coverage:** Adequate coverage of the sample is essential if it is to remain representative. High rates of refusal, unavailability, loss of follow-up, and other missing data can render a sample unrepresentative of the parent population
- **Goal orientation:** Sample selection and estimation procedures should be oriented toward the study objectives and research design and considerations
- **Feasibility:** The design should be simple enough to be carried out in practice
- **Economy and cost efficiency:** The design of the sample should be such that appreciable savings in time and cost can be achieved without determining the study objectives. The sample should therefore yield the desired information within expected but tolerable limits of sampling error for the lowest cost.

Determination of Sample Size

- It is imperative that the sample size be sufficient to be dependable and to allow tests of significance to be applied to the data collected
- The degree of difference or strength of association one wants to be able to detect also influences the required sample size. Sometimes, it is advisable to obtain an idea of the required sample size through a "Pilot study"
- Statisticians should be consulted for methods of calculating sufficient sample size
- There are two basic ways of approaching the problem of determining sample size—the empirical and the analytical
- The empirical approach usually requires sample sizes that have been used by others in similar situations. This approach is least recommended by statisticians
- The analytical method of sample size determination requires an understanding of statistical concepts such as sampling techniques, sampling errors, hypothesis testing, significance levels, and powers of tests. It is a statistically sound method.

Advantages of Sampling

- Sampling reduces the cost of investigation, the time required, and the number of personnel involved
- Sampling is especially important when the tests used are highly technical or detailed or must be administered or interpreted by experts
- Sampling allows through investigation of the units of observation
- It is obvious that a sample can be covered more adequately and in more depth in a research project than in a total population.

Errors in Sampling

Sampling Errors

- Faulty sampling design—method of collection of sample is inappropriate
- Small sample size—the sample size collected is less for the representation of the population

Nonsampling Errors

- *Coverage errors:* Caused by failure to sample the entire population adequately, which may arise from inadequacy of the sampling frame or from unsatisfactory coverage of the sample units. These errors are exaggerated in the use of postal questionnaires, interviews, etc. Inability to make the required observations on all the assigning sampling units is called nonresponse
- *Processing error:* These might arise during data processing. Includes theoretical errors in the methods of statistical analysis, clerical errors in the copying of material, and computational errors
- *Observational errors:* May be introduced by the fault committed by the investigator or through use of imperfect test instruments and techniques.

Pathfinder survey
- Stratified cluster sampling technique used.
- Most important population subgroups (index groups) likely to have differing disease levels are chosen covering a standard number of subjects in a specific group in a selected location
- **Suitable to evaluate:** overall prevalence of various oral diseases
- Variations in disease levels, severity, and treatment needs are evaluated
- Can be pilot survey or national survey

MEASURES OF CENTRAL TENDENCY

Mean

$$\frac{\text{Sum of all the observations}}{\text{Total number of observations}}$$

For grouped data:

$$\text{Mean}=\frac{\text{Total (value of variable} \times \text{frequency)}}{\text{Total frequency}}$$

For grouped data with range:

$$\text{Mean}=\frac{\text{Total (midpoint of class internal} \times \text{frequency)}}{\text{Total frequency}}$$

Median

Arrange the observations in ascending or descending order. The middle observation is the median.

Mode

- It is that value which in a series of observation occurs with greatest frequency
- Mode = 3 median – 2 mean

MEASURES OF VARIABILITY

Measures of Dispersion

- Dispersion is the degree of spread or variation of the variable about a central value.
- A good measure of dispersion should be simple, easy to compute, based on all items, amenable for further analysis and not affected by extreme values.
- Uses:
  - Determine reliability of an average
  - Serve as a basis of control of variability
  - Comparison of two or more series
  - Facilitate further statistical analysis

Measures of Variation or Scatter

- Range
- Interquartile range
- Mean deviation
- Standard deviation
- Coefficient of variation

Range

- Difference between value of smallest and largest item
- Range defines the normal limits of a biologic characteristic
- Simple to calculate
- Not based on all items
- Subjected to fluctuations

Standard Deviation

- Root mean square deviation
- Summary measure of differences of each observations from mean of all observations
- Greater the standard deviation greater will be magnitude of dispersion from the mean
- Small is standard deviation, higher is degree of uniformity of observations
- Calculation of standard deviation

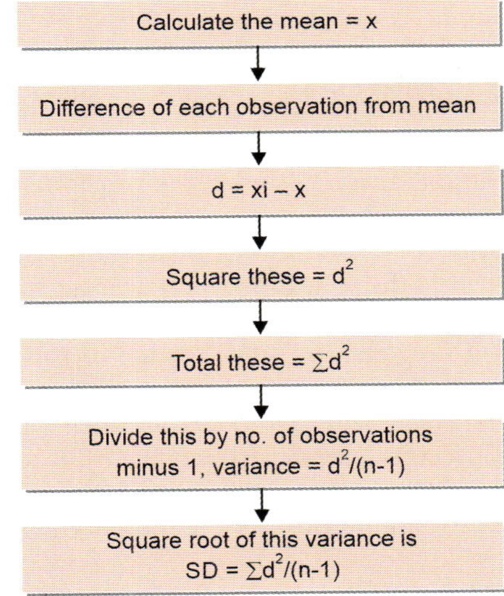

- Uses of standard deviation
  - Summarizes the deviations of a large distribution
  - Indicates whether the variation from mean is by chance or real
  - Helps in finding standard error
  - Helps in finding the suitable size of sample
  - Standard deviation is only interpretable as a summary measure for variations having approximately symmetric preparations

Coefficient of Variation

- The average of differences of values of items
- Can be mean deviation from mean, median or mode
- Compare relative variability
- Variation of same character in two or more series
- Coefficient of variation is used to compare the variability of one character in two different groups having different magnitude of values or two characters in the same group by expressing in percentage
- Coefficient of variation = Standard deviation × 100/mean
- Higher the coefficient of variation, greater is variability

Standard Error

- Standard deviation of a statistic like mean, proportion, etc.
- Different samples from same population have different mean, variability of such mean's is assessed
- Mean of all is population mean
- Standard error of mean = SD of means of several sample from same population
- $SE = SD/\sqrt{n}$
- Standard error of proportion = pq/n, p = probability, q = 1-p

Probability or Chance

- Defined as relative frequency or probable chances of occurrence with which an event is expected to occur on an average
- Uncertainty is numerically expressed as probability
- Expressed as 'p'
- Range zero (0) - one (1): when p = 0 no chance of event happening and when p = 1, 100%

p = no of events occurring/total no of trials

q = negative probability

TESTS OF SIGNIFICANCE

Whatever is the sampling procedure or the care taken while selecting sample, the sample statistics will differ from the population parameters. Also variations between two samples drawn from the same population may also occur, i.e., differences in the results between two research workers for the same investigation may be observed. Thus, it becomes important to find out the significance of this observed variation, i.e., whether it is due to chance or biological variation (statistically not significant) or due to influence of some external factors (statistically significant). To test whether the variation observed is of significance, the various tests of significance are parametric tests and nonparametric tests.

Two Tailed Test

- This test determines if there is a difference between the two groups without specifying whether difference is higher or lower
- It includes both ends or tails of the normal distribution
- Such test is called two tailed test
- For example, when one wants to know if mean IQ in malnourished children is different from well-nourished children but does not specify if it is more or less

One Tailed Test

- In the test of significance when one wants to specifically know if the difference between the two groups is higher or lower
- The direction plus or minus side is specified.
- Then one end or tail of the distribution is excluded
- If one wants to know if mal nourished children have less mean IQ than well nourished then higher side of the distribution will be excluded
- Such test of significance is called one tailed test

Parametric Tests

- Parametric tests are those tests in which certain assumptions are made about the population.
  - Population from which sample is drawn has normal distribution.
  - The variances of sample do not differ significantly.
  - The observations found are truly numerical thus arithmetic procedure such as addition, division, and multiplication can be used.
- Since these tests make assumptions about the population parameters hence, they are called parametric tests. These are usually used to test the difference. They are:
  - Student T test (paired or unpaired)
  - ANOVA
  - Test of significance between two means.

Nonparametric Tests

- In many biological investigations, the research worker may not know the nature of distribution or other required values of the population. Also, some biological measurements may not be true numerical values hence arithmetic procedures are not possible in such cases. In such cases distribution free or nonparametric tests are used in which no assumption are made about the population parameters, e.g.,
  - Mann Whitney test
  - Chi square test
  - Phi coefficient test
  - Fischer's exact test
  - Sign test
  - Freidman's test

Stages in Performing Test of Significance

- State the null hypothesis
  - *Null hypothesis:* It is a hypothesis of no difference between statistics of a sample and parameter of the population or between statistics of two samples
  - It nullifies the claim that the experimental result is different from or better than the one observed already
- State the alternative hypothesis
  - It is hypothesis stating that the sample result is different i.e., larger or smaller than the value of population or statistics of one sample is different from the other
- Accept or reject the null hypothesis
  - Null hypothesis is accepted or rejected depending on whether the result falls in zone of acceptance or zone of rejection

- If the result of a sample falls in the area of mean ± 2SE the null hypothesis is accepted.
- This area of normal curve is called zone of acceptance for null hypothesis
- If the result of sample falls beyond the area of mean ± 2SE
- Null hypothesis of no difference is rejected and alternate hypothesis accepted
- This area of normal curve is called zone of rejection for null hypothesis

❖ Finally determine the p value
- P value is determined using any of the previously mentioned methods
- If $P > 0.05$ the difference is due to chance and not statistically different but if
- $P < 0.05$ the difference is due to some external factor and statistically significant

Chi-square Test
- Chi-square test is a nonparametric test.
- The test involves calculation of a quantity called chisquare.
- Chi-square is denoted by X^2.
- It was developed by Karl Pearson
- The most important application of chi-square test in medical statistics are:
  - Test of proportion—used as an alternate test to find the significance of difference in two or more than two proportions
  - Test of association—to measure the probability of association between two discrete attributes, e.g., smoking and cancer
  - Test of goodness of fit —tests whether the observed values of a character differ from the expected value by chance or due to play of some external factor
- $X^2 = \Sigma$ (O – E) 2/E
- X^2 denotes chi-square, O = observed value, E = expected value.
- Steps in chi-square test
  - State the null hypothesis
  - Determine the chi-square value
  - Find the degree of freedom
  - Refer the chi-square table to find the probability value corresponding to the degree of freedom

ANOVA (Analysis of variance)
- Investigations may not always be confined to comparison of two samples only. In such cases where more than two samples are used ANOVA can be used
- It can also be used when measurements are influenced by several factors
- ANOVA helps to decide which factors are more important
- In such a situation when we to compare among three or more than three groups, analysis of variance (ANOVA) is an appropriate statistics.
- It is an extension of t-test and z-test.
- It is better to say the technique as analysis of means rather than variance as inference about the means are made by analyzing the variances.
- This test is used to test general rather than specific differences among means.
- While performing analysis of variance, we get two variances, between group variance and within group variance. Difference between the means is called between group variance and difference within the means is called within group variance.
- If the difference between the two group variances (i.e., between and within groups) is significant, i.e., between group have large

Contd...

Contd...

variance as compared to within group, we reject the null hypothesis and conclude that our experimental manipulation had a real effect. If the difference between the variance is not significant, we accept the null hypothesis and conclude that experimental manipulation didn't have real effect.
- In analysis of variance, we get the F ratio. The F ratio is computed by dividing the between groups variance estimate by the within group variance.
- Two main requirements for ANOVA are that firstly data for each group are assumed to be independent and normally distributed and secondly sampling should be at random.
- There are different types of ANOVAs such as
  - One way ANOVA randomized
  - One way ANOVA repeated
  - Two way ANOVA randomized
  - Two way ANOVA repeated
  - Factorial ANOVA
- A one way ANOVA is used whenever we have one independent variable with three or more than three levels.
- If separate groups of subjects participate in each condition/level, in a between subject design, a Randomized ANOVA is the appropriate test.
- If the same subjects have participated in each condition, in a within subject design, a repeated measure ANOVA is the appropriate test.
- A two way ANOVA is used whenever two independent variables are manipulated and all the combinations of levels of each of the two variables are used.
- When we have one continuous dependent and two or more categorical independent variables, the factorial ANOVA is the appropriate statistics.

F test
- F = Mean square between samples/mean square within samples
- F = Variance ratio
- The values of mean square are seen from the analysis of variance table if we have the values of sum of squares and degree of freedom (which are calculated)
- Mean square between samples: It denotes the difference between the sample mean of all groups involved in the study with the mean of the population
- Mean square within samples: It denotes the difference between the means in between different samples
- The greater both these value more is the difference between the samples
- The F value observed from the study is compared to the theoretical F value obtained from the Tables at 1% and 5% confidence limits.
- If the observed value is more than theoretical value at 1%, the relation is highly significant; If the observed value is less than the theoretical value at 5% it is not significant; If the observed value is between 1 and 5% of theoretical value it is statistically significant.

T-test
- A statistical test that offers an opportunity to compare between two group means is called t-test. For example, if we want to compare between male and female on health issues or if we want to compare between rural and urban people on the same, t-test is the appropriate statistical test to measure the difference between these groups.
- T-test is used when we have smaller group of data while as z-test is used when we greater group of data (>30).
- It verifies, if the difference between two means is larger than would be expected by chance.
- Common types of t-tests which are frequently used are dependent sample t-test and independent sample t-test.

Contd...

Contd...

- Dependent samples t-test is a statistical test which is used to compare between two sample means on a single variable (dependent variable) is called dependent sample t-test. In this, the participants are meaningfully related with each other as the participants are same in both pre-and post-test. Dependent sample t-test is used to compare the mean of a single sample or paired samples.
  - For example, if a researcher is interested to compare the mental health of the participants before and after the national disaster such as (earthquake, tsunami, etc.). He will first administer the mental health inventory on a group of participants before the national disaster. The same group of participants then participates in the study after the tsunami. Then the researcher can compare the two means. In the dependent sample t-test, each score is matched and because of this matching, the researcher can predict that the scores are interdependent. For such kind of study, dependent sample t-test is the appropriate statistics.
- Independent samples t-test independent sample t-test is used when we have to make a comparison between two sample means who's means are not dependent on each other. Unlike dependent sample t-test (where the participants are meaningfully related with each other), two separate groups of participants participate in the study. One of the commonly used t-test is the independent sample t-test, where each groups are completely independent of each other.
  - Comparision between male and female, urban and rural areas is the simple examples of independent sample t-test. If we want to make a comparision between male and females on mental health, an independent sample t-test is the appropriate statistics. In this test, the sample of men should not be related to the sample of females, and there should not be any kind of overlap between the two groups, i.e., the groups should be independent of each other.

Z-test

- Z-test like t-test, z-test is a statistical test that offers an opportunity between the two groups but unlike t-test, where the variance is unknown and sample size is small, in z-test, there is known variance and sample size larger.
- For example, if we want to compare between male and female on mental health, z-test is the appropriate statistical test to measure the difference between the groups. The condition is that, the data should be greater than thirty and normally distributed, and the standard deviation should be known.
- Besides that, while conducting a z-test, the null and alternative hypotheses, alpha and z-score should be stated.

ERRORS IN BIOSTATISTICS

- **Type I error**
  - This type of error occurs
  - When we conclude that the difference is significant when in fact there is no real difference in the population i.e., we reject the null hypothesis when it is true
  - Denoted by α
- **Type II error**
  - This type of error occurs
  - When we say that the difference is not significant when in fact there is a real difference between the populations, i.e., the null hypothesis is not rejected when it is actually false
  - It is denoted by β
- **Standard error of mean**
  - Used for quantitative data
  - Standard error of mean is the difference between sample mean and population mean given by

$$SE\ x = SD\ of\ sample/\sqrt{n}$$

  - Also, population mean will be sample mean ± two standard error of mean
  - This will enable us to know whether the sample mean is within the limits of population mean
- **Standard error of difference between two means**
  - Used for quantitative data
  - It is the difference between means of two samples drawn from the same population
  - It helps to know what is the significance of difference obtained by two research workers for the same investigation

$$SE\ (X1 - X2) = \sqrt{SD1^2/n1 + SD2^2/n2}$$

- **Standard error of proportion**
  - In case of qualitative data where character remains same but its frequency varies we express it in proportion instead of mean
  - Proportion of individual having special character p
  - q is number of individual not having the character
  - P + q = 1 or 100 if expressed in percentage
  - Standard error of proportion is the unit which measures variation in proportion of a character from sample to population

$$SE\ of\ proportion = \sqrt{p\ X\ q/n}$$

p = proportion of positive character; q = proportion of negative character; n = sample size

The knowledge behind the distribution and determinants of common and rare diseases is fundamental in order for the health professional to orient preventive and treatment strategies at an individual and community level. In order to understand the usual pattern of reasoning in epidemiology it is important to study whether the probability of development of a particular disease in presence of a particular factor or exposure is different from the corresponding probability in its absence after excluding any alternate explanation such draw of lots (chance), errors in data collection or interpretation (bias), effects of additional factors (confounding). Finally interpretation is made on whether the observed association of the determinant and the disease is casual in nature by considering the magnitude of the association, consistency of findings with others studies and biologic credibility. Essentially, therefore, statistics is a scientific approach to analyze the numerical data which enable us to maximize our interpretation, understanding and use. The science of biostatics and its application in clinical epidemiology provides a foundation in understanding patterns of various oral diseases and thus applying appropriate strategies in its prevention and control.

POINTS TO REMEMBER

- Biostatistics is the tool of statistics applied to the data that is derived from biological sciences. John Graunt is known as father of health statistics.
- Uses of biostatistics in dentistry—to define the limits of normality for variable; to find correlation between two variables; to compare the efficiency; to find association between two attributes; in epidemiologic studies and helps in compilation of data, drawing conclusions, and making recommendations.
- Types of sampling are—simple random, systematic random, stratified random, multistage, multiphase and cluster sampling. Standard deviation is root mean square deviation and is a measure of differences of each observation from mean of all observations.
- Tests of significance include—student t-test, ANOVA, Mann–Whitney test, chi-square test, and Fischer's extract test.
- Chi-square test was developed by Karl Pearson and is used as test of proportion, association, and goodness of fit.
- ANOVA (Analysis of variance) is used when there are more than two samples and when measurements are influenced by several factors playing their role.

Questionnaire

1. Define biostatistics and explain its uses in dentistry.
2. What are sampling methods?
3. Write a note on standard deviation.
4. Classify different types of charts of presentation of data.
5. Explain standard deviation.
6. What are tests of significance?
7. What are type 1 and type 2 errors?

FURTHER READING

1. Armitage P, Berry G. Statistical Methods in Medical Research , 2nd edition. London: Blackwell Scintific; 1987.
2. Darby ML, Bowen DM. Research Methods for Oral Health Professionals: CV Mosby; 1980.
3. Dunning JM: Principles of Dental Public Health. Cambridge, Massachusetts,1975.
4. Gupta SC. Fundamentals of Statistics, 6th edition. Himalaya Publishing House, New Delhi;1997.
5. Mahajan BK. Methods in Biostastics, 5th edition. New Delhi: Jaypee Brothers, New Delhi; 1989.
6. World health organization. Oral Health No 318. Geneva;2007.
7. Roncalli AG. Epidemiology and public health dentistry: a shared walkway. 2006;11(1):105-114.

Research Methodology

Rajesh Sharma, Anupma Sharma

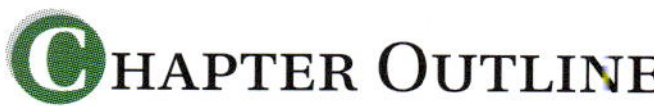

Research: *It is the quest for knowledge through diligent search or investigation or experimentation aimed at the discovery and interpretation of new knowledge.*

Dental research: *It is the study of laws, theories, and hypothesis through a systematic examination of pertinent facts and their interpretation in the field of dentistry.*

Methodology: *It is procedures by which researchers go about describing, explaining, and predicting phenomenon.*

Dissertation/thesis: *A formal or a lengthy discourse or treatise on some subject, especially one based on original research, and written in partial fulfillment of requirements for a doctorate/ Masters degree.*

Scientific paper: *An acceptable primary publication must be the first disclosure containing sufficient information to enable the peers to assess the information and to evaluate the intellectual process.*

CATEGORIES OF RESEARCH

Empirical and Theoretical Research

- It is based upon observation and experience more than theory and abstraction.
- It involves quantifications for the most part.
- This is achieved by three-related numerical procedures:
  1. Measurement of variables.
  2. Estimation of population parameters (the determination and comparison of rates, ratios).
  3. Statistical testing of hypothesis, or the extent to which chance alone may account for our findings. Theoretical research is based solely on theory and abstraction (conceptual, hypothetical, and nonrealistic).

Basic and Applied Research

- Research can be functionally divided into basic research and applied research.
- Basic research is usually considered to involve a search for knowledge without a defined goal of utility or specific purposes.
- Applied research is problem-oriented and is directed toward a defined and a purposeful end; it is frequently generated by a perceived need, and is directed toward the solution of an existing problem.

COMPONENTS OF A RESEARCH PROJECT

Selection and Formulation of the Research Problem

The statement of the research problem is the basis for the development of a research proposal, including the research objectives and hypothesis, the method and the budget. It allows the investigator to describe the problem systematically and to point out why the proposed research should be undertaken. The research hypothesis should be clearly and acceptably stated. The value to scientific work depends on the originality and the logic with which the hypotheses are formulated. Hypotheses may be formulated only if researchers know enough to make predictions about what they are studying. During planning stage, the research variables should be clearly identified and their methods of measurement, as well as the unit of measurement clearly indicated.

Research Design

The selection of the research strategy depends on the study objective. It comprises the following:
- Descriptive, validating, and surveillance strategies, using an interview, survey or mailed questionnaire.
- Observational or analytical strategies including prospective studies (cohort), historical cohort studies, retrospective (case-controlled) studies, cross sectional studies, and follow-up studies.
- Experimental strategies, including animal studies, therapeutic clinical trials, and prophylactic clinical trials
- Operational strategies, which include operation studies.
- The selection of research strategy is the core of the research design and is the single most important decision the investigator has to make. The strategy must include definition of variables, their levels and their relationships to one another.

Sampling

It is the way in which a study population is chosen. When using experimental studies, the inclusion of control groups should be considered when practical. The experimental and control groups should be as similar as possible except for the factors being studied.

Data Collection

A short description of plans for collecting data should be included in the research proposal in order to minimize the possibility of confusion, delays, and errors. Pilot testing of the research methods and research designs when appropriate, should be included as part of the project.

Analysis and Interpretation

Plans for analysis are an integral part of the research design, since they can prevent the investigator from realizing at the end of the study that certain required information has not been collected, or that some data has been gathered in an appropriate form for statistical analysis.

Reporting

Tentative plans for disseminating research results should be clearly outlined. Major emphasis should be placed in these plans and on distribution of the results to potential users.

Limitations of the experimental approach:
- **Lack of reality:** In most human situations, it is impossible to randomize all risk factors, except those under examination. Observational methods deal with more realistic situations.
- **Difficulties in extrapolation:** Results of experiments in animal models, which are rigorously controlled, cannot be extrapolated to human population.
- **Ethical problems:** In human experimentation, people are either deliberately exposed to risk factors or treatment is deliberately withheld from cases. It is equally unethical to test the efficiency or side effects of new treatments without critical evaluation in a small group.
- Difficulties in manipulating the independent variable.
- **Non-representatives of sample:** Many experiments are carried out of captive population or volunteers, who are not necessarily representative of the population at large.

DESCRIPTIVE STUDIES

- When an epidemiological study is not structured formally as an analytical or experimental study, i.e., when it is not aimed specifically to test an etiological hypothesis, it is called a "descriptive study" and belongs to the observational category of studies.
- The wealth of material obtained in most descriptive study allows the generation of hypothesis, which can then be tested by analytical or experimental study designs.
- Descriptive studies are usually the first phase of an epidemiological investigation. These studies are concerned with observing the distribution of disease in human populations and identifying the characteristics with which the disease seems to be associated.
- Such studies ask the following questions:
  - When is the disease occurring?–Time
  - Where is it occurring?–Place
  - Who is getting the disease?–Person
- Descriptive studies entail the collection, analysis and interpretation of data.
- Both qualitative and quantitative techniques may be used, including questionnaires, interviews, and observation of participants, service statistics and documents describing communities, groups, situations, programmes and other individual or ecological units.
- The distinctive feature of this approach is that its primary concern is with the description rather than with the testing of hypothesis or proving causality. The descriptive approach may, nevertheless, be integrated with or supplement methods that address these issues, and may add considerably to the information bases.

Types of Descriptive Studies

1. **Case series:** This kind of study is based on reports of a series of cases of a specific condition or a series of treated cases, with no specifically allocated control group. They represent the numerator of the disease occurrence and should not be used to estimate risks.
2. **Community diagnosis and needs assessment:** This kind of study entails the collection of data on existing health problems, programmes, achievements, constraints, social stratification, leadership patterns, focal points of high resistance or high risk. Their purpose is to identify existing needs and to provide baseline data for the design of further studies or action.
3. **Epidemiological description of disease occurrence:** This common use o descriptive approach entails the collection of data on the occurrence and distribution of disease in population according to specific characteristics of individuals (age, sex, education, marital status, health status, personality etc.) place (rural/urban, local, national, international); and time (epidemic, seasonal, cyclic, secular). A description may also be given by familial

characteristics such as birth order, family size, maternal age, family type etc. This type of information is used in every part of every study.

4. **Descriptive cross:** Sectional studies or community (population) surveys: Cross sectional studies entails the collection of data on, as the term implies, a cross section of the population, which may comprise the whole population or a proportion (a sample). Many cross sectional studies do not aim at testing a hypothesis about an association and are thus descriptive. They provide a prevalence rate at a point in time (point prevalence) or over a period of time (period prevalence). The study population is the denominator for these prevalence rates. Included in this type of studies are surveys, in which the distribution of a disease, disability, pathological condition, immunological condition, nutritional study, fitness, intelligence etc., is assessed.
5. **Ecological descriptive studies:** When the unit of study is an aggregate (e.g., family, clan or school) or an ecological unit (village, town or district), the study becomes a ecological descriptive study.

ANALYTICAL STUDIES

- Analytical studies are observational means used in the epidemiological investigations to test the specific etiologic hypothesis. The term "analytical" implies that the study is designed to establish the cause of the disease by looking for associations between exposure to risk factor and disease occurrence.
- The basic approach in analytical studies is to develop a testable hypothesis and to design the study to control for extraneous variables that could confound the observed relationship between the studied factor and the disease. The approach varies according to the specific strategy used.

Types of Analytical Studies

- **Observational studies:** Investigator simply observes the natural causes of the disease
  - Case control studies
  - Prospective cohort studies
  - Historical cohort studies
  - Analytical cross-sectional studies
- **Interventional studies:** Investigator allocates the exposure and then follows the subject for subsequent development of disease.

Case Control Studies (Retrospective)

- It is an efficient and common experimental strategy.
- It is designed particularly to establish the causes of diseases by investigating associations between the exposure to a risk factor and the occurrence of disease. The design is relatively simple, except that, it is "backward looking" (retrospective), based on the exposure histories of the cases and controls.
- With this type of study, one investigates an association by contrasting the exposure of a series of cases of the specified disease with the exposure pattern of carefully selected control groups free from that particular disease. Thus, the data are analysed to determine whether the exposure was different for the cases and controls. The risk factor was something that happened or began in the past, presumably before disease onset. Information about the exposure is obtained by taking a history or from records. A higher frequency of the risk factor among the cases than among the controls is indicative of the association with the disease condition. In other words, if greater proportion of cases than controls give the history of exposure, or have records or indications of exposure in the past, the factor or attribute can be suspected of being the causative factor.
- **Selection of cases:**
  - What constitutes a case in the study should be clearly defined with regard to histological type and other specifying characteristics, such as date of diagnosis and geographical location.
  - The sources of cases may be cases admitted to or discharged from the hospital within a specified period, cases reported or diagnosed during a survey or surveillance programme within a specified period, Incident or newly diagnosed cases, incident cases in an ongoing cohort study, deaths with a record of causes of death or if the number of cases is too large, a probability sample may be drawn.
- **Selection of controls:** It is crucial to set up control groups of people who don't have the specified disease condition in order to obtain estimates of the frequency of the attribute or risk factor for comparison with its frequency among cases. They may be:
  - A probability sample of a defined population, if the cases are drawn from that population, sample of patients admitted to or attending the same institution as the cases, group of persons selected from the same source of population as the cases and matched with the cases on other risk factor.
- Matching means that the controls are selected which have certain characteristics in common with the cases. The characteristics are those that would confound the effect of the putative risk factors. This can be done on a one to one basis (individual matching) or on a group-matching basis (frequency distribution matching). The major advantage of matching is to cancel out the confounding effects of the competing variables and to guarantee the comparability of cases and controls in that regard. It also guarantees that sufficient numbers will be available in the categories of interest. The disadvantage of matching is the tendency of over matching, i.e., matching on numerous variables.
- It is sometimes desirable to have more than one control group, representing a variety of disease conditions other than that under study. Use of multiple control groups offers three advantages:
  - If the frequency of the attribute or risk factor does not differ from one control group to another, but is consistently lower than that among the cases, this increases the internal consistency of the association.
  - If the control group is taken of patients with another disease, which is independently associated with the risk factor, the difference in the frequency of the factor between cases and controls may be well masked.
  - Multiple controls provide a check on bias.

- **Advantages of case control studies:**
  - Feasible when studying rare diseases.
  - Relatively efficient, requiring a smaller sample than a cohort study
  - Little problem with attrition
  - Earliest practical observational strategy for determining an association.
- **Disadvantages and biases of case control studies**
  - Absence of epidemiological denominators makes the calculation of incidence rates impossible.
  - Temporality is a serious problem in many case control studies where it is not possible to determine whether the attribute led to the disease condition or vice versa.
  - There is a great chance for bias in the selection of cases and controls.
  - It may be difficult or impossible to obtain information on exposure if the recall period is too long.
  - Selective survival, which operates in case control studies, may bias the comparison.
  - Measurement bias may exist, including selective recall or misclassification. There is possibility of the Hawthorne Effect; with repeated interviews, respondents may be influenced by being under study.
  - Case control studies are incapable of disclosing other conditions related to the risk factor.

Prospective Cohort Studies

- The common strategy of cohort studies is to start with a reference population (or a representative population), some of whom have certain characteristics or attributes relevant to the study (exposed groups), and others who don't have those characteristics (unexposed groups). Both the groups, should at the outset of the study, be free of the conditions under consideration. Both the groups are then observed over a period to find out the risk each group has of developing the condition of interest.
- **Selection of a cohort**
  - A community cohort of a specific age or sex.
  - An exposure cohort
  - A birth cohort
  - A military cohort
  - A diagnosed or a treated cohort
- **Data to be collected**
  - Characteristics of cohort
  - Data on the exposure of interest to study
  - Data on the outcome of interest to study
- **Advantages of a cohort study**
  - Because of the presence of a defined epidemiological denominator (population at risk), cohort studies allow the possibility of measuring directly the frequency of developing the condition for those who have the characteristic and for those who don't, on the basis of incidence measures, which can be calculated and compared, for both groups.
  - In a cohort study, it is known that the characteristic precedes in-time the occurrence of the disease; this knowledge of antecedent-consequent relationship is necessary to determine whether or not there is a cause-effect relationship.
  - Because the presence or absence of the risk factor is recorded before the disease occurs, there is no chance of bias being introduced due to awareness of being sick as is encountered in case control studies.
  - There is also less chance of encountering the problem of selective survival or selective recall; although selection bias can still occur because some subjects who contracted the disease will have been eliminated from consideration at the start of the study.
  - Cohort studies are capable of disclosing other diseases related to the same risk factor.
  - If a probability sample is taken from the reference population, it is possible to generalize from the sample to the population with a known degree of precision.
- **Disadvantages of cohort study:**
  - These studies are long term and thus are not always feasible; they are relatively inefficient for studying rare diseases.
  - They are very costly in time, personnel, space and patient follow-up.
  - Sample sizes required for cohort studies are extremely large, especially for infrequent conditions.
  - The most serious problem is that of attrition or loss of people from the sample or control during the course of the study as a result of migration or refusal to continue to participate in the study. Such attrition can affect the validity of the conclusion. The higher the proportion lost (>10-15%) the more serious the potential bias.
  - There may also be attrition among investigators, who may lose interest, leave for another job or become involved in another project.
  - Over a long period, many changes may occur in the environment, among individuals or in the type of intervention, and then these may confuse the issue of association and an attributable risk.
  - Over a long period, study procedures may influence the behavior of the persons investigated in such a way that the development of the disease may be influenced accordingly (Hawthorne effect).
  - A serious ethical problem may arise when it becomes apparent that the exposed population is manifesting significant disease excess, before the follow up period is completed.

Historical Cohort Studies (Retrospective)

- It is also called TROHOC study.
- It is possible to maintain the advantages of the cohort studies without the continuous presence of the investigators, through the use of historical cohort study.
- It depends on the availability of data or records, which allow reconstruction of the exposure of the cohorts to a suspected risk factor and the follow up of their mortality or morbidity over time. In other words, although the investigator is not present when the exposure as first identified, he reconstructs exposed and unexposed populations fro the records and then proceeds as though he had been present throughout the study.
- **Disadvantages of historical cohort studies**
  - All of the relevant variables may not be available in the original records.
  - It may be difficult to ascertain that the study population was free from the condition at the start of the comparison.

- Attrition problems are serious due to the losses of records, incomplete records or difficulties in tracing or locating all of the population for further study.

Analytical Cross-sectional Studies

- In an analytical cross- sectional study, the investigator measures exposure and disease simultaneously in a representative sample of population. By taking a representative sample, it is possible to generalize the results obtained in the sample to the population as a whole.
- Cross-sectional studies measure the association between the exposure variable and the existing disease (prevalence) unlike cohort studies, which measure the rate of developing of the disease (incidence).
- Used for study of rare disease, conditions of short durations or diseases with high case fatality are often not detected by the cross-sectional studies.
- **Advantages of cross-sectional studies:**
  - They have the great advantage over case-control studies of starting with a reference population from which the cases and control are drawn.
  - They can be short-term and therefore less costly than prospective studies.
  - They are the starting point in prospective cohort studies of screening out already existing conditions.
  - They provide a wealth of data that can be of great use in health systems use.
  - They allow a risk statement to be made although not precise.
- **Disadvantages of cross- sectional studies:**
  - They provide no direct estimate of risk.
  - They are prone to bias from selective survival
  - Since exposure and disease are measured at same point in time, it is not possible to establish temporality (whether the exposure preceded the development of disease).

Experimental Studies

- An experiment can be viewed as the final or definitive step in the research process, a mechanism for confirming or rejecting the validity of ideas, assumptions, postulates and hypothesis about the behavior of objects, or effects upon them, which result from interventions under defined sets of conditions.
- An experiment or trial is an investigation in which the researcher studies the effects of exposure to a defined factor.
- As in other designs, the investigator is rarely able to study all the units within a universe; a sample must be drawn from a target population for the purpose of the experiment, which will preserve the integrity of the representatives for generalization. This is done through a probabilistic process of random selection of study units.
- In addition the units must be selected in sufficient numbers to be able to determine the best estimate, and a measure of its reliability from a set of observations or to determine the significance of difference between the outcomes of comparison groups.
- Although the experiments are an important step in establishing causality, it is often neither feasible nor ethical to subject human beings to risk factors in etiological studies. However in one area of epidemiology, experimental strategies are used extensively; this is the area of field and clinical trials and intervention programs.

Ecological Studies

- They can take the form of any strategy, as long as the unit of observation is an aggregate, a geographical administrative locality, a cluster of houses, town.
- Thus these studies may be descriptive, case-control, cross-sectional, cohort or experimental.
- While such studies are of interest as sources of hypothesis and as initial or quick methods of examining association they can't be used as basis for making causal interferences.
- Their most serious flaw is the risk of ecological fallacy, when the characteristics of the geographical unit are incorrectly attributed to individuals.

EXPERIMENTAL DESIGN

- **Completely randomized design:** It is most straightforward design in this context, in which treatment are allocated to the units entirely by chance. It has a number of advantages like complete flexibility in number of treatments and replicates, all the available material can be used and statistical analysis is simple.
- **Block design:** Control for inherent differences between experimental subjects and for differences in experimental conditions is one of the most difficult problems facing experiments in biological sciences. The simplest method for reducing variability between treatment groups by a more homogeneous combination of subject and experimental condition is through 'Block Design'.
- **Latin square block:** It is a further advance upon single grouping. In this design, there are qualitative variables like rows, columns and treatments. In a 4*4 arrangements of groups, we could divide our experimental subjects into groups on the basis of 2 variables and 4 treatments (A, B, C, D), so that each variable and each treatment occurs once and only once in each row and each column.

	1	2	3	4
1	A	B	C	D
2	B	C	D	A
3	C	D	A	B
4	D	A	B	C

Clinical Trials

- Clinical trials are essentially experimental designs used by clinicians. The most common form is the "randomized, controlled, double blind clinical trial".
- Types of clinical trials:
  - Prophylactic trials
  - Therapeutic trials
  - Safety trials
  - Effectiveness trials

- Risk factor trials
- Efficiency trials

Phases of Clinical Trials

- **Phase I clinical trials:** This first phase in humans is preceded by considerable research, including toxicological and pharmacological studies in experimental animals to establish that the new agent is effective and may be suitable for human use and to estimate roughly the dose to be used in man. Phase I trial includes studies of volunteers who receive, initially, a fraction of what the anticipated dose is likely to be and are monitored for effects on body functions. This phase, which may not exceed one or two months, requires high technology in biochemistry, endocrinology and developed laboratory facilities. This trial is carried out under ideal conditions.
- **Phase II clinical trials:** This phase is carried out on volunteers selected according to strict criteria. The purpose of phase II is to assess the effectiveness of the drug or appliance, to determine the dosage and safety. Further information on the pharmacology of the drug is collected. In case of appliance, it effectiveness is assessed.
- **Phase III clinical trials:** This is the classical phase (the one usually referred to when the term Clinical Trials is used). It is performed on patients, who should consent to being in clinical trial. Strict criteria of inclusion and exclusion from the trial are followed. The purpose of this phase is to assess the effectiveness, safety and continued use of the drug or device in a larger and a more heterogeneous population than in phase II. It includes more detailed studies and monitoring than that given in a usual service situation. This phase is usually carried out on hospital in patients, but may be carried out on outpatients with extensive follow up. It requires proper planning, organization and strict coherence to pre-formulated protocols and instructions. Emphasis is also given to record keeping, follow up and supervision.
- **Phase IV trial:** Although it has been customary to approve drugs and devices for general use following phase III trials increasing interest has been shown by Governments, WHO to put drugs and devices through still another phase i.e., a trial in normal field or programme settings. The purpose of phase IV is to reassess the effectiveness, safety and acceptability. Although this phase is carried out under conditions that are as close to normal as possible, phase IV requires additional epidemiological and biostatistical skills as well as research requirements including record keeping and computer facilities.

Factors that Influence the Design and Analysis of Clinical Trials

- **The agent, treatment or experimental factor:** A complete knowledge about the treatment should be available to the researchers. This information usually comes from the phase I and II trials, as well as from many auxiliary sources.
- **Conditions to be treated:** Adequate clinical and epidemiological knowledge about the conditions to be treated should be available to the researchers. This includes the natural history of the condition, diagnostic criteria, and other variables that can influence the progress of the condition. Detailed treatment procedures should be explicitly stated and adhered to.
- **Target population:** The type of cases to be included in the trial should be carefully specified, with explicit criteria for inclusion in and exclusion from the trial. The sample size should be predetermined and if one institution cant provide the required sample, collaborative trials should be carefully planned with rigid protocols. Strict procedures should be used in allocating cases to groups. The ratio preferred is 1:1.
- **Ethical issues:** No clinical trial should be performed without due consideration of ethical issues.
- **Outcome to be measured:** One should specify explicitly what outcomes are expected and what criteria are to be applied for the success or failure of the trial.
- **Side effects:** Criteria for observing and recording side effects should also be made. If side effects would endanger the health of the patient, he/she should be excluded from the trial and treated appropriately.
- **Study instruments:** These are also to be specified including the laboratory tests, clinical diagnostic procedures etc.
- **Blinding:** It is highly desirable to enhance the objectivity of measurements by "blinding", or hiding the identity of whether the person being examined or interviewer belongs to the experimental or the control group.
- **Plans for analysis:** No clinical trial should be undertaken in the absence of epidemiological and statistical talent of the research team. Detailed plans for analysis must be made prior to the trial.
- **Selective attrition:** This is the most serious to clinical trials because the sample size is usually small. Thus, many investigations prior to use as candidates in their captive populations such as hospitalized patients, reliable volunteers, students and colleagues, among whom attrition is minimal. Selective attrition can be due to secondary refusal, death or discharge from hospital, etc.
- **Methods for ensuring the integrity of the data:** Data collection procedures and adequate supervision, record keeping, quality control and blinding are crucial. If these are not guaranteed, no trial should be undertaken.
- **The choice of design:** There are a variety of experimental designs for clinical trials. The choice depends on the nature of the trial components and the composition of the research team. The usual design is the randomized, controlled double blind clinical trial.
- **Time required:** One should allow several months (up to 1 year) for planning the trial, including; preparation of protocol, sampling procedures, determination of sample size, identification of sources for cases and controls, outlining management procedures and planning the analysis. A feasibility study may be needed in the preparatory stage.

FIELD TRIALS

- **Preventive trials:** when one has to derive disease free status in a healthy population using preventive techniques like vaccination one has to resort to large scale Field trials. Here the individuals belonging to such population are selected. The outcome will be the proportion of the disease, which was prevented.

- **Risk factor trial:** here instead of vaccine/drug, specific risk factors are averted in groups of population and the reduction in disease incidence is observed.

ETHICAL ASPECT OF HEALTH RESEARCH

An experiment is an attempt to discover the unknown, or test a principle, but we cannot be sure of an outcome. The experiment involves a chance. It is because of this chance or element of the unknown that ethics becomes a paramount issue in those experiments involving humans. Animal-based studies do not show the same results in humans. Therefore, all scientific interventions should be ultimately evaluated in human subjects. Several codes have been developed for protection of human subjects. The three underlying principles are:

1. *Beneficence:* Which requires that good should result, harm should be avoided.
2. *Respect from rights:* Includes the free choice of the subject.
3. *Justice:* Which requires an equal distribution of burden and benefit.

Guidelines as Per International Declarations

The first code was "the Nuremberg Code of 1947". This was followed by the "Declaration of Helsinki" which was adopted by The World Medical Association and the WHO in 1975.

- Biomedical research should follow scientific principles and should be based on adequately performed laboratory and criminal experimentation.
- The design of each procedure involving humans should be clearly formulated in an experimental protocol. The experiment should be conducted by scientifically qualified persons under supervision of medical experts. The right of the research subject to safeguard his/her integrity must always be respected.
- The accuracy of the research results must be preserved
- In any research on humans, each subject is informed about the aim, methods, benefits, and potential hazards of the study. When obtaining informed consent for research, a doctor should be cautious if the subject is in a dependent relationship to him/her.
- In case of legal competence, informed consent should be obtained from the legal guardian.
- Subjects should be informed that they are free to abstain or to withdraw from participation at any time.

Thus, the study of the research procedures and methods is a very important aspect of all postgraduate studies and at the same time provides guidelines on which our future research will be based. It also shows us the procedures that need to be followed while undertaking research and also shows us the data or findings of our study should be presented for correct interpretation and for publication. As stated by **Beveridge**, a successful research method would be for—"the person who possess the flair for choosing profitable lines of investigation, is able to see further where his work is leading than are other people, because he has the habit of using his investigation to look far ahead, instead of restricting his thinking to established knowledge and immediate problem."

POINTS TO REMEMBER

- Research is the quest for knowledge through diligent search or investigation or experimentation aimed at the discovery and interpretation of new knowledge.
- Dental research is the study of laws, theories, and hypothesis through a systematic examination of pertinent facts and their interpretation in the field of dentistry.
- Empirical research is based upon observation and experience. Theoretical research is based solely on theory and abstraction.
- Components of a research project are selection and formulation of the research problem, research design, sampling, data collection, analysis and interpretation, and reporting.
- Observational studies include case-control studies, prospective cohort studies, and analytical cross-sectional studies.
- Types of clinical trials are—prophylactic trials, therapeutic trial, drug treatment, safety trials, effectiveness trials, risk factor trials, and efficiency trials.
- Factors that influence the design and analysis of clinical trials are—agent, conditions to be treated, target population, ethical issues, side effects, blinding, plans for analysis, selective attrition, integrity of data, choice of design, and time required.
- Classification area sampling of sampling are random sampling, systemic sampling, panels for studying trends, stratified sampling, cluster sampling, multistage sampling, multiphase sampling, sequential sampling.

Questionnaire

1. What are components of research projects?
2. Describe various strategies and designs of research.
3. Explain clinical trials, its phases and designs.
4. Define sampling and explain its types and requisites.
5. What are international declaration guidelines?

FURTHER READING

1. Park K. Park's Textbook of Preventive and Social Medicine. 18th edition. Banarsidas Bhanot Publishers, (2005).
2. Peter S. Essential of Preventive Community Dentistry, 3rd edition. New Delhi: Arya Medical Publishing House Pvt. Ltd.; 2008.
3. World Health Organization. Health Research Methodology: A Guide for Training in Research Methods.

Index

Page numbers followed by *f* refer to figure, *fc* refer to flowchart, and *t* refer to table.

B

C

D

E

F

G

H

I

M

N

O

P

Q

R

S

T

U